SURGERY ESSENCE

SURGERY ESSENCE

Tenth Edition

Pritesh Kumar Singh
MBBS (MAMC) MS (Surgery) FMAS FIAGES
Author of Surgery Essence, AIIMS Essence, NEET Essence
Quick Review of Surgery, INI-CET Essence

Director, **Dr Pritesh Institute**

Chief Advisor of Editorial Board—PGMEE, Jaypee Brothers Medical Publishers
Guest Faculty of Surgery, Ningbo University, China
Stavropol State Medical University, Russia
International School of Medicine, Bishkek (Kyrgyzstan)
Avicenna Tajik State Medical University, Tajikistan

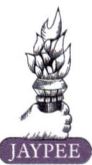

JAYPEE BROTHERS MEDICAL PUBLISHERS
The Health Sciences Publisher
New Delhi | London

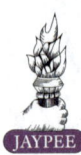 **Jaypee Brothers Medical Publishers (P) Ltd**

Headquarters
Jaypee Brothers Medical Publishers (P) Ltd
EMCA House, 23/23-B
Ansari Road, Daryaganj
New Delhi 110 002, India
Landline: +91-11-23272143, +91-11-23272703
+91-11-23282021, +91-11-23245672
Email: jaypee@jaypeebrothers.com

Corporate Office
Jaypee Brothers Medical Publishers (P)
Ltd 4838/24, Ansari Road, Daryaganj
New Delhi 110 002, India
Phone: +91-11-43574357
Fax: +91-11-43574314
Email: jaypee@jaypeebrothers.com

Overseas Office
JP Medical Ltd
83 Victoria Street, London
SW1H 0HW (UK)
Phone: +44 20 3170 8910
Fax: +44 (0)20 3008 6180
Email: info@jpmedpub.com

Website: www.jaypeebrothers.com
Website: www.jaypeedigital.com

© 2022, Jaypee Brothers Medical Publishers

The views and opinions expressed in this book are solely those of the original contributor(s)/author(s) and do not necessarily represent those of editor(s) or publisher of the book.

All rights reserved. No part of this publication may be reproduced, stored or transmitted in any form or by any means, electronic, mechanical, photocopying, recording or otherwise, without the prior permission in writing of the publishers.

All brand names and product names used in this book are trade names, service marks, trademarks or registered trademarks of their respective owners. The publisher is not associated with any product or vendor mentioned in this book.

Medical knowledge and practice change constantly. This book is designed to provide accurate, authoritative information about the subject matter in question. However, readers are advised to check the most current information available on procedures included and check information from the manufacturer of each product to be administered, to verify the recommended dose, formula, method and duration of administration, adverse effects and contraindications. It is the responsibility of the practitioner to take all appropriate safety precautions. Neither the publisher nor the author(s)/editor(s) assume any liability for any injury and/or damage to persons or property arising from or related to use of material in this book.

This book is sold on the understanding that the publisher is not engaged in providing professional medical services. If such advice or services are required, the services of a competent medical professional should be sought.

Every effort has been made where necessary to contact holders of copyright to obtain permission to reproduce copyright material. If any have been inadvertently overlooked, the publisher will be pleased to make the necessary arrangements at the first opportunity.

Inquiries for bulk sales may be solicited at: jaypee@jaypeebrothers.com

Surgery Essence
Third Edition: 2015
Fourth Edition: 2016
Fifth Edition: 2017
Sixth Edition: 2018
Seventh Edition: 2019
Eighth Edition: 2020
Ninth Edition: 2021
Tenth Edition: 2022, **Reprint: 2024**

ISBN: 978-93-5465-985-0

Printed at: Samrat Offset Pvt. Ltd.

Dedicated to

My Parents and
Uncle, Dr CP Singh

EDITORS

ENDOCRINE SURGERY

- Dr Ashish Jakhetiya (MCh, Surgical Oncology, AIIMS)
- Dr Subham Garg (MCh, Surgical Oncology, TATA)
- Dr Subham Jain (MCh, Surgical Oncology, TATA)
- Dr Niket Harsh (MCh, GI Surgery, AIIMS)

HEPATOBILIARY PANCREATIC SURGERY

- Dr Swati Agarwal (DNB, Surgical Oncology)
- Dr Harsh Shah (MCh, GI Surgery, GB Pant Hospital)
- Dr Vaibhav Varshney (MCh, GI Surgery, GB Pant Hospital)
- Dr Amit Jain (MCh, GI Surgery, GB Pant Hospital)

GASTROINTESTINAL SURGERY

- Dr Vaibhav Varshney (MCh, GI Surgery, GB Pant Hospital)
- Dr Harsh Shah (MCh, GI Surgery, GB Pant Hospital)
- Dr Niket Harsh (MCh, GI Surgery, AIIMS)
- Dr Amit Jain (MCh, GI Surgery, GB Pant Hospital)

UROLOGY

- Dr Gaurav Kochar (MCh, Urology)
- Dr Manoj Kumar Das (MCh, Urology)
- Dr Shiva Navariya (MCh, Urology)
- Dr Animesh Singh (MCh, Urology, AIIMS)

CARDIOTHORACIC VASCULAR SURGERY

- Dr Tarun Raina (MCh, CTVS, GB Pant Hospital)
- Dr Vivek Wadhva (MCh, CTVS, PGI Chandigarh)

PLASTIC SURGERY

- Dr Ritesh Anand (MCh, Plastic Surgery)
- Dr Alok Tiwari (MCh, Plastic Surgery)

NEUROSURGERY

- Dr Amit Kumar Singh (MCh, Neurosurgery, RML Hospital)
- Dr Ishu Bishnoi (MCh, Neurosurgery, GB Pant Hospital)
- Dr Shivender Sobti (MCh, Neurosurgery, RML Hospital)
- Dr Ugan Singh (MCh, Neurosurgery)

HEAD AND NECK

- Dr Ashish Jakhetiya (MCh, Surgical Oncology, AIIMS)
- Dr Subham Garg (MCh, Surgical Oncology, TATA)
- Dr Subham Jain (MCh, Surgical Oncology, TATA)
- Dr Niket Harsh (MCh, GI Surgery, AIIMS)

SURGICAL ONCOLOGY

- Dr Ashish Jakhetiya (MCh, Surgical Oncology, AIIMS)
- Dr Subham Garg (MCh, Surgical Oncology, TATA)
- Dr Subham Jain (MCh, Surgical Oncology, TATA)
- Dr Niket Harsh (MCh, GI Surgery, AIIMS)

GENERAL SURGERY

- Dr Harindra Sandhu (MS, Surgery)
- Dr Mayank Agarwal (MS, Surgery)
- Dr Mohit Garg (MS, Surgery)
- Dr Gunjan Desai (MS, Surgery)

PREFACE TO THE TENTH EDITION

First of all I would like to thank all my students, including the super speciality aspirants, for their constant feedback regarding improvement of the book (*Surgery Essence*) and making the book as the bestseller.

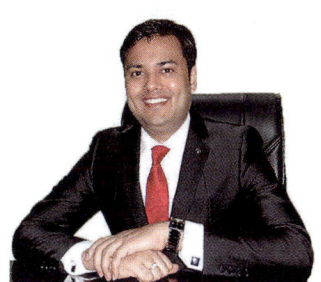

I can proudly say that all my students have contributed a lot to get me to this place, where I am today. They have helped me in becoming a better teacher, a better author and, most importantly, a better human being. I take this opportunity to thank all of you. The happiness you all give me keeps me telling always to work harder, to bring a positive change in the life of my students. This will be reflected in the pages of this book. I always strive to provide a winning edge to my students. This book has become the bestseller chiefly because of the suggestions, love and even critics that I come across and am informed of.

Higher education has become necessary, as graduation alone is found inadequate in this highly competitive and dynamic world. Trends in the way, the questions being asked are changing continuously. **The NEET exam is now the standard exam for both postgraduation and super specialty. As an author, I closely follow the kind of questions being asked and the change of pattern of questions in the NEET exam.** I am pleased to present the *10th* edition of *Surgery Essence* replete with new trends in the field of surgery and recent advances. In most of the PG entrance exams, lots of image-based questions are being asked, especially in INI-CET and NEET. **To provide to an edge, image-based questions are given in the beginning. Triads, signs, investigation of choices and topics based on "most common" type of questions are included in the annexures to save your precious time and to help you in revision at the most crucial hours.** *Synopsis* of the chapter is given in the beginning to develop concepts about the topics. **The recent questions and their concepts are highlighted and have been written in the way that will help the students to remember and reproduce them in the examination hall.** The information provided is cogent but concise to save the precious time, as we all know the clock is ticking. Time is one thing that can never be recovered once gone. Be careful!

I am passionate about excellence. Excellence in the field of education, and in my efforts to groom my students to make them confident enough that they lose the fear of failure. Being the Director of Dr Pritesh Institute, I follow the same principle in this institute so that the students should be benefited most with an extra edge.

I believe that all my students should know the importance of challenges. Challenges are what make life interesting and overcoming them is what makes life meaningful. For the time being, the only challenge that you should be facing is to secure a good rank in the entrance exam. One of the most important keys to success is having the discipline to do what you know you should do, even when you do not feel like doing it. Nobody ever wrote down a plan to be broke, lazy or stupid. These things happen when you do not have a plan.

PG entrance examination has made the medical world very competitive and has made it imperative for the students to acquire all the skills and competencies to deliver results. My aim, as an author and as a teacher, is to provide students with a learning experience which when amalgamated with perseverance and commitment helps them in achieving goals.

I am still not sure about one thing that who is more happy when a student achieves something, the student or the teacher, but I am very sure that the teacher is more satisfied when he sees his students achieving what they deserve and desire. I am working day and night to get that satisfaction and you have to work equally hard so that you do not let me down.

I always tell my students to dream big but not while sleeping. But, these dreams should always be accompanied with intelligence and hard work. To guide your work intelligently, this book and the author, both are there, with you throughout the year. But, the hard work is totally in your hands. Accept responsibility for your life. Know that it is you who will get you where you want to go, no one else.

Extensive revisions have been made to minimize the chances of error but still some mistakes might be there which should be brought to the notice of the authors through e-mail address or in writing.

It is a pleasure now to give outlet to the overflowing appreciation and thanks to all my colleagues, friends, teachers and family because this book is the result of encouragement and guidance from all of them.

I am pleased to acknowledge the overwhelming love I have received from my students, who are my ultimate source of inspiration. Wishing you all the best and looking forward for your feedback and suggestions…

✉ drpritesh@drpriteshsurgeryclasses.com

f drpriteshsingh

🐦 drpriteshsingh

G+ drpriteshsingh

in drpriteshsingh

YouTube /Dr Pritesh Institute

hi drpriteshsingh

📷 drpriteshsingh

www.drpriteshsurgeryclasses.com

Pritesh Kumar Singh

MBBS (MAMC) MS (Surgery) FMAS FIAGES
Author of Surgery Essence
AIIMS Essence, NEET Essence
Quick Review of Surgery, INI-CET Essence
Director, Dr Pritesh Institute
Chief Advisor of Editorial Board—PGMEE
Jaypee Brothers Medical Publishers
Guest Faculty of Surgery, Ningbo University, China
Stavropol State Medical University, Russia
International School of Medicine Bishkek (Kyrgyzstan)
Avicenna Tajik State Medical University Tajikistan

www.drpriteshinstitute.com

ACKNOWLEDGMENTS

I would like to express my greatest gratitude to the people who have helped and supported me throughout my project.

I wish to thank my parents for their undivided support and interest, who inspired me and encouraged me to go my own way, without whom I would be unable to complete my project.

First of all I would like to thank my beloved wife Dr Usica Singh, for her constant support and motivation. She helped me in updating the book from the latest editions of standard textbooks. She helped me throughout this project by giving her valuable advises and feedbacks regarding improvement of the book. Two strongest pillars of my strength are my wife **Usica** and my daughter **Prishika**.

I express my sincere thanks to my friends **Dr Niket Harsh** (MCh, GI Surgery, AIIMS) and **Dr Saurabh Rai** (MS, Orthopedics). They provided me the explanations of difficult and controversial questions.

I am very thankful to **Dr SK Tudu**, Ex. HOD of Surgery, Maulana Azad Medical College, New Delhi, for the valuable help. He was always there to show us the right track when we needed his help. It is with the help of his valuable suggestions, guidance and encouragement, that I was able to complete this project.

I am grateful to **Dr MP Arora,** for the continuous support for the project, from initial advice and contacts in the early stages of conceptual inception and through ongoing advice and encouragement to this day.

I sincerely thank my uncle **Dr SD Maurya** (President SELSI and Ex. Professor of Surgery, SNMC, Agra), for his valuable advice and knowledge regarding the surgery subject and surgical skills, which helped me a lot in preparation of certain topics of surgery given in this book.

I wish to express my sincere thanks to **Dr OP Pathania** and **Dr S Thomas.**

I wish to express my sincere thanks to **Dr Manoj Andley,** Professor of Surgery, LHMC, New Delhi, for helping me throughout this project. His caring and fatherly attitude for the unit as well as towards his residents needs a mention. His excellent way of teaching and presentation helped me a lot in making various explanations in the book. His hard working and caring attitude towards patients is source of inspiration for me and surgery residents.

I am very thankful to **Dr Ashok Kumar,** Professor of Surgery, LHMC, New Delhi, for his valuable and indispensable help. His unique ideas regarding presentation of explanations helped me a lot in this project. It is with the help of his valuable suggestions, guidance and encouragement, that I was able to complete this project.

I wish to express my sincere thanks to **Dr Lalit Aggarwal**, **Dr Gyan Saurabh**, **Dr Sudipta Saha**, **Dr P Rahul,** Assistant Professor of Surgery, Lady Hardinge Medical College, for guiding me to complete general surgery topics.

I wish to express my sincere thanks to **Dr Pawan Kumar, Dr Priya Hazrah, Dr Nikhil Talwar, Dr Ezaz Siddiqui, Dr Ashish Arsia, Dr Sadan Ali, Dr Jitender** and **Dr Kusum Meena,** Assistant Professors of Surgery, Lady Hardinge Medical College, for their indispensable contribution.

I would like to thank **Dr UC Garga**, Professor of Radiology, Dr RML Hospital, New Delhi, for his special guidance for radiology and valuable advices for improvement of the book and boosting my morale to bring this project.

I express my extreme gratitude for immense inspiration from my family members especially:

- Dr Avinash Kumar Singh (Urologist)
- Mr Abhay Kumar Singh (MBA, IMT, Ghaziabad)
- Mr Ritesh Kumar Singh (B Tech, MBA, Symbiosis, Pune)
- Ms Monika Singh (B Tech, Computer Science)
- Mr Rohit Kumar Singh (B Tech, Computer Science)
- Dr Kundan Kumar Patel (DMRD)
- Dr Jigyasa Singh (MS, Gynae IMS, BHU)
- Dr Ambuj Kumar Singh (MD Dermatology)
- Dr Charu Singh (Dermatologist)
- Mrs Deepasha Singh (MBA, IMT, Ghaziabad)
- Ms Pratibha Singh (M Tech, Computer Science)
- Ms Khushboo Singh (B Tech, Computer Science)
- Dr Anita Singh (MD, Pediatrics, KGMC, Lucknow)
- Dr Akanksha Singh (DGO, KGMC)
- Mr Abhishek Kumar Singh (B Tech, IIT Kharagpur)
- Mr Rahul Kumar Singh (B Tech)

I would like to especially thank my friends for their invaluable help and advice from time to time especially:

- **Dr Niket Harsh**
- **Dr Suarabh Rai**

I feel pleasure in conveying my sincere thanks to my friends and colleagues especially:
- Dr Shipra Goel (MD, Microbiology)
- Dr Mayank Agarwal (MS, Surgery)

A special thank of mine goes to **Dr Parul Gautam** (MD, Pathology, MAMC), who helped me in completing the project and exchanged her interesting ideas, thoughts which made this project easy and accurate. Her help for topics related to tumor and pathology is indispensable.

I am equally grateful to my friend **Dr Sushant Bhanja** (MD, Pediatrics), who gave me moral support and guided me in different matters regarding the topics related to Pediatric Surgery. He has been very kind and patient, whilst suggesting me the outlines of this project and correcting my doubts.

I would be failing in my duty if I do not express my thanks to all my friends who have really inspired me to write this book especially:

- Dr Vivek Kumar (MD, Medicine)
- Dr Harwinder (MS, Orthopedics)
- Dr Ugan Singh (MCh, Neurosurgery)
- Dr Bhamini Agal (MS, Gynae, SMS, Jaipur)
- Dr Anant Pachisia (MD, Anesthesia)
- Dr Neha Chaudhary (MD, Pediatrics)
- Dr Nitasha (MS, Ophthalmology)
- Dr Pragati Meena (MS, Gynae, SMS, Jaipur)
- Dr Aniket Malhotra (MD, Pediatrics)
- Dr Anant Shukla (MD, Anesthesia)

I would like to express my sincere thanks to my colleagues at Dr RML Hospital, especially **Dr Amit Kumar Singh** (MCh, Neurosurgery), **Dr Shivender Sobti** (MCh, Neurosurgery), **Dr Humam** (SR, Neurosurgery), **Dr Wazid** (DNB, Neurosurgery), **Dr Uzair** (DNB, Neurosurgery), **Dr Azaz** (DNB, Neurosurgery) and **Dr Neeraj** (DNB, Neurosurgery).

I would like to express my sincere thanks to my colleagues at Lady Hardinge Medical College and Associated Dr RML Hospital, **Dr Sushma Kataria, Dr Gyan Ranjan, Dr Kamal Yadav, Dr Priyank Yadav, Dr Vineet, Dr Munish, Dr Nivedita, Dr Tarun Raina, Dr Sumit Saini** and **Dr Abhinav Veerwal.**

I would like to express my sincere thanks to my colleagues at Lady Hardinge Medical College and Associated Dr RML Hospital, **Dr Meenakshi, Dr Ankur, Dr Prashant, Dr Rigved, Dr Munish Raj, Dr Diwakar Pandey, Dr Vikram Deswal, Dr Gunjan Desai, Dr Vikas, Dr Nikunj Jain, Dr Hari Singh, Dr Vimlesh, Dr Mannu, Dr Anshul, Dr Vikas and Dr Abhijeet Jha, Dr Mayank Aggarwal, Dr Vipul Dogra, Dr Abhishek, Dr Kunjan, Dr Sumit, Dr Kartikey, Dr Rao Bhupender.**

I would like to express my sincere thanks to my colleagues at Lady Hardinge Medical College and Associated Dr RML Hospital, for their valuable advice, especially:

- Dr Divish Saxena (Asst. Prof of Surgery, LMMC, Nagpur)
- Dr Prasad Bhukebag (SR, RML Hospital)
- Dr Anil Gulwani (MCh, Urology)
- Dr Arvinda PS (MCh, GI Surgery)
- Dr Yogender (SR, LHMC)
- Dr Shiv Navariya (MCh, Urology)
- Dr Zuber Khan (FNB, Minimal Invasive Surgery, LHMC)
- Dr Ravindra Gupta (Ex. SR, RML Hospital, MS, Gynae, PMCH)
- Dr Ritesh Pathak (SR, RML Hospital)
- Dr Nitin Sardana (Ex. SR, LHMC)
- Dr Rahul Rai (Ex. SR, LHMC)
- Dr Anand Yadav (Ex. SR, LHMC)
- Dr Nihar (MCh-Hepatobiliary Surgery)

I would like to express my sincere thanks to my colleagues at Maulana Azad Medical College and Associated LNJP Hospital, for their valuable advice, especially:
- Dr Mohit Garg (MS, Surgery)
- Dr Kamal Kishore Gautam (MS, Surgery)
- Dr Anurag Mishra (Assistant Professor, MAMC)
- Dr Ashish Airen (MS, Surgery)

I would also like to thank **Mr Varish Sharma** and **Mr Anurag Sharma** of MAMC Bookshop for their encouragement for writing this book.

I would like to thenk Mr Sahil Mahajan (Manager, Dr Pritesh Institute) and Mr Rajesh Jha (Assistant Marketing Manager, Dr Pritesh Institute) for their contribution.

I would like to thank **Dr Ashish Jakhetiya** and **Dr Inderjeet Yadav**, who helped me a lot in gathering different information, collecting data and guiding me from time to time in completing this project. Despite their busy schedules, they gave me different ideas to help make this project unique.

Last but not the least I want to thank all my students who appreciated me for my work and motivated me and finally to God who made all the things possible.

I convey my sincere thanks to Jaypee Brothers Medical Publishers (P) Ltd, New Delhi, India, for their efforts and suggestions, especially Shri Jitendar P Vij (Group Chairman), for helping me through my idea.

CONTENTS

Recent Questions and Answers with Explanation   p1–p47
Image-based Questions   p49–p72
Annexures   p73–p99

SECTION 1: ENDOCRINE SURGERY

1. Breast★★★★★   3
2. Thyroid★★★★★   49
3. Parathyroid and Adrenal Glands★★★   87

SECTION 2: HEPATOBILIARY PANCREATIC SURGERY

4. Liver★★★★   107
5. Portal Hypertension★★★   143
6. Gallbladder★★★   165
7. Bile Duct★★★   194
8. Pancreas★★★★★   226

SECTION 3: GASTROINTESTINAL SURGERY

9. Esophagus★★★★★   275
10. Stomach and Duodenum★★★★   314
11. Peritoneum★★★★   365
12. Intestinal Obstruction★★★★   381
13. Small Intestine★★★★   409
14. Large Intestine★★★★   435
15. Ileostomy and Colostomy★★★★   468
16. Inflammatory Bowel Disease★★★★★   473
17. Vermiform Appendix★★★★   488
18. Rectum and Anal Canal★★★★   500
19. Hernia and Abdominal Wall★★★★★   525
20. Spleen★★★★   552

SECTION 4: UROLOGY

21. Kidney and Ureter★★★★★   567
22. Urinary Bladder★★★★   626
23. Prostate and Seminal Vesicles★★★★   646
24. Urethra and Penis★★★★   662
25. Testis and Scrotum★★★★   684

SECTION 5: CARDIOTHORACIC VASCULAR SURGERY

26. Arterial Disorders★★★★★   711
27. Venous Disorders★★★★   745
28. Lymphatic System★★★★   761
29. Thorax and Lung★★★★★   770

SECTION 6: PLASTIC SURGERY

30. Burns★★★★★   815
31. Plastic Surgery and Skin Lesions★★★★★   828
32. Wound Healing, Tissue Repair and Scar★★★★   851

SECTION 7: NEUROSURGERY

33.	Cerebrovascular Diseases★★★★	863
34.	CNS Tumors★★★	886

SECTION 8: HEAD AND NECK

35.	Oral Cavity★★★★	907
36.	Salivary Glands★★★★★	922
37.	Neck★★★★	939
38.	Facial Injuries and Abnormalities★★★	952

SECTION 9: ONCOLOGY

39.	Oncology★★★★	963
40.	Sarcoma★★★★	984

SECTION 10: OTHERS

41.	Pediatric Surgery★★★★	993
42.	Trauma★★★★★	996
43.	Transplantation★★★★★	1035
44.	Anesthesia and Perioperative Complications★★★	1052
45.	Robotics, Laparoscopy and Bariatric Surgery★★★★	1055
46.	Sutures and Anastomoses★★★★★	1065
47.	Sterilization and Infection★★★★	1077
48.	Fluid, Electrolyte and Nutrition★★★	1097
49.	Blood Transfusion★★★	1108
50.	Shock★★★★★	1114
51.	Miscellaneous★★★★	1123

★★★★★ Most Important
★★★★ Very Important
★★★ Important

Recent Questions and Answers with Explanation

INI-CET MAY 2022

1. A 37 years old unmarried female, nulliparous having regular sexual intercourse, on OCPs since last 3 years. Mother had carcinoma breast at 50 years of age. Sister had ovarian cancer at 40 years of age. What will you advise as next step?
   (INI-CET May 2022)
   a. Stop taking OCP
   b. Do mammography annually
   c. Genetic counselling & BRCA testing
   d. Immediate prophylactic mastectomy

2. Patient was taking tamoxifen for the last 5 years after breast cancer surgery. When will she stop the tamoxifen if she wants to conceive? *(INI-CET May 2022)*
   a. One month before
   b. 3 months before
   c. Just stop and conceive
   d. Must continue even at pregnancy

3. On the basis of image given below, which of the following statement is incorrect? *(INI-CET May 2022)*

   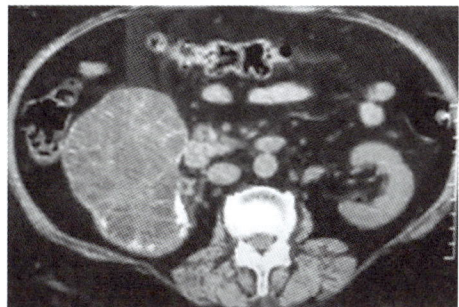

   a. FNAC or biopsy required before surgery
   b. Albendazole is given preoperatively
   c. Caused by Dog tapeworm
   d. Leakage of the cyst can cause anaphylaxis

4. On the basis of given image, what is the diagnosis?
   (INI-CET May 2022)

   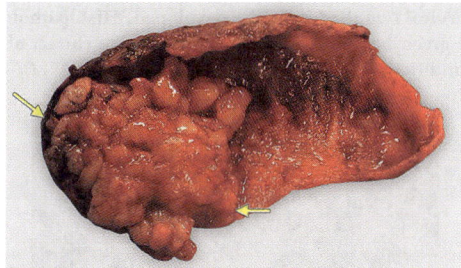

   a. Gall bladder polyp   b. Carcinoma
   c. Cholesterolosis   d. Gallbladder stone

5. A 46 years old alcoholic and smoker male presented with 2 months history of waxing and waning of jaundice. CT shows dilatation of CBD and pancreatic duct dilation. What is the most probable diagnosis? *(INI-CET May 2022)*
   a. CBD stone   b. Periampullary carcinoma
   c. Chronic pancreatitis   d. Cholangiocarcinoma

6. On the basis of given image, which cancer is operated here?
   (INI-CET May 2022)

   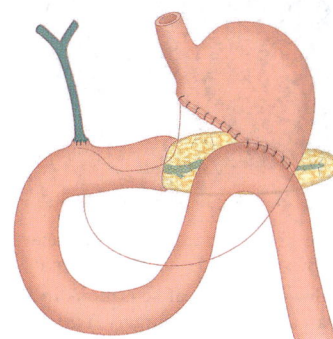

   a. Carcinoma gall bladder
   b. Carcinoma head of pancreas
   c. Cholangiocarcinoma
   d. Carcinoma stomach

7. Which investigation is not commonly used in the condition, whose image is given below? *(INI-CET May 2022)*

   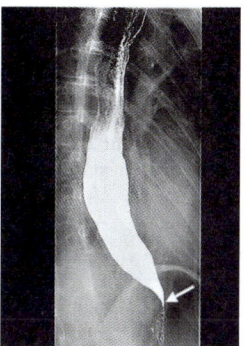

   a. 24-hour pH monitoring   b. Manometry
   c. Upper GI endoscopy   d. Barium swallow

8. What is the investigation of choice to diagnose the above-mentioned disease? *(INI-CET May 2022)*
   a. Manometry   b. 24-hour pH monitoring
   c. Endoscopy   d. CECT

9. Nutritional complications are more with which fistula?
   (INI-CET May 2022)
   a. Pancreatic fistula   b. Ileal fistula
   c. Duodenal fistula   d. Colonic fistula

10. Most common ectopic tissue found in Meckel's diverticulum is/are: *(INI-CET May 2022)*
    1. Gastric   2. Colonic
    3. Pancreatic   4. Thyroid
    a. 1 and 3   b. 1 and 2
    c. 1 and 4   d. 2 and 3

11. All of the following statements are true about inflammatory bowel disease, *except*: *(INI-CET May 2022)*
    a. Crohn's disease has skip lesions
    b. Childhood IBD is genetic
    c. Crohn's disease is mucosal and UC is transmural
    d. Crohn's is fully curable

12. Image showing rectal prolapse in a 45 years old female. Which is not the perineal approach for rectal prolapse?
    (INI-CET May 2022)

    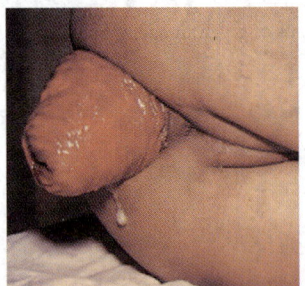

    a. Ripstein
    b. Altemeier
    c. Thiersch
    d. Delorme

13. A patient developed loss of sensations in the root of penis after a laparoscopic hernia surgery. Which of the following nerves would have been damaged? *(INI-CET May 2022)*
    a. Iliohypogastric nerve
    b. Ilioinguinal nerve
    c. Medial cutaneous nerve of thigh
    d. Lateral cutaneous nerve of thigh

14. True statement for clear cell renal carcinoma: (Multiple options) *(INI-CET May 2022)*
    a. Contain glycogen and lipid
    b. Mostly are sporadic
    c. Defect of long arm of chromosome 3
    d. Arises from DCT

15. A 30 years male had a blunt injury to abdomen. There was no blood at the tip of meatus. Foley's catheter was put and urine was collected in the bag for 2 hours. Radiological image is given below. What is the next step in management?
    (INI-CET May 2022)

    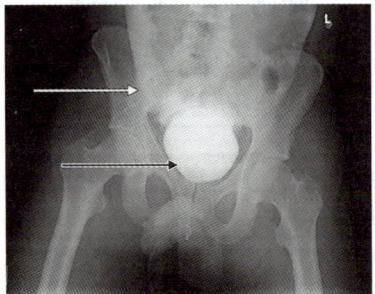

    a. Suprapubic catheterization
    b. Per-urethral catheterization
    c. Laparotomy
    d. Pelvic packing with bilateral nephrostomy

16. True statement for full thickness skin graft and split thickness skin graft: (Multiple choice) *(INI-CET May 2022)*
    a. Primary contraction more with split thickness skin grafting
    b. Secondary contraction more with split thickness skin grafting
    c. Primary contraction more with full thickness skin graft
    d. Secondary contraction more with full thickness skin graft

17. Which of the following are true regarding frost bite?
    (INI-CET May 2022)
    a. Amputation in severe cases
    b. Antibiotics and analgesics are not used
    c. Rewarming not done
    d. Clean and dry the area

18. Psoas abscess presents as all of the following, *except*:
    (INI-CET May 2022)
    a. Fluctuant mass
    b. Pott's spine can present as psoas abscess
    c. Can present in thigh
    d. Hematogenous spread of TB in immunocompromised

19. A trauma patient was brought to the emergency. On examination, no major injuries were detected. CT head was normal, but GCS was only 3. What is the most likely diagnosis? *(INI-CET May 2022)*
    a. Diffuse axonal injury
    b. Concussion
    c. Subdural hematoma
    d. Extradural hematoma

20. A patient of blunt trauma abdomen with grade 3 splenic laceration was being managed conservatively. On second day, for what reason you take the patient for laparotomy?
    (INI-CET May 2022)
    a. Fall in Hb from 12 to 10%
    b. Presence of pneumoperitoneum
    c. Extraperitoneal rupture of bladder
    d. Gall bladder distension

NEET PG 2022

21. A 35 years old female presented to OPD. Physical examination findings are given in the image. Which structure is affected in this condition? *(NEET PG 2022)*

    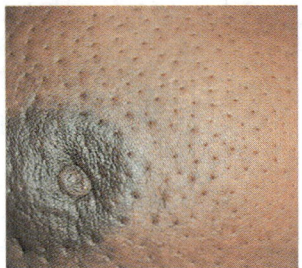

    a. Involvement of chest wall
    b. Involvement of subdermal lymphatics
    c. Involvement of Cooper's ligaments
    d. Involvement of connective tissue

22. A young male presented with slow growing midline swelling in anterior part of neck. After 6 months, bilateral cervical lymphadenopathy developed. Histopathology slide is given below. All of the following are correct about this condition, *except*: *(NEET PG 2022)*

    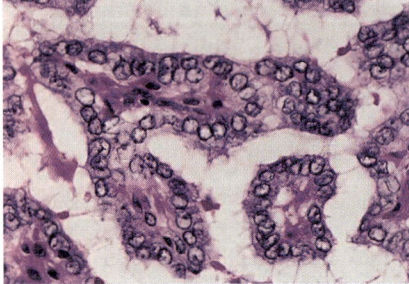

    a. Lymphatic spread is seen
    b. Specific nuclear pattern on histology
    c. Has excellent prognosis
    d. FNAC is not diagnostic

23. A 45 years old female underwent thyroidectomy. On 3rd day, she developed perioral numbness. Further investigation involves:
    a. Free T3, T4
    b. Calcium, phosphate and PTH levels
    c. RAI scan
    d. T3, T4, TSH
    (NEET PG 2022)

24. All of the following are the components of MEN-2B, *except*: *(NEET PG 2022)*
    a. Parathyroid adenoma
    b. Megacolon
    c. Marfanoid habitus
    d. Mucosal neuroma

25. A 35 years old patient presented with severe abdominal pain and vomiting. His vitals are stable. The radiograph is given below. What is the most effective way to treat this patient? *(NEET PG 2022)*

    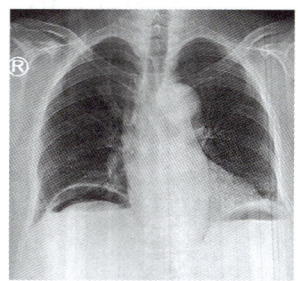

    a. Gastric lavage with cold saline
    b. Tracheostomy
    c. Chest tube insertion
    d. Resuscitation and laparotomy

26. An 11-month-old boy was brought to emergency with pain abdomen and multiple episodes of vomiting. On examination, mass was palpable in right lumbar region. Barium enema image is given below. What is the diagnosis? *(NEET PG 2022)*

    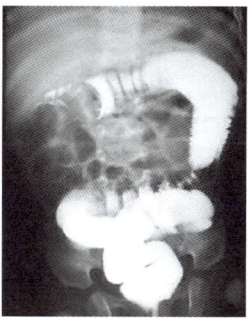

    a. Intussusception
    b. Volvulus
    c. Malrotation
    d. Duodenal atresia

27. A 30 years old male presented with recurrent painful perianal nodules on buttocks with serous discharge. The image is given below. What is the most probable diagnosis? *(NEET PG 2022)*

    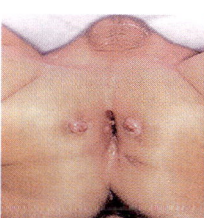
    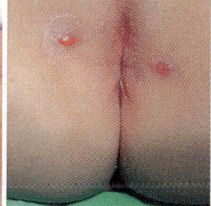

    a. Perianal boils
    b. Carbuncle
    c. Fistula-in-ano
    d. Pilonidal sinus

28. A delayed intravenous urogram of the patient is shown below. What is the most likely diagnosis? *(NEET PG 2022)*

    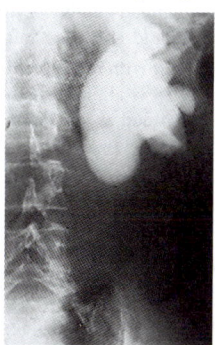

    a. Putty kidney
    b. Staghorn calculus
    c. Pelviureteric junction obstruction
    d. Renal cyst

29. A 6-year-old child presented with recurrent UTI. Micturating cystourethrogram image of the patient is given below. What is the most likely diagnosis? *(NEET PG 2022)*

    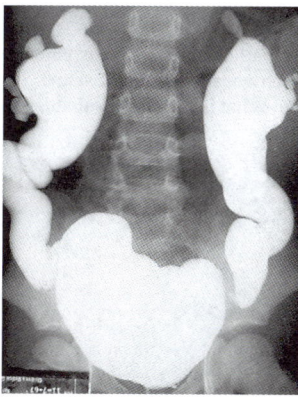

    a. Vesicoureteric reflux
    b. Vesicocolic fistula
    c. Urinary bladder hernia
    d. Urinary bladder diverticula

30. Identify the congenital anomaly shown in the newborn baby: *(NEET PG 2022)*

    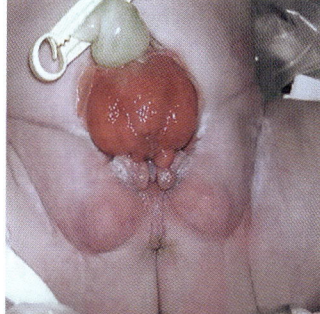

    a. Omphalocele
    b. Gastroschisis
    c. Persistent vitello-intestinal duct
    d. Bladder exstrophy

31. Route of metastasis of prostate cancer to lumbar vertebrae: *(NEET PG 2022)*
    a. Transcoelomic spread b. Lymphatics
    c. Prostatic venous plexus d. Inferior vesical vein

32. A 30 years old patient with motor vehicle accident presented to the causality. His vitals are stable but he is unable to pass urine. He has blood at the tip of meatus. An RGU was performed as shown below. What is the most likely site of urethral injury? *(NEET PG 2022)*

    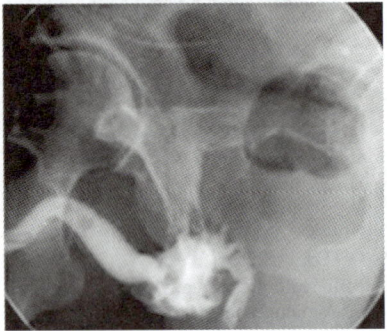

    a. Membranous urethra b. Penile urethra
    c. Bulbar urethra d. Spongy urethra

33. A 55 years patient presented to emergency with scrotal swelling, ecchymosis, fever and serous discharge. Image is given below. What is the most probable diagnosis? *(NEET PG 2022)*

    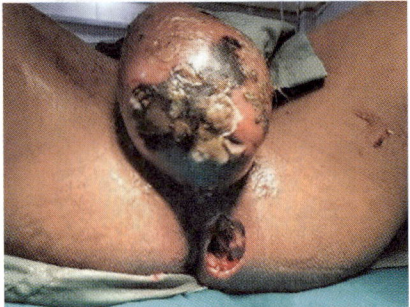

    a. Fournier's gangrene b. Epididymo-orchiditis
    c. Torsion testis d. Carcinoma testis

34. A patient presented to emergency with claudication of calf muscles, numbness in thigh with impotence. Image showing gangrene of foot is given below. Which artery is involved? *(NEET PG 2022)*

    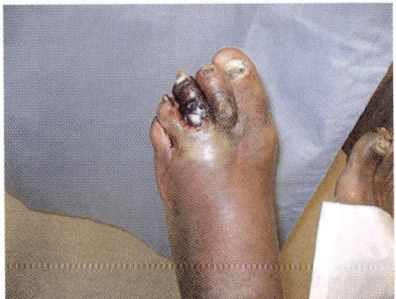

    a. Aortic-iliac bifurcation b. Internal iliac artery
    c. Bilateral popliteal artery d. Femoral artery

35. Following surgery for varicose veins, patient started complaining of numbness along the medial aspect of leg. Which nerve is most commonly affected? *(NEET PG 2022)*
    a. Superficial peroneal b. Deep peroneal
    c. Saphenous nerve d. Sural nerve

36. A 25-year-old patient presents with multiple injuries due to RTA. 2 days later in the hospital he developed dyspnea with petechial rash and altered sensorium. Which of the following is the cause? *(NEET PG 2022)*
    a. Air embolism b. Thromboembolism
    c. Massive hemorrhage d. Fat embolism

37. A 30 years old patient presented to the casualty after a motor vehicle accident. He has bruises on the chest. His pulse is 120 beats per minute. BP is 90/60 mm Hg and respiratory rate is 40/minute. A chest X-ray was performed and shown below. What is the next most appropriate step in the management of this patient? *(NEET PG 2022)*

    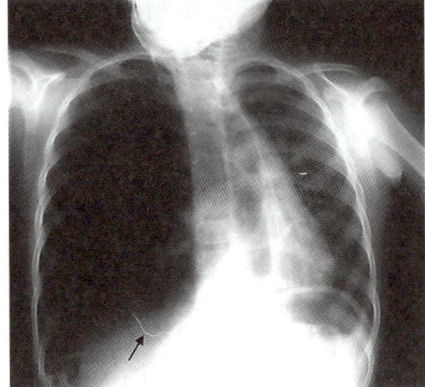

    a. Immediate thoracotomy
    b. Pericardiocentesis
    c. Pleurodesis
    d. Chest drain insertion and drainage

38. A 9 years old child was brought to the hospital after burns. There was involvement of half of chest wall and abdomen towards left side, posterior arm and thigh. Calculate the burnt surface area: *(NEET PG 2022)*
    a. 5–10% b. 15–20%
    c. 25–30% d. 35–40%

39. A 73 years old male was bed ridden for 15 years. The image of bed sore is given below. What is the grade of bed sore? *(NEET PG 2022)*

    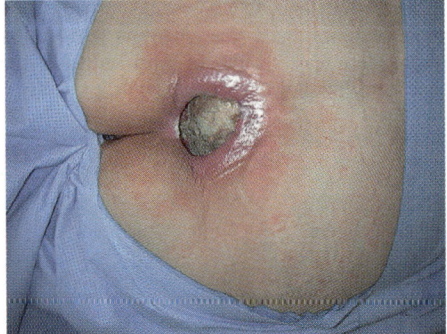

    a. Grade I b. Grade II
    c. Grade III d. Grade IV

40. A patient with history of chronic alcoholism presented to OPD with whitish patch, whose image is given below. What is the most probable diagnosis? *(NEET PG 2022)*

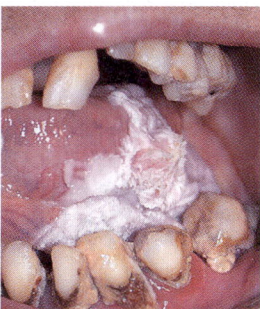

   a. Leukoplakia
   b. Submucosal fibrosis
   c. Erythroplakia
   d. Malakoplakia

41. A 45 years old patient complaints of recurrent swelling in one side of the neck. She is afraid of eating food as it worsens the swelling. Imaging was performed and shown below. What is the most likely diagnosis? *(NEET PG 2022)*

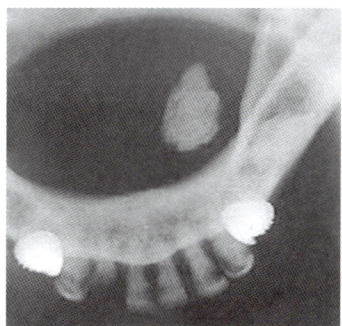

   a. Sialolithiasis
   b. Penetrating irregular foreign body
   c. Isolated osteoma of floor of mouth
   d. Cervical lymphadenopathy

42. A patient came with swelling under the ear lobe as shown below in the image. The swelling was non-tender & firm. What is the most likely diagnosis? *(NEET PG 2022)*

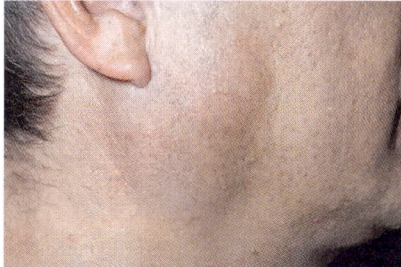

   a. Bezold abscess
   b. Parotid gland swelling
   c. Osteoid osteoma
   d. Deep cervical lymph node enlargement

43. Which of the following is most likely to be seen due to rupture of saccular aneurysm in brain? *(NEET PG 2022)*
   a. Subdural hemorrhage
   b. Subarachnoid hemorrhage
   c. Hydrocephalous
   d. Intracerebral hemorrhage

44. A patient with stab injury was brought to the emergency. Vitals were stable. Image is given below. What is next best step of management? *(NEET PG 2022)*

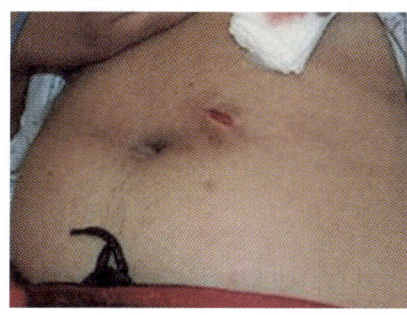

   a. Further investigation
   b. IV fluids
   c. Wait and watch after dressing
   d. Exploratory laparotomy

45. Green color in triage signifies: *(NEET PG 2022)*
   a. Moderate priority
   b. High priority
   c. Ambulatory
   d. Dead

INI-CET NOVEMBER 2021

46. A patient underwent mastectomy and given drain was kept under the flap and flap was closed. What type of drain is this? *(INI-CET November 2021)*

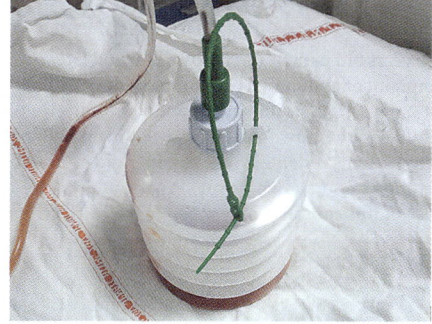

   a. Semi open
   b. Semi closed
   c. Open
   d. Closed

47. During surgery of carcinoma breast, frozen section was done. This procedure will be useful for all, *except*: *(INI-CET November 2021)*
   a. For margins positivity
   b. For sentinel lymph node biopsy
   c. Done in all cases for immediate diagnosis
   d. To identify the metastatic lesion

48. A 30 years old female patient presented with complaints of palpitation and feeling febrile all the time with midline neck swelling. On examination, a diffusely enlarged thyroid is felt and lower border of swelling is seen moving with deglutition. Exophthalmos was also noted. What are the essential investigations to be done? *(INI-CET November 2021)*
   1. Thyroid scan
   2. FNAC
   3. Thyroid function test
   4. USG neck
   5. Anti-Thyroid antibody
   a. 1 and 3
   b. 1, 3, 4 and 5
   c. 1, 4 and 5
   d. 2, 3 and 4

49. Inferior thyroid artery supplies: *(INI-CET November 2021)*
    1. Esophagus
    2. Parathyroid
    3. Thyroid
    4. Thymus
    a. 1 and 3
    b. 1, 2 and 3
    c. 1, 3 and 4
    d. 1, 2, 3 and 4

50. Which of the following statement is correct regarding HCC demographics and treatment? *(INI-CET November 2021)*
    1. Global incidence is rising
    2. NASH and NAFLD are the risk factors
    3. Lenvatinib is used for tumor size <3 cm
    4. TACE is done for multinodular tumor
    a. 1, 2, 4 are correct
    b. 1, 2, 3, 4 are correct
    c. 2 and 3 correct
    d. 1 and 2 correct

51. A patient presented to emergency with abdominal pain, jaundice, fever with chills. Cholangitis was suspected in the patient. Which of the following are the components of Reynold's pentad along with abdominal pain?
    1. Jaundice *(INI-CET November 2021)*
    2. Melena
    3. Mental obtundation
    4. Hypotension
    5. Fever
    6. Hematemesis
    a. 1, 2, 4, 6
    b. 1, 3, 4 and 5
    c. 2, 3, 4 and 5
    d. 1, 3, 4 and 6

52. A patient presented to hospital with jaundice. Ultrasound & CECT was done. There was no stone in the gallbladder but intrahepatic biliary radicle dilatation was detected. What is the next investigation done? *(INI-CET November 2021)*
    a. MRI
    b. PET CT
    c. PTC
    d. ERCP

53. A 30 years old patient was hit by a bull and later presented with complaint of abdominal pain for last 3 days and obstipation for last 2 days along with nausea and vomiting. He was initially stabilized but now presented with increased pain and on examination, abdomen was found rigid. A radiograph was performed and shown below. What could be the most likely cause of this condition? *(INI-CET November 2021)*

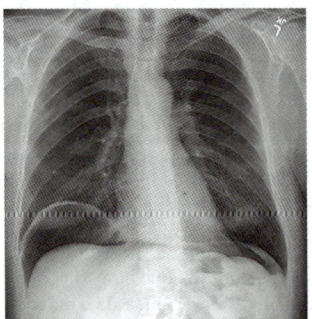

    a. Hollow viscus perforation
    b. Liver laceration
    c. Pneumothorax
    d. Hemoperitoneum

54. Which of the following is true about colon cancer? *(INI-CET November 2021)*
    1. Colon cancer can be prevented by metformin
    2. Right and left colon cancers can have different clinical presentations
    3. Colon cancers can be hereditary
    4. Colon cancers frequently metastasize to liver
    a. 1, 2, 3 and 4
    b. 1, 2 and 3
    c. 1 and 2
    d. 1 and 4

55. Appendicectomy was being performed in a patient of appendicitis. The surgeon first used a Gridiron incision, which was later converted to Rutherford Morrison incision. Which of the following does the surgeon needs to cut further?
    1. External oblique *(INI-CET November 2021)*
    2. Internal oblique
    3. Transversus abdominis
    4. Rectus abdominis
    a. 1, 2, 3
    b. 1 and 2
    c. 2 and 3
    d. 1, 2, 3, 4

56. Patient presented to hospital with hematuria, Urine microscopic examination reveals high-grade transitional cell cancer. CT scan shows 2 × 2 cm mass in bladder. What is the management? *(INI-CET November 2021)*
    a. Transurethral resection of bladder tumor
    b. Radical cystectomy
    c. Hemicystectomy with bladder reconstruction
    d. Neoadjuvant chemotherapy

57. All are lower urinary tract symptoms, *except*:
    a. Incontinence while intercourse *(INI-CET November 2021)*
    b. Sudden urge to urinate
    c. Incontinence while asleep
    d. Check for leak by making the patient cough

58. Most common cause of bladder outlet obstruction in male neonate: *(INI-CET November 2021)*
    a. Posterior urethral valve
    b. Anterior urethral valve
    c. Ureterocele
    d. Urethral atresia

59. An elderly male, age 60 years patient presented with left testicular swelling and ataxia. What is the diagnosis?
    a. Germ cell tumor *(INI-CET November 2021)*
    b. Glioblastoma multiforme
    c. Non-Hodgkin's lymphoma
    d. Hodgkin's lymphoma

60. A patient had chest trauma, whose chest X-ray image is given below. Which of the following procedure is contraindicated? *(INI-CET November 2021)*

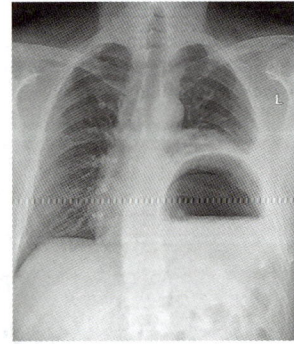

    a. Log roll
    b. ICD tube
    c. Nasogastric tube
    d. Epidural anesthesia

61. A patient presented to hospital after knife injury over arm. Radial and ulnar pulses were not felt. Right brachial artery has a 2.5 cm longitudinal cut. Ideal repair is: *(INI-CET November 2021)*
    a. Primary closure
    b. Repair with prosthetic graft
    c. Ligate
    d. Repair with saphenous vein graft

62. A patient suffered tibia fracture a month ago, and now has his cast removed. There were some ecchymoses on the skin. A few days later, he comes with pain on lifting his great toe and decreased sensation in the first web space. Posterior tibial and dorsalis pedis pulses were felt. What will be the next step to be performed? *(INI-CET November 2021)*
    a. Venous Doppler
    b. Measure anterior compartment pressure
    c. A test related to DIC
    d. Admit and give analgesics and antibiotics

63. Nasogastric tube length is measured by: *(INI-CET November 2021)*
    a. Tip of nose to ear lobule and xiphoid process
    b. Tip of nose to xiphoid process and umbilicus
    c. Tip of nose to ear lobule to mid-distance between xiphisternum and umbilicus
    d. From the angle of mouth to the below the ear lobe till the xiphisternum

64. A patient was brought into emergency department. The intern was asked about flow rate/minute of the cannula shown below: *(INI-CET November 2021)*

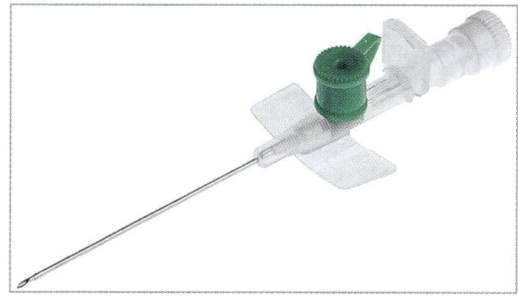

    a. 66 mL   b. 86 mL
    c. 96 mL   d. 106 mL

65. Which phase of cell cycle is least radiosensitive? *(INI-CET November 2021)*
    a. G1   b. S
    c. G2   d. M

INI-CET JULY 2021

66. A female patient presented to the hospital with right breast lump. On examination, lump was located in the upper outer quadrant with negative ipsilateral axillary lymph nodes. Mammography revealed BIRADS 4. Patient underwent breast conservation surgery (BCS). Final histopathology report revealed high-grade DCIS. What is the next step?
    a. Chemotherapy *(INI-CET July 2021)*
    b. Radiotherapy
    c. Trastuzumab
    d. Follow-up 6 monthly for 2 years then yearly

67. A young female with history of renal calculi complains of bone pain, abdominal cramps and psychosis. On investigation, multiple fractures were discovered and serum calcium and PTH was raised. Which of the following will be the best investigation to arrive at a definitive diagnosis? *(INI-CET July 2021, AIIMS May 2017)*
    a. Sestamibi scan
    b. FDG-PET
    c. MRI
    d. USG neck

68. A patient presented to the hospital with intermittent pain in right upper quadrant of abdomen and jaundice. On investigations, multiple gallstones were found without any GB wall thickening. CBD diameter was 12 mm. GGT was elevated 5 times of normal and ALP was 380 IU. What is the next best step? *(INI-CET July 2021)*
    a. MRCP   b. ERCP
    c. Semi-urgent cholecystectomy
    d. Conservative management and send home

69. After laparoscopic cholecystectomy, patient started developing pain after some days of discharge. On evaluation, 5 × 5 cm fluid collection was present under the liver. What should be done next? *(INI-CET July 2021)*
    a. USG guided pigtail catheter drainage
    b. Reopen the wound & T-tube insertion
    c. ERCP with stenting
    d. Give antibiotics and send the patient home

70. A child presented with mild abdominal discomfort and intermittent abdominal pain. The radiograph is given below. What is the most likely diagnosis? *(INI-CET July 2021)*

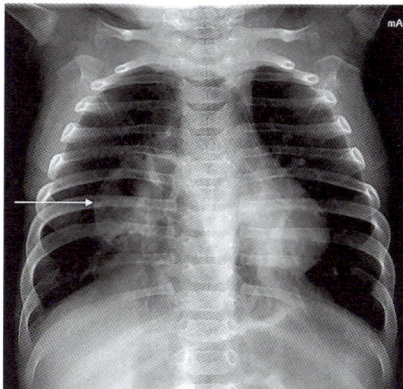

    a. Bochdalek hernia   b. Eventration of diaphragm
    c. Morgagni hernia   d. Gastric volvulus

71. A child presented with mild abdominal discomfort and intermittent abdominal pain. The radiograph is given below. What is the most likely diagnosis? *(INI-CET July 2021)*

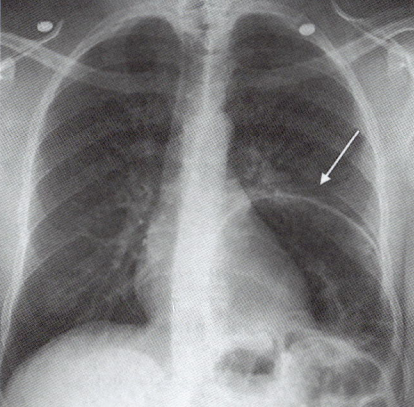

    a. Bochdalek hernia
    b. Eventration of diaphragm
    c. Morgagni hernia
    d. Gastric volvulus

72. A child presented with intermittent abdominal pain and vomiting. The radiograph is given below. What is the most likely diagnosis? *(INI-CET July 2021)*

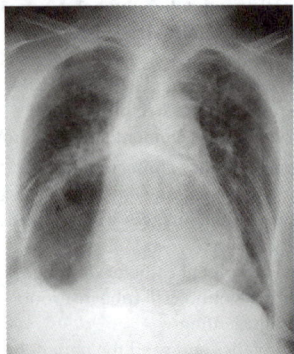

   a. Bochdalek hernia
   b. Eventration of diaphragm
   c. Morgagni hernia
   d. Gastric volvulus

73. Which of the following vaccine can cause intussusception? *(INI-CET July 2021)*

   a. Rotavirus b. Oral polio vaccine
   c. MMR d. DPT

74. A 17 years old male was brought to the hospital with recurrent attacks of intussusception. During surgery, multiple polyps were found in small intestine. One of the polyps was removed, whose histopathological image is given below. What is the pathological change shown in the picture?
(INI-CET July 2021, AIIMS November 2015)

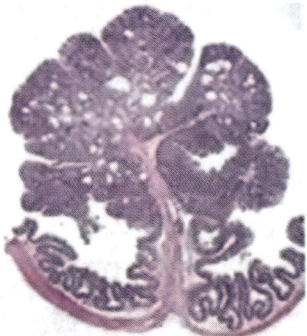

   a. Hamartomatous b. Inflammatory
   c. Adenomatous d. Tubulovillous

75. Which of the following is excreted in urine in carcinoid tumor? *(INI-CET July 2021)*
   a. 5-HIAA
   b. Metanephrines
   c. VMA
   d. Histamine

76. Which of the following matching is correct related to the confirmation of diagnosis? *(INI-CET July 2021)*
   a. Hirschsprung's disease: Rectal biopsy
   b. Carcinoma colon: CECT
   c. Carcinoma breast: Mammography
   d. Carcinoma bladder: MRI

77. Identify the urinary crystal shown below:
(INI-CET July 2021, AIIMS November 2015)

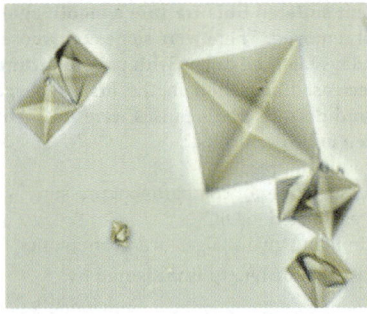

   a. Cystine b. Uric acid
   c. Triple phosphate d. Calcium oxalate

78. A 65 years old male banker came for an ultrasound to renew his medical insurance. In right kidney, 4 × 5 cm Bosniak type 3 complex cyst was found and the picture of CT scan is given below. What is the most likely diagnosis?
(INI-CET July 2021, AIIMS May 2017)

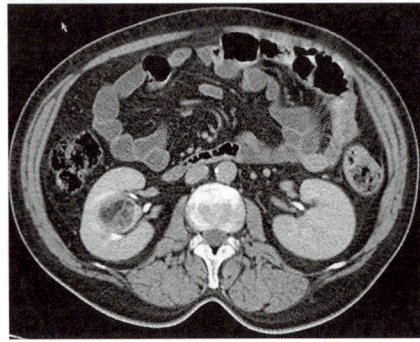

   a. Oncocytoma b. Angiomyolipoma
   c. Perinephric cyst d. Renal cell carcinoma

79. A 65 years old male banker came for an ultrasound to renew his medical insurance. In right kidney, 4 × 5 cm Bosniak type 3 complex cyst was found and the picture of CT scan is given below. What is the most likely diagnosis? *(INI-CET July 2021)*

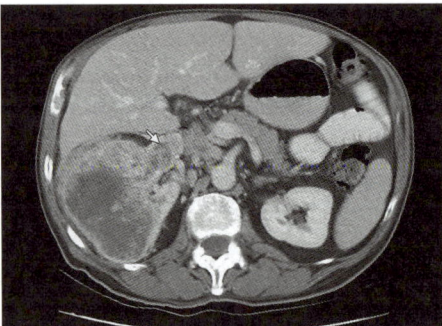

   a. Oncocytoma b. Angiomyolipoma
   c. Perinephric cyst d. Renal cell carcinoma

80. In a 3-year-old child, mother noticed the abdominal lump during giving bath to the baby. There was history of painless hematuria also. On evaluation, the swelling was ballotable with any other organomegaly. Which of the following investigation should be done in this case? *(INI-CET July 2021)*
   a. CECT b. Biopsy
   c. PET-CT d. Urinary VMA level

81. A 10 years old boy with perineal injury brought to the emergency department. After injury, patient did not pass the urine. On examination, blood was present at the meatus and bladder was palpable. What is the next step of management?
    a. Wait and watch *(INI-CET July 2021)*
    b. Wait for bladder to fill and urge to urinate
    c. Suprapubic aspiration
    d. Foley's catheter insertion

82. A 40 years old male presented with painless enlargement of right testis. On examination, right testis was enlarged with hard mass of size 4 × 4 cm. Para-aortic areas were normal. Both LDH & AFP levels were increased. What is the next best step in the management? *(INI-CET July 2021)*
    a. Biopsy   b. FNAC
    c. High inguinal orchidectomy
    d. Tumor marker

83. Most common lacrimal gland tumor: *(INI-CET July 2021)*
    a. Pleomorphic adenocarcinoma
    b. Adenoid cystic carcinoma
    c. Mucoepidermoid carcinoma
    d. Lymphoma

84. Triage means: *(INI-CET July 2021)*
    a. To sort out   b. To classify
    c. To investigate   d. To rehabilitate

85. The most delayed sign of compartment syndrome is: *(INI-CET July 2021)*
    a. Pain on passive stretching   b. Pulselessness
    c. Paralysis   d. Paraesthesia

86. Most common cause of postoperative admission after a day care procedure: *(INI-CET July 2021)*
    a. Nausea & vomiting   b. Respiratory distress
    c. Hypotension   d. Bleeding

87. Angle of needle with the skin for interrupted sutures should be: *(INI-CET July 2021)*
    a. 60 degrees   b. 70 degrees
    c. 80 degrees   d. 90 degrees

88. In a COVID positive patient, who was symptomatic and recovered at home without hospital admission, elective surgery can be planned after: *(INI-CET July 2021)*
    a. 4 weeks   b. 6 weeks
    c. 8 weeks   d. 12 weeks

89. What is the size of given cannula? *(INI-CET July 2021)*

    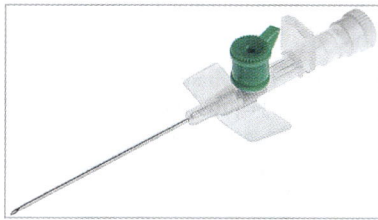

    a. 16 gauge   b. 18 gauge
    c. 20 gauge   d. 22 gauge

90. What is the name of this instrument, used in laparoscopy to insufflate abdomen?

    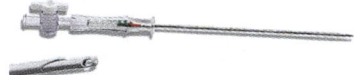

    a. Veress needle   b. Lind needle
    c. Jacob needle   d. Mathew needle

NEET PG 2021

91. A 55 years old woman underwent modified radical mastectomy 3 months back for breast cancer, which was located in upper outer quadrant of left breast. Now, she developed painless swelling in the left upper limb, whose image is given below. What is the most probable cause? *(NEET PG 2021)*

    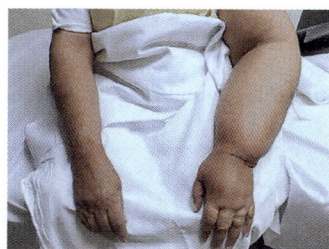

    a. Lymphedema   b. Lymphangiosarcoma
    c. Axillary vein thrombosis d. Cellulitis

92. After total thyroidectomy under GA, anesthetist tried to extubate the patient but he was unable to extubate. When he removes the tube, the patient begins to have recurrent cyanotic spells. What is the most probable reason? *(NEET PG 2021)*
    a. Unilateral recurrent laryngeal nerve damage
    b. Bilateral recurrent laryngeal nerve damage
    c. Hemorrhage
    d. Superior laryngeal nerve damage

93. All of the following statements are true about pheochromocytoma patient, *except*: *(NEET PG 2021)*
    a. Propranolol is the initial drug to be started
    b. Surgery is the treatment of choice
    c. VMA and catecholamines are the diagnostic tests
    d. Can present as hypertension alone and sometimes with vomiting and pain abdomen

94. A 50 years old male presented to the hospital with colicky abdominal pain and bilious vomiting. On evaluation, air was present in the CBD. What is the most probable diagnosis? *(NEET PG 2021)*
    a. Adhesions   b. Gastroenteritis
    c. Outlet obstruction d. Gallstone ileus

95. A 45 years old female patient presented to hospital with obstructive jaundice and CBD stone. Patient has the history of cholecystectomy, done 2 years back. What is the type of stone seen in CBD? *(NEET PG 2021)*
    a. Primary   b. Secondary
    c. Retained   d. Recurrent

96. A 40 years old male patient presented to emergency with acute abdominal pain and distention. A fluid filled lesion is present in the epigastric region. Which of the following parameter will be raised? *(NEET PG 2021)*
    a. Bilirubin   b. GGT
    c. Lipase   d. CEA

97. A 60 years old male patient presented to the hospital with gastric outlet obstruction. On evaluation, there was antral gastric carcinoma extending to head of pancreas with multiple metastasis to right lobe of liver. What is the most appropriate management? *(NEET PG 2021)*
    a. Right lobe hepatectomy with radical gastrectomy
    b. Whipple operation
    c. Palliative gastrojejunostomy with chemotherapy
    d. Radical gastrectomy with chemotherapy

98. An 18 months old male child was brought to the hospital with multiple episodes of non-bilious vomiting and poor feeding. The child was passing dry pellets like stools. Which of the following findings will be seen? *(NEET PG 2021)*
    a. Hypochloremic hypokalemic metabolic alkalosis
    b. Hypochloremic hypokalemic metabolic acidosis
    c. Hypochloremic hyperkalemic metabolic alkalosis
    d. Hypochloremic hyperkalemic metabolic acidosis

99. A patient presented to emergency with pain abdomen and fever for 3 days and dehydrated face. Abdominal X-ray images are shown below. What is the most probable diagnosis? *(NEET PG 2021)*

    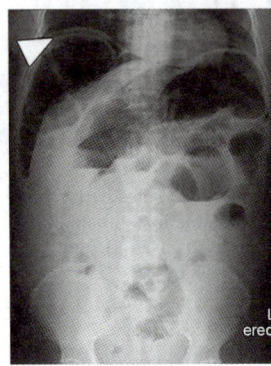 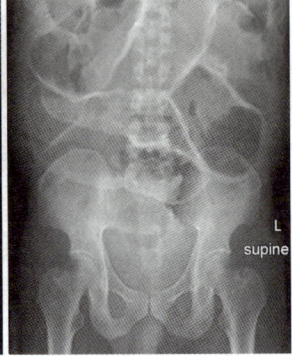

    a. Liver abscess
    b. Gastric volvulus
    c. Empyema thoracis
    d. Hollow viscus perforation

100. A 55 years old patient underwent hysterectomy 2 years back, now presented with colicky abdominal pain and bilious vomiting. On examination, abdomen was tender with exaggerated bowel sounds. On investigations, multiple air fluid levels were seen in the abdomen. What is the most probable diagnosis? *(NEET PG 2021)*
    a. Adhesive small bowel obstruction
    b. Gastroenteritis
    c. Ischemic enterocolitis
    d. Gallstone ileus

101. A 25 years old patient presented with abdominal pain and distension. Abdominal X-ray revealed the below image. Identify the prominent structure seen in the image: *(NEET PG 2021)*

    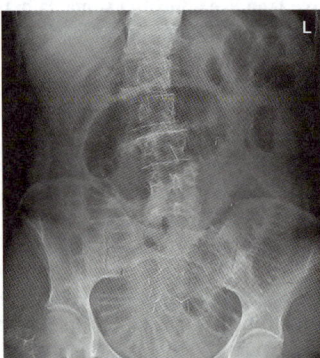

    a. Transverse colon
    b. Ileum
    c. Jejunum
    d. Duodenum

102. A 45 years old male patient with paralysis operated for rectal prolapse as shown in the image. Which of the following procedure is done? *(NEET PG 2021)*

    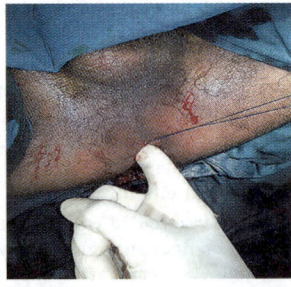

    a. Stapled hemorrhoidopexy
    b. Well's procedure
    c. Thiersch wiring
    d. Altemeier repair

103. A 54 years old male presented with right groin swelling, located below inguinal ligament, medial to inferior epigastric artery. Cough impulse was present. What is the type of hernia and its management? *(NEET PG 2021)*
    a. Direct hernia and Bassini repair
    b. Direct hernia and Lichtenstein repair
    c. Indirect hernia and Bassini repair
    d. Indirect hernia and Lichtenstein repair

104. A 30 years old female presented to the hospital with abdominal pain, weight loss & sterile pyuria. Radiograph is shown below. What is the most probable diagnosis? *(NEET PG 2021)*

    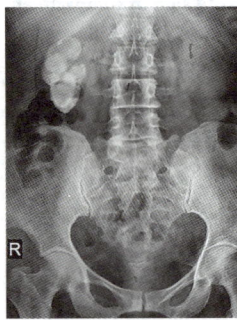

    a. Putty kidney
    b. Pyelonephritis
    c. Nephrocalcinosis
    d. Staghorn calculi

105. A patient of RTA was brought to the hospital with left flank bruise associated with hematuria. Patient was hemodynamically stable. Which of the following investigation should be done for hematuria? *(NEET PG 2021)*
    a. CECT
    b. DPL
    c. RGU
    d. MCU

106. A patient underwent radical cysto-prostatectomy and the specimen is given below. Identify the etiology: *(NEET PG 2021)*

    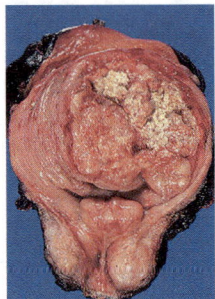

    a. Bladder cancer
    b. Schistosomiasis
    c. Prostate cancer
    d. Malakoplakia

107. What is the preferred treatment option for an 85 years old patient, known case of prostate cancer with Gleason score 6, having 2 × 3 cm nodule in prostate and level of PSA is 8 ng/mL?
    a. Brachytherapy *(NEET PG 2021)*
    b. Palliative external beam radiotherapy
    c. Active surveillance
    d. Radical prostatectomy

108. A 10 years old boy skids while cycling. The child was stable and abdominal examination was normal. Blood was noticed at the tip of meatus. What is he next best step? *(NEET PG 2021)*
    a. Nephrostomy
    b. Suprapubic cystostomy
    c. Foley's catheterization
    d. Bilateral ureteric diversion

109. A 26 years old male was operated for redness over the perineal area. Postoperative day 5 image is given below. Which of the following statement is correct about this condition? *(NEET PG 2021)*

    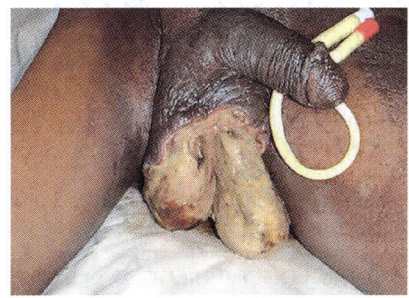

    a. Caused by mixed aerobic anerobic infection
    b. Urinary diversion is required in this patient
    c. Bilateral orchidectomy should be done
    d. Anti-gas gangrene serum should always be considered

110. A 35 years old HIV positive female on ART had a severe migraine headache, for which she was given multiple doses of ergotamine 2 days ago. Now, she presented with claudication of right thigh with some numbness and tingling in the right lower limb and peripheral pulses were feeble. Angiography image is given below. What will be the next step of management? *(NEET PG 2021)*

    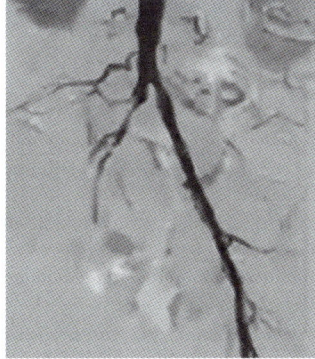

    a. Aortofemoral bypass   b. Aortoiliac bypass
    c. Iliofemoral bypass   d. PTA with stenting

111. A 45 years old male patient presents to the hospital with asymptomatic varicose veins, whose image is given below. Which CEAP classification does the patient fall under? *(NEET PG 2021)*

    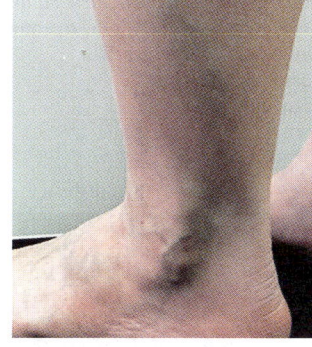

    a. 2a   b. 2b
    c. 3a   d. 3b

112. A 64 years old male patient underwent CABG, for which graft was taken from great saphenous vein. The patient is now complaining of lack of sensation over medial aspect of leg and foot, associated with heel pain. What is the most likely nerve affected in this scenario? *(NEET PG 2021)*
    a. Saphenous nerve   b. Sural nerve
    c. Superficial peroneal nerve   d. Deep peroneal nerve

113. An 80 years old female presented with fatigue and pallor. On chest X-ray, anterior mediastinal mass was seen. Patient was diagnosed with pure red cell aplasia. What is the most probable cause of aplasia? *(NEET PG 2021)*
    a. Thymic neoplasia
    b. Non-Hodgkin's lymphoma
    c. Bronchogenic carcinoma
    d. Germ cell tumor

114. A 9 years old male child was brought to emergency by the mother with difficulty in swallowing for the past few hours. He was noted to play unsupervised. X-ray was taken. Identify the location of foreign body:

    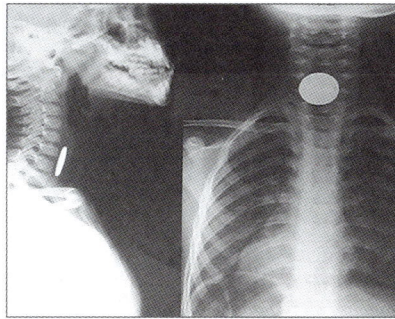

    a. Esophagus   b. Trachea
    c. Soft-tissue of neck   d. Artifact of X-ray

115. A patient presented with a jaw swelling and weight loss. Suspecting a malignancy, the sub-mandibular gland was resected and the Wharton's duct was ligated in the process. Which is the most likely nerve to be damaged during submandibular gland resection? *(NEET PG 2021)*
    a. Lingual nerve   b. Hypoglossal nerve
    c. Inferior alveolar nerve   d. Nerve to mylohyoid

116. A 56 years old man was working in a benzene factory for the long time. He got retired 5 years back. What would be the possible complication in this patient? *(NEET PG 2021)*
    a. Bladder cancer   b. Blood cancer
    c. Lung cancer   d. Skin cancer

117. A child undergoes prophylactic irradiation as a preparation for bone marrow transplant, for the treatment of ALL. Which of the following is affected least? *(NEET PG 2021)*
    a. Spermatogonia
    b. Intestinal epithelial cells
    c. Neurons
    d. Bone marrow

118. What is the maneuver shown below? *(NEET PG 2021)*

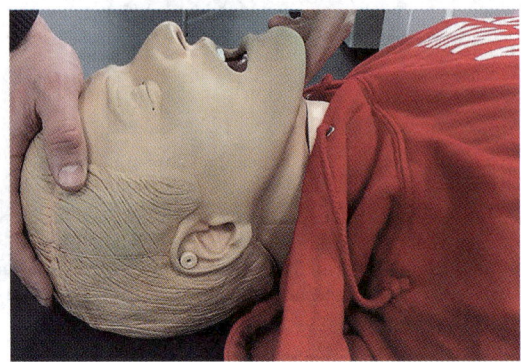

    a. Head extension
    b. Head tilt, chin lift
    c. Jaw thrust
    d. Manual inline stabilisation

119. A 25 years old male patient presented to the emergency with history of road traffic accident. On examination, the patient had subcutaneous emphysema, absence of air entry on the right side of hemithorax & hypotension. Which of the following will be the next step of management? *(NEET PG 2021)*
    a. Needle decompression in 5th intercostal space
    b. Fluid resuscitation with wide bore needle
    c. Plan for intubation
    d. Positive pressure ventilation

120. A 25 years old male patient with alleged history of road traffic accident sustained injury over chest and abdomen. At the time of presentation, systolic BP was 70 mm Hg and pulse rate was 110/minute. Which of the following is the next step? *(NEET PG 2021)*
    a. FAST
    b. CECT
    c. Chest X-ray
    d. MRI

NEET PG 2020

121. A 40 years old women presented to the clinic with a 4 cm mass in the upper outer quadrant. Biopsy from the mass showed densely packed cells with bland nuclei and mucin infiltrating the stroma. Most probable diagnosis is: *(NEET PG 2020)*
    a. Colloid carcinoma
    b. Tubular carcinoma
    c. Papillary carcinoma
    d. Medullary carcinoma

122. Which of the following statements is true regarding retrosternal goitres? *(NEET PG 2020)*
    a. Operated only if patient is symptomatic
    b. Sternal incision is always required
    c. Majority of the goitres derive their blood supply from mediastinal vessels
    d. Majority of the retrosternal goitres can be removed by a neck incision

123. A 25 years old male presented with a 2 cm nodule. Thyroidectomy was done. The histology picture is given below. What is the most likely diagnosis? *(NEET PG 2020)*

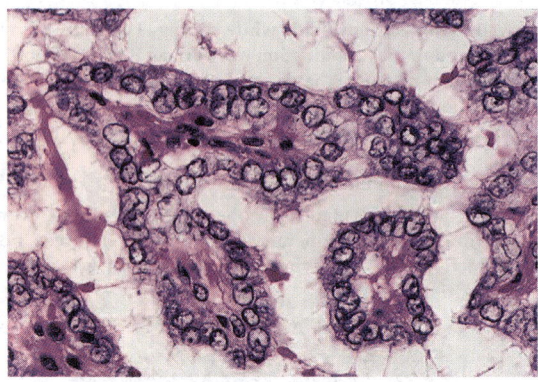

    a. Papillary thyroid carcinoma
    b. Medullary thyroid carcinoma
    c. Toxic nodular goitre
    d. Follicular thyroid carcinoma

124. A 30 years old female presents with a diffuse thyroid swelling. On investigations, TSH levels were elevated. Postoperative HPE reports showed intense lymphocytic infiltration and Hürthle cells. Which of the following is the most likely diagnosis? *(NEET PG 2020)*
    a. Grave's disease
    b. Hashimoto's thyroiditis
    c. Follicular carcinoma
    d. Medullary thyroid carcinoma

125. In a patient with parathyroid adenoma, how do we confirm the removal of the correct gland after surgery?
    a. 50% reduction in PTH within 10 mins of gland removal
    b. 50% reduction in PTH within 5 mins of gland removal
    c. 25% reduction in PTH within 10 mins of gland removal
    d. 25% reduction in PTH within 5 mins of gland removal

126. What is the Child-Pugh class for patient who has a serum bilirubin of 2.5 mg/dL, serum albumin of 3 g/dL, INR of 2 along with mild ascites but no encephalopathy? *(NEET PG 2020)*
    a. CP class A
    b. CP class B
    c. CP class C
    d. CP class D

127. Ligation of common hepatic artery will impair blood supply in: *(NEET PG 2020)*
    a. Right gastric and right gastroepiploic artery
    b. Right gastric and left gastric artery
    c. Right gastroepiploic artery and short gastric vessels
    d. Right gastric and short gastric vessels

128. An 80 years old female presented with colicky pain and jaundice. Serum bilirubin and GGT was raised. MRCP image shows gallstones and CBD stones with dilated biliary radicles. Next step in the management: *(NEET PG 2020)*
    a. Cholecystectomy
    b. ERCP
    c. CECT
    d. PET scan

129. A 35 years old male presented with recurrent episodes of abdominal pain, abdominal tenderness, fever and jaundice. MRCP image of the patient is given below. Most likely diagnosis is: *(NEET PG 2020)*

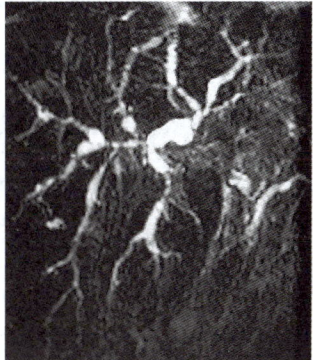

   a. Primary sclerosing cholangitis
   b. Primary biliary cirrhosis
   c. Oriental cholangiohepatitis
   d. Caroli's disease

130. Tumor of the uncinate process of pancreas affects which of the following? *(NEET PG 2020)*
   a. Superior mesenteric artery
   b. Portal vein
   c. Common hepatic artery
   d. Inferior mesenteric artery

131. Most common pancreatic endocrine neoplasm: *(NEET PG 2020)*
   a. Insulinoma   b. Gastrinoma
   c. VIPoma   d. Glucagonoma

132. What is the most common site of gastrinoma in MEN 1 syndrome? *(NEET PG 2020)*
   a. Jejunum   b. Ileum
   c. Duodenum   d. Stomach

133. Patient presents with halitosis and a swelling in the lateral aspect of the neck, which on pressing gives rise to a regurgitant sound. Barium swallow image is shown. What is the diagnosis? *(NEET PG 2020)*

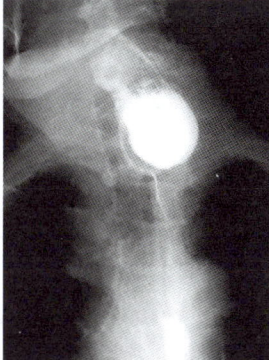

   a. Laryngocele   b. Achalasia cardia
   c. Pharyngeal pouch d. Schatzki's ring

134. On esophageal manometry, abnormal spastic contractions in esophagus >450 mm Hg·s·cm in the body is suggestive of: *(NEET PG 2020)*
   a. Type I achalasia   b. Type II achalasia
   c. Type III achalasia d. Jackhammer esophagus

135. What is the diagnosis based on the given barium swallow image? *(NEET PG 2020)*

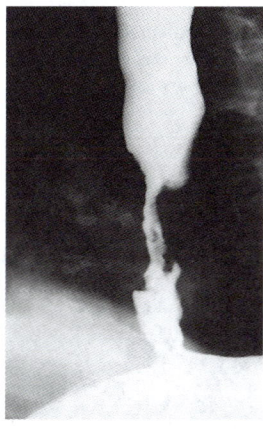

   a. Achalasia cardia   b. Carcinoma esophagus
   c. Esophageal stricture d. GERD

136. A middle-aged man complains of upper abdominal pain after a heavy meal. There is tenderness in the upper abdomen and on X-ray, widening of the mediastinum is seen with pneumo-mediastinum. What is the diagnosis? *(NEET PG 2020)*
   a. Spontaneous perforation of the esophagus
   b. Perforated peptic ulcer
   c. Foreign body in esophagus
   d. Rupture of emphysematous bulla

137. A young man met with a motor bike accident and had injury to ileum and jejunum. Therefore the entire ileum and part of jejunum was resected. Which of the following would the patient suffer from? *(NEET PG 2020)*
   a. Vitamin B_{12} deficiency   b. Constipation
   c. Gastric ulcer   d. Hypogastrinemia

138. A patient presented with abdominal pain, blood in stool and a palpable mass on the abdominal examination. The following barium image was obtained from the patient. What is the most probable diagnosis? *(NEET PG 2020)*

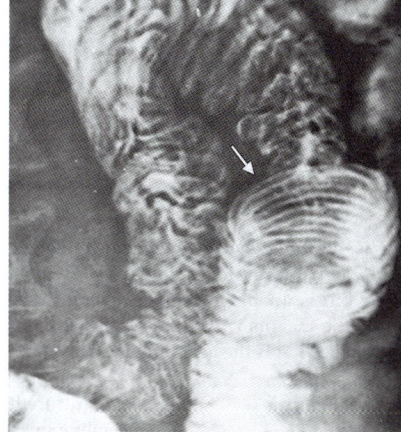

   a. Meckel's diverticulum   b. Intussusception
   c. Volvulus   d. Diverticulitis

139. Patient presents with peritonitis and during surgery a diverticular perforation is seen with fecal peritonitis. What is the Hinchey's stage? *(NEET PG 2020)*
    a. 1
    b. 2
    c. 3
    d. 4

140. A 5 years old child presented with history of blood in stools. On examination, there was a polypoidal mass in the rectum, biopsy of which is shown as below. Most probably diagnosis is: *(NEET PG 2020)*

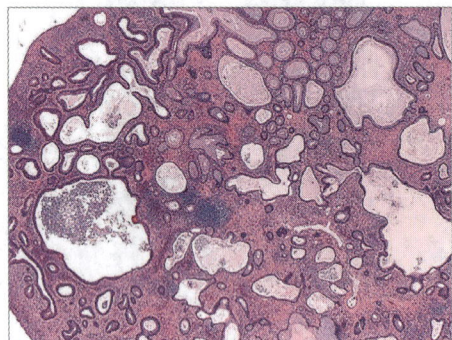

    a. Villous adenoma
    b. Juvenile polyp
    c. Vascular malformation
    d. Serrated adenoma

141. What is the diagnosis based on the given image?
    (NEET PG 2020)

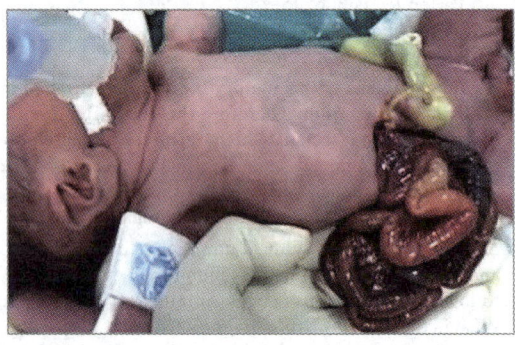

    a. Omphalocele
    b. Gastroschisis
    c. Umbilical hernia
    d. Spigelian hernia

142. Management of RCC less than 4 cm in size: *(NEET PG 2020)*
    a. Radical nephrectomy
    b. Partial nephrectomy
    c. Chemotherapy
    d. Surgery followed by chemotherapy

143. A man is brought to the emergency after he fell into a man-hole and injured his perineum. He feels the urge to micturate but is unable to pass urine and there is blood at the tip of the meatus with extensive swelling of the penis and scrotum. What is the location of the injury? *(NEET PG 2020)*
    a. Bulbar urethra
    b. Prostatic urethra
    c. Bladder
    d. Membranous urethra

144. Identify the investigation being performed and possible diagnosis: *(NEET PG 2020)*

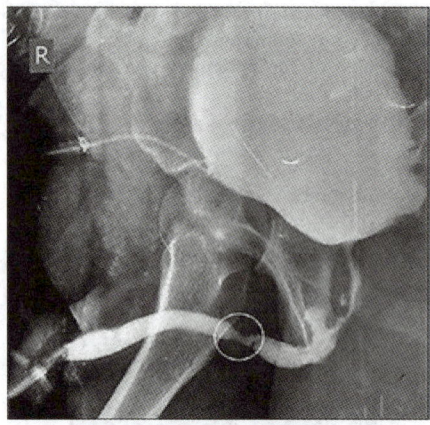

    a. MCU with membranous urethral stricture
    b. MCU with bulbar urethral stricture
    c. RGU with penile urethral stricture
    d. RGU with prostatic urethral stricture

145. True statement about intermittent claudication:
    a. Felt at rest *(NEET PG 2020)*
    b. Most common site is the calf
    c. Claudication distance can vary from day to day
    d. Relieved after getting out of bed and walking

146. A 30 years old man presents with cramping gluteal pain after walking 500 meters. Which is the vessel involved? *(NEET PG 2020)*
    a. Arterial disease with aorto-iliac involvement
    b. Arterial disease with femoral artery involvement
    c. Femoral venous insufficiency
    d. Saphenous venous insufficiency

147. Male patient presents to the hospital with abdominal pain and is incidentally detected with an abdominal aortic aneurysm. What is the appropriate management of this patient? *(NEET PG 2020)*
    a. Immediate surgery
    b. USG monitoring till size of the aneurysm reaches 70 mm
    c. Monitor till size reaches 40 mm
    d. Monitor till size reaches 55 mm

148. Which one of the following is not a component of THORACOSCORE? *(NEET PG 2020)*
    a. Performance status   b. Complication of surgery
    c. ASA grading   d. Priority of surgery

149. What is the T stage of a 2.5 cm lung carcinoma, which is not involving the pleura? *(NEET PG 2020)*
    a. T1a   b. T1b
    c. T1c   d. T2

150. Patient with clinical signs of DVT had tachycardia and history of bladder cancer. According to modified Well's scoring, the probability of pulmonary embolism would be: *(NEET PG 2020)*
    a. Low   b. Moderate
    c. High   d. Severe

151. A child was brought to the emergency with multiple injuries which included a femur fracture as well. He was confused and dyspneic. There was presence of rash all over the body. What is the most probable diagnosis? *(NEET PG 2020)*
    a. Fat embolism   b. Air embolism
    c. Pulmonary embolism   d. DIC

152. What is the most probable cause of this condition?
    (NEET PG 2020)

    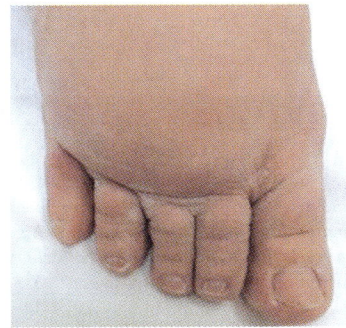

    a. Chronic lymphedema
    b. Chronic arterial blockage
    c. Chronic venous blockage
    d. Chronic venous insufficiency

153. An elderly man with a long standing mole over the face which is increasing in size and showing irregular borders. Diagnosis: *(NEET PG 2020)*
    a. Superficial spreading melanoma
    b. Lentigo maligna
    c. Acral melanoma
    d. Nodular melanoma

154. For frost-bite rewarming, the temperature should be:
    (NEET PG 2020)
    a. 20°C
    b. 25°C
    c. 37°C
    d. 42°C

155. CT scan image showing cystic lesion with suprasellar calcification is suggestive of: *(NEET PG 2020)*

    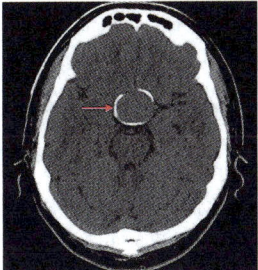 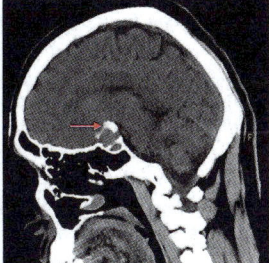

    a. Craniopharyngioma
    b. Meningioma
    c. Astrocytoma
    d. Oligodendroglioma

156. Which of the following is not a surgical landmark for facial nerve identification in parotid surgery? *(NEET PG 2020)*
    a. Inferior belly of omohyoid
    b. Tragal pointer
    c. Posterior belly of digastric
    d. Dissecting from peripheral branches

157. A middle-aged man presented with a swelling over the neck since childhood. Neck swelling has a bag of worm appearance. Most probable diagnosis is: *(NEET PG 2020)*
    a. Plexiform neurofibroma
    b. Toxic nodular goitre
    c. Vasculitis
    d. Lymphangioma

158. Primary survey of ATLS does not include: *(NEET PG 2020)*
    a. CT scan
    b. FAST
    c. Chest X-ray
    d. Pelvic X-ray

159. A 20 years old boy is brought to the emergency following a RTA with respiratory distress and hypotension. He has subcutaneous emphysema and no air entry on the right side. What is the next best step in the management?
    (NEET PG 2020)
    a. Start IV fluids after insertion of wide bore IV line
    b. Needle decompression in the 5th intercostal space
    c. Shift to ICU and intubate
    d. Positive pressure ventilation

160. Patient with stab injury to the lower chest presented with low pulses and BP improved after giving IV fluids. Chest X-ray showed clear lung fields. Next step in the management:
    (NEET PG 2020)
    a. Chest tube insertion
    b. CECT abdomen
    c. CECT chest
    d. E-fast

161. The given below image in a patient with road traffic accident shows: *(NEET PG 2020)*

    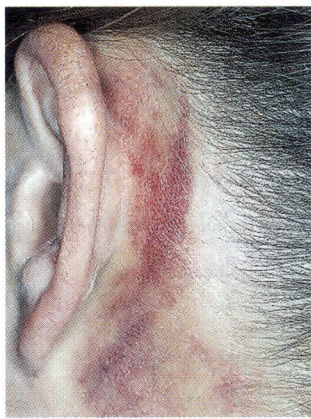

    a. Battle sign
    b. Bezold abscess
    c. Citelli's abscess
    d. Griesinger sign

162. A 5 years old child is having acute liver failure. Which one of the following criteria is not included in the King's college criteria? *(NEET PG 2020)*
    a. Age <11 years
    b. INR >6.5
    c. Bilirubin >300 µmol/L
    d. Jaundice <7 days before development of encephalopathy

163. Which is the most common infection in a transplant patient after 3–4 months? In renal transplant recipients, which is the likely organism causing reactivation disease within 3–4 months after surgery? *(NEET PG 2020)*
    a. HSV
    b. CMV
    c. EBV
    d. VZV

164. Nosocomial infections are diagnosed after how many hours of hospitalization/admission? *(NEET PG 2020)*
    a. 24 hours
    b. 48 hours
    c. 72 hours
    d. 96 hours

165. All of the following are part of the ASEPSIS wound score, *except*: *(NEET PG 2020)*
    a. Serous discharge
    b. Purulent exudate
    c. Induration
    d. Erythema

166. Graft taken from identical twin is called as: *(NEET PG 2020)*
    a. Autograft
    b. Allograft
    c. Isograft
    d. Xenograft

Explanations

INI-CET MAY 2022

1. **Ans. c. Genetic counselling & BRCA testing** *(Ref: Sabiston 21/e p823)*

   "Indications for consideration of genetic testing include breast cancer diagnosed before age 50, bilateral breast cancer, breast and ovarian cancer in the same individual, and breast cancer in men. Other factors that may be indications for testing are a family history (maternal or paternal) of two or more individuals with breast and ovarian cancer, a close male relative with breast cancer, a close relative with early-onset (<50 years) breast or ovarian cancer, and known BRCA1 or BRCA2 mutation in the family."-Sabiston 21/e p823

2. **Ans. b. 3 months before** *(Ref: Breast Cancer by Erban & Smith (2009)/p77)*

   "Because it may take 6 to 8 weeks for tamoxifen metabolites to be cleared from the bloodstream, most women should plan to wait at least 3 months after stopping tamoxifen before attempting to conceive."- Breast Cancer by Erban & Smith (2009)/p77

3. **Ans. a. FNAC or biopsy required before surgery** *(Ref: Sabiston 21/e p1460)*

   Diagnosis of hydatid cyst is highly suggested by ultrasound or CT and confirmed by serology. FNAC or biopsy can cause anaphylaxis, and hence not done in hydatid cyst.

4. **Ans. b. Carcinoma** *(Ref: Sabiston 21/e p1516)*

5. **Ans. b. Periampullary carcinoma** *(Ref: Sabiston 21/e p1554)*

   "The waxing and waning nature of jaundice is due to sloughing of ampullary cancer, resulting in transient resolution of the jaundice."

6. **Ans. b. Carcinoma head of pancreas** *(Ref: Sabiston 21/e p1556)*

   This is a diagrammatic representation of Whipple's procedure, in which pancreaticojejunostomy, hepaticojejunostomy and gastrojejunostomy is done. Whipple's procedure is done for carcinoma head of pancreas.

7. **Ans. a. 24-hours pH monitoring** *(Ref: Sabiston 21/e p1026, 1022)*

   Ambulatory pH monitoring is the "gold standard" test to diagnose GERD, not the achalasia.

   "Manometry is the "gold standard" test for diagnosis and distinguishes achalasia from other potential esophageal motility disorders."- Sabiston 21/e p1026

   "The diagnosis of achalasia is usually made from an esophagram and a motility study. The findings may vary, depending on the degree to which the disease has advanced. The esophagram will often show a dilated esophagus with a distal narrowing referred to as the classic bird beak appearance of the barium-filled esophagus."- Sabiston 21/e p1026

   "Endoscopy must also be performed in all suspected achalasia patients to evaluate the mucosa for esophagitis and rule out secondary causes of distal esophageal narrowing ("pseudoachalasia") such as GEJ tumors, neuropathy, and strictures."- Sabiston 21/e p1026

   "Ambulatory pH monitoring quantifies distal esophageal acid exposure and is the "gold standard" test to diagnose GERD."- Sabiston 21/e p1060

8. **Ans. a. Manometry** *(Ref: Sabiston 21/e p1026)*

   Manometry is the "gold standard" test for diagnosis of achalasia.

9. **Ans. c. Duodenal fistula** *(Ref: Sabiston 21/e p1291)*

   "Enterocutaneous fistulas are classified according to their location and volume of daily output. These factors dictate treatment and morbidity and mortality rates. Proximal fistulas are associated with higher output, greater fluid and electrolyte loss, and greater loss of digestive capacity. Distal fistulas tend to have lower output, making them easier to manage and more likely to close spontaneously."-Sabiston 21/e p1291

10. **Ans. a. 1 and 3** *(Ref: Sabiston 21/e p1864)*

    "Meckel diverticulum is the most common congenital anomaly of the GI tract and occurs in approximately 2% of the population. More than 70% of symptomatic patients have heterotopic gastric mucosa and another 5% have pancreatic tissue."- Sabiston 21/e p1864

11. **Ans. a. Crohn's disease has skip lesions; b. Childhood IBD is genetic** *(Ref: Sabiston 21/e p1162, 1259, 1265)*

"Crohn disease is more typically associated with guaiac-positive diarrhea and mucous stools without gross blood. It can affect any portion of the GI tract and is characterized by skip lesions, transmural thickening and inflammation of the bowel wall, and granulomas."-Sabiston 21/e p1162

"Genetic factors play an important role in the pathogenesis of Crohn disease because the single strongest risk factor for development of disease is having a first-degree relative with Crohn disease."- Sabiston 21/e p1259

"There is no cure for Crohn disease. Therefore, medical therapies are directed toward inducing and maintaining steroid-free remission as well as preventing acute exacerbations or complications of the disease."- Sabiston 21/e p1265

12. **Ans. a. Ripstein** *(Ref: Sabiston 21/e p1395; Bailey 27/e p1323)*

Altemeier, Thiersch and Delorme are perineal approaches, whereas Ripstein is an abdominal approach for rectal prolapse.

13. **Ans. b. Ilioinguinal nerve** *(Ref: Sabiston 21/e p1083)*

*Ilioinguinal nerve fibres are distributed to the skin of upper and medial part of thigh, and to the following locations in the male and female: In the male ("anterior scrotal nerve"): to the **skin over root of penis & upper part of scrotum**; In the female ("anterior labial nerve"): to the **skin covering mons pubis & labia majora**.*

14. **Ans. a. Contain glycogen and lipid; b. Mostly are sporadic** *(Ref: Bailey 27/e p1419)*

Clear cell RCC can be sporadic (>96%) or familial (<4%). VHL disease is an autosomal dominant disorder resulting from a deletion or mutation in the VHL gene located on the short arm of chromosome 3. Clear cell RCC arises from PCT, contains glycogen and lipid.

15. **Ans. c. Laparotomy** *(Ref: Bailey 27/e p1425)*

Extravasation of contrast into peritoneal cavity suggest the diagnosis of intraperitoneal bladder rupture. In the treatment of intraperitoneal bladder rupture, lower midline laparotomy is performed.

"Treatment of intraperitoneal rupture: A lower midline laparotomy should be performed; the edges of the rent are trimmed and sutured with a single-layer 2/0 absorbable suture. A suprapubic and a urethral catheter are placed. Very rarely, the rupture will be through an unsuspected tumour; a biopsy can be taken before suturing the defect."- Bailey 27/e p1425

16. **Ans. b. Secondary contraction more with split thickness skin grafting; c. Primary contraction more with full thickness skin graft**
    (Ref: Schwartz 10/e p1832, 1833)

Primary contraction: Immediate reduction in size of skin graft after it has been harvested, caused by passive recoil of elastin fibers in dermis. As FTSGs have a greater amount of dermis, primary contraction is more significant in FTSG than STSG.
Secondary contraction: Shrinkage of skin graft in wound bed over time, caused by myofibroblasts. Secondary contraction is greater for STSGs than FTSGs, as the additional dermis in FTSGs is resistant to the pull of myofibroblasts.

"Split-Thickness Grafts. Split-thickness skin grafting represents the simplest method of superficial reconstruction in plastic surgery. Many of the characteristics of a split-thickness graft are determined by the amount of dermis present. Less dermis translates into less primary contraction (the degree to which a graft shrinks in surface area after harvesting and before grafting), more secondary contraction (the degree to which a graft shrinks during healing), and better chance of graft survival. Thin split grafts have low primary contraction, high secondary contraction, and high reliability of graft take, often even in imperfect recipient beds."- Schwartz 10/e p1832

"Full-Thickness Grafts. By definition, full-thickness skin grafts include the epidermis and the complete layer of dermis. The subcutaneous tissue is carefully removed from the deep surface of the dermis to maximize the potential for engraftment. Full-thickness grafts are associated with the least secondary contraction upon healing, the best cosmetic appearance, and the highest durability." - Schwartz 10/e p1833

17. **Ans. a. Amputation in severe cases; b. Antibiotics and analgesics are not used; d. Clean and dry the area** *(Ref: Bailey 27/e p422)*

"Frost bite: Warming should be gentle as the heat used may actually cause a burn! Rehydration with warm fluids and use of non-steroidal anti-inflammatory drugs like ibuprofen are beneficial. Demarcation will occur between dead and viable tissue and at this stage no surgery should be undertaken as there is often considerable deep recovery. The injured area should be kept clean and dry and efforts made to prevent further injury, as well as to prevent infection. Definitive surgery to excise dead tissue can be left for many months."-Bailey 27/e p422

18. **Ans. a. Fluctuant mass; b. Pott's spine can present as psoas abscess; c. Can present in thigh; d. Hematogenous spread of TB in immunocompromised** *(Ref: Bailey 27/e p1065)*

"Psoas abscess is a relatively uncommon diagnosis, the true incidence of which is not well described. At the start of the twentieth century, psoas abscess was mainly caused by TB of the spine (Pott's disease)."-Bailey 27/e p1065

"In recent years a primary psoas abscess due to haematogenous spread from an occult source is more common, especially in immunocompromised and older patients, as well as in association with intravenous drug misuse."-Bailey 27/e p1065

"Clinical presentation is with back pain, lassitude and fever. A swelling may point to the groin as it tracks along iliopsoas. Pain may be elicited by passive extension of the hip or a fixed flexion of the hip evident on inspection."-*Bailey 27/e p1065*

19. **Ans. a. Diffuse axonal injury** *(Ref: Bailey 27/e p326; Sabiston 21/e p397)*

"Diffuse axonal injury: This is a form of primary brain injury, seen in high-energy accidents, and which usually renders the patient comatose."-*Bailey 27/e p326*

"Commonly, diffuse axonal injury becomes evident when patients demonstrate poor neurologic status in the setting of underwhelming imaging studies, although ultimate functional prognosis remains difficult to predict based on this finding."-*Sabiston 21/e p397*

20. **Ans. b. Presence of pneumoperitoneum** *(Ref: Sabiston 21/e p415)*

Presence of pneumoperitoneum (hollow viscus injury is an indication for laparotomy.

"Operative management of splenic injuries may be required in the setting of instability at the time of admission or after failed non-operative management."- *Sabiston 21/e p415*

NEET PG 2022

21. **Ans. b. Involvement of subdermal lymphatics** *(Ref: Bailey 27/e p879)*

"Phenomena resulting from lymphatic obstruction in advanced breast cancer (Peau d'orange): Peau d'orange is caused by cutaneous lymphatic oedema. Where the infiltrated skin is tethered by the sweat ducts it cannot swell, leading to an appearance like orange skin."-*Bailey 27/e p879*

22. **Ans. d. FNAC is not diagnostic** *(Ref: Bailey 27/e p818)*

This is a case of papillary carcinoma thyroid, in which the diagnosis is confirmed by FNAC.

23. **Ans. b. Calcium, phosphate and PTH levels** *(Ref: Bailey 27/e p815)*

Perioral numbness on 3rd day of thyroidectomy suggest the parathyroid insufficiency leading to hypocalcemia. So, calcium, phosphate and PTH levels should be assessed.

24. **Ans. a. Parathyroid adenoma** *(Ref: Bailey 27/e 856)*

Parathyroid adenoma is not the component of MEN-2B.

"MEN 2B comprises MTC, phaeochromocytoma and characteristic facial and oral mucosal neurinomas and intestinal ganglioneuromatosis, accompanied by a Marfanoid habitus."- *Bailey 27/e 856*

25. **Ans. d. Resuscitation and laparotomy** *(Ref: Bailey 27/e p1051)*

Chest X-ray is showing air under the right dome of diaphragm, which is seen in perforation peritonitis. In cases of perforation peritonitis, laparotomy is the treatment of choice after fluid resuscitation of the patient and IV antibiotics.

26. **Ans. a. Intussusception** *(Ref: Bailey 27/e p1289)*

"A barium enema may be used to diagnose the presence of an ileocolic intussusception (the claw sign)."- *Bailey 27/e p1289*

27. **Ans. c. Fistula-in-ano** *(Ref: Bailey 27/e p1363, 1364)*

"A fistula-in-ano, or anal fistula, is a chronic abnormal communication, usually lined to some degree by granulation tissue, which runs outwards from the anorectal lumen (the internal opening) to an external opening on the skin of the perineum or buttock (or rarely, in women, to the vagina)."-*Bailey 27/e p1363*

28. **Ans. c. Pelviureteric junction obstruction** *(Ref: Bailey 27/e p1411)*

"PUJ Obstruction: IVU helps only if there is significant function in the obstructed kidney. The extrarenal pelvis is dilated and the minor calyces lose their normal cupping and become 'clubbed'."-*Bailey 27/e p1411*

29. **Ans. a. Vesicoureteric reflux** *(Ref: Bailey 27/e p1404)*

MCU is showing gross dilation of the ureter, pelvis & calyces; loss of papillary impression and ureteral tortuosity, suggestive of bilateral Grade V vesicoureteric reflux.

30. **Ans. d. Bladder exstrophy** *(Ref: Bailey 27/e p1424)*

31. **Ans. c. Prostatic venous plexus** *(Ref: Vishram Singh 3/e p248)*

The prostatic venous plexus drains into the internal iliac vein which connects with the vertebral venous plexus, this is thought to be the route of bone metastasis of prostate cancer. It is sometimes known as "Santorini's plexus," named for the Italian anatomist Giovanni Domenico Santorini.

"Prostatic venous plexus → vertebral venous plexus (of Batson) → intracranial dural venous sinuses. This pathway explains the metastasis of cancer prostate into the vertebral column and brain."-Vishram Singh 3/e p248

32. **Ans. a. Membranous urethra** *(Ref: Bailey 27/e p1481)*

RGU demonstrates the extravasation of contrast from the membranous urethra at the site of a urethral injury.

33. **Ans. a. Fournier's gangrene** *(Ref: Bailey 27/e p1509)*

"Fournier's gangrene is an uncommon and nasty condition characterised by a polymicrobial infection of the soft tissues of the perineum, external genitalia and perianal region. It is a form of necrotising fasciitis. There is rapid onset of gangrene leading to exposure of the scrotal contents."- Bailey 27/e p1509

34. **Ans. a. Aortic-iliac bifurcation** *(Ref: Bailey 27/e p943)*

"Aorto-iliac disease (30% of cases) may cause thigh or buttock claudication. Buttock claudication in association with sexual impotence resulting from arterial insufficiency is eponymously called Leriche's syndrome."-Bailey 27/e p943

35. **Ans. c. Saphenous nerve** *(Ref: Bailey 27/e p982)*

"Complications of standard varicose vein surgery: Complications (minor and major) are reported in up to 20% of patients who undergo traditional varicose vein surgery. Wound infections, the most common complication, are reduced by prophylactic antibiotics. Nerve injury is the most common serious complication. The incidence of saphenous nerve neuralgia is up to 7% following GSV stripping to the knee (the incidence is higher with stripping to the ankle)."-Bailey 27/e p982

36. **Ans. d. Fat embolism** *(Ref: Apley's 9/e p681; Rockwood 6/e p553)*

"Fat embolism is a common phenomenon following limb fractures. Circulating fat globules larger than 10 µm in diameter occur in most adults after closed fractures of long bones and histological traces of fat can be found in the lungs and other internal organs." -Apley's 9/e p681

"Early warning signs of fat embolism (usually within 72 hours of injury) are a slight rise of temperature and pulse rate. In more pronounced cases, there is breathlessness and mild mental confusion or restlessness. Pathognomonic signs are petechiae on the trunk, axillae and in the conjunctival folds and retinae. In more severe cases there may be respiratory distress and coma, due both to brain emboli and hypoxia from involvement of the lungs. The features at this stage are essentially those of ARDS."- Apley's 9/e p681

37. **Ans. d. Chest drain insertion and drainage** *(Ref: Bailey 27/e p367; Schwartz 11/e p186)*

History of trauma with bruises on the chest, pulse rate-120/minute, BP-90/60 mm Hg, respiratory rate-40/minute and chest X-ray showing pneumothorax with depressed diaphragm, collapsed right lung and shift of mediastinum suggest the diagnosis of tension pneumothorax. Treatment of choice for this condition is chest tube insertion and drainage.

"Tension pneumothorax and simple pneumothorax have similar signs, symptoms, and examination findings, but hypotension qualifies the pneumothorax as a tension pneumothorax. Although immediate needle thoracostomy decompression with a 14-gauge angiocatheter in the second intercostal space in the midclavicular line may be indicated in the field, tube thoracostomy should be performed immediately in the ED before a chest radiograph is obtained. Recent studies suggest the preferred location for needle decompression may be the 5th intercostal space in the anterior axillary line due to body habitus."-Schwartz 11/e p186

38. **Ans. b. 15–20%** *(Ref: Sabiston 21/e p488)*

In a 9 years old child, there is involvement of half of chest wall and abdomen (13/2 = 6.5%), posterior arm (4/2 = 2%) and thigh (8%); that is equal to 16.5% (15–20%).

39. **Ans. d. Grade IV** *(Ref: Bailey 27/e p29)*

Staging of Pressure Scores	
Stage	Description
1	Non-blanchable erythema without a breach in the epidermis
2	Partial-thickness skin loss involving the epidermis and dermis
3	Full-thickness skin loss extending into the subcutaneous tissue but not through underlying fascia
4	Full-thickness skin loss through fascia with extensive tissue destruction, maybe involving muscle, bone, tendon or joint

40. **Ans. a. Leukoplakia** *(Ref: Sabiston 21/e p772)*
41. **Ans. a. Sialolithiasis** *(Ref: Bailey 27/e p780)*
42. **Ans. b. Parotid gland swelling** *(Ref: Bailey 27/e p788)*

It's the typical location of parotid swelling, located in-front, below and behind the ear lobule, pushing it up.

43. **Ans. b. Subarachnoid hemorrhage** *(Ref: Sabiston 21/e p1887)*

Rupture of saccular aneurysm in brain leads to subarachnoid hemorrhage.

"Saccular Aneurysms: As the name implies, these aneurysms, also referred to as berry aneurysms, are usually saccular in form and come off the vessel wall or at a bifurcation. Many of these are found incidentally, given the frequency of neuroimaging, but many present with hemorrhage. The classic presentation of subarachnoid hemorrhage due to a cerebral aneurysm is that of sudden onset of a headache, described as the "worst headache of my life.""- *Sabiston 21/e p1887*

44. **Ans. a. Further investigation** *(Ref: Sabiston 21/e p412)*

The patient is having anterior stab wound and patient is stable. So, evaluation for peritoneal violation may be conducted via local wound exploration, ultrasound, CT, or diagnostic laparoscopy. Hence, the answer would be further investigation.

"Abdominal stab wound patients with hemodynamic instability, peritonitis, or evisceration require immediate laparotomy. In patients who are not examinable, evaluation for peritoneal violation may be conducted via local wound exploration, ultrasound, CT, or diagnostic laparoscopy."-*Sabiston 21/e p412*

45. **Ans. c. Ambulatory** *(Ref: Bailey 27/e p412)*

Green color in triage signifies ambulatory patient.

INI-CET NOVEMBER 2021

46. **Ans. d. Closed** *(Ref: Bailey 27/e p99, 100)*

The given drain is Romo Vac drain, which utilise suction to work. So, it is a closed drain.

Drains
• Drains are inserted to **allow fluid or air** that might collect at an operation site or in a wound **to drain freely to the surface**. • Fluid to be drained may include blood, serum, pus, urine, feces, bile or lymph. • **Allow wound irrigation**. • Adequate drainage of fluid collections prevents the development of cavities or spaces that may delay wound healing. • Their use can be regarded as **prophylactic in elective surgery** and **therapeutic in emergency surgery.**

Types of Drains	
Type	**Principles Applied**
Open drains	• Utilizes the principle of **gravity**^{Q}
Semi-open drains	• Work on the principle of the **capillary effect**^{Q}
Closed drain	• Utilise **suction** to work^Q

47. **Ans. c. Done in all cases for immediate diagnosis** *(Ref: Bailey 27/e p238, 877; Schwartz 11/e p590)*

Frozen section is used for assessment of margins positivity, for sentinel lymph node biopsy and to identify the metastatic lesion (Differentiates primary tumor from metastatic tumors intraoperatively). Frozen section is not required in all cases for immediate diagnosis, because in breast cancer, the diagnosis is already done by the tru-cut biopsy.

"Frozen section diagnosis is useful when a very rapid answer is necessary for diagnosis or management. Surgeons are the main users of this service. A representative fresh tissue sample of the area of interest is supplied by the surgeon and frozen quickly in the pathology laboratory, and sections are cut and stained within several minutes. There are a few disadvantages: fresh tissue carries a higher risk of infection than fixed tissue; the quality of a frozen section slide is inferior to that of routinely processed material, reducing the accuracy and precision of diagnosis; small samples are required; certain types of tissue (e.g. fat) are difficult to deal with; and the process is time-consuming and disruptive for the histopathology department."-*Bailey 27/e p238*

48. **Ans. b. 1, 3, 4 and 5** *(Ref: Schwartz 11/e p1636; Sabiston 21/e p881, 887)*

Diffusely enlarged thyroid, complaints of palpitation and exophthalmos suggest the diagnosis of Grave's disease.
The diagnosis of Grave's disease is made by a suppressed TSH with or without an elevated free T_4 or T_3 level. If eye signs are present, other tests are generally not needed. However, in the absence of eye findings, thyroid scan should be performed. Elevated TSH-R or thyroid-stimulating antibodies (TSAb) are diagnostic of Graves' disease. Ultrasound neck is performed to assess the clinical landmarks for surgical planning. FNAC is not required for the diagnosis of Grave's disease.

"The biochemical workup for Grave's disease typically includes thyroid function tests, including TSH, free T_4 and T_3, as well as measurement for TRAb (typically with TSI but also with TSH receptor-binding inhibitory immunoglobulin in selected scenarios). The presence of TRAb is diagnostic for Grave's disease. Imaging may consist of neck ultrasound and/or nuclear medicine thyroid uptake scan, depending on the indications. Sonographic features may include a diffusely hypervascular gland, often with heterogeneous echogenicity; thyroid nodular disease may also be identified. Nuclear scintigraphy using either ^{99m}technetium pertechnetate or ^{123}I may help differentiate TSI-negative Grave's disease from toxic nodular disease based on diffuse versus nodular uptake pattern. Cross-sectional imaging of the head may be useful for the evaluation of orbitopathy."- *Sabiston 21/e p887*

"The diagnosis of hyperthyroidism is made by a suppressed TSH with or without an elevated free T_4 or T_3 level. If eye signs are present, other tests are generally not needed. However, in the absence of eye findings, an ^{123}I uptake and scan should be performed. An elevated uptake, with a diffusely enlarged gland, confirms the diagnosis of Graves' disease and helps to differentiate it from other causes of hyperthyroidism. Technetium scintigraphy (using pertechnetate, which is trapped by the thyroid, but not organified) can also be used to determine etiology. While technetium scans results in low range of normal uptake and high background activity, total-body radiation exposure is less than that of ^{123}I scans. If free T_4 levels are normal, free T_3 levels should be determined, as they often are elevated in early Graves' disease or toxic nodules (T_3 toxicosis). Anti-Tg and anti-TPO antibodies are elevated in up to 75% of patients but are not specific. Elevated TSH-R or thyroid-stimulating antibodies (TSAb) are diagnostic of Graves' disease and are increased in about 90% of patients. MRI scans of the orbits are useful in evaluating Graves' ophthalmopathy."- Schwartz 11/e p1636

49. **Ans. b. 1, 2 and 3** *(Ref: Sabiston 21/e p876, 923, 1016)*

Inferior thyroid artery supplies esophagus, parathyroid and thyroid.

"The thyroid is a highly vascular gland with abundant and redundant blood supply. The arterial supply to the thyroid gland generally derives from two bilateral pairs of arteries. The superior thyroid arteries originate from the external carotid arteries, and divide as they enter the superior poles of the thyroid lobes. The inferior thyroid arteries are branches from the thyrocervical trunks of the subclavian arteries."- Sabiston 21/e p876

"The inferior thyroid artery is the predominant vascular supply for both the superior and inferior parathyroid glands in 80% of cases."- Sabiston 21/e p923

"The cervical esophagus receives most of its blood supply from the inferior thyroid arteries, which branch off of the thyrocervical trunk on the left and the subclavian artery on the right."- Sabiston 21/e p1016

50. **Ans. a. 1, 2, 4 are correct** *(Ref: Harrison 20/e p580, 585)*

The global incidence of HCC is rising. NASH and NAFLD are the risk factors. Lenvatinib is used for advanced and metastatic disease. TACE is done for multinodular tumors.

"There is a growing incidence of HCC world-wide. The growth in U.S. incidence results from the emergence of end-stage liver disease due to hepatitis C, the increase in HBV-related HCC among immigrants from endemic countries, and the accelerating prevalence of obesity and fatty liver disease."- Harrison 20/e p580

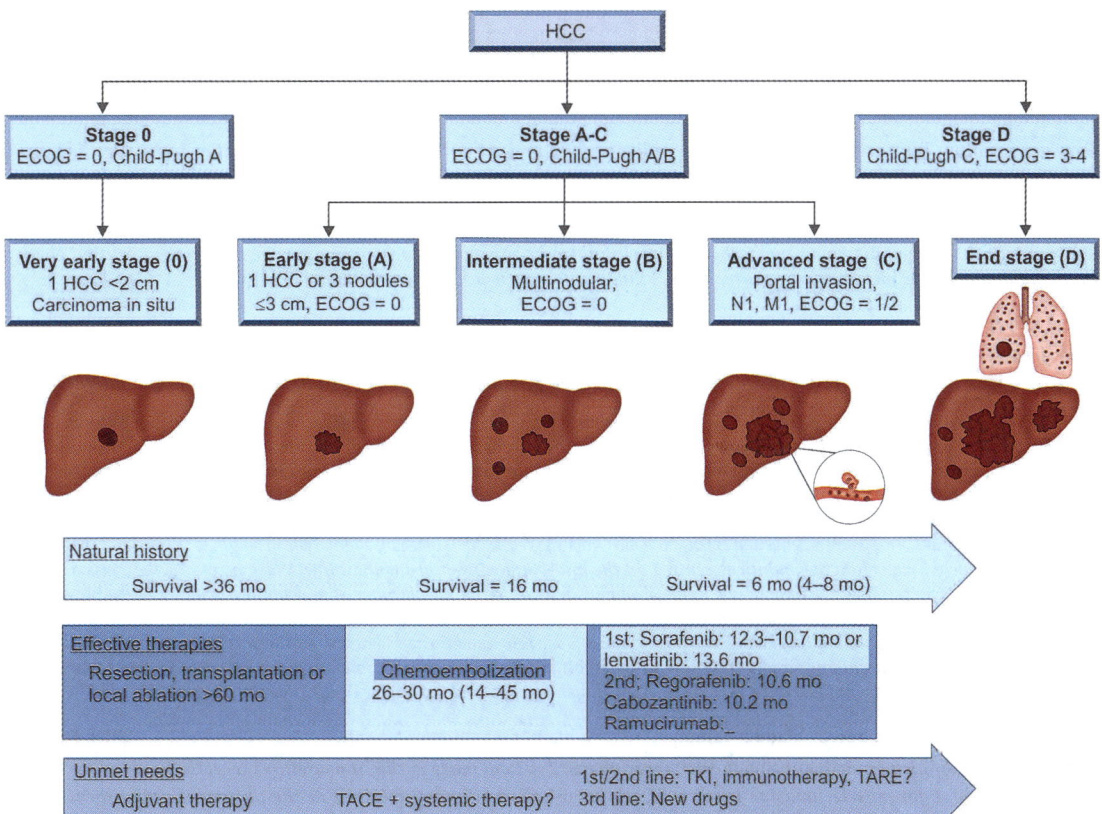

"TACE is the most widely used primary treatment for unresectable HCC worldwide, and the first-line indication for patients with intermediate BCLC B stage. Conventional chemoembolization (c-TACE) consists of the local hepatic artery administration of chemotherapy (either doxorubicin 50 mg/m^2 or cisplatin) mixed with an emulsion of lipiodol followed by obstruction of the feeding artery with sponge particles."- Harrison 20/e p585

51. **Ans. b. 1, 3, 4 and 5** *(Ref: Sabiston 21/e p1500)*

    Reynolds pentad is characterized by Charcot triad (right upper quadrant pain + fever + jaundice), mental obtundation and shock.

    "Cholangitis presents with right upper quadrant pain, fever, and jaundice, known as Charcot triad, and may progress to septic shock with mental status changes, and hypotension, known as Reynolds pentad, which is an ominous sign, and mortality approaches 100% without prompt treatment."- Sabiston 21/e p1500

52. **Ans. a. MRI** *(Ref: Schwartz 11/e p1360)*

    This is a case of obstructive jaundice with intrahepatic biliary radicle dilatation. MRCP (T2 phase of MRI) provides visualization of dilated bile ducts, and the high spatial and contrast resolution often enables accurate assessment of the level of occlusion in the biliary tree.

    "Magnetic resonance cholangiopancreatography (MRCP) enables rapid, non-invasive depiction of both the biliary tree and the pancreatic duct without the use of ionizing radiation or intravenous contrast media. One of the most common clinical indications for MRCP is biliary obstruction. MRCP provides visualization of dilated bile ducts, and the high spatial and contrast resolution often enables accurate assessment of the level of occlusion in the biliary tree. MRCP also can be enhanced with liver-specific MRI contrast agents that are actively secreted into the bile, but the clinical indications for such studies are still a matter of intensive investigation."- Schwartz 11/e p1360

53. **Ans. a. Hollow viscus perforation** *(Ref: Bailey 27/e p210)*

    The given chest X-ray shows free air under right dome of diaphragm, which suggests hollow viscus perforation. Abdominal pain, obstipation and rigid abdomen on palpation are the other findings suggestive of hollow viscus perforation.

    "Perforation: The erect chest X-ray (CXR) is the ideal first test for hollow organ perforation and as little as 10–20 mL of free air can be detected under the diaphragm, with the following caveats: about 10 minutes should be left between sitting the patient upright to allow air time to rise; the free air must be sought under the right hemidiaphragm to prevent misinterpretation of the gastric air bubble; and the reviewer must be able to recognise Chilaiditi's syndrome, the harmless and asymptomatic interposition of large bowel between the liver and diaphragm. Caution must also be exercised in interpreting any free air in the context of recent abdominal surgery, as air can persist for up to 5–7 days in the peritoneal cavity."- Bailey 27/e p210

54. **Ans. a. 1, 2, 3 and 4** *(Ref: Bailey 27/e p1262; Sabiston 21/e p1368)*

    Colon cancer can be prevented by metformin. Right and left colon cancers can have different clinical presentations. Right sided colon cancers bleed whereas left sided colon cancers present with obstruction. Colon cancers can be hereditary. Two classical examples of hereditary colon cancers are FAP & HNPCC. Most common site of metastasis in colon cancer is liver.

    "Carcinoma Colon: Tumours of the left side of the colon usually present with a change in bowel habit or rectal bleeding, while proximal lesions typically present later, with iron deficiency anaemia or a mass."- Bailey 27/e p1262

    "Carcinoma Colon: Haematogenous spread is most commonly to the liver via the portal vein. One-third of patients will have liver metastases at the time of diagnosis and 50% will develop them at some point, accounting for the majority of deaths. The lung is the next most common site; metastasis to ovary, brain, kidney and bone is less common."-Bailey 27/e p1262

55. **Ans. a. 1, 2, 3** *(Ref: Bailey 27/e p1309)*

    Rutherford Morrison incision is the muscle cutting incision. External oblique, internal oblique and transversus abdominis are divided in Rutherford Morrison incision. It has its lower end over McBurney's point and extending obliquely upwards and laterally as necessary.

    *"CONVENTIONAL APPENDICECTOMY: When the preoperative diagnosis is considered reasonably certain, the incision that is widely used for appendicectomy is the so-called **gridiron incision** (gridiron: a frame of cross-beams to support a ship during repairs). The gridiron incision (described first by McArthur) is made at right angles to a line joining the anterior superior iliac spine to the umbilicus, its centre being along the line at McBurney's point. If better access is required, it is possible to convert the gridiron to a Rutherford Morison incision (see below) by cutting the internal oblique and transversus muscles in the line of the incision. In recent years, a **transverse skin crease (Lanz) incision** has become more popular, as the exposure is better and extension, when needed, is easier. The incision, appropriate in length to the size and obesity of the patient, is made approximately **2 cm below the umbilicus centred on the mid-clavicular–mid-inguinal line.** When necessary, the incision may be extended medially, with retraction or suitable division of the rectus abdominis muscle. When the diagnosis is in doubt, particularly in the presence of intestinal obstruction, a lower midline abdominal incision is to be preferred over a right lower paramedian incision. The latter, although widely practised in the past, is difficult to extend, more difficult to close and provides poorer access to the pelvis and peritoneal cavity. Rutherford Morison's incision is useful if the appendix is para- or retrocaecal and fixed. It is essentially an oblique muscle-cutting incision with its lower end over McBurney's point and extending obliquely upwards and laterally as necessary. All layers are divided in the line of the incision."-Bailey 27/e p1309*

56. **Ans. a. Transurethral resection of bladder tumor** *(Ref: Bailey 27/e p1450)*

    The management of high grade transitional cell cancer of size 2 × 2 cm mass is the transurethral resection of bladder tumor. Radical cystectomy is done for muscle invasive tumors. Neoadjuvant chemotherapy is given in the patients having locally advanced or metastatic tumors.

57. Ans. a. Incontinence while intercourse
(Ref: Bailey 27/e p1375)

Lower urinary tract symptoms (LUTS) include urge incontinence (Sudden urge to urinate), nocturnal enuresis (Incontinence while asleep) and stress incontinence (Check for leak by making the patient cough). Incontinence while intercourse is not included in LUTS.

"Urge incontinence (UI) is involuntary urinary leakage, often large volume, immediately preceded by the sensation of urgency. Urgency and episodes of urge incontinence are often associated with an overactive bladder or a bladder neuropathy."- Bailey 27/e p1375

"Stress incontinence is involuntary urinary leakage which occurs when the intra-abdominal pressure rises. This is most common in females who have had vaginal deliveries who describe small-volume urinary leakage associated with activity such as coughing, laughing, sneezing or exercising."- Bailey 27/e p1375

"Nocturnal enuresis is involuntary loss of urine during sleep. A common cause in an elderly male is chronic retention of urine with overflow incontinence."- Bailey 27/e p1375

Lower Urinary Tract Symptoms (LUTS)

- LUTS are classified as either **storage LUTS (frequency, nocturia, urgency & Urge incontinence^Q); voiding LUTS (hesitancy, a reduced stream, straining^Q)** or **post-micturitional LUTS (incomplete emptying & Post micturition dribble^Q).**
- **Storage LUTS** result from **failure of bladder to act as a functioning reservoir** for urine; commonly seen in patients with an **overactive bladder or a bladder neuropathy^Q.**
- **Voiding & post-micturitional LUTS** are commonly seen in **males with bladder outlet obstruction^Q (BOO)**
- A male with **BOO** may also have **storage LUTS** as the **thickened detrusor muscle resulting from outlet obstruction becomes overactive**, resulting in the combination of symptoms.

Definitions for Lower Urinary Tract Symptoms (LUTS)

Frequency	Needing to **void more frequently than is their usual habit** or more frequently than they consider is socially acceptable.
Nocturia	Individual needs to **wake at night at least once to void.**
Strangury	Sensation of **constantly needing to void^Q.**
Urgency	**Sudden compelling desire to pass urine** which is difficult to defer.
Urge incontinence	**Involuntary urinary leakage**, often large volume, immediately **preceded by the sensation of urgency^Q.**
Stress incontinence	**Involuntary urinary leakage** which occurs when the **intra-abdominal pressure rises^Q**. **MC in females** who have had **vaginal deliveries** who describe small-volume urinary leakage associated with activity such as **coughing, laughing, sneezing or exercising^Q.**
Nocturnal enuresis	**Involuntary loss of urine during sleep^Q** A common cause in an elderly male is chronic retention of urine with overflow incontinence.
Hesitancy	Individual describes **difficulty in initiating micturition**, resulting in a delay in the onset of voiding after the individual is ready to pass urine.
Reduced urinary stream	Usually reported compared with previous performance or in comparison with the performance of others. This is often a symptom of bladder outlet obstruction.
Intermittency	When the individual describes **urine flow which stops and starts**, on one or more occasions, during micturition.
Straining	Muscular effort used in order to initiate, maintain or improve the urinary stream.
Incomplete emptying	Incomplete emptying is the sensation that at the end of micturition bladder fullness persists.
Post micturition dribble	When an individual describes the involuntary loss of urine immediately after he/she has finished passing urine. This is a common symptom in the ageing male when the bulbar urethra fails to empty itself of urine at the completion of micturition

58. **Ans. a. Posterior urethral valve** *(Ref: Bailey 27/e p1477)*

Most common cause of bladder outlet obstruction in male neonate is posterior urethral valve.

"Posterior urethral valves occur in around 1 in 5000–8000 live male births. The valves are membranes that have a small posterior slit within them, which typically lie just distal to the verumontanum and cause obstruction to the urethra of boys. They function as flap valves and so although they are obstructive to antegrade urinary flow, a urethral catheter can be passed retrogradely without any difficulty."- Bailey 27/e p1477

59. **Ans. c. Non-Hodgkin's lymphoma** *(Ref: Harrison 20/e p672)*

The most common testicular tumor in elderly is lymphoma (Non-Hodgkin's lymphoma). Lymphomas can lead to paraneoplastic neurological disorders like cerebellar degeneration, which can cause ataxia.

60. **Ans. b. ICD tube** *(Ref: Sabiston 21/e p411)*

The X-ray shows the presence of gastric air bubble in the left hemithorax after trauma. So, it is a case of traumatic diaphragmatic hernia. Intercostal drain (ICD) insertion is contraindicated in diaphragmatic hernia, as it may injure the bowel. After reduction of content and repair of diaphragmatic defect, ICD insertion is done.

61. **Ans. d. Repair with saphenous vein graft** *(Ref: Sabiston 21/e p1800)*

Vessel injuries that cannot be repaired by primary end-to-end technique, require an interposition graft. The most desirable graft is autologous great saphenous vein harvested from an uninjured leg. In this case, brachial artery has a 2.5 cm longitudinal cut. So, the preferred method of repair would be repair with saphenous vein graft. In cases of inadequate size or traumatized saphenous vein or saphenous vein being harvested previously, prosthetic graft may be needed.

"Choice of Repair and Graft Material: Vessel injuries that cannot be repaired by primary end-to-end technique will require an interposition graft. The most desirable graft is autologous great saphenous vein harvested from an uninjured leg. Native vein graft is preferable because it has elastic properties that make it compliant with the normal pulsatile flow of an artery; it has a diameter that approximates that of an extremity artery, producing an adequate size match for grafting in the arm and leg; it is not thrombogenic; and it has superior long-term patency in elective vascular surgery compared with prosthetic material when it is used with smaller vessels (popliteal and tibial). Cephalic vein and lesser saphenous vein have been suggested as suitable second choices, but cephalic vein is less muscular than the greater saphenous and, like the lesser saphenous, may present problems with harvesting in a trauma patient. Also, upper extremity venous access becomes compromised when the cephalic vein is used."- Sabiston 21/e p1800

"Saphenous vein may not be suitable in all instances because of inadequate size or because it has been traumatized or harvested previously. In such cases, a prosthetic conduit may be needed."- Sabiston 21/e p1800

62. **Ans. b. Measure anterior compartment pressure** *(Ref: Bailey 27/e p408; Sabiston 21/e p463)*

History of fracture of lower limb (tibia fracture) with pain on lifting the great toe (Pain on passive stretch) and decreased sensation in the first web space (paraesthesia) are the pointers of compartment syndrome. Compartment pressure monitoring can confirm the diagnosis of compartment syndrome, when the compartment pressure is >30 mm Hg.

"Compartment syndrome is raised pressure in an osseofascial compartment to a level that compromises tissue perfusion. There are several causes of compartment syndrome, fractures being the most common (70%), followed by soft tissue contusions (23%)."- Bailey 27/e p408

"Compartment syndrome is a clinical diagnosis characterised by pain out of proportion, increasing pain and pain on passive stretch. Paralysis, paraesthesia and pallor are late signs and pulselessness is an extremely late sign."- Bailey 27/e p408

"Compartment pressure monitoring may be useful in cases of diagnostic uncertainty and in patients with altered levels of consciousness (intubated, head injury)."- Bailey 27/e p408

"Compartment pressure monitoring is an important adjunct to serial clinical exams. In patients with altered mental status or who are unreliable upon exam, measuring the compartment pressures is an important objective finding (and sometimes the only objective finding), and it can be used to drive treatment decisions."- Sabiston 21/e p463

"First, pressure measurements should be taken using a side-port needle and a pressure measurement system. The most common method of measurement is the Stryker Intra-Compartmental Pressure Monitor System (STIC; Stryker, Mahwah, NJ), which uses the side port needle technique. Alternative measurement systems include a wick or slit catheter or an arterial line setup. Slit catheters can be used in continuous monitoring systems."- Sabiston 21/e p463

63. **Ans. a. Tip of nose to ear lobule and xiphoid process** *(Ref: Jaypee Manual of Surgical Equipments/p96)*

Nose-earlobe-xiphoid (NEX) distance formula is used for determining the required nasogastric tube length. Measure from the tip of nose to earlobe to xiphoid process.

64. **Ans. b. 86 mL** *(Ref: Essential Guide to Acute Care by Nicola Cooper, 2020/p86)*

The flow rate/minute of the green cannula is 90 mL/minute (best option would be 86 mL/minute).

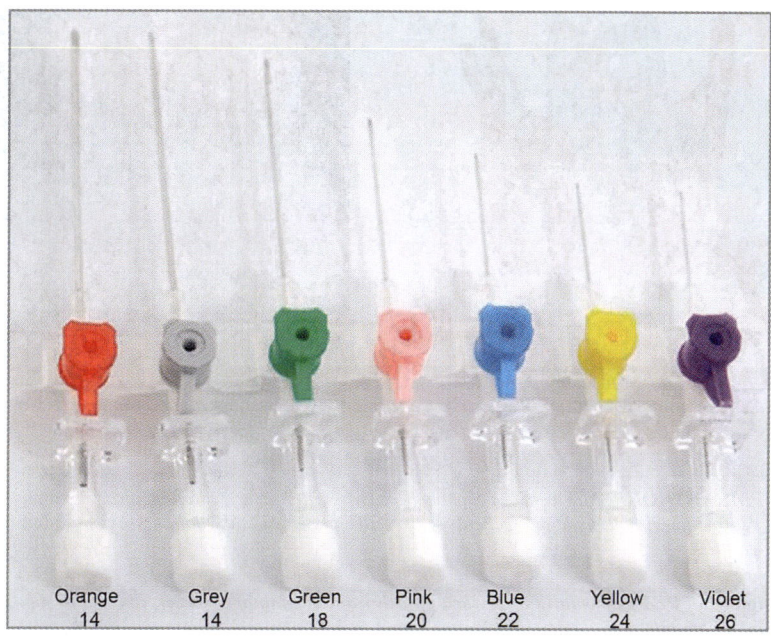

Color Code	Gauge	Flow Rate (mL/min)	Indications
Orange	14G	240	Trauma, surgical procedures
Grey	16G^Q	180^Q	Trauma, surgical procedures
Green	18G^Q	90^Q	Trauma, quick blood transfusion
Pink	20G^Q	60^Q	Normal IV or blood transfusion
Blue	22G^Q	36^Q	Children, older adults
Yellow	24G	20	Neonates, children, elderly
Violet	26G	13	Neonates

65. **Ans. b. S** *(Ref: Bailey 27/e p154; Sabiston 21/e p135)*

Most radiosensitive phase of cell cycle is $G_2M > G_2$ and the least radiosensitive phase is 'S' phase.

"Ionizing radiation has its greatest effect on rapidly dividing cells in phases G_2 through M of the cell cycle."- *Sabiston 21/e p135*

Phase of Cell Cycle	Comment
$G_2M > G_2$	• **Most sensitive** to radiation^Q
End of S phase	• **Most resistant** to radiation^Q
G_1	• Radiation exposure leads to **chromosomal aberration**^Q
G_2	• Radiation exposure leads to **chromatid aberration**^Q
Susceptibility of various phases of cell cycle to radiation: $G_2M > G_2 > M > G_1 >$ Early S > Late S Phase^Q	

INI-CET JULY 2021

66. **Ans. b. Radiotherapy** *(Ref: Schwartz 11/e p580)*

After breast conservation surgery, radiotherapy is given to prevent the recurrence.

"Women with DCIS and evidence of extensive disease (>4 cm of disease or disease in more than one quadrant) usually require mastectomy. For women with limited disease, lumpectomy and radiation therapy are generally recommended."- *Schwartz 11/e p580*

67. **Ans. a. Sestamibi scan** *(Ref: Bailey 27/e p825, 827)*

History of renal calculi, complains of bone pain, abdominal cramps and psychosis suggest the diagnosis of primary hyperparathyroidism (PHPT). The underlying aetiology of PHPT is usually a solitary parathyroid adenoma. Sestamibi scan is regarded as the most accurate and reliable method for imaging the parathyroid glands.

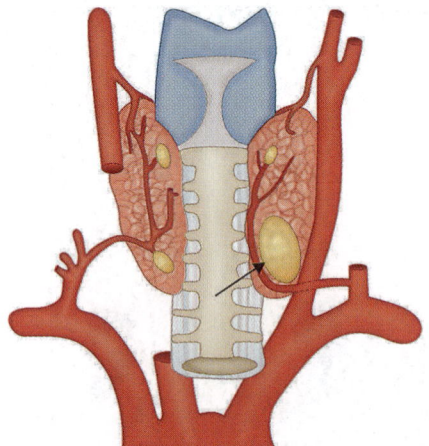
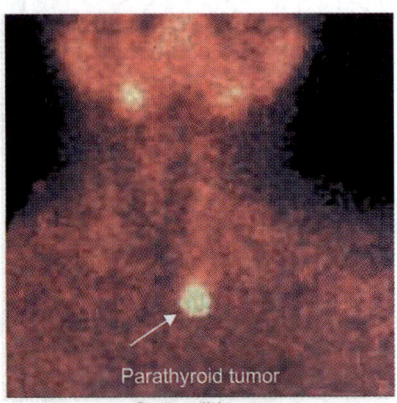

Sestamibi scan (parathyroid adenoma)

> *"**PRIMARY HYPERPARATHYROIDISM:** Over 80% of patients had associated renal stones, significant neuromuscular dysfunction and muscle weakness. This led to the traditional mnemonic that patients with PHPT presented with '**bones, stones, abdominal groans and psychiatric overtones**'."-Bailey 27/e p825*

> *"The underlying aetiology of PHPT is usually a solitary parathyroid adenoma; however, in a small number of patients (2–4%) there are double adenomas."-Bailey 27/e p825*

> *"The use of sestamibi (2-methoxy-2-methylpropylisonitrile (MIBI)) for parathyroid localisation was first described in 1989 and is now regarded as the most accurate and reliable method for imaging the parathyroid glands. It is safe and reproducible and while it has a sensitivity and specificity similar to ultrasound, it may image glands in ectopic positions better."-Bailey 27/e p827*

68. **Ans. a. MRCP**   (Ref: Bailey 27/e p1200; Sabiston 20/e p1495)

    Dilated CBD with raised GGT and ALP suggest CBD obstruction. MRCP provides accurate imaging of the biliary tree.

> *"Gallstones: Ultrasonography is performed to confirm the diagnosis. If jaundice is present MRCP is performed to exclude choledocholithiasis."- Bailey 27/e p1200*

> *"MRCP is highly sensitive (>90%) with an almost 100% specificity for the diagnosis of common duct stones. As a non-invasive test, MRCP provides accurate imaging of the biliary tree, but in the setting of choledocholithiasis, it does not provide a therapeutic solution. A clear cholangiogram by MRCP eliminates the need for ERCP."-Sabiston 20/e p1495*

69. **Ans. a. USG guided pigtail catheter drainage**   (Ref: Sabiston 20/e p1503)

    After laparoscopic cholecystectomy, presence of 5 × 5 cm fluid collection under the liver suggest the possibility of bile duct injury. In such cases, first, control of infection followed by drainage of any fluid collections (USG-guided pigtail catheter drainage).

> *"In the delayed presentation of a bile duct injury, three major goals guide therapy. First, control of infection with drainage of any fluid collections will minimize the inflammatory process. Inflammation in the porta hepatis leads to fibrosis, which acts only to increase stricture formation. Broad-spectrum antibiotics, decompression of the biliary tree, and drainage, whether percutaneous or operative, of any fluid collections will achieve this goal. With control of sepsis, there is no urgency for biliary reconstruction."- Sabiston 20/e p1503*

70. **Ans. c. Morgagni hernia**   (Ref: Bailey 27/e p938; Sabiston 20/e p1863)

    The given X-ray shows the focal opacity along the anterior and medial aspect of the right hemithorax with associated lucency. These findings are consistent with a bowel-containing anteromedial right hemidiaphragm defect, or Morgagni hernia.

> *"The **posterolateral location** of this hernia is known as **Bochdalek hernia**; it is distinguished from a CDH of the **anteromedial location** known as **Morgagni hernia**."-Sabiston 20/e p1863*

> *"**The foramen of Morgagni**: a hernia in the anterior part of the diaphragm with a **defect between the sternal and costal attachments**. The most commonly involved viscus is the **transverse colon**."-Bailey 27/e p938*

> *"The foramen of Bochdalek: Through the dome of the diaphragm posteriorly."- Bailey 27/e p938*

71. **Ans. a. Bochdalek hernia**   (Ref: Bailey 27/e p938; Sabiston 20/e p1863)

    The given frontal view of the chest shows a large air-containing and walled structure in the region of the left lower lobe. It is originating from below the diaphragm. It is suggestive of Bochdalek Hernia.

72. **Ans. d. Gastric volvulus** *(Ref: Shackelford 8/e p872)*

The given Chest X-ray reveals a large intrathoracic gastric volvulus, which appears as a cyst-like retrocardiac mass with a small air-fluid interface.

"Acute gastric volvulus will most commonly present in children less than 5 years old with nonbilious emesis, epigastric pain, abdominal distention, respiratory distress, cyanosis, and hematemesis."-Shackelford 8/e p872

"Chronic gastric volvulus is a more difficult diagnosis, with more subtle symptoms of intermittent volvulus. The most common presentation of chronic gastric volvulus is in an infant less than 1 year old with nonbilious emesis, feeding intolerance, abdominal pain, and respiratory distress."-Shackelford 8/e p872

"Plain radiographs may show a dilated gastric silhouette at or above the level of the diaphragm. The orientation of the stomach may be horizontal if twisted along the organoaxial axis or vertical if volvulized along the mesenteroaxial axis. Definitive diagnosis is confirmed by a UGI study."- Shackelford 8/e p872

73. **Ans. a. Rotavirus** *(Ref: Nelson 20/e p1618)*

Rotavirus vaccine can cause intussusception.

"A trivalent rotavirus vaccine was licensed in the United States in 1998 and was subsequently linked to an increased risk for intussusception, especially during the 3–14 day period after the 1st dose and the 3–7 day period after the 2nd dose."-Nelson 20/e p1618

74. **Ans. a. Hamartomatous** *(Ref: Robbin's 10/e p810)*

Recurrent attacks of intussusception with multiple hamartomatous polyps in small intestine suggest the diagnosis of Peutz-Jegher's syndrome. The pathological change shown in the picture shows arborization.

"The arborization and presence of smooth muscle intermixed with lamina propria are helpful in distinguishing polyps of Peutz-Jeghers syndrome from juvenile polyps."-Robbin's 10/e p810

75. **Ans. a. 5-HIAA** *(Ref: Bailey 27/e p855; Harrison 20/e p604)*

5-Hydroxy indole acetic acid (5-HIAA) is excreted in urine in carcinoid tumor.

"The diagnosis of carcinoid syndrome relies on measurement of urinary or plasma serotonin or its metabolites in the plasma or urine. The measurement of urinary 5-HIAA is used most frequently."-Harrison 20/e p604

"The diagnosis of NET of the small bowel is made by history, physical examination of the abdomen, imaging and an assessment of 5-HIAA in a 24-hour urine sample."- Bailey 27/e p855

76. **Ans. a. Hirschsprung's disease: Rectal biopsy** *(Ref: Bailey 27/e p136; Schwartz 11/e p1734)*

The diagnosis of Hirschsprung's disease is confirmed by rectal biopsy. The diagnosis of carcinoma colon is made by colonoscopy and biopsy. Carcinoma breast is diagnosed by biopsy. Carcinoma bladder is diagnosed by cystoscopy and biopsy.

"Hirschsprung's disease: The diagnosis requires an adequate rectal biopsy and an experienced pathologist."- Bailey 27/e p136

"The definitive diagnosis of Hirschsprung's disease is made by rectal biopsy."-Schwartz 11/e p1734

77. **Ans. d. Calcium oxalate** *(Ref: Smith Urology 17/e p260)*

The given crystals are bipyramidal. Calcium oxalate dihydrate stones are bipyramidal (envelop shaped).

"Cystine crystals are hexagonal; struvite stones appear as coffin lids; brushite ($CaHPO_4$) stones are splinter-like and may aggregate with a spoke-like center; calcium apatite—$(Ca)_5(PO_4)_3(OH)$—and uric acid crystals appear as amorphous powder because the crystals are so small; calcium oxalate dihydrate stones are bipyramids; and calcium oxalate monohydrate stones are small biconcave ovals that may appear as a dumbbell."-Smith Urology 17/e p260

78. **Ans. b. Angiomyolipoma** *(Ref: Smith Urology 17/e p329; Campbell 10/e p1499)*

Presence of fat (Fat imaged by CT has a negative density, –20 to –80 Hounsfield units) in the given CT within a renal lesion is considered the diagnostic hallmark of angiomyolipoma.

"Ultrasonography and CT are frequently diagnostic in lesions with high fat content. Fat visualized on US appears as very high intensity echoes. Fat imaged by CT has a negative density, –20 to –80 Hounsfield units, which is pathognomonic for angiomyolipomas when observed in the kidney."- Smith Urology 17/e p329

"Angiomyolipoma is the only benign renal tumor that is confidently diagnosed on cross-sectional imaging. The presence of fat (confirmed on non-enhanced thin-cut CT by a value of –20 Hounsfield Units [HU] or less) within a renal lesion is considered the diagnostic hallmark."-Campbell 10/e p1499

79. **Ans. d. Renal cell carcinoma** *(Ref: Smith 17/e p334)*

"CT scanning is more sensitive than US or IVU for detection of renal masses. A typical finding of RCC on CT is a mass that becomes enhanced with the use of intravenous contrast media. In general, RCC exhibits an overall decreased density in Hounsfield units compared with normal renal parenchyma but shows a heterogeneous pattern of enhancement or increased attenuation (slightly decreased from the surrounding parenchyma) when contrast is used. In addition to defining the primary lesion, CT scanning is also the method of choice in staging the patient by visualizing the renal hilum, perinephric space, renal vein and vena cava, adrenals, regional lymphatics, and adjacent organs."-Smith 17/e p334

80. **Ans. a. CECT, c. PET-CT** *(Ref: Campbell Urology 11/e p2466; Smith 17/e p341)*

Ballotable abdominal lump in a 3-year-old child with painless hematuria suggest the diagnosis of Wilms' tumor.
CT of the abdomen is performed with suspected Wilms' tumor; useful in providing information regarding tumor extension, the status of the contralateral kidney, and the presence of regional adenopathy. Wilms' tumor lesions are metabolically active and concentrate fluorodeoxyglucose. Regional spread and metastatic lesions can be visualized on positron emission tomography (PET)-CT scanning.

"The most common initial clinical presentation for WT is the incidental discovery of an asymptomatic abdominal mass by parents while bathing or clothing an affected child or by a physician during a routine physical examination."- Campbell Urology 11/e p2466

"Hypertension is present in approximately 25% of tumors at presentation and has been attributed to increased renin activity. Abdominal pain, gross painless hematuria, and fever are other frequent findings at diagnosis."- Campbell Urology 11/e p2466

"Abdominal US and CT scanning are performed initially to evaluate the mass. CT of the abdomen is performed with suspected Wilms' tumor and can be useful in providing information regarding tumor extension, the status of the contralateral kidney, and the presence of regional adenopathy."- Smith 17/e p341

"WT lesions are metabolically active and concentrate fluorodeoxyglucose. Regional spread and metastatic lesions can be visualized on positron emission tomography (PET)-CT scanning."- Campbell Urology 11/e p2466

"Wilms' Tumor: Although biopsy is a reliable diagnostic tool, it is discouraged as it results in disease upstaging. A core needle biopsy obtained via a posterior approach should be performed in cases of unusual presentation (older age, signs of infection, inflammation) or unusual imaging findings (significant adenopathy, no renal parenchyma seen, intratumoral calcification)." - Campbell Urology 11/e p2466

"Preoperative biopsy is indicated routinely only in tumors deemed too large for safe primary surgical resection and for which preoperative chemotherapy or radiation therapy is planned."- Smith 17/e p341

"Wilms' Tumor: All patients should undergo either CT of the abdomen and pelvis with oral and intravenous contrast or MRI of the abdomen and pelvis with gadolinium. MRI avoids radiation but typically requires anesthesia or sedation in young children. These imaging modalities can further define the extent of the lesion."-Campbell Urology 11/e p3573

81. **Ans. c. Suprapubic aspiration** *(Ref: Bailey 27/e p1479, 1480)*

History of perineal injury, retention of urine and blood at the meatus suggests urethral injury. The next best step is suprapubic cystostomy (Suprapubic aspiration).

"Rupture of the bulbar urethra: There is a history of a blow to the perineum, usually due to a fall astride injury. The bulbar urethra is crushed upwards onto the pubic bone, typically with significant bruising."- Bailey 27/e p1479

"Rupture of the bulbar urethra: If the diagnosis is suspected, the patient should be treated with appropriate analgesia and antibiotics should be administered. He should be discouraged from passing urine. A full bladder should be drained with a catheter placed by percutaneous suprapubic puncture using a Seldinger technique. This reduces urinary extravasation and allows investigations to establish the extent of the urethral injury. Diagnosis is made by urethrography using water-soluble contrast."-Bailey 27/e p1480

82. **Ans. c. High inguinal orchidectomy** *(Ref: Bailey 27/e p; Schwartz 11/e p1772; Sabiston 20/e p2102)*

Painless enlargement of testis with presence of hard mass and raised LDH & AFP levels suggest the diagnosis of testicular tumor. Initial treatment of suspected testicular tumor is radical inguinal orchiectomy, which involves removal of the testicle and spermatic cord at the level of the inguinal ring.

"The most common presenting complaint in men with testicular cancer is a painless testicular mass."-Sabiston 20/e p2102

"Testicular Tumors: Standard initial workup includes scrotal ultrasound and serum tumor markers (α-fetoprotein, quantitative human chorionic gonadotropin, and lactate dehydrogenate). Most consider percutaneous biopsy is contraindicated due to the rare but historical risk of disturbing the natural lymphatic drainage to the retroperitoneum and possible seeding of the scrotum. Radical inguinal orchiectomy is the gold standard treatment for excision of the primary tumor."- Schwartz 11/e p1772

"Initial treatment of suspected testicular tumor is radical inguinal orchiectomy, which involves removal of the testicle and spermatic cord at the level of the inguinal ring. Because of the characteristic and well-described lymph drainage of the testicle, there is no role for trans-scrotal biopsy or orchiectomy. If the intrascrotal tissue planes are violated during orchiectomy, the lymphatic drainage can be altered, affecting future treatment. After radical inguinal orchiectomy, the patient should undergo disease staging, including cross-sectional, contrast-enhanced imaging of the abdomen and pelvis and chest imaging, either chest radiography in low-risk patients or cross-sectional chest imaging in patients with high-risk disease."- Sabiston 20/e p2102

83. **Ans. a. Pleomorphic adenocarcinoma** *(Ref: Parson's 22/e p474)*

Most common lacrimal gland tumor is pleomorphic adenocarcinoma.

*"Tumours of the Lacrimal Gland: Tumours of the lacrimal gland show a very marked resemblance to those of the parotid. **Much the commonest is a pleomorphic adenocarcinoma, frequently characterized histologically by myxomatous material (the so-called 'mixed tumour')**. Benign mixed lacrimal gland tumours present in middle life as slowly progressive painless swellings in the upper lid and later proptosis.."-Parson's 22/e p474*

84. **Ans. a. To sort out** *(Ref: Bailey 27/e p412)*

Triage means 'to sort' and is the cornerstone of the management of mass casualties.

"Triage: Derived from the French verb 'trier', triage means 'to sort' and is the cornerstone of the management of mass casualties. It aims to identify the patients who will benefit the most by being treated the earliest, ensuring 'the greatest good for the greatest number'." -Bailey 27/e p412

85. **Ans. b. Pulselessness** *(Ref: Bailey 27/e p28)*

The most delayed sign of compartment syndrome is pulselessness.

"Compartment syndromes: Compartment syndromes typically occur in closed lower limb injuries. They are characterised by severe pain, pain on passive movement of the affected compartment muscles, distal sensory disturbance and, finally, by the absence of pulses distally (a late sign)."- Bailey 27/e p28

86. **Ans. d. Bleeding** *(Ref: https://www.ncbi.nlm.nih.gov/pmc/articles/PMC7436986/)*

MC reasons for hospital admission in adults following ambulatory surgery: Acute pain > Haemorrhage & haematoma > Retention of urine

"Pain and haemorrhage are the most common reasons for emergency department use and hospital admission in adults following ambulatory surgery."- https://www.ncbi.nlm.nih.gov/pmc/articles/PMC7436986/

87. **Ans. d. 90 degrees** *(Ref: Bailey 27/e p91)*

Angle of needle with the skin for interrupted sutures should be 90 degrees.

"Interrupted sutures: Interrupted sutures require the needle to be inserted at right angles to the incision and then to pass through both aspects of the suture line and exit again at right angles."- Bailey 27/e p91

88. **Ans. b. 6 weeks** *(Ref: https://www.asahq.org/about-asa/newsroom/news-releases/2020/12/asa-and-apsf-joint-statement-on-elective-surgery-and-anesthesia-for-patients-after-covid-19-infection)*

The elective surgery for a symptomatic patient, who did not require hospitalization after recovery from COVID-19, can be planned after six weeks.

American Society of Anesthesiologist (ASA)- Anesthesia Patient Safety Foundations (APSF) Joint Statement on Elective Surgery and Anesthesia for Patients after COVID-19 Infection

Timing of elective surgery after recovery from COVID-19 uses both **symptom- and severity-based categories.** That statement includes suggested wait times from the date of COVID-19 diagnosis to surgery as:
- **Four weeks for an asymptomatic patient or recovery** from only mild, non-respiratory symptoms.
- **Six weeks for a symptomatic patient** (e.g., cough, dyspnea) who **did not require hospitalization**.
- **Eight to 10 weeks for a symptomatic patient who is diabetic, immunocompromised, or hospitalized**.
- **Twelve weeks** for a patients admitted to **ICU** due to COVID-19 infection.

89. **Ans. b. 18 gauge** *(Ref: Essential Guide to Acute Care by Nicola Cooper, 2020/p86)*

The size of green cannula is 18 gauge.

90. **Ans. a. Veress needle** *(Ref: Schwartz 11/e p549, 1412)*

The name of given instrument is Veress needle, which is used in laparoscopy to insufflate abdomen.

"Laparoscopic Access: A small incision is made in the umbilicus, and a specialized spring-loaded (Veress) needle is placed in the abdominal cavity. With the Veress needle, two distinct pops are felt as the surgeon passes the needle through the abdominal wall fascia and the peritoneum."- Schwartz 11/e p459

"Pneumoperitoneum is established with carbon dioxide gas, either with an open technique (Hasson) or closed-needle technique (Veress)."-Schwartz 11/e p1412

NEET PG 2021

91. Ans. a. Lymphedema *(Ref: Bailey 27/e p879)*

Painless swelling in the left upper limb after modified radical mastectomy is because of lymphedema.

"Lymphoedema of the arm is a troublesome complication of breast cancer treatment, fortunately seen less often now that radical axillary dissection and radiotherapy are rarely combined. However, it does still occur occasionally after either mode of treatment alone and appears at any time from months to years after treatment. There is usually no precipitating cause but recurrent tumour should be excluded because neoplastic infiltration of the axilla can cause arm swelling as a result of both lymphatic and venous blockage. This neoplastic infiltration is often painful because of brachial plexus nerve involvement."-Bailey 27/e p879

92. Ans. b. Bilateral recurrent laryngeal nerve damage *(Ref: Sabiston 21/e p876)*

After total thyroidectomy, if patient begins to have recurrent cyanotic spells, it is because of bilateral recurrent laryngeal nerve damage. Bilateral RLN injury with resultant resting vocal cord position in the midline can lead to airway compromise and can potentially require temporary or permanent tracheostomy. Unilateral injury to the RLN and resultant vocal cord paralysis can cause hoarse and breathy voice, vocal fatigue, dysphagia, and aspiration. Hemorrhage can lead to tension hematoma leading to respiratory distress, but it occurs in post-operative period, not immediately after the surgery. Superior laryngeal nerve innervates the cricothyroid muscles, and its injury leads to difficulties with achieving high pitch and vocal projection and volume.

"Vocal cord paralysis: Rates of temporary and permanent RLN injury during thyroidectomy are in the 4% to 10% and 0.5% to 2% ranges, respectively; rates in the pediatric population are estimated to be up to fourfold higher. Unilateral injury to the RLN and resultant vocal cord paralysis can cause a spectrum of problems with the voice or swallowing, due to the mixed motor and sensory fibers within the nerve. Symptoms can include hoarse and breathy voice, vocal fatigue, dysphagia, and aspiration. Rarely, bilateral RLN injury with resultant resting vocal cord position in the midline can lead to airway compromise and can potentially require temporary or permanent tracheostomy."- Sabiston 21/e p876

"The RLN is by far the more important nerve and innervates the motor function of all of the intrinsic laryngeal muscles except for the cricothyroid. It carries sensory fibers from the lower larynx, as well as minor motor and sensory fibers from the trachea and esophagus. Unilateral injury to the RLN leads to paralysis of the ipsilateral vocal fold, with typical symptoms ranging from voice complaints such as hoarseness and vocal fatigue to aspiration. Bilateral RLN injury with subsequent bilateral vocal fold paralysis may require tracheostomy for airway control if the paralyzed vocal folds rest in a median position preventing adequate air exchange; alternatively, the risk of persistent aspiration and respiratory tract infections is high if the resting vocal folds remain in an abducted position."-Sabiston 21/e p876

"The EBSLN innervates the cricothyroid muscles, and it contributes to vocal fold tone and tension. EBSLN injury leads to difficulties with achieving high pitch and vocal projection and volume."- Sabiston 21/e p877

93. Ans. a. Propranolol is the initial drug to be started *(Ref: Sabiston 21/e p981; Bailey 27/e p845, 846)*

In pheochromocytoma, beta-blockers (propranolol) should never be the first agent administered because a decrease in peripheral vasodilatory beta receptor stimulation results in unopposed α-adrenergic tone, which may exacerbate hypertension. Pheochromocytoma can present as hypertension alone and sometimes with vomiting and pain abdomen. VMA and catecholamines are the diagnostic tests. Surgery (adrenalectomy) is the treatment of choice for pheochromocytoma.

"Beta blockers may be administered after adequate alpha blockade has been achieved for the subset of patients with persistent tachycardia, who often have predominantly epinephrine-secreting tumors. Beta blockers should never be the first agent administered because a decrease in peripheral vasodilatory beta receptor stimulation results in unopposed α-adrenergic tone, which may exacerbate hypertension."-Sabiston 21/e p981

"The first step in the diagnosis of a phaeochromocytoma is the confirmation of excessive catecholamine levels in the patient either by the measurement of adrenaline and noradrenaline breakdown products, metanephrine and normetanephrine level, in a 12 or 24-hour urine collection, (levels that exceed the normal range by 2–40 times will be found in affected patients) or by determination of plasma-free metanephrine and normetanephrine levels."-Bailey 27/e p845

"Laparoscopic resection is now routine in the treatment of phaeochromocytoma. If the tumour is larger than 8–10 cm or radiological signs of malignancy are detected, an open approach should be considered."- Bailey 27/e p846

"Once a phaeochromocytoma has been diagnosed, an α-adrenoreceptor blocker (phenoxybenzamine) is used to block the effects of catecholamine excess and its consequences during surgery. With adequate medical pretreatment, the perioperative mortality rate has decreased from 20–45% to less than 3%. A dose of 20 mg of phenoxybenzamine initially should be increased daily by 10 mg until a daily dose of 100–160 mg is achieved and the patient reports symptomatic postural hypotension. Additional β-blockade is required if tachycardia or arrhythmias develop; this should not be introduced until the patient is α-blocked."- Bailey 27/e p846

94. Ans. d. Gallstone ileus *(Ref: Bailey 27/e p1282)*

Colicky abdominal pain and bilious vomiting (small bowel obstruction) and pneumobilia (air in the CBD) are the pointers for the diagnosis of Gallstone ileus. Pneumobilia is not seen in adhesions, gastroenteritis or outlet obstruction.

"The characteristic radiological sign of gallstone ileus is Rigler's triad, comprising: Small bowel obstruction, pneumobilia and an atypical mineral shadow on radiographs of the abdomen. The presence of two of these radiological signs has been considered pathognomic of gallstone ileus and is encountered in 40–50% of the cases (note than pneumobilia is common following endoscopic retrograde cholangiopancreatography (ERCP) with sphincterotomy)."-Bailey 27/e p1282

95. **Ans. c. Retained** *(Ref: Sabiston 21/e p1514)*

Retained stones are discovered within 2 years of cholecystectomy & recurrent stones are detected >2 years following cholecystectomy. In the question, it was detected within 2 years of cholecystectomy, so it's a retained stone.

"Retained Biliary Stones: Retained stones or secondary stones, originating in the gallbladder and passing into the common duct, are usually cholesterol stones and frequently become symptomatic within weeks of a cholecystectomy. They can be identified for up to 2 years after cholecystectomy. Hyperbilirubinemia and an elevated alkaline phosphatase level should raise the suspicion of a retained stone. Ultrasound may not show intrahepatic biliary ductal dilation if the stone does not fully occlude the duct or the obstruction is early. Endoscopic removal of these stones through a generous sphincterotomy is almost universally successful."-Sabiston 21/e p1514

96. **Ans. c. Lipase** *(Ref: Blumgart 6/e p355; Bailey 27/e p1214)*

Presence of fluid filled lesion in the epigastric region after acute pancreatitis (history of acute abdominal pain and distention) suggest the acute fluid collection. Acute fluid collections associated with pancreatitis are enzyme-rich collections, contains amylase & lipase.

"Acute fluid collections associated with pancreatitis are enzyme-rich collections, which lack a defined wall."-Blumgart 6/e p355

"Estimation of pancreatic enzymes in body fluids: When the pancreas is damaged, enzymes such as amylase, lipase, trypsin, elastase and chymotrypsin are released into the serum. Measurement of serum amylase is the most widely used test of pancreatic damage (serum lipase is more sensitive and specific, but is not widely available)."-Bailey 27/e p1214

97. **Ans. c. Palliative gastrojejunostomy with chemotherapy** *(Ref: Bailey 27/e p1138; Sabiston 21/e p1230)*

This is a case of unresectable carcinoma stomach, as the malignancy leads to gastric outlet obstruction extending to head of pancreas with multiple metastasis to liver. Most appropriate management is palliative gastrojejunostomy (to relieve gastric outlet obstruction) with chemotherapy (to prolong the survival).

"Carcinoma Stomach: In patients suffering from significant symptoms of either obstruction or bleeding, palliative resection is appropriate."-Bailey 27/e p1138

"Patients with unresectable or metastatic gastric cancer account almost 50% of patients presenting with the disease and have only a 3- to 5-month median survival with the best supportive therapy. While many patients with advanced disease are asymptomatic, a significant subset of patients with unresectable gastric cancer have debilitating symptoms and should be considered for palliative surgical therapy even in the setting of metastatic disease."-Sabiston 21/e p1230

"Obstructing gastric cancers can sometimes be symptomatically improved with the placement of an endoscopic enteral stent. Radiation therapy and systemic chemotherapy can be considered in an attempt to shrink the obstructing tumor. Surgical intervention can also be offered to patients fit to undergo surgery. The most common procedure in this setting is a gastrojejunostomy; however, a palliative gastrectomy can be considered in select patients."- Sabiston 21/e p1230

98. **Ans. a. Hypochloremic hypokalemic metabolic alkalosis** *(Ref: Sabiston 21/e p1855)*

History of multiple episodes of non-bilious vomiting, poor feeding and passage of dry pellets like stools in an 18 months old male child suggest the diagnosis of hypertrophic pyloric stenosis. Loss of hydrochloric acid secondary to persistent emesis leads to hypokalemic, hypochloremic, metabolic alkalosis.

"Hypertrophic pyloric stenosis (HPS) is a disease of newborns, with an incidence of 1 in 300 to 900 live births. It is most common between the ages of 2 and 8 weeks. Boys are affected four times more often than girls, with first-born male infants being at highest risk. Hypertrophy of the circular muscle of the pylorus results in constriction and obstruction of the gastric outlet, leading to nonbilious, projectile emesis. Loss of hydrochloric acid secondary to persistent emesis leads to hypokalemic, hypochloremic, metabolic alkalosis, and dehydration."-Sabiston 21/e p1855

99. **Ans. d. Hollow viscus perforation** *(Ref: Bailey 27/e p210)*

The given abdominal X-ray shows (A) erect view with air fluid levels & free air under right hemidiaphragm (arrow head) and (B) supine view shows significant dilated bowel loops. The findings are suggestive of hollow viscus perforation.

"Perforation: The erect chest X-ray (CXR) is the ideal first test for hollow organ perforation and as little as 10–20 mL of free air can be detected under the diaphragm, with the following caveats: about 10 minutes should be left between sitting the patient upright to allow air time to rise; the free air must be sought under the right hemidiaphragm to prevent misinterpretation of the gastric air bubble; and the reviewer must be able to recognise Chilaiditi's syndrome, the harmless and asymptomatic interposition of large bowel between the liver and diaphragm. Caution must also be exercised in interpreting any free air in the context of recent abdominal surgery, as air can persist for up to 5–7 days in the peritoneal cavity."- Bailey 27/e p210

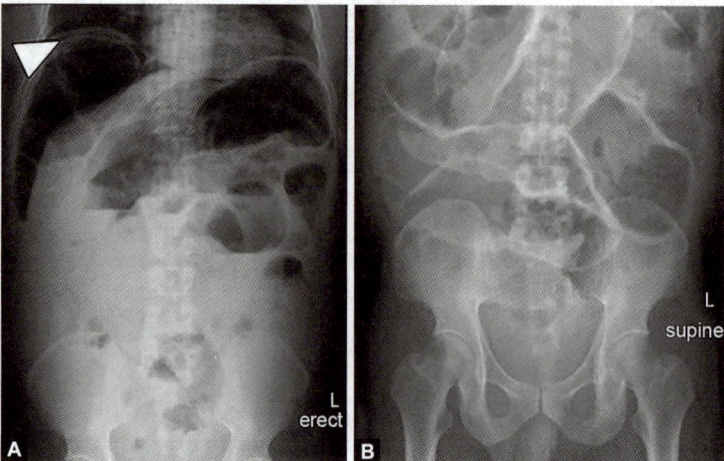

Abdominal X-ray showing (A) erect view with air fluid levels & free air under right hemidiaphragm (arrow head), (B) supine view with significant dilated bowel loops.

100. **Ans. a. Adhesive small bowel obstruction** *(Ref: Bailey 27/e p1060; Sabiston 21/e p262)*

Colicky abdominal pain, bilious vomiting with abdominal tenderness and exaggerated bowel sounds is suggestive of small bowel obstruction. History of hysterectomy 2 years back suggests adhesions as the etiology.

"Adhesions are strands of fibrous tissue that form, usually as a result of surgery, between surgically injured tissues."-Bailey 27/e p1060

"The most common adhesion-related problem is small bowel obstruction (SBO). Adhesions are the most frequent cause of SBO in resource-rich countries and are responsible for 60–70% of SBOs."-Bailey 27/e p1060

"Postoperative adhesions may occur after any intraabdominal surgery but are more likely to cause bowel obstructions after pelvic surgery, especially colorectal and gynecologic procedures."–Sabiston 21/e p262

101. **Ans. c. Jejunum** *(Ref: Bailey 27/e p1288)*

Multiple, centrally placed dilated bowel loops in a patient with abdominal pain and distension suggest the diagnosis of small bowel obstruction. Presence of circumferential ring like pattern (valvulae conniventes) is suggestive of jejunum.

"The jejunum is characterised by its valvulae conniventes, which completely pass across the width of the bowel and are regularly spaced, giving a 'concertina' or ladder effect."-Bailey 27/e p1288

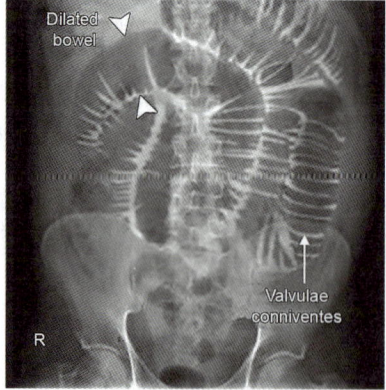

"Ileum: the distal ileum has been piquantly described by Wangensteen as featureless."- Bailey 27/e p1288

102. **Ans. c. Thiersch wiring** *(Ref: Shackleford 8/e p1785; Bailey 27/e p1323)*

In the given image, the suture is being placed around the anal canal for rectal prolapse. This procedure is known as Thiersch wiring.

"Thiersch operation: In this procedure, a steel wire, or silastic or nylon tape, is placed around the anal canal. It has become largely obsolete owing to problems with chronic perineal sepsis, anal stenosis and obstructed defaecation."-Bailey 27/e p1323

Thiersch wiring

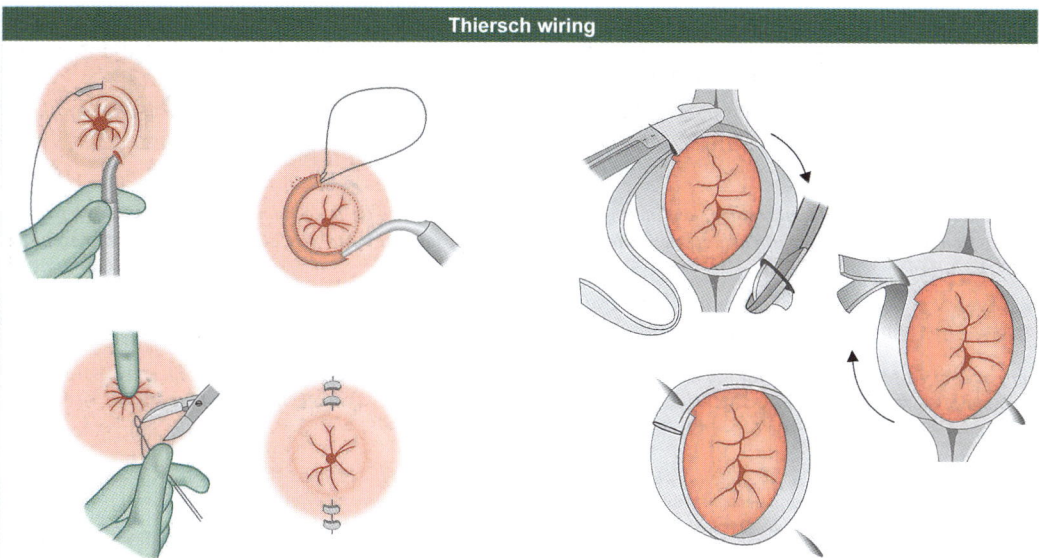

"Anal encirclement for the treatment of rectal prolapse was introduced in 1891 by Thiersch. In the original description, Thiersch used a silver wire to encircle the anus in an effort to provide a mechanical replacement of the relaxed sphincter. The presence of a foreign body would incite an inflammatory reaction and create an adhesive circumferential band to create support of the perineum. The procedure does not correct the prolapse but simply mechanically supports the anal sphincter function by narrowing the anal canal and preventing external rectal prolapse. The procedure can be performed quite quickly. With the patient in prone jackknife or lithotomy position, in reference to the center of the anus, two lateral perianal skin incisions are made 180 degrees apart. The incisions are connected subcutaneously by tunneling through the ischiorectal fossa and perineal body. Next, a piece of polypropylene mesh or silicone roll 1.5 cm in height is tunneled circumferentially around the entire anus. The mesh is tightened to a point that allows only the passage of one finger into the anal canal, and the mesh is sutured to itself at this level of tension."-Shackleford 8/e p1785

103. **Ans. b. Direct hernia and Lichtenstein repair**   *(Ref: Bailey 27/e p1030, 1032; Sabiston 21/e p1106)*

Indirect inguinal hernia is lateral because its origin is lateral to the inferior epigastric vessels. Direct inguinal hernia is medial because its origin is medial to the inferior epigastric vessels. Direct hernia should be treated by Lichtenstein repair.

"An indirect hernia is lateral because its origin is lateral to the inferior epigastric vessels. It is also oblique as the hernia passes obliquely from lateral to medial through the abdominal muscle layers. The second type of inguinal hernia, referred to as direct or medial, is acquired. It is a result of stretching and weakening of the abdominal wall just medial to the inferior epigastric (IE) vessels."-Bailey 27/e p1030

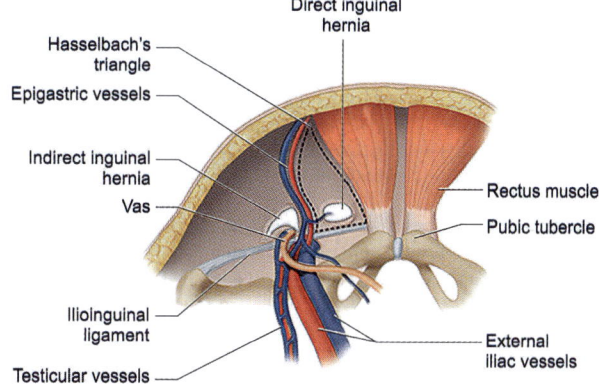

Indirect inguinal hernia (lateral to IEV) & direct inguinal hernia (medial to IEV)

"Inguinal hernias are classified as direct or indirect. The sac of an indirect inguinal hernia passes from the internal inguinal ring obliquely toward the external inguinal ring and ultimately into the scrotum. In contrast, the sac of a direct inguinal hernia protrudes outward and forward and is medial to the internal inguinal ring and inferior epigastric vessels."-Sabiston 21/e p1106

"Lichtenstein's repair is the most common operation for inguinal hernia in resource-rich countries."- Bailey 27/e p1032

104. **Ans. a. Putty kidney** *(Ref: Bailey 27/e p1405)*

History of abdominal pain, weight loss & sterile pyuria suggest the diagnosis of renal tuberculosis. Radiograph is showing calcification involving the entire kidney, known as putty kidney.

"Genitourinary tuberculosis (GUTB): Amorphous dystrophic calcification eventually involves the entire kidney (known as putty kidney)."-Bailey 27/e p1405

105. **Ans. a. CECT** *(Ref: Sabiston 21/e p2078, 424; Bailey 27/e p1414)*

In patients with a history of blunt trauma, key findings of renal injuries include flank ecchymosis, and gross or microscopic hematuria (in the question left flank bruise with hematuria is mentioned). Since the patient is stable CECT should be done to accurately assess the extent of the injury.

"Renal Injuries: In patients with a history of blunt trauma, key findings include location of impact, flank ecchymosis, and gross or microscopic hematuria."-Sabiston 21/e p2078

"The presence of gross hematuria is the most valuable screen for injuries to the genitourinary organs and should prompt further evaluation. As with other abdominal structures, imaging with IV contrast-enhanced CT frequently identifies injuries to the genitourinary organs."- Sabiston 21/e p424

"CT scan with contrast is the investigation of choice. It will accurately assess the extent of the injury, showing laceration, extravasation, surrounding haemorrhage and vessel injury. It also shows non-renal injuries and effectively stages renal pedicle injuries. Arterial occlusion is manifest as rim enhancement of the normal renal contour."-Bailey 27/e p1414

106. **Ans. a. Bladder cancer** *(Ref: Bailey 27/e p1446; Robbin's 10/e p960)*

The given specimen of opened bladder shows advanced stage multinodular carcinoma bladder. So, this radical cysto-prostatectomy was performed for bladder cancer.

107. **Ans. c. Active surveillance** *(Ref: Bailey 27/e p1457, 1472, 1473)*

Low risk prostate cancer (low PSA, small foci of Gleason 6 disease) can be managed by active surveillance. Radical prostatectomy is suitable for localised disease and should be carried out only in men with a life expectancy of >10 years. In the question, since the age of the patient is 85 years, the life expectancy of <10 years, so Radical prostatectomy is ruled out. Since, the prostate cancer is small (2 × 3 cm nodule) with Gleason score 6, and PSA level of 8 ng/mL, it should be managed by active surveillance.

"Men with locally confined prostate cancer usually have serum PSA levels <10–15 ng/mL."-Bailey 27/e p1457

"Low risk prostate cancer (low PSA, small foci of Gleason 6 disease) can be managed by active surveillance. Here, with 3- to 6-monthly digital rectal examination (DRE) and PSA measurement and repeated prostate biopsy, a proportion can safely avoid the toxicity of radical treatment."- Bailey 27/e p1472

"Radical prostatectomy is suitable for localised disease and should be carried out only in men with a life expectancy of >10 years." - Bailey 27/e p1473

108. **Ans. b. Suprapubic cystostomy** *(Ref: Bailey 27/e p1479; Smith Urology 17/e p294)*

History of cycling accident and blood at the tip of meatus suggest the rupture of the bulbar urethra. No attempt should be made to pass a urethral catheter. Percutaneous suprapubic cystostomy can be done as a temporary procedure.

"Rupture of the bulbar urethra: There is a history of a blow to the perineum, usually due to a fall astride injury. The bulbar urethra is crushed upwards onto the pubic bone, typically with significant bruising. In the days of sailing ships, the common cause was falling astride a spar and the modern equivalent is seen among workers losing their footing on scaffolding. Cycling accidents, loose manhole covers and gymnasium accidents astride the beam account for a number of cases."-Bailey 27/e p1479

"The perineum is very tender; a mass may be found, as may blood at the urethral meatus. Rectal examination reveals a normal prostate. The patient usually has a desire to void, but voiding should not be allowed until assessment of the urethra is complete. No attempt should be made to pass a urethral catheter, but if the patient's bladder is overdistended, percutaneous suprapubic cystostomy can be done as a temporary procedure."-Smith Urology 17/e p294

109. **Ans. a. Caused by mixed aerobic anerobic infection** *(Ref: Bailey 27/e p1509, 1510)*

The postoperative image shows exposed bilateral testis with Foley's catheter in-situ. It suggests that debridement was performed for the Fournier's gangrene. Fournier's gangrene is a mixed infection of aerobic and anaerobic bacteria. Urinary diversion is usually not required. Testis is spared, so orchidectomy is not done. Anti-gas gangrene serum is not used.

"Fournier's gangrene is an uncommon and nasty condition characterised by a polymicrobial infection of the soft tissues of the perineum, external genitalia and perianal region. It is a form of necrotising fasciitis. There is rapid onset of gangrene leading to exposure of the scrotal contents."- Bailey 27/e p1509

"There is a mixed infection of aerobic and anaerobic bacteria in a fulminating inflammation of the subcutaneous tissues, which results in an obliterative arteritis of the arterioles to the scrotal skin that in turn results in gangrene. The condition can spread rapidly to involve the fascia and skin of the penis, perineum and abdominal wall."- Bailey 27/e p1509

"Treatment of a case of Fournier's gangrene is a surgical emergency. Initial management involves intravenous fluid resuscitation and early use of broad spectrum intravenous antibiotics. Urgent wide surgical excision of the dead and infected tissue is essential and the extent of the internal necrosis is typically much greater than the external appearances suggest, such that extensive debridement is often necessary. Urinary and faecal diversion may be necessary. Supportive care is essential, because the patients often become severely septic."- Bailey 27/e p1510

110. **Ans. d. PTA with stenting** (Ref: Bailey 27/e p948, 949)

History of claudication of right thigh with numbness, tingling in the right lower limb and feeble peripheral pulses suggest the arterial occlusion, at the level of common iliac artery as shown in the angiography. The next step of management is Percutaneous transluminal angioplasty (PTA) with stenting. PTA has proved very successful in dilating the iliac and femoropopliteal segments. Surgical operations are usually reserved for patients with severe symptoms where angioplasty has failed or is not possible.

"Percutaneous transluminal angioplasty (PTA) has proved very successful in dilating the iliac and femoropopliteal segments; the results below the knee are less successful."-Bailey 27/e p948

"Surgical operations are usually reserved for patients with severe symptoms where angioplasty has failed or is not possible. Aortoiliac occlusion responds well to aorto-femoral bypass using a Dacron graft; although the operation carries a perioperative mortality and systemic morbidity rates of about 5% and 15%, respectively. In unfit patients, an axillofemoral bypass is an alternative, although patency rates are less. If only one iliac system is occluded, an iliofemoral or femorofemoral crossover graft may be performed." - Bailey 27/e p949

"Superficial femoral artery disease can be treated by femoropopliteal bypass; long-term graft patency is determined by the quality of inflow and outflow, graft length (whether the distal anastomosis is above or below the knee) and the conduit used for the bypass. Autologous long saphenous vein (LSV) gives the best results and can be used reversed or in situ after valve disruption. If the LSV is not available from either leg, short saphenous or arm veins may be used. If no vein is available, a prosthetic polytetrafluoroethylene (PTFE) graft may be employed although patency rates are lower; many surgeons construct the lower anastomosis using a small collar of vein (Miller cuff) between the PTFE and the recipient artery, which may improve patency. Isolated common femoral artery or profunda disease can be treated with endarterectomy and patch (vein or prosthetic) or a short bypass in the groin."- Bailey 27/e p949

111. **Ans. a. 2a** (Ref: Gray's 41/e p)

According to 'CEAP' Classification, asymptomatic varicose veins is included in C2a category.

'CEAP' Classification of Chronic Lower Extremity Venous Disease	
C	• **Clinical signs** (grade 0–6), supplemented by **"A"** for **asymptomatic** & **"S"** for **symptomatic** presentation
E	• **Etiologic classification** (**c**ongenital, **p**rimary, **s**econdary)
A	• **Anatomic distribution** (**s**uperficial, **d**eep, or **p**erforator, alone or in combination)
P	• **Pathophysiologic dysfunction** (**r**eflux or **o**bstruction, alone or in combination)

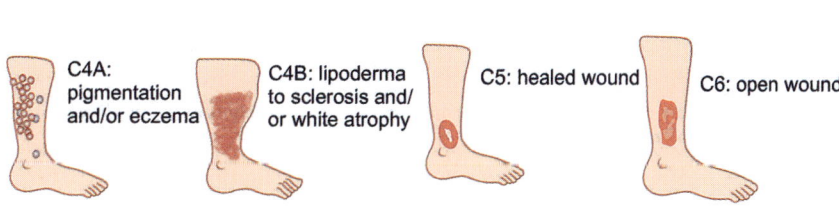

Clinical (C of CEAP) Classification (C0-6)

- **Any limb with possible chronic venous disease** is first placed into **one of seven clinical classes (C0-6)**, according to the **objective signs of disease.**

Class	Features
0	No visible or palpable signs of venous disease
1	Telangiectasia, reticular veins, malleolar flare^Q
2	Varicose veins^Q
3	Edema without skin changes^Q
4	Skin changes ascribed to venous disease (e.g., **pigmentation, venous eczema, lipodermatosclerosis**)^Q
5	Skin changes as defined above **with healed ulceration**
6	Skin changes as defined above **with active ulceration**^Q

112. **Ans. a. Saphenous nerve** *(Ref: Sabiston 21/e p1821, 1822)*

Lack of sensation over medial aspect of leg and foot associated with heel pain after harvesting the great saphenous vein graft is due to saphenous nerve injury. Saphenous neuralgia after harvest of great saphenous vein (GSV) for coronary artery bypass graft (CABG) is common. The main symptom is anaesthesia and certain areas may persist for some considerable time postoperatively.

Saphenous nerve is the terminal sensory branch of the femoral nerve (L 2, 3, 4), supplying the skin of the anteromedial aspect of the leg. It arises anterior to the femoral artery within the adductor canal, and perforates the anterior wall (roof) of the canal, travelling closely associated with the GSV in the subcutaneous tissues of the leg. The mechanism of injury is thought to be from local division of the nerve or its branches, or from compression by post-operative soft tissue swelling.

"Today, traditional surgical treatment of superficial venous reflux involves high ligation as well as stripping of the great saphenous vein from the knee to the groin. Stripping at the ankle has been largely abandoned because of a high incidence of saphenous nerve injury."-Sabiston 21/e p1821

"Saphenous nerve injury is a well-documented complication that occurs more frequently when the great saphenous vein is stripped from the ankle to the groin. The saphenous nerve runs close to the great saphenous vein in the calf compared with the thigh, where the nerve and vein have more separation. This anatomic detail may explain why stripping from the knee to the thigh only reduces the risk of nerve injury."- Sabiston 21/e p1822

"Stripping of the small saphenous should be done only to the level of the midcalf to avoid injury to the closely aligned sural nerve." - Sabiston 21/e p1822

113. **Ans. a. Thymic neoplasia** *(Ref: Sabiston 21/e p1635)*

Thymomas are the most common neoplasm of the anterior compartment of the mediastinum. Pure red cell aplasia is one of the hematological paraneoplastic syndromes associated with thymoma.

"Thymomas are the most common neoplasm of the anterosuperior compartment of the mediastinum."- Sabiston 21/e p1635

"The most common syndrome is myasthenia gravis (in up to 50% of cases); other syndromes include pure red blood cell aplasia, hypogammaglobulinemia, and thymoma-associated multi-organ autoimmunity."-Sabiston 21/e p1635

114. **Ans. a. Esophagus** *(Ref: Nelson 20/e p1793)*

The foreign body appears to be a coin, which appears to be just anterior to vertebrae (location of esophagus) plus there is tracheal air shadow observed in front of the coin. Hence, it is a coin in oesophagus, which is further elucidated by the fact that the patient has presented a bit late with a complaint of difficulty in swallowing (foreign body in gut tube) rather than in acute emergency with difficulty in respiration (foreign body in respiratory tube). The flat surface of a coin in the esophagus is seen on the anteroposterior view and the edge on the lateral view.

"The flat surface of a coin in the esophagus is seen on the anteroposterior view and the edge on the lateral view. The reverse is true for coins lodged in the trachea; here, the edge is seen anteroposteriorly and the flat side is seen laterally."-Nelson 20/e p1793

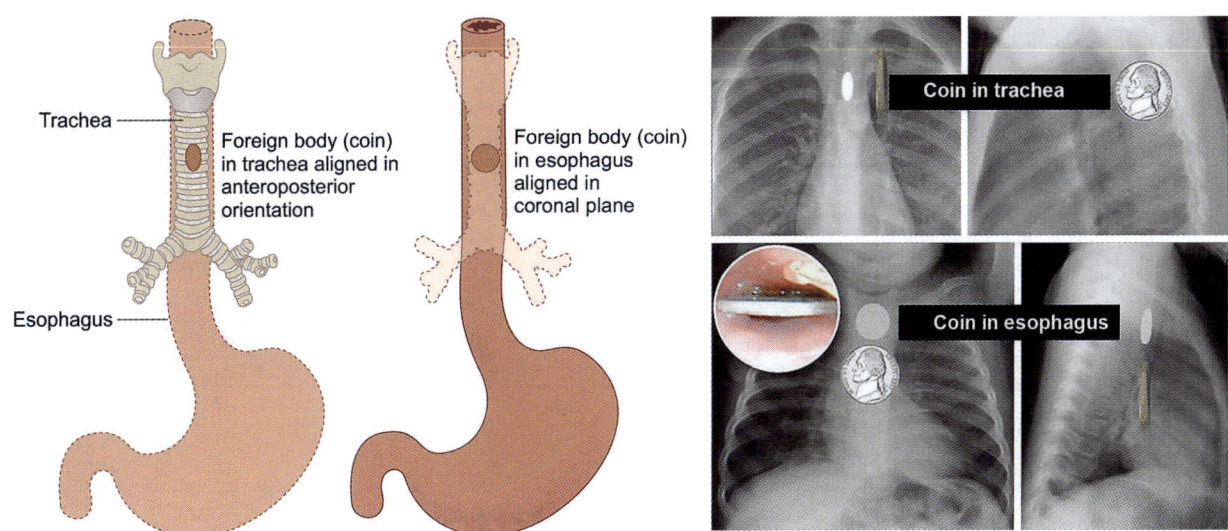

115. **Ans. a. Lingual nerve** *(Ref: Bailey 27/e p780)*

Lingual nerve hooks under submandibular gland duct, and any surgical manipulation of the duct might injure the nerve, as has happened in present case scenario. Inferior alveolar nerve is a branch from the posterior division of trigeminal nerve, which runs protected within the substance of mandible and supplies the lower teeth. Hypoglossal nerve may be damaged in submandibular gland excision, but less commonly. Marginal mandibular branch of facial nerve is the 'most common' nerve to be damaged during submandibular gland excision, but has not been taken as the answer since, there is a mention of a nerve injury while surgical manipulation of submandibular gland duct.

"The submandibular glands are paired salivary glands that lie below the mandible on either side. They consist of a larger superficial and a smaller deep lobe that are continuous around the posterior border of the mylohyoid muscle. Important anatomical relations include the anterior facial vein and artery running over the surface of the gland in close association with the ramus mandibularis (marginal mandibular) of the facial nerve. The deep part of the gland lies on the hyoglossus muscle closely related to the lingual nerve and inferior to the hypoglossal nerve."- Bailey 27/e p780

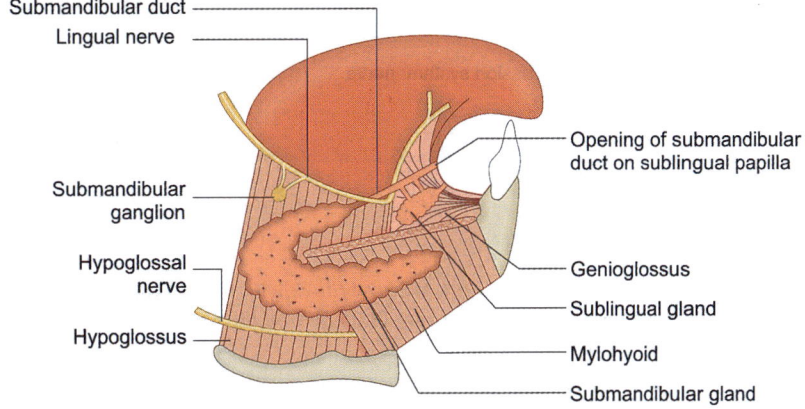

"Important anatomical relationships of the submandibular glands: Lingual nerve; Hypoglossal nerve; Anterior facial vein; Facial artery; Marginal mandibular branch of the facial nerve."- Bailey 27/e p780

116. **Ans. b. Blood cancer** *(Ref: Robbin's 10/e p414)*

Benzene is a carcinogen, which increases the risk of acute myelocytic leukemia (blood cancer).

"Occupational exposure to benzene and 1, 3-butadiene increases the risk of leukemia. Benzene is oxidized to an epoxide through hepatic CYP2E1, a component of the P-450 enzyme system already mentioned. The epoxide and other metabolites disrupt progenitor cell differentiation in the bone marrow and may lead to marrow aplasia and acute myeloid leukemia."- Robbin's 10/e p414

117. **Ans. c. Neurons** *(Ref: Robbin's 10/e p429)*

Rapidly dividing cells of the gastrointestinal mucosa and bone marrow are particularly sensitive to the effects of radiation. Least radiosensitive tissue of body is nervous tissue or brain.

"Because ionizing radiation damages DNA, rapidly dividing cells are more vulnerable to injury than quiescent cells. Except at extremely high doses that impair DNA transcription, irradiation does not kill nondividing cells, such as neurons and muscle cells. However, in dividing cells DNA damage is detected by sensors that produce signals leading to the upregulation of p53, the "guardian of the genome." p53 in turn upregulates the expression of genes that initially lead to cell cycle arrest and, if the DNA damage is too great to be repaired, genes that cause cell death through apoptosis. Understandably, therefore, tissues with a high rate of cell division, such as gonads, bone marrow, lymphoid tissue, and the mucosa of the gastrointestinal tract, are extremely vulnerable to radiation, and the injury is manifested early after exposure."-Robbin's 10/e p429

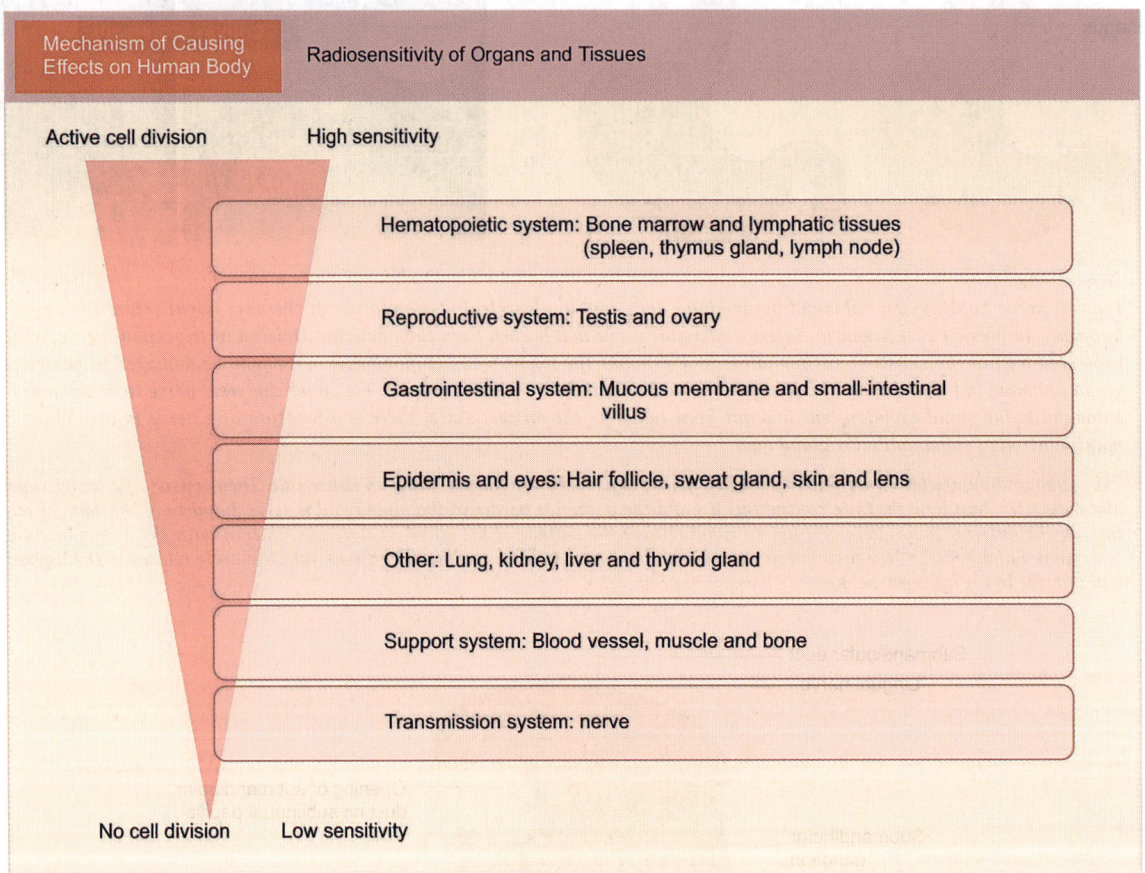

118. **Ans. b. Head tilt, chin lift** *(Ref: Bailey 27/e 271; Miller's 9/e p2718)*

The maneuver shown in the image is head tilt and chin lift. The head tilt-chin lift and jaw-thrust methods are indicated for conscious and unconscious patients who do not have an adequate airway. The purpose of these methods is to open and maintain a patent (clear) airway or to relieve a partial or total airway obstruction.

"Head tilt, chin lift and jaw thrust manoeuvres, along with adjuncts such as oropharyngeal airways, are used to facilitate bag-mask ventilation while induction agents exert full effect."- Bailey 27/e 271

"Bag-mask ventilation with a head tilt–chin lift or head tilt–jaw thrust maneuver is recommended for initial airway control in most circum- stances."-Miller's 9/e p2718

119. **Ans. a. Needle decompression in 5th intercostal space** *(Ref: Schwartz 11/e p186)*

After road traffic accident, presence of subcutaneous emphysema, absence of air entry on the right side of hemithorax & hypotension are pointers towards the diagnosis of tension pneumothorax. Immediate needle thoracostomy decompression should be done. The preferred location for needle decompression is 5th intercostal space in the anterior axillary line in adults.

"Tension pneumothorax and simple pneumothorax have similar signs, symptoms, and examination findings, but hypotension qualifies the pneumothorax as a tension pneumothorax. Although immediate needle thoracostomy decompression with a 14-gauge angiocatheter in the second intercostal space in the midclavicular line may be indicated in the field, tube thoracostomy should be performed immediately in the ED before a chest radiograph is obtained. Recent studies suggest the preferred location for needle decompression may be the 5th intercostal space in the anterior axillary line due to body habitus."-Schwartz 11/e p186

120. **Ans. a. FAST** (Ref: Bailey 27/e p372)

FAST is a technique whereby ultrasound imaging is used to assess the torso for the presence of free fluid, either in the abdominal cavity, and is extended into the thoracic cavities and pericardium (eFAST). This patient, after road traffic accident, developed sustained injury over chest and abdomen with unstable vitals (systolic BP: 70 mm Hg & pulse rate: 110/minute). The next step in this patient to perform the FAST.

"Focused abdominal sonar for trauma (FAST) is a technique whereby ultrasound (sonar) imaging is used to assess the torso for the presence of free fluid, either in the abdominal cavity, and is extended into the thoracic cavities and pericardium (eFAST)."-Bailey 27/e p372

"eFAST is usually a rapid, reproducible, portable and non-invasive bedside test and can be performed at the same time as resuscitation. eFAST is accurate at detecting >100 mL of free blood; however, it is very operator dependent and, especially if the patient is very obese or the bowel is full of gas, it may be unreliable."-Bailey 27/e p372

NEET PG 2020

121. **Ans. a. Colloid carcinoma** (Ref: Bailey 27/e p872; Schwartz 11/e p566; Sabiston 20/e p840)

"The infiltrating cells may secrete copious amounts of mucin and appear to float in this material. These lesions are called mucinous or colloid tumors."-Sabiston 20/e p840

"Mucinous carcinoma (colloid carcinoma), another special-type breast cancer, accounts for 2% of all invasive breast cancers and typically presents in the older population as a bulky tumor. This cancer is defined by extracellular pools of mucin, which surround aggregates of low-grade cancer cells."-Schwartz 11/e p566

122. **Ans. d. Majority of the retrosternal goitres can be removed by a neck incision** (Ref: Bailey 27/e p810, 811; Schwartz 11/e p1642; Sabiston 20/e p892)

The vast majority (>95%) of retrosternal goitres can be removed transcervically.

"Retrosternal goitre tends to arise from the slow growth of a multinodular gland down in to the mediastinum. As the gland enlarges within the thoracic inlet, pressure may lead to dysphagia, tracheal compression and eventually airway symptoms. The vast majority of patients have minimal symptoms. Patient should be considered for surgery if there is significant airway compression, if symptoms are present or in young patients in whom symptoms are likely to develop."-Bailey 27/e p810

"If a decision is made to proceed to surgery, assessment of the extent of disease is critical. The vast majority (>95%) of retrosternal goitres can be removed transcervically. Those at most risk of requiring conversion to an open sternotomy approach include malignant or revision cases, those which extend into the posterior mediastinum and those in which the diameter of the goitre exceeds that of the thoracic inlet. In such cases a joint case with thoracic surgery should be planned."-Bailey 27/e p811

123. **Ans. a. Papillary thyroid carcinoma** (Ref: Schwartz 11/e p1647; Sabiston 20/e p898)

The given HPE image shows optically clear nuclei (Orphan Annie eye nuclei), which is highly suggestive of papillary carcinoma thyroid.

"Papillary Carcinoma Thyroid: The diagnosis is established by characteristic nuclear cellular features. Cells are cuboidal with pale, abundant cytoplasm, crowded nuclei that may demonstrate "grooving," and intranuclear cytoplasmic inclusions (leading to the designation of Orphan Annie nuclei, which allow diagnosis by FNAB). Psammoma bodies, which are microscopic, calcified deposits representing clumps of sloughed cells, also may be present."-Schwartz 11/e p1647

124. **Ans. b. Hashimoto's thyroiditis** (Ref: Bailey 27/e p821; Schwartz 11/e p1640; Sabiston 20/e p891)

History of diffuse thyroid swelling in a female, who is hypothyroid (elevated TSH levels) and HPE reports showing intense lymphocytic infiltration with Hürthle cells is highly suggestive of Hashimoto's thyroiditis.

"Hashimoto's thyroiditis is also more common in women (male-to-female ratio is 1:10 to 20) between the ages of 30 and 50 years old. The most common presentation is that of a minimally or moderately enlarged firm granular gland discovered on routine physical examination or the awareness of a painless anterior neck mass, although 20% of patients present with hypothyroidism, and 5% present with hyperthyroidism (Hashitoxicosis)."-Schwartz 11/e p1640

"On microscopic examination, the gland is diffusely infiltrated by small lymphocytes and plasma cells and occasionally shows well-developed germinal centers. Thyroid follicles are smaller than normal with reduced amounts of colloid and increased interstitial connective tissue. The follicles are lined by Hürthle or Askanazy cells, which are characterized by abundant eosinophilic, granular cytoplasm."-Schwartz 11/e p1640

125. **Ans. a. 50% reduction in PTH within 10 mins of gland removal** (Ref: Bailey 27/e p830; Sabiston 20/e p934)

"The Miami criteria were developed to determine the extent of resection. A drop in the PTH into the normal range and to less than half the maximum preoperative PTH at 10 minutes appears to accurately predict single-gland disease."-Bailey 27/e p830

"Various protocols exist that use intraoperative PTH measurements. The "Miami" criteria developed by Irvin and colleagues describe biochemical cure as a 50% decrease in PTH levels from baseline 10 to 15 minutes after resection of the targeted parathyroid gland." -Sabiston 20/e p934

126. **Ans. b. CP class B** (Ref: Bailey 27/e p1157; Schwartz 11/e p1365; Sabiston 20/e p216)

The Child-Pugh class for patient who has a serum bilirubin of 2.5 mg/dL (2 points), serum albumin of 3 g/dL (2 points), INR of 2 (2 points) along with Mild ascites (2 points) but no encephalopathy (1 point) is class B (total points = 9).

Child-Turcotte-Pugh (CTP) Scoring System

- **CTP score** is a measure to **assess hepatic function**^{Q} in many liver diseases.
- It was **initially devised to classify patients** into **risk groups** prior to **undergoing portosystemic shunt surgeries**^{Q}.
- It is used to **assess prognosis in cirrhosis**^{Q} and many liver diseases.

Child-Turcotte-Pugh (CTP) Score			
Variable	1 Point	2 Points	3 Points
Serum albumin (g/dL)	>3.5	2.8–3.5^Q	<2.8
Bilirubin (mg/dL)	<2	2–3^Q	>3
Prothrombin time (sec above normal) or INR	<4 <1.7	4–6^Q 1.7–2.3^Q	>6 >2.3
Ascites	None	Controlled^Q	Uncontrolled
Encephalopathy	None	Controlled^Q	Uncontrolled

Class A	5–6 points^Q
Class B	7–9 points^Q
Class C	10–15 points^Q

127. **Ans. a. Right gastric and right gastroepiploic artery** (Ref: Bailey 27/e p1106; Schwartz 11/e p1103; Sabiston 20/e p1189)

Ligation of common hepatic artery will impair blood supply in right gastric and right gastroepiploic artery.

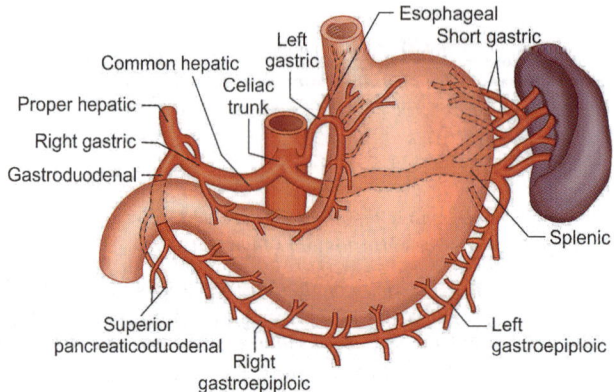

Branches of coeliac trunk

"The stomach has an arterial supply on both lesser and greater curves. On the lesser curve, the left gastric artery, a branch of the coeliac axis, forms an anastomotic arcade with the right gastric artery, which arises from the common hepatic artery. Branches of the left gastric artery pass up towards the cardia. The gastroduodenal artery, which is also a branch of the hepatic artery, passes behind the first part of the duodenum, highly relevant with respect to the bleeding duodenal ulcer. Here it divides into the superior pancreaticoduodenal artery and the right gastroepiploic artery. The superior pancreaticoduodenal artery supplies the duodenum and pancreatic head, and forms an anastomosis with the inferior pancreaticoduodenal artery, a branch of the superior mesenteric artery. The right gastroepiploic artery runs along the greater curvature of the stomach, eventually forming an anastomosis with the left gastroepiploic artery, a branch of the splenic artery."-Bailey 27/e p1106

128. **Ans. b. ERCP** *(Ref: Bailey 27/e p1158; Schwartz 11/e p1400; Sabiston 20/e p1489)*

"ERCP is performed in patients with obstructive jaundice when an endoscopic intervention is anticipated based on prior imaging (endoscopic removal of CBD stones, biliary drainage in septic patient or insertion of a biliary tract stent)."-Bailey 27/e p1158

"However, for cases of choledocholithiasis, obstructive jaundice, biliary strictures, or cholangitis, ERCP has the advantage of being both diagnostic and therapeutic. If ductal stones are identified on the endoscopic cholangiogram, biliary sphincterotomy and stone extraction can be performed, clearing the common bile duct of stones."-Schwartz 11/e p1400

129. **Ans. a. Primary sclerosing cholangitis** *(Ref: Bailey 27/e p1206; Schwartz 11/e p1417; Sabiston 20/e p1509)*

History of recurrent episodes of abdominal pain, abdominal tenderness, fever and jaundice (suggestive of recurrent attacks of cholangitis) in a 35 years old male and MRCP image showing multiple strictures of intrahepatic and extrahepatic bile duct is highly suggestive of primary sclerosing cholangitis.

"The mean age of presentation for PSC is 30 to 45 years, and men are affected twice as often as women. Most patients are symptomatic when diagnosed, and may complain of intermittent jaundice, fatigue, weight loss, pruritus, or abdominal pain."-Schwartz 11/e p1417

"PSC: ERCP is the preferred route for cholangiography and can demonstrate the characteristic multifocal, diffusely distributed dilations and strictures of the intrahepatic and extrahepatic biliary trees."-Sabiston 20/e p1509

130. **Ans. a. Superior mesenteric artery** *(Ref: Bailey 27/e p1213; Schwartz 11/e p1430; Sabiston 20/e p1238, 1520)*

Tumor of the uncinate process of pancreas affects superior mesenteric artery (SMA) due to its close relation with SMA.

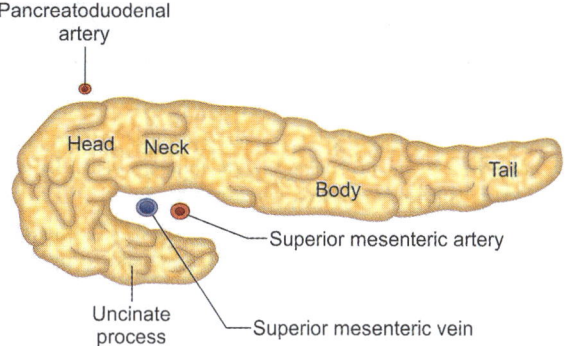

Transverse section of the pancreas (Note the position of the uncinate process behind the vessels)

"The uncinate process extends from the head of the pancreas behind the superior mesenteric vein (SMV) and terminates adjacent to the superior mesenteric artery (SMA)."-Sabiston 20/e p1520

"The uncinate process and the head of the pancreas wrap around the right side of the portal vein and end posteriorly near the space between the superior mesenteric vein and superior mesenteric artery."-Schwartz 11/e p1430

131. **Ans. a. Insulinoma** *(Ref: Bailey 27/e p849; Schwartz 11/e p1480; Sabiston 20/e p952)*

"Insulinomas are the most common functional pancreatic endocrine neoplasms and present with a typical clinical syndrome known as Whipple's triad."-Schwartz 11/e p1480

"Insulinomas are the most frequent of all the functioning PETs with a reported incidence of 2–4 cases per million population per year."-Bailey 27/e p849

132. **Ans. c. Duodenum** *(Ref: Bailey 27/e p857; Schwartz 11/e p1136; Sabiston 20/e p958)*

MC site of gastrinoma in MEN 1 syndrome is duodenum.

"MEN 1 gastrinomas are more often located in the duodenum as multiple small tumours than in the pancreas. For gastrinomas located in the duodenum or pancreatic head (gastrinoma triangle), pylorus-preserving partial pancreaticoduodenectomy is recommended. In rare cases the gastrinoma is located in the body or tail of the pancreas. In such cases distal pancreatectomy with excision of tumours in the pancreatic head is the procedure of choice."-Bailey 27/e p857

133. **Ans. c. Pharyngeal pouch** *(Ref: Bailey 27/e p1101; Schwartz 11/e p1053; Sabiston 20/e p1019)*

History of halitosis and a swelling in the lateral aspect of the neck, which on pressing gives rise to a regurgitant sound along and the given Barium swallow image is highly suggestive of pharyngeal pouch (Zenker's diverticulum).

"Zenker's diverticulum (pharyngeal pouch) is not really an oesophageal diverticulum as it protrudes posteriorly above the cricopharyngeal sphincter through the natural weak point (the dehiscence of Killian) between the oblique and horizontal (cricopharyngeus) fibres of the inferior pharyngeal constrictor. When the diverticulum is small, symptoms largely reflect this in coordination with predominantly pharyngeal dysphagia. As the pouch enlarges, it tends to fill with food on eating, and the fundus descends into the mediastinum. This leads to halitosis and oesophageal dysphagia."-Bailey 27/e p1101

"Diagnosis is made by barium esophagram. At the level of the cricothyroid cartilage, the diverticulum can be seen filled with barium resting posteriorly alongside the esophagus (the "cricopharyngeal bar"). Lateral views are critical because this is usually a posterior structure. Neither esophageal manometry nor endoscopy is needed to diagnose Zenker diverticulum." Sabiston 20/e p1019

134. **Ans. c. Type III achalasia** *(Ref: Bailey 27/e p1096; Sabiston 20/e p1015)*

On esophageal manometry, abnormal spastic contractions in esophagus >450 mm Hg·s·cm in the body is suggestive of Type III achalasia (spastic achalasia).

Type of Achalasia	Criteria
Type I achalasia (classic achalasia)	• **Elevated median IRP (>15 mm Hg), 100% failed peristalsis (DCI <100 mm Hg·s·cm)** • Premature contractions with DCI values <450 mm Hg·s·cm satisfy criteria for failed peristalsis
Type II achalasia (**with oesophageal compression**)	• Elevated median IRP (>15 mm Hg), 100% failed peristalsis, **panoesophageal pressurisation with ≥20% of swallows** • Contractions may be masked by oesophageal pressurisation & DCI should not be calculated
Type III achalasia (**spastic achalasia**)	• **Elevated median IRP (>15 mm Hg), no normal peristalsis, premature (spastic) contractions with DCI >450 mm Hg·s·cm with ≥20% of swallows**^{Q} • May be mixed with panoesophageal pressurisation

DCI, distal contractile integral (mm Hg·s·cm); EGJ, esophaogastric junction; IRP, integrated relaxation pressure (mm Hg); LES, lower esophageal sphincter.

135. **Ans. b. Carcinoma esophagus** *(Ref: Bailey 27/e p1086; Schwartz 11/e p1070; Sabiston 20/e p1028)*

The given barium swallow shows advanced carcinoma esophagus with abrupt, irregular narrowing in the distal esophagus, with more proximal dilation along with shouldered margin and apple core appearance.

"Barium esophagram may demonstrate irregular narrowing or ulceration. The classic "apple-core" filling defect is seen only if there is symmetrical, circumferential narrowing. Instead, there is often an asymmetrical bulge seen with an infiltrative appearance." -Sabiston 20/e p1028

136. **Ans. a. Spontaneous perforation of the esophagus** *(Ref: Bailey 27/e p1072, 1073; Schwartz 11/e p1083; Sabiston 20/e p1025)*

History of upper abdominal pain after a heavy meal along with tenderness in the upper abdomen and on X-ray, widening of the mediastinum with pneumo-mediastinum is highly suggestive of Spontaneous perforation of the esophagus (Boerhaave's syndrome).

"Barotrauma (spontaneous perforation, Boerhaave's syndrome): This occurs classically when a person vomits against a closed glottis. The pressure in the oesophagus increases rapidly, and the oesophagus bursts at its weakest point in the lower third, sending a stream of material into the mediastinum and often the pleural cavity as well."-Bailey 27/e p1072

"The diagnosis can usually be suspected from the history and associated clinical features. A chest radiograph is often confirmatory with air in the mediastinum, pleura or peritoneum. Pleural effusion occurs rapidly either as a result of free communication with the pleural space or as a reaction to adjacent inflammation in the mediastinum. A contrast swallow or CT is nearly always required to guide management."-Bailey 27/e p1072, 1073

137. **Ans. a. Vitamin B_{12} deficiency** *(Ref: Bailey 27/e p1256; Schwartz 11/e p1254; Sabiston 20/e p1291)*

"Short Bowel Syndrome: Length alone, however, is not the only determining factor of complications related to small bowel resection. For example, if the distal two thirds of the ileum, including the ileocecal valve, is resected, significant abnormalities of absorption of bile salts and vitamin B_{12} may occur, resulting in diarrhea and anemia, although only 25% of the total length of the small bowel has been removed."-Sabiston 20/e p1291

"Short Bowel Syndrome: Patients with as little as 100–200 cm of jejunum anastomosed to an intact colon may therefore be able to maintain satisfactory macronutrient, fluid and electrolyte status, although they will, of course, be at risk of fat-soluble and B12 vitamin deficiencies and will also generally need oral nutritional supplements of trace elements, vitamins and minerals."
-Bailey 27/e p1256

138. **Ans. b. Intussusception** *(Ref: Bailey 27/e p129; Schwartz 11/e p1253; Sabiston 20/e p1879; Nelson 20/e p1813)*

History of abdominal pain, blood in stools and a palpable mass on the abdominal examination along with barium enema showing coiled spring sign is highly suggestive of Intussusception.

"Intussusception: Classically, a previously healthy infant presents with colicky pain and vomiting (milk then bile). Between episodes, the child initially appears well. Later, they may pass a 'redcurrant jelly' stool. Clinical signs include dehydration, abdominal distension and a palpable sausage-shaped mass in the right upper quadrant. Rectal examination may reveal blood or rarely the apex of the intussusceptum."-Bailey 27/e p129

"Contrast enemas demonstrate a filling defect or cupping in the head of the contrast media where its advance is obstructed by the intussusceptum. A central linear column of contrast media may be visible in the compressed lumen of the intussusceptum, and a thin rim of contrast may be seen trapped around the invaginating intestine in the folds of mucosa within the intussuscipiens (coiled-spring sign), especially after evacuation."-Nelson 20/e p1813

139. **Ans. d. 4** *(Ref: Bailey 27/e p1274; Schwartz 11/e p1287; Sabiston 20/e p1333)*

Hinchey Classification of Complicated Diverticulitis	
Grade I	Mesenteric or pericolic abscess^Q
Grade II	Pelvic abscess^Q
Grade III	Purulent peritonitis^Q
Grade IV	Faecal peritonitis^Q

140. **Ans. b. Juvenile polyp** *(Ref: Bailey 27/e p1327; Schwartz 11/e p1291; Sabiston 20/e p1372)*

History of bleeding PR in a 5 years old child with presence of a polypoidal mass in the rectum and biopsy showing dilated crypts and inflamed stroma is highly suggestive of juvenile polyp.

"Juvenile polyp: This is a bright red, glistening pedunculated sphere ('cherry tumour'), which is found in infants and children. Occasionally, it persists into adult life. It can cause bleeding, or pain if it prolapses during defecation. It often separates itself, but can be removed easily with forceps or a snare. A solitary juvenile polyp has virtually no tendency to malignant change, but should be treated if it is causing symptoms. It has a unique histological structure with large mucus-filled spaces covered by a smooth surface of thin rectal cuboidal epithelium."-Bailey 27/e p1327

141. **Ans. b. Gastroschisis** *(Ref: Bailey 27/e p135; Schwartz 11/e p1554; Sabiston 20/e p1071)*

In this newborn image, the bowel is exposed and located on the right side of umbilical cord is highly suggestive of gastroschisis.

"Gastroschisis is another congenital defect of the abdominal wall in which the umbilical membrane has ruptured in utero, allowing the intestine to herniate outside the abdominal cavity. The defect is almost always to the right of the umbilical cord, and the intestine is not covered with skin or amnion."-Sabiston 20/e p1071

142. **Ans. b. Partial nephrectomy** *(Ref: Bailey 27/e p1420; Sabiston 20/e p2098)*

"The trend in extirpative surgery is to perform nephron sparing or partial nephrectomy for most T1 tumors (Tumor 7 cm or less in greatest dimension, limited to the kidney). Partial nephrectomy is equivalent to radical nephrectomy in this tumor stage and should be considered for all patients with a T1a tumor (Tumor 4 cm or less) and most with T1b (Tumor more than 4 cm but not more than 7 cm) tumors."-Sabiston 20/e p2098

143. **Ans. a. Bulbar urethra** *(Ref: Bailey 27/e p1479)*

"Rupture of the bulbar urethra: There is a history of a blow to the perineum, usually due to a fall astride injury. The bulbar urethra is crushed upwards onto the pubic bone, typically with significant bruising. In the days of sailing ships, the common cause was falling astride a spar and the modern equivalent is seen among workers losing their footing on scaffolding. Cycling accidents, loose manhole covers and gymnasium accidents astride the beam account for a number of cases."-Bailey 27/e p1479

144. **Ans. b. MCU with bulbar urethral stricture** *(Ref: Schwartz 11/e p2093)*

The given image is of MCU showing bulbar urethral stricture.

145. **Ans. b. Most common site is the calf** *(Ref: Bailey 27/e p943; Schwartz 11/e p953; Sabiston 20/e p1780)*

"Intermittent claudication: Intermittent claudication occurs as a result of anaerobic muscle metabolism and is classically described as debilitating cramp-like pain felt in the muscles that is: reliably brought on by walking; not present on taking the first step (unlike osteoarthritis); reliably relieved by rest both in the standing and sitting positions; usually within 5 minutes. The distance that a patient is able to walk without stopping varies (claudication distance) only slightly from day to day. It is decreased by increasing the work demands and hence oxygen requirements of the muscles affected, e.g. walking up hill, increasing the speed of walking and/or carrying heavy weights, and secondly by general health conditions that reduce the oxygen delivery capacity of the arterial system, e.g. anaemia or heart failure. The muscle group affected by claudication is classically one anatomical level below the level of arterial disease and is usually felt in the calf because the superficial femoral artery is the most commonly affected artery (70% of cases). Aorto-iliac disease (30% of cases) may cause thigh or buttock claudication. Buttock claudication in association with sexual impotence resulting from arterial insufficiency is eponymously called Leriche's syndrome. It is very rare."-Bailey 27/e p943

146. **Ans. a. Arterial disease with aorto-iliac involvement** *(Ref: Bailey 27/e p943; Schwartz 11/e p941; Sabiston 20/e p1738)*

"Aorto-iliac disease (30% of cases) may cause thigh or buttock claudication. Buttock claudication in association with sexual impotence resulting from arterial insufficiency is eponymously called Leriche's syndrome. It is very rare."-Bailey 27/e p943

"Aorto-iliac disease: Symptoms typically consist of bilateral thigh or buttock claudication and fatigue. Men report diminished penile tumescence and may have complete loss of erectile function. These symptoms in the absence of femoral pulses constitute Leriche's syndrome."-Schwartz 11/e p941

147. **Ans. d. Monitor till size reaches 55 mm** *(Ref: Bailey 27/e p961; Schwartz 11/e p920; Sabiston 20/e p1725)*

"An asymptomatic abdominal aortic aneurysm in an otherwise fit patient should be considered for repair if >55 mm in diameter (measured by ultrasonography). The annual incidence of rupture rises from 1% or less in aneurysms that are <55 mm in diameter to a significant level, perhaps as high as 25%, in those that are 70 mm in diameter. Assuming open elective surgery (transabdominal) carries a 5% mortality rate, the balance is in favour of elective operation once the maximum diameter is >55 mm, provided there is no major comorbidity. Regular ultrasonographic assessment is indicated for asymptomatic aneurysms <55 mm in diameter."-Bailey 27/e p961

"Abdominal Aortic Aneurysm: Surgical treatment is generally recommended for aneurysms more than 5.5 cm in maximal diameter, those demonstrating more than 5 mm of growth in 6 months or more than 1 cm in a year, and aneurysms with a saccular rather than the typical fusiform anatomy."-Sabiston 20/e p1725

148. **Ans. b. Complication of surgery** *(Ref: Bailey 27/e p915)*

"The Thoracoscore is the most widely used model to assess risk of operative mortality in thoracic patients. Risk is calculated based on nine variables—age, sex, American Society of Anesthesiologists (ASA) score, performance status, dyspnoea score, priority of surgery, extent of surgery, malignant diagnosis and composite comorbidity score. It is currently the most robust model available to estimate the risk of death when considering patients for thoracic surgery."-Bailey 27/e p915

149. **Ans. c. T1c** *(Ref: Bailey 27/e p927; Schwartz 11/e p690; Sabiston 20/e p1587)*

T1c is Tumor >2 cm but ≤3 cm in greatest dimension.

8th AJCC TNM Classification of Lung Cancer
Tis: Carcinoma in situ
T1a: Tumor **≤1 cm** in greatest dimension^Q
T1b: Tumor **>1 cm** but **≤2 cm** in greatest dimension^Q
T1c: Tumor **>2 cm** but **≤3 cm** in greatest dimension^Q
T2: Tumor **>3 cm** but **≤5 cm** or tumor with any of the following features: Involves **main bronchus**, regardless of **distance to the carina** but **without involvement of carina**^Q • Invades **visceral pleura**^Q • Associated with **atelectasis** or **obstructive pneumonitis** that extends to the hilar region either involving part of or the entire lung^Q • **T2a:** Tumor **>3 cm** but **≤4 cm** in greatest dimension^Q • **T2b:** Tumor **>4 cm** but **≤5 cm** in greatest dimension^Q
T3: Tumor >5 cm but **≤7** cm in greatest dimension or one that **directly invades any of the following: parietal pleura, chest wall** (including superior sulcus tumors), **phrenic nerve, parietal pericardium**; or separate tumor nodule(s) in the same lobe as the primary^Q
T4: Tumor **>7 cm** or of any size that **invades any** of the following: **diaphragm, mediastinum, heart, great vessels, trachea, recurrent laryngeal nerve, esophagus, vertebral body, carina**; or **Separate tumor nodule(s)** in a **different ipsilateral lobe to that of primary**^Q
N1: Metastasis in **ipsilateral peribronchial** and/or **ipsilateral hilar lymph nodes** and **intrapulmonary nodes**, including involvement by direct extension^Q
N2: Metastasis in **ipsilateral mediastinal** and/or **subcarinal lymph node(s)**^Q

Contd…

Contd…

8th AJCC TNM Classification of Lung Cancer
N3: Metastasis in **contralateral mediastinal, contralateral hilar, ipsilateral or contralateral scalene**, or **supraclavicular lymph node(s)**^{Q}
M1a: Separate tumor nodule(s) in a **contralateral lobe**; tumor with **pleural or pericardial nodules** or **malignant pleural (or pericardial) effusion**^{Q}
M1b: Single extra-thoracic metastasis in a single or multiple organs^Q
M1c: Multiple extra-thoracic metastasis in single or multiple organs^Q

150. **Ans. b. Moderate** *(Ref: Bailey 27/e p989)*

The patient with clinical signs of DVT (score 3) has tachycardia (score 1.5) and history of bladder cancer (score 1). According to modified Well's scoring, there would be moderate probability (Score 5.5) of pulmonary embolism.

Modified Wells Criteria for Predicting Pulmonary Embolism (PE)	
Variable	**Score**
Clinical signs & symptoms DVT^Q (minimum of leg swelling & pain on palpation of deep veins)	3
Alternative diagnosis less likely than PE^Q	3
Heart rate >100 bpm^Q	1.5
Immobilisation >3 days or surgery within past 4 weeks^Q	1.5
Previous DVT or PE^Q	1.5
Haemoptysis^Q	1
Malignancy^Q (treatment or palliation within past 6 months)	1
Low risk: <2; Moderate risk: 3-6; High risk: >6	

151. **Ans. a. Fat embolism** *(Ref: Bailey 27/e p956; Sabiston 20/e p501)*

"Fat embolism may follow major bony fractures."-Bailey 27/e p956

"Fat emboli syndrome (FES) is a condition characterized by respiratory distress, altered mental status, and skin petechiae."-Sabiston 20/e p501

152. **Ans. a. Chronic lymphedema** *(Ref: Bailey 27/e p998; Sabiston 20/e p1850)*

In the given image, there is swelling of dorsum of foot and buffalo hump appearance of foot, which is seen in chronic lymphedema.

"Unlike other types of oedema, lymphoedema characteristically involves the foot. The contour of the ankle is lost through infilling of the submalleolar depressions, a 'buffalo hump' forms on the dorsum of the foot, the toes appear 'square' because of confinement of footwear and the skin on the dorsum of the toes cannot be pinched because of subcutaneous fibrosis (Stemmer's sign)."-Bailey 27/e p998

"In most patients with second- or third-stage lymphedema, the characteristic findings on physical examination can usually establish the diagnosis. The edematous limb has a firm and hardened consistency. There is loss of the normal perimalleolar shape, resulting in a "tree trunk" pattern. The dorsum of the foot is characteristically swollen, resulting in the appearance of the "buffalo hump," and the toes become thick and squared."-Sabiston 20/e p1850

153. **Ans. b. Lentigo maligna** *(Ref: Bailey 27/e p609; Schwartz 11/e p530; Sabiston 20/e p729)*

"Lentigo maligna melanoma occurs most commonly on the sun-exposed areas of older individuals and is manifested as a flat, dark, variably pigmented lesion, with irregular borders and a history of slow development."-Sabiston 20/e p729

"Lentigo maligna represents 10% of melanoma cases and is a less aggressive subtype of melanoma in situ that typically arises on sun-exposed areas of the head and neck."-Schwartz 11/e p530

154. **Ans. d. 42°C** *(Ref: Bailey 27/e p632; Schwartz 11/e p523; Harrison 20/e p1930)*

"Frostbite usually affects the distal aspects of the extremities or exposed parts of the face, such as the ears, nose, chin, and cheeks." -Harrison 20/e p1930

*"Initial treatment is rewarming, performed in an environment where reexposure to freezing conditions will not occur. Rewarming is accomplished by immersion of the affected part in a water bath at temperatures of **40°–44°C (104°–111°F)**. Massage, application of ice water, and extreme heat are contraindicated. The injured area should be cleansed with soap or antiseptic, and sterile dressings should be applied. Analgesics are often required during rewarming. Antibiotics are used if there is evidence of infection."-Harrison 20/e p1930*

"Frostbite injuries affect the peripheries in cold climates. The initial treatment is with rapid rewarming in a bath at 42°C. The cold injury produces delayed microvascular dam- age similar to that of cardiac reperfusion injury. The level of damage is difficult to assess, and surgery usually does not play a role in its management, which is conservative, until there is absolute demarcation of the level of injury."-Bailey 27/e p632

"Even so, the standard treatment of frostbite injury begins with rapid rewarming to 40°C to 42°C."-Schwartz 11/e p523

155. **Ans. a. Craniopharyngioma** *(Ref: Schwartz 11/e p1858; Sabiston 20/e p1915; Harrison 20/e p648)*

"Craniopharyngiomas are rare, usually suprasellar, partially calcified, solid, or mixed solid-cystic benign tumors that arise from remnants of Rathke's pouch. They have a bimodal distribution, occurring pre-dominantly in children but also between the ages of 55 and 65 years. They present with headaches, visual impairment, and impaired growth in children and hypopituitarism in adults. Treatment involves surgery, RT, or a combination of the two."-Harrison 20/e p648

156. **Ans. a. Inferior belly of omohyoid** *(Ref: Bailey 27/e p790)*

"LOCATION OF THE FACIAL NERVE TRUNK: The main methods of facial nerve trunk localisation can be divided into antegrade and retrograde. The former utilises anatomical landmarks to identify the nerve trunk after its exit from the stylomastoid foramen, which is then traced distally. Landmarks commonly used are: 1. The inferior portion of the cartilaginous canal. This is termed Conley's pointer (tragal pointer) and indicates the position of the facial nerve, which lies 1 cm deep and inferior to its tip; 2. The upper border of the posterior belly of the digastric muscle. Identification of this muscle not only helps to mobilise the parotid gland, but also exposes an area immediately superior, in which the facial nerve is usually located; 3. The squamotympanic fissure; 4. The styloid process (the nerve is superficial to it); 5. The mastoid process can be drilled and the nerve identified more proximally."-Bailey 27/e p790

157. **Ans. a. Plexiform neurofibroma** *(Ref: Harrison 20/e p655; Neena Khanna 4/e p34)*

"Plexiform neurofibroma: A special type of neurofibroma is the plexiform variant, which involves an entire large nerve and its branches, forming a mass of tangled, ropelike structures that feel like a "bag of worms" on palpation and that can reach an enormous size and be associated with massive soft tissue overgrowth leading to significant functional impairment. A plexiform neurofibroma is considered to be pathognomonic of NF1."-Fitzpatrick 6/e p1159

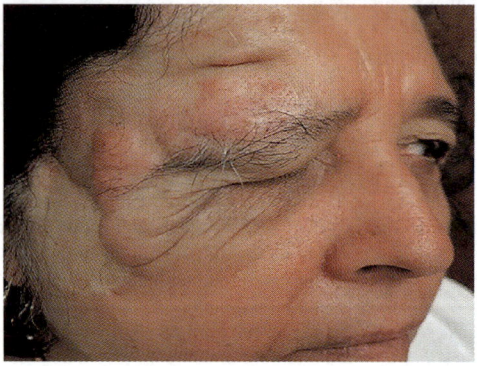

Plexiform neurofibromatosis

"Plexiform neurofibromas: Diffuse plaques that feel knotty or wormy on palpation."-Neena Khanna 4/e p34

158. **Ans. a. CT scan** *(Ref: Sabiston 20/e p413, 414, 416)*

Primary survey of ATLS does not include CT scan.

"Following a defined order of assessment, life-threatening conditions are immediately addressed at the time of identification. This initial assessment, also termed the primary survey, follows the mnemonic ABCDE: Airway and cervical spine protection; Breathing; Circulation; Disability or neurologic condition; Exposure and environmental control"-Sabiston 20/e p413

"Circulation: A chest radiograph can then evaluate for thoracic blood loss, and a pelvic radiograph will identify a pelvic fracture. To evaluate the abdomen, the focused abdominal sonography in trauma (FAST) scan is a rapidly obtainable ultrasound examination that assesses for intraperitoneal fluid."-Sabiston 20/e p416

159. **Ans. b. Needle decompression in the 5th intercostal space** *(Ref: Bailey 27/e p367; Schwartz 11/e p186; Sabiston 20/e p415)*

"Tension pneumothorax: The clinical presentation is dramatic. The patient is increasingly restless with tachypnoea, dyspnoea and distended neck veins (similar to pericardial tamponade). Clinical examination may reveal tracheal deviation; this is a late finding and is not necessary to clinically confirm diagnosis. There will also be hyper-resonance and decreased or absent breath sounds over the affected hemithorax. Tension pneumothorax is a clinical diagnosis and treatment should never be delayed by waiting for radiological confirmation.

Treatment consists of immediate decompression, initially by rapid insertion of a large-bore cannula into the second intercostal space in the mid-clavicular line of the affected side, then followed by insertion of a chest tube through the fifth intercostal space in the anterior axillary line."-Bailey 27/e p367

160. **Ans. d. E-fast** *(Ref: Bailey 27/e p366; Schwartz 11/e p188)*

"Thoracic Injury: Ultrasound can be used to differentiate between contusion and the actual presence of blood. Extended focused assessment with sonar for trauma (eFAST) is becoming the most common investigation. The technique uses sonar assessment in the chest, looking for a cardiac tamponade or free blood and air in the hemithorax on each side, and assessment for blood in the abdominal cavity, in the paracolic gutters, subdiaphragmatic spaces and pelvis."-Bailey 27/e p366

161. **Ans. a. Battle sign** *(Ref: Bailey 27/e p332; Schwartz 11/e p1835)*

"Battle's sign: A skull base fracture may be associated with bruising over the mastoid process."-Bailey 27/e p332

"Extravasation of blood results in ecchymosis behind the ear, known as Battle's sign."-Schwartz 11/e p1835

162. **Ans. d. Jaundice <7 days before development of encephalopathy** *(Ref: Blumgart 6/e p1775)*
Time from onset of jaundice to development of coma >7 days (not <7 days) is included in King's College Criteria).

| King's College Criteria Associated with Poor Prognosis for Acute Liver Failure (ALF) Patients ||
Patients with Non–Acetaminophen-Induced ALF	Patients with Acetaminophen-Induced ALF
INR >6.5^Q *or* **Three of the following five criteria:** • Patient **age <11 or >40 years**^{Q} • Serum **bilirubin >300 µmol/L**^{Q} • **Time from onset of jaundice to development of coma >7 days**^{Q} • **INR >3.5**^{Q} • **Drug toxicity**, regardless of whether it caused ALF	**Arterial pH <7.3** (taken by arterial blood sampling) **All three of the following:** • **INR >6.5**^{Q} • **Serum creatinine >300 µmol/L**^{Q} • **Presence of encephalopathy**^{Q} (grade **III or IV**)

163. **Ans. b. CMV** *(Ref: Bailey 27/e p1541; Schwartz 11/e p363)*

"The risk of viral infection is highest during the first 6 months after transplantation and the most common problem is CMV infection. CMV disease may arise because of either reactivation of latent infection or primary infection that can be transmitted by an organ from a CMV-positive donor."-Bailey 27/e p1541

164. **Ans. b. 48 hours** *(Ref: Sabiston 20/e p291)*

"Nosocomial infections can be defined as those occurring within 48 hours of hospital admission, 3 days of discharge or 30 days of an operation."-Practical Healthcare Epidemiology 3/e p124

165. **Ans. c. Induration** *(Ref: Bailey 27/e p48)*
Induration is not the part of the ASEPSIS wound score.

| The ASEPSIS wound score ||
Criterion	Points
Additional treatment^Q • Antibiotics for wound infection • Drainage of pus under local anaesthesia • Debridement of wound under general anaesthesia	0 10 5 10
Serous discharge^Q	Daily 0–5
Erythema^Q	Daily 0–5
Purulent exudate^Q	Daily 0–10
Separation of deep tissues^Q	Daily 0–10
Isolation of bacteria from wound^Q	10
Stay as inpatient prolonged over 14 days as result of wound infection^Q	5

166. **Ans. c. Isograft** *(Ref: Sabiston 20/e p602)*

"Isografts are organs transplanted between identical twins and are immunologically indistinguishable and thus are not rejected."-Sabiston 20/e p602

IMAGE-BASED QUESTIONS

IMAGE BASED QUESTIONS

Image-based Questions

Multiple Choice Questions

INSTRUMENTS

1. **What is the name of given instrument?**
   a. Kocher's thyroid dissector b. Doyen's retractor
   c. Joll's thyroid retractor d. Deaver's retractor

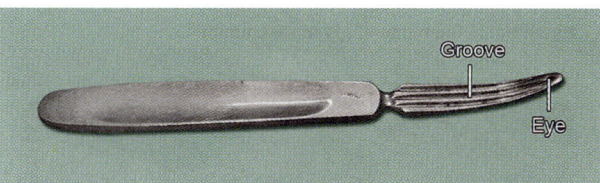

2. **What is the name of given instrument?**
   a. Aneurysm needle b. Veress needle
   c. Tracheal dilator d. Urethral dilator

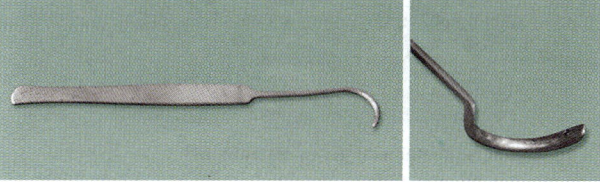

3. **What is the name of given instrument?**
   a. Aneurysm needle b. Veress needle
   c. Tracheal dilator d. Urethral dilator

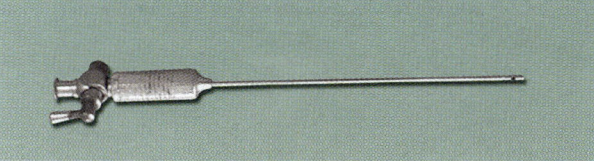

4. **What is the name of given instrument?**
   a. Doyen's towel clip b. Mayo's towel clip
   c. Moynihan's tetra towel clip d. Lanes tissue forceps

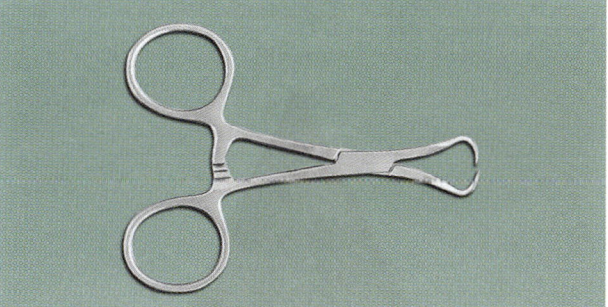

5. **What is the name of given instrument?**
   a. Doyen's towel clip b. Mayo's towel clip
   c. Moynihan's tetra towel clip
   d. Lanes tissue forceps

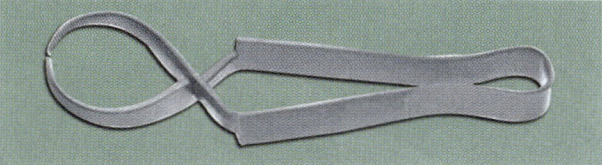

6. **What is the name of given instrument?**
   a. Doyen's towel clip b. Mayo's towel clip
   c. Moynihan's tetra towel clip
   d. Lanes tissue forceps

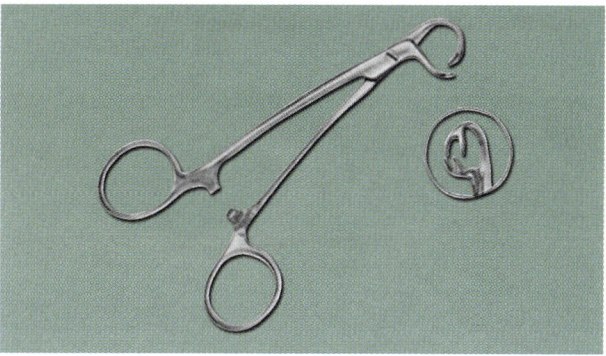

7. **What is the name of given instrument?**
   a. Doyen's towel clip b. Bone curette
   c. Aneurysm needle d. Doyen's coastal elevator

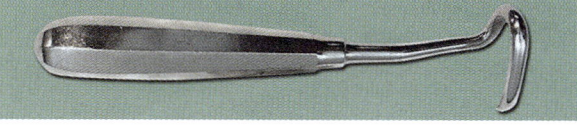

8. **What is the use of given instrument?**
   a. Dissection in thyroid surgeries
   b. Elevation of periosteum
   c. Suturing
   d. Used with blade for skin incision

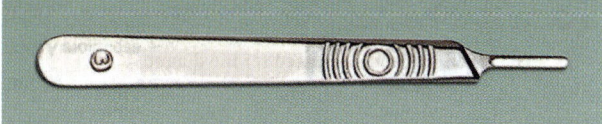

9. Identify the surgical blade used for incision and drainage:
   (Recent Question 2019)

   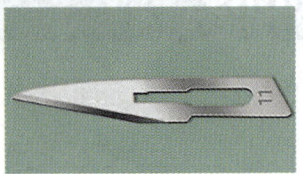

   a. 10 b. 11
   c. 15 d. 23

10. What is the use of instrument? *(Recent Question 2017)*
    a. Elevation of periosteum
    b. Cutting the bone
    c. Harvesting skin graft
    d. Retraction of abdominal wall

    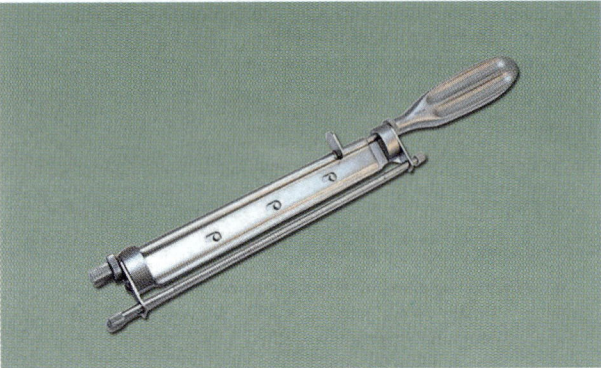

11. What is the name of given instrument?
    a. Artery forceps   b. Needle holder
    c. Kocher's forceps   d. Tissue forceps

    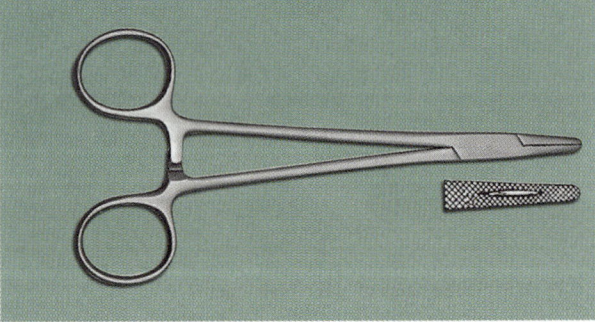

12. What is the name of given instrument?
    a. Osteotome   b. Bone cutter
    c. Bone nibbler   d. Rib shear

    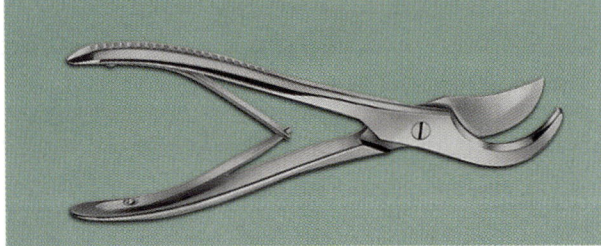

13. The given instrument is used for the diagnosis of:
    (Recent Question 2018)
    a. Hemorrhoids   b. Fissure-in-ano
    c. Pilonidal sinus d. All of the above

    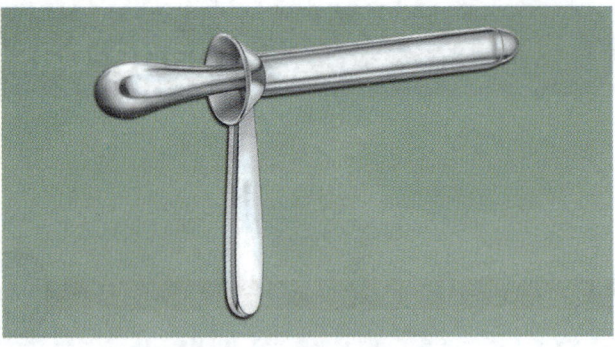

14. What is the name of given instrument?
    a. Bone hook   b. Bone curette
    c. Periosteal elevator d. Kocher's dissector

    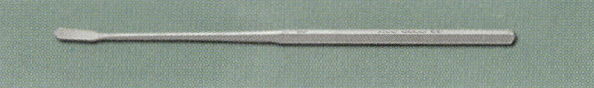

15. What is the name of given instrument?
    a. Gigli saw   b. Mayo's vein stripper
    c. Fogarty balloon catheter d. Long intravenous catheter

    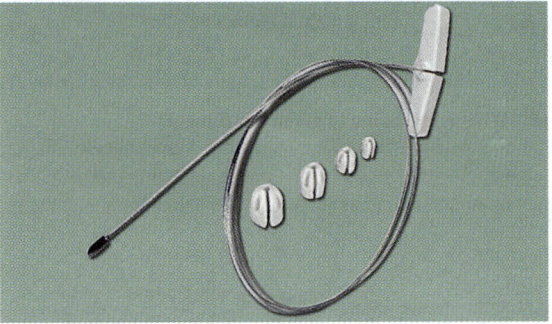

16. What is the name of given instrument?
    a. Gigli saw   b. Mayo's vein stripper
    c. Fogarty balloon catheter d. Long intravenous catheter

    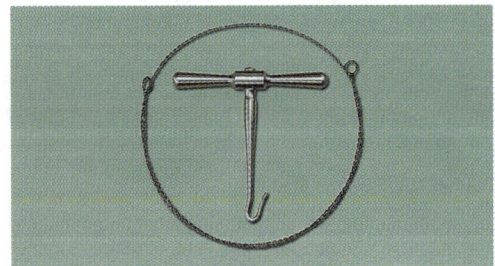

17. The given needle symbol represents:
    a. Taper point needle
    b. Blunt taper point needle
    c. Cutting edge needle
    d. Reverse cutting edge needle

18. What is the name of given instrument?
    (Recent Question 2016)
    a. Aneurysm needle   b. Fistula probe
    c. Veress needle   d. Bone hook

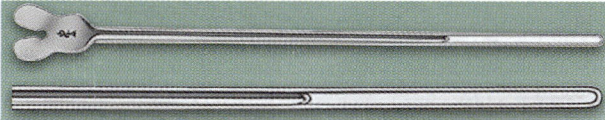

19. What is the name of given instrument?
    a. Gallbladder trocar   b. Bone curette
    c. Gallstone scoop   d. Laparoscopic trocar

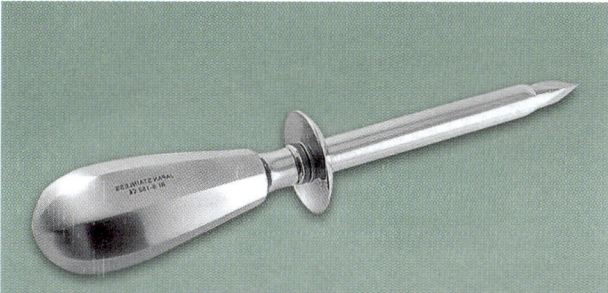

FORCEPS

20. What is the name of given instrument? *(Recent Question 2016)*
    a. Ovum forceps   b. Sponge holding forceps
    c. Cord holding forceps   d. Pile holding forceps

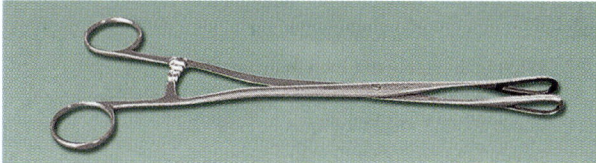

21. What is the name of given instrument?
    a. Lister's sinus forceps
    b. Kocher's hemostatic forceps
    c. Babcock's tissue forceps
    d. Lane's tissue forceps

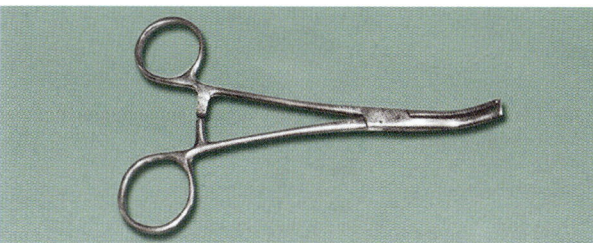

22. What is the name of given instrument?
    a. Lister's sinus forceps
    b. Kocher's hemostatic forceps
    c. Babcock's tissue forceps
    d. Lane's tissue forceps

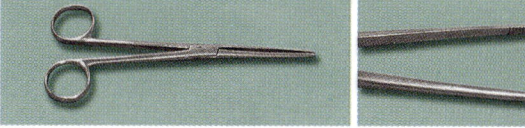

23. What are the uses of given instrument?
    a. Used during laparotomy to retract skin margins
    b. Used to hold neck of bladder during bladder neck resection
    c. Used to hold skin flaps
    d. All of the above

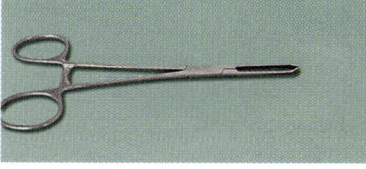 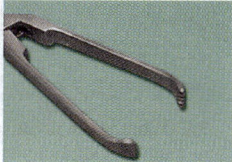

24. What is the name of given instrument? *(Recent Question 2017)*
    a. Lister's sinus forceps
    b. Kocher's hemostatic forceps
    c. Babcock's tissue forceps
    d. Lane's tissue forceps

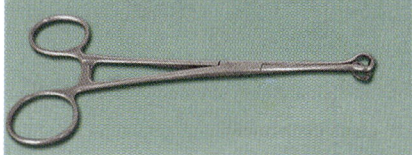 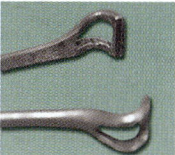

25. What is the name of given instrument?
    a. Lister's sinus forceps
    b. Kocher's hemostatic forceps
    c. Babcock's tissue forceps
    d. Lane's tissue forceps

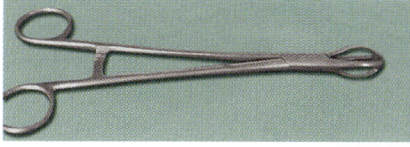 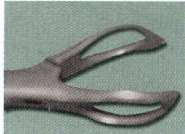

26. What are the uses of given instrument?
    a. Used to hold the cut skin margins during suturing
    b. Used to hold the linea alba or the rectus sheath during closure of abdominal incision
    c. Used to hold the scalp during closure of scalp incision
    d. All of the above

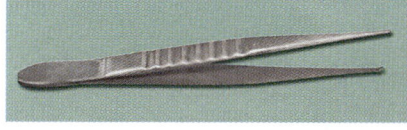 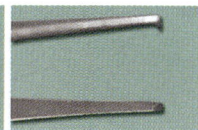

27. What is the name of given instrument?
    a. Ovum forceps   b. Sponge holding forceps
    c. Cord holding forceps   d. Pile holding forceps

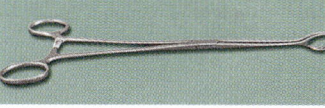 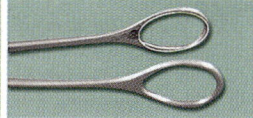

28. What is the name of given instrument?
    a. Pyelolithotomy forceps   b. Sponge holding forceps
    c. Desjardins forceps   d. Pile holding forceps

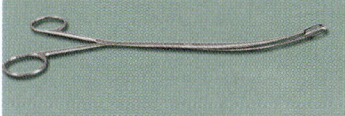 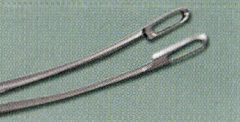

29. What is the name of given instrument?
    a. Pyelolithotomy forceps
    b. Sponge holding forceps
    c. Sprapubic cystolithotomy forceps
    d. Pile holding forceps

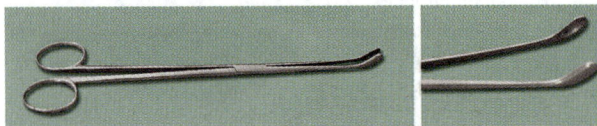

30. What is the name of given instrument?
    a. Pyelolithotomy forceps
    b. Sponge holding forceps
    c. Sprapubic cystolithotomy forceps
    d. Pile holding forceps

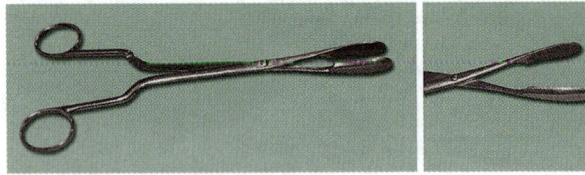

31. What is the use of given instrument?
    a. Used for blunt dissections
    b. Used to clean abscess cavity
    c. Used to hold sponge during cleaning and draping
    d. Used to pick sterilized instruments

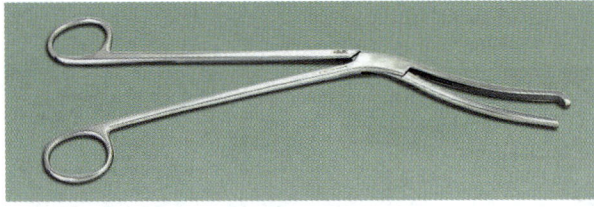

32. What is the name of given instrument?
    a. Rampley's sponge holding forceps
    b. Piles holding forceps
    c. Duval lung holding forceps
    d. Ovum holding forceps

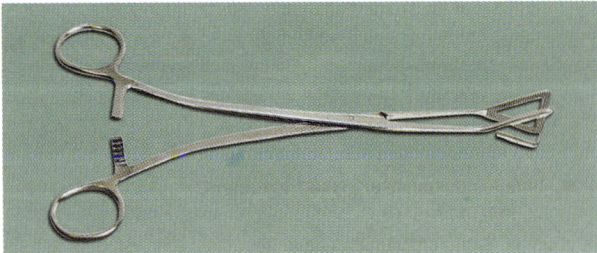

33. What is the name of given instrument?
    a. Rampley's sponge holding forceps
    b. Piles holding forceps
    c. Duval lung holding forceps
    d. Ovum forceps

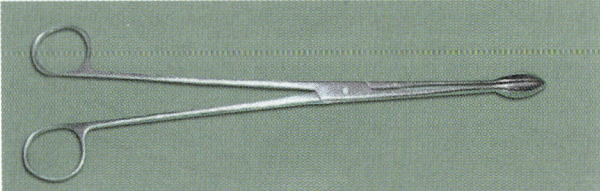

34. What is the name of given instrument?
    a. Lister sinus forceps   b. Lanes tissue forceps
    c. Russian tissue forceps   d. Kocher's forceps

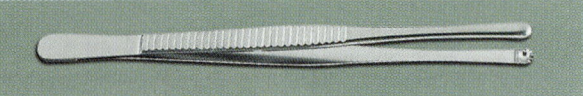

35. What is the name of given instrument?
    a. Kocher's forceps   b. Right angle forceps
    c. Lanes tissue forceps   d. Russian tissue forceps

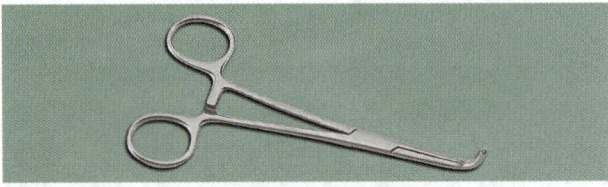

36. What is the name of given instrument?
    a. Mosquito hemostatic forceps
    b. Spencer Wells hemostatic forceps
    c. Kocher's hemostatic forceps
    d. Right angle forceps

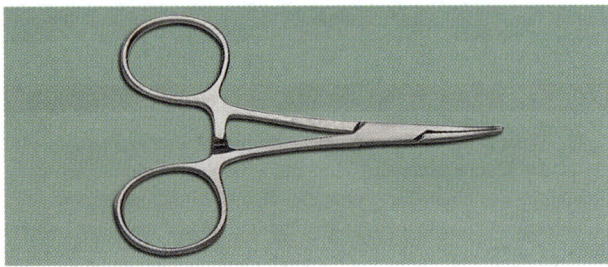

37. What is the name of given instrument?
    a. Mosquito hemostatic forceps
    b. Spencer Wells hemostatic forceps
    c. Kocher's hemostatic forceps
    d. Right angle forceps

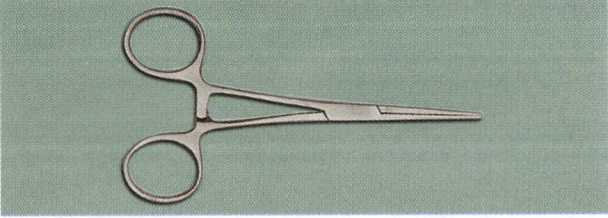

38. Identify the instruments shown here and choose the best combination: *(APPG 2016)*

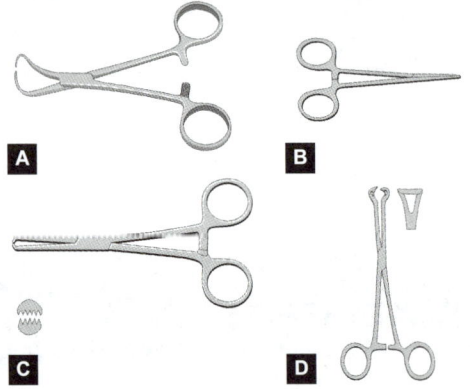

a. A = Dunhill's forceps. B = Halstead mosquito forceps.
   C = Allis forceps. D = Crile's hemostatic forceps
b. A = Crile's hemostatic forceps
   B = Allis intestinal forceps.
   C = Schnidt tonsil forceps. D = Babcock intestinal forceps.
c. A = Backhaus towel clamp. B = Halstead mosquito forceps.
   C = Allis forceps. D = Babcock intestinal forceps.
d. A = Backhaus towel clamp. B = Foerster sponge forceps.
   C = Dunhill's forceps. D = DeBakey forceps.

39. **What is the name of given instrument?**
    a. Desjardins forceps
    b. Yeoman punch biopsy forceps
    c. Lister sinus forceps
    d. Cheatle's forceps

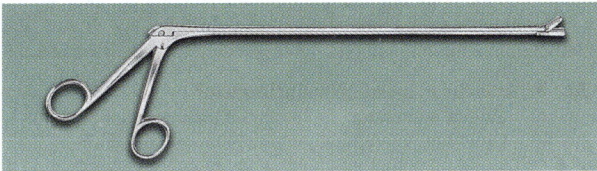

40. **What is the name of given instrument?**
    a. Cord holding forceps
    b. Piles holding forceps
    c. Sponge holding forceps
    d. Duval lung holding forceps

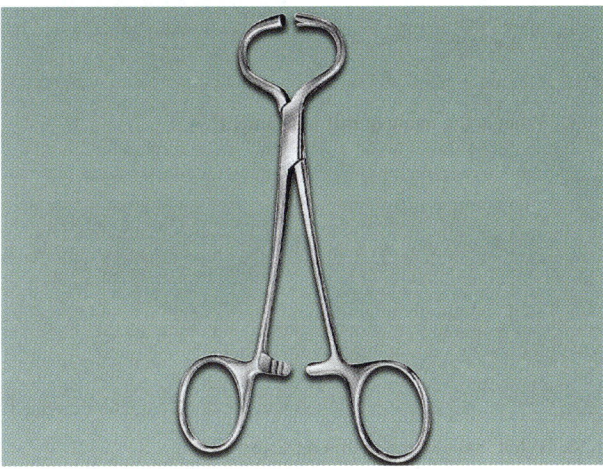

RETRACTOR

41. **What is the name of given instrument?** *(Recent Question 2017)*
    a. Morris retractor   b. Doyen's retractor
    c. Czerney's retractor   d. Deaver's retractor

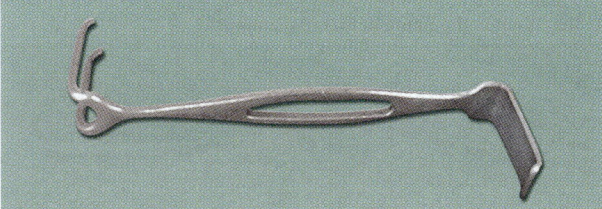

42. **What is the name of given instrument?**
    (Recent Questions 2015)
    a. Morris retractor   b. Doyen's retractor
    c. Czerney's retractor   d. Deaver's retractor

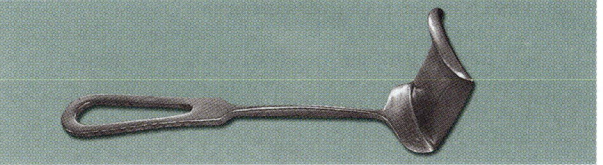

43. **What are the uses of given instrument?**
    a. Used to retract skin flap for excision of sebaceous cyst
    b. Used during venesection for retraction of skin
    c. Used during tracheostomy for retraction of skin and thyroid isthmus
    d. All of the above

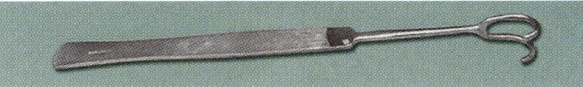

44. **What is the name of given instrument?**
    a. Morris retractor   b. Doyen's retractor
    c. Volkman's retractor   d. Deaver's retractor

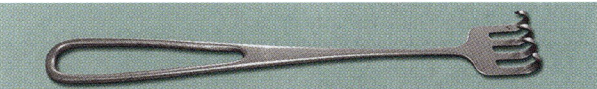

45. **What is the name of given instrument?** *(Recent Question 2017)*
    a. Morris retractor   b. Doyen's retractor
    c. Volkman's retractor   d. Deaver's retractor

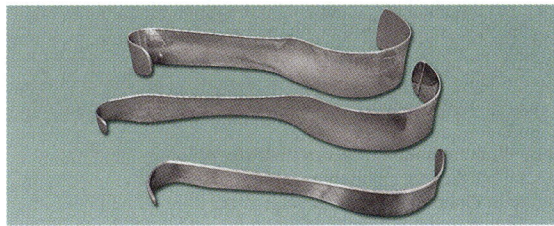

46. **What is the name of given instrument?**
    a. Kocher's thyroid dissector b. Doyen's retractor
    c. Joll's thyroid retractor   d. Deaver's retractor

47. **What is the name of given instrument?**
    a. Doyen's retractor   *(Recent Question 2016)*
    b. Doyen's intestinal occlusion clamp
    c. Doyen's mouth gag   d. Joll's thyroid retractor

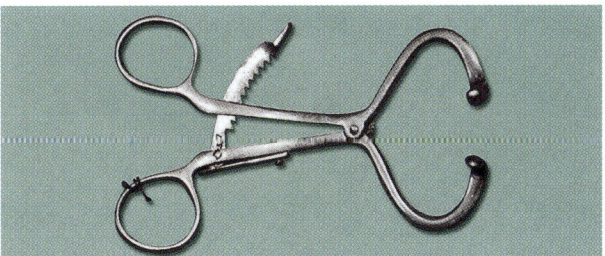

48. What is the name of given instrument?
    a. Morris retractor
    b. Volkman's retractor
    c. Doyen's retractor
    d. Balfours retractor

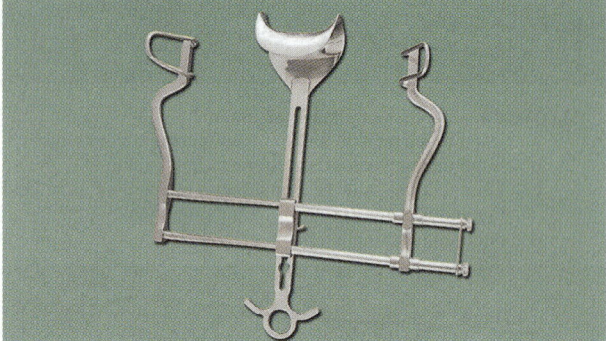

49. What is the name of given instrument?
    a. Doyen's mouth gag
    b. Beckman Weitlaner retractor
    c. Cat's paw retractor
    d. Bladder neck retractor

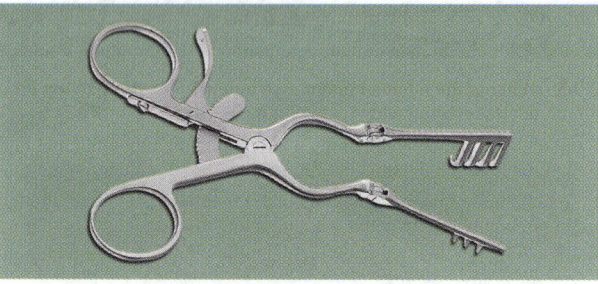

50. What is the use of given instrument?
    a. Retracting skin flaps in thyroid surgery
    b. Opening mouth in oral surgery
    c. Retracting skin in grafting
    d. Retracting bladder neck

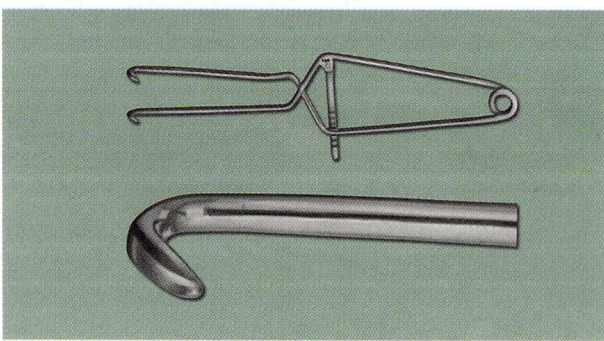

51. What is the name of given instrument?
    a. Morris retractor
    b. Farabeuf retractor
    c. Doyen's retractor
    d. Volkman's retractor

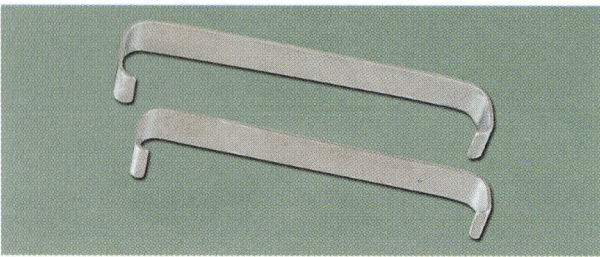

52. What is the name of given instrument?
    a. Liver retractor
    b. Rib retractor
    c. Scapula retractor
    d. Abdominal wall retractor

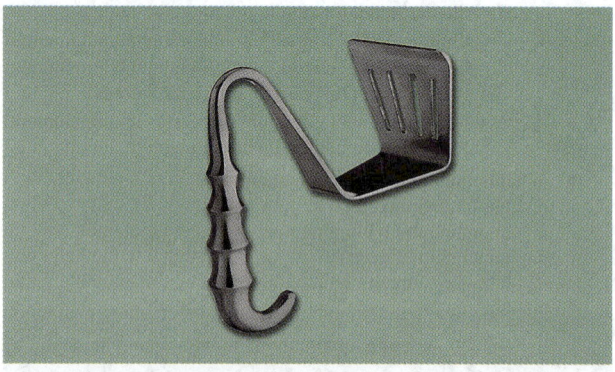

53. What is the name of given instrument?
    a. Czerny's retractor
    b. Morris retractor
    c. Langenbeck's retractor
    d. Doyen's retractor

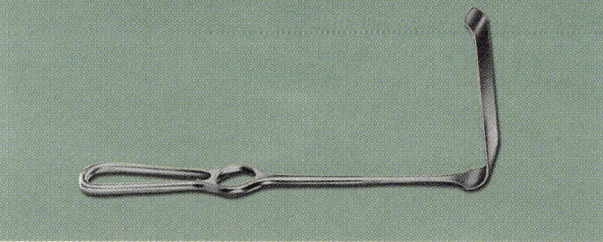

54. What is the name of this instrument?
    a. Scapula retractor
    b. Morris retractor
    c. Kelly retractor
    d. Doyen's retractor

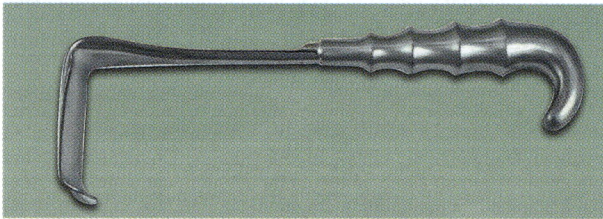

55. What is the name of this retractor?
    a. Cat's paw retractor
    b. Double hook retractor
    c. Single hook retractor
    d. Langenbeck's retractor

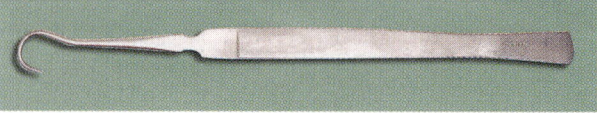

56. What is the name of this instrument?

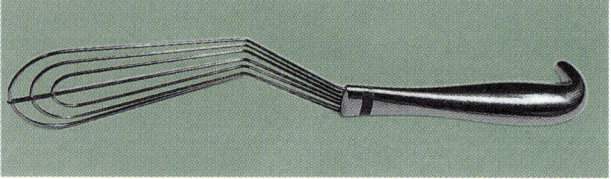

    a. Allison lung retractor
    b. Duval lung holding forceps
    c. Russian tissue forceps
    d. Joll's thyroid retractor

CLAMP

57. What is the name of given instrument?
a. Payr's crushing clamp
b. Doyen's intestinal occlusion clamp
c. Hemostatic clamp
d. Vascular clamp

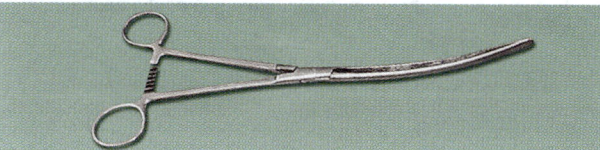

58. What is the name of given instrument?
a. Payr's crushing clamp
b. Doyen's intestinal occlusion clamp
c. Hemostatic clamp
d. Vascular clamp

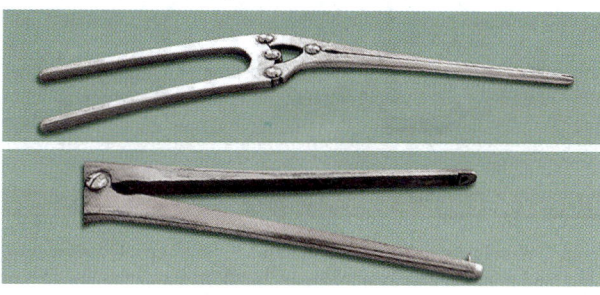

59. What is the name of given instrument?
a. Satinsky vascular clamp   b. Light bulldog clamp
c. Pott's bulldog clamp   d. Well's arterial clamp

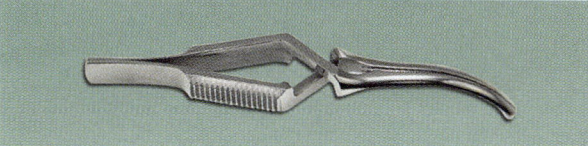

60. What is the name of given instrument?
a. Satinsky vascular clamp
b. Light bulldog clamp
c. Pott's bulldog clamp
d. Well's arterial clamp

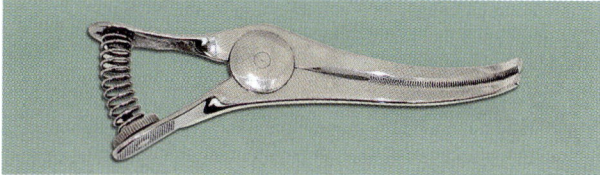

61. What is the name of given instrument?
a. Satinsky vascular clamp   b. Light bulldog clamp
c. Pott's bulldog clamp   d. Well's arterial clamp

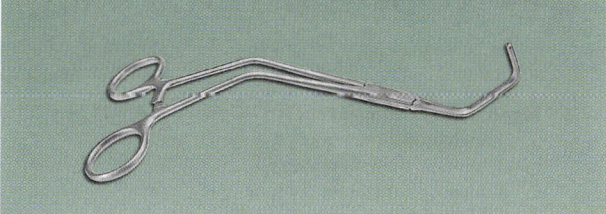

SCISSORS

62. What is the name of given instrument?
a. Mayo scissors   b. Metzenbaum scissors
c. Mcindoe scissors   d. None of the above

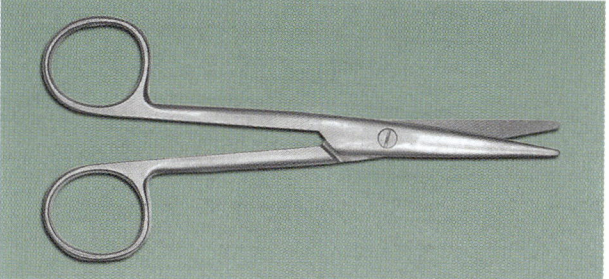

63. What is the name of given instrument?
a. Mayo scissors   b. Metzenbaum scissors
c. Mcindoe scissors   d. None of the above

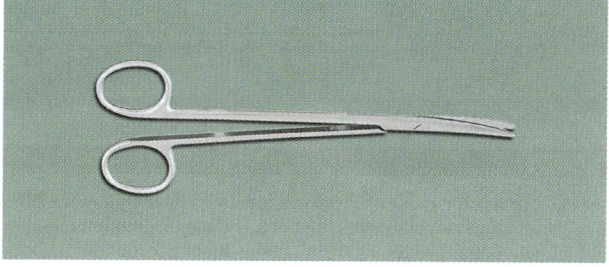

64. What is the name of given scissors?
a. Mayo's scissors
b. Metzenbaum scissors
c. Lister bandage scissors
d. Tenotomy scissors

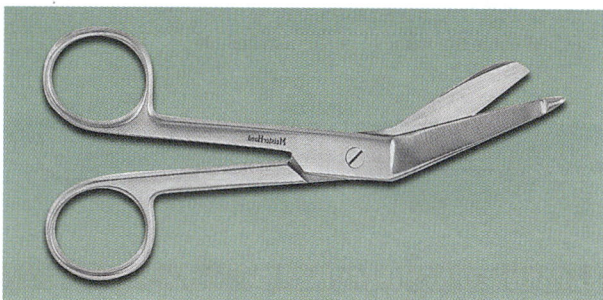

DILATOR

65. What is the name of given instrument?
a. Aneurysm needle   b. Cervical dilator
c. Tracheal dilator   d. Urethral dilator

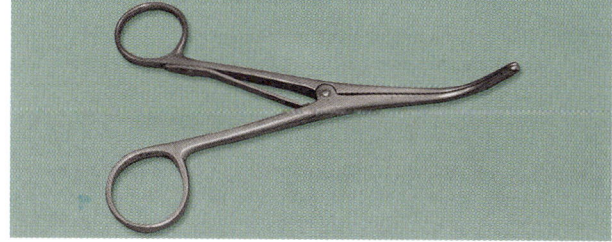

Surgery Essence

66. **What is the name of given instrument?**
    a. Cervical dilator
    b. Urethral dilator
    c. Esophageal dilator
    d. Anal dilator

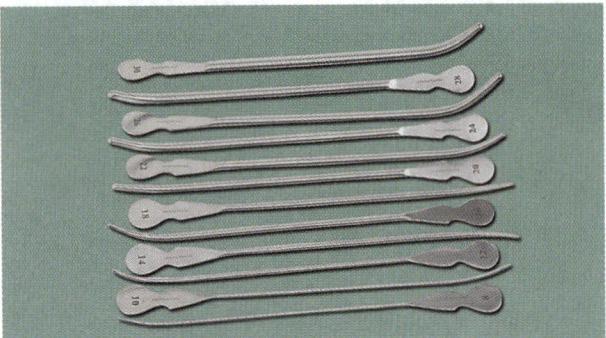

67. **What is the name of given instrument?**
    a. Bile duct dilator
    b. Ureteric dilator
    c. Urethral dilator
    d. Cervical dilator

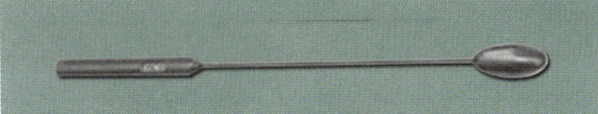

SCOOP

68. **What is the name of given instrument?** *(Recent Question 2016)*
    a. Volkmann scoop
    b. Gallstone scoop
    c. Bone curette
    d. Biopsy scoop

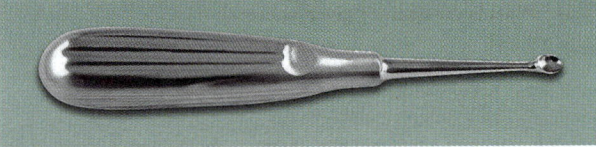

69. **What is the name of given instrument?**
    a. Volkmann scoop
    b. Gallstone scoop
    c. Bone curette
    d. Biopsy scoop

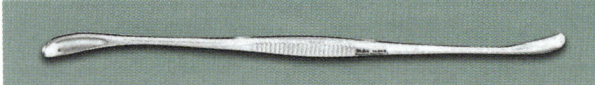

LAPAROSCOPIC INSTRUMENTS

70. **What is the name of given instrument?**
    a. Ureteroscope
    b. Cystoscope
    c. Laparoscope
    d. Sigmoidoscope

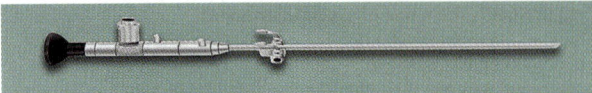

71. **What is the name of given instrument?**
    a. Ureteroscope
    b. Cystoscope
    c. Laparoscope
    d. Sigmoidoscope

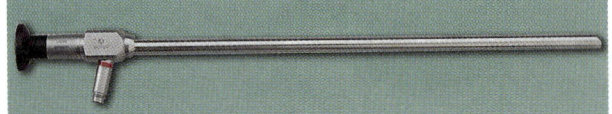

72. **What is the name of given instrument?**
    a. Veress needle
    b. Hasson cannula
    c. Trocar
    d. Laparoscope

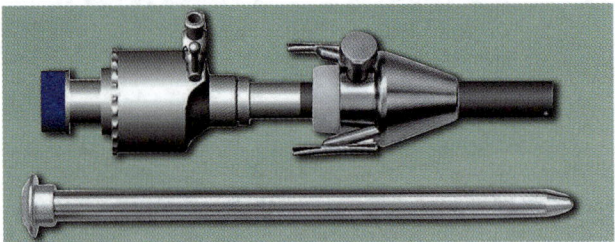

73. **What is the name of given instrument?**
    a. Veress needle
    b. Hasson cannula
    c. Trocar
    d. Laparoscope

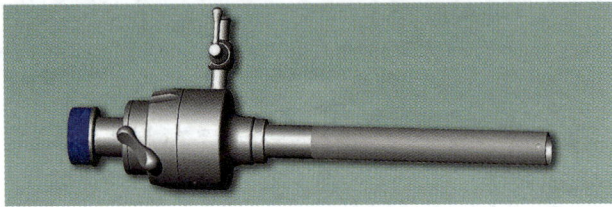

BIOPSY NEEDLE

74. **What is the name of this needle?** *(Recent Question 2016)*
    a. Tru cut biopsy needle
    b. Vim-Silverman needle
    c. Menghini biopsy needle
    d. Salah needle

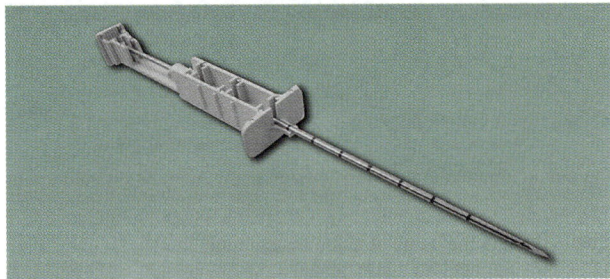

75. **What is the name of this needle?**
    a. Tru cut biopsy needle
    b. Vim-Silverman needle
    c. Menghini biopsy needle
    d. Salah needle

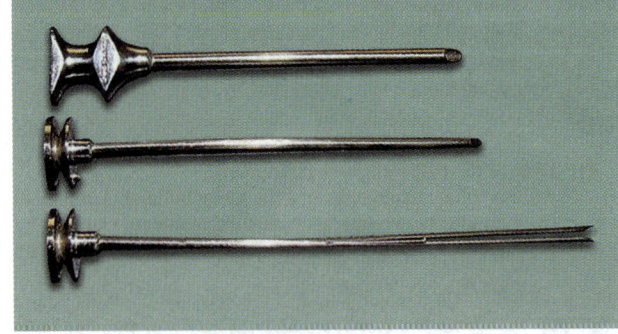

76. **Identify the instrument shown below:** *(AIIMS May 2016)*
    a. Laparoscopic port trocar
    b. Peritoneal dialysis catheter
    c. Endoscopic ultrasound probe
    d. DPL catheter

Image-based Questions | p59

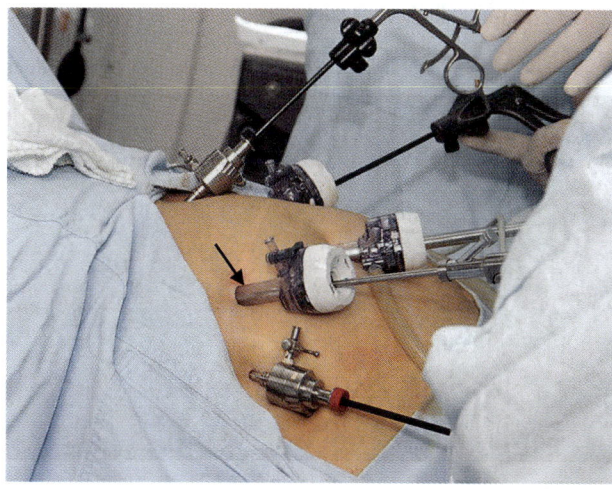

77. A 60 years old male came with bleeding per rectum and was diagnosed to have carcinoma colon. The patient underwent extended right hemicolectomy as shown below. Identify the instrument that the surgeon is using: *(AIIMS May 2016)*
    a. Monopolar cautery
    b. Ligasure vessel ligating system
    c. Harmonic scalpel
    d. Hyfrecator

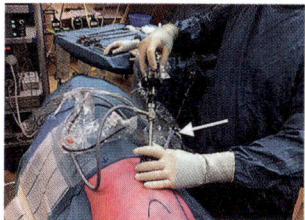 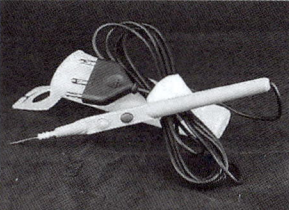

STAPLER

78. What is the name of given stapler?
    a. Linear stapler
    b. Intraluminal stapler
    c. Skin stapler
    d. Linear cutting stapler

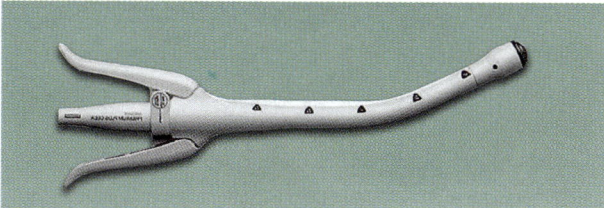

79. What is the name of given stapler?
    a. Linear stapler
    b. Intraluminal stapler
    c. Skin stapler
    d. Linear cutting stapler

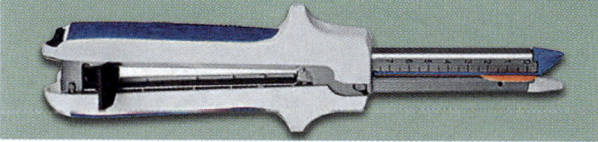

80. What is the name of given stapler?
    a. Intraluminal stapler
    b. Linear cutting stapler
    c. Skin stapler
    d. Linear stapler

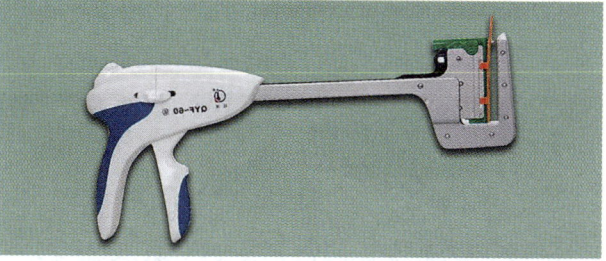

81. What is the name of given stapler?
    a. Linear stapler
    b. Intraluminal stapler
    c. Skin stapler
    d. Linear cutting stapler

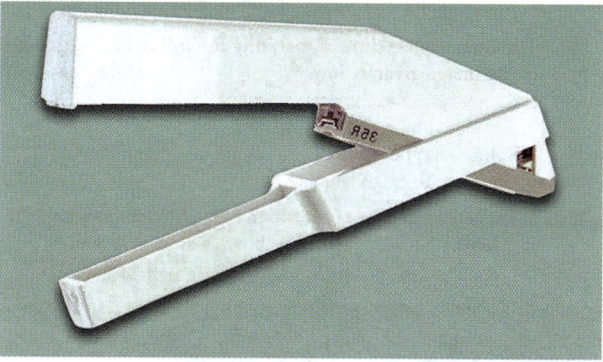

TUBES

82. What is the name of given tube?
    a. Kocher's T-tube   b. Kehr's T-tube
    c. Lanz T-tube   d. Mayo's T-tube

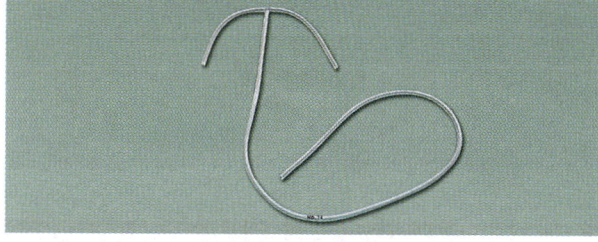

83. What is the name of given tube/catheter?
    a. Nelaton's catheter
    b. Fogarty catheter
    c. Sengstaken-Blakemore tube
    d. Bladder irrigation catheter

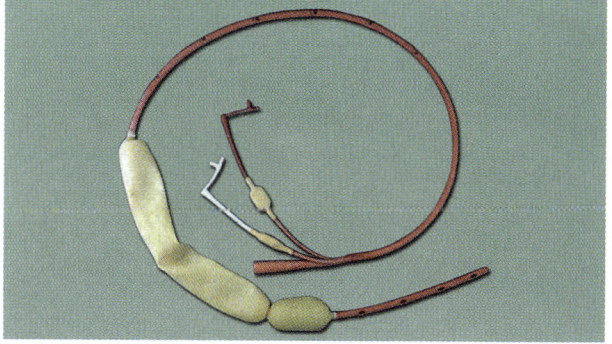

84. What is the name of given tube? *(Recent Question 2017)*
    a. Kehr's T-tube
    b. Flatus tube
    c. Ryle's tube
    d. Infant feeding tube

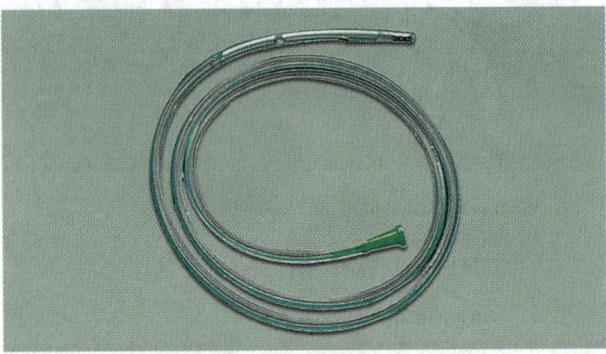

85. The correct procedure of inserting the following equipment in the image given below: *(AIIMS May 2018)*
    a. Supine with flexed neck
    b. Supine with extended neck
    c. Sitting with flexed neck
    d. Sitting with extended neck

86. What is the name of given tube? *(Recent Question 2017)*
    a. Kehr's T-tube
    b. Nelaton's catheter
    c. Ryle's tube
    d. Infant feeding tube

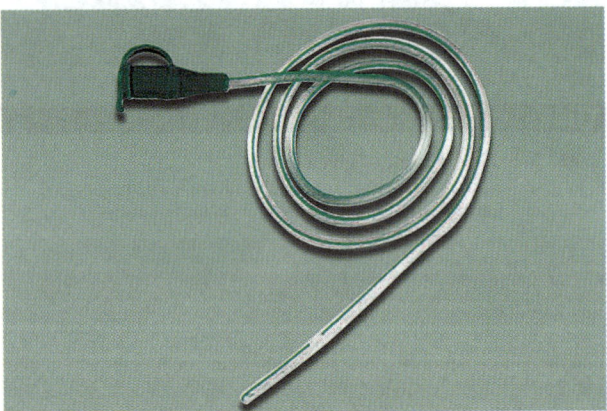

CATHETERS

87. What is the name of given catheter?
    a. Nelaton's catheter
    b. Fogarty catheter
    c. Infant feeding tube
    d. Ryle's tube

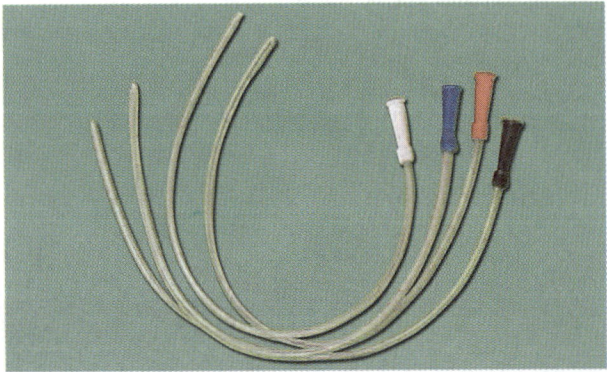

88. This tube/catheter is used in:
    a. Portocaval shunt
    b. Peritoneovenous shunt
    c. Mesocaval shunt
    d. Ventriculoperitoneal shunt

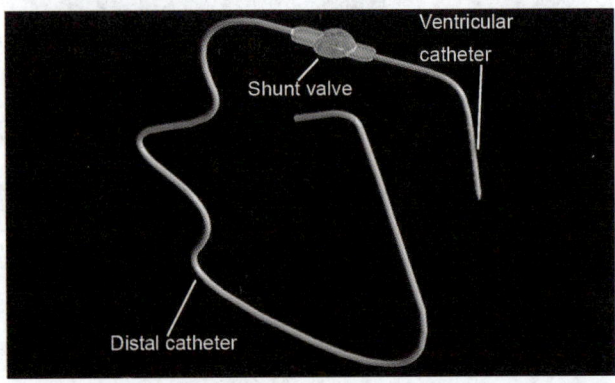

89. What is the name of given tube/catheter?
    a. Nelaton's catheter
    b. Fogarty catheter
    c. Sengstaken Blakemore tube
    d. Bladder irrigation catheter

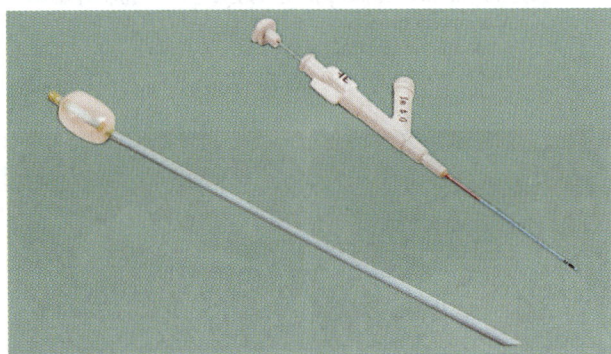

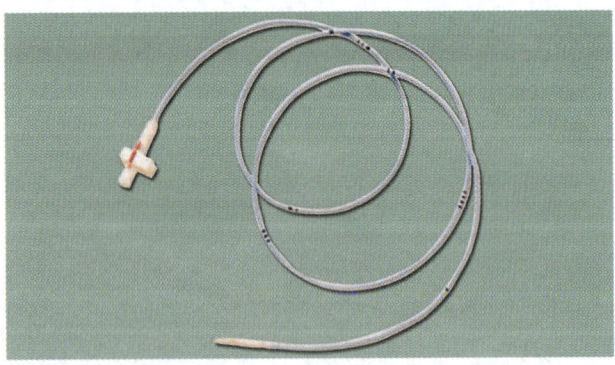

90. What is the name of given catheter?
    a. Nelaton's catheter
    b. Fogarty catheter
    c. Foley's catheter
    d. Malecot's catheter

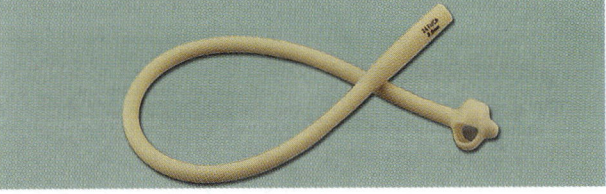

91. What is the name of given tube?
    a. Foley's catheter
    b. Red rubber catheter
    c. Malecot's catheter
    d. Nelaton's catheter

Image-based Questions p61

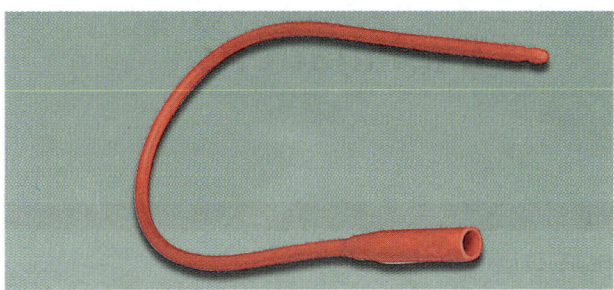

92. What is the name of given catheter?
    a. Fogarty catheter
    b. Central venous catheter
    c. Bladder irrigation catheter
    d. Nelaton's catheter

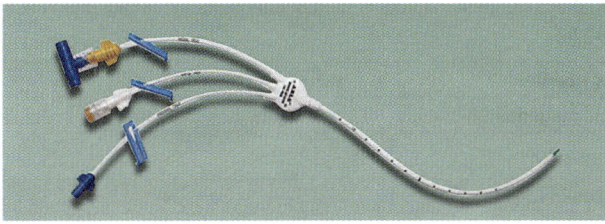

SUCTION AND DRAIN

93. What is the name of this drain?
    a. Penrose drain
    b. Jackson-Pratt drain
    c. Romovac suction drain
    d. Corrugated rubber drain

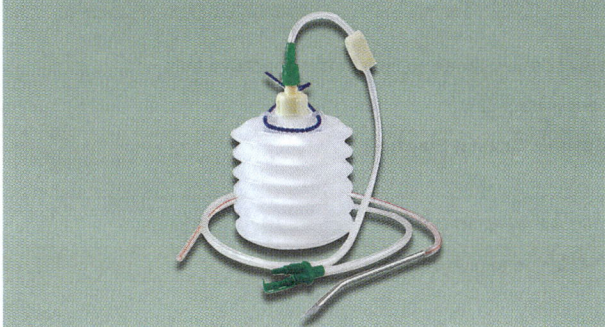

94. What is the name of given instrument?
    a. Frazier suction tip   b. Poole suction tip
    c. Adson suction tip   d. Yankauer suction tip

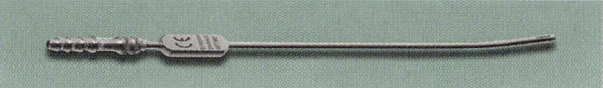

95. What is the name of given instrument?
    a. Frazier suction tip   b. Poole suction tip
    c. Adson suction tip   d. Yankauer suction tip

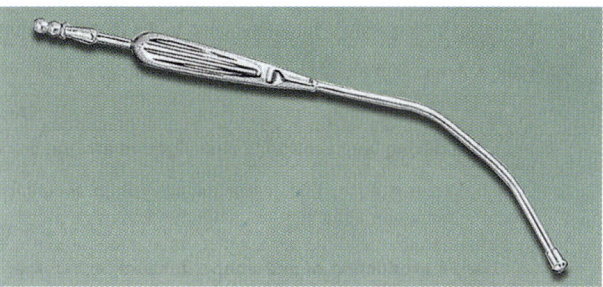

GASTROINTESTINAL SURGERY

96. Identify the labelled structures in the CT abdomen here:
    (APPG 2016)

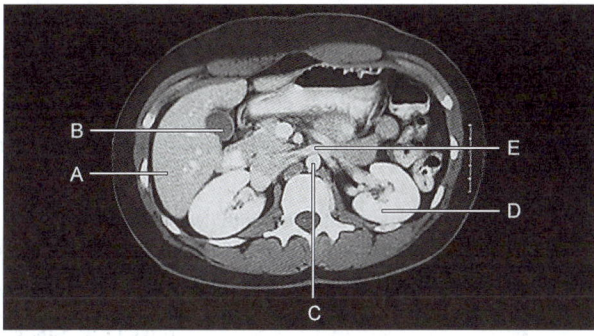

   a. A = liver, B = inferior vena cava, C = head of pancreas, D = left kidney, E = transverse colon
   b. A = right kidney, B = gallbladder, C = aorta, D = stomach E = pancreas
   c. A = right kidney, B = inferior vena cava, C = head of pancreas, D = left psoas muscle, E = transverse colon
   d. A = liver, B = gallbladder, C = aorta, D = left kidney, E = pancreas

Explanations

INSTRUMENTS

1. **Ans. a. Kocher's thyroid dissector** *(Ref: Jaypee Manual of Surgical Equipments/p 178)*

Kocher's thyroid dissector
• Used during thyroid surgeries, used **to dissect the superior thyroid pedicle**

2. **Ans. a. Aneurysm needle** *(Ref: Jaypee Manual of Surgical Equipments/p 135)*

Aneurysm needle
• Used **during venesection** to **pass ligature around the vein**

3. **Ans. b. Veress needle** *(Ref: Jaypee Manual of Surgical Equipments/p 226)*

Veress needle
• Used for **induction of pneumoperitoneum** during laparoscopic surgeries

4. **Ans. b. Mayo's towel clip** *(Ref: Jaypee Manual of Surgical Equipments/p 109)*

Mayo's Towel Clip
• **Curved blades** helps to **hold entire thickness of drapes firmly**
• Used to **fix drapes, suction tubes, laparoscopic cables** and **diathermy wires** on OT table

5. **Ans. a. Doyen's towel clip** *(Ref: Jaypee Manual of Surgical Equipments/p 109)*

Doyen's Towel Clip
• **Short instrument** with **curved blades**, used to **fix the towels during draping**

6. **Ans. c. Moynihan's tetra towel clip** *(Ref: Jaypee Manual of Surgical Equipments/p 110)*

Moynihan's Tetra Towel Clip
• **Curved blades with four teeth** (two teeth in each blade)
• Used to **hold the cut edges of skin incision** to the four corners of draped towels to **isolate the operative field**

7. **Ans. d. Doyen's coastal elevator** *(Ref: Jaypee Manual of Surgical Equipments/p 223)*

Doyen Rib Raspatory (Doyen's Coastal Elevator)
• Used to **remove tissue** and **cartilage from the ribs**

8. **Ans. d. Used with blade for skin incision** *(Ref: Jaypee Manual of Surgical Equipments/p 127)*

Bard Parker Handle (BP Handle): Blades are held in position by BP Handle to give incisions

9. **Ans. b. 11**

Surgical Blade	Uses
10	• For skin incision (to open skin^Q)
11	• Arteriotomy^Q, incision & drainage^Q
15	• Minor surgical procedures^Q, plastic & pediatric surgery^Q
22	• Abdominal incisions^Q
23	• For very thick skin^Q

10. **Ans. c. Harvesting skin graft** *(Ref: Jaypee Manual of Surgical Equipments/p 247)*

Humby Knife
• A knife with a roller attached, **used for cutting skin grafts of varying thickness**
• The **distance** between the roller and blade of the knife **can be varied by means of a calibration device.**

11. **Ans. b. Needle holder** *(Ref: Jaypee Manual of Surgical Equipments/p 136)*

Mayo Hegar Needle Holder
• Smaller distal blades with cross-serrations with a groove in middle • **Ratio of length of handle to blade is 4:1** • **Needle is placed** at junction of **proximal 2/3rd** and **distal 1/3rd of the blade** • Used **for suturing** skin and other organs

12. **Ans. d. Rib shear** *(Ref: Jaypee Manual of Surgical Equipments/p 234)*

Rib Shear	
• Same as bone cutter but it has **one cutting blade**	• Used to **cut the ribs**

13. **Ans. a. Hemorrhoids** *(Ref: Jaypee Manual of Surgical equipments/p189)*

14. **Ans. c. Periosteal elevator** *(Ref: Jaypee Manual of Surgical Equipments/p 233)*

Periosteal Elevator
• Used to **elevate and dissect bone, tissue, nerves,** clean and scrape bone. • Used to **expose fracture sites** or bone in other procedures. • Used to **strip portions of the membrane (periosteum)** covering the exterior surface of a bone.

15. **Ans. b. Mayo's vein stripper** *(Ref: Jaypee Manual of Surgical Equipments/p 175)*

Mayo's Vein Stripper: Used in the stripping of varicose veins

16. **Ans. a. Gigli saw** *(Ref: Jaypee Manual of Surgical Equipments/p 235)*

Gigli's Saw: Used to **cut bones** in amputations

17. **Ans. c. Cutting edge needle** *(Ref: Jaypee Manual of Surgical Equipments/p 58)*

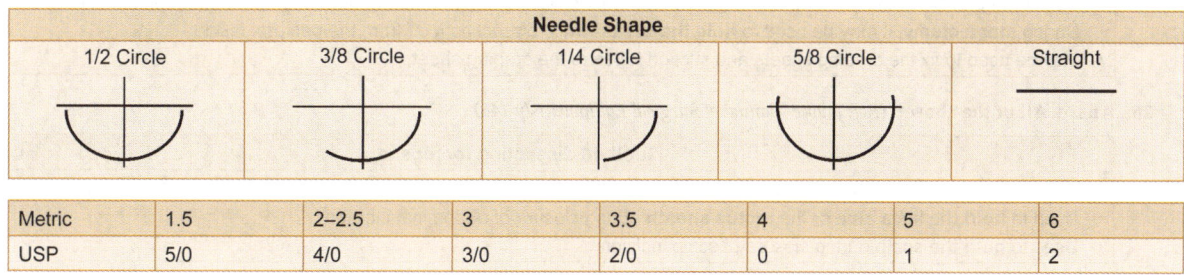

18. **Ans. b. Fistula probe** *(Ref: Jaypee Manual of Surgical Equipments/p 190)*

Brodie's Fistula probe
• **Winged blade, curved shaft** gradually tapered to **pointed tip with groove** along the curvature longitudinally • **Used to probe and treat fistula in ano;** as a guide and protector to release tongue tie

19. **Ans. a. Gallbladder trocar** *(Ref: Scott-Conner & Dawson: Essential Operative Techniques and Anatomy/p 416)*

Gallbladder trocar
• Gallbladder trocar is used to decompress the distended gallbladder during cholecystectomy

FORCEPS

20. Ans. b. Sponge holding forceps *(Ref: Jaypee Manual of Surgical Equipments/p 108)*

Rampley's Sponge Holding Forceps
• Used for **cleansing the skin** with swab dipped in antiseptic solution during all operations • Used for **removing laminated membrane** and the **daughter cysts** during operation of hydatid cyst • Used to **hold the fundus** and **Hartmann's pouch** of gallbladder **during cholecystectomy** • Used to **swab an abscess cavity**

21. Ans. b. Kocher's hemostatic forceps *(Ref: Jaypee Manual of Surgical Equipments/p 154)*

Kocher's hemostatic forceps
• Used during **appendectomy** to **crush the base** • Used to **hold perforating vessels** during **mastectomy** • Used during **subtotal thyroidectomy** • Used to **hold bleeding vessels** while operating on **palm** and **sole**

22. Ans. a. Lister's sinus forceps

Lister's sinus forceps
• Used for **incision and drainage** of abscess by **Hilton's method** • May be used to **hold a guaze swab to clean the abscess cavity**

23. Ans. d. All of the above *(Ref: Jaypee Manual of Surgical Equipments/p 160)*

Allis Tissue Forceps
• Used during **laparotomy** to **retract skin margins** • Used to **hold neck of bladder** during bladder neck resection • Used to **hold skin flaps** while excising lipoma, sebaceous cyst or LN • Used during thyroid operations, neck dissection to **hold the margins of skin** while raising skin flaps

24. Ans. c. Babcock's tissue forceps *(Ref: Jaypee Manual of Surgical Equipments/p 160)*

Babcock's tissue forceps
• Used during **appendectomy** • Used during **gastrectomy**, **gastrojejunostomy** to **hold the margins of stomach** while applying the occlusion clamps • Used during small and large intestine resection anastomosis to **hold the margins of gut** • Used to **hold the cut margins of bladder** during suprapubic cystolithotomy

25. Ans. d. Lane's tissue forceps *(Ref: Jaypee Manual of Surgical Equipments/p 160)*

Lane's tissue forceps
• Used during **submandibular** or **parotid gland excision** to **hold the gland** during dissection from the adjacent structures • During **mastectomy**, it may be used to **hold the breast** while dissecting it off from the pectoral fascia • May be used to fix the draping sheets and suction tubes to the draping sheet

26. Ans. d. All of the above *(Ref: Jaypee Manual of Surgical Equipments/p 146)*

Toothed dissecting forceps
• Used to **hold the cut skin margins** during **suturing** • Used to **hold the linea alba** or the **rectus sheath** during closure of abdominal incision • Used to **hold the scalp** during closure of scalp incision

27. Ans. d. Pile holding forceps *(Ref: Jaypee Manual of Surgical Equipments/p 192)*

Pile holding forceps
• Used during pile operation to **hold the pile mass**

28. Ans. c. Desjardins forceps *(Ref: Jaypee Manual of Surgical Equipments/p 199)*

Desjardins choledocholithotomy forceps
• Used during **choledocholithotomy** for **stone removal** • Used during **laparoscopic cholecystectomy** for **stone removal** • May also be used during removal of kidney, ureteric or bladder stone

29. **Ans. a. Pyelolithotomy forceps** *(Ref: Jaypee Manual of Surgical Equipments/p 199)*

Pyelolithotomy forceps
• Used to **hold the stone** during **nephrolithotomy**, **pyelolithotomy** or **ureterolithotomy**

30. **Ans. c. Suprapubic cystolithotomy forceps** *(Ref: Jaypee Manual of Surgical Equipments/p 195)*

Sprapubic cystolithotomy forceps
• Used for **suprapubic cystolithotomy**, to **hold and bring out the calculi** from urinary bladder

31. **Ans. d. Used to pick sterilized instruments** *(Ref: Jaypee Manual of Surgical Equipments/p 107)*

Cheatle's Forceps
• Used to **pick sterile articles (instruments and drapes) to avoid touching the instruments** while transferring them from the tray to table

32. **Ans. c. Duval lung holding forceps** *(Ref: Jaypee Manual of Surgical Equipments/p 227)*

Duval Lung Holding Forceps
• Used to **grasp lung tissue during lobectomy** or **pneumonectomy**
• **Triangular aperture** and **fine serrations** in the distal blade provide **firm grip without any trauma**

33. **Ans. d. Ovum forceps** *(Ref: Jaypee Manual of Surgical Equipments/p 209)*

Ovum Forceps
• Used to **remove placental fragments, small endometrial polyps** from the uterus.
• Used to **remove gallstone from gallbladder during extraction** of gallbladder

34. **Ans. c. Russian tissue forceps** *(Ref: Jaypee Manual of Surgical Equipments/p 161)*

Russian Tissue Forceps
• **Clubbed tip** in the blades with **serrated inner surface**
• Used to **hold skin while suturing**

35. **Ans. b. Right angle forceps** *(Ref: Jaypee Manual of Surgical Equipments/p 159, 153)*

Right Angle Forceps (Meigster or Lahey)
• Used to **dissect pedicle, pass ligatures, to hold bleeding vessel in depth,** to dissect and pass **ligatures to cystic duct** and **cystic artery** in cholecystectomy

36. **Ans. a. Mosquito hemostatic forceps** *(Ref: Jaypee Manual of Surgical Equipments/p 152)*

Mosquito Hemostatic Forceps
• Used to hold fine bleeding vessels
• Used to puncture the mesoappendix at an avascular site

37. **Ans. b. Spencer Wells hemostatic forceps** *(Ref: Jaypee Manual of Surgical Equipments/p 152)*

Spencer-Wells Hemostatic Forceps
• Used to **hold the bleeding vessel**
• Used to **split internal oblique** and **transversus abdominis during appendectomy**
• Used to do **blunt dissection**

38. **Ans. c. A= Backhaus towel clamp. B = Halstead mosquito forceps. C = Allis forceps. D = Babcock intestinal forceps**

39. **Ans. b. Yeoman punch biopsy forceps** *(Ref: Jaypee Manual of Surgical Equipments/p 217)*

Yeoman punch biopsy forceps
• Two short stout jaws on the tip
• Used to **take biopsy from rectal lesions** like **carcinoma, polyps or ulcers**

40. **Ans. a. Cord holding forceps** *(Ref: Jaypee Manual of Surgical Equipments/p 159)*

Cord holding forceps
• **Cord holding forceps** is used during **hernia surgery to hold the structures of spermatic cord, to keep the cord structures apart from the sac to prevent injury.**

RETRACTOR

41. **Ans. c. Czerny's retractor** *(Ref: Jaypee Manual of Surgical Equipments/p 140)*

Czerny's retractor
- Used for **tissue retraction** in **appendectomy**, **thyroidectomy**, **mastectomy** and **inguinal hernia operation**

42. **Ans. a. Morris retractor** *(Ref: Jaypee Manual of Surgical Equipments/p 141)*

Morris retractor
- Used for tissue retraction **appendectomy**, **thyroidectomy**, **mastectomy** and **inguinal hernia operation**

43. **Ans. d. All of the above** *(Ref: Jaypee Manual of Surgical Equipments/p 143)*

Double hook retractor
- Used to **retract skin flap for excision of sebaceous cyst**
- Used during **venesection** for retraction of skin
- Used during **tracheostomy** for retraction of skin and thyroid isthmus

44. **Ans. c. Volkman's retractor** *(Ref: Jaypee Manual of Surgical Equipments/p 141)*

Cat's paw or Volkman's retractor
- Used for **retraction of skin flaps** or **fascia** for operation at the surface, e.g. excision of the sebaceous cyst, lipoma, dermoid.

45. **Ans. d. Deaver's retractor** *(Ref: Jaypee Manual of Surgical Equipments/p 142)*

Deaver's retractor
- Used during **cholecystectomy** for **retraction of right lobe of liver**
- Used during **pancreaticojejunostomy** for **retraction of stomach**
- Used during kidney operations to retract the abdominal wall

46. **Ans. c. Joll's thyroid retractor** *(Ref: Jaypee Manual of Surgical Equipments/p 178)*

Joll's thyroid retractor
- **Self retaining** retractor used during thyroid operations to **retract skin flaps**

47. **Ans. c. Doyen's mouth gag** *(Ref: Jaypee Manual of Surgical Equipments/p 304)*

Doyen's mouth gag
- Used to **open mouth during intraoral operations** like **glossectomy**, **cleft palate operation**, **excision of intraoral ranula**

48. **Ans. d. Balfours retractor** *(Ref: Jaypee Manual of Surgical Equipments/p 144)*

Balfour Abdominal Retractor
- **Self-retaining retractor** used in **laparotomy procedures, cesarean sections** and **bowel resection.**

49. **Ans. b. Beckman Weitlaner retractor** *(Ref: Jaypee Manual of Surgical Equipments/p 144)*

Beckman Weitlaner retractor: Used to **retract** or **hold back tissue** or **bone** for Surgical exposure

50. **Ans. d. Retracting bladder neck** *(Ref: Jaypee Manual of Surgical Equipments/p 198)*

Bladder Neck Retractor: Used to **retract bladder neck in bladder surgeries**

51. **Ans. b. Farabeuf retractor** *(Ref: Jaypee Manual of Surgical Equipments/p 143)*

Farabeuf Double-Ended Retractor
- Versatile **handheld retractor** used in **dentistry, in wrist** and **hand procedures**, or in **hernia repair**

52. **Ans. c. Scapula retractor** *(Ref: Jaypee Manual of Surgical Equipments/p 228)*

Scapula Retractor: Used to **retract scapula during thoracotomy**

53. **Ans. c. Langenbeck's retractor** *(Ref: Jaypee Manual of Surgical Equipments/p 140)*

Langenbeck's Retractor
- Retractor used in **hernia surgery** and **superficial surgeries** to retract skin, fascia and muscles

54. **Ans. c. Kelly retractor** *(Ref: Jaypee Manual of Surgical Equipments/p 212)*

Kelly retractor
- A **curved right-angled retractor**, used in **deep pelvic surgery** such as rectal dissection.

55. **Ans. c. Single hook retractor** *(Ref: Jaypee Manual of Surgical equipments/p143)*

Single Hook Retractor
• Used for **superficial retraction** specially for **tough structures** like **skin, fascia of sole & palm**

56. **Ans. a. Allison lung retractor** *(Ref: Jaypee Manual of Surgical equipments/p145)*

Allison Lung Retractor
• Used for **retraction of lung in thoracotomy**. • Because of its special design, it **does not damage the lung** & lung can expand in between the wires.

CLAMP

57. **Ans. b. Doyen's intestinal occlusion clamp** *(Ref: Jaypee Manual of Surgical Equipments/p 181)*

Doyen's straight intestinal occlusion clamp: Used for **gut resection** and **anastomosis**

58. **Ans. a. Payr's crushing clamp** *(Ref: Jaypee Manual of Surgical Equipments/p 180)*

Payr's gastric crushing clamp: Used during **partial gastrectomies**

59. **Ans. b. Light bulldog clamp** *(Ref: Jaypee Manual of Surgical Equipments/p 156)*

Light Bulldog Clamp
• It has **pinch cock action** to open and close with **fine transverse serrations** in the blade • Used for **temporary occlusion of small peripheral blood vessels** • Can be used as a **suture tag**

60. **Ans. c. Pott's bulldog clamp** *(Ref: Jaypee Manual of Surgical Equipments/p 156)*

Pott's Bulldog Clamp
• **Paper clip like** instrument with serrations and **spring loaded handle** which permits a **secure grip** of the vessel • Used for **temporary occlusion of small peripheral blood vessels**

61. **Ans. a. Satinsky vascular clamp** *(Ref: Jaypee Manual of Surgical Equipments/p 226)*

Satinsky Vascular Clamp
• Used for **partial occlusion of blood vessel** • Partially occlude the wall of a vessel over a distance; **blood flow to continue through the rest of the vessel.**

SCISSORS

62. **Ans. a. Mayo scissors** *(Ref: Jaypee Manual of Surgical Equipments/p 137, 269)*

Mayo's Scissors: Used for **cutting tough tissues;** used for **cutting ligaments**

63. **Ans. b. Metzenbaum scissors** *(Ref: Jaypee Manual of Surgical Equipments/p 137, 269)*

Metzenbaum Scissor: Used for **cutting delicate tissues like intestine, bladder** (viscera)

64. **Ans. c. Lister bandage scissors** *(Ref: Jaypee Manual of Surgical Equipments/p 137, 269)*

Lister bandage scissors
• **Distal blades** are **bent at angle,** so that it is passed easily under the bandage • **Flat blunt atraumatic tip** in the **lower blade** • Used for **cutting bandages**

DILATOR

65. **Ans. c. Tracheal dilator**

Tracheal dilator: Used during **tracheostomy**

66. **Ans. b. Urethral dilator** *(Ref: Jaypee Manual of Surgical Equipments/p 194)*

Urethral Dilator: Used to **dilate urethra in urethral strictures** and **before cystoscopy**

67. **Ans. a. Bile duct dilator**

Bake Bile Duct Dilator
• Used in **choledocholithotomy**, after removing the stones from the bile duct • Used to **sound the bile duct for any retained stone** • Used to **check the patency of ampulla of Vater**

SCOOP

68. **Ans. a. Volkmann scoop** *(Ref: Jaypee Manual of Surgical Equipments/p 235)*

Volkmann scoop
• This instrument has a working end **similar to curette**   • Used for **debriding** the contents of an **abscess cavity, sinus or fistula** & collection of cancellous bone grafts

69. **Ans. b. Gallstone scoop** *(Ref: Jaypee Manual of Surgical Equipments/p 173)*

Gallstone scoop
• Flat and thin structure with **spoon like shape holder** on both sides   • Spoon like shape helps to **remove stones from gallbladder**

LAPAROSCOPIC INSTRUMENTS

70. **Ans. b. Cystoscope** *(Ref: Jaypee Manual of Surgical Equipments/p 260)*

Cystoscope
• Lighted tube with a **telescopic lens** used to **examine inside of the bladder**

71. **Ans. c. Laparoscope** *(Ref: Jaypee Manual of Surgical Equipments/p 260)*

Laparoscope
• **Laparoscopes** are based on **Hopkins optical** system which uses a **series of glass rods with lenses placed at appropriate intervals** along the shaft of instrument   • Provide **visualization** of Surgical field **with magnification**   • **Oblique viewing (30°) laparoscopes provide larger field of vision** than the end viewing (0°) laparoscopes

72. **Ans. b. Hasson cannula** *(Ref: Jaypee Manual of Surgical Equipments/p 267)*

Hasson cannula
• Used as alternative technique to **create pneumoperitoneum by open technique,** especially in patients with **upper abdominal surgeries** or accompanying ileus   • **Incidence of vessel injury is very less** with Hasson cannula

73. **Ans. c. Trocar** *(Ref: Jaypee Manual of Surgical Equipments/p 267)*

Trocar
• **Trocars** are required **to access the peritoneal cavity during surgery** and for **maintaining pneumoperitoneum when instruments are exchanged**

BIOPSY NEEDLE

74. **Ans. a. Tru cut biopsy needle** *(Ref: Jaypee Manual of Surgical Equipments/p 60)*

Tru cut biopsy needle
• Tru cut biopsy needle consists of **cutting needle encased in a trocar.**   • Cutting needle slides into the trocar to a **preset depth.**   • Cutting needle is advanced rapidly into the organ tissue followed by trocar   • Needle and trocar are removed together and the **biopsy core** is **collected from the cutting needle.**

75. **Ans. b. Vim-Silverman needle** *(Ref: Jaypee Manual of Surgical Equipments/p 60)*

Vim-Silverman needle
• **Vim-Silverman needle** consists of **trocar, a fitting obturator** and a **cutting needle with prongs.**   • Trocar and fitting obturator are introduced together into organ tissue after which the obturator is removed and cutting needle with prongs is introduced through the trocar.   • **Biopsy core is collected between the prongs of cutting needle.**

76. **Ans. a. Laparoscopic port trocar**

   The instrument marked in the laparoscopy image above is the port containing the trocar. It is used for creating pneumoperitoneum and inserting the instruments for the procedure.

77. **Ans. a. Monopolar cautery** *(Ref; Sabiston 20/e p235-236)*

Monopolar Electrocautery	Bipolar Electrocautery	LigaSure	Hyfrecators

Surgical Devices and Energy Sources			
Monopolar Electrocautery	<ul><li>Monopolar electrocautery is used for **cutting, blending, desiccation** and **fulguration**.</li><li>Using a **pencil instrument**, active electrode is placed in the entry site and can be **used to cut tissue and coagulate bleeding**.</li></ul>		
	Cutting	<ul><li>Cautery **activated** with a **constant waveform**^{Q}</li><li>**Heat** is **generated relatively quickly** over the target with **minimal lateral thermal spread**^{Q}.</li></ul>	
	Coagulation	<ul><li>Cautery activated with an **intermittent waveform**^{Q}</li><li>**Less heat** is **generated** on a **slower frequency,** with the potential for **large lateral thermal spread**, resulting in **tissue dehydration** & **vessel thrombosis**^{Q}.</li></ul>	
	<ul><li>**Blended waveform** have the advantage of both cutting and coagulation modes.</li><li>**Grounding pad** is placed securely on the patient **for monopolar cautery** device **to function properly** and **to prevent thermal burn injury** at the current reentry electrode site.</li><li>**MC used** because of **versatility and effectiveness**^{Q}.</li></ul>		
Bipolar Electrocautery	<ul><li>**Bipolar electrocautery** establishes a **short circuit between the tips of instrument** (forceps)^Q</li><li>**Grounding pad** is **not required**^{Q}</li><li>**Grasped tissue** between the **tips of instrument completes** the **circuit**^{Q}</li></ul>		
	<ul><li>It provides **precise thermal coagulation** (generating **heat affects only the tissue within short circuit**)^Q</li><li>**More effective than the monopolar instrument in coagulating vessels** due to **mechanical advantage of compression of tissue between the tips** of the instrument to the thermal coagulation^Q.</li></ul>		
	<ul><li>Particularly useful for procedures in which **lateral thermal injury** or an **arcing phenomenon needs to be avoided**^{Q}.</li></ul>		
LigaSure	<ul><li>**LigaSure** is a **new electrothermal bipolar tissue sealing system**^{Q}</li><li>Applied in **abdominal and pelvic surgery**, mostly **through laparoscopy**^{Q}.</li><li>**Advantage:** It improves **vessel sealing** with **minimal lateral thermal spread**^{Q}.</li></ul>		
Hyfrecators	<ul><li>Hyfrecator functions by **sending electrical impulses into body with the use of a probe**^{Q}.</li></ul>		
	<ul><li>It **works by emitting low-power high-frequency AC** (alternating current) **electrical pulses via a probe**, directly to the affected area of the body^Q.</li></ul>		
	<ul><li>Hyfrecator is used for **removal of warts**, **pearly penile papules**, **desiccation of sebaceous gland disorders**, electrocautery of bleeding, **epilation,** destruction of small cosmetically **unwanted superficial veins**, destruction of skin cancers (**basal cell carcinoma**).</li></ul>		

STAPLER

78. **Ans. b. Intraluminal stapler** *(Ref: Berry & Kohn's Operating Room Technique by Nancymarie Phillips/p 335, 336, 551)*

Staplers used in Surgery	
• **Types of Stapler: Skin, Linear (cutting and stapling), Ligating and Intraluminal types.**	
Skin stapler	• Skin staplers are used to **approximate skin edges during skin closure**.
Linear stapler	<ul><li>Linear staplers are used to **insert two straight, staggered evenly spaced, parallel rows of staples** into tissues.</li><li>Linear staplers are typically used to **staple tissue to be transected within the alimentary tract or thoracic cavity**.</li></ul>
Linear cutter	<ul><li>Linear cutter is used to **staple and transect the tissue,** especially **in GI procedures.**</li><li>Linear cutters **deliver two double staple lines and contain a knife blade** that **passes between the two staple lines, dividing the tissue.**</li></ul>
Ligating clips	• Ligating clip is used to **occlude a single small structure (blood vessel or duct).**
Ligating cutter	• Ligating cutter ejects **two ligating clips side by side** and then **divides the tissue between the clips** with a single activation.
Intraluminal stapler	<ul><li>Intraluminal (circular) staplers are **used to anastomose tubular structures** within the GIT.</li><li>This stapler **fires a double row of circular staples** and then **trims the lumen with a knife** located within the head of the stapler.</li><li>**Used during resection and anastomoses** of the **distal colon or rectum**</li></ul>

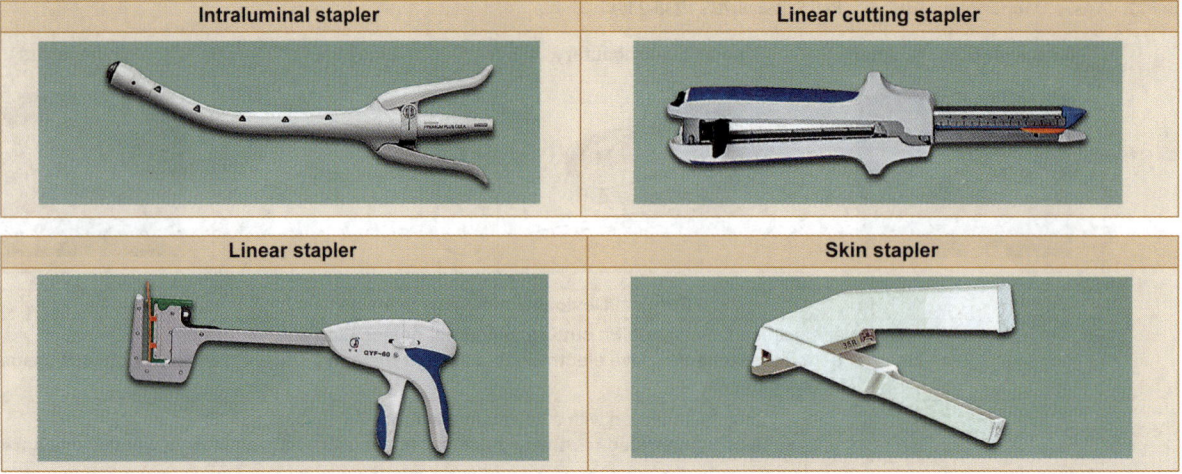

79. **Ans. d. Linear cutting stapler** *(Ref: Berry & Kohn's Operating Room Technique by Nancymarie Phillips/p 335, 336, 551)*
80. **Ans. d. Linear stapler** *(Ref: Berry & Kohn's Operating Room Technique by Nancymarie Phillips/p 335, 336, 551)*
81. **Ans. c. Skin stapler** *(Ref: Berry & Kohn's Operating Room Technique by Nancymarie Phillips/p 335, 336, 551)*

TUBES

82. **Ans. b. Kehr's T-tube** *(Ref: Jaypee Manual of Surgical Equipments/p 97)*

Kehr's T-tube
• Following choledochotomy, the bile duct is closed over a T-tube, as primary closure of bile duct is associated with higher incidence of leakage
• Used to drain bile duct following repair of bile duct injury. The T-tube acts as a stent and is usually kept for 4-6 weeks

83. **Ans. c. Sengstaken Blakemore tube**

Sengstaken Blakemore Tube
• The tube is passed down into esophagus & gastric balloon is inflated inside the stomach.
• **Traction** is applied to the tube so that **gastric balloon** will **compress the GE junction** & **reduce the blood flow to esophageal varices.**
• Used **only in emergencies** where **bleeding from presumed varices is impossible to control with medication alone**.
• **Endotracheal intubation** before the procedure is strongly advised to secure the airway **to prevent aspiration**

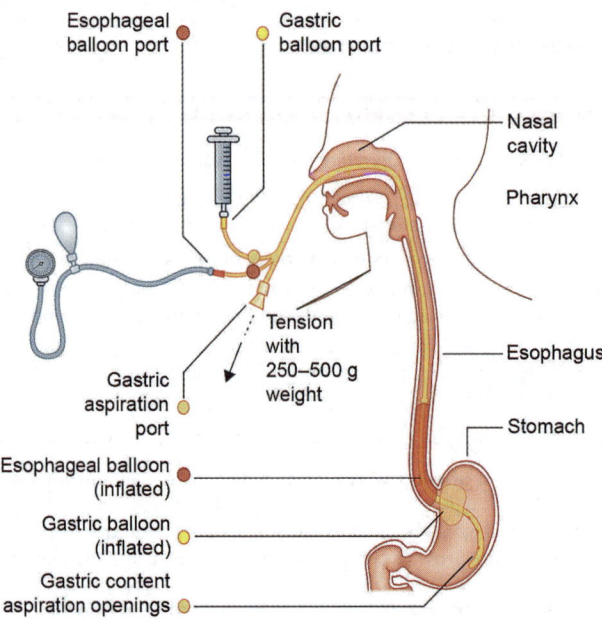

84. **Ans. c. Ryle's tube** *(Ref: Jaypee Manual of Surgical Equipments/p 96)*

Ryle's (Nasogastric) tube

• To measure the required length of tube, measure from the tip of the patient's nose, to their ear, and then down to the xiphisternum.
• Markings of Ryle's tube (**GBPD**)
  – At 40 cm: Indicates the level of **GE junction**^Q   – At 60 cm: Indicates the level of **pylorus**^Q
  – At 50 cm: Indicates the level of **body of stomach**^Q   – At 65 cm: Indicates the level of **duodenum**^Q

Indications of Ryle's Tube Insertion	
Diagnostic	**Therapeutic**
• Saline load test to confirm gastric outlet obstruction • To assess free & total acid in peptic ulcers • To diagnose tracheoesophageal fistula • In Hollander's test for completion of vagotomy	• Decompression in intestinal obstruction, gastric outlet obstruction • In perforation peritonitis, upper GI bleed, abdominal surgeries • Enteral nutrition in head injuries, comatose patients, maxillofacial injuries

85. **Ans. c. Sitting with flexed neck**
86. **Ans. d. Infant feeding tube** *(Ref: Jaypee Manual of Surgical Equipments/p 97)*

Infant feeding tube	
• **No markings** and **no shots** in Infant feeding tube	• Indications are similar to Ryle's tube in **infants & children**

CATHETERS

87. **Ans. a. Nelaton catheter**

Nelaton Catheter
• **Nelaton catheters** can be used for **one-time emptying of the bladder**, for instance **during/after surgery** or to **determine the amount of urine** in the bladder.

88. **Ans. d. Ventriculoperitoneal shunt** *(Ref: Bailey 27/e p655, 26/p-608)*

Ventriculoperitoneal Shunt
• **MC shunt for hydrocephalus**: Ventriculoperitoneal shunt • It involves the **insertion of a catheter**^Q **into the lateral ventricle** (usually **right frontal** or **occipital**) • The catheter is then connected to a shunt valve under the scalp and finally to a distal catheter, which is tunneled subcutaneously down to the abdomen and inserted into the peritoneal cavity. • If the CSF pressure exceeds the shunt valve pressure, then CSF will flow out of the distal catheter and be absorbed by the peritoneal lining. • **Other options for distal catheter placement** include the **right atrium** via the deep facial and jugular vein (**ventriculoatrial shunt**) or the **pleural cavity** (**ventriculopleural shunt**).

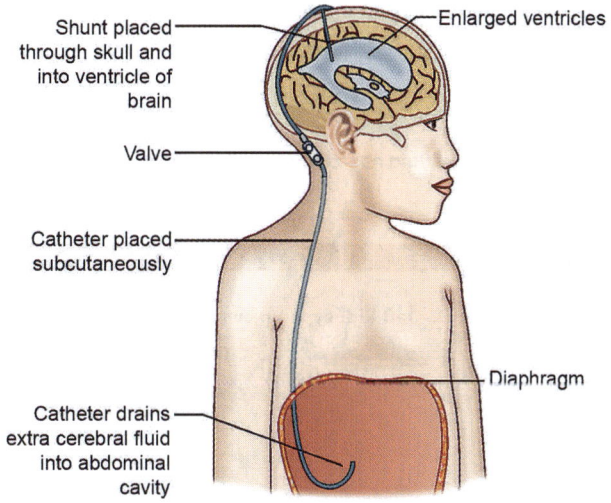

89. **Ans. b. Fogarty catheter**   *(Ref: Bailey 27/e p955)*

Fogarty Embolectomy Catheter
• Used to **remove fresh emboli from vessels**^Q • Consists of a hollow tube with an inflatable balloon attached to its tip. • Inserted into the blood vessel through a clot. The balloon is then inflated to extract it from the vessel.

90. **Ans. d. Malecot's catheter**   *(Ref: Jaypee Manual of Surgical Equipments/p 96)*

Malecot's Catheter
• **Self retaining catheter** with an **umbrella or flower** at the **tip** • **Used for draining urine** from the urinary bladder, when the urethra is damaged as in **suprapubic catheterization**; drainage of urine from the kidney by **percutaneous nephrostomy** • Used for **drainage of fluid collections**, e.g. an abdominal abscess • Used as **intercostal drain**

91. **Ans. b. Red rubber catheter**

Red rubber catheter
• **Non self retaining urinary catheter** with **rounded and blunt tip** • Temporarily used to **drain urine from bladder** and **to estimate the residual urine**

92. **Ans. b. Central venous catheter**   *(Ref: Jaypee Manual of Surgical Equipments/p 105)*

Central venous catheter

• **Central venous catheters are used for fluid, medication and nutrition administration**^Q
• **Used for monitoring pressure or volume changes to detect potential problems or evaluate patient improvement**^Q
 	
   • **Most preferred veins** for central venous catheterization **in operating room: Internal jugular vein**^Q
   • **Most preferred veins** for central venous catheterization **outside operating room: Subclavian vein**^Q
   • **Most preferred veins** for central venous catheterization **in acutely injured, critically ill** patients: **Femoral vein**^Q (Relative ease of insertion)

SUCTION AND DRAIN

93. **Ans. c. Romovac suction drain**   *(Ref: Jaypee Manual of Surgical Equipments/p 98)*

Romovac Suction Drain
• Suction is created by pressing the suction corrugation • Used for **mastectomy, thyroidectomy, flap and reconstructive surgeries**

94. **Ans. c. Adson suction tip**   *(Ref: Jaypee Manual of Surgical Equipments/p 101)*

Adson suction tip
• Angles with a vent or thumb rest to control suction • **Fine suction tip** helps in **fine and meticulous surgeries** like **vascular, plastic or reconstructive surgeries**

95. **Ans. d. Yankauer suction tip**   *(Ref: Jaypee Manual of Surgical Equipments/p 101)*

Yankauer suction tip
• It has **large suction tip** • Used in surgeries in which **large volume of fluid** has to be **sucked** (peritoneal cavity after lavage, in perforation peritonitis, hemoperitoneum)

GASTROINTESTINAL SURGERY

96. **Ans. d. A = liver. B. = gallbladder. C. = aorta. D. = left kidney E. = pancreas**

Annexures

Annexure 1

NAMED CLASSIFICATION FOR TUMORS

Important Tumor Classification	
Chang staging[Q]	Medulloblastoma[Q]
Masaoka staging[Q]	Thymoma[Q]
Shimda index[Q]	Neuroblastoma[Q]
Reiss and **Ellsworth** classification **Esson prognostic index**[Q]	Retinoblastoma[Q]
Bloom-Richardson grading[Q]	CA breast[Q]
Noguchi classification[Q]	Adenocarcinoma lung[Q]
Sullivan modification of **Macfarlane system**[Q]	Adrenocortical carcinoma[Q]
Gleason	CA prostate[Q]
Nevine staging	CA GB[Q]
Duke staging	Colorectal carcinoma[Q]
Robson staging	RCC[Q]
Jackson	CA penis[Q]
Butchart staging	Mesothelioma[Q]

Annexure 2

GENES AND CHROMOSOMES

Syndrome	Genes	Locations
Breast/ovarian syndrome	BRCA1	17[Q]
	BRCA2[Q]	13[Q]
Cowden's disease	PTEN[Q]	10[Q]
FAP	APC[Q]	5[Q]
HNPCC	hMLH1[Q]	3[Q]
	hMSH2[Q]	2[Q]
	hMSH6	2[Q]
	hPMS1	2[Q]
	hPMS2	7[Q]
Hereditary papillary RCC	**MET**[Q]	7[Q]
Li-Fraumeni	**p53**[Q]	17[Q]
	hCHK2	22
MEN-1	MEN1[Q]	11[Q]
MEN-2	RET[Q]	10[Q]
NF-1	NF1[Q]	17[Q]

Contd...

Contd...

Syndrome	Genes	Locations
NF-2	NF2^Q	22^Q
Peutz-Jeghers syndrome	STK11^Q	19^Q
Retinoblastoma	RB^Q	13^Q
Tuberous sclerosis	TSC1^Q	9^Q
	TSC2^Q	16^Q
VHL syndrome	VHL^Q	3^Q
Wilms' tumor	WT^Q	11^Q

Name of Incisions	
Lazy 'S', Sistrunk, Modified Blair's	Parotidectomy
McBurney's, Grid-Iron, McArthur, Lanz	Appendectomy
Pfannenstiel incision	Caesarean section Abdominal hysterectomy
Chevron incision	Whipple's procedure Upper abdominal Malignancies
Cherney incision	**Pelvic surgery** (excellent surgical exposure to the space of Retzius and pelvic side walls)
Kocher's incision	Open cholecystectomy
Kustner's incision	Transverse incision made 5 cm above the symphysis pubis but below the anterior superior iliac spine
Maylard incision	• A variation of Pfannenstiel incision • Rectus abdominis muscles are sectioned transversely to permit wider access to the pelvis
McEvedy's Incision	Lateral paramedian incision
Turner-Warwick's incision	• Placed **2 cm above the symphysis pubis** and within the lateral borders of the rectus muscle • **Good for exposure of retropubic space**

Annexure 3

LYMPH NODES

Most Common Lymph Nodes Involved	
CA Penis	Inguinal LN^Q
CA Testis	On right: Inter-aortocaval^Q LN On left: Paraaortic^Q LN
CA Bladder	Obturator^Q LN
CA Prostate	Obturator^Q LN

Important Lymph Nodes	
Rotter's nodes^Q	• **Interpectoral** nodes (**CA breast**)^Q
Rouvier nodes^Q	• **Retropharyngeal** nodes (**CA Nasopharynx**)^Q
Delphian nodes^Q	• **Pre-cricoid/Pre-tracheal/Pre-laryngeal** lymph nodes^Q
Irish nodes^Q	• Nodes in **left axilla (CA stomach)**^Q
Sister Mary Joseph nodes^Q	• **Periumbilical metastatic cutaneous** nodules
Virchow nodes^Q	• **Left supraclavicular** node^Q
Cloquet node^Q	• **Femoral canal** node^Q
LN of **Lund**^Q	• **Cystic** lymph node^Q
Krouse Lymph node	• **Jugular fossa** lymph node^Q
Giuliano node	• Sentinel LN in carcinoma breast

Annexure 4

NAMED TRIADS

Important Triads

Triad	Seen in	Components
Virchow's Triad[Q]	Thrombosis	Hypercoagulability + Stasis + Endothelial injury[Q]
Galezia's Triad[Q]		Dupuytren's contracture + Retroperitoneal fibrosis + Peyronie's disease of penis[Q]
Cushing's Triad[Q]	Intracranial hypertension	↑ BP + Bradycardia + ↓ respiratory rate
Hutchison's Triad[Q]	Congenital syphilis	Hutchison's teeth (notched upper incisors) + Interstitial keratitis + Nerve deafness[Q]
Trotter's Triad[Q]	Nasopharyngeal Carcinoma	Conductive hearing loss + Immobility of homolateral soft palate + Trigeminal neuralgia[Q]
Saints Triad		Hiatus hernia + Gallstones + Colonic diverticulosis[Q]
Dieulafoy's Triad[Q]	Acute appendicitis	Hypersensitiveness of skin + Reflex muscular contraction + tenderness at McBurney's point[Q]
Quincke's Triad[Q]	Hemobilia	GI hemorrhage + biliary colic + jaundice[Q]
Borchardt's Triad[Q]	Gastric Volvulus	Epigastric pain + Inability to vomit + Inability to pass a NG tube[Q]
Tillaux's Triad[Q]	Mesenteric cyst	Soft fluctuant swelling in umbilical region + Freely mobile perpendicular to mesentery + Zone of resonance all around[Q]
Mackler's Triad[Q]	Boerhaave's syndrome	Thoracic pain + vomiting + cervical subcutaneous emphysema[Q]
Rigler's Triad[Q]	Gallstone ileus	Small bowel obstruction + Pneumobilia + Ectopic gallstone[Q]
Whipple's Triad[Q]	Insulinoma	Symptoms of hypoglycemia + S. glucose <45 mg/dL + Symptomatic relief on glucose ingestion[Q]
Currarino or ASP triad		Anorectal malformations + Sacrococcygeal osseous defect + Presacral mass (Anterior sacral meningocele)

Annexure 5

TREATMENT OF CHOICE

Condition	Treatment of Choice
Duodenal Atresia	Duodenoduodenostomy[Q]
Annular pancreas	Duodenoduodenostomy[Q]
Superior mesenteric artery syndrome	Duodenojejunostomy[Q]

Enucleation is treatment of choice in

1. Hemangioma liver[Q]
2. Leiomyoma esophagus[Q]
3. Chylolymphatic cyst[Q]
4. Insulinoma involving head of pancreas[Q]

Annexure 6

METASTASIS

Carcinoma Thyroid

Type	Mode of spread
Papillary carcinoma	**Lymphatic**^Q spread
Follicular carcinoma	**Hematogenous**^Q spread
Medullary carcinoma	Both **lymphatic** and **hematogenous**^Q spread
Anaplastic carcinoma	**Direct invasion**^Q

Carcinoma Thyroid

Type	MC site of Metastasis
Papillary carcinoma	**Lungs**^Q
Follicular carcinoma	**Bones**^Q
Medullary carcinoma	**Liver**^Q
Anaplastic carcinoma	**Lungs**^Q

Pulsating Secondaries

1. Follicular carcinoma thyroid^Q
2. RCC^Q

Bone Metastasis in Carcinoma Thyroid

Follicular carcinoma	**Osteolytic** metastasis (**Pulsating secondaries** in **flat bones**)^Q
Medullary carcinoma	**Osteoblastic** metastasis^Q

Metastatic Tumors

Metastatic Tumors of Thyroid
- Rare, most cases are found in autopsy
- MC site of primary: **CA Breast**^Q > CA Lung
- If thyroid metastases is detected pre-mortem, MC site of primary: **RCC**^Q > CA Breast > CA Lung

Metastatic Tumors to lung, MC primary: CA breast^Q

Metastatic Tumors to Pancreas
- MC site of primary: **RCC**^Q > Malignant melanoma
- On **autopsy**, MC site of primary: **CA lung**^Q

Metastatic Tumors Adrenal, MC site of primary: **CA Lung**^Q

Metastatic Tumors to Small Bowel
- Metastatic tumors involving small bowel are more common than primary tumors
- MC site of primary: Other intra-abdominal organs
- MC extra-abdominal source: **Melanoma** > CA Breast > CA Lung

Metastatic Tumors to Skin
- MC site of primary in males: **CA Lung**^Q
- MC site of primary in females: **CA Breast**^Q
- **Scalp** is **MC site** for **cutaneous metastatic disease**^Q

Metastatic Tumors to Liver
- MC site of primary: **Colorectal cancer > CA lung** > CA Pancreas > CA Breast > CA Stomach

Metastatic Tumors to CNS
- MC site of primary for **brain** metastases: **CA Lung**^Q > CA Breast
- MC site of primary for **leptomeningeal metastases**: **CA Breast**^Q

Metastatic Tumors to esophagus, MC primary: CA lung^Q

Contd...

Contd...

Metastatic Tumors
Metastatic Tumors to spleen   • MC site of primary: **Malignant Melanoma**   • MC site of primary for Isolated Secondaries to spleen: **CA ovary**
Metastatic Tumors to Heart   • MC primary in **males**: **CA lung**[Q]   • MC primary in **females**: **CA breast**[Q]
Metastatic Tumors to Testis   • MC site of primary: **CA prostate**[Q] > **CA lung** > **GI malignancies** > **melanoma** > **kidney**
Metastatic Tumors to penis, MC site of primary: CA bladder[Q]

Annexure 7

MOST COMMON SYMPTOMS AND CHEMOTHERAPY

Malignancy	Chemotherapy Regimen
CA breast	**CAF** (**C**yclophosphamide + **A**driamycin + 5-**F**U)[Q]
Hepatoblastoma	**VCF** (**V**incristine + **C**isplatin + 5-**F**U)[Q]
CA gall bladder & Cholangiocarcinoma	**G**emcitabine + **C**isplatin[Q]
CA pancreas	**G**emcitabine[Q]
CA esophagus & CA stomach	**ECF** (**E**pirubicin + **C**isplatin + 5-**F**U)[Q]
Small intestinal adenocarcinoma	**FOLFOX**
Small bowel carcinoid	**DEF** (**D**acarbazine + **E**pirubicin + 5-**F**U)[Q]
Colorectal carcinoma	**FOLFOX-IV** (**Fol**inic acid/Leucovorin + 5-**FU** + **Ox**aliplatin)[Q]
CA anal canal	**Nigro regimen** (5-FU + Mitomycin-C + Radiation)[Q]
Wilm's tumor	**VCD** (**V**incristine + **C**yclophosphamide + **D**oxorubicin or **D**actinomycin)[Q]
CA bladder	**MVAC** (**M**ethotrexate + **V**inblastine + **A**driamycin + **C**isplatin)[Q]
Testicular tumors	**BEP** (**B**leomycin + **E**toposide + **C**isplatin)[Q]
Rhabdomyosarcoma	**VAC** (**V**incristine + **A**ctinomycin + **C**yclophosphamide)[Q]
Hodgkin's lymphoma	**ABVD** (**A**driamycin + **B**leomycin + **V**inblastine + **D**acarbazine)[Q] **MOPP** (**M**echlorethamine + **O**ncovin or vincristine + **P**rocarbazine + **P**rednisone)[Q]
Non-Hodgkin's lymphoma	**CHOP** (**C**yclophosphamide + **H**ydroxydaunorubicin or Doxorubicin + **O**ncovin or vincristine + **P**rednisone)[Q]

Most Common Symptom	
CA Esophagus	• **Dysphagia** > weight loss[Q]
CA stomach	• **Abdominal pain** > weight loss[Q]
Periampullary carcinoma (including CA head of pancreas)	• **Jaundice**[Q]
HCC	• **Abdominal pain** > weight loss[Q]
Cholangiocarcinoma	• **Painless progressive jaundice**[Q]
CA Gallbladder	• **Biliary colic**[Q]
CA small bowel	• **Abdominal pain**[Q]
CA colon	• **Abdominal pain**[Q]
CA rectum	• **Bleeding PR**[Q]
CA anal canal	• **Bleeding PR**[Q]

Annexure 8

MOST COMMON SITES

Important Most Common Sites	
• Gastric ulcer[Q]	Lesser curvature (near incisura angularis)
• Peptic ulcer[Q] • Gastric outlet obstruction[Q]	1st part of duodenum
• Small bowel[Q] adenocarcinoma • Atresia[Q]	Duodenum
• Polyps in PJS[Q] • Pneumatosis intestinalis[Q]	Jejunum
• Crohn's disease[Q] • Fistula, perforation and carcinoma in Crohn's disease[Q] • Typhoid ulcer[Q] • Tubercular ulcer[Q] • Small intestinal lymphoma[Q] • Gallstone ileus[Q]	Terminal Ileum
• Amebic colitis[Q] • Bleeding in angiodysplasia[Q] • Bleeding in colonic diverticula[Q]	Cecum and ascending colon
• Ischemic colitis[Q]	Splenic flexure
• Colonic diverticula[Q] • Stricture after ischemic colitis[Q] • Volvulus[Q]	Sigmoid
• Ulcerative colitis[Q] • Colorectal cancer[Q] • Hirschsprung's disease[Q]	Rectum

Annexure 9

NAMED HERNIA

Gibbon's hernia	• Hernia with hydrocele[Q]
Berger's hernia	• Hernia into pouch of Douglas[Q]
Beclard's hernia	• Femoral hernia through opening of saphenous vein[Q]
Amyand's hernia	• Inguinal hernia containing appendix[Q]
Ogilvie's hernia	• Hernia through the defect in conjoint tendon just lateral to where it inserts with the rectus sheath[Q]
Stammer's hernia	• Internal hernia occurring through window in the transverse mesocolon after retrocolic gastrojejunostomy[Q]
Peterson hernia	• Hernia under Roux limb after Roux-en-Y gastric bypass[Q]
Hesselbach's Hernia	• Fatty tissue herniation lateral to the femoral vessels through the lacuna musculorum (lateral compartment of the thigh inferior to the inguinal ligament, for the passage of the iliopsoas muscle)[Q]
Velpeau's Hernia (Prevascular)	• A protrusion of viscera in front of the femoral vessels in the groin[Q]
Serafini's Hernia (Retrovascular)	• The hernial sac emerges behind femoral vessels[Q]
Holthouse hernia	• Inguinal hernia with extension of the loop of intestine along inguinal ligament[Q]

Annexure 10

CHARACTERISTIC RADIOLOGICAL APPEARANCES

Radiological Features	Seen in
• Apple core lesion on barium enema	Carcinoma colon[Q]
• Claw appearance on barium enema	Intussusception[Q]
• Saw tooth appearance	Colonic diverticula
• Bird beak appearance	Achalasia[Q] (on barium swallow) Sigmoid volvulus (on barium enema)
• Cork screw appearance • Rosary bead appearance • Pseudodiverticula appearance	Diffuse esophageal spasm[Q]
• String sign of Kantor • Sterlein sign	Crohn's disease[Q] Tuberculosis
• Thumb print sign	Ischemic colitis[Q]
• Squeeze sign, Cushion sign, Tenting sign, naked fat sign	Colonic lipoma[Q]
• Rat tail appearance	Achalasia[Q]

Characteristic Appearances	
ADPKD	• Spider leg or Bell deformity[Q] • Bubble or Swiss cheese appearance on IVP[Q]
Infantile PKD	• Sunburst pattern on IVP[Q]
Medullary Sponge Kidney	• Bristles on brush appearance[Q] • Bouquet of flower appearance on IVP[Q]
Multicystic Dysplastic Kidney	• Bunch of grapes appearance[Q]
Renal Artery Aneurysm	• Ring like calcification[Q]
Ectopic Ureteric Orifice	• Drooping lily sign on IVP[Q]
Retrocaval Ureter	• Fish hook or Reverse 'J' deformity on IVP[Q]
Retroperitoneal Fibrosis	• Medial pulling of ureter or pipestem ureter[Q] (Pipestem ureter is also seen in TB)
CA Renal Pelvis	• Goblet sign or stipple sign on RGP[Q]

Radiological Feature	Disease
• Rim/crescent sign[Q] • Soap bubble appearance[Q]	Hydronephrosis
• Spider leg appearance[Q]	Polycystic Kidney
• Flower vase appearance of ureter[Q]	Horse shoe Kidney
• Golf hole ureter[Q]	TB bladder
• Drooping lily sign[Q]	Ectopic ureter
• Cobra head or Adder head appearance[Q] • Spring onion appearance[Q]	Ureterocele
• Egg in cup appearance[Q]	Analgesic nephropathy causing papillary necrosis
• Thimble bladder[Q]	Tubercular chronic cystitis
• Sandy patches[Q]	Schistosomiasis of bladder
• Chalice/Bergman sign[Q]	Ureteric dilatation distal to neoplasm
• Fish hook bladder[Q]	BPH

Contd...

Contd...

Radiological Feature	Disease
• B/L spider leg appearance^Q • Swiss-cheese nephrogram^Q • Sun burst nephrogram^Q	Polycystic kidney

Radiological Appearance		
Acute Pancreatitis	**Chronic Pancreatitis**	**CA Pancreas**
• Renal halo sign[Q] • Gasless abdomen[Q] • Ground glass appearance[Q] • Colon cut off sign[Q] • Sentinel loop[Q]	• Chain of lakes appearance[Q] • String of pearl appearance[Q] • Beaded appearance[Q] • Numerous irregular calcifications[Q] are pathognomonic (on X-ray)	• Double contour of medial border of duodenal C loop • Double duct sign[Q] • Dilated/widening of duodenal C loop[Q] • Mucosal irregularity[Q] • Scrambled egg appearance • Inverted/reverse 3 sign of Frostberg[Q] • Rose thorning of medial wall of 2nd part of duodenum[Q] • Antral pad sign

Annexure 11

Suspected Carcinogens	
Carcinogens	**Associated Cancer or Neoplasm**
Alkylating agents	• Acute myeloid leukemia[Q], bladder cancer[Q]
Androgens	• Prostate cancer[Q]
Aromatic amines (dyes)	• Bladder cancer[Q]
Arsenic	• Cancer of the lung[Q], skin[Q]
Asbestos	• Cancer of the lung[Q], pleura[Q], peritoneum[Q]
Benzene	• Acute myelocytic leukemia[Q]
Chromium	• Lung cancer[Q]
Diethylstilbestrol (prenatal)	• Vaginal cancer (clear cell)[Q]
Epstein-Barr virus	• Burkitt's lymphoma[Q], nasal T cell lymphoma[Q]
Estrogens	• Cancer of the endometrium, liver, breast[Q]
Ethyl alcohol	• Cancer of the breast, liver, esophagus, head & neck[Q]
Helicobacter pylori	• Gastric cancer[Q], gastric MALT lymphoma[Q]
Hepatitis B or C virus	• Liver cancer[Q]
HIV	• Non-Hodgkin's lymphoma, Kaposi's sarcoma, squamous cell carcinomas[Q] (especially of the urogenital tract)
Human papilloma virus	• Cancers of the cervix, anus, oropharynx[Q]
Human T cell lymphotropic virus	• Adult T cell leukemia/lymphoma type 1 (HTLV-1)[Q]
Immunosuppressive agents (azathioprine, cyclosporine, glucocorticoids)	• Non-Hodgkin's lymphoma[Q]
Ionizing radiation (therapeutic or diagnostic)	• Breast, bladder, thyroid, soft tissue, bone, hematopoietic[Q]
Nitrogen mustard gas	• Cancer of the lung, head & neck, nasal sinuses[Q]
Nickel dust	• Cancer of the lung, nasal sinuses[Q]
Diesel exhaust (miners)	• Lung cancer[Q]
Phenacetin	• Cancer of the renal pelvis & bladder[Q]
Polycyclic hydrocarbons	• Cancer of the lung, skin (SCC of scrotal skin)[Q]
Radon gas	• Lung cancer[Q]
Schistosomiasis	• Bladder cancer (squamous cell)[Q]
Sunlight (ultraviolet)	• Skin cancer (SCC & melanoma)[Q]
Tobacco (including smokeless)	• Cancer of the upper aerodigestive tract, bladder[Q]
Vinyl chloride	• Liver cancer (angiosarcoma)[Q]

Annexure 12

FAMILIAL CANCER SYNDROMES

Familial Cancer Syndromes

Syndrome	Genes	Locations	Cancer Sites and Associated Traits
Breast/ovarian syndrome	**BRCA1**	**17**q21^Q	Cancer of **breast, ovary, colon, prostate**^Q
	BRCA2	**13**q12.3^Q	Cancer of **breast, ovary, colon, prostate, gallbladder and biliary tree, pancreas, stomach; melanoma**^Q
Cowden's disease	**PTEN**	**10**q23.3^Q	Cancer of **breast, endometrium, thyroid**^Q
FAP	**APC**	**5**q21^Q	Cancer of breast, endometrium, thyroid
Familial melanoma	p16	9p21	Melanoma, pancreatic cancer, dysplastic nevi, atypical moles
	CDK4	12q14	
Hereditary diffuse gastric cancer	CDH1	16q22	Gastric cancer
HNPCC	**hMLH1**^Q	**3**p21^Q	**Colorectal** cancer, **endometrial** cancer, **transitional cell carcinoma** of **ureter** and **renal pelvis, carcinomas** of the **stomach, small bowel, pancreas, ovary**^Q
	hMSH2^Q	**2**p22-21	
	hMSH6	2p16^Q	
	hPMS1	2q31.1	
	hPMS2	7p22.2^Q	
Hereditary papillary RCC	**MET**^Q	**7**q31^Q	Renal cell cancer
Hereditary paraganglioma and pheochromocytoma	SDHB	1p36.1-p35	Paraganglioma, pheochromocytoma
	SDHC	1q21	
	SDHD	11q23	
Juvenile polyposis coli	BMPRIA	10q21-q22	Juvenile polyps of the gastrointestinal tract, gastrointestinal malignancies
	SMAD4/DPC4	18q21.1	
Li-Fraumeni	p53	17p13^Q	**Breast** cancer, **soft tissue sarcoma, osteosarcoma, brain** tumors, **adrenocortical** carcinoma, **Wilms'** tumor, **phyllodes tumor (breast),** pancreatic cancer, **leukemia, neuroblastoma**^Q
	hCHK2	22q12.1	
MEN-1	**MENIN**^Q	**11**q13^Q	**Pancreatic islet cell** tumors, **parathyroid hyperplasia, pituitary adenomas**^Q
MEN-2	**RET**^Q	**10**q11.2	**Medullary thyroid** cancer, **pheochromocytoma, parathyroid hyperplasia**^Q
MYH-associated adenomatous polyposis	MYH	1p34.3-p32.1	Cancer of the colon, rectum, breast, stomach
Neurofibromatosis-1	**NF1**^Q	**17**q11^Q	**Neurofibromas, neurofibrosarcoma, acute myelogenous leukemia, brain** tumors^Q
Neurofibromatosis -2	**NF2**^Q	**22**q12^Q	**Acoustic neuromas, meningiomas, gliomas, ependymomas**^Q
Nevoid basal cell carcinoma	PTC	9q22.3	Basal cell carcinoma
Peutz-Jeghers syndrome	**STK11**^Q	**19**p13.3^Q	**Gastrointestinal carcinomas, breast** cancer, **testicular** cancer, **pancreatic** cancer, **benign pigmentation** of **skin** and **mucosa**^Q
Retinoblastoma	**RB**^Q	**13**q14^Q	**Retinoblastoma, sarcomas, melanoma, malignant neoplasms** of the **brain** and **meninges**^Q
Tuberous sclerosis	**TSC1**	**9**q34	**Multiple hamartomas, RCC, astrocytoma**
	TSC2	**16**p13	
von Hippel-Lindau syndrome	**VHL**^Q	**3**p25^Q	**RCC, hemangioblastomas** of **retina** and **CNS, pheochromocytoma**^Q
Wilms' tumor	**WT**^Q	**11**p13^Q	**Wilms' tumor, aniridia, genitourinary abnormalities, mental retardation**^Q

Annexure 13

SUTURES

Suture	Types	Raw material	Tensile strength	Absorption rate
Silk	Braided or twisted **multifilament**; Coated (with wax or silicone) or uncoated	Natural protein Raw silk from silkworm	Loses 20% when wet; 80–100% lost by 6 months	Fibrous encapsulation in body at 2–3 weeks; **Absorbed** slowly over **1–2 years**[Q]
Catgut	Plain	Collagen derived from healthy **sheep** or cattle	Lost within 7–10 days	**Phagocytosis** and **enzymatic degradation** within **7–10 days**[Q]
Catgut	Chromic	Tanned with **chromium salts** to **improve handling** and **resist degradation** in tissue[Q]	Lost within 21–28 days	Phagocytosis and enzymatic degradation **within 90 days**
Polyglactin (Vicryl)	Braided multifilament	Copolymer of **lactide** and **glycolide**[Q] in a ratio of 90:10, coated with polyglactin and calcium stearate	Approx. 60% remains at 2 weeks; 30% remains at 3 weeks	Hydrolysis minimal until 5-6 weeks; Complete absorption **60–90 days**[Q]
Polyglyconate	Monofilament Dyed or undyed	Copolymer of **glycolic acid** and **trimethylene carbonate**[Q]	Approx. 70% remains at 2 weeks; 55% remains at 3 weeks	Hydrolysis minimal until 8–9 weeks; Complete absorption **180 days**[Q]
Poliglecaprone	Monofilament	Copolymer of **glycolite** and **caprolactone**[Q]	21 days maximum	**90–120 days**[Q]
Polyglycolic acid (Dexon)	Braided multifilament Dyed or undyed Coated or Uncoated	Polymer of **polyglycolic acid**[Q]	Approx. 40% remains at 1 weeks; 20% remains at 3 weeks	**Hydrolysis**[Q] minimal at 2 weeks; significant at 4 weeks; Complete absorption **60–90 days**[Q]
Polydioxanone (PDS)	Monofilament dyed or undyed	**Polyester polymer**[Q]	Approx. 70% remains at 2 weeks; 50% remains at 4 weeks; 14% remains at 8 weeks	**Hydrolysis** minimal at 90 days; Complete absorption **180 days**[Q]

Guidelines for Day of Suture Removal by Area

Body Regions	Removal	Body Regions	Removal
Eyelid	3–4	Chest, abdomen	8–10
Eyebrow	3–5	Ear	10–14
Nose	3–5	Back	12–14
Lip	3–4[Q]	Extremities	12–14
Face (other)	3–4[Q]	Hand	10–14
Scalp	6–8[Q]	Foot, sole	12–14

Annexure 14

NEW DRUGS IN SURGERY

\multicolumn{2}{|c|}{New Drugs in CA Breast}
Ixabepilone	• Used for **anthracycline** and **taxane resistant** breast cancer[Q]
Lapatinib	• Inhibitor of Her-2-neu and EGFR tyrosine kinase • **Second line Her-2-neu therapy**[Q]
Sunitinib	• Approved for **advanced renal cancer** and **refractory metastatic breast cancer**[Q]

\multicolumn{2}{|c|}{New Drugs}
Drug	Indication
Imatinib mesylate	• GIST • CML • 1st line treatment for advanced & unresectable **DFSP** (Dermatofibrosarcoma protuberans)
Sunitinib	• **Imatinib resistant GIST** • **Advanced Renal cancer** • **Refractory metastatic breast cancer**[Q]
Sorafenib	• **Unresectable HCC**[Q]
Geftinib	• **Adenocarcinoma lung in non-smoking females**
Lapatinib	• Inhibitor of Her-2-neu and EGFR tyrosine kinase • **Second line Her-2-neu therapy**[Q]
Vandetanib (EGFR inhibitor)	• Only drug approved by US FDA for treatment of **advanced & progressive MTC**

Annexure 15

INHERITANCE PATTERN

Autosomal Dominant	Autosomal Recessive	X-linked Disorders
• Familial hypercholesterolemia • **HNPCC** • **FAP**[Q] • **BRCA1** and **BRCA2** breast cancer • Hereditary hemorrhagic telangiectasia • **Marfan's syndrome**[Q] • **Hereditary spherocytosis**[Q] • **Adult polycystic kidney disease** • **Huntington's chorea**[Q] • **Acute intermittent porphyria**[Q] • **Osteogenesis imperfecta**[Q] • **von Willebrand's disease**[Q] • **Myotonic dystrophy**[Q] • Familial hypertrophic cardiomyopathy • **Neurofibromatosis**[Q] • **Tuberous sclerosis**[Q] • **Otospongiosis**[Q] • **Achondroplasia**[Q]	• Deafness • **Albinism**[Q] • **Wilson's disease**[Q] • **Hemochromatosis**[Q] • **Sickle cell anemia**[Q] • **β-thalassemia**[Q] • **Cystic fibrosis**[Q] • **Hereditary emphysema** (α_1 **antitrypsin deficiency**) • **Homocystinuria**[Q] • **Friedreich's ataxia**[Q] • **Phenylketonuria**[Q] • **Fanconi's syndrome** • **Gaucher's disease**	• **Hemophilia A**[Q] **(recessive)** • **G6PD deficiency**[Q] **(recessive)** • **Duchenne/Becker muscular dystrophy**[Q] **(recessive)** • Fabry's disease • Ocular albinism • Testicular feminization • Chronic granulomatous disease • **Hypophosphatemic rickets**[Q] **(dominant)** • **Fragile-X syndrome**[Q] **(recessive)** • **Color blindness**[Q]

Annexure 16

MOST COMMON TYPE OF STONES

Most Common Type of Stones	
Gallbladder	Cholesterol^Q (**Mixed** if given in the option)
Pancreas	Calcium carbonate^Q
Kidney	Calcium oxalate^Q
Primary Bladder Stone	Ammonium urate^Q
Secondary Bladder Stone	Uric acid >Struvite^Q
Prostate	Calcium phosphate^Q
Salivary gland (Submandibular)	Calcium carbonate^Q

Annexure 17

IDEAL TIME FOR TREATMENT

Ideal time for Treatment	
Undescended testis	6 months^Q
Hypospadias	6–12 months^Q
Umbilical hernia	5 years^Q
Cleft lip	3–6 months^Q
Cleft palate	6–18 months^Q
Congenital hydrocele	2 years^Q

Annexure 18

IMPORTANT NAMES IN THE FIELD OF SURGERY

Father of **surgery** Father of **Indian surgery**	• Sushruta^Q
Father of **modern surgery**	• Joseph Lister^Q
Father of **modern neurosurgery**	• Harvey Cushing^Q
Father of **modern plastic surgery**	• Harold Gillies^Q
Father of **vascular surgery**	• Rudolph Matas^Q
Father of **pediatric surgery**	• William Edward Ladd^Q
Father of **modern urology**	• Hugh Hampton Young^Q

Annexure 19

INVESTIGATION OF CHOICE

Investigation of Choice			
Barium swallow	Hiatus hernia[Q]	Zenker's diverticula[Q]	Leiomyoma[Q]
Barium meal	Gastric diverticula[Q]		
Barium meal follow-through	Small bowel diverticula[Q]		
Enteroclysis	Crohn's disease[Q]		
Barium enema	Colonic diverticula[Q]		
CECT	Diverticulitis[Q]	Hepatocellular carcinoma[Q] (Triple phase CT)	
	Mesenteric cyst[Q]	Renal cell carcinoma[Q]	
	GI tuberculosis[Q]	Retroperitoneal fibrosis[Q]	
	Acute pancreatitis[Q]	Retroperitoneal sarcoma[Q]	
	Carcinoma pancreas[Q]	Renal tuberculosis[Q]	
	Pancreatic pseudocyst[Q]	ADPKD[Q]	
	Carcinoma gall bladder[Q]	GIST[Q]	
MRI	Brain tumors[Q]		
	Spinal cord tumors[Q]		
	Pancoast tumor[Q]		
	Soft tissue sarcoma[Q]		
	Staging of carcinoma penis[Q]		
Endoscopy with biopsy	Barrett's esophagus[Q]	Carcinoma esophagus[Q]	Carcinoma stomach[Q]
Colonoscopy with biopsy	Carcinoma colon[Q]		
Sigmoidoscopy with biopsy	Carcinoma rectum[Q]		
Proctoscopy with biopsy	Carcinoma anal canal[Q]		
Cystoscopy with biopsy	Carcinoma bladder[Q]		
FNAC	Parotid tumors[Q]	Thyroid malignancies[Q]	
Biopsy	Carcinoma breast	Skin malignancies[Q]	
	Carcinoma penis[Q]	Oral cavity malignancies[Q]	
Manometry	Achalasia cardia[Q] Diffuse esophageal spasm[Q] Nutcrackers esophagus[Q]		
24-hours pH monitoring	GERD[Q]		
Somatostatin receptor scintigraphy (IOC for localization)	All neuroendocrine tumors of pancreas except insulinoma[Q]		
	Carcinoid tumors[Q]		
Ultrasound	Gallstones[Q]	Acute cholecystitis[Q]	Chronic cholecystitis[Q]
MRCP	CBD stone[Q]	PSC	
	Choledochal cyst[Q]	Pancreas divisum	
	Biliary strictures[Q]	Chronic pancreatitis[Q]	

Investigation of Choice	
Acute mesenteric ischemia	• Angiography[Q]
Mesenteric venous thrombosis	• CECT[Q]
Chronic mesenteric ischemia	• Aortography[Q]

Investigation of Choice	
ADPKD	CT scan[Q]
Retroperitoneal Fibrosis	
Medullary Sponge Kidney	IVP[Q]
VUR	MCU[Q]
Retrocaval ureter	MRI[Q]
PUJ Obstruction	DTPA scan[Q]
Renal structure or surface	DMSA scan[Q]

Annexure 20

TUMOR MARKERS

Markers	Associated Cancers	Non-neoplastic Conditions
Hormones		
• Human chorionic gonadotropin • Calcitonin • Catecholamines	• **Trophoblastic tumors**[Q], nonseminomatous testicular tumors • **Medullary carcinoma**[Q] of thyroid • **Pheochromocytoma**[Q]	• Pregnancy
Oncofetal Antigens		
• Alpha-Fetoprotein • CEA	• **Liver**[Q] cell cancer, **nonseminomatous**[Q] germ cell tumor of testis, **lung**[Q] cancer • Adenocarcinoma of the **colon**[Q], **pancreas**[Q], **lung**[Q], **breast**[Q], **ovary**[Q], **prostate**[Q]	• Cirrhosis, hepatitis • Pancreatitis, hepatitis, inflammatory bowel disease, smoking
Isoenzymes		
• Prostatic acid phosphatase • **Neuron-specific enolase** • Lactate dehydrogenase	• Prostate cancer • **Small cell** cancer of **lung**[Q], **Neuroblastoma**[Q] • Lymphoma, Ewing sarcoma	• Prostatitis, prostatic hypertrophy • Hepatitis, hemolytic anemia, many others
Specific proteins		
• **Immunoglobulins** • PSA and prostate specific membrane antigen	• **Multiple myeloma**[Q] and other gammopathies • **Prostate cancer**[Q]	• Infection, MGUS • Prostatitis, prostatic hypertrophy[Q]
Mucins and other Glycoproteins		
• CA-125 • CA-19-9 • CD30 • CD25	• **Cancer of ovary**[Q], fallopian tube, **endometrium**[Q], cervix, **breast**[Q], **lung**[Q], **pancreas**[Q] and **colon**[Q] • **Colon**[Q] cancer, **pancreatic**[Q] cancer • **Hodgkin's disease**[Q], anaplastic large cell lymphoma • **Hairy cell leukemia, adult T cell leukemia/lymphoma**[Q]	• **Pregnancy**[Q], **endometriosis**[Q], **PID**[Q], uterine fibroids[Q] • **Pancreatitis**, Ulcerative colitis

Annexure 21

MOST COMMON

Indications of Liver Transplantation
• **MC indication** for LT: Cirrhosis from Hepatitis C (**HCV**)[Q] • **2nd MC indication** for LT: **Alcoholic liver disease**[Q] • MC indication for LT in **children**: **Biliary atresia**[Q] • MC **metabolic disorder** requiring LT: **Alpha-1 antitrypsin deficiency**[Q] • MC indication for LT following **acute liver failure**: Acetaminophen toxicity[Q]

Pediatric Tumors	
• MC **malignant** tumor of **infancy** • MC **extracranial solid** tumor in **children** • MC **abdominal** malignancy in **children**	Neuroblastoma[Q]
• MC **primary malignant renal** tumor of **childhood**	Wilms' tumor[Q]
• MC **renal tumor** of **infancy**	Congenital mesoblastic nephroma[Q]
• MC **soft tissue** tumor in **infants** and **children**	Rhabdomyosarcoma[Q]
• MC **solid tumor** of **childhood**	Brain tumor[Q]
• MC cancer of childhood	Leukemia[Q] (30%) > Brain tumors[Q] (22%)

MC cancer in **males (PLC)**: Prostate > Lung > Colorectal[Q]
MC cancer in **females (BLC)**: Breast > Lung > Colorectal[Q]
Cancer deaths in **males (LPC)**: Lung > Prostate > Colorectal[Q]
Cancer deaths in **females (LBC)**: Lung > Breast > Colorectal[Q]

Annexure 22

MISCELLANEOUS

- **Widest portion** of colon: **Cecum**^{Q}
- **Narrowest portion** of colon: **Sigmoid**^{Q}
- **MC site** of **colonic rupture** caused **by distal obstruction**: **Cecum**^{Q}
- Colon absorbs water, **NaCl**^{Q}; secretes K^+, HCO_3 and **mucus**^{Q}
- **MC site of ischemic colitis**: Splenic flexure

Sarcomas with Lymph Node Metastasis (MARCES)

- **M**alignant fibrous histiocytoma^Q
- **A**ngiosarcoma^Q
- **R**habdomyosarcoma^Q
- **C**lear cell sarcoma^Q
- **E**pithelial sarcoma^Q
- **S**ynovial sarcoma^Q

Tumors with Spontaneous Regression (NCR MR)

- **N**euroblastoma^Q
- **C**horiocarcinoma^Q
- **R**enal cell carcinoma^Q
- **M**alignant melanoma^Q
- **R**etinoblastoma^Q

Malignancies associated with Migratory Thrombophlebitis

- **CA pancreas (MC)**^{Q}
- **CA lung**^{Q}
- **GI malignancies**^{Q}
- **Prostate cancer**^{Q}
- **Ovarian** cancer^Q
- **Lymphoma**^{Q}

- **Trousseau's syndrome**: Migratory thrombophlebitis^Q
- **Trousseau's sign**: Carpopedal spasm in hypocalcemia^Q
- **Troisier's sign**: Palpable left supraclavicular LN (Virchow's node)^Q

Perineural Spread is seen in

1. **Adenoid cystic carcinoma**^{Q}
2. **CA GB**^{Q}
3. **Cholangiocarcinoma**^{Q}
4. **Ductal adenocarcinoma** of pancreas^Q

Small Round Blue Cell Tumors (WEL PNR)

- Wilms' tumor
- Ewing's sarcoma
- Lymphoma
- Medulloblastoma
- Small cell variant of osteosarcoma
- Primitive neuroectodermal tumor
- Neuroblastoma
- Rhabdomyosarcoma
- Askin tumor
- Desmoplastic small cell tumor

Causes of Postoperative Fever

Day	Cause
2–5 days	**Atelectasis** of the lung^Q
3–5 days	**Superficial** and **deep wound infection**^{Q}
5 days	**Chest infection** including viral respiratory tract infection, **UTI** and **thrombophlebitis**^{Q}
> 5 days	**Wound infection**, anastomotic leakage, intracavitary collections and abscesses^Q

Increased Cancer Risk in Obese Patients (PEEL CP GO KBC)

- Prostate^Q
- Endometrial^Q
- Esophagus^Q
- Liver^Q
- Cervix^Q
- Pancreas^Q
- Gallbladder^Q
- Ovarian^Q
- Kidney^Q
- Bile duct^Q
- Breast^Q
- Colon and rectum^Q

Psammoma Bodies (PSM)
1. **P**apillary carcinoma thyroid[Q]
2. **P**apillary carcinoma (RCC)[Q]
3. **S**erous cystadenoma[Q]
4. **M**eningioma[Q]

Proctoscope	10–12 cm[Q]
Rigid sigmoidoscope	25 cm[Q]
Flexible sigmoidoscope	60 cm[Q]
Colonoscope	160 cm[Q]

• Most radiosensitive **ovarian** tumor	• Dysgerminoma[Q]
• Most radiosensitive **brain** tumor	• Medulloblastoma[Q]
• Most radiosensitive **testicular** tumor	• Seminoma[Q]
• Most radiosensitive **lung** tumor	• Small cell CA[Q]
• Most radiosensitive **kidney** tumor	• Wilms, tumor[Q]
• Most radiosensitive **bone** tumor	• Ewing's Sarcoma[Q] and Multiple myeloma[Q]

Condition	Seen in
• Necrolytic erythema migrans	• Glucagonoma
• Erythema chronicum migrans	• Lyme's disease
• Erythema infectiosum (fifth disease)	• Parvovirus B19
• Erythema marginatum	• Acute rheumatic fever

Screening Immunohistochemistry
• **Epithelial Markers**: **Cytokeratin** (positive in **carcinomas**)[Q]
• **Lymphoid Markers**: **CD-45** (positive in **lymphoma**)[Q]
• **Melanocytic Markers**: **S-100** (positive in **melanoma**)[Q]
• **Mesenchymal Markers**: **Vimentin** (positive in **sarcoma**)[Q]
• **Neuroendocrine Markers**: **Chromagranin** and **neuron-specific enolase**[Q]

Annexure 23

FIRST ORGAN TRANSPLANTATION

First **kidney** transplantation (in **identical twins**)	• **Murray**[Q] (1954)
First **liver** transplantation	• **Starzl**[Q] (1963)
First **pancreas** transplantation	• **Kelly & Lillehei**[Q] (1966)
First **heart** transplantation	• **Christian Barnard**[Q] (1967)
First **lung** transplantation	• **Fritz Derom**[Q] (1968)
First **pancreatic islet cell** transplantation	• **Sutherland**[Q] (1974)
First **heart & lung** transplantation	• **Reitz & Shumway**[Q] (1981)
First successful intestinal transplantation	• Deltz (1988)

Annexure 24

SURGICAL POSITIONS

Supine position	• **MC surgical position**, patient lies with back flat on operating room bed
Trendelenburg position	• Same as supine position but the **upper torso is lowered**^Q
Reverse Trendelenburg position	• Same as supine but **upper torso is raised & legs are lowered**^Q
Fracture Table Position	• **For hip fracture surgery** • **Upper torso** is **in supine position with unaffected leg raised**. Affected leg is extended with no lower support. The leg is strapped at the ankle and there is padding in the groin to keep pressure on the leg and hip
Lithotomy position	• Used for **gynecological, anal & urological procedures**^Q • **Upper torso is placed in the supine position**, legs are raised and secured, **arms are extended**^Q
Fowler's position	• Begins with patient in supine position. **Upper torso is slowly raised to a 90° position**^Q
Semi-Fowler's position	• **Lower torso is in supine position & upper torso is bent at a nearly 85° position**. The patient's head is secured by a restraint
Prone position	• Patient lies with **stomach on the bed**. Abdomen can be raised off the bed
Jackknife position	• Also called the **Kraske position**^Q • Patient's abdomen lies flat on the bed. The **bed is scissored so the hip is lifted & legs & head are low**^Q
Knee-chest position	• Similar to the jackknife except the **legs are bent at the knee at a 90° angle**
Lateral position	• Also called the **side-lying position**, it is like the jackknife except the patient is on his or her side. Other similar positions are Lateral chest & Lateral kidney
Lloyd-Davies position	• Common position for **surgical procedures involving the pelvis & lower abdomen** • **Majority of colorectal & pelvic surgery** is conducted in the **Lloyd-Davis position**^Q
Kidney position	• **Patient's abdomen is placed over a lift in the operating table** that **bends the body to allow access to the retroperitoneal space** • A kidney rest is placed under the patient at the location of the lift
Sims' position	• **Variation of the left lateral position** • Patient will roll to his or her left side. **Keeping the left leg straight, the patient will slide the left hip back and bend the right leg.** This position allows **access to the anus**^Q

Abdominal Examination Signs

Sign	Description	Diagnosis
Aaron sign	**Pain** or pressure **in epigastrium** or **anterior chest** with **persistent firm pressure** applied to **McBurney's point**^Q	**Acute appendicitis**^Q
Bassler sign	Sharp pain created by compressing appendix between abdominal wall and iliacus	Chronic appendicitis
Blumberg's sign	Transient abdominal wall **rebound tenderness**^Q	**Peritoneal inflammation**
Carnett's sign	Loss of abdominal tenderness when abdominal wall muscles are contracted	Intra-abdominal source of abdominal pain
Chandelier sign	Extreme lower abdominal and pelvic pain with movement of cervix	Pelvic inflammatory disease
Claybrook sign	Accentuation of breath and cardiac sounds through abdominal wall	Ruptured abdominal viscus
Courvoisier's sign	**Palpable gallbladder** in presence of **painless jaundice**^Q	**Periampullary tumor**^Q
Cruveilhier sign	**Varicose veins** at **umbilicus (caput medusae)**^Q	**Portal hypertension**^Q
Danforth sign	Shoulder pain on inspiration	Hemoperitoneum
Fothergill's sign	Abdominal wall mass that does not cross midline and remains palpable when rectus contracted	Rectus muscle hematomas
Mannkopf's sign	Increased pulse when painful abdomen palpated	Absent if malingering
Ransohoff sign	**Yellow discoloration** of **umbilical region**	**Ruptured CBD**^Q
Ten Horn sign	**Pain** caused by **gentle traction of right testicle**^Q	**Acute appendicitis**^Q

Annexure 25

IMPORTANT POINTS ABOUT TUMORS

Breast	• **MC type** of breast cancer: **Adenocarcinoma**[Q] • **MC subtype** of breast cancer: **Invasive ductal cancer**[Q] • **Least common type** of breast cancer: **Papillary**[Q] • **Most malignant** type of breast cancer: **Inflammatory breast cancer**[Q] • Breast cancer associated with **best prognosis: Tubular**[Q] • **MC site** of breast cancer: **Upper outer quadrant**[Q] • **Least common site** of breast cancer: **Lower inner quadrant**[Q] • **MC site of metastasis: Bone (Lumbar vertebra >Femur >Thoracic vertebra)**[Q]
Thyroid	• **MC type** of thyroid cancer: **Papillary > Follicular >Medullary > Anaplastic**[Q] • **MC site of metastasis from papillary** carcinoma: **Lungs**[Q] • MC site of metastasis **from follicular carcinoma: Bones**[Q] (Osteolytic secondaries) • MC site of metastasis **from Medullary carcinoma: Liver**[Q] • MC site of metastasis **from anaplastic carcinoma: Lungs**[Q] • **MC primary** responsible **for metastasis to thyroid: CA breast >CA lung**[Q]
Adrenal	• **MC adrenal tumor: Non-functioning adenoma**[Q]
Liver	• **MC malignancy** of liver: **Metastasis**[Q] • **MC primary malignancy** of liver: **HCC**[Q] • MC primary malignancy of liver **in children: Hepatoblastoma**[Q] • **MC benign tumor** of liver: **Hemangioma**[Q]
Spleen	• **MC neoplasm** of spleen: **Lymphoma** (Non-Hodgkin's lymphoma)[Q] • **MC primary tumor** of spleen: **Hemangioma**[Q] • **MC primary malignant tumor** of spleen: **Angiosarcoma**[Q]
Gallbladder	• **MC site** of CA gallbladder: **Fundus (60%) > Body (30%) >Neck (10%)**[Q] • **Maximum incidence** of CA gallbladder: **India > Pakistan**[Q] • **MC histological type** of CA gallbladder: **Diffuse infiltrative** or **sclerosing**[Q]
Bile Duct	• **MC site** of cholangiocarcinoma: **Hilum (65%) >Distal (25%) >Intrahepatic (10%)**[Q] • **MC histological type** of cholangiocarcinoma: **Diffuse infiltrative** or **sclerosing**[Q]
Pancreas	• **MC site** of carcinoma pancreas: **Head**[Q] • **MC site of gastrinoma: Duodenum (1st part) > Pancreas**[Q] • **MC site of insulinoma: Equally distributed in head, body & tail**[Q] • **MC site of glucagonoma & mucinous cystadenoma: Body & tail**[Q] • **MC site of somatostatinoma, PPoma, serous cystadenoma & IPMN: Head**[Q] • **MC site of VIPoma: Tail**[Q]
Esophagus	• **MC type** of carcinoma esophagus: **SCC**[Q] • MC type of carcinoma esophagus **in western population: Adenocarcinoma**[Q] • **MC site of SCC** esophagus: **Middle 1/3rd**[Q] • **MC site of Adenocarcinoma** esophagus: **Lower 1/3rd**[Q] • **MC site of carcinoma esophagus: Middle 1/3rd**[Q]
Stomach	• **MC site of carcinoma stomach, gastric lymphoma: Antrum**[Q] • **MC site of carcinoma stomach in pernicious anemia: Fundus**[Q] • **MC site of diffuse variety of carcinoma stomach: Fundus**[Q]
Small intestine	• **MC tumor** of small bowel: **Stromal tumor >Adenoma**[Q] • **MC tumor of small bowel in children: Lymphoma**[Q] • **MC malignant tumor** of small bowel: **Adenocarcinoma**[Q] **>Carcinoid** • **MC site of carcinoid, adenoma, lipoma, lymphoma, leiomyoma: Ileum**[Q] • **MC site of adenocarcinoma: Duodenum**[Q]
Colon-Rectum	• **MC site of colorectal cancer: Rectum**[Q] • **Least common site** of colorectal cancer: **Hepatic flexure**[Q] • **MC site of colon cancer: Sigmoid**[Q]

Contd...

Contd...

Appendix	• **MC neoplasm** of appendix: **Carcinoid tumor**^Q • **MC malignant neoplasm** of appendix: **Mucinous adenocarcinoma > Adenocarcinoma >Carcinoid tumor**^Q
Anal canal	• **MC type** of carcinoma anal canal: **SCC>BCC>Melanoma**^Q
Kidney	• **MC type** of RCC: **Clear cell** carcinoma^Q • **MC type** of RCC seen **in dialysis associated disease**: **Papillary** carcinoma^Q • Type of RCC with **best prognosis**: **Chromophobe** carcinoma^Q
Urinary bladder	• **MC type** of carcinoma bladder: **TCC >SCC >Adenocarcinoma**^Q • **MC benign mesenchymal tumor** of urinary bladder: **Leiomyoma**^Q • **MC malignant mesenchymal tumor** of urinary bladder: **Leiomyosarcoma**^Q • **MC malignant mesenchymal tumor** of urinary bladder **in children**: **Rhabdomyosarcoma**^Q
Prostate	• **MC type** of carcinoma prostate: **Adenocarcinoma >TCC**^Q • **MC site** of carcinoma prostate: **Peripheral zone (75%) >Transition zone (15%) >Central zone (10%)**^Q
Penis & Urethra	• **MC type** of carcinoma penis: **SCC**^Q • **MC site** of carcinoma penis: **Glans >Prepuce >Shaft (GPS)**^Q • **MC site** of carcinoma male urethra: **Bulbomembranous urethra**^Q • **MC type** of carcinoma **prostatic urethra**: **TCC >SCC**^Q • **MC type** of carcinoma **penile urethra**: **SCC >TCC**^Q
Testis	• MC **histological type** of testicular tumour: **Seminoma**^Q (**Mixed**^Q if given in the option) • MC **bilateral primary testicular tumour**: **Seminoma**^Q • **Most radiosensitive** testicular tumor: **Seminoma**^Q • MC testicular tumor in **infant & children up to 3 years**: **Yolk sac tumour**^Q • Testicular tumour with **best prognosis**: **Yolk sac tumour**^Q • MC testicular tumor in **pre-pubertal children**: **Teratoma**^Q • **MC testicular tumor** in patients **>60 years**: **Lymphoma**^Q • MC **bilateral testicular tumour**: **Lymphoma**^Q • MC **secondary testicular tumour**: **Lymphoma**^Q • MC **histologic type** of testicular lymphoma: **DLBL**^Q • Testicular tumour with **worst prognosis**: **Hurricane tumour (Type of choriocarcinoma)**^Q
Scrotum	• **MC benign lesion** of scrotum: **Sebaceous cyst**^Q • **MC malignant tumor** of scrotum: **SCC**^Q
Lung	**Adenocarcinoma** • MC histological **type**^Q • MC in **non-smokers, young** patients, **females**^Q • Located **peripherally**^Q • **Slow growth** & propensity to **metastasize** to **opposite lung**^Q • **Metastasize** more frequently to **CNS**^Q • Most cells contain **mucin**^Q • **Noguchi classification**^Q is used for adenocarcinoma **Squamous Cell Carcinoma** • MC in **smokers**^Q; MC type in **India**^Q • MC variety associated with **hypercalcemia (produces PTH-rp)**^Q • **Central**^Q in distribution • Prone to undergo **central necrosis & cavitation**^Q • **Pancoast** tumor is histologically **SCC**^Q • Associated with **best prognosis**^Q

Contd...

Contd...

	Small Cell Carcinoma	• Most malignant, central^Q in distribution, strongly related to smoking^Q • Associated with massive hilar or mediastinal lymphadenopathy, mediastinal invasion & perihilar mass^Q • MC variety associated with paraneoplastic syndrome, hypokalemia & SVC syndrome^Q • Most responsive to chemotherapy (cisplatin + etoposide) • Shows response to radiotherapy^Q • Hormones produced by small cell carcinoma: ACTH, AVP (vasopressin), calcitonin, ANF, gastrin releasing peptide^Q
	Large Cell Carcinoma	• Highly undifferentiated with cavitating nature^Q • Metastasize early with poor prognosis^Q
Heart		• MC cardiac tumor: Metastasis^Q • MC primary cardiac tumor: Myxoma^Q • MC primary cardiac tumor in infants & children: Rhabdomyoma^Q
Brain		• MC brain tumor: Metastasis^Q • MC primary brain tumor: Meningioma (35%) > Glial tumors (30%)^Q • MC malignant brain tumor of children: Medulloblastoma^Q • Most radiosensitive brain tumor: Medulloblastoma^Q • MC astrocytoma in children: Pilocytic astrocytoma^Q • MC astrocytoma in adults: Glioblastoma multiforme^Q • Astrocytoma is supratentorial in adults & infratentorial in children^Q • Maximum incidence of calcification in brain tumor: Craniopharyngioma (most) >Oligodendroglioma (90%) >Meningioma (25%)^Q • MC pituitary tumor: Adenoma^Q (arising from anterior lobe)
Oral cavity		• MC site of CA oral cavity: Tongue >Lip^Q • MC histological type of CA oral cavity: Squamous cell carcinoma^Q • MC type of cancer in India: CA oral cavity^Q • MC site of CA oral cavity in India: Buccal mucosa^Q (38%) > Anterior tongue (16%) >Lower alveolus (15.7%) • LN metastasis is most common in: CA tongue^Q >Floor of mouth >Lower alveolus >Buccal mucosa >Upper alveolus >Hard palate >Lip^Q • Bilateral lymphatic spread is common in: Lower lip^Q, supraglottis^Q & soft palate^Q
Salivary gland		• MC neoplasm of salivary gland: Pleomorphic adenoma^Q • MC malignant tumor of salivary gland: Mucoepidermoid carcinoma^Q • MC neoplasm of salivary gland in children: Hemangioma^Q • MC malignant tumor of salivary gland in children: Mucoepidermoid carcinoma^Q • MC malignant tumor of minor salivary glands: Adenoid cystic carcinoma^Q
Sarcoma		• MC site of GIST: Stomach >Small bowel >Colorectum & esophagus^Q • MC soft tissue sarcoma in adults: Liposarcoma >Leiomyosarcoma >Malignant fibrous histiocytoma^Q • MC soft tissue sarcoma of extremities: Malignant fibrous histiocytoma > Liposarcoma^Q • MC soft tissue sarcoma of retroperitoneum: Liposarcoma^Q • MC pediatric soft tissue sarcoma: Rhabdomyosarcoma^Q
Bone		• MC site of primary for bone metastasis: CA Breast > CA Prostate >RCC >CA Lung > CA Thyroid > CA Bladder (BP increased by RL in TB)^Q • MC site of bone metastasis: Thoracic vertebra^Q • MC cause of osteoblastic secondaries in males: CA Prostate^Q • MC cause of osteolytic secondaries in males: RCC^Q • Lytic expansile metastasis is seen in: RCC & follicular carcinoma thyroid^Q • MC cause of osteoblastic & osteolytic secondaries in females: CA Breast^Q • MC tumor metastasize to bone in females: CA Breast^Q

Annexure 26

NAMED OPERATIONS

Named Operations	Done for
• Hadfield's operation^Q	Duct ectasia^Q
• Sistrunk operation^Q	Thyroglossal cyst^Q
• Hartley-Dunhill procedure^Q	Subtotal thyroidectomy^Q (10-12 gm of thyroid remnant is left in the same lobe)
• Puestow procedure^Q • Duval procedure^Q • Beger's procedure^Q • Frey's procedure^Q	Chronic Pancreatitis^Q
• Whipple's procedure^Q • Traverso-Longmire procedure^Q	Periampullary carcinoma^Q
• Kasai procedure^Q	Extrahepatic biliary atresia^Q
• Nissen's fundoplication^Q	GERD^Q
• Heller's cardiomyotomy^Q	Achalasia cardia^Q
• Ivor-Lewis operation^Q • Orringer transhiatal esophagectomy^Q • Mckeon en-bloc esophagectomy^Q	Carcinoma esophagus^Q
• Shoemaker procedure^Q • Pouchet procedure^Q • Kelling-Madlener procedure^Q • Csendes procedure^Q	Type IV gastric ulcer^Q
• Ramstedt-Fredet pyloromyotomy^Q	Infantile hypertrophic pyloric stenosis^Q
• Bishop-Koop operation^Q	Meconium ileus^Q
• Bianchi procedure^Q	Short bowel syndrome^Q
• Ladd's operation^Q	Malrotation of gut^Q
• Swenson operation^Q • Duhamel operation^Q • Soave operation^Q	Hirschsprung's disease^Q
• Hartmann's procedure^Q	Carcinoma sigmoid colon^Q
• Kocher's maneuver^Q	Mobilization of duodenum^Q
• Extended Kocher's maneuver^Q	Right sided medial visceral rotation^Q
• Mattox maneuver^Q	Left sided medial visceral rotation^Q
• Cattell-Braasch maneuver^Q	For extensive retroperitoneal exposure^Q
• Mitrofanoff's procedure^Q	Appendicovesicostomy^Q
• Malone procedure^Q	Appendicolostomy^Q
• Milligan-Morgan open hemorrhoidectomy^Q • Ferguson closed hemorrhoidectomy^Q • Whitefield submucosal hemorrhoidectomy^Q • Longo's stapler hemorrhoidectomy^Q	Hemorrhoidectomy^Q
• Well's procedure^Q • Ripstein procedure^Q • Frykman & Goldberg procedure^Q	Abdominal rectopexy^Q
• Delorme's mucosectomy^Q • Thiersch anal encirclement^Q • Altmier's rectosigmoidectomy^Q	Perineal rectopexy^Q
• Lord's procedure^Q • Notara's lateral sphincterostomy^Q	Fissure in ano^Q
• Bascom procedure^Q • Karydakis procedure^Q	Pilonidal sinus^Q

Contd...

Contd...

Named Operations	Done for
• **Bassini** repair, **Shouldice** repair^Q • **McVay** repair^Q • **Lichtenstein** repair^Q	**Inguinal hernia**^Q
• **Lockwood** operation^Q • **Lothiessen** operation^Q • **McEvedy** operation^Q • **Henry** procedure^Q	**Femoral hernia**^Q
• **Dowd's** operation^Q	**Lumbar hernia**^Q
• **Mayo's** repair^Q	**Umbilical hernia**^Q
• **Rovsing's** operation^Q	**Deroofing of cyst in ADPKD**^Q (**Rovsing's sign**: Pain in right lower quadrant during palpation of left lower quadrant in **acute appendicitis**) (**Rovsing's syndrome**: Abdominal pain, nausea & vomiting on hyperextension of spine in **horse shoe kidney**)
• **Anderson Hynes dismembered pyeloplasty**^Q	**PUJ obstruction**^Q
• **Lich-Gregoir** technique^Q • **Leadbetter-Politano** technique^Q	**Methods of ureteric implantation in VUR**^Q
• **Boari's** operation^Q	**Lower ureteric reconstruction** with a strip of bladder wall
• **Frayer's suprapubic** prostatectomy^Q • **Millin's retropubic** prostatectomy^Q • **Young's perineal** prostatectomy^Q	**Open prostatectomy for BPH**^Q
• **Dennis-Brown** technique^Q • **MAGPI**^Q • **Mathiew** procedure^Q • **Asopa or Duckett** technique^Q • **Thiersch-Duplay or Bracka** technique^Q	**Hypospadias**^Q
• **Winter** shunt^Q • **Al-Ghorab** shunt^Q • **Quackel or Sacher** shunt^Q • **Grayhack** shunt^Q • **Barry** shunt^Q	**Surgical management of ischemic priapism**^Q
• **Nesbitt** operation^Q	**Peyronie's disease**^Q
• **Fowler-Stephens** orchiopexy^Q • **Ladd & Gross** orchiopexy^Q • **Ombridann's** orchiopexy^Q • **Keetley-Torek** orchiopexy^Q	**Undescended Testis**^Q
• **Lord's plication of sac**^Q	**Small hydrocele**^Q
• **Jaboulay's eversion of sac**^Q	**Medium sized hydrocele**^Q
• **Palomo's** operation^Q	**Varicocele**^Q
• **Trendelenberg** operation^Q	**Varicose vein**^Q
• **Gilles, Neibulowitz & Kinmonth** procedure^Q	**Reconstructive operation for lymphedema**^Q
• **Kontoleons, Homans, Thompson & Charles** procedure^Q	**Excisional operation for lymphedema**^Q
• **Moh's micrographic surgery**^Q	**BCC or SCC** involving **vital areas, cosmetic areas** or **recurrent tumors**^Q
• **COMMANDO's** operation^Q	**COM**bined **M**andibulectomy **A**nd **N**eck **D**issection **O**peration for **carcinoma tongue fixed to mandible** with **infiltration of floor of mouth**^Q.
• **Newman & Seabrocks'** operation^Q	**Parotid fistula**^Q
• **Millard rotation advancement technique**^Q • **Thompson, Le Musurier & Tennison-Randall** operation^Q	**Cleft lip repair**^Q

Annexure 27

DIFFUSE LARGE B CELL LYMPHOMA (DLBL) IS MC TYPE OF LYMPHOMA IN

- **Primary CNS lymphoma**[Q] (in immunocompetent patients)
- **Orbital** lymphoma[Q]
- **Thyroid** lymphoma[Q]
- **Breast** lymphoma[Q]
- **Gastric** lymphoma[Q]
- **Small intestinal** lymphoma[Q]
- **Appendicular** lymphoma[Q]
- **Colorectal** lymphoma[Q]
- **Testicular** lymphoma[Q]

Annexure 28

TRIANGLES IN SURGERY

Calot's triangle	- Superiorly: **Cystic artery**[Q] - Medially: **Common hepatic duct**[Q] - Laterally: **Cystic duct**[Q]
Hepatocystic triangle	- Superiorly: **Inferior surface** of **liver**[Q] - Medially: **Common hepatic duct**[Q] - Laterally: **Cystic duct**[Q]
Femoral triangle	- Superiorly: **Inguinal ligament**[Q] - Medially: Medial border of **adductor longus** muscle[Q] - Laterally: Medial border of **sartorius** muscle[Q] (**Femoral artery pulsations** are felt at this site[Q])
Inferior triangle of Petit	- Inferiorly: **Iliac crest**[Q] - Medially: **Latissimus dorsi muscle**[Q] - Laterally: **External oblique muscle**[Q]
Superior triangle of Grynfeltt	- Superiorly: **12th rib**[Q] - Medially: **Paraspinal muscles**[Q] - Laterally: **Internal oblique muscle**[Q]
Scalene triangle	- Anteriorly: **Scalenus anticus**[Q] - Posteriorly: **Scalenus medius**[Q] - Inferiorly: **First rib**[Q] (Trunk of **Brachial plexus & subclavian vessels** are **compressed** at Scalene triangle causing **thoracic outlet syndrome**[Q])
Sherren's triangle	- Bounded by lines joining **anterior superior iliac spine, pubic tubercle & umbilicus**[Q] - Area of **skin hyperaesthesia in acute appendicitis**[Q]
Simon's triangle	- Superiorly: **Inferior thyroid artery**[Q] - Laterally: **Common carotid artery**[Q] - Medially: **Esophagus**[Q] (**Simon's triangle** aids in **identification of recurrent laryngeal nerve**[Q])
Joll's triangle	- Laterally: **Upper pole** of thyroid gland & **superior thyroid vessels**[Q] - Superiorly: Attachment of **strap muscles & deep investing layer of fascia to hyoid**[Q] - Medially: **Midline**[Q] - Floor: **Cricothyroid muscle**[Q] (**External branch of superior laryngeal nerve** lies **in Joll's triangle**[Q])

Contd...

Contd...

Triangle of **Auscultation**	• Superiorly & medially: **Inferior portion of trapezius** • Inferiorly: **Upper border of latissimus dorsi** • Laterally: **Medial border of scapula** (Only part of back **not covered by muscles, respiratory sounds** are better heard)
Triangle of **Doom**	• Bounded **laterally** by the **gonadal vessels**[Q] • **Medially** by the **vas deferens**[Q] • **Apex** oriented superiorly at the **internal ring**[Q] (Contain **external iliac vessels**[Q], deep circumflex iliac vein, the femoral nerve & genital branch of the genitofemoral nerve)
Triangle of **Hesselbach**[Q]	• Laterally: **Epigastric artery**[Q] • Medially: **Lateral border** of **rectus abdominis**[Q] where it is attached to pubic crest • Inferiorly: **Inguinal ligament**[Q]

Triangle of **Pain**	• Medially: **Gonadal vessels**[Q]
	• Superiorly: **Iliopubic tract**[Q]
	• Laterally: **Peritoneum**[Q]
	• This triangle **contains** from lateral to medial:
	  – **Lateral femoral cutaneous nerve**[Q] (MC injured nerve[Q])
	  – **Anterior femoral cutaneous**[Q]
	  – **Femoral branch** of the **genitofemoral nerve**[Q]
	  – **Femoral nerve**[Q]

Annexure 29

PREOPERATIVE & PREPROCEDURE MEDICATION INSTRUCTION GUIDELINES (PPAC FORM 5)

Preoperative & Preprocedure Medication Instruction Guidelines (PPAC Form 5)	
Instruct patients to take the following medications with a small sip of water EVEN IF OTHERWISE NPO:	
Antihypertensive medications	• **Continue** on the day of the operation or procedure[Q]
Diuretics	• **Continue** on the day of the operation or procedure[Q]
Cardiac medications (digoxin)	• **Continue** on the day of the procedure[Q]
Antidepressant, antianxiety & psychiatric medications	• **Continue** on the day of the operation or procedure[Q]
Thyroid medications	• **Continue** on the day of the operation or procedure[Q]
Birth control pills	• **Continue** on the day of the operation or procedure[Q]
Eye drops	• **Continue** on the day of the operation or procedure[Q]
Heartburn or reflux medications (Prilosec, Zantac)	• **Continue** on the day of the operation or procedure[Q]
Narcotic pain medications	• **Continue** on the day of the operation or procedure[Q]
Antiseizure medications	• **Continue** on the day of the operation or procedure[Q]
Asthma medications	• **Continue** on the day of the operation or procedure[Q]
Steroids (oral & inhaled)	• **Continue** on the day of the operation or procedure[Q]
Statins (e.g., Zocor, Lipitor)	• **Continue** on the day of the operation or procedure[Q]
Aspirin	• **Usually continue; discontinue 7 days before plastic surgery & surgery on retina**[Q]
COX-2 inhibitors	• **Continue** on the day of the operation or procedure unless the surgeon specifies[Q] (usually concerned about bone healing)
NSAIDs	• **Usually continue; discontinue 48 hours before plastic surgery & surgery on retina**[Q]
Vitamins, iron, Premarin	• **Discontinue** on the day of the operation or procedure[Q]

Contd...

Contd...

Preoperative & Preprocedure Medication Instruction Guidelines (PPAC Form 5)	
Topical medications (creams & ointments)	• **Discontinue** on the day of the operation or procedure^Q
Oral hypoglycemic drugs	• **Discontinue on** the day of the operation or procedure^Q
Insulin	• **For all patients, discontinue all regular or combination** (70/30 preparations) insulin on the day of the operation or procedure^Q • **Type 2 diabetics should discontinue *all*** insulins of any type^Q • **Type 1 diabetics** should take **a small amount (usually ⅓) of their usual AM longacting insulin** (e.g., Lente or NPH) **on the day of the operation or procedure**^Q • **Type 1 diabetics should not take any short-acting insulin such as regular insulin** on the day of the procedure^Q • Patients with an **insulin pump should continue** their **basal rate *only***^Q
Viagra, Levitra, Cialis or similar drugs	• **Discontinue 36 hours before surgery**^Q
Warfarin (Coumadin)	• **Discontinue 4 days before surgery** except for patients undergoing cataract surgery without a bulbar block^Q
Plavix (**clopidogrel**)	• **Discontinue 7 days before surgery** except for vascular patients or those undergoing cataract surgery^Q
Herbals & nonvitamin supplements	• **Discontinue 7 days before surgery**^Q
MAOIs	• Patients taking these antidepressant medications need an **anesthesia consultation before surgery** (preferably **3 weeks before surgery**)^Q
COX, cyclooxygenase; MAOIs, monoamine oxidase inhibitors; NPO, nothing by mouth; NSAIDs, nonsteroidal anti-inflammatory drugs.	

Annexure 30

Condition	Most Commonly occurs on
Parathyroid insufficiency	2nd–5th day^Q
Duodenal stump blowout	4th–7th day^Q
Bowel anastomotic leak	7th day^Q
Wound dehiscence	5th–8th day^Q
T-tube cholangiogram	7th–10th day^Q
Perforation in typhoid ulcer	3rd week^Q

Condition	Location
Hemorrhoids	3, 7 & 11'O clock position^Q
Vascular supply of bile duct	Co-axial 3'O clock & 9'O clock position^Q
TUIP (Transurethral incision of prostate)	Incision at 5 & 7'O clock position^Q
Fissure-in-ano	6'O clock position^Q
Endoscopic sphincterotomy	11'O clock position^Q
Optical internal urethrotomy	12'O clock position^Q
MC position of appendix	12'O clock position^Q (Retrocecal)

Annexure 31

Condition	MC Organism Responsible
- Breast abscess - Splenic abscess - Acute pyelonephritis (hematogenous spread) - Carbuncle - Hand infections	- Staphylococcus aureus^Q
Acute suppurative thyroiditis	- Staphylococcus aureus^Q > Streptococcus^Q
- Pyogenic liver abscess	- In Western countries: E. coli^Q - In Asian countries: Klebsiella pneumoniae^Q - In children with chronic granulomatous disease: Staphylococcus aureus^Q
Amoebic liver abscess	- Entamoeba histolytica^Q
Hydatid cyst	- Echinococcus granulosus^Q
Emphysematous cholecystitis	- Clostridium welchii^Q (anaerobe) > E. coli^Q (aerobe)
- Emphysematous pyelonephritis - Acute pyelonephritis (ascending form) - Chronic pyelonephritis - Perinephric abscess - UTI - Acute & chronic bacterial prostatitis - Prostatic abscess - Infected pancreatic necrosis	- E. coli^Q
Xanthogranulomatous pyelonephritis	- Proteus^Q
Cholangitis	- E. coli^Q > Klebsiella^Q
Peptic ulcer MALT lymphoma	- H. pylori^Q
Spontaneous bacterial peritonitis	- In adults: E. coli^Q - In children: Group 'A' Streptococci^Q
Secondary bacterial peritonitis	- Bacteroides^Q (anaerobe) > E. coli^Q (aerobe)
Peritonitis in CAPD	- Staphylococcus epidermidis^Q
Acute mesenteric lymphadenitis	- Yersinia enterocolitica^Q
Gastrointestinal tuberculosis Genitourinary tuberculosis	- Mycobacterium tuberculosis^Q
Appendicular perforation	- Bacteroides^Q (anaerobe) > E. coli^Q (aerobe)
Anorectal abscess	- E. coli^Q > Bacteroides^Q
OPSI (Overwhelming post-splenectomy infection)	- Streptococcus pneumoniae^Q
Struvite stone (Staghorn calculi)	- Proteus^Q
Schistosomiasis	- Schistosoma hematobium^Q
Acute epididymo-orchitis	- Sexually active male <35 years: Chlamydia^Q - Children, elderly males, homosexuals: E. coli^Q
Mycotic aneurysm	- Staphylococcus aureus^Q > Salmonella^Q
Lymphedema	- Wuchereria bancrofti^Q
Burn sepsis	- Pseudomonas^Q
Cellulitis	- Streptococcus pyogenes^Q
Erysipelas	- Beta-hemolytic group 'A' Streptococci^Q
Gas gangrene	- Clostridium perfringens^Q
Chronic burrowing ulcer (Meleney gangrene)	- Microaerophilic non-hemolytic Streptococci^Q

Annexure 32

Etiology	Type of Renal Calculus
• Laxative abuse	**Ammonium urate**[Q]
• Thiazide • Ileostomy	**Uric acid**[Q]
• Primary hyperparathyroidism • Crohn's disease • Short bowel syndrome • Excess intake of spinach, rhubarb, tea, chocolate & pepper	**Calcium oxalate**[Q]
• Ethylene glycol	**Oxalate stone**[Q]
• Inflammatory bowel disease	**Calcium oxalate > Uric acid**[Q]
• Allopurinol	**Xanthine stone**[Q]
• Renal tubular acidosis	**Calcium phosphate**[Q]

SECTION 1

Endocrine Surgery

CHAPTERS

- ☐ Breast
- ☐ Thyroid
- ☐ Parathyroid and Adrenal Glands

CHAPTER 1

Breast

NIPPLE DISCHARGE

Nipple Discharge

- **Unilateral, spontaneous, serous** or **serosanguinous discharge** from a **single duct** is usually caused by an **intraductal papilloma**[Q], or rarely by an **intraductal cancer.**
- **Mostly** the underlying **cause** is a **duct papilloma** or **duct ectasia**[Q], but since the **chances** of **malignancy** are high, it must be investigated further.
- **Risk of malignancy** increases if an **underlying mass**[Q] is present.[Q]

Causes of Nipple Discharge	
Colour	**Cause**
Blood-stained	• **Duct papilloma**[Q] **(MC)** • Intraductal carcinoma[Q] • Duct ectasia[Q]
Serous	• **Fibrocystic disease**[Q] • Duct ectasia[Q] • Carcinoma[Q]
Black, green, paste like or grumous discharge	• Duct ectasia[Q]

Investigations
- **Mammography:** Can show underlying suspicious lesions
- **Cytological examination:** (may identify malignant cells, but a negative finding does not rule out cancer)

Ductography

- **Primary indication:** Nipple discharge[Q] (particularly when the fluid contains **blood**)
- Radiopaque contrast media is injected into one or more of the major ducts and mammography is performed
- **Intraductal papillomas: Small filling defects**[Q] surrounded by contrast media
- **Cancers: Irregular masses** or as **multiple intraluminal filling defects**[Q]
- **Duct ectasia: Dilated cystic structure**[Q]

- **Ultrasound:** May show presence of an underlying mass or duct ectasia

Final Diagnosis
- Final diagnosis is made by **excising** the **involved duct (Microdochectomy)**[Q] and any **underlying mass** if present and subjecting then for a histopathological diagnosis.
- **Radical duct excision** (removal of all lactiferous ducts) is **not done**[Q].

Treatment
- Firstly **exclude a carcinoma** by **occult blood test** and **cytology.**
- **Simple reassurance** may then be sufficient but, if the **discharge** is proving **intolerable,** an **operation** to remove the **affected duct** or **ducts** can be performed **(microdochectomy).**

CARCINOMA BREAST: RISK FACTORS

Risk Factors for Breast Cancer

1. **Age:** Incidence **increases with age**[Q]
2. **Country of birth:** More common in **western countries**[Q]
3. **Family history** and **genetic risk factors** (BRCA)[Q]
4. **Hyperestrogenemia:**
   - **Early menarche**[Q], **late menopause**[Q]
   - **Nulliparity**[Q]
   - **Obesity**[Q]
5. **Late first** full term **pregnancy**[Q]
6. **Alcohol** and **high fat diet**[Q]
7. **Personal history** of malignancy:
   - Contralateral breast cancer[Q]
   - **Ovarian** and **endometrial cancer**[Q]
8. Previous **benign breast disease**[Q]
9. **High socioeconomic status**[Q]
10. **Radiation** exposure[Q]
11. **Hormone replacement therapy**[Q]

- Combined (estrogen + progesterone) HRT is associated with **increased risk** of CA breast.^{Q}
- Only estrogen HRT is **not associated** with increased **risk of CA breast**^{Q}.

> - **Smoking**^{Q} and **OCPs**^{Q} does not appear to **increase risk** of **breast cancer**
> - **Longer duration** of **breast feeding** has a **protective effect**^{Q}

BRCA-1	BRCA-2
• Chromosome: **17**^{Q}	• Chromosome: **13**^{Q}
• **BRCA-1 associated** breast cancers:	• **BRCA-2 associated** cancers:
– Invasive **ductal carcinomas**	– Invasive ductal carcinomas
– **Poorly differentiated**^{Q}	– **Well differentiated**^{Q}
– **Hormone-receptor negative**^{Q}	– **Hormone-receptor positive**^{Q}.
– **Early age** of **onset**	– **Early age** of onset
– **Bilateral**	– **Bilateral**
• Associated **ovarian, colon and prostate cancers**^{Q}.	• Associated **ovarian, colon, prostate, pancreas, gall-bladder, stomach** cancers and **melanoma**^{Q}.

Carcinoma Breast Risk Assessment Models

Gail Model^Q	Claus Model^Q

• **Most frequently used** model
• Incorporates:
  1. **Age** at **menarche**
  2. **Number** of **breast biopsies**
  3. **Age** at **first live birth**
  4. **Number** of **first-degree relatives** with breast cancer
• Predicts the **cumulative risk of breast cancer** according to decade of life
	• Based on assumptions about the prevalence of high-penetrance breast cancer susceptibility genes.
	• Incorporates **more information about family history** but excludes other risk factors.
	• Estimates of breast cancer risk according to: **decade of life** based on presence of **1st** and **2nd-degree relatives** with breast cancer and their **age** at **diagnosis**.

- Risk factors that are less consistently associated with breast cancer (diet, use of OCPs, lactation) or are rare in the general population (radiation exposure) are not included in either the Gail or Claus risk assessment model
- None of these models accounts for the risk associated with mutations in BRCA-1 & BRCA-2

CARCINOMA IN SITU

Ductal Carcinoma in Situ

- Although **DCIS** is **predominantly** seen in the **female breast**, it accounts for 5% of **male breast** cancers.
- DCIS carries a **high risk for progression** to an **invasive cancer**^{Q}.
- DCIS is **classified** on the basis of **nuclear grade & presence of necrosis**^{Q}

Pathology
- Proliferation of epithelium that lines the minor ducts, resulting in **papillary growths within** the **duct lumina**.
- Papillary growths (**papillary growth pattern**) eventually coalesce & fill the duct lumina so that only scattered, rounded spaces remain between the clumps of atypical cancer cells, which show **hyperchromasia** and **loss of polarity (cribriform growth pattern)**.
- Eventually pleomorphic cancer cells with **frequent mitotic figures obliterate** the **lumina & distend** the **ducts (solid growth pattern)**.
- With continued growth, these cells outstrip their blood supply and become **necrotic (comedo growth pattern)**.

Histological Types of DCIS
- **Low Grade:** Cribriform, Papillary & Micropapillary^Q
- **High Grade:** Solid & Comedocarcinoma^Q

Diagnosis
- **Calcium deposition** occurs in the areas of necrosis and is a common feature seen on mammography^Q.
- **DCIS** most frequently **presents** as **mammographic calcifications**^{Q}.

Treatment
- **Non-palpable DCIS:** Section by **needle localisation** technique with **specimen mammography** to ensure that all visible evidence of cancer is excised
- **Low grade DCIS** (cribriform or papillary subtype <0.5 cm in diameter): **Lumpectomy** alone if margins are widely free of disease
- **DCIS with limited disease:** Lumpectomy + Radiotherapy^Q
- **DCIS with Extensive disease** (>4 cm in diameter or disease in >1 quadrant): **Mastectomy**^{Q}

	LCIS	DCIS
• Age (years)	• 44–47 (Early)	• 54–58 (Late)^Q
• Incidence	• 2–5% (Less common)	• 5–10% (More common)^Q
• Clinical signs	• None	• Mass, pain, nipple discharge
• Mammographic signs	• None	• **Microcalcifications**^Q
• Premenopausal	• 2/3^Q	• 1/3
• Incidence of synchronous invasive carcinoma	• 5%	• 2–46%^Q
• Multicentricity	• 60–90%^Q	• 40–80%
• Bilaterality	• 50–70%^Q	• 10–20%
• Axillary metastasis	• 1%	• 1–2%^Q
• **Subsequent carcinomas:**		
• Incidence	• 25–35%	• 25–70%^Q
• Laterality	• **Bilateral**^Q	• Ipsilateral
• Interval to diagnosis	• **15–20 years**^Q	• 5–10 years
• Histologic type	• Ductal	• Ductal

LOBULAR CARCINOMA

- LCIS originates from the **terminal duct lobular units** and develops **only in** the **female breast**^Q.
- LCIS is mostly multicentric & bilateral
- Increased **risk of invasive carcinoma** is in the **both breasts**^Q.

Histopathology
- Characterized by **distention & distortion** of **terminal duct lobular units**^Q by cancer cells
- **Cytoplasmic mucoid globules**^Q are a distinctive cellular feature.
- **Histologic hallmark** of **invasive** lobular carcinoma is **tendency** of **tumor cells** to **invade in linear strands (Indian file pattern)**^Q

Clinical Characteristics
- **Presenting symptom** in most cases is **breast mass with ill-defined margins**
- Usually presents as an **incidental finding**^Q, on breast biopsy performed for other indication.
- Average age at diagnosis: **44-47 years**; more common in **white women**^Q
- **Invasive breast cancer** develops in **25-35%** of women with LCIS, **in either breast**, regardless of which breast harbored the initial focus of LCIS, and is **detected synchronously** with **LCIS** in 5% of cases.
- In women with LCIS, up to **65%** of subsequent **invasive cancers** are **ductal**, not lobular, in origin.
- **Marker** of **increased risk** for **invasive breast cancer**^Q rather than as an anatomic precursor.
- **Invasive lobular carcinoma: Different pattern** of metastases, propensity to **involve peritoneal surface & meninges**^Q, less likely to metastasize to lungs or bone.

Diagnosis
- **Calcifications** associated with LCIS typically **occur in adjacent tissues (neighborhood calcification)**^Q
- **Neighborhood calcification** is a **unique feature** of **LCIS**^Q and contributes to its diagnosis.

Treatment
- **Observation/Chemoprevention/Prophylactic bilateral mastectomy**^Q

CARCINOMA BREAST

BREAST CANCER

- MC cancer in **women** in the **world**^Q and **MC** cancer in **urban**^Q women in India
- MC type is **adenocarcinoma**^Q and most carcinoma arises from **terminal duct lobular unit**^Q
- MC type of CA breast: **Invasive ductal (schirrous) carcinoma**^Q
- **Least common type** of CA breast: **Papillary**^Q

  - **Most malignant** type of CA breast: **Inflammatory breast cancer**^Q
  - **Best prognosis** is seen in: **Tubular**^Q
  - **MC site** of CA breast: Upper outer **quadrant**^Q (left^Q breast >right)
  - **Least common** site of CA breast: **Lower inner quadrant**^Q
  - **MC site of metastasis** is **Bone**^Q (Osteolytic deposits in Lumbar vertebra >Femur >Thoracic vertebra >Rib >Skull)

- Metastatic disease (Malignant pleural effusion^Q) is the **principal cause of death** from **breast cancer**.
- **2nd MC cause** of **cancer related death in women**^{Q} (MC is **CA lung** in both **males** and **females**)^Q
- **Pathway of metastasis in breast cancer:** Cancer cells from breast → Posterior intercostal veins → Batson veretebral venous plexus → intracranial dural venous sinus → Brain

Clinical Features
- Early breast cancer may be **asymptomatic**^{Q}

Symptoms indicating possibility of breast cancer	
• **Change in size** or **shape** of breast^Q	• **Single duct discharge**, particularly **blood stained**^{Q}
• **Skin dimpling, nipple retraction**^{Q}	• **Axillary node** enlargement^Q

- **Peau-d-orange:** Due to **obstruction of subdermal lymphatics** (lymphatic permeation by tumor cells^Q) leading to **cutaneous lymphatic edema**^{Q}
- **Symptoms** indicating possibility of **Metastasis:**
  - Breathing difficulty, bone pain, symptoms of **hypercalcemia**^{Q}, abdominal distention, jaundice

- **Multifocality:** Second cancer in the **same quadrant (within 4 cm)**
- **Multicentricity:** Second cancer outside the quadrant of primary cancer (away at least 4 cm)
- **Dimpling:** Small depression over skin of breast due to **infiltration of ligament of Cooper** by carcinoma^Q
- **Puckering:** Small fold or wrinkle of skin over the breast due to **infiltration of ligament of Cooper** by carcinoma^Q
- **Cancer en-cuirasse:** Infiltration of breast skin & chest wall with **multiple nodules & ulceration** by the carcinoma^Q

Evaluation

Triple Assessment		
• **Clinical examination**^{Q}	• **Imaging (USG** or **mammography)**^{Q}	• **Tissue sampling (FNAC** or **true cut biopsy)**^{Q}
• **Confident diagnosis** by **triple assessment** in **99.9%**		

- **First investigation** for suspected case of breast cancer: **Mammography**^{Q}
- **Best and diagnostic investigation: Biopsy**^{Q}

- MC cancer in women in India: CA cervix^Q
- MC cancer in urban women in India: CA breast^Q
- MC cancer in women in the world: CA breast^Q
- MC cause of cancer related death in men and women: CA lung^Q > CA breast

CARCINOMA BREAST INVESTIGATIONS

INVESTIGATIONS IN CA BREAST	
FNAC	**True-cut (core-cut) Biopsy**
• **FNA** is **easily performed**, but **requires** a **trained cytopathologist**^{Q} for accurate specimen interpretation.	• Core cutting needle biopsy provides a **histologic specimen** suitable for **interpretation by any pathologist**^{Q}.
• **False-negative results**^{Q} are **most common** in **fibrotic** or **well-differentiated tumors.**	• **ER, PR status** and **presence of HER-2 overexpression** can be **routinely determined**^{Q} from core biopsy specimens.
• **FNA does not reliably distinguish invasive cancer from DCIS**^{Q}, potentially leading to the overtreatment of gross DCIS.	• **Diagnostic technique of choice** for patients who will **receive preoperative systemic therapy**^{Q}.

Biopsy Techniques for Breast Lesions		
Technique	**Advantages**	**Disadvantages**
FNAC	• Rapid, painless, inexpensive. • No incision prior to selection of local therapy	• **Does not distinguish invasive from in situ cancer**^{Q}. • **Markers (ER, PR, HER-2) not routinely available**^{Q}. • Requires **experienced cytopathologist**^{Q}. • False negatives and insufficient specimens occur.
True-cut (core-cut) Biopsy	• Rapid, relatively painless, inexpensive. No incision. • Can be **read by any pathologist**^{Q}, markers **(ER, PR, HER-2) routinely available**^{Q}.	• False-negative results, incomplete lesion characterization can occur.
Excisional biopsy	• False-negative results rare. • Complete histology before treatment decisions. • May serve as definitive lumpectomy.	• **Expensive, more painful.** • Creates an **incision** to be incorporated into definitive surgery. • Unnecessary surgery with potential for cosmetic deformity in patients with benign abnormalities.

Ultrasonography in Breast Disease

- Initial investigation for palpable lesions in **women <35 years**^{Q}
- **Young woman's breast** contains a **large proportion** of glandular tissue which appears as a **soft tissue density**^{Q} and **lowers the sensitivity of mammogram**^{Q}.
- The **sensitivity of ultrasound** for **detecting DCIS** is **significantly lower than mammography**^{Q} that is why USG is not a useful screening test for breast cancer.
- Ultrasonography is an important method of:
  - **Resolving equivocal mammographic findings**
  - Defining cystic masses
  - Demonstrating the echogenic qualities of specific solid abnormalities

• Breast cysts	• **Smooth margins** and echo-free center
• Benign breast masses	• **Smooth contours,** round or oval shapes, weak internal echoes **Well-defined anterior and posterior margins**^{Q}.
• Breast cancer	• **Irregular walls**^{Q} but may have smooth margins with acoustic enhancement

Mammography

- **Delivers** a radiation dose of **0.1 cGy**^{Q} per study (**chest radiography** delivers 25% of this dose)^Q.
- **Bremsstrahlung type of X-ray** is used in mammography.
- **No increased breast cancer risk**^{Q} associated with the radiation dose delivered with screening mammography.
- Used to detect **unexpected breast cancer** in **asymptomatic women**.
- Two views of the breast are obtained, the **craniocaudal view** & **mediolateral oblique view**.

> - **MLO view** images the **greatest volume**^{Q} of breast tissue, including **upper outer quadrant** & **axillary tail** of Spence
> - **CC view** provides better visualization of **medial aspect** of the breast & permits **greater breast compression**^{Q}

- Mammography also is used to guide interventional procedures, including needle localization & needle biopsy.
- **Sensitivity** is much **reduced in younger** or **dense breasts**, considered **inappropriate** in patients **<35 years**^{Q}.

Mammographic Features Suggestive of Breast Cancer

- A **solid mass** with or without **stellate features**^{Q}
- **Asymmetric thickening**^{Q} of breast tissues
- **Clustered microcalcifications**^{Q}

> - Presence of **fine, stippled calcium** in and around a suspicious lesion is suggestive of breast cancer and occurs in as many as 50% of **nonpalpable cancers**^{Q}
> - These microcalcifications are an **especially important** sign of cancer **in younger women**, in whom it may be the **only mammographic abnormality**^{Q}

Advantages

- Around **33% reduction in mortality**^{Q} for women after screening mammography.
- **Mammography** was **more accurate than clinical examination** for the detection of **early breast cancers**, providing a true-positive rate of 90%.
- Starting at age **40 years**, breast examinations should be performed **yearly** and a **yearly mammogram** should be taken^Q.
- Mammography helps in **40% reduction in stage II, III, and IV cancer** in the screened population, with a **30% increase in overall survival**^{Q}.

	Mammography	
	Benign	**Malignant**
Opacity	• **Smooth** margin	• **Ill defined**^{Q} margin, **irregular stellate, spiculated**^{Q} margin, **comet tail**^{Q}
	• **Low density**	• **High density**^{Q}
	• Homogeneous	• Heterogeneous
	• Thin halo	• **Wide halo**^{Q}
Calcification	• **Macrocalcification**^{Q} (>0.5 mm in diameter)	• **Microcalcification**^{Q} (<0.5 mm in diameter)
Breast Parenchyma	• Normal	• **Architectural distortion**^{Q}
Nipple/areola	• Normal	• **± Retracted**
Skin	• Normal	• **Thickened**^{Q}
Cooper ligaments	• Normal	• **Thickened**^{Q}, increased number
Subcutaneous retro mammary space	• Normal	• **Obliterated**^{Q}

Endocrine Surgery

BIRADS (Breast Imaging Reporting And Data System)		
Category	Definition	Likelihood of Malignancy
0	**Incomplete assessment**, need **additional imaging** evaluation^Q	Not applicable
1	**Negative**, **routine mammogram** in 1 year is recommended^Q	0%
2	**Benign** findings, **routine mammogram** in 1 year is recommended^Q	0%
3	**Probably benign** findings, short term **follow-up** suggested^Q	>0 to ≤2%
4	**Suspicious** abnormality, **biopsy** should be considered^Q (**4A**-Low suspicion; **4B**-Moderate suspicion; **4C**-High suspicion)	4A: >2-≤10% 4B: >10-≤50% 4C: >50-≤95%
5	**Highly suggestive** of malignancy, **appropriate action** should be taken^Q	>95%
6	Known **biopsy-proven malignancy**	Not applicable

MRI

- Screening with MRI is **superior to mammography** in **detecting invasive breast cancer in younger women**^Q, where the **sensitivity of mammography is low** due to **presence of mammographically dense breast parenchyma**^Q

Indications for Breast MRI
1. **Lobular carcinoma**^Q: Difficult to detect and measure by conventional method because of multifocal and infiltrating
2. **Staging of primary breast cancer**^Q
3. **Occult primary tumour** with malignant axillary lymphadenopathy and **normal mammogram** and **breast USG**^Q
4. **Screen younger women** with **high familial risk** of breast cancer^Q
5. Assessing the **integrity of breast implant**^Q

Pattern of Calcification in Breast Diseases	
Carcinoma	**Microcalcification**, punctate, branching^Q
Fibroadenoma	**Popcorn**^Q (coarse, granular, crushed stone)
Fibrocystic disease	Powdery
Fat necrosis	Curvilinear

CLASSIFICATION OF BREAST CANCER

WHO Classification of Breast Cancer		
In-situ Carcinoma	Invasive Carcinoma (MC)	Paget's Disease of Nipple
• Ductal carcinoma in-situ • Lobular carcinoma in-situ	• Ductal carcinoma (**MC**) • Lobular carcinoma • **Tubular (Cribiform)** carcinoma • **Mucinous (Colloid)** carcinoma • **Medullary** carcinoma • **Papillary** carcinoma • Metaplastic carcinoma • Inflammatory carcinoma	

INVASIVE BREAST CARCINOMA

Invasive Ductal Carcinoma
- **Invasive ductal carcinoma** of the breast with **productive fibrosis** (**scirrhous**^Q, simplex, NST) accounts for **80%** of breast cancers
- Presents with macroscopic or microscopic **axillary LN metastases** in up to **60%**^Q of cases.
- Usually occurs in **perimenopausal** or **postmenopausal women** in the **5th to 6th** decades of life
- Presents as a **solitary, firm mass**^Q.

Medullary Carcinoma
- **Special-type** breast cancer, accounts for 4% of all invasive breast cancers
- Frequent phenotype of **BRCA-1** hereditary breast cancer.
- Grossly, the cancer is **soft** & **hemorrhagic**.
- A **rapid increase in size** may occur secondary to necrosis and hemorrhage.
- On physical examination, it is **bulky** and often **positioned deep** within the breast.

Medullary Carcinoma is Characterized Microscopically by
• **Dense lymphoreticular infiltrate** of **lymphocytes** and **plasma cell**
• **Large pleomorphic nuclei**
• **Sheet-like growth pattern**

- **Better 5-year survival rate** than those with NST or invasive lobular carcinoma.

Mucinous Carcinoma (Colloid Carcinoma)
- **Special-type** breast cancer, accounts for 2% of all invasive breast cancers
- Typically presents in the **elderly population** as a **bulky tumor**.
- Characterized by **extracellular pools of mucin**
- **Analysis of multiple sections** is essential **to confirm the diagnosis**
- **LN metastases** occur in 33% of cases, and 5- and 10-year survival rates are 73 and 59%, respectively.

Papillary Carcinoma
- **Special-type** cancer of the breast that accounts for 2% of all invasive breast cancers.
- Presents in the **7th decade** of life and occurs in a disproportionate number of **nonwhite women.**
- Typically **small**.
- Defined by **papillae with fibrovascular stalks** and **multilayered epithelium**.
- **Low frequency** of axillary **LN metastases** and had 5- and 10-year survival rates similar to those for mucinous and tubular carcinoma.

Tubular Carcinoma
- **Special-type** breast cancer and accounts for 2% of all invasive breast cancers.
- Usually diagnosed in the **perimenopausal** or **early menopausal periods**.

> • **Distant metastases** are **rare** in tubular carcinoma with **long-term survival approaches 100%**.^{Q}

Invasive Lobular Carcinoma
- Accounts for 10% of breast cancers.

> • **Invasive lobular carcinoma** is frequently **multifocal, multicentric, and bilateral.**^{Q}

CARCINOMA BREAST STAGING

8th AJCC (2017) TNM Staging for Breast Cancer
T: Primary tumor
T1: Tumor ≤2 cm^Q
T2: Tumor >2 cm & ≤5 cm^Q
T3: Tumor >5 cm^Q
T4a: Extension to **chest wall**, not including pectoralis muscle^Q
T4b: **Edema** (including peau d'orange) or **ulceration** of skin, or **satellite skin nodules** confined to the same breast^Q
T4c: Both **T4a & T4b**^{Q}
T4d: Inflammatory carcinoma^Q
Note
• Invasion of dermis alone does not qualify as T4^Q.
• Chest wall includes ribs, intercostal muscles & serratus anterior but not the pectoral muscles^Q.
• Dimpling of the skin, nipple retraction, or other skin changes, except those in T4b & T4d, may occur in T1, T2 or T3 without affecting the classification^Q.
N: Regional lymph nodes
N1: Metastasis to **movable ipsilateral level I, II axillary LNs**^{Q}
N2a: Metastasis in **ipsilateral level I, II axillary LNs fixed or matted**^{Q}
N2b: Metastasis only in **clinically apparent ipsilateral internal mammary LNs** and in the absence of clinically evident axillary LNs metastasis^Q
N3a: Metastasis in **ipsilateral infraclavicular LNs**^{Q}
N3b: Metastasis in **ipsilateral internal mammary LNs & axillary LNs**^{Q}
N3c: Metastasis in **ipsilateral supraclavicular LNs**^{Q}
M: Distant metastases
M0: No distant metastasis; M1: Distant metastasis

[Note: Clinically apparent is defined as detected by **imaging studies** (excluding lymphoscintigraphy) or by **clinical examination** or **grossly visible pathologically**^{Q}.]

Stage I	Stage IIA	Stage IIB	Stage IIIA	Stage IIIB	Stage IIIC	Stage IV
T1 N0M0	T0N1 M0 T1N1 M0 T2 N0M0	T2N1 M0 T3 N0M0	T0 N2 M0 T1-2 N2 M0 T3 N1-2 M0	T4 N0-2 M0	AnyT N3 M0	AnyT anyN M1

Special Conditions in Staging	
• Positive LN in opposite axilla	• Metastasis
• Two mass in same breast	• Staging according to big mass
• Mass in both breasts	• Separate staging for both breasts

CARCINOMA BREAST MANAGEMENT

BREAST CANCER TREATMENT

A. Early Invasive Breast Cancer (Stage I, IIA, IIB):
- Mastectomy + Axillary LN status assessment^Q or
- BCT + Axillary LN status assessment + RT^Q
- If sentinel LN can not be identified or found to harbor metastatic disease, axillary LN dissection (**Level I+II**) should be done

Indications of Adjuvant Chemotherapy
1. **LN positive**^{Q}
2. **Tumor >1 cm**^{Q}
3. **LN negative, >0.5 cm** with **adverse prognostic factors**: – **Blood vessel** or **lymph vessel** invasion^Q – **High** nuclear or histologic **grade**^{Q} – **Her-2-neu** over expression^Q – **Negative hormone receptor** status^Q

- **Tamoxifen** should be given for **hormone receptor positive**, cancer **>1 cm**^{Q}
- **Trastazumab** should be given for **Her-2-neu positive** cancer^Q

B. Locally Advanced Breast Cancer (Stage IIIA, IIIB, IIIC)^Q:
- **Neoadjuvant chemotherapy + MRM + Adjuvant RT**^{Q}
- **BCT** for IIIA with N1 with patients who achieve **good response** to **neoadjuvant chemotherapy**^{Q}
- Systemic **chemotherapy + radiotherapy** are indicated in treatment of grossly involved internal mammary nodes (**N3b**)

C. Distant Metastases (Stage IV):
- **Prolong survival** and **improve quality** of life^Q
- **Hormonal therapies** are **preferred** to cytotoxic therapy as it is associated with **minimal toxicity**^{Q}

Indications of Hormonal Therapy	Indications of Systemic Chemotherapy
1. Hormone receptor positive (**ER/PR positive**)^Q	1. Hormone receptor **negative**^{Q}
2. **Bone** or **soft tissue metastases only**^{Q}	2. Hormone **refractory**^{Q} (after 3 endocrine regimens)
3. **Limited** or **asymptomatic** visceral metastases	3. **Symptomatic visceral metastases**^{Q}

Local Regional Recurrence
• Who had **mastectomy**: **Resection** of local regional recurrence **with reconstruction + chemotherapy + hormonal therapy + RT** (if not received RT previously)^Q
• Who had **lumpectomy**: Mastectomy with reconstruction + chemotherapy + hormonal therapy^Q

INDICATIONS OF RADIOTHERAPY IN CARCINOMA BREAST

- **Locally Advanced Breast Cancer**^{Q} (to decrease recurrence rate)
- **Margin** is **positive** after mastectomy^Q
- After **breast conservation surgery**^{Q}
- Metastases to **4** or **more lymph nodes**^{Q}

CHEMOTHERAPY IN CARCINOMA BREAST

Chemotherapy in CA Breast

- **First-generation regimen** such as a 6-monthly cycle of **cyclophosphamide, methotrexate and 5-fluorouracil (CMF)**[Q] will achieve a **25% reduction** in the **risk of relapse** over a 10- to 15-year period[Q].
- CMF is **no longer** considered **adequate adjuvant chemotherapy**[Q]
- Modern regimens include an **anthracycline** (**doxorubicin** or **epirubicin**) and **taxanes**.

> - Effect of **combining hormone & chemotherapy** is **additive** although **hormone therapy** is **started after completion** of **chemotherapy** to reduce side-effects.

- Most popular combinations were **CMF & CAF**[Q] (Cyclophosphamide, Adriamycin [doxorubicin], and 5-fluorouracil.
- In the United States, a **combination** of **Adriamycin (doxorubicin)** and **cyclophosphamide (AC)** or **AC plus a taxane** (docetaxel, paclitaxel) are likely to be used as **polychemotherapy**[Q].
- For **HER-2–positive breast cancer**, adding **trastuzumab**[Q] to polychemotherapy is approved for use as a surgical adjuvant.
- **Anthracycline-containing combinations** are significantly **better than** no treatment, **single-agent treatment**, or **CMF**[Q].

New Drugs in CA Breast	
Ixabepilone	• Used for **antracycline & taxane resistant** breast cancer[Q]
Lapatinib	• Inhibitor of Her-2-neu & EGFR tyrosine kinase • Second line Her-2-neu therapy[Q]
Sunitinib	• Approved for **advanced renal cancer & refractory metastatic breast cancer**[Q]

HORMONE THERAPY IN CARCINOMA BREAST

Hormonal Therapy in Carcinoma Breast

1. **Ovarian suppression or ablation:**
   - Bilateral oophorectomy[Q]
   - Medically by LHRH agonist (**Goserelin, Leuperolide**)[Q]
2. **SERM: Tamoxifen** and **Raloxifene**[Q]
3. **Aromatase Inhibitors:**
   - Non-steroidal: **Letrozole** and **Anastrazole**[Q]
   - Steroidal: **Exmestane**[Q]
4. **Anti-estrogens: Fulvestrant**[Q]
5. **Progestins:** Megesterol & Medroxyprogesterone acetate

Aromatase Inhibitors

- **No increased risk** of endometrial carcinoma[Q]
- **Decreases bone mineral density** & increases risk of **fracture**[Q]
- Used in postmenopausal patients[Q]

Hormonal Therapy in Carcinoma Breast

- **Tamoxifen** is DOC in **premenopausal** patients[Q]
- **Aromatase inhibitors** are DOC in **postmenopausal** patients

Tamoxifen

- **Tamoxifen** is a **standard hormonal treatment** of breast cancer in both **premenopausal & postmenopausal women**[Q]
- Tamoxifen is **effective in Estrogen Receptor (ER) positive** breast carcinoma but some ER negative tumors also respond to tamoxifen[Q].

> - Tamoxifen is **approved for primary prophylaxis** of breast cancer in **high risk women**[Q]
> - It **reduces the recurrence rate** of breast cancer in **ipsilateral** as well **contralateral breast**[Q]
> - **Tamoxifen** is associated with **reduced risk of cancer** in the **contralateral breast**[Q].

- **Dose:** 10 mg BD × 5-years[Q]
- While tamoxifen blocks estrogen receptors on the breast, it stimulates these receptors in the uterus (because tamoxifen is a **partial against of ER**), may **lead** to **endometrial hyperplasia & endometrial cancer**[Q]

Tamoxifen
• **Potent antagonist** in **breast carcinoma cells**, **blood vessels** and at some peripheral sites[Q]
• **Partial agonist** in the **pi**tuitary, **b**one, **u**terus and **l**iver **(Pit Bul)**

- Tamoxifen causes **retinal deposits, decreased visual acuity & cataracts** in occasional patients[Q]
- Tamoxifen **increases** the **risk of thromboembolic events**[Q]

Adverse Effects of Tamoxifen	
• **Hot flushes**, nausea & vomiting **(MC)**[Q] • **Menstrual irregularities**[Q], vaginal bleeding, discharge, pruritus vulvae & dermatitis • **Endometrial cancer**[Q]	• **Thromboembolism**[Q] • **Cataract**[Q] • Retinal deposits & decreased visual acuity

LYMPH NODE METASTASIS IN CARCINOMA BREAST

LYMPHATIC METASTASIS IN CA BREAST

- **Lymphatic spread** in CA breast occurs **through subareolar lymphatic plexus of Sappey's** lymphatic plexus, **cutaneous lymphatics & inflammatory lymphatics**[Q].

> - **Lymphatic metastasis** occurs **primarily** to the **axillary (75%)**[Q] & **internal mammary lymph nodes**[Q].
> - **Tumors** in the **posterior one third** of breast are more likely to drain to the **internal mammary nodes**[Q].

- Involvement of LNs has both biological & chronological significance.
- It represents not only an evolutional event in the spread of the carcinoma but is also a **marker for** the **metastatic potential**[Q] of that tumour.
- Involvement of **supraclavicular nodes** and of **any contralateral lymph nodes** represents **advanced disease**[Q].
- LN metastasis is treated by **surgical dissection** or **radiotherapy**

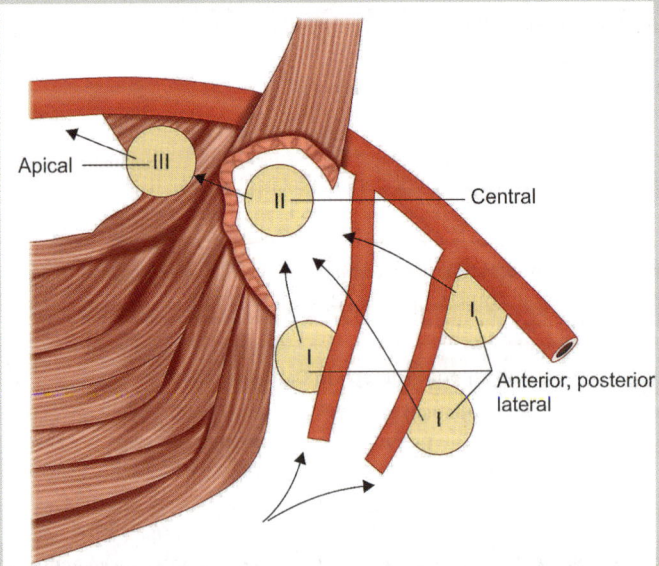

Axillary LN Levels in relation with Pectoralis minor		
Level	Relation with Pectoralis minor	Axillary LNs Included
I	Below or lateral	Anterior, posterior, lateral[Q]
II	Posterior (behind)	Central, Interpectoral[Q] (Rotter's nodes)
III	Medial or above	Apical[Q]

MASTECTOMY

Types of Mastectomy	
Simple or total mastectomy	Removal of **breast tissue, nipple-areola complex, & skin**^{Q}.
Extended simple mastectomy	Simple mastectomy + removal of **level I** axillary LNs.
Modified radical mastectomy	Removes all **breast tissue, nipple-areola complex, skin** and level **I & II** axillary LNs^Q.
Halsted's radical mastectomy	Removes all **breast tissue** and **skin, nipple areola complex, pectoralis major** and **minor** muscles and the level **I, II & III** axillary LNs^Q.
Extended radical mastectomy	Radical mastectomy + Removal of **internal mammary LNs**
Super radical mastectomy	Radical mastectomy + Removal of **internal mammary, mediastinal & supraclavicular LNs**

Variants of MRM	
Auschincloss Procedure	Removes all **breast tissue, nipple-areola complex, skin** and level **I & II** axillary LNs^Q.
Patey's Procedure	**Pectoralis minor** is **removed** to allow complete dissection of **level III** axillary LNs^Q
Scanlon's Modification of Patey's Procedure	**Pectoralis minor** is **divided** instead of removing^Q. Division of pectoralis minor allows **complete removal** of **level III** axillary LNs^Q

COMPLICATIONS OF MASTECTOMY

Complications of Mastectomy

- **Seroma**
  - MC complication^Q, beneath skin flaps & axilla, occurs in **30%** cases
  - Catheter is retained until drainage is <30 mL/day
- **Wound Infection**
  - Majority are due to **skin flap necrosis**
- **Lymphedema**
  - Occurs less frequently with the standard axillary dissections.
  - Extensive LN dissection, radiation therapy, presence of positive LNs, obesity are predisposing factors^Q.
- Injury to Long Thoracic (Motor) Nerve
  - Seen in **10%** of all cases.
  - Result in a palsy of the Serratus anterior muscle (classical **winged scapula**)
- Injury to Thoracodorsal Nerve
  - Leads to palsy of the latissimus dorsi muscle.
- Redundant Axillary Fat Pad

Post-Mastectomy Pain

- Breast, axilla upper arm are innervated by variety of nerves; lateral cutaneous branch of T2 (**intercostobrachial nerve**), T3 & T4 provides innervation to anterior chest wall and upper back, torso and nipple.
- **Sympathetic innervation** of cutaneous structures of breast is provided by **medial & lateral branches** of ventral ramus of **3rd to 6th intercostal nerves**.
- While both nociceptive pain (due to damage of muscle & ligaments) and neuropathic pain can occur after surgery for breast cancer, **neuropathic pain is more likely to persist after wound healing** has occurred.

Four Pain Syndromes have been Distinguished

1. **Phantom Breast Pain:** Painful (often knife like or shooting) sensation that the removed breast is still present
2. **Intercostobrachial neuralgia:** Usually known as **post-mastectomy pain syndrome (PMP)**, consists of **pain in axilla, medial upper arm and anterior chest wall** and is often is caused by nerve damage during axillary node dissection.
3. **Neuroma Pain:** Can occur from scars from either mastectomy or lumpectomy but is more common if surgery is followed by radiotherapy.
4. **Other Nerve Injury Pain:** Can occur even if intercostobrachial nerve is spared and is more common in breast reconstruction and implants.

ANGIOSARCOMA

- Classified as **de novo**, as **postradiation**, or as arising in **association with postmastectomy lymphedema**.
- Stewart and Treves described **lymphangiosarcoma** of **upper extremity** in women with **ipsilateral lymphedema** after **radical mastectomy**. (Stewart-Treves Syndrome)^Q
- Angiosarcoma is now the preferred name.
- **Average interval** between MRM or radical mastectomy and the development of an angiosarcoma is **10.5 years**^{Q}.
- **60% of women** developing this cancer have a **history of adjuvant radiation therapy**^{Q}.

Clinical Features
- **Acute worsening** of edema
- Appearance of **subcutaneous nodules** with propensity towards **hemorrhage and ulceration**

Radiation-induced Angiosarcoma	Angiosarcoma (in the absence of previous radiation therapy or surgery)
• **Reddish brown** to **purple raised rash** within the radiation portals and on the skin of the breast	• May form a **mass within** the **parenchyma of the breast**

Treatment
- **Preoperative chemotherapy** & **radiotherapy** followed by **surgical excision (radical amputation)**^{Q}
- Associated with **poor prognosis**^{Q}
- **Forequarter amputation** may be necessary to palliate the ulcerative complications and advanced lymphedema.

BREAST CONSERVATIVE SURGERY

Breast Conservative Surgery (BCT)

- Involves **resection** of **primary breast cancer** with a margin of normal appearing breast tissue, **adjuvant radiation therapy** with or without **assessment** of axillary LN status^Q.
- Surgical procedures employed: **wide local excision, lumpectomy, quadrantectomy**
- BCT is currently treatment for women with **DCIS, Stage I and Stage II invasive breast cancer**^{Q}.

Suitable Candidates for BCT
- Cancer is **solitary**, with no clinical or mammographic evidence of cancer elsewhere in the breast.
- Tumour can be **excised with tumor free surgical margins** without producing a cosmetically unacceptable breast.
- There are **no contraindications to radiation**
- Patients is **willing** & **motivated** for breast conservation

Contraindications for BCT

Absolute contraindications	Relative contraindications
1. **Pregnancy**^{Q} is an absolute contraindication to the use of breast irradiation.	1. History of **collagen vascular disorders**^{Q} (Scleroderma and **active lupus erythematosus** but not the rheumatoid arthritis)
2. Women with **two** or **more primary tumors** in **separate quadrants** of the breast or with **diffuse malignant** appearing **micro calcifications**^{Q}.	2. Presence of **multiple gross tumours** in the **same quadrant** and **indeterminate calcifications**^{Q}
3. A **history** of prior **therapeutic irradiation**^{Q} to the breast region that would require treatment to an excessively high total-radiation dose to a significant volume	3. **Large tumour** in **small breast**^{Q}
4. **Persistent positive margins**^{Q} after reasonable surgical attempts	4. **Breast size, large pendulous breast**^{Q} presents difficulty in delivering uniform radiation dose
	5. **Centrally located tumour**^{Q}, for which removal of nipple-areola complex is required to obtain a tumour free margin

CARCINOMA BREAST PROGNOSTIC INDICATORS

Prognostic Factors in Carcinoma Breast

- **Most important prognostic factor** in CA breast: **Stage >Axillary LN status**^{Q}
- **In case of metastasis**, the **prognosis no more depends** upon the **lymph node status**^{Q}

  - In **breast carcinoma metastasis**, prognosis **best depends** upon **estrogen & progesterone receptor status**^{Q} (ER & PR status)

- Prognostic markers like **PCNA, Ki-67, bcl-2, bax:bcl-2, VEGF, HER 2/neu, EGFr expressions** are associated with **poor prognosis**[Q].

Prognostic and Predictive Factors for Invasive Breast Cancer	
Tumor Factors	**Host Factors**
Nodal status	Age
Tumor **size**	Menopausal status
Histologic/nuclear **grade**	Family history
Lymphatic/vascular invasion	Previous breast cancer
Pathologic **stage**	Immunosuppression
Hormone receptor status	Nutrition
DNA content (**ploidy, S-phase fraction**)	Prior chemotherapy
Extent of **intraductal component**	Prior radiation therapy
HER-2/*neu* expression	

ONCOTYPE DX

- Oncotype DX is a **genomic test that predicts the likelihood of a cancer recurrence, likelihood of benefit from chemotherapy, & likelihood of survival in patients with newly diagnosed breast cancer** that **has not spread to LNs (node negative)** and is **hormone receptor-positive**.
- Oncotype DX evaluates the **activity of 21 genes** from a sample of the patient's cancer **to determine the patient's Recurrence Score**.
- **Recurrence Score** ranges from **0 to 100**, with a **higher score indicating a greater risk of recurrence**.
- Oncotype DX diagnostic tests help individualize treatment planning for breast, colon and prostate cancer patients.

Oncotype DX may be used to guide chemotherapy decisions among certain women with:		
Node-negative[Q]	Hormone receptor-positive[Q]	HER2-negative breast cancer[Q]

For Breast Cancer	For Colon Cancer	For Prostate Cancer
• It helps physicians and patients to **decide on the best course of treatment**. • For invasive breast cancer, it **predicts chemotherapy benefit** and **likelihood of distant breast cancer recurrence**. • For **DCIS** patients, it **predict the risk of local recurrence**.	• For Colon Cancer, it quantifies **recurrence risk in stage II** and **stage III colon cancer**, beyond traditional qualitative measures. • This enables an **individualized approach to treatment planning**. • It measures a group of cancer genes in the tumor, **providing a quantitative Recurrence Score** so physicians & patients can have a **more complete discussion of recurrence risk**.	• For prostate Cancer, it provides a **more precise** & **accurate assessment of risk based on individual tumor biology**. • Provides additional, clinically relevant insight into underlying prostate tumor biology, enabling physicians & their patients **to make treatment decisions** with greater confidence.

Name of Test	Brief Description	Scoring/Measurement	Tissue Needed
Oncotype DX	A genomic test that uses a **21-gene assay** to provide an **individual, quantitative assessment of the likelihood of disease recurrence**.	Recurrence Score, a number between **0 and 100** that **correlates to a specific likelihood of breast cancer recurrence within 10 years** of initial diagnosis	Fixed-tissue blocks
Mamma Print	A unique **70-gene assay** that has the ability to **identify which early-stage breast cancer patients are at risk of distant recurrence following surgery, independent of Estrogen Receptor status** and any **prior treatment**.	Low risk or high risk	Paraffin embedded or fresh tissue
PAM50	A **50-gene test** in development that is designed to be performed in local routine hospital pathology laboratories and has been optimized **to separate intrinsic disease subtypes that are used to generate a ROR score**.	Risk of Recurrence (ROR) score	Fixed-tissue blocks

GENE EXPRESSION PROFILING IN BREAST CANCER

- "*Gene expression profiling, which can measure the relative quantities of mRNA for essentially every gene, has* identified **five major patterns of gene expression** in the NST group: **luminal A, luminal B, normal, basal-like**, and **HER2 positive**. These molecular classes **correlate with prognosis** and **response to therapy**, and thus have taken on clinical importance."

Luminal Criteria	
Type	Properties
Luminal A (MC)	ER & PR +ve, Her-2-neu –ve[Q] (MC type[Q]; Best prognosis[Q])
Luminal B	ER, PR & Her-2-neu +ve (Triple positive)[Q]
Normal breast-like	Well-differentiated, ER-positive
Basal cell type	**Triple negative, positive** for **myoepithelial markers**[Q] (basal keratins, P-cadherin, p63, or laminin), **CK-5, 6 & 17, EGFR**
Her-2 type	Her-2-neu +ve, ER & PR –ve[Q] (worst prognosis)

Immunohistochemistry in CA Breast
• **Most widely used** test for **ER & PR** receptor status[Q] • Immunohistochemistry analysis of **heat-treated paraffin sections** (**of tumor tissue**) has largely superseded ELISA ligand-binding assay. • **ER and PR positive status** (>10 fmol on ELISA; >15 H-score on Immunohistochemistry)[Q] predict **improved response** to **endocrine treatment**, **time to relapse** and **overall survival**[Q].

Heat Map
• **Portrayal of global gene expression**[Q] is called heat map • This illustration provides an **unbiased look at breast cancer** according to **gene expression**[Q]

TRIPLE-NEGATIVE BREAST CANCER (TNBC)

Triple-negative Breast Cancer (TNBC)

- TNBC: Breast cancer that **does not express** the genes for **ER, PR & Her-2-neu**[Q]
- Accounts for **15–25%** of breast cancer cases.
- More common in **premenopausal women**[Q]

Pathology
- **Germline mutations** of **BRCA1 & BRCA2 genes**[Q] are the causative factor
- Also known as **basal-like**[Q] (75% of basal-type breast cancers are **triple negative**)
- Some TNBC **overexpresses EGFR** & **transmembrane glycoprotein NMB**[Q] (GPNMB).

Treatment
- Standard treatment: Surgery (Mastectomy/BCS) + Adjuvant chemotherapy + Radiotherapy[Q]

> - **Didox** (**synthetic antioxidant**) in addition to chemotherapy **reduces drug resistance**[Q].
> - Didox inhibits ribonucleotide reductase M2 (RRM2)[Q]
> - RRM2 contributes to **cells resistance of the chemotherapy** resulting in relapse[Q].

- TNBCs are very **susceptible to chemotherapy**[Q].
- **BRCA1-related TNBC** is particularly susceptible to **platinum-based agents & taxanes**[Q].

Prognosis
- **High risk of recurrence**[Q] after treatment

BREAST RECONSTRUCTION

Breast Reconstruction		
Autogenous	Alloplastic	Combined
• TRAM flap (MC)[Q] • Lattisimus dorsi flap[Q] • Gluteal flap • Ruben's flap[Q] • Thoracoepigastric flap • Lateral thigh flap	• Silicone gel implant[Q] • Silicone implant with saline refill[Q]	• Lattisimus dorsi flap with implant[Q] • TRAM flap with implant[Q]

- Placement of **implant in a submuscular plane** beneath **pectoralis major**[Q], superior portion of **rectus abdominis**, & **serratus anterior muscles** provides **better protection** against **implant extrusion**, as well as **decreased risk for capsular contracture & implant displacement**[Q]

Type	Advantages	Disadvantages
Common Reconstructive Options after Mastectomy		
Implant	**One stage** procedure, minimal prolongation, hospitalization, or recovery, low cost	**Poor symmetry**[Q] if skin removed or in large ptotic breasts. **Capsular contracture, leakage, rupture**[Q] possible.
Tissue expander	Short operative time, hospitalization, recovery not prolonged, low cost	**Multiple** physician **visits** post-op. **Poor symmetry** large or ptotic breasts. **Capsular contracture, leakage rupture**[Q] possible.
Latissimus dorsi flap	Short operative time, hospitalization, recovery not prolonged, low cost	**Donor site scar**[Q] Usually **requires an implant**[Q] Moderate prolongation hospitalization and recovery.
TRAM flap	Natural contour. Good match for large or ptotic breasts. Abdominoplasty.	**Donor site scar**[Q] **Fat necrosis, flap loss** possible. **Abdominal wall weakness** and **hernia**[Q]. Significant prolongation hospitalization plus recovery.

- **MC method** of **breast reconstruction**: Implants (**silicon implants**)[Q]
- **Surgical breast reconstruction** should **never done prior to RT**[Q].
- **Best flap** for breast reconstruction: **DIEP flap**[Q] (Deep inferior epigastric perforator flap) > **TRAM FLAP**[Q]

INFLAMMATORY BREAST CARCINOMA (MASTITIS CARCINOMATOSA)

- IBC (stage **IIIB**) accounts for <3% of breast cancers.
- Characterized by the skin changes of **brawny induration**, **erythema** with a raised edge, & **edema** (**rapid onset** peau d'orange) involving >33% of **skin** of breast[Q].

Pathology
- **Permeation** of the **dermal lymph vessels** by **cancer cells** is seen in skin biopsy specimens[Q].
- There **may be** an associated **breast mass**[Q].

Clinical Features
- Characterized by skin changes of **brawny induration**, **erythema** with a raised edge, and **edema** (peau d'orange)[Q].
- IBC may be **mistaken for** a **bacterial infection**[Q] of the breast.
- More than **75%** of women present with **palpable axillary lymphadenopathy**[Q]
- **Distant metastases at diagnosis** in **25%** of white women with IBC.

Diagnosis
- IOC for diagnosis is **skin biopsy**[Q].

Treatment
- Multimodal approach (NACT + Mastectomy + RT ± Hormonal therapy)[Q]
- **Chest wall**, **supraclavicular**, **internal mammary** and **axillary** lymph node basins receive **adjuvant radiation therapy**.
- This **multimodal approach** results in 5-year survival rates that approach **30%**[Q].

- Both **inflammatory breast cancer** & **Paget's disease** may or may not be **associated** with **breast mass**.

BREAST CANCER DURING PREGNANCY

BREAST CANCER DURING PREGNANCY

- Occurs in **1 of every 3000**[Q] pregnant women
- **MC non-gynecologic malignancy** associated with **pregnancy**[Q].
- **Ductal carcinoma** is MC type, accounting for **75–90%**[Q] of breast cancer in pregnancy.

Clinical Features
- Presents as **painless palpable mass**[Q] with or without nipple discharge
- **Axillary LN metastases** in up to **75%** patients
- Approx. **<25% nodules** developing during **pregnancy** and **lactation** will be **cancerous**[Q]
- **Present at a later stage** of disease because breast changes occurring in hormone-rich environment of pregnancy obscure early cancer

Diagnosis
- **USG** and **needle biopsy**[Q] are used for diagnosis
- **Mammography** is rarely indicated due to its **decreased sensitivity** during **pregnancy** and **lactation**

Treatment: Mainstay of therapy is surgical resection

• Stage I and II	• Mastectomy with axillary dissection[Q]
• LABC	• NACT after 1st trimester + MRM in 2nd trimester + RT after delivery[Q]

LABC in Pregnancy
• **MRM** can be performed during **first & second** trimester (increased risk of spontaneous abortion after first-trimester anesthesia), **chemotherapy after first trimester** and **radiotherapy after delivery**. • **Chemotherapy** during **first trimester** carries a risk of **spontaneous abortion** and **12%** risk of **birth defects, given after first trimester.** • No evidence of teratogenecity by chemotherapy during second and third trimester.

Remember
- Breast cancer in pregnancy have **prognosis stage by stage similar** to that of non-pregnant patient
- **Elective termination of pregnancy** to receive appropriate therapy without the risk for fetal malformation is **no longer routinely recommended** because no improvement in survival has been demonstrated.

PAGET'S DISEASE OF NIPPLE

PAGET'S DISEASE OF NIPPLE

- **Chronic eczematous eruption** of **nipple** which may progress to an ulcerated weeping lesion.
- Differentiated by superficial spreading melanoma by **CEA positivity**[Q]

Histopathology
- Paget cell is **large**, pale staining with **round nuclei & large nucleoli**[Q]
- Paget cells **spread into lactiferous sinuses**[Q] under the nipple and upward to invade overlying epidermis of the nipple
- Paget cells **does not invade dermal basement membrane**[Q] (carcinoma in situ)

Clinical Features
- Most (>97%) patients with Paget's disease have an **underlying ductal carcinoma**[Q] (in situ or invasive)
- Paget's disease **may (54%)** or **may not (46%)** be accompanied by a **mass**[Q]
- **Invasive breast cancer coexists** with Paget's disease in **93% of patients with mass** and in **38% of patients without mass**[Q]

Diagnosis
- **Complete mammography** and **biopsy** is required to rule out occult multicentric disease
- **Biopsy** showing **Paget cell is diagnostic**[Q]

Treatment
- Most commonly utilized procedure is **simple mastectomy**[Q]
- Wide excision of nipple and areola to achieve clear ,margins + Radiotherapy + Axillary staging
- Lumpectomy + Radiotherapy + Axillary LN dissection

CARCINOMA OF MALE BREAST

CARCINOMA OF MALE BREAST

- Peak in **6th decade**[Q] of life, accounts for less than **1%** of all cases of breast cancer.
- MC Type: Infiltrating ductal carcinoma[Q].

• Male breast cancer is **preceded by gynecomastia in 20% of men**[Q]. • **Hormone receptor positive: 80%; Her-2-neu positive: 35%**

- **Lobular carcinoma** (both in-situ and invasive) is **rarely seen** due to **absence of lobules** in males.

Predisposing Factors
- Excess endogenous or exogenous **estrogen** (Testicular disease, **infertility, obesity, cirrhosis**)[Q]
- Radiation therapy, **Klinefelter's syndrome** and **testicular feminizing syndromes**[Q].
- **BRCA2 mutations**[Q]

• **Gynecomastia** is **not a risk factor** for **carcinoma male breast**[Q].

Clinical Features
- MC presentation is **lump**[Q].
- Local pain, axillary adenopathy, nipple retraction, ulceration, bleeding, & discharge.

> • Breast cancer in men more commonly **involves** the **pectoralis major muscle**^Q due to **scanty breast tissue**.

Diagnosis
- Evaluation includes **breast imaging** studies and diagnostic **needle** or **surgical biopsy**.

Treatment
- Treatment of male breast cancer is **surgical** (Most common procedure: **MRM**)^Q
- **Adjuvant radiation therapy** is in **high risk cases** for local-regional recurrence.
- **Eighty per cent** of male breast cancers are **hormone receptor positive**, and adjuvant **tamoxifen** is considered.

Prognosis
- Stage >**Lymph node status** is the **best prognostic indicator**^Q as in female breast carcinoma.
- Stage by stage prognosis is **same** as female **CA breast**^Q

CYSTOSARCOMA PHYLLODES

PHYLLODES TUMORS

- Tumors of **mixed connective tissue** & **epithelium** (biphasic proliferation of **stroma** & mammary **epithelium**)^Q
- Also known as **serocystic disease of Brodie**^Q
- Classified as benign, borderline, or malignant.
- **Borderline tumors** have a greater potential for **local recurrence**.

Pathology
- Sharply demarcated from surrounding breast tissue, which is compressed & distorted.
- **Connective tissue** composes the **bulk** of these tumors, which have mixed gelatinous, solid & cystic areas.
- **Cystic areas** represent sites of **infarction** & **necrosis**.
- Gross cut tumor surface: **Classical leaf-like (phyllodes) appearance**^Q.
- **Stroma** of a phyllodes tumor has **greater cellular activity** than fibroadenoma.

Stromal cells of **fibroadenomas**	Either **polyclonal** or **monoclonal**^Q
Stromal cells of **phyllodes tumors**	Always **monoclonal**^Q

- Most **malignant phyllodes tumors** contain **liposarcomatous** or **rhabdomyosarcomatous elements** rather than fibrosarcomatous elements^Q.
- Evaluation of **number of mitoses** & **presence or absence of invasive foci** at the tumor margins may help to identify a **malignant tumor**^Q.

Clinical Features
- **Smooth, rounded**, usually **painless** multinodular lesions
- Average **age: 4th decade**.
- Large, mostly **massive size** but always **mobile over chest wall**^Q
- **Bosselated surface** with **pressure necrosis** of overlying skin^Q
- Diagnosis is suggested by **larger size**, a history of **rapid growth**^Q, and occurrence in **older patients**.
- **Differentiated from carcinoma** by: No fixity to skin and pectoralis, no nipple retraction, no LN involvement^Q

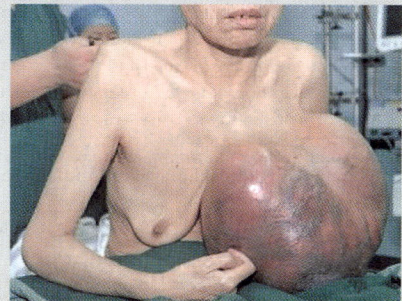

Diagnosis
- Mammographic evidence of **calcifications** & **morphologic evidence** of **necrosis do not distinguish** between benign, borderline, and malignant phyllodes tumors.
- **Ultrasound:** Discrete structure with **cystic spaces**
- Diagnosis is best made by **biopsy**^Q

Treatment

Small phyllodes tumors	Wide local excision^Q
Large phyllodes tumors	Mastectomy^Q
Phyllodes tumor with **suspicious malignant elements**	**Re-excision** of biopsy site **to ensure complete excision** of tumor with a **1 cm margin**

- **Axillary dissection** is **not recommended** because axillary LN metastases rarely occur^Q.
- **Metastases** from malignant phyllodes tumors occur **via hematogenous spread**, with common sites including **lung, bone**, abdominal viscera and mediastinum.

BREAST LEIOMYOSARCOMA

BREAST LEIOMYOSARCOMA

- Leiomyosarcomas are **malignant tumors**[Q] composed of cells showing smooth muscle features
- Locally aggressive tumor and **hematogenous metastasis**[Q]
- Palpable axillary lymphadenopathy is **uncommon**[Q] and when encountered usually represents **reactive LNs uninvolved by metastatic disease**[Q]
- A **clinically negative axilla** in presence of **large tumor** may be indicative of breast sarcoma
- Tumor is **well-circumscribed** or **encapsulated**[Q]

Treatment
- **Simple mastectomy** is **gold standard**[Q] of treatment
- **Axillary lymph node dissection** is **not indicated**[Q]
- **Postoperative radiation** may be used in patient undergoing mastectomy because chest wall recurrence are observed

BENIGN DISORDERS OF BREAST

ABERRATIONS OF NORMAL DEVELOPMENT AND INVOLUTION

- ANDI classification encompasses all aspects of breast condition, including pathogenesis and degree of abnormality.

Early Reproductive Years
- **Fibroadenomas** in younger women aged **15–25 years**
- Nipple inversion is a disorder of development of the major ducts, which prevents normal protrusion of the nipple.
- Mammary duct fistulas arise when nipple inversion predisposes to major duct obstruction, leading to recurrent subareolar abscess and mammary duct fistula.

Later Reproductive Years
- **Cyclical mastalgia** and **nodularity** usually are associated with **premenstrual enlargement** of the breast and are regarded as normal.
- In epithelial hyperplasia of pregnancy, papillary projections sometimes give rise to bilateral bloody nipple discharge.

Involution
- **Macrocysts** are common, are often **subclinical**, and do not require specific treatment.
- **Sclerosing adenosis** is considered a disorder of both the proliferative and the involutional phases of the breast cycle.
- **Duct ectasia** (dilated ducts) and periductal mastitis are other important components.
- **Sixty per cent** of women **70 years** of age exhibit some degree of **epithelial hyperplasia**.
- **Atypical** proliferative diseases include **ductal** and **lobular hyperplasia**, both of which display **some features** of **carcinoma in situ**.
- Women with **atypical ductal** or **lobular hyperplasia** have a **fourfold increase** in **breast cancer risk**.

ANDI Classification of Benign Breast Disorders			
	Normal	**Disorder**	**Disease**
Early reproductive years (age 15–25 years)	Lobular development Stromal development Nipple eversion	**Fibroadenoma**[Q] Adolescent hypertrophy Nipple inversion	Giant fibroadenoma Gigantomastia Subareolar abscess Mammary duct fistula
Later reproductive years (age 25–40 years)	Cyclical changes of menstruation Epithelial hyperplasia of pregnancy	**Cyclical mastalgia**[Q] Nodularity Bloody nipple discharge	**Incapacitating mastalgia**[Q]
Involution (age 35–55 years)	Lobular involution Duct involution Dilatation Sclerosis Epithelial turnover	Macrocysts Sclerosing lesions Duct ectasia Nipple retraction **Epithelial hyperplasia**	Periductal mastitis **Epithelial hyperplasia with atypia**[Q]

FIBROADENOMA

- **MC benign tumor** of **female breast**^{Q};
- **MC age group: 15–30 years**^{Q};
- Known as **breast mouse**^{Q}
- Etiology: **Increased sensitivity** of **focal areas** of breast tissue **to estrogen**^{Q}

Pathology
- **Encapsulated** spherical lesion, composed of **fibrous and glandular tissue**^{Q}
- Arise from interlobular stroma, stromal cells can be monoclonal or polyclonal

Types
- **Pericanalicular (Hard):** Due to proliferation of connective tissue **inside** the **elastic lamina**
- **Intracanalicular (Soft):** Due to proliferation of connective tissue **outside** the **elastic lamina**

Clinical Feature
- **Painless**, slowly growing **solitary mobile lump** in the breast (**Breast mouse**)^Q

Diagnosis
- IOC is FNAC^Q (**Antler horn configuration**^{Q} of ductal epidermal cells)
- Characteristic **popcorn calcification**^{Q} on mammography

Treatment
- **No treatment**^{Q} is necessary when diagnosis is confirmed.
- **Excision biopsy** is the treatment of choice for **suspicious lesion**^{Q} and for cosmetic indications.

BREAST CYST

- Occur most commonly in the **last decade** of **reproductive life**^{Q} as a result of a non-integrated involution of stroma and epithelium.

Clinical Features
- Often **multiple**, may be **bilateral**^{Q} and can mimic malignancy.
- Typically **present suddenly** and cause great alarm; **prompt diagnosis** and **drainage** provides **immediate relief**^{Q}.

Diagnosis
- Diagnosis can be confirmed by **aspiration** and/or **ultrasound**^{Q}.

Treatment
- **Aspiration** for Solitary cyst: If they **resolve completely**, and if the fluid is **not blood-stained, no further treatment** is required (30% will **recur** and require **reaspiration**)^Q
- **Core biopsy** or **local excision**^{Q}: If there is a **residual lump** or if the fluid is **blood-stained**, **for histological diagnosis** (exclude cystadenocarcinoma, which is more common in elderly women)

GALACTORRHEA

- Secretion of **milk looking discharge** from **one** or **both breasts unrelated to pregnancy**^{Q} is called galactorrhea.
- Physiological galactorrhea is the continued production of milk after lactation has ceased and menses resumed and is often caused by continued mechanical stimulation of the nipple.
- In both **men** and **women**^{Q}, galactorrhea may **vary in colour** and **consistency**.
- Galactorrhea is commonly **associated with prolactinoma**^{Q}.

Treatment
- Treatment is aimed at **normalizing prolactin level**^{Q}.
- **Bromocriptine**^{Q} (dopamine agonist) is the **drug of choice**.
- **Surgery** is considered when there is **failure of medical therapy**^{Q} (Trans-nasal trans-sphenoidal excision of pituitary adenoma is done^Q)

AMAZIA

- **Congenital absence** of the **breast**^{Q} may occur on one or both sides.
- It is sometimes **associated with absence** of the **sternal portion** of the **pectoralis major (Poland's syndrome)**^{Q}
- It is **more common in males**^{Q}.

MONDOR'S DISEASE

- A variant of **thrombophlebitis** involving the **superficial veins** of the **anterior chest wall**^{Q} and breast.
- Also known as "**string phlebitis**," a thrombosed vein presenting as a **tender, cord-like structure**^{Q}.
- Frequently involved veins: **Lateral thoracic vein, thoracoepigastric vein**, superficial epigastric vein.
- **Benign**, self-limited disorder.

Clinical Features
- **Acute pain** in the **lateral aspect** of the **breast** or the **anterior chest wall**^{Q}.
- A **tender, firm cord** is found to follow the distribution of one of the major superficial veins.

Diagnosis
- When the diagnosis is **uncertain**, or when a **mass** is present near the tender cord, **biopsy** is indicated.

Treatment
- NSAIDs and application of **warm compresses**^{Q} along the symptomatic vein with **restriction of motion** and **brassiere support** of the breast
- Usually **resolves** within **4–6 weeks**.
- When symptoms **persist** or are **refractory to therapy**, **excision** of the involved vein segment

DUCT PAPILLOMA

- Intraductal pailloma are true polyps of epithelium lined breast ducts.
- **Benign**^{Q} lesions (**not pre-cancerous**)
- **Mostly solitary**^{Q}, located under the areola (within 4-5 cm of nipple orifice)
- Generally **<1 cm**, can grow up to 4–5 cm

Clinical Features
- MC presentation: Bloody nipple discharge^Q
- **Intraductal papilloma** is MC cause of **bloody nipple discharge**^{Q}

Diagnosis
- **Ductography:** Small filling defects^Q surrounded by contrast media

Treatment
- **Microdochectomy:** Complete **excision** of the **involved duct** along with **tumor**^{Q}

DUCT ECTASIA (PERIDUCTAL MASTITIS)

- **Dilatation** of the **breast ducts**, which is often associated **with periductal inflammation**.
- Pathogenesis is obscure, **more common in smokers**^{Q}.

Pathology
- First stage in the disorder is a **dilatation** in **one or more** of the **larger lactiferous ducts**, which fill with a stagnant **brown** or **green secretion**^{Q}, this may discharge.
- These fluids then set up an **irritant reaction** in surrounding tissue leading to periductal **mastitis** or even abscess and fistula formation.
- **Dilatation** of the **breast ducts**, which is often associated **with periductal inflammation**.
- Pathogenesis is obscure, **more common in smokers**^{Q}.

Clinical Features
- **Nipple discharge** (of **any colour**), a subareolar mass, abscess, mammary duct fistula and/or **nipple retraction**^{Q} are the most common symptoms.

Diagnosis
- **Ductography:** Dilated cystic structure^Q in duct Ectasia
- In the case of a **mass** or **nipple retraction**, a **carcinoma** must be **excluded** by obtaining a **mammogram** and **negative cytology** or histology.

Treatment
- **Hadfield's operation**^{Q}: Excision of all of the major ducts
- Shave the back of the nipple to ensure that **all terminal ducts** are **removed** to prevent recurrence.
- **Cessation of smoking**^{Q} increases the chance of a long-term cure.
- Antibiotic therapy may be tried.

BREAST ABSCESS

- Typically seen in **staphylococcal infections**^{Q}
- Present with point **tenderness, erythema,** and **hyperthermia**
- **Related to lactation** and occur **within** the **first few weeks** of **breastfeeding**^{Q}.
- **S. aureus** are transmitted via suckling neonate^Q

Staphylococcal infections (MC)	Localized and situated deep in the breast tissues
Streptococcal infections	Diffuse superficial involvement

Diagnosis
- Preoperative **ultrasonography** is effective in **delineating the required extent** of the drainage procedure

Treatment
- Local wound care, including application of warm compresses, & IV antibiotics.
- For **mastitis, first line antibiotics** are **dicloxacillin**^{Q} or **Cloxacillin**^{Q} (given for **10-14 days**).
- **Drainage procedure** is best accomplished via **circumareolar incisions** or incisions **paralleling Langer's lines**^{Q}.
- **Biopsy** of **abscess cavity wall** at the time of incision and drainage **to rule out** underlying or coexisting **breast cancer** with **necrotic tumor**^{Q}.

GYNECOMASTIA

PHYSIOLOGIC GYNECOMASTIA

- **Excess** of circulating **estrogens** in relation to circulating testosterone: Neonatal period, adolescence and senescence.

Neonatal Gynecomastia
- Action of **placental estrogens**^Q on neonatal breast tissues
- Usually disappear in few weeks

Adolescent Gynecomastia
- Excess of **estradiol** relative to testosterone^Q
- **Usually unilateral**, asymmetrical if bilateral, occurs between **12–15 years**^Q
- **Regresses spontaneously**^Q within 3 years

Senescent Gynecomastia
- Circulating testosterone level falls resulting in **relative hyperestrinism**^Q
- **Usually bilateral**^Q

PATHOLOGICAL GYNECOMASTIA

- Causes: Idiopathic (MC)^Q, Relative estrogen excess, Absolute estrogen excess, Drugs

Relative Estrogen Excess
- Occurs because of **failure** of **testosterone synthesis or action**^Q

Congenital Defects	Secondary Testicular Failure

• Anorchia
• **Klinefelter's syndrome**
• Androgen resistance
   – Testicular feminization syndrome
   – Reinfenstein syndrome
• Defects in testosterone synthesis
	• Viral **orchitis** (mumps)
	• Trauma
	• **Castration**
	• **Leprosy**
	• Myotonic dystrophy, spinal cord injury
	• **Renal failure**

Absolute Estrogen Excess

1. Increased Testicular Estrogen Secretion:
   – Testicular tumors (**Leydig** cell, **sertoli** cell, **granulos/etheca cell** tumors)^Q
   – **Bronchogenic carcinoma** and **TCC** of urinary tract (secrete hCG)^Q
   – True hermaphroditism (Both testicular and ovarian components are active)
2. Increased Substrate for Peripheral Aromatization:
   – **Adrenal carcinoma** and **congenital adrenal hyperplasia**^Q (increased adrenal androgens)
   – Exogenous androgen administration
   – **Cirrhosis**^Q (decreased hepatic catabolism)
   – Starvation with refeeding (decreased hepatic catabolism)
   – Thyrotoxicosis (increased production by adrenals)
3. Increase in Extraglandular aromatization

Drugs

Estrogen Related Drugs	Drugs Enhancing Endogenous Estrogen Formation	Drugs Inhibiting Testosterone Synthesis/Action (MACKS)	Unknown Mechanism (CBI inquires PMT)
• DES^Q • OCPs^Q • Digitalis^Q	• Gonadotropins^Q • Clomiphene^Q	• Metronidazole^Q • Alkylating agents^Q • Cimetidine^Q • Cisplatin^Q • Ketoconazole^Q • Spironolactone^Q • Flutamide^Q	• Captopril^Q • CCB^Q • Busulphan^Q • INH^Q • Penicillamine^Q • Methyldopa^Q • TCA^Q

GYNECOMASTIA

- **Enlarged male breast** due to growth of **ductal tissue** and **stroma**^Q
- Basic mechanism: **Excess of estrogen** (relative or absolute)^Q

Clinical Classification of Gynecomastia	
Grade I	**Mild** breast enlargement without skin redundancy
Grade IIa	**Moderate** breast enlargement without skin redundancy
Grade IIb	**Moderate** breast enlargement with **skin redundancy**
Grade III	**Marked** breast enlargement with **skin redundancy** and **ptosis**, which simulates a female breast

Diagnosis
- In the **nonobese male**, **breast tissue** measuring **at least 2 cm** in diameter[Q]

Treatment
- **Most cases resolve spontaneously**[Q]
- **Non-surgical management**: Correction of underlying cause, cessation of offending drug
- **Pharmacological agents**: Antiestrogens (Tamoxifen), Aromatase inhibitors and danazol to inhibit gonadotropin secretion

Indications of Surgery in Gynecomastia	
1. Gynecomastia of **longer duration** (>1 year)[Q]	4. **Tenderness**[Q]
2. **Continued growth**[Q]	5. **Suspected malignancy**[Q]
3. **Psychological** or **cosmetic** problem[Q]	

- Surgical Procedures: **Mastectomy, subtotal mastectomy, subcutaneous mastectomy, reduction mammoplasty**[Q].

Suction Assisted Lipectomy
• **Removes only adipose tissue**[Q], if performed as a sole method
• Performed as an **adjunct surgical procedure**[Q]
• Use is limited in cases that are severe or in fibrous breasts
• **Reduces overall breast size** and may result improved appearance, but it **does not remove** the **glandular tissue** (does not correct gynecomastia)[Q]

- **Most cases** of gynecomastia are **amenable** to **simple liposuction** with minimal glandular resection through **periareolar incision** as necessary[Q].

Multiple Choice Questions

NIPPLE DISCHARGE

1. **Blood stained nipple discharge is seen in:**
   (Recent Question 2017, DNB 2013, 2011, Orissa 2011, PGI June 2009, UPPG 2010, AIIMS Nov 2003, All India 2005)
   a. Breast abscess
   b. Fibroadenoma
   c. Ductal papilloma
   d. Fat necrosis of breast

2. **Green discharge is most commonly seen with:**
   (Recent Question 2016, Kerala PG 2015, WBPG 2015, AIIMS Nov 98)
   a. Duct papilloma
   b. Duct ectasia
   c. Retention cyst
   d. Fibroadenosis

3. **A 25 years old female complains of discharge of blood from a single duct in her breast. The most appropriate treatment is:** *(All India 2008)*
   a. Radical excision
   b. Microdochectomy
   c. Radical mastectomy
   d. Biopsy to rule out carcinoma

4. **True statement (s) about nipple discharge is/are:**
   a. Mammography *(PGI June 2004)*
   b. Cone excision done in single intraductal tumour
   c. Mammography done when duct papilloma is <4.5cm
   d. Red discharge indicate malignancy
   e. Blue-black discharge indicate duct ectasia

5. **A 25 years old lady presents with spontaneous nipple discharge of 3-months duration. On examination the discharge is bloody and from a single duct. The following statements about management of this patient are true except:**
   a. Ultrasound can be a useful investigation *(AIIMS Nov 2004)*
   b. Radical duct excision is the operation of choice
   c. Galactogram, though useful, is not essential
   d. Majority of blood stained nipple discharges are due to papillomas or other benign condition

CARCINOMA BREAST INVESTIGATIONS

6. **Triple assessment for CA Breast includes:** *(Kerala PG 2015)*
   a. History, clinical examination and mammogram
   b. History, clinical examination and FNAC
   c. USG, mammogram and FNAC *(DNB 2010, All India 2009)*
   d. Clinical examination, mammogram and FNAC

7. **Best diagnostic method for breast lump is:** *(AIIMS June 95)*
   a. USG
   b. Mammogram
   c. Biopsy
   d. FNAC

8. **A 45-years old woman presents with a hard and mobile lump in the breast. Next investigation is:** *(All India 2001)*
   a. FNAC
   b. USG
   c. Mammography
   d. Excision biopsy

9. **A female patient present with a hard mobile lump in her right breast. Which investigation would be most helpful in making the diagnosis?** *(AIIMS Nov 2001)*
   a. FNAC
   b. Needle biopsy
   c. Excision biopsy
   d. Mammography

10. **Investigation of choice for high risk breast cancer in female is:** *(DNB 2014)*
    a. MRI
    b. CT-PET
    c. Mammography
    d. USG

11. **Gold standard investigation for screening of breast carcinoma in patients with breast implant:** *(Recent Question 2015)*
    a. MRI
    b. USG
    c. Mammography
    d. CT Scan

12. **A 60-year-old lady comes with blood stained discharge from the nipple with family history of breast cancer. Next best step for her will be:** *(AIIMS May 2015)*
    a. Ductoscopy
    b. Sono-mammogram
    c. Nipple discharge cytology
    d. MRI

13. **Best investigation to differentiate scar from recurrence after mastectomy done for carcinoma breast:** *(Recent Question 2016)*
    a. MRI
    b. CT
    c. PET scan
    d. Mammography

14. **All of the following are indications for MRI in breast carcinoma except:** *(Recent Question 2017)*
    a. Microcalcification
    b. High-risk cases
    c. Breast-implant patients
    d. Lobular carcinoma in situ

15. **What is the sensitivity of axillary ultrasound in identifying axillary metastases in clinically node negative carcinoma breast?** *(AIIMS May 2017)*
    a. 10–20%
    b. 20–30%
    c. 30–40%
    d. 55–60%

MAMMOGRAPHY

16. **Most sensitive imaging for ductal carcinoma in situ of breast is:** *(AIIMS Nov 2010)*
    a. Mammography
    b. MRI
    c. PET
    d. USG

17. **Dose of radiation per study in mammography:**
    a. 0.1cGy
    b. 0.2 *(Recent Question 2016)*
    c. 0.3
    d. 0.4

18. **True about screening mammography:** *(PGI June 2004)*
    a. Indicated in 50–70 years of age
    b. Mortality reduced by 30%
    c. Radiation due to mammography can cause carcinoma
    d. MRI is better than mammography
    e. USG is better than mammography

19. **On mammogram all of the following are the features of a malignant tumor except:** *(AIIMS Nov 2003)*
    a. Spiculation
    b. Microcalcification
    c. Macrocalcification
    d. Irregular mass

20. **BIRADS stands for:** *(AIIMS Nov 2012)*
    a. Breast Imaging Reporting and Data System
    b. Best Imaging Reporting and Data System
    c. Brain Imaging Reporting and Data System
    d. Best Imaging Reporting and Data System

21. **All are indicators of malignancy in a mammography except:**
    a. Nodular calcification *(PGI Dec 99)*
    b. Speckled margin
    c. Attenuated architecture
    d. Irregular mass

22. **Popcorn calcification in mammography is seen in:**
    (Recent Question 2016, AIIMS June 2000)
    a. Fibroadenoma   b. Fat necrosis
    c. Cystosarcoma phyllodes   d. CA Breast

23. **A 55-year-old post menopausal woman, on hormone replacement therapy (HRT), presents with heaviness in both breasts. A screening mammogram reveals a high density speculated mass with cluster of pleomorphic microcalcification and ipsilateral large axillary lymph nodes. The mass described here most likely represents:** *(AIIMS Nov 2003)*
    a. Cystosarcoma phyllodes   b. Lymphoma
    c. Fibroadenoma   d. Carcinoma

24. **With reference to mammography, which one of the following statements is correct?** *(UPSC 2005)*
    a. A baseline study should be done for all women at age 30
    b. It uses less radiation energy than a chest X-ray
    c. It should be part of the regular follow up of a woman following therapy for unilateral breast cancer
    d. It provides an effective substitute for biopsy of suspicious lesions

25. **What is the age of routine screening mammography?**
    a. 20 years   b. 30 years   *(DNB 2014)*
    c. 40 years   d. 50 years

26. **BIRADS score 4 suggests:** *(Recent Question 2018)*
    a. Normal lesion   b. Suspicion of malignancy
    c. Mostly benign   d. Proven malignancy

27. **BIRADS score 5 is:** *(Recent Question 2015)*
    a. Negative   b. Probably benign
    c. Suspicious abnormality
    d. Highly suggestive of malignancy

28. **Risk of malignancy in BIRADS II:** *(Recent Question 2017)*
    a. 0–2%   b. 2–4%
    c. 10%   d. 50%

29. **Radiation dose in mammography:** *(Recent Question 2017)*
    a. 0.1 Gray/study   b. 0.01 cGray/study
    c. 0.1 cGray/study   d. 0.01 Gray/study

30. **Which of the following is seen in carcinoma breast?**
    (Recent Question 2017)
    a. Powdery calcification   b. Popcorn calcification
    c. Nodular calcification   d. Pleomorphic calcification

CARCINOMA BREAST RISK FACTORS

31. **Risk factor for carcinoma breast:** *(PGI Nov 2011, Nov 2010)*
    a. Nulliparity   b. OCP
    c. Family history   d. BRCA-1 mutation
    e. Estrogen

32. **Which of the following is a predisposing factor for carcinoma of breast?** *(MHSSMCET 2005)*
    a. Sclerosing adenosis   b. Epithelial hyperplasia
    c. Fibrocystic disease of breast
    d. Fibroadenoma

33. **Following condition has no increased risk of invasive breast carcinoma except:** *(MHCET 2016)*
    a. Hyperplasia atypical   b. Sclerosing adenosis
    c. Apocrine metaplagia   d. Duct ectasia

34. **Moderately increased risk for invasive breast carcinoma is associated with which of the following?**
    a. Sclerosing adenoma   *(DNB 2010, Kerala 2000)*
    b. Apocrine metaplasia
    c. Duct ectasia
    d. Atypical ductal hyperplasia
    e. Fibro adenoma

35. **All of the following are predisposing factors for breast carcinoma except:** *(DNB 2008, MCI Sept 2008)*
    a. Family history of breast carcinoma
    b. First child at a younger age
    c. Early menarche and late menopause
    d. Nulliparous women

36. **BRCA-1 positive woman have _____% increased risk of breast carcinoma:** *(JIPMER 2011)*
    a. 10   b. 20
    c. 40   d. 60

37. **Gail model of risk assessment is used for:**
    (Recent Question 2013)
    a. CA stomach   b. CA esophagus
    c. CA breast   d. CA prostate

38. **Which of the following cancer is least associated with genetic and familial cause?** *(DNB 2008)*
    a. Ovarian   b. Prostate
    c. Lung   d. Breast

39. **Least risk of CA breast is seen in:** *(AIIMS Nov 2006)*
    a. BRCA-1   b. BRCA-2
    c. Li-Fraumeni syndrome   d. Ataxia telangiectasia

40. **BRCA-1 gene is associated with:** *(DPG 2008)*
    a. Ductal carcinoma   b. Lobular carcinoma
    c. Medullary carcinoma   d. Colloid carcinoma

41. **Type of fibroadenosis most likely to undergo malignant change is:** *(AIIMS June 93)*
    a. Adenosis   b. Epitheliosis
    c. Sclerosing adenosis   d. Cystic

42. **Doesn't lead to carcinoma breast:** *(DPG 2006)*
    a. Sclerosing adenosis   b. Epithelial hyperplasia
    c. Fibrocystic change   d. Papillomatosis

43. **Which of the following is an increased risk of breast cancer?** *(PGI Dec 2005)*
    a. Sclerosing adenosis   b. Atypical hyperplasia
    c. Fibroadenoma   d. Florid hyperplasia

44. **BRCA-1 gene is located on which chromosome?**
    a. 11   b. 13   *(MHCET 2016)*
    c. 17   d. 22

45. **BRCA-2 gene is located on chromosome:**
    (Recent Question 2017)
    a. 17   b. 13
    c. 7   d. 11

46. **All of the following are true about tumors associated with BRCA-1 except:** *(Recent Question 2017)*
    a. Hormone receptor positive
    b. Poorly differentiated
    c. Chromosome 17   d. Early age onset

47. **Which of the following is the most significant risk factor for developing breast cancer is?** *(Karnataka 96)*
    a. The presence of sclerosing adenosis
    b. Nullipartiy
    c. Atypical lobular hyperplasia
    d. Atypical ductal hyperplasia

48. All the following are risk factors for development of carcinoma breast except: *(APPG 2016)*
    a. BRCA 1 gene mutation
    b. Multiparity & prolonged lactation
    c. History of contralateral breast carcinoma
    d. Early age of menarche and multiparity

49. All are risk factors for carcinoma breast except: *(Recent Question 2013)*
    a. Early menarche
    b. Late menopause
    c. Ovarian cancer
    d. Early full term pregnancy

50. % of malignancy in duct ectasia is: *(Recent Question 2015)*
    a. No risk
    b. 15:1
    c. 7:1
    d. 10:1

51. Premalignant lesion with high-risk for malignancy:
    a. Atypical ductal hyperplasia *(Recent Question 2017)*
    b. Sclerosing adenosis
    c. Duct ectasia
    d. Papilloma

CARCINOMA BREAST

52. In which of the following types of carcinoma breast, comedo growth pattern is seen?
    a. Ductal carcinoma in-situ
    b. Medullary carcinoma
    c. Lobular carcinoma in-situ
    d. Infiltrating lobular carcinoma

53. False about lobular carcinoma breast is: *(DNB 2008)*
    a. Present as breast mass
    b. Frequently bilateral
    c. Poor prognosis
    d. Multicentric

54. True about histology in infiltrating lobular breast carcinoma:
    a. Single file pattern *(JIPMER 2012, 2011)*
    b. Pleomorphic cells in sheets
    c. Cribiform pattern
    d. Pin wheel pattern

55. Lymph node first involved in CA breast is/are: *(PGI Nov 2009)*
    a. Axillary LN
    b. Internal mammary LN
    c. Supraclavicular LN
    d. Contralateral axillary LN

56. In breast cancer following are expressed: *(PGI Dec 2007)*
    a. Her-2-neu
    b. p53
    c. BRCA-1
    d. BCL-1
    e. CEA

57. Most common presentation of lobular carcinoma breast is:
    a. Nipple discharge *(DNB 2012)*
    b. Breast mass
    c. Mammographic calcification
    d. Nipple retraction

58. Carcinoma breast is most commonly seen in which quadrant of breast: *(MHSSMCET 2005)*
    a. Upper outer
    b. Upper inner
    c. Lower inner
    d. Lower outer

59. Nottingham Prognostic Index for CA breast is:
    a. I = (0.2 x size) + grade + nodes *(MHSSMCET 2008)*
    b. I = (0.4 x size) + grade + nodes
    c. I = (0.6 x size) + grade + nodes
    d. I = (0.8 x size) + grade + nodes

60. Rare histological variants of carcinoma breast with better prognosis include all except: *(DPG 2009 March)*
    a. Colloid carcinoma
    b. Medullary carcinoma
    c. Inflammatory carcinoma
    d. Tubular carcinoma

61. In which of the following types of carcinoma breast, comedo growth pattern is seen? *(Karnataka 2006)*
    a. Ductal carcinoma in situ
    b. Medullary carcinoma
    c. Lobular carcinoma in-situ
    d. Infiltrating lobular carcinoma

62. Histological variety of breast carcinoma with best prognosis is: *(DNB 2012, 2008, 2005, 2002)*
    a. Medullary
    b. Colloid
    c. Lobular
    d. Tubular

63. Breast cancer which is multicentric and bilateral? *(DPG 2008, AIIMS Feb 97, May 95, All India 96, PGI June 95)*
    a. Ductal carcinoma
    b. Lobular carcinoma
    c. Mucoid carcinoma
    d. Colloid carcinoma

64. Single file pattern is seen breast cancer type: *(APPG 2004)*
    a. Intraductal
    b. Infiltrating lobular
    c. Infiltrating ductular
    d. None

65. In which of the following type of carcinoma of the breast, is a biopsy of the opposite breast advised? *(UPSC 2002)*
    a. Inflammatory carcinoma
    b. Medullary carcinoma
    c. Lobular carcinoma
    d. Scirrhous carcinoma

66. In which of the following type of breast carcinoma, would you consider biopsy of opposite breast? *(All India 2006)*
    a. Adenocarcinoma poorly differentiated
    b. Medullary carcinoma
    c. Lobular carcinoma
    d. Comedo carcinoma

67. The type of mammary ductal carcinoma is situ (DCIS) most likely to result in a palpable abnormality in the breast is: *(All India 2006)*
    a. Apocrine DCIS
    b. Neuroendocrine DCIS
    c. Well differentiated DCIS
    d. Comedo DCIS

68. Not true about CA breast in India: *(AIIMS June 98)*
    a. Incidence is 20/1,00,000
    b. Average age 42 years
    c. Positive family history is a risk factor
    d. More common in muslims

69. Best prognosis amongst the following histological variants of breast carcinoma is seen with: *(All India 98)*
    a. Intraductal
    b. Colloid (Mucinous)
    c. Lobular
    d. Medullary

70. Which of the following carcinoma is familial? *(All India 99)*
    a. Breast
    b. Prostate
    c. Cervix
    d. Vaginal

71. Which one of the following familial carrier syndromes is associated with mutation in BRCA genes? *(APPG 2016)*
    a. Hereditary non-polyposis colorectal cancer
    b. Von Hippel Lindau disease
    c. Peutz-Jegher syndrome
    d. Familial breast/ovarian cancer

72. A 45-year-old female presented to your OPD with this lesion in the left breast. What is the most probable diagnosis?
    a. DCIS
    b. LCIS
    c. Peau-d'orange
    d. Paget's disease of nipple

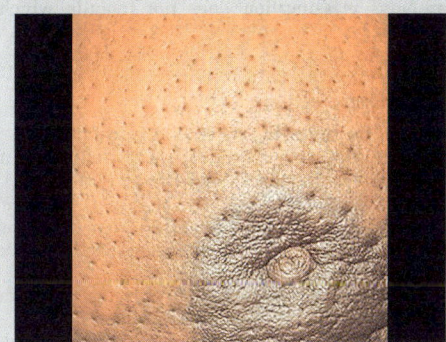

73. 'Peau-d-orange' appearance of the mammary skin is due to:
    (DNB 2012, PGI June 95, Dec 95)
    a. Intra-epithelial cancer   b. Sub-epidermal cancer
    c. Lymphatic permeation   d. Vascular embolisation
74. Which is the most conspicuous sign in breast cancer? (AIIMS November 2018)
    A. Nipple retraction   b. Peau-d'orange
    c. Puckering
    d. Both nipple retraction and puckering
75. Most common site of metastasis from breast carcinoma:
    a. Thoracic vertebra   b. Pelvis   (DNB 2012)
    c. Femur   d. Lumbar vertebra
76. Carcinoma breast with high incidence of involving opposite breast is: (Recent Question 2016, AIIMS Nov 94)
    a. Lobular carcinoma   b. Medullary carcinoma
    c. Scirrhous adenocarcinoma
    d. Atrophic scirrhous carcinoma
77. All are true about CA breast, except: (AIIMS May 93)
    a. Affected sibling is a risk factor
    b. Paget's disease of nipple is intraductal type of CA
    c. Common in aged nulliparous
    d. Increased incidence with prolonged breast feeding
78. 'Peau-d-orange' is due to: (DNB 2009, 2008, AIIMS Nov 93)
    a. Arterial obstruction   (AIIMS November 2015)
    b. Blockage of subdermal lymphatics
    c. Invasion of skin with malignant cells
    d. Secondary infection
79. True about lymphatic spread of CA breast: (PGI June 2005)
    a. Axillary nodes are most commonly involved
    b. Internal mammary nodes are also involved
    c. If supraclavicular lymph node is involved then it is N3
    d. Axillary nodes are treated by surgical resection
80. Secondary deposits from carcinoma breast is commonest in:
    (DNB 2010, 2001, All India 89)
    a. Lung   b. Liver
    c. Brain   d. Bone
81. Most common type of breast carcinoma: (WBPG 2014, 2015)
    a. LCIS   b. DCIS
    c. Phyllodes tumour   d. Invasive ductal carcinoma
82. Carcinoma breast is least commonly seen in:
    a. Superior outer quadrant   (Recent Question 2013)
    b. Inferior outer quadrant
    c. Subareolar   d. Lower inner quadrant
83. Nipple inversion occurs due to involvement of: (DNB 2014)
    a. Cooper's ligament   b. Subareolar duct
    c. Parenchyma of breast   d. Subdermal lymphatics
84. Van Nuys grading system is used for: (DNB 2014)
    a. LCIS   b. DCIS
    c. Inflammatory
    d. Medullary Carcinoma breast
85. Van-Nuys classification does not include which of the following?   (Recent Question 2018)
    a. Patients age   b. Size of tumor
    c. Presence of microcalcification
    d. Her-2-neu receptor status
86. Which of the following statements is fully true?
    a. Paget's disease of the nipple is a type of breast cancer with prominent Paget cells and presence of S-100 Ag immunostaining   (APPG 2015)
    b. BRCA 1 and 2 gene mutations cause breast cancer and are passed from mother to daughter by mitochondrial inheritance
    c. Raloxifene is an SERM that prevents breast cancer but increases risk of endometrial cancer
    d. Lobular carcinoma in situ arises from epithelial lining of the minor ducts and 10% occur in males
87. Dimpling in carcinoma breast is due to:
    a. Edema   (Recent Question 2016)
    b. Contraction of Cooper's ligaments
    c. Subdermal lymphangitis
    d. Scarring
88. Most common site of metastases in carcinoma breast:
    (Recent Question 2017)
    a. Bone   b. Lung
    c. Liver   d. Brain

CARCINOMA BREAST STAGING

89. A 45 years old postmenopausal lady presents with an 8-cm breast lump that is adherent to the skin, with one firm apical lymph node in the axilla and one more node in the ipsilateral supraclavicular area with no clinical evidence of distant metastasis. The staging is: (COMEDK 2010)
    a. T3 N2 M1   b. T4 N3c M0
    c. T4 N2c M1   d. T3 N3 M0
90. The clinician was palpating with tips of finger except thumb started from 2 o'clock posteriorly, palpated at 3 points on line joining periphery to nipple. Then again went to 3 o'clock point directly and came back centripetally while palpating at 3 points again on the line joining periphery and nipple. What is the method of breast examination depicted in the video?   (AIIMS November 2018)
    a. Vertical strip method   b. Concentric method
    c. Dial of clock method   d. Quadrant method
91. In patients with breast cancer, chest wall involvement means involvement of any one of the following structures except: (DPG 2010, AIIMS Nov 2005)
    a. Serratus anterior   b. Pectoralis major
    c. Intercostal muscles   d. Ribs
92. Ipsilateral supraclavicular lymph nodes are positive in a patient of CA breast. Stage is:
    (Recent Question 2013, AIIMS Nov 2008)
    a. II   b. III B
    c. III C   d. IV
93. CA breast stage T4b involves all except: (AIIMS May 2012)
    a. Nipple retraction
    b. Skin ulcer over the swelling
    c. Dermal edema   d. Satellite nodule
94. Which of the following stage of breast cancer corresponds with following feature: Breast mass of 6×3 cm size with hard mobile ipsilateral axillary lymph node and ipsilateral supraclavicular lymph node: (AIIMS June 2000)
    a. T4N2M0   b. T3N1M1
    c. T4N1M1   d. T3N3M0
95. A 43-year-old lady presents with a 5cm lump in right breast with a 3cm node in the supraclavicular fossa. Which of the following TNM stage she belongs to as per the latest AJCC staging system?   (AIIMS June 2004)
    a. T2N0M1   b. T1N0M1
    c. T2N3M0   d. T2N2M0
96. Patient with 1.2 cm breast lump with three lymph nodes in the axilla with no metastasis is in which stage as per AJCC?
    (COMEDK 2014)
    a. T1N0M0   b. T1bN1bM0
    c. T1cN1bM0   d. T2N1cM0
97. TNM staging of breast carcinoma with positive bilateral supraclavicular lymph nodes is?   (DNB 2014)
    a. N3a   b. N3b
    c. N3c   d. M1

CARCINOMA BREAST MANAGEMENT

98. True about modified radical mastectomy is: *(Punjab 2007)*
    a. Pectoralis major is removed
    b. Axillary lymph nodes are preserved
    c. Pectoralis minor is divided
    d. Internal mammary lymph nodes are removed

99. Contraindication for radical mastectomy in CA breast:
    a. Distant metastasis *(PGI Dec 2006)*
    b. Fixity to chest wall
    c. Axillary LN involvement
    d. Supraclavicular LN involvement

100. Breast conservation surgery indicated in: *(PGI Nov 2011)*
    a. Tumor size < 4 cm   b. Central
    c. Mobile   d. Pendulous breast
    e. Diffuse microcalcification

101. All of the following are removed in radical mastectomy except: *(MHPGMCET 2005, AIIMS 92)*
    a. Pectoralis major
    b. Pectoralis minor
    c. Axillary lymph node
    d. Supraclavicular lymph node

102. In Patey's modified mastectomy, which of the following is preserved? *(Recent Question 2014, MHSSMCET 2006)*
    a. Intercostobrachial nerve   b. Pectoralis major
    c. Pectoralis minor   d. Axillary fascia

103. Patey's mastectomy following are preserved except: *(Recent Question 2014, MHSSMCET 2009)*
    a. Teres major   b. Teres minor
    c. Axillary vein   d. Breast

104. Drug used in estrogen dependent breast cancer: *(AIIMS May 2012)*
    a. Tamoxifen   b. Clomiphene citrate
    c. Estrogen   d. Adriamycin

105. Components of QUARTZ except: *(MHSSMCET 2009)*
    a. Quadrantectomy   b. Axillary dissection
    c. Radiotherapy   d. Tamoxifen

106. Chronic treatment with tamoxifen can cause carcinoma of: *(COMEDK 2010, 2007)*
    a. Ovary   b. Endometrium
    c. Cervix   d. Vulva

107. Use of tamoxifen for breast cancer can cause all of the following adverse effects, except: *(AIIMS May 2011, DPG 2011, PGI Dec 2001)*
    a. Thromboembolism
    b. Endometrial carcinoma
    c. Carcinoma in contralateral breast
    d. Cataract

108. True about treatment of early breast cancer: *(AIIMS May 2008)*
    a. Aromatase inhibitors are replacing tamoxifen in premenopausal women
    b. Postmastectomy radiation therapy is given when 4 or more lymph nodes are positive
    c. Tamoxifen is not useful in post-menopausal women
    d. In premenopausal women, multidrug chemo-therapy is given in selected patients

109. Superolateral boundary of axillary dissection is: *(DNB 2010)*
    a. Clavipectoral fascia   b. Brachial plexus
    c. Axillary artery   d. Axillary vein

110. A 50-years old female has under gone mastectomy for CA breast. After mastectomy patient is not able to extend adduct and internally rotate the arm. Now supply to which of the following muscle is damaged? *(AIIMS May 2012)*
    a. Pectoralis major   b. Teres minor
    c. Lattisimus dorsi   d. Long head of triceps

111. In Patey's mastectomy, the step not done is: *(PGI 95)*
    a. Nipple and areola removed
    b. Surrounding normal tissue of tumor is removed
    c. Pectoralis major removed
    d. Pectoralis minor removed

112. Which is used in CA Breast? *(DPG 2007)*
    a. Daunorubicin   b. Doxorubicin
    c. Cisplatin   d. Actinomycin D

113. Malti, a 45-year-female patient with a family history of breast carcinoma, showed diffuse microcalcifi-cation on mammography. Indraductal carcinoma is situ was seen on biopsy. Most appropriate management is: *(Recenrt Question 2013, AIIMS June 2001)*
    a. Quadrantectomy   b. Radical mastectomy
    c. Simple mastectomy   d. Chemotherapy

114. For CA breast best chemotherapeutic regimen: *(AIIMS Sept 96, PGI June 96)*
    a. Cyclophosphamide, methotrexate, 5-fluorouracil
    b. Methotrexate, cisplatin
    c. Cisplatin, adrimaycin, steroid
    d. Methotrexate, adriamycin, steroid

115. A 30-year-old female presented with unilateral breast cancer associated with axillary lymph node enlargement. Modified radical mastectomy was done, further treatment plan will be: *(AIIMS May 2007)*
    a. Observation and follow-up
    b. Adriamycin based chemotherapy followed by tamoxifen depending on estrogen/progesterone receptor status
    c. Adriamycin based chemotherapy only
    d. Tamoxifen only

116. Breast conservative surgery is done in all except:
    a. Young patients *(DPG 2010, UPPG 2000)*
    b. Ductal carcinoma in situ
    c. Lobular carcinoma
    d. Infiltrative ductal carcinoma

117. In breast conservation surgery, the healthy margin excised is typically: *(DNB 2013)*
    a. 1 cm   b. 2 cm
    c. 3 cm   d. 5 cm

118. In the breast conservation surgery, which of the following investigation is required: *(DNB 2002)*
    a. Serum calcium   b. Total body scan
    c. Sentinel node biopsy   d. Tumor markers

119. Post operative radiotherapy in breast is given for:
    a. To prevent metastasis *(JIPMER 95)*
    b. For ablation of remnant of cancer tissue
    c. To prevent recurrence
    d. Prevents distant metastasis

120. A 40-year-old female with a 2 cms nodule in the breast and a proved metastatic node in the axilla, treatment is: *(PGI 96)*
    a. Quadrantectomy
    b. Mastectomy with local radiotherapy
    c. Patey's with adjuvant chemotherapy
    d. Halstedt's operation with tamoxifen

121. **Treatment of hormone dependent fungating carcinoma of breast with secondaries in the lung in a female patient aged 30 years is:** *(MAHE 2005)*
    a. Simple mastectomy followed by oophorectomy
    b. Radical mastectomy followed by oophorectomy
    c. Adrenalectomy
    d. Lumpectomy followed by castration

122. **A premenopausal lady presents with pulmonary metastasis. She underwent mastectomy 3 years back. True statement regarding her management:** *(PGI Nov 2011)*
    a. It was better if she took adjuvant therapy after mastectomy
    b. First analyze estrogen and progesterone receptor levels on the tumor
    c. Response of chemotherapy is dose dependent
    d. Combined chemotherapy is better than monotherapy
    e. She should now be given chemotherapy with radiotherapy

123. **Aromatase inhibitors used in CA breast are:** *(PGI June 2007)*
    a. Letrozole   b. Anastrozole
    c. Exemestane   d. Tamoxifen

124. **According to NSABP tamoxifen given in breast carcinoma for:** *(WBPG 2014)*
    a. 5 years   b. 3 years
    c. 10 years   d. Lifelong

125. **In radical mastectomy, the structures preserved are all except:** *(Recent Question 2015)*
    a. Axillary vein   b. Cephalic vein
    c. Nerve to Serratus anterior   d. Pectoralis minor

126. **Treatment of choice for locally advanced breast cancer:** *(Recent Question 2016)*
    a. Neoadjuvant chemotherapy followed by MRM followed by radiotherapy
    b. Surgery alone
    c. Radiation alone
    d. Surgery followed by chemotherapy

127. **A 36-year-old patient underwent breast conservation therapy and chemotherapy for a 1.5 × 1.2 cm ER positive breast cancer with one positive axillary lymph node. She is now on tamoxifen. How will you follow up the patient?** *(AIIMS May 2017)*
    a. Annual bone scan
    b. Assessment of tumor markers 6 monthly
    c. Routine clinical examination 3 monthly in 1st year with annual mammogram
    d. Routine clinical examination 3 monthly and 6 monthly liver function tests

128. **A 45 years old female presented with a history of painless breast lump of size 6 × 5 cm in left upper quadrant with no axillary lymph nodes. A true-cut biopsy was suggestive of ductal carcinoma in situ. She undergoes surgery with resection of all tumor tissue with adequate margins and postoperative HPE showing DCIS with high-grade necrosis with 4 mm clearance on margins. Which of the following is needed?** *(AIIMS May 2017)*
    a. Adjuvant chemotherapy
    b. Adjuvant chemoradiotherapy
    c. Adjuvant radiotherapy   d. No additional treatment

129. **Ixabepilone is used in:** *(Recent Question 2017)*
    a. Melanoma   b. Breast carcinoma
    c. Oat cell carcinoma d. Small cell carcinoma lung

130. **Adjuvant therapy after mastectomy is needed in all of the following except:** *(Recent Question 2017)*
    a. High risk, node positive   b. Low risk, no node
    c. HR –ve   d. Her-2-neu +ve

131. **Prophylactic mastectomy is done in:** *(Recent Question 2017)*
    a. BRCA-1 and BRCA-2 carrier
    b. History of breast cancer in mother
    c. After surgery in opposite breast
    d. Invasive ductal cancer

132. **Level II axillary lymph node:** *(Recent Question 2017)*
    a. Lateral to pectoralis major and minor
    b. Behind pectoralis minor
    c. Medial to pectoralis minor
    d. Superomedial to pectoralis major

133. **Which of the following statements is not true about tamoxifen?** *(Recent Question 2019)*
    a. It is used for visceral metastasis
    b. Tamoxifen is useful in post-menopausal and aromatase inhibitors in premenopausal patients
    c. Dose is 20 mg for 5 years
    d. It can cause endometrial carcinoma

134. **A patient underwent breast conservation surgery for a 3 cm lesion along with sentinel lymph node biopsy, which showed one third of sentinel lymph nodes are positive for macro-metastasis. Next step is:** *(Recent Question 2017)*
    a. Completion axillary lymph node dissection, chemotherapy and radiotherapy
    b. MRM with level I lymphadenectomy
    c. MRM with level III lymphadenectomy
    d. Only chemotherapy and radiotherapy

CARCINOMA BREAST PROGNOSTIC INDICATORS

135. **The most important prognostic factor of carcinoma breast is:** *(COMEDK 2010)*
    a. Tumor size   b. DNA content of tumour
    c. Histologic subtype d. Tumor grade

136. **True regarding axillary lymph node dissection in breast cancer:** *(PGI November 2017)*
    a. Axillary dissection can be carried out through the incision for a mastectomy
    b. Level I, II and III nodes are removed in modified radical mastectomy
    c. In Halsted radical mastectomy, all breast tissue and skin, the nipple, areola complex, the pectoralis major and pectoralis minor muscles, and the level I, II and III axillary lymph nodes are removed
    d. Arm is kept abducted at 90⁰ during axillary dissection
    e. Halsted radical mastectomy preserves pectoralis major and the lateral pectoral nerve

137. **Not a poor prognostic factor in breast carcinoma:** *(PGI May 2011)*
    a. Her-2-neu +ve   b. Progesterone receptor +ve
    c. Extranodal metastasis d. Vascularity of tumor
    e. ER +ve

138. **Good prognosis in carcinoma breast are all except:**
    a. Positive estrogen progesterone hormone receptor
    b. High HER-2-neu oncogene   *(UPPG 2010)*
    c. DNA flow cytometry shows-diploidy
    d. Low cathepsin-D
    e. Tumour labeling index <3%

139. **The most important prognostic factor in carcinoma breast is:** *(DPG 2009 Feb)*
    a. Size of tumour   b. Skin involvement
    c. Involvement of muscles d. Axillary LN involvement

140. **Prognosis of breast cancer is best determined by:** *(APPG 2008)*
    a. Estrogen/progesterone receptors
    b. Axillary lymph node status
    c. Clinical assessment
    d. CT

141. In case of CA breast most important prognostic factor is:
    a. Size of tumor (WB PG 2015, AIIMS Nov 96, Feb 97)
    b. Lymph node status
    c. Presence of estrogen receptor
    d. Age of menopause

142. The risk factor for increased incidence of relapse in stage I carcinoma breast includes all except:
    a. Negative estrogen/progesterone receptor status
    b. High 'S' phase (All India 98)
    c. Aneuploidy
    d. Decreased Her-2-neu oncogene

143. In breast cancer following are expressed: (PGI Dec 2007)
    a. Her-2-neu
    b. p53
    c. BRCA-1
    d. BCL-1
    e. CEA

144. Features, which are evaluated for histological grading of breast carcinoma, include all of the following except: (AIIMS Nov 2005)
    a. Tumour necrosis
    b. Mitotic count
    c. Tubule formation
    d. Nuclear pleomorphism

145. The most important prognostic factor in breast carcinoma is:
    a. Histological grade of the tumour (All India 2006)
    b. Stage of the tumour at the time of diagnosis
    c. Status of estrogen and progesterone receptors
    d. Over expression of p53 tumor suppressor gene

146. Molecular classification of breast cancer is based on: (AIIMS November 2014)
    a. Serum hormone levels
    b. Expression of hormone receptors (ER/PR)
    c. In-vitro response to chemotherapeutic agents
    d. Gene expression profiling

147. Estrogen receptor studies in carcinoma breast is done on:
    a. Blood
    b. Urine (JIPMER 87)
    c. Tumour tissue
    d. Ovary

148. Oncotype Dx test is done to for the following in breast cancer: (AIIMS May 2015)
    a. Chemotherapy in hormone receptor positive patients
    b. Hormone therapy in hormone positive
    c. Chemotherapy in hormone receptor negative patients
    d. Herceptin in Her-2-neu +ve

149. In the cases of carcinoma breast with Her-2 neu immunohistochemistry staining, which of the following score needs further FISH study? (AIIMS November 2017)
    a. 0
    b. 1+
    c. 2+
    d. 3+

150. Most common histo-immunological type of breast cancer: (Recent Question 2017)
    a. Luminal A
    b. Luminal B
    c. Basal cell type
    d. Her-2-neu type

151. Luminal A breast cancer shows following feature: (PGI May 2018)
    a. Low-grade tumor
    b. Her-2-neu amplification
    c. Good prognosis
    d. High-grade tumor
    e. ER-negative

152. Poor prognosis of breast carcinoma is associated with: (PGI May 2018)
    a. Over expression of Her-2-neu
    b. Increased estrogen & progesterone receptor expression
    c. Triple negative tumor
    d. Decreased percentage of cells in 'S' phase of mitosis
    e. Increased percentage of cells expressing Ki-67 marker

TRIPLE NEGATIVE BREAST CANCER

153. Which of the following is incorrect about triple negative breast cancer? (Recent Question 2016)
    a. Does not express the genes for ER, PR and Her-2-neu
    b. More common in postmenopausal women
    c. Germline mutations of BRCA1 and BRCA2 genes increases the risk
    d. Very susceptible to chemotherapy

COMPLICATIONS OF MASTECTOMY

154. Distressing complication after modified radical mastectomy? (Kerala PG 2015, APPG 2008, Orissa 90)
    a. Lymphedema
    b. Axillary vein thrombosis
    c. Seroma
    d. Death

155. The tumour, which may occur in the residual breast or overlying skin following wide local excision and radiotherapy for mammary carcinoma is: (Recent Question 2016, All India 2004)
    a. Leiomyosarcoma
    b. Squamous cell carcinoma
    c. Basal cell carcinoma
    d. Angiosarcoma

156. Complication of post mastectomy lymphedema is:
    a. Metastases of cancer
    b. Recurrence (JIPMER 95)
    c. Lymphosarcoma
    d. Pain

157. Pain along medial aspect of arm in a post-mastectomy patient is due to: (DNB 2009, 2008)
    a. Phantom breast pain
    b. Intercostobrachial neuralgia
    c. Neuroma pain
    d. Other nerve injury pain

158. Winging of scapula is seen after mastectomy due to injury of: (Recent Question 2017)
    a. Musculocutaneous nerve
    b. Long thoracic nerve of Bell
    c. Intercostobrachial nerve
    d. Thoracodorsal nerve

159. Most common complication of mastectomy:
    a. Intercostobrachial nerve palsy (Recent Question 2017)
    b. Long thoracic nerve palsy
    c. Thoracodorsal palsy
    d. Angiosarcoma

160. In a post mastectomy patient, the suction drain is accidentally removed on 2nd postoperative day and the lady started to have ooze with swelling in the chest. Next option in management in this case is: (Recent Question 2018)
    a. Open incision and pack with saline gauze
    b. Aspiration followed by pressure dressing and one more aspiration only
    c. Re-insert the drain
    d. Wait and watch

BREAST RECONSTRUCTION

161. Reconstruction surgery in breast carcinoma, best myocutaneous flap is: (UPPG 2009)
    a. Pectoralis minor
    b. Pectoralis major
    c. Latissimus dorsi
    d. Transverse rectus abdominis

162. Flap commonly used in breast reconstruction is: (Recent Question 2014)
    a. Serratus anterior
    b. TRAM
    c. Flap from arm
    d. Delto pectoral flap

163. All of the following are used for reconstruction of breast except: *(AIIMS Nov 2000)*
    a. Transverse rectus abdominis myocutaneous flap
    b. Latissimus dorsi myocutaneous flap
    c. Pectoralis major myocutaneous flap
    d. Transversus rectus abdominis free flap

164. Which of the following flaps gives best cosmetic results for breast reconstruction? *(MHPGMCET 2008)*
    a. Pectoralis major muscle flap
    b. Latissimus dorsi flap
    c. Transversus rectus abdominis muscle flap
    d. Serratus anterior muscle flap

INFLAMMATORY CARCINOMA BREAST

165. Most malignant type of carcinoma breast is: *(Recent Question 2015)*
    a. Paget's disease
    b. Anaplastic carcinoma
    c. Scirrhous carcinoma
    d. Atrophic Scirrhous carcinoma
    e. Mastitis carcinomatosa

166. In inflammatory carcinoma breast with metastasis of axilla, treatment of choice is: *(PGI Dec 96)*
    a. Radical mastectomy + chemotherapy
    b. Radical mastectomy + radiotherapy
    c. Simple mastectomy + radiotherapy
    d. Chemotherapy + radiotherapy

MALE BREAST CANCER

167. True about breast carcinoma in men: *(Recent Question 2016)*
    a. Estrogen receptor positive
    b. Associated with gynaecomastia
    c. Radiotherapy contraindicated due to close proximity to chest wall
    d. Seen in young males

168. What is true about male breast carcinoma? *(DPG 2008)*
    a. Gynaecomastia is a predisposing factor
    b. More common on right side
    c. Tamoxifen is not given   d. No estrogen present

169. True regarding male breast cancer: *(PGI June 2009)*
    a. MC lobular type
    b. Estrogen receptor positive
    c. History of gynaecomastia may be present
    d. Paget's disease of nipple is more common in male than female
    e. Undescended testis is a risk factor

170. True about male breast cancer is all except: *(MHPGMCET 2009)*
    a. Less than 2% of all cases of breast cancer
    b. Most commonly it is infiltrating duct carcinoma
    c. Most commonly it is infiltrating lobular carcinoma
    d. Exocrine or endocrine estrogen exposure can predispose to it

171. True abort male breast cancer: *(Recent Question 2014)*
    a. Invasive lobular carcinoma is most common type
    b. ER is negative
    c. Seen in young males
    d. BRCA-2 mutation is associated with increased risk

172. Most common carcinoma breast in male is: *(Recent Question 2014)*
    a. LCIS   b. DCIS
    c. Invasive ductal cancer   d. Invasive lobular cancer

CARCINOMA BREAST IN PREGNANCY

173. True about breast cancer in pregnancy:
    a. Occurs in 1 of every 3000 pregnant women
    b. MC non-gynecologic malignancy associated with pregnancy
    c. Ductal carcinoma is MC type, accounting for 75-90% of breast cancer in pregnancy
    d. All of the above

MONDOR'S DISEASE

174. Mondor's disease is: *(MCI June 2018, Recent Question 2015, 2014)*
    a. Thrombophlebitis of the superficial veins of breast
    b. Carcinoma of the breast *(DNB 2014, All India 96)*
    c. Premalignant condition of the breast
    d. Filariasis of the breast

175. Mondor's disease is superficial thrombophlebitis of: *(COMEDK 2005)*
    a. Axillary vein   b. Long saphenous vein
    c. Veins of the breast   d. Internal mammary vein

DUCTAL ANOMALIES

176. Treatment of choice in duct papilloma of breast is: *(Kerala PG 2015, All India 98, All India 96)*
    a. Simple mastectomy   b. Microdochectomy
    c. Local wide excision   d. Chemotherapy

177. Treatment for duct ectasia:
    a. Hadfield's operation *(Recent Question 2014, MAHE 2008)*
    b. Patey's mastectomy
    c. Modified radical mastectomy
    d. Radical mastectomy

178. Slit shaped nipple is seen in: *(Recent Question 2015)*
    a. Duct ectasia   b. Duct papilloma
    c. Paget's disease   d. CA breast

179. A woman noticed mass in her left breast with bloody discharge. Histopathology revealed duct ectasia. Treatment is: *(AIIMS Nov 2008)*
    a. Simple mastectomy   b. Microdochotomy
    c. Lobectomy   d. Hadfield's operation

180. Using a small fine probe, single lactiferous duct is excised. What is the name of the procedure? *(Recent Question 2018)*
    a. Macrodochectomy   b. Microdochectomy
    c. Webster operation   d. Hadfield operation

181. Sign seen in large duct papilloma is: *(DNB 2012)*
    a. Nipple discharge   b. Breast mass
    c. Skin excoriation   d. Lymph node involvement

CYSTOSARCOMA PHYLLODES

182. Treatment of cystosarcoma phyllodes in a young woman:
    a. Wide excision with a margin *(JIPMER 2011)*
    b. Wide excision with chemotherapy
    c. Wide excision with radiotherapy
    d. MRM

183. A 50 years old female presented with the given tumor in the OPD. The tumor was found to be malignant on biopsy. What is the best treatment option?
    a. Breast conservation surgery
    b. Simple mastectomy   c. Wide local excision
    d. Modified radical mastectomy

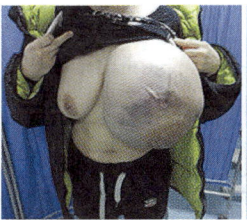
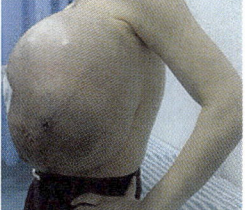

184. Cystosarcoma phyllodes is treated by:
    a. Simple mastectomy *(Recent Question 2015, AIIMS May 93)*
    b. Radical mastectomy
    c. Modified radical mastectomy
    d. Antibiotic with conservative treatment

185. Which one of the following statements is true of cystosarcoma phyllodes? *(UPSC 96)*
    a. It is a malignant tumour
    b. It often metastasizes to axillary nodes
    c. It is usually bulky and may fungate through the skin
    d. It is treated by radical mastectomy

186. A mobile, variegated large lump in the breast of a 20-years old female is most likely to be due to: *(UPSC 97)*
    a. Medullary carcinoma   b. Inflammatory carcinoma
    c. Cystosarcoma phyllodes   d. Lobular carcinoma

187. True about cystosarcoma phyllodes is: *(DNB 2007)*
    a. Calcification   b. Cystic compondent
    c. Tendency to recur   d. All of the above

188. Most common sarcoma of breast: *(Recent Question 2015)*
    a. Angiosarcoma   b. Phyllodes tumor
    c. Kaposi sarcoma   d. None

189. True about phyllodes tumor is: *(PGI May 2018)*
    a. Associated with BRCA1
    b. FNAC can diagnose reliability
    c. Treated with mastectomy
    d. Axillary lymph nodes are commonly involved
    e. Associated with BRCA2

GYNECOMASTIA

190. Gynecomastia may be seen in all of the following conditions except: *(All India 98)*
    a. Klinefelter's syndrome   b. Cirrhosis of liver
    c. Cryptorchidism
    d. Sex-cord tumour of sertoli cells

191. All of the following statements about gynecomastia are true except: *(All India 2007)*
    a. Subcutaneous mastectomy is the initial treatment of choice
    b. Seen in liver disease
    c. There may be estrogen/testosterone imbalance
    d. Can be drug induced

192. All are true regarding gynaecomastia except:
    a. May be seen in Addison's disease *(AIIMS Nov 93)*
    b. Usually unilateral in young males
    c. Acini are not involved
    d. Bilaterality is due to endocrinopathy

193. Gynaecomastia may be seen in patient with all except: *(Recent Question 2016)*
    a. Cimetidine therapy   b. Cirrhosis of liver
    c. Klinefelter's syndrome   d. Turner's syndrome

194. An adolescent boy presents with bilateral prominence of breasts and wants the breasts to be removed. Which one of the following incisions would be ideal? *(UPSC 97)*
    a. Radial
    b. Incision along the areolar margin
    c. Submammary incision
    d. Elliptical incision

195. Which of the following is least likely to be associated with gynecomastia? *(All India 2012)*
    a. Prolactinoma   b. Adrenal tumors
    c. hCG secreting tumors   d. Estrogen secreting tumors

PAGET'S DISEASE OF NIPPLE

196. Paget's disease of breast, true statements are: *(PGI Nov 2009)*
    a. Intraductal carcinoma   b. Mastectomy needed
    c. Malignant   d. Bilateral

197. A 40-year-old female presented to your OPD with this lesion in the left breast. What is the most probable diagnosis?
    a. DCIS   b. LCIS
    c. Peau-d'orange   d. Paget's disease of nipple

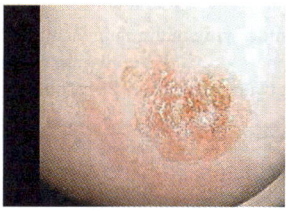
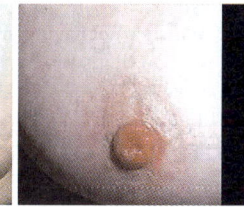

198. Consider the following statements regarding Paget's disease of the breast: *(UPSC 2008)*
    1. It is a malignant disease
    2. Diagnosis can be established by scrape cytology
    3. Lymph nodes involvement is an associated clinical feature
    4. Treatment of choice is simple mastectomy
    Which of the statements given above is/are correct?
    a. 1, 2 and 4 only   b. 1, 2 and 3 only
    c. 3 and 4 only   d. 1, 2, 3 and 4

199. Paget's disease: *(DPG 2006)*
    a. Incidence is 1:1000
    b. Has underlying intralobular carcinoma
    c. May have underlying carcinoma
    d. Blood stained discharge

200. Primarily a disease of nipple and areola: *(DNB 2007)*
    a. Duct papilloma   b. Paget's disease
    c. Periductal mastitis   d. Fibroadenoma

201. Paget's disease of breast following are true except:
    a. Treated by simple mastectomy *(Recent Question 2015)*
    b. Represents underlying malignancy
    c. Presents as eczema
    d. Cytology diagnostic

202. Characteristic feature of Paget's cell is: *(Kerala 94)*
    a. Eosinophilic cytoplasm   b. Abundant clear cytoplasm
    c. Glycogen mass   d. Multinucleated giant cell

203. True about Paget's disease of the nipple is: *(Kerala 95)*
    a. Always there is underlying carcinoma
    b. Often bilateral eczema of nipple seen
    c. Histology reveals giant cells
    d. Highly malignant

204. All are true about Paget disease of breast except: *(DNB 2014)*
    a. 1% associated with underlying invasive carcinoma of breast
    b. Hormone receptor negative
    c. Poor prognosis
    d. Wedge or punch is biopsy taken from nipple for diagnosis

205. Following are true of Paget's disease of breast except:
    a. Usually bilateral   *(Karnataka 98)*
    b. Associated intraductal carcinoma
    c. Prognosis good in absence of lump
    d. Treatment simple mastectomy with axillary clearance

206. Which of the following is the first line drug for mastitis? *(Recent Question 2019)*
    a. Cloxacillin   b. Cefazolin
    c. Ampicillin   d. Metronidazole

207. A lady primigravida developed fluctuant painful mass of breast and fever after 14 days of delivery. Preferred treatment option is: *(Recent Question 2019)*
    a. Stop lactation
    b. Analgesics and continue breastfeeding
    c. Antipyretic   d. Incision and drainage

208. Which is not having underlying malignancy? *(APPG 2008)*
    a. Paget disease of bone   b. Paget disease of nipple
    c. Paget disease of vulva   d. Paget disease of anal region

MASTITIS AND BREAST ABSCESS

209. Retromammary abscess arises from:
    a. Tuberculous rib   b. Infected hematoma
    c. Chronic empyema   d. All of the above

210. Acute mastitis commonly occurs during: *(DNB 2000)*
    a. Pregnancy   b. Puberty
    c. Lactation   d. Infancy

211. A lactating female presented with breast abscess. Most common organism responsible for her mastitis and abscess formation is: *(Recent Queston 2014, Punjab 2011)*
    a. S. aureus   b. E. coli
    c. Streptococci   d. Anaerobes

ANDI FIBROADENOMA AND FIBROADENOSIS

212. Fibroadenoma of the breast are:
    a. Fixed mass   b. Diffuse mass
    c. Multiple diffuse mass   d. Solitary mobile mass

213. A young female came to the surgery OPD with bilateral breast mass. On examination, mass was firm and mobile. What is the diagnosis on the basis of findings?
    a. Breast cyst   b. Fibroadenoma
    c. DCIS   d. LCIS

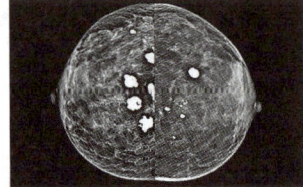

214. Pre-menstrual fullness in breast in 21-years old unmarried female is: *(AIIMS 98)*
    a. Galactocele   b. Fibroadenoma
    c. Fibroadenosis   d. Breast cancer

215. Regarding cystic disease of breast, which one is true?
    a. Common in 25 years of age   *(AIIMS Nov 97)*
    b. Excision is the treatment
    c. May turn into malignant   d. Aspiration is the treatment

216. The following are suitable for simple mastectomy except: *(Recent Question 2013)*
    a. Pagets disease   b. Fibroadenoma
    c. Cystosarcoma phyllodes   d. None

217. A 17-year-old female underwent Fine Needle Aspiration cytology (FNAC) for a lump in the breast which was non-tender, firm and mobile. Which of the following features would suggest finding of a benign breast disease? *(AIIMS November 2014, May 2013)*
    a. Dyscohesive ductal epithelial cells without cellular fragments
    b. Tightly arranged ductal epithelial cells with dyscohesive bare nuclei
    c. Stromal predominance with spindle cells
    d. Polymorphism with single or arranged ductal epithelial cells

MISCELLANEOUS

218. Cracked nipple may be:
    a. Due to syphilitic chancre   b. Cause of retention cyst
    c. Paget's disease of nipple   d. Forerunner of breast abscess

219. A 50 years old lady presented with lump in the left breast, which has developed suddenly in weeks. Perimenstrual symptoms are present. No associated family history. On examination, the lump is well circumscribed, fluctuant, 1.5 cm oval in shape. Most likely diagnosis: *(JIPMER May 2018)*
    a. Breast cyst   b. Galactocele
    c. Fibroadenoma   d. Breast cancer

220. Lymphatic drainage of breast: *(PGI Dec 2003)*
    a. Axillary   b. Supraclavicular
    c. Internal mammary   d. Mediastinal
    e. Celiac

221. Breast examination is done yearly in patients with: *(PGI 88)*
    a. Multiple fibroadenoma
    b. Family history of CA breast
    c. Carcinoma cervix   d. Endometrial carcinoma

222. A 50 years old woman complains of intermittent bleeding from the left nipple over the past 3 months. No mass is palpable, but a bead of blood can be expressed from the nipple. The ideal procedure in this case would be: *(UPSC 97)*
    a. Cytological examination of discharge and if no malignant cells, to be kept under careful observation
    b. Segmental excision of breast
    c. Microdochotomy   d. Simple mastectomy

223. Tylectomy literally means: *(DNB 91)*
    a. Excision of a lump   b. Excision of LN
    c. Excision of breast   d. Excision of skin

224. True about galactorrhoea: *(PGI Dec 2008)*
    a. Always bilateral
    b. Found in pregnancy and lactation
    c. Associated with prolactinoma and other endocrinopathies
    d. Surgery is done
    e. Hypothyroidism can cause galactorrhoea

225. Large breast is not seen in: *(AIIMS Dec 95)*
    a. Filariasis
    b. Giant fibroadenoma
    c. Cystosarcoma phylloides
    d. Schirrhous carcinoma

226. A 14 years old healthy girl of normal height and weight for age, complains that her right breast has developed twice the size of her left breast since the onset of puberty at the age of 12. Both breasts have a similar consistency on palpation with normal nipples areolae. The most likely cause for these findings is: *(AIIMS Nov 2003)*
    a. Cystosarcoma phyllodes
    b. Virginal hypertrophy
    c. Fibrocystic disease
    d. Early state of carcinoma

227. Haagensen's sing of inoperability of carcinoma include all except: *(DNB 91)*
    a. Edema of skin of breast or arm
    b. Satellite tumor nodules in skin of breast
    c. Proved supraclavicular or distant metastases
    d. Parasternal tumorous growth
    e. None of the above

228. Unilateral amastia is associated 90% of the time with absence or hypoplasia of following muscle: *(COMEDK 2004)*
    a. Latissimus doris
    b. Subclavian
    c. Pectoral
    d. Serratus anterior

229. True about leiomyosarcoma breast: *(PGI Nov 2010)*
    a. Axillary lymph node dissection is mandatory
    b. Well encapsulated
    c. Follow up not required
    d. Mastectomy is mainstay treatment
    e. Metastasize by lymphatic channel

230. Most frequent site of accessory breast: *(Orissa 2011)*
    a. Axilla
    b. Groin
    c. Buttock
    d. Thigh

231. Zuska's disease common is smokers causes: *(DNB 2012, 2007)*
    a. Acute mastitis
    b. Chronic areolar abscess
    c. Fibroadenosis
    d. Acute abscess formation

232. Lymphatic from left upper quadrant of breast brain into all of the following group of lymphnodes except: *(DNB 2001)*
    a. Anterior axillary
    b. Central
    c. Apical
    d. Parasternal

233. A lady 35 years old lactating mother presented with a painful breast lump. Most appropriate initial investigation should be: *(AIIMS Nov 2012)*
    a. Mammography
    b. USG
    c. MRI
    d. X-ray

234. In patients of breast pain, primrose oil is used for how many months? *(Recent Question 2017)*
    a. 1
    b. 2
    c. 3
    d. 4

SENTINEL LYMPH NODE BIOPSY

235. In sentinel node biopsy for breast cancer, the most commonly injured nerve is: *(AIIMS May 2013)*
    a. Lateral pectoral nerve
    b. Nerve to lattissimus dorsi
    c. Intercostobrachial nerve
    d. Long thoracic nerve (Nerve to serratus anterior)

236. Intraoperative sentinel lymph node detection in axilla is done by using: *(Recent Question 2013)*
    a. Mammography
    b. Isosulfan blue dye
    c. MRI
    d. CT

237. Sentinel lymph node biopsy in carcinoma breast is done if: *(Recent Question 2013)*
    a. LN palpable
    b. Breast mass but no lymph node palpable
    c. Breast lump with palpable axillary node
    d. Metastatic CA breast

238. Radioisotope used in sentinel lymph node biopsy in breast: *(Recent Question 2017)*
    a. Technetium iodine
    b. Technetium labeled colloid sulfur
    c. Tc99
    d. Iodine-131

Explanations

NIPPLE DISCHARGE

1. **Ans. c. Ductal papilloma** *(Ref: Schwartz 10/e p554, 9/e p467; Sabiston 20/e p824-826; 19/e p828; Bailey 27/e p863, 26/e p802)*

   - **MC cause** of greenish discharge: **Duct ectasia**[Q]
   - **MC cause** of blood-stained discharge: **Duct papilloma**[Q]

2. **Ans. b. Duct ectasia.**
3. **Ans. b. Microdochectomy** *(Ref: Bailey 27/e p863, 26/e p802; CSDT 12/e p299; Schwartz 10/e p526, 9/e p448)*
4. **Ans. a. Mammography, b. Cone excision done in single intraductal tumour, d. Red discharge indicate malignancy, e. Blue-black discharge indicate duct ectasia**
5. **Ans. b. Radical duct excision is the operation of choice.**

CARCINOMA BREAST INVESTIGATIONS

6. **Ans. d. Clinical examination, Mammogram and FNAC** *(Ref: Schwartz 10/e p522-523, 9/e p444-446; Sabiston 20/e p826-828; 19/e p840-842; Bailey 27/e p863, 26/e p799-801)*

   - **Triple Assessment** includes a combination of **clinical assessment, radiological imaging** (USG/ Mammography) and **tissue sample analysis** (FNAC/Biopsy)[Q]
   - The **positive predictive value** of Triple Assessment should **exceed 99.9%**[Q]

7. **Ans. c. Biopsy** *(Ref: Schwartz 10/e p529-530, 9/e p450; Sabiston 20/e p826-828; 19/e p830-831; Bailey 27/e p862, 26/e p800)*

   CA Breast

   - First investigation for tissue sampling: **FNAC**[Q]
   - Best and diagnostic investigation: **Biopsy**[Q]

8. **Ans. c. Mammography** *(Ref: Schwartz 10/e p523-529, 9/e p447-450; Sabiston 20/e p826-827; 19/e p830-832; Bailey 27/e p861, 26/e p799-801)*

   - First investigation: Mammography
   - Best and diagnostic investigation: Biopsy[Q]

Investigations in CA Breast	
Mammography	• **Initial investigation** for symptomatic breast in **women >35 years** and for **screening**[Q] • **IOC** for **microcalcification**[Q]
Ultrasound	• **Initial investigation** for **palpable lesions** in **women <35 years**[Q] • Not useful in screening
MRI	• Indicated in scarred breast, implants and borderline lesions for breast conservation • **IOC** for **implant related complications**[Q] • Gold standard for **imaging breast** in females **with implants**[Q]
PET scan	• **IOC** for **detecting recurrences** in **scarred breast**[Q] • Useful in multifocal disease and in helping detect axillary involvement

9. **Ans. b. Needle biopsy**
10. **Ans. a. MRI**
11. **Ans. a. MRI**
12. **Ans. d. MRI** *(Ref: Schwartz 10/e p527, 9/e p447-450; Harrison 20/e p557,19/e p526; Sabiston 20/e 828; 19/e p830-832; Bailey 26/e p799-801)*

    A 60-year-old lady comes with blood stained discharge from the nipple with family history of breast cancer. Next best step for her (high risk female) will be MRI for screening of breast cancer.

    > "There is **current interest in the use of MRI to screen the breasts of high-risk women** and of women with a newly diagnosed breast cancer. In the first case, women who have a strong family history of breast cancer or who carry known genetic mutations require screening at an early age, but mammographic evaluation is limited because of the increased breast density in younger women. In the second case, an MRI study of the contralateral breast in women with a known breast cancer has shown a contralateral breast cancer in 5.7% of these women."- *Schwartz 10/e p527, 9/e p450*

13. **Ans. c. PET scan**
14. **Ans. a. Microcalcification** *(Ref: Schwartz 10/e p527; Sabiston 20/e p828; Bailey 27/e p862)*

15. **Ans. d. 55–60%** *(Ref: Schwartz 10/e p527; De Vita 10/e p1122)*

> "The status of the regional lymph nodes is one of the most important prognostic factors in early stage breast cancer. Ultrasound may add to clinical examination and improve the sensitivity of node detection (combined sensitivity ranges from 60–80% in various trials, as it is based on subjective findings and operator dependence), but surgical staging using US guided FNA or SLNB/ALND is required for all patients."-De Vita 10/e p1122

MAMMOGRAPHY

16. **Ans. b. MRI** *(Ref: Grainger 5/e p1190, 1188)*

    - Screening with **MRI** is **superior to mammography** in **detecting invasive breast cancer in younger women**^{Q}, where the **sensitivity of mammography is low** due to **presence of mammographically dense breast parenchyma**^{Q}

17. **Ans. a. 0.1cGy**
18. **Ans. a. Indicated in 50–70 years of age, b. Mortality reduced by 30%** *(Ref: Schwartz 10/e p523-525, 9/e p447; Sabiston 20/e p828; 19/e p831-832; Bailey 27/e p861, 26/e p799)*
19. **Ans. c. Macrocalcification** *(Ref: Schwartz 10/e p523-525, 9/e p447; Sabiston 20/e p828, 19/e p831-832; Bailey 27/e p861, 26/e p799)*
20. **Ans. a. Breast Imaging Reporting and Data System** *(Ref: Sabiston 20/e p831, 19/e p834)*
21. **Ans. a. Nodular calcification**
22. **Ans. a. Fibroadenoma** *(Ref: Robbins 9/e p1069)*

Pattern of Calcification in Breast Diseases	
Carcinoma	**Microcalcification,** punctate, branching^Q
Fibroadenoma	**Popcorn**^{Q} (coarse, granular, crushed stone)
Fibrocystic disease	Powdery
Fat necrosis	Curvilinear

23. **Ans. d. Carcinoma**
24. **Ans. c. It should be part of the regular follow-up of a woman following therapy for unilateral breast cancer**
25. **Ans. c. 40 years**
26. **Ans. b. Suspicion of malignancy** *(Ref: Sabiston 20/e p831)*
27. **Ans. d. Highly suggestive of malignancy**
28. **Ans. a. 0–2%** *(Ref: Sabiston 20/e p831)*
29. **Ans. c. 0.1 cGray/study** *(Ref: Schwartz 10/e p523; Sabiston 20/e p828; Bailey 27/e p861)*
30. **Ans. d. Pleomorphic calcification** *(Ref: Schwartz 10/e p526; Sabiston 20/e p828)*

CARCINOMA BREAST RISK FACTORS

31. **Ans. a. Nulliparity, c. Family history, d. BRCA-1 mutation, e. Estrogen** *(Ref: Schwartz 10/e p511-512, Sabiston 20/e p831, Bailey 27/e p871)*
32. **Ans. b. Epithelial hyperplasia** *(Ref: Schwartz 10/e p508, Sabiston 20/e p832, Bailey 27/e p871)*

Proliferative Lesions Relative Risks for Developing Invasive Breast Cancer	
• **Nonproliferative changes: 70%** • Relative Risk = 1.0	• Adenosis • Cysts and apocrine change • Ductal ectasia • Mild epithelial hyperplasia of usual type
• **Proliferative disease** without atypia: **26%** • Relative Risk = 1.5–2.0	• **Hyperplasia** of usual type, moderate or florid • **Papilloma** • **Sclerosing adenosis**
• **Proliferative disease** with atypia: **4%** • Relative Risk = 4–5	• **Atypical ductal hyperplasia**^{Q} • **Atypical lobular hyperplasia**^{Q}

33. **Ans. a. Hyperplasia atypical** *(Ref: Schwartz 10/e p508, Sabiston 20/e p832, Bailey 26/e p809)*

Cancer Risk Associated (with Benign Breast Disorders and In Situ Carcinoma of the Breast)	
Abnormality	**Relative Risk**
Nonproliferative lesions of the breast	No increased risk
Sclerosing adenosis	No increased risk

Intraductal papilloma	No increased risk
Florid hyperplasia	1.5 to 2-fold
Atypical lobular hyperplasia^Q	4–fold
Atypical ductal hyperplasia^Q	4–fold
Ductal involvement^Q by cells of atypical ductal hyperplasia	7–fold
Lobular carcinoma in situ^Q	10–fold
Ductal carcinoma in situ^Q	10–fold

34. Ans. d. Atypical ductal hyperplasia
35. Ans. b. First child at a younger age
36. Ans. d. 60 *(Ref: Schwartz 10/e p514-515; Sabiston 20/e p832; Bailey 26/e p817-818; Harrison 20/e p556, 19/e p523-524, 18/e p754-755; Devita 9/e p1373)*

- Harrison says "Women who inherit a mutated allele of **BRCA-1 gene** from either parent have at least a **60–80% lifetime chance of developing breast cancer** and about a **33% chance of developing ovarian cancer.**"
- Schwartz says "Germline mutations in BRCA1 represent a predisposing genetic factor in as many as 45% of hereditary breast cancers and in at least 80% of hereditary ovarian cancers. Female mutation carriers have up to a 90% lifetime risk for developing breast cancer and up to a 40% lifetime risk for developing ovarian cancer."

37. Ans. c. CA breast
38. Ans. c. Lung
39. Ans. d. Ataxia telangiectasia *(Ref: Schwartz 10/e p514-515; Sabiston 20/e p832; Bailey 26/e p817)*

Incidence of Sporadic, Familial and Hereditary Breast Cancer	
• Sporadic breast cancer^Q	65–75%
• Familial breast cancer^Q	20–30%
• Hereditary breast cancer	5–10%
• BRCA1^Q	**45%**
• BRCA2^Q	**35%**
• p53 (**Li-Fraumeni** syndrome)^Q	1%
• STK11/LKB1a (**Peutz-Jeghers** syndrome)^Q	<1%
• PTENa (**Cowden** disease)^Q	<1%
• MSH2/MLH1a (**Muir-Torre** syndrome)^Q	<1%
• ATMa (**Ataxia-telangiectasia**)^Q	<1%
• Unknown	20%
Hereditary Breast Cancer	
• **BRCA** and **PLACH**: PJS, Li-Fraumeni, Ataxia telangiectasia, Cowden's, HNPCC	

40. Ans. a. Ductal carcinoma *(Ref: Schwartz 10/e p514-515; Sabiston 20/e p832; Bailey 27/e p880)*
41. Ans. b. Epitheliosis
42. Ans. c. Fibrocystic change *(Ref: Robbins 9/e p1048)*

- Fibrocystic change doesn't lead to carcinoma breast.
- Robbins says "**Fibrocystic changes** (**Non-proliferative breast changes**): Non-proliferative changes are most likely part of the **spectrum of histologic features** that can be **observed in normal breast.**"

43. Ans. b. Atypical hyperplasia, d. Florid hyperplasia
44. Ans. c. 17
45. Ans. b. 13 *(Ref: Schwartz 10/e p515; Sabiston 20/e p832; Bailey 27/e p880)*
46. Ans. a. Hormone receptor positive *(Ref: Schwartz 10/e p514; Sabiston 20/e p832; Bailey 27/e p880)*
47. Ans. c. Atypical lobular hyperplasia, d. Atypical ductal hyperplasia
48. Ans. b. Multiparity & prolonged lactation
49. Ans. d. Early full term pregnancy
50. Ans. a. No risk
51. Ans. a. Atypical ductal hyperplasia *(Ref: Schwartz 10/e p508; Sabiston 20/e p831; Bailey 27/e p871)*

CARCINOMA BREAST

52. Ans. a. Ductal carcinoma in-situ *(Ref: Schwartz 10/e p520; Sabiston 20/e p837; Bailey 27/e p872)*
53. Ans. c. Poor prognosis
54. Ans. a. Single file pattern
55. Ans. a. Axillary LN, b. Internal mammary LN *(Ref: Bailey 27/e p873)*
56. Ans. a. Her-2-neu, b. p53, c. BRCA-1, e. CEA *(Ref: Schwartz 9/e p438; Sabiston 20/e p840; Bailey 27/e p875)*

- BCL-1 gene is expressed in **mantle cell lymphoma**^{Q}.
- Her-2-neu, p53, BRCA-1 and CEA is expressed in **CA breast**^{Q}.

57. Ans. b. Breast mass
58. Ans. a. Upper outer
59. Ans. a. {I= (0.2 x size) + grade + nodes} *(Ref: Bailey 27/e p875)*

Nottingham Prognostic Index (NPI)

- NPI = (0.2 X **tumor size** in cm) + **Tumor grade** (1–3) + **LN stage** (1–3)^Q
- Used to select patients for **adjuvant treatment**

60. Ans. c. Inflammatory carcinoma *(Ref: Schwartz 10/e p520-522; Sabiston 20/e p860)*

Inflammatory Carcinoma

- **Ominous clinical category**^{Q} associated with **diffuse tumor involvement of the lymphatic channels**^{Q} within the breast and overlying skin

61. Ans. a. Ductal carcinoma in situ
62. Ans. d. Tubular
63. Ans. b. Lobular carcinoma
64. Ans. b. Infiltrating lobular
65. Ans. c. Lobular carcinoma
66. Ans. c. Lobular carcinoma
67. Ans. d. Comedo DCIS
68. Ans. d. More common in Muslims
69. Ans. b. Colloid (Mucinous)
70. Ans. a. Breast *(Ref: Sabiston 20/e p691)*
71. Ans. d. Familial breast/ovarian cancer
72. Ans. c. Peau-d'orange
73. Ans. c. Lymphatic permeation *(Ref: Bailey 27/e p873)*

Peau-d-orange

- Peau-d-orange is due to **cutaneous lymphatic edema**, where the infiltrated skin is tethered by sweat ducts, it can not swell, leading to an appearance like **orange skin**^{Q}.
- Due to **obstruction** of **subdermal lymphatics** (**lymphatic permeation** by **tumor cells**)
- Seen in **advanced breast cancer** (may be seen in **chronic abscess**)

74. Ans. b. Peau-d'orange *(Ref: Schwartz 10/e p518; Sabiston 20/e p860; Bailey 27/e p873)*
75. Ans. d. Lumbar vertebra *(Ref: Bailey 27/e p873)*

- Most common site of metastasis from breast carcinoma is lumbar vertebra.

Bailey says that "It is by this route (**spread by the bloodstream**) that **skeletal metastases** occur, although the initial spread may be via the lymphatic system. **In order of frequency** the **lumbar vertebrae, femur, thoracic vertebrae, rib and skull are affected** and these deposits are generally **osteolytic**."

76. Ans. a. Lobular carcinoma
77. Ans. d. Increased incidence with prolonged breastfeeding
78. Ans. b. Blockage of subdermal lymphatics
79. Ans. a. Axillary nodes are most commonly involved, b. Internal mammary nodes are also involved, c. If supraclavicular lymph node is involved then it is N3, d. Axillary nodes are treated by surgical resection *(Ref: Bailey 27/e p873)*
80. Ans. d. Bone
81. Ans. d. Invasive ductal carcinoma
82. Ans. d. Lower inner quadrant *(Ref: Bailey 27/e p874)*

- Upper inner (12–15%) • Upper outer (~ 50%) • Lower inner (3–5%) • Lower outer (6–10%) • Central/areolar (20%)

83. Ans. b. Subareolar duct *(Ref: Bailey 27/e p873)*

- Retraction of nipple is due to fibrosis in and around subareolar duct
- Retraction/dimpling of skin is due to involvement of cooper's ligament
- Peau-D-orange is due to blockage of subdermal lymphatics

84. **Ans. b. DCIS** *(Ref: Sabiston 20/e p853, Bailey 27/e p872, p838)*

Van Nuys Prognostic Index (VNPI)

- Van Nuys prognostic index (VNPI) is widely used to classify ductal carcinoma in situ (DCIS) into dissimilar risk categories that may be treated accordingly. Attempts have been made to identify subsets of DCIS for which wide excision without irradiation would provide sufficient local control.
- Silverstein and colleagues derived the **Van Nuys criteria** from a series of DCIS patients treated by wide excision with and without radiation therapy and proposed a system to **identify patients** who do **not need radiation therapy based on:**
  1. Patient's age^Q
  2. DCIS nuclear **grade**^{Q} and presence of **microcalcification**^{Q}
  3. **Size**^{Q} of the lesion
  4. **Width**^{Q} of the surgical margin.

85. **Ans. d. Her-2-neu receptor status** *(Ref: Sabiston 20/e p853; Bailey 27/e p872)*
86. **Ans. c. Raloxifene is an SERM that prevents breast cancer but increases risk of endometrial cancer**
87. **Ans. c. Subdermal lymphangitis**   88. **Ans. a. Bone** *(Ref: Schwartz 10/e p543; Sabiston 20/e p838; Bailey 27/e p873)*

CARCINOMA BREAST STAGING

89. **Ans. d. T3 N3 M0** *(Ref: Schwartz 10/e p532; Sabiston 20/e p843)*
90. **Ans. c. Dial of clock method** *(Ref: https://www.ncbi.nlm.nih.gov/pmc/articles/PMC5473793/)*

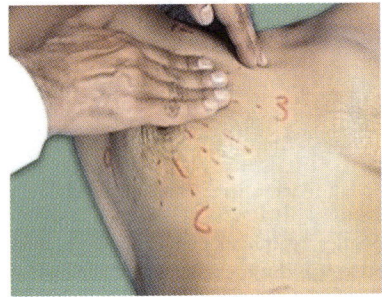

"Dial of Clock" Method of Breast Examination

"Dial of Clock" Method of Breast Examination
- In **dial of clock method**, palpation is **performed in segmental manner** until entire breast is **examined with "pads of middle three fingers" (index, middle, and ring)** with hand held in slightly bowed position.
- **Whole breast** is palpated as if it was **"dial of a clock":**
– **12 o'clock: Highest point at upper edge of breast** just below mid-clavicular point
– **6 o'clock: At infra-mammary crease**.
- **Palpation begins at 12 o'clock** from **periphery to nipple** by describing **small circles of about 3 cm in diameter**.
- Breast is palpated by making **circular movements of the "pad of fingers", three times with increasing pressure** & without lifting the fingers.
- **Next circle** is **palpated towards nipple**, overlapping with the previous circle to about half in diameter. Once areola & nipple area is reached, the next segment/sector is palpated at 1 o'clock.
- **Inner half of mammary gland** is **palpated in supine position**.
- Patient is requested to **roll over the opposite side** for **palpation of outer half of mammary gland**. This allows the mammary tissue to fall towards the midline by gravity resulting in **flattening of lateral half of mammary gland**, making a **lump in lateral half more discernible**.

91. **Ans. b. Pectoralis major** *(Ref: Schwartz 9/e p452; Sabiston 20/e p843)*

- **Chest wall involvement** means involvement of **ribs**^{Q}, **intercostal muscles**^{Q} or **Serratus anterior**^{Q} as **chest wall** is formed by these structures **not** the **pectoralis major.**

92. Ans. c. IIIC
93. Ans. a. Nipple retraction
94. Ans. d. T3N3M0
95. Ans. c. T2N3M0
96. Ans. c. T1cN1bM0
97. Ans. d. M1

CARCINOMA BREAST MANAGEMENT

98. Ans. c. Pectoralis minor is divided *(Ref: Schwartz 10/e p547-549; Sabiston 20/e p848-850; Bailey 27/e p876)*
99. Ans. a. Distant metastasis *(Ref: Breast diseases by Jay R. Harris 2/e p354; Bailey 27/e p876)*

Radical Mastectomy	
Indications	**Contraindications**
• Large, bulky tumor involving the pectoralis major muscle or the fascia • Bulky axillary LN involvement • Grossly involved interpectoral nodes in whom posterior fascia of muscle is also involved	• Non-palpable or small tumor^Q • Advanced disease with distant metastasis^Q • Who wants reconstructive surgery • Need of improved cosmetic result that is achieved by MRM^Q • Co-existing severe systemic diseases like DM, CHF or CRF^Q

100. Ans. a. Tumor size < 4 cm c. Mobile.
101. Ans. d. Supraclavicular lymph node *(Ref: Schwartz 9/e p461; Bailey 27/e p876)*

Halstead's Radical Mastectomy	
Structures Removed	**Structures Preserved (ABC)**
• Whole **breast, skin** and **nipple-areola complex**^{Q}. • Subcutaneous fat, deep fascia **vertically** from **lower border** of the **clavicle** upto the **upper quarter of** the sheath of the **rectus** abdominis and **horizontally** from **sternum** to **anterior border** of **lattissimus dorsi**. • **Pectoralis major** and **minor** muscle^Q with **clavipectoral fascia**^{Q} • Level **I, II** and **III** axillary LNs^Q	• **Axillary vein** and **cephalic vein**^{Q} • **Long thoracic nerve** of Bell (Nerve to serratus anterior)^Q.

102. Ans. b. Pectoralis major
103. Ans. d. Breast
104. Ans. a. Tamoxifen *(Ref: Schwartz 10/e p552; Goodman and Gillman's 12/e p1179)*
105. Ans. d. Tamoxifen
   • QUARTZ: Quadrantectomy + Axillary LN dissection + Radiotherapy^Q
106. Ans. b. Endometrium *(Ref: Goodman and Gillman's 12/e p1179)*
107. Ans. c. Carcinoma in contralateral breast
108. Ans. b. Postmastectomy radiation therapy is given when 4 or more lymph nodes are positive *(Ref: Schwartz 10/e p550; Sabiston 20/e p853-854; Bailey 27/e p877)*

INDICATIONS OF RADIOTHERAPY IN CARCINOMA BREAST	
• Locally Advanced Breast Cancer^Q (to decrease recurrence rate) • Margin is positive after mastectomy^Q	• After breast conservation surgery^Q • Metastases to 4 or more lymph nodes^Q

• **Metastatic disease** is the **principal cause of death** from **breast cancer**^{Q}.

109. Ans. d. Axillary vein *(Ref: Gray's 39/e p841)*

AXILLARY NODE CLEARANCE

• Axillary node clearance can be defined as clearing the axillary contents bounded by:
   – **Laterally:** Axillary skin
   – **Posteriorly:** Lattissimus dorsi, Teres major and Subscapularis
   Superiorly: Lower border of **axillary vein**^{Q}
   – **Anteriorly:** Pectoralis muscle
   – **Medially:** Chest wall

110. **Ans. c. Latissimus dorsi**

- **Latissimus dorsi** is active in **adduction, extension** and especially in **medial rotation** of the humerus.

111. **Ans. c. Pectoralis major removed**
112. **Ans. b. Doxorubicin** *(Ref: Bailey 27/e p878; Schwartz 10/e p550-551)*
113. **Ans. c. Simple mastectomy**
114. **Ans. a. Cyclophosphamide, methotrexate, 5-fluorouracil**
115. **Ans. b. Adriamycin based chemotherapy followed by tamoxifen depending on estrogen/progesterone receptor status**
116. **Ans. c. Lobular carcinoma** *(Ref: Schwartz 10/e p520; Sabiston 20/e p833-834; Bailey 27/e p872)*

- **Lobular carcinoma** is frequently **multifocal, multicentric** and **bilateral** and is **contraindication** for **breast conservative surgery**[Q].

117. **Ans. a. 1 cm** *(Ref: Mastery of Surgery 5/e p525)*

Breast Conservation Surgery

- The amount of breast tissue excised with the lesion may vary with the clinical situation, but is **typically 5 mm to 10 mm in all directions**.
- BCS may consist of **removal of tumor with 1 cm margin of normal tissue** (wide local excision) or a more extensive excision of a whole quadrant of breast (Quadrantectomy).

118. **Ans. c. Sentinel node biopsy**
119. **Ans. c. To prevent recurrence**
120. **Ans. b. Mastectomy with local radiotherapy**
121. **Ans. a. Simple mastectomy followed by oophorectomy**
122. **Ans. a. It was better if she took adjuvant therapy after mastectomy, b. First analyze estrogen and progesterone receptor levels on the tumor**
123. **Ans. a. Letrozole, b. Anastrozole, c. Exemestane** *(Ref: Schwartz 10/e p552-553; Sabiston 20/e p857-858)*

Hormonal Therapy in Carcinoma Breast

- **Tamoxifen** is **DOC** in **pre-menopausal** patients[Q]
- **Aromatase inhibitors are DOC in post-menopausal patients**

124. **Ans. a. 5 years**
125. **Ans. d. Pectoralis minor**
126. **Ans. a. Neoadjuvant chemotherapy followed by MRM followed by radiotherapy**
127. **Ans. c. Routine clinical examination 3 monthly in 1st year with annual mammogram** *(Ref: De Vita 10/e p1145 (ASCO 2006 Updated guidelines); Bailey 27/e p879; MD Anderson Handbook of Surgical Oncology 5/e p71-72)*

*"Follow-up of breast cancer: Patients with breast cancer used to be followed for life to detect recurrence and dissemination. This led to large clinics with little value for either patient or doctor. **It is current practice to arrange yearly or two-yearly mammography of the treated and contralateral breast.** There is a move to return the patient early to the care of the general practitioner with fast-track access back to the breast clinic if suspicious symptoms appear. **There is currently no routine role for repeated measurements of tumor markers or imaging other than mammography."*- Bailey 27/e p879*

Breast Cancer Follow-Up	
Recommended for Routine Surveillance	
History/physical examination	Every 3 to 6 months for the first 3 years, every 6 to 12 months, 4 and 5 years, annually thereafter[Q]
Mammography	Annually, beginning no earlier than 6 months after radiation therapy[Q]
Breast self-examination	All women should be counseled to perform monthly[Q]
Pelvic examination	Annually[Q]
Coordination of care	Continuity of care with breast cancer specialist and appropriate other health care providers

Not Recommended for Routine Surveillance	
Routine blood test	Complete blood count & LFT are **not recommended**[Q]
Imaging studies	CXR, bone scans, liver USG, CT scans, FDG-PET scans & breast MRI are **not recommended** for routine breast cancer surveillance[Q]
Tumor markers	Cancer antigen 15.3, 27.29 & **CEA** are **not recommended**[Q]

128. **Ans. c. Adjuvant radiotherapy** *(Ref: Sabiston 20/e p851-855; Schwartz 10/e p537; Bailey 27/e p877)*

    In this case, patient is 45 years old (Score 2) with size 5 cm (Score 3), margin of 4 mm (Score 2), necrotic features without high grade (Score 2), the total score is 9. Usually for score 7-9, if local excision is done radiotherapy should be given. If simple mastectomy is done, there is no need of adjuvant treatment. In this patient next best step would be adjuvant radiotherapy.

129. **Ans. b. Breast carcinoma** *(Ref: Goodman Gilman 12/e p1709)*

    > *"Ixabepilone is approved for breast cancer treatment."-Goodman Gilman 12/e p1709*

130. **Ans. b. Low risk, no node** *(Ref: Schwartz 10/e p550; Sabiston 20/e p853)*
131. **Ans. a. BRCA-1 and BRCA-2 carrier** *(Ref: Schwartz 10/e p516; Sabiston 20/e p835; Bailey 27/e p881)*
132. **Ans. b. Behind pectoralis minor** *(Ref: Schwartz 10/e p502; Sabiston 20/e p819)*
133. **Ans. b. Tamoxifen is useful in post-menopausal and aromatase inhibitors in premenopausal patients** *(Ref: Schwartz 10/e p552; Sabiston 20/e p857; Bailey 27/e p878)*
134. **Ans. a. Completion axillary lymph node dissection, chemotherapy and radiotherapy** *(Ref: Schwartz 10/e p541; Sabiston 20/e p853)*

CARCINOMA BREAST PROGNOSTIC INDICATORS

135. **Ans. a. Tumor size** *(Ref: Schwartz 10/e p535-536; Bailey 27/e p875; Harrison 20/e p19/e p528)*

    - The **most important** prognostic variables are provided by **tumor staging**^{Q}.
    - The **size** of the tumor and status of the **axillary LN** provide resonably **accurate information** on the likelihood of **tumor relapse**^{Q}.

136. **Ans. a. Axillary dissection..., b. Level I, II and III..., c. In Halsted, d. Arm is kept....** *(Ref: Schwartz 10/e p547; Sabiston 20/e p851; Bailey 27/e p877)*
137. **Ans. b. Progesterone receptor +ve, e. ER +ve**
138. **Ans. b. High HER-2-neu oncogene**
139. **Ans. d. Axillary LN involvement**
140. **Ans. b. Axillary lymph node status**
141. **Ans. b. Lymph node status**

    ### PROGNOSIS IN MALE BREAST CANCER

    - Stage >**Lymph node status** is the **best prognostic indicator**^{Q} as in female breast carcinoma.

142. **Ans. d. Decreased Her-2-neu oncogene**
143. **Ans. a. HER-2-neu, b. p53, c. BRCA-1, e. CEA**
144. **Ans. a. Tumour necrosis** *(Ref: Bailey 27/e p872)*

Bloom-Richardson Grading (TNM)		
1. Tubule formation^Q	2. Nuclear pleomorphism^Q	3. Mitotic count^Q

145. **Ans. b. Stage of the tumour at the time of diagnosis**
146. **Ans. d. Gene expression profiling** *(Ref: Harrison 19/e p526; Schwartz 9/e p453; Sabiston 20/e p839, 19/e p842-845)*

    Molecular classification of breast cancer is based on gene expression profiling.

    > **Gene expression profiling,** *which can measure the relative quantities of mRNA for essentially every gene, has* identified **five major patterns of gene expression** in the NST group: **luminal** A, **luminal** B, **normal, basal-like,** and **HER2 positive.** These molecular classes **correlate with prognosis** and **response to therapy**, and thus have taken on clinical importance. *-Robbins 8/e p1084*

    > One of the most exciting aspects of breast cancer biology has been its recent subdivision into at least five subtypes based upon gene expression profiling. *-Harrison 19/e p526*

147. **Ans. c. Tumour tissue** *(Ref: Schwartz 9/e p453; Sabiston 19/e p842-845; Sabiston 20/e p840, 19/e p844; Bailey 27/e p878, 26/e p816)*
148. **Ans. a. Chemotherapy in hormone receptor positive patients** *(Ref: Harrison 19/e p528; http://www.oncotypedx.com/http://education.nccn.org/node/11346. http://www.cancercare.on.ca/common/pages/UserFile.aspx?fileId=291504)*

    > Oncotype DX may be used to guide chemotherapy decisions among certain women with:
    > - Node-negative^Q
    > - Hormone receptor-positive^Q
    > - HER2-negative breast cancer^Q

    The Oncotype DX, PAM5O, and Mamma Print are multigene tests that are being used clinically for early-stage breast cancer to predict recurrence risk and guide adjuvant chemotherapy decisions.

149. Ans. c. 2+ *(Ref: Sabiston 20/e p840, 857; Diagnostic Histopathology of Tumors By Christopher D. M. Fletcher 4/e p1117)*

> "**Scoring of HER-2 Immunohistochemistry Assays:** Only membrane staining of the invasive tumor should be considered when scoring IHC tests. If a commercial kit assay system is used, it is recommended that laboratories adhere strictly to the kit assay protocol and scoring methodology. Local modifications of techniques can lead to false-positive and false-negative assay results. **The scoring method recommended is a semi quantitative system based on the intensity of reaction product and percentage of membrane positive cells, giving a score of 0 to 3+. Samples scoring 3+ are regarded as positive and those scoring 0/1+ as negative. Borderline scores of 2+ require confirmation with use of another analysis system, ideally FISH.**"-*Diagnostic Histopathology of Tumors By Christopher D. M. Fletcher 4/e p1117*

150. Ans. a. Luminal A *(Ref: Sabiston 20/e p840)*
151. Ans. a. Low-grade tumor, c. Good prognosis *(Ref: Sabiston 20/e p840)*
152. Ans. a. Over expression.., c. Triple negative, e. Increased percentage of cells expressing Ki-67 marker *(Ref: Schwartz 10/e p535-536; Bailey 27/e p875)*

TRIPLE NEGATIVE BREAST CANCER

153. Ans. b. More common in postmenopausal women *(Ref: Bailey 27/e p878; Schwartz 10/e p515)*

Triple-Negative Breast Cancer
• Tends to be **more aggressive**^{Q} than other types of breast cancer.
• Tends to be **higher grade**^{Q} than other types of breast cancer.
• Usually is a cell type called **"basal-like"**^{Q}

COMPLICATIONS OF MASTECTOMY

154. Ans. a. Lymphedema *(Ref: Schwartz 10/e p549; Sabiston 20/e p852; Bailey 27/e p879)*
155. Ans. d. Angiosarcoma *(Ref: Schwartz 10/e p549; Sabiston 20/e p848; Bailey 27/e p879)*
156. Ans. c. Lymphosarcoma
157. Ans. b. Intercostobrachial neuralgia *(Ref: Medical Care of Cancer Patients by Sai-Ching Jim Yeung, Carmen P. Escalanate, Robert F)*
158. Ans. b. Long thoracic nerve of Bell *(Ref: Schwartz 10/e p548; Sabiston 20/e p848)*
159. Ans. a. Intercostobrachial nerve palsy *(Ref: Schwartz 10/e p502)*
160. Ans. a. Open incision and pack with saline gauze *(Ref: Schwartz 10/e p549; Sabiston 20/e p852; Bailey 27/e p879)*

BREAST RECONSTRUCTION

161. Ans. d. Transverse rectus abdominis *(Ref: Schwartz 10/e p549-550; Sabiston 20/e p867; Bailey 26/e p816-817)*
162. Ans. b. TRAM *(Ref: Schwartz 10/e p549-550; Sabiston 20e/ p867; Bailey 27/ep 879)*
163. Ans. c. Pectoralis major myocutaneous flap
164. Ans. c. Transversus rectus abdominis muscle flap

INFLAMMATORY CARCINOMA BREAST

165. Ans. e. Mastitis carcinomatosa *(Ref: Schwartz 10/e p555; Sabiston 20/e p860)*

- **MC type** of CA breast: **Invasive ductal carcinoma**^{Q}
- **Most malignant** type of CA breast: **Inflammatory breast cancer**^{Q}

166. Ans. None *(Ref: Schwartz 10/e p555; Sabiston 20/e p860)*

MALE BREAST CANCER

167. Ans. a. Estrogen receptor positive, b. Associated with gynaecomastia *(Ref: Schwartz 10/e p555; Sabiston 20/e p861; Bailey 27/e p862)*
168. Ans. a. Gynaecomastia is a predisposing factor *(Ref: Schwartz 9/e p468; Sabiston 20/e p861; Bailey 25/e p848)*
    - Male breast cancer is preceded by gynecomastia in 20% of men^Q.
169. Ans. b. Estrogen receptor positive, c. History of gynaecomastia may be present, e. Undescended testis is a risk factor
170. Ans. c. Most commonly it is infiltrating lobular carcinoma
171. Ans. d. BRCA-2 mutation is associated with increased risk
172. Ans. c. Invasive ductal cancer

CARCINOMA BREAST IN PREGNANCY

173. Ans. d. All of the above *(Ref: Schwartz 10/e p554; Sabiston 20/e p2059-2060; Bailey 27/e p881)*

MONDOR'S DISEASE

174. Ans. a. Thrombophlebitis of the superficial veins of breast *(Ref: Schwartz 10/e p507; Sabiston 19/e p1594; Bailey 27/e p867)*
175. Ans. c. Veins of the breast

DUCTAL ANOMALIES

176. Ans. b. Microdochectomy *(Ref: Bailey 27/e p865)*
177. Ans. a. Hadfield's operation *(Ref: Bailey 27/e p865)*
178. Ans. a. Duct ectasia 179. Ans. d. Hadfield's operation
180. Ans. b. Microdochectomy *(Ref: Bailey 27/e p865)*

"Microdochectomy: A lacrimal probe or length of stiff nylon suture is inserted into the duct from which the discharge is emerging. A tennis racquet incision can be made to encompass the entire duct or a periareolar incision used and the nipple flap dissected to reach the duct. The duct is then excised."- *Bailey 27/e p865*

181. Ans. a. Nipple discharge

CYSTOSARCOMA PHYLLODES

182. Ans. a. Wide excision with a margin *(Ref: Schwartz 10/e p555; Sabiston 20/e p841-842; Bailey 27/e p870)*
183. Ans. b. Simple mastectomy *(Ref: Schwartz 10/e p555; Sabiston 20/e p841; Bailey 27/e p870)*

On the basis of clinical findings, patient is having malignant cystosarcoma phyllodes, which is best treated by simple mastectomy.

184. Ans. a. Simple mastectomy 185. Ans. c. It is usually bulky and may fungate through the skin
186. Ans. c. Cystosarcoma phyllodes 187. Ans. d. All of the above
188. Ans. b. Phyllodes tumor
189. Ans. c. Treated with mastectomy *(Ref: Schwartz 10/e p555; Sabiston 20/e p841-842; Bailey 27/e p870)*

GYNECOMASTIA

190. Ans. c. Cryptorchidism *(Ref: Schwartz 10/e p505-506; Sabiston 20/e p824; Bailey 27/e p882)*
191. Ans. a. Subcutaneous mastectomy is the initial treatment of choice *(Ref: Schwartz 10/e p505-506; Sabiston 20/e p824; Bailey 27/e p882; Williams Endocrinology 10/e p741)*
192. Ans. a. May be seen in Addison's disease, b. Usually unilateral in young males
193. Ans. d. Turner's syndrome 194. Ans. b. Incision along the areolar margin
195. Ans. a. Prolactinoma *(Ref: Harrison 20/e 92676, 19/e p2267)*

PROLACTINOMA

- **Prolactinomas** are essentially **associated with galactorrhea**, not the gynecomastia[Q].
- Gynecomastia does not result from either excess or deficiency of prolactin.

PAGET'S DISEASE OF NIPPLE

196. Ans. a. Intraductal carcinoma, b. Mastectomy needed, c. Malignant *(Ref: Schwartz 10/e p506-521; Sabiston 20/e p860-861; Bailey 27/e p873)*
197. Ans. d. Paget's disease of nipple 198. Ans. d. 1, 2, 3 and 4
199. Ans. c. May have underlying carcinoma 200. Ans. b. Paget's disease
201. Ans. d. Cytology diagnostic 202. Ans. b. Abundant clear cytoplasm
203. Ans. a. Always there is underlying carcinoma
204. Ans. a. 1% associated with underlying invasive carcinoma of breast
205. Ans. a. Usually bilateral 206. Ans. a. Cloxacillin *(Ref: Sabiston 20/e p836; Bailey 27/e p866)*
207. Ans. d. Incision and drainage *(Ref: Schwartz 10/e p506; Sabiston 20/e p836; Bailey 27/e p866)*
208. Ans. a. Paget disease of bone

MASTITIS AND BREAST ABSCESS

209. Ans. d. All of the above *(Ref: http://nobleboss.awardspace.com/mednotes/surgnotes/operativ/ebreast_abscess.htm)*

RETROMAMMARY BREAST ABSCESS

- It may an **extension of Breast abscess**, **Empyema thoracis**, **Osteomyelitis** of the **ribs**^{Q}
- **No need to drain** retromammary abscess, **only conservative treatment**^{Q}

210. Ans. c. Lactation *(Ref: Schwartz 10/e p506; Sabiston 20/e p836; Bailey 27/e p866)*

NONEPIDEMIC (SPORADIC) PUERPERAL MASTITIS

- **Involvement** of the **interlobular connective tissue** of the breast by an infectious process.
- The patient develops **nipple fissuring** and **milk stasis**, which initiate a **retrograde bacterial infection**^{Q}.
- **Emptying of the breast** using breast suction pumps **shortens** the **duration** of symptoms^Q and **reduces** the incidence of **recurrences**.
- The addition of **antibiotic therapy**^{Q} results in a satisfactory outcome in >95% of cases.

211. Ans. a. S. aureus *(Ref: Schwartz 10/e p506; Sabiston 20/e p836; Bailey 27/e p866)*

ANDI FIBROADENOMA AND FIBROADENOSIS

212. Ans. d. Solitary mobile mass *(Ref: Bailey 27/e p870; Schwartz 10/e p510; Sabiston 20/e p836)*
213. Ans. b. Fibroadenoma *(Ref: Schwartz 10/e p510; Bailey 27/e p870)*

Pattern of Calcification in Breast Diseases	
Carcinoma	**Microcalcification**, punctate, branching^Q
Fibroadenoma	**Popcorn**^{Q} (coarse, granular, crushed stone)
Fibrocystic disease	Powdery
Fat necrosis	Curvilinear

214. Ans. c. Fibroadenosis *(Ref: Schwartz 10/e p507; Sabiston 20/e p824; Bailey 27/e p869)*

- **Fibroadenosis** or **fibrocystic disease** is the cause of pre-menstrual fullness in breast in 21 years old unmarried female.
- Rest of the options are highly unlikely.

215. Ans. d. Aspiration is the treatment *(Ref: Schwartz 10/e p51; Bailey 27/e p869)*
216. Ans. b. Fibroadenoma
217. Ans. b. Tightly arranged ductal epithelial cells with dyscohesive bare nuclei *(Ref: Winfred Grays diagnostic cytopathology 2/e p279-280)*

Fibroadenoma:
- Diagnostic findings on needle biopsy consist of:
  - **Abundant stromal cells** which appear as **bare bipolar nuclei**
  - **Sheets of fairly uniform-size epithelial** cells that are typically arranged in either an antler like pattern or a honeycomb pattern.
  - Foam cells and apocrine cells may also be seen, although these are less diagnostic features.

MISCELLANEOUS

218. Ans. d. Forerunner of breast abscess *(Ref: Bailey 27/e p863)*

CRACKED NIPPLE

- This may occur **during lactation** and be the **forerunner of acute infective mastitis**^{Q}.
- If the **nipple** becomes **cracked during lactation**, it **should be rested for 24–48 hours** and the breast should be **emptied with** a **breast pump**^{Q}.
- Feeding should be resumed as soon as possible.

219. **Ans. a. Breast cyst** *(Ref: Bailey 27/e p869)*

BREAST CYSTS

- Mostly occur in **last decade of reproductive life**, as a result of **non-integrated involution of stroma & epithelium**.

Clinical Features
- Often **multiple, may be bilateral** & can mimic malignancy; Typically **present suddenly**

Diagnosis
- Diagnosis can be confirmed by **aspiration and/or ultrasound**.

Treatment
- **Aspiration**: In cases of **solitary cyst or cyst with small collection** (Reaspiration in cases of recurrence)

220. **Ans. a. Axillary, b. Supraclavicular, c. Internal mammary**

221. **Ans. b. Family history of CA breast**

222. **Ans. c. Microdochotomy**

223. **Ans. a. Excision of a lump**
- **Lumpectomy (Tylectomy):** Surgical procedure designed to remove a discrete lump

224. **Ans. c. Associated with prolactinoma and other endocrinopathies, d. Surgery is done, e. Hypothyroidism can cause galactorrhoea** *(Ref: Harrison 20/e p2676, 19/e p2267; Dutta Gynecology 5/e p548-549)*

225. **Ans. d. Schirrhous carcinoma** *(Ref: Norman Brows/e p277)*

Causes of Massive Breast Enlargement	
1. **Benign hypertrophy**^{Q} (usually bilateral)	4. **Sarcoma**^{Q}
2. **Cystosarcoma phyllodes**^{Q}	5. **Colloid carcinoma**^{Q}
3. **Giant fibroadenoma**^{Q}	6. **Filarial elephanitiasis**^{Q}

226. **Ans. b. Virginal hypertrophy** *(Ref: CPDT 16/e p1128)*

VIRGINAL HYPERTROPHY

- **Massive enlargement** of usually both breasts^Q
- It **can** also **be unilateral**
- Usually occurs due to an **alteration** in the **normal sensitivity** of the **breast to estrogenic hormones**^{Q}
- Treatment: Reduction mammoplasty^Q

227. **Ans. e. None of the above** *(Ref: NMS surgery 4/e p456)*

Haagensen's Criteria of Inoperability	
1. **Extensive edema** of the **breast**^{Q}	5. A **parasternal tumor**^{Q}, indicating spread to the internal mammary LNs
2. **Satellite nodule**^{Q} of carcinoma	6. **Edema of arm**^{Q}
3. **Inflammatory carcinoma**^{Q}	7. **Distant metastasis**^{Q}
4. **Supraclavicular metastasis**^{Q}	

228. **Ans. c. Pectoral** *(Ref: Bailey 27/e p865)*

229. **Ans. b. Well encapsulated, d. Mastectomy is mainstay treatment** *(Ref: Cancer of Breast by Donegau 5/e p933-936; Breast Cancer by Roses 2/e p207-208)*

230. **Ans. a. Axilla** *(Ref: Bailey 27/e p865)* 231. **Ans. b. Chronic areolar abscess** *(Ref: Schwartz 10/e p506)*

ZUSKA'S DISEASE (RECURRENT PERIDUCTAL MASTITIS)

- Condition of **recurrent retroareolar infections** and **abscesses**
- **Smoking** has been implicated as a **risk factor**
- Managed symptomatically by **antibiotics** with **incision** and **drainage**

Prognosis
- The prognosis is favorable, with **5-** and **10-year** survival rates of **74** and **51%**, respectively.

232. **Ans. d. Parasternal** *(Ref: Bailey 27/e p873)*
233. **Ans. b. USG** *(Ref: Sutton's Radiology 7/e p1456; Schwartz 9/e p467; Sabiston 20/e p828; Bailey 27/e p861)*

INDICATIONS OF BREAST ULTRASOUND	
• Symptomatic breast lump in women <35 years • Breast lump during lactation and pregnancy • Assessment of mammographic abnormality • Assessment of MRI or scintimammography detected lesions (± further mammographic views) • Guidance of needle biopsy or localization • Clinical breast mass with negative mammogram	• Breast inflammation • Augmented breast (together with MRI) • Breast lumps in males (together with MRI) • Follow-up of breast carcinoma treated with adjuvant chemotherapy

234. **Ans. c. 3** *(Ref: Bailey 27/e p869)*

> "Treatment of mastalgia: Oil of evening primrose, in adequate doses given over 3 months, will help more than half of these women"
> —*Bailey 27/e p869*

SENTINEL LYMPH NODE BIOPSY

235. **Ans. c. Intercostobrachial nerve**
236. **Ans. b. Isosulfan blue dye** *(Ref: Schwartz 10/e p545)*
237. **Ans. b. Breast mass but no lymph node palpable** *(Ref: Schwartz 10/e 545)*
238. **Ans. b. Technetium labeled colloid sulfur** *(Ref: Schwartz 10/e p545; Sabiston 20/e p850; Bailey 27/e p877)*

> "Lymphatic mapping can be performed with a combination of ^{99m}Tc-labeled sulfur colloid and a vital blue dye, isosulfan blue (Lymphazurin), or with a single agent for localization of the sentinel node."-*Sabiston 20/e p850*

CHAPTER 2

Thyroid

THYROGLOSSAL CYST

THYROGLOSSAL CYST

- **Cystic swelling** developed in the remnant of the **thyroglossal duct** or **tract**
- **Present** in **any part** of the **thyroglossal tract**[Q] (thyroglossal tract extends from foramen caecum to isthmus of thyroid)

Common Sites
- **Subhyoid (MC)**[Q]
- Region of the thyroid cartilages
- Suprahyoid
- Floor of mouth
- Beneath the foramen caecum

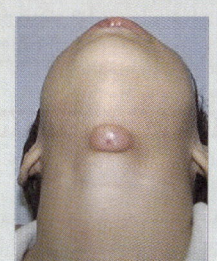

Clinical Features
- It is a **midline swelling**[Q], except in the region of thyroid cartilage, where thyroglossal tract is pushed to one side, usually to the left.
- Though it's a **congenital swelling**[Q] MC **age of presentation** is between **15 and 30 years**[Q].
- Cyst can be **moved sideways** but not vertically.
- Peculiar characteristic which helps in distinguishing thyroglossal cyst from other neck swelling
  - **Moves up with protrusion of tongue**[Q] as the thyroglossal tract is attached to the tongue.
  - **Moves with deglutition**[Q] so do all thyroid swellings, subhyoid bursitis.
- Cyst is lined by pseudostratified columnar epithelium and squamous epithelium with **heterotopic thyroid tissue** present in **20%** of cases.

Complications
- **Recurrent infections**[Q]
- Formation of **thyroglossal fistula**[Q]
- Carcinomatous change (**papillary carcinoma**[Q])

Treatment
- **Sistrunk operation**: En-bloc cystectomy and excision of **central hyoid bone**[Q] to minimize recurrence.

RETROSTERNAL GOITER

RETROSTERNAL (SUBSTERNAL/MEDIASTINAL/INTRATHORACIC GOITER)

- A goiter is said to be **retrosternal, substernal** or **mediastinal** if > 50% of **thyroid tissue** is below the **opening** of **thoracic cage**[Q].
- Usually arises from **lower pole** of a **nodular goiter**[Q].

Types

Primary Mediastinal Goiters	Secondary Mediastinal Goiters
• Constitute approximately **1%** of all mediastinal goiters • Arise from **accessory (ectopic)**[Q] **thyroid tissue** located in the **chest** • Supplied by **intrathoracic blood vessels**[Q] • Do not have any connection to thyroid tissue in the **neck**[Q].	• Constitute **majority**[Q] of mediastinal goiters • Arise from **downward extension** of **cervical thyroid tissue**[Q] along the fascial planes of the neck • Derive their **blood supply from superior inferior thyroid arteries**[Q].

Clinical Features
- Often **symptomless**, discovered on a routine **chest X-ray**[Q].
- Can lead to **tracheal deviation** and **scabbard trachea**[Q] (flattening of trachea caused by compression)

Severe Symptoms due to Mass Effect on the Trachea, Esophagus, Great Vessels and Nerves

1. **Dyspnea (MC symptom)** particularly at night, **cough** and **stridor**[Q]
2. Dysphagia
3. Enlargement of neck veins and superficial veins on the chest wall
4. Recurrent nerve palsy
5. **Pemberton's sign**[Q]: Symptoms of faintness with evidence of facial congestion and external jugular venous obstruction when the arms are raised above the head.

Treatment
- Virtually **all intrathoracic goiters** can be **removed via a cervical incision**[Q].

Indications of Median Sternotomy
Patients who have:
1. **Invasive thyroid cancers**[Q]
2. Had **previous thyroid operations** and may have developed **parasitic mediastinal vessels**[Q]
3. **Primary mediastinal goiters** with **no thyroid tissue in the neck**[Q]

INVESTIGATIONS IN THYROID DISORDERS

THYROID SCAN

- Whereas ultrasound allows anatomic evaluation, **radionuclide scans** allow assessment of **thyroid function**[Q].
- ^{123}I and ^{131}I iodine scintigraphy is also used to evaluate the functional status of the gland.
- Advantages of scanning with ^{123}I include a **low dose of radiation** (30 mrad) and **short half-life**[Q].
- ^{131}I has a **longer half-life** (8 days) and **emits higher levels of β-radiation**[Q].
- ^{131}I is optimal for **imaging thyroid carcinoma**. It is the **screening modality of choice** for the **evaluation of distant metastasis**[Q].

Isotope	$t_{1/2}$
I^{132}	2.3 hours[Q]
I^{123}	13 hours[Q]
I^{131}	8 days[Q]

RADIOACTIVE IODINE (I^{131}) THERAPY

- I^{131} is an **effective agent** for **delivering high radiation doses** to thyroid tissue[Q].
- It **emits mainly beta radiation (90%)**, which **penetrates** only **0.5 mm**[Q] of the **tissue** & allow therapeutic effects on thyroid **without any damage** to the surrounding structures, particularly **parathyroids**.

Mechanism of Action
- I^{131} emits **beta particles**[Q] and **γ-rays**.
- **Beta rays** are utilized for their **destructive effects** on **thyroid**[Q] cells.
- **X-rays** are useful for **tracer studies**.

Indications in Carcinoma Thyroid	Contraindications of I^{131} Therapy
1. **Distant metastasis**[Q] at diagnosis	1. **Childhood**[Q]
2. Incomplete tumor resection[Q]	2. **Pregnancy**[Q]
3. Patients at **high risk** for **mortality** or **recurrence**[Q]	3. **Lactation**[Q]

SOLITARY THYROID NODULE

SOLITARY THYROID NODULE

- MC **solitary thyroid nodule** is **benign colloid nodule**[Q], it accounts for **60%** cases of solitary thyroid nodule.
- **2nd MC cause** of solitary thyroid nodule is **follicular adenoma (30%)**[Q].

History
- Details regarding the nodule, such as time of onset, change in size, and associated symptoms such as pain, dysphagia, dyspnea, or choking, should be elicited.

- **Risk factors** for **malignancy**, such as exposure to **ionizing radiation** and **family history of thyroid** and **other malignancies**[Q] associated with thyroid cancer.

External Beam Radiation
• **Low-dose therapeutic radiation**[Q] has been used to treat conditions such as tinea capitis, thymic enlargement, enlarged tonsils and adenoids, acne vulgaris, and other conditions such as hemangioma and scrofula.
• **History of exposure** to **low-dose ionizing radiation**[Q] to the thyroid gland places the patient at **increased risk for** developing **papillary thyroid cancer**[Q].
• Risk is **maximum 20 to 30 years** after **exposure**[Q]

Physical Examination

- Thyroid gland is **best palpated from behind** the patient and with the **neck in mild extension**[Q].
- Nodules that are **hard, gritty,** or **fixed to surrounding structures** such as the trachea or strap muscles are **more likely to be malignant**[Q].

Diagnostic Investigations

Laboratory Studies
• **Most patients** with **thyroid nodules** are **euthyroid**[Q]. Determining the **blood TSH level**[Q] is helpful.
• **Tg levels in patients** who have undergone total thyroidectomy for thyroid cancer and **for serial evaluation** of patients undergoing nonoperative management of thyroid nodules.
• **Serum calcitonin** in patients with **MTC** or a family history of MTC or **MEN2**.

FNAC
• **Single most important test** in the evaluation of **thyroid masses**[Q]
• **Ultrasound guidance** is recommended for nodules that are **difficult to palpate** and for **cystic or solid-cystic nodules** that **recur**[Q] after the initial aspiration.
• A **23-gauge needle** is used. If a FNAC is reported as **nondiagnostic**, it generally **should be repeated**.
• When **FNAC** is used in **complex nodules**, the **solid portion** should be **sampled**[Q].
• The **risk of malignancy** in the setting of a **suspicious cytology** is about **20%**.

Imaging
• **Ultrasound** is helpful for detecting **nonpalpable thyroid nodules**, differentiating **solid from cystic nodules,** and **identifying adjacent lymphadenopathy**.
• Ultrasound evaluation can identify features of a nodule that increase the **risk of malignancy**, such as **fine stippled calcification** and **enlarged regional nodes**; however, a **tissue diagnosis is strongly recommended before thyroidectomy**[Q].
• **Scanning** the thyroid with ^{123}I or ^{99m}Tc is **rarely necessary**, and thyroid scanning currently is **recommended in** the assessment of **thyroid nodules** only in patients who have **follicular thyroid nodules** on **FNAC** and a **suppressed TSH**[Q].

Management

- Total thyroidectomy for malignant tumors[Q]

Thyroid Cyst
• **Simple thyroid cysts** resolve with **aspiration**[Q] in about 75% of cases
• **Hemithyroidectomy:**
– If the cyst **persists after three attempts** at aspiration[Q]
– **Cysts >4 cm** in diameter[Q]
– **Complex cysts** with solid and cystic components (higher incidence of malignancy, 15%).

Colloid Nodule
• **Observation** with serial **ultrasound** and **Tg** measurements[Q].
• **Hemithyroidectomy:** If a **nodule enlarges** on **TSH suppression**, causes **compressive symptoms**, or for **cosmetic reasons**[Q].
• **Total thyroidectomy:** Patient who has had **previous irradiation** of the **thyroid gland** or has a **family history of thyroid cancer**, because of the **high incidence of thyroid cancer** and **decreased reliability of FNAC** in this setting[Q].

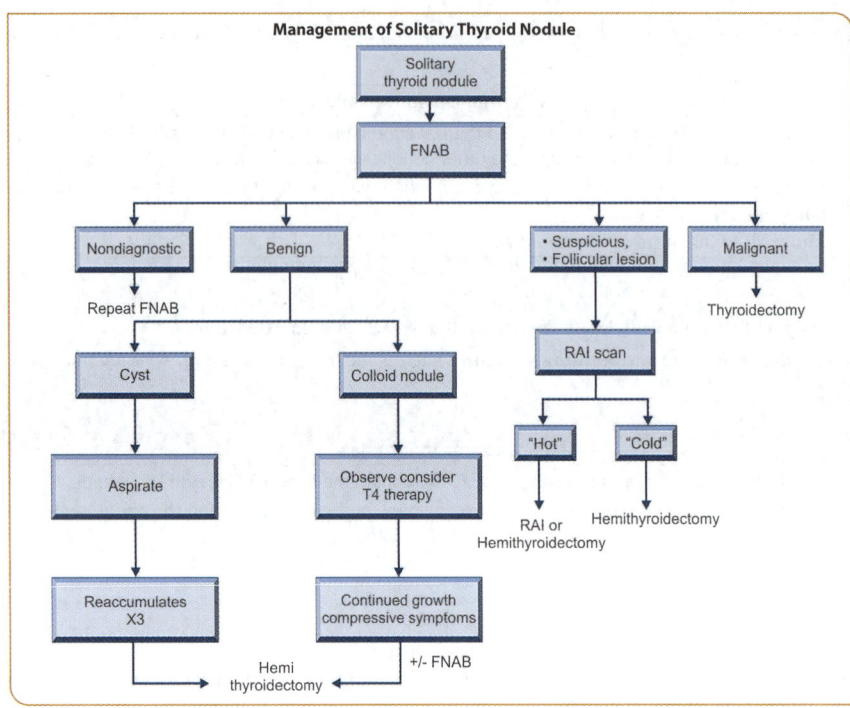

Bethesda System for Reporting Thyroid Cytopathology (TBSRTC)	
Thy1	• Non-diagnostic
Thy1c	• Non-diagnostic **cystic**
Thy2	• Non-neoplastic
Thy3	• Follicular
Thy4	• Suspicious of malignancy
Thy5	• Malignant

ACUTE (SUPPURATIVE) THYROIDITIS

Acute (Suppurative) Thyroiditis

- Acute thyroiditis is rare and due to **suppurative infection** of the **thyroid**[Q].
- **More common** in **children** and often is **preceded by** an **upper respiratory tract infection** or **otitis media**[Q].

Etiology
- Thyroid gland is inherently resistant to infection due to its extensive blood & lymphatic supply, high iodide content, and fibrous capsule.

Infectious Agents Can Seed Thyroid
1. Via **hematogenous** or **lymphatic route**[Q]
2. Via direct **spread** from **persistent pyriform sinus fistulae** or **thyroglossal duct cysts**[Q]
3. As a result of **penetrating trauma**[Q]
4. Due to **immunosuppression**[Q]

- **MC organism** responsible: **Staph. aureus > Streptococcus**[Q]
- In **children & young adults**, **MC cause** is presence of a **pyriform sinus**[Q] (remnant of the **fourth branchial pouch** that connects the oropharynx with thyroid), such sinuses are predominantly **left-sided**[Q].
- **Long-standing goiter** and **degeneration** in **thyroid malignancy** are risk factors in **elderly**[Q]

Clinical Features
- **Thyroid pain**, often referred to the throat or ears, and a **small, tender goiter**[Q]
- **Fever, dysphagia** and **erythema** over the thyroid.
- Systemic symptoms of a **febrile illness** and **lymphadenopathy**[Q].
- Complications such as systemic sepsis, tracheal or esophageal rupture, jugular vein thrombosis, laryngeal chondritis, and perichondritis or sympathetic trunk paralysis may also occur.

Diagnosis

- **ESR** and **WBC count** are usually **increased**, but **thyroid function** is **normal**.
- **FNA biopsy** shows infiltration by **polymorphonuclear leukocytes**.
- **Culture** of the sample can identify the organism.
- **Persistent pyriform sinus fistula** should be suspected in **children** with recurrent acute thyroiditis. A **barium swallow** demonstrates the anomalous tract with **80% sensitivity**^{Q}.

Treatment

- **Parenteral antibiotics** and **drainage** of **abscesses**^{Q}.
- Patients with **pyriform sinus fistulae** require **complete resection**^{Q} of the sinus tract, including the area of the thyroid where the tract terminates, **to prevent recurrence**.

SUBACUTE THYROIDITIS

SUBACUTE/DE QUERVAIN'S/GRANULOMATOUS/VIRAL THYROIDITIS/GIANTCELL THYROIDITIS

- Also termed de Quervain's thyroiditis, granulomatous thyroiditis, or viral thyroiditis.
- Peak incidence: **30–50 years**; **women** are affected three times more frequently than men.
- Usually follows **upper respiratory tract infection**^{Q}
- A **viral etiology** has been proposed
- **Strong association** with the **HLA-B35 haplotype**^{Q}

> **The Disorder Classically Progresses through Four Stages.**
> 1. Initial **hyperthyroid phase**, due to release of thyroid hormone
> 2. **Euthyroid** phase
> 3. **Hypothyroidism**, occurs in about 20 to 30% of patients
> 4. **Resolution** and return to the **euthyroid state** in 90% of patients.

- In the **early stages** of the disease, **TSH** is **decreased**, and **Tg, T4**, and **T$_3$** levels are **elevated** due to the release of preformed thyroid hormone from destroyed follicles.
- **ESR** is typically **>100 mm/h**^{Q}.
- **RAIU** also is **decreased**^{Q} (<2% at 24 hours), even in euthyroid patients, due to the release of thyroid hormones from destruction of the thyroid parenchyma.

Clinical Features

- **Painful** and **enlarged thyroid**, sometimes accompanied by fever.
- Features of **thyrotoxicosis** or **hypothyroidism**, depending on the phase of the illness.
- Malaise and symptoms of an **upper respiratory tract infection** may **precede** the **thyroid-related features**^{Q} by several weeks.
- The patient typically complains of a **sore throat** and **small exquisitely tender goiter**^{Q}
- Pain is often referred to the jaw or ear.
- **Complete resolution** is the **usual outcome**^{Q}
- Permanent hypothyroidism can occur, particularly in those with coincidental thyroid autoimmunity.

Laboratory Findings

- **ESR** is **markedly elevated**^{Q}
- **Antithyroid antibodies** are **low** with T4, T3 and TSH levels depend on the stage of disease.

> - **RAIU** is **decreased** during the hyperthyroid stage (distinguishes from Grave's disease)
> - In doubt: **FNAC** (shows characteristic **giant multinucleated cells**)^Q

Treatment

- Treatment is **primarily symptomatic**, as disease is **self-limited**^{Q}.
- **Aspirin** or other **NSAIDs** are sufficient to control symptoms in most cases.
- **Severe cases** with marked local or systemic symptoms may require **glucocorticoids**.
- **Short-term thyroid replacement** may be needed in the **hypothyroid phase**.
- **Thyroidectomy** is reserved for the **rare patients** who have a prolonged course **not responsive** to **medical measures**.

RIEDEL'S THYROIDITIS

RIEDEL'S THYROIDITIS

- A rare variant of thyroiditis also known as **Riedel's struma**^{Q} or **invasive fibrous thyroiditis**
- Characterized by the **replacement of** all or part of the **thyroid parenchyma** by **fibrous tissue**
- Also **invades** into **adjacent tissues**^{Q}.
- **Etiology**: Primary **autoimmune etiology** (probably)

Riedel's Thyroiditis is Associated with
• **Mediastinal** and **retroperitoneal** fibrosis • **Periorbital** and **retro-orbital** fibrosis • **Sclerosing cholangitis**

Clinical Features
- Occurs predominantly in **women, 30–60 years**.
- Presents as a **painless, hard anterior neck mass**^{Q}, which progresses over weeks to years to produce **symptoms** of **compression**, including dysphagia, dyspnea, choking, and hoarseness.
- Patients may present with symptoms of **hypothyroidism** and **hypoparathyroidism**^{Q} as the **gland** is **replaced** by **fibrous tissue**.
- Physical examination: **Hard, "woody" thyroid gland** with **fixation**^{Q} to surrounding tissues.

Treatment
- **Surgery**^{Q} is the **mainstay** of the treatment (decompress the trachea by **wedge excision of isthmus**)
- Some patients show dramatic improvement with **tamoxifen** & **corticosteroids**.

HASHIMOTO'S THYROIDITIS

HASHIMOTO'S THYROIDITIS

- First described by Hashimoto as **struma lymphomatosa**^{Q}, i.e. a transformation of thyroid tissue to lymphoid tissue.
- MC inflammatory disorder of the thyroid and **leading cause** of **hypothyroidism**^{Q}.

• **Thyroid lymphoma**^{Q} is a rare but **well-recognized complication**
• **Papillary thyroid carcinoma**^{Q} may be occasionally associated

- **Genetic association** has been noted with **HLA B8, DR3** and **DR5**^{Q}.
- More common in **women** (Male:female, 1:10), near menopause (**30-50 years**).

Etiopathogenesis
- **Autoimmune** disease
- Thought to be initiated by **activation** of **CD4+T (helper) lymphocytes** which further recruit cytotoxic CD8+T cells.
- Thyroid tissue is destroyed by **cytrotoxic T cells** and **autoantibodies**^{Q}.

Autoantibodies are Directed against		
1. Thyroglobulin (Tg): 60%	2. **Thyroid peroxidase** (TPO): **95%**^{Q}	3. TSH-R: 60%

- It is also thought to be **associated with:**
  - Increased intake of **iodine**
  - Drugs such as **interferon alpha, lithium, amiodarone**

Pathology
- **Gross examination**: Mildly enlarged **thyroid**^{Q} with pale, gray-tan cut surface
- **Microscopic examination:**
  - Gland is **diffusely infiltrated** by **small lymphocytes** and **plasma cells**^{Q} and occasionally shows well-developed germinal centers.
  - **Smaller** thyroid **follicles** with **reduced colloid** and increased interstitial connective tissue.
  - Follicles are lined by **Hürthle** or **Askanazy cells**^{Q} (characterized by abundant eosinophilic, granular cytoplasm).

Clinical Features
- **MC presentation:** **Minimally** or **moderately enlarged firm gland**^{Q}.
- On examination an **enlarged pyramidal lobe** is often palpable.
- Mild hyperthyroidism may be present initially (due to destruction of thyroid tissue).
- **Hypothyroidism** is inevitable and **usually permanent**^{Q}.

Laboratory Findings
- Elevated TSH and presence of thyroid **autoantibodies confirm** the **diagnosis**^{Q}.
- Elevated TSH, reduced T4 and T3 levels^Q.

- Presence to thyroid autoantibodies (particularly **TPO antibody**)^Q.
- In case of doubt, diagnosis is confirmed by **FNA biopsy**.

Management
- **Thyroid hormone replacement therapy** for overtly **hypothyroid** patients or in euthyroid patients to **shrink large goiters**^{Q}.
- Treatment is advised especially for middle-aged patients with **cardiovascular risk factors** such as hyperlipidemia or hypertension and in **pregnant patients**.
- **Surgery** may occasionally be indicated for **suspicion of malignancy** or for **goiters** causing **compressive symptoms** or cosmetic deformity.

PAINLESS OR SILENT THYROIDITIS

Painless or Silent Thyroiditis

- Painless thyroiditis, or "silent" thyroiditis, occurs in patients with **underlying autoimmune thyroid disease** and has a **clinical course similar to that of subacute thyroiditis**.
- Occurs in up to **5% of women 3–6 months after pregnancy** termed as **postpartum thyroiditis**.
- **Associated with presence of TPO antibodies antepartum**, three times **more common in women with type 1 DM**.

Clinical Features
- Characterised by **brief phase of thyrotoxicosis lasting 2–4 weeks, followed by hypothyroidism for 4–12 weeks, and then resolution**.

Diagnosis
- **Uptake of ^{99m}Tc pertechnetate or radioactive iodine is initially suppressed**.
- In addition to the **painless goiter**, silent thyroiditis can be **distinguished from subacute thyroiditis by a normal ESR & presence of TPO antibodies**.

Treatment
- Glucocorticoid treatment is not indicated for silent thyroiditis.
- **Severe thyrotoxic symptoms: Propranolol**
- **Thyroxine replacement** for hypothyroid phase but **should be withdrawn after 6–9 months, as recovery is the rule**.

Prognosis
- **Annual follow-up** thereafter is recommended, because a proportion of these individuals develop permanent hypothyroidism.
- The condition **may recur in subsequent pregnancies.**

GRAVE'S DISEASE (DIFFUSE TOXIC GOITER)

Grave's Disease (Diffuse Toxic Goiter)

- **MC cause** of hyperthyroidism, caused by **stimulatory autoantibodies** to TSH-R^Q.
- **Autoimmune disease** with strong **familial predisposition**^{Q}.
- More common in **females** with peak incidence between **40–60** years.
- Characterized by **thyrotoxicosis, diffuse goiter & extrathyroidal conditions**^{Q} (ophthalmopathy, dermopathy, thyroid acropachy and gynecomastia).

Etiopathogenesis
- **Autoimmune process** with possible **triggers** (post-partum state, iodine excess, lithium therapy and bacterial or viral infections)
- Associated with HLA-B8, HLA-DR3, HLA-DQA1*0501 and CTLA-4^Q
- HLA-DRB1*0701 is **protective** against it
- **Thyroid stimulating antibodies**^{Q} stimulate thyrocytes to grow and synthesize excess thyroid hormone, which is **hallmark** of Grave's disease
- Associated with **type I diabetes mellitus, Addison's disease, pernicious anemia** and **myasthenia gravis**.

Histopathology
- **Hyperplastic gland** with columnar epithelium and minimal colloid
- Nuclei exhibit **mitosis**
- **Papillary projections** of hyperplastic epithelium^Q.

Clinical Features
- **Hyperthyroid symptoms**^{Q} (heat intolerance, increased sweating and thirst, weight loss despite adequate caloric intake)

- **Symptoms of adrenergic stimulation**^{Q} (palpitations, nervousness, fatigue, emotional lability, hyperkinesis and tremors)
- **MC GI symptom** is **increased frequency** of **bowel movements** and **diarrhea**^{Q}

> - **Female patients** often develop **amenorrhea, decreased fertility** and **increased** incidence of **miscarriage**^{Q}
> - **Children** experience **rapid growth** with **early bone maturation**^{Q}
> - **Older patients** present with **CVS complications (AF and CHF)**^{Q}
> - **Overt cardiac failure** occurs in only **6–19%**, in Grave's disease

- Weight loss, facial flushing, warm and moist skin, tachycardia, cutaneous vasodilatation, **collapsing pulse** is seen on examination
- A **fine tremor, muscle wasting** and **proximal muscle** group **weakness** with **hyperactive tendon reflexes** often are present^Q

> - Overlying **bruit** or **thrill** at **upper pole**^{Q} due to **increased vascularity**
> - **Loud venous hum**^{Q} in supraclavicular space
> - **Ophthalmopathy** (orbital proptosis) occurs in **50%**, **dermopathy** in **1–2%**.^{Q}
> - Dermopathy is characterized by deposition of **glycosaminoglycans** leading to **thickened skin** in **pretibial region** and **dorsum of foot**^{Q} (pretibial myxedema).

- **Gynecomastia** is common in **young men**^{Q}
- Rare bony involvement leads to **subperiosteal bone formation** and **swelling in metacarpals**^{Q} (thyroid acropathy).

Diagnosis
- **Suppressed TSH** with or without an elevated free T4 or T3 level. **If eye signs are present,** other tests are generally not needed^Q.
- In absence of eye signs, elevated RAIU with **diffusely enlarged gland**^{Q} confirms the diagnosis.
- Elevated TSH-R or **thyroid-stimulating antibodies (TSAb)** are **diagnostic**^{Q} of Grave's disease and increased in about **90%** patients.
- Anti-Tg and Anti-TPO antibodies are **non-specific** and elevated in upto **75%** cases.
- **MRI of orbits** are useful in evaluating **Grave's ophthalmopathy**.

Treatment
- Treatment modalities: **Antithyroid drugs**, thyroid ablation with radioactive ^{131}I and **thyroidectomy**^{Q}.

TREATMENT OF GRAVE'S DISEASE

Treatment of Grave's Disease

- Treatment modalities are antithyroid drugs, thyroid ablation with radioactive ^{131}I, and thyroidectomy.

Antithyroid Drugs
- Administered in **preparation for RAI ablation** or **surgery**^{Q}.
- Drugs commonly used: **Propylthiouracil** and **methimazole**^{Q}.
- **Propylthiouracil** can cause **liver failure in pregnancy**.
- **Methimazole** is associated with **aplasia cutis & choanal atresia**.

> - **Antithyroid drug of choice in Graves: Methimazole**^{Q}
> - Antithyroid drug of choice **in pregnancy: Carbimazole**^{Q}
> - Antithyroid drug of choice **in thyroid storm: Propylthiouracil**^{Q}

- Most patients have **improved symptoms** in **2 weeks** and become **euthyroid** in about **6 weeks**^{Q}.
- Treatment is associated with a **high relapse rate** when these drugs are discontinued, with 40-80% of patients developing recurrent disease after a 1- to 2-year course.

Treatment for Curative Intent is Reserved for
1. **Small, nontoxic goiters** <40 gms^Q
2. **Mildly elevated** thyroid hormone levels^Q
3. **Rapid decrease** in gland size with antithyroid medications^Q

- **Catecholamine response** of thyrotoxicosis can be **alleviated** by **propranolol**^{Q}.

Radioactive Iodine Therapy (^{131}I)
- ^{131}I emits **beta (90%)** and **gamma rays**^{Q}

Radioactive Iodine Therapy	
Advantages	**Disadvantages**
Avoidance of a **surgical procedure**^{Q} and its concomitant risks	**Progression** of **Grave's ophthalmopathy**^{Q}
Reduced overall treatment **costs**^{Q}	Small increased **risk** of **nodular goiter, thyroid cancer** and **hypoparathyroidism**^{Q}
Ease of treatment^Q	**Unexplained increase** in overall and **cardiovascular mortality**^{Q}
	Higher initial dose of ^{131}I: Earlier onset and higher incidence of **hypothyroidism**^{Q}

Indications of RAI Therapy
1. **Older patients** with **small** or **moderate-sized goiters**[Q]
2. Patients **relapsed after medical** or **surgical therapy**[Q]
3. **Antithyroid drugs** or **surgery** are **contraindicated**[Q]

- After standard treatment with RAI, most patients become euthyroid within 2 months.
- Only 50% of patients treated with RAI are euthyroid 6 months after treatment, and the remaining are still hyperthyroid or already hypothyroid.

Contraindications of RAI	
Absolute Contraindications	**Relative Contraindications**
• **Pregnancy**[Q] • **Lactation**[Q]	• **Young patients** (children and adolescents)[Q] • **Thyroid nodules**[Q] • **Ophthalmopathy**[Q]

Surgical Treatment
- Surgery is recommended when **RAI is contraindicated**[Q]

Indications of Surgery	
When RAI is Contraindicated	**Relative Indications**
• Confirmed **cancer** or **suspicious thyroid nodules**[Q] • **Young patients**[Q] • **Pregnancy and Lactation**[Q] • **Severe reactions** to antithyroid medications • **Large goiters** causing compressive symptoms • Reluctant to undergo RAI therapy	• **Smokers**, with **moderate to severe Grave's ophthalmopathy**[Q] • Patients desiring **rapid control of hyperthyroidism** with a chance of being euthyroid • **Poor compliance** to **antithyroid medications**.

- Patients should be **rendered euthyroid before operation**[Q]
- **Antithyroid drugs** should be continued **up to the day of surgery**[Q].

Lugol's Iodide Solution or Saturated Potassium Iodide
• Administered **7–10 days preoperatively** (three drops twice daily)[Q] • **Reduce vascularity** of the gland and **decrease** the **risk** of **precipitating thyroid storm**. • The **major action** of iodine in this situation is to **inhibit release** of **thyroid hormone**[Q].

Indications of Total or Near-total Thyroidectomy
• Patients with **coexistent thyroid cancer**[Q] • Who **refuse RAI therapy**[Q] • Have **severe ophthalmopathy**[Q] • **Life-threatening reactions** to **antithyroid medications**[Q] (vasculitis, agranulocytosis, or liver failure)

- A **subtotal thyroidectomy**, leaving a **4–7 gm remnant**[Q], is recommended for all remaining patients.
- Remnants <4 g are associated with a **2–10% recurrence rate** but a **high (>40%) rate of hypothyroidism**[Q].

TOXIC ADENOMA

Toxic Adenoma (Plummer's Disease)

- Hyperthyroidism from a **single hyperfunctioning nodule**[Q] typically occurs in **younger patients**
- Usually occurs in the setting of a patient with endemic goiter.
- Increased thyroid hormone production occurs **independent of TSH control**[Q].
- **Recent growth** of a **long-standing nodule** along with the symptoms of **hyperthyroidism**[Q].
- Characterized by **somatic mutations** in the **TSH-R gene**[Q]
- Most nodules have attained a **size** of at least **3 cm before hyperthyroidism** occurs.

Clinical Features
- **Recent growth** of a **long-standing nodule** along with the symptoms of **hyperthyroidism**[Q].
- Hyperthyroidism from a **single hyperfunctioning nodule** typically occurs in **younger patients**
- Physical examination: **Solitary thyroid nodule** without palpable thyroid tissue on the contralateral side.
- Eye signs are not common, mainly **CVS dysfunction**
- These nodules are **rarely malignant**[Q].

Diagnosis
- **RAI scanning** shows a **"hot" nodule**[Q] with suppression the rest of the thyroid gland.

Treatment
- **Smaller nodules** may be managed with **antithyroid medications** and **RAI**[Q].
- Most patients are **euthyroid** after **radioiodine therapy**[Q] (radioiodine preferentially accumulates in hyperfunctioning nodules)
- Surgery (**Hemithyroidectomy**) is preferred in **young** patients with **larger nodules**[Q].

DIFFERENTIAL DIAGNOSIS OF HYPERTHYROIDISM

Differential Diagnosis of Hyperthyroidism	
Increased Hormone Synthesis (Increased RAIU) **TSH GATT**	**Release of Preformed Hormone (Decreased RAIU)** **HIT**
• **T**SH secreting adenoma • **T**hyroid cancer, **S**truma ovarii, **H**ydatidiform mole (TSH) • **G**rave's disease[Q] (diffuse toxic goiter) • **A**miodarone, iodine (Drug induced) • **T**oxic multinodular goiter[Q] • **T**oxic adenoma	• **H**amburger thyrotoxicosis • **I**atrogenic (Factitious) thyrotoxicosis • **T**hyroiditis: Acute phase of **Hashimoto's** thyroiditis, **subacute** thyroiditis[Q]

THYROTOXICOSIS

CVS FINDINGS IN THYROTOXICOSIS

- MC cardiovascular manifestation is **sinus tachycardia**[Q], often associated with **palpitations**, occasionally caused by **supraventricular tachycardia**[Q].
- **Exertional dyspnea**[Q]
- Hyperactive precordium with **loud first heart sound**, an accentuated pulmonic component of the second heart sound, and a **thirds heart sound**[Q].
- **Systolic ejection click**[Q]
- The high cardiac output produces a **bounding pulse**, **widened pulse pressure**[Q], and an **aortic systolic murmur** and can lead to worsening of angina or heart failure in the elderly or those with preexisting heart disease.
- **Atrial fibrillation** is more common in patients >50 years of age[Q].
- A systolic scratch, also known as **Means-Lerman scratch**[Q], is occasionally heard in 2nd left intercoastal space during expiration.
- Systolic hypertension

Cardiovascular Manifestations of Thyrotoxicosis	
Increased Atrial Irritability	**High Cardiac Output**
• **Sinus tachycardia (MC)**[Q] • Palpitations[Q] • Supraventricular tachycardia[Q] • Atrial fibrillations[Q]	• Bounding pulse • Wide pulse pressure[Q] • Hyperdynamic precordium[Q] • **Loud first heart sound**[Q], an accentuated pulmonic component of the second heart sound, and a **thirds heart sound**[Q]. • **Aortic systolic murmur**[Q] • **Means-Lerman scratch**[Q]

THYROID STORM (THYROTOXIC CRISIS)

- It is an **emergency** due to **decompensated hyperthyroidism**[Q].

Treatment
- Non-selective beta blocker (Propranolol):
  - Most valuable measure in **thyroid storm**[Q].
  - In thyroid storm most of the symptoms are because of adrenergic over activity due to **increased tissue sensitivity** to **catecholamines** in hyperthyroidism.
  - This **increased sensitivity** is due to **increased** number of **beta receptors**[Q].
- Quick relief is obtained by blocking **beta** receptors.
- Propylthiouracil:
  - **Antithyroid drug of choice** for **thyroid storm**[Q]
  - **Reduces hormone synthesis** as well as **peripheral conversion** of T_4 to T_3[Q]

- **Corticosteroids (Hydrocortisone):**
  - Inhibits both **release of thyroid hormone** from the gland and **peripheral conversion** of T_4 to T_3.^{Q}
- **Iodides (Potassium iodide** or **ipanoic acid):**
  - Used to **inhibit** further **hormone release**^{Q} from the gland.
- **Other Measures:**
  - **Diltiazem,** if **tachycardia** is not controlled by propranolol alone.
  - **Rehydration, anxiolytics, external cooling** and appropriate antibiotics

CARCINOMA THYROID

Familial Cancer Syndromes Involving Nonmedullary Thyroid Cancer			
Syndrome	**Gene**	**Manifestation**	**Thyroid Tumor**
Cowden's syndrome	PTEN	Intestinal hamartomas, benign and malignant breast tumors	**FTC,** rarely PTC and Hürthle cell tumors
FAP	APC	Colon polyps and cancer, duodenal neoplasms, desmoids	**PTC** cribriform growth pattern
Werner's syndrome	WRN	**Adult progeroid syndrome**^{Q}	PTC, FTC, anaplastic cancer
Carney complex type 1	PRKAR1	**Cutaneous** and **cardiac myxomas, breast** and **adrenal tumors**^{Q}	PTC, FTC
McCune-Albright syndrome	GNAS1	**Polyostotic fibrous dysplasia,** endocrine abnormalities, **café-au-lait spots**^{Q}	**PTC** clear cell

Type of Thyroid Carcinoma	Prevalence
Papillary (**MC**)	**80–90%**
Follicular	5–10%
Medullary	10%
Anaplastic	Rare
Lymphoma	1%

Well Differentiated Thyroid Cancer	
1. **Papillary** carcinoma of thyroid^Q	2. **Follicular** carcinoma of thyroid^Q
3. **Follicular variant** of **papillary** carcinoma thyroid^Q	4. **Hurthle cell carcinoma** (variant of follicular carcinoma thyroid)^Q

Carcinoma Thyroid		
Type	**Mode of spread**	**MC site of metastasis**
Papillary carcinoma	**Lymphatic**^{Q} spread	Lungs
Follicular carcinoma	**Hematogenous**^{Q} spread	Bones
Medullary carcinoma	Both **lymphatic** and **hematogenous**^{Q} spread	Liver
Anaplastic carcinoma	**Direct invasion**^{Q}	Lungs

Pulsating Secondaries	
1. **Follicular carcinoma thyroid**^{Q}	2. **RCC**^{Q}

Bone Metastasis in Carcinoma Thyroid	
Follicular carcinoma	**Osteolytic** metastasis (**Pulsating secondaries** in **flat bones**)^Q
Medullary carcinoma	**Osteoblastic** metastasis^Q

PAPILLARY CARCINOMA OF THYROID

Papillary Carcinoma of Thyroid

- Accounts for **80%** of all thyroid malignancies in **iodine-sufficient areas**^{Q}
- **MC** thyroid cancer in **children** & **individuals** exposed to **external radiation**^{Q}.
- More often in **women, 30–40** years.

Pathology
- Grossly: **Hard** & **whitish remain flat** on sectioning with a blade with macroscopic **calcification, necrosis**, or **cystic changes**

> - **Multifocality**^{Q} is **common** (up to **85% of cases**) on **microscopic examination**.
> - **Multifocality** is associated with an **increased risk** of **cervical nodal metastases**^{Q}, rarely **invade adjacent structures** such as the trachea, esophagus & RLNs.

- **Rarely encapsulated**^{Q} (PCT are **seldom encapsulated**)
- Other variants: **Tall cell**^{Q}, **insular**^{Q}, columnar, diffuse sclerosing, clear cell, **trabecular**, and poorly differentiated types; account for about 1%; associated with a **worse prognosis**.

Histological Characteristics of Papillary Carcinoma Thyroid
- **Papillary projections**^{Q}: PTC contains branching papillae of cuboidal epithelial cells
- **Orphan Annie eye nuclei:**
  - The nuclei contain finely dispersed chromatin, which imparts an **optically clear** or **empty appearance**, giving rise to term **ground glass** or **Orphan Annie eye nuclei**^{Q}.
  - **Invaginations** of **cytoplasm** in cross-sections: **Intranuclear inclusions**^{Q} (**pseudo-inclusion**) or **intranuclear grooves**^{Q}.
  - **Diagnosis** of PTC is **based on** these **nuclear characteristics**^{Q} even in the absence of papillary structures.
- **Psammoma bodies**^{Q}: Microscopic, calcified deposits representing clumps of sloughed cells

Clinical Features
- Most patients are **euthyroid** & present with a **slow-growing painless mass**^{Q} in the neck.
- Dysphagia, dyspnea dysphonia are associated with locally advanced invasive disease.
- **Lymph node metastases** are **common**^{Q}, especially in **children young adults**, and may be the presenting complaint.

> - **"Lateral aberrant thyroid"** denotes a **cervical lymph node** that has been **invaded by metastatic cancer**^{Q}.

- **Distant metastases** are **uncommon** at initial presentation, but may ultimately develop in up to **20%** of patients.
- MC sites of metastasis: **Lungs**^{Q} > bone > liver > brain.

Diagnosis
- **Diagnosis is** established by **FNAC** of the **thyroid mass** or **lymph node**^{Q}.
- Once thyroid cancer is diagnosed on FNAC, a **complete neck ultrasound** to evaluate the **contralateral lobe** and for **LN metastases** in the central & lateral neck compartments.

Treatment
- Total or near-total **thyroidectomy**^{Q}
- During thyroidectomy, **enlarged central neck nodes** should be **removed**^{Q}.
- **Biopsy-proven lymph node metastases** detected clinically or by imaging in the lateral neck in patients with papillary carcinoma are managed with **modified radical neck dissection**.

Prognosis
- PTC have an **excellent prognosis** with a **>95% 10-year survival rate**^{Q}.

FOLLICULAR CARCINOMA THYROID

Follicular Carcinoma of Thyroid
- FTC account for **10% of thyroid cancers**
- Occurs more commonly in **iodine-deficient areas**^{Q}.
- More common in **women** with mean age of **50 years**
- **Genes** implicated in **FCT: p53**^{Q}, **PTEN**^{Q}, **Ras**^{Q}, **PAX8/PPAR1**

Pathology
- Usually **solitary lesion** surrounded by **capsule**^{Q}.
- Histologically, **follicles** are present, but the **lumen** may be **devoid of colloid**^{Q}.
- **Malignancy** is defined by the presence of **capsular** and **vascular invasion**^{Q}.
- **Tumor infiltration** and **invasion**, as well as **tumor thrombus** within the **middle thyroid** or **jugular vein**s, may be apparent at operation.

Clinical Features
- Usually present as **solitary thyroid nodules**, occasionally with a history of **rapid size increase**, and **long-standing goiter**^{Q}.
- Pain is uncommon, unless hemorrhage into the nodule has occurred.
- **Cervical lymphadenopathy** is **uncommon** at initial presentation (about 5%)

- Preoperative clinical diagnosis of cancer is difficult unless distant metastases are present.
- Large follicular tumors (>4 cm) in older men are more likely to be malignant^Q.

> - MC site of metastasis is bone (Osteolytic metastasis with pulsating secondaries in flat bones)^Q
> - MC site of metastasis: Vertebra^Q >Ribs >Pelvis Bones >Skull

Diagnosis
- FNAC is unable to distinguish benign follicular lesions from follicular carcinomas^Q.
- Intraoperative frozen-section examination usually is not helpful, but should be performed when there is evidence of capsular or vascular invasion, or when adjacent lymphadenopathy is present.

Treatment
- Follicular lesion: Hemithyroidectomy^Q (80% of these patients will have benign adenomas)
- Thyroid cancer: Total thyroidectomy^Q
- Total thyroidectomy in older patients with follicular lesions >4 cm because of the higher risk of cancer in this setting (50%)^Q.
- Prophylactic nodal dissection is unwarranted^Q because nodal involvement is infrequent.

Prognosis
- Cumulative mortality: 15% at 10 years and 30% at 20 years.
- Most important prognostic factor: Age and distant metastasis.

Poor Long-term Prognosis	
• Age >50 years^Q	• Marked vascular invasion^Q
• Tumor size >4 cm^Q	• Extrathyroidal invasion^Q
• Higher tumor grade^Q	• Distant metastases^Q

HÜRTHLE CELL CARCINOMA

Hürthle Cell Carcinoma

- Account for 3% of all thyroid malignancies
- Considered to be a subtype of follicular thyroid cancer^Q

Hürthle Cell Tumors Differ from Follicular Carcinomas in
• More often multifocal and bilateral (about 30%)^Q
• Usually do not take up RAI (about 5%)^Q
• More likely to metastasize to local nodes (25%) and distant sites^Q
• Associated with a higher mortality rate^Q (about 20% at 10 years)

Pathology
- Characterized by vascular or capsular invasion and can't be diagnosed by FNAC^Q.
- Tumors contain sheets of eosinophilic cells packed with mitochondria, which are derived from the oxyphilic cells of the thyroid gland.

Treatment
- Unilateral Hürthle cell adenomas: Hemithyroidectomy^Q
- Invasive Hürthle cell neoplasms: Total thyroidectomy + Routine central neck node removal^Q (MRND when lateral neck nodes are palpable)
- Retinoic acid, PPAR agonists have shown some utility in treating these tumors in vitro

MEDULLARY CARCINOMA THYROID

Medullary Carcinoma Thyroid

- Neuroendocrine carcinoma arising from parafollicular 'C' cells^Q of thyroid
- Parafollicular 'C' cells are derived from the ultimobranchial bodies^Q & secrete calcitonin^Q
- 'C' Cells are concentrated superolaterally in thyroid lobes, from where MTC usually develops
- Most MTCs (75–80%) arise sporadically^Q
- Spread is both lymphatic & hematogenous^Q
- MC site of metastasis: Liver^Q

Medullary Carcinoma Thyroid	
Sporadic: 80%^Q	Familial: 20%^Q (Non-MEN setting/MEN-2A/MEN-2B)
• Originate in **one lobe**^Q • Seen in **6th decade** • **RET protoncogene**^Q mutation	• **Multicentric** and **bilateral**^Q • Occur in **younger age**^Q • Associated with **C-cell hyperplasia**^Q • **RET protoncogene**^Q mutation

Clinical Features

Medullary Carcinoma Should Be Suspected
• **High level** of serum **Calcitonin**^{Q} & **CEA**^{Q} • **Cervical lymph nodes** at time of presentation (**LN involvement**, thyroid and **blood borne metastases** occurs **early**)^Q • **Diarrhea**^{Q} at the time of presentation. • **Amyloid**^{Q} in stroma histologically. • **MEN setting**: Evidence of Pheochromocytoma/Hyperparathyroidism/Thyroid cancer in family. • (Discovery of **medullary carcinoma thyroid** makes **family surveillance advisable**)^Q

Diagnosis
- Diagnosed by **FNAC**^{Q}
- I^{131} scan is of **no use** as MTC is **TSH independent**^{Q}.
- **Tumor marker: Calcitonin** is raised in **almost all cases** of MTC
- **Calcitonin excess** in MTC is **not associated** with **hypocalcemia**

Treatment
- Total thyroidectomy + Central LN dissection ± Ipsilateral MRND if tumor >1 cm^Q
- If **nodes** are **positive** on **ipsilateral side**: Bilateral MRND
- **Vandetanib (EGFR inhibitor)** is the only drug approved by US FDA for treatment of **advanced & progressive MTC**

Follow-up
- Level of **Calcitonin** falls after resection and is raises again in cases of recurrence, **used for follow up**^{Q}.

Prognosis
- MTC is **associated** with **poor prognosis**^{Q}.

ANAPLASTIC CARCINOMA

Anaplastic Carcinoma

- Accounts for **1%** of all thyroid malignancies
- Mainly affect **women in 7th and 8th decade**^{Q}
- The typical patient has a **long-standing neck mass**, which **rapidly enlarges** and may be **painful**^{Q}.
- Most aggressive form of **thyroid cancer**^{Q}

Pathology
- **Grossly: Firm & whitish** in appearance.
- Microscopically, sheets of cells with marked heterogeneity & characteristic **giant & multinucleated cells**^{Q}.

Clinical Features
- **Typical manifestation**: An **older patient** with **dysphagia, cervical tenderness** & a **painful, rapidly enlarging neck mass**^{Q}.
- **Superior vena cava syndrome** can also be part of the findings.
- The clinical situation **deteriorates rapidly** into **tracheal obstruction** & **rapid local invasion**^{Q} of surrounding structures.
- Associated symptoms: **Dysphonia, dysphagia & dyspnea**

> - **Lymph nodes** usually are **palpable** at presentation.
> - **Evidence** of **metastatic spread** also may be present.
> - **MC site** of metastasis: **Lungs**^{Q}

Diagnosis
- Confirmed by **FNAC** revealing characteristic **giant & multinucleated cells**^{Q}.
- **Incisional biopsy** occasionally is needed to **confirm** the **diagnosis**

Treatment
- **Thyroidectomy** for **resectable mass**^{Q} (may lead to a small improvement in survival, especially in younger individuals)
- Combined **radiation** & **chemotherapy** in an adjuvant setting in patients with resectable disease has been associated with **prolonged survival**^{Q}.
- **Tracheostomy**^{Q} to alleviate **airway obstruction**.

Prognosis
- Most aggressive thyroid malignancies^Q, with **<6 months** survival

> **Anaplastic Carcinoma**
> - On **gross inspection**, anaplastic tumors are **firm & whitish** in appearance.
> - **Microscopically**, sheets of cells with **marked heterogeneity** are seen. Cells may be spindle shaped, polygonal, or large, multinucleated cells.
> - **Foci of** more differentiated thyroid tumors, either **follicular** or **papillary**^{Q}, may be seen, suggesting that **anaplastic tumors arise from** more **well-differentiated tumors**^{Q}.

METASTATIC TUMORS OF THYROID

Metastatic Tumors of Thyroid

- Rare, most cases are found in autopsy
- MC site of primary: **CA Breast**^{Q} > CA Lung
- If thyroid metastases is detected pre-mortem, MC site of primary: **RCC**^{Q} > CA Breast > CA Lung

THYROID LYMPHOMA

Thyroid Lymphoma

- MC type is **NHL B cell**^{Q} type, of **intermediate** grade.
- Majority of patients have thyroid disease plus **cervical** or **mediastinal lymph nodes**^{Q}.
- More common in **females**.
- Most thyroid lymphomas **develop in** patients with **Chronic Lymphocytic Thyroiditis**^{Q}

Clinical Features
- **Lymphomas** are **rapidly growing tumours,** present with **rapidly enlarging neck mass** which is often **painless.**
- Patients may present with **acute respiratory distress & dysphagia**
- About **10–30%** present with symptoms relating to local invasion, including **hoarseness**, **dyspnoea** with stridor, or **dysphagia**.

> - **Painless**^{Q} and associated with **fever**^{Q}
> - Patients with thyroid lymphoma virtually **never have hyperthyroidism** but frequently have **hypothyroidism**^{Q}.
> - Hypothyroid patients have evidence of **autoimmune thyroiditis** or **Hashimoto's thyroiditis**^{Q}.

Diagnosis
- Diagnosis is confirmed by **core-needle biopsy**^{Q}.

Treatment: External Beam Radiotherapy + Chemotherapy^Q
- Patients with **thyroid lymphoma** respond rapidly to chemotherapy (**CHOP**—cyclophosphamide, doxorubicin, vincristine, and prednisone) and associated with **improved survival**.
- Combined treatment with **radiotherapy** & **chemotherapy** often is recommended.
- To alleviate **pressure symptoms**, **surgical resection** (Thyroidectomy and nodal dissection) is recommended.

THYROIDECTOMY

Steps of Thyroidectomy

- A Kocher transverse collar incision, typically **4 to 5 cm** in length, is placed in or parallel to a **natural skin crease 1 cm below cricoid cartilage**.
- Subcutaneous tissues & platysma are incised sharply and subplatysmal **flaps are raised superiorly** to the level of **thyroid cartilage** and **inferiorly** to the **suprasternal notch**^{Q}
- **Strap muscles** are **divided in the midline** along the entire length of mobilized flaps, & thyroid gland is exposed.
- **Middle thyroid veins** are ligated and **divided**^{Q}.

- **Dissection plane** is kept as **close** to the **thyroid** as possible & **superior pole** vessels are individually identified, skeletonized, ligated, & divided low on the thyroid gland **to avoid injury** to external branch of **superior laryngeal nerve**^{Q}.

- RLNs can be most consistently identified at the **level of cricoid cartilage**.
- **Parathyroids** usually can be identified **within 1 cm of** the crossing of the **inferior thyroid artery** and **the RLN**^{Q}

  - **Inferior thyroid vessels** are **dissected, skeletonized, ligated**, and **divided as close to the surface of thyroid gland as possible** to minimize devascularization of the parathyroids (**extracapsular**^{Q} **dissection**) or **injury to the RLN**^{Q}.

- **RLN** is **most vulnerable to injury in** the vicinity of the **ligament of Berry**. Any **bleeding** in this area should be **controlled with gentle pressure** before carefully identifying the vessel & ligating it. Use of the **electrocautery should be avoided** in proximity to the RLN^Q.
- Once the ligament is divided, the thyroid can be separated from the underlying trachea by sharp dissection.

  - **Parathyroid glands** that have been **inadvertently removed** during the thyroidectomy should be resected, confirmed as parathyroid tissue by frozen section, **divided into 1-mm fragments**, and **reimplanted into** individual pockets in the **sternocleidomastoid**^{Q} muscle. The sites should be **marked with silk sutures** and a **clip**^{Q}.

COMPLICATIONS OF THYROIDECTOMY

COMPLICATIONS OF THYROIDECTOMY

- **Hemorrhage**
  - Due to **slipping of ligature** on the **superior thyroid artery**^{Q}, bleeding from muscular artery
  - **Hematomas** may cause airway compromise and **must be evacuated immediately**^{Q}.
  - Hematomas may occur immediately or later on.
  - An **immediate bleed** occurs after or shortly before extubation when the patient lightens from anaesthesia and may **begin to cough**, causing a vessel to open.
- **Respiratory obstruction: Causes include**
  - **Tension hematoma**^{Q}
  - **Laryngeal edema (by anesthetic intubation): MC cause of respiratory obstruction**^{Q}
  - **Bilateral recurrent laryngeal nerve paralysis**^{Q}
- **Recurrent laryngeal nerve paralysis**
  - May be unilateral or bilateral, transient or permanent.
  - Bilateral paralysis causes respiratory obstruction - Dyspnea, stridor.
- **Injury to other nerves**
  - **External branches of superior laryngeal nerve**^{Q} (MC injured nerve during thyroid surgery: **External laryngeal nerve**^{Q})
  - Cervical sympathetic trunk - may cause Horner's syndrome.
- **Parathyroid insufficiency**
  - Due to **removal of the parathyroid glands** or **infarction due to vascular injury**^{Q}.
  - **Vascular injury**^{Q} is more important.
  - Cases usually present **2–5 days after operation**^{Q} with symptoms of **hypocalcemia** (circumoral and fingertip numbness and tingling tetany, carpopedal spasm and laryngeal stridor)^Q
  - Treatment with **oral calcium & vitamin D supplements**^{Q}
  - **IV calcium gluconate**^{Q} may be required in severe cases.
- **Thyroid insufficiency**
- **Thyrotoxic crisis**
  - Occurs if the thyrotoxic patient has been **inadequately prepared for thyroidectomy**^{Q}.

Multiple Choice Questions

PAPILLARY CARCINOMA

1. A 35 years old female presented with a swelling in the neck for the past 2 months, she had the treatment for Hodgkin's lymphoma when she was 22 years with irradiation. On, examination, her vitals were normal, there was a single, firm, irregular nodule, moving with deglutition in the left side of midline. Clinical examination also revealed a single node in the left side of the neck. The most likely clinical diagnosis of this condition is: *(COMEDK 2011)*
   a. Recurrence of lymphoma
   b. Malignant goiter
   c. Benign multinodular goiter
   d. Toxic nodular goiter

2. Most probable pathological diagnosis would be: *(COMEDK 2011)*
   a. Anaplastic carcinoma
   b. Follicular carcinoma
   c. Medullary carcinoma
   d. Papillary carcinoma

3. The FNAC of the lesion should reveal: *(COMEDK 2011)*
   a. 'Orphan-Annie eye' nucleus cells
   b. Amyloid deposits
   c. Epitheloid cells and giant cells
   d. Follicular cells

4. The ideal treatment of the above condition would be:
   a. Total thyroidectomy with lymph nodal dissection of the same side *(COMEDK 2011)*
   b. Radiotherapy
   c. Lobectomy
   d. Lobectomy with isthmusectomy

5. About papillary carcinoma what is/are true? *(PGI Dec 2008)*
   a. Often encapsulated
   b. Prognosis is bad
   c. Lymph node metastases is common
   d. Can metastasize to lung
   e. Multiple foci of tumour is seen

6. Variant of papillary carcinoma thyroid: *(PGI June 2007)*
   a. Medullary
   b. Warthin
   c. Columnar
   d. Insular
   e. Diffuse sclerosing

7. Which of the following would be the best treatment for a 2 cm thyroid nodule in a 50-year-old man with FNAC revealing it to be a papillary carcinoma? *(AIIMS May 2011)*
   a. Hemithyroidectomy
   b. Total thyroidectomy with left sided modified neck dissection
   c. Near total thyroidectomy with radiotherapy
   d. Hemithyroidectomy with modified neck dissection

8. Psammoma bodies may be seen in all of the following, except: *(Recent Question 2016, All India 2011)*
   a. Follicular carcinoma of thyroid
   b. Papillary carcinoma of thyroid
   c. Meningioma
   d. Serous cystadenocarcinoma of ovary

9. Features of papillary carcinoma includes: *(PGI May 2011)*
   a. FNAC easy
   b. Almost always unifocal
   c. Psammoma body
   d. Spread to cervical LN
   e. Bad prognosis

10. About papillary carcinoma true statement is/are:
    a. Radiation is a risk factor *(PGI Nov 2010)*
    b. Multifocal
    c. Hematogenous spread is common
    d. Distant metastasis is seen

11. Most common thyroid malignancy is: *(DNB 2012, MHPGMCET 2002)*
    a. Anaplastic carcinoma
    b. Follicular carcinoma
    c. Medullary carcinoma
    d. Papillary carcinoma

12. Which thyroid malignancy is common after radiation exposure? *(Recent Question 2016, MHSSMCET 2005)*
    a. Follicular
    b. Papillary
    c. Medullary
    d. Anaplastic

13. A 10 years old boy presented with cervical lymph adenopathy. Needle biopsy from the nodes revealed secondaries from papillary carcinoma of thyroid. The child under went complete removal of tumor near total thyroidectomy and radical neck dissection. What should be the immediate next line of management? *(All India 2012)*
    a. Start thyroxine suppression therapy
    b. I-131 whole body scan to assess the extent of disease
    c. Bone scan to evaluate secondaries
    d. CECT scan to assess any residual disease

14. Orphan Annie-eye nuclei seen in: *(Orissa 2011)*
    a. Papillary carcinoma of thyroid
    b. Medullary carcinoma of thyroid
    c. Anaplastic carcinoma of thyroid
    d. Follicular carcinoma of thyroid

15. Psammoma bodies are seen in following except: *(PGI 2002)*
    a. Serous cystadenoma of ovary
    b. Mucinous cystadenoma of ovary
    c. Meningioma
    d. Papillary carcinoma of thyroid

16. Which of the following would be the best treatment for a 2 cm thyroid nodule in a 50 years old man with FNAC revealing it to be a papillary carcinoma? *(All India 2009)*
    a. Hemithyroidectomy *(Recent Question 2015)*
    b. Subtotal thyroidectomy with modified neck dissection
    c. Near total thyroidectomy with modified neck dissection
    d. Hemithyroidectomy with modified neck dissection

17. True regarding papillary carcinoma of thyroid:
    a. Undifferentiated carcinoma *(MCI March 2006)*
    b. Blood-borne metastasis is commoner
    c. Excellent prognosis
    d. Capsulated

18. Which type of thyroid carcinoma has the best prognosis? *(DNB 2010, All India 96)*
    a. Papillary carcinoma
    b. Anaplastic carcinoma
    c. Follicular carcinoma
    d. Medullary carcinoma

19. Compared to follicular carcinoma, papillary carcinoma of thyroid have: *(PGI Dec 2007, June 2005, Dec 2006)*
    a. More male preponderance
    b. Bilaterality
    c. Local recurrence common
    d. Increased lymph node metastasis
    e. Increased mortality

20. **Occult thyroid malignancy with nodal metastasis is:**
    (DNB 2005, 2001, AIIMS Sept 96)
    a. Medullary carcinoma
    b. Follicular carcinoma
    c. Papillary carcinoma
    d. Anaplastic carcinoma

21. **Least malignant thyroid cancer is:** (AIIMS Nov 2003)
    a. Papillary carcinoma
    b. Follicular carcinoma
    c. Anaplastic carcinoma
    d. Medullary carcinoma

22. **Lateral aberrant thyroid refers to:** (AIIMS June 2002)
    a. Congenital thyroid abnormality
    b. Metastatic foci from primary in thyroid
    c. Struma ovarii
    d. Lingual thyroid

23. **Which of the following is used in the treatment of differentiated thyroid cancer?** (All India 2006)
    a. I-131
    b. 99mTc
    c. P-32
    d. I-131 MIBG

24. **In treatment of papillary carcinomas thyroid, radioiodine destroys the neoplastic cells predominantly by:**
    (AIIMS Nov 2005)
    a. X-rays
    b. Beta rays
    c. Gamma rays
    d. Alpha particles

25. **A 21 years old woman has 3 cm node in the lower deep cervical chain on the left. The biopsy is interpreted as revealing normal thyroid tissue in a lymph node. The most likely diagnosis is:** (DNB 2012, DPG 2009 Feb)
    a. Subacute thyroiditis
    b. Metastatic carcinoma thyroid
    c. Hashimoto's disease
    d. Lateral aberrant thyroid

26. **All of the following regarding papillary carcinoma thyroid is true except:** (All India 90)
    a. Multicentric origin
    b. Secondaries to lymph nodes
    c. Slowing growing
    d. Bony metastasis in early stage

27. **Most common type of carcinoma thyroid having least chances of hematogenous spread:** (Recent Question 2015)
    a. Follicular
    b. Papillary
    c. Anaplastic
    d. Medullary

28. **Chance of metastasis to lymph nodes in PTC:**
    (Recent Question 2017)
    a. <10%
    b. 10–20%
    c. 20–40%
    d. >60%

29. **Orphan-Annie eye nuclei is seen in:** (Recent Question 2017)
    a. Papillary carcinoma thyroid
    b. Follicular carcinoma thyroid
    c. Medullary carcinoma thyroid
    d. Anaplastic carcinoma thyroid

30. **Psammoma bodies are seen in:** (Recent Question 2017)
    a. Papillary carcinoma thyroid
    b. Follicular carcinoma thyroid
    c. Medullary carcinoma thyroid
    d. Thyroid lymphoma

31. **A 27-year-old lady with 20 weeks pregnancy presented with a thyroid nodule on right side. FNAC from the nodule was suggestive of papillary carcinoma. Which of the following is contraindicated in her management?** (AIIMS May 2017)
    a. Total thyroidectomy plus neck node dissection
    b. Right lobectomy
    c. Radioactive iodine ablation
    d. Total thyroidectomy

FOLLICULAR CARCINOMA

32. **All of the following are true for follicular carcinoma of thyroid except:** (COMEDK 2006)
    a. Lymph node involvement rare
    b. Vascular involvement common
    c. Younger patients have good prognosis
    d. Diagnosis by FNAC

33. **Thyroid carcinoma with pulsating vascular skeletal metastasis is:** (COMEDK 2007, All India 95)
    a. Follicular
    b. Anaplastic
    c. Medullary
    d. Papillary

34. **Follicular carcinoma of thyroid is due to mutation of:**
    a. RAS
    b. HGF (JIPMER 2010)
    c. RET
    d. ABL

35. **A well differentiated follicular carcinoma of thyroid can be best differentiated from a follicular adenoma by:**
    a. Hurthle cell change (All India 2011, 2009)
    b. Lining of tall columnar and cuboidal cells
    c. Vascular invasion
    d. Nuclear features

36. **FNAC is useful in all the following types of thyroid carcinoma except:** (UPPG 2010, MCI March 2005, All India 95)
    a. Papillary
    b. Follicular
    c. Anaplastic
    d. Medullary

37. **Most probable malignancy that develops in a case of long-standing goiter is:** (MCI June 2018, Recent Question 2015, Kerala PG 2015, AIIMS Feb 97, Nov 2001)
    a. Follicular carcinoma
    b. Anaplastic carcinoma
    c. Papillary carcinoma
    d. Medullary carcinoma

38. **Bone metastasis is common in which thyroid tumor:**
    a. Follicular
    b. Papillary (AIIMS Nov 99)
    c. Hurthle cell tumour
    d. Anaplastic

39. **Thyroid nodule of 4 cm size, mobile but causing compressive symptoms. All are true except:** (DNB 2011)
    a. FNAC is investigation of choice
    b. FNAC cannot distinguish follicular adenoma from carcinoma
    c. Managed by sub-total thyroidectomy
    d. Cold nodules are diagnostic of malignancy

40. **In case of adenomatoid goiter which carcinoma is commonest to occur:** (AIIMS Nov 98)
    a. Medullary carcinoma
    b. Follicular carcinoma
    c. Papillary carcinoma
    d. Anaplastic carcinoma

41. **Carcinoma thyroid with blood borne metastasis is:**
    a. Follicular
    b. Papillary (AIIMS Feb 97)
    c. Medullary
    d. Anaplastic

42. **Lymph node metastasis is least commonly seen with:**
    a. Papillary CA Thyroid (All India 94)
    b. Medullary CA Thyroid
    c. Follicular CA Thyroid
    d. Anaplastic CA Thyroid

43. **A 20 years old female patient presented with a thyroid swelling. Most probably, the fine needle aspiration cytology will not diagnose:** (AIIMS Nov 97)
    a. Papillary carcinoma of thyroid
    b. Medullary carcinoma of thyroid
    c. Non-Hodgkin's lymphoma of thyroid
    d. Follicular carcinoma of thyroid

44. Hurthle cells tumour is: *(WBPG 2012, DPG 2007)*
    a. Papillary carcinoma thyroid
    b. Follicular carcinoma thyroid
    c. Medullary carcinoma thyroid
    d. Anaplastic carcinoma

45. Metastasis from follicular carcinoma should be treated by:
    a. Radioiodine
    b. Surgery *(MCI Sept 2006)*
    c. Thyroxine
    d. Observation

46. True regarding follicular carcinoma of thyroid:
    a. Hematogemous spread *(JIPMER 2014, 2013)*
    b. Commonly multifocal
    c. Readily diagnosed by face
    d. Most commonly carcinoma of thyroid

47. The microscopic feature that differentiates a follicular carcinoma from a follicular adenoma: *(COMEDK 2014)*
    a. Nuclear pleomorphism
    b. Hurthle cell change
    c. Capsular invasion
    d. Absence of colloid

48. FNAC cannot detect which of the following? *(AIIMS November 2014)*
    a. Follicular carcinoma
    b. Papillary carcinoma
    c. Colloid goiter
    d. Hashimoto's thyroiditis

MEDULLARY CARCINOMA

49. Screening method of medullary carcinoma thyroid is:
    a. Serum calcitonin *(All India 97, AIIMS Nov 95)*
    b. Serum calcium
    c. Serum alkaline phosphate
    d. Serum acid phosphatase

50. Treatment of medullary carcinoma thyroid:
    a. Surgery and Radiotherapy *(AIIMS May 2011)*
    b. Radiotherapy and Chemotherapy
    c. Surgery only
    d. Radioiodine ablation

51. False statement about feature of MTC: *(PGI Nov 2011)*
    a. Familial MTC may presents in 2nd decade
    b. It has characteristic amyloid stroma
    c. Secrete serotonin
    d. Take up radioiodine
    e. Secrete calcitonin

52. Thyroid radioiodine ablation therapy is useful in all except:
    a. Recurrent papillary carcinoma *(PGI May 2011)*
    b. Residual papillary carcinoma
    c. Anaplastic carcinoma
    d. Follicular carcinoma
    e. Medullary carcinoma

53. Age for prophylactic thyroidectomy in MEN IIB syndrome? *(MHSSMCET 2009)*
    a. 1 month
    b. 2 months
    c. 4 months
    d. 6 months

54. Recommended age for prophylactic thyroidectomy for MEN-2 is: *(Recent Question 2015)*
    a. 5 years
    b. Before 1 year
    c. At the time of diagnosis
    d. Any time

55. Thyroid carcinoma associated with hypocalcemia is: *(AIIMS Dec 94)*
    a. Follicular carcinoma
    b. Medullary carcinoma
    c. Anaplastic carcinoma
    d. Papillary carcinoma

56. Medullary carcinoma thyroid arises from: *(AIIMS Nov 93)*
    a. Parafollicular cells
    b. Cells lining the acini
    c. Capsule of thyroid
    d. Stroma of the gland

57. A biopsy from a mass in front of the neck revealed parafollicular cells. How do you follow up? *(JIPMER November 2017)*
    a. Calcitonin
    b. T4
    c. Thyroxine
    d. Thyroglobulin

58. Treatment of medullary carcinoma thyroid:
    a. Surgery and radiotherapy *(AIIMS Nov 2008)*
    b. Radiotherapy and chemotherapy
    c. Surgery only
    d. Radioiodine ablation

59. Needle biopsy of solitary thyroid nodule in a young woman with palpable cervical lymph nodes on the same sides demonstrates amyloid in stroma of lesion. Likely diagnosis is:
    a. Medullary carcinoma thyroid *(All India 2002)*
    b. Follicular carcinoma thyroid
    c. Thyroid adenoma
    d. Multinodular goiter

60. In medullary carcinoma thyroid tumour marker is: *(WBPG 2014, AIIMS June 98)*
    a. TSH
    b. Calcitonin
    c. T3, T4 and TSH
    d. Alpha Fetoprotein

61. After thyroidectomy for medullary carcinoma of thyroid, which is important for determining recurrence of tumour?
    a. Thyroglobulin
    b. TSH *(MCI Sept 2009)*
    c. CEA
    d. Thyroxine levels

62. The expression of the following oncogene is associated with a high incidence of medullary carcinoma of thyroid: *(AIIMS Nov 2005)*
    a. p53
    b. Her-2-neu
    c. Ret proto-oncogene
    d. Rb gene

63. A 26 years old women presents with a palpable thyroid nodule, and needle biopsy demonstrates amyloid in the stroma of the lesion. A cervical lymph node is palpable on the same side as the lesion. The preferred treatment should be:
    a. Removal of the involved node, the isthmus, a portion of the opposite bone and he enlarged lymph node
    b. Removal of the involved lobe, the isthmus, a portion of the opposite lobe, and he enlarged lymph node
    c. Total thyroidectomy and modified neck dissection on the side of the enlarged lymph node
    d. Total thyroidectomy and irradiation of the cervical lymph nodes *(BIHAR PG 2014, All India 2002)*

64. Amyloid stroma is seen in which carcinoma thyroid:
    a. Papillary carcinoma *(AIIMS June 2000)*
    b. Medullary carcinoma
    c. Anaplastic carcinoma
    d. Follicular carcinoma

65. A patient has pituitary tumour and pheochromocytoma and a thyroid nodule. Which carcinoma is most likely to occur? *(AIIMS Nov 2000)*
    a. Follicular carcinoma
    b. Medullary carcinoma
    c. Papillary carcinoma
    d. Anaplastic carcinoma

66. A 52 years old female patient presents with symptoms of pheochromocytoma. She also has a thyroid carcinoma. Her thyroid carcinoma is of which type: *(AIIMS June 99)*
    a. Anaplastic
    b. Medullary
    c. Follicular
    d. Papillary

67. MEN-2 is seen with the following type of thyroid carcinoma:
    a. Papillary   b. Medullary   (All India 97)
    c. Anaplastic   d. Follicular

68. Serum calcitonin is a marker for: (DNB 2003, All India 94)
    a. Anaplastic carcinoma   b. Papillary carcinoma
    c. Medullary carcinoma   d. Follicular carcinoma

69. Treatment of choice for medullary carcinoma of thyroid is:
                                           (AIIMS May 2005)
    a. Total thyroidectomy   b. Partial thyroidectomy
    c. I-131 ablation   d. Hemithyroidectomy

70. All of the following are helpful for diagnosis of medullary carcinoma thyroid except: (PGI 2000)
    a. Spindle cell stroma with few follicles
    b. Amyloid deposition
    c. Calcitonin in stroma
    d. Histological mitochondria is essential for diagnosis

71. Which of the following gene defects is associated with development of medullary carcinoma of thyroid?
    a. Ret proto-oncogene   b. FAP gene   (All India 2004)
    c. Rb gene   d. BRCA-1 gene

72. Commonest presenting complaints of medullary carcinoma thyroid: (PGI 84)
    a. Diarrhea   b. Dysphagia
    c. Hoarseness   d. Flushing

73. Which of the following is true about medullary carcinoma?
    a. Calcitonin is not a marker   (DPG 2008)
    b. Arises from parafollicular C cells
    c. Produces PTH
    d. Take up radioiodine

74. True about medullary carcinoma thyroid: (DPG 2007)
    a. Good prognosis
    b. Associated with MEN-1
    c. Increased calcitonin is not associated with hypocalcemia
    d. Treated by near total thyroidectomy

75. All are true regarding medullary carcinoma of thyroid except: (JIPMER 2014, 2013)
    a. It arises from 'C' cells
    b. Secrete high levels of calcitonin
    c. It is dependent on TSH
    d. Most cases are familial

76. Which of the following does not take radioactive iodine?
                                           (Recent Question 2017)
    a. Medullary carcinoma thyroid
    b. Papillary carcinoma thyroid
    c. Follicular carcinoma thyroid
    d. Hürthle cell carcinoma thyroid

77. Calcitonin is the marker for: (Recent Question 2017)
    a. Papillary carcinoma thyroid
    b. Follicular carcinoma thyroid
    c. Medullary carcinoma thyroid
    d. Anaplastic carcinoma thyroid

78. Medullary carcinoma thyroid is associated with which mutation?
                                           (Recent Question 2017)
    a. RET   b. MET
    c. p53   d. PTEN

79. RET proto-oncogene is associated with development of:
    a. Medullary carcinoma thyroid   (Recent Question 2018)
    b. Astrocytoma
    c. Paraganglioma
    d. Hürthle cell tumor thyroid

ANAPLASTIC CARCINOMA

80. Not true about anaplastic thyroid carcinoma:
    a. Local infiltration common   (PGI May 2011)
    b. Spread by lymphatic route
    c. Long term survival in patient undergoing surgery
    d. Surgery is of limited value
    e. Highly chemosensitive

81. A patient with long standing multinodular goitre develops hoarseness of voice and swelling undergoes sudden increase in size. Likely diagnosis is:
                                  (Recent Question 2014, All India 2001)
    a. Follicular carcinoma   b. Papillary carcinoma
    c. Medullary carcinoma   d. Anaplastic carcinoma

82. The treatment of choice for anaplastic carcinoma of thyroid infiltrating trachea and sternum will be: (AIIMS Nov 2005)
    a. Radical excision   b. Chemotherapy
    c. Radiotherapy
    d. Palliative/Symptomatic treatment

83. Least common thyroid malignancy is: (Recent Question 2015)
    a. Papillary   b. Follicular
    c. Medullary   d. Anaplastic

THYROID METASTASIS

84. Metastasis in thyroid gland come most commonly from carcinoma of: (PGI June 98)
    a. Testis   b. Prostate
    c. Breast   d. Lungs

THYROID LYMPHOMA

85. All of the following are true about lymphoma of the thyroid except: (All India 2007)
    a. More common in females
    b. Slow growing
    c. Clinically confused with undifferentiated tumors
    d. May present with respiratory distress and dysphagia

CARCINOMA THYROID

86. False statement regarding thyroid carcinoma: (PGI Nov 2011)
    a. Medullary thyroid carcinoma is associated with MEN-2A
    b. Follicular carcinoma -Most common type of carcinoma
    c. Papillary carcinoma -Multifocal
    d. Thyroid lymphoma is often associated with Hashimoto thyroiditis
    e. Anaplastic carcinoma occur in old age women

87. True about thyroid carcinoma: (PGI Dec 2006)
    a. Follicular carcinoma have worse prognosis than papillary carcinoma
    b. Papillary carcinoma spreads by hematogenous route more frequently than follicular carcinoma
    c. Papillary carcinoma have increased mortality than follicular carcinoma
    d. Follicular carcinoma are more bilateral than papillary carcinoma
    e. Follicular carcinoma have more male incidence than papillary carcinoma

88. Low risk in carcinoma thyroid: (PGI Dec 2006)
    a. Men <50 years   b. Women <40 years
    c. Papillary carcinoma <4 cm   d. Metastasis
    e. Follicular carcinoma >5c m

89. The most common histologic type of thyroid cancer is:
    (Recent Question 2015, All India 2008, 2004, AIIMS Nov 05, PGI Dec 2005)
    a. Medullary type   b. Follicular type
    c. Papillary type   d. Anaplastic type

90. Which of the following is not a histological variant of thyroid neoplasm? *(All India 2007)*
    a. Follicular   b. Merkel cell
    c. Insular   d. Anaplastic

91. Thyroid carcinoma:
    a. Is often associated with hypothyroidism
    b. Often produces hyperthyroidism
    c. Is usually euthyroid
    d. Occurs in toxic nodules

92. Amount of I-131 given for carcinoma thyroid: *(DPG 2006)*
    a. 5 micro curie   b. 50 micro curie
    c. 5 milli curie   d. 50 milli curie

93. Thyroxine can be given in which thyroid carcinoma: *(MCI Sept 2009)*
    a. Papillary   b. Medullary
    c. Anaplastic   d. Undifferentiated

94. Thyroid carcinoma causes laryngeal paralysis due to:
    a. Recurrent laryngeal nerve palsy *(PGI June 96)*
    b. Vagus nerve palsy
    c. Glossopharyngeal nerve palsy
    d. Hypoglossal nerve palsy

95. Which of the following is used in the treatment of thyroid malignancy? *(PGI June 2001)*
    a. I-131   b. I-125
    c. Tc-99   d. P-32
    e. Strontium

96. Which of the following is used in the treatment of well differentiated thyroid carcinoma: *(Recent Question 2013)*
    a. I^{131} b. 99m Tc
    c. 32P   d. MIBG

SOLITARY THYROID NODULE

97. Most sensitive investigation of thyroid nodule:
    a. MRI   b. PET Scan *(Punjab 2011)*
    c. USG   d. Clinical examination

98. True about solitary thyroid nodule: *(PGI Dec 2006)*
    a. THR-Antibody
    b. Lined by columnar epithelium
    c. Diffuse hyperplasia of thyroid
    d. Common in female
    e. Thyroidectomy done

99. A case of solitary thyroid nodule, investigation of choice is:
    (PGI June 97, 96, AIIMS Nov 97)
    a. T3, T4 estimation   b. Thyroid scan
    c. FNAC   d. Excision biopsy

100. Initial preferred investigation for thyroid nodule is:
     a. FNAC   b. Radionucleide test
     c. Thyroid function test d. USG *(DPG 2008)*

101. Investigation of choice in discrete thyroid swelling is:
     (Recent Question 2014)
     a. Isotope scans   b. Ultrasonography
     c. Autoantibody titres d. FNAC

102. A patient came with a small solitary nodule in right lobe of thyroid. FNAC shows follicular adenoma. The best surgery is: *(DNB 2002)*
     a. Enucleation   b. Sub-total thyroidectomy
     c. Right hemithyroidectomy d. Near-total thyroidectomy

103. A 53-year-old female with multinodular goiter underwent radioisotope scan, whose report shows warm nodules. Her chances of warm nodules being malignant is:
     a. 5%   b. 10% *(MHCET 2016)*
     c. 15%   d. 20%

104. A 45-year-old male presents with 4 × 4 cm, mobile right solitary thyroid nodule of 5 months. The patient is euthyroid. The following statements about his management are true except: *(AIIMS Nov 2005)*
     a. Cold nodule on thyroid scan is diagnostic of malignancy
     b. FNAC is the investigation of choice
     c. The patient should undergo hemithyroidectomy if FNAC report is inconclusive
     d. Indirect laryngoscopy be done in the preoperative period to assess mobility of vocal cords

105. Most common solitary thyroid nodule is:
     a. Follicular adenoma *(AIIMS Nov 2004, June 93)*
     b. Hurthle cell carcinoma
     c. Papillary carcinoma d. Solitary idiopathic goiter

106. What is the most appropriate operation for a solitary nodule in one lobe of thyroid? *(All India 2003, AIIMS Nov 95)*
     a. Lobectomy   b. Hemithyroidectomy
     c. Nodule removal
     d. Partial lobectomy with 1 cm margin around nodule

107. Which of the following is true about subtotal thyroidectomy?
     a. Removal of one lobe and isthmus *(Recent Question 2018)*
     b. Removal of both lobes leaving behind 6-8 grams of tissue
     c. Removal of entire lobe with cervical lymph nodes
     d. Removal of one lobe with isthmus

108. Percentage of cold nodules that becomes malignant are?
     a. 5%   b. 15% *(DNB 2014)*
     c. 20%   d. 40%

109. Which is the investigation of choice to differentiate between benign and malignant thyroid nodule? *(DNB 2014)*
     a. USG   b. FNAC
     c. Scintigraphy   d. Biopsy

110. Management of a single 1 cm non-functioning dominant nodule of thyroid in an asymptomatic patient:
     (Recent Question 2017)
     a. Observation   b. Radioiodine ablation
     c. Hemithyroidectomy d. Antithyroid drugs

GOITER

111. Multi-nodular goiter (MNG) secondary thyrotoxicosis is seen how much percentage of patient with MNG:
     a. 10%   b. 20% *(MHSSMCET 2005)*
     c. 30%   d. 40%

112. The most common presentation of endemic goiter is:
     (All India 96)
     a. Hypothyroid   b. Diffuse goiter
     c. Hyperthyroid   d. Solitary nodule

113. Thoracic extension of cervical goitre is usually approached through: *(AIIMS May 2005)*
     a. Neck   b. Chest
     c. Combined cervico-thoracic d. Thoracoscopic

114. A 20-year-old girl presents with 9 months history of neck swelling with thyrotoxic symptoms. On investigation increased T4 and decreased TSH with palpable 2 cm nodule was found. Next investigation will be: (AIIMS May 2007)
    a. USG
    b. Thyroid scan
    c. Radioactive iodine uptake
    d. CT scan

115. Indication of surgery in a case of thyroid swelling is/are:
    a. Cosmetic
    b. Pressure symptoms
    c. Myxedema
    d. Pain (PGI June 2004)
    e. Swelling with symptoms

116. In a patient presenting with a swelling of the thyroid, the radionuclide scan showed a cold nodule and the ultrasound showed a non cystic solid mass. The management of this patient would be: (AIIMS June 2002)
    a. Lobectomy
    b. Hemithyroidectomy
    c. Eltroxin
    d. Radio Iodine therapy

117. Symptoms of endemic goitre are all except:
    a. Cold intolerance
    b. Hoarseness
    c. Dysphagia
    d. Heat intolerance

118. What percentage of cold thyroid nodules are malignant?
    a. 70–80%
    b. 50–60% (MHCET 2016)
    c. 40–50%
    d. 10–20%

119. Treatment of choice in cold nodule of thyroid: (JIPMER 93)
    a. Subtotal thyroidectomy
    b. Wait and watch
    c. I-131
    d. Hemithyroidectomy

120. Which of the following is true? (AIIMS May 2011)
    a. Colloid goiter mostly presents as hyperthyroidism
    b. Thyroid storm, the clinical features are primarily due to increased thyroxine
    c. Excess calcium intake can lead to hyperthyroidism
    d. Goiter more than 5% of population is endemic goiter

121. A 12-year old girl presents with nodular goiter. Which of the following statements regarding her evaluation and management is incorrect? (AIIMS May 2014)
    a. 99 m-Tc scan should be performed to determine whether the nodules are hypofunctioning or hyperfunctioning
    b. Functional thyroid nodules are usually benign
    c. All nodules > 4 cm should be resected irrespective of cytology
    d. FNAC should be performed for allnodules > 1 cm in diameter

RETROSTERNAL GOITER

122. Most common symptom of retrosternal goiter:
    a. Dysphagia
    b. Stridor (Punjab 2010, PGI June 97)
    c. Dyspnea
    d. Superior vena cava syndrome

123. Retrosternal goiter is characterized by: (DPG 2005)
    a. Stridor
    b. Always malignant
    c. Bilateral
    d. None of the above

124. Most commonly used approach for retrosternal goitre:
    a. Transthoracic via second intercostal space
    b. Transthoracic via fourth intercostal space
    c. Trans-sternal through anterior mediastinum
    d. Transcervical (Recent Question 2019)

THYROTOXICOSIS

125. Thyroid storm after operation is due to: (COMEDK 2007)
    a. Inadequate control of hyperthyroidism
    b. Massive bleeding
    c. Recurrent laryngeal nerve injury
    d. Postoperative infection

126. Which of the following is the agent of choice for treating thyrotoxicosis during pregnancy? (COMEDK 2010)
    a. Carbimazole
    b. Propylthiouracil
    c. Methimazole
    d. Radioactive I-131

127. All of the following are features of thyrotoxicosis, except:
    a. Diastolic murmur (Recent Question 2016)
    b. Soft non-ejection systolic murmur
    c. Irregularly, irregular pulse
    d. Scratching sound in systole

128. Dancing carotid is seen in: (AIIMS Dec 98)
    a. Thyrotoxicosis
    b. Hypothyroidism
    c. AV Fistula
    d. Blow out carotid

129. The best marker to diagnose thyroid related disorder is:
    a. T3
    b. T4
    c. TSH
    d. Thyroglobulin

130. The occurrence of hypothyroidism following administration of supplemental iodine to subjects with endemic iodine to subjects with endemic iodine deficiency goiter is known as:
    a. Jod-Basedow effect (All India 2004)
    b. Wolff-Chaikoff effect
    c. Thyrotoxicosis factitia
    d. De Quervain's thyroiditis

131. In thyrotoxicosis, β-blockers do not control: (All India 94)
    a. Anxiety
    b. Tremors
    c. Tachycardia
    d. Oxygen consumption

132. All of the following are associated with thyroid storm, except: (All India 2002)
    a. Surgery for thyroiditis
    b. Surgery for thyrotoxicosis
    c. Stressful illness in thyrotoxicosis
    d. I-131 therapy for thyrotoxicosis

133. Cardiovascular findings in an elderly thyrotoxicosis patient are all, except: (All India 2000)
    a. Early diastolic murmur
    b. Systolic ejection murmur
    c. Scratch in left 2nd intercostal space
    d. Irregularly irregular pulse

134. Treatment of thyroid storm includes all, except: (AIIMS Nov 2003)
    a. Propranolol
    b. Radioactive iodine
    c. Hydrocortisone
    d. Lugol's iodine

135. Difference between thyrotoxicosis and malignant hyperthermia is: (AIIMS June 2001)
    a. Hyperthermia
    b. Tachycardia
    c. Muscle rigidity
    d. Elevated serum CPK level

136. In thyrotoxicosis, which of the following is seen?
    a. Pretibial myxedema
    b. Glycosuria
    c. Unilateral exophthalmos
    d. All

137. Toxic adenoma on scanning appear as: (JIPMER 98)
    a. Hot nodule
    b. Cold nodule
    c. Warm nodule
    d. Neutral

138. Thyroid storm after operation is due to: (COMEDK 2007)
    a. Inadequate control of hyperthyroidism
    b. Massive bleeding
    c. Recurrent laryngeal nerve injury
    d. Postoperative injection

139. A 48-year-old woman underwent subtotal thyroidectomy. She has vague family history of malignant hyperthermia. She develops agitation, restlessness, fever, tremor, shivering, and tachypnea. Thyrotoxic crises can be best distinguished from malignant hyperthermia by estimating: (Kerala 2004)
    a. Temperature variation
    b. Increased CPK levels
    c. LDH
    d. Muscular rigidity

140. A 55-year-old male patient underwent cholecystectomy for Gall stone calculus. During surgery the patient's pulse was irregularly irregular, 160/min, BP = 80/50 mm of Hg, temp. 40°C. On examination a swelling in the neck was found. Most likely diagnosis is: *(MAHE 2007)*
    a. Thyroid storm
    b. Myocardial infarction
    c. Arrythmias
    d. Stridor

141. All of the following conditions are associated with hyperthyroidism, except: *(All India 2011)*
    a. Hashimoto's thyroiditis
    b. Grave's disease
    c. Toxic multinodular goiter
    d. Struma ovary

142. Hyperthyroidism occurs in: *(PGI Nov 2011)*
    a. Hashimoto thyroiditis
    b. Graves' disease
    c. Medullary thyroid carcinoma
    d. Plummer's disease
    e. Struma ovarii

143. Which of the following is a symptom of hypothyroidism? *(JIPMER 2014, 2007)*
    a. Hyperactivity
    b. Palpitation
    c. Diarrhoea
    d. Hair loss

144. Reduction of size and vascularity prior to thyroidectomy is done by: *(Recent Question 2015)*
    a. Iodides
    b. Propylthiouracil
    c. Radioiodine
    d. Propranolol

145. A patient underwent thyroidectomy for Hyperthyroidism. Two days later he presented with features of thyroid storm. What is the most likely cause? *(AIIMS November 2015)*
    a. Poor antibiotic coverage
    b. Rough handling during surgery
    c. Removal of parathyroid
    d. Inadequate preoperative preparation

146. Treatment of choice for recurrent thyrotoxicosis after surgery is: *(MCI June 2018)*
    a. Further surgery
    b. Radioiodine followed by surgery
    c. Radioiodine
    d. Observation & follow-up

GRAVE'S DISEASE

147. All of the following are features of Grave's disease except: *(MCI Sept 2005)*
    a. More common in males
    b. Tremor
    c. Pretibial myxoedema
    d. Intolerance to heat

148. Complications of therapy with radioactive iodine includes:
    a. Thyroid malignancy
    b. Hypothyroidism
    c. Leukemia
    d. All of the above

149. Which of the following conditions is most common complication of radioiodine treatment of Grave's disease? *(COMEDK 2005, 2004)*
    a. Thyroid storm
    b. Subacute thyroiditis
    c. Thyroid cancer
    d. Hypothyroidism

150. In which of the following conditions radioactive iodine (Irradiation) can be used in Grave's disease: *(PGI Nov 2010)*
    a. Recurrence
    b. Age >40 years
    c. Elderly
    d. Pregnant
    e. Presence of associated co-morbidities

151. Pretibial myxedema is seen in: *(MHPGMET 2005)*
    a. Thyrotoxicosis
    b. Hypothyroidism
    c. Hyperparathyroidism
    d. All

152. Therapy of choice for diffuse toxic goiter in a patient over 45 years:
    a. Surgery
    b. Antithyroid drugs
    c. Radioiodine
    d. Antithyroid drugs first followed by surgery

153. Which of the following statements about Grave's disease is false? *(Recent Question 2018)*
    a. Results in hyperthyroidism
    b. Autoimmune disorder
    c. Common in male
    d. Referred as diffuse toxic goiter

154. All of the following are true about Graves disease except:
    a. Cardiac failure is common *(JIPMER 2013)*
    b. Hypertrophy and hyperplasia or thyroid gland is due to TSH-Rab
    c. Remissions and exacerbations are not infrequent
    d. It is highly vascular with audible bruit

HYPOTHYROIDISM

155. In case of hypothyroidism which investigation is most informative and most commonly used: *(AIIMS June 98)*
    a. Serum TSH level
    b. Serum T3, T4 level
    c. Serum calcitonin assay
    d. Serum TRH assay

156. Hypothyroidism with increased TSH level is seen in all except: *(PGI 90)*
    a. Sheehan's syndrome
    b. Lithium carbonate therapy
    c. Post radioiodine ablation
    d. Endemic goitre

POST THYROIDECTOMY COMPLICATIONS

157. During thyroidectomy, inferior thyroid artery is ligated at:
    a. Maximally away from the gland *(MCI Sept 2005)*
    b. Close to the gland
    c. Half way from the gland
    d. None of the above

158. Complications of total thyroidectomy include all except: *(AIIMS May 2005)*
    a. Hoarseness
    b. Airway obstruction
    c. Hemorrhage
    d. Hypercalcemia

159. Two hours after subtotal thyroidectomy for thyrotoxicosis, young woman rapidly becomes agitated and complains of increasing difficulty in breathing. Her pulse rate rises and central cyanosis is noticed on examination, her neck is found to be tensely swollen beneath the stitches. The most appropriate management in this case would be: *(DPG 2011)*
    a. Intranasal oxygen
    b. Passing an endotracheal tube in the ward
    c. Removing sutures from all layers in the ward and evacuation of hematoma
    d. Immediate transfer of the patient to the operation theatre for tracheostomy

160. Horner's syndrome, all are true except: *(AIIMS May 2011)*
    a. Miosis
    b. Anhydrosis
    c. Hyperchromatic iris
    d. Apparent exophthalmos

161. Horner's syndrome is seen in all except: *(AIIMS Nov 2010)*
    a. Carotid artery aneurysm
    b. Medial medullary syndrome
    c. Can occur following surgery for Raynaud's syndrome
    d. Multiple sclerosis

162. Horner's syndrome does not include: *(COMEDK 2004)*
    a. Ptosis
    b. Anhydrosis
    c. Flushing
    d. Mydriasis

163. During thyroidectomy, inferior thyroid artery ligation is done at what level? *(MHPGMCET 2003)*
    a. As close to the thyroid gland as possible
    b. As far away as possible from the thyroid gland
    c. In the trachea-esophageal groove
    d. Any of the above

164. About thyroid surgery all are true except: *(Punjab 2008)*
    a. Superior thyroid artery is ligated near the gland
    b. Capsule is removed
    c. Inferior thyroid artery is ligated away from gland
    d. Capsule is kept intact

165. Hypoparathyroidism following thyroid surgery occurs within: *(AIIMS Nov 2004, Nov 2003)*
    a. 24 hours
    b. 2–5 days
    c. 7–14 days
    d. 2–3 weeks

166. Complications of hemithyroidectomy include all of the following except? *(All India 2008)*
    a. Hypocalcemia
    b. Wound hematoma
    c. Recurrent laryngeal nerve palsy
    d. External branch of superior laryngeal nerve palsy

167. A patient undergoes thyroid surgery, following which he develops perioral tingling. Blood calcium is 8.9 meq/L. Next step is: *(All India 2001)*
    a. Vitamin D orally
    b. Oral calcium and vitamin D
    c. Intravenous calcium gluconate and serial monitoring
    d. Wait for calcium to decrease to < 7.0 before talking further action

168. Patient after thyroid surgery presents with perioral paresthesia. Serum calcium level is 7 mg/dl. What will be the best management: *(AIIMS Nov 2000)*
    a. Oral vitamin D3
    b. Oral vitamin D3 with calcium
    c. IV calcium gluconate
    d. Oral calcium

169. A post-thyroidectomy patient develops signs and symptoms of tetany. The management is: *(All India 2000)*
    a. IV calcium gluconate
    b. Bicarbonate
    c. Calcitonin
    d. Vitamin D

170. In postoperative room after thyroid surgery patient developed sudden respiratory distress, dressing was removed and it was found to be slightly blood stained and wound was bulging. What will be first thing to be done?
    a. Tracheostomy *(AIIMS June 2000, Nov 2000)*
    b. Cricothyroidotomy
    c. Laryngoscopy and intubation
    d. Remove the stitch and take the patient to O.T.

171. A patient presents with swelling in the neck following a thyroidectomy; what is the most likely resulting complication?
    a. Respiratory obstruction *(All India 2001)*
    b. Recurrent laryngeal nerve palsy
    c. Hypovolemia
    d. Hypocalcemia

172. Patient presents with neck swelling and respiratory distress few hours after a thyroidectomy surgery. Next management would be: *(All India 2001)*
    a. Open immediately
    b. Trecheostomy
    c. Wait and watch
    d. Oxygen by mask

173. Most dangerous complication in a patient who had undergone thyroid surgery and develop hematoma at the operative site: *(AIIMS Nov 99)*
    a. Respiratory obstruction
    b. Recurrent laryngeal nerve palsy
    c. Dysphagia
    d. Shock

174. After thyroidectomy, patient developed stridor within 2 hours. All are likely cause of stridor except:
    a. Hypocalcemia *(AIIMS Nov 2001, Nov 2000)*
    b. Recurrent laryngeal nerve palsy
    c. Laryngomalacia
    d. Wound hematoma

175. A 50-year-old male is suffering from severe dyspnea after thyroid surgery, treatment of choice is: *(AIIMS June 97)*
    a. Tracheostomy
    b. Open the operative site
    c. Wait and watch
    d. Cricothyroidotomy

176. A patient operated for thyroid surgery for a thyroid swelling, later in the evening developed difficulty in breathing. There was swelling in the neck. The immediate management would be: *(AIIMS June 2002)*
    a. Epinephrine injection
    b. Tracheostomy
    c. IV calcium gluconate
    d. Open the wound sutures in the ward

177. Replacement dose of thyroxine is: *(All India 93)*
    a. 0.1–0.2 mg
    b. 0.3–0.4 mg
    c. 1–2 mg
    d. 3–4 mg

178. All of the following are early life threatening complications of thyroid operation except: *(DPG 2010, SGPGI 2005)*
    a. Tracheomalacia and collapse of the larynx
    b. Wound hematoma with compression of the trachea
    c. Hypocalcemia
    d. Thyroid storm

179. Vocal cord palsy in thyroid surgery is due to injury to:
    a. Superficial laryngeal nerve *(COMEDK 2008, UPSC 2008)*
    b. Recurrent laryngeal nerve
    c. Ansa cervicalis
    d. Vagus nerve

180. Hemorrhage after thyroidectomy is due to: *(Recent Question 2014)*
    a. External carotid artery
    b. Internal carotid artery
    c. Superior thyroid artery
    d. Inferior thyroid artery

THYROIDITIS

181. Thyroid biopsy of a patient showed the presence of Hurthle cells. Antibodies found in this condition are: *(Punjab 2011)*
    a. Anti-TPO
    b. Anti-mitochondrial
    c. Anti-RNP
    d. Anti-dsDNA

182. A 40-year-old female presents with fever, fatigue, diffuse painful swelling in the midline of the neck, FNAC of the same reveals epitheloid cells and giant cells, the likely diagnosis is:
    a. Acute thyroiditis
    b. Subacute thyroiditis
    c. Tubercular lymphadenitis
    d. Hashimotos thyroiditis

183. A patient with autoimmune thyroiditis present with hypothyroidism. Which of the following is true?
    a. Thyroid peroxidase antibodies *(JIPMER 2011)*
    b. Painless enlargement of thyroid
    c. Common in men
    d. No malignant risk

184. A person has fever and pain in thyroid gland. True statement(s) is/are: *(PGI June 2009)*
    a. T3 and T4 level normal
    b. ↑ESR
    c. ↑TSH
    d. It is due to TB
    e. Radioactive iodine uptake is ↑ed

185. Hashimoto's thyroiditis, all are true except: *(AIIMS May 2011)*
    a. Follicular destruction
    b. Increase in lymphocytes
    c. Oncocytic metaplasia
    d. Orphan Annie eye nuclei

186. The laboratory investigation of a patient shows ↓T4, and ↑TSH. Which of the following is the most likely diagnosis: *(All India 2011)*
    a. Grave's disease
    b. Hashimoto's disease
    c. Pituitary failure
    d. Hypothalamic failure

187. Which of the following conditions is associated with hypothyroidism? *(All India 2011)*
    a. Hashimoto's thyroiditis
    b. Grave's disease
    c. Toxic multinodular goiter
    d. Struma ovary

188. Most common cause of thyroiditis is: *(All India 2000)*
    a. Reidel's thyroiditis
    b. Subacute thyroiditis
    c. Hashimoto's thyroiditis
    d. Viral thyroiditis

189. All of the following are true of de-Quervain's thyroiditis except: *(All India 1996)*
    a. Pain
    b. Increased ESR
    c. Increased radioactive iodine uptake
    d. Fever

190. Not a feature of de-Quervain's disease: *(All India 2002)*
    a. Autoimmune in etiology
    b. ↑ESR
    c. Tends to regress spontaneously
    d. Painful and associated with enlargement of thyroid

191. Which of the following is wrong about subacute thyroiditis?
    a. Usually presents with painful enlargement of thyroid gland *(Orissa 2011)*
    b. There may be features of hyperthyroidism or hypothyroidism
    c. In the thyrotoxic phase radioiodine uptake is increased
    d. High ESR

192. 'Hurthle cells' are seen in: *(All India 95)*
    a. Agranulomatous thyroiditis
    b. Hashimoto's thyroiditis
    c. Papillary carcinoma of the thyroid
    d. Thyroglossal cyst

193. A patient presents with bilateral proptosis, heat intolerance and palpitations. Most unlikely diagnosis here would be: *(All India 2001)*
    a. Hashimoto's thyroiditis
    b. Thyroid adenoma
    c. Diffuse thyroid goitre
    d. Reidel's thyroiditis

194. A 25-years-old male presents with ophthalmologic signs of thyrotoxicosis. All are possibilities, except: *(All India 2002)*
    a. Diffused thyroid goitre
    b. Hashimoto's thyroiditis
    c. Riedel's thyroiditis
    d. Adenomatous goitre

195. A young patient has a midline, tender swelling in neck occurring after an attack of sore throat. The diagnosis is: *(AIIMS Nov 93)*
    a. Acute thyroiditis
    b. Thyroglossal cyst
    c. Subacute thyroiditis
    d. Toxic goiter

196. In Hashimoto's disease serum antibodies are mainly against: *(Recent Question 2016)*
    a. Thyroid follicles
    b. Thyroxine
    c. Thyroglobulins
    d. Iodine

197. The only reason for operating in case thyroiditis:
    a. To prevent cancerous degeneration
    b. For relief of pain in neck and ear
    c. To overcome pressure on trachea or esophagus
    d. To cure the toxic reaction
    e. If there is auto immune reaction

198. All are true abut Hashimoto's thyroiditis except: *(Kerala 95)*
    a. Antithyroid microsomal antibodies
    b. Antithyroid nuclear antibodies
    c. Anti-TSH receptor antibodies
    d. Increased level of thyroid hormones

199. The thyroiditis also known as "Painless Thyroiditis":
    a. Subacute lymphocytic thyroiditis *(MAHE 2007)*
    b. de-Quervain's thyroiditis
    c. Hashimoto's thyroiditis
    d. Riedel's thyroiditis

200. A patient present with bilateral proptosis, heat intolerance and palpitations; most unlikely diagnosis here would be: *(All India 2001, 2000)*
    a. Hashimoto's thyroiditis
    b. Thyroid adenoma
    c. Diffuse thyroid goiter
    d. Reidel's thyroiditis

201. DeQvervain's thyroiditis is characterised by:
    a. Mononuclear cell infiltration *(COMEDK 2014)*
    b. Histiocyte reaction
    c. Giant cell infiltration
    d. Eosinophilia

THYROGLOSSAL CYST AND FISTULA

202. Hyoid bone is closely associated with: *(Orissa 2011)*
    a. Bronchogenic cyst
    b. Cystic hygroma
    c. Branchial cyst
    d. Thyroglossal cyst/fistula

203. True about thyroglossal cyst is all except:
    a. Does not move with deglutition *(MHPGMCET 2003)*
    b. Move with protrusion of tongue
    c. Sistrunk's operation is treatment of choice
    d. Most common site is subhyoid region

204. A 10-year-old child presented with midline swelling in anterior position of neck. Most probable diagnosis is:
    a. Thyroglossal cyst
    b. Thyroglossal fistula
    c. Cold abscess
    d. Acute lymphadenitis

205. Sistrunk's operation is done in: *(WBPG 2015, MHPGMCET 2008, 2006)*
    a. Parotid tumor
    b. Thyroglossal fistula
    c. Thyroglossal cyst
    d. Branchial fistula

206. Most common site of thyroglossal cyst: *(Recent Question 2013, DNB 2009, 2007, 2005, 2003, MHSSMCET 2005, AIIMS June 97)*
    a. Suprahyoid
    b. Hyoid
    c. Subhyoid
    d. Intra-thyroid

207. The following statements about thyroglossal cyst are true, except: *(All India 2006)*
    a. Frequent cause of anterior midline neck masses in the first decade of life
    b. The cyst is located within 2 cm of the midline
    c. Incision and drainage is the treatment of choice
    d. The swelling moves upwards on protrusion of tongue

208. Thyroglossal cyst may occasionally give rise to carcinoma:
    a. Papillary   b. Medullary
    c. Anaplastic   c. Follicular

209. Sistrunk's operation consists of: *(DPG 2009 March)*
    a. Excision of hyoid bone and cone of tongue muscle
    b. Excision of hyoid bone and the cyst
    c. Excision of central part of hyoid bone and cone of tongue muscles upto foramen caecum
    d. Excision of cyst only

210. A central midline neck swelling is noted in a 4 years old girl posted for tonsillectomy. The swelling is, painless, mobile, and cystic, just below the hyoid bone of size 2x1.1x1cm. USG showed a thick walled cystic lesion. Management would include: *(AIIMS Nov 97)*
    a. Surgical removal   b. Antibiotics
    c. Percutaneous aspiration d. Chest X-ray

THYROID ANATOMY AND PHYSIOLOGY

211. The occurence of hyperthyroidism following administration of supplemental iodine to subject with endemic iodine deficiency goitre is known as: *(All India 2012)*
    a. Jod-Basedow effect   b. Wolff-Chaikoff effect
    c. Thyrotoxicosis factitia d. De-Quervains thyroiditis

212. Which of the following most closely represents the lowest detection limit for third generation TSH assays?
    a. 0.4 mIU/L   b. 0.04 mIU/L *(All India 2012)*
    c. 0.004 mIU/L   d. 0.0004 mIU/L

213. Recurrent laryngeal nerve is in close association with: *(AIIMS Nov 93)*
    a. Superior thyroid artery   b. Inferior thyroid artery
    c. Middle thyroid vein   d. Superior thyroid vein

214. Normal thyroid weight varies .... with dietary iodine content:
    a. Directly proportional   b. Inversely
    c. Inverse cubically   d. Not fixed

215. Average weight of thyroid gland where diet is rich in iodine is:
    a. 10–12 gm   b. 14–16 gm
    c. 18–20 gm   d. 28–30 gm

216. Protein bound iodine measures secretary function of thyroid in all of the following circumstances except: *(All India 90)*
    a. Nephrotic syndrome
    b. Following hemithyroidectomy
    c. During ampicillin therapy
    d. Asthamatics on ephedrine

217. Isthmus of thyroid gland overlies the: *(DPG 97)*
    a. 1st tracheal cartilage
    b. 1st and 2nd tracheal cartilage
    c. 2nd and 3rd and 4th tracheal cartilage
    d. 3rd and 4th tracheal cartilage

MISCELLANEOUS

218. Scabard trachea is seen in: *(Karnataka 99)*
    a. Thyroid cancer   b. Thyroiditis
    c. Goitre   d. All of the above

219. A new born with a goiter large enough to cause dyspnoea is best treated with:
    a. Sulfonamides   b. Tracheostomy
    c. T3   d. Iodides

220. Which of the following factors contribute to the development of duodenal ulcer? *(PGI 2001)*
    a. I-131   b. I-125
    c. Tc-99   d. P-32

221. In pregnancy: *(APPG 2004)*
    a. Radioiodine contraindicated
    b. Thiouracil is contraindicated
    c. Surgery is contraindicated
    d. None

222. Pendred's syndrome is due to a defect in: *(MCI June 2018, COMEDK 2007, 2008)*
    a. Chromosome 7p   b. Chromosome 7q
    c. Chromosome 8p   d. Chromosome 8q

223. Reddish swelling in the region of foramen caecum: *(DPG 2007)*
    a. Lingual thyroid   b. Lingual tonsil
    c. Ranula   d. Thyroglossal cyst

224. True about Struma Ovarii: *(PGI June 2007)*
    a. Ectopic thyroid
    b. Ectopic ovary
    c. Malignancy
    d. Benign lesion
    e. Included in teratoma

225. Absent parathyroid, thymic aplasia with immuno-deficiency and cardiac defects are features of: *(MHPGMCET 2009)*
    a. Autoimmune polyglandular syndrome
    b. Pendred syndrome
    c. Di George syndrome
    d. Lesch-Nyhan syndrome

226. This picture depicts .... of examination of the thyroid gland. Choose the correct answer: *(APPG 2016)*
    a. Kocher's method
    b. Lahey's method
    c. Crile's method
    d. Pizzillo's method

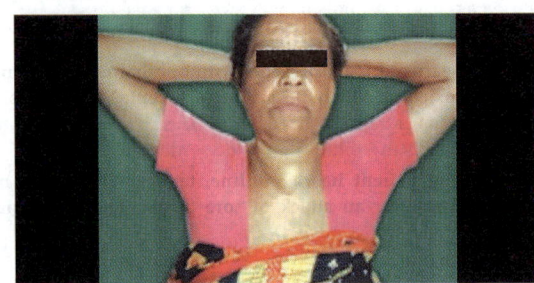

Explanations

PAPILLARY CARCINOMA

1. Ans. b. Malignant goiter *(Ref: Schwartz 10/e p1542-1544; Sabiston 20/e p902; Bailey 27/e p818; Harrison 20/e p2715, 19/e p2305)*
2. Ans. d. Papillary carcinoma
3. Ans. a. 'Orphan-Annie eye' nucleus cells
4. Ans. a. Total thyroidectomy with lymph nodal dissection of the same side
5. Ans. c. Lymph node metastases is common; d. Can metastasize to lung; e. Multiple foci of tumour is seen

> Papillary carcinoma are rarely encapsulated^Q

6. Ans. c. Columnar d. Insular; e. Diffuse sclerosing *(Ref: Schwartz 10/e p1542, 9/e p1361-1363; Sabiston 20/e p902, 19/e p906-909; Bailey 27/e p818, 26/e p765, 25/e p793-796)*

Types of Papillary Carcinoma Associated with Poor Prognosis	
1. Tall cell^Q	5. Clear cell^Q
2. Insular^Q	6. Trabecular^Q
3. Columnar^Q	7. Poorly differentiated type
4. Diffuse sclerosing^Q	

7. Ans. b. Total thyroidectomy with left sided modified neck dissection
8. Ans. a. Follicular carcinoma of thyroid *(Ref: Schwartz 10/e p1542; Sabiston 20/e p902; Bailey 27/e p818)*

Psammoma Bodies (PSM)	
1. Papillary carcinoma thyroid^Q	2. Papillary carcinoma (RCC)^Q
3. Serous cystadenoma^Q	4. Meningioma^Q

9. Ans. a. FNAC easy; c. Psammoma body; d. Spread to cervical LN
10. Ans. a. Radiation is a risk factor; b. Multifocal; d. Distant metastasis is seen
11. Ans. d. Papillary carcinoma   12. Ans. b. Papillary
13. Ans. a. Start thyroxine suppression therapy *(Ref: Schwartz 10/e p1549; Sabiston 20/e p906; Bailey 27/e p819)*

Well Differentiated Thyroid Cancer	
1. **Papillary** carcinoma of thyroid^Q	2. **Follicular** carcinoma of thyroid^Q
3. **Follicular variant** of **papillary** carcinoma thyroid^Q	4. **Hurthle cell** carcinoma (variant of follicular carcinoma thyroid)^Q

POSTOPERATIVE MANAGEMENT OF WELL-DIFFERENTIATED THYROID CANCER

Radioiodine Therapy

- Postoperative RAI therapy **reduces recurrence** and provides a small **improvement in survival**, even in low-risk patients^Q.
- **Metastatic differentiated thyroid carcinoma** can be **detected** and **treated by** ^{131}I in about **75%** of patients^Q.
- RAI **effectively treats >70% of lung micrometastases**^{Q} that are detected by RAI scan in the presence of a normal chest x-ray, whereas the success rates drop to <10% with pulmonary macrometastases. Early detection therefore appears to be very important to improve prognosis.

RAI Ablation Currently is Recommended for
• All patients with **stage III or IV disease**^{Q}
• All patients with **stage II** disease **<45 years**^{Q}
• Most patients 45 years or older with **stage II disease**^{Q}
• Patients with **stage I disease** who have **aggressive histologies**, **nodal metastases, multifocal disease,** and **extrathyroid** or **vascular invasion**^{Q}

- **T4 therapy** should be **discontinued for 6 weeks** before scanning with ^{131}I. Patients should **receive T$_3$** during this time period to decrease the period if hypothyroidism. T$_3$ has a shorter half-life than T$_4$ (**1 day vs. 1 week**) and needs to be **discontinued for 2 weeks** to allow **TSH levels to rise** before treatment^Q.

- A **low-iodine diet** also is recommended **during this 2-week period**[Q].
- The usual protocol involves administering a **screening dose** of **1 to 3 mCi** of ^{123}I and measuring uptake 24 hours later. **After a total thyroidectomy**, this value should be **<1%**. A "**hot**" spot in the neck after initial screening usually represents **residual normal tissue** in the thyroid bed.
- If there is **significant uptake**, then a **therapeutic dose** of ^{131}I, **30 to 100 mCi**[Q] should be administered **to low-risk patients** and **100 to 200 mCi in high-risk patients**[Q].
- Approximately **one third** of these patients **demonstrate uptake** on posttreatment imaging, and **Tg levels usually decrease** in these patients, **documenting therapeutic benefit**[Q].
- Patients with **previously positive scans** and patients with **serum Tg levels >2 ng/mL**[Q] usually need **another** ^{131}I treatment after **6 to 12 months** until one or two negative scans are obtained.
- The **follow-up scan** can be done **after hormone withdrawal** or **after recombinant TSH**. The **latter is more expensive**[Q] but is preferred by patients.

External Beam Radiotherapy and Chemotherapy

- **EBRT** is occasionally required to **control unresectable**, **locally invasive** or **recurrent disease** and to **treat metastases** in **support bones**[Q] to decrease the risk of fractures.
- EBRT is of value for the **treatment** and **control of pain** from **bony metastases**[Q] when there is **minimal** or **no RAIU**[Q].
- **Single** and **multidrug chemotherapy** has been used with **little success**[Q] in disseminated thyroid cancer, and there is **no role for routine chemotherapy**
- **Doxorubicin** (Adriamycin) and **paclitaxel** (Taxol) are the **most frequently use**d agents.

Thyroid Hormone

- **T4** is necessary as **replacement therapy**[Q] in patients after total or near-total thyroidectomy.
- Has the **additional effect** of **suppressing TSH**[Q] and **reducing the growth stimulus**[Q] for any **possible residual thyroid cancer cells**[Q].
- **TSH suppression reduces tumor recurrence** rates[Q].
- T_4 should be administered to ensure that the **patient remains euthyroid**[Q], with circulating TSH levels at about 0.1 U/L in low-risk patients, or <0.1 U/mL in high-risk patients.

14. Ans. a. Papillary carcinoma of thyroid
15. Ans. b. Mucinous cystadenoma of ovary
16. Ans. c. Near total thyroidectomy with modified neck dissection
17. Ans. c. Excellent prognosis
18. Ans. a. Papillary carcinoma
19. Ans. b. Bilaterality; c. Local recurrence common; d. Increased lymph node metastasis *(Ref: Schwartz 10/e p1542-1545; Sabiston 20/e p902, 904)*

	Papillary	Follicular
Male incidence	+	++[Q]
Lymph node metastasis	+++[Q]	+
Blood vessel invasion	+	+++[Q]
Recurrence rate	+	++[Q]
Overall mortality	+	++[Q]
Location of recurrent carcinoma		
Distant metastasis	+	++
Nodal metastasis	+++[Q]	+
Local recurrence	++[Q]	+
Bilaterality	+++[Q]	+

20. Ans. c. Papillary carcinoma
21. Ans. a. Papillary carcinoma
22. Ans b. Metastatic foci from primary in thyroid *(Schwartz 10/e p1542; Sabiston 20/e p903)*

LATERAL ABERRANT THYROID

- Any thyroid tissue found laterally separate from the thyroid gland, is always considered to be a **metastasis in a cervical lymph node**[Q], as aberrant thyroid tissue never occurs in lateral position.
- Aberrant thyroid tissues are **found along the course of** the **thyroglossal tract**:
  - Lingual[Q]
  - Cervical[Q]
  - Thoracic[Q]
- **Papillary carcinoma** of thyroid is **MC associated**[Q] with lateral aberrant thyroid

23. **Ans. a. I-131**
24. **Ans. b. Beta rays** *(Schwartz 10/e p1546; Sabiston 20/e p908; William's Endocrinology 10/e p479)*
25. **Ans. d. Lateral aberrant thyroid**
26. **Ans. d. Bony metastasis in early stage** *(Ref: Schwartz 9/e p1362, 1363, 1367, 1368; Sabiston 20/e p902, 904, 909, 910; Bailey 27/e p818)*
27. **Ans. b. Papillary**
28. **Ans. d. >60%** *(Ref: Schwartz 10/e p1542; Sabiston 20/e p904)*
29. **Ans. a. Papillary carcinoma thyroid** *(Ref: Schwartz 10/e p1542; Sabiston 20/e p903)*
30. **Ans. a. Papillary carcinoma thyroid** *(Ref: Schwartz 10/e p1542; Sabiston 20/e p903)*
31. **Ans. c. Radioactive iodine ablation** *(Ref: Schwartz 10/e p1546; Sabiston 20/e p906; Bailey 27/e p819)*

FOLLICULAR CARCINOMA

32. **Ans. d. Diagnosis by FNAC** *(Fef: Schwartz 10/e p1544, 1357; Sabiston 20/e p906; Bailey 27/e p818)*

LIMITATIONS OF FNAC IN THYROID DISEASES

1. **Not able** to **distinguish follicular adenoma** from **follicular carcinoma**^{Q}
2. Not able to distinguish **Hurthle cell adenoma** from **Hurthle cell carcinoma**^{Q}
3. **Useless** in **Reidel's thyroiditis**^{Q} (Biopsy is preferred)^Q
4. FNAC is **less reliable** in patients who have **history** of **head** and **neck irradiation** or **family history** of **thyroid cancer** due to higher likelihood of **multifocal lesions** and **occult cancer**^{Q}

33. **Ans. a. Follicular**
34. **Ans. a. RAS** *(Ref: Schwartz 10/e p1541; Sabiston 20/e p901)*
    - Genes implicated in FCT: p53^Q, PTEN^Q, Ras^Q, PAX8/PPAR1

Oncogenes and Tumor-Suppressor Genes Implicated in Thyroid Tumorigenesis		
Gene	**Function**	**Tumor**
Oncogenes		
RET^Q	Membrane receptor with tyrosine kinase activity	Sporadic and familial **MTC, PTC** (RET/PTC rearrangements)
MET^Q	Same	Overexpressed in **PTC**
TRK1	Same	Activated in some **PTC**
TSH-R	Linked to heterotrimeric G protein	Hyperfunctioning adenoma
Gs (gsp)	Signal transduction molecule (GTP binding)	Hyperfunctioning adenoma, follicular adenoma
Ras^Q	Signal transduction protein	**Follicular adenoma** and **carcinoma, PTC**
PAX8/PPAR1	Oncoprotein	**Follicular adenoma**, follicular **carcinoma**
B-Raf (BRAF)^Q	Signal transduction	**PTC, tall cell** and **poorly differentiated, anaplastic**
Tumor suppressors		
p53^Q	Cell cycle regulator, arrests cells in G$_1$, induces apoptosis	De-differentiated **PTC, FTC, anaplastic cancers**
p16^Q	Cell cycle regulator, inhibits cyclin dependent kinase	Thyroid cancer cell lines
PTEN^Q	Protein tyrosine phosphatase	**Follicular adenoma** and **carcinoma**

35. **Ans. c. Vascular invasion** *(Ref: Schwartz 10/e p1544; Sabiston 20/e p904; Bailey 27/e p818; Harrison 20/e p2715, 19/e p2305)*
36. **Ans. b. Follicular**
37. **Ans. a. Follicular carcinoma**
38. **Ans. a. Follicular**
39. **Ans. d. Cold nodules are diagnostic of malignancy**
40. **Ans. b. Follicular carcinoma**
41. **Ans. a. Follicular; c. Medullary**
42. **Ans. c. Follicular CA Thyroid**
43. **Ans. d. Follicular carcinoma of thyroid**

44. Ans. b. Follicular carcinoma thyroid *(Ref: Schwartz 10/e p1546; Sabiston 20/e p910)*
45. Ans. a. Radioiodine
46. Ans. a. Hematogenous spread
47. Ans. c. Capsular invasion
48. Ans. a. Follicular carcinoma

MEDULLARY CARCINOMA

49. Ans. a. Serum calcitonin *(Ref: Schwartz 10/e p1549-1550; Sabiston 20/e p909; Bailey 27/e p820; Harrison 20/e p2716, 19/e p2307)*
50. Ans. c. Surgery only *(Ref: Schwartz 10/e p1550; Sabiston 20/e p909; Bailey 27/e p820)*
51. Ans. d. Take up radioiodine
    - I^{131} scan is of no use as MTC is TSH independent^Q, so MTC does not take up radioiodine (I^{131}).
52. Ans. c. Anaplastic carcinoma, e. Medullary carcinoma
    - Radioactive iodine is used to destroy residual thyroid tissue (thyroid ablation) in well differentiated thyroid cancer.
53. Ans. d. 6 months *(Ref: Schwartz 9/e p1368; Sabiston 20/e p909)*

Prophylactic Thyroidectomy in RET Mutation Carriers	
MEN-2A	Before **5 years**^{Q}
MEN-2B	Before **1 year**^{Q}
• **Central neck dissection** is **avoided** in **children**^{Q}. • **Indications of central neck dissection** in children: 1. **Raised calcitonin**^{Q} 2. **USG suggesting thyroid cancer**^{Q} **>5 mm** 3. **Evidence of LN metastasis**	

54. Ans. a. 5 years
55. Ans. None *(Ref: Sabiston 20/e p909)*
    - Sabiston says "The **calcitonin excess** in **MTC** is **not associated with hypocalcemia.**"^{Q}
    - Robbins says "Notably **hypocalcemia** is **not a prominent feature** despite the **presence** of **raised calcitonin levels.**"^{Q}

56. Ans. a. Parafollicular cells
57. Ans. a. Calcitonin *(Ref: Schwartz 10/e p1549; Sabiston 20/e p909; Bailey 27/e p820)*
58. c. Surgery only
59. Ans. a. Medullary carcinoma thyroid
60. Ans. b. Calcitonin
61. Ans. c. CEA
62. Ans. c. Ret proto-oncogene
63. Ans. c. Total thyroidectomy and modified neck dissection on the side of enlarged lymph node
64. Ans. b. Medullary carcinoma
65. Ans. b. Medullary carcinoma
66. Ans. b. Medullary
67. Ans. b. Medullary
68. Ans. c. Medullary carcinoma
69. Ans. a. Total thyroidectomy
70. Ans. d. Histological mitochondria is essential for diagnosis
71. Ans. a. Ret proto-oncogene
72. Ans. a. Diarrhea
73. Ans. b. Arises from parafollicular C cells
74. Ans. c. Increased calcitonin is not associated with hypocalcemia
75. Ans. c. It is dependent on TSH
76. Ans. a. Medullary carcinoma thyroid *(Ref: Schwartz 10/e p1550; Sabiston 20/e p909; Bailey 27/e p820)*
77. Ans. c. Medullary carcinoma thyroid *(Ref: Schwartz 10/e p1550; Sabiston 20/e p909; Bailey 27/e p820)*
78. Ans. a. RET *(Ref: Schwartz 10/e p1541; Sabiston 20/e p909)*
79. Ans. a. Medullary carcinoma thyroid *(Ref: Schwartz 10/e p1541; Sabiston 20/e p909)*

ANAPLASTIC CARCINOMA

80. Ans. c. Long term survival in patient undergoing surgery; e. Highly chemosensitive *(Ref: Schwartz 10/e p1551, Sabiston 20/e p910)*
81. Ans. d. Anaplastic carcinoma
82. Ans. d. Palliative/Symptomatic treatment
83. Ans. d. Anaplastic

THYROID METASTASIS

84. Ans. c. Breast *(Schwartz 10/e p1551)*

METASTATIC TUMORS OF THYROID

- Rare, most cases are found in autopsy
- MC site of primary: **CA Breast**[Q] > CA Lung
- If thyroid metastases is detected pre-mortem, MC site of primary: **RCC**[Q] > CA Breast > CA Lung

THYROID LYMPHOMA

85. **Ans. b. Slow growing** *(Ref: Schwartz 10/e p1551; Sabiston 20/e p910; Bailey 27/e p821; Harrison 19/e p2307)*

- Lymphomas of the thyroid gland are rapidly growing tumors and usually present with goiter that has grown significantly over a short period.

CARCINOMA THYROID

86. **Ans. b. Follicular carcinoma—Most common type of carcinoma** *(Ref: Schwartz 9/e p1361; Sabiston 20/e p900; Bailey 27/e p818)*
87. **Ans. a. Follicular carcinoma have worse prognosis than papillary carcinoma; e. Follicular carcinoma have more male incidence than papillary carcinoma**
88. **Ans. b. Women <40 years; c. Papillary carcinoma <4 cm** *(Ref: Schwartz 9/e p1362-1363; Sabiston 20/e p903; Bailey 27/e p818)*

Prognostic Risk Classification for Well Differentiated Thyroid Cancer (AMES or AGES)		
Features	**Low Risk**	**High Risk**
Age	<40[Q] years	>40 years
Metastasis	None	**Regional or distant**[Q]
Size	<4 cm[Q]	>4 cm
Grade	Well differentiated	**Poorly differentiated**[Q]
Extent	No local extension, intrathyroidal, no capsular invasion	**Capsular invasion, extrathyroidal extension**[Q]

PROGNOSTIC INDICATORS OF DIFFERENTIATED THYROID CANCER (PTC, FTC)

AGES Scoring System[Q]
- Age, histologic Grade, Extrathyroidal invasion, and metastases and tumor Size to predict the risk of dying from papillary cancer.
- **Low-risk** patients are **young**, with **well-differentiated tumors, no metastases**, and **small primary lesions**
- High-risk patients are older, with poorly differentiated tumors, local invasion, distant metastases, and large primary lesions.

The MACIS Scale[Q]
- This scale incorporates distant Metastases, Age at presentation (<40 or >40 years old), Completeness of original surgical resection, extrathyroidal Invasion, and Size of original lesion.

AMES System[Q]
- To classify differentiated thyroid tumors into low- and high-risk groups using Age (men <40 years old, women <50 years old), Metastases, Extrathyroidal spread, and Size of tumors (<5 or >5 cm).

89. **Ans. c. Papillary type**   90. **Ans. b. Merkel cell**   91. **Ans. c. Is usually euthyroid**
92. **Ans. d. 50 milli curie** *(Schwartz 9/e p1365-1366; Sabiston 20/e p908; Bailey 25/e p797; Harrison 20/e p2716, 19/e p2306)*

- Amount of I^{131} given for carcinoma thyroid is 50 milli curie (30-100 mCi).
- Schwartz says "If there is significant uptake, then a therapeutic dose of ^{131}I, 30 to 100 mCi should be administered to low-risk patients and 100 to 200 mCi in high-risk patients."

93. **Ans. a. Papillary**   94. **Ans. a. Recurrent laryngeal nerve palsy**

- The **nerves** found in **close relationship to thyroid gland** and therefore likely to be **involved in malignant spread** and **thyroid surgery** are **recurrent laryngeal nerve** and **superior laryngeal nerve**.

95. **Ans. a. I-131** *(Ref: Schwartz 10/e p1546; Sabiston 20/e p908; Bailey 27/e p819; Harrison 20/e p2716, 19/e p2306; William's Endocrinology 10/e p479)*
96. **Ans. a. I^{131}**

SOLITARY THYROID NODULE

97. Ans. c. USG *(Ref: Schwartz 10/e p1540; Sabiston 20/e p895)*

- PET scans are not routinely used in the evaluation of thyroid nodules, however, they may show clinically occult thyroid lesions.
- Emedicine-Medscape says "**USG is the most sensitive method** for **diagnosing intrathyroid lesions**"
- CT and MRI are neither specific nor sensitive in diagnosing the intrathyroid lesions.

Ultrasound in STN

- Ultrasound is helpful in assessing a thyroid nodule.
- **Advantages**: Portability, cost-effectiveness, and lack of ionizing radiation.
- It is **extremely useful** in patients who are being **managed conservatively**^{Q} because it can easily determine whether a nodule has increased in size.
- Ultrasound is **used routinely**^{Q} in the office setting and is also available for intraoperative evaluation.
- It has proved **highly effective** in determining the **location** and characteristics (**cystic versus solid**)^Q of nodules but is unable to accurately predict the diagnosis of solid nodules.

Ultrasound features of carcinoma in a Thyroid Nodule	
Feature	**Carcinoma/Malignancy**
Structure	**Hypoechoic/Nonhomogeneous**/*Solid*^{Q}
Regressive changes	Rare
Microcalcifications	**Common**^{Q}
Peripheral rim	Variable
Internal vascularity	**Common**^{Q} (70-100 percent)
Lymph nodes	Relatively common^Q

98. Ans. d. Common in female; e. Thyroidectomy done *(Ref: Schwartz 10/e p1537-1539; Harrison 20/e p2711, 19/e p2303)*

Solitary Thyroid Nodule

- **Palpable discrete swelling** within an otherwise apparently normal thyroid gland.
- Incidence in adults is **1–10%.**
- STN are **4 times more common** in **women**^{Q} than in men.
- There is **nodular hyperplasia**^{Q} (not the diffuse hyperplasia)
- **THR-Ab** is **not found** in STN.
- STN are more likely to be neoplastic than multiple nodules.
- Nodules in **younger patients** are **more likely** to be **neoplastic**^{Q} than those in older patients.
- History of **radiation exposure increases** the **risk** of **malignancy**^{Q}.
- **Cold nodules** (don't take up radioactive iodine) are **more likely** to be **malignant (15–20%)**^{Q} than **hot** (take up radioactive iodine) nodules (1–3%)^Q.
- **STN** are **removed surgically**^{Q} to exclude malignancy.

99. Ans. c. FNAC *(Ref: Schwartz 10/e p1538; Sabiston 20/e p897)*

- **FNAC** is the **investigation of choice in discrete thyroid swellings,** offers excellent patient compliance and is easy and quick to perform^Q.
- **FNAC cannot distinguish** between **benign follicular adenoma** and **follicular carcinoma**^{Q}.

100. Ans. c. Thyroid function test *(Ref: Sabiston 20/e p890; Harrison 20/e p2711, 19/e p2303)*

- **Initial investigation** done in STN is **thyroid function test** (TFT)^Q.
- **Investigation of choice** in STN for diagnosis is **FNAC**^{Q}.

Solitary Thyroid Nodule

- **Initial investigation** done in STN is **thyroid function test** (TFT)^Q.
- If **TFT** is **raised**, next investigation is **thyroid scan**, (For **hot nodules, RAI ablation** or **surgery** is done; For **warm or cold nodules**, **follow-up** or **surgery**)^Q
- If **TFT** is **normal**, **USG** is **done** (Aspiration in **cystic lesions**, FNAC for **solid** or **heterogenous lesions**)^Q.
- **Investigation of choice** in STN for diagnosis is **FNAC**^{Q}.

101. Ans. d. FNAC   102. Ans. c. Right hemithyroidectomy   103. Ans. a. 5%
104. Ans. a. Cold nodule on thyroid scan is diagnostic of malignancy *(Ref: Schwartz 10/e p1537; Sabiston 20/e p890; Chandrasoma Taylor 3/e p849-850; Harrison 20/e p2711, 19/e p2303)*
105. Ans. a. Follicular adenoma

- MC STN is colloid goiter > follicular adenoma.

106. Ans. b. Hemithyroidectomy *(Ref: Schwartz 10/e p1540; Harrison 20/e p2711, 19/e p2303)*

HEMITHYROIDECTOMY

- Hemithyroidectomy is **removal of one lobe** with **isthmus**.
- Hemithyroidectomy is **treatment of choice** for **follicular adenoma** and **solitary thyroid nodule**.

107. Ans. b. Removal of both lobes leaving behind 6-8 grams of tissue *(Ref: Sabiston 20/e p906; Bailey 27/e p814; Schwartz 10/e p1551)*

Surgery	Structure Removed
Hemithyroidectomy (Thyroid lobectomy)	Removal of **one lobe with isthmus**^{Q}
Subtotal thyroidectomy	Removal of **both lobes leaving** behind **3-4 gms** of tissue **in each lobe**^{Q}
Near-total thyroidectomy	Leaving **<1 gm** of tissue **adjacent to RLN at ligament of Berry** on **one side**^{Q}
Total thyroidectomy	Removal of **all visible thyroid tissue**^{Q}
Hartley-Dunhill procedure	Removal of **one lobe with isthmus & second lobe partially (leaving 4-6 gms** of thyroid tissue)^Q

108. Ans. c. 20% *(Ref: Bailey 27/e p804)*

- About 80% of discrete swellings are cold. The **risk of malignancy** is higher in **"cold" lesions (20%)** compared to **"hot"** or **"warm" lesions (< 5%)**.

109. Ans. b. FNAC   110. Ans. a. Observation *(Ref: Schwartz 10/e p1540; Sabiston 20/e p890; Bailey 27/e p810)*

GOITER

111. Ans. c. 30% *(Ref: Bailey 27/e p807)*

COMPLICATIONS OF MULTI-NODULAR GOITER

- **Secondary Thyrotoxicosis:** Transient episodes of mild hyperthyroidism are common, occurring in up to **30%**^{Q} of patients.
- **Carcinoma:** An increased incidence of cancer (usually **follicular**) has been reported from **endemic areas**^{Q}.

112. Ans. b. Diffuse goiter *(Ref: Harrison 20/e p2711, 19/e p2301)*

ENDEMIC GOITER

- Worldwide, **diffuse goiter** is most commonly caused by **iodine deficiency** and is termed **endemic goiter** when it affects **>5%**^{Q} of the population.
- Endemic goiter occurs in **geographical areas** where the **soil, water** and **food** supply contains **low levels of iodine**^{Q}.
- The **lack of iodine** leads to decreased synthesis of thyroid hormones and a **compensatory increase in TSH** which in turn leads to **follicular cell hypertrophy** and **hyperplasia** and goitrous enlargement leading to **diffuse hyperplastic goiter**^{Q}.
- Mostly, **patients** are **euthyroid**^{Q}.

113. Ans. a. Neck *(Ref: Schwartz 10/e p1554)*

- Virtually **all intrathoracic goiters** can be **removed via a cervical incision**^{Q}.

114. Ans. b. Thyroid scan *(Ref: Sabiston 20/e p897; Schwartz 10/e p1537)*
115. Ans. a. Cosmetic; b. Pressure symptoms; e. Swelling with symptoms *(Ref: Schwartz 9/e p1358; Sabiston 20/e p899)*

INDICATIONS OF SURGERY IN THYROID SWELLING

1. Neoplasia (FNAC positive, clinical suspicion)^Q
2. Toxic adenoma^Q
3. Pressure symptoms^Q
4. Cosmetic reason or patient's preference^Q

116. Ans. b. Hemithyroidectomy 117. Ans. None 118. Ans. d. 10–20%

- **Cold nodules** (don't take up radioactive iodine) are **more likely** to be **malignant (15–20%)**[Q] than **hot** (take up radioactive iodine) **nodules (1–3%)**[Q]

119. Ans. d Hemithyroidectomy
120. Ans. d. Goiter more than 5% of population is endemic goitre *(Ref: Harrison 19/e p2301, 18/e p2931)*
121. Ans. c. All nodules > 4 cm should be resected irrespective of cytology *(Ref: Schwartz 9/e p1358; Sabiston 20/e p895-899, 19/e p899; Harrison 20/e p2711, 19/e p2301)*

All nodules > 4 cm should be resected irrespective of cytology, is an incorrect statement.

RETROSTERNAL GOITER

122. Ans. c. Dyspnea *(Ref: Schwartz 10/e p1537; Sabiston 20/e p893-894; Bailey 27/e p810)*
123. Ans. a. Stridor
124. Ans. d. Transcervical *(Ref: Schwartz 10/e p1537; Sabiston 20/e p894; Bailey 27/e p810)*

THYROTOXICOSIS

125. Ans. a. Inadequate control of hyperthyroidism *(Ref: Schwartz 10/e p1534; Sabiston 20/e p920; Bailey 27/e p811, 758; Harrison 20/e p2712, 19/e p2297)*
126. Ans. a. Carbimazole *(Ref: Harrison 20/e p2706)*   127. Ans. a. Diastolic murmur *(Ref: Harrison 20/e p2704, 19/e p2294)*
128. Ans. a. Thyrotoxicosis *(Ref: Harrison 20/e p2704, 19/e p2294)*

DANCING CAROTIDS MAY BE SEEN IN
• Aortic regurgitation[Q]   • Thyrotoxicosis[Q]

129. Ans. c. TSH *(Ref: Schwartz 10/e p1529; Sabiston 20/e p895; Bailey 27/e p/802; Harrison 20/e p2697, 19/e p2288)*

The **ultrasensitive TSH assay** has become the **most sensitive** and **specific test** for the **diagnosis of hyper-** and **hypothyroidism** and **for optimizing T_4 therapy**[Q].

The **enhanced sensitivity** and **specificity** of **TSH assays** have **greatly improved laboratory assessment** of **thyroid function**[Q].

130. Ans. b. Wolff-Chaikoff effect *(Ref: Schwartz 10/e p1526; Sabiston 20/e p886; Harrison 20/e p2710, 19/e p2286)*

Wolff-Chaikoff effect	• Iodine induced hypothyroidism[Q] (Iodine dependent transient thyroid suppression)
Jod-Basedow's effect	• Iodine induced hyperthyroidism[Q]

131. Ans. d. Oxygen consumption *(Ref: Harrison 20/e p2712, 19/e p2296)*

- **Beta-blockers do not correct** the underlying **metabolic abnormalities** (i.e. does not affect the **oxygen consumption**)

Beta Blockers in Thyrotoxicosis	
Advantages	Limitations
Alleviates adrenergic manifestations: • Sweating, tremor[Q] • Tachycardia, palpitations[Q] • Nervousness, anxiety[Q]	• Beta blockers **do not significantly affect the thyroid status**[Q], it reduces to some extent the conversion of T_4 to T_3. • Beta blockers **do not correct**[Q] the underlying **metabolic abnormalities** (i.e. does not affect the **oxygen consumption**)[Q]

132. Ans. a. Surgery for thyroiditis   133. Ans. a. Early diastolic murmur   134. Ans. b. Radioactive iodine
135. Ans. d. Elevated serum CPK level

- Both thyrotoxicosis and malignant hyperthermia may cause myopathy, but in hyperthyroidism serum CPK is often normal.

136. Ans. d. All
137. Ans. a. Hot nodule *(Ref: Schwartz 10/e p1533; Sabiston 19/e p896; Bailey 27/e p804; Harrison 20/e p2713, 19/e p2302)*
138. Ans. a. Inadequate control of hyperthyroidism   139. Ans. b. Increased CPK levels
140. Ans. a. Thyroid storm   141. Ans. a. Hashimoto's thyroiditis
142. Ans. b. Graves' disease; d. Plummer's disease; e. Struma ovarii *(Ref: Harrison 20/e p2703, 19/e p2293)*

143. Ans. d. Hair loss
144. Ans. a. Iodides
145. Ans. d. Inadequate preoperative preparation
146. Ans. c. Radioiodine

GRAVE'S DISEASE

147. Ans. a. More common in males *(Ref: Schwartz 10/e p1531-1533; Sabiston 20/e p892; Bailey 27/e p811; Harrison 20/e p2703, 19/e p2293)*
148. Ans. d. All of the above *(Ref: William's Endocrinology 10/e p479)*

Complications of Radioactive Iodine (I^{131}) Therapy	
Acute	**Long-term**
• **Bone marrow suppression**[Q] • **Cerebral edema & hemorrhage**[Q] (brain metastasis) • Nausea & vomiting[Q] • Neck pain, swelling • Sialedenitis, thyroiditis • **Vocal cord paralysis**[Q]	• Chronic sialedenitis, taste dysfunction • Fertility: Ovarian & testicular damage leading to infertility & increased abortion rate • **Hematologic: Bone marrow suppression**[Q], **Leukemia**[Q] • **Hypoparathyroidism**[Q] • **Increased risk of cancer: Anaplastic carcinoma thyroid**[Q], carcinoma stomach, carcinoma bladder lung & breast, HCC • Pulmonary fibrosis

149. Ans. d. Hypothyroidism
150. Ans. b. Age >40 years; c. Elderly; e. Presence of associated co-morbidities *(Ref: Schwartz 10/e p1532-1533; Sabiston 20/e p892-893; Bailey 27/e p812; Harrison 20/e p2706, 19/e p2296)*
151. Ans. a. Thyrotoxicosis
152. Ans. c. Radioiodine
153. Ans. c. Common in male *(Ref: Schwartz 10/e p; Sabiston 20/e p; Bailey 27/e p)*
154. Ans. c. Remissions and exacerbations are not infrequent

HYPOTHYROIDISM

155. Ans. a. Serum TSH level *(Ref: Schwartz 10/e p1529; Sabiston 20/e p895; Bailey 27/e p802; Harrison 20/e p2701, 19/e p2288)*

> • The **ultrasensitive TSH assay** has become the **most sensitive** and **specific test** for the **diagnosis of hyper-** and **hypothyroidism** and **for optimizing T_4 therapy**[Q].
> • The **enhanced sensitivity** and **specificity** of **TSH assays** have greatly improved laboratory assessment of **thyroid function**[Q].

156. Ans. a. Sheehan's syndrome *(Harrison 20/e p2734, 19/e p2257)*
     Sheehan's syndrome causes **hypopituitarism** leading to **decreased TSH**[Q].

POST THYROIDECTOMY COMPLICATIONS

157. Ans. b. Close to the gland *(Schwartz 10/e p1551-1554; Sabiston 20/e p913; Bailey 27/e p813)*
     • Both **superior** and **inferior thyroid vessels** should be **ligated close to the thyroid**[Q].
     • Superiorly, **to avoid injury** to the **external branch** of the **superior laryngeal nerve**.
     • Inferiorly, to **minimize devascularization of the parathyroids** (extracapsular[Q] dissection) or **injury to the RLN**[Q].

> **THYROIDECTOMY: SCHWARTZ 10/E P1553**
>
> • The **dissection plane** is kept as **close to the thyroid** as possible and the **superior pole vessels** are individually identified, skeletonized, ligated, and **divided low on the thyroid gland to avoid injury** to the **external branch** of the **superior laryngeal nerve**[Q]
> • The **inferior thyroid vessels** are **dissected, skeletonized, ligated**, and **divided as close to the surface of the thyroid gland as possible** to **minimize devascularization of the parathyroids** (extracapsular dissection) or **injury to the RLN**[Q].

158. Ans. d. Hypercalcemia *(Ref: Schwartz 10/e p1556; Sabiston 20/e p920; Bailey 27/e p815)*
159. Ans. c. Removing sutures from all layers in the ward and evacuation of hematoma
160. Ans. d. Apparent exophthalmos *(Ref: Harrison 20/e p3173, 19/e p196, 208)*

Horner's Syndrome	
Clinical Features	**Less Common Features**
• Ptosis[Q] • Miosis (constricted pupil)[Q] • Anhydrosis[Q] • Enopthalmos[Q] • Loss of ciliospinal reflexes[Q]	• Hyperactive accommodation • Hypochromic heterochromia • Hypotony • Hyperaemia

161. Ans. b. **Medial medullary syndrome** *(Ref: Harrison 20/e p3173, 19/e p196, 208)*
162. Ans. d. **Mydriasis**
163. Ans. a. **As close to the thyroid gland as possible** *(Ref: Schwartz 10/e p1553; Sabiston 20/e p913)*
164. Ans. c. **Inferior thyroid artery is ligated away from gland; d. Capsule is kept intact** *(Ref: Schwartz 10/e p1553)*

- The **inferior thyroid vessels** are **dissected, skeletonized, ligated,** and **divided as close to the surface of the thyroid gland as possible** to minimize devascularization of the parathyroids (extracapsular dissection) or injury to the RLN^Q.
- Dissection is extracapsular (**Capsule is removed**)^Q.

165. Ans. b. **2–5 days**
166. Ans. a. **Hypocalcemia**
167. b. **Oral calcium and vitamin D** *(Ref: Sabiston 20/e p919, 19/e p921; Bailey 27/e p815)*

Management of Post-operative Hypocalcemia	
Transient Hypocalcemia	**Prolonged or Permanent Hypocalcemia**
• **Asymptomatic** with calcium level **>8 mg/dL: No treatment**^Q • **Mild symptoms** or calcium level **<8 mg/dL: Oral calcium**^Q • **Severe Symptoms: IV calcium**^Q	• **Oral calcium** with **vitamin D**^Q

- If **hypocalcemia** is expected to be **prolonged** or **permanent** (as following a 3 and 1/2 gland parathyroid resection or following total parathyroidectomy with autograft) then **oral calcium** should be started as soon as possible **with vitamin D**.

168. Ans. d. **Oral calcium**
169. Ans. a. **IV calcium gluconate**
170. Ans. d. **Remove the stitch and take the patient to O.T.**
171. Ans. a. **Respiratory obstruction**
172. Ans. a. **Open immediately**
173. Ans. a. **Respiratory obstruction**
174. Ans. a. **Hypocalcemia**
175. Ans. b. **Open the operative site**
176. Ans. d. **Open the wound sutures in the ward**
177. Ans. a. **0.1–0.2 mg** *(Ref: Harrison 19/e p2306)*

- **Daily replacement dose** of **thyroxine: 1.6 µg/kg** body weight (**0.1–0.15 gm**)^Q
- For **TSH suppression** (in **PTC** and **FTC**), dose of thyroxine: **2.7 µg/kg** body weight^Q

178. Ans. c. **Hypocalcemia**

- **Tracheomalacia** and **collapse** of the **larynx, wound hematoma** with **compression** of the **trachea** and **thyroid storm** are **early life threatening complications** of thyroidectomy^Q.
- **Hypocalcemia** which occurs after **2–5 days** after operation and severity of causing life threatening situation is least with hypocalcemia as compared to the given options.

179. Ans. b. **Recurrent laryngeal nerve**
180. Ans. c. **Superior thyroid artery**

THYROIDITIS

181. Ans. a. **Anti-TPO** *(Ref: Schwartz 10/e p1535; Sabiston 20/e p891; Bailey 27/e p821; Harrison 20/e p2699, 19/e p2290)*
182. Ans. b. **Subacute thyroiditis** *(Ref: Schwartz 10/e p1535; Sabiston 20/e p891; Bailey 27/e p822; Harrison 20/e p2708, 19/e p2298)*
183. Ans. a. **Thyroid peroxidase antibodies**
184. Ans. b. **↑ESR**
185. Ans. d. **Orphan Annie eye nuclei**
186. Ans. b. **Hashimoto's disease**
187. Ans. a. **Hashimoto's thyroiditis**
188. Ans. c. **Hashimoto's thyroiditis**
189. Ans. c. **Increased radioactive iodine uptake**
190. Ans. a. **Autoimmune in etiology**
191. Ans. c. **In the thyrotoxic phase radioiodine uptake is increased**
192. Ans. b. **Hashimoto's thyroiditis**
193. Ans. d. **Reidel's thyroiditis** *(Ref: Schwartz 10/e p1536; Sabiston 20/e p891; Bailey 27/e p822)*
194. Ans. c. **Riedel's thyroiditis**
195. Ans. c. **Subacute thyroiditis** *(Ref: Schwartz 10/e p1535; Sabiston 20/e p891)*

Diagnosis in this case is subacute thyroiditis. Symptoms are more severe in acute thyroiditis with complications and acute thyroiditis is more common in children.

196. Ans. c. **Thyroglobulins**
197. Ans. c. **To overcome pressure on trachea or esophagus**
198. Ans. b. **Antithyroid nuclear antibodies**
199. Ans. a. **Subacute lymphocytic thyroiditis**
200. Ans. d. **Reidel's thyroiditis**
201. Ans. c. **Gaint cell infiltration**

Thyroid

THYROGLOSSAL CYST AND FISTULA

202. **Ans. d. Thyroglossal cyst/fistula** *(Ref: Schwartz 10/e p1521; Sabiston 20/e p1861)*
203. **Ans. a. Does not move with deglutition**
204. **Ans. a. Thyroglossal cyst** *(Ref: Schwartz 10/e p1521; Sabiston 20/e p1861)*
205. **Ans. c. Thyroglossal cyst**   206. **Ans. c. Subhyoid**
207. **Ans. c. Incision and drainage is the treatment of choice**   208. **Ans. a. Papillary**
209. **Ans. c. Excision of central part of hyoid bone and cone of tongue muscles upto foramen caecum**
210. **Ans. a. Surgical removal**

THYROID ANATOMY AND PHYSIOLOGY

211. **Ans. a. Jod-Basedow effect** *(Ref: Schwartz 10/e p1526; Sabiston 20/e p886; Harrison 20/e p2710, 19/e p2286)*
212. **Ans. b. 0.04 mIU/L** *(Ref: The thyroid: a Fundamental and Clinical Text (Lippincott Williams) 2008/329-330)*

    The lower functional limit for third generation TSH assays is about 0.01 to 0.02 mIU/L.

213. **Ans. b. Inferior thyroid artery**   214. **Ans. b. Inversely**   215. **Ans. c. 18–20 gm**
216. **Ans. a. Nephrotic syndrome**
    - In Nephrotic syndrome, iodine binding proteins are decreased.
217. **Ans. c. 2nd and 3rd and 4th tracheal cartilage** *(Ref: Schwartz 10/e p1523; Sabiston 20/e p880-882)*

    Isthmus that is located just inferior to the cricoid cartilage, usually anterior to the 2nd and 3rd tracheal cartilages.

THYROID GLAND

- **Normal weight** of thyroid gland: **20–25 gms**^{Q}
- Thyroid is storage site of **> 90% of body's iodine content**^{Q}
- **Daily iodine requirement: 100–150 µg**^{Q}
- Father of thyroid surgery: **Theodor Kocher**^{Q}
- **Gland weight** varies **inversely with iodine intake**^{Q}.
- **Isthmus** that is **located just inferior** to the **cricoid cartilage**, usually anterior to **2nd & 3rd (mainly)** and **4th tracheal rings**^{Q}.
- A **pyramidal lobe** is present in about **50%** of patients.
- **Thyroid capsule** is **condensed into the posterior suspensory** or **Berry's ligament**^{Q} near the cricoid cartilage & upper tracheal rings.
- **Thyroid gland** has a **thin capsule** of connective tissue, which extends into glandular parenchyma & divides each lobe into irregularly shaped and sized lobules.
- **External laryngeal nerve** runs **close** to the **superior thyroid artery** and the **recurrent laryngeal nerve runs close** to the **inferior thyroid artery**^{Q}.

Coverings of the Gland

- **True capsule:** Thin capsule of connective tissue, which **extends into the glandular parenchyma** & divides each lobe into irregularly shaped & sized lobules.
- **False capsule** is derived from **pretracheal fascia.**

Beahr's Triangle

- **Boundaries: Base: Common carotid artery; Superiorly: Inferior thyroid artery; Inferiorly: RLN**^{Q}
- Helps in **identifying RLN** & avoiding its injury^Q

MISCELLANEOUS

218. **Ans. d. All the above** *(www.medixon.com)*

SCABARD (SABER-SHEATH) TRACHEA

- **Flattening of trachea** caused **by lateral compression**^{Q} by swellings or tumors
- **Causes:** Carcinoma thyroid, thyroiditis, carcinoma larynx, goitre^Q

219. **Ans. b. Tracheostomy** *(Ref: Nelson 19/e p2284)*

    Partial thyroidectomy is preferred over tracheostomy.

220. Ans. a. I-131
221. Ans. a. Radioiodine is contraindicated
222. Ans. b. Chromosome 7q *(Ref: Harrison 20/e p2693, 19/e p2284; Schwartz 10/e p1534)*

Pendred's Syndrome

- Consists of **congenital sensorineural hearing loss + goitre**[Q]
- Due to defect in sulfate transport protein (chromosome **7q**[Q]) to the thyroid gland and cochlea

| Rafetoff Syndrome | End organ resistance to T4[Q] |

223. **Ans. a. Lingual thyroid** *(Ref: Schwartz 10/e p1522)*

Reddish swelling in the region of foramen caecum is Lingual thyroid.

Lingual Thyroid

- Forms a **rounded swelling** at the **back of tongue** at the **foramen caecum**[Q]
- It may represent the **only thyroid tissue present**[Q]
- May cause dysphasia, impairment of speech, respiratory obstruction or hemorrhage
- **Medical treatment** options include administration of **exogenous thyroid hormone** to **suppress TSH** and **RAI ablation** followed by **hormone replacement**.
- **Surgical excision** is **rarely needed** but, if required, should be preceded by an evaluation of normal thyroid tissue in the neck to avoid inadvertently rendering the patient hypothyroid.

224. **Ans. d. Benign lesion; e. Included in Teratoma** *(Ref: Shaws Gynecology 14/e p336-337)*

Struma Ovarii

- Highly specialized variety of **teratoma**
- A **benign ovarian tumor** containing **thyroid tissue**[Q]
- The tumor is solid and consisting entirely of thyroid tissue
- Some cases develop **thyrotoxicosis**[Q]
- Most of the tumor is **innocent**, but malignant transformation have been recorded

225. **Ans. c. Di George syndrome** *(Ref: Schwartz 10/e p1574)*

Di-George Syndrome

Characterized by
- **Congenital cardiac defects**, particularly those involving great vessels[Q]
- Hypocalcemic tetany due to **failure of parathyroid development**[Q]
- **Absence of normal thymus**, T-cell immunodeficiency[Q]

226. **Ans. d. Pizzillo's method.**

CHAPTER 3

Parathyroid and Adrenal Glands

MULTIPLE ENDOCRINE NEOPLASIA

	MEN-1	MEN-2 (MEN-2A or Sipple syndrome)	MEN-3 (MEN-2B)	MEN-4 (MEN-X)
Components	• Parathyroid hyperplasia or adenoma^Q • Pancreatic NET^Q • Pituitary adenoma^Q • Bronchial & thymic carcinoids^Q • Adrenocortical tumors • Subcutaneous or visceral lipomas^Q • Facial cutaneous angiofibromas^Q • Collagenomas^Q	• Medullary carcinoma thyroid^Q • Pheochromocytoma^Q • Parathyroid hyperplasia or adenoma^Q • Hirschsprung's disease^Q • Cutaneous lichen amyloidosis^Q	• Medullary carcinoma thyroid^Q • Pheochromocytoma^Q • Intestinal ganglioneuroma^Q • Mucosal neuromas^Q • Megacolon^Q • Marfanoid features^Q	• Hyperparathyroidism • Pituitary adenoma • Pancreatic NET • Gonadal, adrenal, renal & thyroid tumors • (MEN-1 not having mutation of MEN1 gene is known as MEN-4)
Gene/Defect	MEN1 gene^Q	RET oncogene (cysteine^Q codon)	RET oncogene (tyrosine kinase^Q domain)	Cyclin dependent kinase inhibitor (CDNKIB) gene
Chromosome	11	10^Q	10^Q	12
Transmission	Autosomal dominant^Q	Autosomal dominant^Q	Autosomal dominant^Q	Autosomal dominant^Q

MEN-1 (WERMER'S SYNDROME)

- Autosomal dominant^Q
- Defect: MEN1 gene^Q on chromosome 11^Q (encodes tumour suppressor protein, menin^Q)

Characteristic Features

Common Manifestations	Less Common Manifestations
• Parathyroid hyperplasia or adenoma^Q • Pancreatic NET^Q • Pituitary adenoma^Q	• Bronchial and thymic carcinoids^Q • Adrenocortical tumors • Subcutaneous or visceral lipomas^Q • Facial cutaneous angiofibromas^Q • Collagenomas^Q

Parathyroid Gland
- MC endocrine abnormality (>98% of affected individuals) in MEN-1 is **multiglandular parathyroid tumors**^{Q}.
- **Hyperparathyroidism** is MC manifestation (cardinal sign of MEN-1 is **parathyroid adenoma** of **multicentricity**)^Q.
- **Parathyroid hyperplasia** is the MC cause of **hyperparathyroidism** in MEN-1.
- **Hypercalcemia** is **first biochemical abnormality**^{Q} detected in MEN 1 and may precede the clinical onset of a pancreatic NET or pituitary neoplasm by several years.

Pancreatic Neuro-endocrine Tumors
- Pancreatic NET is **2nd MC manifestation**^{Q}.
- **Nonfunctioning** or that secrete **pancreatic polypeptide** are MC pancreatic NET in MEN-1^Q.
- MC **functional NET** in patients with MEN-1 is **gastrinoma**^{Q} followed by insulinoma.
- MC increased pancreatic hormone: Pancreatic polypeptides >Gastrin >Insulin^Q. (PGI)

Pituitary Adenoma
- **MC tumor**: Prolactinoma > Somatotrophinoma > Corticotrophinoma (PSC)

PRIMARY HYPERPARATHYROIDISM

PRIMARY HYPERPARATHYROIDISM

- PHPT arises from **increased PTH production**^{Q} from abnormal parathyroid glands and results from a disturbance of normal feedback control exerted by serum calcium.
- More common in **women**^{Q}

> - **Solitary adenoma**^{Q} is the **MC cause** (in **80%**)
> - **Parathyroid adenomas** are **most commonly located** in **inferior** parathyroid glands.

- Increased PTH production leads to **hypercalcemia** via:
  - **Increased GI absorption** of calcium
  - **Reduced renal calcium clearance**
  - **Increased** production of **vitamin D3**

Etiology
- Exposure to **low-dose therapeutic ionizing radiation** and **familial predisposition**^{Q}
- Renal leak of calcium
- **Declining renal function** with age
- **Alteration in** the **sensitivity** of parathyroid glands to suppression by calcium
- **Lithium** therapy

Genetics
- **Most cases** of PHPT are **sporadic**
- Also associated with **MEN1, MEN2A,** isolated familial HPT, and familial HPT with jaw-tumor syndrome.

Clinical Features
- Patients with PHPT formerly presented with the **"classic" pentad** of symptoms:
  - Kidney stones^Q
  - Painful bones^Q
  - Abdominal groans^Q
  - Psychic moans^Q
  - Fatigue overtones^Q
- Alteration in the "typical" patient with PHPT due to widespread use of automated blood analyzers.
- Patients are more likely to be minimally symptomatic or asymptomatic.
- Currently, **most patients** present with **weakness,** fatigue, **polydipsia, polyuria, nocturia, bone** and **joint pain, constipation**^{Q}, decreased appetite, nausea, heartburn, pruritus, depression, and memory loss.
- Renal **calculi** are typically composed of **calcium phosphate** or **oxalate**^{Q}.

> **Osteitis Fibrosa Cystica in Advanced PHPT**
>
> **Pathognomonic radiologic findings** on **X-rays** of **hands**, characterized by:
> - **Subperiosteal resorption**^{Q} (most apparent on the **radial aspect**^{Q} of **middle phalanx**^{Q} of **2nd** and **3rd** fingers)
> - Bone cysts^Q
> - **Tufting** of **distal phalanges**^{Q}

Diagnosis
- **Elevated serum calcium & intact PTH** or two-site PTH levels, **without hypocalciuria** establishes the **diagnosis of PHPT** with virtual certainty^Q.
- **Decreased serum phosphate** (50%) & **elevated 24-hour urinary calcium** (60%) in **PHPT**^{Q}

Localization
- ^{99m}Tc-labeled sestamibi: Most widely used & accurate modality^Q (sensitivity >80% for detection of parathyroid adenomas)

Treatment
- **Parathyroidectomy** for patients having **"classic" symptoms** of PHPT or **<50 years**^{Q}
- **SERM** and **bisphosphonates** are used to **lower serum calcium** and **increase BMD** in **PHPT.**

> **Indications for Parathyroidectomy in Asymptomatic Primary HPT**
>
> 1. Serum **calcium >1 mg/dL above** the **upper limits** of normal
> 2. **Life-threatening hypercalcemic** episode
> 3. **Creatine clearance** reduced by **30%**
> 4. **Kidney stones** on abdominal X-rays
> 5. Markedly **elevated 24-h urinary calcium excretion (≥400** mg/d)
> 6. Substantially **decreased bone mineral density** at the lumbar spine, hip, or distal radius
> 7. Age **<50 years**
> 8. Long-term medical surveillance not desired or possible

SECONDARY HYPERPARATHYROIDISM

- Secondary HPT **commonly occurs** in **chronic renal failure**[Q]
- May occur in hypocalcemia secondary to **inadequate calcium** or **vitamin D intake**, or **malabsorption**[Q].

Pathophysiology of HPT in Chronic Renal Failure
- Related to **hyperphosphatemia**[Q] (and resultant hypocalcemia)
- Deficiency of 1,25-dihydroxy vitamin D due to loss of renal tissue
- Low calcium intake
- Decreased calcium absorption
- Abnormal parathyroid cell response to extracellular calcium or vitamin D in vitro and in vivo.

Clinical Feature
- Patients generally are **hypocalcemic** or normocalcemic.

Treatment
- Patients generally are **hypocalcemic** or normocalcemic.

> - These patients generally are **treated** medically with a **low-phosphate diet**, **phosphate binders**, adequate intake of **calcium** and **1,25-dihydroxy vitamin D** and a **high calcium, low-aluminum dialysis bath**[Q].

- **Parathyroidectomy** should be considered if **PTH levels remain** high **despite optimal therapy**[Q].

TERTIARY HYPERPARATHYROIDISM

Tertiary Hyperparathyroidism

- Development of autonomous parathyroid gland function, after long standing secondary hyperparathyroidism, most often in renal disease
- Cause problems similar to PHPT, such as pathologic fractures, bone pain, renal stones, peptic ulcer disease, pancreatitis, and mental status changes.
- **Operative intervention** is indicated in:
  - **Symptomatic disease**[Q]
  - If **autonomous PTH secretion** persists for >1 year after a successful **transplant**[Q].

Treatment
- **Subtotal** or **total parathyroidectomy** with **Autotransplantation + Upper thymectomy**[Q].

PARATHYROID CARCINOMA

Parathyroid Carcinoma

- Accounts for approximately **1%** of **PHPT** cases.

Clinical Features

Parathyroid Carcinoma is suspected preoperatively by	
• Presence of **severe symptoms**[Q]	• Serum **calcium levels > 14**[Q] mg/dL
• Significantly **elevated PTH**[Q] levels (5 × normal)	

- **Palpable parathyroid**[Q] gland
  - **Local invasion**[Q] is most common; LN metastases in 15% & distant metastases in 33% at presentation.
  - **Intraoperatively:** Presence of a large, gray-white to gray-brown parathyroid **tumor adherent to** or **invasive into surrounding tissues**[Q] and enlarged LN.

Diagnosis
- Accurate diagnosis necessitates **histologic examination** that reveals **local tissue invasion, vascular or capsular invasion**[Q], trabecular or fibrous stroma, and frequent mitoses.

Treatments
- Parathyroid cancer: **Bilateral neck exploration + En-bloc excision** of **tumor** and ipsilateral **thyroid lobe ± MRND** in presence of LN metastases[Q]
- **Reoperation** for **locally recurrent** or **metastatic disease** to **control hypercalcemia**.
- **Cinacalcet**[Q] (reduce PTH levels by directly **binding** to **CASR cells** on parathyroid) is useful in **controlling hypercalcemia** in **refractory parathyroid carcinoma**.

INCIDENTALOMA

INCIDENTALOMA

- **Incidentally discovered adrenal masses** through imaging performed for unrelated/nonadrenal disease.
- Differential diagnosis includes both secreting & nonsecreting neoplasms.
- In patients with a **history of malignancy**, **metastatic disease** is the **most likely cause** of adrenal masses, particularly **when bilateral**[Q].
- In those **without a clear history of malignancy**, at least **80% of incidentalomas** will turn out to be **nonfunctioning cortical adenomas** or other **benign lesions** that **do not require surgical management**[Q].

Clinical Evaluation

- **Diagnostic work-up** of an incidentaloma is aimed at **identifying patients** that would **benefit from adrenalectomy**
- Workup for adrenal incidentaloma integrates **hormonal evaluation** with **size criteria**[Q].
- Evaluation begins with **history** taking, with a focus on **previous malignancy**, **hypertension**, and symptoms of **glucocorticoid** or **sex steroid excess**.
- **Biochemical investigations** for hormonally active tumors are followed by consideration of **size criteria**.
- Tumors **>6 cm** carry a **>25% risk for malignancy**[Q].

> - **CT-guided FNAC** is **rarely helpful**[Q] in the evaluation of adrenal masses and may be **hazardous**.
> - The **diagnosis** of **primary adrenal malignancy cannot be reliably based** on **cytologic criteria alone**[Q].

- Use of **FNAC** is generally confined to patients with a **history of extra-adrenal malignancy**[Q] in whom the clinician seeks to establish the diagnosis of **metastatic disease**[Q].
- **Pheochromocytoma must be excluded**[Q] before attempting such a procedure to avoid precipitating potentially fatal hypertensive crisis.

Treatments

- **Surgery** for **hormonally active tumors** and masses carrying **significant risk** for **malignancy**[Q].
- **Most incidentalomas** can be **removed laparoscopically**[Q], except for those displaying obvious malignant features on imaging.
- **Remove all incidentalomas** measuring **>5 cm** and to strongly consider removal of those measuring 3–5 cm, **follow up** with CT, every 6 months for <3 cm.

Indications of Surgery in Incidentaloma 3–5 cm	
1. **Suspicious** imaging characteristics (**heterogeneity**, **high attenuation**, or **irregular margins**)[Q]	3. Few surgical risk factors[Q]
2. **Young age**[Q]	4. Interval tumor growth[Q]
	5. Patient preference

Adrenal Incidentalomas	
Tumor Types	Percentage
• **Presumed non-functional adenoma (MC)**	**82%**[Q]
• **Preclinical Cushing's**[Q]	5%
• **Pheochromocytoma**[Q]	5%
• Adrenocortical carcinoma	5%
• **Metastatic** carcinoma	2%
• Aldosterone producing adenoma	1%

ADRENOCORTICAL CARCINOMA

ADRENOCORTICAL CARCINOMA

- Adrenocortical carcinoma is a **rare tumor**
- **More than half** of adrenocortical carcinomas **are functional**[Q].
- **Cushing's syndrome**[Q] is **most commonly seen**, followed by virilization.

Pathology

- Microscopically: **Hyperchromatic cells** with and have **large nuclei**, prominent nucleoli.
- It is very difficult to distinguish benign adrenal adenomas from carcinomas by histologic examination alone.
- **Capsular** or **vascular invasion**[Q] is the **most reliable sign of cancer**.

Clinical Features

- Almost **all cases** occur in patients **40–50 years** of age
- No gender predilection

- More than half of adrenocortical carcinomas **are functional**.
- **Cushing's syndrome**^{Q} is **most commonly seen**, followed by virilization.
- **Very large**^{Q} at **initial evaluation** (mean tumor size, **9–12 cm**)
- Metastases to the lymph nodes, **liver**^{Q}, and lungs may be found.

Diagnosis
- CT: Heterogeneous mass with **irregular/indistinct borders**, **central necrosis**^{Q}, and invasion of adjacent structures.
- **Size** of adrenal mass is the **single most important criterion** to **diagnose malignancy**^{Q}

Treatment
- **Radical open surgery:** En-bloc resection of **adjacent organs** or regional **lymphadenectomy**^{Q} (or both).
- **Ketoconazole, aminoglutethimide** or **metyrapone (KAM):** control **steroid hypersecretion**^{Q}.

Mitotane
• Principal chemotherapeutic agent, **derivative of** insecticide **DDT**^{Q}
• Mitotane: Used as an **adjuvant to surgery** and as **primary therapy** in **unresectable** or **metastatic disease**^{Q}.
• Use is limited by **significant gastrointestinal** and **neurologic toxicity**^{Q}.

Prognosis
- **Most important predictor** of **survival: Adequacy of resection**^{Q}
- **Poor** prognosis, **5-year survival is 15–20%**
- Patients who undergo **incomplete resection** have **extremely limited life expectancy**^{Q} (median survival, <1 year).
- Prone to develop **local recurrence** and metastases, typically **within 2 years**.

PHEOCHROMOCYTOMA

Pheochromocytoma

- Tumors arise from **chromaffin cells**^{Q} in adrenal medulla and elsewhere
- Peak incidence in **4th and 5th** decade without any gender predilection
- MC site of extra-adrenal tumor is **organ of Zuckerkandl**^{Q}
- Extra-adrenal pheochromocytoma is known as **paraganglioma**^{Q}.

Also Called 10% Tumor Because	
• 10% are **bilateral**^{Q}	• 10% are **extra-adrenal**^{Q}
• 10% are **malignant**^{Q}	• 10% are **familial**^{Q}
• 10% occur in **pediatric patients**^{Q}	

Etiology and Risk Factors
- Either familial or sporadic. Familial can be syndromic or non-syndromic.

Syndromes Associated with Pheochromocytoma (MVVS)	
• MEN-2A and MEN-2B^Q	• Von-Recklinghausen syndrome^Q (NF-1: MC)
• VHL syndrome^Q	• Sturge-Weber syndrome^Q

- **Non-syndromic familial pheochromocytomas** are most commonly associated with **succinyl dehydrogenase D and B mutations**^{Q}.

Pathology
- Most are **unilateral & solitary**^{Q}
- When pheochromocytoma develop in **MEN syndrome**, they are **rarely malignant**^{Q}
- In contrast, patients with germline **SDHB mutation** appear to have **higher propensity** for **extra-adrenal** and **malignant tumors**^{Q}
- Tumors are **not innervated**^{Q}, so catecholamines doesn't result from neural stimulation
- Tumors also secrete **endogenous opioids, adrenomedullin, erythropoietin, PTHrp, neuropeptide Y & chromogranin A**^{Q}.

> - **Most pheochromocytoma** produce both NA and Adr with **NA>Adr**^{Q}.
> - **Extra-Adrenal pheochromocytoma** secretes **NA exclusively**^{Q} (Deficiency of enzyme PNMT-Phenylethanolamine-N-Methyltransferase).
> - Pheochromocytoma associated with **MEN** secretes **Adr alone**^{Q}.
> - Increased production of **dopamine and homovanillic acid** is usually seen in **malignant lesions**^{Q}.

Histologically Tumor Consists of
- Polygonal to spindle chromaffin cells clustered in small nests or alveoli (Zelballen) by a rich vascular network
- Nuclei are round with **salt & pepper chromatin**^{Q}

> Criteria for **malignancy** are based **exclusively** on **presence of metastases**^{Q} (because **capsular** or **vascular invasion** can be present in **benign tumors**)^Q

Clinical Features

- Classic triad: **Headache + Diaphoresis + Palpitation**[Q]
- **MC symptom** is **headache**[Q]
- **MC manifestation** is **hypertension**[Q] (remember hypertension is not a symptom)
- **Weight loss**[Q] due to increased energy expenditure
- **Cardiac manifestations:** Sinus tachycardia, sinus bradycardia, supraventricular arrhythmia and ventricular premature contractions
- **Carbohydrate intolerance** and increased hematocrit (**volume depletion**)

Diagnosis

Biochemical test:

- **Most sensitive screening test:** Urinary catecholamines and **VMA level**[Q]
- **Best test for diagnosis:** Fractionated plasma metanephrines[Q]

Pharmacological Test

- Positive response to **phentolamine** is reduction of BP of at least 35/25 mm Hg after 2 min. It is not diagnostic and biochemical confirmation is necessary.
- **Glucagon infusion** increases catecholamine release and causes **paroxysm of hypertension**[Q]

Imaging

- MRI is IOC for **adrenal**[Q], **extra adrenal pheochromocytoma**[Q] and in **pregnancy**[Q].
- MRI is **95% sensitive** and **100% specific** for pheochromocytoma[Q].
- CT scan should be performed **without contrast administration**[Q] to avoid hypertensive crisis.
- **MIBG scan** is useful for **extra-adrenal pheochromocytoma** but IOC is **MRI**[Q] even for extra adrenal pheochromocytoma.

Biopsy is contraindicated as it precipitates hypertensive crisis[Q]

Treatment

- **Adrenalectomy** is TOC[Q].
- **Laparoscopic adrenalectomy** is preferred for **<5 cm tumors**[Q].
- **Pre-operatively alpha-blockers (phenoxybenzamine)**[Q] should be given.
- **Beta-blockers** are indicated **only if tachycardia develops** and should not be given until patient if **fully alpha blocked**[Q] to avoid hypertensive crisis due to unopposed alpha stimulation.

MALIGNANT PHEOCHROMOCYTOMA

Malignant Pheochromocytoma

- Risk of malignancy increases with **size**[Q].
- Malignant tumors are more likely to express **p53, Bcl-2** and have **activated telomerase**[Q].

- **Capsular** and **vascular invasion** may be seen in **benign lesions as well.**
- **Malignancy** usually is **diagnosed** when there is evidence of **invasion** into **surrounding structures** or **distant metastasis**[Q].

- Increased production of **dopamine** and **homovanillic acid** is usually seen in **malignant lesions**[Q]
- **MC site of metastases** is **bone**[Q] > liver > lymph nodes.
- **Treatment:** Resection followed by **chemotherapy**[Q] (cyclophosphamide + vincristine + dacarbazine)

MDH: Malignant pheochromocytoma secrete **Dopamine** and **HVA**[Q]

NEUROBLASTOMA

Neuroblastoma

- Arise from **neural crest**[Q] and may originate anywhere along the distribution of sympathetic chain
- **MC tumor** diagnosed in **infants <1 year of age**[Q]
- **MC intra-abdominal malignancy** in **children**[Q]
- **Sporadic** in **majority** of cases

- **MC site**: Adrenal (30%)^Q > Paravertebral reteroperitoneum^Q (28%) > Posterior mediastinum^Q (15%) > Pelvis (5%) > Cervical area^Q
- Associated with neurofibromatosis, Hirschsprung's disease, heterochromia, fetal hydantoin, featal alcohol syndrome and Freidreich's ataxia
- **Spontaneous regression** is unique behaviour especially in **stage 4S^Q**.

Pathology
- **Classic neuroblastomas**: Small, primitive-appearing cells with dark nuclei, scant cytoplasm
- **Mitotic activity**, nuclear breakdown ("**karyorrhexis**")^Q, and **pleomorphism** may be prominent
- **Homer-Wright pseudorosettes**^{Q} can be found
- Immunochemical detection of **neuron-specific enolase**^{Q}

Clinical Features
- **MC presentation**: Fixed, lobular mass extending from the flank **toward the midline**^{Q} of the abdomen
- Most (80%) cases present **before 4 years** and **peak incidence** is **2 years**^{Q} of age
- Metastasis is present in 60–70% of patients **at the time of diagnosis**^{Q}

> - **Orbital metastasis** commonly present with **periorbital ecchymoses** and **proptosis** called as **Raccoon eyes**^{Q}.
> - Infants with **stage 4S** may display **cutaneous metastasis** called as **blueberry muffin lesions**^{Q}.
> - **Chronic watery diarrhea**^{Q} (due to secretion of **VIP**) and **opsoclonus-myoclonus**^{Q} (**dancing eyes, dancing feet**^{Q}) are unusual paraneoplstic manifestations.

- **MC site** of metastasis in older children are **bones**^{Q} (**Long bones–MC**, facial bones, skull particularly **sphenoid**), bone marrow and LN.
- In **infants** metastasis is confined to **liver** or **subcutaneous tissue**^{Q}.
- Lung metastasis are **rare**^{Q} in neuroblastoma

Diagnosis
- Anemia, thrombocytopenia or **thrombocytosis** (more common)
- Increased LDH, ferritin, urinary catecholamines and neuron specific enolase
- **X-ray or CT**: **Stippled calcification**^{Q} (MC abdominal tumor to demonstrate calcification prior to chemotherapy)

> - **Drooping Lily sign**: Neuroblastoma displaces **kidney inferolaterally**^{Q}
> - **MRI**^{Q} is superior to CT in assessing **vessel encasement**, vessel **patency**, **spinal cord compression** and **bone marrow involvement**.

- **MIBG scan** or **SRS** are used in the diagnosis of primary, residual and metastatic neuroblastoma.
- MIBG is one of the **single best studies** to document the **presence of metastatic**^{Q} disease.
- **Appearance** of neuroblastoma **in bone marrow** may **simulate** the appearance of **ALL**^{Q}, differentiation can be done by monoclonal antibody phenotype^Q.

Treatment
- **Localized neuroblastoma**: Excision^Q
- **Unresectable tumor**: **Biopsy**, initially treated by **chemotherapy** and **radiotherapy** followed by **surgical resection** of residual tumor^Q
- **Disseminated disease**: Chemotherapy^Q (Cyclophosphamide, vincristine, dacarbazine, doxorubicin, Cisplatin)

Prognosis
- **Shimada classification**^{Q} describes prognosis based on the **degree of differentiation**, mitosis-karyorrhexis index, presence or absence of **Schwannian stroma**^{Q}.

International Neuroblastoma Staging System	
Stage	**Definition**
1	**Localized tumor** with **complete gross excision**, with or without microscopic residual disease; representative ipsilateral LNs negative for tumor microscopically (nodes attached to and removed with the primary tumor may be positive)
2A	Localized tumor with **incomplete gross excision**; representative ipsilateral nonadherent LNs negative for tumor microscopically
2B	Localized tumor with or without complete gross excision, with **ipsilateral nonadherent LNs**
3	**Unresectable unilateral tumor** with **contralateral regional LN involvement**; or midline tumor with **bilateral extension** by infiltration (unresectable) or by LN involvement
4	Any primary tumor with **dissemination** to **distant** LNs, bone, bone marrow, liver, skin, and/or other organs (except as defined for stage 4S)
4S	**Localized primary tumor** (as defined for stage 1, 2A, or 2B), with **dissemination limited to skin**, **liver**, and/or **bone marrow** (limited to infant **<1 year** of age)

Neuroblastoma Prognostic Factors

Favorable Prognosis
- Age <1 year^Q
- **Thoracic** primary lesion
- **Shimada index** showing **well differentiated stromal rich tumor**^Q
- **Increased ratio** of **VMA/HVA**
- **Normal** serum **ferritin**
- **Hyperdiploid**^Q or **near triploid**^Q
- **High level** of expression of **Trk-A gene**^Q

Unfavorable Prognosis
- **N-myc amplification**^Q (>10)
- **Deletion** of **1p**^Q (most characteristic cytogenetic abnormality) and **Gain** of **17q**^Q
- Expression of multidrug resistance protein
- **Overexpression** of **telomerase**^Q
- **Increased** serum **ferritin**
- Diploid^Q
- **Older patients** of **stages III** and **IV**^Q

ESTHESIONEUROBLASTOMA

ESTHESIONEUROBLASTOMA (OLFACTORY NEUROBLASTOMA)

- Esthesioneuroblastoma is a **rare** unique tumor of **neural crest origin**^Q
- Arises from the **basal neural cells** of the **olfactory mucosa** of the **cribiform plate**, upper nasal wall and superior turbinate^Q
- Seen in **either sex** and most common in **3rd** and **4th** decade

Clinical Features
- Presents as a **unilateral polypoidal mass** in the **upper third** of the **nasal cavity** with symptoms of nasal obstruction, epistaxis and anosmia^Q
- It is a **vascular tumor** that **bleeds profusely on biopsy**^Q
- LN and systemic metastases can occur

Treatment
- Favored treatment is **surgical excision followed by radiation**^Q.

Multiple Choice Questions

MULTIPLE ENDOCRINE NEOPLASIA

1. A 20-year-old male presents with chronic constipation, headache and habitus, neuromas of tongue, medullated corneal nerve fibers and nodule of 2X2 cm size in left lobe of thyroid. This patient is a case of: *(All India 2004)*
   a. Sporadic medullary carcinoma of thyroid
   b. Familial medullary carcinoma of thyroid
   c. MEN-2A
   d. MEN-2B

2. True about MEN-1: *(PGI June 2004)*
   a. ↑ VMA in urine
   b. ↑ Calcitonin
   c. Hypergastrinemia
   d. Hyperprolactinemia
   e. Hypocalcemia

3. The most common organ involved in MEN-1 is: *(COMEDK 2010)*
   a. Parathyroid
   b. Thyroid
   c. Adrenal
   d. Testis

4. True about MEN-2A (Sipple syndrome): *(PGI Dec 2006)*
   a. Pheochromocytoma
   b. Hyperparathyroidism
   c. Mucocutaneous neuromas
   d. Medullary carcinoma of thyroid

5. Intestinal obstruction with jejunal neuromas are found in:
   a. MEN-1 *(MHSSMCET 2006)*
   b. MEN-2A
   c. MEN-2B
   d. Familial intestinal polyposis

6. An infant is diagnosed with MEN-2B trait. Which the following will be best line of management?
   (Recent Question 2016, MHSSMCET 2007)
   a. Prophylactic surgery
   b. Clinical observation and follow up
   c. Regular FNAC
   d. All of the above

7. Common feature to MEN1 and MEN2?
   a. Hyperparathyroidism *(MHSSMCET 2010, 2006)*
   b. Medullary carcinoma of thyroid
   c. Pheochromocytoma
   d. Carcinoids

8. Most common NET of pancreas seen in MEN-1:
   (Recent Question 2017)
   a. Gastrinoma
   b. Glucagonoma
   c. Insulinoma
   d. Somatostatinoma

9. All of the following are true about MEN-I except:
   (Recent Question 2017)
   a. Pituitary tumors
   b. Parathyroid hyperplasia
   c. Medullary carcinoma
   d. Pancreatic endocrine tumors

10. In MEN-2B prophylactic surgery in a child is indicated at:
    (Recent Question 2017)
    a. 1 year
    b. 3 years
    c. 5 years
    d. 10 years

PARATHYROID GLAND

11. Primary hyperparathyroidism is caused by: *(PGI June 2002)*
    a. Parathyroid hyperplasia
    b. Adenosis
    c. MEN-1
    d. Thyrotoxicosis
    e. CRF

12. Treatment for parathyroid hyperplasia is: *(UPSC 2001)*
    a. Removal of all four glands
    b. Calcitonin
    c. Removal of 3½ glands
    d. Enlarged glands to be removed

13. Parathyroid adenoma most commonly involves which of the following site: *(AIIMS June 2002)*
    a. Thyroid substance
    b. Superior parathyroid lobe
    c. Inferior parathyroid lobe
    d. In the mediastinum

14. Features to differentiate parathyroid adenoma from hyperplasia would include which of the following?
    a. Presence of excess chief cells *(AIIMS June 2002)*
    b. High levels of parathormone
    c. Infiltration of capsule
    d. Identifying hyperplasia of all 4 glands at surgery in parathyroid hyperplasia

15. True about parathyroid carcinoma:
    a. Parathyroid gland is palpable
    b. High calcium lebel
    c. Cinacalcet is used
    d. All of the above

16. In case of parathyroid adenoma, treatment is: *(AIIMS Nov 95)*
    a. Calcitonin and steroid
    b. Removal of adenoma
    c. Total parathyroidectomy and implantation in arm
    d. Total parathyroidectomy

17. Kamli Rani, 75-year-old woman present with post myocardial infarction after 6 weeks mild CHF. There was past H/O neck surgery for parathyroid adenoma 5 years ago, ECG shows slow atrial fibrillation. Serum Ca^{2+} 13.0 mg/L and urinary Ca^{2+} is 300 mg/24 hr. On examination there is small mass in the Para tracheal position behind the right clavicle. Appropriate management at this time is: *(All India 2002)*
    a. Repeat neck surgery
    b. Treatment with technetium-99
    c. Observation and repeat serum Ca^{2+} in two months
    d. Ultrasound-guided alcohol injection of the mass

18. Commonest cause for hyperparathyroidism is:
    (MHCET 2016, All India 89)
    a. Single adenoma
    b. Multiple adenomas
    c. Single gland hyperplasia
    d. Multiple gland hyperplasia

19. Most common cause of hypercalcemic crisis is:
    a. Parathyroid adenoma
    b. Parathyroid hyperplasia
    c. Carcinoma breast
    d. Paget's disease

20. Hypoparathyroidism occurs as a result of:
    (Recent Question 2015)
    a. Idiopathic atrophy of parathyroids
    b. Following surgery
    c. Thyroiditis with secondary atrophy of parathyroids
    d. All of the above

21. **Hypoparathyroidism can occur in:** *(PGI May 2018)*
    a. After thyroid surgery
    b. DiGeorge syndrome
    c. Radical resection of head & neck cancer
    d. MEN1

22. **Hypocalcemia in immediate post-op period following excision of parathyroid adenoma is due to:** *(Recent Question 2015)*
    a. Stress
    b. Increased uptake by bones
    c. Hypercalciuria
    d. Increased calcitonin

23. **In parathyroid crisis with sudden elevations of calcium over 16 mg/dL; the treatment consist of:**
    a. Intravenous vitamin D
    b. Parathyroidectomy for removal of adenoma
    c. Thyrocalcitonin
    d. Intravenous bicarbonate
    e. All of the above

24. **Hyperparathyroidism is characterized by the following except:** *(Recent Question 2016)*
    a. Generalized osteoporosis
    b. Renal calculi
    c. Hypercalcemia
    d. Osteosclerosis

25. **A patient has hypocalcaemia which was the result of a surgical complication. Which operation could it possibly have been?** *(Recent Question 2015)*
    a. Nephrectomy
    b. Thyroidectomy
    c. Gastrectomy
    d. Vocal cord tumour biopsy

26. **The symptoms of hyperparathyroidism include:**
    a. Constipation and muscle weakness
    b. Anorexia and weight loss
    c. Polydipsia and polyuria
    d. All of the above

27. **A known patient with renal stone disease developed pathological fractures along with abdominal pain and certain psychiatric symptoms. He should be investigated for:** *(Recent Question 2016)*
    a. Polycystic kidney
    b. Renal tubular acidosis
    c. Hyperparathyroidism
    d. Paget's disease of bone

28. **Hypocalcemia is a feature of all of the following except:** *(UPSC 2000)*
    a. Chronic renal failure
    b. Hypoparathyroidism
    c. Pseudo hypoparathyroidism
    d. Total thyroidectomy

29. **Which of the following is true about secondary hyperparathyroidism?** *(Recent Question 2015)*
    a. Commonly occurs in CRF
    b. Related to hyperphophatemia
    c. Patients are generally hypocalcemic
    d. All of the above

30. **Which of the following is true about parathyroid?**
    a. Post parathyroid glands are within junction of inferior thyroid artery and RLN
    b. Most common location of ectopic parthyroid glands is paraesophageal
    c. Lower parathyroid is anterior to RLN
    d. All of the above

31. **Parathyroid gland was implanted into forearm muscle. What is the type of transplantation?** *(Recent Question 2016)*
    a. Orthotopic
    b. Heterotopic
    c. Auxiliary
    d. None

32. **Parathyroid autotransplantation is done in which of the following muscle?** *(Recent Question 2019)*
    a. Brachioradialis
    b. Biceps
    c. Triceps
    d. Sartorius

33. **A young female with history of renal calculi complains of bone pain and abdominal cramps. On investigation, multiple fractures were discovered and serum calcium and PTH was raised. Which of the following will be the best investigation to arrive at a definitive diagnosis?** *(AIIMS May 2017)*
    a. CECT neck
    b. Sestamibi scan
    c. Radioiodine scan
    d. Ultrasound neck

34. **Which of the following is least sensitive for parathyroid imaging?** *(Recent Question 2017)*
    a. USG
    b. Sestamibi
    c. Sestamibi-SPECT
    d. MRI

ADRENAL GLANDS

35. **During bilateral adrenalectomy, intra-operative dose of hydrocortisone should be given after:** *(AIIMS Nov 2004)*
    a. Opening the abdomen
    b. Ligation of left adrenal vein
    c. Ligation of right adrenal vein
    d. Excision of both adrenal glands

36. **Parathyroid autotransplantation is done in which of the following muscle?** *(Recent Question 2019)*
    a. Hyperparathyroidism
    b. Cushing's syndrome
    c. Zollinger-Ellison syndrome
    d. Adrenogenital syndrome

37. **A 35-year-old woman has had recurrent episodes of headache and sweating. Her mother had renal calculi and died of thyroid cancer. Physical observations revealed a thyroid nodule and ipsilateral enlarged cervical lymph nodes. Before performing thyroid surgery the woman's physician should order:**
    a. Thyroid scan *(All India 2002)*
    b. Estimation of hydroxyl indole acetic acid in urine
    c. Estimation of urinary metanephrines, VMA and catecholamines
    d. Estimation of TSH, and TRH levels in serum

38. **Young female presents with hypertension with VMA >14 mg/day, associated with:** *(PGI Dec 2002)*
    a. Medullary carcinoma thyroid
    b. Von-Hippel Lindau disease
    c. Sturge-Weber syndrome
    d. Grave's disease
    e. Neurofibromatosis

39. **Palpation on the costovertebral angle produces pain and tenderness in acute adrenal insufficiency. This is:**
    a. Rotch's sign
    b. Rossolimo's sign
    c. Rogoff's sign
    d. Osler's sign

40. **Commonest cause of Cushing syndrome is:** *(Kerala 95)*
    a. Adrenal adenoma
    b. Carcinoma
    c. Hyperplasia
    d. Atrophy

41. Most common cause of Addison's disease in India: *(AIIMS Nov 2011)*
    a. Tuberculosis
    b. Post-partum
    c. Autoimmune
    d. HIV
42. Indication for surgery in a case of adrenal incidentaloma:
    a. Size >5 cm *(MAHE 2008, 2007)*
    b. Bilateral adrenal metastasis
    c. Functional tumor
    d. All of the above
43. Incidental finding in CT scan, a 3 cm adrenal mass, which of the following is not done? *(UPPG 2008)*
    a. Adrenalectomy
    b. Dexamethasone suppression test
    c. Measurement of catecholamines
    d. Midnight plasma cortisol
44. Accidental finding of incidentaloma (Adrenal mass) on USG is detected. Following is/are to be ruled out: *(PGI Dec 2006)*
    a. Cushing's disease
    b. Metastasis
    c. Adrenal adenoma
    d. Carcinoma
    e. Adrenal hyperplasia
45. True about adrenocortical carcinoma: *(Recent Question 2016)*
    a. Rare tumor
    b. More than half are functional
    c. Most commonly associated with Cushing syndrome
    d. All of the above
46. A 50-year-old male presents with severe refractory hypertension, weakness, muscle cramps and hypokalemia, the most likely diagnosis is: *(COMEDK 2011)*
    a. Hypoaldosteronism
    b. Hyperaldosteronism
    c. Cushing syndrome
    d. Pheochromocytoma
47. Which one of the following is not a CT feature of adrenal adenoma? *(AIIMS Nov 2010)*
    a. Low attenuation
    b. Homogeneous density and well defined borders
    c. Enhances rapidly, contrast stays in it for relatively longer time and washes out late
    d. Calcification is rare
48. After bilateral adrenalectomy, patient developed gradual loss of vision, with hyperpigmentation of skin, and headache. Likely cause is: *(MHSSMCET 2006)*
    a. Addison's disease
    b. Nelson's syndrome
    c. Cushing's disease
    d. Hypopituitarism
49. Nonfunctional adrenal tumors are operated at what size:
    a. >3 cm
    b. >5 cm *(MHSSMCET 2009)*
    c. >6 cm
    d. >10 cm
50. In renal agenesis, the adrenal gland is: *(MHSSMCET 2006)*
    a. Absent
    b. Present on contralateral side
    c. Ectopic in the iliac fossa
    d. Present at the usual location
51. Most prevalent incidentacoma is: *(MHCET 2016)*
    a. Cushing's adenoma
    b. Pheochromocytoma
    c. Adrenocortical carcinoma
    d. Non-functioning adenoma

PHEOCHROMOCYTOMA

52. Which one of the following clinical features is not seen in pheochromocytoma? *(COMEDK 2011)*
    a. Hypertension
    b. Episodic palpitations
    c. Weight loss
    d. Diarrhea
53. Episodic hypertension is a feature of: *(JIPMER 2010)*
    a. Carcinoid tumor
    b. Insulinoma
    c. Pheochromocytoma
    d. Zollinger-Ellison syndrome
54. The investigation of choice for extra adrenal pheochromocytoma: *(PGI Dec 2007)*
    a. MIBG scan
    b. MRI
    c. CT
    d. X-ray
    e. USG
55. All are true about pheochromocytoma except:
    a. 90% are malignant *(All India 2011)*
    b. 95% occur in the abdomen
    c. They secrete catecholamines
    d. They arise from sympathetic ganglions
56. Investigation useful for detecting extra-adrenal pheochromocytoma: *(PGI May 2011)*
    a. USG
    b. CT
    c. T2-weighted MRI with gadolinium contrast
    d. MIBG
57. True about pheochromocytoma is: *(MHPGMCET 2002)*
    a. Arises from chromaffin cells of adrenal medulla
    b. Bilateral in 20% of all cases
    c. Hypotension rules out pheochromocytoma
    d. Almost always a malignant tumor
58. Pheochromocytoma with malignant potential exclusively secretes: *(MHPGMCET 2008)*
    a. Dopamine
    b. Epinephrine
    c. Metanephrine
    d. Norepinephrine
59. False regarding pheochromocytoma:
    a. 10% of nonfamilial adrenal pheochromocytomas are bilateral *(MHSSMCET 2006)*
    b. Only 10% of hypertensive patients have an underlying pheochromocytoma
    c. 10% of adrenal pheochromocytomas arise in childhood
    d. FNAC is must for diagnosis
60. Commonest symptom of pheochromocytoma is: *(Recent Question 2015)*
    a. Palpitation
    b. Headache
    c. Sweating
    d. Dyspnea
61. In pheochromocytoma, the urine will contain: *(UPPG 96)*
    a. VMA
    b. HIAA
    c. Both
    d. None
62. False statement about pheochromocytoma:
    a. 10% are bilateral *(All India 97)*
    b. Arises from chromaffin cells
    c. Extra adrenal tumor - increased nor adrenaline levels
    d. Increased VMA levels in urine
63. Radionuclide used in pheochromocytoma is:
    a. Radioactive iodine I-131 *(COMEDK 2005)*
    b. Technitium pertechnate
    c. Radiolabelled chromium
    d. I^{123} Metaiodobenzylguanidine (MIBG)
64. The most common site of ectopic pheochromo-cytoma is: *(COMEDK 2008)*
    a. Organ of Zuckerkandl
    b. Bladder
    c. Filum terminale
    d. Celiac plexus

65. A patient presented with headache and flushing. He has a family history of his relative having died of a thyroid tumour. The investigation that would be required for this patient would be: *(AIIMS June 99)*
    a. Chest X-ray
    b. Measurement of 5 HIAA
    c. Measurement of catecholamine
    d. Intravenous pyelography

66. Investigation of choice in case of a patient with episodic hypertension, headache and thyroid nodule: *(AIIMS Nov 97)*
    a. Urinary HIAA
    b. Urinary catecholamine and aspiration of nodule
    c. Thyroid function test only
    d. Urinary basic amino acid metabolite

67. Best way to localize extra-adrenal pheochromocytoma: *(MCI June 2018)*
    a. X-ray
    b. Nucleotide scan
    c. VMA excretion
    d. Clinical examination

NEUROBLASTOMA

68. Neuroblastomas: Good prognostic factor is: *(PGI June 2000)*
    a. N-myc amplification
    b. RAS oncogene
    c. Hyperdiploidy
    d. Translocations

69. Opsoclonus-Myoclonus is a phenomenon seen in: *(PGI 97)*
    a. Wilms' tumor
    b. Neuroblastoma
    c. Meningioma
    d. Cortical tuberculoma

70. All of the following are correct about neuroblastoma except:
    a. Arises from adrenal cortex *(Recent Question 2017)*
    b. Can cause paraplegia
    c. May cause hypertension
    d. Secretes hormones

71. Not seen in neuroblastoma is: *(UPPG 96)*
    a. Diarrhea
    b. Proptosis
    c. Splenomegaly
    d. Bone involvement

72. True about neuroblastoma: *(PGI Dec 2006)*
    a. Seen in adrenal glands
    b. ↑VMA/HVA
    c. Lymphatic metastasis more common than blood metastasis
    d. Presents with abdominal mass
    e. Old age presentation implies good prognosis

73. Which of the following statements about neuro-blastoma is not true? *(All India 2009)*
    a. Most common extra cranial solid tumor in childhood
    b. >50% present with metastasis at time of diagnosis
    c. Lung metastasis are common
    d. Often encase aorta and its branches at time diagnosis

74. Mrs. Neena noted an abdominal mass in left side of her 6 months old child, which showed calcification near the left kidney. What will be the cause? *(AIIMS Nov 2000)*
    a. Leukemia
    b. Neuroblastoma
    c. RCC
    d. Lymphoma

75. Tumor arising from olfactory nasal mucosa is:
    a. Nasal glioma *(All India 2012)*
    b. Adenoid cystic carcinoma
    c. Nasopharyngeal carcinoma
    d. Esthesioneuroblastoma

Explanations

MULTIPLE ENDOCRINE NEOPLASIA

1. **Ans. d. MEN-2B:** *(Ref: Schwartz 10/e p289; Sabiston 20/e p993, 1003, 1006; Bailey 27/e p856-857; Harrison 20/e p2752, 19/e p2335)*

MEN-1 (WerMer's Syndrome)

Parathyroid Adenoma	Pancreatic NET (PGI)	Pituitary Adenoma
• MC endocrine abnormality (>98% of affected individuals) in MEN-1 is **multiglandular parathyroid tumors**[Q]. • Hyperparathyroidism is **MC manifestation** (cardinal sign of MEN-1 is parathyroid adenoma of **multicentricity**)[Q]. • Hypercalcemia is **first biochemical abnormality**[Q] detected in MEN-1 and may precede the clinical onset of a pancreatic NET or pituitary neoplasm by several years.	• Pancreatic NET is **2nd MC manifestation**[Q]. • **Nonfunctioning** or that secrete **pancreatic polypeptide**[Q] are MC pancreatic NET in MEN-1. • MC **functional NET** in patients with MEN-1 is **gastrinoma**[Q] followed by insulinoma. • MC increased pancreatic hormone: **P**ancreatic polypeptides >**G**astrin >**I**nsulin[Q] (**PGI**)	• **Prolactinoma** is **most common**[Q]. • Diagnosed by increased prolactin (>200 µg/l) and MRI.

	MEN-2A (Sipple syndrome MEN)	MEN-2B (MEN-3)
Components	• Medullary carcinoma thyroid[Q] • Pheochromocytoma[Q] • Parathyroid hyperplasia or adenoma[Q] • Hirschprung's disease[Q] • Cutaneous lichen amyloidosis[Q]	• Medullary carcinoma thyroid[Q] • Pheochromocytoma[Q] • Intestinal ganglioneuromas[Q] • Mucosal neuromas[Q] • Megacolon[Q] • Marfanoid features[Q]
Defect	• **RET** oncogene (**cysteine**[Q] codon) • Chromosome: **10**[Q]	• **RET** oncogene (**tyrosine kinase**[Q] domain) • Chromosome: **10**[Q]
Transmission	• Autosomal dominant[Q]	• Autosomal dominant[Q]

2. **Ans. a. ↑ VMA in urine, c. Hypergastrinemia, d. Hyperprolactinemia** *(Ref: Schwartz 10/e p289; Sabiston 20/e p993; Bailey 27/e p856-857; Harrison 20/e p2747, 19/e p2335)*

3. **Ans. a. Parathyroid** *(Ref: Schwartz 10/e p289; Sabiston 20/e p993; Bailey 27/e p856-857; Harrison 20/e p2747, 19/e p2335)*

4. **Ans. a. Pheochromocytoma, b. Hyperparathyroidism, d. Medullary carcinoma of thyroid**

5. **Ans. c. MEN-2B**

6. **Ans. a. Prophylactic surgery** *(Ref: Schwartz 10/e p1550; Sabiston 20/e p1008)*

Prophylactic Thyroidectomy in RET Mutation Carriers	
MEN-2A	Before **5 years**[Q]
MEN-2B	Before **1 year**[Q]

7. **Ans. a. Hyperparathyroidism**

8. **Ans. a. Gastrinoma** *(Ref: Sabiston 20/e p1000; Schwartz 10/e p1071; Bailey 27/e p857)*

9. **Ans. c. Medullary carcinoma** *(Ref: Sabiston 20/e p998; Schwartz 10/e p289; Bailey 27/e p857)*

10. **Ans. a. 1 year** *(Ref: Sabiston 20/e p1008; Schwartz 10/e p1550; Bailey 27/e p858)*

PARATHYROID GLAND

11. **Ans. a. Parathyroid hyperplasia, b. Adenosis, c. MEN-1** *(Ref: Schwartz 10/e p1559-1563; Sabiston 20/e p927; Bailey 27/e p825; Harrison 20/e p2925, 19/e p2470-2475)*

12. **Ans. c. Removal of 3½ glands** *(Ref: Harrison 20/e p2928, 19/e p2473-2475; Schwartz 10/e p156; Sabiston 20/e p931)*

TREATMENT OF PRIMARY HYPERPARATHYROIDISM

- **Initial correction** of **hypercalcemia** (Rapid IV Normal saline with **furosemide**)^Q
- **Neck exploration** is done and treatment is done accordingly

A **single parathyroid adenoma (85%)**^{Q}	• Resection^Q
Two adenomas (5%)	• Resection^Q
Hyperplasia of all four glands (10-15%)	• Resection of 3½ glands^Q • **Resection** of **all four glands** with **autotransplantation** of a parathyroid gland in the forearm (**brachioradialis**) or **SCM muscle**^{Q}

PARATHYROID AUTOTRANSPLANTATION

- Whenever **multiple parathyroids** are **resected**, it is preferable to **cryopreserve tissue**, so that it may be autotransplanted should the patient become hypoparathyroid^Q.
- Approx. **12–14 pieces** of 1 mm are transplanted into the **nondominant forearm** in belly of **brachioradialis**^{Q} muscle

13. **Ans. c. Inferior parathyroid lobe** *(Ref: Harrison 20/e p2925, 19/e p2470)*
    - Parathyroid adenomas are **most commonly located** in **inferior**^{Q} parathyroid glands.

14. **Ans. d. Identifying hyperplasia of all 4 glands at surgery in parathyroid hyperplasia** *(Ref: Harrison 20/e p2928, 19/e p2470)*
    - **Parathyroid adenoma** can be **differentiated from hyperplasia** only at the **time of surgery**^{Q}.
    - In case of **adenoma**, **only one gland** is found to be **enlarged**^{Q}, the other three are normal.
    - In **hyperplasia**, **all four glands** are **enlarged**^{Q}.

15. **Ans. d. All of the above** *(Ref: Schwartz 10/e p1560; Sabiston 20/e p937; Bailey 27/e p835)*

16. **Ans. b. Removal of adenoma**

17. **Ans. d. Ultrasound-guided alcohol injection of the mass** *(Ref: Harrison 20/e p2929, 19/e p2470)*
    - Patient is a case of **recurrent hyperparathyroidism**, as she was operated previously for parathyroid adenoma.
    - In the setting of recent myocardial infarction, CHF and atrial fibrillation, any operation carries a **high risk**.
    - **Ultrasound-guided alcohol injection** in the mass is preferred in this setting.

18. **Ans. a. Single adenoma**

19. **Ans. c. Carcinoma breast** *(Ref: Harrison 20/e p2925, 19/e p2470)*
    - **Parathyroid adenoma** is the **MC cause of hypercalcemia**^{Q}.
    - **Malignant tumors** are the **MC cause of hypercalcemic crisis**, of which **CA breast**^{Q} is the common cause.

20. **Ans. b. Following surgery** *(Ref: Schwartz 10/e p1574; Sabiston 20/e p936; Bailey 27/e p825)*

PARATHYROID INSUFFICIENCY OR HYPOPARATHYROIDISM

- Mostly due to **removal of the parathyroid glands** or infarction due to vascular injury^Q.
- **Vascular injury**^{Q} is more important.
- Cases usually present **2–5 days after operation**^{Q} with symptoms of **hypocalcemia** (circumoral and fingertip numbness and tingling tetany, carpopedal spasm and laryngeal stridor)^Q
- Treatment with **oral calcium** and **vitamin D supplements**^{Q}
- **IV calcium gluconate**^{Q} may be required in severe cases.

21. **Ans. a. After thyroid surgery, b. DiGeorge syndrome, c. Radical resection of head & neck cancer** *(Ref: Harrison 20/e p2935; Schwartz 10/e p1574; Sabiston 20/e p925)*

22. **Ans. b. Increased uptake by bones** *(Ref: Schwartz 10/e p73)*

HUNGRY BONE SYNDROME

- **Hypocalcemia** in **immediate postoperative period** following excision of parathyroid adenoma is due to **increased uptake by bones**^{Q}.
- It is known as **Hungry Bone Syndrome**

23. **Ans. b. Parathyroidectomy for removal of adenoma, c. Thyrocalcitonin** *(Ref: Harrison 20/e p2935, 19/e p2478)*

HYPERCALCEMIC CRISIS

- Patients with PHPT may occasionally **present acutely** with **nausea, vomiting, fatigue, muscle weakness, confusion**^{Q}, and a decreased level of consciousness; a complex referred to as hypercalcemic crisis.
   - These symptoms **result from severe hypercalcemia** from uncontrolled PTH secretion, **worsened by polyuria, dehydration,** and **reduced kidney function**^{Q} and may occur with other conditions causing hypercalcemia.
- **Calcium levels** are **markedly elevated** and may be as high as **16 to 20 mg/dL**^{Q}.
- **Parathyroid glands** tend to be **large** or **multiple**, and the tumor may be palpable.
- Patients with **parathyroid cancer** or **familial HPT** are **more likely**^{Q} to present with hypercalcemic crisis.

Treatment
- Treatment consists of **therapies to lower serum calcium levels** followed by **surgery** to correct HPT.
- **Mainstay of therapy:** Rehydration with a **0.9% saline** and diuresis with **furosemide**^{Q}
- Other drugs used to lower serum calcium levels:
   - **Bisphosphonates, Calcitonin**^{Q}
   - **Mithramycin** (plicamycin), **Gallium nitrate**^{Q}
   - **Glucocorticoids** (Hydrocortisone)^Q

24. **Ans. d. Osteosclerosis**
25. **Ans. b. Thyroidectomy**
26. **Ans. d. All of the above**
27. **Ans. c. Hyperparathyroidism**
28. **Ans. d. Total thyroidectomy** *(Ref: Harrison 20/e p2937, 19/e p314)*

Chronic renal failure, Hypoparathyroidism, Pseudo hypoparathyroidism are causes of hypocalcemia.

29. **Ans. d. All of the above** *(Ref: Schwartz 10/e p1572-1573; Sabiston 20/e p927-928; Bailey 27/e p833; Harrison 20/e p2933, 19/e p2478-2479)*
30. **Ans. d. All of the above** *(Ref: Schwartz 10/e p1568; Sabiston 20/e p929-930; Bailey 27/e p829)*

IDENTIFICATION OF PARATHYROIDS

- Approximately **85%** of the **parathyroid glands** are found **within 1 cm** of the **junction** of the **inferior thyroid artery** and RLNs^Q.

Upper parathyroid glands	• **Superior** to junction of inferior thyroid artery and RLNs^Q • **Dorsal (posterior)** to RLN^Q
Lower parathyroid glands	• **Inferior** to junction of inferior thyroid artery and RLNs^Q • **Ventral (anterior)** to RLN^Q

- The thin fascia overlying a "suspicious" fat lobule should be incised using a sharp curved hemostat and scalpel. This maneuver often causes the **parathyroid** gland to **"pop" out**.
- Alternatively, gentle, **blunt peanut sponge dissection** between the carotid sheath and the thyroid gland often reveals a **"float" sign**, suggesting the site of the abnormal parathyroid gland.
- **Normal parathyroids** are **light beige** and only **slightly darker** or **brown** compared to adjacent fat.
- **MC location** of ectopic parathyroid gland: **Paraesophageal**^{Q} >Mediastinal >Intrathymic

31. **Ans. b. Heterotopic**
32. **Ans. a. Brachioradialis** *(Ref: Schwartz 10/e p1569; Sabiston 20/e p936; Bailey 27/e p830)*

"Total parathyroidectomy requires complete resection of all glands combined with immediate heterotopic transplantation of several 1- to 3-mm slices of fresh parathyroid tissue into individual pockets created in the brachioradialis muscle of the nondominant forearm." Sabiston 20/e p936

33. **Ans. b. Sestamibi scan** *(Ref: Sabiston 20/e p930; Schwartz 10/e p1565; Bailey 27/e p827)*
34. **Ans. d. MRI** *(Ref: Sabiston 20/e p930; Schwartz 10/e p1565; Bailey 27/e p828)*

ADRENAL GLANDS

35. **Ans. d. Excision of both adrenal glands** *(Ref: Schwartz 10/e p1590-1590)*

- Patients undergoing surgical treatment of endogenous hypercortisolism require glucocorticoid replacement.
- Steroids are not given pre-operatively because these patients are already hypercortisolemic.
- Instead **hydrocortisone** 100 mg IV is **given after** the **removal** of **second hyperplastic adrenal gland**.

36. **Ans. a. Hyperparathyroidism** *(Ref: Harrison 20/e p2923; Sabiston 20/e p925)*
37. **Ans. c. Estimation of urinary metanephrines, VMA and catecholamines**

    The combination of symptoms suggests **MEN-2A (Sipple syndrome)**, so the patient should be investigated for **pheochromocytoma** by estimation of **urinary metanephrines, VMA** and **catecholamines.**

MEN-2A (Sipple Syndrome)		
• Medullary carcinoma thyroid[Q]	• Pheochromocytoma[Q]	• Parathyroid hyperplasia or adenoma[Q]
• Hirschprung's disease[Q]	• Cutaneous lichen amyloidosis[Q]	

38. **Ans. a. Medullary carcinoma thyroid, b. Von-Hippel Lindau disease, c. Sturge-Weber syndrome, e. Neurofibromatosis** *(Ref: Schwartz 9/e p1399-1400; Sabiston 20/e p985; Bailey 26/e p784-785)*

Syndromes Associated with Pheochromocytoma (MVVS)	
• MEN-2A and MEN-2B[Q]	• Von-Recklinghausen syndrome[Q]
• VHL syndrome[Q]	• Sturge-Weber syndrome[Q]

39. **Ans. c. Rogoff's sign** *(Ref: www.medhelp.org)*

    ROGOFF'S SIGN

    - **Costovertebral angle pain** and **tenderness** in **acute adrenal insufficiency** is known as **Rogoff's sign**[Q].

40. **Ans. c. Hyperplasia** *(Ref: Harrison 20/e p2724, 19/e p2314)*
    - **MC cause** of **Cushing's syndrome** is **iatrogenic** exogenous administration of **steroids**[Q].
    - **MC endogenous cause** of Cushing's syndrome is **bilateral adrenal hyperplasia**[Q] secondary to hypersecretion of **ACTH** from pituitary or from an ectopic non-pituitary source.

Causes of Cushing's Syndrome	
Endogenous	**Exogenous**

ADRENAL HYPERPLASIA
• **Pituitary ACTH overproduction:**
  – **Microadenoma**[Q] >Macroadenoma
• **Ectopic ACTH overproduction:**
• **Small cell carcinoma lung**[Q]
  – Thymus carcinoid
  – Carcinoma pancreas
  – Bronchial adenoma
	• **Iatrogenic** exogenous administration of **steroids (MC cause)**[Q]

ADRENAL NEOPLASIA • Adenoma[Q] • Carcinoma[Q]	

41. **Ans. a. Tuberculosis** *(Ref: ASI 7/e p1073)*
    - **Most common cause** of **adrenal insufficiency** (**Addison's disease**) in **developing countries** is **Tuberculosis**[Q] followed by autoimmune disorders.
42. **Ans. d. All of the above** *(Ref: Schwartz 10/e p1589; Sabiston 20/e p985-987; Bailey 27/e p839; Harrison 20/e p2731, 19/e p2321)*
43. **Ans. a. Adrenalectomy**
44. **Ans. All** *(Ref: CSDT 11/e p811-812; Bailey 27/e p839; Schwartz 10/e p1589; Sabiston 20/e p986; Harrison 20/e p2731, 19/e p2321)*
45. **Ans. d. All of the above** *(Ref: Schwartz 10/e p1588; Sabiston 20/e p979-980; Bailey 27/e p843; Harrison 20/e p2732, 19/e p2322)*
46. **Ans. b. Hyperaldosteronism** *(Ref: Harrison 20/e p2729, 19/e p1618-1619)*

Manifestation of Conn's Syndrome (Primary Hyperaldosteronism)	
Clinical	**Laboratory**
• **Muscle weakness** and **fatigue** (due to hypokalemia) • **Hypertension without edema** • **Polyuria** and **polydipsia**	• **Hypokalemia** • **Metabolic alkalosis** • **Hypernatremia** • Increased Aldosterone • **Low rennin**

47. **Ans. c. Enhances rapidly, contrast stays in it for a relatively longer time and washes out late** *(Ref: Grainger Radiology 4/e p1388; Dahnert Wolfgang Radiology Review Manual 6/e p919)*
    - **Adrenal adenoma** on **contrast enhanced CT/MRI** show **rapid uptake** and relatively **rapid washout** of **contrast**[Q] material than do non adenomas.

CT Features of Adrenal Adenoma	
• Well defined /sharply defined^Q • <5 cm in size^Q • Low attenuation (<10 HU) due to lipid content^Q • Mild homogenous enhancement	• Relatively rapid washout of contrast material (due to lack of large interstitial spaces) ^Q • Relatively rapid washout is characteristic of adenoma^Q

48. **Ans. b. Nelson's syndrome** *(Ref: Harrison 20/e p2682, 19/e p2273)*

NELSON'S SYNDROME

- **Adrenalectomy** in the setting of **residual corticotroph adenoma** tissue predisposes to the development of Nelson's syndrome^Q.
- Characterized by **rapid pituitary tumor enlargement** and **increased pigmentation** secondary to **high ACTH** levels^Q.
- **Radiation therapy** may be indicated **to prevent** the development of **Nelson's syndrome** after adrenalectomy^Q.

> Primary adrenal Cushing's syndrome → **Adrenalectomy** → **Loss of negative feedback** to pituitary → Development of **pituitary adenoma** → Nelson's syndrome.

49. **Ans. b. >5 cm**

50. **Ans. d. Present at the usual location** *(Ref: Grainger Radiology 4/e p1722)*

- **Embryological development** of **kidneys** and **adrenal** is **different**, hence even in **renal agenesis, adrenal glands** will be in **normal position**^{Q}.

51. **Ans. d. Non-functioning adenoma**

PHEOCHROMOCYTOMA

52. **Ans. d. Diarrhea** *(Ref: Schwartz 10/e p1586; Sabiston 20/e p980-985; Bailey 27/e p845; Harrison 20/e p2740, 19/e p2329-2331)*

53. **Ans. c. Pheochromocytoma**   54. **Ans. b. MRI**   55. **Ans. a. 90% are malignant**

Management of Pheochromocytoma

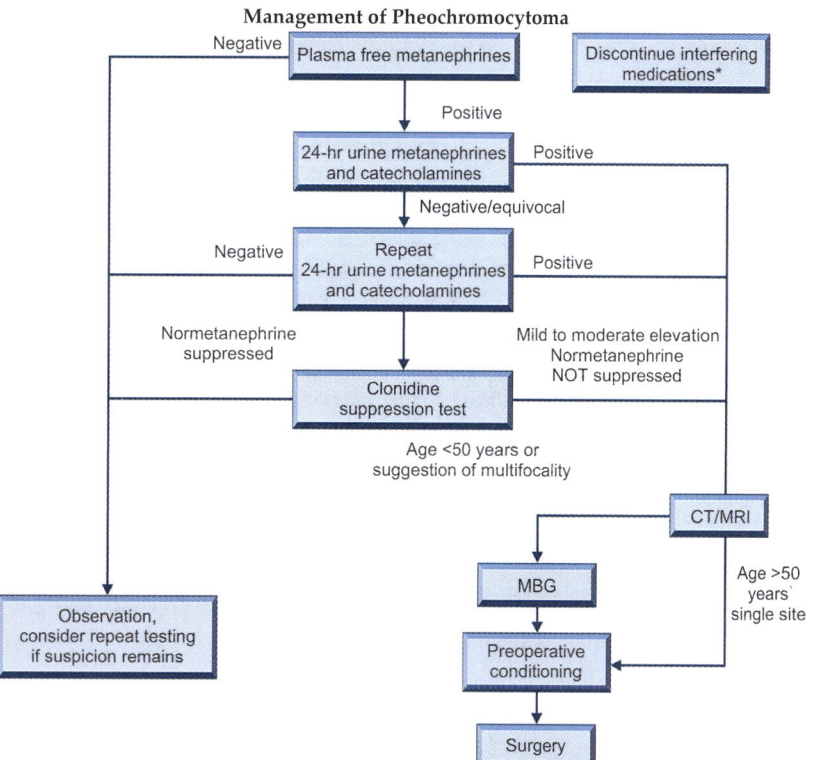

56. Ans. c. T2-weighted MRI with gadolinium contrast
57. Ans. a. Arises from chromaffin cells of adrenal medulla
58. Ans. a. Dopamine *(Ref: Schwartz 10/e p1587; Sabiston 20/e p985; Bailey 27/e p846; Harrison 20/e p2744, 19/e p2331)*
59. Ans. d. FNAC is must for diagnosis
60. Ans. b. Headache
61. Ans. a. VMA
62. Ans. None
63. Ans. d. I^{123} Metaiodobenzylguanidine (MIBG)
64. Ans. a. Organ of Zuckerkandl
65. Ans. c. Measurement of catecholamine
66. Ans. b. Urinary catecholamine and aspiration of nodule
67. Ans. b. Nucleotide scan *(Ref: Schwartz 10/e p1586; Sabiston 20/e p980; Harrison 20/e p2741)*

NEUROBLASTOMA

68. Ans. c. Hyperdiploidy *(Ref: Schwartz 10/e p1639-1640; Sabiston 20/e p1887-1888; Bailey 27/e p847; Harrison 20/e p443, 19/e p618; Robbins 9/e p477)*

Prognostic Factors in Neuroblastomas		
Variable	Favorable	Unfavorable
Stage	Stage 1, 2A, 2B, 4S^Q	Stage 3, 4^Q
Age	<18^Q months	>18 months
Evidence of **schwannian stroma** and **gangliocytic differentiation**	Present^Q	Absent
Mitosis-karyorrhexis index	<200/5000 cells	>200/5000 cells
DNA ploidy	**Hyperdiploid** or **near-triploid**^{Q}	Near-diploid
N-MYC	Not amplified	Amplified^Q
Chromosome 17q gain	Absent	Present^Q
Chromosome 1p loss	Absent	Present^Q
Chromosome 11q loss	Absent	Present^Q
TRKA expression	Present^Q	Absent
TRKB expression	Absent	Present^Q
Telomerase expression	Low or absent	Highly expressed^Q

69. Ans. b. Neuroblastoma *(Ref: Schwartz 10/e p1639-1640; Sabiston 20/e p1887-1888; Bailey 27/e p847; Harrison 20/e p443, 19/e p618; Robbins 9/e p475-479)*
70. Ans. a. Arises from adrenal cortex *(Ref: Sabiston 20/e p1887; Schwartz 10/e p1639; Bailey 27/e p847)*
71. Ans. c. Splenomegaly
72. Ans. a. Seen in adrenal glands, b. ↑ VMA/HVA, d. Presents with abdominal mass
73. Ans. c. Lung metastasis are common *(Ref: Sabiston 20/e p1887-1888; Robbins 9/e p475-479)*

NEUROBLASTOMA

- **Lung metastasis** are **rare** in **neuroblastoma**
- **Metastasis** is present in **60–70%** of patients **at the time of diagnosis**^{Q}
- **Common sites of metastasis**: **Long bones (MC)**, Liver, Lymph nodes and Skin
- **Encasement of abdominal aorta** and **IVC** by tumor is common
- Some neuroblastomas are sharply demarcated with a **fibrous pseudocapsule** but others are far more infiltrative and **invade surrounding strictures** including the **kidney, renal vein, IVC** and **envelop the aorta**

> - Neuroblastoma is the MC extracranial solid tumor in childhood
> - Neuroblastoma is the 2nd MC solid malignancy of childhood after brain tumors.
> - MC solid tumor in childhood: Brain tumors^Q
> - MC intra abdominal solid tumor in childhood: Neuroblastoma^Q

Feature	Neuroblastoma	Wilms' Tumor
Common tumor	MC intra-abdominal solid tumor in children^Q	MC renal tumor in children
At the time of diagnosis	Already metastatic in >50% of patients^Q	Generally confined to the kidney
Lung Metastasis	Rare^Q	Common
Encasement of Aorta	Characteristic^Q	Uncommon
Calcification	Common (Stippled calcification^Q)	Rare

74. Ans. b. Neuroblastoma
75. Ans. d. Esthesioneuroblastoma *(Ref: Dhingra 5/e p217-218; Washington Manual of Surgical Pathology 2/e p45; Harrison 20/e p656, 19/e p199-e4)*

SECTION 2

Hepatobiliary Pancreatic Surgery

CHAPTERS

- Liver
- Portal Hypertension
- Gallbladder
- Bile Duct
- Pancreas

CHAPTER 4

Liver

PYOGENIC LIVER ABSCESS

Pyogenic Liver Abscess

- Liver is MC site of abdominal visceral abscess[Q]
- PLA accounts for **majority** of hepatic abscesses[Q]
- Higher incidence of **cryptogenic abscess** occur in **Asian series**[Q]
- No significant gender, ethnic or geographic differences in disease frequency[Q]
- Associated comorbid conditions: **Cirrhosis, CRF**, history of **malignancy**

E. coli	MC in **western countries**[Q]
Klebsiella pneumoniae	MC in **Asian countries**[Q]
Staphylococcus	MC in **children**, suffering from **chronic granulomatous disease**[Q]

- **Multiple abscesses** occur in patients with a **biliary origin**[Q]
- **Solitary abscesses** are more likely than multiple abscesses to be **polymicrobial**.

Routes of Infection in PLA

- **Biliary tract (MC):**[Q]
  - **CBD stones** leading to cholangitis (in **Asia**)[Q]
  - **Hilar cholangiocarcinoma** in **western countries**[Q]
  - CBD strictures
- **Portal vein (2nd MC)**[Q]
- **Hepatic artery:**[Q]
  - Hematogenous spread, usually monomicrobial, staphylococcus or streptococcus
- **Direct extension:**
  - From subdiaphragmatic abscess
  - From empyema in chest
  - From suppurative cholecystitis
  - From perinephric abscess
- Penetrating or blunt trauma
- Cryptogenic

Clinical Features
- MC presenting symptom is **fever**[Q].
- MC LFT abnormality is an elevation of **ALP**[Q].
- **Classic presentation**: Fever, **jaundice (25%)**[Q], and right upper quadrant pain & tenderness
- **Fever, chills**, & **abdominal pain** are the most common presenting symptoms
- Usually **single**, involve **right lobe**[Q]
- Malignancy, jaundice, deranged LFT and sepsis are associated with poor prognosis.

Endogenous Endophthalmitis in PLA
- A rare complication specific to **Klebsiella**[Q] hepatic abscesses
- Occurring in 3% of cases.
- More common in **diabetic patients**[Q].
- **Early diagnosis** and **treatment** represent the best chance to **preserve visual function**[Q].

Diagnosis
- USG & CT are the **main diagnostic modalities**[Q]
- **Diagnosis is confirmed** by aspiration & culture[Q]
- CXR: Elevated hemidiaphragm, right sided pleural effusion or atelectasis

Treatment
- **Percutaneous catheter drainage + IV antibiotics** has become the **treatment of choice**[Q].
- After 2 weeks of parenteral antibiotics, oral agents should be used for further 4 weeks.

AMOEBIC LIVER ABSCESS

Amoebic Liver Abscess

- Caused **by Entamoeba histolytica** whose cysts are acquired through the **feco-oral route**^{Q}.
- Trophozoites reach the liver through **portal venous system**^{Q}.

> - **Solitary** and **more common** in **right lobe of liver**^{Q}.
> - **Low incidence** of **invasive amoebiasis in menstruating women**^{Q}.

- Majority of patients are **young men** (may be due to heavy alcohol consumption)

Pathogenesis
- MC form of invasive disease is **colitis**, frequently affects the **cecum & ascending colon**^{Q}
- In colon: **Flask-shaped ulcers**^{Q} **(MC site: Cecum & ascending colon)**^{Q}
- **Synchronous hepatic abscess** is found in **one third** of patients with **active amebic colitis.**

Clinical Features
- MC symptom is **abdominal pain**^{Q}
- **Typical clinical picture**: Patient of **20-40 yrs of age,** with history of travel to **endemic area**, presents with **fever**, chills, anorexia, **right upper quadrant pain**^{Q}.
- Results from an obligatory colonic infection, a **recent history** of **diarrhea** are **uncommon**^{Q}.

> - **Active colitis** and **amoebic liver abscess** rarely occur simultaneously, as a rule **colonic lesions** are **silent**^{Q}
> - **Jaundice is rare**^{Q}
> - **Raised PT** is **MC LFT abnormality**^{Q}.

Diagnosis
- **USG** and **CT** are the **main diagnostic modalities**^{Q}

> - **Diagnosis** is **confirmed** by **serological tests**^{Q} **(ELISA)** for antiamoebic antibodies.
> - **Cultures** of amoebic abscess are **usually sterile** or **negative**^{Q}.

- **CXR:** Elevated hemidiaphragm, right sided pleural effusion or atelectasis
- **ALA:** Reddish-brown anchovy paste^Q; **more reliable characteristic** than color is the **odour** of the fluid.

Treatment
- **Metronidazole** (750 mg orally TDS × 10-14 days) is the **mainstay of treatment** and is **curative in** over **90%** of patients^Q, clinical improvement is seen within 3 days.
- **Luminal agents** include **iodoquinol, paromomycin & diloxanide furoate**^{Q}.
- Average time to **radiologic resolution** of abscess is **3-9 months**

Indications of Aspiration in ALA	
1. Diagnostic uncertainty^Q	4. **High risk of rupture** (size **>5 cm**, **left lobe abscess**)^Q
2. **Failure to respond** to therapy in 3-5 days^Q	5. **Pregnancy**^{Q} (Therapeutic trial with high dose Metronidazole is deemed inappropriate)
3. **Pyogenic superinfection**^{Q}	

Complications
- Most frequent complications: Rupture into the **peritoneum (MC)**^{Q}, pleural cavity, or pericardium.
- **Size** of **abscess** appears to be the **most important risk factor** for rupture
- **Laparotomy** is indicated in cases of doubtful diagnosis, **hollow viscus perforation**, **fistulization** resulting in hemorrhage or sepsis, and **failure of conservative therapy.**
- Treatment of rupture into the pleural space: **Thoracentesis**^{Q}
- **Rupture into bronchi** is **self-limited** with **postural drainage & bronchodilators**^{Q}.

HYDATID DISEASE

Hydatid Disease

- Hydatid disease is a **zoonosis**, occurs primarily in **sheep-grazing areas**^{Q} of the world
- Endemic in Mediterranean countries, Middle East, Far East, South America, Australia, New Zealand, & East Africa.

> - **Humans** contract the **disease from dogs**, and there is **no human-to-human transmission**^{Q}.
> - **Hydatid cyst** is caused by **Echinococcus granulosus**^{Q}.
> - Other species affecting human beings: E. **multilocularis**, E. **vogelli**, E. **oligarthus**^{Q}
> - **Malignant hydatidosis** is caused by **E. multilocularis**^{Q}

Life-cycle
- **Dogs** are the **definitive host**[Q] of E. granulosus
- Eggs are passed (up to thousands of ova daily) and deposited with the dog's feces.

> - **Sheep**: Usual **intermediate host**[Q]
> - **Human**: Accidental dead end intermediate host[Q] without human to human transmission

- In the **human duodenum**, parasitic embryo releases an **oncosphere**, that **penetrate mucosa**, allowing access to **bloodstream**[Q].
- In the blood, **oncosphere** reaches liver (MC)[Q] or lungs, develops its **larval stage**, **hydatid cyst**.
- Organs most commonly involved are: **Liver >Lungs >Spleen >Kidney >Brain >Bone**[Q].

> **Hydatid Cyst**
> - Three weeks after infection, a visible hydatid cyst develops
> - The cyst wall has two layers:
>   – **Ectocyst**: outer **gelatinous** membrane[Q]   – **Endocyst**: inner **germinal** membrane[Q]
> - **Pericyst**: Fibrous capsule **derived from host tissues**, develops around the hydatid cyst.

- Scoleces develop into an **adult tapeworm in definitive host**[Q]
- Scoleces **differentiate into** a **new hydatid cyst in intermediate host**[Q]
- **Hydatid sand**: **Freed brood capsules** and **scoleces** in the hydatid fluid

Clinical Features
- **Equally common** in males & females, age of **45 years**.
- Most (75%) are **singular**, located in **right liver** (VII & VIII)[Q].
- Mostly **asymptomatic**[Q] until complications occur

> - **MC presenting symptoms**: Abdominal pain, dyspepsia & vomiting.
> - **MC sign: Hepatomegaly**[Q]

- **Complications**: Rupture of the cyst into the **biliary tree (MC)**[Q] or **bronchial tree**, or free rupture into **peritoneal, pleural**, or **pericardial cavities**.
- **Intrabiliary rupture** is MC complication of **hydatid liver cysts**[Q]
- Free ruptures can result in disseminated echinococcosis and a potentially fatal anaphylactic reaction.

Diagnosis
- USG and CT are the **main diagnostic modalities**[Q]
  – **Daughter cyst** within the **large cyst** (rosette appearance) & **calcification** of **wall** are **highly suggestive** of **hydatid cyst**[Q].

> - Diagnosis is **confirmed** by **serological tests**[Q] (ELISA, Immunoblot, Arc-5, IHA) for antibodies.
> - **Ring like calcification on CECT** is seen in hydatid cyst[Q]

- In cases of **suspected biliary involvement (Jaundice)**, **ERCP (gold standard)**[Q] or PTC is necessary.

Treatment
- Most cysts are **treated surgically**[Q]
- **Conservative management** is appropriate in **elderly** patients with **small, asymptomatic, densely calcified cysts**[Q].
- **Treatment options**: PAIR, pericystectomy, marsupialization, leaving the cyst open, drainage of the cyst, omentoplasty, or partial hepatectomy to encompass the cyst.
- Currently, **PAIR** is the **preferred method** of **treatment**[Q] for **anatomically & surgically appropriate lesions**

> **Surgery remains the treatment of choice for cysts where**
> - **PAIR** is **not possible** or cysts are **refractory to PAIR**[Q]
> - For **complicated cysts** (communicating with biliary tract)[Q]

- **Radical** (resection) and **conservative** (drainage & evacuation) surgical approaches appear to be **equally effective** at controlling disease.
- **Pericystectomy** is the **preferred surgical approach**[Q] (complete cyst with surrounding fibrous tissue are removed)
- If surgical **cystectomy** is **not** technically feasible, then formal **liver resection** can be done.

> **Chemotherapy in Hydatid Disease**
> - Chemotherapy with **albendazole** or **mebendazole** is effective at **shrinking** the **cysts**
> - **Cyst disappearance** occurs in **fewer than 50%** of patients[Q].
> - **Preoperative treatment** may **decrease the risk for spillage**[Q] and is a reasonable and safe practice.
> - **Chemotherapy without definitive resection** or drainage is only considered **for**:
>   – **Widely disseminated disease**[Q]   – Patients with **poor surgical risk**[Q]

Treatment of E. multilocularis
• E. multilocularis cyst is **always multiloculated**[Q].   • Treatment is **surgical resection**[Q].

PAIR

PAIR (Puncture, Aspiration of cyst content, Injection of scolicidal agent, and Reaspiration)

- Currently, **PAIR** is **preferred method** of **treatment**[Q] for **anatomically & surgically appropriate lesions**
- The **efficacy of PAIR** in managing hydatid cysts is **>75%**.
- During PAIR, patient is given **prophylactic coverage of albendazole**

Scolicidal Agents
- **Hypertonic (20%) saline**[Q]: 100% scolicidal with contact time of 6 minutes
- 0.5% cetrimide with 0.05% **chlorhexidine**[Q]
- **Absolute alcohol**[Q]
- **10% povidone iodine**[Q]

Contraindications of PAIR
- **Superficially located cysts**[Q]
- **Inaccessible** or **hazardous location**[Q] of cyst
- Cysts with **multiple internal septal**[Q] divisions (**honeycombing** pattern)
- **Dead** or **inactive cysts**[Q]
- Cysts **communicating with biliary tree**[Q]
- **Lung** or **brain cysts**[Q]

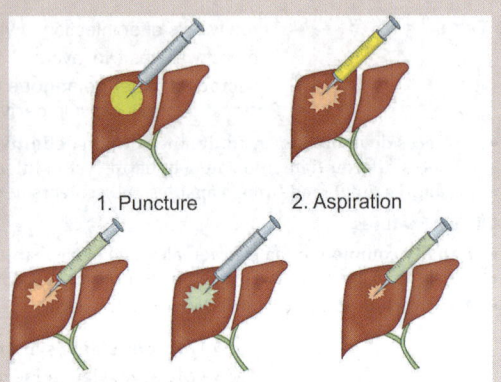

1. Puncture   2. Aspiration
3. Injection (Scolicidal agent)   4. Reaspiration

	Most Common		
	Symptom	**Sign**	**Laboratory abnormality**
Pyogenic abscess	**Fever**[Q]	RUQ **tenderness**[Q]	Raised **ALP**[Q]
Amebic abscess	Abdominal **pain**[Q]	**Hepatomegaly**[Q]	Raised **PT**[Q]
Hydatid cysts	No symptom or Abdominal **pain**[Q]	RUQ **mass**[Q]	Eosinophilia

ACTINOMYCOSIS OF LIVER

Actinomycosis of Liver

- Most commonly, Actinomyces **reaches liver through portal vein**[Q].
- **Liver** is gradually replaced by **multiple abscesses**, typical **honey comb liver**[Q]

Diagnosis
- Needle aspiration: **Actinomyces in pus**[Q]

Treatment
- Antibiotic **(Penicillin)** is the **DOC**[Q].

HEPATIC CYST

Simple Hepatic Cyst

- Contain **serous fluid**, **do not communicate** with the biliary tree, and **do not have septations**[Q]
- **Single in 50% cases**[Q]

Treatment
- Nonsurgical treatment: **Aspiration** and **injection** of a **sclerosing agent** (most frequently **ethanol**)[Q].
- Surgical therapy: **Fenestration** or **unroofing** the **extrahepatic** portion of **cyst**[Q].

Complication
- MC complication: **Intracystic bleeding**[Q].

POLYCYSTIC LIVER DISEASE

- **Autosomal dominant**[Q] disorder, often found is association with polycystic renal disease
- MC extra-renal manifestation of **ADPKD**[Q]
- Liver cysts are **always preceded by kidney cysts**[Q].

> - **Renal function** and **hepatic cyst load** are **correlated**[Q].
> - Associated condition: **Berry aneurysm** and **mitral valve prolapse**[Q].

Types
- **Type I:** Few large cysts (>7-10 cm)
- **Type II:** Multiple medium cysts (5-7 cm)
- **Type III:** Diffuse small to medium cysts (<5 cm)

Treatment
- **Laparoscopic unroofing**[Q] for small number of large cysts
- A combination of **cyst unroofing + liver resection**[Q] for reducing liver volume.
- **MC complication** specific to **surgery**: Ascites

Complications
- The **main complication** is **bacterial infection**[Q] of a cyst.
- Other complications: Intracystic bleeding, cholestasis, portal hypertension
- **Liver failure** has **not been observed** in these patients.

LIVER TUMORS

- MC malignancy of liver: Metastasis[Q]
- MC primary malignancy of liver: HCC[Q]
- MC primary malignancy of liver in children: Hepatoblastoma[Q]
- MC benign tumor of liver: Hemangioma[Q]

LIVER HEMANGIOMA

Liver Hemangioma

- **MC benign tumor** of the **liver**[Q].
- Mainly seen in **women** of **45 years**[Q].
- Small capillary hemangiomas (no clinical significance), larger cavernous hemangiomas
- **Usually single** and **<5 cm** in diameter, occur **equally in right** & **left liver**[Q].
- **Giant hemangioma**: Lesions >5 cm

Pathology
- Microscopically: Endothelium-lined, blood-filled spaces that are separated by thin, fibrous septa.
- **Enlargement** of hemangiomas are **by ectasia**[Q] rather than neoplasia.

Clinical Features
- Most commonly **asymptomatic** and **incidentally found**[Q] on imaging studies.
- Large compressive masses may cause **vague upper abdominal symptoms**[Q].
- **Kasabach-Merritt syndrome**[Q]: Syndrome of thrombocytopenia & consumptive coagulopathy, rarely seen
- **LFTs** & **tumor markers** are **normal**[Q]

Diagnosis
- Diagnosis is made radiologically.
- **CT** and **MRI** are diagnostic if a **typical peripheral nodular enhancement**[Q] pattern is seen.
- Percutaneous **biopsy** is potentially **dangerous & inaccurate, not recommended**[Q].

Treatment
- **Observation** for asymptomatic cases[Q]
- **Enucleation** with inflow control is **TOC** for **symptomatic cases**[Q]

FOCAL NODULAR HYPERPLASIA

Focal Nodular Hyperplasia

- FNH is **second MC benign tumor**[Q] of the liver.
- Usually a **small (<5 cm) nodular mass** arising in a normal liver, involves right & left liver equally.
- Mainly seen in **young women,** associated with **OCPs use**[Q]

Pathology
- **Central fibrous scar**[Q] with **radiating septa** in the mass
- **Typical hepatic vascularity** is **not seen** with **atypical biliary epithelium**[Q]

  - **Central scar** contains a **large artery** that branches out into multiple smaller arteries in a **spoke-wheel pattern**[Q] (on angiography)

Clinical Features
- **Incidental finding** at laparotomy or more commonly on imaging studies in most patients,.
- **Vague abdominal pain** in symptomatic cases
- **AFP** levels are **normal.**

Diagnosis
- Most cases of FNH can be diagnosed radiologically, on **CECT** or **MRI**
- **Homogeneous mass** with a **central scar**[Q] that rapidly enhances during the arterial phase of contrast administration.
- Histologic confirmation and resection for definitive diagnosis if radiologic diagnosis is difficult

Treatment
- **No treatment**[Q] in asymptomatic patients with typical radiologic features
- **Resection** in cases of **diagnostic uncertainty**, for **histologic confirmation**[Q].

HEPATIC ADENOMA

Hepatic Adenoma

- **Benign** proliferative disorder of hepatocytes
- Predominantly found in **young women (20-40 years)**, associated with **OCPs**[Q]
- Usually **single**[Q] (multiple lesions in 12-30%)

Pathology
- Composed of **cords** of **benign hepatocytes** containing **increased glycogen & fat**, without bile ductules, fibrous septa, portal tracts or **central vein**[Q].

  - **Bile ductules** are **not seen**, only few or **no Kupffer cells** are seen[Q].
  - **Normal architecture** of the liver is **not present**[Q] in these lesions.

- Contain large plates of hepatocytes separated by **dilated sinusoids** which are **perfused solely** by **peripheral arterial feeding vessels** (lack portal venous supply), under **arterial pressure**[Q].
- **Hemorrhage & necrosis**[Q] are commonly seen

Clinical Features
- Symptomatic (upper **abdominal pain**) in **50-75%**[Q], related to hemorrhage or local compressive symptoms.
- Tumor markers (**AFP**) are **normal**[Q].

  - Two major risks: **Rupture** (with potentially life-threatening **intraperitoneal hemorrhage**) & **malignant transformation**[Q].
  - Risk for **rupture** is **30-50%, related to size**[Q].
  - **Risk for transformation** into HCC is **low**[Q].

Diagnosis
- **MRI:** Well-demarcated heterogeneous mass containing **fat** or **hemorrhage**.

CT Findings in Hepatic Adenoma
• **Hypervascular & heterogeneous** on the **arterial phase** and become isodense or hypodense on the portal phase as a result of **arteriovenous shunting**
• Distinctive findings from FNH: **Smooth surface** (95%), presence of **necrosis & hemorrhage** (25%), and **tumor capsule** (25%)[Q].

- **Angiography:** Hypervascular well circumscribed tumor **supplied by peripheral arteries**[Q].
- **Resection** may be necessary to **secure a diagnosis** in **difficult cases**[Q].

Treatment
- **Acute hemorrhage**: Hepatic artery embolization^Q, after stabilization, resection of the mass.
- **Resection** for **symptomatic masses**^{Q}
- **Resection before a planned pregnancy**, as behavior during pregnancy has been unpredictable

PELIOSIS HEPATITIS

PELIOSIS HEPATITIS

- It is an uncommon disorder characterized by **multiple, small, blood-filled sinuses**^{Q}
- Commonly occurs in **immunocompromised** postpartum patients, **AIDS** patients, and patients taking long term **steroids**^{Q}.

Etiology
- Drugs causing it are **androgens, azathioprine, tamoxifen, estrogen** & **vitamin A**^{Q}.

Diagnosis
- Radiographically these lesions present as **diffuse hypodense areas** spread **throughout the liver**^{Q}
- CT and MRI show enhancement on early images, which may progress from central to peripheral on delayed imaging.

Treatment
- The **treatment** for bleeding lesion has been **angiographic embolization**^{Q}.

RISK FACTORS FOR HEPATOCELLULAR CARCINOMA

Conditions Associated with Hepatocellular Carcinoma					
1. Cirrhosis		**2. Metabolic diseases**		**3. Environmental**	
Condition	Risk	Condition	Risk	Condition	Risk
• HBV^Q	High	• Hereditary **hemochromatosis**^{Q}	High	• Thorotrast	Moderate
• HCV^Q	High	• Hereditary **tyrosinemia**^{Q}	High	• Androgenic steroids^Q	Moderate
• Alcohol^Q	High	• **Alpha-1 antitrypsin deficiency**	Moderate	• Cigarette smoking^Q	Low to moderate
• Autoimmune chronic active hepatitis	High	• **Ataxia telangiectasia**^{Q}	Moderate	• Aflatoxin^Q	Moderate
• Cryptogenic cirrhosis		• Types 1 & 3 glycogen storage disease	Moderate		
		• **Galactosemia**^{Q}	Moderate		
• Cirrhosis due to NAFLD^Q	Moderate	• **Citrullinemia**	Moderate		
	Moderate	• Hereditary hemorrhagic telangiectasia	Moderate		
• **Primary biliary cirrhosis**^{Q}	Low	• **Porphyria cutanea tarda**	Moderate		
		• **Wilson's disease**^{Q}	Low		
		• Orotic aciduria	Moderate		
		• **Alagille's syndrome**^{Q} (congenital cholestatic syndrome)	Moderate		

HEPATOCELLULAR CARCINOMA

HEPATOCELLULAR CARCINOMA

- **MC primary liver malignancy is HCC**^{Q}
- HCC represents **MC solid organ cancers**^{Q}.
- HCC: MC malignancy responsible for **death in patients with cirrhosis.**

  - More prevalent in **Asia** & **sub Saharan Africa**^{Q} (high frequency of **chronic infection** with **HBV** & **HCV**^{Q})
  - **100 folds increase** in risk in individuals with **HBV infection**^{Q}

- More common in **males, 60-90%** arise in **cirrhotic liver**^{Q}
- **Post necrotic cirrhosis** has **highest risk**^{Q} of developing into HCC
- **Alcoholic cirrhosis** & Primary biliary cirrhosis has **lower risk**^{Q}

  - **Strong propensity** for **invasion of vascular channels**^{Q}

Pathology
- **Gross Morphology: Hanging, pushing** & **invasive** tumors[Q].
- **Histologic patterns:** Trabecular, pseudoglandular or acinar, compact pattern and scirrhous pattern

Clinical Features
- MC symptom is **abdominal pain** >**weight loss**[Q]

> Significant weight loss: 5% in 1 month or 10% in 6 months or 20% in 1 year[Q]

- Usually presents at **late stage**[Q], symptoms at advanced stage are **vague**
- Non-specific symptoms (anorexia, weight loss) and **Hepatomegaly**[Q]

> **Paraneoplastic Syndromes in HCC**
> - **Hypercholesterolemia (MC)**[Q] >**hypoglycemia**[Q], erythrocytosis, hypercalcemia

- **Vascular bruit** (25%), GI bleed (10%), tumor rupture (2-5%), jaundice due to biliary obstruction (10%), paraneoplastic syndrome (<5%).

Tumor Markers
- Protein induced by Vitamin K Absence (**PIVKA**; Des-gamma-Carboxy Prothrombin); **glypican-3**; **AFP** fractions[Q]

> - Lectin fraction-3 of AFP (**AFP-L3**) is **highly specific to HCC** and also an indicator of **poorly-differentiated** histology and **unfavorable prognosis**[Q]
> - Serum **AFP** level is elevated above **20 ng/mL** in >**70%** of patients with HCC.

- Monoclonal antibody **HepPar-1 (hepatocyte paraffin-1)** identifies a unique antigen on **hepatocyte mitochondria** and is used to identify hepatocytes or HCC.

Diagnosis

> **Non-invasive Diagnostic Criteria for HCC**
> - **Focal lesion 1-2 cm: Two** imaging **techniques** with **arterial hypervascularization** & **venous washout**[Q].
> - **Focal lesion >2 cm: One** imaging **technique** with **arterial hypervascularization** & **venous washout**[Q].
> - Techniques to be considered: Dynamic CT & MRI.

- **Screening** is based on regular **ultrasound scanning** in **high risk population**[Q]
- **Biopsy** proof of HCC is **not required**[Q]

Treatment
- **Complete excision**[Q] by **partial hepatectomy** or by **total hepatectomy** and **transplant** is the only treatment modality with **curative** potential[Q].

> Remember: Only 15-20% of HCC is resectable, because rest of the tumors have
> - Multicentricity, Bilobar involvement[Q]
> - Portal vein invasion, Lymphatic metastasis[Q]

Okuda Staging System for HCC (BATA)[Q]		
Clinical parameter	Cut-off value	Points
Serum **B**ilirubin	<3	0
	>3	1
Serum **A**lbumin	>3	0
	<3	1
Tumor size	<50%	0
	>50%	1
Ascites	Absent	0
	Present	1
Stage I = 01; Stage II = 1–2 points; Stage III = 3–4 points.		

Cancer of the Liver Italian Program (CLIP)
- Components: **PACT** (**P**ortal vein thrombosis, **A**FP levels, **C**hild-Pugh stage, **T**umor extension)[Q]
- CLIP system is applicable to **Hepatitis C-related** HCC cases[Q]

Chinese University Prognostic Index
- Components: **BA$_3$TS** (**B**ilirubin; **A**$_3$: **A**scites, AFP, ALP; **T**NM stage; **S**ymptoms)[Q]
- Applicable to **HBV** related HCC in **China**[Q].

Barcelona Clinic Liver Cancer Staging System
- It was developed to allow for the **indication** of the **best therapy** for **each stage of HCC**[Q] and is **best suited** for **treatment guidance** and to **select early-stage patients** who could benefit from **curative therapies**.
- It divides patients into four major groups (early, intermediate, advanced and end stage)
- It considers variables related to **tumor stage, liver functional status, physical status** and **cancer related symptoms**[Q].

Treatment Options for Hepatocellular Carcinoma	
1. Surgical: • Resection • Orthotopic liver transplantation	**4. Transarterial:** • Embolization • Chemoembolization • Radiotherapy
2. Ablative: • Ethanol injection • Acetic acid injection • Thermal ablation (**cryotherapy**, **radiofrequency ablation**, **microwave**)	**5. Systemic:** • Chemotherapy • Hormonal • Immunotherapy
3. Combination Transarterial and Ablative	**6. External-beam Radiation Therapy**

FIBROLAMELLAR HEPATOCELLULAR CARCINOMA

Fibrolamellar HCC

- Occurs in **young adults without underlying cirrhosis**[Q]
- **Non-encapsulated** but well, circumscribed, so **high resectability rate**[Q]
- **Grows slowly** and & has **better prognosis**[Q]

Pathology
- **Well demarcated** & **non-encapsulated** and may have a **central fibrotic area**[Q].
- Composed of **large polygonal tumor cells** embedded in a **fibrous stroma** forming **lamellar structures**

> • **Calcification**[Q] differentiates FHCC from FNH in **35-55%** of **FHCC; heterogeneous enhancement**[Q] is also an important imaging finding.

Clinical Features
- Occurs in **younger patients**[Q] without a history of cirrhosis.

> • FHCC does not produce **AFP**[Q]
> • Associated with **elevated neurotensin**[Q] & Vitamin B_{12} binding globulin levels[Q]

Treatment
- **Better prognosis** than HCC due to **high resectability rates, lack of chronic liver disease**, and a more **indolent course**[Q].
- **Long-term survival** can be expected in about **50-75%** of patients **after complete resection**[Q]
- **Recurrence** is **common** and occurs in at least **80% of patients**[Q].
- Presence of **lymph node metastases** predicts a **worse outcome**[Q].

COLORECTAL LIVER METASTASIS

Colorectal Liver Metastasis

- About **20%** of these patients are candidates for a potentially **curative liver resection** with a **5-year survival rates** range from **25-58%**[Q].
- About **two-third** of cases **recur**, but in high-risk situations (**four** or **more** tumors, **extrahepatic** disease), recurrence rates are generally **80% or higher**[Q].
- Resections of **extrahepatic metastases** that appear to be associated with the **best outcome** are limited lung metastases, locoregional recurrences of the primary tumor, and **portal lymph nodes**.

Factors most influential on outcome of Colorectal liver metastasis		
• Size **>5 cm**[Q] • **Lymph node-positive** primary lesion[Q]	• Disease free interval **<1 year**[Q] • CEA **>200 ng/mL**[Q]	• More than one tumor[Q]

- **Synchronous liver metastasis** is associated with poor prognosis

Local Ablative therapy for liver secondaries

Mechanism	Technique	Zone of Necrosis	Advantages	Disadvantages
Freezing	Cryotherapy	3-5 cm	**Large zone** of necrosis Easily followed by ultrasound	Requires laparotomy Large size probe size
Hyperthermic coagulative necrosis	**Radiofrequency or microwave ablation**	2 cm	**Percutaneous** technique	Small size of necrosis
Local injection therapy	Ethanol, **acetic acid**, chemotherapy, **hot saline**	3 cm	Simple, inexpensive	Inhomogenous distribution

HEPATOBLASTOMA

Hepatoblastoma

- MC **primary hepatic tumor** of **childhood**, more common in **males**^{Q}.
- **Low birth weight** may represent a **risk factor**^{Q}.
- Most cases are **sporadic**, also associated with Beckwith-Wiedemann syndrome & **FAP**^{Q}
- **No** evidence of **association** with **HBV** or **HCV** infection or any other **chronic viral hepatitis**^{Q}.
- These patients usually do **not have cirrhosis** or **inborn errors of metabolism**^{Q}.

Pathology
- Five histologic subtypes: Fetal, embryonal, mixed mesenchymal, macrotubular, and anaplastic or small cell.

Clinical Features
- **Median age** of presentation is **18 months**, and almost **all cases occur** before **3 years**^{Q}.
- MC presenting sign is an **asymptomatic abdominal mass**^{Q}.
- Mild **anemia** & **thrombocytosis**^{Q} are commonly found at presentation.

> - Serum **AFP levels** are **elevated in 85-90%** of patients and can serve as a useful **marker for therapeutic response**^{Q}.

Diagnosis
- CT scan reveals a **vascular mass** that is often (50%) **speckled with calcification**^{Q}.
- To **confirm the diagnosis**, an **initial biopsy**^{Q} is required.

Treatment

> - **For unresectable tumors**, the initial surgical procedure should include a **diagnostic biopsy** and **placement of a vascular access device for chemotherapy**^{Q}.
> - A **second laparotomy** is performed after **four cycles of chemotherapy**, if imaging studies show a good response, and the tumor appears resectable.

- **Neoadjuvant chemotherapy** (cisplatin, 5-fluorouracil, vincristine) followed by **resection**^{Q}
- 50% of patients with **pulmonary metastases** can be **cured with resection**^{Q} of the hepatic tumor and **chemotherapy** or resection of the pulmonary metastases^Q.

Prognosis
- Survival appears to be **dependent** on **complete resection**^{Q}.
- Long-term survival rates of **60-70%** can be expected with **complete resection**^{Q}.

EPITHELIOID HEMANGIOENDOTHELIOMA

Epithelioid Hemangioendothelioma

- Malignant soft tissue tumor of **endothelial origin**^{Q}.
- **Infantile variety** is **benign**, **adult** one is **malignant** & **highly aggressive**^{Q}.
- **Female predominance** is related to **vinyl chloride** exposure & **OCPs**^{Q}.
- In approximately one **half of cases, cutaneous hemangiomas** are also present (45%)^Q.

Pathology
- **Factor VIII staining**^{Q} differentiates it from other nonvascular tumors.
- Liver **parenchymal architecture** is **preserved**^{Q}.

Diagnosis
- Percutaneous **biopsy**[Q] is performed for diagnosis.
- CT scan: Irregular hypodense lesions that may have **hypervascular enhancement**[Q] in the periphery following injection of intravenous contrast.

Treatment
- **Total hepatectomy** and **liver transplantation**[Q] (disease is diffuse & multifocal).

BILIARY CYSTADENOMA

Cystadenoma

- Mostly **intrahepatic**[Q] (83%), may occur within the **extrahepatic bile ducts** (13%) or **GB** (0.02%).
- Located in the **right lobe (50%)**[Q]
- Cystadenoma with **mesenchymal stroma** occurs exclusively in **young** and **middle-aged women**[Q]

Pathology
- Cyst has a globular external surface with **multiple protruding cysts** and **locules** of various sizes.
- **Fluid** content is **mucinous**.
- Lined with **columnar epithelium** and have **papillary infoldings.**

Clinical Features
- Usually presents as a **large cystic mass**[Q] (10-20 cm).
- Mainly affects **women**[Q] older than 40 years.
- **Majority of patients** present with a **history of abdominal pain** or **mass**

Diagnosis
- **Ultrasound: Cystic structure** with varying wall thickness, **nodularity, septations**, and fluid-filled locules.
- **CECT: Enhancement** of the **cyst wall** and **septa**[Q]
- **ERCP:** Displacement of the intrahepatic bile ducts by the tumor and **no communication** between the **biliary tree** and **cystadenoma**.

Treatment
- **Enucleation** for neoplastic cysts with **no** signs of **malignancy**[Q]
- **Formal hepatic resection** for neoplastic cysts with signs of **malignancy**[Q]

BILIARY CYSTADENOCARCINOMA

Biliary Cystadenocarcinoma

- Rare malignancy, typically **intrahepatic**[Q] in location.
- May arise from preexisting **biliary cystadenomas**.
- **Female**[Q] to male ratio is 2 : 1; **CA 19-9** is **raised**[Q]

Pathology
- The presence of an **associated ovarian-like stroma**[Q] in **female** patients appears to signify a **favorable prognosis**
- Tends to be **multilocular**, fluid from the cyst can be blood stained, clear, or bile tinged.
- **Preoperative cyst aspiration** is **not recommended** because there is a risk for **peritoneal tumor seeding**[Q]

Clinical Features
- Cystadenocarcinoma tends to be **larger than cystadenoma**, but clinical features are similar

Diagnosis
- **Radiologic findings: Thick or irregular wall**, **peripheral enhancement**, associated **mass**, or **papillary tumor projections**[Q] into the cyst cavity.

Treatment
- The only **potentially curative treatment** is **complete removal**, by a **major liver resection with clear margins**[Q].
- **Survival rates** for this disease have been reported in the range of **25% to 100%** at 5 years.

WILSON'S DISEASE

WILSON'S DISEASE

- Wilson's disease is an **autosomal recessive**^{Q} inherited disorder of copper metabolism.
- Characterized by **excessive deposition** of **copper** in the **liver, brain,** and other tissues^Q.
- **Major physiologic aberration**: Excessive absorption of **copper** from the **small intestine** and **decreased excretion** of copper by the **liver**^{Q}.
- Defect on chromosome 13q (ATP7B gene)^Q

Pathology
- Kayser-Fleischer rings consist of **electron-dense granules** rich in **copper** and **sulfur**.
- Rings form **bilaterally, initially** appearing at **superior pole**^{Q} of cornea, then inferior pole, &, ultimately, circumferentially.

Clinical Features
- Patients with Wilson's disease usually present with **liver disease** during **first decade** of life or with **neuropsychiatric illness** during **third decade**^{Q}.

  - Any young patient with **unexplained chronic** or **fulminant liver disease** should be investigated for Wilson's disease^Q.
  - **Kayser-Fleischer rings** are formed by **deposition of copper** in **Descemet's membrane** in limbus of cornea. The color may range from **greenish gold** to **brown**^{Q}
  - When well developed, rings may be **readily visible** to the **naked eye** or with an ophthalmoscope
  - When not visible to the unaided eye, rings may be identified using **slit-lamp** examination or **gonioscopy**.

- **Kayser-Fleischer rings** are observed in up to **90%** of individuals with **symptomatic** Wilson's disease and are almost invariably present in those with **neurologic manifestations**^{Q}.

Diagnosis
- Approximately 90% of patients have **ceruloplasmin levels** of **<20 mg/d**^{Q} (reference range, 20-40 mg/dL).

  - **Urinary copper excretion rate** is **>100 mg/d**^{Q} (reference range, <40 mg/d) in most patients with symptomatic Wilson's disease.
  - **Hepatic copper concentration** is regarded as the criterion **standard for diagnosis** of Wilson's disease.

- A liver biopsy with sufficient tissue reveals levels of **>250 µg/g of dry weight**^{Q} even in asymptomatic patients.

Treatment
- **Zinc**^{Q} is the **treatment of choice** for **maintenance therapy** in **Wilson's disease**.

COURVOISIER'S LAW

COURVOISIER'S LAW

- In **obstruction** of the **common bile duct** due to a **stone**, distention of gallbladder seldom occurs; the **organ** usually **is shriveled**^{Q}.
- If there is no disease in the gallbladder and the **obstruction is due to cancer of ampulla, pancreas or bile duct**, then **gallbladder will be distended**^{Q}.

Exceptions to Courvoisier's Law
- **Double impaction of stones**^{Q} (one in **cystic duct** & other in **CBD**).
- Oriental cholangiohepatitis^Q
- **Pancreatic calculus obstructing** the **ampulla** of **Vater**^{Q}
- **Mucocele** due to **stone** in the **cystic duct**^{Q}

LIVER ANATOMY

Functional Anatomical Divisions of Liver
- Functional anatomy of the liver is based on Couinaud's division of liver into eight (subsequently nine) functional segments, based upon the distribution of **portal venous branches** & location of **hepatic veins** in the parenchyma **(Couinaud 1957)**.

  - **Segment IX** is a **recent subdivision of segment I**, and describes that **part of segment that lies posterior to segment VIII**^{Q}.

- Liver is **divided into four portal sectors** by **four main branches of portal vein**. These are **right lateral, right medial, left medial & left lateral** (sometimes the term posterior is used in place of lateral & anterior in place of medial).
- Three main hepatic veins lie between these sectors as intersectorial veins. These **intersectoral planes** are also called **portal fissures (scissures)**. Fissures containing portal pedicles are called **hepatic fissures**.
- Each sector is sub-divided into segments (usually two) based on their supply by tertiary divisions of vascular biliary sheaths.

Fissures of the liver:
- **Three major fissures**, not visible on the surface, run through the liver parenchyma and **harbor the three main hepatic veins** (**main, left & right portal fissures**)^Q.
- **Three minor fissures** are visible as **physical clefts of the liver surface** (**umbilical, venous & fissure of Gans**)^Q.

Sectors and segments of the liver:
- Sectors of liver are made up of between one & three segments: right lateral sector = segments VI & VII; right medial sector = segments V & VIII; left medial sector = segments III & IV (and part of I); left lateral sector = segment II.

  - **Segments are numbered in an ante-clockwise spiral centered on the portal vein** with the **liver viewed from beneath**, starting with segment I up to segment VI, and then back clockwise for the most cranial two segments VII & VIII.

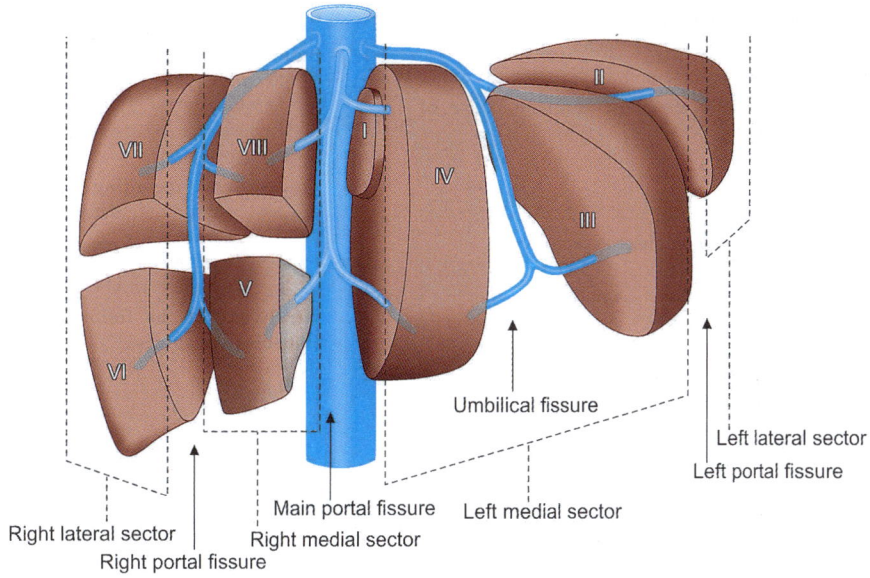

The fissures and sectors of the liver. (Right lateral = right posterior; right medial = right anterior)

Segmental Nomenclature			
I	Caudate lobe^Q	V	Right **anterior inferior** segment
II	Left **lateral superior** segment	VI	Right **posterior inferior** segment
III	Left **lateral inferior** segment	VII	Right **posterior superior** segment
IV	Left medial segment or **Quadrate lobe**^{Q}	VIII	Right **anterior superior** segment

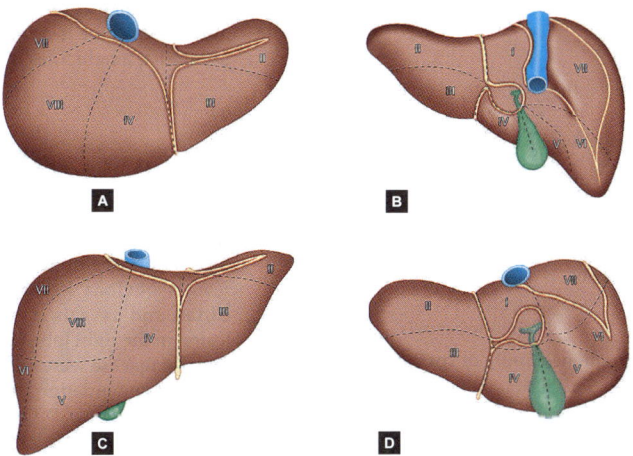

Segments of the liver (after Couinaud). (A) superior view; (B) posterior view; (C) anterior view; (D) inferior view.

Multiple Choice Questions

LIVER ABSCESS

1. **Most common cause of liver abscess in chronic granulomatous disease:** *(ILBS 2012)*
   a. Klebsiella
   b. Staph. aureus
   c. Peptostreptococcus
   d. E. coli

2. **Most common cause of liver abscess:** *(AIIMS GIS May 2011)*
   a. E. coli
   b. Proteus
   c. Klebsiella
   d. Staphylococcus

3. **Which of the following is the most common cause of pyogenic liver abscess?** *(All India 2012, AIIMS GIS Dec 2009) (Recent Question 2014)*
   a. Trauma
   b. Biliary tract infection
   c. Colonic Diverticulitis
   d. Appendicitis

4. **All are true about pyogenic liver abscess except:** *(JIPMER GIS 2011)*
   a. Most common route of infection is biliary tree
   b. Most common site is right lobe
   c. Klebsiella is most common in gas forming abscess
   d. Percutaneous drainage is least cured

5. **All are true about amoebic liver abscess except:**
   a. Metronidazole is mainstay of treatment *(PGI Nov 2010)*
   b. Multifocal abscess can not be treated by aspiration
   c. More common in left side
   d. More common in female

6. **Liver abscess ruptures most commonly in:** *(AIIMS GIS 2003)*
   a. Pleural cavity
   b. Peritoneal cavity
   c. Pericardial cavity
   d. Bronchus

7. **True about amebic liver abscess:** *(AIIMS GIS May 2008)*
   a. Male:female >10:1
   b. Not predisposed by alcohol
   c. More common in diabetics
   d. E. histolytica is isolated in >50% from blood culture

8. **Not an indication for percutaneous aspiration in amebic liver abscess:** *(AIIMS GIS May 2008)*
   a. Radiographically unresolved lesion after 6 months
   b. Suspected diagnosis
   c. Left lobe liver abscess
   d. Compression or outflow obstruction of hepatic or portal vein

9. **Commonest cause of pyogenic liver abscess:** *(AIIMS Sept 96)*
   a. Aspiration
   b. Hematogenous spread from a distant site
   c. Direct contact
   d. Lymphatic spread

10. **Anchovy sauce pus is a feature of:** *(All India 99)*
    a. Amebic liver abscess
    b. Lung abscess
    c. Splenic abscess
    d. Pancreatic abscess

11. **In pyogenic liver abscess commonest route of spread is:** *(AIIMS Nov 98, AIIMS Nov 95)*
    a. Hematogenous through portal vein
    b. Ascending infection through biliary tract
    c. Hepatic artery
    d. Local spread

12. **True statement regarding pyogenic liver abscess is/are:** *(PGI May 2018)*
    a. More common on left side of liver
    b. Surgical drainage is the treatment of choice
    c. Most common organism responsible is E. coli
    d. X-rays are diagnostic
    e. Diagnosis is confirmed by aspiration and culture

13. **Indications for needle aspiration in liver abscess are:**
    a. Recurrent *(PGI June 2006)*
    b. Left lobe
    c. Refractory to treatment after 48–72 hours
    d. >10 cm size
    e. Multiple

14. **True treatment regarding hepatic amoebiasis:** *(PGI 96)*
    a. More common in females
    b. Multiple lesions
    c. Mostly treated conservatively
    d. Jaundice is common

15. **Which one of the following is not corrected regarding amoebic liver abscess?** *(ICS 2005)*
    a. Its usual occurrence is in the right lobe
    b. Patient is toxic
    c. Surgical drainage is always indicated
    d. Extension of abscess from liver to pericardium is the most dreaded complication

16. **All are used in treatment of amoebic liver abscess except:**
    a. Diloxanide furoate *(MAHE 2007)*
    b. Chloroquine
    c. Metronidazole
    d. Emetine

17. **Not true about amebic liver abscess is:** *(DPG 2006)*
    a. Adult forms are seen
    b. Conservative treatment is generally seen
    c. Larvae are seen
    d. USG can diagnose it

18. **A patient with 8 cm × 8 cm abscess in right lobe of liver was treated with aspiration multiple times (3 times) and with systemic amebicide. Now cavity is remaining in right lobe of liver but there is nothing in the cavity. Seven days course of luminal amebicides is given. How will you follow-up?**
    a. Stool examination only *(AIIMS Nov 2012)*
    b. USG weekly for 1 month followed by monthly USG till 1 year
    c. USG weekly for 3 months followed by CT scan at 3 months
    d. USG or CT scan monthly and stool examination weekly

19. **A young patient presents to the emergency department with fever and right upper quadrant pain. Clinical examination reveals obvious hepatomegaly but there is no jaundice. Ultrasound reveals a solitary, homogeneous, hypoechoic lesion in the right lobe measuring 5 cm × 5 cm × 4 cm. Tests for hydatid disease were negative. Which of the following is the best recommendation for initial treatment?** *(All India 2011)*
    a. Multiple aspirations and antiamoebics/antibiotics
    b. Catheter drainage and antiamoebics/antibiotics
    c. Antiamoebics/antibiotics alone
    d. Hepatectomy followed by antiamoebics/antibiotics

20. Flask shaped ulcers in colon is caused by:
 (Recent Question 2019)
 a. Giardia lamblia
 b. Entamoeba histolytica
 c. H. pylori
 d. Enterobius vermicularis

HYDATID CYST

21. Water lily appearance in a chest radiograph suggests:
 (COMEDK 2005, 2004)
 a. Metastasis
 b. Cavitating metastasis
 c. Aspergilloma
 d. Ruptured hydatid cyst

22. Which of the following is not a sign of pulmonary hydatidosis? *(COMEDK 2010)*
 a. Water lily sign
 b. Rising sun sign
 c. Meniscus sign
 d. Drooping lily sign

23. Ultrasound was performed in a patient of hydatid cyst. What is the name of this sign?
 a. Water lily sign
 b. Honeycomb sign
 c. Spoke wheel sign
 d. Triradiate sign

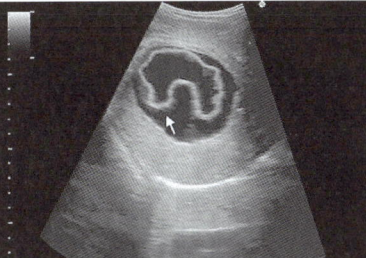

24. False about hydatid cyst of liver: *(PGI Nov 2010)*
 a. Hepatic resection is never done
 b. Laparoscopic aspiration of cyst is performed
 c. Most commonly located in the right liver
 d. Mostly asymptomatic
 e. Most common causative organism is Echinococcus granulosus

25. Not an indication for PAIR treatment in hydatid cyst:
 (PGI Nov 2010)
 a. Size >5 cm
 b. Multiloculated
 c. Cyst in lung
 d. Recurrence after surgery
 e. Perforated cyst

26. Capitonnage is used in treatment of: *(MHSSMCET 2008)*
 a. Choledochal cyst
 b. Dermoid cyst
 c. Hydatid cyst
 d. Renal cyst

27. A 40-year-old female presented with abdominal discomfort, dyspepsia and palpable abdominal mass. USG and CECT was performed. What is the diagnosis based on this ultrasound image?
 a. Hydatid cyst
 b. Multiple HCC
 c. Liver secondaries
 d. Polycystic liver disease

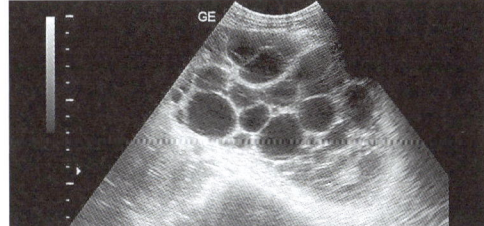

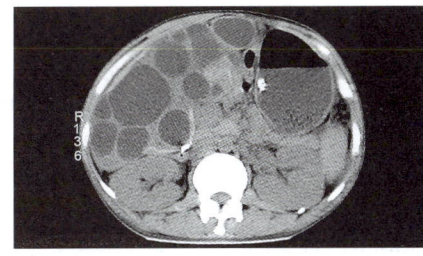

28. In the treatment of hydatid cyst, PAIR is contraindicated in:
 (PGI Dec 2006)
 a. Lung cyst
 b. Size > 5 cm
 c. Not amenable to treatment with albendazole
 d. Multiple
 e. Inaccessible location

29. A 40-year-old male presents with a painless cystic liver enlargement of four years duration without fever or jaundice. The most likely diagnosis is: *(UPSC 96)*
 a. Amoebic liver abscess
 b. Hepatoma
 c. Hydatid cyst of liver
 d. Choledochal cyst

30. All are complications of hydatid cyst in the liver except:
 a. Jaundice
 b. Suppuration *(APPG 97)*
 c. Cirrhosis
 d. Rupture

31. During surgical exploration for hydatid cyst of the liver, any of the following agents can be used as scolicidal agent except: *(UPSC 2004)*
 a. Hypertonic sodium chloride
 b. Formalin
 c. Cetrimide
 d. Povidone iodine

32. Ring like calcification on CECT is seen in:
 (Recent Question 2016)
 a. HC
 b. FNH
 c. Liver metastasis
 d. Hydatid cyst

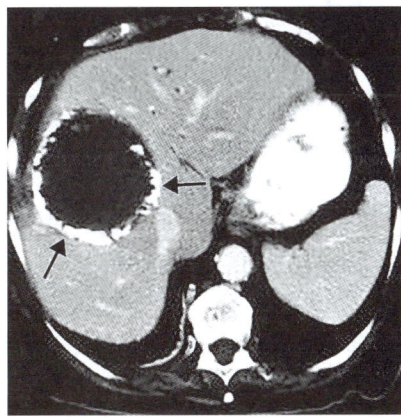

33. Which of the following is true about hydatid cyst of liver?
 (Recent Question 2014, DPG 2007)
 a. Surgical management is done always
 b. Conservative treatment is effective
 c. Aspiration is safe
 d. E. multilocularis is the most common cause

34. Treatment of hydatid cyst: *(APPG 2008)*
 a. Excision of cyst
 b. Percutaneous drainage
 c. Conservative management
 d. None

35. Investigation of choice for hydatid disease is:
    a. CT scan   b. ELISA   *(MCI Sept 2009)*
    c. Biopsy   d. USG
36. Medical management of hydatid disease is indicated in:
    a. Pregnancy
    b. Infected hydatid cyst
    c. Moribund patients
    d. Multiple peritoneal cyst
37. The sensitivity of Casoni's test is: *(Recent Question 2016)*
    a. 50%   b. 60%
    c. 75%   d. 90%
38. Malignant hydatidosis is caused by: *(Recent Question 2016)*
    a. Echinococcus granulosus
    b. Echinococcus multilocularis
    c. Echinococcus vogelli
    d. Echinococcus oligarthus
39. Malignant hydatid disease is caused by:
    (Recent Question 2017)
    a. E. granulosus   b. E. oligarthus
    c. E. vogelli   d. E. multilocularis
40. What is the name of this sign seen on CT chest?
    (Recent Question 2017)
    a. Rising sun sign   b. Water lily sign
    c. Meniscus sign   d. Serpent sign

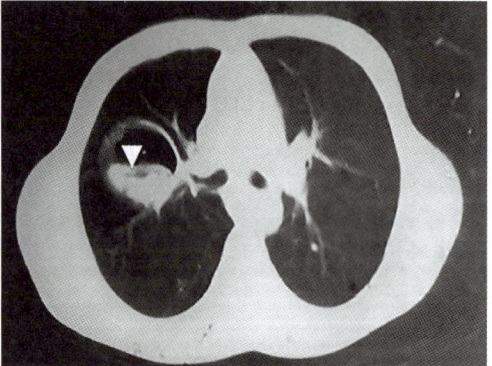

HEPATIC ADENOMA

41. False about hepatic adenoma: *(ILBS 2012)*
    a. Chances of malignancy in 10% cases
    b. Rupture in 20% cases
    c. Hepatic architecture is maintained
    d. Most patients are symptomatic
42. All are true about liver adenoma except:
    (AIIMS GIS May 2011)
    a. Normal liver architecture b. Increased fat
    c. Increased glycogen   d. Cells arranged in cords
43. About hepatic adenoma, all are true except:
    a. Increased glycogen and fat in hepatocytes
    b. Normal liver architecture   *(AIIMS GIS Dec 2009)*
    c. Bile ductules are not seen
    d. Tumor markers are normal
44. Most common cause of non-traumatic hemo-peritoneum:
    a. Hepatic adenoma   b. FNH   *(AIIMS GIS 2003)*
    c. HCC   d. Hemangioma

45. Most common liver tumor in those on OCPs:
    (MHSSMCET 2007)
    a. HCC   b. Liver cell adenoma
    c. Bile duct adenoma d. Focal nodular hyperplasia
46. All are true about hepatic adenoma except:
    a. Usually multiple   *(JIPMER GIS 2011)*
    b. OCP is a predisposing factor
    c. Has cords of benign hepatocytes
    d. 50-75% are symptomatic
47. Which of the following liver tumors always merit surgery?
    (DPG 2009 March)
    a. Hemangioma   b. Hepatic adenoma
    c. Focal nodular hyperplasia
    d. Peliosis hepatis

FOCAL NODULAR HYPERPLASIA

48. Central stellate scar is seen in: *(AIIMS GIS May 2011)*
    a. FNH   b. Hemangioma
    c. Hepatic adenoma   d. HCC
49. Radiographic image of a benign tumor is given below. What is the most probable diagnosis?
    a. Hemangioma   b. Focal nodular hyperplasia
    c. Hepatic adenoma   d. Peliosis hepatis

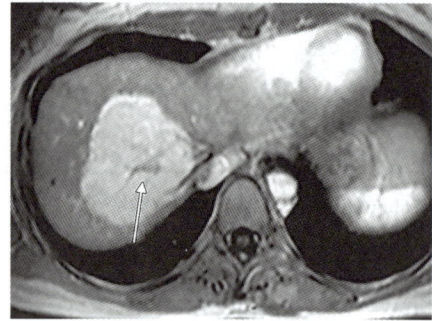

50. All of the following are true regarding FNH except:
    (AIIMS GIS Dec 2010)
    a. Not frequently associated with OCPs
    b. Surgical resection is required due to risk of malignancy
    c. Stellate scar is diagnostic
    d. Typical hepatic vascularity is not seen with spoke wheel pattern
51. True statement regarding focal nodular hyperplasia:
    a. More common in young women   *(PGI Nov 2011)*
    b. Associated with OCP use
    c. May present with abdominal pain
    d. Excision biopsy may aid in diagnosis
    e. Progress to cirrhosis
52. Similarity between FNH and hepatic adenoma are all except: *(AIIMS GIS 2003)*
    a. Hemoperitoneum is common
    b. Biliary abnormalities are seen
    c. More common in females
    d. Associated with OCPs
53. Which one of the following hepatic lesions can be diagnosed with high accuracy by using nuclear imaging?
    (AIIMS Nov 2004)
    a. Hepatocellular carcinoma
    b. Hepatic adenoma
    c. Focal nodular hyperplasia
    d. Hemangioma

HEMANGIOMA

54. All are true about liver hemangioma except:
    a. CHF is very common   *(AIIMS GIS Dec 2006)*
    b. Incidental detection
    c. Consumptive coagulopathy can occur
    d. Spontaneous regression is seen

55. Most common benign tumor of liver is:
    (DNB 2005, 2000, JIPMER GIS 2011)
    a. Hemangioma   b. Hepatic adenoma
    c. Hepatoma   d. Hamartoma

56. CECT with nodular enhancement is suggestive of:
    a. Hepatic adenoma   b. FNH *(AIIMS GIS Dec 2006)*
    c. Hemangioma   d. HCC

57. Most common nodule found in the liver is:
    a. Hepatoma   b. Hamartoma
    c. Hemangioma   d. Cholangiodenoma

58. Which is the commonest incidentaloma detected in the liver? *(Karnataka 94)*
    a. Focal nodular hyperplasia b. Hemangioma
    c. Hepatocellular adenoma   d. Hydatid cyst

59. Most common liver tumor in children: *(Recent Question 2017)*
    a. Hemangioma   b. Non-parasitic cyst
    c. Adenoma   d. Focal nodular hyperplasia

HEPATIC CYST

60. Solitary Hypoechoic lesion of the liver without septa or debris is most likely to be: *(AIIMS Nov 2005)*
    a. Hydatid cyst   b. Caroli's disease
    c. Liver abscess   d. Simple cyst

61. Simple hepatic cyst, all are true except: *(AIIMS GIS Dec 2006)*
    a. Asymptomatic
    b. Lined by columnar epithelium
    c. Intracystic bleeding is common and deroofing is mandatory
    d. Congenital

62. What is the diagnosis based on this ultrasound image?
    a. Simple hepatic cyst b. HCC
    c. Liver secondaries
    d. Intrahepatic cholangiocarcinoma

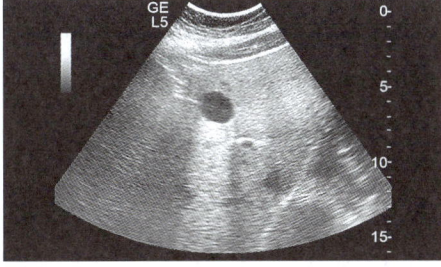

63. Treatment of choice for simple cyst of liver:
    (JIPMER November 2017)
    a. Percutaneous drainage   b. Cysto-enterostomy
    c. Deroofing   d. Aspiration

POLYCYSTIC LIVER DISEASE

64. Treatment of symptomatic polycystic liver disease is:
    (DPG 2008)
    a. Deroofing of the cyst   b. Injection of sclerosant
    c. Hepatic resection   d. Liver transplantation

HEPATOCELLULAR CARCINOMA
RISK FACTORS

65. All are risk factors for HCC except: *(AIIMS GIS Dec 2006)*
    a. HBV   b. HCV
    c. Alcohol   d. IBS

66. Which of the following most significantly increases the risk of HCC? *(AIIMS May 2012)*
    a. HBV   b. HAV
    c. CMV   d. EBV

67. True regarding HCC: *(JIPMER 2010)*
    a. Non alcoholic steatohepatitis is a risk factor
    b. OCP's are a cause
    c. Focal nodular hyperplasia may turn malignant
    d. Chromosomal abnormalities are common

HEPATOCELLULAR CARCINOMA

68. Tumor marker of HCC: *(AIIMS GIS 2003)*
    a. AFP   b. Alpha fucosidases
    c. DCGP   d. Carbohydrate antigen

69. In high risk population, HCC is best detected by:
    a. USG   b. CT *(AIIMS GIS 2003)*
    c. MRI   d. PET scan

70. All are true about AFP except: *(AIIMS GIS 2003)*
    a. Not return to normal after hepatic resection
    b. Levels >400 ng/mL with typical radiological findings is diagnostic of HCC
    c. Can be raised in other benign conditions
    d. Fibrolamellar HCC has normal levels

71. AFP is elevated in: *(PGI May 2011)*
    a. HCC   b. Hepatoblastoma
    c. Infant hemangioendothelioma
    d. Amoebic liver abscess   e. Embryonic sarcoma

72. Okuda staging contains all except: *(ILBS 2012)*
    a. Bilirubin   b. Tumor size
    c. Ascites   d. AFP

73. What is the most probable diagnosis based on this triple-phase CT?
    a. Hemangioma   b. Focal nodular hyperplasia
    c. Hepatic adenoma   d. Hepatocellular carcinoma

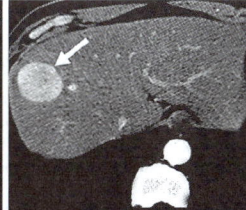
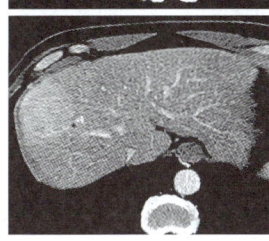
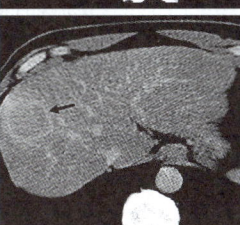

74. In HCC: *(AIIMS GIS 2003)*
    a. Arterial bruit is present in 80% cases
    b. Two third patients present with signs of liver disease
    c. Hemoperitoneum in 7% patients
    d. Percutaneous biopsy is mandatory for diagnosis

75. Most common paraneoplastic syndrome of HCC: (AIIMS GIS 2003)
    a. Hypoglycemia   b. Hypertension
    c. Hypercalcemia   d. Erythrocytosis

76. Oncological outcome in HCC is described by all except: (AIIMS GIS Dec 2010)
    a. MELD   b. BCLC
    c. CLIP   d. OKUDA

77. The following are true about HCC except: (AIIMS Nov 2003)
    a. It has a high incidence in East Africa and South East Asia
    b. Its worldwide incidence parallels the prevalence of hepatitis B
    c. Over 80% of tumors are surgically resectable
    d. Liver transplantation offers the only chance of cure in those with unresectable disease

78. The most unlikely clinical feature of hepatocellular carcinoma is: (All India 94)
    a. Hepatomegaly
    b. Raised AFP levels
    c. Raised alkaline phosphatase
    d. Jaundice

79. True about Hepatocellular carcinoma: (PGI Dec 2002)
    a. Most common tumor of liver
    b. Resectable only in 1% cases
    c. AFP increased in 70% cases
    d. USG guided aspiration biopsy is used for diagnosis

80. Spontaneous rupture of the liver occurs in:
    a. Hepatoma   b. Portal hypertension
    c. Spherocytosis   d. Secondary deposits

81. Tumor marker for primary hepatocellular carcinoma are all except: (AIIMS May 2007)
    a. Alpha-feto protein   b. Alpha-2 macroglobulin
    c. PIVKA-2   d. Neurotensin

82. All of the following are modalities of therapy for hepatocellular carcinoma except: (AIIMS Nov 2005)
    a. Radiofrequency ablation
    b. Transarterial catheter embolization
    c. Percutaneous acetic acid
    d. Nd-YAG laser ablation

83. Which of the following liver tumour has a propensity to invade the portal or hepatic vein? (AIIMS June 2004)
    a. Cavernous hemangioma
    b. Hepatocellular carcinoma
    c. Focal nodular hyperplasia
    d. Hepatic adenoma

84. Ramu, 40-year old male, chronic alcoholic, diagnosed as cirrhosis, presents with a lump in the right lobe of liver. Serum AFP level is normal. Most probable diagnosis is:
    a. Fibrohyperplasia   (AIIMS June 2001)
    b. Hepatocellular carcinoma
    c. Secondaries   d. Hepatocellular adenoma

85. Least common presentation of HCC: (AIIMS GIS 2003)
    a. PUO   b. Mass
    c. Jaundice   d. Weakness

86. Hypercalcemia is seen in: (AIIMS GIS May 2011)
    a. Pancreatic cancer   b. HCC
    c. CA stomach   d. CA GB

87. All are tumor markers of HCC except: (PGI SS Dec 2010)
    a. Neurotensin   b. AFP
    c. CA 19-9   d. PIVKA-2

88. New drug in HCC: (GB Pant 2010)
    a. Sorafenib   b. Bevacizumab
    c. Sunitinib   d. Cetuximab

89. Consider the following features - Asian Male, alcoholic cirrhosis, hypervascular lesion during arterial phase of CT & Portal vein thrombosis. The above features are mostly suggestive of: (APPG 2016)
    a. Cholangiocarcinoma
    b. Hepatocellular carcinoma
    c. Metastatic colorectal carcinoma
    d. Neuroendocrine tumors

90. The screening for HCC in chronic liver disease is: (MHCET 2016)
    a. Serial USG + AFP   b. Serial LFT + AFP
    c. Serial LFT + CT scan d. Serial USG + Serial LFT

91. Which of the following is not true about Milan's criteria? (Recent Question 2017)
    a. Single tumor <5 cm in size
    b. 3 nodules <3 cm in size
    c. >5 nodules
    d. No extrahepatic disease

92. True statement regarding hepatocellular carcinoma is/are: (PGI May 2018)
    a. Frequently associated with raised AFP
    b. Good prognosis even without resection
    c. Ultrasound guided biopsy is diagnostic
    d. There is extensive vascular invasion
    e. Most cases present with resectable tumor

FIBROLAMELLAR HCC

93. All are true about fibrolamellar HCC except:
    a. AFP is not raised   (AIIMS GIS Dec 2009)
    b. Recurrence is common
    c. Raised neurotensin levels
    d. Well demarcated and encapsulated

94. True statement about fibrolamellar carcinoma: (GB Pant 2010)
    a. Young adults, children   b. More in males
    c. Related to OCP use   d. Bad prognosis

95. All are true about fibrolamellar HCC except:
    a. Associated with cirrhosis   (AIIMS GIS 2003)
    b. Recurrences are seen despite of better prognosis
    c. Increased neurotensin and vitamin B12 binding factor
    d. Lymph node metastasis is seen

96. All of the following are true about fibrolamellar carcinoma of the liver except: (JIPMER 2012, All India 2001)
    a. More common in females
    b. Better prognosis than HCC
    c. AFP levels always >1000 pg/ml
    d. Occur in younger individuals

97. Which of the following is having better prognosis?
    a. HCC
    b. Cholangiocarcinoma
    c. Fibrolamellar variant of HCC
    d. Angiosarcoma

LIVER SECONDARIES

98. All of the following modalities can be used for in situ ablation of liver secondaries, except: (All India 2006)
    a. Ultrasonic waves   b. Cryotherapy
    c. Alcohol   d. Radiofrequency

99. Multiple liver secondaries are most common in the following cancers:
    a. Head of pancreas   b. Stomach
    c. Gallbladder   d. Periampullary

Liver

100. **All are considered to be poor prognostic factors in liver metastasis except:** *(JIPMER GIS 2011)*
    a. Synchronous lesions
    b. Metachronous lesions
    c. Extra-hepatic metastasis
    d. CEA >200 ng/ml

101. **Calcific hepatic metastases are seen in:** *(COMEDK 2009)*
    a. Adenocarcinoma of the colon
    b. Carcinoid tumours
    c. Renal cell carcinoma
    d. Lymphoma

102. **Which of the following liver metastasis appear hypoechoic on ultrasound?** *(All India 2012)*
    a. Breast cancer
    b. Colon cancer
    c. RCC
    d. Mucinous adenocarcinoma

HEPATOBLASTOMA

103. **All are true about hepatoblastoma except:**
    a. Associated with FAP *(AIIMS GIS May 2008, Dec 2006)*
    b. Most cases <3 years
    c. Prognosis is very poor with pulmonary metastasis
    d. Treatment is chemotherapy followed by surgical resection

104. **All are true about hepatoblastoma except:** *(PGI SS June 2005)*
    a. Present in childhood
    b. Common in cirrhosis of liver due to HBV
    c. Chemosensitive
    d. Surgical resection is treatment of choice

105. **AFP is raised in:** *(KGMC 2011)*
    a. 100% of hepatoblastoma
    b. 90% of hepatoblastoma
    c. 100% of HCC
    d. 90% of HCC

HEMANGIOENDOTHELIOMA

106. **All are true about hemangioendothelioma except:**
    a. Adult variant is benign *(ILBS 2012)*
    b. More common in females
    c. Multiple and involve bilateral lobe
    d. An indication for liver transplant

107. **All of the following are true regarding epitheloid hemangioendothelioma except:** *(AIIMS GIS Dec 2010)*
    a. Most common in males
    b. Liver transplantation is treatment of choice
    c. Associated with vinyl chloride
    d. Factor VIII staining is used for diagnosis

CYSTADENOMA AND CYSTADENOCARCINOMA

108. **False in cystadenoma:** *(ILBS 2012)*
    a. More common in females due to OCP use
    b. Cystadenocarcinoma presents as hemorrhagic fluid
    c. Internal septations are better delineated by USG than CT
    d. Most patients are symptomatic

109. **True about biliary cystic adenocarcinoma:** *(PGI Nov 2009)*
    a. CT scan is used for diagnosis
    b. CA 19-9 is elevated
    c. Intrahepatic location
    d. Extrahepatic location
    e. Common in males

110. **All are true about hepatic cystadenoma except:**
    a. Age >40 years and asymptomatic *(AIIMS GIS Dec 2006)*
    b. Malignant predisposition
    c. Surgical resection is required
    d. Large projection with thickened wall is suggestive of malignancy

LIVER TRANSPLANTATION

111. **Most common indication for liver transplantation in children is:** *(JIPMER GIS 2011)*
    a. Biliary atresia
    b. Indian childhood cirrhosis
    c. HCC
    d. Hepatitis C infection

112. **Place of first liver transplant:** *(ILBS 2011)*
    a. Pittsburgh
    b. Boston
    c. Colarado
    d. Cambridge

113. **Auxiliary orthotopic liver transplant is indicated for:**
    a. Metabolic liver disease *(AIIMS May 2008)*
    b. As a standby procedure until finding a suitable donor
    c. Drug induced hepatic failure
    d. Acute fulminant liver failure for any cause

114. **In orthotropic liver transplantation, which is the best way to get bile drainage in donor liver?**
    a. Donor bile duct with recipient bile duct or Roux-en-Y choledochojejunostomy
    b. Donor bile duct with duodenum of recipien
    c. Donor bile duct with jejunum of recipient
    d. External drainage for few days followed by choledochojejunostomy

115. **Reduced liver transplants:** *(GB Pant 2011)*
    a. Given to two recipients after dividing into two parts
    b. Left lateral lobe divided and given to child
    c. Left lateral segment divided from segment 2 and given to child
    d. Part of liver segment transplanted into recipient depending upon requirement

116. **Liver after transplantation enlarges by:** *(Recent Question 2015)*
    a. Increase in size of cell
    b. Increase in number of cells
    c. Both of the above
    d. None of the above

117. **All are indications of liver transplantation except:** *(Recent Question 2014)*
    a. Cholangiocarcinoma
    b. Cirrhosis
    c. Biliary atresia
    d. Fulminant hepatitis

HEPATIC RESECTION

118. **Contraindications to major hepatic resection for metastatic disease includes all of the following except:** *(COMEDK 2006, Karnataka 2006)*
    a. Total hepatic involvement
    b. Advanced cirrhosis
    c. Extrahepatic tumour involvement
    d. Jaundice from extrinsic ductal obstruction

119. **The minimum amount of normal perfused liver parenchyma to be left intact when a hepatic resection is planned is:**
    a. 10%
    b. 20% *(COMEDK 2008, 2007)*
    c. 50%
    d. 75%

120. **Regarding hepatic artery ligation which statement is false?**
    a. The best results are obtained in case of hemobilia
    b. Not useful in primary hepatoma *(Karnataka 96)*
    c. Can cure secondary carcinoma
    d. Must be covered by massive antibiotic administration

121. **Vascular inflow occlusion of the liver is by:**
    a. Clamping the hepatic artery *(DNB 2012)*
    b. Occluding the portal vein
    c. Clamping the hepatic veins
    d. The Pringle maneuver

122. **Pringle maneuver may be required for treatment of:**
    a. Injury to tail of pancreas
    b. Mesenteric ischemia
    c. Bleeding esophageal varices
    d. Liver laceration *(APPG 2015, Recent Question 2014)*

123. **Left trisegmentectomy involves removal of:** *(GB Pant 2010)*
    a. Segment II III IV V VIII
    b. Segment II III IV
    c. Segment IV V VI VII VIII
    d. Segment V VI VII VIII

HEPATIC REGENERATION

124. **Following resection of 2/3rd of the liver, regeneration is complete within:**
    a. 2-3 months
    b. 8-10 weeks
    c. 4-6 months
    d. 4-5 weeks

LIVER TRAUMA

125. **A 17-years old boy is admitted to the hospital after a road traffic accident. Per abdomen examination is normal. After adequate resuscitation, his pulse rate is 80/min and BP is 110/70 mmHg. Abdominal CT reveals 1 cm deep laceration in the left lobe of the liver extending from the done more than half way through the parenchyma. Appropriate management at this time would be:** *(DPG 2011, UPSC 2005)*
    a. Conservative management
    b. Abdominal exploration and packing of hepatic wounds
    c. Abdominal exploration and ligation of left hepatic artery
    d. Left hepatectomy

126. **'Beer-Claw' appearance on CECT abdomen is seen in:** *(MHCET 2016)*
    a. Hepatic laceration
    b. Pancreatic laceration
    c. HCC
    d. RCC

LIVER ANATOMY

127. **Left posterior sector of liver consists of:** *(JIPMER GIS 2011)*
    a. Segment II and III
    b. Segment II, III and IV
    c. Segment II only
    d. Segment I only

128. **All of the following are true about caudate lobe except:** *(AIIMS GIS Dec 2010)*
    a. Blood supply from both right and left hepatic artery
    b. Ductal drainage from both right and left duct
    c. Venous drainage is mainly by left and middle hepatic vein
    d. Supply by both branches of portal vein

129. **Which is not true regarding the basis of functional divisions of liver?** *(AIIMS May 2015)*
    a. Based on portal vein and hepatic vein
    b. Divided into 8 segments
    c. There are three major and three minor fissures
    d. 4 sectors

130. **Left medial sector contains segment:** *(GB Pant 2010)*
    a. III, IV
    b. II, III
    c. I, II
    d. I, IV

131. **Portal triad is not formed by:** *(Punjab 2008)*
    a. Hepatic artery
    b. Portal Vein
    c. Bile duct
    d. Hepatic vein

132. **Function of hepatic Kupffer cells is:** *(COMEDK 2004)*
    a. Formation of sinusoids
    b. Vitamin A storage
    c. Increase blood perfusion
    d. Phagocytosis

133. **Which of the following is false about portal vein?**
    a. Formed behind the neck of pancreas *(JIPMER 2011)*
    b. Bile duct lies anterior and right to it
    c. Gastro duodenal artery lies to the left and anterior to it
    d. Ascends behind the 2nd part of duodenum

134. **Surgeon excises a portion of liver to the left of the attachment of the falciform ligament. The segments that have been resected are:** *(All India 2011, 2008)*
    a. Segment 1a and 4
    b. Segment 1 and 4b
    c. Segment 2 and 3
    d. Segment 1 and 3

135. **False about hepatic duct:** *(AIIMS May 2011, 2009)*
    a. Left hepatic duct formed in umbilical fissure
    b. Caudate lobe drains only left hepatic duct
    c. Right hepatic duct formed by V and VIII segments
    d. Left hepatic duct crosses IV segment

136. **Surgical lobes of liver are divided on the basis of:**
    a. Hepatic artery
    b. Hepatic vein
    c. Bile ducts
    d. Portal vein *(PGI June 2002)*
    e. Central veins

137. **In Couinaud's classification, segment IV of liver is:** *(AIIMS Nov 2007)*
    a. Caudate lobe
    b. Quadrate lobe
    c. Right lobe
    d. Left lobe

138. **Line of surgical division of the lobes of the liver is:**
    a. Falciform ligament to the diaphragm *(AIIMS 85, 87)*
    b. Gall bladder bed to IVC
    c. Gall bladder bed to the left crus of diaphragm
    d. One inch to the left of falciform ligament to the IVC

139. **With Couinaud's nomenclature, which one of the following segments of liver has an independent vascularization?**
    a. Segment I
    b. Segment II *(UPSC 2002)*
    c. Segment IV
    d. Segment VIII

140. **The Couinaud's segmental nomenclature is based on the position of the:** *(All India 2004)*
    a. Hepatic veins and portal vein
    b. Hepatic veins and biliary ducts
    c. Portal vein and biliary ducts
    d. Portal vein and hepatic artery

141. **Quadrate lobe of liver is present between:** *(DPG 97)*
    a. Groove for ligamentum teres and gallbladder
    b. Inferior vena cava and fissure for ligamentum venosum
    c. Groove for inferior vena cava and fissure for ligamentum venosum
    d. Porta hepatis and falciform ligament

142. **Boundary of Morrison's pouch is formed by:** *(DPG 2008)*
    a. Kidney
    b. Falciform ligament of liver
    c. Spleen
    d. Pancreas

143. **The right lobe of liver consists of which of the following segments:** *(AIIMS 2004)*
    a. V, VI, VII and VIII
    b. IV, V, Vi, VII and VIII
    c. I, V, VI, VII and VIII
    d. I, IV, V, VI, VII and VIII

144. **Liver is divided in 2 halves by all except:** *(AIIMS 2004)*
    a. Right hepatic vein
    b. Portal vein
    c. Hepatic artery
    d. Common bile duct

145. **Which of the following is not a capsular plate?** *(AIIMS Nov 2011)*
    a. Portal plate
    b. Hilar plate
    c. Umbilical plate
    d. Cystic plate

146. **Right hepatic duct drains all, except:** *(AIIMS May 2009)*
    a. Segment I
    b. Segment III
    c. Segment V
    d. Segment VI

LIVER FUNCTION TESTS AND JAUNDICE

147. **A patient has a surgical cause of obstructive jaundice. USG can tell all of the following except:** *(AIIMS Nov 2012)*
    a. Biliary tree obstruction
    b. Peritoneal deposits
    c. Gall bladder stones
    d. Ascites

148. **Cholecystocaval line:** *(Recent Question 2019, 2018)*
    a. Separate right and left hepatic lobes
    b. Separate gallbladder from portal vein
    c. Separate right anterior and right posterior sectors
    d. Separate left medial and left lateral sectors

149. Which is wrong about Crigler-Najjar syndrome Type-I?
    a. Very high level of unconjugated bilirubin occurs in neonatal period *(Orissa 2011)*
    b. Kernicterus is usual
    c. It responds well to phenobarbitone
    d. Hepatic histology is normal

150. Conjugated hyperbilirubinemia is seen in:
    a. Dubin-Johnson syndrome
    b. Criggler-Najjar syndrome
    c. Criggler-Najjar syndrome- II
    d. Gilbert syndrome *(COMEDK 2011)*

151. **Most common surgical cause of obstructive jaundice:**
    a. Periampullary carcinoma *(NEET 2013, Punjab 2007)*
    b. Carcinoma gallbladder
    c. Carcinoma head of pancreas
    d. CBD stones

152. True about Criggler-Najjar syndrome II: *(PGI Nov 2011)*
    a. Autosomal dominant
    b. Kernicterus is frequently present
    c. Child may alive to adolescence
    d. Cause unconjugated hyperbilirubinemia
    e. Phenobarbitone therapy is ineffective

153. True about obstructive jaundice: *(PGI May 2011)*
    a. Unconjugated bilirubin
    b. Positive indirect Vanden Bergh test
    c. Pruritus   d. Pale stools
    e. Icterus

154. In non hemolytic jaundice, urobilinogen is seen in: *(PGI 99)*
    a. Obstructive jaundice   b. Hepatic fibrosis
    c. Fatty liver   d. Infective hepatitis

155. **Courvoisier's law is related to:** *(Recent Question 2016)*
    a. Jaundice   b. Ureteric calculi
    c. Portal hypertension
    d. The length of skin flap in skin grafting

156. **Which of the following is an exception of Courvoisier's law?** *(Recent Question 2015)*
    a. Double impaction   b. Portal lymphadenopathy
    c. Periampullary Carcinoma d. None of above

157. Which is not elevated in a child presenting with jaundice, icterus, pruritus and clay colored stools?
    (AIIMS Nov 2011, Nov 2006)
    a. Gamma glutamyl transpeptidase
    b. Alkaline phosphatase
    c. 5'-nucleotidase
    d. Glutamate dehydrogenase

158. One is not the feature of obstructive jaundice:
    a. Pruritus   *(AIIMS Nov 95)*
    b. Elevated level of serum bilirubin
    c. Raised alkaline phosphatase
    d. Raised urinary urobilinogen

159. Vitamin to be corrected in obstructive jaundice: *(DNB 2009)*
    a. Vitamin K   b. Vitamin C
    c. Vitamin D   d. Vitamine B12

160. A 50 years old patient presented with progressive jaundice. Liver function test was done in which conjugated serum bilirubin-4.8% and total bilirubin-6.7%, alkaline phosphatase-550 IU, SGOT-50, SGPT-65. Most probable diagnosis is: *(AIIMS Nov 2013)*
    a. Jaundice due to choledocholithiasis
    b. Dubin-Johnson syndrome
    c. Viral hepatitis
    d. Malignant obstructive jaundice

161. In a patient with obstructive jaundice, what is the possible explanation for a bilirubin level of 40 mg/dL?
    a. Malignant obstruction   *(AIIMS November 2016)*
    b. Complete obstruction of common bile duct
    c. Renal failure   d. Liver failure

MISCELLANEOUS

162. **Liver biopsy is done through 8th ICS midaxillary line to avoid:** *(All India 97)*
    a. Lung   b. Pleural cavity
    c. Subdiaphragmatic space   d. Gallbladder

163. **"Crumbled egg appearance" in liver is seen in:**
    (Recent Question 2016)
    a. Hepatic adenoma
    b. Chronic amoebic liver abscess
    c. Hydatid liver disease   d. Hemangioma

164. **"Honey-comb liver is seen in:** *(Recent Question 2016)*
    a. Micronodular cirrhosis
    b. Dubin Johnson's syndrome
    c. Actinomycosis   d. Hydatidosis

165. Primary sinusoidal dilatation of liver is also known as:
    (COMEDK 2010)
    a. Hepar lobatum   b. Peliosis hepatic
    c. Von-Meyerburg complex d. Caroli's disease

166. Obstruction of IVC leads to: *(Punjab 2008)*
    a. Dilatation of thoracoepigastric veins
    b. Caput medusae
    c. Hemorrhoids   d. Esophageal varices

167. Middle aged man presents with complaints of weakness, fatigue and hyperpigmentation. On examination hepatomegaly and hypoglycemia are present. Diagnosis:
    (JIPMER 2011)
    a. Addison's disease   b. Hemochromatosis
    c. IDDM   d. Cushing's syndrome

168. A 20 years old male presents with extrapyramidal symptoms and liver damage. Diagnosis:
    a. Wilson's disease   b. Huntington's disease
    c. Parkinson's disease   d. Hemochromatosis

169. Risk factor for angiosarcoma of liver: *(MHSSMCET 2008)*
    a. OCPs   b. Phenacetin
    c. Vinyl chloride   d. All of the above

170. Focal lesion of liver is best detected by: *(AIIMS GIS 2003)*
    a. MRI   b. CT
    c. USG   d. PET scan

Explanations

LIVER ABSCESS

1. **Ans. b. Staph. aureus** *(Ref: Sabiston 20/e p1445-1449; Schwartz 10/e p1284-1285; Bailey 27/e p1168; Blumgart 6/e p1074, 5/e p1006-1115; Shackelford 8/e p1434, 7/e p1464-1471)*

   ### PYOGENIC LIVER ABSCESS IN CHILDREN

   - In **children, Staphylococcus PLA**[Q] is most common
   - Occurs in the setting of **chronic granulomatous disease**[Q], disorder of granulocyte function and **hematologic malignancies**.
   - In chronic granulomatous conditions, abscess are **dense and thick**, **early excision** and **treatment** with **antibiotics against Staphylococcus** aureus is recommended[Q].

2. **Ans. a. E. coli**
3. **Ans. b. Biliary tract infection**
4. **Ans. d. Percutaneous drainage is least cured**
5. **Ans. c. More common in left side, d. More common in female** *(Ref: Sabiston 20/e p1449-1452; Schwartz 10/e p1285; Bailey 27/e p1168; Blumgart 6e/ p1074-1076, 5/e p1016-1024; Shackelford 8/e p1431, 7/e p1471-1478)*
6. **Ans. b. Peritoneal cavity**
7. **Ans. a. Male:female >10:1**
8. **Ans. a. Radiographically unresolved lesion after 6 months** *(Ref: Sabiston 20/e p1452)*

   ### AMOEBIC LIVER ABSCESS

   - Although **clinical improvement after adequate treatment** with antiamebic agents **is the rule**, **radiologic resolution** of the abscess cavity is **usually delayed**.
   - The **average time to radiologic resolution** is **3 to 9 months** and can take as long as years in some patients.
   - Studies have shown that **more than 90%** of the **visible lesions disappear radiologically**, but a small percentage of patients are left with a clinically irrelevant residual lesion.

9. **Ans. b. Hematogenous spread from a distant site**

   Hematogenous spread is most common among the given options.

10. **Ans. a. Amebic liver abscess**
11. **Ans. b. Ascending infection through biliary tract**
12. **Ans. c. Most common organism responsible is *E. coli*, e. Diagnosis is confirmed by aspiration and culture** *(Ref: Schwartz 10/e p1284-1285; Sabiston 20/e p1445-1449; Bailey 27/e p1168)*
13. **Ans. b. Left lobe, d. >10 cm size**
14. **Ans. c. Mostly treated conservatively**
15. **Ans. c. Surgical drainage is always indicated**
16. **Ans. a. Diloxanide furoate** *(Ref: Goodman Gilman 12/e p1420)*

    ### DILOXANIDE FUROATE

    - **Diloxanide furoate** is **highly effective luminal amebicide**[Q] but has **no systemic anti-amebic activity**[Q], because furoate ester is hydrolysed in the intestine and the released diloxanide is absorbed.
    - Diloxanide is a weaker amebicide than its furoate ester and no systemic antiamebic activity is seen despite its absorption.

17. **Ans. c. Larvae are seen** *(Ref: Bailey 27/e p1169; Schwartz 10/e p1285)*

    Larvae are not seen in amoebic liver abscess.

18. **Ans. b. USG weekly for 1 month followed by monthly USG till 1 year** *(Ref: Sabiston 20/e p1451; Schwartz 10/e p1284; Blumgart 6/e p 1087, 5/e p1016-1024; Shackelford 8/e p1440, 7/e p1471-1478)*

    In **uncomplicated cases of amebic liver abscess**, follow-up is done with ultrasound.

19. **Ans. c. Antiamebics/antibiotics alone**

   - Presence of a **solitary homogeneous, hypoechoic lesion** in the **right lobe** of the liver in a **young patient** with **fever** and **right upper quadrant pain** suggests a diagnosis of **amebic liver abscess**.
   - The **initial treatment of choice** for amebic liver abscess is **metronidazole alone**.
   - **Multiple aspirations** and/or **catheter drainage** or **hepatectomy** have **no role** in the "initial" management of **amebic liver abscess**.

20. **Ans. b. Entamoeba histolytica** *(Ref: Schwartz 10/e p1285; Bailey 27/e p58)*

HYDATID CYST

21. **Ans. d. Ruptured hydatid cyst** *(Ref: Sabiston 20/e p1452-1455; Schwartz 10/e p1285-1286; Bailey 27/e p1169; Blumgart 6/e p1108, 5/e p1035-1048; Shackelford 8/e p1425, 7/e p1459-1462)*

22. **Ans. d. Drooping lily sign** *(Ref: Wolfgang 2/e p309)*

   - **Drooping lily sign** is seen in **neuroblastoma** and **duplication of ureter**[Q].
   - Duplication of ureter: **Drooping lily sign**[Q] **on IVP** (Nonvisualized upper pole of a duplex system displaces the lower pole down, looking like a drooped down lily flower on IVP)

Characteristic Signs of Pulmonary Hydatidosis	
• Meniscus sign[Q]	• Water lily sign[Q]
• Double arc sign[Q]	• Crescent sign[Q]
• Moon sign[Q]	

WHO Classification of Hydatid Cyst	
CL Type	• Well-circumscribed liquid image with a **clearly defined wall**
CE 1	• Concentric hyperechogenic halo around the cyst which may contain free-floating hyperechogenic foci called **hydatid sand**[Q]
CE 2	• Multivesicular cyst with the daughter and grand-daughter cysts identified by **honeycomb, rosette, spoke wheel** or **cluster images**[Q]
CE 3	• Partial or total detachment of the laminated layer with floating undulated hyperechogenic membranes showing the dual wall, **water lilly** and **water snake signs**[Q].
CE 4	• **Cystic** and **solid components**[Q] together without visible daughter cysts.
CE 5	• Matrix or amorphous mass with a **solid** or **semisolid appearance**; limited amount of calcification; **least common** type.

- Only **completely calcified cyst** (eggshell appearance) is accepted as a **dead cyst**.
- CL, CE 1, and CE 2 are active fertile cysts; CE 3 is a **transitional cyst** with degeneration started; CE 4 is a degenerated cyst; CE 5 is a calcified cyst; CE 4 and CE 5 is **inactive cyst**.

Gharbi Classification of Hydatid Cyst	
Type I	Pure (clear) **fluid collection**[Q]
Type II	Fluid collection with a **split wall** (Floating membrane)[Q]
Type III	Fluid collection with septa (**Honeycomb** image)[Q]
Type IV	Heterogeneous complex mass[Q]
Type V	Calcified mass (eggshell)[Q]

23. **Ans. a. Water lily sign** *(Ref: Bailey 27/e p66)*
24. **Ans. a. Hepatic resection is never done**
25. **Ans. b. Multiloculated, c. Cyst in lung, d. Recurrence after surgery, e. Perforated cyst**
26. **Ans. c. Hydatid cyst:** *(Ref: Blumgart 6/e p1114, 5/e p1045)*

Methods of Management of the Residual Cavity after Cyst Evacuation		
• External tube drainage	• Omentoplasty[Q]	• Introflexion plus omentoplasty
• Capsulorrhaphy	• Internal collapse[Q]	• Cystojejunostomy or Cystogastrostomy
• **Capitonnage**[Q]	• **Introflexion**[Q]	
• Myoplasty	• Marsupialization[Q]	

27. **Ans. a. Hydatid cyst**

28. **Ans. a. Lung cyst, e. Inaccessible location** *(Ref: Sabiston 20/e p1454; Bailey 27/e p1169; Blumgart 6/e p1117, 5/e p1047-1048; Shackelford 8/e p1425, 7/e p1461)*
29. **Ans. c. Hydatid cyst of liver**
30. **Ans. c. Cirrhosis**
31. **Ans. b. Formalin**
32. **Ans. d. Hydatid cyst** *(Ref: Sabiston 20/e p1452)*
    - Ring like calcification on CECT is seen in hydatid cyst.
33. **Ans. c. Aspiration is safe** *(Ref: Bailey 27/e p1169)*
    Aspiration is safe in Hydatid cyst of liver.
34. **Ans. b. Percutaneous drainage**
35. **Ans. b. ELISA**
36. **Ans. d. Multiple peritoneal cyst, c. Moribund patients** *(Ref: Sabiston 20/e p1453)*
37. **Ans. b. 60%**
    - The sensitivity of Casoni's test varies from 55 to 65%^{Q}.
38. **Ans. b. Echinococcus multilocularis**
39. **Ans. d. E. multilocularis** *(Ref: Sabiston 20/e 1452p; Schwartz 10/e p1286)*
40. **Ans. b. Water lily sign** *(Ref: Wolfgang 2/e p309)*

    "The **water-lily sign** is seen in **hydatid cyst** when there is **detachment of the endocyst membrane** which results in **floating membranes within the pericyst** that mimic the **appearance of a water lily**. It is classically described on **plain radiographs** (mainly **chest X-ray**) when the **collapsed membranes are calcified** but may be seen on **ultrasound and CT**."

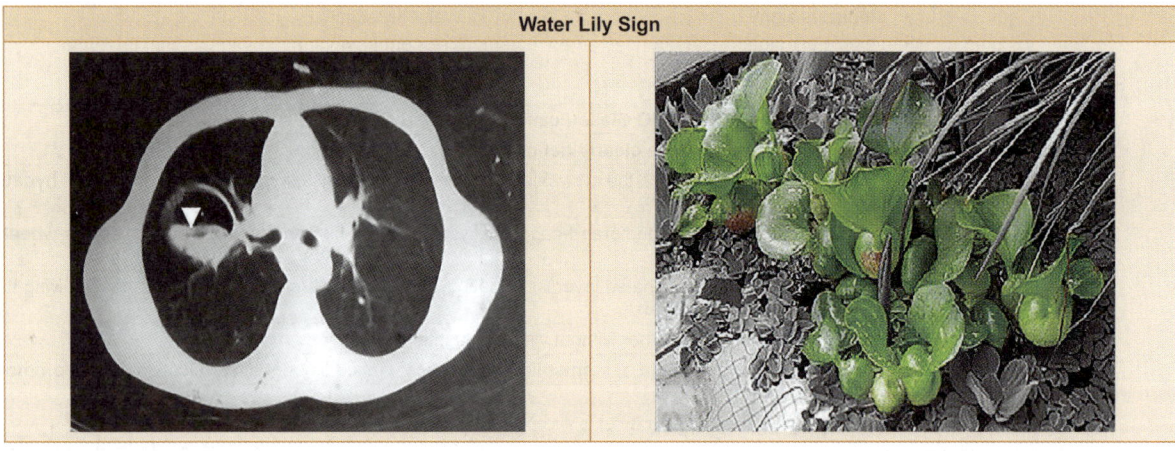

HEPATIC ADENOMA

41. **Ans. c. Hepatic architecture is maintained** *(Ref: Sabiston 20/e p1455; Schwartz 10/e p1290-1291; Bailey 26/e p1083; Blumgart 6/e p1284, 5/e p1258-1262; Shackelford 8/e p1537, 7/e p1564-1565)*
42. **Ans. a. Normal liver architecture**
43. **Ans. b. Normal liver architecture**
44. **Ans. a. Hepatic adenoma**
45. **Ans. b. Liver cell adenoma**
46. **Ans. a. Usually multiple**
47. **Ans. b. Hepatic adenoma** *(Ref: Bailey 27/e p1172; Taber's Medical Dictionary 19/e p1600)*

    Hepatic adenoma always merits surgery. As **no characteristic radiological features to differentiate** these lesions **from malignant tumor**. These tumors are thought **to have malignant potential** and **resection** is therefore the **treatment of choice**^{Q}.

FOCAL NODULAR HYPERPLASIA

48. **Ans. a. FNH** *(Ref: Sabiston 20/e p1456; Schwartz 10/e p1291; Bailey 27/e p1172; Blumgart 6/e p1306, 5/e p1255-1258; Shackelford 8/e p1536, 7/e p1563-1564)*
49. **Ans. b. Focal nodular hyperplasia** *(Ref: Sabiston 20/e p1456; Schwartz 10/e p1291; Bailey 27/e p1172)*

    The given image shows central stellate scar, which is seen in focal nodular hyperplasia.

50. **Ans. b. Surgical resection is required due to risk of malignancy**

51. Ans. a. More common in young women, b. Associated with OCP use, c. May present with abdominal pain, d. Excision biopsy may aid in diagnosis
52. Ans. a. Hemoperitoneum is common
53. Ans. c. Focal Nodular Hyperplasia

HEMANGIOMA

54. Ans. a. CHF is very common *(Ref: Sabiston 20/e p1456-1457; Schwartz 10/e p1289-1290; Bailey 27/e p1172; Blumgart 6/e p1300, 5/e p1250-1255; Shackelford 8/e p1532, 7/e p1560-1563)*
55. Ans. a. Hemangioma
56. Ans. c. Hemangioma
57. Ans. c. Hemangioma
58. Ans. b. Hemangioma *(Ref: Schwartz 10/e p1288-1289; Bailey 27/e p1172; Blumgart 6/e p1300, 5/e p1250-1262)*

Hemangioma	Hepatic Adenoma	Focal Nodular Hyperplasia	Peliosis Hepatis
• MC hepatic neoplasm^Q • **Benign** in nature • CT scan showing characteristic appearance of **slow contrast enhancement** due to **small vessel uptake**^{Q} in the hemangioma • Little malignant potential, hemangioma is **not an indication** for **surgery**^{Q}	• Rare benign liver tumors • **No** characteristic **radiological features** to **differentiate** these lesions **from malignant tumors**^{Q} • These tumors are thought to have **malignant potential** and **resection** is the **treatment of choice**^{Q}	• **Benign condition**^{Q} of unknown etiology • **Focal overgrowth**^{Q} of functioning liver tissue supported by fibrous stroma • Patients are **middle aged females**^{Q}, no association with underlying liver disease • **Sulphur colloid scan** of liver is useful for diagnosis. **FNH contain** both **hepatocytes** and **Kupffer cells**^{Q}. The **latter take up** the **colloid**, differentiating FNH from either a benign **adenoma** or a **primary** or metastatic cancer, none of which **contains** a significant number of **Kupffer cells**^{Q}.	• **Multiple cystic blood filled spaces**^{Q} in the liver associated with **dilatation of the sinusoids**^{Q}. • Leads to **hepatic enlargement** and **pain**^{Q} • Associated with use of **OCPs, anabolic steroids** and **Bartonella**^{Q} • If due to **infection**, treatment requires **parenteral doxycycline**^{Q} (surgery is not required in every case)

59. Ans. a. Hemangioma *(Ref: Sabiston 20/e p1456; Schwartz 10/e p1289; Bailey 27/e p1171)*

HEPATIC CYST

60. Ans. d. Simple cyst: *(Ref: Sabiston 20/e p1469; Schwartz 10/e p1288-1289; Blumgart 6/e p530, 5/e p1052-1054; Shackelford 8/e p1421, 7/e p1453-1457)*
61. Ans. c. Intracystic bleeding is common and deroofing is mandatory
62. Ans. a. Simple hepatic cyst *(Ref: Sabiston 20/e p1469; Schwartz 10/e p1288; Blumgart 6/e p530, 5/e p1052-1054; Shackelford 8/e p1421, 7/e p1453-1457)*

Simple Hepatic Cyst
• Contain **serous fluid**, **do not communicate** with the biliary tree, and **do not have septations**^{Q} • **Diagnosis: USG (Posterior acoustic enhancement)**

63. Ans. c. Deroofing *(Ref: Schwartz 10/e p1289; Sabiston 20/e p1469)*

POLYCYSTIC LIVER DISEASE

64. Ans. a. Deroofing of the cyst *(Ref: Sabiston 20/e p1469; Schwartz 10/e p1288-1289; Blumgart 6/e p1140, 5/e p1054-1062; Shackelford 8/e p1424, 7/e p1457-1458; Maingot 11/e p776)*

Treatment of **symptomatic polycystic liver disease** is **deroofing** of the **cyst**.

HEPATOCELLULAR CARCINOMA: RISK FACTORS

65. Ans. d. IBS *(Ref: Sabiston 20/e p1458; Schwartz 10/e p1291, 1294-1296; Bailey 27/e p1173; Blumgart 6/e p1334, 5/e p1284; Shackelford 8/e p1542, 7/e p1565-1568)*
66. Ans. a. HBV
67. Ans. a. Non alcoholic steatohepatitis is a risk factor *(Ref: Shackelford 8/e p1542, 7/e p1567)*
   • Cirrhosis due to NAFLD (**Non-alcoholic fatty liver disease**) mainly **caused by obesity** is a **risk factor for HCC**.

HEPATOCELLULAR CARCINOMA

68. Ans. a. AFP *(Ref: Sabiston 20/e p1458-1463; Schwartz 10/e p1294-1296; Bailey 27/e p1175; Blumgart 6/e p1335, 5/e p1283-1289; Shackelford 8/e p1544, 7/e p1567-1576)*

69. **Ans. a. USG**
70. **Ans. a. Not return to normal after hepatic resection**
71. **Ans. a. HCC, b. Hepatoblastoma**
72. **Ans. d. AFP** *(Ref: Sabiston 20/e p1460; Blumgart 6/e p1335, 5/e p1286-1287; Shackelford 8/e p1544, 7/e p1567-1576)*
73. **Ans. d. Hepatocellular carcinoma** *(Ref: Sabiston 20/e p1459; Schwartz 10/e p1291; Bailey 27/e p1173-1174)*

> *In the given triple-phase CT, there is arterial hyper vascularization with venous washout, diagnostic of HCC.*

74. **Ans. c. Hemoperitoneum in 7% patients** *(Ref: Sabiston 20/e p1459)*

Clinical Features of HCC

- **Vascular bruit (25%)**^{Q}, GI bleed (**10%**), tumor rupture (**2-5%**)^Q, jaundice due to biliary obstruction (**10%**), paraneoplastic syndrome (<**5%**).

75. **Ans. a. Hypoglycemia** *(Ref: Sabiston 20/e p1459)*

Paraneoplastic Syndromes in HCC

- **Hypercholesterolemia (MC)**^{Q} > **hypoglycemia**^{Q}, erythrocytosis, hypercalcemia

76. **Ans. a. MELD**
77. **Ans. c. Over 80% of tumors are surgically resectable**
78. **Ans. d. Jaundice**
79. **Ans. c. AFP is increased in 70% cases**
80. **Ans. a. Hepatoma**
81. **Ans. b. Alpha-2 macroglobulin**
82. **Ans. d. Nd-YAG laser ablation** *(Ref: Sabiston 20/e p1461; Schwartz 10/e p1291, 1294-1296; Bailey 27/e p1174; Blumgart 6/e p1338, 5/e p1287-1288; Shackelford 8/e p1547, 7/e p1571-1577)*

Treatment of HCC

- **Hepatic resection** as the **first-line treatment** for cirrhotic patients with small HCC and **preserved liver function** and reserve salvage **transplantation** for **recurrence** or **deterioration of liver function** after hepatic resection^Q
- Only patients with **normal bilirubin** concentration and **absence of portal hypertension** should be considered for **resection**^{Q}.
- If not candidate for surgery offer **percutaneous ablation**; patients with more advanced disease (**large** or **multifocal HCC**) **without portal vein invasion** are candidates for **transarterial chemoembolization** if liver function is preserved (the sole palliative approach that has been shown to have a **positive impact** in **survival** is transarterial chemoembolization)^Q.

> - For **patients without cirrhosis** who develop **HCC**, resection is the treatment of choice^Q.
> - For those patients with **Child's class A cirrhosis** with **preserved liver function** and **no portal hypertension, resection** also is considered^Q.
> - If **resection** is **not possible** because of **poor liver function** and the HCC meets the **Milan criteria** (one nodule <5 cm, or two or three nodules all <3 cm, no gross vascular invasion or extrahepatic spread), **liver transplantation** is the **treatment of choice**^{Q}.

Milan Criteria (Mazzafero)		
• One nodule <5 cm	• Two or three nodules all <3 cm	• No gross vascular invasion or extrahepatic spread

83. **Ans. b. Hepatocellular carcinoma** *(Ref: Sabiston 20/e p1459; Schwartz 10/e p1291-1294-1296; Blumgart 6/e p1334, 5/e p1344; Shackelford 8/e p1547, 7/e p1573-1574)*

Hepatocellular Carcinoma

- **HCC derive its blood supply** from **hepatic artery**^{Q}.
- **HCC** is characterized by being **hyperdense** on the **arterial phase** of contrast imaging, meaning that they have **more arterial perfusion**^{Q}.
- Arterial perfusion of HCC also allows for **treatment** of the **lesions via embolization** of feeding artery^Q.
- Characteristic of HCC: Propensity to invade the **portal vein**^{Q}.
- **Risk of portal vein invasion** appears to **correlate with tumor size** & **differentiation**^{Q}.
- **Outcome** of patients with **portal venous invasion** is **worse** than that of patients whose tumor does not invade the portal vein.

84. **Ans. b. Hepatocellular carcinoma**

This is a **typical case of HCC**, remember **AFP is raised** in about **75% of Africans** and only **30% of patients in US** and **Europe**.

85. **Ans. a. PUO** *(Ref: Sabiston 20/e p1459; Schwartz 10/e p1291, 1294-1296)*

Rare Presentations of HCC

- On **rare occasions**, HCC can present as a **rupture** with the sudden onset of abdominal pain followed by **hypovolemic shock** secondary to **intraperitoneal bleeding**.
- Other rare presentations include **hepatic vein occlusion (Budd-Chiari syndrome)**, **obstructive jaundice, hemobilia**, or **fever of unknown origin (PUO)**^{Q}.

86. Ans. b. HCC
87. Ans. c. CA 19-9
88. Ans. a. Sorafenib *(Ref: Sabiston 20/e p1462; Blumgart 6/e p1513, 5/e p1289; Shackelford 8/e p1547, 7/e p1568)*

Sorafenib

- **Sorafenib** inhibits serine/threonine kinase Raf-1, **vascular endothelial growth factor receptor** 1, 2, 3; **platelet-derived growth factor receptor -β**; and **tumorigenic receptor tyrosine kinases** (RTKs; RET, Flt-3, and c-Kit)^Q.
- **Sorafenib** is **approved** as a standard therapy **for unresectable HCC**^{Q}.

89. Ans. b. Hepatocellular carcinoma
90. Ans. a. Serial USG + AFP
91. Ans. c. >5 nodules *(Ref: Shackelford 8/e p1551, 7/e p1576; Sabiston 20/e p645; Schwartz 10/e p1295; Bailey 27/e p1175)*
92. Ans. a. Frequently associated with raised AFP, c. Ultrasound guided biopsy is diagnostic, d. There is extensive vascular invasion *(Ref: Schwartz 10/e p1294-1296; Sabiston 20/e p1461; Bailey 27/e p1174)*

FIBROLAMELLAR HCC

93. Ans. d. Well demarcated and encapsulated *(Ref: Sabiston 20/e p1462-1463; Blumgart 6/e p1337-1338, 5/e p1227-1228)*
94. Ans. a. Young adults, children
95. Ans. a. Associated with cirrhosis *(Ref: Sabiston 20/e p1463)*

Characteristic Feature	HCC	Fibrolamellar Variant of HCC
Age	55-60 years^Q	25-30 years^Q
Sex	Male^Q >Female	Male=Female^Q
HBV positivity	60-70%^{Q}	Rare^Q
Presence of cirrhosis	90%^{Q}	Rare^Q
Tumor Markers	AFP^Q PIVKA-2^Q	Neurotensin^Q Vitamin B12 binding globulin^Q
Tumor	Multicentric, bilobar & invasive^Q	Well-circumscribed^Q
Resectability	Unresectable in 70-75% cases^Q	Resectable in 70-75% cases^Q
Prognosis	Poor^Q	Good^Q

96. Ans. c. AFP level always >1000 pg/ml
97. Ans. c. Fibrolamellar variant of HCC

LIVER SECONDARIES

98. Ans. a. Ultrasonic waves *(Ref: Sabiston 20/e p1464-1465; Schwartz 10/e p1123; Bailey 27/e p1172; Blumgart 6/e p1665, 5/e p1290-1305; Shackelford 8/e p1568, 7/e p1585-1591)*

   Ultrasonic waves are not described as a method of local ablative therapy for liver secondaries.

99. Ans. c. Gallbladder

   CA GB leads to **multiple secondaries to liver** in **advanced stage**, and is the most common cause among the given option.

100. Ans. b. Metachronous lesions *(Ref: Sabiston 20/e p1465; Schwartz 10/e p1293-1294; Bailey 27/e p1172; Blumgart 6/e p1643, 5/e p1290-1305; Shackelford 8/e p1566, 7/e p1585-1589)*
101. Ans. a. Adenocarcinoma of the colon *(Ref: www.learningradiology.com)*

Calcified Hepatic Metastases

- **Calcified hepatic metastases** are most frequently associated with **mucin-producing neoplasms** such as **colon carcinoma**^{Q} or less likely **ovarian carcinoma**.

102. **Ans. a. Breast cancer** *(Ref: Focal Liver Lesions (Springer) 2006/266)*

HEPATIC METASTASES

- Metastases from **breast cancer** are typically **hypoechoic (echopoor)**[Q] on ultrasonography.
- Metastases from **carcinoma colon** and **RCC** are typically **hyperechoic (echogenic)**[Q].
- Metastases from **mucinous adenocarcinoma** of colon are typically **calcified**[Q].

Sonographic Pattern of Hepatic Metastases

Echogenic (NCR)	Echopoor (BPL)
• **Neuroendocrine tumors**	• **Breast cancer**[Q]
• **Colonic carcinoma**[Q]	• Carcinoma pancreas
• Choriocarcinoma	• Lung cancer
• **RCC**[Q]	• Lymphoma
• Multifocal HCC	

HEPATOBLASTOMA

103. **Ans. c. Prognosis is very poor with pulmonary metastasis** *(Ref: Sabiston 20/e p1464; Schwartz 10/e p1641-1642; Blumgart 5/e p1328-1334; Shackelford 7/e p2037-2038)*

104. **Ans. b. Common in cirrhosis of liver due to HBV**   105. **Ans. b. 90% of hepatoblastoma**

HEMANGIOENDOTHELIOMA

106. **Ans. a. Adult variant is benign** *(Ref: Blumgart 6/e p1395, 5/e p1246)*
     - **Infantile variety** is **benign**, **adult** one is **malignant** and **highly aggressive**[Q].

107. **Ans. a. Most common in males**
     Epitheloid hemangioendothelioma is **more common in females.**

CYSTADENOMA AND CYSTADENOCARCINOMA

108. **Ans. a. More common in females due to OCP use** *(Ref: Sabiston 20/e p1469; Schwartz 10/e p1409-1413; Blumgart 6/e p1326, 5/e p1268-1276; Shackelford 8/e p1426, 7/e p1459)*

109. **Ans. a. CT scan is used for diagnosis, b. CA 19-9 is elevated, c. Intrahepatic location** *(Ref: Sabiston 20/e p1469, 19/e p1464; Blumgart 6/e p1327-1328, 5/e p1277-1280; Shackelford 8/e p1426, 7/e p1459)*

110. **Ans. a. Age > 40 years and asymptomatic**
     Majority of patients of biliary cystadenoma present with a **history of abdominal pain** or **mass**[Q].

LIVER TRANSPLANTATION

111. **Ans. a. Biliary atresia** *(Ref: Sabiston 20/e p637-638; Schwartz 10/e p1277; Bailey 27/e p1554; Blumgart 6/e p661, 5/e p1662-1663; Shackelford 8/e p1365, 7/e p1519-1520)*

112. **Ans. c. Colorado** *(Ref: Sabiston 20/e p637, 19/e p655-664; Schwartz 10/e p1277, 9/e p295; Bailey 27/e p1554, 26/e p1427, 25/e p1408; Blumgart 6/e p1848, 5/e p1662)*

113. **Ans. a. > d. Metabolic liver disease >Acute fulminant liver failure for any cause** *(Ref: Blumgart 6/e p 1779, 5/e p1689-1693)*
     APOLT is **used in acute fulminant liver failure** mainly **caused by metabolic liver diseases**, not in liver failure from any cause.

INDICATIONS OF AUXILIARY PARTIAL ORTHOTOPIC LIVER TRANSPLANTATION (APOLT)

1. Reversible fulminant hepatic failure[Q]
2. Small-for-size grafts[Q]
3. Non-cirrhotic metabolic liver disease[Q]
4. ABO-incompatibility[Q]

Auxiliary Partial Orthotopic Liver Transplantation (APOLT)

- In fulminant hepatic failure, **APOLT** provides **temporary support** until the **native liver** recovers and then immunosuppression can be withdrawn.
- **APOLT** can **compensate** for **enzyme deficiency** in **non-cirrhotic metabolic liver disease** (most commonly Criggler-Najjar syndrome) without complete removal of native liver.
- Transplants of **ABO-incompatible grafts** are often unavoidable due to **limited number of potential donor** candidates. A **high incidence** of **early graft failure** with a high rate of **biliary** and **vascular complications** in ABO-incompatible liver transplantation is reported. The **remnant liver** could **sustain a patient's life** if the anticipated **graft failure** occurred in an ABO-incompatible case.
- In **small-for-size graft**, the **remnant liver** is expected to **support** the function of **implanted graft** during the **early post-op period**. The graft liver expands its function in proportion to volume growth. After the graft liver has grown sufficiently, it can be expected to meet the hepatic functional demands of the recipient.

114. **Ans. a. Donor bile with recipient bile duct or Roux-en-Y choledochojejunostomy** *(Ref: Blumgart 6/e p1807, 5/e p1727-1728)*

The **preferred method biliary drainage** during **orthotropic liver transplantation** is **direct end-to-end anastomosis** between **donor common bile duct** and **recipient common bile duct**.

Bile duct anastomosis in orthotropic liver transplantation

Choledochocholedochostomy (CDCD)
- This is **end-to-end anastomosis** between **donor common bile duct** and **recipient common bile duct**
- This is **preferred bile duct anastomosis** and is **used** when the **recipient bile duct not diseased**.

Choledochojejunostomy (CDJ)
- This is an **Roux-en-Y configuration anastomosis** between the end of the common bile duct and the side of a loop of jejunum
- This is an **alternative bile duct anastomosis** and is **performed when CDCD anastomosis** is **not feasible**. This may be the case when the **recipient extrahepatic bile duct is diseased** or **small** or when there is **significant recipient donor duct size mismatch**.

Five sequential anastomosis of OLT (SIPH-B)
1. **S**uprahepatic IVC
2. **I**nfrahepatic IVC
3. **P**ortal vein
4. **H**epatic artery
5. **B**ile duct

115. **Ans. d. Part of liver segment transplanted into recipient depending upon requirement**

116. **Ans. b. Increase in number of cells**   117. **Ans. a. Cholangiocarcinoma**

HEPATIC RESECTION

118. **Ans. d. Jaundice from extrinsic ductal obstruction** *(Ref: Sabiston 20/e p1470; Blumgart 5/e p1462)*

    Jaundice from extrinsic ductal obstruction is not a contraindication to major hepatic resection.

119. **Ans. b. 20%** *(Ref: Blumgart 5/e p1462; Shackelford 7/e p1494)*

- Up to **70% to 75%** of the **hepatic volume** may be **resected with good recovery in patients with relatively normal hepatic parenchyma**^{Q} (without active hepatitis, cirrhosis, or metabolic defects), as long as the remnant liver has adequate portal venous and hepatic arterial inflow, adequate hepatic venous outflow, and adequate biliary drainage.

120. **Ans. b. Not useful in primary hepatoma, c. Can cure secondary carcinoma** *(Ref: Sabiston 20/e p1470; Blumgart 6/e p1925, 5/e p1344)*

Hepatic Artery Ligation

- Used in **management of hemobilia, hepatic artery aneurysm** and **pseudoaneurysm**
- **Hepatic artery ligation** or embolization is a **method of ablation** for **HCC** and liver **secondaries**, as these tumors are **exclusively supplied by hepatic artery** but it **does not cure** the **malignancy**^{Q}.
- In each case **massive antibiotic therapy** should be given **post-operatively**^{Q}.

121. **Ans. d. The Pringle maneuver** *(Ref: Sabiston 20/e p439; Blumgart 6/e p1581, 5/e p1547; Shackelford 8/e p1417, 7/e p1450-1451)*

Pringle Maneuver (Total Inflow Occlusion)

- **Total clamping** of the **hepatic pedicle**, by placing an **atraumatic clamp** across the **foramen of Winslow**[Q].
- **Appropriate-sized vascular clamp** or **loop snare** easily **controls hemorrhage** from either the **portal vein** or the **hepatic arteries**[Q].
- Inflow occlusion durations of up to **30 minutes** can be **tolerated safely** in **cirrhotic livers** and possibly up to **60 minutes** in **early disease**.
- If prolonged occlusion is required, intermittent clamping can be used with **repeated clampings** of **10-20 minutes** duration, each followed by **5 minutes declamping**.

122. Ans. d. Liver Laceration

123. Ans. a. Segment II III IV V VIII *(Ref: Blumgart 6/e p1548, 5/e p1512-1513; Shackelford 8/e p1466, 7/e p1501-1503)*

Trisegmentectomy

- **Right trisegmentectomy** or **extended right hepatectomy**: Complete resection of **segment IV** with the **right liver** (removal of segment IV, V, VI, VII, VIII)[Q].
- **Left trisegmentectomy** or **extended left hepatectomy**: Complete resection of **segments V** and **VIII** with the **left liver** (removal of segment II, III, IV, V, VIII)[Q].

HEPATIC REGENERATION

124. Ans. c. 4-6 months

Liver Regeneration

- Following **resection of 2/3rd of the liver**, regeneration is **complete within 5-6 months**.

LIVER TRAUMA

125. Ans. a. Conservative management *(Ref: Sabiston 20/e p437-439; Schwartz 10/e p173-174, 1642; Bailey 27/e p1161; Blumgart 6/e p1890-1891, 5/e p1806-1814; Shackelford 8/e p1448, 7/e p1479-1487)*

    In stable patients, conservative management is preferred option.

126. Ans. a. Hepatic laceration

LIVER ANATOMY

127. Ans. c. Segment II only *(Ref: Sabiston 20/e p1421-1422; Schwartz 10/e p1264-1269; Bailey 27/e p161)*

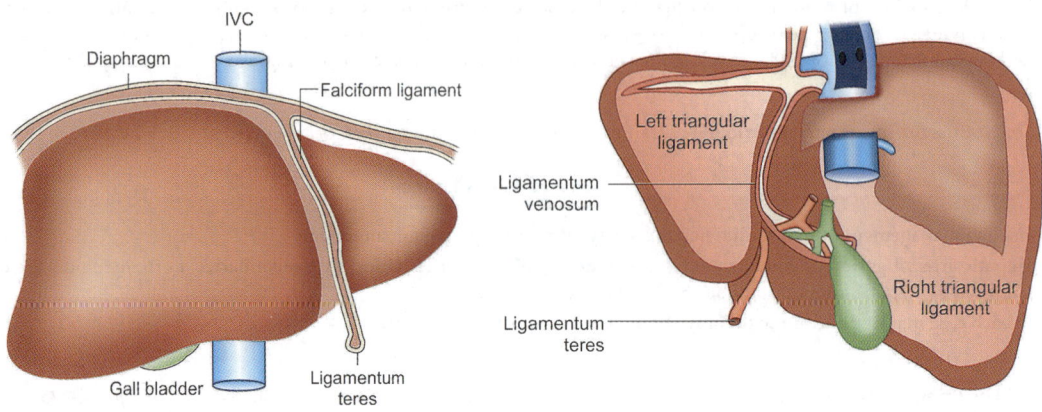

LOBAR ANATOMY OF THE LIVER

- Liver is divided into **two lobes by** the **main portal fissure** (scissura), known as **Cantlie's line**[Q].
- **Physiological right & left lobe** are **equally divided by** an imaginary line **(cholecysto-vena caval line**[Q]) running from GB fossa to groove for **IVC**[Q].

> - **Cantlie's line** describes a **75⁰ angle** with a **horizontal plane**[Q]
> - It extends from the **gallbladder fossa** to the **left side** of the **IVC**[Q].

- **Right & left halves** of the liver is **delineated by a plane** through the **MHV** and **IVC**[Q].
- **Right portal fissure** divides the right lobe into an **anteromedial** and **posterolateral sector**. RHV courses **along this fissure**[Q].
- **Right portal fissure** describe an **angle of 40⁰** with the **transverse plane**[Q].
- **Left portal fissure** divides the **left lobe** into an **anterior** and **posterior sector**, LHV courses **along this fissure**[Q].

> - In the **right lobe**:
>   - **Anteromedial sector**: Segment **V anteriorly** & segment **VIII posteriorly**[Q]
>   - **Posterolateral sector**: Segment **VI anteriorly** & segment **VII posteriorly**[Q]
> - In the **left lobe**:
>   - **Anterior sector** is divided by the umbilical fissure into **segment IV** and **segment III**[Q]
>   - **Posterior sector** is comprised of **only one segment, segment II**[Q]

- **Umbilical fissure** is **not a scissura**[Q], does not contain a hepatic vein, but **contains** the **left portal triad**.
- **Left scissura** runs **posterior** to the **ligamentum teres** and contains the **LHV**; the left liver is split into an **anterior** (segments III and IV)[Q] and **posterior** (segment II- the **only sector** composed of a **single segment**)[Q] sector by the left scissura.

128. **Ans. c. Venous drainage is mainly by left and middle hepatic vein** (Ref: Sabiston 20/e p1422; Schwartz 10/e p1267; Bailey 27/e p1154; Blumgart 6/e p37, 5/e p36; Shackelford 8/e p1250, 7/e p1431)

CAUDATE LOBE

- **Caudate lobe (segment I)**, lies between left portal vein & IVC and extends to hepatic venous confluence[Q].

> **Caudate lobe is unique**
> - It receives **blood supply** from **both right** & **left portal pedicles**[Q]
> - **Bile drain** into **both right** & **left hepatic duct**[Q]
> - **Venous drainage is directly into IVC**[Q]

- **Caudate lobe** is anatomically divided into three parts,
  1. **Spigel lobe** (Segment I)
  2. **Paracaval portion** (segment 9)
  3. **Caudate process**

129. **Ans. b. Divided into 8 segments** (Ref: Gray's 40/e p1165, 1166,1178; Sabiston 20/e p1421-1423; Blumgart 6/e p37, 5/e p31-37; Shackelford 8/e p1250, 7/e p1426-1430)

All of the given options are true. If we have to choose one answer, most preferred option is 'liver is divided into 8 segments', because sometimes segment IX is described. Segment IX is a recent subdivision of segment I, and describes that part of the segment that lies posterior to segment VIII.

> "Current understanding of the functional anatomy of the liver is based on Couinaud's division of the liver into eight (subsequently nine) functional segments, based upon the distribution of portal venous branches and the location of the hepatic veins in the parenchyma (Couinaud 1957)."-Gray's 40/e p1165

> "Segment IX is a recent subdivision of segment I, and describes that part of the segment that lies posterior to segment VIII."-Gray's 40/e p1166

130. **Ans. a. III, IV**

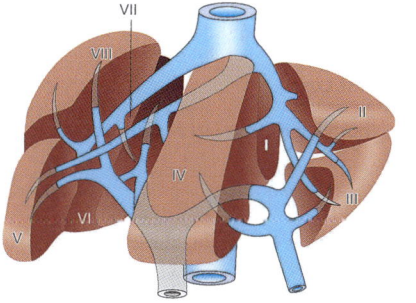
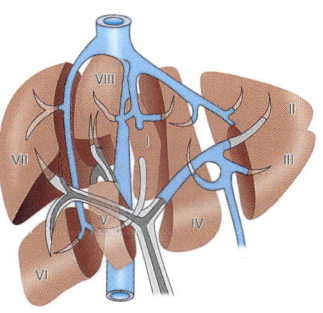

- Left medial sector contains segment **III & IV**
- Left lateral sector contains **only one segment, II**.

131. **Ans. d. Hepatic vein**

PORTAL TRIAD RELATIONS

- CBD laterally[Q]
- Portal vein posteriorly[Q]
- Hepatic artery medially[Q]

Mickey Mouse View: Ultrasound image of **hepatic artery, bile duct & portal vein** is in a **configuration**, referred as **Mickey Mouse View**[Q].

132. **Ans. d. Phagocytosis** (Ref: Sabiston 20/e p1430)

KUPFFER CELLS

- Kupffer cells, **derived from** the **macrophage-monocyte system**[Q]
- Are **irregular stellate-shaped cells** that also **line the sinusoids**, insinuating between endothelial cells.
- **Phagocytic**, play a **major role** in the **trapping of foreign substances**[Q] and initiating an inflammatory response.
- **MHC-II antigens** are **expressed on Kupffer cells** but do not confer efficient antigen presentation compared with macrophages elsewhere in the body.

HEPATIC STELLATE CELLS

- **Hepatic stellate cells** (also known as **Ito cells** or **lipocytes**) are cells **high** in **lipid content** (accounting for their phenotypic identification)[Q]
- Found **in** the **space of Disse**[Q]
- Have **dendritic processes** that contact hepatocyte microvilli and also wrap around endothelial cells.
- **Major function**: Vitamin A storage and **synthesis** of **extracellular collagen**[Q].

133. **Ans. d. Ascends behind the 2nd part of duodenum** (Ref: Gray's 40/e p1170)

Portal vein ascends behind the 1st part, not the 2nd part of duodenum.

Portal Vein		
Part	Position	Structure
Infraduodenal Part	Anterior	Neck of pancreas
	Posterior	**IVC**
Retroduodenal Part	Anterior	Duodenum (first part)[Q]
	Posterior	Common Bile duct[Q]
		Gastroduodenal artery[Q]
		IVC
Supraduodenal Part	Anterior	Hepatic artery[Q]
	Posterior	Bile duct[Q]
		IVC[Q] (separated by **epiploic foramen**)

134. **Ans. c. Segment 2 and 3** (Ref: Sabiston 20/e p1421; Schwartz 10/e p1264-1265; Bailey 27/e p1154)

FALCIFORM LIGAMENT

- Falciform ligament is the **most obvious external landmark** on the **liver surface**.
- Plane passing through the falciform ligament **passes through** the left lobe
- It **divides** the **left lobe** into a **medial segment** (segment IV) and **lateral segment** (segment II and III)[Q]

135. **Ans. b. Caudate lobe drains only left hepatic duct** (Ref: Blumgart 6/e p37, 5/e p36)

CAUDATE LOBE

- In approx. **80%** of the individuals, **caudate lobe drains** into **both** the **right** & **left** hepatic ducts[Q]
- In **15%**, caudate lobe drains **only** into **left** hepatic duct
- In **5%**, caudate is drained **exclusively by right** hepatic duct.

136. **Ans. b. Hepatic vein, d. Portal vein**   137. **Ans. b. Quadrate lobe**

138. **Ans. b. Gallbladder bed to IVC**

Liver

- Weight: **1800 gm** in **men** and **1400 gm** in **women**[Q]
- **Total blood flow**: **1.5 L/min**[Q]
- **Free pressure** in a **hepatic vein: 1-2 mm Hg**[Q]
- Liver can **store** up to maximum of **65 gm** of **glycogen/kg** of liver tissue[Q].
- Account for **4%** of **body weight**, consumes about **28%** of **total body blood flow** and **20%** of the **total oxygen** consumed by the body[Q].
- Expends **20%** of the **total kilocalories** used by the whole body.

Hepatic Vascular Supply	
Hepatic artery	**Portal vein**
• **Hepatic artery** supplies about **30 mL/min per 100 gm** of liver tissue[Q] • Approx. **25%** of the total blood flow to the liver[Q]. • Provide **30-50%** of the **oxygen requirement**[Q]. • The **intrahepatic bile ducts** are exclusively perfused by the **hepatic arterial blood** via the **peribiliary plexus**[Q].	• **Portal vein** carries **90 mL/min per 100 gm** liver tissue[Q] • It carries about **75%** of the **total blood flow** to the liver[Q]. • It may provide **50% to 70%** of the **oxygen requirement**[Q]. • Normal portal pressure is **5-10 mm Hg**[Q].

Relationship between Hepatic Artery and Portal vein Blood Flow
- There is an **increase in hepatic arterial blood flow** after **portal flow reduction** but the converse is not observed[Q].

139. Ans. a. Segment I
140. Ans. a. Hepatic veins and portal vein
141. Ans. a. Groove for ligamentum teres and gallbladder

    Quadrate lobe of liver is present **between groove** for **ligamentum teres** and **gallbladder**.

142. Ans. a. Kidney *(Ref: Gray's 40/e p1101, 1108)*

    Boundary of Morrison's pouch is formed by kidney.

Boundaries of Morrison's pouch (Hepatorenal pouch)			
Anteriorly	**Posteriorly**	**Superiorly**	**Inferiorly**
• **Inferior surface** of **right lobe** of the liver • **Gall bladder**	• **Right suprarenal** gland • Upper part of **right kidney** • **2nd part** of **duodenum** • **Hepatic flexure** of colon • Transverse **mesocolon** • Part of **head** of pancreas	• **Inferior layer** of **coronary ligament**	• Opens into general peritoneal cavity

143. Ans. a. V, VI, VII and VIII

Couinaud's Classification

- **Caudate lobe: I**[Q]
- **Left lobe: II, III, IV**[Q]
- **Right lobe: V, VI, VII, VIII**[Q]

144. Ans. a. Right hepatic vein
145. Ans. a. Portal plate *(Ref: Sabiston 20/e p1423; Bailey 27/e p1154; Blumgart 6/e p574, 5/e p41; Shackelford 8/e p2077, 7/e p1430)*

Fascial Plates of Liver Hilus

- **Fascial plates** of liver hilus, represents a fusion of **endoabdominal fascia** around the **portal structures**
- **Fascial plate** is formed by: **cystic, hilar** & **umbilical** plate[Q]
- **Hepatic veins lack endoabdominal fascial investment**[Q].

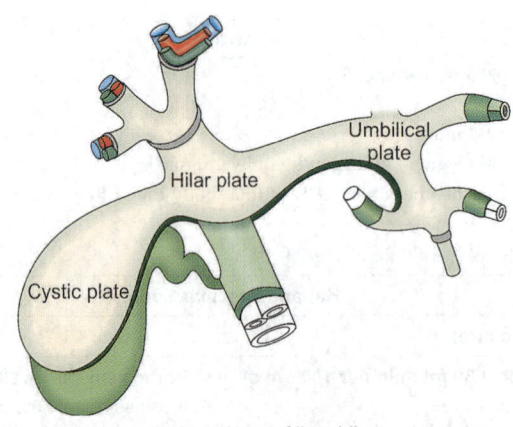

Fascial plates of liver hilus

146. **Ans. b. Segment III**

LIVER FUNCTION TESTS AND JAUNDICE

147. **Ans. b. Peritoneal deposits** *(Ref: Sabiston 20/e p1081; Schwartz 9/e p1140)*

- Peritoneal deposits are **not detected by ultrasound**. Even **CECT can miss** the **peritoneal deposits**.
- Best investigation for diagnosis of peritoneal deposits is **Diagnostic laparoscopy**.

148. **Ans. a. Separate right and left hepatic lobes**

149. **Ans. c. It responds well to phenobarbitone** *(Ref: Harrison 20/e p2344, 19/e p2001)*

Crigler-Najjar Syndromes		
Feature	Type I	Type II
Total **serum bilirubin** (mg/dL)	18-45 (usually **>20**)[Q]	6-25 (usually **20**[Q])
Routine liver tests	Normal[Q]	Normal
Response to Phenobarbital	None[Q]	Decreases bilirubin by >25%[Q]
Kernicterus	Usual[Q]	Rare[Q]
Hepatic histology	Normal[Q]	Normal[Q]
Bile characteristics		
Color	Pale or colorless	Pigmented
Bilirubin fractions	>90% unconjugated[Q]	Largest fraction (mean: 57%) **monoconjugates**[Q]
Bilirubin **UDP-glucuronosyl transferase activity**	Typically **absent**[Q]; traces in some patients	Markedly **reduced**: 0-10% of normal
Inheritance (all autosomal)	Recessive[Q]	Predominantly recessive (AR>AD)[Q]

150. **Ans. a. Dubin-Johnson syndrome** *(Ref: Harrison 20/e p2345, 19/e p2003)*

Causes of Hyperbilirubinemia		
Indirect (unconjugated) Hyperbilirubinemia		Direct (conjugated) Hyperbilirubinemia
Hemolytic disorders		Inherited Conditions: 1. Dubin-Johnson syndrome[Q] 2. Rotor's syndrome[Q]
Inherited	Acquired	
• Spherocytosis[Q] • Elliptocytosis • **G-6-PD** and pyruvate kinase deficiencies[Q] • Sickle cell anemia[Q]	• Microangiopathic hemolytic anemia • **PNH**[Q] • Immune hemolysis	
• Ineffective erythropoesis in cases of vitamin B and iron deficiencies • **Drugs: Rifampicin, ribavarin**[Q], probenicid		
Inherited conditions: • **Criggler-Najjar and Gilbert's syndrome**[Q]		

151. **Ans. d. CBD Stones**
152. **Ans. a. Autosomal dominant, c. Child may alive to adolescence, d. Cause unconjugated hyperbilirubinemia**
153. **Ans. c. Pruritus, d. Pale stools, e. Icterus** *(Ref: Harrison 20/e p2343-2345, 19/e p1998)*

OBSTRUCTIVE JAUNDICE

- **MC surgical cause** of obstructive jaundice is **CBD stones**[Q]
- Characterized by **dark urine, clay colored stools, icterus** and **pruritus**[Q].
- Presence of **urobilinogen** in **urine rules out obstructive jaundice**[Q].
- **USG** is the **best test** to **differentiate medical** from **surgical jaundice**.

Parameter	Hemolytic	Hepatocellular	Obstructive
Blood			
Hemoglobin (12-18 gm/dl)	Decreased	N	N
Unconjugated bilirubin (0.2-0.7 mg/dl)	↑	N or ↑	N
Conjugated bilirubin (0.1-0.3 mg/dl)	N	N or ↑	↑
ALP (3-13 KAU; 30-120 IU/L)	N	↑	↑
Aminotransferases	N	↑	N
Cholesterol	N	N	↑
Stool			
Colour of stool	N	N	Pale
Fecal urobilinogen	Increased	Decreased	Trace to absent
Urine			
Bilirubin	Nil		
Urobilinogen	↑	↑	↓

154. **Ans. d. Infective hepatitis**
155. **Ans. a. Jaundice** *(Ref: Saiston 20/e p1544)*
156. **Ans. a. Double impaction**
157. **Ans. d. Glutamate dehydrogenase** *(Ref: Harrison 19/e p1997, 18/e p2529)*

ENZYMES ELEVATED IN CHOLESTASIS

- **ALP**[Q]
- **5′-Nucleotidase**[Q]
- **Gamma glutamyl transpeptidase**[Q]

158. **Ans. d. Raised urinary urobilinogen**
159. **Ans. a. Vitamin K**
160. **Ans. a. Jaundice due to choledocholithiasis** *(Ref: Sabiston 20/e p1495; Schwartz 9/e p1113; Blumgart 5/e p1129-1146; Schackelford 7/e p1599-1604; Harrison 20/e p2431, 19/e p1998)*
161. **Ans. c. Renal failure** *(Ref: Bailey 27/e p213; Textbook of hepatology 6/e p206)*

All causes of **cholestatic jaundice**, i.e. malignant obstruction, complete CBD obstruction **can cause high jaundice** but presence of concomitant **renal failure leads to increase in bilirubin beyond 30 mg/dL**. This is because **conjugated bilirubin is soluble** and **can be excreted in urine**. But **in renal failure**, this mechanism is absent and the **serum bilirubin can rise up to very high levels**. Usually even in the **presence of total absence of bile flow the bilirubin levels reach a plateau of around 25-30 mg/dl as there is continuous excretion of conjugated bilirubin the bile**. When there is such **high bilirubin (>30/40 mg/dl) in obstructive jaundice**, then suspect associated **renal failure** or **ongoing hemolysis** (**Sepsis with DIC** which may be the case in **ascending cholangitis**, **sickle cell anemia**, etc.).

MISCELLANEOUS

162. **Ans. a. Lung** *(Ref: Shackelford 7/e p1491-1492)*
    - **Liver biopsy** is done through **8th ICS** in **midaxillary line** to **avoid Lung**.

LIVER BIOPSY

- **Needle biopsy** has proved to be **most useful**[Q] technique to obtain representative liver tissue for analysis.
- For accurate and reliable grading and staging of **chronic viral hepatitis**; a biopsy specimen of **2 cm**[Q] **in length** or longer containing **at least 11 complete portal tracts**[Q] is needed.
- **Liver biopsy** is done through **8th ICS** in **midaxillary line** to **avoid Lung**[Q].

163. **Ans. c. Hydatid liver disease**
     - **Crumbled egg appearance** in liver is seen in **hydatid disease**[Q].
164. **Ans. c. Actinomycosis** *(Ref: Harrison 20/e p1221, 19/e p1089)*
165. **Ans. b. Peliosis hepatic** *(Ref: Shackelford 7/e p1556-1557)*
166. **Ans. a. Dilatation of thoracoepigastric veins**
     - **IVC obstruction** can lead to **dilatation of thoracoepigastric veins**.
167. **Ans. b. Hemochromatosis** *(Ref: Harrison 20/e p2980, 19/e p2516)*

Manifestation of Hemochromatosis

- **Liver:** Hepatomegaly, cirrhosis, HCC[Q]
- **Pancreas: Diabetes mellitus**[Q]
- **Heart: CHF,** cardiomyopathy[Q]
- **Skin: Hyperpigmentation**[Q] (bronzing of skin)
- **Joints:** Arthropathy[Q]
- **Hypogonadism**[Q]

168. **Ans. a. Wilson's disease** *(Ref: Harrison 20/e p2982, 19/e p2519)*
169. **Ans. c. Vinyl chloride**
     - **Vinyl chloride** is a **risk factor** for **hepatic angiosarcoma**.
170. **Ans. a. MRI** *(Ref: Shackelford 8/e p1545, 7/e p1560, 1571)*

MRI in Liver Lesions

- **MRI** gas emerged as the **best imaging test** for **liver lesion detection** and **characterization**[Q]
- MRI provides **high lesion-to-liver contrast** and **does not use radiation**[Q].
- **Liver-specific contrast media**, such as **mangofodipir trisodium**[Q] (taken up by **hepatocytes**) and **ferrumoxides** (taken up by **Kupffer cells**)[Q] demonstrate **selective uptake** in the **liver** and are primarily **used for lesion detection**.
- These two **contrast agents** are also **useful in characterizing specific liver tumors**, such as **FNH, hepatic adenoma** and **HCC**[Q].

CHAPTER 5

Portal Hypertension

ETIOLOGY OF PORTAL HYPERTENSION

Etiology of Portal Hypertension		
Presinusoidal	**Sinusoidal**	**Postsinusoidal**
Extrahepatic or sinistral: • Splenic vein thrombosis^Q • Splenomegaly^Q • Splenic arteriovenous fistula^Q	**Intrahepatic: Cirrhosis** due to- • **HBV, HCV, Alcohol**^Q • Metabolic abnormality • Autoimmune hepatitis • Primary biliary cirrhosis & **PSC**	**Intrahepatic:** • Veno-occlusive disease^Q
Intrahepatic: • **Schistosomiasis**^Q • Congenital hepatic fibrosis • Nodular regenerative hyperplasia • Idiopathic portal fibrosis • **Myeloproliferative disorder**^Q • **Sarcoid** and **GVHD**		**Posthepatic** • **Budd-Chiari syndrome**^Q • **Congestive heart failure** • **IVC web**^Q • **Constrictive pericarditis**^Q

- MC cause of **intrahepatic presinusoidal** portal hypertension: **Schistosomiasis**^Q
- MC cause of **sinusoidal** portal hypertension: **Cirrhosis**^Q

PORTAL HYPERTENSION

PORTAL PRESSURE

- Normal portal vein pressure: **5–10 mm Hg**^Q
- Normal portal vein pressure: **10–15 cm saline**^Q
- **Variceal formation** occurs when portal pressure is **>10 mm Hg**^Q.
- **Variceal bleeding** occurs when portal pressure is **>12 mm Hg**^Q.

PORTAL HYPERTENSION

- Definition: Portal pressure >10 mm Hg^Q
- **MC cause** of portal hypertension in **United States**: Cirrhosis^Q.
- Consequence of **both increased portal vascular resistance & increased portal flow**^Q.
- Portal hypertension results in **splenomegaly** with enlarged, tortuous, & even aneurysmal splenic vessels.

> • **Cruveilhier-Baumgarten murmur**^Q: Audible **venous hum in caput medusa**

- **Hyperdynamic portal venous circulation** seems to be **related to severity of liver failure**^Q.
- **Upper GI bleeding** is caused by **portal hypertension** in about **90%** of instances.
- Most bleeding episodes occur during the **first 1 to 2 years** after **identification of varices**^Q.
- **Colour Doppler** is **investigation of choice** for evaluation of **PHT**.

> • About **one third** of **deaths** in patients with known esophageal varices are due to **upper GI bleed**^Q
> • A **larger proportion** dies as a result of **liver failure**^Q.

- **MC causes** of death in **cirrhosis** patients: **Hepatic failure**^Q
- **2nd MC causes** of **death in cirrhosis** patients: **variceal hemorrhage**^Q

LABORATORY ABNORMALITIES IN CIRRHOSIS

- Cirrhosis is often accompanied by **anemia, leukopenia**, & **thrombocytopenia**[Q].
- **Degree of thrombocytopenia** has been found to be a quite **accurate predictor** of **presence of esophageal varices**[Q].
- **Hypoalbuminemia** and a **prolonged INR** are reliable indices of **chronic** rather than acute liver disease[Q].
- **ALT/AST >2** is **highly suggestive** of **alcohol** as the cause of liver disease[Q].
- Common serum **electrolyte abnormalities** in **cirrhosis** are **hyponatremia, hypokalemia & metabolic alkalosis**[Q].

HEPATOPULMONARY SYNDROME

Hepatopulmonary Syndrome

- Patients with long-standing cirrhosis and portal hypertension are prone to develop HPS.
- It is defined as a **triad of signs: Liver disease**[Q] + increased alveolar-arterial gradients (**hypoxemia**[Q]) + evidence of intrapulmonary vascular resistance (**intra-pulmonary vascular dilatation**)[Q].
- **Severity** depends upon **liver disease, oxygenation defect** and **pulmonary vascular dilatation**[Q]

Clinical Features
- Clinical features are **orthodeoxia, platypnea**[Q], and insidious & slow progression of dyspnea, clubbing, distal cyanosis and spider angiomas.

Diagnosis
- **Contrast echocardiography** is the **study of choice** to diagnose **HPS** by demonstrating the presence of **intra-pulmonary vascular dilatations**[Q].

Treatment
- **Liver transplant reverses HPS** in **most** of the **patients**[Q].

PORTOPULMONARY HYPERTENSION

Portopulmonary Hypertension

- PPH is **pulmonary artery hypertension** in **portal hypertension**[Q].
- Portopulmonary Hypertension (**PPH**) occurs when there is **pulmonary vasoconstriction** and **increased pulmonary artery pressure**[Q].

Clinical Features
- Asymptomatic PPH predisposes to **intra-operative cardiac arrhythmias** and **arrest**[Q].

Diagnosis
- Patients with pulmonary artery pressure gradient (PAPG) >25 mm Hg should undergo **right heart catheterization** for further assessment[Q].
- With **right heart catheterization**, a mean **pulmonary artery pressure** of >25 mm Hg with a **capillary wedge pressure <15 mm Hg** confirm the **diagnosis**[Q].

> - PAPG >25 mm Hg, pulmonary capillary wedge pressure <15 mm Hg and pulmonary vascular resistance >240 dynes S. cm^{-5} occurring in setting of portal hypertension is **diagnostic of PPH**[Q].

Treatment
- **Best treatment**: Combination of **medical therapy** and **liver transplantation**[Q].
- Moderate to severe PPH (PAP > 50 mm Hg) is a contraindication for liver transplantation; first consider prostanid therapy (**epoprostenol**) to **reduce pulmonary hypertension**[Q].

CHILD-TURCOTTE-PUGH (CTP) SCORING SYSTEM

Child-Turcotte-Pugh (CTP) Scoring System

- **CTP score** is a measure to **assess hepatic function**[Q] in many liver diseases.
- It was **initially devised to classify patients** into **risk groups** prior to **undergoing porto-systemic shunt surgeries**[Q].
- It is used to **assess prognosis in cirrhosis**[Q] and many liver diseases.

Child-Turcotte-Pugh (CTP) Score			
Variable	1 Point	2 Points	3 Points
Serum albumin (g/dL)	>3.5	**2.8–3.5**^{Q}	<2.8
Bilirubin (mg/dL)	<2	2–3^Q	>3
Prothrombin time (sec above normal) or **INR**	<4	**4–6**^{Q}	>6
	<1.7	1.7–2.3^Q	>2.3
Ascites	None	**Controlled**^{Q}	Uncontrolled
Encephalopathy	None	**Controlled**^{Q}	Uncontrolled

Class A	5–6 points^Q
Class B	7–9 points^Q
Class C	10–15 points^Q

- **Major surgeries** can be done **only in Class A**^{Q}
- **Only minor surgical procedures** can be performed in **Class B**^{Q}
- **No surgical intervention** should be done in **Class C** (**Best treatment** is **liver transplantation**)^Q.

LEFT SIDED PORTAL HYPERTENSION

LEFT SIDED PORTAL HYPERTENSION

- Portal hypertension **due to isolated splenic vein thrombosis**^{Q} is known as left sided portal hypertension or **sinistral hypertension**^{Q}.
- **Pressure** in **portal vein** and **SMV** are **normal**^{Q}
- There is **gastrosplenic venous hypertension** leading to **formation of gastric varices**^{Q}

Causes
- **Pancreatitis (MC)**^{Q} leading to splenic vein thrombosis
- Neoplasm
- Trauma

Treatment
- **Splenectomy** is the **treatment of choice**^{Q}.

ESOPHAGEAL VARICES

ESOPHAGEAL VARICES

- **Most significant clinical finding** associated with **PHT** is development of **GE varices**^{Q}.
- **Major blood supply** to GE varices is **anterior branch** of **left gastric** or **coronary vein**^{Q}.
- **Variceal bleeding** is **leading cause** of **morbidity & mortality** associated with PHT^Q

  - Approximately **30%** of patients with **compensated cirrhosis** and **60%** of patients with **decompensated cirrhosis** have **esophageal varices**^{Q}.
  - **One third** of all patients with **varices** experience **variceal bleeding**^{Q}.
  - **Each episode** of **bleeding** is associated with a **20–30% risk** of **mortality**^{Q}.

- Seventy per cent of **patients who survive** the initial bleed will experience **recurrent variceal hemorrhage within 1 year,** if left **untreated**^{Q}.

Prevention of Variceal Bleeding
- Current measures aimed at preventing variceal bleeding include:
  - Improvement of liver function (**abstention from alcohol**)^Q
  - **Avoidance** of **aspirin & NSAIDs**^{Q}
  - Administration of **propranolol** or **nadolol** (**nonselective beta blockers**)^Q

  - **Beta blockers** reduce the **index variceal bleed** by **45%** and reduce **bleeding mortality** by **50%**^{Q}.
  - **20%** of patients **do not respond** to **beta blockers** and **20% cannot tolerate beta blockers** due to medication **side effects**^{Q}.

- **Prophylactic endoscopic variceal ligation (EVL)** is associated with a **lower incidence** of **first variceal bleed**^{Q}.
- **EVL** is recommended for **medium to large varices**, performed **every 1 to 2 weeks**^{Q} until obliteration, followed by endoscopy 1 to 3 months later and surveillance endoscopy every 6 months to monitor for recurrence of varices.

Management of Acute Variceal Bleeding

- Patients should be **admitted to** an ICU for **resuscitation** and management[Q].
- **Blood resuscitation** should be performed to a **hemoglobin** level of **8 g/dL**[Q].
- **Over-replacement** of packed **red blood cells** and the overzealous administration of **saline** can lead to both **rebleeding** and **increased mortality**[Q].
- Administration of **FFP** and **platelets** in patients with **severe coagulopathy**[Q].

> - **Cirrhotic patients** with variceal bleeding have a **high-risk** of developing **bacterial infections**[Q]
> - **Bacterial infections** are **associated with rebleeding** and a **higher mortality rate**[Q].
> - Use of **short-term prophylactic antibiotics** has been shown both to **decrease** the **rate of bacterial infections** and to **increase survival**[Q].
> - **Ceftriaxone 1 g/day IV** is often given[Q].

Pharmacologic therapy for Variceal Hemorrhage

- Pharmacologic therapy can be initiated as soon as the diagnosis of variceal bleeding is made.
- **Vasopressin**, administered IV at a dose of **0.2–0.8 units/min**, is the **most potent vasoconstrictor**, its use is **limited by** its large number of **side effects**, and it should be administered for **only a short period** to prevent ischemic complications[Q].
- **Somatostatin** and **octreotide** (initial bolus of **50 µg IV** followed by continuous infusion of **50 µg/h**) also cause **splanchnic vasoconstriction**[Q].
- **Octreotide** is the **preferred pharmacologic agent** for **initial management** of acute variceal bleeding[Q].

- In addition to pharmacologic therapy **endoscopy** should be carried out **as soon as possible** and **EVL** should be performed.
- Combination of **pharmacologic and EVL therapy improve** initial **control of bleeding** and **increase the 5-day hemostasis rate**[Q].
- **Shunt therapy (surgical shunts** or **TIPS)** has been shown to **control refractory variceal bleeding** in >90% of treated individuals[Q].
- **Shunt surgery** is considered only in patients with **preserved hepatic function (CTP class A)**[Q]
- **TIPS** is used in patients with **decompensated liver disease (CTP class B or C)**[Q].

Sengstaken-Blakemore Tube

- Balloon tamponade using will **control refractory variceal bleeding** in **>80% of patients**[Q].
- Its **application** is **limited** due to complications (**aspiration** and **esophageal perforation**)[Q]
- Use of a Sengstaken-Blakemore tube should be **limited** to **short-term therapy (<24 hours)** in those patients awaiting definitive care[Q].

BALLOON TAMPONADE

Balloon Tamponade

- Sengstaken and Blakemore designed a **triple-lumen**[Q] (esophageal balloon, gastric balloon, & gastric aspiration) tube.

Modifications
- Addition of a **fourth port** above the esophageal balloon for aspiration of oral and esophageal secretions (more effective for bleeding esophageal varices)[Q]
- Development of a **single balloon Linton-Nachlas tube** (for **gastric varices**)[Q].

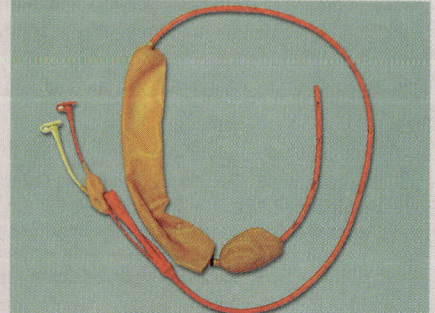

- Airway should be protected by placement of an **endotracheal tube**[Q].
- Use of **water** or **oily contrast** media to inflate the balloon is **contraindicated**[Q].
- In the case of Sengstaken–Blakemore tube, the **gastric balloon** is inflated with **50 mL of air**[Q] and **after proper positioning**, the gastric balloon inflated with **250 mL of air** and plugged snug against the GE junction.

> - If bleeding does not stop promptly, the **gastric balloon** may be inflated to at least a volume of **300 mL**, or the **esophageal balloon** may be inflated to a pressure of **40 mm Hg**[Q].

- **Linton-Nachlas tube** is inflated with **400–700 mL of air**[Q].

Complication
- **MC complication** of balloon tamponade is **aspiration**[Q] pneumonia.

TRANSJUGULAR INTRAHEPATIC PORTAL-SYSTEMIC SHUNT (TIPSS)

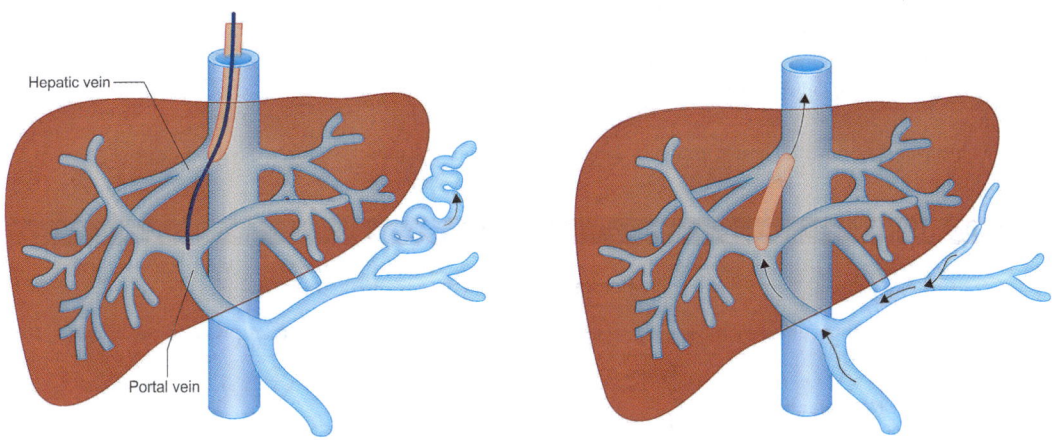

TIPS (Transjugular intrahepatic portosystemic shunt)

Transjugular Intrahepatic Portal-Systemic Shunt (TIPSS)

- TIPSS is a **non-selective shunt**, created between **portal** and **hepatic vein**^{Q}
- TIPSS is **portahepatic** or **intrahepatic shunt**^{Q}
- **TIPS** in the **acute situations** should be **avoided** in patients requiring **ventilation** and with evidence of **sepsis** & **renal failure**^{Q}.

Technique of Placement
- Initial venous access is through the **right internal jugular vein** because this is the **shortest** and **most direct path** to catheterize the hepatic veins^Q.
- **Right hepatic vein** is **MC used** because it is the **largest hepatic vein** and usually has the **most favourable orientation**^{Q}.
- Portal vein is cannulated by **Rosch needle**.
- Portal vein is **localized** by **carbon dioxide wedge hepatic venography**^{Q}.
- **Portal venogram** before dilating parenchymal tract is **crucial**, provides **confirmation** that **portal vein** has been **accessed**.

Stent
- **VIATORR** is a **stent-graft**^{Q} specifically designed for TIPSS.
- Device has a **2 cm** long bare stent segment that sits in the portal vein; the **covered portion** consists of **three PTFE layers**^{Q}, one of which is an impermeable film **to prevent bile leak** into the shunt.

Indications of TIPSS	
1. **Prevention of rebleeding** from varices (**MC**)^Q	5. Refractory hepatic hydrothorax^Q
2. Acute variceal bleeding^Q	6. Budd-Chiari syndrome^Q
3. Refractory ascites^Q	7. Hepatic veno-occlusive disease^Q
4. Hepatorenal syndrome^Q	8. Portal hypertensive gastropathy^Q

Contraindications of TIPSS	
Absolute	**Relative**
1. Right-sided heart failure^Q	1. Portal vein thrombosis^Q
2. Polycystic liver disease^Q	2. Hypervascular liver tumors^Q
3. Pulmonary hypertension^Q	3. Encephalopathy^Q
4. Hepatopulmonary syndrome^Q	

Complications
- **Encephalopathy (10–20%)**^{Q}:
  - Usually occurs **within 1 month** of procedure
  - Relatively easy to manage with **protein restriction** & **lactulose**^{Q}
  - **Declines after the first 3 months** as the stent develops spontaneous closure
- **Stenosis** or **thrombosis (5–15%)**^{Q}:
  - Half of the **stenoses** occur in the **hepatic vein**, & half are due to **intimal hyperplasia** in the parenchymal segment^Q.
  - **Shunt stenosis** is usually secondary to **neointimal hyperplasia** and is **more common than thrombosis**^{Q}.

- **Shunt thrombosis** occur in **<30 days**, whereas **stenosis after 30 days**[Q].
- **Embolization** of the stent to the pulmonary artery
- Inadvertent puncture of the gallbladder or laceration of the liver capsule
- Hemobilia, bacteremia with septic shock, intravascular hemolysis
- Contrast induced oliguric renal failure, worsening hepatic function, right heart failure.

Surveillance
- **Doppler duplex ultrasonography** at 24 hours, 1 month, 3 months, and 6 months after the initial TIPS procedure.

PORTOSYSTEMIC SHUNTS

PORTOSYSTEMIC SHUNTS

- **Portosystemic shunts** are the **most effective** means of **preventing recurrent hemorrhage**[Q] in patients with portal hypertension.

Types of Portosystemic Shunts		
Nonselective	**Selective**	**Partial**
1. **Eck fistula**[Q] 2. Side-to-side PCS (**SSPCS**)[Q] 3. Interposition graft (**portacaval, mesocaval, mesorenal**)[Q] 4. Proximal splenorenal shunt (**Linton shunt**[Q])	1. **Distal** splenorenal shunt (**Warren shunt**[Q]) 2. **Inokuchi shunt**[Q]	1. Diameter of shunt **<10 mm**[Q]

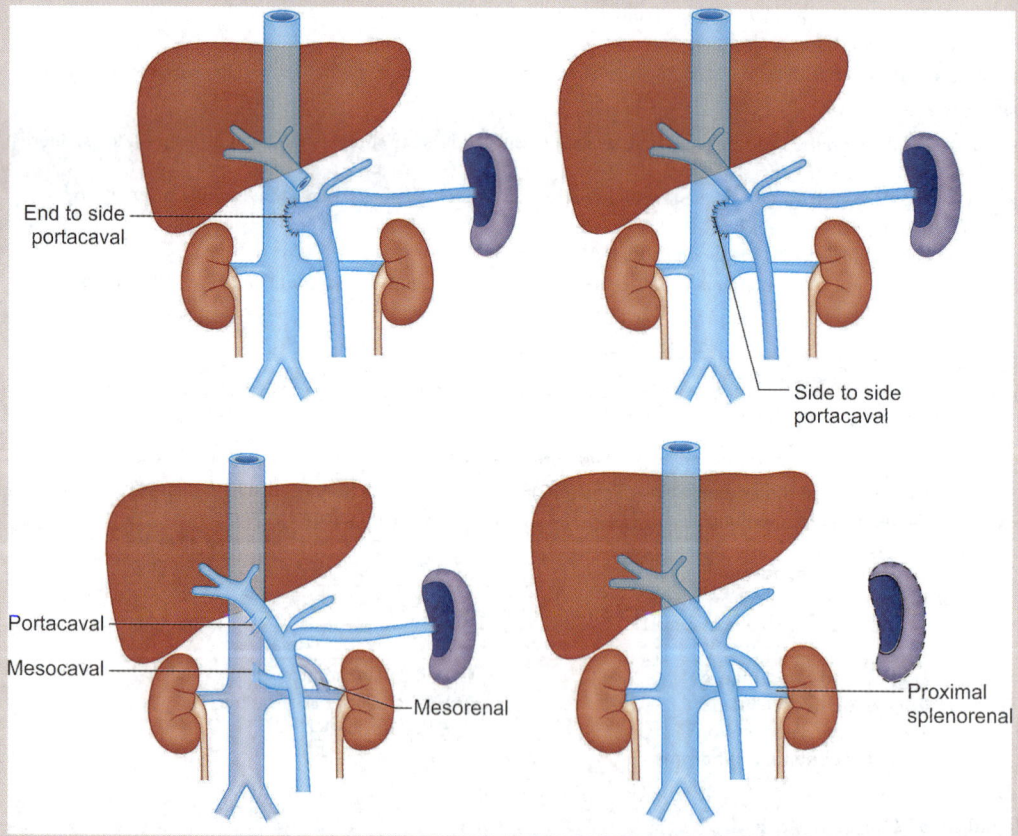

Non-selective shunts

- In the current era, indications for a **nonselective shunt** would include an **emergency shunt** for **variceal hemorrhage**, an **elective shunt** in the presence of **significant ascites** and treatment of **Budd-Chiari syndrome**[Q].
- Patients in whom a **future liver transplant** is required should be treated with a **shunt** in which **dissection** is **performed outside** of the **porta hepatis**.

- Choice (TIPS or shunt) is based on the predicted time to transplantation:
  - TIPS if transplant is **delayed <1 year**^{Q}
  - **Portosystemic shunt** if transplant is **delayed >1 year**^{Q}.
- Patients who live in **remote locations** and those who **fail endoscopic** and **drug therapy** receive a **selective shunt**.

Types of Portosystemic Shunts		
Nonselective	**Selective**	**Partial**
• Divert all portal flow away from the liver^Q • End-to-side or side-to-side anastomosis >11 mm^Q • Side-to-side shunts decompress varices and decompress the obstructed sinusoids, alleviate ascites^Q.	• Only decompresses the gastroesophageal and splenic segments^Q • Distal splenorenal shunt (Warren shunt)^Q • Inokuchi shunt consists of interposition of a vein graft between the left gastric or coronary vein and IVC^Q	• Only diverts part of portal venous flow^Q • Side-to-side anastomosis <10 mm^Q diameter

- MC causes of **death** in:
  - **Medically treated** patients: **Rebleeding**^{Q}
  - **Shunted** patients: **Accelerated hepatic failure**^{Q}
- **Rex shunt** is an **internal jugular vein graft (mesenteric-left portal vein bypass)**^{Q} used in **EHPVO**^{Q}.
- **Eck's Fistula** is an **end-to-side portacaval shunt**^{Q}.

PERITONEOVENOUS SHUNT

Peritoneovenous Shunt

- **Le-Veen shunt** is designed for the **relief of ascites due to chronic liver disease**^{Q}.
- One end of the silastic tube is inserted into the ascites within the peritoneal cavity and the other end is tunneled subcutaneously to the neck, where it is **inserted under direct vision into the internal jugular vein** and **fed into the SVC**^{Q}.

Mechanism of Action
- Owing to a one-way valve within the tubing, peritoneal fluid is drawn from the abdomen and drained to the circulation due to the lower pressure in the SVC in comparison with the abdomen during the respiratory cycle^Q.

Complications
- Occlusion, displacement & infection^Q.

> - In an attempt to prevent the high occlusion rate, a further development was the **insertion of a chamber placed over the costal margin to allow digital pressure and evacuation of any debris within the peritoneovenous shunt (Denver shunt)**^{Q}.

ENCEPHALOPATHY

Encephalopathy

- Cerebral toxins include ammonia, mercaptans and GABA. **Severity** of encephalopathy **does not correlate** with blood **ammonia** levels.

> - **MC cause** is **azotemia**^{Q}; most episodes are **acute**^{Q}
> - **MC setting** for the development of encephalopathy is in patients with **cirrhosis** who undergo a **procedural shunt**^{Q}.

- Only drugs with proven effectiveness:
  - **Neomycin**^{Q}: A poorly absorbed antibiotic that **suppresses urease containing bacteria**
  - **Lactulose**^{Q}: A nonabsorbable disaccharide that **acidifies colonic contents** and also has **cathartic effects**
- **Unproven therapies** include the enteral or parenteral administration of **branch chain amino acids** and the drug **flumazenil**, a selective antagonist of benzodiazepine receptor.

Factors Precipitating Hepatic Encephalopathy			
Nitrogenous causes		**Non-nitrogenous causes**	
• Uremia/Azotemia (MC)^Q • GI bleeding^Q • Dehydration • Metabolic alkalosis^Q	• Hypokalemia^Q • Constipation^Q • Excessive dietary protein^Q • Infection^Q	• Sedative, benzodiazepines • Barbiturates^Q • Hypoxia^Q • Hypoglycemia^Q	• Hypothyroidism • Anemia

GASTRIC VARICES

Gastric Varices

- Classified by **Sarin** into two types:
  1. **Gastroesophageal varices**
  2. **Isolated gastric varices**.
     Type 1: Varices located in the fundus of the stomach^Q
     Type 2: Isolated ectopic varices located anywhere in the stomach^Q.

Pathophysiology
- Gastric varices can develop **secondary to portal hypertension**, in conjunction with esophageal varices, or **secondary to sinistral hypertension** from splenic vein thrombosis^Q.
- **Isolated gastric varices** tend to occur **secondary to splenic vein thrombosis**^{Q}.

Clinical Features
- The **incidence of bleeding** from gastric varices is **<10%**^{Q}.

Diagnosis
- **USG** to **document splenic vein thrombosis** before surgical intervention because gastric varices are most often associated with generalized portal hypertension.
- Gastric varices may be **difficult to recognize endoscopically** even in non-bleeding patients.

> - **Endoscopic ultrasound** is a **more sensitive diagnostic test** than endoscopy alone **for detection** of gastric varices^Q.

Treatment
- Gastric varices in **splenic vein thrombosis**: Splenectomy^Q.
- Gastric varices in the setting of **portal hypertension** should be managed like **esophageal varices**^{Q}.

> - As gastric varices arise in the **submucosa**, a common complication associated with gastric variceal **sclerotherapy** is **ulceration**^{Q}.

NON CIRRHOTIC PORTAL HYPERTENSION

Noncirrhotic Portal Hypertension

- **Noncirrhotic portal hypertension** encompasses two distinct pathological condition that present with similar clinical features.
  - Non cirrhotic portal fibrosis (NCPF)
  - Extra-Hepatic Portal Venous Obstruction (EHPVO)
- Distinction between the two conditions should ideally be made by further investigations as the similarly in presentation makes clinical criteria unreliable.

NCPF	EHPVO

• NCPF presents in **young adults**^{Q}
• Most commonly during the **2nd & 3rd decade**^{Q}
	• EHPVO may present in two age groups:
	  – **Children: 1st and 2nd** decade due to congenital malformations^Q
	  – **Adults: 4th and 5th** decade due to thrombotic event^Q

Clinical Presentation: • Gradual onset of symptoms • **Splenomegaly** is about **4 times more common in NCPF** than EHPV^Q	**Clinical Presentation:** • **Gradual onset** in **children**, where the cause is **congenital malformation**^{Q} • **Acute onset** in adults where the cause is a **thrombotic event**^{Q} • Splenomegaly is 4 times less common in patients with EHPV^Q

EXTRA-HEPATIC PORTAL VENOUS OBSTRUCTION (EHPVO)

Extra-Hepatic Portal Venous Obstruction (EHPVO)

- EHPVO is a **vascular disorder** of the liver.
- **Obstruction** of the **extra-hepatic portal vein**^{Q} with or without involvement of the intra-hepatic portal veins or splenic or SMV.

> - **MC site** of obstruction is at the **confluence** of **splenic vein and SMV**^{Q}
> - **Common cause** of **portal hypertension** in the **developing countries** (up to **30%** of all variceal bleeders) and is **second to cirrhosis** in the West (up to **5–10%**)^Q.

- EHPVO is **MC cause** of **upper gastrointestinal bleeding** in **children**^{Q}.
- Accounts for almost **70%** of **pediatric patients** with **portal hypertension**^{Q}.

Etiology
- **Children:** Etiology is not clear in majority (Evidence of **umbilical sepsis, umbilical catheterization** and **intra-abdominal sepsis** in a small percentage of patients)^Q
- **Adults:** Hypercoagulable and prothrombotic states^Q

Pathology
- Grossly, **original portal vein** is **difficult to identify** as it is **replaced by a cluster of variable-sized vessels arranged haphazardly** within a connective tissue support^Q.
- Histology: **Architectural pattern** of the **liver** is **preserved.**

Clinical Features
- EHPVO can present in two clinical forms:
  - **Recent EHPVO: Abdominal pain, ascites** or **fever**, may be asymptomatic.
  - **Chronic EHPVO: Repeated, well-tolerated bleeding episodes** from esophageal varices.

> - **Ectopic varices** are common (**duodenum, anorectal region, biliary tree** and **gallbladder**), manifest as **obscure GI bleed, bleeding per rectum** or **biliary obstruction**^{Q}

- **Moderate splenomegaly**^{Q} is universal, and may be a presenting feature.
- A proportion of children have **growth retardation**^{Q}.

Diagnosis
- **Liver biopsy** is necessary in a patient with EHPV^O if the **liver functions** are **deranged**.
- **Doppler US, CT** or **MRI:** Demonstrates **portal vein obstruction**, presence of **intraluminal thrombus** in the portal vein and/or **portal vein cavernoma**^{Q}.
- **ERCP** is the **definitive method for diagnosis** of **portal biliopathy**^{Q}.

Treatment

Acute variceal bleeding	Endoscopic variceal ligation^Q
Gastric varices	**Glue injection**^{Q}
Ectopic varices	**Pharmacotherapy, shunts or TIPS**^{Q}.
Hypercoagulable states	**Life-long oral anticoagulants** should be administered
Symptomatic hypersplenism	Shunt surgery^Q Splenectomy without a shunt is not recommended^Q

- **Surgery, shunt** or **non-shunt**, is indicated in patients with **variceal bleeding** who **fail endoscopic therapy**^{Q}.
- **Children with EHPV**^{O}: Rex shunt (mesenterico-left portal shunt)^Q

NONCIRRHOTIC PORTAL FIBROSIS (NCPF)

NONCIRRHOTIC PORTAL FIBROSIS (NCPF)

- Condition of liver characterized by **widespread fibrosis of liver** (mainly **portal, subcapsular** & rarely perisinusoidal) causing **wide variation in normal architecture**^{Q}
- There is **no true cirrhosis**^{Q}.

Etiology
- Chronic ingestion of **Arsenic (As), Copper (Cu)** & **Vinyl chloride**^{Q} is incriminated in causing NCPF.

Pathology
- Characterized by **fibrous intimal thickening** of the **portal vein or its branches**^{Q}.

> - **Hallmark** of diseases is **thrombosis/sclerosis** of the **portal vein branches**^{Q}.
> - **Portal** & **periportal fibrosis** of varying extent (**No bridging fibrosis**)^Q

- **Portal vein** is **dilated with sclerosis of the walls**^{Q} and in autopsy thrombin in the medium or small portal vein branches with accompanying areas of ischemic necrosis.
- **Aberrant intrahepatic vessels** may be present in the **periportal area**, which correspond to dilated terminal portal vein branches or venules, termed as **megasinusoids** or **periportal angiomatosis**^{Q}.

Clinical Features
- **Young age patient** with features of **portal hypertension** with conspicuous **absence of liver cell failure**^{Q}.

- Patients are usually in **2nd or 3rd decade**^Q.
- Onset of symptoms is **gradual**^Q
- MC presenting symptom is **GI bleed (90% cases)**^Q.
- **Splenomegaly**^Q
- **Jaundice, Hepatomegaly, ascites** and **stigmata** of **liver cell failure** are **uncommon**^Q.

Diagnosis
- Site of block is smaller branches (**3rd or 4th order branches**)^Q

> - **Ultrasound** shows **normal splenoportal axis. Withered tree appearance** & **periportal fibrosis** is seen in **NCPF**^Q.

MELD SCORE AND PELD SCORESS

MODEL FOR END-STAGE LIVER DISEASE (MELD) SCORE

- **MELD score** is used to **assess** the **severity of chronic liver disease**^Q
- It was **initially developed** to **predict death within 3 months** of surgery in patients that had **undergone TIPS.**^Q
- It is calculated by using **3 variables (CBI)**: S. Creatinine, S. Bilirubin, INR^Q

> - MELD score is **currently used** by United Network for Organ Sharing (**UNOS**) for **prioritizing allocation of liver transplant**^Q.

- It is **6–40 point** scale
- **Relative risk of mortality** increases by **14% for each 1point increase in MELD score.**
- MELD score = 3.8log(e) (S. bilirubin mg/dL) + 11.2Log(e) (INR) + 9.6Log(e) (S. creatinine mg/dL)

PEDIATRIC END-STAGE LIVER DISEASE (PELD) SCORE

- **PELD score** utilizes following variables (**NABIA**)^Q:
  1. Nutritional status^Q
  2. Age^Q
  3. Bilirubin^Q
  4. INR^Q
  5. Albumin^Q

MELD score (CBI)	**C**reatinine, **B**ilirubin, **I**NR^Q
PELD score (NABIA)	**N**utritional status, **A**ge, **B**ilirubin, **I**NR, **A**lbumin^Q

BUDD-CHIARI SYNDROME

BUDD-CHIARI SYNDROME

- BCS is caused by **obstruction of hepatic venous outflow**^Q producing intense congestion of the liver.

Etiology
- **Polycythemia rubra vera** is the MC etiology^Q.
- In the **West, thrombosis of the major hepatic veins**^Q is more common.
- In BCS, **all three major hepatic veins** usually are occluded.
- Small hepatic veins that joins the reterohepatic IVC, particularly **veins draining the caudate lobe** are **spared**^Q.

> - **Membranous obstruction** of IVC is MC cause of BCS in **Japan, China, India** and **South Africa**^Q.

- Infections causing BCS: Filariasis, **amebic liver abscess, aspergillosis, schistosomiasis,** syphilitic gumma & hydatid disease.
- **MC cancers** associated with BCS: **HCC, RCC, adrenal carcinoma & leiomyosarcoma** of the IVC.

Pathology
- **Centrilobular congestion**
- Centrilobular **hepatocyte loss** and **necrosis, fibrosis** & **cirrhosis**

Clinical Features
- Characterised by triad of **A**scites + **H**epatomegaly + **A**bdominal pain **(AsHA)**
- Abdominal **pain**, abdominal **distention**, weakness, anorexia and jaundice^Q
- Signs are **massive ascites, hepatomegaly** (with **hypertrophied caudate lobe**)^Q, wasting, abdominal venous distention, **splenomegaly,** jaundice and edema of thighs, legs & feet.

- **Jaundice & abdominal venous distention** is more common in **hepatic vein occlusion**[Q].
- **Edema** of thighs, legs & feet is seen only in **IVC occlusion**[Q].

- **Striking & progressive weakness** occur as a manifestation in **acute form** but not in chronic forms of BCS[Q].

Diagnosis
- Diagnostic study of greatest value in BCS is **angiographic examination** of **IVC & hepatic veins** with **pressure measurements**[Q].

  - **Patency of IVC** is a **pre-requisite** for side-to-side portacaval shunt (**SSPCS**)[Q].

- Injection of dye in wedged position often shows a characteristic **spider-web pattern** of small hepatic venous **collaterals** connecting to portal or systemic veins.
- **Most**, but not all, **patients** with **thrombosis** of IVC also have **occlusion** of **hepatic veins**[Q].

Hepatic Scintiscanning in BCS
- **Decreased & non-homogenous hepatic uptake** of radiocolloid
- **Increased uptake** of radiocolloid by **spleen & bone marrow**
- **Central hot spot** due to healthy & **hypertrophied caudate lobe** is **diagnostic**[Q]

Treatment
- **Thrombolysis** of **hepatic vein** clot is largely **ineffective** because the **window** for **effective clot lysis** is only **2–3 weeks**, and most patients present after months of symptoms;
- **Side to Side Porto-Caval Shunt: SSPCS** is the **most effective therapy** for **BCS** caused by **thrombosis of hepatic veins**[Q].

Ideal Circumstances for Shunt Surgery Include in BCS
- **Absence** of **cirrhosis** or significant **fibrosis** on biopsy[Q]
- **Absence** of a **significant gradient** between the suprahepatic and infrahepatic IVC[Q]
- Relatively **short duration** of disease

- In cases of BCS caused by **thrombosis or occlusion** of **IVC**, combined **SSPCS & CAS**[Q] (Cavoatrial Shunt) has replaced mesoatrial shunt as the **preferred treatment**[Q].

Surgical Treatment of Membranous Obstruction of IVC in BCS
- **Percutaneous transluminal angioplasty** & **transcardiac membranotomy**[Q] (preferred one) when the membrane is **thin**
- When a **long area of stenosis** is involved treatment consists of **direct excision** & **repair** of involved area of IVC (endovenotomy) or **cavoatrial bypass graft**[Q].

Indications of OLT in BCS
- **Cirrhosis with progressive liver failure** (MC indication)[Q]
- **Failure of a portal-systemic shunt,** usually because of thrombosis[Q]
- **Unshuntable portal hypertension** due to thrombosis of the portal vein, splenic vein or SMV[Q]
- **Acute fulminant hepatic failure**; rarest indication[Q]

VENO-OCCLUSIVE DISEASE

VENO-OCCLUSIVE DISEASE

- It is a group of disorders in which **hepatic venous outflow obstruction** is due to **subendothelial sclerosis** of **sublobular hepatic veins** & **terminal hepatic venules**[Q] within the liver.

Risk Factors
- In the **western hemisphere, MC cause** of VOD is **bone marrow transplantation**[Q].
- **Chemotherapy: Cytosine arabinoside**, Thioguanine, **Carmustine**, Gemtuzumab ozogamocin[Q]
- Long term immunosuppression with **azathioprine** in renal and **liver transplantation**[Q]
- Ingestion of **bush teas (pyrrolizidine alkaloids)**[Q] from plants of **Crotalaria** & **Scenacio** genera. These plants and plants of **Heliotropium genus**[Q] produce liver failure in herbivores.

Pathology
- Involves **sinusoids, central** & **sublobular hepatic vein**[Q]
- **Subendothelial sclerosis** of sublobular hepatic vein & sinusoids secondary to endothelial injury
- **Centrilobular necrosis,** ultimately leading to **diffuse fibrosis & cirrhosis**[Q]

Clinical Features
- **Hallmark** of **VOD:** Hyperbilirubinemia, tender hepatomegaly and **fluid retention**[Q].
- **Onset** of VOD usually occurs **within 3 weeks** after bone marrow transplantation, with a **peak 12 days post-transplantation**[Q].
- **Major cause** of **death** is **bleeding esophageal varices**[Q].

Modified Seattle Criteria
Two or more of the following must be present prior to 20 days after stem cell transplantation for diagnosis of VOD: • **Bilirubin >2 mg/dL**[Q]   • **Tender hepatomegaly**[Q]   • **Ascites** and/or **unexplained weight gain** of **>2%** above reference range[Q]

Diagnosis
- **Percutaneous needle liver biopsy** is **diagnostic**[Q], showing specific abnormality of extensive occlusion of small hepatic veins in liver.

• **Angiography: Major hepatic veins** and **IVC** are **normal**, but **WHVP** is **increased**[Q].   • LFT is abnormal with **elevated plasminogen activator inhibitor-1 (PAI-1)**[Q].

- PAI-1 has been **implicated** in the **pathology of VOD** and is a **useful marker** in **distinguishing VOD** from the several **other causes** of post-transplant hepatic dysfunction.

Treatment
- Acute stages of VOD: **Withdrawal of causative agent** and **supportive treatment**[Q] to damaged liver.

Indications of SSPCS in VOD in Acute Phases
• Patients who **bleed from esophageal varices**[Q]   • Patients who show **no signs of recovery** within **4–8 weeks**[Q] (e.g. Disappearance of ascites, improvement in LFT, improvement in lesion on percutaneous needle biopsy)

Defibrotide
• **Most promising agent** undergoing trial in the treatment of **severe VOD** is **defibrotide**[Q]   • A polydeoxyribonucleotide with adenosine receptor activity which **modulates endothelial cell injury** and **protects sinusoidal endothelium**[Q].

Multiple Choice Questions

PORTAL HYPERTENSION

1. Which of the following is not associated with left sided portal hypertension? *(COMEDK 2006)*
   a. Secondary to pancreatic inflammation or neoplasm
   b. Normal superior mesenteric and portal venous pressure
   c. Easily reversed by splenectomy
   d. Isolated esophageal varices present

2. Normal portal vein pressure is:
   (Recent Question 2016, COMEDK 2008)
   a. < 3 mm Hg   b. 3–5 mm Hg
   c. 5–10 mm Hg   d. 10–12 mm Hg

3. Which of the following causes minimal porto-hepatic compromise? *(JIPMER GIS 2011)*
   a. Non-selective shunts   b. TIPSS
   c. Distal splenorenal shunt   d. Sclerotherapy

4. Most common metabolic disturbance of cirrhosis is:
   (ILBS 2012, JIPMER GIS 2011)
   a. Metabolic acidosis   b. Metabolic alkalosis
   c. Respiratory acidosis d. Respiratory alkalosis

5. All are true about hepatopulmonary syndrome except:
   (JIPMER GIS 2011)
   a. Frequency in ESLD is between 8–29%
   b. Characterized by hypoxemia and anatomical shunting of blood
   c. Only established treatment at present is OLT
   d. A pre-operative oxygen tension of < 30 mmHg alone is a predictor of disease

6. Metabolic complication of cirrhosis are all except:
   (AIIMS GIS Dec 2006)
   a. Hypokalemia   b. Hyponatremia
   c. Hypoglycemia   d. Hypoammonemia

7. In a patient with compensated liver cirrhosis presented with history of variceal bleed. The treatment of choice in this patient is: *(AIIMS June 2002)*
   a. Propranolol
   b. Liver transplantation
   c. TIPS (Transjugular intrahepatic portal shunt)
   d. Endoscopic sclerotherapy

8. Left sided portal hypertension is best treated by:
   (Recent Question 2016, AIIMS June 2001)
   a. Splenectomy   b. Portocaval shunt
   c. Lieno-renal shunt d. Spleno-renal shunt

9. Portal hypertension following portal vein thrombosis are guided by: *(PGI Dec 2003)*
   a. ↑ in splenic pulp pressure
   b. ↑ in portal vein pressure
   c. ↑ in hepatic vein pressure
   d. Portal vein Doppler study

10. Child criteria include all except: *(PGI May 2011)*
    a. Nutritional status   b. S. Bilirubin
    c. S. Creatinine   d. Acid phosphate
    e. Ascites

11. Child-Pugh criteria does not include: *(Punjab 2010)*
    a. Encephalopathy   b. ALT
    c. Ascites   d. Albumin

12. According to Child-Pugh staging, child's B is:
    a. 5–6   b. 7–9   *(JIPMER GIS 2011)*
    c. 10–11   d. 9–12

13. According to Pughs classification moderate to severe hepatic insufficiency is managed by: *(AIIMS Nov 2000)*
    a. Sclerotherapy
    b. Conservative
    c. Orthotopic liver transplantation
    d. Shunt surgery

14. The Sengstaken tube must maintain a pressure of ...... to stop bleeding from varices:
    a. 20 mm Hg   b. 25 mm Hg
    c. 35 mm Hg   d. 45 mm Hg

15. Drug induced portal hypertension is seen with:
    a. Vitamin A toxicity   b. Methotrexate
    c. Aldomet   d. Hydatid cyst

16. In Child's criteria partial encephalopathy, bilirubin 2.5 mg/dL albumin 3 gm/dl, controlled ascites indicates: *(PGI 96)*
    a. Grade A   b. Grade B
    c. Grade C   d. More information needed

17. Which one of the following is not a treatment of gastroesophageal variceal hemorrhage? *(UPSC 2001)*
    a. Sclerotherapy
    b. Sengstaken tube
    c. Transjugular intrahepatic portacaval shunt
    d. Gastric freezing

18. In portal hypertension the sites of portosystemic anastomosis includes: *(DPG 2010)*
    a. Lower end of esophagus
    b. Around umbilicus
    c. Lower third of rectum and anal canal
    d. All of the above

19. A 50-year-old male presented with history of hematemesis-500 mL of blood and on examination shows BP-90/60, PR-110/min and splenomegaly 5cm below lower costal margin. Most probable diagnosis is: *(All India 2012, AIIMS Nov 2006)*
    a. Mallory-Weiss tear   b. Duodenal ulcer
    c. Gastritis   d. Portal hypertension

20. MELD score doesn't include:
    (Recent Question 2017, AIIMS GIS Dec 2011, Dec 2006)
    a. INR   b. S. bilirubin
    c. S. creatinine   d. Blood urea

21. A 40-year-old male presented with hematemesis. On examination his BP was 90/60 mm Hg and heart rate was 120/min. Splenomegaly was also present. The most probable cause of his bleeding is: *(AIIMS May 2012)*
    a. Portal hypertension   b. Gastric ulcer
    c. Duodenal ulcer   d. Drug induced GI injury

22. Child's Criteria is used in: *(DNB 2005, 2001, 2000)*
    a. Pancreatitis   b. Cirrhosis
    c. Multiple myeloma d. AIDS

23. **Child-Pugh score is used for:** *(Recent Question 2017)*
    a. Hepatic encephalopathy b. Uremic encephalopathy
    c. Chronic liver disease   d. Head injury

24. **All of the following are true in case of chronic liver disease except:** *(Recent Question 2019)*
    a. MELD score is used frequently to see whom needs liver transplant early
    b. MELD score includes serum albumin, creatinine, and INR
    c. Child Pugh score includes PT-INR, albumin and bilirubin
    d. Child Pugh score has class A, B, C

ESOPHAGEAL VARICES

25. **Worm-like filling defect is seen in:** *(MHCET 2016, COMEDK 2005)*
    a. Erosive gastritis   b. Esophageal varices
    c. CA esophagus   d. Schatzki's ring

26. **What is the most probable diagnosis on the basis of given endoscopy image?** *(Recent Question 2016)*
    a. GAVE   b. Schatzki ring
    c. Barrett's esophagus d. Esophageal varices

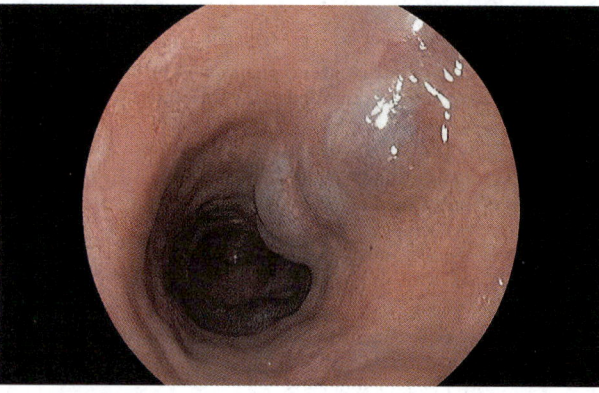

27. **Which one of the following treatment modalities is not used for management of acute blood loss due to ruptured esophageal varices?** *(UPSC 2004)*
    a. Endoscopic sclerotherapy b. Endoscopic band ligation
    c. Octreotide   d. Propranolol

28. **On barium swallow the grade IV esophageal varices appear as:** *(AIIMS June 2001)*
    a. Mucosal folds above the carina
    b. Mucosal folds below the carina
    c. Mucosal folds at the carina
    d. A thick band

29. **Best test for esophageal varices is:** *(UPPG 2009)*
    a. CT-scan   b. Gastro-esophagoscopy
    c. Tomography   d. Ultrasound

30. **The balloons of Sengstaken-Blakemore tube should be temporarily deflated after how many hours to prevent pre-necrosis of the oesophagus?** *(MHSSMCET 2011)*
    a. 12 hours   b. 24 hours
    c. 36 hours   d. 48 hours

31. **To stop variceal bleeding pressure in Sengstaken B lackmore tube should be:** *(MHSSMCET 2007)*
    a. 40 mm   b. 50 mm
    c. 60 mm   d. 70 mm

32. **Treatment of choice for bleeding esophageal and gastric varices:** *(MHSSMCET 2007)*
    a. Injection sclerotherapy b. Banding (Endoscopic)
    c. Shunt surgery   d. Devascularization

33. **Variceal banding was invented by:** *(MHSSMCET 2006)*
    a. Borema and Crile
    b. Stiegmann and Goff
    c. Sugiura and Futagawa
    d. Crafoord and Frenckner

34. **Which of the following agents is recommended for medical treatment of variceal bleed?** *(All India 2011)*
    a. Octreotide   b. Desmopressin
    c. Vasopressin   d. Nitroglycerine

35. **Sclerotherapy failure is defined as:** *(JIPMER GIS 2011)*
    a. Unresponsiveness to consecutive 2 energy sclerotherapies
    b. Unresponsiveness to consecutive 3 energy sclerotherapies
    c. Remnant bleeding even after sclerotherapy for successive 2 hospital admissions
    d. Failure to heal after a single treatment

GASTRIC VARICES

36. **Most common cause of gastric varices is:** *(AIIMS GIS Dec 2011)*
    a. Splenic vein thrombosis b. Splenectomy
    c. Cirrhosis   d. Mesenteric thrombosis

37. **Isolated gastric varices:** *(AIIMS GIS May 2011)*
    a. Profuse bleeding
    b. Most commonly due to splenic vein thrombosis
    c. EUS is better than endoscopy
    d. Single treatment can lead to eradication

38. **Veins involve in stomach varices are:** *(PGI Dec 2008)*
    a. Coronary vein   b. Short gastric vein
    c. Right gastroepiploic vein d. Left gastroepiploic vein
    e. Left gastric vein

TIPS

39. **Contraindications of TIPS:** *(ILBS 2012)*
    a. HPS   b. HRS
    c. VOD   d. BCS

40. **False about TIPS:** *(AIIMS GIS May 2008)*
    a. Shunt thrombosis is more common than stenosis
    b. Encephalopathy is more common
    c. Improves ascites and hydrothorax
    d. Much better control of bleeding than variceal ligation

41. **TIPS means creating anastomosis between which of the following?** *(WB PG 2015, MHSSMCET 2009, Karnataka 2006)*
    a. Portal vein and hepatic artery
    b. Portal vein and IVC
    c. Portal vein and hepatic vein
    d. Hepatic vein and hepatic artery

42. **TIPS is a type of:** *(JIPMER GIS 2011)*
    a. Non-selective shunt
    b. Selective shunt
    c. Both selective and non-selective shunt
    d. Systemic shunt

43. **True about TIPS:** *(PGI June 98)*
    a. It is a type of portocaval shunt
    b. It is intrahepatic shunt
    c. Performed by passing endoscopes
    d. Most suitable for patient going for liver transplant

Portal Hypertension

44. **TIPS is used in all except:** *(AIIMS GIS Dec 2011)*
    a. Refractory ascites
    b. BCS
    c. Hepatopulmonary syndrome
    d. Refractory hepatic hydrothorax

45. **Early complication of TIPS procedure:** *(JIPMER November 2017)*
    a. Shunt stenosis and blockage
    b. Capsular haemorrhage
    c. Metabolic encephalopathy
    d. Recurrent variceal bleed

SURGICAL SHUNTS

46. **Coronary-Caval fistula is:** *(ILBS 2011)*
    a. Inokuchi
    b. Warren's
    c. Eck's fistula
    d. Shamik

47. **Mesocaval shunt what incision approach is used?** *(MHSSMCET 2009)*
    a. Midline
    b. Paramedian
    c. Subcoastal
    d. Chevron

48. **Which is a non-selective shunt?** *(AIIMS GIS May 2008)*
    a. DSRS
    b. Inokuchi shunt
    c. 12 mm interposition shunt
    d. 8 mm interposition shunt

49. **What is the type of this shunt?**

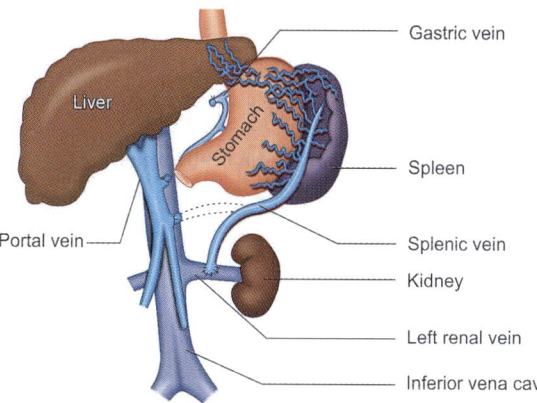

    a. Non-selective shunt
    b. Selective shunt
    c. Partial shunt
    d. None of the above

50. **For bleeding varices of the esophagus, the common operation operations is/are:**
    a. Portocaval shunt
    b. Gastrectomy
    c. Splenectomy
    d. All of the above

51. **Prognosis of portocaval shunt depends on all except:** *(AIIMS Sept 96)*
    a. Serum bilirubin
    b. Serum albumin
    c. Refractory ascites
    d. Type of shunt

52. **Contraindications of portal systemic shunting include:**
    a. Serum albumin less than 3 mg%
    b. Massive ascites
    c. Significant jaundice
    d. All of the above

53. **Denver shunt is used in:** *(DNB 2012)*
    a. Ascites
    b. Dialysis
    c. Raised ICT
    d. Raised IOP

54. **The Le-Veen shunt in ascites is done between peritoneum and:** *(Recent Question 2016, AIIMS November 2014)*
    a. Cisterna chyli
    b. Renal pelvis
    c. Superior vena cava
    d. Gall bladder

55. **The operation that precipitates portosystemic encephalopathy is:** *(MAHE 2005)*
    a. Splenorenal shunt
    b. Suguira operation
    c. Talmal-marison operation
    d. Portacaval anastomosis

56. **Which of the following is a selective shunt?**
    a. Proximal splenorenal shunt *(Recent Question 2017)*
    b. Warren shunt
    c. Side-to-side portocaval shunt
    d. Mesocaval shunt

EXTRA-HEPATIC PORTAL VENOUS OBSTRUCTION

57. **A 20-year-old male presented with repeated episodes of hematemesis. There is no history of jaundice or liver decompensation. On examination the significant findings include splenomegaly (8 cms below costal margin), and presence of esophageal varices. There is no ascites or peptic ulceration. The liver function tests are normal. The most likely diagnosis is:** *(AIIMS Nov 2004)*
    a. Extrahepatic portal venous obstruction
    b. Non-cirrhotic portal fibrosis
    c. Cirrhosis
    d. Hepatic venous outflow tract obstruction

58. **A 12-year-old boy presents with hematemesis, melena and mild splenomegaly. There is no obvious jaundice or ascites. The most likely diagnosis is:** *(All India 2011)*
    a. EHPVO
    b. NCPF
    c. Cirrhosis
    d. Malaria with DIC

59. **Treatment of choice for extrahepatic portal thrombosis:** *(MHSSMCET 2009)*
    a. Mesocaval shunt
    b. Porto caval shunt
    c. Mesorenal shunt
    d. Splenorenal shunt

60. **This shunt is used in which condition?**
    a. NCPF
    b. EHPVO
    c. Budd-Chiari syndrome
    d. Veno-occlusive disease

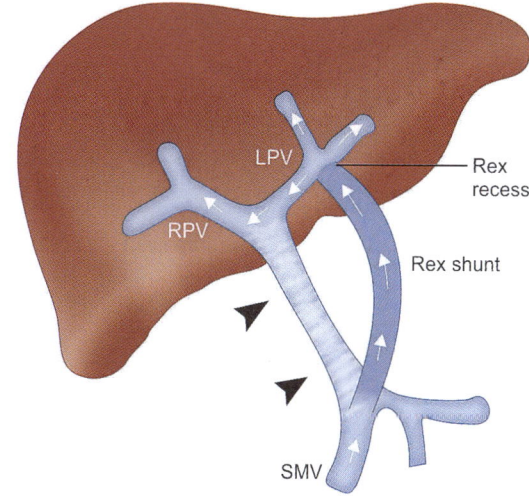

NON-CIRRHOTIC PORTAL FIBROSIS

61. Which of the following is the most common presenting symptom of non-cirrhotic portal hypertension?
    a. Chronic liver disease *(All India 2006)*
    b. Ascites
    c. Upper gastrointestinal bleeding
    d. Encephalopathy

62. NCPF is due to: *(AIIMS GIS Dec 2010)*
    a. Extrahepatic obstruction
    b. Intrahepatic pre-sinusoidal obstruction
    c. Intrahepatic sinusoidal obstruction
    d. Intrahepatic post-sinusoidal obstruction

BUDD-CHIARI SYNDROME

63. True about Budd-Chiari syndrome is the following except:
    a. Can occur due to web in IVC *(MHPGMET 2005)*
    b. Thrombosis of hepatic veins
    c. Causes prehepatic portal hypertension
    d. Intractable ascites

64. The obstruction of two or more major hepatic veins is seen in:
    a. Budd-Chiari syndrome *(MHCET 2016)*
    b. Reye's syndrome
    c. Rotor syndrome
    d. Crigler-Najjar syndrome

65. Budd-Chiari syndrome is due to thrombosis of:
    a. Infra renal IVC *(Orissa 2011)*
    b. Renal part of IVC
    c. Superior mesenteric vein thrombosis
    d. Hepatic veins

66. Classical triad of Budd-Chiari syndrome:
    a. Fever, jaundice, abdominal pain *(Recent Question 2016)*
    b. Fever, ascites, jaundice
    c. Hepatomegaly, abdominal pain, ascites
    d. Abdominal pain, jaundice, hepatomegaly

67. Most commonly performed hepatobiliary shunt in Budd-Chiari syndrome: *(Recent Question 2016)*
    a. Rex shunt
    b. Lienorenal shunt
    c. Mesocaval shunt
    d. Side to side portocaval shunt

68. In a patient of portal hypertension, venography was performed and the image is given below. What is the most probable diagnosis?
    a. Veno-occlusive disease   b. NCPF
    c. Budd Chiari syndrome   d. EHPVO

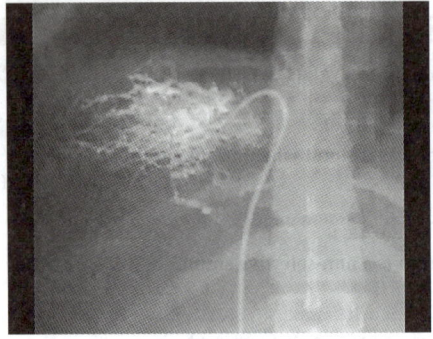

VENO-OCCLUSIVE DISEASE

69. Veno-occlusive disease in hepatic vein is characterized by:
    a. Central venous congestion *(PGI Dec 2007)*
    b. Hepatomegaly
    c. Portal vein obstruction
    d. Budd-Chiari syndrome
    e. Hepatic fibrosis

70. Veno-occlusive disease is seen in all except:
    a. Bone marrow transplant *(AIIMS GIS Dec 2011)*
    b. Bush teas
    c. Mushroom poisoning
    d. Cytosine arabinoside

Explanations

PORTAL HYPERTENSION

1. **Ans. d. Isolated esophageal varices present** *(Ref: Sabiston 20/e p1436-1437; Schwartz 10/e p1281; Harrison 20/e p2411, 19/e p2063)*
2. **Ans. c. 5–10 mm Hg** *(Ref: Sabiston 20/e p1436-1437; Schwartz 10/e p1280-1281; Harrison 20/e p2410, 19/e p2062)*
3. **Ans. d. Sclerotherapy**
4. **Ans. b. Metabolic alkalosis** *(Ref: Sabiston 20/e p565; Harrison 20/e p2410, 19/e p2064)*

ELECTROLYTE ABNORMALITIES IN CIRRHOSIS

- **Hyponatremia, hypokalemia** and **metabolic alkalosis**^{Q} (↓PNH)

5. **Ans. d. A preoperative oxygen tension of < 30 mm Hg alone is a predictor of disease** *(Ref: Shackelford 8/e p1588, 7/e p1606-1608; Sabiston 20/e p639)*

- **Severity in HPS** depends upon **liver disease, oxygenation defect** and **pulmonary vascular dilatation**^{Q}.

6. **Ans. d. Hypoammonemia**
   - In cirrhosis, there is hyperammonemia.

7. **Ans. d. Endoscopic sclerotherapy** *(Ref: Sabiston 20/e p1444; Blumgart 6/e p1201, 5/e p1129-1134; Shackelford 8/e p1582, 7/e p1597, 1599-1601; Harrison 20/e p2411, 19/e p2064)*

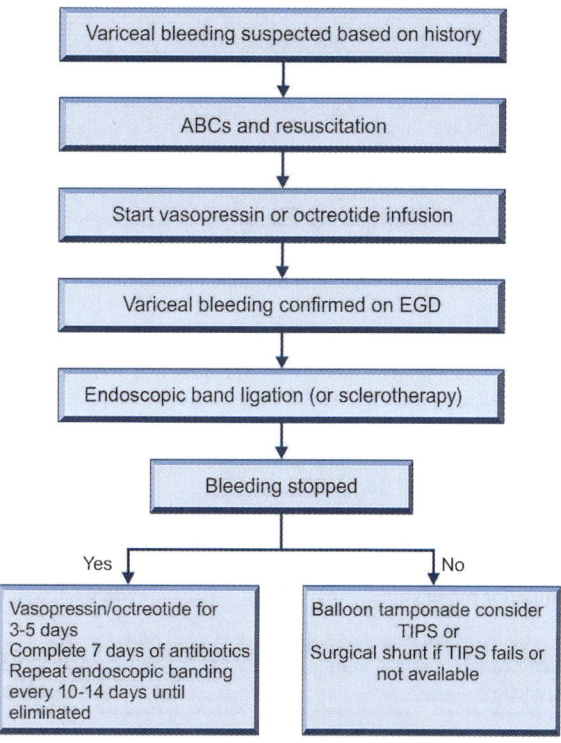

Management of Variceal Bleeding

VARICEAL BLEEDING

- In addition to pharmacologic therapy **endoscopy** should be carried out **as soon as possible**
- If varices are found they are treated with either **endoscopic variceal ligation** or **sclerotherapy**^{Q}.
- **EVL** is the **treatment of choice** for **variceal bleeding**^{Q}.

8. **Ans. a. Splenectomy**
9. **Ans. a. ↑ in splenic pulp pressure, b. ↑ in portal vein pressure, d. Portal vein Doppler study**

   - **Splenic pulp pressure** gives a **measure of** the **portal vein pressure**; it can be measured by **inserting a needle percutaneously**[Q].
   - **Portal vein Doppler study** is the **most useful non-invasive investigation** for assessing **thrombosis** of the **main portal vein branches**[Q].

10. **Ans. a. Nutritional status, c. S. Creatinine, d. Acid phosphate** *(Ref: Sabiston 20/e p1436; Schwartz 10/e p1280; Harrison 20/e p2416, 19/e 1995)*
11. **Ans. b. ALT**
12. **Ans. b. 7–9**
13. **Ans. c. Orthotopic liver transplantation**

    - Patient of cirrhosis with variceal bleeding or ascites can be controlled by shunt surgery only if he falls in CTP class A or B.
    - **Moderate to severe grade liver insufficiency** can only be **managed by liver transplantation**[Q].

14. **Ans. c. 35 mm Hg** *(Ref: Sabiston 20/e p1438; Schwartz 9/e p1113; Blumgart 6/e p1172, 5/e p1136-1137; Harrison 20/e p2411, 19/e p2063)*

    - If bleeding does not stop promptly, the **gastric balloon** may be inflated to at least a volume of **300 mL**, or the **esophageal balloon** may be inflated to a pressure of **40 mm Hg**[Q].

15. **Ans. a. Vitamin A toxicity** *(Ref: livertox.nlm.nih.gov)*

    ### VITAMIN A INDUCED HEPATOTOXICITY

    - **Normal doses** of vitamin A are **not associated with liver injury** or liver test abnormalities, but **higher doses can be toxic**[Q].

    > **Mechanism of Injury**
    >
    > - **Excess vitamin A** is **stored in stellate cells**[Q] in the liver and accumulation can lead to their **activation** and **hypertrophy**, **excess collagen production**, **fibrosis**[Q] and liver injury.

    - **Serum bilirubin** is typically only **mildly elevated**[Q].
    - **Liver biopsy** is **diagnostic**[Q]

16. **Ans. b. Grade B, d. More information needed**
17. **Ans. d. Gastric freezing**
18. **Ans. d. All of the above** *(Ref: Sabiston 20/e p1437)*

    In portal hypertension the sites of portosystemic anastomosis includes lower end of esophagus, around umbilicus, lower third of rectum and anal canal, posterior abdominal wall, bare area of liver.

Porto-Systemic Anastomosis		
Location	**Portal Component**	**Systemic Component**
Esophagus (lower end) **Esophageal varices**	Left gastric vein[Q]	Azygous vein[Q] and accessory hemiazygous vein
Rectum and anal Canal Hemorrhoids	Superior rectal vein[Q]	Middle and inferior rectal vein[Q]
Umbilicus Caput medusa	Left branch of portal vein (paraumblical branches)	Superficial (superior and inferior) epigastric veins[Q]
Posterior abdominal wall	Colic and omental veins[Q]	Retroperitoneal veins[Q] of abdominal wall, renal capsule, splenic and hepatic flexure
Bare area of liver	Hepatic venules[Q] Right branch of portal vein	Phrenic and intercostal veins Retroperitoneal veins draining into lumbar, azygous and hemiazygous veins
Liver (rarely)	Patent ductus venosus[Q] Left branch of portal vein	Inferior vena cava

19. **Ans. d. Portal hypertension** *(Ref: Sabiston 20/e p1142)*

Common Causes of Upper Gastrointestinal Hemorrhage			
Non-variceal Bleeding	(80%)[Q]	Portal Hypertensive Bleeding	(20%)[Q]
Peptic ulcer disease (MC)[Q]	30–50%[Q]	Gastroesophageal varices[Q]	>90%[Q]
Mallory-Weiss tears	15–20%	Hypertensive portal gastropathy	<5%
Gastritis or **duodenitis**	10–15%	Isolated gastric varices	Rare
Esophagitis	5–10%		
Arteriovenous malformations	5%		
Tumors	2%		
Other	5%		

- **Splenomegaly** and **massive bleeding** leading to **hypotension** are in favor of **portal hypertension**[Q].

20. **Ans. d. Blood urea** *(Ref: Sabiston 20/e p640; Schwartz 10/e p1280; Harrison 20/e p2416, 19/e p2069)*

MELD score (CBI)	**C**reatinine, **B**ilirubin, **I**NR[Q]
PELD score (NABIA)	**N**utritional status, **A**ge, **B**ilirubin, **I**NR, **A**lbumin[Q]

21. **Ans. a. Portal hypertension**   22. **Ans. b. Cirrhosis**
23. **Ans. c. Chronic liver disease** *(Ref: Sabiston 20/e p1436; Schwartz 10/e p1280; Bailey 27/e p1156)*
24. **Ans. b. MELD score includes serum albumin, creatinine, and INR**

ESOPHAGEAL VARICES

25. **Ans. b. Esophageal varices** *(Ref: Wolfgang Radiology 2/e p509)*

   ESOPHAGEAL VARICES

   - On USG:
     - **Thickened sinus, interrupted mucosal folds (earliest sign)**[Q]
     - Tortuous radiolucencies of variable size
     - The **"worm-eaten"** smooth **lobulated filling defects**[Q]

26. **Ans. d. Esophageal varices** *(Ref: Sabiston 20/e p1437; Schwartz 10/e p1281; Bailey 27/e p1126; Harrison 20/e p2411, 19/e p1890)*

Esophageal Varices

- **Most significant clinical finding** associated with **PHT** is development of **GE varices**[Q].
- **Major blood supply** to GE varices is **anterior branch** of **left gastric** or **coronary vein**[Q].
- **Variceal bleeding** is **leading cause** of **morbidity** and **mortality** associated with PHT[Q]
- Approximately **30%** of patients with **compensated cirrhosis** and **60%** of patients with **decompensated cirrhosis** have **esophageal varices**[Q].

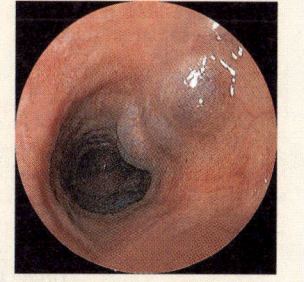

27. **Ans. d. Propranolol** *(Ref: Sabiston 20/e p1437-1440; Blumgart 6/e p1200, 5/e p1129-1146; Shackelford 8/e p1581, 7/e p1599-1604; Harrison 20/e p2411, 19/e p2063-2064)*
28. **Ans. b. Mucosal folds below the carina** *(Ref: Surgical Diseases in Tropical countries/130)*

- **Esophageal varices** presents as **serpiginous filling defects**[Q] (arrows) in the esophagus **below** the level of the **carina**[Q].

Radiological Grading of Varices	
Grade I	**Straight varices** seen only on **inspiration**
Grade II	Straight varices seen in **all phases of respiration**
Grade III	**Tortuous varices** in **lower half** of esophagus
Grade IV	Tortuous varices in **entire esophagus**

29. **Ans. b. Gastro-esophagoscopy**
30. **Ans. a. 12 hours** *(Ref: Bailey 27/e p1164)*

- The **balloons** should be **temporarily deflated after 12 hours**[Q] to **prevent pressure necrosis** of the esophagus.

SENGSTAKEN-BLAKEMORE TUBE

- If the **rate of blood loss prohibits endoscopic evaluation**, a **Sengstaken–Blakemore tube** may be **inserted** to **provide temporary hemostasis**[Q].
- Once inserted, the **gastric balloon** is inflated with **300 mL of air**[Q] and retracted to the gastric fundus, where the varices at the esophagogastric junction are tamponaded by the subsequent inflation of the **esophageal balloon** to a pressure of **40 mmHg**[Q].
- The **two remaining channels** allow **gastric** and **esophageal aspiration**[Q].
- A **radiograph** is used to **confirm the position of the tube**[Q].
- The **balloons** should be **temporarily deflated after 12 hours** to **prevent pressure necrosis** of the esophagus[Q].

31. **Ans. a. 40 mm**
32. **Ans. b. Banding (Endoscopic)** *(Ref: Sabiston 20/e p1439; Blumgart 6/e p1201, 5/e p1135-1138; Shackelford 8/e p1581-1582, 7/e p1600-1601; Harrison 20/e p2411, 19/e p2063-2064)*

Injection Sclerotherapy	Endoscopic Variceal Ligation
• Tetradecyl sodium (**1–3%**), sodium morrhuate (5%), ethanolamine oleate (**5%**) and **3% phenol** are most common sclerosing agents[Q].	• For control of **acute variceal bleeding EVL** has been found to be **as effective as EST**[Q]
• A **combined para** and **intravariceal technique** is used for the management of **acute variceal bleeding** and a predominantly intravariceal technique for long term management[Q].	• Technically **more difficult than EST**[Q] in presence of massive bleeding due to reduction in field of view
• **Variceal eradication** is considered the **end point of EST**[Q]	• **Variceal recurrence** rate is **higher in EVL** since, **paraoesophageal varices**[Q] (perforating veins) are **not obliterated**.
• **Variceal obliteration** can be achieved in **80–95%** patients with a mean of **4–6.8 sessions**[Q].	• **Not suitable** for **small varices** (grade I, II)
• **Esophageal stricture**[Q] is a common **complication**	• EVL is associated with **lesser complications** and **rebleeding**[Q]
	• Variceal eradication in **fewer sessions** but **higher recurrence** of varices[Q].

33. **Ans. b. Stiegmann and Goff** *(Ref: Bailey 24/e p1071)*

Van Steigmann and Goff	Endoscopic esophageal variceal ligation[Q]
Crile and Borema	**Transesophageal ligation** of bleeding esophageal varices[Q]
Suguira and Futagawa	**Esophageal transections** with **paraesophago-gastric devascularization** in the treatment of esophageal varices[Q]
Crafoord and Freckner	Endoscopic sclerotherapy[Q]

34. **Ans. a. Octreotide** *(Ref: Harrison 20/e p2411, 19/e p2063-2064)*

- **Somatostatin** and/or its analog **octreotide** are the **agents of choice** for **medical management** of **variceal bleed**[Q].
- **Octreotide** and **Somatostatin** have been found to be effective in **achieving hemostasis** and **preventing early rebleeding**[Q].
- **Terlipressin** is released in sustained and slow manner. It does not share several systemic side effects of vasopressin and **may be used** to **control variceal bleeding**[Q].

Drugs used in Portal Hypertension	
Drugs Decreasing portal blood flow	**Drugs decreasing intrahepatic resistance**
• Non-selective beta blockers	• Nitrates
• Vasopressin and **Terlipressin**	• Alpha1-blockers (Prazosin)
• Somatostatin and **Octreotide (DOC)**[Q]	• Angiotensin receptor blockers

35. **Ans. a. Unresponsiveness to consecutive 2 energy sclerotherapies**
- **Failure of endoscopic treatment** is declared when **two sessions fail to control hemorrhage**[Q].

GASTRIC VARICES

36. **Ans. c. Cirrhosis** *(Ref: Sabiston 20/e p1232; Schwartz 10/e p1088)*

- MC cause of gastric varices: **Cirrhosis**[Q]
- MC cause of **isolated gastric varices**: Splenic vein thrombosis[Q]

Portal Hypertension

37. **Ans. b.** Most commonly due to splenic vein thrombosis
38. **Ans. All** *(Ref: Sabiston 20/e p1232)*

> **GASTRIC VARICES**
>
> - Gastric varices can develop **secondary to portal hypertension**, in conjunction **with esophageal varices**^{Q}, or secondary to **sinistral hypertension** from **splenic vein thrombosis**^{Q}.
> - In generalized portal hypertension, the **increased portal pressure** is **transmitted by** the **left gastric vein**^{Q} to **esophageal varices** and by the **short** and **posterior gastric veins**^{Q} to the **fundic plexus** and **cardia veins**.
> - **Isolated gastric varices** tend to occur secondary to **splenic vein thrombosis**.
> - **Splenic blood flows** retrograde through the **short** and **posterior gastric veins** into the **varices**, then **hepatopetally through** the **coronary vein**^{Q} into the **portal vein**.
> - **Left-to-right retrograde flow** through the **gastroepiploic vein**^{Q} to the **superior mesenteric vein** can explain the development of **ectopic varices** in the stomach.

TIPS

39. **Ans. a. HPS** *(Ref: Sabiston 20/e p1439; Schwartz 10/e p347; Blumgart 6/e p439, 5/e p1180-1188; Shackelford 8/e p1584, 7/e p1602-1603; Harrison 20/e p2412, 19/e p2064-2065)*
40. **Ans. a.** Shunt thrombosis is more common than stenosis

> - **Shunt stenosis** is usually secondary to **neointimal hyperplasia** and is **more common than thrombosis**^{Q}.

41. **Ans. c.** Portal vein and hepatic vein   42. **Ans. a.** Non-selective shunt

> - TIPS is a **non-selective shunt**, created between **portal** and **hepatic vein**^{Q}
> - TIPS is **portahepatic** or **intrahepatic shunt**^{Q}

43. **Ans. b.** It is intrahepatic shunt, **d.** Most suitable for patient going for liver transplant
44. **Ans. c.** Hepatopulmonary syndrome
45. **Ans. c.** Metabolic encephalopathy *(Ref: Schwartz 10/e p1282; Sabiston 20/e p1440; Bailey 27/e p1164)*

SURGICAL SHUNTS

46. **Ans. a. Inokuchi** *(Ref: Sabiston 20/e p1440; Shackelford 8/e p1575, 7/e p1603-1604)*

> **INOKUCHI SHUNT**
>
> - Interposition of a **vein graft** between the **left gastric** (Coronary) vein and the **IVC**^{Q}.
> - Also known as **coronary-caval fistula**^{Q}
> - Choice (TIPS or shunt) is based on the predicted time to transplantation:

47. **Ans. a. Midline** *(Ref: Mastery of Surgery 2007/1352; Atlas of GI Surgery by John L. Cameron 2007/194)*

> **MESOCAVAL SHUNT**
>
> - A **mesocaval shunt** can be performed through either a **bilateral subcostal** or **midline incision**.
> - **Midline incision** is **preferred**^{Q}.

48. **Ans. c.** 12 mm interposition shunt   49. **Ans. b. Selective shunt** *(Ref: Sabiston 20/e p1442; Schwartz 10/e p1283)*

> *The given shunt is distal splenorenal shunt, which is a selective shunt.*

50. **Ans. a.** Portocaval shunt   51. **Ans. d.** Type of shunt

> - **Prognosis** of **portacaval shunt** depend on **Child's criteria** (Bilirubin, albumin, ascites, PT, encephalopathy)^Q.

52. **Ans. d.** All of the above

    Porto-systemic shunting is avoided in CTP class C. All the options belong to Class C.

53. **Ans. a. Ascites** *(Ref: Textbook of Hepatology by Erwin Kuntz/317)*
54. **Ans. c. Superior vena cava** *(Ref: Bailey 26/e p1077; Textbook of Hepatology by Erwin Kuntz/317)*

    The Le-Veen shunt in ascites is done between peritoneum and superior vena cava.

> *"The Le-Veen shunt is designed for the relief of ascites due to chronic liver disease. One end of the silastic tube is inserted into the ascites within the peritoneal cavity and the other end is tunneled subcutaneously to the neck, where it is inserted under direct vision into the internal jugular vein and fed into the SVC."- Bailey 26/e p1077*

Surgery Essence

55. **Ans. d. Portacaval anastomosis** *(Ref: Blumgart 5/e p1110; Harrison 20/e p2420, 19/e p 2066, 1773)*
56. **Ans. b. Warren shunt** *(Ref: Sabiston 20/e p1442; Schwartz 10/e p1283)*

EXTRA-HEPATIC PORTAL VENOUS OBSTRUCTION

57. **Ans. b. Non-cirrhotic portal fibrosis** *(Ref: Blumgart 6/e p1216, 5/e p1099-1105)*
58. **Ans. a. EHPVO** *(Ref: Blumgart 6/e p1216, 5/e p1099-1105)*
59. **Ans. a. > d. Mesocaval shunt > Splenorenal shunt**

   - Since obstruction is in the portal vein, to bypass the obstruction the shunt should be preferably **Rex shunt (mesenterico-left portal shunt)**[Q] or a **mesocaval shunt.**
   - Splenorenal shunt is also done in EHPVO but in **50%** of patients of **EHPVO, splenic vein is thrombosed**, not available for **splenorenal shunt**[Q].

60. **Ans. b. EHPVO** *(Ref: Fundamentals of Pediatric Surgery by Peter Mattei 2/e p655)*

   The name of the given shunt is Rex shunt (between superior mesenteric vein and left branch of portal vein). This is used for EHPVO.

   "In the subset of patient with EHPVO, PHT, and recurrent variceal bleeding, the treatment of choice is the meso-Rex bypass (MRB)."
   -Fundamentals of Pediatric Surgery by Peter Mattei 2/e p655

NON-CIRRHOTIC PORTAL FIBROSIS

61. **Ans. c. Upper gastrointestinal bleeding** *(Ref: Blumgart 6/e p1216, 5/e p1088)*
62. **Ans. b. Intrahepatic pre-sinusoidal obstruction**

BUDD-CHIARI SYNDROME

63. **Ans. c. Causes prehepatic portal hypertension** *(Ref: Schwartz 10/e p1283-1284; Bailey 27/e p1166; Blumgart 6/e p1248, 5/e p1189-1198; Shackelford 8/e p1521, 7/e p1547-1548)*
64. **Ans. a. Budd-Chiari syndrome**
65. **Ans. d. Hepatic veins**
66. **Ans. c. Hepatomegaly, abdominal pain, ascites**
67. **Ans. d. Side to side portocaval shunt**
68. **Ans. c. Budd Chiari syndrome** *(Ref: Sabiston 20/e p1780; Schwartz 10/e p1083, 1822; Harrison 20/e p2415, 19/e p1645)*

   Spider web collaterals on venography are seen in Budd Chiari syndrome.

Budd Chiari syndrome	Buerger disease
Spider web collaterals on Venography[Q]	*Corkscrew collaterals on Arteriography*[Q]

VENO-OCCLUSIVE DISEASE

69. **Ans. b. Hepatomegaly, e. Hepatic fibrosis** *(Ref: Blumgart 6/e p1268, 5/e p1189-1198; Shackelford 8/e p1528, 7/e p1556)*
70. **Ans. c. Mushroom poisoning**

CHAPTER 6

Gallbladder

GALLSTONES: PATHOGENESIS

PATHOGENESIS OF CHOLESTEROL GALLSTONES

- **Cholesterol** is **insoluble** in **water** (water is major constituent of bile, **85-95%**)^Q.
- **Bile acid** & **phospholipids** in bile keep cholesterol in solution by the formation of **micelles**^{Q}.
- An **excess of cholesterol** relative to bile acids & phospholipids allows cholesterol to form crystals and such bile is called **lithogenic** or **supersaturated bile**^{Q}.

Factors Responsible for Formation of Gallstones		
Lithogenic bile	**Nucleation**	**Stasis or GB hypomotility**

• **Increased Biliary Cholesterol:**
  – **Obesity**^{Q}
  – **Cholesterol rich diet**^{Q}
  – **Clofibrate** therapy^Q
• **Decreased Bile Acids:**
  – Primary biliary cirrhosis
  – **OCPs**^{Q}
  – Mutation of **CYP7A1** gene^Q
  – **Impaired enterohepatic circulation** of bile acids: **Ileal disease** or **resection, cholestyramine** or **colestipol** (bile acid sequestrants)^Q
• **Decreased Biliary Lecithin:**
  – **MDR-3** gene **mutation**^{Q} leads to defective lecithin secretion in bile
	• Cholesterol monohydrate crystal agglomerate to become macroscopic crystal by nucleation
	• **Pro-nucleating Factors:**
	  – **Mucin**^{Q}
	  – Non-mucin glycoprotein^Q
	  – Infection^Q
	• **Anti-nucleating Factors:**
	  – Apolipoprotein **A-I & A-II**^{Q}
	• **Excess** of **pro-nucleating factors** or **deficiency** of **anti-nucleating factors** results in formation of gallstones
		• Prolonged **TPN**^{Q}
		• Prolonged **fasting**^{Q}
		• **Pregnancy**^{Q}
		• **Octreotide**^{Q}
		• **OCPs**^{Q}
		• Massive **burns**^{Q}

- **Cholesterol gallstones** are made up of **crystalline cholesterol monohydrate**^{Q}.

Pigmented Stones	
Black Stones	**Brown Stones**

• **Black stones** are composed of **insoluble bilirubin pigment polymer**^{Q} mixed with **calcium phosphate** & **calcium bicarbonate**^{Q}.
• **Predisposing Factors:**
  – **Hemolytic disorders**^{Q} (Hereditary spherocytosis, sickle cell anemia)
  – Mechanical **prosthetic heart valves**^{Q}
  – Cirrhosis
  – **Gilbert's syndrome**^{Q}
  – **Cystic fibrosis**^{Q}
  – Ileal disease or resection
	• **Brown pigment** stones contain **calcium bilirubinate**, calcium **palmitate** & calcium **stearate** as well as cholesterol^Q.
	• Typically found in **Asia**^{Q}
	• Rare in **GB**^{Q}
	• Formed in bile duct^Q
	• Related to the **bile stasis and infection:**
	  – Gram negative bacteria (**E. coli** & **Klebsiella**)^Q secretes **beta-glucuronidase**^{Q}, which **deconjugate** soluble **conjugated bilirubin**
	  – Free unconjugated bilirubin precipitates & combines with **calcium** and **bile** to form **brown pigment stones**.
	  – Stones form whenever static foreign bodies are present in the bile duct (**stents** or parasites such as **Clonorchis sinensis** & **Ascaris lumbricoides**)^Q

GALLSTONES INVESTIGATIONS

Oral Cholecystography (Graham Cole Test)

- Once considered the diagnostic test of choice for gallstones, oral cholecystography has been **replaced by ultrasonography**.
- It involves **oral administration** of a **radiopaque compound** that is **absorbed, excreted** by the **liver**, and **passed into** the **gallbladder**[Q].

Successful Visualization of GB in Oral Cholecystography depends on	
• **Blood flow** to the **liver**[Q]	• **Patency**[Q] of hepatic and cystic duct system
• **Ability** of the **liver cells** to **excrete** dye into the bile (**functioning liver**)[Q]	• **Ability of GB** to **concentrate** the excreted **dye**[Q] (by absorbing water)

- **Stones** are noted on a film as **filling defects** in a visualized, **opacified gallbladder**.

Oral cholecystography is of no value in patients with			
• Intestinal malabsorption[Q]	• Vomiting[Q]	• Obstructive jaundice[Q]	• Hepatic failure[Q]

Ultrasonography

- Initial imaging modality of choice in obstructive jaundice[Q]
- It is **operator dependent** and may be **suboptimal due to excessive body fat** and **intraluminal bowel gas**[Q].

USG can demonstrate		
• **Biliary calculi**[Q]	• **Size** of GB and CBD[Q]	• Presence of **inflammation**[Q] around GB
• **Thickness** of GB wall[Q]		• Occasionally, **presence of stones within** the **biliary tree**[Q]

- It may even show a **carcinoma** of the **pancreas** occluding the **CBD**[Q].

USG in obstructive jaundice
• **Initial imaging modality** of **choice** in **obstructive jaundice**[Q]
• It **can identify intra-** and **extrahepatic biliary dilatation**[Q]
• Identify the **level of obstruction**[Q]
• **Cause of the obstruction**[Q] may also be identified
(**Gallstones** in the gallbladder, common hepatic or **CBD stones** or lesions in the wall of the duct suggestive of a **cholangiocarcinoma** or enlargement of the pancreatic head indicative of a **pancreatic carcinoma**)[Q]

- **Iopanoic acid** is used in **oral cholecystography**[Q].
- **Biligraffin** is used in **IV cholangiography**[Q].

Radioisotope Scanning

- **Technetium-99m labelled derivatives** of **iminodiacetic acid** (HIDA, IODIDA) are, when injected intravenously, **selectively taken up** by the **reticuloendothelial cells** of the liver and **excreted into bile**[Q].

HIDA Scan
• Allows **visualization** of the **biliary tree** and **gallbladder**[Q]
• Presence of **inflammation**[Q] around GB
• Occasionally, **presence of stones within** the **biliary tree**[Q]
• **GB** is **visualized within 30 min** of isotope injection in 90% of normal individuals and within 1 hour in the remainder.
• The **bowel** is usually **seen within 1 hour** in the majority of patients.
• **Nonvisualization** of the **GB** is suggestive of **acute cholecystitis**[Q].
• If the patient has **contracted gallbladder**, as often occurs in **chronic cholecystitis**, **GB visualization** may be **reduced** or **delayed**[Q].

- **Biliary scintigraphy** may also be **helpful in diagnosing bile leaks** and **iatrogenic biliary obstruction**[Q].
- **Scintigraphy can confirm** the **presence & quantify the leak**[Q].

ACUTE CHOLECYSTITIS

Acute Cholecystitis

- Acute cholecystitis is **related to gallstones** in **90–95%**[Q] of cases.
- **Characteristic triad: RUQ pain + Fever + Leukocytosis**[Q]

Etiopathogenesis
- **Obstruction** of **cystic duct** leading to **biliary colic** is the initial event in acute cholecystitis.
- An inflammatory process with a thickened & **reddish wall** with **subserosal hemorrhage**[Q].
- Mostly the **gallstone dislodges**, & inflammation will gradually resolve.
- In the **most severe cases**, this process can lead to **ischemia** & **necrosis** of the GB wall (**5–10%**[Q]).

Clinical Features
- RUQ pain of **much longer duration** than biliary colic, is the **MC symptom**[Q]
- Other common symptoms: Fever, nausea, and vomiting.
- **Physical examination**: RUQ tenderness and guarding are usually present **inferior to** the **right costal margin**, distinguishing the episode from simple biliary colic.
- A **mass** (**gallbladder** & **adherent omentum**) is occasionally palpable[Q]
- **Murphy's sign**[Q]: Inspiratory arrest with **deep palpation** in the **RUQ** in acute cholecystitis (also known as **Naunyn's sign**)
- **Boa's sign**[Q]: Hyperesthesia below right scapula in acute cholecystitis.

> - A **mild leukocytosis** is **usually present** (12,000–14,000 cells/mm^3).
> - Mild elevations in serum bilirubin (>4 mg/dL), ALP, transaminases, & amylase may be present.

Diagnosis

> - **USG**: **IOC** for diagnosing **acute cholecystitis**[Q] (sensitivity 85%, specificity 95%).
> - **HIDA scan**: **Gold standard**[Q] for diagnosing **acute cholecystitis**

- **USG findings**: Presence of **gallstones**, **thickening** of GB wall (**> 4 mm**), pericholecystic fluid, GB distention, impacted stone, and a **sonographic Murphy's sign**[Q] (focal tenderness directly over the GB).
- **HIDA scan**: **No filling** of GB with the radiotracer (^{99m}Tc-HIDA) **after 4 hours** indicates an **obstructed cystic duct**[Q]

> **Tokyo guidelines** provide guidance regarding **diagnosis, severity assessment & management** of acute cholecystitis & acute cholangitis[Q].

- A **normal** HIDA scan **excludes acute cholecystitis**[Q].

Treatment
- **IV fluids, antibiotics**, and **analgesia** should be initiated[Q].
- **Cholecystectomy** is the **definitive treatment**[Q] for patients with acute cholecystitis.

> - **Early cholecystectomy** performed **within 2 to 3 days (within 72 hours)**[Q] of presentation **is preferred over interval** or **delayed cholecystectomy** that is performed 6 to 10 weeks after initial medical therapy.
> - **Laparoscopic cholecystectomy** is the **preferred approach** to patients with **acute cholecystitis**[Q].

- **Morbidity rate, hospital stay**, and **time to return to work** are **lower** in patients undergoing **laparoscopic cholecystectomy** than open cholecystectomy.

> - **Early laparoscopic cholecystectomy**, due to a **reduced length of hospital stay** and **readmissions**, is a **more cost-effective approach** than open cholecystectomy for acute cholecystitis.

MEDICAL THERAPY FOR GALLSTONES

MEDICAL THERAPY FOR GALLSTONES

- Medical therapy for gallstones utilizes bile acids: **Chenodeoxycholic acid (CDCA)** & **Ursodeoxycholic acid (UDCA)**[Q]

Mechanism of Action
- They **inhibit HMG-CoA reductase**[Q], rate limiting enzyme for cholesterol synthesis, thus **decreases cholesterol saturation of bile**[Q]
- They cause **dispersion** of **cholesterol** from the **stones** by **physicochemical means**[Q]

Prerequisites for Medical Treatment	Drawbacks of Medical Treatment
- **Radioluscent (cholesterol) stones**[Q] - **Stones <10 mm** in diameter[Q] - **Functioning GB**[Q] - **Non-acute symptoms**[Q]	- **Low rates** of **complete resolution**[Q] - **High recurrence rate**[Q] - **Not cost-effective** (expensive drug has to be taken for up to 2 years)[Q] - **Need** of **maintenance therapy** to prevent recurrence[Q]

GALLSTONE ILEUS

Gallstone Ileus

- Passage of **stone** through a **spontaneous biliary-enteric fistula** leading to a **mechanical bowel obstruction**[Q]
- **MC site** of fistula: Between the **gallbladder** and **duodenum**[Q]
- **2nd MC site**: Between **gallbladder** and **transverse colon**[Q].

Clinical Features

> - **Rigler's triad**[Q]: Classic plain abdominal film triad of **small bowel obstruction, pneumobilia, & ectopic gallstone** is considered **pathognomonic**[Q].

- Most **cholecystoduodenal fistula** does **not** result in Gallstone ileus[Q]. Rather, they are **asymptomatic**[Q] or occur in associated with usual digestive complaints consistent with gastric or biliary tract disease.
- Occurs **most commonly** in the **elderly (>70 years)**[Q]
- Accounts for **1%** of all cases of **small bowel obstruction** and occur in fewer than 1% of patients with gallstones.

> **Bouveret's Syndrome**
> - **Duodenal obstruction** due to gallstones, usually in the **bulb** is known as **Bouveret's syndrome**[Q].
> - It is treated by **duodenostomy** or **pyloroplasty**[Q].

- **Nausea, vomiting**, and **abdominal pain**, signs & symptoms of intestinal obstruction
- A history of **gallstone-related symptoms** may be present in only **50%** of patients.
- **Pain** may be **episodic** and **recurrent** as the impacted stone temporarily obstructs the bowel lumen and then dislodges and moves distally, known as **tumbling obstruction**[Q].
- **MC site** of obstruction is **ileum**[Q] (60%); **jejunum** (15%); **stomach** (15%) colon (5% > sigmoid colon); & **duodenum** (5%).

Diagnosis

- **Abdominal X-ray**: Evidence of an **intestinal obstruction** with **pneumobilia** or a **calcified stone**[Q] distant from the gallbladder.
- **MC site** of obstruction is the **terminal ileum**[Q] because of its narrow lumen.

Treatment

- It is a **surgical emergency**[Q] without a period of waiting in the hope that stone will pass
- In case of **obstruction in the ileum calculus** can be **manipulated proximally** to a **healthy jejunum**[Q] where a **safe enterotomy** and stone removal may be executed.
- **Stable patients**: Takedown of the **biliary-enteric fistula** and **cholecystectomy**[Q] during the same procedure is warranted because recurrent cholecystitis and cholangitis are common.

> - **Unstable patients** or a **significant inflammation** in RUQ: Unstable to withstand a prolonged **operative procedure**, the fistula can be addressed at a second laparotomy[Q].

MUCOCELE

Mucocele (Hydrops)

- **Hydrops** or **mucocele** result from **prolonged obstruction** of the **cystic duct**, usually by a **large solitary calculus**[Q].
- **Obstructed GB lumen** is progressively **distended** by **mucus** (mucocele) or by a **clear transudate** (hydrops) produced by mucosal epithelial cells[Q].

Clinical Features

- A **visible, easily palpable, nontender gallbladder**[Q] sometimes extending from the RUQ into the right iliac fossa may be found on physical examination.
- The patient with hydrops of the gallbladder **frequently remains asymptomatic**[Q], although chronic RUQ pain may also occur.

Treatment

- **Early cholecystectomy**[Q], because empyema, perforation, or gangrene may complicate the condition.

Gallbladder Empyema

- GB empyema results from **progression of acute cholecystitis** with **persistent cystic duct obstruction** to **superinfection**[Q] of the stagnant bile with a pus-forming bacterial organism.

Clinical Features

- Clinical picture resembles that of **cholangitis** with **high fever**; **severe RUQ pain**; marked **leukocytosis**; and often, **prostration**[Q].
- Empyema carries a **high risk of gram-negative sepsis** and/or **perforation**[Q].

Treatment

- **Emergency surgical intervention** with **antibiotic coverage** is required as soon as the diagnosis is suspected.

PROPHYLACTIC CHOLECYSTECTOMY

Indications of Prophylactic Cholecystectomy	
• Cardiac transplant recipients^Q • Lung transplant recipients^Q • Chronic TPN requirement^Q • Recipients of biliopancreatic diversion^Q (bariatric patient) • Children with hemoglobinopathy^Q (sickle cell, thalassemia and spherocytosis) • Asymptomatic gallstone ≥3 cm^Q • Stone associated with the polyp	• Family history of GB cancer and asymptomatic stones^Q • Cholelithiasis encountered during elective abdominal procedures^Q • Nonfunctioning GB^Q • Typhoid carrier with positive bile culture^Q • Trauma to GB^Q • Porcelain GB

- Many **heart/lung transplant** recipients use **cyclosporine** as maintenance immunotherapy; **chronic cyclosporine use**[Q] (>2 years) has been associated with the prevalence of **gallstones**.

ACALCULOUS CHOLECYSTITIS

ACALCULOUS CHOLECYSTITIS

- Acute **inflammation of gallbladder without stones**[Q]
- Accounts for 5-10% of all patients of acute cholecystitis
- **More fulminant course**[Q] than the acute calculous cholecystitis.
- **More commonly progresses** to **gangrene, empyema, or perforation**[Q].
- **Visceral ischemia** is common in acute acalculous cholecystitis and may explain the high incidence of GB gangrene.

Predisposing Factors
- **Elderly** and **critically ill patients** after **trauma**[Q]
- **Burns**[Q]
- **Long-term TPN**[Q]
- **Major operations** (**abdominal aneurysm repair** & **cardiopulmonary bypass**[Q])

Etiopathogenesis
- Exact etiology is not clear

> - **GB stasis & ischemia**[Q] have been implicated as causative factors.

- **Stasis** (disturbed micro-circulation) is **common** in **critically ill patients** not being fed enterally and **may** lead to **colonization** of the GB with **bacteria**[Q].
- **Decreased arteriolar** and **capillary filling** is present in contrast with the dilatation of these vessels in acute calculous cholecystitis.

Clinical Features
- **Similar** to acute **calculous cholecystitis**[Q].
- Patients may present with only **unexplained fever, leucocytosis** and **hyperamylasemia and right upper quadrant tenderness**[Q].
- If untreated, **rapid progression to gangrene and perforation**[Q] may occur.

Diagnosis
- **Ultrasonography** is the **diagnostic test of choice**[Q], especially because it can be done at the bed side.
- **Cholescintigraphy** demonstrates **absent gallbladder filling**

Treatment
- **Emergency cholecystectomy**[Q] for **stable**[Q] patients
- Because of high incidence of gangrene, perforation and empyema, **open cholecystectomy**[Q] is often the **preferred approach**.

> **Percutaneous Cholecystostomy**
> - If patients are **unfit for surgery**, percutaneous, ultrasound guided, or **CT guided cholecystostomy** is the **treatment of choice**[Q].
> - About **90% patients improve** with **percutaneous cholecystostomy**.

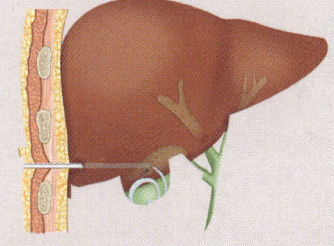

XANTHOGRANULOMATOUS CHOLECYSTITIS

XANTHOGRANULOMATOUS CHOLECYSTITIS

- **XGC:** Inflammatory disease characterized by a **focal or diffuse destructive inflammatory process** with **lipid-laden macrophages**[Q]

Pathology
- Inflammatory response to **extravasated bile**, possibly from **ruptured Rokitansky-Aschoff sinuses**[Q].
- Presence of **hypoechoic nodules** or **bands** in **thickened GB wall**[Q] together with calculi (cholesterol or mixed gallstones) in patient of chronic disease.
- There is **extension of yellow tissue** into **adjacent organs**, **fistulas** from GB to **skin** or **duodenum** may develop, may be **mistaken for cancer**[Q].

Clinical Features
- Similar to acute cholecystitis

Diagnosis
- **Thickening** of GB wall is **most common radiological finding**, sometimes presence of **hypoattenuated bands**[Q].

Treatment
- Surgical treatment **(Laparoscopic cholecystectomy)** remains **the most** effective and **feasible option for XGC**

EMPHYSEMATOUS CHOLECYSTITIS

EMPHYSEMATOUS CHOLECYSTITIS

- Thought to begin with acute cholecystitis (calculous or acalculous), followed by ischemia or gangrene of GB wall and **infection** by **gas producing organisms**[Q].
- Occur most frequently in **elderly men** and patients with **diabetes mellitus**[Q].
- **Gallstones** are observed in **28–80% of patients with emphysematous cholecystitis.**
- Emphysematous cholecystitis in the presence of acalculous cholecystitis is well established.

Causative organisms of Emphysematous Cholecystitis
• **Anaerobes: Cl. welchii** or **Cl. perfringens (MC)**[Q]
• **Aerobes: E. coli**[Q]

Clinical Features
- Clinical manifestations are essentially indistinguishable from those of nongaseous cholecystitis.

Diagnosis
- **Diagnosis** is usually made on **abdominal X-ray**[Q]
- **Abdominal X-ray** findings: **Gas** within the **GB lumen**, dissecting within GB wall to form a **gaseous ring** or in **pericholecystic tissues**[Q].
- **IOC for diagnosis: CT scan**[Q]

Treatment
- Morbidity & mortality rates with emphysematous cholecystitis are considerable.
- **Prompt surgical drainage** coupled with appropriate **antibiotics** is mandatory[Q].
- **Cholecystectomy** is **best treatment** of complicated acute cholecystitis[Q].
- **Unstable patients**: Percutaneous cholecystostomy under **LA**[Q] can be performed to drain GB.

MIRIZZI'S SYNDROME (FUNCTIONAL HEPATIC SYNDROME)

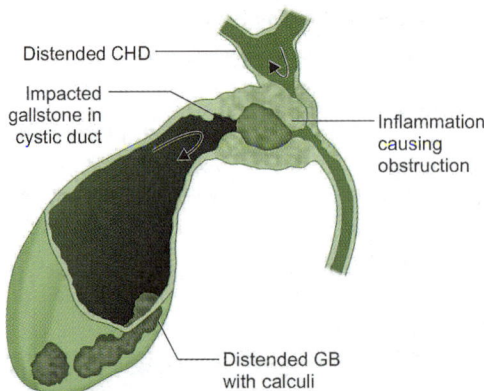

MIRIZZI'S SYNDROME (FUNCTIONAL HEPATIC SYNDROME)

- It is defined as **obstruction** of the **common hepatic duct** or **CBD** by **external compression** or by **erosion** of stone in the **Hartmann pouch** or **cystic duct**[Q].
- **External compression** has been classified as **type 1** whereas **erosion** as **type 2** Mirizzi syndrome by **McSherry**[Q].

- **Csendes** subclassified type 2 into three categories based on the percentage of the wall of CBD eroded by offending calculus.

Csendes Classification of Mirizzi's Syndrome	
Type I	**Obstruction** of common duct by **external compression only** (no erosion)^Q
Type II	Erosion of **less than one-third** circumference of common duct^Q
Type III	Erosion of **up to two-third** circumference of common duct^Q
Type IV	**Total/near total** circumferential destruction of common duct^Q
Type V	**Erosion of GB in common duct** with **cholecystoenteric fistula**

Treatment

Type I	Partial cholecystectomy^Q
Type II & Type III	**Partial cholecystectomy** leaving behind a cuff of gallbladder for reconstruction of bile duct (**choledochoplasty**) with **T-tube drainage**^{Q}
Type IV & V	Bilioenteric anastomosis^Q

- **Stenosis** of the **biliary tree** often **resolves spontaneously** in the **postoperative period**, and **choledochotomy** is **seldom indicated**^{Q}.

STRAWBERRY GALLBLADDER (CHOLESTEROLOSIS)

Strawberry Gallbladder (Cholesterolosis)

- It is an **acquired**^{Q} histologic abnormality of gallbladder epithelium that results in an **excessive accumulation** of lipid (**cholesterols esters & triglyceride**)^Q **within epithelial macrophage** of GB wall.
- **Cholesterol stones** are found in **half** of the **cases**^{Q}.

Pathology
- **Gross Appearance:** Mucosa has **pale, yellow streaks** running longitudinally giving rise to the term **strawberry gallbladder**^{Q} (although the mucosa is usually bile stained rather than red).
- **Diffuse form** ("strawberry gallbladder"): GB mucosa is **brick red** and speckled with **bright yellow flecks** of lipid^Q.
- **Localized form: Solitary** or multiple "**cholesterol polyps**" studding the gallbladder wall^Q.

Treatment
- **Cholecystectomy** is indicated in **symptomatic cholesterolosis** or when **cholelithiasis** is present^Q.

GALLBLADDER POLYPS

Polypoid Lesions of the Gallbladder	
Cholesterol polyps	**Adenomatous polyp**

• **Cholesterol polyps** are the **most common**^{Q}
• Usually **<10 mm** in size^Q
• Have a characteristic echogenic **pedunculated**^{Q} appearance on USG
• **Multiple (30% of cases)**^{Q}
	• Adenomatous polyp has **malignant potential**^{Q}.
	• Adenoma may be **difficult to distinguish from adenocarcinoma** of GB
	• Main differentiating feature is a **lack of transmural invasion** on USG^Q
	• **Risk factors** associated with **malignancy:**
	  – **Age > 60 years**^{Q} – Coexistence of gallstones^Q
	  – Documented **increase in size**^{Q} – **Size > 10 mm**^{Q}

GALLBLADDER ADENOMYOMATOSIS

Gallbladder Adenomyomatosis

- **Adenomyomatosis** is a benign condition characterized by **hyperplastic changes**^{Q} of unknown etiology involving the GB wall.
- It causes **overgrowth of mucosa, thickening of muscular wall,** and **formation of intramural diverticula** or **sinus tracts** termed as **Aschoff-Rokitansky sinuses**^{Q}.
- These sinuses may contain **cholesterol crystals**^{Q}.
- The disease can be **focal** or **diffuse**.
- It has **no malignant potential**^{Q}.

Diagnosis

- **USG:** The presence of cholesterol crystals in these sinuses can result in "**diamond ring sign**"^{Q}, "**V-shaped**"^{Q}, or "**comet-tail**" **artifacts**^{Q} on USG.
- **Adenomyomatosis** appears as a **sessile polyp** with characteristic **microcysts** on USG and is often **>10 mm**^{Q}.
- **Cholecystography** is more specific for diagnosis.

Treatment

- **Cholecystectomy** is indicated in **symptomatic adenomyomatosis** or when **cholelithiasis** is present^Q.

RISK FACTORS FOR CARCINOMA GALLBLADDER

Risk Factors for Carcinoma Gallbladder	
• Gallstones >3 cm^Q	• Adenomatous polyps^Q
• Porcelain gallbladder^Q	• Primary sclerosing cholangitis^Q
• Anomalous pancreaticobiliary junction^Q	• Obesity^Q
• Choledochal cysts^Q	• Salmonella typhi infection^Q

PORCELAIN GALLBLADDER

PORCELAIN GALLBLADDER

- Porcelain GB is characterized by **extensive calcium encrustation** of **GB wall**^{Q}.
- The term porcelain gallbladder has been used to emphasize the **blue discoloration** & **brittle consistency** of GB wall at surgery^Q.

Pathology

- **Calcium salt deposition** within the wall of a **chronically inflamed gallbladder**^{Q}

Clinical Features

- Most porcelain GB (**90%**) are **associated** with **gallstones**^{Q}.
- Mean **age** of patients is **54 years** (38–70 years).
- Patients are usually **asymptomatic** and the condition is usually **found incidentally** on **plain abdominal radiographs,** sonograms or CT images.
- **Incidence of CA GB: 6%**
- **Surgery** should not be delayed even if the patient is asymptomatic, because the occurrence of carcinoma is remarkably high.

Diagnosis

- In porcelain GB, **plain radiographic findings** are usually **straight forward**^{Q}.
- **CT scan** is **diagnostic** in cases of **doubt**

Treatment

- **Cholecystectomy** in **all patients**^{Q} with porcelain GB (high incidence of development carcinoma GB).

CARCINOMA GALLBLADDER

CARCINOMA GALLBLADDER

- **Highest incidence** of CA GB in **India** and **Pakistan**^{Q}
- More common in **women** of **6th** & **7th** decade^Q
- **Cholelithiasis** is seen in **75–98%** of all patients with CA GB^Q.
- **Incidence** of CA GB **in** a population of **patients with gallstones** is from **0.3–3%**^{Q}.
- CA GB is an aggressive malignancy with **poor prognosis**^{Q}
- **Nevin classification**^{Q} is used for **CA GB staging**.

  - **Calcified GB** is associated with cancer in **10**^{Q} of cases.
  - **Helicobacter pylori** & **H. bilis** demonstrated to **increase** the **risk of CA GB** by 6 fold^Q.
  - **Increased risk** of CA GB in **FAP** & **HNPCC**^{Q}.

- MC gene mutation in CA GB: **p53> K-ras>BRAF**^{Q}
- MC mode of CA GB spread: **Direct invasion**^{Q} into the adjacent organs

Pathology

- **MC Site: Fundus (60%)**^{Q} >Body (30%) >Neck (10%)

- **Histological types:**
  - **Diffuse Infiltrative: MC type**^{Q}
  - **Nodular** or **mass forming**
  - **Papillary:** Exhibits **polypoid** or cauliflower appearance and have **best prognosis**^{Q}.
- **Adenocarcinoma**^{Q} is the MC histologic subtype of CA GB.
- In CA GB: **Direct hepatic invasion** in **59%**^{Q}, **LN metastasis** in **45%**, **perineural invasion** in **42%** cases.

Clinical Features
- Most commonly presents with **RUQ pain** often **mimicking cholecystitis** and cholelithiasis^Q.
- **Weight loss, jaundice,** and an **abdominal mass** are less common presenting symptoms.
- **Chronic cholecystitis** with a **recent change** in **quality** or **frequency** of the **painful episodes** in 40% patients^Q
- Malignant biliary obstruction with jaundice, weight loss, and RUQ pain.

Diagnosis
- **USG** is **first diagnostic modality**^{Q} used in evaluation of patients with **RUQ pain**.

  - **USG:** A **heterogeneous mass replacing** the GB lumen and an **irregular gallbladder wall**^{Q}
  - **CT scan:** Mass replacing the **gallbladder (MC finding)**; focal or diffuse gallbladder **wall thickening**; and an **intraluminal polypoidal mass.**^{Q}

- **Typical cholangiographic finding: Long stricture** of the **common hepatic duct**^{Q}.
- Triple phase CT is used to identify hepatic arterial or portal venous involvement.
- **Unresectable** or **incurable CA GB:** Percutaneous biopsy or FNAC for **confirmatory tissue diagnosis.**^{Q}

Tumor Markers
- **Best tumor marker** for CA GB is **CA19-9**^{Q} (CA19-9 >20 U/ml-**75%** of sensitivity and specificity).
- **CEA >4 ng/mL** is associated with **93% specificity** but **50% sensitivity**.

TNM CLASSIFICATION OF CARCINOMA GALLBLADDER

8th AJCC (2017) TNM Classification of Carcinoma Gallbladder	
T1a	**Lamina propria** invasion^Q
T1b	**Muscular invasion**^{Q}
T2	Invade the **perimuscular connective tissue**^{Q} **T2a:** Invade the **perimuscular connective tissue** on the **peritoneal side** with **no extension to serosa**^{Q} **T2b:** Invade the **perimuscular connective tissue** on the **hepatic side with no extension into the liver**^{Q}
T3	**Serosal perforation** and/or **direct invasion of the liver** (regardless of extent) and/or invasion of any other **single extrahepatic organ**^{Q}.
T4	Tumor invades the main **portal vein, hepatic artery** or **two or more extrahepatic organ**^{Q}
N1	Metastasis to **1-3 regional nodes**^{Q}
N2	Metastasis to **4 or more regional nodes**^{Q}
M1	Distant metastasis

Stage IA	Stage IB	Stage IIA	Stage IIB	Stage IIIA	Stage IIIB	Stage IVA	Stage IVB
T1a N0M0	T1b N0M0	T2a N0M0	T2b N0M0	T3 N0M0	T1-3 N1M0	T4 N0-1M0	Tany N2M0 Tany Nany M1

TREATMENT OF CARCINOMA GALLBLADDER

TREATMENT OF CARCINOMA GALLBLADDER
- Gallbladder cancer: Incidental pathological finding after Laparoscopic cholecystectomy
- **T1a** with **negative cystic duct margin:** No further therapy^Q
- **T1a** with **positive cystic duct margin:** Reresection of **cystic duct** or **CBD** to negative margin^Q

  - **T1b, T2, T3** tumor with no evidence of metastasis: Reresection, **extended cholecystectomy** (possible CBD or extended hepatic resection)^Q

- **T4:** Extended cholecystectomy with **extended right hepatectomy**[Q]
- **N2 or M1 disease: Clinical trial** (chemoradiation or chemotherapy) in good performance status[Q]
- Laparoscopic **trocar site scars** are **excised for staging purpose** to identify **M1** disease than for any potential therapeutic benefit[Q].

Preoperatively diagnosed CA GB
- **T2, T3:** Extended cholecystectomy[Q]
- **T4 N0:** Extended cholecystectomy with **extended right hepatectomy**[Q]
- **N1 or hilar invasion:** Extended cholecystectomy with **CBD resection**[Q]
- **N2 or M1: Clinical trial** (chemoradiation or chemotherapy) in good performance status, **palliative care** in poor performance status[Q]

Surgical Technique
- For patients suspected of having resectable gallbladder cancer, begin **surgical exploration with laparoscopy**, in the absence of disseminated disease, proceed with open laparotomy.

  > - **Extended cholecystectomy** consists of **cholecystectomy with en bloc resection** of segments **IVB** and **V**; including **lymphadenectomy** of the **cystic duct, pericholedochal, periportal,** and **posterior pancreaticoduodenal** and **local interaortocaval** lymph nodes.

- During a **standard cholecystectomy** the **serosa** of the gallbladder is **typically opened** and the avascular subserosal layer is used as the surgical plane of dissection.
- In case of **suspected carcinoma** the **plane of dissection** is along the **cystic plate** of the liver to avoid violation of the gallbladder subserosa.
- Only **15%** of patients develop **loco-regional recurrence** while most (**85%**) had **recurrence** involving a **distant site**.

Gallbladder Cancer with Obstructive Jaundice
- **Percutaneous external biliary drainage** offers a minimally invasive and effective means of palliation.

INDICATIONS FOR REPEAT OPERATIVE INTERVENTION IN CA GB DIAGNOSED INCIDENTALLY AFTER LAPAROSCOPIC CHOLECYSTECTOMY

- Pathologic analysis identifies **T2** or **greater** degree invasion[Q]
- Cystic duct **margins** are **positive**[Q]
- Presence of intra-operative **bile spillage**[Q]

UNRESECTABLE CARCINOMA GALLBLADDER

- **Median survival** for patients presenting with unresectable disease is **2-4 months** with **1-year survival** is less than **5%**[Q].
- Goal of palliation is to relieve jaundice, pain, bowel obstruction and prolongation of life.
- **Percutaneous stents** are effective **for relieving jaundice** and should be used, as expected survival does not usually warrants a surgical bypass[Q].
- **Gemcitabine** plus **cisplatin** (reference regimen) is used for **palliation** of **unresectable disease**[Q].

GALLBLADDER: ANATOMY AND PHYSIOLOGY

GALLBLADDER: ANATOMY AND PHYSIOLOGY

- It is lined by a single, highly-folded, **tall columnar epithelium**
- The **mucus** originates in **tubuloalveolar glands**[Q] found in mucosa lining the infundibulum & **neck**, but are **absent** from the **body & fundus**.
- It is **covered by** the **serosa** except where it is embedded in the liver

  > - GB lacks a muscularis mucosa & submucosa[Q].

- Normal capacity of the gallbladder is **30–50 mL**[Q].
- Mucosa contain **crypt of Luschka**[Q].

Cystic Duct
- **Cystic duct** measures **2–4 cm** in length & contains prominent **concentric folds** known as **spiral valves of Heister**[Q].
- Cystic duct frequently exhibits a **tortuous** or **serpentine course**[Q].
- Diameter of the cystic duct ranges from **1–5 mm**.
- Mucosa of the **cystic duct** is arranged in **spiral folds** known as **valves of Heister**[Q] surrounded by a sphincteric structure called **sphincter of Lutkans**[Q].

- **Cystic artery** is nearly **found within** the **Hepatocystic triangle**^{Q}, the area bound by the cystic duct, common hepatic duct and the liver margin.
- GB mucosa has the **greatest absorptive capacity**^{Q} per unit of any structure in the body.
- **Hartmann's pouch** is an **acquired diverticulum**^{Q} of the infundibulum or **neck** of the gallbladder.

Functions of Gallbladder
• Reservoir of bile
• **Concentration of bile 5-10 times**^{Q}
• Secretion of **mucus, 20 mL/day** by **tubuloalveolar glands**
• **Acidification of bile**

LIMEY BILE

- **Calcium salts** in the lumen of the GB in sufficient concentration may produce **calcium precipitation** and **diffuse, hazy opacification of bile** or a **layering effect** on plain abdominal X-ray^Q.
- Filled with a mixture of **calcium carbonate** and **calcium phosphate** usually, the consistency of toothpaste.^{Q}
- Caused by **gradual obstruction** of the **cystic duct** or **CBD** by chronic pancreatitis or carcinoma pancreas^Q.
- **Organisms** are **rarely grown** from emulsion.

Diagnosis
- Best revealed on **plain radiography**^{Q}

Treatment
- **Limey bile**, or milk of calcium bile, is usually **clinically innocuous**^{Q}
- **Cholecystectomy** is recommended when it occurs in a **hydropic gallbladder**^{Q}.

Composition of Bile		
Characteristic	Hepatic Bile	GB Bile
Na$^+$	160.0	270.0
K$^+$	5	10
Cl$^-$	90	15
HCO$_3^-$	45	10
Ca^{2+}	4	25
Mg^{2+}	2	—
Bilirubin	1.5	15
Protein	150	—
Bile acids	50	150
Phospholipids	8	40
Cholesterol	4	18
Total solids	—	125
pH	7.8	7.2

- The **inorganic solute** has a **concentration in bile** that is **similar to plasma** and account for the bile **osmolality of 300 mOsm/kg**.

COURVOISIER'S SIGN

- A **palpable, nontender gallbladder**^{Q}
- Usually results from a **distal common duct obstruction** secondary to a **peripancreatic malignancy**^{Q}

PHRYGIAN CAP

- This **anomaly** is **most common** of gallbladder^Q
- Created by an **infolding** of a **septum** between **body & fundus**^{Q}
- GB functions normally, and this anomaly is **not an indication** for **cholecystectomy**^{Q}.

MOYNIHAN'S HUMP (CATERPILLAR'S TURN)

- **Most dangerous anomaly** (for cholecystectomy)
- **Right hepatic artery** takes a **tortuous turn**.

Multiple Choice Questions

GALLSTONES: PATHOGENESIS

1. **All of the following are essential for formation of gallstones except:** *(MHSSMCET 2008)*
   a. Bile stasis
   b. Nucleation
   c. Crystallization
   d. Lithogenic bile

2. **Cholesterol gallstones are made up of:** *(Recent Question 2019)*
   a. Crystalline cholesterol monohydrate
   b. Crystalline cholesterol dihydrate
   c. Amorphous cholesterol monohydrate
   d. Amorphous cholesterol dihydrate

3. **All are true about pigmented stones except:** *(AIIMS GIS Dec 2006)*
   a. Seen in cholangiohepatitis
   b. Secondary CBD stones
   c. Primary CBD stones
   d. More common in Asians

4. **False about brown pigmented stones:** *(AIIMS GIS May 2008)*
   a. Associated with disorders of biliary motility and associated bacterial infection
   b. More common in Caucasians
   c. Soft and earthy in texture
   d. High content of cholesterol and calcium palmitate

5. **Lithogenic bile has the following properties:** *(All India 96)*
   a. ↑ Bile and cholesterol ratio
   b. ↓ Bile and cholesterol ratio
   c. Equal bile and cholesterol ratio
   d. ↓ Cholesterol only

6. **Stone formation in gallbladder is enhanced by all except:** *(All India 96)*
   a. Clofibrate therapy
   b. Ileal resection
   c. Cholestyramine therapy
   d. Vagal stimulation

7. **Gallbladder stone formation is influenced by all except:** *(All India 98)*
   a. Clofibrate therapy
   b. Hyper alimentation
   c. Primary biliary cirrhosis
   d. Hypercholesterolemia

8. **Incidence of gallstone is high in:** *(AIIMS Nov 93)*
   a. Partial hepatectomy
   b. Ileal resection
   c. Jejunal resection
   d. Subtotal gastrectomy

9. **True statement about gallstones are all except:** *(AIIMS Nov 99)*
   a. Lithogenic bile is required for stone formation
   b. May be associated with carcinoma gallbladder
   c. Associated with diabetes mellitus
   d. More common in males between 30–40 years of age

10. **Which among the following does not lead to pigment gallstones?** *(PGI June 99)*
    a. TPN
    b. Clonorchis sinensis
    c. Hemolytic anemia
    d. Alcoholic cirrhosis

11. **True about gallstones:** *(PGI Dec 2002)*
    a. More common in females
    b. Gallstones, hiatus hernia, CBD stones form Saints triad
    c. Limey bile precipitated
    d. Lithotripsy always done

12. **All are component of Saint's triad except:** *(AIIMS Nov 95)*
    a. Renal stones
    b. Hiatus hernia
    c. Diverticulosis of colon
    d. Gallstones

13. **Commonest type of gallstone is:** *(DNB 2011)*
    a. Cholesterol stone
    b. Pigment
    c. Mixed
    d. All are equally common

14. **Percentage of gallstones which are radiopaque:** *(NEET 2013, JIPMER 86)*
    a. 10%
    b. 20%
    c. 30%
    d. 40%

15. **Which of the following statement is correct about gallstones?**
    a. 1-Cholesterol, 2-Black, 3-Brown
    b. 1-Cholesterol, 2- Brown, 3- Black
    c. 1- Brown, 2-Black, 3- Cholesterol
    d. 1- Black, 2- Brown, 3- Cholesterol

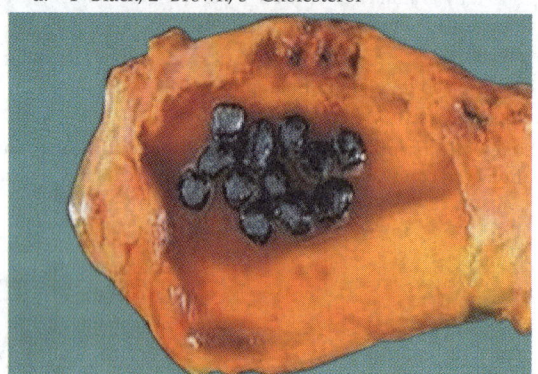

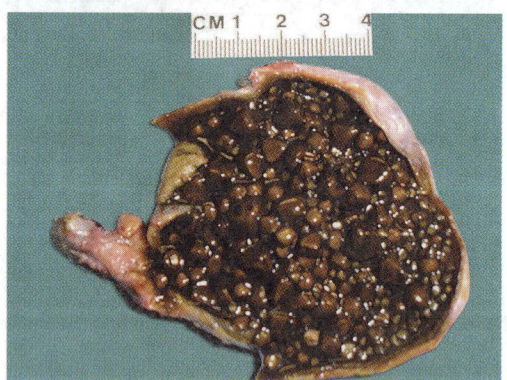

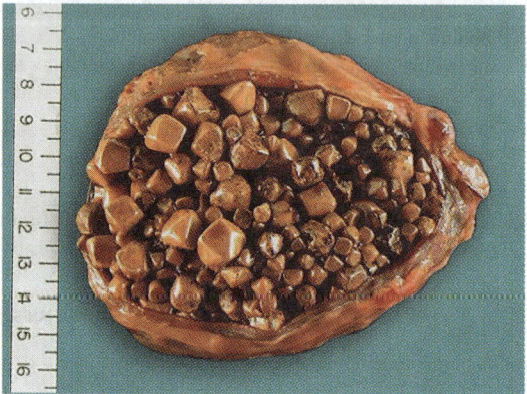

Gallbladder

16. **A gallstone gets impacted most commonly in which part of common bile duct?** *(JIPMER 87)*
    a. Supraduodenal
    b. Retroduodenal
    c. Ampulla of Vater
    d. Common hepatic duct

17. **Gallstones do not contain:** *(Recent Question 2014)*
    a. Oxalate
    b. Cholesterol
    c. Phosphate
    d. Carbonate

18. **Cholesterol gallstones are due to:** *(JIPMER 95)*
    a. Decreased motility of gallbladder
    b. Hyposecretion of bile salts
    c. Hypercholesterolemia
    d. All of the above

19. **True color of cholesterol stone is:** *(DNB 2012)*
    a. Black
    b. Brown
    c. Dark yellow
    d. Pale yellow

20. **The predominant constituent of the pale yellow gallstones in the gallbladder is:** *(COMEDK 2007)*
    a. Mucin glycoprotein
    b. Calcium carbonate
    c. Cholesterol
    d. Calcium phosphate

21. **Most common type of gallstone in India is:** *(MCI March 2009)*
    a. Cholesterol
    b. Pigment
    c. Mixed
    d. Both A and C

22. **Calculous cholecystitis is associated with all of the following except:** *(MCI March 2005)*
    a. Oral contraceptives
    b. Estrogen
    c. Obesity
    d. Diabetes

23. **Which is true about gallstones?** *(Punjab 2010)*
    a. Pigment stones are most common
    b. Bacterial nidus of infection may be seen
    c. Even if asymptomatic gallbladder should be removed
    d. They are mostly solitary

24. **By definition pigment stone contain how much % of cholesterol?** *(MHSSMCET 2005)*
    a. <10
    b. <20
    c. <30
    d. <60

25. **80% of gallstones contain:** *(Recent Question 2015)*
    a. Bile pigments
    b. Cholesterol
    c. Calcium salts
    d. Phospholipids

GALLSTONES: INVESTIGATIONS

26. **Investigation of choice in acute cholecystitis:** *(PGI Dec 2005)*
    a. OCG
    b. HIDA scan
    c. USG
    d. CT

27. **The given image is suggestive of:**

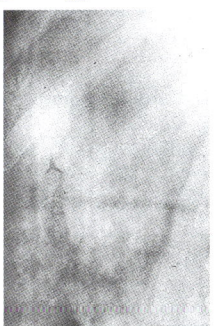

    a. Gallstone
    b. Renal stone
    c. Ureteric stone
    d. Pancreatic stone

28. **Mercedes Benz sign or Seagull sign is seen in:** *(Recent Quetion 2015 MHSSMCET 2006)*
    a. Gallstones
    b. Renal stones
    c. CBD stones
    d. Hydatid cyst

29. **Which is not required for visualization of gallbladder in oral cholecystograph?** *(AIIMS Nov 95, All India 97)*
    a. Functioning liver
    b. Motor mechanisms of gallbladder
    c. Patency of cystic duct
    d. Ability to absorb water

30. **What is the diagnosis based on the given HIDA-scan?**

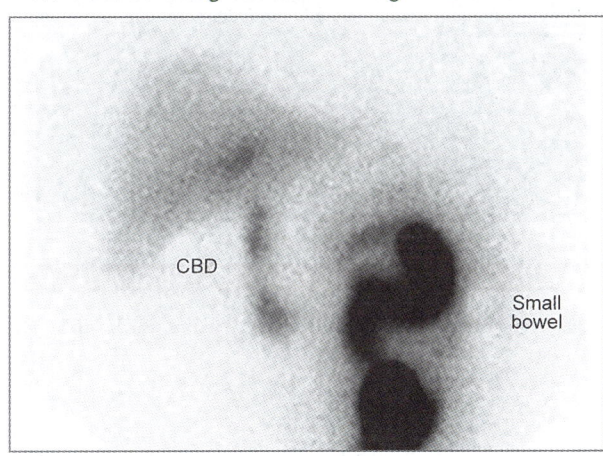

    a. Chronic cholecystitis
    b. Mucocele
    c. Acute cholecystitis
    d. Normal scan

31. **Best investigative modality for gallbladder:**
    a. OCG
    b. PTC
    c. Ultrasound
    d. Intravenous cholangiogram

32. **Graham Cole test refers to:**
    a. Oral cholecystography
    b. Intravenous cholangiography
    c. Pre-operative cholangiography
    d. Post-operative cholangiography
    e. Tomography

33. **Initial investigation of choice for biliary obstruction:**
    a. CT Abdomen
    b. ERCP *(JIPMER 2013)*
    c. MRCP
    d. USG

34. **The substance used in OCG is:**
    a. Iopanoic acid
    b. Sodium diatrozite
    c. Meglumine iodothalamate
    d. Biligraffin
    e. Dianosil

35. **Dye used in IV cholangiography is:** *(Recent Question 2016)*
    a. Diansoil
    b. Conray
    c. Biligraffin
    d. Myodil

36. **Investigation of choice in suspected gallbladder stone is:** *(Recent Question 2017, UPPG 2010, MCI March 2010)*
    a. Ultrasound
    b. X-ray
    c. Barium study
    d. Oral cholecystography

37. **Investigation for assessing proper functioning of biliary system:** *(MCI March 2007)*
    a. USG
    b. CT scan
    c. HIDA scan
    d. All of the above

38. What is the diagnosis based on this ultrasound image?
    a. Gallstone
    b. Gallbladder polyp
    c. Porcelain gallbladder
    d. Adenomyomatosis

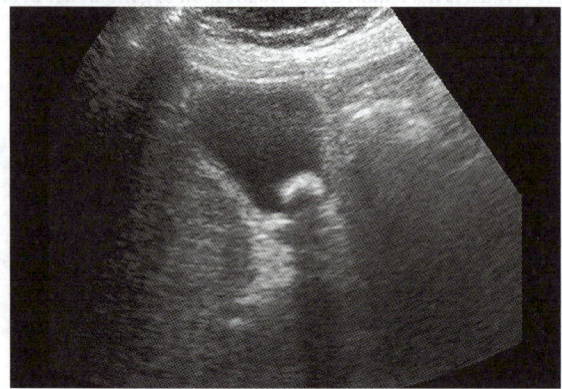

GALLSTONES COMPLICATIONS AND TREATMENT

39. Not a complication of gallstones: *(JIPMER 2010)*
    a. Mucocele
    b. Diverticulosis
    c. Acute cholangitis
    d. Empyema of the gallbladder

40. True about Gallstone disease: *(PGI SS Dec 2009)*
    a. Acute cholecystitis presents with GB perforation
    b. Acute cholecystitis presents with mucosal ulceration of GB
    c. 80% cases of cholilithiasis are symptomatic
    d. Mucocele of GB contains infected bile

41. Ursodeoxycholic acid is a: *(PGI June 95)*
    a. Urinary stone dissolving drug
    b. Thrombolytic drug
    c. Gallstone dissolving drug
    d. Antifibrinolytic

42. In which condition, medical treatment of Gallstone is indicated? *(AIIMS Nov 96, All India 98)*
    a. Stone is < 15 mm size
    b. Radiopaque stone
    c. Calcium bilirubinate stone
    d. Non functioning gallbladder

43. Which one of the following statements is incorrect regarding gallbladder stones?
    a. Pigment stones are due to increased excretion of conjugated bilirubin
    b. Are considered a risk factor for the development of gallbladder carcinoma
    c. 10% gallstones are radiopaque
    d. A mucocele of the gallbladder is caused by a stone impacted in Hartmann's pouch

44. Regarding stones in gallbladder the following are true except: *(Kerala 2000)*
    a. Mixed stones are common in the west
    b. In Saint's triad diverticulosis of colon and hiatus hernia coexist
    c. Is a risk factor in the development of GB carcinoma
    d. 90% of GB stones are radiopaque
    e. A mucocele of GB is caused by a stone impacted in the Hartmann's pouch

45. About gallstone, false is: *(DPG 2006)*
    a. Intervention should be done if gallstones are present in the bile duct irrespective of the duct diameter
    b. Operation should be done in most cases
    c. Can be caused due to parasitic infestation
    d. Can lead to cholecystitis

46. Which of the following is a contraindication for medical management of gallstones? *(Karnataka 2012)*
    a. Radiopaque stones
    b. Radioluscent stones
    c. Normal functioning gallbladder
    d. Small stones

GALLSTONE ILEUS

47. In gallstone ileus, obstruction is seen at: *(Recent Question 2014, AIIMS GIS Dec 2009)*
    a. Jejunum   b. Proximal ileum
    c. Distal ileum   d. Colon

48. All are true about gallstone ileus except: *(AIIMS GIS 2003)*
    a. May be diagnosed with abdominal X-ray
    b. Most common fistula is to duodenum
    c. Tumbling obstruction
    d. Cholecystectomy should be done in same episode

49. False about gallstone ileus: *(AIIMS GIS May 2008)*
    a. 90% patients give history of biliary disease
    b. Causes 1% of all SBO; around 25% cases in >70 years
    c. Tumbling obstruction
    d. Fistula is mostly formed between duodenum and gallbladder

50. Most common site of fistula in fallstone ileus is between: *(AIIMS GIS Dec 2006)*
    a. GB and duodenum
    b. GB and transverse colon
    c. GB and stomach
    d. GB and ileum

51. Rigler's triad consists of: *(PGI May 2011, Nov 2009)*
    a. Intestinal obstruction
    b. Gas in bile duct
    c. Cholangitis
    d. Ectopic gallstone
    e. Biliary stenosis

52. The treatment of fallstone ileus is: *(PGI June 99, UPSC 2008)*
    a. Cholecystectomy alone
    b. Removal of obstruction
    c. Cholecystectomy, closure of fistula and removal of stone by enterotomy
    d. Cholecystectomy with closure of fistula

MUCOCELE

53. The treatment of choice for a mucocele of gallbladder is:
    a. Aspiration of mucous *(AIIMS June 2004)*
    b. Cholecystectomy
    c. Cholecystostomy
    d. Antibiotics and observation

54. Which of the following is false about mucocele of gallbladder? *(Recent Question 2015)*
    a. Complication of gallstones
    b. Treatment is early cholecystectomy
    c. Obstruction at neck of gallbladder
    d. Gallbladder is never palpable

CHOLECYSTITIS AND CHOLECYSTECTOMY

55. Indications of prophylactic cholecystectomy are all except:
    a. Diabetes
    b. Hemoglobinopathy
    c. Gallstone size >3 cm
    d. Porcelain GB *(ILBS 2012)*

56. Which of the following is not an indication for cholecystectomy? *(ILBS 2011)*
    a. GB polyp with stone
    b. Asymptomatic polyp >1 cm
    c. Multiple GB polyps
    d. Symptomatic GB polyps

57. Not an indication for cholecystectomy for asymptomatic gallstones: *(AIIMS GIS May 2011)*
    a. Diabetes
    b. Sickle cell anemia
    c. Porcelain GB
    d. In high prevalence area of CA GB

58. The indications of cholecystectomy are:
    a. Strawberry gallbladder *(PGI Dec 2007, Dec 2006)*
    b. Mucocele of the gallbladder
    c. Gallbladder polyp
    d. Asymptomatic Gallstone disease
    e. Symptomatic cholelithiasis

59. The technique of laparoscopic cholecystectomy was first described by? *(AIIMS May 2011)*
    a. Erich Muhe
    b. Phillip Moure
    c. Kurt Semm
    d. Eddie Reddick

60. All are indications for cholecystectomy except:
    a. Emphysematous cholecystitis *(JIPMER GIS 2011)*
    b. Biliary dyskinesia
    c. Perforation of gallbladder
    d. Adenomyomatosis

61. Prophylactic cholecystectomy is done in: *(AIIMS GIS 2003)*
    a. Calcified GB
    b. Diabetes
    c. Asymptomatic gallstones
    d. Family history of gallstones

62. After surgery, there was 50 ml bile output from abdominal drain on 1st postoperative day. Management is: *(JIPMER GIS 2011)*
    a. Intrabiliary stent
    b. Immediate exploration
    c. T-tube drainage
    d. Observation

63. Indication of cholecystectomy for gallstones disease is/are: *(PGI Nov 2011)*
    a. Asymptomatic gallstones with DM
    b. Porcelain gallbladder
    c. Asymptomatic with history of single attack of acute pancreatitis
    d. Asymptomatic Gallstone disease
    e. Symptomatic cholecystitis

64. Which of the following is the absolute contraindication for laparoscopic cholecystectomy?
    a. Clotting factor deficiency *(NEET 2013, MHSSMCET 2005)*
    b. Perforation peritonitis
    c. Empyema of the gallbladder
    d. Adhesions

65. Contraindications of laparoscopic cholecystectomy is:
    a. Coagulopathy *(Recent Question 2015, DNB 2011)*
    b. Obstructive pulmonary disease
    c. End stage liver disease
    d. All of the above

66. Which of the following is not an indication for cholecystectomy? *(AIIMS May 2005)*
    a. A 70 years old male with symptomatic gallstones
    b. A 20 years old male with sickle cell anemia and symptomatic gallstones
    c. A 65 years old female with a large gallbladder polyp
    d. A 55 years old with an asymptomatic gallstone

67. A 45 years old female presents with symptoms of acute cholecystitis. On USG there is a solitary gallstone of size 1.5 cm. Symptoms are controlled with medical management. Which of the following is the next most appropriate step in the management of this patient? *(All India 2008)*
    a. Regular follow up
    b. IV Antibiotics
    c. Laparoscopic cholecystectomy immediately
    d. Open cholecystectomy immediately

68. Antegrade cholecstectomy: *(PGI Dec 2000)*
    a. Starts from fundus
    b. Starts from cystic duct identification
    c. Starts from hilar dissection
    d. Considered unsafe

69. A 69 years old male patient having coronary artery disease was found to have gallbladder stones while undergoing a routine ultrasound of the abdomen. There was no history of biliary colic or jaundice at any time. What is the best treatment advice for such a patient for his gallbladder stones? *(AIIMS Nov 2003, All India 2003)*
    a. Open cholecystectomy
    b. Laparoscopic cholecystectomy
    c. No surgery for gallbladder stones
    d. ERCP and removal of gallbladder stones

70. The treatment of choice for silent gallbladder stones is:
    a. Observation *(All India 97)*
    b. Chenodeoxycholic acid
    c. Cholecystectomy
    d. Lithotripsy

71. Features of healthy gallbladder on laparotomy are:
    a. Typical "sea-green" colored *(PGI Dec 2000)*
    b. Wall is thin and elastic
    c. Cannot be emptied
    d. Not easily visible

72. Contraindication for laparoscopic cholecystectomy is all except: *(Kerala 95)*
    a. Shrunken liver
    b. Previous laparotomy
    c. Emphysema
    d. Obese individual

73. Most common malignancy after cholecystectomy is of:
    a. Colon
    b. Stomach
    c. Pancreas
    d. Ileum *(PGI SS Dec 2005)*

74. Laparoscopic cholecystectomy is largely preferred for all of the following reasons to conventional laparotomy except:
    a. Decrease pain *(SGPGI 2004)*
    b. Decreased incidence of bile duct injuries
    c. Smaller scar
    d. Decreased stay in hospital

75. A 50-year-old with history of jaundice in the past has presented with right upper quadrant abdominal pain. Examination and investigations reveal chronic calculous cholecystitis. The liver functions tests are within normal limits and on ultrasound examination, the common bile ducts is not dilated. Which of the following will be the procedure of choice in her? *(J and K 2005)*
    a. Laparoscopic cholecystectomy
    b. Open choledocholithotomy with CBD exploration
    c. ERCP + choledocholithotomy followed by laparoscopic cholecystectomy
    d. Laparoscopic cholecystectomy followed by ERCP + choledocholithotomy

76. A 88 years old male patient presented with end stage renal disease with coronary artery block and metastasis in the lungs. Now presents with acute cholecystitis, patient's relatives need treatment to do something: *(UPPG 2008)*
    a. Open cholecystectomy
    b. Tube cholecystostomy
    c. Laparoscopic cholecystectomy
    d. Antibiotics then elective cholecystectomy

77. An otherwise normal female presents with symptoms of flatulent dyspepsia. She was started on proton pump inhibitors, which controlled her symptoms. The next step in management of this condition should be: *(All India 2008)*
    a. Immediate laparoscopic cholecystectomy
    b. Laparotomy after 1 or 2 months
    c. Wait and watch
    d. ERCP

78. In cholecystectomy, fresh plasma should be given: *(UPPG 2008)*
    a. Just before operation
    b. At the time of operation
    c. 6 hours before operation
    d. 12 hours after operation

79. A patient underwent laparoscopic cholecystectomy and was discharged on the same day. On postoperative day 3, he presented to the hospital with fever. Ultrasonography showed a 5 × 5 cm collection in the right subdiaphragmatic region. What will be the management? *(AIIMS May 2017)*
    a. Observe with antibiotic cover
    b. Re-explore the wound with T-tube insertion
    c. Pigtail insertion and drainage
    d. ERCP and proceed

80. Referred pain to inferior angle of right scapula in acute cholecystitis is known as: *(Recent Question 2017)*
    a. Murphy's sign
    b. Naunyn's sign
    c. Boa's sign
    d. Cullen's sign

ACALCULOUS CHOLECYSTITIS

81. All are true about acute acalculous cholecystitis except:
    a. Distended GB is seen in scintigraphy
    b. Vascular cause *(AIIMS GIS May 2011)*
    c. Seen in bed ridden patients
    d. Rapid course

82. Acalculous cholecystitis can be seen in all except: *(Punjab 2008, AIIMS Nov 2005)*
    a. Dengue hemorrhagic fever
    b. Malaria
    c. Leptospirosis
    d. Enteric fever

83. Acalculous cholecystitis are caused by: *(PGI Dec 2006, Dec 2001)*
    a. DM
    b. TPN
    c. Leptospirosis
    d. Estrogen therapy

84. Acalculous cholecystitis is caused by: *(PGI Dec 2001)*
    a. Diabetes mellitus
    b. Total parenteral nutrition
    c. Tuberculosis
    d. Anemia
    e. Malignancy

85. Which of the following statements about acalculous cholecystitis is incorrect? *(DPG 2009 March)*
    a. Manifestation of disturbed microcirculation in critically ill patient
    b. Prolonged parenteral nutrition can be causative
    c. It is life threatening condition
    d. Cholecystectomy is not indicated

86. All of the following are causes of acalculous cholecystitis except: *(Recent Question 2013)*
    a. Bile duct stricture
    b. Schistostoma
    c. Prolonged TPN
    d. Major operations

XANTHOGRANULOMATOUS CHOLECYSTITIS

87. All of the following statements about Xanthogranulomatous inflammation are true except: *(NEET Pattern)*
    a. Foam cells are seen
    b. Yellow nodules are seen
    c. Multinucleated giant cells are seen
    d. Associated with tuberculosis

EMPHYSEMATOUS CHOLECYSTITIS

88. Acute emphysematous cholecystitis is caused by:
    a. Pseudomonas aeuroginosa *(JIPMER 2012, 2010)*
    b. Staphylococcus
    c. Clostridium perfringens
    d. Streptococcus pyogenes

89. All of the following are correct regarding emphysematous cholecystitis except: *(NEET Pattern, DNB 2010)*
    a. More common in males
    b. More common in diabetics
    c. In many cases the gallbladder does not contain stone
    d. It is caused most commonly by Pseudomonas

90. What is the most probable diagnosis based on the given X-ray finding?

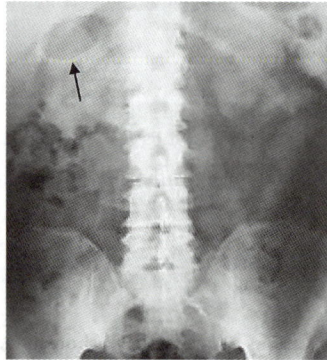

    a. Emphysematous cholecystitis
    b. Emphysematous pyelonephritis
    c. Xanthgranulomatous cholecystitis
    d. Xanthgranulomatous pyelonephritis

MIRIZZI'S SYNDROME

91. **Type II Mirizzi's syndrome:**
    a. Obstruction of common duct by external compression only (no erosion)
    b. Erosion of one-thirds circumference of common duct
    c. Erosion of up to two-third circumference of common duct
    d. Total/near total circumferential destruction of common duct

92. **Mirizzi syndrome is:** *(Recent Question 2015, 2014, DNB 2011)*
    a. GB stone compressing common hepatic duct
    b. GB carcinoma invading IVC
    c. GB stone causing cholecystitis
    d. Pancreatic carcinoma

STRAWBERRY GALLBLADDER

93. **Cholesterolosis is:** *(Karnataka 94)*
    a. Disease of defective metabolism of choline
    b. Concerned with epithelial tumors of brain
    c. Diffuse deposition of cholesterol in mucosa of gallbladder
    d. Disease concerned with obstructive jaundice

94. **Gross appearance of gallbladder specimen is suggestive of:**
    a. Emphysematous cholecystitis
    b. Xanthogranulomatous cholecystitis
    c. Gallbladder cholesterolosis
    d. Adenomyomatosis

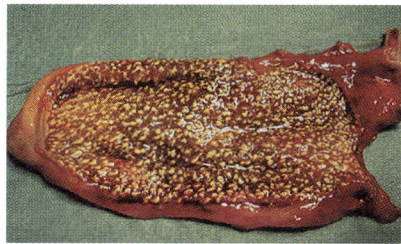

GALLBLADDER POLYP AND ADENOMYOMATOSIS

95. **Indications of cholecystectomy in GB polyp removal are all except:** *(ILBS 2012)*
    a. Size >1 cm
    b. With stone
    c. >3 in number
    d. Locally invasive

96. **Risk factors for malignant change in an asymptomatic patient with a gallbladder polyp on ultrasound include all of the following, except:** *(AIIMS May 2011, All India 2009)*
    a. Age > 60 years
    b. Rapid increase in size of polyp
    c. Size of polyp > 5 mm
    d. Associated gallstones

97. **Identify the diagnosis of the given gross specimen:** *(AIIMS November 2017)*

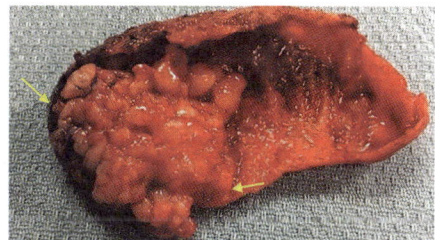

    a. Cancer gallbladder
    b. Cholesterolosis
    c. Strawberry gallbladder
    d. Polyps in gallbladder

98. **False about GB polyps:** *(AIIMS GIS May 2008)*
    a. Adenomyomatosis < 1 cm, pedunculated
    b. Cholesterol polyps are most common
    c. Symptomatic polyps are indication for cholecystectomy
    d. Polyp with stone is an increased risk of malignancy

99. **On abdominal ultrasound gallbladder shows diffuse wall thickening with hyperechoic nodules at neck and comet tail artifacts. The most likely diagnosis will be:**
    a. Adenomyomatosis *(AIIMS May 2011)*
    b. Adenocarcinoma of gallbladder
    c. Xanthogranulomatous cholecystitis
    d. Cholesterol crystals

100. **All of the following are risk factors for CA GB except:** *(JIPMER GIS 2011)*
    a. Gallstones
    b. Adenomyomatosis
    c. Porcelain gallbladder
    d. Choledochal cyst

101. **This incidental finding on ultrasound abdomen is suggestive of:**
    a. Gallbladder stone
    b. Gallbladder polyp
    c. Adenomyomatosis
    d. Xanthogranulomatons cholecystitis

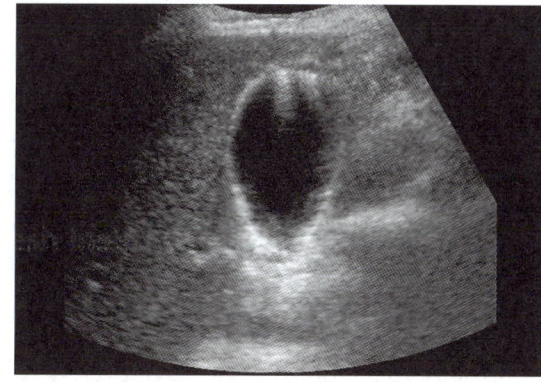

CARCINOMA GALLBLADDER PREDISPOSING FACTORS

102. **True about CA GB and gallstones:** *(GB Pant 2011)*
    a. 3% association
    b. 30% association
    c. 50% association
    d. 90% association

103. **Precancerous lesions of GB are all except:** *(AIIMS GIS Dec 2010)*
    a. Porcelain GB
    b. Typhoid carrier
    c. ABPDJ
    d. Biliary ascariasis

104. **Organism associated with fish consumption and also causes carcinoma gallbladder:** *(AIIMS Nov 2012, AIIMS Nov 2010)*
    a. Gnathostoma
    b. Anglostrongyloidosis cantonensis
    c. Clonorchis sinensis
    d. H. dimunata

105. **Risk factor for carcinoma gallbladder:** *(PGI Nov 2011)*
    a. Female sex
    b. Choledochal cysts
    c. Xanthogranulomatous cholecystitis
    d. Calcification of gallbladder
    e. Gallstone

106. **All are risk factors for CA GB except:** *(GB Pant 2011)*
    a. Adenomyosis
    b. ABPDJ
    c. Gallstones
    d. Adenomatous polyps

107. **All of the following are risk factors for carcinoma gallbladder, except:** *(AIIMS June 2004)*
    a. Typhoid carriers
    b. Adenomatous gallbladder polyps
    c. Choledochal cyst
    d. Oral contraceptives

108. **Precancerous lesion of gallbladder is:** *(AIIMS June 98)*
    a. Porcelain gallbladder
    b. Mirizzi's syndrome
    c. Cholesterosis
    d. Acalculous Cholecystitis

109. **All of the following are the risk factors for carcinoma gallbladder except:** *(Recent Question 2017)*
    a. Primary sclerosing cholangitis
    b. Porcelain gallbladder
    c. Multiple 2 cm gallstones
    d. Choledochal cyst

110. **All of the following are true about porcelain gallbladder except:** *(Kerala PG 2015)*
    a. May be seen on plain X-ray
    b. More commonly diagnosed on CT
    c. It is an indication for cholecystectomy
    d. Always denotes benign etiology

111. **Incidental finding in a female patient of age 56 years who underwent the CECT abdomen is suggestive of:**
    a. Carcinoma gallbladder
    b. Gallbladder polyp
    c. Porcelain gallbladder
    d. Gallstone

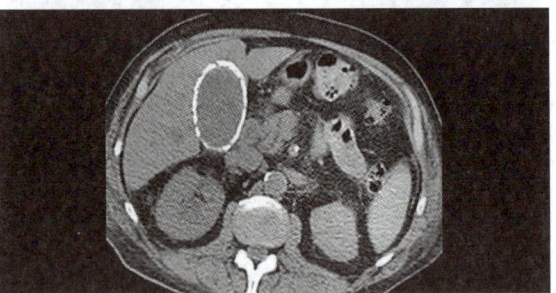

CARCINOMA GALLBLADDER

112. **In a male after laparoscopic cholecystectomy, specimen is sent for histopathology which shows carcinoma gallbladder stage T1a. Appropriate management is:** *(AIIMS May 2011)*
    a. Conservative and follow-up
    b. Extended cholecystectomy
    c. Excision of all port sites
    d. Radiotherapy

113. **After laparoscopic cholecystectomy, if biopsy reveals in-situ cancer of gallbladder (Stage-I), then the appropriate management is:** *(Orissa 2011)*
    a. Follow-up
    b. Extended cholecystectomy
    c. Excision of all port sites
    d. Radiotherapy

114. **Survival in unresectable GB carcinoma is?** *(AIIMS May 2011)*
    a. 4–6 months
    b. 8–10 months
    c. 1 year
    d. 12–24 months

115. **T2N1 of CA GB represents which stage?** *(KGMC 2011)*
    a. IA
    b. IB
    c. II
    d. III

116. **True about CA GB:** *(ILBS 2012)*
    a. T1a can be treated and cured by laparoscopic cholecystectomy
    b. T1b needs radical operation in all cases
    c. Port site metastasis is localized disease
    d. Pre-operative diagnosis of CA GB has different survival according to stage

117. **Most common gallbladder malignancy?** *(MHSSMCET 2008)*
    a. Adenocarcinoma
    b. Squamous cell carcinoma
    c. Mucinous cystadenocarcinoma
    d. Serous cystadenocarcinoma

118. **All are true about CA GB except:** *(GB Pant 2011)*
    a. Redo surgery is radical or extended cholecystectomy increases significant survival advantage
    b. Inter-aortocaval node involvement potentially rule out cure
    c. <25% 5-year survival for all stages
    d. Pancreaticoduodenectomy has 5-year survival of 25%

119. **True about CA GB:** *(PGI SS Dec 2009)*
    a. Most commonly presents with obstructive jaundice
    b. 90% are associated with gallstones
    c. 5-year survival is 35%
    d. 30% are squamous cell carcinoma

120. **Best prognosis in CA GB is seen in:** *(PGI SS Dec 2009)*
    a. Papillary
    b. Adenocarcinoma
    c. Squamous
    d. Melanoma

121. **False regarding CA GB:** *(PGI SS Dec 2010)*
    a. T1a: simple cholecystectomy
    b. T1b: extended cholecystectomy
    c. T1a: extended cholecystectomy if carcinoma in neck of gallbladder
    d. Excision of port sites improves survival

122. **Laparoscopic cholecystectomy was done, on histopathology, stage was T2. Next line of treatment:** *(AIIMS GIS 2003)*
    a. Observation
    b. Extended cholecystectomy
    c. Port site excision
    d. Chemotherapy

123. **Commonest type of carcinoma gallbladder with gallstones is:** *(AIIMS Nov 95)*
    a. Adenocarcinoma
    b. Anaplastic carcinoma
    c. Squamous cell carcinoma
    d. Transitional cell carcinoma

124. **A 40-year-old woman has undergone a cholecystectomy. The histopathology reveals that she has a 3 cm adenocarcinoma in the body of the gallbladder infiltrating up to the serosa. Which of the following further management would you advise her?** *(AIIMS Nov 2004)*
    a. Chemotherapy
    b. Radiotherapy
    c. Radical cholecystectomy
    d. Follow up with regular ultrasound examinations

125. **Regarding carcinoma gallbladder:** *(PGI June 2002)*
    a. Squamous cell carcinoma is the most common
    b. Present with jaundice
    c. Good prognosis
    d. Gallstones predispose
    e. 65% survival after surgery

126. **Commonest association seen in carcinoma gallbladder:** *(AIIMS 91)*
    a. Peritoneal deposits
    b. Duodenal infiltration
    c. Secondaries to liver
    d. Cystic node involvement

127. **Most common type of cancer gallbladder in a patient with gallstone:** *(APPG 2005)*
    a. Adenocarcinoma
    b. Squamous carcinoma
    c. Sarcoma
    d. None

128. **Most appropriate treatment option for the carcinoma gallbladder with invasion of perimuscular connective tissue, diagnosed after laparoscopic cholecystectomy:** *(Recent Question 2017)*
    a. Resection of segment IVb & V of liver with nodal clearance
    b. Resection of segment IVb & V of liver with nodal clearance with port site excision
    c. Wedge excision of liver with lymphadenectomy
    d. Wedge excision of liver with lymphadenectomy and port-site excision

129. In a male after laparoscopic cholecystectomy, specimen is sent for histopathology which shows carcinoma gallbladder stage IB. Appropriate management is: *(AIIMS Nov 2008)*
    a. Conservative and follow up
    b. Extended cholecystectomy
    c. Excision of all port sites   d. Radiotherapy

GALLBLADDER ANATOMY AND PHYSIOLOGY

130. Bile is concentrated in the gallbladder to .... times: *(PGI Dec 2006, Dec 2001)*
    a. 5   b. 10
    c. 20   d. 50

131. The gallbladder is capable of distending… mL: *(Recent Question 2016)*
    a. 10   b. 20
    c. 40   d. 50

132. Sentinel node of gallbladder is: *(MAHE 2006)*
    a. Virchow's nodes   b. Iris nodes
    c. Clouquet node   d. Lymph node of Lund

MISCELLANEOUS

133. Sump syndrome occurs most commonly after:
    a. Cholecystojejunostomy   *(COMEDK 2008)*
    b. Choledochoduodenostomy
    c. Mirizzi's syndrome
    d. Choledochojejunostomy

134. True about cystic duct stump stone are all except:
    a. Stone cause of postoperative pain   *(PGI Nov 2009)*
    b. Re-cholecystectomy is the definite treatment of choice
    c. ERCP is the investigation of choice to diagnose
    d. Basket extraction is the treatment of choice
    e. Oral ursodeoxycholic acid relieves symptoms remarkably

135. Sphincter of Oddi consists of: *(AIIMS May 2011)*
    a. 2 sphincters   b. 3 sphincters
    c. 4 sphincters   d. 5 sphincter

136. Bleeding adjacent to the "Triangle of Calot" should be controlled by: *(MHPGMCET 2009)*
    a. Pressing the artery manually
    b. Blind clipping
    c. Kocher's artery forceps
    d. Stitching

137. "Limey bile" is: *(Karnataka 94)*
    a. Present in the CBD
    b. Thin and clear
    c. Like toothpaste emulsion in the gallbladder
    d. Bacteria rich

138. Pain at the tip of shoulder is due to all except: *(DNB 2008)*
    a. Peptic ulcer   b. Pancreatitis
    c. Cholecystitis   d. Appendicitis

139. A middle aged patients presents with the complained of right hypochondrial pain. On X-ray, elevated right hemidiaphragm was seen. All of the following are the possible diagnoses except: *(AIIMS Nov 2012)*
    a. Subphrenic abscess
    b. Acute cholecystitis
    c. Pyogenic liver abscess
    d. Amoebic liver abscess in right lobe

140. What is the name of this congenital anomaly seen on ultrasound?
    a. Moynihan's hump   b. Phrygian cap
    c. Duplication   d. None of the above

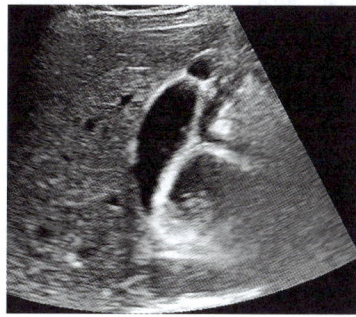

Explanations

GALLSTONES: PATHOGENESIS

1. **Ans. c. Crystallization** *(Ref: Sabiston 20/e p1492; Schwartz 10/e p1318-1319; Bailey 27/e p1198; Blumgart 6/e p551, 5/e p483-487; Shackelford 8/e p1262, 7/e p1298-1299)*

2. **Ans. a. Crystalline cholesterol monohydrate** *(Ref: Robbins 9/e p876; Sleisenger & Fordtran 9/e p1098)*

   "There are two general classes of gallstones: cholesterol stones, containing more than 50% of crystalline cholesterol monohydrate, and pigment stones composed predominantly of bilirubin calcium salts."(Robbins 9/e p876)

3. **Ans. b. Secondary CBD stones** *(Ref: Sabiston 20/e p2078, 19/e p1485-1486; Schwartz 10/e p1318-1319; Bailey 27/e p1198; Blumgart 6/e p551-553, 5/e p483-487)*

4. **Ans. b. More common in Caucasians**
   Brown pigment stones are common in **Asians**^{Q}, not the caucasians.

5. **Ans. b. (↓Bile and cholesterol ratio)**

6. **Ans. d. Vagal stimulation** *(Ref: Sabiston 20/e p1491; Bailey 26/e p1107; Harrison 20/e p2424, 19/e p2077)*
   - Vagal stimulation increases GB motility and prevents Gallstone formation^Q.

7. **Ans. d. Hypercholesterolemia**
   - **Hyperalimentation decreases GB motility promotes stasis** and Gallstone formation.
   - **Primary biliary cirrhosis decreases bile salt secretion** in bile.
   - **Clofibrate** therapy **increases biliary cholesterol.**

8. **Ans. b. Ileal resection**
9. **Ans. d. More common in males between 30–40 years of age**
10. **Ans. a. TPN**
11. **Ans. a. More common in females**
12. **Ans. a. Renal stones**
13. **Ans. c. Mixed** *(Ref: Bailey 27/e p1198)*

MIXED GALLSTONES
- **Most common gallstones**, account for **90% calculi**^{Q}

14. **Ans. a. 10%**
    - Most (90%) gallstones are radioluscent^Q.
    - Most (90%) kidney stones are radiopaque^Q.

15. **Ans. d. 1- Black, 2- Brown, 3- Cholesterol** *(Ref: Sabiston 20/e p1491-1492; Schwartz 10/e p1318-1319; Bailey 27/e p1198)*

16. **Ans. c. Ampulla of Vater** *(Ref: digestive.niddk.nih.gov)*
    - Most gallstones pass out of the body unnoticed, but some become lodged in the **common bile duct**, causing **jaundice**^{Q}.
    - A **frequent site of gallstone impaction** is the **ampulla of Vater**^{Q}, where the common channel meets the small intestine.
    - **Blockage of the common channel** by a **gallstone** can induce **acute pancreatitis**^{Q}.

17. **Ans. a. Oxalate**
18. **Ans. d. All of the above**
19. **Ans. d. Pale yellow**
20. **Ans. c. Cholesterol**
    - **Cholesterol stones** contain almost **entirely cholesterol** and are often **solitary, pale yellow** in color^Q.

21. **Ans. b. Pigment** *(Ref: Bailey 27/e p1198)*
    - In the **USA** and **Europe**, **80%** are **cholesterol** or **mixed stones**, whereas in **Asia**, 80% are **pigment stones**^{Q}.

    - **MC gallstone: Mixed (90%)**^{Q}
    - **MC gallstones in USA and Europe: Cholesterol stones**^{Q} **(Mixed,** if given in the option)
    - **MC gallstones in India (Asia): Pigment stones** (80%)^Q

22. **Ans. d. Diabetes**

23. **Ans. b. Bacterial nidus of infection may be seen** *(Ref: www.ncbi.nlm.nih.gov/pubmed/2213913)*

- Recently, **bacterial infection** has been shown to play the **role in pathogenesis of gallstone**, this adds to the growing pool of studies finding an **infectious nidus** in these **gallstones**[Q].

24. **Ans. c. <30** *(Ref: Bailey 26/e p1106)*

- **Pigment stone** is the name used for stones **containing <30% cholesterol**[Q].

Classification of Gallstones			
	Cholesterol	**Black pigment**	**Brown pigment**
Location	Gallbladder and bile duct	Gallbladder and bile duct	Bile ducts[Q]
Major constituent	Cholesterol	Bilirubin pigment **polymer**[Q]	Calcium bilirubinate[Q]
Consistency	Crystalline with nucleus	Hard[Q]	Soft, friable[Q]
% Radiopaque	15%	60%[Q]	0%[Q]

25. **Ans. b. Cholesterol**

GALLSTONES: INVESTIGATIONS

26. **Ans. c. USG** *(Ref: Sabiston 20/e p1493; Schwartz 10/e p1319; Bailey 27/e p1199; Shackelford 8/e p1269-1270, 7/e p1303, 1306)*

- **IOC** for **acute cholecystitis: USG**[Q]
- **Gold standard** for **diagnosis** of **acute cholecystitis: HIDA scan**[Q]
- **USG** is **IOC** for **acute calculous cholecystitis, chronic cholecystitis** and **cholelithiasis**[Q].

27. **Ans. a. Gallstone** *(Ref: Gastrointestinal Radiology By Ronald L. Eisenberg 4/e p785)*

In this X-ray, triradiate fissure (Mercedes-Benz sign) is seen, which is present in gallstones. Triradiate fissure on X-ray give rise to Mercedes-Benz sign and biradiate fissure give rise to seagull sign.

"*Stones* can also become trapped in the neck of the gallbladder or cystic duct. Although infrequently seen, a *characteristic finding of gallstones* is the "*Mercedes Benz*" sign. Stellate radiolucencies reflecting gas containing fissures or faults within the gallstone produce a *triradiate* pattern similar to that of the German automobile trademark." *(Gastrointestinal Radiology By Ronald L. Eisenberg 4/e p785)*

28. **Ans. a. Gallstones** *(Ref: Bailey 27/e p1199)*

29. **Ans. b. Motor mechanisms of gallbladder** *(Ref: Schwartz 9/e p1141; Bailey 27/e p1200)*

- **Motor mechanism of GB** is a **requirement for medical treatment** of **gallstones**, not for oral cholecystography.

30. **Ans. c. Acute cholecystitis** *(Ref: Sabiston 20/e p1488; Schwartz 10/e p1315, 1320; Bailey 27/e p1192)*
Non-visualization of gallbladder in hepatic scintigraphy is suggestive of acute cholecystitis.

"*Ultrasonography is the most useful radiologic test for diagnosing acute cholecystitis. It has a sensitivity and specificity of 95%. In addition to being a sensitive test for documenting the presence or absence of stones, it will show the thickening of the gallbladder wall and the pericholecystic fluid. Focal tenderness over the gallbladder when compressed by the sonographic probe (sonographic Murphy's sign) also is suggestive of acute cholecystitis. Biliary radionuclide scanning (HIDA scan) may be of help in the atypical case. Lack of filling of the gallbladder after 4 hours indicates an obstructed cystic duct and, in the clinical setting of acute cholecystitis, is highly sensitive and specific for acute cholecystitis. A normal HIDA scan excludes acute cholecystitis.*" *(Schwartz 10/e p1320)*

HIDA Scan	
Normal HIDA Scan	**HIDA Scan in Acute Cholecystitis**
Tracer in GB, in CBD & small bowel	Non-filling of GB, Tracer in CBD & small bowel

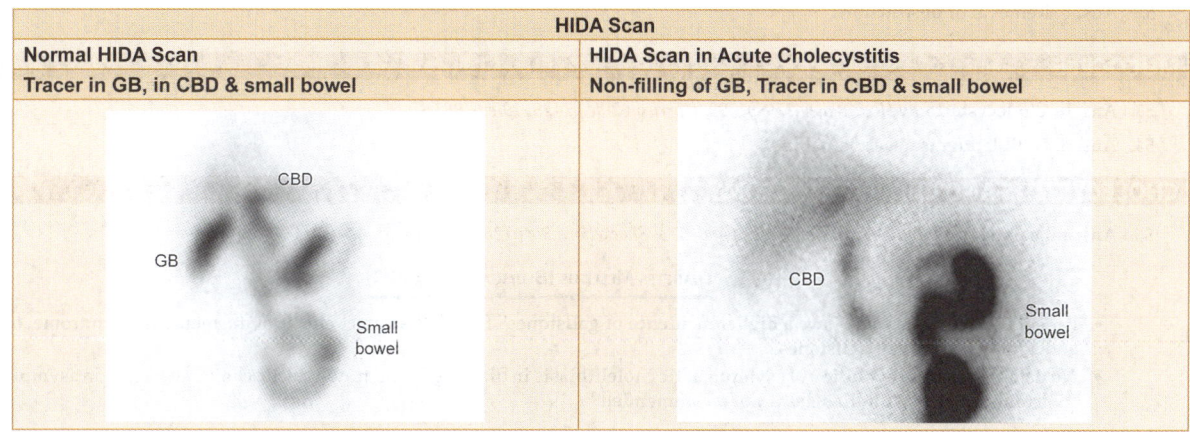

31. **Ans. c. Ultrasound** *(Ref: Sabiston 20/e p1487; Schwartz 10/e p1319; Bailey 26/e p1100; Blumgart 5/e p223; Shackelford 7/e p1303)*
    - **USG** is **IOC** for **acute calculous cholecystitis, chronic cholecystitis** and **cholilithiasis**.
32. **Ans. a. Oral cholecystography**   33. **Ans. d. USG**   34. **Ans. a. Iopanoic acid**
    - **Iopanoic acid** is used in **oral cholecystography**^Q.
    - **Biligraffin** is used in **IV cholangiography**^Q.
35. **Ans. c. Biligraffin**   36. **Ans. a. Ultrasound**
37. **Ans. c. HIDA scan** *(Ref: Sabiston 20/e p1488; Schwartz 10/e p1320; Bailey 27/e p1199; Blumgart 5/e p254-270; Shackelford 7/e p1306)*
38. **Ans. a. Gallstone**
    - USG in Gallstone: Posterior acoustic shadow.

GALLSTONES COMPLICATIONS AND TREATMENT

39. **Ans. b. Diverticulosis** *(Ref: Sabiston 20/e p1492-1493; Bailey 27/e p1199; Blumgart 6/e p554, 5/e p483-487)*

Effects and Complications of Gallstones		
In gallbladder	**In Bile duct**	**In Intestine**
• Silent stones • Acute cholecystitis • Chronic cholecystitis • Mucocele	• Empyema • Perforation • Gangrene • Carcinoma	• Obstructive jaundice • Cholangitis • **Acute pancreatitis**
		• Gallstone ileus

40. **Ans. b. Acute cholecystitis presents with mucosal ulceration of GB** *(Ref: Sabiston 20/e p1493-1494; Schwartz 10/e p1321; Bailey 27/e p1199; Blumgart 6/e p556, 5/e p487-494; Shackelford 7/e p1315-1317)*
41. **Ans. c. Gallstone dissolving drug** *(Ref: Sabiston 20/e p1494)*
42. **Ans. a. Stone is <15 mm size**   43. **Ans. a. Pigment stones are due to increased excretion of conjugated bilirubin**
44. **Ans. d. 90% of GB stones are radiopaque**
45. **Ans. b. Operation should be done in most cases**
    - **Operation** is not done in most cases of gallstones, done **in symptomatic cases**.
46. **Ans. a. Radiopaque stones**

GALLSTONE ILEUS

47. **Ans. c. Distal ileum** *(Ref: Sabiston 20/e p1506-1507; Blumgart 6/e p563, 5/e p649-655; Shackelford 8/e p844, 7/e p865)*
48. **Ans. d. Cholecystectomy should be done in same episode**
    - Most patients in Gallstone ileus are **unstable to withstand a prolonged operative procedure**, so **cholecystectomy should not be done** in **same episode**.
    - **Fistula** can be **addressed** at a **second laparotomy**^Q
49. **Ans. a. 90% patients give history of biliary disease**   50. **Ans. a. GB and duodenum**
51. **Ans. a. Intestinal obstruction, b. Gas in bile duct, d. Ectopic gallstone**
52. **Ans. b. Removal of obstruction**

MUCOCELE

53. **Ans. b. Cholecystectomy** *(Ref: Bailey 27/e p1199; Harrison 20/e p2428, 19/e p2081)*
54. **Ans. d. Gallbladder is never palpable**

CHOLECYSTITIS AND CHOLECYSTECTOMY

55. **Ans. a. Diabetes** *(Ref: Blumgart 6/e p623, 5/e p486, 513; Shackelford 8/e p1281, 7/e p1316)*

DIABETES MELLITUS (BLUMGART 6/e p623)

- Patients with diabetes may have a **higher incidence of gallstones**^Q from the **indirect effects** of the metabolic syndrome, obesity, and a **family history of gallstones**^Q.
- **No data show worse evolution** of asymptomatic cholelithiasis in diabetics^Q, and **prophylactic cholecystectomy** in asymptomatic gallstones carriers with diabetes is **not recommended**^Q

56. **Ans. c. Multiple GB polyps** *(Ref: Sabiston 20/e p1511; Bailey 27/e p1203)*
57. **Ans. a. Diabetes**
58. **Ans. b. Mucocele of the gallbladder, e. Symptomatic cholelithiasis**
59. **Ans. a. Erich Muhe** *(Ref: Blumgart 6/e p6,551, 5/e p512)*

History of Laparoscopic Cholecystectomy

- Dr. **Kurt Semm**, the **father of "pelviscopy,"** performed the **first laparoscopic appendectomy** in 1980[Q].
- **Eric Muhe**[Q] performed the **first laparoscopic cholecystectomy** in **1982**. He used a **modified operating laparoscope** placed at the umbilicus after establishing pneumoperitoneum.
- In 1987, **Phillipe Mouret** performed the **first video laparoscopic cholecystectomy** by using a **camera attached to the laparoscope**[Q].

60. **Ans. d. Adenomyomatosis**

- **Cholecystectomy** is indicated in **symptomatic adenomyomatosis** or when **cholelithiasis** is present[Q].

61. **Ans. a. Calcified GB**
62. **Ans. d. Observation** *(Ref: Blumgart 5/e p524-525)*

- "A **small amount of biliary drainage** following cholecystectomy should cause **no alarm** because it **usually disappears within 1 or 2 days**[Q]. However, **excessive biliary drainage** through the **wound** or **drain site**, jaundice, sepsis or a combination of these events early in the **post-operative period** should suggest a **bile duct injury**, as should **copious biliary drainage** for **more than few post-op days**[Q]."

63. **Ans. b. Porcelain gallbladder, c. Asymptomatic with history of single attack of acute pancreatitis, e. Symptomatic cholecystitis**
64. **Ans. a. Clotting factor deficiency** *(Ref: Blumgart 6/e p575, 5/e p514)*

Contraindications to Laparoscopic Cholecystectomy	
Absolute	**Relative**
• Unable to **tolerate general anesthesia**[Q] • **Refractory coagulopathy**[Q] • Suspicion of **carcinoma**[Q]	• Previous **upper abdominal surgery**[Q] • **Cholangitis**[Q] • **Diffuse peritonitis**[Q] • **Cirrhosis** or **portal hypertension**[Q] • Chronic obstructive pulmonary disease • **Cholecystenteric fistula**[Q] • **Morbid obesity**[Q] • **Pregnancy**[Q]

Indications of Open Cholecystectomy	
• Poor pulmonary or cardiac reserve[Q] • Cirrhosis and portal hypertension[Q] • Combined procedure	• Suspected or known gallbladder cancer[Q] • Third-trimester pregnancy[Q]

65. **Ans. d. All of the above**   66. **Ans. d. A 55 years old with an asymptomatic gallstone**

Boundaries of Callot's Triangle	Boundaries of Hepatocystic Triangle
• Superiorly **cystic artery**[Q] • Medially, **common hepatic duct**[Q] • Laterally, **cystic duct**[Q]	• Superiorly, **inferior surface** of **liver**[Q] • Medially, **common hepatic duct**[Q] • Laterally, **cystic duct**[Q]

67. **Ans. c. Laparoscopic cholecystectomy immediately** *(Ref: Sabiston 20/e p1494; Schwartz, 10/e p1325; Bailey 25/e p1121; Blumgart 6/e p557-558, 5/e p488-489; Shackelford 8/e p1282, 7/e p1316)*

Treatment of Acute Cholecystitis

- **Early cholecystectomy** performed **within 2 to 3 days (within 72 hours)**[Q] of presentation **is preferred over interval** or **delayed cholecystectomy** that is performed 6 to 10 weeks after initial medical therapy.
- **Laparoscopic cholecystectomy** is the **preferred approach** to patients with **acute cholecystitis**[Q].

68. **Ans. a. Starts from fundus** *(Ref: Mastery of Surgery 5/e p1128)*

Types of Cholecystectomy

Retrograde	Antegrade or Fundus-first or Top-down
• Hilar structure dissection occurs first followed by the **removal of gallbladder** in the triangle of Callot's^Q	• **Separates GB from the liver before** the **cystic duct** and **artery** are **ligated**^Q • Considered **safer** because it allows for the **progressive demonstration of the anatomy down to the infundibulocystic junction**^Q.

69. **Ans. c. No surgery for gallbladder stones** *(Ref: Blumgart 6/e p623, 5/e p486)*

- "There was **no clear cost benefit** and **no life-years** were **gained from prophylactic cholecystectomy**, indicating **no clear-cut advantages** of **prophylactic cholecystectomy** in **asymptomatic cholelithiasis**. As a result, in patients with asymptomatic gallstones, **expectant management** is **recommended**^Q."

70. **Ans. a. Observation**   71. **Ans. a. Typical "sea-green" colored, b. Wall is thin and elastic**

Healthy Gallbladder

- **Greenish blue** or **sea green color**^Q
- **Thin** and **elastic wall**^Q
- Can be **emptied by squeezing**^Q

72. **Ans. a. Shrunken liver**   73. **Ans. a. Colon** *(Ref: Maingot 11/e p628)*

- **Bile acids** can induce **hyperproliferation** of the **intestinal mucosa**^Q via a number of intracellular mechanisms.
- **Cholecystectomy**, which alters the enterohepatic cycle of bile acids, has been associated with a **moderately increased risk** of **proximal colon cancers**^Q.

- It cannot be ruled out, however, that it is less the effect of the cholecystectomy than the impact of other, not yet identified factors in the lithogenic bile of such patients.
- A number of **cofactors** have been identified that **may enhance** or **neutralize the carcinogenic effects of bile acids**, e.g. the amount of **dietary fat**, **fiber**, or **calcium**^Q.
- **Calcium**, in fact, **binds bile acids** and thus may **reduce their negative impact**^Q.

74. **Ans. b. Decreased incidence of bile duct injuries**

Bile Duct Injury

- **Most benign strictures** follow **iatrogenic bile duct injury**^Q
- **Most commonly** during **laparoscopic cholecystectomy**^Q
- **Incidence** of bile duct injury during **open** cholecystectomy is **0.1–0.2%**^Q
- **Incidence** of bile duct injury during **laparoscopic** cholecystectomy is **0.3–0.85%**^Q

    • **Morbidity rate, hospital stay,** and **time to return to work** are **lower** in patients undergoing **laparoscopic cholecystectomy** than open cholecystectomy^Q.

75. **Ans. a. Laparoscopic cholecystectomy**

In the given question, there was an episode of jaundice, but **at present, LFT is normal** and **CBD is not dilated**. The best option is **laparoscopic cholecystectomy** only.

Management of CBD Stones Associated with GB Stones	
Pre-operatively Detected Stones	**Unsuspected stones found at the time of Cholecystectomy**
Experienced Laparoscopic Surgeon	**Experienced Laparoscopic Surgeon**
• **Cholecystectomy** and **choledochotomy** in **same sitting**^Q	• **Laparoscopic CBD exploration** and **stone retrieval** through the **cystic duct**^Q • **Laparoscopic choledochotomy** and **stone extraction**^Q
Inexperienced Laparoscopic Surgeon	**Inexperienced Laparoscopic Surgeon**
• **Pre-op ERCP** with **stone removal** and **laparoscopic cholecystectomy** later^Q.	• **Convert** to **open procedure** and **remove CBD stone**^Q • **Complete** the **cholecystectomy** and **refer the patient for ERCP**^Q **Conversion** to an **open procedure** is preferred over **ERCP**^Q, because the **success rate** of **ERCP** is **not 100%**^Q.

76. **Ans. b. Tube cholecystostomy**

- If patients are **unfit for surgery**, percutaneous, **ultrasound guided**, or **CT guided cholecystostomy** is the **treatment of choice**[Q].

77. **Ans. c. Wait and Watch**

FLATULENT DYSPEPSIA

- Flatulent dyspepsia is usually described as **symptom of Gallstone disease**[Q].
- However, **flatulent dyspepsia** (in an otherwise **normal female**), that **responds to PPI** is **more likely** to result **from reflux** or **peptic ulcer disease** (rather than Gallstone disease) and **does not require surgical management** or **invasive investigations**[Q] for gallbladder disease.
- Patients with these symptoms **should be observed** (**wait and watch**)[Q] or investigated by **endoscopy to exclude reflux** or **peptic ulcer disease**[Q].

78. **Ans. a. Just before operation**

The question is incomplete. It should be "A cirrhotic patient with abnormal coagulation needs cholecystectomy, FFP should be given:"

FRESH FROZEN PLASMA

- Transfusions with **FFP** are given to **replenish clotting factors**[Q].
- The **effectiveness** of the **transfusion** in maintaining hemostasis is **dependent on** the **quantity** of each factor delivered and its **half-life**.
- The **half-life** on the **most stable clotting factor**, factor **VII**, is **4 to 6 hours**[Q].
- A reasonable transfusion scheme would be to **give FFP on call** to the **operating room**.
- This way the **transfusion** is **complete prior** to the **incision**, with **circulating factors** to **cover** the **operative** and **immediate postoperative period**[Q].

79. **Ans. c. Pigtail insertion and drainage** *(Ref: Sabiston 20/e p1506; Schwartz 10/e p1332; Bailey 27/e p1203)*

80. **Ans. c. Boa's sign**

ACALCULOUS CHOLECYSTITIS

81. **Ans. a. Distended GB is seen in scintigraphy** *(Ref: Sabiston 20/e p1508; Schwartz, 10/e p1327-1330; Bailey 27/e p1200; Blumgart 6/e p561, 5/e p491-492; Shackelford 8/e p1281, 7/e p1315-1316)*

- **Cholescintigraphy** demonstrates **absent gallbladder filling** in **acalculous cholecystitis**[Q].

82. **Ans. b. Malaria**

- Both malaria and dengue are uncommon causes of acalculous cholecystitis.
- **Malaria**[Q] seems to be more common between the two.

83. **Ans. a. DM, b. TPN, c. Leptospirosis** *(Ref: Harrison 20/e p2428, 19/e p2081)*

Causes of Acalculous Cholecystitis	
Common Causes	**Uncommon Causes**

• **Elderly** and **critically ill patients** after **trauma**[Q]
• **Burns**[Q]
• **Longterm TPN**[Q]
• Major operations (**abdominal aneurysm repair** and **cardiopulmonary bypass**[Q])
• Diabetes mellitus
	• Vasculitis
	• Obstructing GB adenocarcinoma
	• GB torsion
	• Parasitic infestation
	• Unusual bacterial infection:
	  – **Leptospira**[Q]
	  – **Streptococcus**
	  – **Salmonella**
	  – **Vibrio cholera**

84. **Ans. a. Diabetes mellitus, b. Total parenteral nutrition**

85. **Ans. d. Cholecystectomy is not indicated**

86. **Ans. b. Schistostoma**

XANTHOGRANULOMATOUS CHOLECYSTITIS

87. **Ans. d. Associated with tuberculosis** *(Ref: www.medscape.com/viewarticle/449665)*

EMPHYSEMATOUS CHOLECYSTITIS

88. **Ans. c. Clostridium perfringens** *(Ref: Sabiston 20/e p1493; Blumgart 6/e p562, 5/e p492)*
89. **Ans. d. It is caused most commonly by Pseudomonas**
90. **Ans. a. Emphysematous cholecystitis** *(Ref: Sabiston 20/e p1493; Schwartz 10/e p1320; Bailey 27/e p1190-1191)*

> *In the given X-ray, there is ring of air around gallbladder suggestive of emphysematous cholecystitis.*

MIRIZZI'S SYNDROME

91. **Ans. b. Erosion of one-thirds circumference of common duct** *(Ref: Sabiston 20/e p1510; Schwartz; 10/e p1320-1331; Blumgart 6/e p562, 5/e p493; Shackelford 8/e p1328, 7/e p1370)*
92. **Ans. a. GB stone compressing common hepatic duct**

STRAWBERRY GALLBLADDER

93. **Ans. c. Diffuse deposition of cholesterol in mucosa of gallbladder** *(Ref: Bailey 27/e p1201)*
94. **Ans. c. Gallbladder cholesterolosis** *(Ref: Bailey 27/e p1201)*

GALLBLADDER POLYP AND ADENOMYOMATOSIS

95. **Ans. c. >3 in number** *(Ref: Sabiston 20/e p1511; Bailey 27/e p1201; Blumgart 6/e p266, 5/e p751)*
96. **Ans. c. Size of polyp > 5 mm**
97. **Ans. d. Polyps in gallbladder** *(Ref: Sabiston 20/e p1511; Bailey 27/e p1210)*
98. **Ans. a. Adenomyomatosis < 1 cm, pedunculated**
99. **Ans. a. Adenomyomatosis** *(Ref: Sabiston 19/e p1505; Bailey 27/e p1201)*
100. **Ans. b. Adenomyomatosis**
101. **Ans. c. Adenomyomatosis** *(Ref: Sabiston 20/e p1511)*
    - The presence of cholesterol crystals in these sinuses in adenomyomatosis can result in **"diamond ring sign"**[Q], **"V-shaped"**[Q], or **"comet-tail" artifacts**[Q] on **USG**.

CARCINOMA GALLBLADDER PREDISPOSING FACTORS

102. **Ans. d. 90% association** *(Ref: Blumgart 6/e p787, 5/e p742)*

    - **Cholelithiasis** is seen in **75–98%** of all patients with **CA GB**[Q].
    - The **incidence** of CA GB **in** a population of **patients with gallstones** is from **0.3–3%**[Q].

103. **Ans. d. Biliary ascariasis** *(Ref: Blumgart 6/e p787, 5/e p742)*
104. **Ans. c. Clonorchis sinensis** *(Ref: www.ncbi.nlm.gov/pubmed/3993073)*

> **CLONORCHIS SINENSIS**
> - Clonorchis sinensis is a **liver fluke**, **acquired** by **ingestion of raw** or inadequately cooked **freshwater fishes**[Q].
> - In human body, it **lives within bile ducts** and causes **inflammatory reaction** leading to **cholangiohepatitis** and **biliary obstruction**[Q].
> - It is a well known **risk factor** for **cholangiocarcinoma**[Q].
> - It is a **rare**, but mentioned **risk factor** for **carcinoma gallbladder**[Q].

105. **Ans. b. Choledochal cysts, d. Calcification of gallbladder, e. Gallstone**   106. **Ans. a. Adenomyosis**
107. **Ans. d. Oral contraceptives**
108. **Ans. a. Porcelain gallbladder** *(Ref: Sabiston 20/e p1512; Schwartz 10/e p1317-1318; Blumgart 6/e p787, 5/e p742)*
109. **Ans. c. Multiple 2 cm gallstones** *(Ref: Sabiston 20/e p1512; Schwartz 10/e p1334; Bailey 27/e p1210)*

Gallbladder

110. Ans. d. Always denotes benign etiology
111. Ans. c. Porcelain gallbladder *(Ref: Sabiston 20/e p1512; Schwartz 10/e p1317; Bailey 27/e p1190)*

CARCINOMA GALLBLADDER

112. **Ans. a. Conservative and follow up** *(Ref: Sabiston 20/e p1512-1514; Schwartz 10/e p1334-1335; Bailey 27/e p1211; Blumgart 6/e p797, 5/e p748-754; Shackelford 8/e p1323, 7/e p1364-1370)*
113. Ans. a. Follow-up
114. Ans. a. 4–6 months
115. Ans. d. III
116. Ans. a. T1a can be treated and cured by laparoscopic cholecystectomy
117. Ans. a. Adenocarcinoma
118. Ans. d. Pancreaticoduodenectomy has 5 year survival of 25%
119. Ans. b. 90% are associated with gallstones
120. Ans. a. Papillary
121. Ans. d. Excision of port sites improves survival

- **Port site excision** is done **for staging purposes** to identify **M1** disease[Q]
- Port site excision is **not having any potential therapeutic benefit**[Q].

122. **Ans. b. Extended cholecystectomy** *(Ref: Blumgart 6/e p797, 5/e p754)*

- **T1b, T2, T3** tumor with no evidence of metastasis: Re-resection, **extended cholecystectomy** (possible CBD or extended hepatic resection)[Q]
  - **Extended cholecystectomy** consists of **cholecystectomy with en-bloc resection** of segments **IVB** and **V**; including **lymphadenectomy** of the **cystic duct, pericholedochal, periportal,** and **posterior pancreaticoduodenal** and **local interaortocaval** lymph nodes.

PORT SITE RECURRENCES (BLUMGART 6/E P799)

- There is a **theoretical risk** of **port site seeding after laparoscopic cholecystectomy** for what is eventually diagnosed as **gallbladder cancer**. This problem may be **exacerbated by spillage** of **bile** or **stones inside** the **peritoneal cavity**.
- One study looked at 409 patients who underwent laparoscopic cholecystectomy for presumed benign gallbladder disease but were diagnosed with gallbladder cancer on final pathology. Seventeen percent of patients at a median of 180 days were diagnosed with laparoscopic port site recurrences. As a result of this high percentage, **some surgeons recommend port site excision during reoperation for gallbladder cancer.**
- It is important to note, however, that it is **rare for port site recurrences** to **occur** as the **sole site** of **disease**.
- Given that it is **more a marker of aggressive disease than a single site of resectable disease**, our general practice does not include empirically resecting prior port sites during reexploration for gallbladder cancer.

123. Ans. a. Adenocarcinoma
124. Ans. c. Radical cholecystectomy
125. Ans. b. Present with jaundice, d. Gallstones predispose
126. Ans. c. Secondaries to liver

METASTASIS IN CARCINOMA GALLBLADDER

- **Direct hepatic invasion** in **59%**[Q], **LN metastasis** in **45%**, **perineural invasion** in **42%** cases.

127. Ans. a. Adenocarcinoma
128. **Ans. b. Resection of segment IVb & V of liver with nodal clearance with port site excision** *(Ref: Sabiston 20/e p1514; Schwartz 10/e p1335; Bailey 27/e p1211)*
129. Ans. b. Extended cholecystectomy
   - **T1b, T2, T3** tumor with no evidence of metastasis: Re-resection, **extended cholecystectomy** (possible CBD or extended hepatic resection)[Q]

GALLBLADDER ANATOMY AND PHYSIOLOGY

130. **Ans. a. 5, b. 10** *(Ref: Sabiston 20/e p1482; Schwartz 10/e p1309-1310; Bailey 26/e p1097-1098)*
131. Ans. d. 50
132. Ans. d. Lymph node of Lund

MISCELLANEOUS

133. Ans. b. Choledochoduodenostomy *(Ref: Blumgart 6/e p711, 5/e p632; Shackelford 8/e p1356, 7/e p1355)*

SUMP SYNDROME

- **Sump syndrome:** **Particulate matter**, **stones**, and **food debris accumulate** and **stagnate** in the **distal, "blind" end of the common duct**[Q]
- **Sump syndrome** occurs after **choledochoduodenostomy**[Q]
- Occasional cause of **recurrent cholangitis** that can result in anastomotic stricture

Management

- Endoscopic management, consisting of **sphincterotomy** with or without **balloon dilation** of the **anastomosis**[Q]
- **End-to-side hepaticojejunostomy**, **Roux-en-Y**, to prevent persistent regurgitation of intestinal contents and to **remove the "sump" permanently**, is preferred surgical procedure[Q]

134. Ans. b. Re-cholecystectomy is the definite treatment of choice, e. Oral ursodeoxycholic acid relieves symptoms remarkably *(Ref: Sabiston 20/e p1501-1504)*

POSTCHOLECYSTECTOMY SYNDROME

- The **remnant of** the **cystic duct** or **gallbladder** (in subtotal cholecystectomy) has historically been implicated as the **source of pain, nausea**, and **vomiting** in postcholecystectomy patients[Q]
- An **increase in choledochal pressure** resulting in **cystic stump distension**, **inflammation** or **stone obstruction** within the **remnant of the cystic duct** or **gallbladder**[Q], and an increase in the sphincter of Oddi pressure have all served as causes of postcholecystectomy problems

  - However, various studies have confirmed that **symptomatic improvement** only occurs when **a stone is present in the CBD** or cystic duct and is **subsequently removed endoscopically** or **via operative reintervention**[Q]

- In general, **persistent symptoms following a cholecystectomy** in which no cholangiogram was performed warrants analysis of the **liver function profile** and/or **noninvasive imaging** with either **ultrasound** or **MRCP** to **assess for retained stone**
- If **CBD stone** are **present, therapeutic ERCP** is suggested[Q]

135. Ans. c. 4 sphincters *(Ref: Shackelford 8/e p1253, 7/e p1290; Bailey 27/e p1214)*

- The **entire sphincter mechanism is actually composed of four sphincters**[Q] containing **both circular** and **longitudinal smooth muscle fibers**.

SPHINCTER OF ODDI

- The **entire sphincteric system** of the **distal bile duct** and the **pancreatic duct** is commonly referred to as the **sphincter of Oddi**.
- The sphincter mechanism functions **independently from** the surrounding **duodenal musculature** and has **separate sphincters** for the **distal bile duct**, the **pancreatic duct**, and the **ampulla**.
- In **more than 90%** of the population, the **common channel**, where the biliary and pancreatic ducts join, is **<1.0 cm** in **length** and lies within the ampulla.

The four sphincters are	
1. Superior sphincter choledochus[Q]	3. Sphincter pancreaticus[Q]
2. Inferior sphincter choledochus[Q]	4. Sphincter of the ampulla[Q]

136. Ans. a. Pressing the artery manually *(Ref: Blumgart 6/e p574, 5/e p525)*

GOLDEN RULES TO BE FOLLOWED IN CASE OF DIFFICULT CHOLECYSTECTOMY

- When the **anatomy of Callot's triangle** is **not clear**, blind dissection should not be done[Q]
- **Bleeding adjacent to** the **Callot's triangle** should be **controlled by pressure** and not by clipping or clamping[Q]
- When there is **doubt about** the **anatomy**, a **fundus first cholecystectomy** dissecting on gallbladder wall down to the cystic duct can be helpful[Q].
- If the **cystic duct** is **densely adherent to CBD** and there is possibility of **Mirizzi's syndrome**, the **infundibulum** of the GB should be **opened**, the **stone removed** and **infundibulum oversewn**[Q].

137. **Ans. c. Like toothpaste emulsion in the gallbladder** *(Ref: Harrison 20/e p2428, 19/e p2082)*
138. **Ans. d. Appendicitis** *(Ref: Examination of Shoulder by Tae Kyun Kim/4)*

Referred Shoulder Pain

Right Shoulder
- Peptic ulcer
- Myocardial ischemia
- Acute cholecystitis
- Liver disease (Abscess, cirrhosis, hepatitis)
- Pulmonary (Pleurisy, pneumothorax, Pancoast tumor)
- Kidney diseases

Left Shoulder
- Ruptured spleen
- Myocardial ischemia
- Pancreatic diseases
- Ruptured ectopic
- Pulmonary (Pleurisy, pneumothorax, Pancoast tumor)
- Kidney diseases
- Postoperative laparoscopy

139. **Ans. b. Acute cholecystitis** *(Ref: Sabiston 20/e p1493; Schwartz 9/e p1115-1116; http://radiopaedia.org/articles/elevated-hemidiaphragm)*

Causes of Elevated Hemidiaphragm

Above the diaphragm
Decreased lung volume:
- **Atelectasis** / collapse
- **Lobectomy** / pneumonectomy
- **Pulmonary hypoplasia**

Diaphragm
- **Phrenic nerve palsy**
- Diaphragmatic eventration
- Contralateral CVA: usually **MCA distribution**

Below the Diaphragm
- Abdominal tumour
- **Subphrenic abscess**
- **Liver abscess** (**Amebic** and pyogenic)

140. **Ans. b. Phrygian cap** *(Ref: Bailey 27/e p1195)*

Phrygian cap

- MC anomaly of the gallbladder[Q]
- Created by an **infolding** of a **septum** between the **body** & **fundus**[Q]
- GB functions normally
- This anomaly is **not an indication** for **cholecystectomy**[Q].

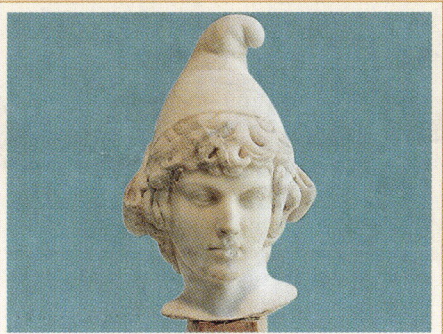
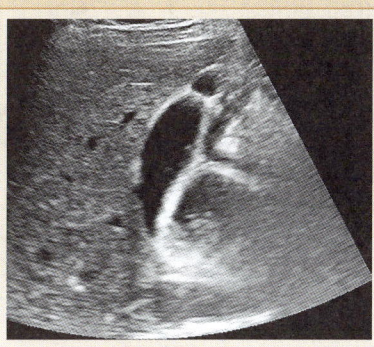

CHAPTER 7

Bile Duct

CHOLEDOCHAL CYST

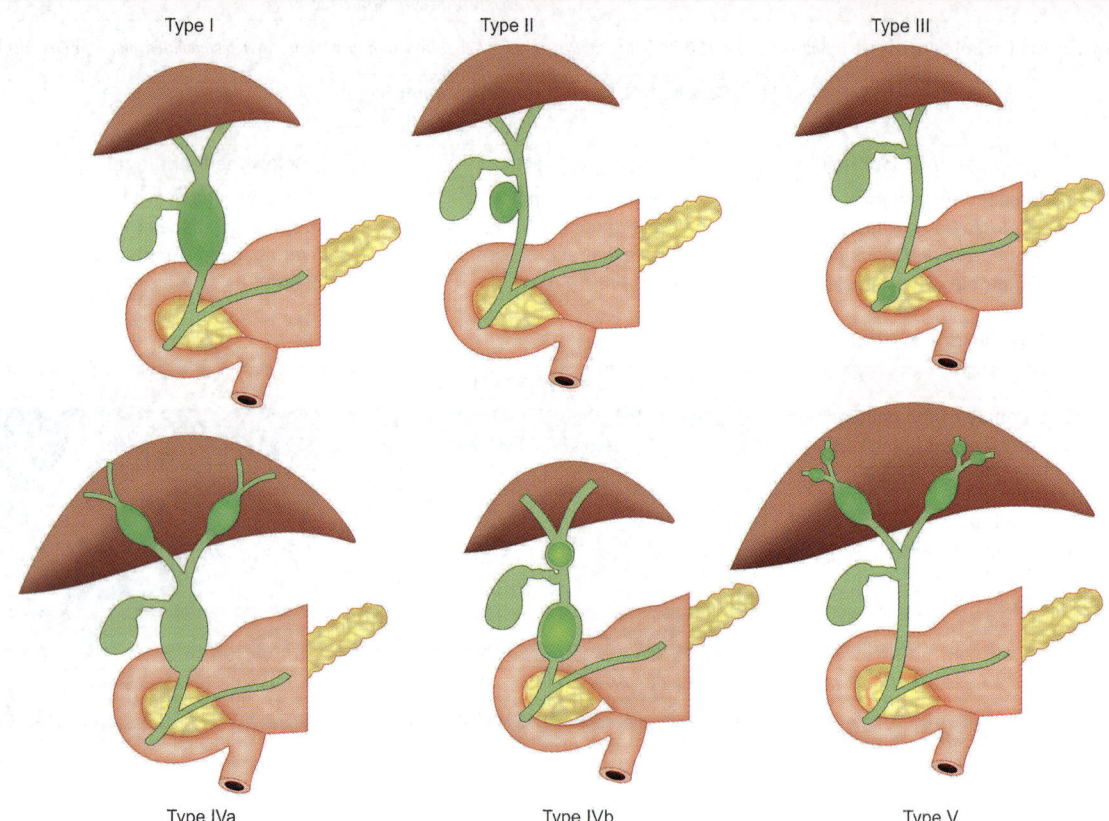

Todani modification of Alonso-Lej classification

CHOLEDOCHAL CYST

- Cystic dilation of the biliary ducts, more common in **females**[Q]
- Association of choledochal cyst with biliary atresia is seen, with **type 1 biliary atresia**[Q] is present in most cases.
- It may be discovered on **antenatal ultrasound**[Q]

Etiology

- Most widely accepted hypothesis: **Abnormal pancreaticobiliary ductal junction (APBDJ)**[Q]
- **APBDJ** results in **reflux of pancreatic fluid** into the distal common hepatic duct and results in mucosal injury, chronic inflammation, and **weakening of the bile duct wall**[Q].

Classification

- Bile duct cysts are classified on the basis of site, extent, and shape of the cystic anomaly of the ductal system.
- MC choledochal cyst: **Type I** > Type **IV** > Type **III (143)**[Q]

Todani Modification of Alonso-Lej Classification[Q]	

Type I (MC)	• Dilation of extrahepatic biliary tree
	  – Type Ia: **cystic dilation**[Q] (MC type)
	  – Type Ib: **focal segmental dilation**[Q]
	  – Type Ic: **fusiform dilation**[Q]

Type II	• **Diverticular dilation**[Q] of extrahepatic biliary tree
Type III	• Cystic dilation of intraduodenal portion of common bile duct (**choledochocele**)[Q]
Type IVA	• Dilation of the **extrahepatic & intrahepatic biliary tree**[Q]
Type IVB	• Dilation of multiple sections of **extrahepatic bile ducts**[Q]
Type V	• Dilation confined to intrahepatic bile ducts (**Caroli's disease**[Q])
Type VI	• **Cystic dilatation of cystic duct**[Q] (not included in Todani's modification)

Clinical Features
- Classic triad: Pain, jaundice (intermittent) & abdominal **mass (10%)**[Q].

> - **MC symptom in Infants: Jaundice (in 80%)**[Q]
> - **MC symptom in patients >2 years of age: Abdominal pain**[Q]

- In **children**, the major clinical symptoms are recurrent **abdominal pain (81.8%)**, nausea & vomiting (65.5%), mild jaundice (43.6%), an abdominal mass (29.0%), and fever (29.0%).
- In **adults**, **abdominal pain (87%)** and **jaundice (42%)** are present frequently. Less common clinical findings include nausea (29%), cholangitis (26%), pancreatitis (23%), and an **abdominal mass (13%)**.

Diagnosis
- IOC for **choledochal cyst: MRCP** (non-invasive)
- ERCP: More useful in defining the distal ductal anatomy and the presence of APBDJ
- PTC: Useful in defining the proximal ductal anatomy and the presence of intrahepatic disease.

Treatment of Choledochal Cyst	
Type I	• **Roux-en-Y hepaticojejunostomy**[Q]
Type II	• **Excision** with **T-tube repair**[Q] • **Roux-en-Y hepaticojejunostomy**[Q]
Type III	• **Endoscopic sphincterotomy** and **cyst unroofing**[Q]
Type IVA	• **Hepatic resection** for **localized** disease[Q] • **Liver transplantation** for **diffuse disease**[Q]
Type IVB	• Transduodenal sphincteroplasty and **Roux-en-Y hepaticojejunostomy**[Q]
Type V	• **Hepatic resection** for **localized disease**[Q] • **Liver transplantation** for **diffuse disease**[Q]

Complications of Choledochal Cyst	
• Recurrent cholangitis[Q] • Pancreatitis[Q] • Gallstones[Q]	• Cirrhosis with portal hypertension • Portal vein thrombosis • Malignancy[Q]

LILLY TECHNIQUE

- **Lilly technique**: Serosal surface of the duct is **left adhering** to **portal vein**, while the mucosa of cyst wall is obliterated by curettage or cautery, when **cyst** is **densely adhered** to the **portal vein** secondary to long-standing inflammatory reaction[Q].
- In this situation, a complete, full-thickness excision of the cyst may not be possible.

CHOLEDOCHOLITHIASIS

CHOLEDOCHOLITHIASIS

- **CBD stones** are classified by **point of origin**
- Found in **6–12%** of patients with GB stones[Q]

- Retained stones discovered within 2 years of cholecystectomy^Q
- Recurrent stones detected >2 years following cholecystectomy^Q

Primary CBD stone	Secondary CBD stone
• **Formed** within the **biliary tract**^Q • Associated with biliary **Stasis and infection**^Q • More commonly seen in **Asian**^Q populations • **Soft, friable, light-brown stones** or **sludge** in the common duct^Q	• **Formed** initially in the **GB**^Q • **Migrate through** the **cystic duct** into CBD^Q • Most common bile duct stones in **Western countries**^Q • Usually **cholesterol stones**^Q

Clinical Features
- CBD stones may be **silent** and are often **discovered incidentally**^Q. In these patients, biliary obstruction is transient, and laboratory tests may be normal.
- Clinical features suspicious for **biliary obstruction** due to **CBD stones** include **biliary colic, jaundice, clay colored stools**, and **darkening of the urine**^Q.
- **Fever** and **chills** may be present in patients with choledocholithiasis and **cholangitis**.
- Serum **bilirubin** (>3.0 mg/dL), **aminotransferases**, and **ALP** are commonly elevated in patients with biliary obstruction but are **neither sensitive nor specific** for the presence of common duct stones.
- Among these, serum **bilirubin** has the **highest positive predictive value**^Q (28%–50%) for the presence of **choledocholithiasis**.
- **Laboratory values** may be **normal** in **one third**^Q of patients with choledocholithiasis.

Diagnosis
- **USG: First test**, can document **GB stones** and estimate the **CBD diameter**^Q
- A **dilated bile duct** (>8 mm in diameter) in a patient with **gallstones, jaundice** and **biliary pain** is **highly suggestive** of choledocholithiasis.
- **MRCP**: Provides excellent anatomic detail, with **sensitivity** and **specificity** of 95% and 98%, respectively, for **CBD stones**^Q.

> • **ERCP**: Diagnostic and therapeutic test of choice for patients with suspected CBD stones^Q.

Treatment
- Treatment options are **ERCP**, laparoscopic or **open CBD Exploration**.

CHOLANGITIS

Cholangitis
- **Ascending bacterial infection**^Q of the biliary ductal system with obstruction
- **MC cause** of acute cholangitis is **choledocholithiasis**^Q
- **MC organisms** present in the bile in patients with cholangitis: **E. coli**^Q, **Klebsiella pneumoniae**^Q, Streptococcus faecalis, & Bacteroides fragilis.

Etiology
- **Choledocholithiasis (MC)**^Q
- Biliary-enteric anastomotic strictures
- Benign strictures
- Cholangiocarcinoma and periampullary cancer

Clinical Features
- Characterized by **Charcot's triad**^Q: Abdominal pain + jaundice + fever
- Cholangitis may be either **self-limited** or **toxic** with severe illness, including **jaundice, fever, abdominal pain, mental status changes**, and **hypotension (Reynold's pentad)**^Q.

> • **Fever & chills** are the **MC presentation** (due to **cholangiovenous & cholangiolymphatic reflux**)^Q

- **Fever** is the **most consistent sign**, generally **intermittent**, spiking and associated **with shaking chills**^Q.

Diagnosis
- Leukocytosis, hyperbilirubinemia, and raised ALP and transaminases^Q
- **Positive blood culture** is **more common** in **partial obstruction**^Q than with complete obstruction

> • **Cholangiography** (If **ERCP** is not available, **PTC** should be performed) is **mandatory** as a **diagnostic** and **potentially therapeutic intervention**^Q.

Treatment
- Initial treatment: IV antibiotics & aggressive hydration^Q

- **Septic shock** with **toxic cholangitis**: **ICU monitoring** and **vasopressors** to support blood pressure.
- **Most patients** will **respond** to **these measures** alone.
- **Urgent biliary decompression** will be necessary in 15% cases^Q.
- Biliary decompression may be performed endoscopically or by a percutaneous transhepatic route based on the level of the obstruction.

Methods of Biliary Decompression

ERCP with Sphincterotomy and Stone Extraction	Percutaneous Transhepatic Cholangiography (PTC)	Surgical Decompression
• **Procedure of choice**^{Q} • Early endoscopy is **diagnostic & therapeutic**^{Q} • Permits biliary decompression by **sphincterotomy & stone extraction**^{Q} • If stone can't be removed, a **nasobiliary catheter** or stent is inserted to decompress biliary tract^Q	• PTC is performed if: • **ERCP** has **failed** or not available^Q • **Proximal** or hilar obstruction^Q • **Stricture** of **biliary enteric anastomosis**^{Q}	• Surgical decompression is indicated when **neither ERCP nor PTC is possible**^{Q}. • Consists of CBD **decompression** with a **T-tube**^{Q}

Elective Definitive Treatment in Stabilized Patients

- **Cholecystectomy** with **choledochotomy** and **CBD exploration**^{Q}
- **T-tube** is left in place for **cholangiography** and **removal** of any **retained stone**^{Q}
- **T-tube cholangiogram** is done on **7th-10th day post-operatively**^{Q}
- **Remove** the T-tube if **cholangiogram is normal**^{Q}
- If **residual stone** is discovered **on** the **post-operative cholangiogram, T-tube** should be **left in place** for **4-6 weeks** for the **tract to mature**^{Q}.
- The **stones** are **removed percutaneously** through the **matured tract** by **Burhenne's technique**^{Q}.

ERCP

ERCP

- Endoscopic clearance of CBD stones can **avoid** the **need for an open operation**^{Q} if expertise in laparoscopic common bile duct exploration is not available.

Indications of preoperative ERCP

• Patients with **worsening cholangitis**^{Q}	• **Biliary pancreatitis**^{Q}
• **Ampullary stone impaction**^{Q}	• **Cirrhosis**^{Q}

- If clearance is not possible because of multiple stones, intrahepatic stones, impacted stones, difficulty with cannulation, duodenal diverticula, or biliary stricture, this information is known before surgery.
- **Endoscopic sphincterotomy** with **stone extraction** is **well tolerated** in most patients, with a **5–8% complication rate**^{Q}.
- **Complete clearance** is achieved in **71–75%** of patients at the **first procedure** and in **84–95%** of patients after **multiple endoscopic procedures**^{Q}.
- **Prompt cholecystectomy** after endoscopic clearance of the CBD should be performed during the hospital admission if the **patient is fit for surgery**^{Q}.
- Patients **> 70 years** should have their **ductal stones cleared endoscopically** as their **sole therapy**; only about **15%** become symptomatic from their Gallstones in their remaining lifetime, which can then be treated as symptoms arise^Q.

Contraindications of Endoscopic sphincterotomy

- CBD diameter **>2 cm**^{Q}
- Long suprasphincteric **stricture, >15 mm**^{Q}
- **Peri-vaterian diverticulum**^{Q}
- **Duodenal wall** and **head** of the pancreas **severely inflamed**^{Q}

BILE DUCT INJURY AND LIGATION

BILE DUCT INJURY AND LIGATION

- **Most benign strictures** follow **iatrogenic bile duct injury**^{Q}
- **Most commonly** during **laparoscopic cholecystectomy**^{Q}
- **Incidence** of bile duct injury during **open** cholecystectomy is **0.1–0.2%**^{Q}
- **Incidence** of bile duct injury during **laparoscopic** cholecystectomy is **0.3–0.85%**^{Q}

Pathogenesis

Risk Factors for Bile Duct Injury	
• Acute or chronic inflammation[Q]	• Anatomic variation[Q]
• Obesity[Q]	• Bleeding[Q]

- **Bile duct injury** rate increased in **acute cholecystitis, pancreatitis, cholangitis, & obstructive jaundice**[Q].

> - As **surgeon experience** increases **beyond 20 cases**, bile duct **injury rate decreases**[Q].
> - **Errors** leading to laparoscopic bile duct injuries stem from '**misperception**'[Q], not errors of skill, knowledge or judgment.
> - **Primary cause of error** in **97% cases** was a '**visual perceptual illusion**'[Q], whereas only **3% injuries** were due to **faults of technical skills**[Q].

- Surgical technique with **inadequate exposure** and **failure to identify** structures **before ligating** or **dividing** them are the most common cause of **significant biliary injury**[Q].
- **Routine** use of **intra-operative cholangiography** may **limit the extent** of **bile duct injury**, but does **not** seem to **prevent it**[Q].
- If a **bile duct injury** is **suspected** during cholecystectomy, a **cholangiogram must be obtained** to identify the anatomy[Q].
- **Classic Laparoscopic Injury:** A long length of the **common duct** is excised up to the **proximal common hepatic duct**, which is either occluded or left to drain bile into the peritoneal cavity.

Clinical Features
- About **25%** of **major ductal injuries** are **recognized intraoperatively**[Q] because of bile leakage, an abnormal cholangiogram, or late recognition of the anatomy.
- **MC presentation** of a **complete occlusion** of the common hepatic or bile duct is **jaundice** with or without **abdominal pain**[Q].
- Patients may also present **months or years after** prior surgery with **cholangitis** or **cirrhosis** secondary to a biliary tract injury.

Diagnosis
- **USG** or **CT** should be performed in patients with signs of **abdominal pain** or **peritonitis, sepsis**, or any other clinical suspicion of **biloma**[Q].
- Patients must be stabilized with **immediate parenteral antibiotics** and **image-guided percutaneous drainage** of any fluid collections[Q].
- **Cholangiography** should be performed to establish the **presence of ductal stricture**, identify the **level** of the stricture, and identify the **nature of the injury** when necessary[Q].
- **PTC** is the **imaging method of choice** for **most postoperative biliary strictures**[Q]

> - **ERCP** may be easier to obtain in a patient with a biliary stricture and cholangitis who **requires urgent cholangiography** and **biliary decompression**.
> - However, this is **only useful** in patients **with bile duct continuity**.
> - **Cystic duct leaks** or **small tangential injuries** can be treated with **endoscopic stenting**.
> - In situations in which the **biliary stricture** is **too tight** to pass with ERCP, **PTC** may be performed for proximal biliary decompression.

- **CT arteriography** should be considered in the **preoperative evaluation** of patients with benign biliary strictures.
- **Unrecognized injury** to the **hepatic artery** or a **portal vein branch** occurs with a frequency of **12–47%** concomitant with a bile duct injury.
- In patients presenting with **late strictures** with evidence of **liver dysfunction**, a **CT arteriogram** should be performed to evaluate for **evidence of portal hypertension**.

BISMUTH CLASSIFICATION OF BILE DUCT STRICTURES

Bismuth Classification of Bile Duct Strictures	
Type 1	**Low** common hepatic duct stricture; hepatic duct **stump >2 cm**[Q]
Type 2	Mid common hepatic duct **stump < 2 cm**[Q]
Type 3	**High** stricture **(hilar)**, no hepatic duct stump; **confluence intact**[Q]
Type 4	**Destruction of** the hilar **confluence**; right and left hepatic ducts separated[Q]
Type 5	Involvement of **aberrant right sectoral hepatic duct** alone **with or without** a concomitant **hepatic duct stricture**[Q]

- The **shortcomings** in **Bismuths classification** were that firstly it did not stipulate the **length** of the stricture, and secondly, and more importantly it did not take into account the presence of **biliary leaks**, which are more common after laparoscopic cholecystectomy.
- This, **latter fact** has been incorporated **in Strasberg's classification**; also patients with limited strictures, isolated right hepatic duct strictures or cystic duct leaks cannot be classified.

STRASBERG CLASSIFICATION OF LAPAROSCOPIC BILIARY INJURIES

	Strasberg Classification of Laparoscopic Biliary Injuries
Type A	• **Bile leaks** from **minor ducts** still in continuity with the CBD[Q] • Includes **leakage from cystic duct** stump and from a **subvesical duct of Luschka**[Q] • **MC causes of biliary leaks** seen after laparoscopic cholecystectomy[Q]
Type B	• **Occlusion** of a part of the biliary tree, almost always an **aberrant right sectoral duct**[Q]
Type C	• **Transection without ligation** of an aberrant right sectoral duct[Q]
Type D	• A **lateral injury** to an **extrahepatic duct**[Q]
Type E	• Includes biliary strictures, divided into **E1 to E5** as classified by **Bismuth**

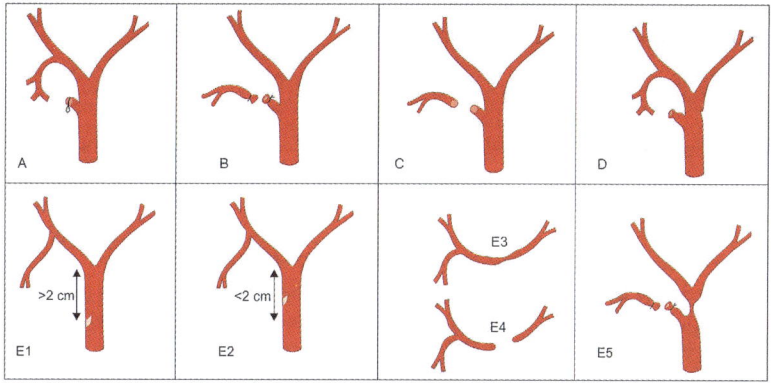

Strasberg classficiation of postoperative bile duct strictures

OTHER CLASSIFICATION SYSTEMS FOR BILE DUCT INJURIES

- Amsterdam Academic Medical Center's classification
- **Neuhaus' classification**
- **Csendes' classification**
- **Stewart-Way's** classification of laparoscopic bile duct injuries
- **Chinese University** of Hong Kong (CUHK) classification

MANAGEMENT OF THE BILE DUCT INJURY RECOGNIZED AFTER CHOLECYSTECTOMY

MANAGEMENT OF THE BILE DUCT INJURY RECOGNIZED AFTER CHOLECYSTECTOMY

- Patients with a **bile leak** will **present early**[Q]
- Patients with **postoperative biliary strictures** alone often present with jaundice or cholangitis **months to years** after the initial injury[Q].

Intraoperative Considerations

- Management of postoperative biliary strictures following ductal injury depends on the degree **of injury**, the presence of **stricture-induced complications**, and the **operative risk** of the patient.

Planning of the following specific goals
- **Control** the **infection** (abscess or cholangitis)[Q]
- **Drain the biloma**[Q]
- Complete the **cholangiography**[Q]
- Provide definitive therapy with **controlled reconstruction** or **stenting**[Q]

- Independent predictors of stricture recurrence after an initial operative repair:
  - **Cholangitis** before the initial repair
  - **Primary repair within 3 weeks** of the bile duct injury
  - Incomplete cholangiography
- If **immediate repair** is to be attempted, consultation with **more experienced surgeons** should be made.
- In those cases in which **expertise** is **not available** at the time of a recognized injury, or **difficult circumstances** preclude elaborate reconstructive attempts, **external biliary drains** will allow patient recovery and **transfer** to a **center of excellence**[Q].

Successful repair of biliary strictures requires adherence to specific surgical principles
- Use of **proximal bile duct** with **minimal inflammation**[Q]
- Creation of a **tension-free anastomosis** with the use of a **Roux-en-Y jejunal limb**[Q]
- Direct **mucosa-to-mucosa anastomosis**[Q]

- **Direct operative biliary-enteric bypass** is the **gold standard procedure**[Q] for the long-term treatment of biliary strictures. These procedures have low operative mortality and acceptable morbidity.
- **Hepp-Couinaud approach** to **bile duct reconstruction** is the **best option**[Q] in most circumstances. This technique requires dissection of the hilar plate to expose the left hepatic duct and allow for a side-to-side anastomosis of the left hepatic duct to the Roux-en-Y jejunal limb.

> **Successful repair of biliary strictures requires adherence to specific surgical principles**
> - Use of **proximal bile duct** with **minimal inflammation**[Q]
> - Creation of a **tension-free anastomosis** with the use of a **Roux-en-Y jejunal limb**[Q]
> - Direct **mucosa-to-mucosa anastomosis**[Q]

- **Direct operative biliary-enteric bypass** is the **gold standard procedure**[Q] for the long-term treatment of biliary strictures. These procedures have low operative mortality and acceptable morbidity.

Interventional Radiologic and Endoscopic Techniques

- These techniques allow:
  - **Percutaneous drainage** of abdominal fluid collections
  - **Preoperative identification** of the **ductal anatomy** through PTC
  - **Stricture dilation** with or without placement of **palliative stents** for bile drainage in the patient whose overall physiologic status precludes a major operation.
- **Percutaneous transhepatic dilation** can be employed in patients with intrahepatic ductal disease and in patients in whom **ERCP is not possible**.

> - Success rate of **percutaneous transhepatic dilation** is **50–70%**[Q].
> - Patients with **anastomotic strictures** (including **biliary-enteric anastomotic strictures**) have the **highest success rates**[Q].
> - Treatment of biliary strictures with **interventional radiologic methods**, requires **multiple sessions of dilations**, and **nonischemic strictures (anastomotic strictures) respond best**[Q].

- **Endoscopic stenting** and **drainage** is a **successful treatment** option for **cystic duct leak** or **small common bile duct leaks** following laparoscopic cholecystectomy.
- **Ischemic biliary strictures** will **not respond permanently to dilation**. **Early retreatment** (through **repeat dilation** or **biliary-enteric reconstruction**) of postdilation recurrent strictures is **essential** to prevent secondary biliary cirrhosis[Q].

GOALS OF THERAPY IN IATROGENIC BILE DUCT INJURY

- **Control of infection limiting inflammation:**
  - Parenteral antibiotics[Q]
- **Clear and thorough delineation of entire biliary anatomy:**
  - MRCP/PTC[Q]
- **Re-establishment of biliary enteric continuity:**
  - Tension-free, mucosa-to-mucosa anastomosis[Q]
  - Long-term transanastomotic stents if involving bifurcation or higher[Q]
- Percutaneous drainage of periportal fluid collection[Q]
- ERCP (especially if cystic duct stump leak suspected)[Q]
- Roux-en-Y hepaticojejunostomy[Q]

BILIARY FISTULA

BILIARY FISTULA

- **Internal fistulas** are spontaneous, rare, and occur without a significant collection of bile.
- **External fistulas** are more common and are often caused by iatrogenic injury after operations, invasive procedures, or trauma involving the biliary tract.

EXTERNAL BILIARY FISTULA

- **External fistulas** are more common and are often caused by iatrogenic injury after operations, invasive procedures, or trauma involving the biliary tract.

Etiology
- **Bile leakage** from the **cystic duct remnant**[Q]
- **Central hepatectomy** and **caudate resection**[Q]
- **Difficult** cases of **open cholecystectomy**[Q]
- Hepatic **cryotherapy** or **harmonic** scalpel use[Q]

Treatment
- Patients with **leaks from** the **cystic duct,** duct of **Luschka,** and **T-tube tract** are optimal candidates for **endoscopic treatment**[Q].
- Patients treated with **stents alone** experience equally good outcomes as patients treated with a combination of **stents** and **sphincterotomy**[Q].

INTERNAL BILIARY FISTULA

- **Internal fistulas** are spontaneous, rare, and occur without a significant collection of bile.
- **Cholecystoduodenal** fistulas (72–80%) are **MC** biliary-enteric fistulas followed by **cholecystocolic** fistulas (8-12%)[Q]
- Most cholecystoduodenal fistula are **asymptomatic**[Q].
- The site of fistula most commonly located in the **vaterian segment** of the **CBD** in case of the **choledochoduodenal fistula**[Q].

Etiology
- **Calculous biliary tract disease (90%)**[Q]
- **Duodenal ulcer (6%)**
- **Neoplasm**, trauma, parasitic infestation, and congenital anomalies (4%)

Diagnosis
- Only **one-third** of biliary-enteric fistulas will present with **air** in the **biliary tree**[Q].
- A **negative upper gastrointestinal series** in the presence of **pneumobilia** is an indication for a **barium enema**, which discloses greater than 95% of **cholecystocolic fistulae**[Q].

Management
- In the **absence of obstruction, residual stones**, or **symptoms**, except for **cholecystogastric** and **cholecystocolic** fistulas, **no operation** should be performed because most fistulas **close spontaneously**[Q].
- For **cholecystocolic fistula, choledochotomy** is recommended as a **first step**, followed by **cholecystectomy**, and **finally takedown** and **repair** of the **fistula** to reduce bacterial contamination[Q].
- In other cases, the usual approach is repair of the fistula, then cholecystectomy and closure of the bowel.

SPHINCTER OF ODDI DYSFUNCTION

Sphincter of Oddi Dysfunction

- Pain similar to **biliary colic** with **normal LFT** and episodes of **acute pancreatitis** have been attributed to a poorly defined syndrome known as Sphincter of Oddi dysfunction[Q].
- The **pathogenesis** is unclear
- Postulated theories include gallstone migration inducing fibrosis of the sphincter, trauma, pancreatitis, and congenital anomalies.
- **Modified Milwaukee classification** is used for Biliary **Sphincter of Oddi dysfunction**[Q]

Types
- **Sphincter of Oddi Stenosis:**
  - Also known as **papillitis**[Q]
  - Benign intrinsic obstruction of the CBD outlet[Q]
- **Sphincter of Oddi Dyskinesis:**
  - It is an **intermittent functional blockage** of the high-pressure zone of the sphincter[Q]
  - **Basal pressure** is **elevated**, but administration of smooth muscle relaxants (**nitrates**) causes **decrease of the basal sphincter pressure** in functional dyskinesis[Q]

Clinical Features
- Pain similar to **biliary colic** with **normal LFT** and episodes of **acute pancreatitis**[Q]

Diagnosis
- A dilated CBD (>12 mm diameter) or **increase in CBD diameter in response** to CCK is a **typical ultrasound finding**[Q].
- **Endoscopic manometry** is considered **gold standard** [Q] for diagnosis
- **Nardi Test**[Q]: The most widely used **pharmacologic test** to assess sphincter function is the **morphine-prostigmine provocation test**[Q]

Treatment
- Treatment of choice: **Transduodenal sphincteroplasty** with **transampullary septectomy**[Q]

BILIARY ATRESIA

Biliary Atresia

- Characterized by **progressive obliteration** of the **extrahepatic** and **intrahepatic** bile ducts[Q].
- **Etiology** is **unknown; incidence 1 in 12,000** live births[Q].
- Presently, there is **no medical therapy** to **reverse the obliterative process**[Q]

  - Patients who are **not offered surgical treatment** uniformly develop biliary cirrhosis, portal hypertension, and **death** by **2 years of age**[Q].

- **MC indication** for **pediatric liver transplantation**[Q]

Pathology
- **Bile duct proliferation**, **severe cholestasis** with **plugging**, and **inflammatory cell infiltrate** are the **pathologic hallmarks** of this disease^Q.
- Over time, these changes **progress to fibrosis** with **end-stage cirrhosis**^{Q}.
- Positive for neural cell adhesion molecule (**CD56**) staining

Classification

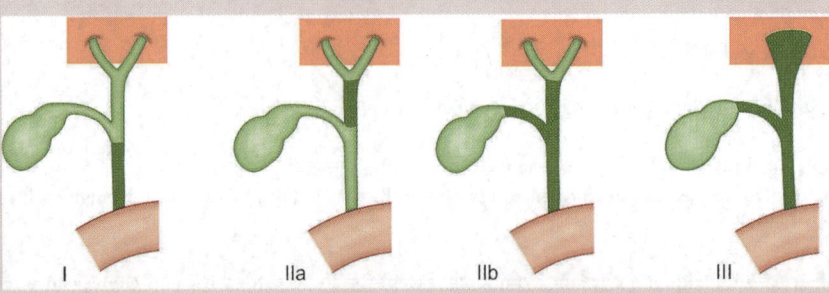

Kasai Classification of Biliary Atresia	
Type I	CBD is **obliterated**, proximal bile ducts are patent^Q
Type IIa	Atresia of common hepatic duct (**CHD**) with patent cystic duct & CBD^Q
Type IIb	Obliteration of CHD, cystic duct & CBD^Q
Type III	Atresia of CBD, cystic duct & hepatic ducts upto porta hepatis^Q (**MC type**, responsible for > **90% cases**^{Q})

Clinical Features
- Infants with biliary atresia present with **jaundice at birth** or **shortly thereafter**^{Q}.
- Infants with biliary atresia characteristically have **acholic, pale gray stools**, secondary to obstructed bile flow.
- With passage of time, **progressive failure to thrive** and, if untreated, develop **stigmata of liver failure** and **portal hypertension** (splenomegaly and esophageal varices)
- **Associated malformations in 25%**: Polysplenia, malrotation, preduodenal portal vein, and **intrahepatic vena cava**^{Q}.

Diagnosis
- USG of the liver and GB is important in the evaluation of the infant with cholestasis.

- **USG**: GB is shrunken and CBD is **not visible**^{Q}. A **triangle cord sign**^{Q} found on ultrasound has a **predictive accuracy** of **95%**, the **gallbladder ghost triad**^{Q} in which the **gallbladder** is **short** (<1.9 cm) and **irregular** and **lacks an echogenic inner lining** also got good sensitivity.

- **Next diagnostic step**: Percutaneous **liver biopsy**^{Q} if the hepatic synthetic function is normal (diagnostic accuracy 90%).
- **Hepatobiliary scintigraphy**: In cases in which the **USG** and **biopsy** findings are **inconclusive (absent excretion into the intestine)**^{Q}

- **Gold standard for diagnosing biliary atresia**: Intraoperative cholangiography^Q (Blumgart 6/e p658)
- Although **percutaneous liver biopsy** is **highly accurate**, there are **no histologic findings** that are **pathognomonic for BA**

Treatment
- **Exploratory laparotomy**: If the needle biopsy or abdominal ultrasound is consistent with BA
- **Intra-operative cholecystocholangiography**: **To confirm** the **diagnosis**, demonstration of the **fibrotic biliary remnant** and definition of **absent proximal** and **distal bile duct patency**^{Q}

- **Treatment of choice**: **Kasai hepatoportoenterostomy**^{Q} (Roux-en-Y hepaticojejunostomy)

Postoperative Management
- **Ursodeoxycholic acid** (facilitate bile flow) + **Methylprednisolone** (anti-inflammatory agent) + **TMP-SMX** (antimicrobial prophylaxis)^Q

- **Cholangitis** is the **MC** post-operative **complication**^{Q}.

Prognosis
- About 30% of infants undergoing hepatoportoenterostomy **before 60 days** of age will have a **long-term successful outcome** and **not require liver transplantation**^{Q}.
- **Liver transplantation** in the patients who develop **progressive hepatic fibrosis** with resultant **portal hypertension** and progressive cholestasis^Q.
- **Serum bilirubin at 3 months** after surgery seems to be **strongly predictive** of **long-term survival**^{Q}.

PRIMARY SCLEROSING CHOLANGITIS

Primary Sclerosing Cholangitis

- PSC is a **cholestatic liver disease** characterized by **fibrotic strictures** involving **intrahepatic & extrahepatic biliary tree**[Q] in the absence of a known precipitating cause.
- More common in HLA **B8/DR3**[Q]

> - **Incidence** of UC in PSC ranges from **75–80%**[Q].
> - PSC is **present** in 5.5% of patients with **chronic UC**[Q].

- Patients with PSC are at **increased risk** for developing **cholangiocarcinoma**[Q].
- **Smoking** is protective in **UC & PSC**[Q].

Pathology

- **Cholangiocytes**[Q], epithelial cells that lines the bile duct are **target cell** of injury in PSC.
- Histologic finding of "**onion skin appearance**"[Q] is **pathognomic** of PSC, but seen in <10% cases.

> - Involvement of **large intrahepatic** and **extrahepatic duct**[Q] distinguishes PSC from PBC.
> - **Absence of the smallest intrahepatic ducts** leading to a **reduction in the branching** of biliary tree (give rise to **pruned-tree appearance**[Q] on direct cholangiography).

- Histologic changes in the same liver can be **markedly varied** from **segment to segment**[Q] at any given time.

Clinical Features

- More common in **males**[Q], mean age at presentation is **40–45 years**[Q]
- About **75% of patients** are **symptomatic**[Q] at presentation with evidence of cholestatic liver disease such as **jaundice, pruritus**, and **fatigue**[Q].
- Symptoms of bacterial cholangitis are uncommon.
- Condition is characterized by **relapses & remissions**[Q], with quiescent periods.

Diagnosis

- **Asymptomatic elevation** of GGT is the **earliest finding**[Q], ALP and bile acids are also increased.
- **Normal ALP** does not always rule out diagnosis of **PSC**[Q].
- **Cholangiography confirms** the **diagnosis of PSC** with evidence of **diffuse multifocal strictures** found in both **intrahepatic & extrahepatic bile ducts**[Q].

> **ERCP Findings in PSC**
> - **ERCP** is the **gold standard**[Q] for diagnosis of PSC.
> - Typical cholangiographic findings of PSC: **Multifocal stricturing & beading**[Q] throughout the biliary tree
> - **Beaded** or **pruned tree appearance**[Q] is characteristic on cholangiography.
> - On ERCP **pseudodiverticula**[Q] (tiny diverticulum like outpouchings) of the extrahepatic bile ducts are **nearly pathognomonic** of **PSC**, seen in **one fourth** of the cases.
> - **Hepatic duct bifurcation** is the **most severely strictured**[Q] segment of biliary tree.

Treatment

- Medical therapy for PSC include **high dose UDCA**[Q] (25–30 mg/kg/day).
- **Recurrent biliary sepsis**: Managed with **antibiotics** & surveillance
- **Biliary strictures**: Dilated or stented using either the percutaneous or endoscopic route.
- **Liver transplantation** has produced **excellent results** in PSC and **end-stage liver disease**[Q]
- **Cholestyramine, Phenobarbital, Ursodeoxycholic acid**, Hydroxyzine, Rifampin and Naltrexone are the drugs approved for the **treatment of pruritus**[Q].

> - **Colectomy** has **no effect on the course of PSC**[Q].

> - **Smoking** is **protective** in: **PSC** and **UC**[Q]
> - **PBC** is more common in **females**[Q].
> - **PSC** and **Cholangiocarcinoma** is more common in **males**[Q].
> - **Colectomy** has **no effect** on the course of **PSC**[Q].

PRIMARY BILIARY CIRRHOSIS

Primary Biliary Cirrhosis

- Believed to be an **autoimmune etiology**, leading to **progressive destruction** of intrahepatic bile ducts[Q]
- More common in **females**[Q]
- Associated with autoimmune disorders (**CREST, Sicca syndrome, Autoimmune thyroiditis, Renal tubular acidosis**)[Q].

Pathology
- **Florid duct lesion** is characterized by **lymphocytic** or **granulomatous bile duct infiltration**[Q].
- In the setting of **positive AMA**, florid duct lesion is **essentially diagnostic**[Q].

Clinical Features
- Most patients are asymptomatic, pruritus is the **commonest & earliest symptom**[Q].
- Pruritus precedes jaundice in PBC[Q], Pruritus is **most bothersome in evening**[Q].
- Jaundice, fatigue, melanosis[Q] (gradual darkening of exposed areas of skin), deficiency of fat soluble vitamins due to malabsorption.
- Xanthomas & xanthelesmas[Q] due to protracted elevation of serum lipids.

Laboratory Findings
- Increased ALP, hyperlipidemia & positive antimitochondrial antibody[Q].

Diagnosis
- Diagnosis can be **made by AMA**[Q].
- IOC for diagnosis: Biopsy[Q]

Treatment
- **Cholestyramine** is **mainstay** of treatment of **pruritus**[Q].
- **Ursodeoxycholic acid** is associated with **significant delay** to time of transplantation[Q].
- Transplantation in PBC may also be indicated for **intolerable lethargy** or **intractable pruritus**[Q].

Prognosis
- **Serum bilirubin** is the **best guide** to **prognosis**[Q].

RECURRENT PYOGENIC CHOLANGITIS

RECURRENT PYOGENIC CHOLANGITIS

- **Cholangiohepatitis** or **intrahepatic stones** are endemic in **East Asia**[Q].
- **More common** in people with **poor economic status**[Q] and living standards.
- **Increases risk** for **cholangiocarcinoma**[Q]

Etiopathogenesis
- Infection is caused by **bacterial contamination**, usually **biliary pathogens**, and **biliary parasites**, such as **Clonorchis sinensis, Opisthorchis viverrini, and Ascaris lumbricoides**[Q].
- **Partial obstruction** of biliary tree caused by **biliary sludge** and **dead bacterial cell bodies, which** form **brown pigment stones**[Q]

Clinical Features
- Patients present with frequent episodes of pain, fever, and jaundice.
- **Biliary strictures** and **repeated episodes of cholangitis**[Q] are the common, may lead to liver abscesses and cirrhosis.
- **GB stones** are present in **<50% cases**[Q]

Diagnosis
- MRCP and PTC:
  - **Primary imaging modalities** for monitoring of **disease progression**[Q]
  - Identifying **location** and **severity** of stones and **strictures**[Q]
  - Allow decompression of the biliary tree in a septic patient.

Treatment
- Treated with a **multidisciplinary approach** (endoscopy, interventional radiology, and surgery)
- The long-term goal of therapy is to **extract stones, remove debris,** and **relieve strictures**.
- **Roux-en-Y hepaticojejunostomy**[Q] with a subcutaneous afferent limb (**Hudson loop**[Q]) is a safe and effective way to provide **access to the biliary tree** for **stone extractions**[Q].

RISK FACTORS FOR CHOLANGIOCARCINOMA

Risk Factors for Cholangiocarcinoma	
Choledochal cyst[Q]	RPC or hepatolithiasis[Q]
Primary sclerosing cholangitis[Q]	Biliary enteric anastomosis[Q]
Ulcerative colitis[u]	HBV, HIV, HCV[u]
Choledocholithiasis[Q]	Radon
Clonorchis sinensis & Opisthorchis viverrini[Q]	Asbestos, Nitrosamines, Dioxin (AND)[Q]
Cirrhosis[Q]	Diabetes, Obesity, OCPs, Smoking, Thorotrast, Isoniazid (DOSTI)[Q]

CHOLANGIOCARCINOMA

CHOLANGIOCARCINOMA

- Tumors arising from bile duct epithelium
- MC type is **adenocarcinoma**[Q]
- Differentiated by anatomic site of origin: **Intrahepatic** (10%), **hilar (65%)**[Q] and **distal** (25%).
- Hilar cholangiocarcinoma is also known as **Klatskin tumor**[Q]
- MC gene mutation: **K-ras >p16 (KRAP-16)**[Q]

Pathology

- Based on **macroscopic growth pattern** divided into:

Sclerosing	Nodular	Papillary
• MC type[Q] • Causes **intense desmoplastic reaction**[Q] • Seen as **diffuse thickening** of the **ducts** without a defined mass[Q]. • This form is **most difficult to treat**[Q].	• Result in **mass lesion**[Q] • Usually **intrahepatic**[Q]	• Rare • **Low grade** adenocarcinoma • Represented by **polypoidal mass filling the lumen of bile duct**[Q] • **Minimal invasion** and **no desmoplastic reaction**[Q]. • More common in **distal CBD**[Q] • Associated with **favorable outcome**[Q].

Clinical Features

- **Painless jaundice (70–90%)** is **MC symptom**[Q] of cholangiocarcinoma, followed by **pruritus** (66%), **abdominal pain**, **weight loss** (30–50%), **fever** (20%).
- **Distant metastasis** occurs in **one third**[Q] of patients.
- MC site of metastasis: **Lung** or **mediastinum**, liver and peritoneum.
- Tumor markers: **CA19-9**[Q], **CEA**, MUC1, MUC5AC, CK19, and CK7.
- Raised CA19-9 is a **poor prognostic factor**[Q] in cholangiocarcinoma.

Diagnosis

- MRI/MRCP is an **ideal imaging**[Q] modality for cholangiocarcinoma.
- **Duplex ultrasonography** and **MRCP** are the principal radiographic techniques used to image hilar cholangiocarcinoma.
- **MDCT** is the **first examination** in the pre-operative management of **hilar cholangiocarcinoma**[Q]

Radiological Features of Cholangiocarcinoma
• **Concentric stricturing**[Q], which sometimes appears **shouldered**, polypoid appearance is rare • Mucin producing cholangiocarcinoma can produce **strand-like filling defects**[Q] caused by mucin • Length of stricture is **at least 1 cm** • **Golf-tree appearance** is seen in **papillary cancer**[Q] involving extra-hepatic bile duct

Treatment

Perihilar cholangiocarcinoma	CBD resection + Lymphadenectomy + Hepatic resection[Q]
Intrahepatic cholangiocarcinoma	Hepatic resection[Q]
Distal cholangiocarcinoma	Pancreaticoduodenectomy (Whipple's procedure)[Q]

Prognosis

- Predictors of improved survival are: **well-differentiated** tumors; **negative-resection margin** and the performance of a **concomitant hepatic resection**[Q].
- **Pattern of failure after curative resection** includes peritoneal spread, hepatic metastasis, local extra-hepatic recurrence and distant metastasis (**most commonly lung**)[Q].
- **Surgery** is generally **not indicated** for **recurrent cholangiocarcinoma**[Q].

Palliation

- **Chemotherapy: Gemcitabine + Cisplatin**[Q] is the reference regimen

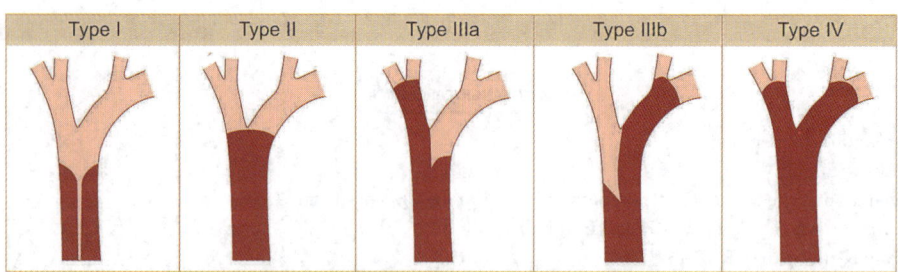

Bismuth-Corlette classification of tumor involvement.

Bismuth-Corlette Classification of Hilar Cholangiocarcinoma	
Type	Criteria
I	Tumor **confined to hepatic duct**, not involving the main biliary confluence[Q]
II	Tumor involving the **main biliary confluence** but not extending to the right or left ducts[Q]
IIIa	Tumor **extending upto** the **right secondary biliary confluence**[Q]
IIIb	Tumor extending upto the **left** secondary biliary confluence[Q]
IV	Tumor extending **bilaterally** to the secondary biliary confluence[Q]

CRITERIA OF UNRESECTABILITY IN HILAR CHOLANGIOCARCINOMA

- **Hepatic duct involvement** up to **secondary radicals bilaterally**[Q]
- **Encasement** or occlusion of the **main portal vein** proximal to its bifurcation[Q]
- **Atrophy** of one lobe with **encasement** of **contralateral portal vein** branch[Q]
- **Atrophy** of one lobe with **contralateral** involvement of **secondary biliary radicals**[Q]
- Histologically proven **metastasis to N2** lymph nodes[Q]
- **Liver, lung** or **peritoneal metastasis**
- In hilar cholangiocarcinoma, several **early branches of left hepatic duct drain the caudate lobe** and can be **involved early** with the tumor.
- Consideration for routine **caudate lobectomy** should be made in these cases.

PALLIATION IN CHOLANGIOCARCINOMA

Surgical Bypass
- Unresectable disease at the time of open exploration- **surgical biliary bypass** offers **more durable palliation**[Q]
- Segment 3 or 5 bypass is used in patients with **advanced perihilar cholangiocarcinoma** with predominantly **right**-or-**left sided** disease respectively[Q].
- **Segment III bypass** yield 1-year patency rate of 80% and it is usually **far from** the **main tumor** and remains **patent for a long time** despite disease progression[Q].

Stenting
- **Hilar obstructions** are best approached through the **percutaneous transhepatic route**[Q]
- **Distal CBD obstruction** is **stented** through endoscopy (ERCP[Q])
- 30% of the **hepatic parenchyma drained** and functional to alleviate jaundice and pruritus[Q]

Indications for Biliary Decompression in Inoperable Cholangiocarcinoma	
• Intractable pruritus	• The need of access for **intra-luminal radiotherapy**[Q]
• Cholangitis[Q]	• To allow **recovery of hepatic function** in patients receiving chemotherapeutic agents[Q]

HEMOBILIA

HEMOBILIA

- Bleeding into the biliary tract from an **abnormal arterial source** to **intrahepatic biliary tract** fistula
- Portal venous bleeding into the biliary tree is rare, minor, and self-limited
- **Arterial hemobilia** is the **MC source**[Q]

Etiology

- **Trauma:**
  - **Iatrogenic trauma (PTC)** is the **MC cause**^Q
  - **Blunt trauma** is more common cause than penetrating trauma
- Gallstones
- Vascular pathology: Aneurysm, angiodysplasia, hemangioma
- Uncommon causes: Malignancy, parasitic infestation, liver abscess, cholangitis

Clinical Features

- Characterized by **Quinck's triad (Sandblom's**^Q **triad)**: GI hemorrhage + biliary colic + jaundice^Q.
- **Presentation**: Melena (90%)^Q, hematemesis (60%), biliary colic (70%), and jaundice (60%).
- Tendency for **delayed presentations** (up to weeks) and **recurrent brisk** but **limited bleeding** over months and even years^Q.

Diagnosis

- **Endoscopy: First investigation**^Q to be done (visualize bleeding from the ampulla of Vater)
- **Angiography: Investigation of choice**^Q (reveal the source of bleeding in 90%)
- **Transarterial embolization** is curative in **major hemobilia**^Q

Treatment

- Treatment is focused on **stopping bleeding** and **relieving biliary obstruction**^Q.
- Most cases of **minor hemobilia** can be **managed conservatively**^Q with correction of coagulopathy, adequate biliary drainage and close observation.

> - **First line therapy** for **major hemobilia**: **Transarterial embolization (TAE)**^Q
> - **TAE** is **curative** in **major hemobilia** (success rates of 80-100%)^Q
> - **Surgery**: When **conservative therapy** and **TAE** have **failed**.

- **Surgical approaches**: Ligation of bleeding vessels, excision of aneurysm, or nonselective ligation of a main hepatic artery^Q.

BILHEMIA

BILHEMIA

- Bilhemia is an **extremely rare condition**
- Bile flows into the **bloodstream** either through the **hepatic veins** or **portal vein branches**^Q

Etiology

- **High intrabiliary pressure**, exceeding that of the venous system (**CBD stone**)^Q
- **Gallstones** eroding into the portal vein
- Accidental or iatrogenic **trauma**

Clinical Features

- **Rapidly increasing jaundice, marked direct hyperbilirubinemia** (without elevation of hepatocellular enzymes) and **septicemia**^Q.
- The condition **can be fatal** secondary to **embolization** of large amounts of **bile into** the **lungs**^Q.
- Most often, **bile flow is low**, and the **fistula spontaneously closes**^Q.

Diagnosis

- **ERCP** is investigation of choice (**diagnostic** and **therapeutic**)^Q

Treatment

- Treatment is directed at **lowering intrabiliary pressures** either through **stents** or **sphincterotomy**^Q

BILE DUCT: ANATOMY AND PHYSIOLOGY

BILE DUCT: ANATOMY AND PHYSIOLOGY

Anatomy

- It lies in front of the portal vein and to the **right of** the **hepatic artery**^Q.
- Common hepatic duct is **1–4 cm** in **length** and has a **diameter** of approx. **4 mm**^Q.
- CBD is about **7–11 cm** in length & **5–10 mm** in diameter^Q.
- A **fibroareolar tissue** containing **scant smooth muscle** surround the mucosa (a **distinct muscle layer** is **absent**)^Q.
- Most important **arteries** to the supraduodenal bile duct run parallel to the duct at the **3 & 9 o' clock**^Q positions.

- Approximately **60%** of the blood supply to the supraduodenal bile duct originates **inferiorly** from the **pancreaticoduodenal** and **retroduodenal arteries**^{Q}.
- Whereas **38%** of the blood supply originate **superiorly** from the **right hepatic artery** and **cystic duct artery**^{Q}.

- Epithelial surface of the duct is generally flat except for **tiny pits** in the mucosa known as **sacculi of Beale**^{Q}, which are luminal openings for the intramural mucous glands.

Physiology
- **Wall** of the CBD contain only **thin, longitudinally oriented** layers of **smooth muscle** of which major tissue component seems to be **elastic fibers**^{Q}.

  - The human **CBD** does **not have** a primary **propulsive function**, the **elastic fibers** and the **longitudinally oriented smooth muscle** provides a **tonic pressure** which help to overcome the tonic resistance of the sphincter of Oddi^Q.

- After the ingestion of a meal, bile flow across the sphincter of Oddi is promoted by inhibition or reduction in the amplitude of the phasic contraction and a decrease in the sphincter of Oddi basal pressure.
- Phasic contractions propel small volumes of bile into the duodenum but the **main function** is to **prevent reflux** of **duodenal contents** into either the **bile** or the **pancreatic ducts** and to maintain the ducts **free** of **small debris**^{Q}.

- **Ultrasound** measurement records the **nondistended lumen**, whereas at **ERCP**, contrast material produces **distension, intraoperative measurements** include **wall thickness**^{Q}.
- In general, the normal diameter of the common bile duct as determined by **ultrasound** is **<6 mm**, by **ERCP <10 mm**, and by **intraoperative** extraluminal measurements **<12 mm**^{Q}.

Vascular Supply of Biliary Tract

- **Supraduodenal** & **infrahilar bile ducts** are predominantly **supplied by two axial vessels** that run in a 3- and 9-o'clock position^Q.

  - These vessels are **derived from** the **superior pancreaticoduodenal, right hepatic, cystic, gastroduodenal, and retroduodenal arteries**^{Q}.

- It has been estimated that **only 2%** of the **arterial supply** to this portion of the bile duct is **segmental** and **arises directly** off of the **proper hepatic artery**.
- **Bile duct** and its **bifurcation** in the hilum **derive their arterial supply** from a rich network of **multiple small branches** from surrounding vessels.
- **Retropancreatic bile duct** derives its **arterial supply** from the **retroduodenal artery**.
- **Venous drainage** of the bile duct parallels the **arterial supply** and **drains into** the **portal venous system**.

  - **Venous drainage** of the **gallbladder** empties into the **veins** that **drain the bile duct** and **does not flow directly** to the **portal vein**^{Q}.

Multiple Choice Questions

CHOLEDOCHAL CYST

1. Choledochal cyst in intrahepatic biliary tree: *(AIIMS GIS Dec 2006)*
   a. I
   b. II
   c. IVa
   d. IVb

2. Caroli's disease is: *(AIIMS GIS Dec 2006)*
   a. Type I choledochal cyst
   b. Type III choledochal cyst
   c. Type IV choledochal cyst
   d. Type V choledochal cyst

3. According to to Alonso-Lej classification, type IVb is: *(JIPMER GIS 2011)*
   a. Both extra and intra-hepatic duct dilatation
   b. Extra-hepatic duct dilatation
   c. Intra-hepatic duct dilatation
   d. Sub-hepatic duct dilatation

4. True about Todani's modification of Alonso-Lej classification include the following except: *(MHSSMCET 2008)*
   a. Type I = saccular dilation of common bile duct
   b. Type II = diverticulum of supraduodenal bile duct
   c. Type IVa = choledochocele
   d. Type IVb = multiple saccular dilatations of extrahepatic ducts only

5. Most commonly seen choledochal cyst: *(PGI May 2011)*
   a. Type I
   b. Type II
   c. Type III
   d. Type IVa
   e. Type V

6. Saccular diverticulum of extrahepatic bile duct in choledochal cyst is classified as: *(COMEDK 2009)*
   a. Type I
   b. Type II
   c. Type III
   d. Type IV

7. Reconstructive surgery for choledochal cyst is not done in: *(MHSSMCET 2009)*
   a. Type I
   b. Type II
   c. Type III
   d. Type IV

8. Choledochal cyst: *(AIIMS GIS 2003)*
   a. Resection decreases the incidence of malignancy but risk persists
   b. 80% cases have stones
   c. Treated by Roux-en-Y cystojejunostomy
   d. Type IV is most common

9. Treatment of choice in choledochal cyst: *(AIIMS GIS 2003)*
   a. Roux-en-Y hepaticojejunostomy
   b. Cystojejunostomy
   c. Choledochoduodenostomy
   d. Choledochojejunostomy

10. A 10-year-female presents with pain in the right hypochondrium, fever, jaundice and a palpable mass in the right hypochondrium. The probable diagnosis is: *(COMEDK 2011)*
    a. Hepatitis
    b. Hepatoma
    c. Choledochal cyst
    d. Mucocele gallbladder

11. A 10 years old female presented with recurrent attacks of cholangitis. CECT was done, the diagnosis on the basis of CECT is: *(Recent Question 2017)*
    a. Type 1 choledochal cyst
    b. Type 3 choledochal cyst
    c. Type 4 choledochal cyst
    d. Type 5 choledochal cyst

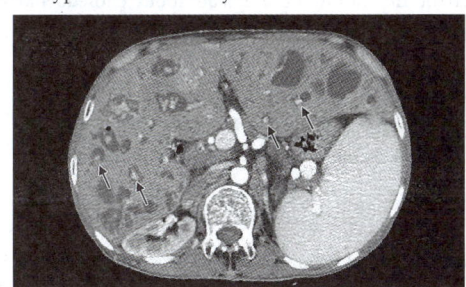

12. Central dot sign is seen in:
    (Recent Question 2016, AIIMS May 2011, Nov 2008, ILBS 2012)
    a. Primary sclerosing cholangitis
    b. Liver Hamartoma
    c. Caroli's disease
    d. Polycystic liver disease

13. True about choledochal cyst is: *(WBPG 2015, AIIMS Sep 96)*
    a. Always extrahepatic
    b. Treatment is cystojejunostomy
    c. Excision is ideal treatment
    d. Drainage is treatment of choice

14. Not true regarding choledochal cyst: *(AIIMS Nov 95)*
    a. Epigastric mass
    b. Jaundice
    c. Pain in abdomen
    d. Cystojejunostomy is treatment of choice

15. In case of choledochal cyst, bile diversion into the small intestine is not done because of the risk of:
    a. Malignancy
    b. Pancreatitis
    c. Recurrent cholangitis
    d. Gallstones

16. Clinical features of choledochal cyst in adult are:
    a. Pain, lump and intermittent jaundice *(UPSC 2004)*
    b. Pain, fever and intermittent jaundice
    c. Pain, lump and progressive jaundice
    d. Pain, fever and progressive jaundice

17. Choledochal cyst develops due to: *(DNB 2006)*
    a. Stenosis of sphincter
    b. Dysfunction of long circular fibre
    c. Congenital
    d. Iatrogenic

18. Choledochal cyst: *(DPG 2006)*
    a. Mostly presents in adulthood
    b. Excision is infrequently done
    c. Presents as slowly progressive jaundice
    d. Can lead to carcinoma

19. **Not true about choledochal cyst is:** *(AIIMS May 2009)*
    a. Associated with anomalous junction of the pancreatic and biliary duct
    b. Type II is most common
    c. Surgical removal is the treatment of choice
    d. If ruptures can cause biliary peritonitis

20. **Multiple intrahepatic bile duct dilation with bile lakes and concurrent sepsis is suggestive of:** *(MHSSMCET 2006)*
    a. Caroli's disease
    b. Watson Algali syndrome
    c. Primary sclerosing cholangitis
    d. Klatskin tumor

21. **All of the following are true about choledochal disease except:** *(Recent Question 2017)*
    a. Type IV is Caroli's disease
    b. Type I is most common
    c. Type III is also called choledochocele
    d. Type II is diverticular disease

22. **Choledochocele is which type of choledochal cyst?** *(Recent Question 2017)*
    a. II   b. III
    c. IV   d. V

23. **Both intra and extrahepatic choledochal cyst is seen in:** *(Recent Question 2017)*
    a. II   b. III
    c. IV   d. V

CHOLEDOCHOLITHIASIS AND CHOLANGITIS

24. **The procedure of choice for elective removal of CBD stones for most patients is:** *(COMEDK 2006)*
    a. Open choledocholithotomy
    b. Endoscopic papillotomy
    c. Laparoscopic choledocholithotomy
    d. Percutaneous choledocholithotomy

25. **The Reynold's pentad of fever, jaundice, right upper quadrant pain, septic shock and mental status change is typical of:** *(COMEDK 2008)*
    a. Cholangitis   b. Hepatitis
    c. Cholecystitis   d. Pancreatitis

26. **Association of choledocholithiasis in cholilithiasis:**
    a. < 5%   b. 15%   *(GB Pant 2011)*
    c. 20–35%   d. 50%

27. **All are true about CBD stones except:** *(AIIMS GIS 2003)*
    a. Associated with GB stones in 10% cases
    b. Primary stones are usually brown
    c. Laboratory values may be normal in one third cases of choledocholithiasis
    d. Retained stones are discovered after 2 years of cholecystectomy

28. **Which of the following calculi are rare in gallbladder, but common in common bile duct?** *(MHPGMCET 2008)*
    a. Cholesterol stone   b. Brown stone
    c. Black stone   d. None

29. **What is the treatment of choice for recurrent CBD stones with multiple strictures in common bile duct?**
    a. Hepaticojejunostomy
    b. Cutaneous hepaticojejunostomy
    c. Cholecystectomy
    d. ERCP and sphincterotomy

30. **Treatment of CBD stone includes:** *(PGI May 2010)*
    a. Endoscopic papillotomy   b. ERCP
    c. Ursodeoxycholic acid   d. Hepaticojejunostomy
    e. Choledochotomy

31. **Charcot's triad:** *(Recent Question 2014, JIPMER 2010, All India 96, 95)*
    a. Fever, abdominal pain, jaundice
    b. Fever, vomiting, jaundice
    c. Fever, jaundice, abdominal distension
    d. Fever, diarrhea, jaundice

32. **Sphincterotomy of sphincter of Oddi is performed at:** *(DNB 2006)*
    a. 3 O'clock position   b. 6 O'clock position
    c. 9 O'clock position   d. 11 O'clock position

33. **Most common cause of cholangitis:** *(AIIMS June 94)*
    a. Viral infection   b. CBD stone
    c. Surgery   d. Amebic infection

34. **A patient of post-cholecystectomy biliary stricture has undergone an ERCP three days ago. Following this, she has developed acute cholangitis. The most likely organism is:** *(All India 2006)*
    a. Escherichia coli   b. Bacillus fragilis
    c. Streptococcus viridians
    d. Pseudomonas aeruginosa

35. **Which of the following statements is true regarding cholangitis?** *(PGI Dec 2001)*
    a. Increased leucocyte count
    b. Increased transaminases
    c. Increased alkaline phosphatase
    d. Association with fever and chills

36. **Not a feature of CBD stone:** *(AIIMS June 98)*
    a. Pain   b. Fever
    c. Jaundice   d. Septic shock

37. **A 50-year-old woman presented with history of recurrent episodes of right upper abdominal pain for the last one year. She presented to casualty with history of jaundice and fever for 4 days. On examination, the patient appeared toxic and a blood pressure of 90/60 mmHg. She was started on intravenous antibiotics. Ultrasound of the abdomen showed presence of stones in the common bile duct. What would be the best treatment option for her?** *(AIIMS Nov 2003)*
    a. ERCP and bile duct stone extraction
    b. Laparoscopic cholecystectomy
    c. Open surgery and bile duct stone extraction
    d. Lithotripsy

38. **What is more appropriate for diagnosis of CBD stones?** *(PGI June 97)*
    a. Ultrasonography   b. ERCP
    c. OCG   d. IV cholangiography

39. **A patient having multiple gallstones and shows 8 mm dilation and 4 stones in CBD. Best treatment modalities are:**
    a. Cholecystectomy with choledocholithotomy at same setting   *(PGI Dec 2002)*
    b. ESWL
    c. Cholecystectomy and wait for ERCP
    d. Sphincterotomy and then cholecystectomy
    e. Cholecystectomy and after 14 days sphincterotomy done

40. **Best treatment modality for common bile duct stone is:**
    a. Endoscopic sphincterotomy   *(AIIMS Nov 94)*
    b. Observation
    c. Chenodeoxycholic acid
    d. Percutaneous removal

41. The treatment of choice for an 8 mm retained common bile duct (CBD) stone is: *(DNB 2011, AIIMS May 2005, Nov 2003)*
    a. Laparoscopic CBD exploration
    b. Percutaneous stone extraction
    c. Endoscopic stone extraction
    d. Extracorporeal shock wave lithotripsy

42. A patient presented 1 year after cholecystectomy with a CBD stone of 2.5 cm in size. Treatment of choice is:
    (KGMC 2011, AIIMS Nov 97, All India 99)
    a. Supraduodenal choledochotomy with exploration
    b. Transduodenal choledochojejunostomy
    c. Transduodenal sphincterotomy
    d. Endoscopic sphincterotomy with stone extraction

43. Which one of the following statement is incorrect regarding stone in the common bile duct? *(All India 2006)*
    a. Can present with Charcot's triad
    b. Are suggested by a bile duct diameter >6 mm of ultrasound
    c. ERCP, sphincterotomy and balloon clearance is now the standard treatment.
    d. When removed by exploration of the common bile duct the T-tube can be removed after 3 days

44. Treatment for common bile duct stone is by: *(PGI Dec 2001)*
    a. ESWL
    b. Exploration of bile duct and recovery of stones
    c. Bile duct stenting
    d. Nasobiliary drainage
    e. Percutaneous drainage

45. Absolute indication for choledochotomy: *(PGI June 2006)*
    a. Gallstone ileus   b. Gallstone pancreatitis
    c. Fever   d. Jaundice
    e. Palpable CBD stone

46. Ramu presents with recurrent attacks of cholelithiasis, USG examination shows a dilated CBD of 1 cm. The next line of management is: *(AIIMS June 2001)*
    a. ERCP
    b. PTC
    c. Cholecystostomy
    d. Intravenous cholangiogram

47. Most common surgical cause of obstructive jaundice:
    (AIIMS Nov 94, AIIMS Nov 96, All India 98, 2000)
    a. Periampullary carcinoma
    b. Carcinoma gallbladder
    c. Carcinoma head of pancreas
    d. CBD stones

48. What is more appropriate for diagnosis of CBD stones?
    a. Ultrasonography   b. ERCP   *(PGI 97)*
    c. OCG   d. IV cholangiography

49. In cholangiography CBD stone appears as:
    a. Meniscus sign   *(AIIMS June 98)*
    b. Cut off sign
    c. Slight flow of dye from the sides
    d. Ability to absorb water

50. Common bile duct stones will manifest all except:
    (MCI March 2008, All India 89)
    a. Distended gallbladder   b. Jaundice
    c. Itching   d. Clay colored stools

51. In cholangitis, the organism mostly responsible is:
    (Recent Questions 2016)
    a. E. coli   b. Streptococcus
    c. E. histolytica   d. Clostridium

52. An ultrasound examination shows dilated intrahepatic biliary channels with a small gallbladder. The most likely possibility is: *(DPG 2010, Karnataka 94)*
    a. Gallbladder stone
    b. Pancreatic calculus
    c. Common bile duct stone
    d. Carcinoma of the head of the pancreas

53. The most common cause of suppurative cholangitis is:
    a. Stone in common bile duct   *(UPPG 97)*
    b. Cancer of the ampulla of vater
    c. Choledochal cyst
    d. Empyema of gallbladder

54. The procedure of choice for elective removal of CBD stones for most patients is: *(Karnataka 2006)*
    a. Open choledocholithotomy
    b. Endoscopic choledocholithotomy
    c. Laparoscopic choledocholithotomy
    d. Percutaneous choledocholithotomy

55. Which of the following is not a component of Reynolds' Pentad in toxic cholangitis? *(DPG 2009 March)*
    a. Right upper quadrant pain
    b. Confusion
    c. Septic shock
    d. Markedly elevated transaminases

56. Best treatment of acute suppurative cholangitis is:
    a. Laparoscopic cholecystectomy   *(DPG 2006)*
    b. Open cholecystectomy
    c. Endoscopic papillotomy
    d. Choledochotomy

57. Leucine aminopeptidase is elevated in obstruction of:
    a. Ureter
    b. Urethra   *(BHU 88)*
    c. Common bile duct
    d. Spermatic cord

58. All of the following are seen with bile duct stone except:
    a. Obstructive jaundice   *(MCI March 2008)*
    b. Distended and palpable gallbladder
    c. Pruritus
    d. Clay colored stools

59. Management of stone in CBD includes following except:
    a. Observation   *(PGI Nov 2011)*
    b. Laparoscopic CBD exploration
    c. Medical dissolution of stone
    d. Endosphincteric removal

CHOLEDOCHOTOMY AND CBD EXPLORATION

60. A surgeon with less experience of laparoscopic cholecystectomy while doing laparoscopic surgery found some stone in CBD. What should he ideally do?
    (AIIMS Nov 2011, AIIMS GIS Dec 2010)
    a. Open cholecystectomy with choledochoduodeno-stomy
    b. Lap CBD exploration and stone removal
    c. Lap CBD exteraction through the cystic duct
    d. Convert to open cholecystectomy and CBD stone removal

61. Choledochotomy is indicated in all of the following except in patients with: *(COMEDK 2010)*
    a. Palpable CBD stones
    b. History of jaundice or cholangitis
    c. Abnormal alkaline phosphatase
    d. Abnormal gamma glutamyl transferase

212 Surgery Essence

62. Best suture for common bile duct is: *(JIPMER 95)*
   a. Synthetic absorbable
   b. Synthetic non-absorbable
   c. Non-synthetic absorbable
   d. Non-synthetic non-absorbable

63. After exploration of common bile duct, the T-tube is removed on which of the following days? *(Karnataka 96)*
   a. 3rd postoperative day   b. 4th postoperative day
   c. 12th postoperative day   d. 6th postoperative day

64. What is the name of this investigation?

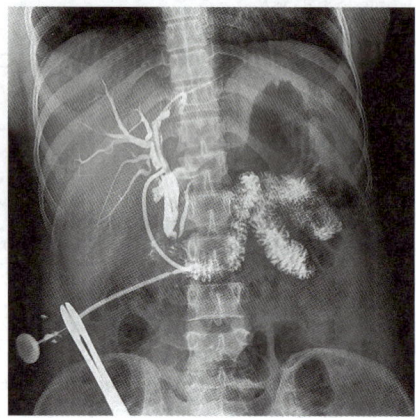

   a. ERCP   b. MRCP
   c. T-tube cholangiogram   d. PTC

65. Cholangiography via T-tube done after how many days of cholecystectomy: *(TN 99)*
   a. 1–5 days   b. 5–9 days
   c. 10–14 days   d. 15–20 days

66. After cholecystectomy a 2.5 cm calculus was found in CBD, treatment for this should be: *(MHSSMCET 2006)*
   a. Supraduodenal choledochotomy
   b. Transduodenal choledochotomy
   c. Dormia basket removal
   d. Choledochotomy and T tube

67. A retained stone impacted in distal common bile duct is seen on T- tube cholangiogram. What is the best management of stone? *(UPSC 2004)*
   a. Dissolution therapy
   b. Operative removal
   c. Endoscopic sphincterotomy and stone extraction
   d. No active treatment is required

68. Most common complication of common bile duct exploration: *(DPG 2008)*
   a. Retained stone
   b. Pancreatitis
   c. Stricture of common bile duct
   d. T-tube displacement

69. Endoscopic sphincterotomy is not successful in the following except: *(MHSSMCET 2008)*
   a. Multiple duodenal diverticuli
   b. Choledocholithiasis
   c. Billroth type II Gastrostomy
   d. None

70. ERCP failure occurs in following except: *(MHSSMCET 2008)*
   a. Smaller stone in CHD   b. Stenosis of papilla
   c. High stricture   d. Malignant obstruction

BILE DUCT INJURY AND BILIARY STRICTURES

71. All are true about bile duct injury except: *(AIIMS GIS 2003)*
   a. Incidence is equal in laparoscopic and open cholecystectomy
   b. After experience of 20 cases, bile duct injury rate decreases
   c. Errors leading to laparoscopic bile duct injuries stem from misperception, not errors of skill, knowledge or judgment
   d. Primary cause of error in most of the cases is visual perceptual illusion

72. False about CBD injury: *(AIIMS GIS May 2008)*
   a. Incidence in open cholecystectomy is 0.1-0.2%
   b. Incidence in laparoscopic cholecystectomy is 0.5-0.8%
   c. After 20 cases of laparoscopic cholecystectomy incidence of bile duct injury decreases
   d. Most common reason for bile duct injury is lack of techniques and errors of judgment

73. Biliary stricture developing after laparoscopic cholecystectomy usually occurs at which part of common bile duct? *(Punjab 2008, All India 2006)*
   a. Upper   b. Middle
   c. Lower   d. All with equal frequency

74. According to Strasberg classification, lateral CBD injuries are classified as: *(JIPMER GIS 2011)*
   a. Type B   b. Type C
   c. Type D   d. Type E

75. According to Bismuth Strasberg classification of bile duct injury, causing occlusion of a branch of biliary tree would be which type? *(MHSSMCET 2010)*
   a. Type A   b. Type B
   c. Type C   d. Type D

76. Strasburg's class 'B' bile injury means: *(MHSSMCET 2010)*
   a. Bile leak from a minor duct
   b. Occlusion of a branch of biliary tree
   c. Injury of bile duct not in communication with CBD
   d. Circumferential injury to major bile ducts

77. In Strasberg Classification of bile duct injury, type C is: *(MHSSMCET 2008)*
   a. Bile leak form a minor duct still in continuity with CBD
   b. Injury form bile duct not in communication with CBD
   c. Sectoral duct injury with consequent leak
   d. Circumferential injury to major bile ducts

78. Bile duct strictures are seen in: *(PGI Dec 2008)*
   a. CBD stone   b. Cholangiocarcinoma
   c. Chronic pancreatitis   d. Trauma
   e. Acute pancreatitis

79. A 40-year-old patient has undergone an open cholecystectomy. The procedure was reported as uneventful by the operating surgeon. She has 100 ml of bile output from the drain kept in the gallbladder bed on the first post operative day. On examination she is afebrile and anicteric. The abdomen is soft and bowel sounds are normally heard. As an attending physician, what should be your best possible advice: *(AIIMS Nov 2003)*
   a. Order an urgent endoscopic retrograde cholangiography and biliary stenting
   b. Urgent laparotomy
   c. Order an urgent hepatic imino diacetic acid scintigraphy (HIDA)
   d. Clinical observation

80. On 7th postoperative day after laparoscopic cholecystectomy, patient developed right upper abdominal pain and 10 cm × 8 cm collection. Treatment consists of: *(PGI Dec 2003)*
    a. Immediate laparotomy
    b. Percutaneous drainage
    c. Laparotomy and surgical exploration of bile duct and T-tube insertion
    d. Laparoscopic cystic duct ligation and percutaneous drainage
    e. Roux-en-Y loop hepaticojejunostomy

81. On 5th postoperative day after laparoscopic cholecystectomy, a 50-year-old lady presented with right upper quadrant pain with fever and 12 cm subhepatic collection on CT and ERCP shows cystic duct leak. The best management is:
    a. Immediate laparotomy *(PGI June 2003)*
    b. Percutaneous drainage of fluid
    c. Laparotomy and surgical exploration of bile duct and T-tube insertion
    d. Laparoscopic cystic duct ligation and percutaneous drainage
    e. Roux-en-Y loop hepaticojejunostomy

82. 5 days after CBD surgery there is a small leak. What will be the best treatment? *(AIIMS June 98)*
    a. Ultrasound guided aspiration
    b. ERCP and stenting
    c. Re-exploration and hepaticojejunostomy
    d. Re-exploration and primary repair

83. The initial investigation of choice for a post cholecystectomy biliary stricture is: *(AIIMS May 2005)*
    a. Ultrasound scan of the abdomen
    b. Endoscopic cholangiography
    c. Computed tomography
    d. Magnetic resonance cholangiography

84. Regarding bile duct injuries following cholecystectomy which of the following statement is false? *(AIIMS Nov 2005)*
    a. The incidences following open cholecystectomy is in the range of 0.2 to 0.3%
    b. The incidence rate following laparoscopic cholecystectomy is three times higher than the rates following open cholecystectomy
    c. Untreated cases may develop secondary biliary cirrhosis
    d. Routine use of 'open' technique of laparoscopic port insertion has resulted in a decline in the incidence of post laparoscopic cholecystectomy bile duct injuries

85. Common bile duct injuries are most commonly seen in:
    a. Radical gastrectomy *(UPSC 2008)*
    b. Penetrating injuries of abdomen
    c. ERCP and sphincterotomy
    d. Laparoscopic cholecystectomy operation

86. Most common cause of biliary stricture is: *(AIIMS June 94)*
    a. CBD stone   b. Trauma
    c. Asiatic cholangitis   d. Congenital

BILIARY FISTULA

87. Most common cause of gallbladder fistula is: *(DPG 2008)*
    a. Liver abscess aspiration   b. Laparoscopic surgery
    c. Gallstones   d. Trauma

88. Which does not contribute to enterobiliary fistula? *(Punjab 2008)*
    a. Gastric ulcer   b. Duodenal ulcer
    c. Carcinoma gallbladder d. Gallstones

SPHINCTER OF ODDI DYSKINESIA

89. The ideal treatment of stenosis of sphincter of Oddi is:
    a. Transduodenal sphincteroplasty *(SGPGI 2004)*
    b. Endoscopic sphincteroplasty
    c. Choledochojejunostomy
    d. Choledochoduodenostomy

90. Milwakukee classification is used for: *(Recent Question 2016)*
    a. Sphincter of Oddi dysfunction
    b. Abnormal pancreaticobiliary duct junction
    c. Acute pancreatitis
    d. Chronic pancreatitis

BILIARY TRACT DISEASES

91. Vanishing bile duct syndrome is seen in: *(PGI June 2003)*
    a. Chronic viral hepatitis
    b. Sarcoidosis
    c. Lymphoma
    d. Non-cirrhotic portal fibrosis
    e. Alcoholism

92. Bile ductopenia seen in: *(PGI Dec 2003)*
    a. GVHD   b. Alcoholic hepatitis
    c. Autoimmune hepatitis d. Cirrhosis
    e. Sclerosing cholangitis

BILIARY ATRESIA

93. Which of the following are histopathological features of Extra hepatic biliary atresia? *(PGI June 2001)*
    a. Bile lakes
    b. Hepatocyte ballooning degeneration
    c. Marked bile duct degeneration
    d. Fibrosis of hepatic duct
    e. Parenchymal cholestasis

94. The gold standard for the definitive diagnosis of the extrahepatic biliary atresia is:
    (Recent Question 2016, AIIMS, Nov 2002)
    a. Per-operative cholangiography
    b. Hepatobiliary scintigraphy
    c. Alkaline phosphatase level
    d. Liver biopsy

95. Better prognostic factor for operation of biliary duct obstruction in newborn are: *(PGI June 2001)*
    a. No passage of bile
    b. Size of ductule >200 micron
    c. Weight of baby >3 kg
    d. Preterm baby
    e. Age of 8 weeks

96. Kasai's procedure is the treatment of choice for:
    (Recent Question 2017, Recent Question 2013, Orissa 2011)
    a. Congenital hypertrophic pyloric stenosis
    b. Duodenal atresia
    c. Biliary atresia
    d. Hirschprung's disease

PRIMARY SCLEROSING CHOLANGITIS

97. Association of PSC with all except: *(ILBS 2012)*
    a. UC   b. ITP
    c. Sarcoidosis d. Retroperitoneal fibrosis

Surgery Essence

98. **False about PSC:** *(AIIMS GIS May 2008)*
    a. PSC in UC, the association is 30%
    b. Low incidence of cholangitis
    c. Increased incidence of colonic carcinoma in PSC + UC
    d. Despite the presence of diffuse disease, hepatic duct bifurcation is most severely strictured segment

99. **A 50-year-old male presents with pain upper abdomen, pruritus, jaundice and weight loss, elevated ANA, the likely diagnosis is:** *(COMEDK 2011)*
    a. Primary sclerosing cholangitis
    b. Klatskin tumor
    c. Secondary sclerosing cholangitis
    d. Choledocholithiasis

100. **A 45 years old male presented with recurrent attacks of cholangitis. MRCP and ERCP findings are given below. What is the most probable diagnosis?**

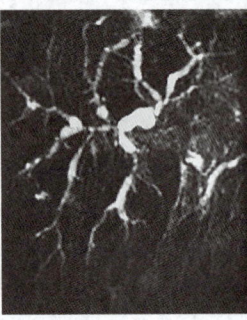 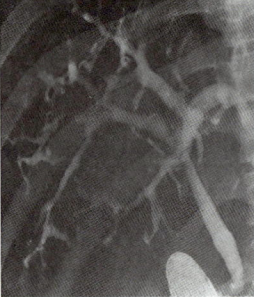

    a. Primary biliary cirrhosis
    b. Primary sclerosing cholangitis
    c. Oriental cholangiohepatitis
    d. Caroli's disease

101. **Primary sclerosing cholangitis is likely to be associated with:** *(JIPMER 2012, 2011)*
    a. Adenocarcinoma of pancreas
    b. Cholangiocarcinoma
    c. Hepatocellular carcinoma
    d. Adenocarcinoma of gallbladder

102. **"Onion skin" fibrosis of bile duct is seen in:**
    a. Primary biliary cirrhosis *(COMEDK 2009)*
    b. Primary sclerosing cholangitis
    c. Extrahepatic biliary fibrosis
    d. Congenital hepatic fibrosis

103. **Regarding PSC, all are true except:** *(AIIMS GIS Dec 2010)*
    a. Cholangiocarcinoma is always intrahepatic
    b. Management of PSC/UC does not alter the course of either disease
    c. Patients with PSC or UC have pancolitis on majority
    d. Patients with PSC or UC have more chances of CRC than UC alone

104. **All are true about PSC except:** *(AIIMS GIS May 2011)*
    a. Commonly affect 40-45 years of age
    b. More common in males
    c. Most patients presents with advanced disease
    d. Survival after diagnosis is 10–15 years

105. **True about primary sclerosing cholangitis are all except:**
    a. Fibrosing cholestasis of bile duct *(PGI June 2005)*
    b. Periductal onion skin fibrosis
    c. Cirrhosis never occurs
    d. Jaundice is seen
    e. Associated with UC

106. **All of the following are true for patients of ulcerative colitis associated with primary sclerosing cholangitis, except:**
    a. They may develop biliary cirrhosis *(All India 2005)*
    b. May have raised alkaline phosphatase
    c. Increased risk of hilar cholangiocarcinoma
    d. PSC reverts after a total colectomy

107. **A patient presenting with history of diarrhea for several years with recent onset pruritus and raised alkaline phosphatase, normal SGOT/PT and USG shows no gallstones and biliary tract abnormality, the diagnosis is:** *(PGI June 2004)*
    a. Hodgkin's Lymphoma b. Sclerosing cholangitis
    c. Autoimmune Hepatitis d. Viral Hepatitis

108. **True regarding primary sclerosing cholangitis associated with ulcerative colitis are all of the following except:** *(MCI March 2007)*
    a. Biliary cirrhosis is a known complication
    b. Increased risk of hilar cholangiocarcinoma
    c. May have raised levels of alkaline phoshphatase
    d. Primary sclerosing cholangitis resolves after total colectomy

PRIMARY BILIARY CIRRHOSIS

109. **Pruritus precedes jaundice in:** *(ILBS 2011)*
    a. Primary biliary cirrhosis
    b. Secondary biliary cirrhosis
    c. Primary sclerosing cholangitis
    d. CBD stone

110. **The earliest symptom in primary biliary cirrhosis is:** *(COMEDK 2008, 2007)*
    a. Jaundice b. Pruritus
    c. Melanosis d. Vomiting

111. **Two most important clinical features of primary biliary cirrhosis:** *(PGI June 2003)*
    a. Generalized pruritus b. Jaundice
    c. Fatigue d. Clubbing
    e. Hematemesis

112. **Which is not true about PBC?** *(APPG 2008)*
    a. No increase in risk of hepatocellular carcinoma
    b. Often asymptomatic
    c. Elevated IgM
    d. Positive anti-mitochondrial antibody

113. **Commonest presentation of primary biliary cirrhosis:**
    a. Pruritus b. Pain *(All India 98)*
    c. Jaundice d. Fever

RECURRENT PYOGENIC CHOLANGITIS

114. **All of the following are true regarding RPC except:**
    a. Equal incidence in males and females
    b. More common in left lobe of liver
    c. All are pigmented stones *(AIIMS GIS Dec 2010)*
    d. GB stones are present in >50% cases

CHOLANGIOCARCINOMA PREDISPOSING FACTORS

115. **Which of the following is not a risk factor for cholangiocarcinoma?** *(AIIMS GIS Dec 2011)*
    a. Thorotrast b. Radon
    c. Dioxin d. Aflatoxin

116. **Not a predisposing factor for cholangiocarcinoma:**
    a. Asiatic cholangio-hepatitis *(Punjab 2007)*
    b. Cholelithiasis
    c. Ulcerative colitis
    d. Choledochal cyst

117. APBDJ is associated with: *(AIIMS GIS 2003)*
    a. Cholangiocarcinoma   b. CA GB
    c. Choledochal cyst   d. All of the above

118. Predisposing factor for cholangiocarcinoma: *(MHSSMCET 2009)*
    a. PSC   b. Gallstones
    c. Ankylostomiasis   d. All of the above

119. Cholangiocarcinoma has been associated with infection by: *(Recent Question 2016, 2015, COMEDK 2004)*
    a. Paragonimus westermani   b. Clonorchis sinensis
    c. Loa Loa   d. Schistosoma haematobium

120. Which of the following does not predispose to cholangiocarcinoma? *(All India 96, AIIMS Feb 97)*
    a. Ulcerative colitis   b. Clonorchis sinensis
    c. Choledochal cyst   d. Chronic pancreatitis

121. All of the following are known predisposing factors for cholangiocarcinoma except:
    a. CBD stones   *(Recnet Question 2016, All India 97)*
    b. Clonorchis sinensis
    c. Ulcerative colitis
    d. Primary sclerosing cholangitis

122. All the following increase risk for cholangiocarcinoma except: *(DPG 2010)*
    a. Ulcerative colitis   b. Gallstones in CBD
    c. Sclerosing cholangitis   d. Clonorchis

CHOLANGIOCARCINOMA

123. Non-resectability criteria in hilar cholangiocarcinoma are all except: *(ILBS 2012)*
    a. Involvement of secondary biliary radicals bilaterally
    b. Metastasis to celiac nodes
    c. Involvement of right branch of portal vein
    d. Contralateral involvement of bile duct

124. Type II cholangiocarcinoma involve: *(DNB 2011)*
    a. Division of both ducts and not extending outside
    b. Common hepatic duct only
    c. Secondary hepatic duct
    d. Extending beyond hilum

125. All are true about prognosis of cholangiocarcinoma except: *(AIIMS GIS 2003)*
    a. Scirrhous type has better prognosis than papillary
    b. Major prognostic factors are margin status and tumor stage
    c. Bile duct resection alone is associated with high chances of recurrence
    d. Curative resection includes hepatic resection + bile duct resection + lymphadenectomy

126. Klatskin tumor is: *(JIPMER 2010)*
    a. Merkel cell carcinoma of skin
    b. Primitive neuroectodermal tumor of chest wall
    c. Common hepatic duct tumor
    d. Adenocarcinoma of anal canal

127. Most common site of cholangiocarcinoma: *(AIIMS Nov 2011, May 2011, Nov 2008)*
    a. Distal biliary duct   b. Hilum
    c. Intrahepatic duct   d. Multifocal

128. True regarding cholangiocarcinoma: *(PGI SS Dec 2010)*
    a. Sclerosing variety is most common
    b. Multifocal in 40%
    c. Jaundice typically precedes pruritus
    d. Adjuvant therapy improves survival

129. Cholangiocarcinoma histologically resembles:
    a. Squamous cell type   b. Colloid cell type
    c. Schirrhous type   d. Columnar cell type

130. All are criteria of non-resectability in patients with hilar cholangiocarcinoma except: *(JIPMER GIS 2011)*
    a. Hepatic duct involvement upto secondary radicals bilaterally
    b. Encasement or occlusion of main portal vein proximal to its bifurcation
    c. Atrophy of one lobe with encasement of contralateral portal vein branch
    d. Atrophy of one lobe with ipsilateral involvement of secondary biliary radicals

131. Contraindication of resection in cholangiocarcinoma are all except: *(ILBS 2011)*
    a. Involvement of main trunk of portal vein
    b. Hepatic atrophy with contralateral bile duct encasement
    c. Hepatic atrophy with contralateral portal vein encasement
    d. Hepatic atrophy with ipsilateral bile duct involvement

132. ERCP is indicated for the following except:
    a. Distal CBD tumor   *(Recent Question 2013)*
    b. Hepatic porta tumor
    c. Proximal cholangiocarcinoma
    d. Gallstone pancreatitis

133. According to Bismuth classification, type IV cholangiocarcinoma involves: *(Recent Question 2015)*
    a. Common hepatic duct
    b. Bifurcation only
    c. Bifurcation and bilateral secondary intrahepatic ducts
    d. Bifurcation and unilateral secondary intrahepatic ducts

134. Most common site of metastasis in cholangiocarcinoma: *(Recent Question 2016)*
    a. Liver   b. Bones
    c. Lung   d. Pancreas

135. A 60-year-old male Shambhu presented with painless progressive jaundice. On examination, gallbladder was palpable. MRCP image is given. On the basis of findings of MRCP, most probable diagnosis is:
    a. Hilar cholangiocarcinoma
    b. Distal cholangiocarcinoma
    c. Carcinoma gallbladder
    d. Carcinoma pancreas

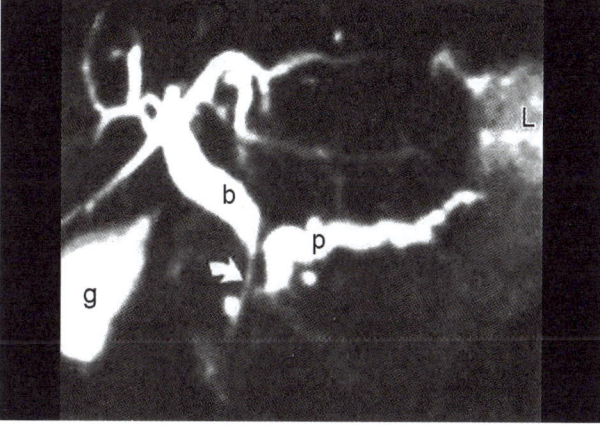

HEMOBILIA

136. Most common cause of hemobilia:
(DNB 2005, 2000, AIIMS GIS 2003)
a. Trauma
b. Iatrogenic
c. Parasites
d. Tumors

137. Not true of hemobilia:
(DNB 2010, Punjab 2009, COMEDK 2007)
a. GI bleeding
b. Fever
c. Jaundice
d. Colicky RUQ pain

138. A patient presents with abdominal pain, jaundice and melena. The diagnosis is: *(All India 2000)*
a. Hemobilia
b. Acute cholangitis
c. Carcinoma gallbladder
d. Acute pancreatitis

139. Cause of hemobilia are all except: *(AIIMS June 2000)*
a. Trauma to abdomen
b. Malignancy
c. Rupture of hepatic artery aneurysm
d. Hepatitis

140. True regarding hemobilia: *(DPG 2007)*
a. Triad of jaundice, pain, melena
b. MC cause- rupture of portal vein into biliary system
c. MR angiography is the IOC
d. None of the above

BILHEMIA

141. Best investigation for bilhemia is: *(JIPMER GIS 2011)*
a. ERCP
b. MRCP
c. CT
d. EUS

142. All are true about bilhemia except: *(AIIMS GIS May 2008)*
a. Biliary pressure > portal pressure
b. Diagnosed by ERCP
c. Death due to embolism of bile in lungs
d. Patient has hyperbilirubinemia with raised enzymes

MISCELLANEOUS

143. False statement about common bile duct: *(PGI May 2011)*
a. Lies in free margin of lesser omentum
b. Anterior to first part of duodenum
c. Right to hepatic artery
d. Anterior to portal vein
e. Open in second part of duodenum

144. True regarding common bile duct is all except:
a. Opens 10 cm distal to the pylorus *(All India 2000)*
b. Lies anterior to IVC
c. Portal vein lies posterior to it
d. Usually opens into duodenum separate from the main pancreatic duct

145. Which of the following statements is true regarding the relation of bile duct? *(PGI Dec 2005)*
a. Posteriorly related to 1st part of duodenum
b. Related posteriorly to the tunnel of pancreatic head
c. Anteriorly related to 1st part of duodenum
d. Related to IVC posteriorly
e. It lies left to hepatic artery in the free border of lesser omentum

146. Predominant blood supply to the supraduodenal bile duct is derived from: *(All India 2012)*
a. Vessels that run upward along the bile duct from the duodenal end of the duct such as the retroduodenal and gastroduodenal arteries
b. Vessels that run downward along the bile duct from the hepatic end of the duct such as the right hepatic artery
c. Vessels that arise from the hepatic artery proper run up along the CBD and supplies it with twigs in non-axial distribution
d. Vessels that arise from the cystic artery

147. All of the following conditions are associated with pneumobilia except:
a. Sphincterotomy
b. Rupture of hydatid cyst
c. Mirizzi's syndrome
d. Gallstone ileus

148. Pneumobilia is seen in: *(DNB 2001)*
a. Gallstone ileus
b. Mirizzi's syndrome
c. TPN
d. Volvulus

149. Normal length of CBD is: *(DNB 2001)*
a. 7 cm
b. 5 cm
c. 3 cm
d. 2 cm

150. Which of the following is true regarding the principle of use of MRCP? *(AIIMS Nov 2012)*
a. Intraluminal dye is used to create the three dimension view of the structures
b. Dye is instilled percutaneously first then MRI is used
c. Use of heavily T2-weighted image without contrast to create the three dimensional image of the biliary tree using MIP algorithm
d. Use of systemic Gadolinium as a contrast agent to create the three dimensional image of the biliary tree

151. Best method to visualize the proximal bile duct is by: *(JIPMER November 2017)*
a. Percutaneous transhepatic cholangiogram
b. EsUS
c. ERCP
d. Transabdominal USG

Explanations

CHOLEDOCHAL CYST

1. **Ans. c. IVa** *(Ref: Sabiston 20/e p1510-1511; Schwartz 10/e p1630; Bailey 27/e p1198; Blumgart 6/e p753, 5/e p707-719; Shackelford 8/e p1368, 7/e p1397-1403)*
2. **Ans. d. Type V choledochal cyst** *(Ref: Sabiston 20/e p 1511; Schwartz 10/e p1289, 1630; Bailey 27/e p1197; Blumgart 6/e p762, 5/e p717; Shackelford 8/e p1374, 7/e p1402-1403)*

> ### CAROLI'S DISEASE (TYPE V CHOLEDOCHAL CYST)
>
> - Congenital malformation, consists of multiple **sacular dilatations** limited to the **intrahepatic**^{Q} bile ducts (segmental bile ducts).
> - **About half** the cases are **associated with congenital hepatic fibrosis**^{Q} (affect **interlobular** bile ducts).
> - Cyst with congenital hepatic fibrosis is known as **Grumbach's disease**^{Q}.
> - **Portal hypertension** is present in Caroli's disease associated **with congenital hepatic fibrosis**^{Q}.
>
> **Clinical Features**
> - Symptoms include **cholangitis (64%)**^{Q}, portal hypertension (22%), and abdominal pain (18%)
> - More common in **male**s
> - Septa containing portal veins protrude into the lumen of the ectatic bile ducts (**central dot sign**)^Q.
> - The main and often the only symptom of **bacterial cholangitis** secondary to **Caroli's** disease is **fever without abdominal pain** and **jaundice**.
> - Frequent episodes of **cholangitis** indicates **poor prognosis**^{Q}.
> - Most **stones** are **pigmented** in Caroli's disease.
>
> **Diagnosis**
> - CT findings: Portal vein radicals can be seen after enhancement within dilated intra-hepatic bile ducts (**central dot sign**)^Q.
>
> **Treatment**
> - **Hepatic resection** for **localized disease**^{Q}.
> - **Liver transplantation** for **diffuse disease**^{Q}.

3. **Ans. b. Extra hepatic-duct dilatation**
4. **Ans. c. Type IVa = choledochocele**
5. **Ans. a. Type I**
6. **Ans. b. Type II**
7. **Ans. c. Type III**
8. **Ans. a. Resection decreases the incidence of malignancy but risk persists** *(Ref: Sabiston 20/e p1511; Bailey 27/e p1197; Blumgart 6/e p758, 5/e p713; Shackelford 7/e p1399)*

> ### CARCINOMA IN CHOLEDOCHAL CYST
>
> - **More than half** tumors occur within the cyst itself (**intracystic**) and **may recur after cyst excision**^{Q}.
> - **Risk** of **malignancy** is **decreased** after **cyst excision**, but **risk persist** even **after cyst excision** (**life long surveillance** is required)
> - Type **I** and **IV** cysts have the **highest risk of cancer**.
> - When malignancy is present it is most commonly found along the **posterior cyst wall**^{Q}.
> - Incidence of **cyst malignancy** is **age related**^{Q}.
>
> | Increased risk of following cancers | | | | |
> |---|---|---|---|---|
> | Biliary tree (MC)^Q | Pancreas^Q | Duodenum^Q | Gallbladder^Q | Liver^Q |
>
> - **Cholangiocarcinoma** is the **MC malignancy**^{Q} associated with bile duct cysts.

9. **Ans. a. Roux-en-Y hepaticojejunostomy**
10. **Ans. c. Choledochal cyst**
11. **Ans. d. Type 5 choledochal cyst** *(Ref: Sabiston 20/e p15; Schwartz 10/e p1289; Bailey 27/e p1168; Blumgart 6/e p762, 5/e p717; Shackelford 8/e p1374, 7/e p1402-1403)*
    - Central dot sign is seen in **Caroli's disease (Type V Choledochal cyst)**.
12. **Ans. c. Caroli's disease**
13. **Ans. c. Excision is ideal treatment**
14. **Ans. d. Cystojejunostomy is treatment of choice**

15. Ans. c. Recurrent cholangitis
16. Ans. a. Pain, lump and intermittent jaundice

CHOLEDOCHAL CYST

- **Classic triad: Pain, jaundice (intermittent)** and abdominal **mass (10%)**^{Q}.

17. Ans. c. Congenital
18. Ans. d. Can lead to carcinoma
19. Ans. b. Type II is most common
20. Ans. a. Caroli's disease
21. Ans. a. Type IV is Caroli's disease *(Ref: Sabiston 20/e p1510; Schwartz 10/e p1289; Bailey 27/e p1168)*
22. Ans. b. III *(Ref: Sabiston 20/e p1510; Schwartz 10/e p1330; Bailey 27/e p1198)*
23. Ans. c. IV *(Ref: Sabiston 20/e p1510; Schwartz 10/e p1330; Bailey 27/e p1198)*

CHOLEDOCHOLITHIASIS AND CHOLANGITIS

24. Ans. b. Endoscopic papillotomy *(Ref: Sabiston 20/e p1494-1496; Schwartz 10/e p1321-1322; Bailey 27/e p1205)*

- **ERCP: Diagnostic** and **therapeutic test of choice** for patients with suspected **CBD stones**^{Q}.

25. Ans. a. Cholangitis *(Ref: Sabiston 20/e p1507; Schwartz 10/e p1322-1323; Bailey 27/e p1205)*
26. Ans. b. 15% *(Ref: Sabiston 20/e p1494; Schwartz 10/e p1321-1322; Bailey 27/e p1205)*
27. Ans. d. Retained stones are discovered after 2 years of cholecystectomy
28. Ans. b. Brown stone
29. Ans. b. Cutaneous hepaticojejunostomy

This is a case of recurrent pyogenic cholangitis. Cutaneous hepaticojejunostomy is preferred treatment modality.

TREATMENT OF RECURRENT PYOGENIC CHOLANGITIS

- Treated with a **multidisciplinary approach** (endoscopy, interventional radiology, and surgery)
- The long-term goal of therapy is to **extract stones, remove debris**, and **relieve strictures**.
- **Roux-en-Y hepaticojejunostomy** with a **subcutaneous afferent limb (Hudson loop**^{Q}**)** is a safe and effective way to provide **access to the biliary tree** for **stone extractions**^{Q}.

30. Ans. a. Endoscopic papillotomy, b. ERCP, e. Choledochotomy
31. Ans. a. Fever, abdominal pain, jaundice

- **Charcot's triad**^{Q}: Abdominal pain + jaundice + fever^Q
- **Reynold's pentad**^{Q}: Charcot's triad + altered mental status + shock (hypotension)^Q

32. Ans. d. 11 O'clock position *(Ref: Sabiston 20/e p1496; Schwartz 10/e p1327)*

TRANSDUODENAL SPHINCTEROPLASTY

- This cut is made superiorly (at the **11 o'clock position**)^Q for **4 to 5 mm**.
- The **sphincter** is **incised at the 11–O'clock position** to avoid injury to the pancreatic duct^Q.

33. Ans. b. CBD stone
34. Ans. a. Escherichia coli
35. Ans. a. Increased leucocyte count, b. Increased transaminases, c. Increased alkaline phosphatase, d. Association with fever and chills
36. Ans. d. Septic shock
37. Ans. a. ERCP and bile duct stone extraction *(Ref: Sabiston 20/e p1496, 1489; Schwartz 10/e p1321; Bailey 27/e p1205)*
38. Ans. b. ERCP
39. Ans. d. Sphincterotomy and then cholecystectomy

Cholecystectomy with choledocholithotomy at same setting should not be done, as diameter of CBD is < 1 cm.

40. Ans. a. Endoscopic sphincterotomy
41. Ans. c. Endoscopic stone extraction
42. Ans. a. Supraduodenal choledochotomy with exploration
43. Ans. d. When removed by exploration of the common bile duct the T-tube can be removed after 3 days
44. Ans. a. ESWL, b. Exploration of bile duct and recovery of stones, c. Bile duct stenting, d. Nasobiliary drainage, e. Percutaneous drainage *(Ref: Shackelford 8/e p1287-1290, 7/e p1326-1331)*

> **CHOLEDOCHOLITHIASIS: TREATMENT OPTIONS**
>
> - **ERCP stone extraction** is successful 80–90% of the time using the techniques of **sphincterotomy** and **balloon catheter** or **Dormia basket stone retrieval**. The addition of **mechanical, electrohydraulic, laser**, or **extracorporeal shockwave lithotripsy** for **large stones increases** the **success rate to over 95%**[Q].
> - The placement of **pancreatic stents** has been found to **reduce the incidence of postbiliary sphincterotomy pancreatitis**[Q] in patient suspected of sphincter of Oddi dysfunction.
> - In patients for whom ERCP is not available, not possible secondary to anatomic considerations, or not successful, an alternative method of cholangiography and nonsurgical therapy is **percutaneous transhepatic cholangiography** (PTC) followed **by transhepatic methods of stone removal**.

45. **Ans. e. Palpable CBD stone** *(Ref: Shackelford 8/e p1290, 7/e p1326-1331)*

Choledochotomy	
Absolute Indications (High suspicion of CBD calculi)	**Relative Indications (Low suspicion of CBD calculi)**
• **Palpable CBD stones**[Q] • **Jaundice with cholangitis**[Q] • Demonstration of **stone** on **intra-operative cholangiography**[Q] • **CBD diameter >12 mm**[Q]	• Jaundice without cholangitis • History of pancreatitis • Dilated CBD • White bile on aspiration • Dilated cystic duct

46. **Ans. a. ERCP**   47. **Ans. d. CBD stones**   48. **Ans. b. ERCP**
49. **Ans. a. Meniscus sign** *(Ref: Sutton 6/e p971)*

> - **MR cholangiography**: Typical **"meniscus sign"** is seen when CBD stone[Q] is wedged at the level of the papilla.

50. **Ans. a. Distended gallbladder**   51. **Ans. a. E. coli**
52. **Ans. c. Common bile duct stone** *(Ref: Bailey 27/e p1234)*

> - In **obstruction** of the **CBD** due to a **stone, distention** of gallbladder seldom occurs; the **organ** usually is **shriveled**[Q].

53. **Ans. a. Stone in common bile duct**   54. **Ans. b. Endoscopic choledocholithotomy**
55. **Ans. d. Markedly elevated transaminases**   56. **Ans. c. Endoscopic papillotomy**
57. **Ans. c. Common bile duct** *(Ref: American Journal of Gastroenterology; Dec 1963, Vol. 41 Issue 6, p620)*

> **LEUCINE AMINOPEPTIDASE**
>
> - **Increased Leucine aminopeptidase (LAP) activity** is seen in:
>   - Carcinoma of the pancreas, choledocholithiasis, acute pancreatitis[Q]
>   - Viral hepatitis, cirrhosis, carcinoma with **liver metastases**[Q]
> - In **common bile duct obstruction**, whether due to **carcinoma pancreas** or **choledocholithiasis**, the **elevated serum LAP levels returned** to **normal following relief of the obstruction**. This is in agreement with the hypothesis that the increased serum LAP activity in these conditions is the result of bile duct obstruction.

58. **Ans. b. Distended and palpable gallbladder**
59. **Ans. a. Observation, c. Medical dissolution of stone** *(Ref: Bailey 27/e p1200; CSDT 11/e p1163)*

> - **Medical dissolution** is used **for Gallstones**, not the CBD stones.
> - **CBD stones** are **rarely asymptomatic**, often **present with complications**. CBD stones should be treated, if diagnosed. Treatment options are **ERCP, laparoscopic** or **open CBD exploration**.

CHOLEDOCHOTOMY AND CBD EXPLORATION

60. **Ans. d. Convert to open cholecystectomy and CBD stone removal** *(Ref: Shackelford 8/e p1290-1291, 7/e p1326-1331)*

Management of CBD Stones Associated with GB Stones	
Pre-operatively Detected Stones	**Unsuspected stones found at the time of Cholecystectomy**
Experienced Laparoscopic Surgeon	**Experienced Laparoscopic Surgeon**
• **Cholecystectomy and choledochotomy in same sitting**[Q]	• **Laparoscopic CBD exploration and stone retrieval** through the **cystic duct**[Q] • Laparoscopic **choledochotomy** and **stone extraction**[Q]

Inexperienced Laparoscopic Surgeon	Inexperienced Laparoscopic Surgeon
• Pre-op ERCP with stone removal and laparoscopic cholecystectomy later[Q].	• Convert to open procedure and remove CBD stone[Q] • Complete the cholecystectomy and refer the patient for ERCP[Q] • Conversion to an open procedure is preferred over ERCP[Q], because the success rate of ERCP is not 100%[Q].

61. Ans. d. Abnormal gamma glutamyl transferase
62. Ans. a. Synthetic absorbable *(Ref: Shackelford 8/e p1290-1291, 7/e p2222-2224)*

- **Synthetic absorbable suture** such as **Vicryl** is preferred for **CBD**[Q].
- **Vicryl sutures** are used in **general soft tissue approximation** and **vessel ligation**[Q].
- **Non absorbable sutures** ordinarily **remain** where they are **buried within the tissues**. This can cause **late complications** such as the development of **Gallstones around non-absorbable sutures** in the **common bile duct** or bladder stones in the **urinary bladder**. **In these situations** it is **best to use absorbable materials**[Q].

63. Ans. c. 12th postoperative day
64. Ans. c. T-tube cholangiogram *(Ref: Sabiston 20/e p1501; Schwartz 10/e p1322)*
65. Ans. b. 5–9 days   66. Ans. a. Supraduodenal choledochotomy
67. Ans. c. Endoscopic sphincterotomy and stone extraction
68. Ans. a. Retained stone *(Ref: Sabiston 20/e p1496)*

Most common complication of common bile duct exploration retained stone.

- **Clearance** of all **common bile duct stones** is achieved **in 75–95%** of patients with **laparoscopic CBD exploration**[Q].
- The rate of **retained CBD stone** is <5%.
- **MC complication** of **laparoscopic CBD exploration**[Q] is retained stone.

Laparoscopic CBD Exploration (LCBDE)

- An **intraoperative cholangiogram** at the time of cholecystectomy will also document the presence of **CBD stones**[Q].
- **LCBDE** through the **cystic duct** or with **formal choledochotomy** allows the stones to be retrieved during the same procedure.
- If the **expertise** and **instrumentation** for laparoscopic CBD exploration are **not available**, a **drain should be placed** and left adjacent next to the cystic duct and an endoscopic cholangiogram performed the following day.
- An **open CBD exploration** should be performed if endoscopic intervention is not available or not feasible because of anatomic restrictions or expertise.
- If a choledochotomy is performed, a T tube is left in place.
- The purpose of the **T tube** is to **provide access to the biliary system** for **postoperative radiologic stone extraction**[Q] and allow spasm or edema of sphincter to settle.
- The size of the tube is therefore of importance, in that **tubes <16 French do not allow for postoperative radiologic instrumentation** without dilation of the tract; a minimum of **4 to 6 weeks** should pass for the **tract to mature**[Q] before instrumentation.

69. Ans. b. Choledocholithiasis   70. Ans. a. Smaller stone in CHD

BILE DUCT INJURY AND BILIARY STRICTURES

71. Ans. a. Incidence is equal in laparoscopic and open cholecystectomy *(Ref: Sabiston 20/e p1501-1504; Schwartz 10/e p1332; Bailey 27/e p1204)*
72. Ans. d. Most common reason for bile duct injury is lack of techniques and errors of judgment *(Ref: Sabiston 19/e p1495)*

- As **surgeon experience** increases **beyond 20 cases**, the bile duct **injury rate decreases**[Q].
- **Errors** leading to laparoscopic bile duct injuries stem from **'misperception'**[Q], not erorrs of skill, knowledge or judgment.
- The **primary cause of error** in **97% cases** was a **'visual perceptual illusion'**[Q], whereas only **3% injuries** were due to **faults of technical skills**[Q].

73. Ans. a. Upper *(Ref: Sabiston 20/e p1502*

- **Most common duct injuries** occur **during attempted dissection** of the **cystic duct** when the **CBD is mistaken for cystic duct**[Q].
- These injuries involve **transection** of the **upper part** of the **CBD**[Q] and excision of a variable portion of the CBD proximal to first transection, including cystic duct-common duct junction.

The Stewart-Way Classification of Laparoscopic Bile Duct Injury

- The **Stewart-Way classification** is based primarily on the **anatomic pattern** and **mechanism** of a particular injury and the presence of associated **vascular injury**.

Class	Criteria
I.	**CBD mistaken** for **cystic duct** but **recognized**; cholangiogram incision of cystic duct extended into CBD
II.	**Lateral damage** to **common hepatic duct** from cautery or clips placed on duct; associated bleeding, poor visibility
III.	**CBD mistaken** for **cystic duct, not recognized**; CBD, CHD, RHD, LHD transected or resected
IV.	**RHD mistaken** for **cystic duct, RHA mistaken** for **cystic artery**, RHD and RHA transected; lateral damage to the RHD from cautery or clips placed on ducts

74. **Ans. c. Type D** *(Ref: Sabiston 20/e p1502; Shackelford 8/e p1355, 7/e p1381-1382)*

75. **Ans. b. Type B**   76. **Ans. b. Occlusion of a branch of biliary tree**

77. **Ans. c. Sectoral duct injury with consequent leak**

78. **Ans. a. CBD stone, b. Cholangiocarcinoma, c. Chronic pancreatitis, d. Trauma** *(Ref: Sabiston 20/e p 1509-1510)*

Causes of Biliary Strictures		
Benign		Malignant

• **Congenital:**
  – **Biliary atresia**[Q]
• **Operative injury:**
  – **Cholecystectomy**[Q]
  – **Choledochotomy**[Q]
  – Gastrectomy
  – Hepatic resection
  – Transplantation
	• **Inflammatory:**
	  – **Stones**[Q]
	  – **Cholangitis**
	  – Parasitic
	  – **Pancreatitis**[Q]
	  – **Sclerosing cholangitis**[Q]
	  – Radiotherapy
	• **Trauma**
	• **Idiopathic**
		• **Cholangiocarcinoma**[Q]
		• CA head of pancreas
		• Ampullary carcinoma
		• Metastasis to liver or biliary tract

- **MC cause** of **benign biliary stricture** is **laparoscopic cholecystectomy**.

79. **Ans. d. Clinical observation** *(Ref: Sabiston 20/e p1503; Schwartz 10/e p1333; Bailey 27/e p1204)*

  - "A small amount of biliary drainage following cholecystectomy should cause **no alarm** because it **usually disappears within 1 or 2 days**[Q]. However, **excessive biliary drainage** through the **wound** or **drain site, jaundice, sepsis** or a **combination of these events** early in the **post-operative period** should suggest a **bile duct injury**, as should **copious biliary drainage** for more than few post-op days[Q]."

80. **Ans. b. Percutaneous drainage** *(Ref: Sabiston 20/e p1502-1503; Schwartz 10/e p1333; Bailey 27/e p1204)*

81. **Ans. b. Percutaneous drainage of fluid** *(Ref: Sabiston 20/e p1503; Schwartz 10/e p1333; Bailey 27/e p1204)*

82. **Ans. a. Ultrasound guided aspiration** *(Ref: Blumgart 6/e p701, 5/e p627)*

  - Many bile leaks resolve with percutaneous drainage alone, and ERCP is probably unnecessary in the absence of radiographic or clinical evidence of ongoing bile drainage.

83. **Ans. c. Computed tomography** *(Ref: Blumgart 6/e p701, 5/e p627)*

  CT is **probably the best initial study**, the results of which **help direct further investigations**.

Radiological Investigations in Post-Cholecystectomy Bile Duct Injury

Duplex ultrasonography
- Excellent, noninvasive means of **showing intrahepatic ductal dilation** and may reveal a **subhepatic fluid collection** or **evidence of vascular damage**.
- May provide **valuable information** regarding the **level of biliary injury**, it is of **little value** in **assessing the extent of a stricture** and is of **no value** if the **biliary tree** is **decompressed**.

Computed tomography
- CT is **probably the best initial study**^{Q}, the results of which **help direct further investigations**.
- A **good quality CT scan** shows a **dilated biliary tree** and helps **localize the level of ductal obstruction** in patients with strictures.
- CT identifies **fluid collections** or **ascites**, which may suggest the **possibility of vascular damage**, and it **reveals lobar atrophy**^{Q}.

Percutaneous transhepatic cholangiography
- **PTC** is much more likely than ERCP to provide this information, and PTC remains the **standard investigation in this setting**^{Q}.

Magnetic resonance cholangiopancreatography
- **MRCP** has emerged as a valuable tool in **evaluating proximal bile duct injuries**
- This noninvasive modality provides striking images of the biliary tree and yields anatomic information in a single study that was previously obtainable only with CT and PTC

ERCP
- ERCP is **seldom of value** in the **precise diagnosis** of **complete proximal bile duct strictures** because there is **often discontinuity** of the **CBD** preventing visualization of the intrahepatic ductal system^Q.
- ERCP may be **more helpful for incomplete strictures (stenoses)**^{Q}
- ERCP also has a **role in the diagnosis** and **treatment of patients** with **bile leakage from the cystic duct stump** or from a **laceration** of the **common duct**^{Q}

Isotopic scanning techniques
- **HIDA scanning** offers a **dynamic** and **quantitative assessment of liver function** and of the **clearance of bile across anastomosis** and **stenosis**.
- In patients with **hepatocellular disease**, **HIDA scanning** may be valuable in **distinguishing** the contribution of the **biliary obstruction** from that of the **intrinsic liver disease** to the overall biochemical of isotope from a portion of the liver.

Arteriography and delayed-phase portography
- Can be obtained **to confirm vascular injury** on the initial studies, a **suspicion of portal hypertension** from the history and physical examination, or a **history of excessive bleeding** at the **time of cholecystectomy**.

84. **Ans. d. Routine use of 'open' technique of laparoscopic port insertion has resulted in a decline in the incidence of post laparoscopic cholecystectomy bile duct injuries** *(Ref: Sabiston 20/e p1498; Bailey 27/e p1203)*

- **Pneumoperitoneum** is created by use of **Hasson's canula** in **open technique** of laparoscopic port insertion.
- **Open technique** has resulted in **reduction of trocar induced vascular** and **bowel injuries**, not the incidence of post laparoscopic cholecystectomy bile duct injuries.
- **Open cholecystectomy** is associated with **reduced incidence** of post laparoscopic cholecystectomy bile duct injuries as compared to laparoscopic cholecystectomy.

85. **Ans. d. Laparoscopic cholecystectomy operation**   86. **Ans. b. Trauma**

- MC cause of **benign biliary stricture** is **laparoscopic cholecystectomy (operative trauma)**^{Q}.

BILIARY FISTULA
87. **Ans. c. Gallstones** *(Ref: Blumgart 6/e p682, 5/e p645-669; Shackelford 8/e p1309, 7/e p1385)*
88. **Ans. a. Gastric ulcer** *(Ref: Blumgart 6/e p685, 5/e p644-657)*

SPHINCTER OF ODDI DYSKINESIA
89. **Ans. a. Transduodenal sphincteroplasty** *(Ref: Sabiston 20/e p1497; Shackelford 8/e p1297, 7/e p1333-1336)*
90. **Ans. a. Sphincter of Oddi dysfunction**

BILIARY TRACT DISEASES
91. **Ans. b. Sarcoidosis** *(Ref: Harrison 20/e p280,1305, 19/e p2027-2028)*

VANISHING BILE DUCT SYNDROME
- Rare condition characterized by **decreased number of bile ducts** seen in **liver biopsy specimens**^{Q}

Causes of Vanishing Bile Duct Syndrome	
• **Chronic rejection**^{Q} after liver transplantation	• **Sarcoidosis**^{Q}
• **Graft-versus-host disease**^{Q} after BM transplantation	• Drugs: **Chlorpromazine**^{Q}
	• **Idiopathic**^{Q}

92. **Ans. a. GVHD**

BILIARY ATRESIA

93. **Ans. c. Marked bile duct degeneration, d. Fibrosis of hepatic duct, e. Parenchymal cholestasis** *(Ref: Sabiston 20/e p639, 1880; Schwartz; 10/e p1628-1630; Bailey 27/e p1196; Blumgart 6/e p656, 5/e p595-603; Shackelford 8/e p1361, 7/e p1390-1396)*

94. **Ans. a. Per-operative cholangiography** *(Ref: Blumgart 6/e p658)*

> *"Despite these advancements in noninvasive imaging of hepatobiliary anatomy, **intraoperative cholangiography remains the gold standard for diagnosing biliary atresia**. Although endoscopic retrograde **cholangiopancreatography (ERCP) may be possible, equipment and expertise in performing ERCP in infants is limited**. Preoperative liver biopsy has become an increasingly safe and used method to help exclude other causes of neonatal jaundice. **Although percutaneous liver biopsy is highly accurate, there are no histologic findings that are pathognomonic for BA. Findings suggestive of BA** include portal or bridging fibrosis, bile duct proliferation, inflammation, or giant cell hepatitis, some of which may not be evident on samples taken from very young infants, thereby necessitating repeat biopsy at a later date."*- Blumgart 6/e p658

95. **Ans. e. Age of 8 weeks** *(Ref: Blumgart 6/e p659, 5/e p600; Shackelford 8/e p1365, 7/e p1394)*

Major Factors in Successful Outcome after Portoentreostomy	
• **Age** in days at diagnosis and initial surgery (30–60 days)[Q]	• Degree and extent of **fibrotic changes** in the liver[Q]
• **Length of time jaundice** was present before surgery[Q]	• **Need for phototherapy** as a neonate[Q]
• **Successful** and **persistent bile flow** postoperatively[Q]	• Technical aspects of the portoenterostomy and anastomosis[Q]
• **Size** and nature of the microscopic ducts **(>150 μm)**[Q]	• Presence of bile in hepatic lobular zone 1

96. **Ans. c. Biliary atresia**

PRIMARY SCLEROSING CHOLANGITIS

97. **Ans. b. ITP** *(Ref: Sabiston 20/e p1508-1509; Schwartz 10/e p1331; Bailey 27/e p1206; Blumgart 6/e p663, 5/e p603-615; Shackelford 8/e p1378, 7/e p1405-1414)*

Diseases Associated with PSC		
• **Chronic ulcerative colitis**[Q]	• Hypereosinophilia	• Sarcoidosis[Q]
• **Crohn's disease**[Q]	• Riedel's thyroiditis[Q]	• Glomerulonephritis
• Autoimmune hepatitis	• Celiac disease	• Retroperitoneal fibrosis[Q]
• Chronic pancreatitis	• Autoimmune hemolytic anemia	• Systemic sclerosis
	• Sicca syndrome	

- **Smoking** is **protective** in: **PSC** and **UC**[Q]
- **PBC** is more common in **females**[Q].
- **PSC** and **Cholangiocarcinoma** is more common in **males**[Q].
- **Colectomy** has **no effect on the course of PSC**[Q].

98. **Ans. a. PSC in UC, the association is 30%**
99. **Ans. a. Primary sclerosing cholangitis**
100. **Ans. b. Primary sclerosing cholangitis** *(Ref: Sabiston 20/e p1508-1509; Schwartz 10/e p1292; Bailey 27/e p1206)*

> *In the MRCP and ERCP image, there is presence of multiple strictures involving both intrahepatic and extrahepatic bile duct and history of repeated attacks of cholangitis is highly suggestive of primary sclerosing cholangitis.*

101. **Ans. b. Cholangiocarcinoma**
102. **Ans. b. Primary sclerosing cholangitis**
103. **Ans. a. Cholangiocarcinoma is always intrahepatic**
104. **Ans. c. Most patients presents with advanced disease**
105. **Ans. c. Cirrhosis never occurs**
106. **Ans. d. PSC reverts after a total colectomy**

- Patients with **PSC** and **ulcerative colitis** typically have a **more quiescent disease course**[Q]
- The **risk for colon cancer** in these patients is **up to five times greater** than in patients with **ulcerative colitis alone**. These tumors are **more likely to arise proximal** to the **splenic flexure**.
- **PSC** is **progressive** and **ultimately fatal unless liver transplantation** is undertaken[Q]. **Colectomy** has **no effect on the course of PSC**[Q].

107. **Ans. b. Sclerosing cholangitis**
108. **Ans. d. Primary sclerosing cholangitis resolves after total colectomy**

PRIMARY BILIARY CIRRHOSIS

109. **Ans. a. Primary biliary cirrhosis** *(Ref: Sabiston 20/e p639; Blumgart 6/e p1155, 5/e p1085-1086, Shackelford 8/e p1406, 7/e p1441)*
110. **Ans. b. Pruritus**
111. **Ans. a. Generalized pruritus, c. Fatigue**
112. **Ans. a. No increase in risk of hepatocellular carcinoma**
113. **Ans. a. Pruritus**

RECURRENT PYOGENIC CHOLANGITIS

114. **Ans. d. GB stones are present in >50% cases** *(Ref: Sabiston 20/e p1507-1508; Blumgart 6/e p727, 5/e p680-697)*
   GB stones are present in **<50% cases**[Q].

CHOLANGIOCARCINOMA PREDISPOSING FACTORS

115. **Ans. d. Aflatoxin** *(Ref: Sabiston 20/e p1514; Schwartz 10/e p1335-1338; Bailey 27/e p1205; Shackelford 8/e p1328, 7/e p1370)*
116. **Ans. b. Cholelithiasis**

- **Choledocholithiasis, not the cholelithiasis** is a **risk factor** for **cholangiocarcinoma**[Q].

117. **Ans. d. All of the above** *(Ref: Sabiston 20/e p1514)*

ANOMALOUS PANCREATICOBILIARY DUCT JUNCTION (APBDJ)

- An anomalous pancreaticobiliary union is considered to be present when the **common channel** is **longer than 15 mm**.

Three Types of APBDJ
- **Bp Type or Type 2: Insertion of** the **bile duct is in** the **pancreatic duct**
- **Pb Type or Type 1: Pancreatic duct** appears to **join** the **common bile duct**
- **Y type: Long common channel**

- **Choledochal cyst is the MC associated abnormality**[Q].
- **APBDJ** is seen **gallbladder cancer; gallbladder adenomyomatosis; cholangiocarcinoma;** and **pancreatitis**[Q].

118. **Ans. a. PSC**
119. **Ans. b. Clonorchis sinensis**
120. **Ans. d. Chronic pancreatitis**
121. **Ans. None**
122. **Ans. None**

CHOLANGIOCARCINOMA

123. **Ans. c. Involvement of right branch of portal vein** *(Ref: Sabiston 20/e p1514-1518; Schwartz 10/e p1335-1338; Bailey 27/e p1208; Blumgart 6/e p826, 5/e p771-788; Shackelford 8/e p1331, 7/e p1370-1378)*
124. **Ans. a. Division of both ducts and not extending outside**
125. **Ans. a. Scirrhous type has better prognosis than papillary**
126. **Ans. c. Common hepatic duct tumor**
127. **Ans. b. Hilum**
128. **Ans. a. Sclerosing variety is most common**
129. **Ans. c. Schirrhous type**
130. **Ans. d. Atrophy of one lobe with ipsilateral involvement of secondary biliary radicals**
131. **Ans. d. Hepatic atrophy with ipsilateral bile duct involvement**
132. **Ans. c. Proximal cholangiocarcinoma**
133. **Ans. c. Bifurcation and bilateral secondary intrahepatic ducts**
134. **Ans. a. Liver**
135. **Ans. b. Distal cholangiocarcinoma** *(Ref: Sabiston 20/e p1514-1518; Schwartz 10/e p1335; Bailey 27/e p1208)*

HEMOBILIA

136. **Ans. b. Iatrogenic** *(Ref: Sabiston 20/e p1472-1474; Blumgart 6/e p1915, 5/e p1832-1843; Shackelford 8/e p1275, 7/e p1487)*
137. **Ans. b. Fever**
138. **Ans. a. Hemobilia**
139. **Ans. d. Hepatitis**
140. **Ans. a. Triad of jaundice, pain, melena**

BILHEMIA

141. **Ans. a. ERCP** *(Ref: Sabiston 20/e p1473-1474; Blumgart 6/e p1926, 5/e p1843-1844; Shackelford 8/e p1453, 7/e p1488)*
142. **Ans. d. Patient has hyperbilirubinemia with raised enzymes**

MISCELLANEOUS

143. **Ans. b. Anterior to first part of duodenum** *(Ref: Sabiston 20/e p1482-1484; Schwartz 10/e p1268, 1310-1311; Bailey 27/e p1188)*
144. **Ans. d. Usually opens into duodenum separate from the main pancreatic duct**
145. **Ans. c. Anteriorly related to 1st part of duodenum** *(Ref: Sabiston 20/e p1482-1484)*
146. **Ans. a. Vessels that run upward along the bile duct from the duodenal end of the duct such as the retroduodenal and gastroduodenal arteries** *(Ref: Sabiston 20/e p1482-1483)*
147. **Ans. b. Rupture of hydatid cyst** *(Ref: Sabiston 18/e p1570)*

Causes of Pneumobilia	
• Previous surgery (Papillotomy, choledochojejunostomy, ERCP with sphincterotomy) • Gallstone ileus • Emphysematous cholecystitis	• Choledochoduodenal or cholecystocolic fistula • Tracheobiliary fistula • Suppurative cholangitis • Mirizzi's syndrome (due to cholecystoenteric fistula)

148. **Ans. a. Gallstone ileus > b. Mirizzi's syndrome**
149. **Ans. a. 7 cm** *(Ref: Grays 39/e p1228)*
150. **Ans. c. Use of heavily T2-weighted image without contrast to create the three dimensional image of the biliary tree using MIP algorithm** *(Ref: Blumgart 6/e p359-361, 5/e p315-315)*

    MRI cholangiography and **MRI cholangiopancreatography** (**MRCP**) are imaging techniques used to **evaluate** the **biliary system**.
    Heavily T2-weighted images are used to **provide an overview of the biliary system** and **pancreatic duct**.
    Excellent diagnostic-quality images are obtainable, with **high sensitivity and specificity** for evaluation of **biliary duct dilation, strictures, and intraductal abnormalities**.

    > **MAGNETIC RESONANCE CHOLANGIOPANCREATOGRAPHY**
    >
    > - The **basic principle of MRCP** is to use **T2-weighted images**, in which **stationary or slowly moving fluid, including bile**, is **high in signal intensity; all the surrounding tissues**, including **retroperitoneal fat** and the **solid visceral organs**, are **lower in signal**.
    > - MR-specific techniques for obtaining cholangiographic images include two-dimensional and three-dimensional sequences, breath-hold or non–breath-hold techniques, and respiratory gated techniques.
    > - MRCP plays an **important role in imaging benign disorders of the biliary and pancreatic system**, and it is **part of a comprehensive imaging evaluation of malignancies of the biliary system**.
    > - MRCP is noninvasive, eliminating the morbidity associated with ERCP or PTC.
    > - An **additional advantage of MRCP** includes **visualization of the extrabiliary anatomy, allowing for exclusion** or **inclusion of alternative diagnoses**.
    > - **Surgical clips** may **create an artifact** known as susceptibility, which may obscure the region of interest by producing areas of signal void. **This artifact may mimic a stone**, so caution must be used in evaluating MRCP images in postoperative patients to avoid a false-positive diagnosis.

    MIP (Maximum Intensity Projection) Algorithm
    - CE FAST (Fourier-acquired steady state) or FSE (Fat spinal echo) require **image processing** with a **maximum intensity projection** (MIP) algorithm, allowing **rotation of summed image** and **display of the cholangiogram to best advantage**.

151. **Ans. a. Percutaneous transhepatic cholangiogram** *(Ref: Schwartz 10/e p1315; Sabiston 20/e p1489; Bailey 27/e p1193)*

CHAPTER 8

Pancreas

PANCREAS DIVISUM

Pancreas Divisum

- MC congenital anomaly of the pancreas^Q
- It occurs when the ductal systems of the **dorsal & ventral pancreatic duct fail to fuse**^Q during the second month of gestation.

Types
- **Type 1** has two **completely separate pancreatic ducts**.
- **Type 2** has **only a dorsal duct**, with no evidence of a ventral duct of Wirsung.
- **Type 3** has a **dominant dorsal duct** with only a small, narrow filamentous connection between the dorsal and ventral ducts.
  - Common to all variants of pancreas divisum is that **all** or **most pancreatic secretion** flows **through** the **accessory papilla**^Q.

Diagnosis
- **IOC** for diagnosis of **pancreas divisum: MRCP**^Q
- **Gold standard** investigation for diagnosis: **ERCP**^Q

Treatment
- Operative **dorsal duct sphincterotomy, with or without sphincteroplasty**^Q, is the preferred surgical treatment.
- Patients with **pancreas divisum** and **acute recurrent pancreatitis** are **good candidates for endoscopic therapy**^Q whereas patients with chronic pancreatitis or chronic pain alone (or both) do not appear to do as well.

ANNULAR PANCREAS

Annular Pancreas

- **Circumferential** or near-circumferential **band of pancreas tissue** surrounding the **2nd part of duodenum**^Q
- It is of **ventral pancreas origin** and is usually **proximal to ampulla**^Q.

  - **Duodenal stenosis** or **atresia** is present at the site of annulus in **40%**^Q
  - **Down's syndrome**^Q (trisomy 21) is present in **15-25%**.

- Intestinal malrotation, tracheoesophageal fistula, & congenital heart defects, Meckel's diverticulum and imperforate anus are also not uncommon.

Diagnosis
- **Definitive diagnosis** is made by **ERCP**.

Treatment
- Treatment of choice: **Duodenoduodenostomy**^Q >Duodenojejunostomy.
- Duodenoduodenostomy has **replaced duodenojejunostomy** as the **treatment of choice** because it has a **lower incidence of postoperative complications**, particularly **obstruction & blind-loop syndromes**^Q.

PANCREATIC CYST

Pancreatic Cyst

- **Solitary** (**congenital,** duplication, or dermoid) **cysts** of the **pancreas** are **rare**^Q.
- **Multiple pancreatic cysts**, lined with cuboidal epithelium, **are more common**^Q.
- They are frequently **associated with polycystic disease** of the **liver** or **kidney**^Q.
- Can be seen in **up to half of patients** with **von Hippel-Lindau disease**^Q.
- Pancreatic cysts **only rarely become symptomatic**, and **no treatment** is **indicated**^Q.

NESIDIOBLASTOSIS

NESIDIOBLASTOSIS

- Also known as **persistent hyperinsulinemic hypoglycemia** of **infancy**^{Q}
- Characterized by **diffuse hyperfunction** of pancreatic **beta cells** with **enlargement of** their **nuclei**^{Q}
- **Neither** the **beta cell proliferation rate nor** the **overall beta cell mass is increased**^{Q}.

Clinical Features
- **Early recognition** of congenital hyperinsulinism is critical because, if untreated, profound hypoglycemia may lead to brain damage.
- Babies may be described as **jittery, floppy, or lethargic; seizures** are common^Q

Diagnosis
- **Inappropriately elevated insulin** in the setting of **hypoglycemia**^{Q}, along with the **need for continuous glucose infusion** (<15 mg/kg/min) to maintain normoglycemia confirms the diagnosis.
- **Pancreatic venous** sampling is used to make the **diagnosis**^{Q}.

Treatment
- **Continuous glucose administration** with **suppression** of **insulin secretion** by **diazoxide** or **somatostatin**^{Q}.
- Treatment consists of **near total (95-98%) pancreatectomy**^{Q}.

ETIOLOGY OF ACUTE PANCREATITIS

Causes of Acute Pancreatitis	
Common Causes	**Uncommon Causes**
• **Gallstones** including microlithiasis (**MC**)^Q • **Alcohol (2nd MC)**^{Q} • **Hypertriglyceridemia**^{Q} • **ERCP**^{Q} • Blunt abdominal trauma • Postoperative • Drugs • Sphincter of Oddi dysfunction **Rare Causes:** • Infections (**C**MV, **C**oxsackie, **M**umps, **E**chovirus, (**CME**) parasites)^Q • Autoimmune (Sjogren syndrome)	• Vascular causes and vasculitis (ischemic-hypoperfusion states after cardiac surgery) • Connective tissue disorders • **TTP**^{Q} • **CA pancreas**^{Q} • **Hypercalcemia (Hyperparathyroidism)**^{Q} • Periampullary diverticulum • **Pancreas divisum**^{Q} • Hereditary pancreatitis • **Cystic fibrosis**^{Q} • Renal failure

Causes in Recurrent Bouts of Acute Pancreatitis without an Obvious Etiology	
• Occult disease of the biliary tree or pancreatic ducts, especially **microlithiasis, sludge**^{Q} • Drugs • **Hypertriglyceridemia**^{Q}	• **Pancreas divisum**^{Q} • Pancreatic cancer^Q • Sphincter of Oddi dysfunction^Q • Cystic fibrosis^Q • Idiopathic

Drugs Associated with Pancreatitis		
Definite Cause (MAD CAT PET TV FM)		**Probable Cause (PILAAS)**
• **6-Mercaptopurine**^{Q} • **A**zathioprine^Q • **D**ideoxyinosine • **C**ytosine arabinoside • **5-A**minosalicylate^Q • **T**etracycline • **P**entamidine^Q	• **E**strogens^Q • **T**rimethoprim-sulfamethoxazole^Q • **T**hiazide^Q • **V**alproic acid^Q • **F**urosemide • **M**etronidazole^Q	• **P**henformin • **P**rocainamide • **I**soniazid • **L**-Asparaginase^Q • **A**cetaminophen^Q • **A**lpha-Methyl-dopa • **S**ulindac

ACUTE PANCREATITIS

ACUTE PANCREATITIS

- AP is **mild & self-limited** in most patients^Q
- **Rapidly progressive inflammatory response** associated with prolonged length of hospital stay and significant morbidity & mortality occur in **10-20%**^{Q} of patients
- **Mortality rate:** Mild pancreatitis <1%; Severe pancreatitis 10-30%^{Q}.

- **MC cause of death** in this group of patients is **multiorgan dysfunction syndrome**^{Q}.
- **First sign of Multi-system organ failure** in AP commonly is **impaired lung function** caused by **ARDS**^{Q}.

- Mortality in the **first 2 weeks (early phase)**: Due to **multiorgan dysfunction**^{Q}
- Mortality **after 2 weeks (late period)**: Caused by **septic complications**^{Q}

Pathophysiology

- AP is the final result of **abnormal pancreatic enzyme activation** inside acinar cells^Q.
- **Colocalization hypothesis:** Cathepsin B-mediated intra-acinar cell activation of the digestive enzymes leads to acinar cell injury and triggers an inflammatory response.

  - **Intra-acinar pancreatic enzyme activation** induces **autodigestion** of normal pancreatic parenchyma.
  - Acinar cells release **proinflammatory cytokines,** which propagate the response locally and systemically.

- **Local inflammatory response** further **aggravates** the **pancreatitis** because it increases the permeability & damages the microcirculation of pancreas.
- In **severe cases**, inflammatory response causes **local hemorrhage & pancreatic necrosis**^{Q}.
- **Inflammatory cascade** is self-limited in 80-90% of patients^Q.

Risk Factors

- **Gallstones (MC) & ethanol abuse (2nd MC)** account for **70-80%** of AP cases^Q.
- In **pediatric patients, abdominal blunt trauma & systemic diseases**^{Q} are the two most common conditions that lead to pancreatitis.

Clinical Features

- **Cardinal symptom:** Epigastric and/or periumbilical **pain** that **radiates to the back, relieved by sitting & leaning forward**^{Q}.
- Up to **90%** of patients have **nausea** and/or **vomiting** that typically does not relieve the pain.
- Nature of the **pain is constant**^{Q}.
- Dehydration, poor skin turgor, tachycardia, hypotension, & dry mucous membranes are commonly seen in patients with AP.
- **Mild pancreatitis:** Abdomen may be normal or reveal only **mild epigastric tenderness**.
- **Severe pancreatitis:** Significant abdominal distention, associated with generalized rebound tenderness and abdominal rigidity.

  - **Flank (Grey Turner)**^{Q}, **periumbilical (Cullen's sign)**^{Q} & **inguinal ecchymosis (Fox sign)**^{Q} are indicative of **retroperitoneal bleeding** associated with **severe pancreatitis.**

- Associated with **left sided pleural effusion**^{Q}

Diagnosis

- Cornerstone of the diagnosis of AP: Clinical findings + elevation of pancreatic enzyme levels in the plasma^Q.

Pancreatic Enzymes

- A **threefold or higher** elevation of **amylase & lipase** levels **confirms** the **diagnosis**^{Q}.
- **Amylase's** serum **half-life** is **shorter** as compared with lipase.
- Lipase is also a **more specific marker of AP**^{Q} because serum amylase levels can be elevated in peptic ulcer disease, mesenteric ischemia, salpingitis, and macroamylasemia.
- Patients with AP are typically **hyperglycemic**; they can also have **leukocytosis** and **abnormal elevation of liver enzyme** levels.
- **Elevation of ALT** levels in the serum in the context of AP has a **positive predictive value** of **95%** in the diagnosis of **acute biliary pancreatitis**^{Q}.

- **X-ray Abdomen:** Localized ileus of **duodenum** and **proximal jejunum (sentinel loop)**^{Q} or that of **transverse colon** up to **its mid point (colon cut off sign)**^{Q}.
- **IOC for acute pancreatitis: CECT**^{Q} (Should be performed **after 72 hours of acute pancreatitis**^{Q})

Treatment

- **Cornerstone of the treatment: Aggressive fluid resuscitation**^{Q} (Fluid of choice: **RL**^{Q}) with **supplementary oxygen**
- **Narcotics** are usually preferred, especially **Buprenorphine >morphine**^{Q} as analgesics.

In Acute Pancreatitis	
NSAIDs of choice	Metamizole^Q
Opiate of choice	Buprenorphine^Q

- **Nutritional support: Enteral nutrition**^{Q} is associated with less infectious complications and reduces the need for pancreatic surgery as compared to TPN.
- **Enteral nutrition** is **started within 24 hours** via NG tube.

- **TPN** can be given if patient is in **shock** & having **severe pancreatitis**.
- **Prophylactic antibiotic** should **not be given**^Q.

  - **ERCP:** Beneficial for patients with **severe acute biliary pancreatitis** and **cholangitis**^Q
  - **Laparoscopic cholecystectomy:** Indicated for **all patients** with **mild acute biliary pancreatitis**^Q with the **exception** of **older** patients and those with **poor performance status**^Q

ASSESSMENT OF SEVERITY OF ACUTE PANCREATITIS

Assessment of Severity of Acute Pancreatitis

- **Severe pancreatitis** is diagnosed if **three or more**^Q of the **Ranson's criteria** are fulfilled.
- Main disadvantage is that it does not predict the severity of disease at the time of the admission because six parameters are only assessed after 48 hours of admission.
- An **APACHE II score** of ≥8^Q defines **severe pancreatitis**. The main advantage is that it can be used on admission and repeated at any time.
- A **CRP level ≥130 mg/mL**^Q defines **severe pancreatitis**.

Tools for Predicting Severity in Acute Pancreatitis Ready for Clinical Use		
On Admission	**At 24 Hours**	**At 48 Hours**
• APACHE-II Score ≥8^Q • IL-6 • Urea >60 mmol/L	• Polymorphonuclear **elastase** • Urinary **trypsinogen 2** • Urinary **trypsinogen** activation peptide	• Ranson/Glasgow score ≥ 3^Q • CRP ≥130^Q mg/mL

- A **CRP level ≥130 mg/mL**^Q defines **severe pancreatitis**.

Ranson's Prognostic Criteria for Non-Gallstone Pancreatitis	
At Admission	**During Initial 48 Hours**
• Age >**55 years**^Q • WBC >**16,000**^Q cells/mm³ • Blood glucose >**200**^Q mg/dL • Serum LDH >**350**^Q IU/L • AST >**250**^Q U/L	• Hematocrit fall >**10**^Q percentage points • BUN elevation >**5**^Q mg/dL • Serum calcium fall to <**8**^Q mg/dL • Arterial **PO$_2$** <**60**^Q mm Hg • Base deficit >**4**^Q mEq/L • Estimated fluid sequestration >**6**^Q **Litres**

Ranson's Prognostic Criteria for Gallstone Pancreatitis	
At Admission	**During Initial 48 Hours**
• Age >**70** years • WBC >**18,000** cells/mm • Glucose >**220** mg/dL • Serum LDH >**400** IU/L • AST >**250** U/L	• Hematocrit fall >10 percentage points • BUN elevation >**2** mg/dL • Serum calcium fall to <8 mg/dL • Base deficit >**5** mEq/L • Arterial PO$_2$ <60 mm Hg • Estimated fluid sequestration >**4 litres**

- Patients with **one or two** criteria have a predicted mortality of less than **1%**, with **three** criteria (**10%**) or **four** criteria (**15%**); with more than **seven** criteria **50%**

Modified Glasgow Criteria

- This system comprises eight factors. The presence of any **3 or more** within 48 hours of admission defines the patient as having **severe disease**.

Criteria during Initial 48 Hours	
• Age >**55** years • WBC count >**15,000** cell/mm • Blood urea nitrogen >**45** mg/dL • Arterial PO$_2$ <**60** mm Hg	• Blood glucose >**180** mg/dL • Serum LDH >**600** IU/L • Serum calcium <**8** mg/dL • Serum albumin <**3.3** g/dL

Acute Physiology and Chronic Health Evaluation (APACHE)-II Scoring System

- **APACHE-II scoring system** incorporates 12^Q physiological and laboratory parameters as well as age and comorbid conditions to estimate severity of any disease process.

The 12 physiologic variables are BT ↑ HR at CWG SHOP-2		
1. Mean arterial **Blood pressure**^{Q}	5. **C**reatinine	9. **H**ematocrit
2. **T**emperature	6. **W**BC count^Q	10. **O**xygenation
3. **H**eart rate	7. **G**lasgow Coma Scale^Q	11. Arterial **pH**^{Q}
4. **R**espiratory rate	8. **S**odium	12. Serum **p**otassium

- Score ≥8 signifies **severe, acute pancreatitis**^{Q}
- It can be determined on a **daily basis**^{Q}.
- Recently modification of the APACHE-II scoring system with **addition of obesity** has been proposed.
- The **APACHE-O** scale, which adds one point for **body mass index** (BMI) between 25 and 30, and two points for BMI larger than 30.

Computed Tomography Severity Index (CTSI) for Acute Pancreatitis

- **CTSI (CT severity index scoring system)** = Balthazar grade score + necrosis score
- Highest attainable score = 10^Q

Pancreatic Inflammation		Pancreatic Necrosis	
Normal pancreas	0	None	0
Focal or diffuse pancreatic **enlargement**	1	≤ 30%	2
Intrinsic pancreatic alterations with **peripancreatic fat inflammatory** changes	2	30–50%	4
Single fluid collection/or phlegmon	3	>50%	6
Two or **more** fluid collections or **gas**, in or adjacent to the pancreas	4		

- CTSI score:
  - 0-3: Mortality 3%, morbidity 8%
  - 4-6: Mortality 6%, morbidity 35%
  - 7-10: Mortality 17%, morbidity 92%

BISAP score: Bedside Index for Severity of Acute Pancreatitis

- BUN > 25 mg/dL
- Impaired mental status
- SIRS ≥ 2 of 4 present
- Age > 60 years
- Pleural effusion

(Score 0–2: Mortality < 2%; Score 3–5: Mortality > 15%)

COMPLICATIONS OF ACUTE PANCREATITIS

Complications of Acute Pancreatitis	
• Sterile and infected peripancreatic fluid collections	• Pancreaticopleural fistulas
• Pancreatic necrosis and infected necrosis	• Vascular complications
• Pancreatic pseudocysts	• Pancreatocutaneous fistula
• Pancreatic ascites	

Vascular Complications of Acute Pancreatitis

- Acute pancreatitis is **rarely associated with arterial vascular complications**.
- MC vessel affected: **Splenic artery**^{Q}
- Other vessels: Superior mesenteric, cystic, and gastroduodenal arteries^Q

Vascular Thrombosis
• Pancreatic inflammation can produce **vascular thrombosis**
• MC affected vessel: **Splenic vein**^{Q}
• in severe cases, it can **extend into** the **portal venous system**
• Imaging demonstrates **splenomegaly, gastric varices**, and **splenic vein occlusion**
• **Thrombolytics** have been described in the **acute early phase**
• Most patients can be managed with **conservative treatment**
• **Recurrent episodes** of **upper gastrointestinal bleeding** caused by venous hypertension should be **treated with splenectomy**^{Q}

Pathogenesis

- It has been proposed that **pancreatic elastase** damages the **vessels**, leading to **pseudoaneurysm formation**.

Clinical Features
- **Spontaneous rupture**^{Q} results in massive bleeding.
- Clinical manifestations include sudden onset of **abdominal pain, tachycardia**, and **hypotension**.

Treatment
- If possible, **arterial embolization** should be attempted **to control the bleeding**^{Q}.
- **Refractory cases** require **ligation of** the **affected vessel**.
- The **mortality** ranges from **28-56%**.

> - **MC affected vessel** in **acute pancreatitis**: Splenic artery (pseudoaneusysm formation)^Q
> - **MC affected vessel** leading to **vascular thrombosis** caused by acute pancreatitis: **Splenic vein**^{Q}

PANCREATIC FISTULA

- Output via an intra-operatively placed drain (or percutaneous drain) of any measurable volume or drain fluid on or after post-operative day 3, amylase >3 times of normal serum value.
- Pancreatic fistula classified into **low output (<200 mL/day)** and **high output (>200 mL/day)**.

Factors Known to Influence the Outcome of a Pancreatic Anastomosis	
• **Texture** of the **pancreatic remnant**^{Q}	• **Caliber** of the **main** pancreatic **duct**^{Q}
• **Exocrine** pancreatic juice **output**^{Q}	• **Surgical technique** applied^Q

- **Texture of Pancreatic Remnant:** Performing an **anastomosis** on a **soft pancreas** is **more difficult** than on a firm or hard pancreas. Thus, a **pancreatic anastomosis** in **chronic pancreatitis** has a **lower risk** of anastomotic failure compared to **pancreatic cancer**^{Q}.
- **Pancreatic Juice Output:** Decreased juice output is associated with a **lowered risk** of anastomotic failure^Q.
- **Surgical Technique:** An **end-to-side pancreaticojejunostomy** irrespective of the caliber of the main pancreatic duct and the texture of the pancreatic parenchyma.

Management
- **Most cases resolve spontaneously** by **conservative treatment**^{Q}
- Benefit of **prophylactic octreotide** in the **prevention** of **pancreatic fistula**^{Q}
- Role **of octreotide**, once a fistula is **established remains unclear**^{Q}.

PSEUDOPANCREATIC CYST

PSEUDOPANCREATIC CYST

- A chronic collection of pancreatic fluid surrounded by a **nonepithelialized wall of granulation tissue** and **fibrosis**^{Q}
- Pseudocysts account **75%** of **cystic lesions**^{Q} of the **pancreas**.
- **MC complication** of **chronic pancreatitis**^{Q}

> - Located anywhere from the **mediastinum** to the **scrotum**^{Q}
> - **MC site of pseudocyst: Lesser sac**^{Q}
> - **Traumatic pseudocysts** tend to occur **anterior to** the **body**^{Q} of the gland
> - **Chronic pancreatitis pseudocysts** are commonly located **within the substance** of the gland

- **Incidence of Pseudocysts:**
  - Acute pancreatitis: **10-20%** of patients^Q
  - Chronic pancreatitis: **20-40%** of patients
- **Multiple** in **17%**^{Q} cases
- **Alcohol** is MC cause of **pancreatitis related pseudocysts**^{Q}.

Pathophysiology
- **Pancreatic duct leak** with extravasation of pancreatic juice results in a pancreatic fluid collection (PFC).
- **Acute pseudocyst:** Over a period of **3 to 4 weeks**^{Q}, the PFC is sealed by an inflammatory reaction that leads to development of a wall of acute granulation tissue without much fibrosis.
- Acute pseudocysts may **resolve spontaneously** in up to **50% of cases**, over a course of **6 weeks** or longer^Q.
- **Pseudocysts >6 cm resolve less frequently** than smaller ones but may regress over a period of weeks to months^Q.

Clinical Features
- Pseudocysts usually cause symptoms of pain, fullness, or early satiety.

> - **Abdominal pain** is **MC symptom**^{Q}, occurs in up to 90% of patients
> - Other common symptoms include **early satiety**, **nausea** and **vomiting** (50% to 70%), **weight loss** (20% to 50%), **jaundice** (10%), and low-grade fever (10%)^Q

- **Physical examination:** Upper abdominal tenderness in the majority of patients, and **25-45%** will have a **palpable abdominal mass**Q.
- Symptoms of early satiety, nausea, and vomiting may be secondary to gastroduodenal obstruction caused by a mass effect of the pseudocyst.

Pseudocyst Complications (Shackelford 7th/1159)	
• **Infection (MC)**Q: **14%**	• Duodenal obstruction
• Pain due to expansion	• Rupture
• Hemorrhage: up to 10%	• Abscess

Diagnosis
- No definitive laboratory findings are available to establish a diagnosis of pancreatic pseudocyst.
- **Elevated serum amylase & lipase**Q concentrations may occur in **half** of these patients.
- **Persistently elevated amylase** after resolution of atitis should prompt investigation for a pseudocyst.
- **CECT abdomen** is **investigation of choice**Q for diagnosis of a pancreatic pseudocyst.

Treatment
- Pseudocyst 5 cm in diameter and **<6 weeks** old should be **observed**Q, as they tend to **resolve spontaneously**Q.
- Pseudocyst **>5 cm** diameter is an indications for **drainage**Q

> - If **infection** is suspected, the pseudocyst should be **aspirated**Q (not drained) by CT- or US-guided FNA, and the contents examined for organisms by Gram's stain and culture
> - If **infection** is present, and the **contents** resemble **pus**, **external drainage** is employed, using either surgical or percutaneous techniques

- Pseudocysts **communicate with the pancreatic ductal system** in up to **80% of cases**, so external drainage creates a pathway for pancreatic duct leakage to and through the catheter exit site.
- **Methods of Internal drainage:**
  - **Percutaneous** catheter-based methods (transgastric puncture and stent placement to create a cystogastrostomy)
  - **Endoscopic** methods (**transgastric** or **transduodenal puncture** and **multiple stent placements**, with or without a nasocystic irrigation catheter)
  - **Surgical methods** (a true cystoenterostomy, biopsy of cyst wall, and evacuation of all debris and contents)
- **Surgical options: Cystogastrostomy, Roux-en-Y cystojejunostomy, cystoduodenostomy.**
- **Preferred modality:** Internal drainage of cyst by **cystojejunostomy**Q

- **Cystojejunostomy** has a **slightly lower recurrence rate**, but it is associated with significantly **more blood loss** and operative time

The D'EGIDIO Classification of Pancreatic Pseudocyst				
	Context	**Pancreatic Duct**	**Duct-pseudocyst Communication**	**Treatment**
Type I	**Acute post-necrotic pancreatitis**	Normal	No	**Percutaneous drainage**
Type II	**Acute-on Chronic pancreatitis**	Abnormal (no stricture)	50:50	**Internal drainage** or **resection**
Type III	**Chronic pancreatitis**	Abnormal (**stricture**)	Yes	**Internal drainage** with **duct decompression**

HEREDITARY PANCREATITIS

Hereditary Pancreatitis

- **Autosomal dominant**Q disease
- Due to a **missense mutation** on **cationic trypsinogen**, or **PRSS1**Q (Protease, Serine 1) results in **premature, intrapancreatic activation** of **trypsinogen**.
- The incidence is **equal in both sexes**.

Clinical Features
- Characterized by **recurrent episodes** of **acute pancreatitis** or familial aggregation of chronic pancreatitis**Q**
- Typically, patients **first present in childhood** or **adolescence** with **abdominal pain** and are found to have **chronic calcific pancreatitis** on imaging studies.
- **Progressive pancreatic dysfunction** is common, and many patients present with symptoms due to **pancreatic duct obstruction**Q.
- The **risk of subsequent carcinoma formation**Q is upto 40%, **age of onset** for **carcinoma** is **>50** years old.

Clinical Pancreatic Syndromes and Associated Genetic Mutations	
• Hereditary Pancreatitis	• PRSS1^Q (Cationic trypsinogen) gene
• Idiopathic chronic Pancreatitis	• CFTR^Q
• Tropical calcific Pancreatitis	• SPINK1 (PTSI)^Q

TROPICAL (NUTRITIONAL) PANCREATITIS

Tropical (Nutritional) Pancreatitis

- Tropical chronic pancreatitis is **highly prevalent** among **adolescents** and **young adults** raised in **Indonesia, southern India**, and **tropical Africa**[Q].
- Associated with **mutations of PSTI or SPINK1 gene**[Q]
- It is subdivided into:
  - Tropical calcific pancreatitis, characterized by severe, recurrent, chronic abdominal pain and extensive pancreatic calcifications[Q].
  - Fibrocalculous pancreatic diabetes, which is characterized by significant pancreatic endocrine insufficiency[Q]

Etiopathogenesis

- **Protein-caloric malnutrition** and **toxic products** of some **indigenous foodstuffs**[Q] may contribute to the disease.

> • **Cassava root** contains **toxic glycosides**, increases susceptibility to **free radical injury** of the **pancreas**[Q]

Clinical Features

- **Abdominal pain** develops in **adolescence**, followed by the development of a **brittle form of pancreatogenic diabetes**[Q].
- **Parenchymal** and **intraductal calcifications** are seen, and the **pancreatic duct stones** may be quite large[Q].
- The **accelerated deterioration** of **endocrine and exocrine function**, the **chronic pain due to obstructive disease**, and the **recurrence of symptoms** despite decompressive procedures **characterize the course of disease**[Q].

CHRONIC PANCREATITIS

Chronic Pancreatitis

- Characterized by the **persistent inflammation** & **irreversible fibrosis** associated with **atrophy** of pancreatic parenchyma[Q].
- Associated with **chronic pain** and **endocrine & exocrine insufficiency**[Q]

> • In most cases of chronic pancreatitis, **exocrine insufficiency precedes endocrine insufficiency** by **many years**[Q]

- **Exocrine insufficiency** is more **closely related with morphologic changes**[Q].
- Approximately **90%** of **beta cell mass must be lost** before clinical **diabetes** develops.
- Classification of various causes of chronic pancreatitis based on the **TIGAR-O system**[Q] (TIGAR-O consist of toxic-metabolic, idiopathic, genetic, autoimmune, recurrent severe, obstructive).

Etiology

- **Heavy alcohol consumption** is MC cause of CP (**70-80%**)[Q]
- **Smoking increases** the **risk**[Q] of alcohol-induced CP.
- **Other causes**: Chronic duct obstruction, trauma, pancreas divisum, cystic dystrophy of the duodenal wall, **hyperparathyroidism, hypertriglyceridemia, autoimmune pancreatitis, tropical pancreatitis**, & **hereditary pancreatitis** (account for <10% of all cases)

Pathology

- **Fibrosis:** Pancreatic **stellate cells** become activated and **proliferate** and transform into myofibroblast-like cells.
- **Stone Formation:** Pancreatic stones are composed largely of **calcium carbonate crystals**[Q]

Clinical Features

- **Classic triad**: DM + Pancreatic calcification + Steatorrhea **(DPS)**
- **Abdominal pain** is the primary manifestation and **MC symptom** of CP[Q].
- **Intensity, frequency,** & **duration** of pain gradually **increase with worsening disease**[Q].
- Pancreatic **inflammation** and **fibrosis** decrease the number & function of acinar cells.

> • At least **90%** of the **gland** needs to be **dysfunctional** before **steatorrhea, diarrhea**, and other symptoms of **malabsorption** develop[Q]
> • **Exocrine insufficiency** occurs in 80-90% of patients with **long-standing CP**[Q]

- **Diabetes** is developed in **40-80%** of patients, typically occurs **many years after** the onset of **abdominal pain** and **pancreatic exocrine insufficiency**[Q].

Diagnosis

- **X-ray abdomen: Diffuse pancreatic calcification** is seen in **30-40%** cases of CP[Q]

  - **CT scan**: **Dilated pancreatic duct** (68%), **parenchymal atrophy** (54%), & **pancreatic calcifications**[Q] (50%). Other findings include peripancreatic fluid, focal pancreatic enlargement, biliary duct dilation, and irregular pancreatic parenchyma contour

- **MRI**: Detect changes in the pancreatic parenchyma suggestive of chronic inflammation, such as changes in intensity, pancreatic atrophy, and irregularities in the contour.
- **MRCP** with **secretin injection**: To evaluate **intraductal strictures** and **pancreatic duct disruption**[Q].

  - **ERCP**: Considered the **gold standard** for the diagnosis of CP, the advent of **secretin MRCP** and **EUS** have **significantly decreased its role** as a **diagnostic test**[Q]

- **Indications of ERCP**: Other diagnostic tests are **contraindicated** or **have failed** to corroborate the diagnosis. ERCP should be considered a **therapeutic modalities** in patients who develop **pancreatic duct complications** amenable to endoscopic therapy, such as **stricture, stone, pseudocysts,** and **biliary stenosis**.
- **EUS**: **Most accurate technique** to diagnose CP in patients with **minimal-change disease** or in the **early stages**[Q].

  - **Rosemont criteria**[Q]: Criteria on EUS required **to diagnose chronic pancreatitis**

- Measurement of the **fecal elastase-1** level is the **preferred noninvasive study** to **diagnose pancreatic exocrine insufficiency**[Q].
- **Steatorrhea**: If the **stool fat** content **exceeds 7 gm/day**[Q]

Treatment

- Patients should be strongly encouraged to stop drinking and smoking.
- **NSAIDs** are the first line of treatment, patients with severe pain should be treated with potent long-acting **narcotics**[Q].
- **Pancreatic enzyme replacement**[Q] in patients with pancreatic exocrine insufficiency.
- **ERCP**: Primary modality for **treating symptomatic pancreatic duct obstruction** with **dilation and polyethylene stent placement**[Q].
- **Endoscopic stone extraction** should be considered for patients with **pain and pancreatic duct dilation secondary to stones**[Q].

  - Patients with a **dilated pancreatic duct** (diameter **>7 mm**) require a **decompressing procedure** and patients with **normal pancreatic duct** require a **resectional procedure**[Q]

Cambridge Criteria for Chronic Pancreatitis on ERCP	
Stage	**Typical Changes**
Normal	**Normal** appearance of side branches and main pancreatic duct
Equivocal	**Dilatation/obstruction** of **< 3 side branches**; normal main pancreatic duct
Mild	Dilatation/obstruction of **> 3** side branches; normal main pancreatic duct
Moderate	Additional **stenosis** and **dilatation of main pancreatic duct**
Severe	Additional **obstructions, cysts, stenosis** of main pancreatic duct; **calculi**

RESECTION PROCEDURES IN CHRONIC PANCREATITIS

Resection Procedures in Chronic Pancreatitis

- It is believed that **inflammatory process** in the **pancreatic head** controls both the severity of symptoms and further progression of disease in remainder of the gland
- **Pancreatic head** is **pacemaker of chronic pancreatitis**[Q].
- Because of this **resection of pancreatic head** has been shown to **completely relieve** the **pain** of chronic pancreatitis in **70-80%**[Q] patients.
- **Distal pancreatectomy** is the ideal procedure for patients whose **chronic pancreatitis** is confined to **pancreatitis tail**[Q].
- Usually, **distal pancreatectomy** is combined **with splenectomy** for technical reasons, but spleen can be preserved if its vascular supply is secure.

Surgical Procedures in Chronic Pancreatitis	
Drainage Procedure	**Resection Procedure**
• **Puestow Procedure**[Q] (Longitudinal Pancreaticojejunostomy): **Resection of** the **tail** followed by a longitudinal pancreaticojejunostomy[Q] • **Partington** and **Rochelle Modification** of **Puestow Procedure**: **Elimination** of the **resection** of the **pancreatic tail**[Q]. • **Duval Procedure**: Distal pancreatectomy with Roux-en-Y pancreaticojejunostomy (**caudal PJ**)[Q]	• **Beger's Procedure** (Duodenal Preserving Pancreatic Head Resection **DPPHR**[Q]) • **Warren's modification** of Beger's procedure • **Frey's Procedure** (Local Resection of the Head of the Pancreas Combined with Longitudinal Pancreaticojejunostomy **LR-LPJ**)[Q] • **Berne modification**: (Combines some aspects of **Beger's** and **Frey's**) • **Hamburg modification of Frey's**

SURGICAL PROCEDURES IN CHRONIC PANCREATITIS

- Ideal procedure: DPPHR^Q (Beger's)
- In presence of **portal vein thrombosis**: **Frey's**^Q
- **Small duct disease**: **V-shaped excision**^Q
- **Disease recurrence** in **body** and **tail** (after DPPHR, Whipples or Longmire-Traverso procedure): **V-shaped drainage**^Q
- **Disease limited to tail**: Spleen-preserving **distal pancreatectomy**^Q

SEROUS CYSTADENOMA OF PANCREAS

SEROUS CYSTADENOMA OF PANCREAS

- SCNs usually occur in the **head**^Q of the pancreas; Affect **women** almost **exclusively**^Q
- Most are **benign** and have **no malignant potential**^Q

Pathology
- SCNs are **large**^Q, well-circumscribed masses (**microcystic**)
- Microscopic examination reveals **multiloculated**, **glycogen-rich** small cysts^Q
- Typically have **small cyst**^Q filled with clear fluid with **spongelike** or **honeycomb appearance**^Q.

Clinical Features
- Most are **asymptomatic**^Q
- Patients commonly present with **vague abdominal pain**^Q and less frequently with weight loss & obstructive jaundice.

Diagnosis
- Aspiration from cyst yields **non-viscous fluid** with **low CEA & low amylase** levels^Q.

> - **Central calcification** gives rise to a characteristic **central sunburst**^Q, **radial**, or **stellate scar pattern** on **CT scan**^Q (10-20%)

Treatment
- SCN is benign, **resection** is indicated when **diagnosis** is **in doubt** or when they become **symptomatic**^Q, size > 4 cm

MUCINOUS CYSTADENOMA OF PANCREAS

MUCINOUS CYSTADENOMA OF PANCREAS

- MCN: **MC cystic neoplasm**^Q of the pancreas
- Frequently seen in **young women**, mean age **5th decade**^Q; More common in the **body & tail** of the pancreas

Pathology
- MCNs contain **mucin-producing epithelium**^Q, **macrocystic**
- Histology: Presence of **mucin-rich cells** and **ovarian-like stroma**^Q
- Estrogen & progesterone staining are positive in most cases^Q

Clinical Features
- Up to **50%** of patients present with **vague abdominal pain**.
- A **history of pancreatitis** may be found in up to **20%** of patients, which explains the common misdiagnosis of pseudocyst.

Diagnosis
- CT scan: Presence of a **solitary cyst** with **fine septations & rim of calcification**^Q
- **Cross-sectional imaging** may **not** be able to **distinguish** between **benign** and **malignant MCNs**

> - Presence of **eggshell calcification**, **larger** tumor **size**, or a **mural nodule** on cross-sectional imaging is **suggestive of malignancy**^Q
> - Cyst fluid analyses: **Mucin-rich** aspirate, **high CEA** & **low amylase** levels^Q

Treatment
- **Surgical excision** is indicated for **all mucinous cystic neoplams**^Q
- **Pancreatic resection** is the **standard treatment** for MCNs^Q.

INTRADUCTAL PAPILLARY MUCINOUS NEOPLASM (IPMN)

INTRADUCTAL PAPILLARY MUCINOUS NEOPLASM

- IPMN is also known as **mucin-secreting carcinoma**^{Q}, villous adenoma of the duct of Wirsung
- Seen in **6th to 7th** decade of life; **Equal sex distribution**^{Q}
- More common in **head & uncinate process**^{Q} of the pancreas

Types of IPMN
- Side branch IPMN: Involves dilation of the pancreatic duct side **branches**
- Main duct IPMN: Abnormal cystic dilation of the **main pancreatic duct**
- Mixed-type IPMN: **Side branch** IPMN that has extended to **involve** the **main pancreatic duct**

Pathology
- **Ductal epithelium** forms a **papillary projection** into the duct
- **Mucin production** causes **intraluminal cystic dilation**^{Q} of the pancreatic ducts
- Careful histologic examination of the entire specimen (**invasive component** in 35-40%)^Q

Clinical Features
- Present with **abdominal pain** or **recurrent pancreatitis**, (caused by obstruction of pancreatic duct by **thick mucin**^{Q}).
- Some patients (5-10%) have **steatorrhea, diabetes,** & **weight loss** secondary to pancreatic insufficiency.

> - **Predictors of malignancy:** Jaundice, elevated serum ALP, mural nodules, diabetes, & main pancreatic **duct diameter ≥ 7 mm**^{Q}

Diagnosis
- **Endoscopy:** Mucus extruding through a large, **fish-mouth** like papillary orifice is **virtually diagnostic of IPMN**^{Q}
- **CT scans:** Dilated main pancreatic duct, cysts of varying sizes, and possibly **mural nodules**^{Q}
- **Aspirated fluid:** Mucinous content with **elevated CEA & amylase level**^{Q}

> **Pre-operative localization is problematic in IPMN**
> - **Over production of mucous**, dilation can occur **proximal & distal** to the tumor^Q
> - **Propensity** of tumor **to spread microscopically** along the duct^Q

Treatment
- **Partial pancreatectomy:** For main duct, symptomatic, and **large branch-type IPMNs (>3 cm)**, or IPMNs with an **invasive component**^{Q}
- **Observation:** For **asymptomatic small** (< 3 cm) **branch duct IPMNs** without **associated nodularity**.

RISK FACTORS FOR PANCREATIC CARCINOMA

RISK FACTORS FOR PANCREATIC CARCINOMA

- There is **association** between risk of **pancreatic cancer, H. pylori** colonization, and **ABO** blood groups^Q.
- Older age, African American race, low socioeconomic status, Ashkenazic jewish heritage are associated with increased risk of pancreatic cancer.
- **Host etiologic factors** associated with increased risk of pancreatic cancer include history of **diabetes mellitus, chronic cirrhosis** and **pancreatitis,** a **high fat** or **cholesterol diet,** and **prior cholecystectomy**^{Q}.

> **Familial Pancreatic Cancer**
> - **Predisposing Conditions: H**ereditary pancreatitis, HNPCC, **H**ereditary Breast Cancer associated with the BRCA2 mutation, **A**taxia Telangiectasia, **F**AMMM, and **P**eutz-Jegher syndrome. (**H3-AFP**)^Q
> - **BRCA-2 mutation** is the **MC germline mutation** in patients with **hereditary pancreatic cancer**^{Q}
> - **K-ras** is the **MC somatic mutation** in patients with **carcinoma pancreas**^{Q}
> - **Peutz-Jegher syndrome** carries the **highest relative risk** of **pancreatic cancer**^{Q}
> - Patients with pancreatic cancer with **DNA mismatch repair mutations** have a **better prognosis**
> - **K-ras mutations** & **HER2/neu over expression** are the **earliest changes** to occur

Risk Factors for Pancreatic Carcinoma			
Established	Tobacco^Q	Inherited susceptibility^Q	
Associated	Chronic pancreatitis^Q	Diabetes mellitus type 2^Q	Obesity^Q
Possible	Physical inactivity^Q	Certain pesticides	High carbohydrate/sugar intake

Genetic Mutation in Pancreatic Cancer (KRAP-16: K-ras >p16))	
Gene	Pancreatic Cancer %
• p16^Q	• 82
• K-ras^Q	• 95-100 (MC)
• p53^Q	• 75
• DPC4	• 55
• BRCA2	• 7

Predisposing Conditions for Familial Pancreatic Cancer (H₃-AFP)	
• Hereditary pancreatitis^Q	• Ataxia Telangiectasia^Q
• HNPCC^Q	• FAMMM (Familial atypical multiple mole melanoma) syndrome^Q
• Hereditary Breast Cancer associated with the BRCA2 mutation^Q	• Peutz-Jegher syndrome^Q **(Highest risk)**

CARCINOMA PANCREAS

CARCINOMA PANCREAS

- MC type is **pancreatic ductal adenocarcinoma (PDAC)**^Q; MC site: **Head (75%) > Body (15%) >Tail (10%)**^Q
- More common in **Men, African Americans**, mean age at diagnosis is **72 years**^Q

  - **Association** between risk of **pancreatic cancer, H. pylori** colonization, and **ABO** blood groups
  - **Established risk factors**: Smoking (Tobacco) and Inherited susceptibility^Q

- **Hereditary risk factors:** Hereditary pancreatitis, HNPCC, Hereditary Breast Cancer associated with the BRCA2 mutation, Ataxia Telangiectasia, FAMMM, and Peutz-Jegher syndrome. **(H3-AFP)**^Q

  - **K-ras2** oncogene is **activated** (by point mutation) in >95% of pancreatic cancers **(MC gene mutation)**^Q

Pathology

- Macroscopically, ductal adenocarcinoma is a **scirrhous (scar forming)**^Q type of carcinoma
- It is associated with **abundant desmoplastic stroma**^Q, in which the **neoplastic glands** are **widely scattered**^Q

Clinical Features

- MC symptom for patients with PDACs in the periampullary region is **jaundice**^Q.
- **Pain** typically arising in epigastrium & radiating to the back.
- **Weight loss** affecting more than 50% of individuals.
- For tumors of **body** & **tail** of pancreas, **pain** & **weight loss** become more common at presentation.
- A **palpable distended gallbladder** in **1/3rd of patients** with periampullary PDAC **(Courvoisier Law)**^Q
- With widespread disease, a left supraclavicular node **(Virchow's node)**^Q may be palpable. Periumbilical lymphadenopathy may be palpable **(Sister Mary Joseph's node)**^Q.
- In cases of **peritoneal dissemination**, perirectal tumor involvement may be palpable via DRE, referred to as **Blumer's shelf**^Q.

Presenting Symptoms of Periampullary Tumors	
• **Jaundice (75%)**^Q	• Pruritus (11%)
• **Weight loss (51%)**^Q	• Fever (3%)
• **Abdominal pain (39%)**	• Gastrointestinal bleeding (1%)
• Nausea/vomiting (13%)	

Diagnosis

- Tumor markers: **CA19-9 (most sensitive)**^Q & **CEA**.

  - Individuals with **blood Lewis antigen–negative status (10-15%)** do **not** develop **elevation of** the **CA19-9**

- **MDCT** is **investigation of choice** for the evaluation of **lesions arising** in the **pancreas**^Q.

  - **ERCP:** Reserved for cases requiring **therapeutic** or **palliative intervention**^Q
  - **Double duct sign** on ERCP is highly suggestive of **pancreatic head cancer**^Q

- **EUS:** For identifying lesions **<2 cm**^Q that do not appear on CT scans
- **Tissue diagnosis** is **not necessary prior to** routine **resection**^Q.

Treatment

- **Surgical resection** remains the **only potentially curative treatment** of pancreas cancer.

• Tumors of **head** of the pancreas	• **Pylorus preserving pancreaticoduodenectomy or Longmire-Traverso procedure** is preferred[Q]
• Tumors of **body & tail** of the pancreas	• **Distal pancreatectomy and en-bloc splenectomy**[Q]

- MC complication of pancreaticoduodenectomy is delayed gastric emptying[Q]
- MC cause of **death** following **pancreaticoduodenectomy** is cardiopulmonary complications[Q].
- Most important predictor of post-operative survival is R0 resection.
- Most important margin in pancreaticoduodenectomy is retroperitoneal or uncinate margin[Q].

Palliative Therapy for Pancreatic Cancer	
• Biliary obstruction	• **ERCP** with **metal stent placement (Best)**[Q] • Roux-en-Y hepaticojejunostomy
• Gastric outlet obstruction	• **Endoscopic stenting (Preferred)**[Q] • Double bypass (Roux-en-Y hepaticojejunostomy + gastrojejunostomy)
• Pain	• **NSAIDs** or **opiates**[Q] • **Celiac nerve block**[Q]

Chemotherapy

- **Gemcitabine**[Q] is currently the standard of care for patients with **metastatic pancreatic cancer**.

Prognosis

- **Five-year** survival **after curative resection** (pancreaticoduodenectomy) approaches **15-20%**[Q].
- Overall, 5 year survival rate **with pancreatic cancer** is **5%**[Q].

Median Survival in Carcinoma Pancreas	
• **Resectable** disease (stage **I** and **II**)	• **15-20** months[Q]
• **Locally advanced** disease (stage **III**)	• **6-10** months[Q]
• **Metastatic** disease (stage **IV**)	• **3-6** months[Q]

- But in specific patients a **tissue diagnosis** may be **needed** such as in **patients entering** a **clinical trial, prior to neoadjuvant chemotherapy**, and **prior to chemotherapy** in **advanced tumors**. In these patients, an EUS is highly accurate.

Indications for Staging Laparoscopy (Routine use of laparoscopy is not warranted)	
1. **Tumor >3 cm** in diameter[Q]	3. **Equivocal findings** of metastasis on CT[Q]
2. **Body** or **tail tumors**[Q]	4. **CA19-9** levels **>100 U/mL**[Q]

TNM CLASSIFICATION OF PANCREATIC CANCER

8th AJCC (2017) TNM Classification of Pancreatic Cancer	
Tis	Carcinoma in situ
T1	Tumor limited to pancreas **upto 2 cm** in greatest dimension
	T1a: Tumor **≤0.5 cm** in greatest dimension
	T1b: Tumor **>0.5 cm** but **≤1 cm** in greatest dimension
	T1c: Tumor **>1 cm** but **≤2 cm** in greatest dimension
T2	Tumor limited to pancreas **>2-4 cm** in greatest dimension
T3	Tumor **>4 cm** in greatest dimension
T4	Tumor involves **celiac axis**, **superior mesenteric artery** and/or **common hepatic artery**
N1	Metastasis in **1-3** regional LN
N2	Metastasis in **4 or more** regional LN
M1	Distant metastasis

Stage 0	Stage IA	Stage IB	Stage IIA	Stage IIB	Stage III	Stage IV
Tis N0 M0	**T1** N0 M0	**T2** N0 M0	**T3** N0 M0	**T1-T3 N1** M0	**T1-T3 N2** M0 **T4** AnyN M0	Any T AnyN **M1**

CARCINOMA PANCREAS: TREATMENT

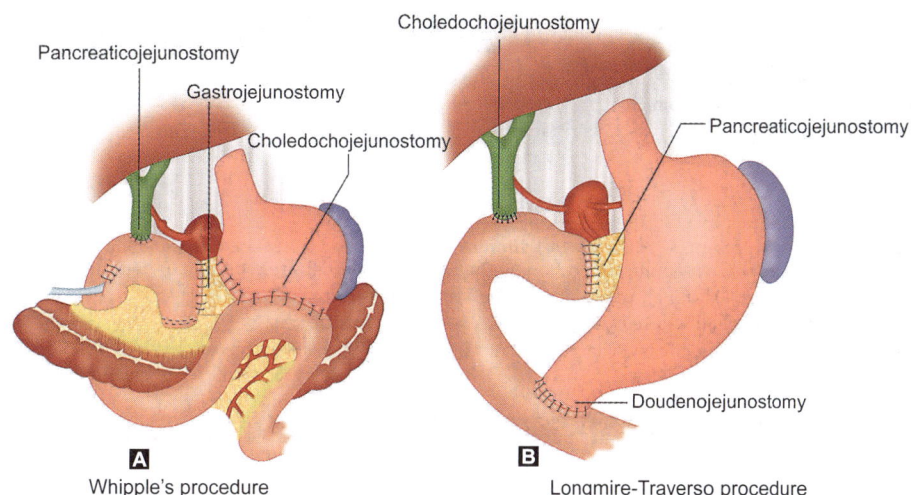

A. Whipple's procedure
B. Longmire-Traverso procedure

WHIPPLE'S PROCEDURE (PANCREATICODUODENECTOMY)

- It consists of complete **removal of the pancreatic** and **hepatoduodenal ligament lymph nodes**, the **duodenum with a short segment of the proximal jejunum** and the **distal half to two-thirds of the stomach with the right half of the greater omentum**.

Whipple's Procedure Involves Resection of	
• Distal stomach[Q]	• Duodenum[Q]
• Gallbladder[Q]	• Proximal jejunum[Q]
• CBD[Q]	• Regional lymphatics
• Head of pancreas[Q]	

Restoration of GI Continuity Requires
• Pancreaticojejunostomy[Q] • Hepaticojejunostomy[Q] • Gastrojejunostomy[Q]

- Pylorus Preserving Pancreaticoduodenectomy (PPPD) or Longmire-Traverso procedure is the **preferred surgery** for **carcinoma head** of **pancreas**[Q].
- The **Whipple procedure** is now **reserved for situations** in which the **entire duodenum has to be removed** (e.g. in FAP) or where the **tumour encroaches** on the **1st part** of the **duodenum** or the **distal stomach** and a **PPPD would not achieve a clear resection margin**[Q].

Pylorus Preserving Pancreaticoduodenectomy or Longmire-Traverso Procedure
- To retain a functioning pylorus, the entire stomach and 2cm of the first part of duodenum and their neurovascular supply are preserved[Q].
- Pylorus Preserving Pancreaticoduodenectomy (PPPD) or Longmire-Traverso procedure is the **preferred surgery** for **carcinoma head** of **pancreas**[Q].

SOLID PSEUDOPAPILLARY TUMOR (PAPILLARY CYSTIC CANCER OR FRANTZ TUMOR)

SOLID PSEUDOPAPILLARY TUMOR (PAPILLARY CYSTIC CANCER OR FRANTZ TUMOR)

- Approximately **90%** of solid pseudopapillary tumor harbor **APC/beta-catenin mutation**[Q].
- Regarded as **low grade malignant potential**[Q] tumor.

Pathology
- Lesions may be **large, encapsulated, evenly distributed**[Q] throughout the pancreas.
- **Strongly positive** for **beta-catenin, progesterone receptors, vimentin, CD-10** and **CD-56**[Q].
- It can mimic the histologic appearance of NET but **lacks** the **nuclear features** of NET and **lacks** the neuroendocerine markers such as **chromagranin and synaptophysin**.

Clinical Features
- **Non-specific** signs and symptoms related to size of tumor at the time of presentation
- Typically occur in **women** in the **second** or **third decade**[Q] of life

Diagnosis
- CT scan: **Hypodense** areas representing **hemorrhage or necrosis**
- **Diagnosis is based on** presence of typical histological characteristics such as **foamy macrophages, cholesterol clefts, nuclear grooves, and aggregate of hyaline globules**[Q].

Treatment
- **Complete resection** is associated with **long-term survival**[Q] even in presence of metastatic disease.
- **Incomplete removal** result in **local recurrence**.

NEURO ENDOCRINE TUMORS (NET) OF PANCREAS

NET of Pancreas

- MC NET of Pancreas: Non-functional (Mostly malignant) >Insulinoma^Q
- MC benign NET of Pancreas: Insulinoma^Q
- MC malignant functional NET of Pancreas: Gastrinoma^Q

Localization of NET of Pancreas

- **Somatostatin receptors** are present in **>90% of gastrinomas**; in contrast, pancreatic adenocarcinomas do not possess somatostatin receptors. They are **also present in** a significant portion of **glucagonomas** and **nonfunctioning endocrine tumors**^{Q}.
- The **sensitivity for SRS** is **over 80%** for all pancreatic NET excluding insulinomas^Q
- SRS has an **overall sensitivity** of **80% to 100%** and **specificity >90%** for **gastrinomas**^{Q}.
- SRS is also **useful for detecting hepatic metastases** from **noninsulinoma endocrine tumors**

INSULINOMA

Insulinoma

- Insulinoma is **MC functioning tumor** of the **endocrine pancreas**^{Q}
- The average age at diagnosis is **45 years**.

Location of Insulinoma
• **97%** in **pancreas** (**equal distribution** in the head, body, and tail)^Q
• **3%** in **duodenum, splenic hilum,** or **gastrocolic ligament**^{Q}

- **Typically small**, with an average size of **1.0 to 1.5 cm**.
- **Diagnostic hallmark is Whipple's triad**: **Symptoms** of hypoglycemia + **Low blood glucose** levels (40-50 mg/dL) + **Relief of symptoms** after the administration of **glucose**^{Q}.

Clinical Features

- **Diagnostic hallmark is Whipple's triad**^{Q}: Fasting-induced **neuroglyopenic symptoms** of hypoglycemia (diaphoresis, shaking, mental confusion, obtundation, and seizures), **low blood glucose** levels (40 to 50 mg/dL), and **relief of symptoms** after the administration of glucose.
- **Sympathetic overactivity**^{Q} in response to hypoglycemia: Fatigue, weakness, fearfulness, hunger, tremor, diaphoresis, and tachycardia.
- **CNS disturbance**: Apathy, irritability, anxiety, confusion, excitement, loss of orientation, blurred vision, delirium, stupor, coma, and/or seizures.
- **Significant weight gain**: Patients eat frequently to prevent hypoglycemia.
- It is a **painless condition**.

Diagnosis

- **Gold standard test** for the **diagnosis** of insulinoma is the **72-hour fasting**^{Q} test
- An **insulin-to-glucose** ratio **> 0.4** is consistent with **insulinoma**^{Q}

- Provocative testing with **tolbutamide, glucagon**; or **intravenous calcium** is rarely required.
- **CECT** or **MRI**: Hyperattenuating as compared with surrounding pancreatic tissue because of **rich vascular supply**^{Q}

Localization

- **Angiography** will detect approximately **70%** of **insulinomas >5 mm**, showing a characteristic **vascular blush**^{Q}

- **Portal venous sampling** for insulin with or without **arterial stimulation** with **calcium** is the **best pre-operative method** of **localization**^{Q}
- **EUS** with **intra-operative palpation** is **best localization technique** for **Insulinoma**^{Q}

Treatment

- **Diazoxide** decreases beta cell release of insulin, used to prevent or attenuate symptoms of hypoglycemia prior to surgical intervention once the diagnosis is made^Q.
- Insulinomas are well suited for **laparoscopic resection** or **enucleations**^{Q}.

• **Insulinoma** of **head** of pancreas	• **Enucleation** is TOC^Q
• **Insulinoma** of **body** or **tail** of pancreas	• **Distal pancreatectomy** is TOC^Q

- **Streptozotocin,** with or without **5-fluorouracil**, is associated with **improved survival in metastatic pancreatic endocrine tumors**^{Q}.

GASTRINOMA/ZOLLINGER-ELLISON SYNDROME

ZOLLINGER-ELLISON SYNDROME

- Gastrinoma is **MC functioning malignant**^{Q} pancreatic endocrine tumor.
- **More common in men**, mean age **50 years**^{Q}
- ZES occur in **two forms: Sporadic (75%) & MEN-1 association (25%)**^{Q}
- Those associated with **MEN-1** are almost always **multiple, early onset**, more common in **duodenum**^{Q}

> - **MC site** of Gastrinoma: **Duodenum > Pancreas**^{Q}
> - **Duodenal primary** tends to spread to **local lymph nodes**^{Q}
> - **Pancreatic primary** tends to spread to the **liver**

- All gastrinomas also produce **chromagranin A**^{Q}

> - Gastrinoma → increased gastrin secretion → marked gastric **acid hypersecretion** → Peptic ulcer

Location

- MC site is **duodenum (50-70%)** followed by **Pancreas (20-40%)**^{Q}
- In **Duodenum**, MC in **1st part**^{Q} (71%) > 2nd part (21%) > 3rd part (8%)
- About **70-90%** of gastrinomas are located **within** the **Passaro's triangle**^{Q}.

> **Boundaries of Passaro's Triangle**
> - **Junction** of **cystic duct** and **CBD**^{Q}
> - **Junction** of **2nd & 3rd part** of **duodenum**^{Q}
> - **Junction** of **neck & body** of **pancreas**

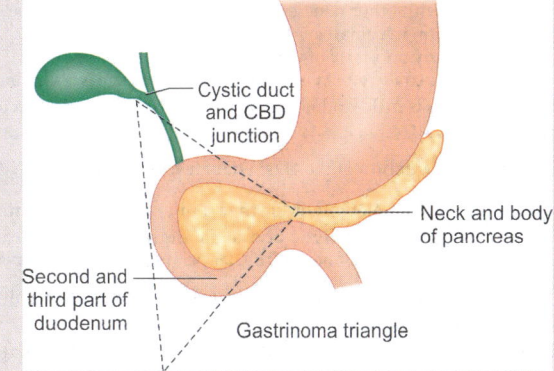

Clinical Features

- Gastric acid hypersecretion causes **peptic ulcer disease** often **refractory severe diarrhea**
- **MC presenting symptoms** are **abdominal pain**^{Q} (70-100%), **diarrhea** (50-70%) & **GERD** (30-35%).
- **Causes of Diarrhea:** Inability of the intestinal tract to absorb the **large volumes** of **fluid secreted** by the **stomach**, **acid-induced injury** to the mucosa of the upper **small intestine**, precipitation of bile salts, inactivation of pancreatic lipase by low pH

> - **Unique characteristic** of acid-induced diarrhea: **Halted by nasogastric aspiration** of gastric secretions^Q

- Most patients have peptic ulcers (MC are **duodenal ulcers**)^Q
- ZES must be excluded in all patients with intractable peptic ulcers, severe esophagitis, or persistent secretory diarrhea.
- MC cause of death in ZES: **Liver metastasis**^{Q}

Diagnosis

- **Hypergastrinemia** with **increased secretion of gastric acid** confirms the diagnosis
- Elevated gastrin alone is not sufficient to diagnose ZES (**Basal gastric acid hypersecretion** must be demonstrated).

> **Zollinger-Ellison Syndrome**
> - 100% patients will have a fasting serum gastrin level >100 pg/mL
> - **BAO >15 mEq/hr** in most patients and **>5 mEq/hr** in patients with **prior surgery** to decrease gastric acid secretion
> - Levels **>1000 pg/mL** are **diagnostic**^{Q}

- Elevated serum gastrin level with a **pH <2** in the gastric aspirate is **almost diagnostic** of ZES^Q.

Provocative Test in Gastrinoma

- If the **diagnosis is in doubt**, the **provocative tests** are highly useful.
- Provocative diagnostic tests for ZES:
  - Secretin stimulation test
  - Bombesin test
  - Calcium stimulation test
  - Protein meal test
  - Secretin-plus-calcium stimulation test
- **Secretin provocation test is best.**

> - **Secretin Provocation Test**: An increase of **>200 pg/mL** in the **gastrin value** after administration of secretin is **diagnostic**^{Q}

Localization
- Somatostatin receptor scintigraphy (**SRS**) is **imaging test of choice** for **localizing** both **primary** and **metastatic gastrinomas**^Q.

Treatment
- **Acid secretion** is controlled by **PPIs**^Q
- Pharmacologic control of acid secretion with PPIs has rendered **total gastrectomy** and other surgical acid-reducing procedures **unnecessary**^Q.

> - **ZES in MEN-1**: **Hyperparathyroidism** should be **treated first** because it can complicate the management of their gastrinoma, **neck exploration** should be performed **before resection** of **gastrinoma**^Q.

- **Distal pancreatectomy**: Gastrinoma involving **body** or **tail**^Q of pancreas
- **Pancreaticoduodenectomy**: Gastrinoma involving **head**^Q of pancreas

Prognosis
- **Best predictor** of survival for patients with gastrinoma is the **presence of liver metastases**^Q
- **LN metastases** are **not predictive**^Q
- **Resection** of all **gross disease and metastases** may provide **palliation** of symptoms and may **prolong survival**^Q.

GLUCAGONOMA

GLUCAGONOMA (HYPERGLYCEMIC CUTANEOUS SYNDROME)

- Compared with other pancreatic NET, they tend to be **larger**^Q, averaging **5-10 cm**^Q in **size** at the time of diagnosis.
- More common in **females**; 70% are **malignant**^Q.
- **MC site: Body** and **tail**^Q of pancreas.
- Tumors are usually >3 cm in diameter and are **highly vascular (tumor blush)**^Q.
- The **diabetes** is **mild** and **not associated** with diabetic **ketoacidosis** because insulin secretion by beta cell is preserved^Q.

Clinical Features
- **Classic presentation** of the 4Ds: **Diabetes, dermatitis, DVT,** and **depression**^Q.

> - **Necrolytic erythema migrans** are MC **manifestations** of the disease, seen in **2/3rd** of **patients**^Q.
> - **Necrolytic erythema migrans**: The characteristic rash occur in **areas of friction**; rash is **migratory, red,** and **scaling,** associated with **intense pruritus**^Q

- **Parenteral administration** of **amino acids** was found to result in the **disappearance** of the **skin lesions**^Q
- **Deep vein thrombosis** occurs in **30%**^Q of patients.
- Neurologic manifestations include ataxia, dementia, scotomata, and proximal muscle weakness.

Diagnosis
- **Fasting glucagon** level >50 pmol/L is considered **diagnostic**^Q.
- **VIPomas, glucagonomas**, and **somatostatinomas** are usually **larger** and **easily localized** by **CT**^Q.
- **SRS** can be performed **if CT is not informative**.

Treatment
- **Resection** is the **treatment of choice** for **VIPomas, glucagonomas, somatostatinomas**, and **nonfunctional pancreatic NET** and remains the **only curative option**^Q.
- **Dacarbazine** is **uniquely effective** against **glucagonoma**^Q as compared with other pancreatic NET and complete remission has been reported in several cases.

PPOMAS/NON-FUNCTIONING PANCREATIC ENDOCRINE TUMOR

PPomas/Non-functioning Pancreatic Endocrine Tumor

- Approximately **10-25%** of all neuroendocrine pancreatic tumors are **nonfunctional**^Q.
- Tumors are **large (>5 cm)** and almost all (80%) are **malignant** and **metastatic**;
- Usually **solitary**, mostly in the **head**^Q

Clinical Feature
- Plasma elevation of PP is not associated with specific symptom.

Diagnosis
- Elevated plasma levels of **chromagranin A** and **B** are found in **69-100%**^Q of patients; **neuron specific enolase** in 31%; **PP** in 50-75%; alpha-HCG in 40%; beta-HCG in 20%.
- **Atropine Suppression Test:** Atropine (1 mg intramuscularly) **does not suppress** the levels of **plasma PP with PETs** but did suppress the level by 50% or more in all patients without tumors.
- **Adenocarcinoma** can be **distinguished** from NETs **by** immunohistochemical staining with **chromagranin A**^Q.

Treatment

- Mostly located in the **head** of the pancreas and require a **pancreaticoduodenectomy**.
- **Dopamine agonists decrease** circulating levels of **PP** and **chromogranin A** in patients with **large, unresectable** islet cell **tumors**[Q].

VIPOMAS (VERNER-MORRISON SYNDROME)

VIPomas (Verner-Morrison Syndrome)

- Also known as WDHA syndrome (**w**atery **d**iarrhea, **h**ypokalemia, **a**chlorhydria) or **pancreatic cholera**[Q]
- Usually **solitary**; MC site is **tail of pancreas**[Q]
- **Two-thirds** are **malignant**[Q].

Clinical Features

- Diagnostic triad: Secretary diarrhea + **High** levels of circulating **VIP** + **Pancreatic tumor**[Q].
- **Profuse, watery, iso-osmotic secretary diarrhea** is **MC presenting symptom** and may exceed a volume of 3 to 5 liters/day.
- The **diarrhea persists despite fasting**, which qualifies it as a secretory diarrhea and, **despite nasogastric aspiration,** which differentiates it from the diarrhea of ZES.

> - Characterized by: **Hypokalemia, hypercalcemia**, **hypochlorhydria** & **hyperglycemia**[Q].

- The **tetany** has been attributed to **hypomagnesemia** from chronic diarrhea.

Diagnosis

- **Constant features** are **diarrhea, hypovolemia, hypokalemia** and **acidosis**, variable features are **achlorhydria** or hypochlorhydria, **hyperglycemia** and **flushing with rash**[Q].
- **VIPomas, glucagonomas,** and **somatostatinomas** are usually **larger** & easily **localized** by **CT**[Q].

Treatment

- **Aggressive preoperative hydration** and **correction of electrolyte abnormalities** & acid-base disturbances[Q].
- **Octreotide** is commonly used preperatively **to reduce diarrhea volume** and facilitate fluid & electrolyte replacement.
- **Resection** is the **treatment of choice** for **VIPomas, glucagonomas, somatostatinomas,** and **nonfunctional pancreatic NET** and remains the **only curative option**[Q].

SOMATOSTATINOMA

Somatostatinoma

- **MC site** is **head** of the **pancreas**[Q].
- Most somatostatinomas are **solitary** and located within the **pancreatic head (MC)**[Q] or duodenum
- **Equally common** in males and females, of about **50 years**.

Clinical Features

- Somatostatin excess causes **steatorrhea** (30-68%), **mild diabetes** (60%), **cholelithiasis** (70%), and **hypochlorhydria** (86%)[Q].

Diagnosis

- **VIPomas, glucagonomas,** and **somatostatinomas** are usually **larger** and easily **localized** by **CT**[Q].

Treatment

- **Resection** is the **treatment of choice** for **VIPomas, glucagonomas, somatostatinomas,** and **nonfunctional pancreatic NET** and remains the **only curative option**[Q].
- In **75% cases**, somatostatinomas are **metastatic** and **>5 cm** at the time of diagnosis.
- **Whipple's procedure** in localized tumor is curative.
- In unresectable disease, **octreotide** and **interferon alfa** may improve symptoms.

Neurotensinoma

- Neurotensinoma cause **hypokalemia**, weight loss, **hypotension**, **cyanosis**, flushing and **diabetes**[Q].
- They are usually **malignant**[Q].

GRFoma

- It occurs **most often in** the **lung** (**bronchus**)^Q, then pancreas, jejunum, adrenal glands and retroperitoneum.
- Patient presents with **acromegaly** and a **pancreatic mass**^{Q}.
- **Pancreatic GRFomas** are **large** (>6 cm).
- One third will have metastasized at the time of diagnosis.
- Approximately **50%** of patients with GRFomas also have **ZES** and **33%** have **MEN-1**.

PANCREATIC TRAUMA

Pancreatic Trauma

- Pancreatic injuries are uncommon.
- **Penetrating injuries** into the abdomen are the **MC injuries** seen in **adults**^{Q}.
- Isolated pancreatic injuries are not common.
- Up to 90% of patients present with associated hepatic, gastric, splenic, renal, colonic, or vascular lesions.
- **MC associated injury** is to a **hollow viscus (38%)**^{Q}; followed by the liver (19%); and spleen (11%).

Pancreatic Trauma in Children

- **MC mechanism** in **children** is **abdominal blunt trauma**^{Q}.
- Direct compression of the epigastrium against the vertebral column and a blunt object (**handlebar**) is typically seen after **bicycle injuries**^{Q}.
- **MC segment** of the pancreas affected is the **body**^{Q}.

Pancreatic Organ Injury Scale

Grade		Type of Injury
I	Hematoma	**Minor contusion** without duct injury
	Laceration	**Superficial laceration** without duct injury
II	Hematoma	**Major Contusion** without duct injury or tissue loss
	Laceration	**Major Laceration** without duct injury or tissue loss
III	Laceration	**Distal transaction** or parenchymal injury with duct injury
IV	Laceration	**Proximal transaction** or parenchymal injury involving ampulla
V	Laceration	**Massive disruption** of pancreatic head

Diagnosis

- **CT scan**: **Investigation of choice** to evaluate patients with **abdominal trauma**^{Q}.
- **CT findings**: Peripancreatic hematomas, free fluid in the lesser sack, or abnormal thickening of Gerota's fascia suggest pancreatic injury.

  - **ERCP**: **Most reliable test** to demonstrate **pancreatic duct integrity**^{Q}

- **Isolated pancreatic amylase** level measurement is **not recommended** because up to 40% of patients with pancreatic duct transected have normal serum amylase levels. **Serial quantification levels**^{Q} increase the sensitivity of the assay.

Treatment

- Definitive treatment is based on surgical findings.
- **Major pancreatic resections** in **stable patients** with **isolated pancreatic injury**^{Q}.
- **Damage control surgery** is indicated for **complex injuries** or **unstable patients**^{Q}.
- **Most** (up to 75%) of **deaths occur within** the **48 to 72 hours** after trauma, and most are related to **hypovolemic shock**^{Q}.

Complication

- A **persistent drain output** or **pancreatic fistula** is the MC complication after **pancreatic trauma**^{Q}.

Grading	Treatment of Pancreatic Injuries
• Grade I	• Observation alone^Q
• Grade II	• Debridement, drainage, possible repair^Q
• Grade III	• Distal resection, possible Roux-en-Y drainage^Q
• Grades IV and V	• Damage control^Q, hemostasis/drainage
	• Resection and possible **Roux-en-Y drainage**^{Q}
	• Triple-tube decompression^Q
	• Pyloric exclusion technique
	• Duodenal diverticularization^Q
	• Pancreaticoduodenectomy

Multiple Choice Questions

ACUTE PANCREATITIS: ETIOLOGY AND RISK FACTORS

1. Which of the following is the most common non-alcoholic cause of acute pancreatitis? *(COMEDK 2008, 2007)*
   a. Thiazides
   b. Hypercalcemia
   c. Hyperlipidemia
   d. Gallstones

2. The commonest cause of acute pancreatitis is: *(COMEDK 2008)*
   a. Biliary calculi
   b. Alcohol abuse
   c. Infective
   d. Idiopathic

3. Pancreatitis may be produced by following drug: *(PGI Dec 96)*
   a. Colchicine
   b. L-Asparaginase
   c. Ciprofloxacin
   d. Nalidixic acid

4. Most common complication after ERCP is: *(AIIMS May 2007)*
   a. Acute pancreatitis
   b. Acute cholangitis
   c. Acute cholecystitis
   d. Duodenal perforation

5. Post-operative pancreatitis is seen in which type of surgery? *(MHSSMCET 2005)*
   a. Billroth type I
   b. Splenectomy
   c. Nephrectomy
   d. Cardiopulmonary bypass

6. Which of the following is not an etiological factor for pancreatitis? *(AIIMS May 2014)*
   a. Abdominal trauma
   b. Hyperlipidemia
   c. Islet cell hyperplasia
   d. Germline mutations in the cationic trypsinogen gene

7. Which of the following drug causes acute pancreatitis? *(Recent Question 2017)*
   a. L-Asparaginase
   b. Metronidazole
   c. Ciprofloxacin
   d. Penicillin

ACUTE PANCREATITIS: CLINICAL FEATURES, DIAGNOSIS AND TREATMENT

8. Which of the following does not cause an increase in serum amylase? *(COMEDK 2008)*
   a. Pancreatitis
   b. Carcinoma lung
   c. Renal failure
   d. Cardiac failure

9. Poor prognostic factor in a patient with acute pancreatitis: *(NEET Pattern, JIPMER 2011)*
   a. Leucocytosis >20,000/μL
   b. ↓ serum amylase
   c. ↓ serum lipase
   d. Diastolic BP >90 mm Hg

10. A lady presents with three day history of epigastric pain radiating to back serum amylase levels were observed to be normal while USG abdomen reveals gallbladder stones and an enlarged pancreas. CT scan was done which clinched the diagnosis. Which of the following is the most likely diagnosis? *(All India 2011)*
    a. Acute cholecystitis
    b. Acute pancreatitis
    c. Acute appendicitis
    d. Acute peritonitis

11. Medical treatment of acute pancreatitis includes:
    a. Calcium
    b. Glucagon *(PGI Nov 2011)*
    c. Aprotinin
    d. Cholestyramine
    e. Antibiotics

12. Which of the following criteria is/are not included in Ranson's scoring? *(PGI Nov 2011)*
    a. WBC >16,000/μl
    b. Serum amylase >350 IU
    c. Age > 55 years
    d. Serum LDH >700 IU
    e. Serum AST >250 U/dL

13. Hyperamylasemia is seen in all except: *(PGI May 2011)*
    a. Peritonitis
    b. Acute pancreatitis
    c. Carcinoma esophagus
    d. Ruptured ectopic pregnancy
    e. Perforated peptic ulcer

14. Ranson's scoring for acute pancreatitis includes: *(PGI May 2011)*
    a. Age >55 years
    b. WBC >16,000/μL
    c. Sequestration of fluid >6L
    d. BUN >10 mg/dl
    e. LDH >700 IU

15. Which of the following is most diagnostic investigation for acute pancreatitis? *(MHPGMCET 2003)*
    a. Serum amylase
    b. Serum lipase
    c. Serum P-isoamylase
    d. Serum LDH

16. Which of the following is not a feature of acute pancreatitis? *(DNB 2011, Orissa 2011)*
    a. Hyperbilirubinemia
    b. Hypercalcemia
    c. Hyperglycemia
    d. Increased serum LDH level

17. Which of the following types of pancreatitis has the best prognosis? *(APPG 2005, All India 2004)*
    a. Alcoholic pancreatitis
    b. Gallstone induced pancreatitis
    c. Post operative pancreatitis
    d. Idiopathic pancreatitis

18. Which one is not the bad prognostic sign for pancreatitis?
    a. TLC >16,000/μL *(AIIMS June 2000)*
    b. Calcium <8 mmol/L
    c. Glucose >200 mg%
    d. Prothrombin >2 times the control

19. Which one is not poor prognostic factor for acute pancreatitis? *(AIIMS Nov 99)*
    a. Hyperglycemia
    b. Hypocalcemia
    c. Raised LDH level in blood
    d. Hyperamylasemia

20. Poor prognostic factor in acute pancreatitis is: *(PGI Dec 96)*
    a. Increased serum amylase
    b. Decreased calcium
    c. Decreased blood sugar
    d. Decreased PaO_2

21. Destruction of fat in acute pancreatitis is due to:
    a. Lipase and trypsin *(MHCET 2016)*
    b. Secretin
    c. Lipase and elastase
    d. Cholecystokinin and trypsin

22. All the following can be used to predict severe acute pancreatitis except:
    a. Glasgow score ≥ 3   b. APACHE II score ≥ 8
    c. CT severity score ≥ 6   d. C-reactive protein <100

23. Monu, a 30-years old male, a chronic alcoholic presents with sudden onset of epigastric pain that radiates to the back. All are seen except: *(AIIMS June 2001)*
    a. Low serum lipase   b. Increased LDH
    c. Hypocalcemia   d. Increased serum amylase

24. A 21-years old patient attended a party the previous night and gives the following symptoms, pain in abdomen radiating to back, pulse 100/min, BP 100/76; Temp 39°C and vomiting before coming. Most probable diagnosis is: *(AIIMS Nov 99)*
    a. Acute appendicitis   b. Acute cholecystitis
    c. Acute diverticulitis   d. Acute pancreatitis

25. The following conditions are indications of surgery in acute pancreatitis, except: *(UPSC 2004)*
    a. Acute fluid collection
    b. Persistent pseudocyst pancreas
    c. Pancreatic abscess
    d. Infective pancreatic necrosis

26. All of the following patients presenting with abdominal pain and shock need immediate laparotomy except: *(DPG 2009 March)*
    a. Ruptured ectopic pregnancy
    b. Hemorrhagic pancreatitis
    c. Rupture abdominal aortic aneurysm
    d. Ruptured liver hemangioma

27. Acute pancreatitis is associated with all except: *(DPG 2005)*
    a. Steatorrhoea   b. Epigastric tenderness
    c. Upper abdominal pain   d. Cullen's sign

28. A patient is admitted with severe pain in the abdomen, nausea, vomiting and fever. The most likely diagnosis is: *(UPSC 97)*
    a. Perforated peptic ulcer b. Intestinal obstruction
    c. Acute pancreatitis   d. Acute cholecystitis

29. A 40-years-old male was brought to the hospital with acute pain in the upper abdomen. Patient was in shock with feeble pulse and tachycardia. There was tenderness present in the epigastrium. There is no blood in the gastric aspirate and the patient felt better after aspiration. X-ray abdomen showed no free gas under the diaphragm. Investigations revealed TLC 13500 serum bilirubin 2.0 mg and serum amylase 800 I.U. The most likely diagnosis is:
    a. Acute cholecystitis   b. Acute pancreatitis
    c. Acute appendicitis   d. Acute hepatitis

30. Gasless abdomen in X-ray is a sign of: *(Recent Question 2019)*
    a. Acute pancreatitis   b. Necrotizing enterocolitis
    c. Ulcerative colitis   d. Intussusception

31. Which of the following is not a component of APACHE score? *(DNB 2012)*
    a. Serum potassium   b. Serum sodium
    c. Serum calcium   d. Creatinine

32. Acute pancreatitis causes all except: *(DNB 2007)*
    a. Pleural effusion   b. Pseudocyst
    c. Gallbladder stone   d. Pancreatic necrosis

33. Most common causes of death due to acute pancreatitis: *(DNB 2001)*
    a. Shock   b. Infection
    c. Hypocalcemia   d. Diabetes

34. Which of the following does not correlate with severity of acute pancreatitis? *(AIIMS Nov 2011, GB Pant 2010)*
    a. Serum glucose   b. Serum amylase
    c. Serum calcium   d. AST

35. A 76-year-old male presents to the emergency with abdominal pain and an episode of binge drinking in shock with a BP of 70/50 mm Hg and HR of 115/min. The oxygen saturation of the patient is 70 mm Hg. Serum creatinine levels was 2.4 mg/dL. The patient had raised transaminases. What is the likely diagnosis based on the CT image shown below? *(AIIMS May 2016)*
    a. Liver abscess   b. Acute pancreatitis
    c. Acute pyelonephritis   d. Severe acute pancreatitis

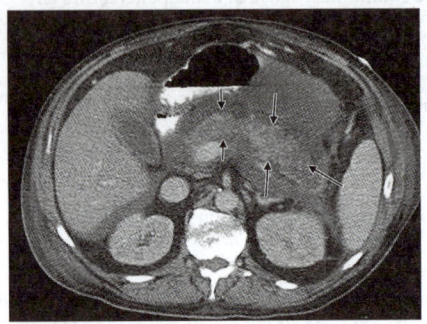

36. Which of the following is not associated with Pancreatitis? *(JIPMER 2014, 2011)*
    a. Raised serum amylase   b. Raised serum lipase
    c. Hypocalcemia   d. Hypoglycemia

37. CT severity index is a measure for: *(Recent Question 2013)*
    a. Hepatitis   b. Pancreatitis
    c. Cerebral trauma   d. Meningitis

38. Balthazar scoring system is used for: *(DNB 2014)*
    a. Acute pancreatitis   b. Acute appendicitis
    c. Acute cholecystitis   d. Cholangitis

39. Ideal fluid of choice in a 35 years old man presenting with acute pancreatitis: *(Recent Question 2018)*
    a. Isotonic crystalloid by IV line
    b. Hypertonic saline by IV line
    c. Hypotonic saline by central line
    d. Vasopressin

40. A patient presented to the emergency with pain in epigastrium radiating to left back. X-ray abdomen was done. The finding seen in the X-ray is:
    a. Sentinel loop   b. Colon cut off sign
    c. Renal Halo sign   d. Ground glass appearance

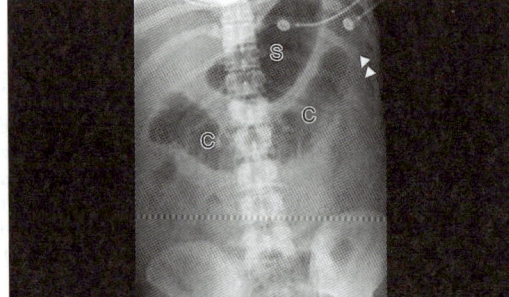

ACUTE PANCREATITIS: COMPLICATIONS

41. **Grey Turner's sign (flank discoloration) is seen in:**
    (MCI June 2018, COMEDK 2008)
    a. Acute pyelonephritis
    b. Acute cholecystitis
    c. Acute pancreatitis
    d. Acute peritonitis

42. **The given signs are seen in which of the following condition?**

    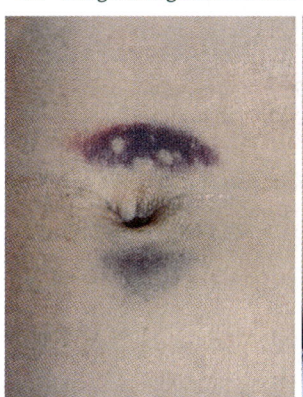
    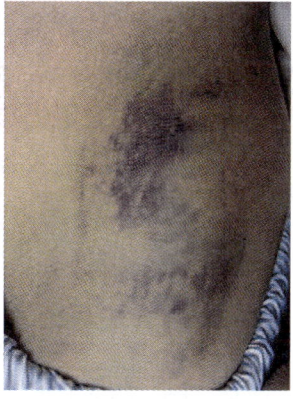

    a. Mild acute pancreatitis
    b. Severe acute pancreatitis
    c. Mild chronic pancreatitis
    d. Severe chronic pancreatitis

43. **Management of pancreatic abscess is:**
    (UPSC 2008, AIIMS Nov 93)
    a. Needle aspiration
    b. Cystogastrostomy
    c. External drainage
    d. Cystojejunostomy

44. **Which is not a feature of pancreatic ascites?** *(PGI June 99)*
    a. Low protein
    b. Somatostatin is the drug of choice
    c. Communication with pancreatic duct in 80%
    d. Raised amylase levels

45. **When to do surgery in pancreatic ascites?**
    (JIPMER May 2018)
    a. Symptomatic
    b. Recurrent ascites following abdominal drainage
    c. Not responding to medical therapy
    d. Leak from the stented duct

46. **Cullen's sign:** *(UPPG 2007)*
    a. Bluish discoloration of the flanks
    b. Bluish discoloration around umbilicus
    c. Migratory thrombophlebitis
    d. Subcutaneous fat necrosis

47. **Vascular complications of acute pancreatitis include the following except:** *(UPSC 2007)*
    a. Splenic vein thrombosis
    b. Splenic artery aneurysm
    c. Gastroduodenal artery aneurysm
    d. Middle colic artery thrombosis

48. **Cullen's sign is seen in:** *(Bihar PG 2014, Kerala 94)*
    a. Acute cholecystitis
    b. Acute pancreatitis
    c. Acute hemorrhagic pancreatitis
    d. Blunt injury abdomen

49. **All are true about acute fluid collection except:**
    a. Not associated with fibrous wall *(AIIMS GIS May 2008)*
    b. Most are extra-pancreatic
    c. Commonly associated with hemosuccus pancreaticus
    d. Most resolve spontaneously

50. **Most common metabolic complication of acute pancreatitis:**
    (AIIMS GIS May 2008)
    a. Hyperglycemia
    b. Hypocalcemia
    c. Hypomagnesemia
    d. Hyponatremia

51. **Hemorrhagic pancreatitis, bluish discoloration of flank:**
    (Recent Question 2013)
    a. Grey Turner sign
    b. Cullen sign
    c. Trousseau sign
    d. None

52. **An infected necrosis is treated with:** *(Recent Question 2017)*
    a. IV antibiotics
    b. Laparotomy and surgical debridement
    c. USG guided drainage
    d. TPN

CHRONIC PANCREATITIS: ETIOLOGY, CLINICAL FEATURES AND DIAGNOSIS

53. **Hereditary chronic pancreatitis is caused by mutation of:**
    a. Cationic trypsinogen or PRSS1 *(GB Pant 2010)*
    b. CFTR
    c. PTSI
    d. SPINK1

54. **All are true about chronic pancreatitis except:**
    a. Characterized by irregularities of pancreatic ducts, duct strictures and areas of dilatation *(JIPMER GIS 2011)*
    b. 60–80% will give history of acute episodes
    c. CT scan showing pancreatic calcification is diagnostic of chronic pancreatitis
    d. Serum amylase is always raised

55. **True regarding chronic pancreatitis is/are:** *(PGI May 2018)*
    a. Can present with steatorrhea and malabsorption
    b. Present with mid epigastric pain radiating to back
    c. Markedly raised level of amylase & lipase
    d. Predisposes to carcinoma
    e. Complete pancreatectomy relieves pain in majority of patients

56. **Most common symptom of chronic pancreatitis is:**
    (JIPMER GIS 2011)
    a. Abdominal pain
    b. Cachexia
    c. Weight loss
    d. Steatorrhea

57. **All are seen in chronic calcific pancreatitis except:** *(Kerala 96)*
    a. Diabetes mellitus
    b. Fat malabsorption
    c. Hypercalcemia
    d. Recurrent abdominal pain
    e. Increased incidence of pancreatic carcinoma

58. **Causes of chronic tropical pancreatitis is:**
    a. Parasitic infection
    b. Cassava ingestion
    c. Idiopathic
    d. Genetic

59. **Below mentioned ERCP is highly suggestive of:**
    a. Acute pancreatitis
    b. Chronic pancreatitis
    c. Carcinoma pancreas
    d. Cholangiocarcinoma

    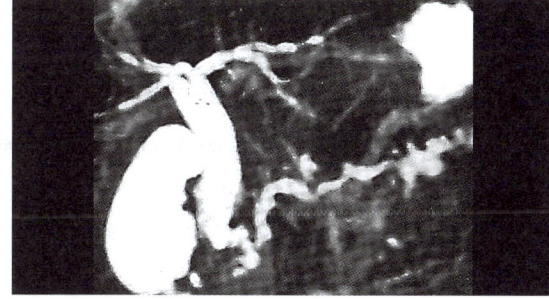

60. "Chain of lakes" appearance seen in: *(MHCET 2016, UPPG 2007, 2005)*
    a. Acute pancreatitis
    b. Chronic pancreatitis
    c. Carcinoma pancreas
    d. Strawberry gallbladder

61. Chronic calcific pancreatitis is associated with all of the following except: *(MCI Sept 2005)*
    a. Hypercalcemia
    b. Diabetes mellitus
    c. Malabsorption of fat
    d. Diabetes associated complications are uncommon

62. Chronic pancreatitis seen in all except: *(PGI Dec 2011)*
    a. Chronic renal failure
    b. Intraductal mucinous carcinoma
    c. Alcohol
    d. Gallstones
    e. Pancreatic divisum

63. What is the most probable diagnosis based on the given X-ray? *(Recent Question 2017)*

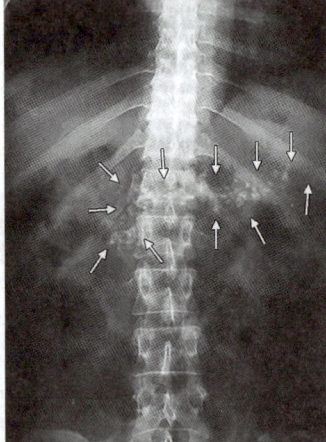

    a. Chronic pancreatitis   b. Acute pancreatitis
    c. Trichobezoar   d. Phytobezoar

64. Feature of chronic pancreatitis w.r.t. pancreatic cancer:
    a. Smooth pancreatic duct dilation with an abrupt interruption *(PGI May 2011)*
    b. Calcification
    c. Duct penetrating sign
    d. Duct/gland width ration <0.5
    e. Dilation of bile and pancreatic duct

65. TIGAR-O classification is for: *(MHSSMCET 2008)*
    a. Acute pancreatitis   b. Chronic pancreatitis
    c. Pancreatic cancer   d. Pancreatic injuries

66. Most common cause of chronic pancreatitis: *(Recent Question 2018)*
    a. Gallstones   b. Alcohol
    c. Hereditary   d. ERCP

67. All of the following are true about tropical pancreatitis except: *(Recent Question 2017)*
    a. Caused by tapioca ingestion
    b. Dilatation of pancreatic ducts with large stones with fibrosis
    c. Increase the risk of pancreatic cancer
    d. Treatment is mainly surgical

68. Gold standard investigation for chronic pancreatitis: *(DNB 2014)*
    a. MRI   b. ERCP
    c. Pancreatic function tests d. Fecal fat estimation

69. Hereditary pancreatitis is characterized by all *except*:
    a. 80% penetrance   *(JIPMER November 2017)*
    b. 30% leads to chronic pancreatitis
    c. Autosomal recessive inheritance
    d. Pancreatic cancer risk is high

CHRONIC PANCREATITIS: TREATMENT AND COMPLICATIONS

70. All are true about pancreatic fistula in chronic pancreatitis except: *(AIIMS GIS May 2008)*
    a. Most caseas resolve spontaneously by conservative treatment
    b. Somatostatin is effective in fistula closure
    c. In prevention of fistula, adherence to standardized and meticulous technique is more important than the pancreatic texture or the type of anastomosis used
    d. Early intervention is required if associated with hemorrhage or sepsis

71. Beger's procedure: *(Recent Question 2016, AIIMS GIS May 2008)*
    a. DPPHR   b. LRLPJ
    c. Caudal pancreaticojejunostomy
    d. Longitudinal pancreaticojejunostomy

72. Duval procedure in case of chronic pancreatitis involves:
    a. Distal resection of tail of pancreas with end to end pancreaticojejunostomy *(AIIMS GIS Dec 2009)*
    b. Distal resection of tail of pancreas with longitudinal opening of duct and pancreaticojejunostomy
    c. Duodenum preserving pancreatic head resection
    d. Local section of pancreatic head with longitudinal pancreaticojejunostomy

73. A 50-year old lady presents with two years history of recurrent abdominal pain with radiation to her back. Pain is severe in intensity, and refractory to simple analgesics. Ultrasound and contrast enhanced CT scan (CECT) confirmed the diagnosis and showed a dilated pancreatic duct. Which of the following is the likely recommended surgical procedure of choice? *(All India 2011)*
    a. Vagotomy with Antrectomy
    b. Vagotomy with Gastrojejunostomy
    c. Whipple's Procedure
    d. Longitudinal Pancreaticojejunostomy

74. A chronic alcoholic presents with abdominal pain radiating to the back that responds to analgesics. At evaluation the pancreatic duct was found to be dilated and stones were noted in the tail of pancreas. The most appropriate management is: *(All India 2008)*
    a. Pancreatic tail resection   b. Pancreaticojejunostomy
    c. Percutaneous removal of stone
    d. Medical management

75. Patient with chronic pancreatitis gives chain of lakes appearance in ERCP examination. Management is:
    a. Total pancreatectomy   *(AIIMS Nov 2000)*
    b. Sphincteroplasty
    c. Side to side pancreaticojejunostomy
    d. Resecting the tail of pancreas and performing a pancreatojejunostomy

76. Pain relief in chronic pancreatitis can be obtained by destruction of: *(Recent Question 2016)*
    a. Celiac ganglia
    b. Vagus nerve
    c. Anterolateral column of spinal cord
    d. None of the above

77. In a patient with chronic pancreatitis limited to tail and body with MPD diameter 4 mm, ideal treatment would be: *(MHSSMCET 2007)*
    a. Stenting
    b. Puestow's operation
    c. Frey's operation
    d. Distal pancreatectomy

78. Operation for chromic pancreatitis are the following except: *(MHSSMCET 2009)*
    a. Beger's procedure
    b. Longitudinal pancreatojejunostomy
    c. Frey procedure
    d. None

79. Complication of chronic pancreatitis include all except: *(Recent Question 2013)*
    a. Renal artery stenosis
    b. Pseudocyst
    c. Splenic vein stenosis
    d. Fistulae

80. All of the following are true about chronic pancreatitis is except: *(DNB 2014)*
    a. Damage to exocrine part with damage to endocrine part
    b. Can lead to malignancy
    c. Whipple's procedure can be done
    d. Gallbladder stone is the most common cause

81. Most common complication of both acute and chronic pancreatitis: *(Recent Question 2017)*
    a. Portal vein thrombosis
    b. Pancreatic abscess
    c. Pseudocyst
    d. Pancreatic necrosis

PSEUDOPANCREATIC CYST

82. True about pseudocyst pancreas: *(PGI SS Dec 2009)*
    a. Cyst wall is lined by squamous epithelium
    b. Endoscopic treatment may be curative
    c. Always found in lesser sac
    d. Always occur due to alcoholic pancreatitis

83. A chronic alcoholic presented with repeated episodes of nonbilious vomiting after meals. On the basis of CECT findings, what is the diagnosis? *(Recent Question 2016)*
    a. Gastric outlet obstruction
    b. Pseudocyst
    c. Carcinoma pancreas
    d. Chronic pancreatitis

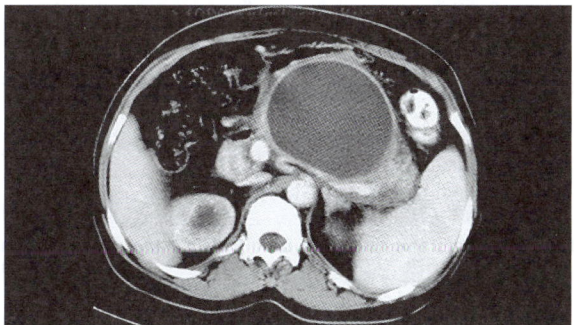

84. Most common complication of pseudocyst: *(DNB 2003, PGI SS Dec 2009)*
    a. Infection
    b. Rupture
    c. Hemorrhage
    d. Compression

85. Major complication of cysto-gastrostomy for pseudopancreatic cyst is: *(DPG 2011, COMEDK 2005)*
    a. Infection
    b. Obstruction
    c. Fistula
    d. Hemorrhage

86. Most common cause of pancreatic pseudocyst: *(JIPMER 2010)*
    a. Blunt abdominal trauma
    b. Pancreatic carcinoma
    c. Pancreatitis
    d. Post pancreatic surgery

87. Most common artery involved in pancreatic pseudoaneurysm:
    a. Gastroduodenal artery *(PGI Nov 2009)*
    b. Inferior pancreatico-duodenal artery
    c. Gastric artery
    d. Splenic artery
    e. Hepatic artery

88. Pseudocyst of pancreas is: *(MHPGMCET 2003)*
    a. Post traumatic cyst
    b. Post inflammatory cyst
    c. Congenital cyst
    d. Neoplastic cyst

89. Most common cause of pseudopancreatic cyst in children is: *(All India 99)*
    a. Choledochal cyst
    b. Annular pancreas
    c. Drug induced pancreatitis
    d. Traumatic pancreatitis

90. After 3 weeks of duration pancreatic pseudocyst 5 cm in size should be managed by which method? *(AIIMS Nov 2000)*
    a. Cystogastrostomy
    b. Needle aspiration
    c. External drainage
    d. USG and follow up

91. Which one is not true regarding pseudocyst of pancreas?
    a. Epigastric mass *(AIIMS Nov 95)*
    b. Increase level of amylase
    c. Cystogastrostomy is the ideal treatment
    d. Percutaneous aspiration is the treatment

92. All of the following statements about pseudopan-creatic cysts are true except: *(All India 97)*
    a. Percutaneous aspiration is treatment of choice
    b. Cystojejunostomy is treatment of choice
    c. Serum amylase levels are increased
    d. Presents as an epigastric mass

93. All of the following are true about pseudopancreatic cyst of pancreas except: *(All India 98)*
    a. Common after acute pancreatitis
    b. Presents as an abdominal mass
    c. Serum amylase is increased
    d. Most common site is in head of pancreas

94. Treatment of choice for asymptomatic pseudocyst pancreas is: *(DNB 2010)*
    a. Marsupialization
    b. Conservative
    c. Drainage
    d. Cystogastrostomy

95. The complication least likely to occur in a pseudocyst of the pancreas is: *(Kerala 90)*
    a. Hemorrhage
    b. Torsion
    c. Infection
    d. Carcinomatous change

96. All are features of pseudopancreatic cyst, except:
    a. Follows acute pancreatitis *(All India 97)*
    b. Lined by false epithelium
    c. May regress spontaneously
    d. Treatment of choice is percutaneous aspiration

97. **Serious complication in pancreatic pseudocyst include all of the following except:** *(UPSC 97)*
    a. Intracystic hemorrhage
    b. Secondary infection
    c. Calcification in the cyst wall
    d. Rupture of the cyst

98. **Commonest complication of pseudocyst of the pancreas is:**
    a. Commonest into peritoneum *(DPG 2009 Feb)*
    b. Rupture into colon
    c. Hemorrhage
    d. Infection

99. **A 20-year old football player received a hard kick in the epigastrium. A large cystic swelling appeared in the epigastrium two weeks later. The most likely diagnosis is:**
    a. Hydatid cyst of liver *(UPSC 96)*
    b. Amoebic liver abscess
    c. Pseudopancreatic cyst
    d. Hematoma of rectus sheath

CYSTIC NEOPLASMS OF PANCREAS

100. **Increased amylase, mucin and CEA is seen in:** *(ILBS 2012)*
    a. IPMN
    b. Mucinous cystadenoma
    c. Serous cystadenoma
    d. Solid pseudopaillary tumor

101. **Not true about mucinous cystadenoma pancreas:**
    a. Microcystic adenoma *(AIIMS May 2011)*
    b. Lined by columnar epithelium
    c. Premalignant
    d. Focus of ovarian stroma in it

102. **A 60-year old female present with history of recurrent abdominal pain. Imaging shows multiple small cystic lesions like bunch of grapes in the head of pancreas with a grossly dilated main pancreatic duct. The most likely diagnosis is:**
    a. SCN   b. MCN *(All India 2012)*
    c. IPMN   d. Pancreatic pseudocyst

103. **Regarding IPMN, all are true except:** *(AIIMS GIS May 2011)*
    a. Treatment is enucleation
    b. Can involve either main or branch duct
    c. Mostly involve pancreatic head
    d. Men and women are equally affected

104. **All of the following are true about mucinous cystic neoplasm except:** *(Recent Question 2017)*
    a. Less amylase in fluid
    b. Enucleation is performed
    c. Estrogens receptors are positive
    d. More common in females

105. **Serous cystadenoma, all are true except:**
    a. 30% are associated with malignancy
    b. Mainly microcystic *(AIIMS GIS May 2008)*
    c. More commonly located in the head
    d. Glycogen rich cells on cytologic examination with central calcified stellate scar

106. **A 60-year-old female presented with dull aching pain in central abdomen. On laboratory evaluation, amylase and CEA was normal. The image of CECT abdomen and tumor cut section after surgery is given below. What is the most probable diagnosis?**
    a. Mucinous cystadenoma   b. Serous cystadenoma
    c. IPMN   d. Pseudocyst pancreas

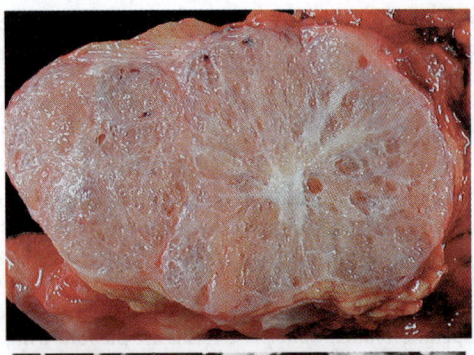
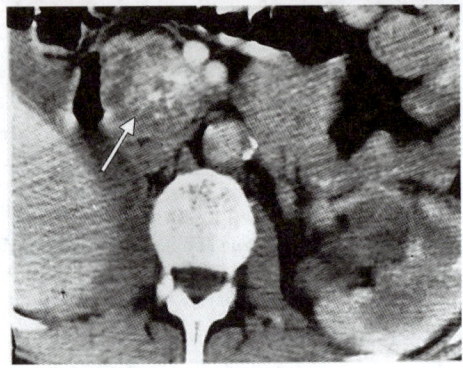

107. **All are true about IPMN except:** *(JIPMER GIS 2011)*
    a. Always involves main pancreatic duct
    b. Involvement of head is most common form
    c. Men and women are equally affected
    d. Patients can experience acute pancreatitis

CARCINOMA PANCREAS: ETIOLOGY AND RISK FACTORS

108. **Earliest genetic change in carcinoma pancreas:** *(ILBS 2012)*
    a. Her-2-neu   b. p53
    c. p16   d. DCC

109. **Not a risk factor for carcinoma pancreas:** *(ILBS 2012)*
    a. Acute pancreatitis   b. Diabetes
    c. Smoking   d. Obesity

110. **Most common mutation in pancreatic adenocarcinoma:**
    a. K-ras   b. p16 *(GB Pant 2010)*
    c. p53   d. BRAF

111. **Which of the following does not predispose to CA pancreas?** *(Recent Question 2017, AIIMS GIS May 2008)*
    a. Familial breast cancer   b. HNPCC
    c. PJS   d. Cronkhite-Canada syndrome

112. **Hereditary pancreatic carcinoma is associated with all except:** *(AIIMS GIS Dec 2009)*
    a. Ataxia Telengiectasia
    b. Peutz-Jegher's syndrome
    c. Hereditary pancreatitis
    d. FAP

113. **Most common oncogene involved in pancreatic carcinoma is:** *(AIIMS GIS Dec 2009)*
    a. p53   b. K-ras
    c. APC   d. DCC

114. Risk factors for carcinoma of pancreas include the following except: *(MHSSMCET 2006)*
    a. Obesity
    b. Alcohol abuse
    c. Peutz-Jegher's syndrome
    d. History of partial gastrectomy

115. What will be your advice to a 60 years moderately obese patient with history of 4–6 cup of coffee per day, 4–6 glass of wine/day with 20 cigarettes per day. He is engaged as a salesman in a computer company. His brother died of pancreatic carcinoma: *(PGI June 2004)*
    a. Urgent weight reduction
    b. Strict vegetarian diet
    c. Stop alcohol
    d. Stop coffee
    e. Stop cigarette smoking

116. False about pancreatic cancer association: *(AIIMS GIS May 2008)*
    a. p53 inactivated
    b. K-ras activated
    c. BRCA activated
    d. EGF overexpression

117. Maximum risk of carcinoma pancreas is seen in which of these? *(AIIMS May 2017)*
    a. Hereditary atypical multiple mole melanoma syndrome
    b. Hereditary pancreatitis
    c. Peutz-Jegher's syndrome
    d. Familial adenomatous polyposis

118. First gene mutated in pancreatic adenocarcinoma is: *(Recent Question 2017)*
    a. K-ras
    b. p53
    c. p16
    d. BRAF

119. Most common oncogene mutated in CA head of pancreas:
    a. K-ras
    b. p53   *(AIIMS GIS 2003)*
    c. C-myc
    d. BRCA 2

120. Which is not autosomal dominant? *(AIIMS GIS May 2011)*
    a. HNPCC
    b. FAMMM
    c. PJS
    d. Ataxia telangiectasia

CARCINOMA PANCREAS: CLINICAL FEATURES AND DIAGNOSIS

121. Most common symptom of CA head of pancreas: *(ILBS 2012, AIIMS GIS Dec 2011, Dec 2006)*
    a. Weight loss
    b. Pain
    c. Jaundice
    d. Anorexia

122. In carcinoma head of pancreas, nausea and vomiting is due to: *(JIPMER May 2018)*
    a. External compression of duodenum
    b. Portal vein infiltration
    c. Proliferation infiltration of tumor into duodenum
    d. Chemotherapy related

123. Diagnostic investigation in carcinoma pancreas: *(ILBS 2012)*
    a. MDCT
    b. PET scan
    c. ERCP
    d. MRCP

124. According to AJCC 8th edition, staging of 2 cm size pancreatic cancer if it involves portal vein in: *(JIPMER May 2018)*
    a. T1
    b. T2
    c. T3
    d. T4

125. Not true about pancreatic ductal adenocarcinoma:
    a. Most common site is body and tail
    b. Associated with desmoplastic changes with scattering of neoplastic glands *(AIIMS GIS May 2008)*
    c. Body tumors are larger
    d. Perineural invasion is characteristic feature

126. Most appropriate initial method of investigation for carcinoma head of pancreas: *(Recent Question 2018)*
    a. Laparoscopic guided biopsy
    b. MRI guided biopsy
    c. CECT guided biopsy
    d. EUS guided transgastric biopsy

127. Scrambled egg appearance is seen in: *(COMEDK 2007)*
    a. Carcinoma stomach
    b. Carcinoma gallbladder
    c. Pancreatic carcinoma
    d. Renal carcinoma

128. The most likely cause of fluctuating jaundice in a middle aged or elderly man is: *(COMEDK 2010)*
    a. Periampullary carcinoma
    b. Liver fluke infestation
    c. Choledochal cyst
    d. Carcinoma head of pancreas

129. Migratory thrombophlebitis seen in: *(PGI Dec 2006)*
    a. Pancreatic cancer
    b. Bladder cancer
    c. Stomach cancer
    d. Breast cancer
    e. Liver cancer

130. True about pancreatic carcinoma: *(PGI Dec 2000)*
    a. Head is the most common site
    b. Pain is the most common symptom
    c. Obstruction of bile and pancreatic secretion is common
    d. 80% cases respond well to resection

131. Investigation to diagnose carcinoma head of pancreas are/is: *(PGI Dec 2000, PGI Dec 2003)*
    a. Hypotonic duodenogram
    b. X-ray abdomen
    c. USG
    d. Endoscopy
    e. CT Scan

132. A 55-year-old male presents with features of obstructive jaundice. He also reports a weight loss of seven kilograms in last two months. On CT scan, the CBD is dilated till the lower end and the main pancreatic duct is also dilated. Pancreas is normal. The most likely diagnosis is: *(AIIMS Nov 2004)*
    a. Choledocholithiasis
    b. Carcinoma gallbladder
    c. Hilar cholangiocarcinoma
    d. Periampullary carcinoma

133. Inverted "3" sign seen in: *(PGI Dec 97)*
    a. Ampullary carcinoma
    b. Insulinoma
    c. CA head pancreas
    d. CA stomach

134. This characteristic appearance is seen in:
    a. Duodenal adenocarcinoma
    b. Distal cholangiocarcinoma
    c. Ampullary carcinoma
    d. Carcinoma head of pancreas

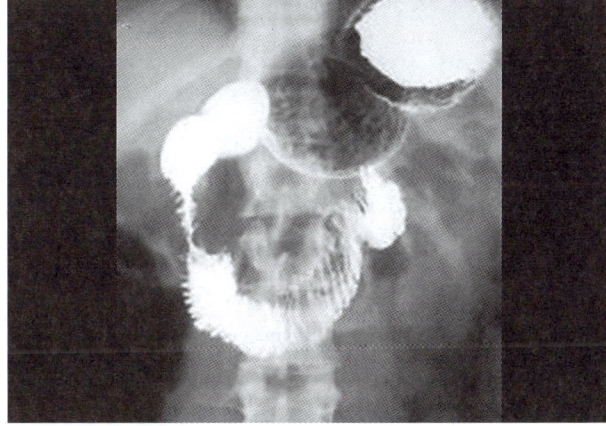

135. Most common tumor of pancreas is: (UPPG 2007)
    a. Adenocarcinoma
    b. Squamous cell carcinoma
    c. Adeno-squamous cell carcinoma
    d. Ductal adenocarcinoma

136. The commonest pancreatic tumor is: (Recent Question 2016)
    a. Ductal adenocarcinoma
    b. Cystadenoma
    c. Insulinoma
    d. Non islet cell tumor

137. Most sensitive investigation of pancreatic carcinoma is: (Recent Question 2016)
    a. Angiography
    b. ERCP
    c. Ultrasound
    d. CT scan

138. Carcinoma of pancreas is associated with: (UPPG 2008)
    a. Hypoglycemia
    b. Syndrome of inappropriate secretion of ADH
    c. Erythropoiesis is due to erythropoietin
    d. Hypercalcemia

139. Elderly male with icterus having large painless gallbladder lump, diagnosis is: (UPPG 2010)
    a. Acute hepatitis
    b. Carcinoma head of pancreas
    c. CBD stone
    d. Cholelithiasis
    e. Hepatocellular carcinoma

140. Most appropriate initial method of investigation for carcinoma head of pancreas: (Recent Question 2018)
    a. EUS guided transgastric biopsy
    b. CECT guided biopsy
    c. MRI guided biopsy
    d. Laparoscopic biopsy

141. A 60-year-old chronic smoker presented with jaundice, anorexia and weight loss. ERCP was done. The diagnosis on the basis of ERCP findings:
    a. Choledochal cyst
    b. Cholangiocarcinoma
    c. Carcinoma pancreas
    d. Chronic pancreatitis

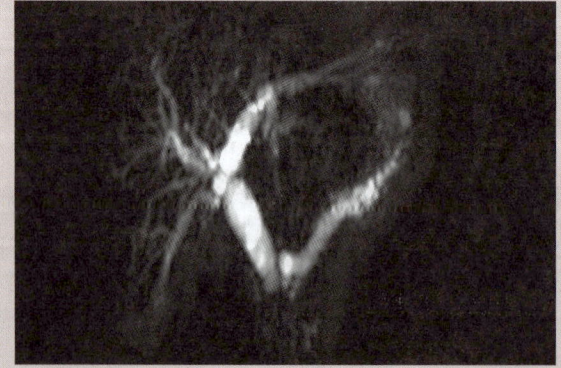

142. Double duct sign is seen in: (Recent Question 2017)
    a. Periampullary carcinoma
    b. Chronic pancreatitis
    c. HCC
    d. Carcinoma gallbladder

143. Most common site for carcinoma pancreas is: (Recent Question 2013)
    a. Head
    b. Body
    c. Tail
    d. Neck

144. A 60-year-old chronic smoker presented with progressive jaundice, pruritus and clay colored stools for 2 months. History of waxing and waning of jaundice was present. A CT scan revealed dilated main pancreatic duct and common bile duct. What is the likely diagnosis?
    a. Carcinoma head of pancreas (AIIMS November 2015)
    b. Periampullary carcinoma
    c. Chronic pancreatitis
    d. Hilar cholangiocarcinoma

145. What is the diagnosis based on the image given below?
    a. Acute pancreatitis
    b. Chronic pancreatitis
    c. Cystic neoplasm of pancreas
    d. Carcinoma head of pancreas

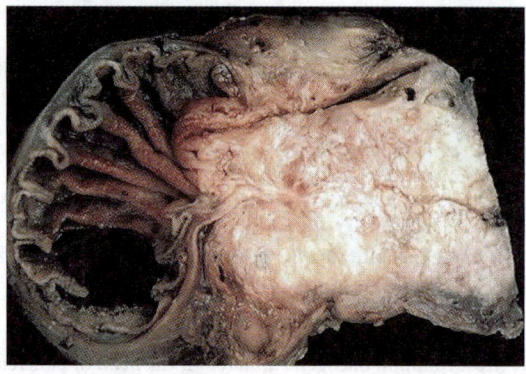

CARCINOMA PANCREAS: TREATMENT AND PROGNOSIS

146. Most important predictor of post-operative survival in CA pancreas: (AIIMS GIS May 2008)
    a. R0 resection
    b. DNA content
    c. Tumor size
    d. LN status

147. Most common primary leading to secondaries in pancreas: (AIIMS GIS May 2008)
    a. Lung
    b. Breast
    c. Colon
    d. Stomach

148. Most common complication of Whipple's procedure is:
    a. Delayed gastric emptying (AIIMS GIS Dec 2010)
    b. Bleeding
    c. Exocrine insufficiency
    d. Anastomotic leak

149. A patient with obstructive jaundice due to pancreatic cancer might have all of the following clinical findings except:
    a. A palpable gallbladder (COMEDK 2004)
    b. Pain is early in the course of the disease
    c. Pulmonary metastasis
    d. Thrombocytopenia

150. Which of the following drugs has been found to increase the survival in locally advanced pancreatic cancer? (COMEDK 2006)
    a. Doxorubicin
    b. Streptozocin
    c. Gemcitabine
    d. Paclitaxel

151. Middle segment pancreatectomy avoided in: (PGI Nov 2009)
    a. Cystadenoma
    b. Tumors of head pancreas
    c. Tumors of tail of pancreas
    d. Tumor of neck of pancreas

152. Which of the following statements is not true about pancreatic carcinoma? *(AIIMS May 2011, All India 2009)*
    a. Mutation in p53 gene is associated in 75% of cases
    b. Hereditary Pancreatitis significantly increase the risk
    c. Median survival in locally advanced (stage III) disease is 3-6 months
    d. Five year survival after curative pancreaticoduo-denectomy is 20%

153. Components of Whipple's operation are following except: *(MHSSMCET 2009)*
    a. Gastrojejunostomy   b. Duodenojejunostomy
    c. Choledochojejunostomy   d. Pancreaticoduodenostomy

154. All are resected in Whipple's operation except: *(AIIMS Nov 98, AIIMS Feb 97, All India 96)*
    a. Duodenum   b. Head of pancreas
    c. Portal vein   d. Common bile duct

155. The preferred bypass procedure in case of non resectable carcinoma of head of pancreas is: *(MAHE 2005)*
    a. Cholecystojejunostomy   b. Cholecystogastrostomy
    c. Choledochoduodenostomy   d. Choledochojejunostomy

156. Best prognosis for carcinoma of pancreas is in the region of:
    a. Head   b. Tail   *(UPPG 2007)*
    c. Body   d. Periampullary

157. What is the most common surgical complication following Whipple's procedure? *(UPSC 2007)*
    a. Disruption of pancreatic anastomosis
    b. Biliary peritonitis
    c. Disruption of gastric anastomosis
    d. GI bleeding

158. Treatment in periampullary carcinoma is by: *(DPG 2008)*
    a. Endoscopic stent   b. Ampullectomy
    c. Pancreaticoduodenectomy   d. Cholecystojejunostomy

159. Kocher's maneuver means:
    a. Mobilization of gallbladder during cholecystectomy
    b. Mobilization of 2nd part of duodenum
    c. Mobilization of pancreas during pancreatectomy
    d. Mobilization of ascending colon

160. Pancreaticoduodenectomy is the treatment of choice for:
    a. Duodenal carcinoma   b. Pancreatic carcinoma
    c. Gallbladder carcinoma   d. Gastric carcinoma

161. 5-FU is the chemotherapeutic agent of choice for all except:
    a. CA breast   b. CA stomach
    c. CA pancreas   d. CA colon

162. All are true about pancreatic carcinoma except:
    a. Ductal adenocarcinoma is the most common type
    b. K-ras mutation and Her-2-neu overexpression are the earliest change *(JIPMER GIS 2011)*
    c. Good prognosis   d. Most cases present late

163. False about CA pancreas: *(KGMC 2011)*
    a. Most common site is head and uncinate process
    b. Pain suggests unresectability
    c. Two third patients present with diabetes
    d. Acute pancreatitis never occurs in CA pancreas

164. Best tumor marker for CA head of pancreas:
    a. CA 19-9   b. CEA   *(AIIMS GIS 2003)*
    c. CA 125   d. AFP

165. Best prognosis after Whipple's is seen in: *(AIIMS GIS Dec 2006)*
    a. Cholangiocarcinoma   b. CA duodenum
    c. CA pancreas   d. Ampullary carcinoma

166. Most important margin for pancreati-coduodenectomy: *(PGI SS June 2001)*
    a. Retroperitoneal margin
    b. CBD
    c. Pancreatic duct
    d. Intestinal margin

167. Most common cause of death after Whipple's procedure:
    a. Pancreatic anastomotic leak   *(PGI SS 2004)*
    b. Biliary anastomotic leak
    c. Cardiopulmonary complications
    d. Gastric leak

168. Asymptomatic, solid 4 cm tumor of distal pancreas. Treatment: *(PGI SS Dec 2010)*
    a. Observation
    b. Distal pancreatectomy with splenectomy
    c. Near total pancreatectomy with splenectomy
    d. Distal pancreatectomy alone

169. Which of the following is not a contraindication for resection of head of pancreas: *(Recent Question 2015)*
    a. Liver metastasis
    b. Ascites
    c. Peritoneal seedings
    d. Involvement of major artery

170. Which of the following is not resected in pylorus preserving pancreaticoduodenectomy? *(Recent Question 2016)*
    a. Pyloric antrum   b. CBD
    c. Duodenum   d. Gall bladder

171. Most common complication after Whipple's procedure: *(Recent Question 2017)*
    a. Delayed gastric emptying
    b. Pancreatic fistula
    c. Wound infection
    d. Anastomotic leak

172. Median survival in carcinoma pancreas after surgery and adjuvant therapy: *(Recent Question 2017)*
    a. 12 months   b. 22 months
    c. 32 months   d. 44 months

173. Order of anastomosis in Whipple's procedure: *(Recent Question 2016, JIPMER SS 2016)*
    a. Pancreaticojejunostomy, gastrojejunostomy, hepaticojejunostomy,
    b. Hepaticojejunostomy, pancreaticojejunostomy, gastrojejunostomy
    c. Gastrojejunostomy, pancreaticojejunostomy, hepaticojejunostomy,
    d. Pancreaticojejunostomy, hepaticojejunostomy, gastrojejunostomy

PSEUDOPAPILLARY TUMOR

174. All are true about pseudopapillary tumors of pancreas except:
    a. Most commonly occurs in young women
    b. Both benign and malignant varieties are seen
    c. These are small tumors   *(JIPMER GIS 2011)*
    d. Local resection is usually curative

175. All are true about Frantz tumor except:
    a. Seen in young females   *(AIIMS GIS Dec 2011)*
    b. Vimentin and CD 56 is positive
    c. Indolent tumor with <15% incidence of metastasis
    d. Chromagranin is positive

INSULINOMA

176. **Best method of localization of insulinoma:** *(ILBS 2011)*
    a. EUS with intra-operative palpation
    b. MRI with dynamic CT
    c. SRS
    d. CECT

177. **Localization in insulinoma is best with:** *(COMEDK 2011)*
    a. Contrast CT
    b. Magnetic Resonance Imaging
    c. Somatostatin Receptor Scintigraphy
    d. Selective arteriography

178. **A 55-year old male presents with tachycardia, sweating, palpitation, giddiness. Most probable diagnosis:**
    a. Insulinoma *(JIPMER 2011)*
    b. Zollinger-Ellison syndrome
    c. Carcinoma pancreas
    d. Carcinoid

179. **All are true about insulinoma except:** *(PGI Nov 2009)*
    a. Usually asymptomatic and need no treatment
    b. Usually small and multiple
    c. Diazoxide and octreotide reduce insulin synthesis
    d. Most common site is pancreas
    e. 90% tumors are benign

180. **True about insulinoma is all except:** *(MHPGMCET 2003)*
    a. Common equally in the pancreatic head, body and tail
    b. Hypoglycemic attacks occur
    c. Weight loss is important feature
    d. Attacks respond to glucose infusion

181. **Gold standard test for insulinoma:** *(AIIMS May 2011)*
    a. 72-hours fasting test
    b. Plasma insulin levels
    c. C-peptide levels
    d. Low glucose levels < 30 mg/dL

182. **Which of the following tests is not used in the diagnosis of insulinoma?** *(All India 2011)*
    a. Fasting blood glucose
    b. Xylose test
    c. C-peptide levels
    d. Insulin/Glucose Ratio

183. **Best modality for diagnosis of insulinoma:** *(PGI SS June 2007)*
    a. Intra-operative USG
    b. Scintigraphy
    c. Arteriography
    d. Venous sampling

184. **A lady presented with recurrent attacks of giddiness and abdominal pain since three months. Endoscopy was normal. Her fasting blood glucose was 40 mg% and insulin levels were elevated. CT abdomen showed a well defined 8 mm enhancing lesion in the head of pancreas, with no other abnormal findings. What should be the treatment plan for this patient?** *(All India 2010)*
    a. Whipple's operation
    b. Enucleation
    c. Enucleation with radiotherapy
    d. Administratiaon of streptozocin

185. **Which of the following is the most common endocrine tumor of pancreas?** *(AIIMS June 2004, PGI June 2006)*
    a. Insulinoma
    b. Gastrinoma
    c. VIPoma
    d. Glucagonoma

186. **Insulinoma is most commonly located in which part of the pancreas?** *(AIIMS June 2002)*
    a. Head
    b. Body
    c. Tail
    d. Equally distributed

187. **Whipples triad is seen in:** *(APPG 2015, WBPG 2012, DNB 2011, AIIMS Feb 97)*
    a. Insulinoma
    b. Somatostatinoma
    c. Glucagonoma
    d. CA pancreas

188. **Most common site of insulinoma:** *(Recent Question 2017)*
    a. Head
    b. Body
    c. Tail
    d. Equally distributed in head, body and tail

189. **Which is not true regarding insulinoma?** *(AIIMS Nov 95)*
    a. Hypoglycemic attacks
    b. Weight loss
    c. Usually solitary tumor
    d. Mostly benign tumor

ZOLLINGER-ELLISON SYNDROME

190. **MC site of gastrinoma:** *(GB Pant 2011)*
    a. Duodenum
    b. Pancreas
    c. Stomach
    d. Colon

191. **All are true about gastrinoma except:** *(GB Pant 2011)*
    a. Abnormal peptic ulcer location
    b. Diarrhea
    c. Decreased BAO and MAO
    d. Best treatment is omeprazole

192. **Localization of gastrinoma is best done by:** *(GB Pant 2011)*
    a. USG
    b. CT
    c. MRI
    d. SRS

193. **All are true about gastrinoma except:** *(AIIMS GIS Dec 2006)*
    a. Mostly found in gastrinoma triangle
    b. Increases acid production
    c. Most common site is pancreas
    d. Lymphadenectomy is not required as there is no improvement in survival

194. **Least common site of gastrinoma:** *(AIIMS GIS May 2008)*
    a. 1st part of duodenum
    b. 2nd part of duodenum
    c. 3rd part of duodenum
    d. 4th part of duodenum

195. **All are true about Zollinger-Ellison syndrome except:** *(DNB 2007, AIIMS GIS Dec 2011)*
    a. Recurrent ulceration after acid reducing surgery
    b. Raised gastrin levels in all cases
    c. Decreased BAO/MAO
    d. Diarrhea

196. **All are true about gastrinoma except:** *(AIIMS GIS May 2011)*
    a. 50% are associated with adrenal malignancy
    b. Duodenum is the most common site
    c. Diarrhea can be prevented by NG aspiration
    d. Total gastrectomy should be avoided

197. **All of the following are features of Zollinger-Ellison syndrome except:** *(AIIMS Nov 2005)*
    a. Intractable peptic ulcers
    b. Severe diarrhea
    c. Beta cell tumors of the pancreas
    d. Very high acid output

198. **Treatment of Zollinger-Ellison syndrome:**
    a. Total gastrectomy with removal of tumor
    b. Partial gastrectomy *(DNB 2004, All India 88)*
    c. Excision of tumor alone
    d. H_2 receptor antagonist

199. The investigation of choice to detect gastrinoma <5 mm size is: (COMEDK 2014)
    a. Endoscopic vctrasound   b. Octreotide scan
    c. CT scan   d. Portal venous sampling

200. What is the name of this triangle? (Recent Question 2019)

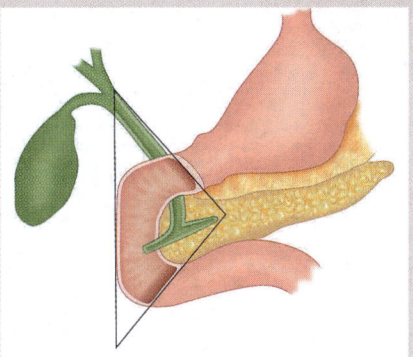

    a. Gastrinoma triangle
    b. Calot's triangle
    c. Doom's triangle
    d. Cholecystohepatic triangle

201. Not a boundary of gastrinoma triangle: (DNB 2011, DPG 2007)
    a. Junction of 2nd and 3rd part of duodenum
    b. Junction of 3rd and 4th part of duodenum
    c. Junction of head with body of pancreas
    d. Junction of cystic duct with common bile duct

202. Which of the following organs is the most common site of origin of the tumor associated with the Zollinger-Ellison syndrome? (COMEDK 2011 2008, 2007)
    a. Duodenum   b. Lymph nodes
    c. Spleen   d. Pancreas

203. A 45-year-old gentleman has undergone truncal vagotomy and pyloroplasty for bleeding duodenal ulcer seven years ago. Now he has intractable recurrent symptoms of peptic ulcer. All of the following suggest the diagnosis of Zollinger Ellison syndrome, except: (AIIMS May 2006)
    a. Basal acid output of 15 mEq/hour
    b. Serum gastrin value of 500 pg/ml
    c. Ulcers in proximal jejunum and lower end of esophagus
    d. Serum gastrin value of 200 pg/ml with secretin stimulation

204. Zollinger-Ellison syndrome is characterized by all of the following except: (All India 94)
    a. Post bulbar ulcer
    b. Recurrent duodenal ulcer
    c. Severe diarrhea
    d. Massive HCl secretion in response to histamine injection

205. True about ZES (gastrinoma): (PGI June 2001)
    a. Gastrin levels >1000 pg/mL
    b. BAO (Basal acid output) >15 mEq/hr
    c. Somatostatin is inhibitor of HCL secretion
    d. Omeprazole is helpful
    e. Secretin increases gastrin secretion in Zollinger-Ellison syndrome

206. Zollinger-Ellison syndrome, all are true except: (PGI June 2008)
    a. Surgery is to be done   b. Exocrine tumor
    c. Endocrine disorder   d. Secretary diarrhea seen
    e. Metastasis seen

207. Which of the following is not true for Zollinger-Ellison syndrome? (DNB 2002, MCI June 2018, Sept 2008)
    a. Recurrence after operation
    b. Reduced BAO: MAO ratio
    c. Gastrin producing tumour
    d. Diarrhea may be a presenting features

208. Diarrhoea with non-healing Gastric ulcer with PPI is due to: (DNB 2014)
    a. MEN 1 syndrome
    b. Zollinger-Ellison syndrome
    c. H. pylori infection   d. VIPoma

209. Which of the following does not form the boundary of gastrinoma triangle? (Recent Question 2017)
    a. Pylorus
    b. Junction of neck and body of pancreas
    c. Cystic duct and CBD junction
    d. Junction of 2nd and 3rd part of duodenum

210. A patient presented with pain in left hypochondrium, vomiting, diarrhea, melena and weight loss. Most probable diagnosis is: (Recent Question 2015)
    a. Cholangitis
    b. Enterocolitis
    c. Zollinger-Ellison syndrome
    d. Amoebiasis

ENDOCRINE TUMORS OF PANCREAS

211. Metastatic glucagonoma is best detected by:
    a. SRS   b. CT   (AIIMS GIS 2003)
    c. MRI   d. USG

212. Most common endocrine tumor of pancreas is: (AIIMS GIS Dec 2006)
    a. Insulinoma   b. Gastrinoma
    c. Somatostatinoma   d. VIPoma

213. Best investigation for neuroendocrine tumors of pancreas: (AIIMS GIS Dec 2006)
    a. Portal venous sampling
    b. CECT
    c. EUS   d. SRS

214. Migratory skin necrosis in a diabetic patient is due to: (AIIMS GIS Dec 2006)
    a. Somatostatinoma   b. Glucagonoma
    c. Insulinoma   d. VIPoma

215. Which is not true about non-functioning NET of pancreas?
    a. Most PPomas are benign   (AIIMS GIS May 2008)
    b. Slow growing tumors
    c. Constitute 30% of all pancreatic NET
    d. Prognosis is better than other exocrine tumors

216. In VIPoma, not seen: (AIIMS GIS May 2008)
    a. Watery diarrhea
    b. Hypokalemia
    c. Hypercalcemia and hyperglycemia
    d. Increased acid secretion

217. Gallstones are associated with which NET: (AIIMS GIS Dec 2010)
    a. Insulinoma   b. VIPoma
    c. Somatostatinoma   d. Glucagonoma

218. The given manifestation is the most common symptom of which of the following neuroendocrine tumor of pancreas?
    a. Insulinoma   b. Glucagonoma
    c. Gastrinoma   d. Somatostatinoma

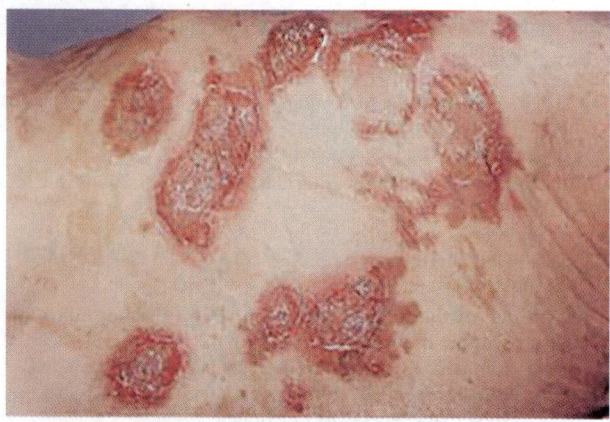

219. **Necrolytic migratory erythema is seen in:**
     (Recnet Question 2016, AIIMS GIS May 2011)
     a. Glucagonoma
     b. Somatostinoma
     c. VIPoma
     d. Insulinoma

220. **The triad of diabetes, gallstones and steatorrhoea is associated with which one of the following tumors?**
     (COMEDK 2014, 2009, 2007)
     a. Gastrinomas   b. Somaststationomas
     c. VIPomas   d. Glucagonomas

221. **Neurotensinoma causes:** *(COMEDK 2010)*
     a. Cyanosis   b. Hypertension
     c. Hyperkalemia   d. Weight gain

222. **Most cases of neuroendocrine tumors are diagnosed by:**
     (AIIMS GIS May 2008)
     a. SRS
     b. Portal venous sampling
     c. Arteriography
     d. CT

223. **WDHA syndrome is associated with:**
     (Recent Question 2017)
     a. VIPoma   b. Somatostatinoma
     c. Glucagonoma   d. Gastrinoma

224. **Which of the following is known as 4D (DVT, Depression, Dermatitis & Diarrhoea) syndrome:**
     (Recent Question 2017)
     a. Glucagonoma
     b. VIPoma
     c. Somatostinoma
     d. Gastrinoma

225. **All are true about neuroendocrine tumor of pancreas:**
     a. Insulinoma is MC *(PGI May 2011)*
     b. VIP cause diarrhea
     c. Diarrhea is MC symptom of gastrinoma
     d. Somatostinoma cause gallstone formation
     e. Gastrinoma has high chance of malignancy

PANCREAS DIVISUM

226. **Pancreas divisum:** *(AIIMS GIS May 2008)*
     a. Most common congenital anomaly
     b. Most are symptomatic
     c. Failure of fusion of dorsal and ventral pancreas
     d. Dorsal duct dilation at lesser papilla is curative

227. **What is the most probable diagnosis based on the given image?**

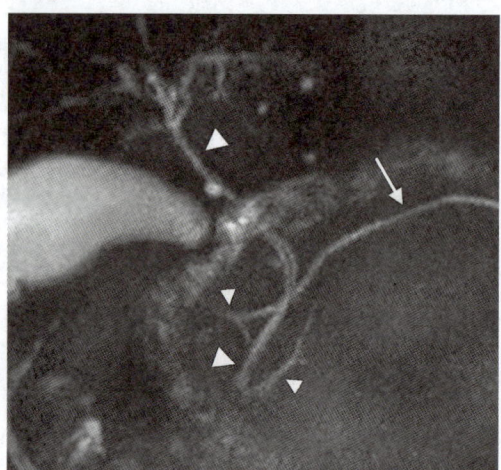

     a. Annular pancreas   b. Pancreas divisum
     c. Chronic pancreatitis d. None of the above

ANNULAR PANCREAS

228. **All are true for annular pancreas except:** *(PGI Nov 2009)*
     a. Upper GI series is IOC
     b. Duodenal obstruction present
     c. ERCP is done
     d. Non-rotation of gut
     e. Treatment is division of ring

229. **Treatment of choice for annular pancreas:**
     (NEET Pattern, MHSSMCET 2006)
     a. Duodenojejunostomy
     b. Distal pancreatectomy
     c. Proximal pancreatectomy
     d. Duodenoduodenostomy

230. **Treatment of choice for annular pancreas is:** *(All India 2010)*
     a. Division of pancreas
     b. Duodenoduodenostomy
     c. Doudenojejunostomy
     d. Roux-en-Y loop

PANCREATIC TRAUMA

231. **True about pancreatic trauma:** *(AIIMS GIS 2003)*
     a. Hyperamylasemia is not specific
     b. Most common is type III and IV
     c. Type II is MPD disruption
     d. ERCP should be done in all patients

232. **Which of the following is true about pancreatic injury?**
     a. Most cases are iatrogenic *(Recent Question 2015)*
     b. Blunt trauma is the most common cause
     c. Urine amylase is diagnostic
     d. HRCT is investigation of choice

233. **Regarding injury to pancreas, which is not true?**
     a. Majority of postoperative complications are due to missed duct injury *(AIIMS Nov 94)*
     b. Fracture is common at the junction of head and body
     c. Commonly associated with vascular injury
     d. Peritoneal lavage is good for making the diagnosis

234. True in pancreatic trauma: *(PGI June 2006)*
    a. Solitary involvement common
    b. Blunt injury usual cause
    c. Always surgery needed
    d. Amylase increases in 90% cases
    e. HRCT is investigation of choice

PANCREATIC TRANSPLANTATION

235. The advantage of bladder drainage over enteric drainage after pancreatic transplantation is better monitoring of: *(All India 2009)*
    a. HBA IC levels
    b. Amylase levels
    c. Glucose levels
    d. Electrolyte levels

MISCELLANEOUS

236. Treatment of congenital cyst of head of pancreas:
    a. Total excision
    b. Partial excision
    c. Marsupialization
    d. Observe and medical treatment

237. In mucoviscidosis of the pancreas the commonest defect is in the:
    a. Jejunum
    b. Ileum
    c. Ascending colon
    d. Descending colon

238. Leukocytic infiltration in islet cells of pancreas is characteristically seen in some cases of:
    a. Juvenile diabetes
    b. Diabetic ketosis
    c. Systemic mucoviscidosis
    d. Hemorrhagic pancreatic necrosis

239. Ectopic pancreatic tissue is present in all except: *(ILBS 2012)*
    a. Stomach
    b. Meckel's diverticulum
    c. Mesentery
    d. Umbilicus

240. The neck of pancreas is related on its posterior surface to: *(AIIMS May 2005)*
    a. Gastroduodenal artery
    b. Superior mesenteric vein
    c. Inferior vena cava
    d. Bile duct

241. Increased amylase levels in pleural fluid are seen in:
    a. Malignancy
    b. Pancreatitis *(Bihar 2003)*
    c. Esophageal rupture
    d. All

242. True increase in islet cell: *(PGI Dec 2002)*
    a. Nesidioblastoma
    b. Type II DM
    c. Insulinoma
    d. None

243. All of the following statements about Nesidioblastosis are true, except: *(All India 2011)*
    a. Hypoglycemic episodes may be seen
    b. Occurs in adults more than children
    c. Histopathology shows hyperplasia of islet cells
    d. Diazoxide may be used for treatment

244. All of the following are true about diazoxide except:
    a. K+ channel opener *(AIIMS May 2011)*
    b. Can be used as antihypertensive agent
    c. Causes severe hypoglycemia
    d. Used in insulinoma

245. Open sphincteroplasty is done at: *(MHSSMCET 2009)*
    a. 12 O' clock position
    b. 11 O' clock position
    c. 6 O' clock position
    d. 2 O' clock position

246. Ectopic pancreatic tissue with islet cells are seen in: *(AIIMS GIS May 2008)*
    a. Stomach
    b. Meckel's diverticulum
    c. Omentum
    d. Appendix

247. Which of the following is not true about polycystic disease of pancreas? *(AIIMS GIS May 2008)*
    a. Associated with liver and renal cyst
    b. 50% associated with VHL syndrome
    c. Surgical intervention is required in most because of features of chronic pancreatitis
    d. Lining of cyst wall is cuboidal

248. Which of the following types of islet cells secrete amylin?
    a. Alpha cells
    b. Beta cells *(All India 2012)*
    c. Delta cells
    d. F cells

249. Investigation of choice to visualise pancreas is: *(DNB 2006)*
    a. MRI
    b. CT Scan
    c. USG abdomen
    d. ERCP

250. Which structure is marked in the given ERCP image? *(Recent Question 2016)*
    a. Gallbladder
    b. Cystic duct
    c. Common hepatic duct
    d. Common bile duct

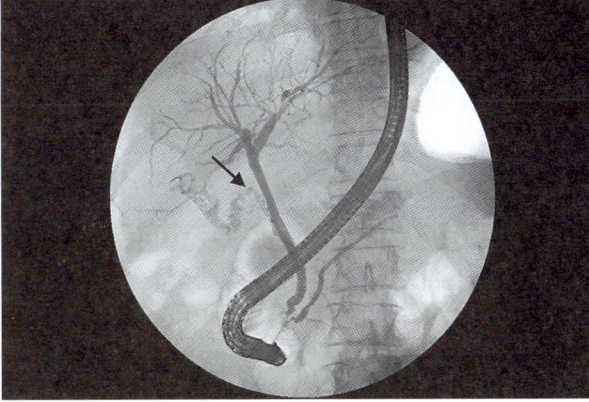

Explanations

ACUTE PANCREATITIS: ETIOLOGY AND RISK FACTORS

1. **Ans. d. Gallstones** *(Ref: Sabiston 20/e p1525-1526; Schwartz 10/e p1351-1360; Bailey 27/e p1222; Blumgart 6/e p883, 5/e p836-845; Shackelford 8/e p1128, 7/e p1123; Harrison 20/e p2438, 19/e p2091)*

2. **Ans. a. Biliary calculi**

3. **Ans. b. L-Asparaginase** *(Ref: Sabiston 20/e p1526; Schwartz 10/e p1351-1360; Bailey 27/e p1222)*

4. **Ans. a. Acute pancreatitis** *(Ref: Sabiston 20/e p1526; Bailey 27/e p1222; Blumgart 6/e p889, 5/e p840; Shackelford 8/e p1076, 7/e p1123)*

> ### COMPLICATIONS OF ERCP
>
> - **Complications**: Pancreatitis, hemorrhage, cholangitis and **perforation**.
> - MC complication is **acute pancreatitis (5%)**[Q]
> - **Hemorrhage** requires **surgical intervention most commonly**, **sphincterotomy** usually is **converted into** formal surgical **sphincteroplasty**, which includes the bleeding artery[Q].
> - **Cholangitis** is confined to patients in whom **CBD clearance** has **not been achieved**, and measures should be directed at providing **adequate bile drainage** and administering **parenteral antibiotics**. Emergency surgery for cholangitis carries high risk, but is indicated in **patients who do not improve within 24 hours**[Q].
> - **Perforation** may be asymptomatic and noticed only as **retroperitoneal gas** or **extravasation of** radiographic **contrast** material, but **even in symptomatic patient, conservative treatment** is often effective with spontaneous resolution and avoidance of potentially difficult surgery[Q].

5. **Ans. b. Splenectomy, d. Cardiopulmonary bypass** *(Ref: Schwartz 10/e p1352)*

> ### IATROGENIC PANCREATITIS
>
> - Acute pancreatitis can be associated with a number of surgical procedures, most commonly those performed on or close to the pancreas, such as **pancreatic biopsy, biliary duct exploration, distal gastrectomy**, and **splenectomy**.
> - Acute pancreatitis is associated postoperatively with **Billroth II gastrectomy** and **jejunostomy**, in which increased intraduodenal pressure can cause backflow of activated enzymes into the pancreas.
> - **Pancreatitis** also can occur in association with surgery that **uses low systemic perfusion**, such as **cardiopulmonary bypass** and **cardiac transplantation**.

6. **Ans. c. Islet cell hyperplasia**

7. **Ans. b. Metronidazole** *(Ref: Sabiston 20/e p1526; Schwartz 10/e p1353; Bailey 27/e p1222)*

ACUTE PANCREATITIS: CLINICAL FEATURES, DIAGNOSIS AND TREATMENT

8. **Ans. d. Cardiac failure** *(Ref: Sabiston 20/e p1524-1528; Schwartz 10/e p1351-1360; Bailey 27/e p1223)*

Non-Pancreatic Causes of Hyperamylasemia		
• Burns	• **Renal transplantation**[Q]	• **Salivary Gland Disorders:** Mumps, Calculus, Maxillofacial surgery[Q]
• Pregnancy	• Perforated Ulcer	• **Tumors:** Carcinoma of the **Lung, Esophagus, Breast, Ovary (LEBO)**[Q]
• Cholecystitis[Q]	• **Chronic liver disease**[Q]	
• **Aortic aneurysm**[Q]	• Intestinal obstruction[Q]	
• **Ruptured ectopic**	• Renal failure[Q]	
• **Diabetic ketoacidosis**	• Drugs: **Morphine**[Q]	

9. **Ans. a. Leucocytosis >20,000/μL** *(Ref: Sabiston 20/e p1527-1528; Schwartz 10/e p1351-1360; Bailey 27/e p1223)*

10. **Ans. b. Acute pancreatitis**

11. **Ans. a. Calcium, e. Antibiotics** *(Ref: Harrison 20/e p2443 19, p2095-2096)*

12. **Ans. b. Serum amylase >350 IU, d. Serum LDH >700 IU**

13. **Ans. None**

14. **Ans. a. Age >55 years, b. WBC >16000/μL, c. Sequestration of fluid >6L**

15. **Ans. b. Serum lipase**

16. **Ans. b. Hypercalcemia**

Pancreas

17. **Ans. b. Gallstone induced pancreatitis** *(Ref: Oxford textbook of surgery 2/e p1766)*

   - The **prognosis is best** in patients where **pancreatitis** is caused by a **remediable cause** such as **cholelithiasis**[Q].
   - **Eradication** of gallstones prevents further attacks of **pancreatitis**[Q].

18. **Ans. d. Prothrombin >2 times the control**   19. **Ans. d. Hyperamylasemia**
20. **Ans. b. Decreased calcium, d. Decreased PaO_2**   21. **Ans. a. Lipase and trypsin**
22. **Ans. d. C-reactive protein <100** *(Ref: Sabiston 20/e p1527; Bailey 27/e p1223)*

Tools for Predicting Severity in Acute Pancreatitis Ready for Clinical Use		
On Admission	**At 24 Hours**	**At 48 Hours**
• APACHE-II Score ≥8[Q] • IL-6 • Urea >60 mmol/L	• Polymorphonuclear **elastase** • Urinary **trypsinogen 2** • Urinary **trypsinogen** activation peptide	• Ranson/Glasgow score ≥ 3[Q] • CRP ≥130[Q] mg/mL

23. **Ans. a. Low serum lipase**   24. **Ans. d. Acute pancreatitis**
25. **Ans. a. Acute fluid collection** *(Ref: Sabiston 20/e p1528-1529)*

   INDICATIONS FOR OPERATIVE TREATMENT IN ACUTE PANCREATITIS

   - Failure of non-operative management with at least 48 hours of maximal ICU support[Q]
   - **Infected necrosis**[Q]
   - Extravisceral **air**[Q]
   - **Hemorrhage** uncontrolled by interventional technique[Q]
   - **Colonic complications**[Q]
   - Operation is indicated for **documented infection** or for **sterile pancreatic necrosis**[Q] with persistent systemic illness.

26. **Ans. b. Hemorrhagic pancreatitis** *(Ref: Bailey 25/e p1144; Sabiston 20/e p1528; Maingot's 11/e p786,977)*

   - All of the following patients presenting with abdominal pain and shock need immediate laparotomy except hemorrhagic pancreatitis.

   Bailey says "In **peritonitis due to pancreatitis** or **salpingitis**, or in cases of **primary peritonitis** of **streptococcal** or **pneumococcal origin**, **non-operative treatment is preferred**[Q] (if diagnosis can be made with certainty)."
   Sabiston says "**Ruptured ectopic is a surgical emergency**[Q]."
   Definitive treatment of ruptured aortic aneurysm is **operation**, not monitoring and **rescuscitation**[Q]
   Maingot's says regarding **liver hemangioma** "**Intra-abdominal hemorrhage** is extremely uncommon, but when does it occur, it should be **considered** as a **life threatening emergency** and **treated with** combination of **angiography with embolization and surgery**[Q]."

27. **Ans. a. Steatorrhoea**

   - **Steatorrhoea** is seen in **chronic pancreatitis**, not in acute pancreatitis.

28. **Ans. c. Acute pancreatitis**   29. **Ans. b. Acute pancreatitis**
30. **Ans. a. Acute pancreatitis** *(Ref: Sabiston 20/e p1527; Schwartz 10/e p1351-1360; Bailey 26/e p1128, 1135, 1138)*

Radiological Appearance		
Acute Pancreatitis	**Chronic Pancreatitis**	**CA Pancreas**
• Renal halo sign[Q] • Gasless abdomen[Q] • Ground glass appearance[Q] • Colon cut off sign[Q] • Sentinel loop[Q]	• **Chain** of **lakes appearance**[Q] • **String** of **pearl appearance**[Q] • **Beaded appearance**[Q] • Numerous **irregular calcifications**[Q] are pathognomonic (on X-ray)	• **Double contour** of medial border of duodenal C loop • **Double duct sign**[Q] • **Dilated /widening** of duodenal C loop[Q] • **Mucosal irregularity**[Q] • **Scrambled egg appearance** • **Inverted /reverse 3 sign** of **Frostberg**[Q]: Seeing CA head of pancreas • **Rose thorning** of **medial wall** of 2nd part of duodenum[Q]

31. **Ans. c. Serum calcium**   32. **Ans. c. Gallbladder stone**
33. **Ans. b. Infection**   34. **Ans. b. Serum amylase**
35. **Ans. d. Severe acute pancreatitis** *(Ref: Sabiston 19/1522-1523; Bailey 27/e p1223)*

   The CT image showing extensive pancreatic necrosis in combination with the acute clinical presentation is typical of severe acute pancreatitis.

36. **Ans. d. Hypoglycemia**   37. **Ans. b. Pancreatitis**   38. **Ans. a. Acute pancreatitis**
39. **Ans. a. Isotonic crystalloid by IV line** *(Ref: Sabiston 20/e p1528; Schwartz 10/e p1358; Bailey 27/e p1225)*

> *"While there are proponents for aggressive fluid therapy and for specific resuscitation goals, it is probably best to resuscitate with a balanced crystalloid and to restore normal blood volume, blood pressure, and urine output. On the basis of recent data it appears that lactated Ringer's solution may be superior to normal saline in reducing the systemic inflammatory response."*
> —*Schwartz 10/e p1358*

40. **Ans. b. Colon cut off sign**

ACUTE PANCREATITIS: COMPLICATIONS

41. **Ans. c. Acute pancreatitis**
42. **Ans. b. Severe acute pancreatitis** *(Ref: Sabiston 20/e p1526; Schwartz 10/e p1356; Bailey 27/e p1019)*

Signs seen in Retroperitoneal bleeding associated with Severe Pancreatitis		
Grey Turner Sign	**Cullen's sign**	**Fox sign**
Ecchymosis in flank	**Periumbilical** ecchymosis	Ecchymosis in **inguinal region**

43. **Ans. a. Needle aspiration, c. External drainage** *(Ref: Sabiston 20/e p1529; Schwartz 10/e p150-151; Bailey 27/e p1227; Blumgart 6/e p902 5/e p858; Shackelford 8/e p1079 7/e p1127-1128)*

STERILE AND INFECTED PERIPANCREATIC FLUID COLLECTIONS (PANCREATIC ABSCESS)

- The presence of **acute abdominal fluid** during an episode of **AP** has been described in **30-57%** of patients[Q].
- In contrast to pseudocysts and cystic neoplasias of the pancreas, **fluid collections are not surrounded** or encased by epithelium or fibrotic capsule[Q].
- **Treatment** is **supportive** because **most fluid collections** will be **spontaneously reabsorbed**[Q] by the peritoneum.
  - **Pancreatic abscess:** The presence of **fever, elevated WBC count**, and **abdominal pain** suggest **infection** of this fluid and **percutaneous aspiration** is **confirmatory**[Q]
  - **Percutaneous drainage** and **IV administration** of **antibiotics** should be instituted if infection (**pancreatic abscess**)[Q] is present

44. **Ans. a. Low protein** *(Ref: Schwartz 9/e p1204; Bailey 27/e p1228; Shackelford 7/e p1128)*

PANCREATIC ASCITES: MANAGEMENT

- **Pancreatic ascites** occurs from a **pancreatic duct disruption** or from a **leaking pseudocyst**.
- **High amylase levels** are found in the **ascitic fluid**[Q].
- Initial treatment: **Non-operative** (**elimination of enteral feeding**, institution of **nasogastric drainage**, and administration of **somatostatin**)[Q]
- **Repeat paracentesis** may also be helpful.
- Roughly **50% to 60%** of patients can be **expected to respond** to this treatment with **resolution** of pancreatic ascites **within 2 to 3 weeks**[Q].

Persistent or recurrent ascites: endoscopic or surgical treatment
• **Endoscopic pancreatic sphincterotomy** with or without placement of a **transpapillary pancreatic duct stent**[Q]. • **Resection** (for **leaks in the pancreatic tail**) or **internal Roux-en-Y drainage** (for leaks in the **head and neck region**)[Q]

45. Ans. d. Leak from the stented duct *(Ref: Schwartz 10/e p1378; Sabiston 20/e p1531; Bailey 27/e p1228)*
46. Ans. b. Bluish discoloration around umbilicus
47. Ans. d. Middle colic artery thrombosis *(Ref: Sabiston 20/e p1531; Schwartz 10/e p1351-1360; Bailey 27/e p1228)*
48. Ans. c. Acute hemorrhagic pancreatitis   49. Ans. c. Commonly associated with hemosuccus pancreaticus
50. Ans. b. Hypocalcemia
    - Most common metabolic complication of acute pancreatitis is hypocalcemia^Q.
51. Ans. a. Grey Turner sign   52. Ans. b. Laparotomy and surgical debridement

CHRONIC PANCREATITIS: ETIOLOGY, CLINICAL FEATURES AND DIAGNOSIS

53. Ans. a. Cationic trypsinogen or PRSS1 *(Ref: Sabiston 20/e p1532; Schwartz 10/e p1362; Bailey 27/e p1230; Blumgart 6/e p915 5/e p861; Shackelford 8/e p1087, 7/e p1134)*
54. Ans. d. Serum amylase is always raised *(Ref: Sabiston 20/e p1531-1536; Schwartz 10/e p1360-1390; Bailey 27/e p1231)*
    - **Amylase** and lipase levels are **not always elevated in chronic pancreatitis, making the diagnosis often clinical.**
55. Ans. a. Can present with steatorrhea, b. Present with mid epigastric pain radiating to back, d. Predisposes to carinoma, e. Complete pancreatectomy relieves pain in majority of patients *(Ref: Schwartz 10/e p1371-1382; Sabiston 20/e p1531-1535; Bailey 27/e p1230-1233)*
56. Ans. a. Abdominal pain
    - **Abdominal pain** is the primary manifestation and **MC symptom** of chronic pancreatitis^Q.
57. Ans. c. Hypercalcemia *(Ref: Sabiston 20/e p1532; Schwartz 10/e p1360, 1366-1367; Bailey 27/e p1230; Harrison 20/e p2445, 19/e p2098)*
58. Ans. b. Cassava ingestion
59. Ans. b. Chronic pancreatitis *(Ref: Sabiston 20/e p1535, 19/e p1521; Schwartz 10/e p1383; Bailey 27/e p1231)*
    - **Chain** of **lakes appearance**^{Q} **or String** of **pearl appearance**^{Q} or **Beaded appearance**^{Q} is characteristic of chronic pancreatitis.
60. Ans. b. Chronic pancreatitis   61. Ans. a. Hypercalcemia
62. Ans. None *(Ref: Harrison 20/e p2445, 19/e p2098)*
    - Chronic pancreatitis is seen in all the given conditions
63. Ans. a. Chronic pancreatitis *(Ref: Sabiston 20/e p1533; Schwartz 10/e p1369; Bailey 27/e p1231)*

    In this X-ray, calcification is seen in epigastric region mainly towards left, along the course of pancreatic duct, seen in chronic pancreatitis.

64. Ans. b. Calcification, c. Duct penetrating sign, e. Dilation of bile and pancreatic duct *(Ref: Bailey 25/e p1157; Sabiston 20/e p1533)*
    - **Irregularity of the pancreatic duct**, **intraductal** or **parenchymal calcifications**, **diffuse pancreatic involvement**, and **normal or smoothly stenotic pancreatic duct penetrating through** the **mass (duct penetrating sign)** ^{Q} favor the **diagnosis of chronic pancreatitis** over cancer.

65. Ans. b. Chronic pancreatitis   66. Ans. b. Alcohol *(Ref: Sabiston 20/e p1531; Schwartz 10/e p1362; Bailey 27/e p1230)*
67. Ans. d. Treatment is mainly surgical *(Ref: Sabiston 20/e p1532; Schwartz 10/e p1366; Bailey 27/e p1230)*
68. Ans. b. ERCP
69. Ans. c. Autosomal recessive inheritance *(Ref: Schwartz 10/e p1352; Sabiston 20/e p1882; Bailey 27/e p1230)*

CHRONIC PANCREATITIS: TREATMENT AND COMPLICATIONS

70. Ans. b. Somatostatin is effective in fistula closure *(Ref: Blumgart 6/e p1010, 5/e p965; Shackelford 8/e p894, 7/e p1278-1280)*
    - Trials have demonstrated the **benefit of prophylactic octreotide** in the **prevention of pancreatic fistula;** however the **role of octreotide, once fistula is established** remains **unclear**^{Q}. In such situations, the octreotide administration is continued for upto 2 weeks, while in those who do not seem to respond, it is discontinued.

71. Ans. a. DPPHR *(Ref: Sabiston 20/e p1535; Schwartz 10/e p1360-1390; Blumgart 6/e p934, 5/e p875-881; Shackelford 8/e p1198 7/e p1138-1142)*

Resection Procedures in Chronic Pancreatitis

- It is believed that **inflammatory process** in the **pancreatic head** controls both the severity of symptoms and further progression of disease in remainder of the gland
- **Pancreatic head** is **pacemaker of chronic pancreatitis**^{Q}.
- Because of this **resection of pancreatic head** has been shown to **completely relieve** the **pain** of chronic pancreatitis in **70-80%**^{Q} patients.
- **Distal pancreatectomy** is the ideal procedure for patients whose **chronic pancreatitis** is confined to **pancreatitis tail**^{Q}.
- Usually, **distal pancreatectomy** is combined **with splenectomy** for technical reasons, but spleen can be preserved if its vascular supply is secure.

72. Ans. a. Distal resection of tail of pancreas with end to end pancreaticojejunostomy
73. Ans. d. Longitudinal Pancreaticojejunostomy

- **Drainage procedure** in the form of **longitudinal pancreaticojejunostomy** is the surgical **treatment of choice** for **chronic pancreatitis with dilated ducts**^{Q}.

74. Ans. d. Medical management

- The patient has **non-disabling pain** that has **responded to analgesia**. Such patients should be best **managed by non-operative means**. **Medical management** is the best option.
- In the patients having **severe pain**, **not relieved by analgesics** with similar situation should be best **managed with longitudinal pancreaticojejunostomy**.

75. Ans. c. Side to side pancreaticojejunostomy
76. Ans. a. Celiac ganglia *(Ref: Sabiston 20/e p1534; Schwartz 10/e p1380; Bailey 27/e p1231)*

Chronic Pancreatitis

- **Pain from** the **pancreas** is carried in **sympathetic fibers** that traverse the **celiac ganglia**, reach the sympathetic chain through the splanchnic nerves, and then ascend to the cortex
- **Celiac plexus nerve blocks**^{Q} performed either **percutaneously** or **endoscopically** have been employed to **abolish this pain** with inconsistent results

77. Ans. d. Distal pancreatectomy
78. Ans. d. None
79. Ans. a. Renal artery stenosis
80. Ans. d. Gallbladder stone is the most common cause
81. Ans. c. Pseudocyst *(Ref: Sabiston 20/e p1530)*

PSEUDOPANCREATIC CYST

82. Ans. b. Endoscopic treatment may be curative *(Ref: Sabiston 20/e p1530; Schwartz 10/e p1377; Bailey 27/e p1231; Shackelford 8/e p1100, 7/e p1144-1148)*
83. Ans. b. Pseudocyst
84. Ans. a. Infection
85. Ans. d. Hemorrhage *(Ref: CSDT 11/e p638)*

- Serious post-op hemorrhage from cyst occurs from cystogastrostomy^Q.

86. Ans. c. Pancreatitis
87. Ans. d. Splenic artery *(Ref: Maingot 11/e p977)*

Artery Involved in Pseudoaneurysm associated with Pancreatic Pseudocyst

- **Splenic artery (30-50%): Most common**^{Q}
- Gastroduodenal artery (10-15%)
- Inferior and superior pancreaticoduodenal artery (10%)

88. Ans. b. Post inflammatory cyst
89. Ans. d. Traumatic pancreatitis

- Trauma is the most common cause of acute pancreatitis in children.

Pancreatic Trauma in Children

- **MC mechanism in children** is **abdominal blunt trauma**^{Q}.
- Direct compression of the epigastrium against the vertebral column and a blunt object (**handlebar**) is typically seen after **bicycle injuries**^{Q}.
- **MC segment** of the pancreas affected is the **body**^{Q}.

90. Ans. d. USG and follow up
91. Ans. d. Percutaneous aspiration is the treatment
92. Ans. a. Percutaneous aspiration is treatment of choice
93. Ans. d. Most common site is in head of pancreas

- **Most common site** of **pancreatic pseudocyst** is **lesser sac**^{Q}

94. Ans. b. Conservative
95. Ans. d. Carcinomatous change

96. Ans. d. Treatment of choice is percutaneous aspiration
97. Ans. c. Calcification in the cyst wall
98. Ans. d. Infection
99. Ans. c. Pseudopancreatic cyst

CYSTIC NEOPLASMS OF PANCREAS

100. Ans. a. IPMN *(Ref: Sabiston 20/e p1538-1539; Schwartz 9/e p1234; Blumgart 6/e p960, 5/e p903-905; Shackelford 8/e p1162 7/e p1220-1222)*
101. Ans. a. Microcystic adenoma *(Ref: Sabiston 20/e p1537; Schwartz 10/e p 1410-1413; Blumgart 5/e p902-903; Shackelford 7/e p1218-1220)*
    - **Mucinous cystadenoma** is **macrocystic**, not the microcystic adenoma.
102. Ans. c. Intraductal papillary mucinous neoplasm
103. Ans. a. Treatment is enucleation
104. Ans. b. Enucleation is performed *(Ref: Sabiston 20/e p1537; Schwartz 10/e p1410; Bailey 27/e p1234)*
105. Ans. a. 30% are associated with malignancy *(Ref: Sabiston 20/e p1538; Schwartz 10/e p 1409-1410)*
106. Ans. b. Serous cystadenoma *(Ref: Sabiston 20/e p1538; Schwartz 10/e p1409)*
107. Ans. a. Always involves main pancreatic duct *(Ref: Sabiston 20/e p1538)*

Cystic Neoplasm of Pancreas			
Characteristics	SCN	MCN	IPMN
Sex	F >> M^Q (4:1)	F >>> M^Q (10:1)	F = M^Q
Age (years)	60-70	50-60	60-70
MC site	**Head**^{Q}	**Body** and **tail**^{Q}	**Head**^{Q}
Pathology	Multiple **small cysts (microcyst)** separated by **internal septations**	Thick-walled, **septated macrocyst**^{Q} with smooth contour; ± **solid** component	Poorly demarcated, lobulated, **polycystic mass** with **dilation** of main or branch **ducts**^{Q}
Radiology/Investigations	**Central sunburst calcifications**^{Q} on CECT	**Egg-shell calcifications**^{Q} on CECT	**Mucin protruding from fish mouth opening on endoscopy**
Cytology	Scant **glycogen-rich cells**, with positive **Periodic Acid Schiff stain**^{Q}	Sheets and clusters of columnar, mucin-containing cells	Tall, columnar mucin-containing cells
Communication with ducts	No	No	**Yes**^{Q}
Amylase level	Low	Low	**High**^{Q}
CEA level	Low	**High**^{Q}	**High**^{Q}
Mucin stain	Negative	**Positive**^{Q}	**Positive**^{Q}

CARCINOMA PANCREAS: ETIOLOGY AND RISK FACTORS

108. Ans. a. Her-2-neu *(Ref: Sabiston 20/e p1541-1542; Schwartz 10/e p1395; Bailey 27/e p1234)*
    - **K-ras mutations** and **HER2/neu over expression** are the **earliest changes** to occur in **pancreatic carcinoma**^{Q}
109. Ans. a. Acute pancreatitis *(Ref: Sabiston 20/e p1541-1542; Schwartz 10/e p1395; Bailey 27/e p1234)*
110. Ans. a. K-ras *(Ref: Sabiston 20/e p1542; Schwartz 10/e p1395; Bailey 27/e p1234)*
111. Ans. d. Cronkhite-Canada syndrome
112. Ans. d. FAP
113. Ans. b. K-ras
114. Ans. d. History of partial gastrectomy
115. Ans. a. Urgent weight reduction, b. Strict vegetarian diet, c. Stop alcohol, e. Stop cigarette smoking
116. Ans. c. BRCA activated
117. Ans. c. Peutz-Jegher's syndrome *(Ref: Sabiston 20/e p1542)*
118. Ans. a. K-ras *(Ref: Sabiston 20/e p1543; Schwartz 10/e p1395; Bailey 27/e p1234)*
119. Ans. a. K-ras
120. Ans. d. Ataxia-Telangiectasia

CA PANCREAS: CLINICAL FEATURES AND DIAGNOSIS

121. Ans. c. Jaundice *(Ref: Sabiston 20/e p1544; Schwartz 10/e p 1394; Bailey 27/e p1234; Blumgart 6/e p979, 5/e p919-925; Shackelford 8/e p1138, 7/e p1190-1196)*

122. **Ans. a. External compression of duodenum** *(Ref: Schwartz 10/e p1395; Sabiston 20/e p1544; Bailey 27/e p1234)*
123. **Ans. a. MDCT**

- **Diagnostic investigation** in **carcinoma pancreas** is **MDCT**[Q]
- **MDCT** is **investigation of choice** for the evaluation of **lesions arising** in the **pancreas**[Q]
- **IOC** for **diagnosis, staging** and **follow-up** in **CA pancreas: MDCT**[Q]

124. **Ans. a. T1** 125. **Ans. a. Most common site is body and tail**
126. **Ans. d. EUS guided transgastric biopsy** *(Ref: Schwartz 10/e p1397-1399; Sabiston 20/e p1544; Bailey 27/e p1235)*

- "EUS is useful if CT fails to demonstrate a tumour, if tissue diagnosis is required prior to surgery (e.g. a mass has developed on a background of chronic pancreatitis and a distinction needs to be made between inflammation and neoplasia), if vascular invasion needs to be confirmed, or in separating cystic tumours from pseudocysts. Transduodenal or transgastric FNA or Trucut biopsy performed under EUS guidance avoids spillage of tumour cells into the peritoneal cavity. Percutaneous transperitoneal biopsy of potentially resectable pancreatic tumours should be avoided as far as possible. Histological confirmation of malignancy is desirable but not essential, particularly if the imaging clearly demonstrates a resectable tumour. The lack of a tissue diagnosis should not delay appropriate surgical therapy. In patients judged to have unresectable disease, tissue diagnosis should be obtained prior to starting palliative therapy." —*Bailey 27/e p1235*

127. **Ans. c. Pancreatic carcinoma** *(Ref: Grainger 4/e p1356-64)* 128. **Ans. a. Periampullary carcinoma**
129. **Ans. a. Pancreatic cancer, c. Stomach cancer** *(Ref: Robbins 9/e p332, 126)*

Malignancies Associated with Migratory Thrombophlebitis	
• CA **pancreas (MC)**[Q]	• Prostate cancer[Q]
• CA **lung**[Q]	• **Ovarian** cancer[Q]
• GI malignancies[Q]	• **Lymphoma**[Q]

- **Trousseau's syndrome: Migratory thrombophlebitis**[Q]
- **Trousseau's sign: Carpopedal spasm in hypocalcemia**[Q]
- **Troisier's sign: Palpable left supraclavicular LN (Virchow's node)**[Q]

130. **Ans. a. Head is the most common site, c. Obstruction of bile and pancreatic secretion is common**
131. **Ans. a. Hypotonic duodenogram, c. USG, d. Endoscopy, e. CT Scan**
132. **Ans. d. Periampullary carcinoma** 133. **Ans. c. CA head of pancreas**
134. **Ans. d. Carcinoma head of pancreas** *(Ref: radiopaedia.org/articles/frostburg-inverted-3-sign-1)*

- **Frostburg inverted 3 sign** is a sign seen on a **barium examination** where there is **effacement and distortion of the mucosal pattern** on the **medial wall of the second part of the duodenum** due to **focal mass and local edema**. It is **most commonly associated with carcinoma of the head of the pancreas**.

135. **Ans. d. Ductal adenocarcinoma** 136. **Ans. a. Ductal adenocarcinoma**
137. **Ans. d. CT scan** *(Ref: CSDT 11/e p645; Schwartz 10/e p1398)*

- **Investigation of choice** for carcinoma pancreas: **MDCT**[Q]
- Currently **CT** is probably the single **most versatile** and **cost effective** tool **for diagnosis of pancreatic cancer**

138. **Ans. b. Syndrome of inappropriate secretion of ADH** *(Ref: Harrison 20/e p2690, 19/e p2280)*

Causes of Syndrome of Inappropriate Antidiuresis (SIADH)		
Neoplasms	Infections	Neurologic
• Lung[Q]	• **Pneumonia**[Q], bacterial or viral	• Guillain-Barré syndrome[Q]
• **Duodenum**[Q], **Pancreas**[Q]	• **Abscess**[Q], lung or brain	• Multiple sclerosis[Q]
• **Ovary**[Q], **Bladder**[Q], **ureter**[Q]	• Cavitation (**aspergillosis**)	• Delirium tremens[Q]
• Thymoma[Q], Mesothelioma[Q]	• **Tuberculosis**, lung or brain	• Amyotrophic lateral sclerosis[Q]
• **Bronchial adenoma**[Q]	• Meningitis, bacterial or viral	• Hydrocephalus, Psychosis
• Carcinoid	• **Encephalitis**[Q], **AIDS**[Q]	• Peripheral neuropathy[Q]
• Gangliocytoma, Ewing's sarcoma		

Metabolic	Vascular	Drugs
• Acute intermittent porphyria	• Cerebrovascular occlusions, hemorrhage	• Vasopressin[Q] or desmopressin
Pulmonary	• Cavernous sinus thrombosis[Q]	• Chlorpropamide[Q]
		• Oxytocin, high dose[Q]
• Asthma, Pneumothorax[Q]	**Congenital malformations**	• Vincristine, Carbamazepine[Q]
• Positive-pressure respiration		• Nicotine, Phenothiazines[Q]
Head trauma	• Agenesis corpus callosum	• Cyclophosphamide[Q]
• Closed and penetrating[Q]	• Cleft lip/palate[Q]	• Tricyclic antidepressants[Q]
	• Other midline defects	• Monoamine oxidase inhibitors[Q]
		• Serotonin reuptake inhibitors[Q]

139. Ans. b. Carcinoma head of pancreas
140. Ans. a. EUS guided transgastric biopsy *(Ref: Sabiston 20/e p1544; Schwartz 10/e p1399; Bailey 27/e p1235)*
141. Ans. c. Carcinoma pancreas *(Ref: Sabiston 20/e p1544; Schwartz 10/e p1397; Bailey 27/e p1235)*
    - **Double duct sign** on **ERCP** is highly suggestive of **pancreatic head cancer**[Q].
142. Ans. a. Periampullary carcinoma *(Ref: Shackelford 7/e p1183)*   143. Ans. a. Head
144. Ans. b Periampullary carcinoma *(Ref: Sabiston 20/e p1544; Schwartz 10/e p1395; Bailey 27/e p1234)*

> • "The waxing and waning nature of jaundice is due to sloughing of ampullary cancer, resulting in transient resolution of the jaundice."

145. Ans. d. Carcinoma head of pancreas

CARCINOMA PANCREAS: TREATMENT AND PROGNOSIS

146. Ans. a. R0 resection *(Ref: Sabiston 20/e p1546; Schwartz 10/e p1394; Blumgart 6/e p 983, 5/e p819-825; Shackelford 8/e p1144, 7/e p1192-1202)*
147. Ans. a. Lung *(Ref: Sabiston 20/e p1544)*

Metastatic Tumors to Pancreas
• **MC site of primary**: **RCC**[Q] > Malignannt melanoma
• On **autopsy**, MC site of primary: **CA lung**[Q]

148. Ans. a. Delayed gastric emptying *(Ref: Sabiston 20/e p1548; Schwartz 10/e p1406; Blumgart 6/e p464, 5/e p819-825; Shackelford 8/e p 1144, 7/e p1200)*

Morbidity Following Pancreaticoduodenectomy	
• **Delayed gastric emptying (18%)**[Q]	• Cardiac events (3%)
• **Pancreas fistula (12%)**	• Bile leak (2%)
• **Wound infection (7%)**	• Overall reoperation (3%)
• Intra-abdominal abscess (6%)	

149. Ans. b. Pain is early in the course of the disease *(Ref: Sabiston 20/e p1544)*

Carcinoma Pancreas
• Symptoms include **unexplained episodes of pancreatitis**[Q], **painless jaundice**, nausea, vomiting, steatorrhea, and **unexplained weight loss**
• With **further spread beyond the pancreas**, these patients may **note upper abdominal** or **back pain** when **peripancreatic nerve plexuses** are **involved** and **ascites** when **peritoneal carcinomatosis** or **portal vein occlusion** develops[Q]

150. Ans. c. Gemcitabine *(Ref: Bailey 27/e p1237; Blumgart 6/e p 1040, 5/e p925; Shackelford 8/e p 1146, 7/e p1202)*
    - **Gemcitabine**[Q] is currently the standard of care for patients with **metastatic pancreatic cancer**.
151. Ans. b. Tumors of head pancreas *(Ref: Blumgart 6/e p 1020, 5/e p959-960)*

MIDDLE OR CENTRAL OR SEGMENTAL PANCREATECTOMY
• Middle pancreatectomy is a **safe, effective procedure** for **treatment of benign and low grade malignant neoplasms** of the **mid pancreas**[Q]

Advantages of Middle or Segmental Pancreatectomy
• **Preserves pancreatic parenchyma**
• **Reduces** the risk of **exocrine** and **endocrine insufficiency**
• Consists of a **limited resection** of the **mid portion** of the pancreas

- Can be performed in selected patients affected by tumors of the **pancreatic neck**^{Q}
- In experienced hands it is associated with **no mortality** but with **high morbidty**, even if the rate of "clinical" panreatic fistula is about 20%
- Middle pancreatectomy is **avoided in** patients affected by **main duct IPMN**.

Indications of Middle or Segmental Pancreatectomy

- **Benign** or **low grade** malignant tumor (**Neuroendocrine tumors, serous cystadenoma, branch duct IPMNs**)^Q
- Location in the **neck**^{Q} or its contiguous portion
- A **distal** pancreas **stump** of at least **5cm** in length^Q

152. **Ans. c. Median survival in locally advanced (stage III) disease is 3-6 months** *(Ref: Sabiston 20/e p1547; Blumgart 6/e p 963, 5/e p922; Shackelford 8/e p 1144, 7/e p1195-1196)*

153. **Ans. b. Duodenojejunostomy** *(Ref: Sabiston 20/e p1546; Bailey 27/e p1237; Shackelford 8/e p1185, 7/e p1196)*
   - **Duodenojejunostomy** is done **in PPPD**, not in Whipple's procedure.
   - **Gastrojejunostomy** is done **in Whipple's procedure**.

154. **Ans. c. Portal vein**   155. **Ans. d. Choledochojejunostomy** *(Ref: Devita 9/e p979)*

Palliative Surgery in Advanced, Non-resectable Pancreatic Adenocarcinoma

- **Surgery** for **advanced, non-resectable pancreatic adenocarcinoma** can **palliate obstruction** of **CBD** or **duodenum**, as well as **control visceral pain**^{Q}
- **Hepaticojejunostomy, choledochojejunostomy** or **choledochoduodenostomy** offers **durable drainage** of an obstructed bile duct.^{Q}
- **Cholecystojejunostomy** is **less reliable** but can be employed when tumor bulk precludes common duct procedure
- **Gastrojejunostomy** (**antecolic** anastomosis) palliates gastric outlet obstruction^Q
- **Antecolic anastomosis**^{Q} is done to **avoid complications** from an **expanding lesser sac tumor**

156. **Ans. d. Periampullary** *(Ref: Shackelford 8/e p 1138, 7/e p1187-1206)*

Periampullary Carcinoma

1. Adenocarcinoma of **head** of the pancreas (**40-60%**)^Q
2. Adenocarcinoma of **ampulla** of vater (10-20%)
3. **Distal bile duct** adenocarcinoma (10%)
4. **Duodenal** adenocarcinoma (5-10%)

- Patients with **pancreas adenocarcinoma** involving the **body or tail** of the gland are more likely to have **weight loss** and **abdominal pain** as their **initial complaints**.
- These lesions can **grow to a larger size before producing symptoms** and are often **diagnosed at a later stage** with a **poorer prognosis**.
- Most **body** and **tail** cancers have **already metastasized to distant sites** or extended locally to involve nodes, nerves, or **major vessels** by the **time of diagnosis**.
- Best prognosis: Duodenal adenocarcinoma >Ampullary carcinoma >Distal Bile duct adenocarcinoma >Head of pancreas >Body and tail of Pancreas (**DAD Head Body** and **Tail**)^Q

157. **Ans. a. Disruption of pancreatic anastomosis**   158. **Ans. c. Pancreaticoduodenectomy**
159. **Ans. b. Mobilization of 2nd part of duodenum**
   - **Kocher** maneuver is a technique for **mobilization of the duodenum**^{Q}.
160. **Ans. b. Pancreatic carcinoma**   161. **Ans. c. CA pancreas**
162. **Ans. c. Good prognosis**
163. **Ans. d. Acute pancreatitis never occurs in CA pancreas** *(Ref: Sabiston 20/e p1544)*

Clinical Features of Carcinoma Pancreas

- **MC site** is **head and uncinate process**^{Q}
- Patients with lesions that occur near the bile duct, such as those near the **ampulla**, **head** of the pancreas, and **uncinate process**, are much more likely to have **obstructive jaundice**^{Q}.
- Those with **lesions in the body or tail of the pancreas** are more likely to complain of **pain**.

- **Pain** suggests **unresectability**^Q in carcinoma pancreas
- **Two third (65%)** patients present with **diabetes in carcinoma pancreas**^Q
- Patients may also have **acute pancreatitis secondary to obstruction of the pancreatic duct**^Q.
- **Elderly patients with acute pancreatitis** but **without a history of alcohol use** or **gallbladder stones** should be **screened for a neoplasm**^Q.

164. Ans. a. CA 19-9   165. Ans. b. CA duodenum *(Ref: Shackelford 8/e p1138, 7/e p1201)*

- **Best prognosis**: **Duodenal** adenocarcinoma >**Ampullary** carcinoma >**Distal Bile duct** adenocarcinoma >**Head** of **pancreas** >**Body** and **tail** of Pancreas (**DAD Head Body** and **Tail**)

166. Ans. a. Retroperitoneal margin *(Ref: Shackelford 7/e p1196-1200)*   167. Ans. c. Cardiopulmonary complications
168. Ans. b. Distal pancreatectomy with splenectomy *(Ref: Sabiston 20/e p1547; Schwartz 9/e p1226; Bailey 27/e p1236; Shackelford 8/e p1186, 7/e p1198-199)*

RESECTIONAL SURGERY FOR PANCREATIC BODY AND TAIL TUMORS

- Most **body and tail cancers** have **already metastasized to distant sites** or extended locally to **involve nodes, nerves**, or **major vessels** by the time of diagnosis.
- **Splenic vein involvement** or **occlusion** is **not a sign of nonresectability**^Q.
- Involvement of the **splenic and SMV confluence** generally **precludes resection**.
- **Resection** involves a **distal pancreatectomy** either **with** or **without concomitant splenectomy**^Q.
- **Splenectomy** is usually **performed with distal pancreatectomy** in patients suspected of **having carcinoma** to obtain **better margins**, to **remove the lymph nodes** at the tip of the pancreas and the hilum of the spleen, and to avoid tedious dissection of the splenic artery and vein.

169. Ans. b. Ascites   170. Ans. a. Pyloric antrum
171. Ans. a. Delayed gastric emptying *(Ref: Sabiston 20/e p1548; Schwartz 10/e p1406; Bailey 27/e p1236)*
172. Ans. b. 22 months *(Ref: Sabiston 20/e p1547)*

"After surgical resection and adjuvant therapy for pancreatic cancer, the median survival is approximately 22 months, with 5-year survival of 15% to 20%. Most patients experience relapse of disease in the form of metastatic disease (85%) and, less commonly, local recurrence (40%). In the absence of surgical resection, those with locally advanced disease who receive palliative chemotherapy may survive 10 to 12 months, whereas those with metastases rarely survive beyond 6 months."-Sabiston 20/e p1547

173. Ans. d. Pancreaticojejunostomy, hepaticojejunostomy, gastrojejunostomy

PSEUDOPAPILLARY TUMOR

174. Ans. c. These are small tumors *(Ref: Blumgart 6/e p968, 5/e p908-909; Shackelford 8/e p1173, 7/e p1268)*
175. Ans. d. Chromagranin is positive

INSULINOMA

176. Ans. a. EUS with intra-operative palpation *(Ref: Sabiston 20/e p947, 952; Schwartz 10/e p1391; Bailey 27/e p849; Blumgart 6/e p 1001, 5/e p935-937; Shackelford 8/e p1150, 7/e p1206-1210)*

LOCALIZATION OF INSULINOMA

- A small portion of insulinomas remain unlocalizable despite extensive studies and are therefore considered occult.
- When the **diagnosis is certain** based on the result of a **72-hour fast**, **surgical exploration** with careful inspection, **palpation**, and **intraoperative ultrasound (IOUS)** is **indicated**^Q.
- Studies have shown that the **combination of surgical exploration** with **IOUS identifies almost all insulinomas**^Q.

177. Ans. d. Selective arteriography

- **Portal venous sampling** for insulin with or without **arterial stimulation** with **calcium** is the **best pre-operative method** of **localization**^Q.
- **EUS** with **intra-operative palpation** is **best localization technique** for **Insulinoma**^Q.

178. Ans. a. Insulinoma
179. Ans. a. Usually asymptomatic and need no treatment
180. Ans. c. Weight loss is important feature
181. Ans. a. 72-hours fasting test
182. Ans. b. Xylose test
183. Ans. a. Intra-operative USG
184. Ans. b. Enucleation
185. Ans. a. Insulinoma

NET OF PANCREAS

- MC NET of Pancreas: Non-functional (Mostly malignant) >Insulinoma[Q]
- MC benign NET of Pancreas: Insulinoma[Q]
- MC malignant functional NET of Pancreas: Gastrinoma[Q]

186. Ans. d. Equally distributed
187. Ans. a. Insulinoma
188. Ans. d. Equally distributed in head, body and tail *(Ref: Sabiston 20/e p952; Schwartz 10/e p1391; Bailey 27/e p849)*
189. Ans. b. Weight loss

ZOLLINGER-ELLISON SYNDROME

190. Ans. a. Duodenum *(Ref: Sabiston 20/e p954; Schwartz 10/e p1071-1073; Bailey 27/e p850; Blumgart 6/e p999, 5/e p937-941; Shackelford 8/e p702, 7/e p749-756)*
191. Ans. c. Decreased BAO and MAO
   - Basal acid output is increased in Gastrinoma[Q].
192. Ans. d. SRS
193. Ans. c. Most common site is pancreas
194. Ans. d. 4th part of duodenum
195. Ans. c. Decreased BAO/MAO
196. Ans. a. 50% are associated with adrenal malignancy
197. Ans. c. Beta cell tumors of the pancreas
198. Ans. d. H$_2$ receptor antagonist
199. Ans. a. Endoscopic ultrasound
200. Ans. a. Gastrinoma triangle *(Ref: Schwartz 10/e p1392; Sabiston 20/e p954; Bailey 27/e p1141)*
201. Ans. b. Junction of 3rd and 4th part of duodenum
202. Ans. a. Duodenum
203. Ans. d. Serum gastrin value of 200 pg/ml with secretin stimulation
204. Ans. d. Massive HCl in response to histamine injection
205. Ans. a. Gastrin levels >1000 pg/mL, b. BAO (Basal acid output) >15 meq/hr, c. Somatostatin is inhibitor of HCL secretion, d. Omeprazole is helpful, e. Secretin increases gastrin secretion in Zollinger-Ellison syndrome
206. Ans. b. Exocrine tumor
207. Ans. b. Reduced BAO: MAO ratio
208. Ans. b. Zollinger-Ellison syndrome
209. Ans. a. Pylorus *(Ref: Sabiston 20/e p1210; Schwartz 10/e p1392; Bailey 27/e p851)*
210. Ans. c. Zollinger-Ellison syndrome

ENDOCRINE TUMORS OF PANCREAS

211. Ans. a. SRS *(Ref: Sabiston 20/e p957; Schwartz 10/e p1393; Bailey 27/e p849; Blumgart 6/e p1001, 5/e p940-941; Shackelford 8/e p1150, 7/e p1211-1212)*
212. Ans. a. Insulinoma
213. Ans. d. SRS *(Ref: Sabiston 20/e p947)*
214. Ans. b. Glucagonoma
215. Ans. a. Most PPomas are benign *(Ref: Sabiston 20/e p958; Schwartz 10/e p1393; Bailey 27/e p852; Shackelford 8/e p1155, 7/e p1213-1214)*
216. Ans. d. Increased acid secretion *(Ref: Sabiston 19/e p954, 956, 960; Schwartz 10/e p1392-1393; Bailey 27/e p850)*
217. Ans. c. Somatostatinoma *(Ref: Sabiston 20/e p957; Schwartz 10/e p1393; Bailey 27/e p849)*
218. Ans. b. Glucagonoma *(Ref: Sabiston 20/e p957; Schwartz 10/e p1393; Bailey 27/e p849)*
   - Necrolytic erythema migrans is the most common symptom of glucagonoma.
219. Ans. a. Glucagonoma
220. Ans. b. Somaststationomas
221. Ans. a. Cyanosis *(Ref: Sabiston 20/e p956)*
222. Ans. a. SRS
223. Ans. a. VIPoma *(Ref: Sabiston 20/e p965; Schwartz 10/e p1392; Bailey 27/e p849)*
224. Ans. a. Glucagonoma *(Ref: Sabiston 20/e p957; Schwartz 10/e p1393; Bailey 27/e p849)*
225. Ans. a. Insulinoma is MC, b. VIP cause diarrhea, d. Somatostatinoma cause gallstone formation, e. Gastrinoma has high chance of malignancy

NET of Pancreas	
Tumor	MC site
• Gastrinoma	• Duodenum (1st part) >Pancreas[Q]
• Insulinoma	• Equally distributed[Q] in head, body and tail
• Glucagonoma	• Body and Tail[Q]
• Somatostatinoma and PPoma	• Head[Q]
• VIPoma	• Tail[Q]

All pancreatic cancers and neoplastic cysts are most common in pancreatic head except:
• Mucinous cystic neoplasm and Glucagonoma: MC in body and tail[Q]
• VIPoma: MC in Tail[Q]
• Insulinoma: Equally distributed[Q] in head, body and tail

PANCREAS DIVISUM

226. **Ans. a. Most common congenital anomaly** *(Ref: Sabiston 20/e p1522; Schwartz 10/e p1365-1366; Bailey 27/e p1219; Blumgart 6/e p861, 5/e p818-819; Shackelford 8/e p1127, 7/e p1134-1135)*

227. **Ans. b. Pancreas divisum** *(Ref: Sabiston 20/e p1522; Schwartz 10/e p1366; Bailey 27/e p1219)*

   In this ERCP, major part of pancreas is drained by accessory duct of Santorini via minor papilla and head and uncinate process is drained by duct of Wirsung via ampulla suggestive of pancreas divisum.

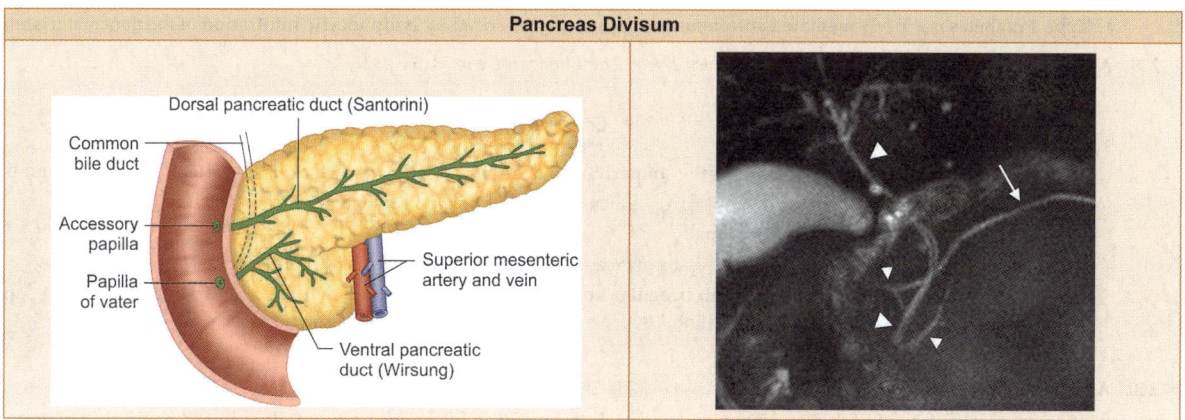

Pancreas Divisum

ANNULAR PANCREAS

228. **Ans. e. Treatment is division of ring** *(Ref: Sabiston 20/e p1522; Bailey 27/e p1219; Blumgart 6/e p870, 5/e p823-826; Shackelford 8/e p1215, 7/e p1179-1180)*

229. **Ans. d. Duodenoduodenostomy** *(Ref: Blumgart 6/e p860, 5/e p823-826)*
   - Read the text from the latest edition of **Blumgart**, surgery of liver, biliary tract and pancreas. It clears that **duodenoduodenostomy** is the **treatment of choice** for **annular pancreas**, not the **duodenojejunostomy** given in Harrison or Maingot.
   - **Duodenoduodenostomy** has **replaced duodenojejunostomy** as the **treatment of choice**[Q] because it has a **lower incidence** of **postoperative complications**, particularly **obstruction** and **blind-loop syndromes**[Q].

   TREATMENT OF ANNULAR PANCREAS
   - A review of the **existing literature published in 1980** concluded that "**while there** is **no single operative procedure of choice, experience militates against any direct attack on the offending annulus**". This conclusion stands, and any attempt to divide the annulus itself risks the formation of a pancreatic fistula.
   - **Early pediatric series established duodenal bypass as the treatment of choice**, although mortality rates remained high, likely related to the presence of other congenital malformations and the lack of supportive care.
   - **Duodenoduodenostomy** has **replaced duodenojejunostomy** as the **treatment of choice** because it has a **lower incidence** of **postoperative complications**, particularly **obstruction** and **blind-loop syndromes**[Q].

230. **Ans. b. Duodenoduodenostomy**

PANCREATIC TRAUMA

231. Ans. a. Hyperamylasemia is not specific *(Ref: Sabiston 20/e p440, 1552; Schwartz 9/e p179)*
232. Ans. d. HRCT is investigation of choice
233. Ans. b. Fracture is common at the junction of head and body, d. Peritoneal lavage is good for making the diagnosis
234. Ans. d. Amylase increases in 90% cases, e. HRCT is investigation of choice

PANCREATIC TRANSPLANTATION

235. Ans. b. Amylase levels *(Ref: Sabiston 20/e p644-665; Schwartz 10/e p340-344; Bailey 27/e p1553; Blumgart 6/e p1881, 5/e p1796-1805; Shackelford 8/e p1230, 7/e p1251-1260)*
    - Bailey 25/e p1425: '**Urinary drainage** of the pancreas has the **advantage** that **urinary amylase levels can be used to monitor graft rejection**'^{Q}

MISCELLANEOUS

236. Ans. d. Observe and medical treatment *(Ref: Blumgart 6/e p873, 5/e p827; Bailey 27/e p120)*
237. Ans. b. Ileum
    - Terminal ileum is filled with meconium in mucoviscidosis.
238. Ans. a. Juvenile diabetes
    - **Type 1 diabetes** is a **T cell-mediated autoimmune disease**, characterized by **lymphocytic infiltration** of the pancreatic **islets**^{Q}.
239. Ans. c. Mesentery *(Ref: Sabiston 20/e p1522; Bailey 27/e p1219; Blumgart 6/e p873, 5/e p827)*

ECTOPIC PANCREAS

- The most common sites are in the **walls of the stomach**^{Q}, **duodenum**^{Q}, or **ileum**, in a **Meckels diverticulum**^{Q}, or at the **umbilicus**^{Q}
- Less common sites include the colon, appendix, gallbladder, omentum, and mesentery.
- **Most ectopic pancreatic tissue** is **functional**^{Q}.
- **Islet tissue** is frequently **present** when ectopic pancreas is located **in the stomach** and **duodenum.**
- Ectopic pancreatic tissue is a **submucosal, irregular nodule** of firm, yellow tissue that has a **central umbilication**^{Q}; pancreatic secretions often exit through this umbilication.
---

240. Ans. b. Superior mesenteric vein *(Ref: BDC 4/e pvol-II/284-285)*
    - The **posterior surface of neck** of **pancreas** is related to the **termination of superior mesenteric vein** and **beginning of portal vein**^{Q}.
241. Ans. d. All
242. Ans. c. Insulinoma
243. Ans. b. Occurs in adults more than children
244. Ans. c. Causes severe hypoglycemia *(Ref: Goodman Gilman 12/ep1271)*

DIAZOXIDE

- **K$^+$ channel opener**, causes **arteriolar dilatation**^{Q}
- Diazoxide **produces hyperglycemia** by **decreasing insulin**^{Q} Used in **insulinoma**^{Q}
- When used as **intravenous antihypertensive agent**^{Q}, it causes excessive hypotension
---

245. Ans. b. 11 O' clock position *(Ref: Sabiston 20/e p1396; Schwartz 10/e p1327)*

TRANSDUODENAL SPHINCTEROPLASTY

- This **cut is made superiorly** (at the **11' O clock position**)^Q for **4 to 5 mm**.
- The **sphincter** is **incised at the 11' O clock position** to **avoid injury to the pancreatic duct**^{Q}.
---

246. Ans. a. Stomach
247. Ans. c. Surgical intervention is required in most because of features of chronic pancreatitis
248. Ans. b. Beta cells *(Ref: Sabiston 20/e p943)*

Islet Cells	Content
• Alpha cells	• Glucagon, **glicentin**[Q], **pancreastatin**[Q]
• Beta cells	• Insulin, **amylin**[Q], **pancreastatin**[Q]
• D cells	• Somatostatin
• D_2 cells	• VIP
• G cells	• Gastrin
• PP cells	• Pancreatic polypeptide

249. Ans. b. CT scan *(Ref: Sutton 7/e p796)*

- **CT is the mainstay of pancreatic imaging**, able to demonstrate **focal masses within the gland calcifications, duct dilatation, cysts, abscesses** and associated abnormalities in upper abdominal organs (hepatic metastases), lymph nodes and peri-pancreatic vascular structures.
- **CT** is a useful tool **for guiding percutaneous pancreatic biopsy** and **cyst aspiration** or **drainage**.

250. Ans. b. Cystic duct *(Ref: Sabiston 20/e p1482)*

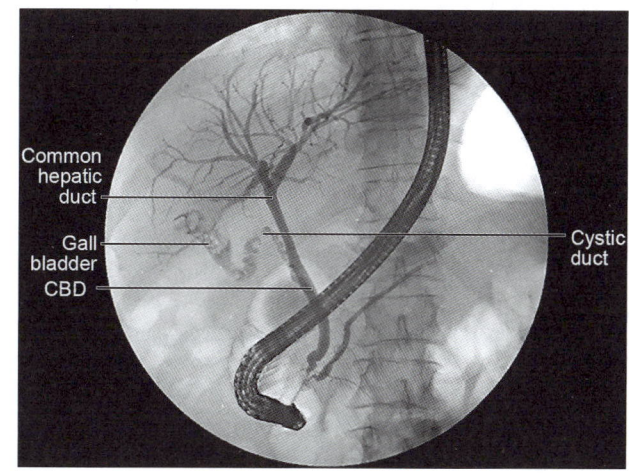

SECTION 3

Gastrointestinal Surgery

CHAPTERS

- ☐ Esophagus
- ☐ Stomach and Duodenum
- ☐ Peritoneum
- ☐ Intestinal Obstruction
- ☐ Small Intestine
- ☐ Large Intestine
- ☐ Ileostomy and Colostomy
- ☐ Inflammatory Bowel Disease
- ☐ Vermiform Appendix
- ☐ Rectum and Anal Canal
- ☐ Hernia and Abdominal Wall
- ☐ Spleen

section 3

Gastrointestinal Surgery

CHAPTER 9

Esophagus

CONGENITAL DIAPHRAGMATIC HERNIA (BOCHDALEK HERNIA OR POSTEROLATERAL HERNIA)

Congenital Diaphragmatic Hernia (Bochdalek Hernia or Posterolateral Hernia)

- CDH term is used for **Bochdalek hernia**^{Q}

  > - Incidence 1 in 2000 to 5000^Q live births.
  > - Most CDH defects are on the **left side (80%)**; up to **20% on right side**^{Q}.
  > - Rarely bilateral.

- Survival rate for CDH **70–90%**^{Q}.
- **Bag & Mask ventilation** is **contraindicated** in **CDH**^{Q}.

Pathogenesis

- The cause is thought to result from **failure of normal closure** of the **pleuroperitoneal canal**^{Q} in the developing embryo.
- As a result, **abdominal contents herniate** through the resultant defect in the **posterolateral diaphragm** and **compress** the **ipsilateral developing lung**^{Q}.
- **Compression** of the lung results in **pulmonary hypoplasia** involving both lungs, with the **ipsilateral lung** being the **most affected**^{Q}.
- **Pulmonary vasculature** is distinctly abnormal in that the **medial muscular thickness** of the **arterioles** is excessive and extremely sensitive to the **multiple local** and **systemic factors** known to **trigger vasospasm**^{Q}.

  > - **Main factors** affecting morbidity and mortality: **Pulmonary hypoplasia & pulmonary hypertension**^{Q}.

Clinical Features

  > - Classic triad: **Respiratory distress + Dextrocardia + Scaphoid abdomen**^{Q}

- **MC** presentation is **respiratory distress** due to severe hypoxemia.
- Infant appears dyspneic, tachypneic, & cyanotic, with severe retractions.
- **Anteroposterior diameter** of the **chest** may be **large**, & abdomen may be **scaphoid**^{Q}.

Diagnosis

- **Diagnosis** is made at the time of a **prenatal ultrasound** during pregnancy.
- **Postnatal diagnosis** by a **plain chest radiograph** demonstrates the **gastric air bubble** or **loops of bowel** within the **chest**^{Q}.
- There may also be a **mediastinal shift away** from the **side of hernia** or **polyhydramnios**^{Q} from the obstructed stomach.
- **Pneumothorax** always occurs on **contralateral** to the **side of CDH**^{Q}.

Treatment

- **Physiologic stress** associated with **early repair** probably **adds more insult** and that **survival is not improved**^{Q} when compared with delayed repair.
- A variable period of time (**24–72 hours**) to allow **for stabilization** before **surgical repair**^{Q}.

  > - The **viscera** are **reduced** into the abdominal cavity, & **posterolateral defect** in diaphragm is **closed** using **interrupted, nonabsorbable sutures**^{Q}.

- In **most cases (80%–90%)**, a **hernia sac** is **not present**. If **identified**, it is **excised** at the time of repair^Q.
- Advantage of a **prosthetic patch** is that a **tension-free repair** can be frequently obtained in **large defects**^{Q}.

MORGAGNI HERNIAS (RETROSTERNAL HERNIAS OR LARREY'S HERNIA^Q)

MORGAGNI HERNIAS (RETROSTERNAL HERNIAS OR LARREY'S HERNIA^Q)

- **Congenital hernia** of **anteromedial, retrosternal diaphragm**
- Occur in the **triangular space** between the muscle fibers that make up the diaphragm
- They extend from the **xiphisternum** and **costal margin** to the central tendon of diaphragm.

> - **Ninety percent** are **right sided**^Q because the pericardium itself prevents left-sided hernias
> - **Superior epigastric vessels** may **pass through Morgagni space**^Q
> - Most commonly involved viscus is **transverse colon**^Q

Clinical Feature
- Patients are **usually asymptomatic**^Q

Diagnosis
- **Anterior mediastinal masses** are found incidentally on **chest radiographs**^Q.

Treatment
- **Prompt surgical repair** after diagnosis is prudent **to avoid incarceration** or **strangulation** of abdominal organs.
- A **transabdominal route**^Q is the preferred choice.
- **Prosthetic mesh** is generally required **to repair the defect**^Q.

HIATUS HERNIA

Types of Hiatal hernia	
Type I	**Sliding** hiatal hernia (**MC**)^Q
Type II	**True** paraesophageal hernia^Q
Type III	**Mixed** paraesophageal hernia (**I and II**)^Q
Type IV	Paraesophageal hernia containing other **intra abdominal organs**^Q

Types of Hiatal Hernia

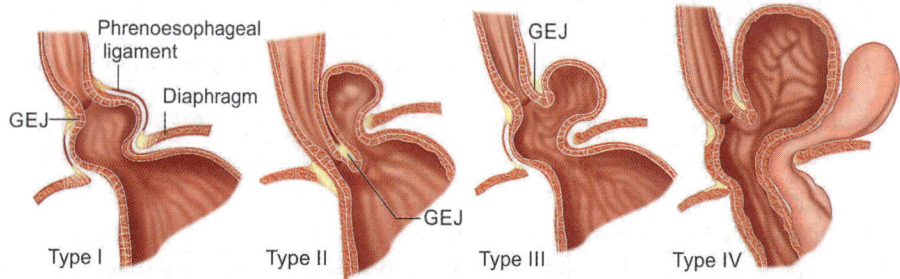

PATHOPHYSIOLOGY OF HIATUS HERNIA

Type I Hernia or Sliding HH
- Characterized by **upward displacement** of the **GE junction** into the **posterior mediastinum**^Q.
- The **stomach** remains in its **usual longitudinal alignment**^Q.
- A **higher incidence of HH** has also been found in people with **inguinal hernias**^Q.
- **Majority** of patients with HH are **asymptomatic**^Q
- The **prevalence** and **size** of the sliding HH **correlate with** increasing **severity of reflux disease**^Q.

Type II Hernia
- **True PEH**: Defined by a **normally positioned intra abdominal GE junction** with **upward herniation** of the **stomach**^Q alongside it.
- A **PEH** develops when there is a **defect**, possibly **congenital**, in the **hiatus anterior** to the esophagus.
- **Persistent posterior fixation** of the **GE junction** is the essential difference between a PEH and a sliding HH.

Type III Hernia
- **Mixed hernia:** Characterized by **displacement** of **both** the **GE junction** and a **large portion** of the **stomach** cephalad into the posterior mediastinum^Q.
- **Starts** as a **sliding HH**, and over time as the **hiatus enlarges**, and more of **fundus** and **body** of the stomach **herniate** into the chest.

Type IV Hernia
- Esophageal hiatus has dilated to such an extent that the **hernia sac** also **contains** other organs such as the **spleen, colon,** or **small bowel**[Q].
- **Bowel obstruction** and **complications**[Q] due to altered anatomy.

FACTORS AFFECTING LES PRESSURE

Lower Esophageal Sphincter (LES) Pressure

Decreased by	Increased by
• Prostaglandin E1 and E2, **P**rogesterone[Q] • **M**orphine and **M**eperidine[Q] • **T**heophylline[Q] • **B**arbiturates, **D**iazepam[Q], **D**opamine • **C**CB, **A**tropine, **N**itrates[Q] • **C**hocolate, **C**offee[Q] • **A**lcohol, **P**ippermint[Q] • **S**moking, **F**at[Q]	• **B**ombesin, **A**ngiotensin II[Q] • **PP**, **S**ubstance P, **M**otilin[Q] • **G**astrin[Q] • Antacids[Q] • Cholinergics[Q] • Domeperidone • Metoclopramide[Q] • Prostaglandin $F_{2\alpha}$

- **PMT BD CAN decrease LES pressure**: Prostaglandin E1 and E2, Progesterone, Morphine and Meperidine, Theophylline, Barbiturates, Diazepam, Dopamine, CCB, Atropine, Nitrates
- **CAPS Fat decrease LES pressure**: Chocolate, Coffee, Alcohol, Pippermint, Smoking, Fat.
- **PSM BAG increase LES pressure**: PP, Substance P, Motilin, Bombesin, Angiotensin II, Gastrin

GASTROESOPHAGEAL REFLUX DISEASE (GERD)

GASTROESOPHAGEAL REFLUX DISEASE (GERD)

- **Classical triad** of symptoms is **retrosternal burning pain, epigastric pain** & **regurgitation**[Q].
- GERD is associated with **complications** such as **esophageal ulcerations** (5%), **peptic strictures** (4–20%), & **Barrett's esophagus** (8–20%).

Pathophysiology
- LES has the **primary role** of **preventing reflux** into the esophagus.

Factors Contributing to the High-pressure Zone in the Lower Esophagus
• **Intrinsic musculature**[Q] of the distal esophagus which are in a state of tonic contraction
• **Sling fibers** of the **cardia**[Q] which are at the same anatomic depth of the circular muscle fibers of the esophagus but are oriented in a different direction
• **Diaphragm**[Q]: during inspiration the anteroposterior diameter of the **crural opening** is decreased, compressing the esophagus and increasing the measured pressure at the LES
• **Transmitted pressure**[Q] of the abdominal cavity

- GERD is often associated with a **hiatal hernia** (MC type is **type I** or **sliding** hernia[Q]).

> - A hiatal hernia is **neither necessary nor sufficient** to make the **diagnosis** of **GERD**, and the **presence** of such a **hernia does not constitute an indication for operative correction**[Q].
> - **Many patients** with **hiatal hernias do not have symptoms** and **do not require treatment**[Q].

Clinical Features
- **Classical triad** of symptoms is **retrosternal burning pain, epigastric pain** and **regurgitation**.
- **MC presentation** of GERD: **Long-standing history** of **heartburn** and a **shorter history of regurgitation**[Q].

> • **Symptoms of GERD**: Heartburn (80%)[Q], Regurgitation (54%), Abdominal pain (29%), **Cough** (27%), Dysphagia for solids (23%), Belching (15%), Bloating (15%), Aspiration (14%), Wheezing (7%).

Diagnosis
- **Endoscopy**: Exclude other diseases, especially a tumor, and to **document** the presence of **peptic esophageal injury**. An **essential step** in the **evaluation of GERD**, who are being **considered for operative intervention**[Q].

> • **Manometry**: For **information about** the **function of** the **esophageal body** and **LES**[Q]

24-hour pH Monitoring

- **Gold standard** for **diagnosing** and **quantifying acid reflux** is the **24-hour pH test**^Q.
- **Information from the study:** Total **number of reflux** episodes (pH < 4), **longest episode** of reflux, number of episodes **lasting >5 minutes**, **extent of reflux** in the **upright** and **supine** position.
- **DeMeester score**^Q: An overall score is obtained with the use of a formula that assigns a **weight to each item** according to its capacity **to cause esophageal injury.**
- **DeMeester score** needs to be **<14.7**^Q.

- **Esophagogram:** For evaluation of **symptoms of GERD** when an **operation is contemplated** or when the **symptoms do not respond as expected**. Presence and size of a hiatal hernia may be **characterized**^Q.

Treatment

- **Lifestyle modifications:** Cessation of smoking, decreased caffeine intake, and **avoidance** of **large meals** before lying down^Q
- **Medical Management:** Double dose of PPI is the **initial approach**^Q
- Compared with H_2 blockers, **PPIs** are **more effective** at **healing** esophageal **ulceration** secondary to acid exposure.

Indications of Surgical Therapy
• **Severe esophageal injury (ulcer, stricture, or Barrett's mucosa)**^Q
• **Incomplete resolution** of **symptoms** or **relapses** while on medical therapy
• **Long duration** of **symptoms**^Q
• **Symptoms** persist **at a young age**^Q

- **Antireflux surgery:** Laparoscopic Nissen fundoplication is gold standard for GERD^Q.
- Patients who have **>10 years** of **life expectancy** and are **in need of lifelong therapy** due to a **mechanically defective sphincter**, surgical therapy may be considered the **treatment of choice**^Q.
- The principles of **modern Nissen fundoplication** include **secure crural closure** and creation of a **short (≤2 cm), 360-degree "floppy" fundoplication** designed to **most closely replicate** the **normal physiology** of the gastroesophageal flap valve^Q.

TYPES OF FUNDOPLICATION

Type of Fundoplication	Degree of Wrap
Watson	• **90-degree anterior** fundoplication^Q
Dor	• **180-degree anterior** fundoplication^Q
Toupet	• 180-degree **posterior** fundoplication subsequently modified to a **270-degree wrap**^Q
Belsey Mark IV	• **270-degree anterior** fundoplication^Q
Nissen	• **360-degree** fundoplication^Q

ACHALASIA CARDIA

Achalasia Cardia

- MC motility disorder of esophagus^Q
- MC hypomotility disorder of esophagus^Q
- Achalasia means **"failure to relax"**^Q (sphincter remains in a **constant state of tone** with periods of relaxation)
- Both the **muscle** of **esophagus** & **LES** are **affected**^Q.
- **Prevailing theory:** Destruction of the nerves to **LES** is **primary pathology** & degeneration of **neuromuscular function** of **body of esophagus** is secondary^Q.
- **Premalignant condition** leading to **squamous cell carcinoma**

> • **Triple A-syndrome** or **Allgrove disease**^Q: Achalasia, Alacrima and ACTH-resistant Adrenal insufficiency.

Pathogenesis

> • **Progressive inflammation** & **selective loss** of **inhibitory myenteric neurons** in **Auerbach's plexus** of esophagus that normally secrete VIP & nitric oxide^Q.

- This results in **failure of relaxation of LES** and **aperistalsis** of esophageal body with subsequent **functional obstruction** at the level of **GE junction** & **gradual dilatation** of esophagus^Q.

Clinical Features

- Classic triad of symptoms consists of **dysphagia, regurgitation**, and **weight loss**.
- Heartburn, postprandial choking, & nocturnal coughing are seen commonly.

> • **Men** & **women** are **equally affected**, with **no ethnic predisposition** to the disease^Q.

- **Regurgitation** of undigested, foul-smelling foods is common, and with **progressive disease**, **aspiration** can become life-threatening[Q].
- **Pneumonia, lung abscess,** & bronchiectasis often result from **long-standing achalasia**.
- **Dysphagia progresses slowly** over years[Q].

Diagnosis
- **Barium swallow:**

> - **Dilated esophagus** with a **distal narrowing**[Q]
> - **"Bird's beak", "Pencil-tip"** or **"Rat's tail"** appearance[Q]

- **Hurst phenomenon:** Thin stream of barium flows beyond bird beak due to increased esophageal pressure[Q]
- **Lack of a gastric air bubble**[Q] on the upright portion is a result of the tight LES not allowing air to pass easily into the stomach.
- Massive esophageal dilation, tortuosity, and a **sigmoidal esophagus (megaesophagus)** in **advanced stage**[Q]

> - **Mecholyl test** is **positive** in **Achalasia**[Q]
> - **CCK test** is **positive** in **Achalasia**[Q]

- **Manometry** is gold standard test for diagnosis.
  - Absence of **body peristalsis** & **poor LES relaxation** is **mandatory**[Q] for diagnosis.

Manometry Findings of Typical Achalasia	
Abnormalities of LES	**Abnormalities of Esophageal Body**
• Incomplete or **absent LES relaxation**[Q] • **Elevated LES pressure**[Q]	• **Elevated intraesophageal pressure**[Q] (pressurization of the esophagus) from incomplete air evacuation • **Simultaneous mirrored contractions** with **no evidence** of **progressive peristalsis**[Q] • **Low-amplitude waveforms**[Q] indicating a lack of muscular tone

Treatment
- **Early stage:** Sublingual **nitroglycerin, nitrates,** or **calcium channel blockers**[Q] may offer hours of relief of chest pressure before or after a meal.
- **Bougie dilation**[Q] up to 54 French may offer several months of relief but requires repeated dilations to be sustainable.
- **Botulinum toxin:**
  - Injection of **botulinum toxin (Botox)** directly into the LES **blocks acetylcholine release**, preventing smooth muscle contraction, and effectively **relaxes the LES**[Q].
  - With **repeated treatments**, Botox may offer **symptomatic relief** for years
  - **Symptoms recur** more than **50%** of the time **within 6 months**[Q].

> - **Laparoscopic Heller myotomy** is now the **operation of choice**[Q].
> - Extent of Heller's myotomy: 2 cm above GE junction to 1 cm below[Q], over stomach.

- **Partial antireflux procedure (Toupet** or **Dor fundoplication)**[Q] will restore a barrier to reflux and decrease postoperative symptoms.
- **Esophagectomy** is considered **megaesophagus**, **sigmoid esophagus**, failure of **more than one myotomy**, or an **undilatable reflux stricture**[Q].

DIFFUSE ESOPHAGEAL SPASM

Diffuse Esophageal Spasm

- Esophageal contractions are **repetitive, simultaneous,** and of **high amplitude**[Q].
- Basic pathology is related to a **motor abnormality** of the **esophageal body** that is most notable in the **lower two thirds** of the esophagus.
- More common in **women** and is often found in patients with multiple complaints[Q].

Clinical Features
- Clinical presentation: **Chest pain** and **dysphagia**[Q] (may be related to eating or exertion and may mimic angina)
- Complain of a squeezing pressure in the chest that may radiate to the jaw, arms, and upper back.
- The **symptoms** are often pronounced during times of **heightened emotional stress**[Q].

Diagnosis
- Barium swallow:
  - **Corkscrew** or **rosary bead** esophagus, **segmental spasm** or **pseudodiverticulosis** appearance[Q]
  - Due to presence of **tertiary contractions**[Q]
  - Indicative of **advanced disease**[Q]

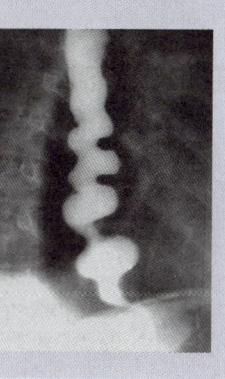

- **Manometry** is **gold standard test** for diagnosis^Q.
  - Classic manometry findings: **Simultaneous, multipeaked contractions** of **high amplitude** (>120 mm Hg) or **long duration** (>2.5 sec).

Treatment

- **Mainstay of treatment** for DES is **nonsurgical**, and **pharmacologic** (Nitrates, calcium channel blockers) or **endoscopic intervention** (Bougie dilation) is preferred^Q.
- Indications of surgery (long esophagomyotomy):
  - **Incapacitating chest pain** or **dysphagia** who have **failed medical** and **endoscopic therapy**^{Q}
  - Presence of a **pulsion diverticulum** of the thoracic esophagus

NUTCRACKER ESOPHAGUS

Nutcracker Esophagus

- **Hypermotility disorder** also known as **supersqueeze esophagus**^{Q}.
- Esophagus with **hypertensive peristalsis** or **high-amplitude peristaltic contractions**.
- **Most common and most painful** esophageal **hypermotility disorder**^{Q}.
- Associated with **hypertrophic musculature** resulting in high-amplitude contractions of the esophagus

Clinical Feature

- **Chest pain** and **dysphagia** are typical symptoms.

Diagnosis

- **Gold standard of diagnosis** is the subjective complaint of **chest pain** with simultaneous objective evidence of **peristaltic esophageal contractions 2 standard deviations above the normal**^{Q} values on manometric tracings.
- On manometry, **amplitude >180 mm Hg** and **duration of contraction >6 seconds**

Treatment

- The treatment of nutcracker esophagus is medical (**Calcium channel blockers**, **nitrates**, and **antispasmodics**)^Q

HYPERTENSIVE LES

Hypertensive LES

- The **LES pressure** is **above normal**, motility of esophageal body may be **hyperperistaltic** or **normal**.

Clinical Feature

- Patients with **hypertensive LES** present with **chest pain** or **dysphagia**^{Q}.

Diagnosis

- Diagnosis is made by **manometry**.
  - **Elevated LES pressure** (>26 mm Hg) and **normal relaxation** of the LES.
  - Esophageal body may be **hyperperistaltic** or **normal**.

Treatment

- **Botox injections** alleviate symptoms temporarily, and **hydrostatic balloon dilation** may provide long-term symptomatic relief.
- **Surgery** in patients who **fail interventional treatments** and those with **significant symptoms**.
- A **laparoscopic modified Heller esophagomyotomy** is the **operation of choice**.

ZENKER'S OR PHARYNGOESOPHAGEAL DIVERTICULA

Zenker's or Pharyngoesophageal Diverticula

- Mucosal outpouching (pulsion diverticulum) occurring **through** the triangular bare area (**Killian's triangle**)^Q, between the **upper oblique fibers (thyropharyngeus muscle)** and **lower horizontal fibers (cricopharyngeus muscle)** of the **inferior constrictor muscle**^{Q}
  - **Increased intraluminal pressures** (secondary to **abnormal esophageal motility**)^Q pushes **mucosa and submucosa** through a muscular defect in the wall of the esophagus creating a **pulsion diverticulum**^{Q}
  - It is a **pseudodiverticula**^{Q}
  - It **arises posteriorly** in the midline of the neck, **mouth is in midline** but **sac projects laterally**^{Q} (usually left laterally)

- It is **not a true esophageal diverticula**^{Q}, as it arises above the upper esophageal sphincter (the cricopharyngeus sphincter)
- MC esophageal diverticula^Q

Pathology
- **Neuromuscular incordination**^{Q} in this region
- May be due to **different nerve supply** of the **two parts of inferior constrictor muscle**^{Q}
  - The **thyropharyngeus (oblique fibers)** supplied by the **pharyngeal plexus**
  - **Cricopharyngeus (horizontal fibers)** by **recurrent laryngeal nerve**

Clinical Features
- Usually seen in patients over **50 years**^{Q}
- MC symptom is **dysphagia**^{Q}
- **Undigested food** is **regurgitated into the mouth**, especially when the patient is in **recumbent position**^{Q}
- Swelling of the neck, gurgling noise after eating, halitosis, and a sour metallic taste in the mouth are common symptoms
- **Cervical webs** are seen **associated in 50%**^{Q} of patients with Zenker's diverticula, can cause dysphagia post-operatively if not treated.

Diagnosis
- **Barium swallow** is **diagnostic**

Complications
- **Pneumonia** and **lung abscess** due to **aspiration**^{Q} **(MC)**
- Perforation, Bleeding • Carcinoma

Management
- Surgical therapy **(Cricopharyngeal myotomy + Diverticulopexy)** is **treatment of choice**^{Q}

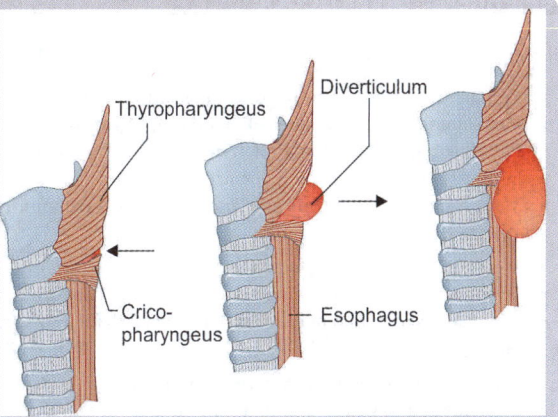

Treatment Options for Zenker's Diverticula
• **Cricopharyngeal myotomy** - a myotomy alone is sufficient for small diverticula
• **Myotomy with excision of sac** - done for large (>4 cm) diverticula
• **Diverticulopexy**
• **Diverticulo-esophagostomy** using a linear cutting staple gun
– The septum between the esophagus and the diverticula is divided
– Also known as **Dohlman procedure**^{Q}

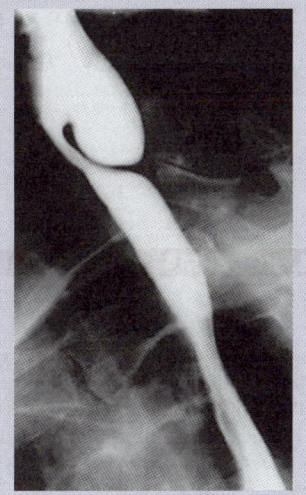

MIDESOPHAGEAL OR TRACTION DIVERTICULA

MIDESOPHAGEAL OR TRACTION DIVERTICULA

- **Inflammation** of the **lymph nodes** exerts **traction** on the wall of the esophagus leading to the formation of a **true diverticulum** in the midesophagus.

> • Caused by **inflamed mediastinal lymph nodes** from **tuberculosis, histoplasmosis**^{Q} and resultant fibrosing mediastinitis.

- Typically present on the **right** owing to the overabundance of structures in the midthoracic region of the left chest and **wide mouthed**.

Clinical Features
- Most patients are **asymptomatic**, incidentally found during a workup for some other complaint.
- **Dysphagia**, **chest pain**, and **regurgitation** can be present and are usually indicative of an **underlying primary motility disorder**.

Diagnosis
- **Investigation of choice** is **barium swallow**^{Q} (**lateral views** to determine side)
- **CT scan** is helpful to identify any **mediastinal lymphadenopathy** and may help to **lateralize the sac**.
- **Manometry in all patients**, symptomatic or not, **to identify** a **primary motor disorder**.

Treatment
- In **asymptomatic patients** who have inflamed mediastinal lymph nodes from **tuberculosis or histoplasmosis: ATT or antifungal agents**^{Q}
- **Diverticulopexy** for **symptomatic** or **2 cm or larger** diverticulum
- **Esophagomyotomy** in severe chest pain or dysphagia and a documented **motor abnormality**^{Q}

EPIPHRENIC DIVERTICULA

Epiphrenic Diverticula

- Epiphrenic diverticula are found **adjacent to diaphragm** in the **distal third** of the esophagus, within 10 cm of the GEJ.
- Most often related to **thickened distal esophageal musculature** or **increased intraluminal pressure**.
- **Pulsion** or **false diverticula**, often **associated with DES**, **achalasia**, and **most commonly NEM** (non-specific esophageal motility) **disorders**.
- In patients in whom a motility abnormality cannot be identified, a congenital (**Ehlers-Danlos syndrome**) or **traumatic cause** is considered.
- More common on the **right side** and tend to be **wide-mouthed**[Q].

Clinical Features
- Most patients are **asymptomatic**.
- **Dysphagia** or **chest pain** indicative of a **motility disturbance**.
- The diagnosis is often made during the workup for a motility disorder, and the diverticulum is **found incidentally**.

Diagnosis
- **Investigation of choice** is **barium swallow** (**lateral views** to determine side)
- **Manometry** to identify a **primary motor disorder**.

Treatment
- **Diverticulopexy**
- **Long esophagomyotomy** in severe chest pain, dysphagia, or a **documented motor abnormality**

Killian-Jamieson Diverticula
- **Lateral cervical** esophageal diverticula
- Located **just below cricopharyngeus**
- Mostly **asymptomatic**

SCLERODERMA

Scleroderma

- Systemic disease accompanied by **esophageal abnormalities** in **80% of patients**.
- In most, the disease follows a **prolonged course**[Q].
- **Renal involvement** occurs in a small percentage of patients and signals a **poor prognosis**.
- The onset of the disease is usually in the **third** or **fourth decade** of life
- Occurring twice as frequently in **women**[Q] as in men.

Pathophysiology
- In the **GI tract**, the predominant feature is **smooth muscle atrophy**[Q].

> **Smooth muscle atrophy** in **lower two-thirds** of esophagus →Incompetent LES →GERD →Stricture[Q]

- **Normal peristalsis** in the **proximal striated esophagus**, with **absent peristalsis** in the **distal smooth muscle portion**[Q].
- The **LES pressure** is **progressively weakened** as the disease advances.
- **Gastroesophageal reflux** commonly occurs in patients with scleroderma, because they have both **hypotensive sphincters** and **poor esophageal clearance**.
- This combined defect can lead to **severe esophagitis** and **stricture formation**[Q].

Clinical Features
- **Dysphagia** and **GERD**
- **Postural dysphagia** for **liquids**: Dysphagia for liquids **in recumbent position**, not in upright position
- Dysphagia for solids is unrelated to posture

Diagnosis
- **Manometry:**
  - **Normal peristalsis** in the **proximal striated esophagus**, with **absent peristalsis** in the distal smooth muscle portion
  - **LES pressure** is **decreased** but sphincter relaxation to deglutition is **normal**

> - **Barium Swallow: Dilated**, barium-filled **esophagus, stomach,** and **duodenum**, or a **hiatal hernia** with **distal esophageal stricture** and **proximal dilatation**[Q].

Treatment
- PPIs, antacids, elevation of the head of the bed, and multiple dilations for strictures for reflux
- **Esophageal shortening** may require a **Collis gastroplasty** in combination with a **partial fundoplication**[Q].

> - **Surgery reduces esophageal acid exposure**, but **does not return it to normal** because of the **poor clearance function of** the **body** of the **esophagus**[Q].

BARRETT'S ESOPHAGUS

BARRETT'S ESOPHAGUS

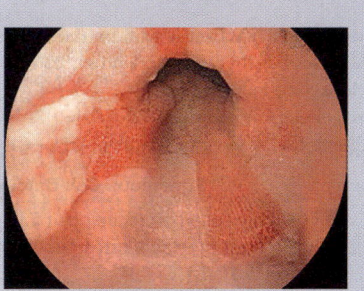

- Distal squamous mucosa is replaced by metaplastic specialized (intestinalized columnar) epithelium, e.g. goblet cells, as a response to chronic injury; may regress after treatment[Q]
- Also called columnar lined esophagus[Q]
- Metaplasia of esophageal squamous epithelium into columnar in distal[Q] esophagus
- MC type of columnar epithelium is intestinal epithelium (Intestinal metaplasia[Q])

Etiology
- Usually due to chronic GERD[Q]
- Columnar epithelium of Barrett's may be more resistant to acid, pepsin & bile[Q]
- Often associated with sliding hiatal hernia[Q]

Clinical Features
- Higher incidence in whites, males & obese
- Symptoms: long history of heartburn & other reflux symptoms; more massive reflux with more numerous and longer episodes than most reflux patients
- Major risk factor for esophageal adenocarcinoma[Q]

Diagnosis
- Characteristic endoscopic appearance plus characteristic histologic findings[Q]
- 8 random biopsies recommended
- Report should include type of epithelium present and presence/absence of dysplasia, grade of dysplasia, & extent of dysplasia[Q]

> - Barrett's esophagus requires both endoscopically visible segment of columnar lining of distal esophagus and intestinal metaplasia showing goblet cells on biopsy[Q]

Endoscopy
- Red velvety GI type mucosa between pale squamous mucosa of lower esophagus & lush pink gastric mucosa[Q]
- May have tongues extending up from GE junction or a broad band displacing GE junction proximally

Positive Stains
- Goblet cells contain acid mucin, usually sialomucin[Q] (Alcian blue+ at pH 2.5, although stain generally not needed or recommended), columnar cells contain neutral mucins (PAS+); intestinal metaplastic cells are often CK7+/CK20−; also CDX2+.
- Guanylyl cyclase C+, Hep+
- In routine practice, only H&E is used for diagnosis

Treatment
- Antireflux therapy[Q]
- Endoscopy every 1-2 years to detect dysplasia or early adenocarcinoma with 4 quadrant biopsies using jumbo forceps at intervals of 2 cm or less throughout the length of the Barrett's segment plus any suspicious lesions[Q].

PREDISPOSING FACTORS FOR CARCINOMA ESOPHAGUS

Predisposing Factors for Carcinoma Esophagus	
Squamous Cell Carcinoma	**Adenocarcinoma**

- Alcohol[Q]
- Smoking[Q]
- Ingested carcinogens:
  - Nitrates[Q], nitrites, nitrosamines[Q]
  - Smoked opiates[Q]
  - Fungal toxins in pickled vegetables
- Mucosal damage:
  - Chronic Achalasia[Q]
  - Lye (caustic) ingestion
  - Long term ingestion of hot liquids
  - Radiation induced strictures[Q]
- Plummer-vinson syndrome[Q]
- Tylosis palmaris et plantaris[Q]: Congenital Hyperkeratosis[Q] and pitting of palms and soles[Q]
- Human papilloma virus[Q]
- Esophageal diverticula[Q]
- Bulimia[Q]
- Deficiency: Vitamin A, zinc, molybdenum
	- GERD (leading to Barrett's esophagus[Q])
	- Obesity[Q]
	- Scleroderma[Q]
	
	> Scleroderma: Smooth muscle atrophy in lower 2/3rd of esophagus → Incompetent LES → GERD → Stricture
	
	- Diet deficient in fruits and vegetables
	- Diet high in animal protein and cholesterol[Q]

CARCINOMA ESOPHAGUS

CARCINOMA ESOPHAGUS

- MC esophageal cancer worldwide: **Squamous cell carcinoma**^{Q}
- MC esophageal cancer in United States (Western countries): **Adenocarcinoma**^{Q}
- More common in **males**^{Q}
- MC site of CA esophagus: **Middle 1/3rd (Overall)**^{Q}
- Chemotherapy regimen: Epirubicin + Cisplatin^Q + 5-FU (ECF)

Squamous Cell Carcinoma	Adenocarcinoma
• Rarely seen before the age of 30 years • **Highest mortality rates** seen in **men** between **60-70 years**^{Q} of age. • Predominantly affects **African American men**^{Q} • **MC site: Middle 1/3rd**^{Q} • Obesity is protective • H. pylori CAG-A strain is a **risk factor**^{Q} • Usually appears as an **exophytic lesion** with a **large fungating mass**^{Q} • More sensitive to **chemoradiotherapy**^{Q} • Treated aggressively with **nonsurgical therapy**^{Q}	• Seen infrequently before the age of 40 years • **Increases in incidence** with **age**^{Q} • Disease affecting **white men**^{Q} • **Barrett's esophagus: 40-fold**^{Q} **increased risk** for adenocarcinoma • **MC site: Lower 1/3rd**^{Q} • **Obesity** is a **risk factor** • **H. pylori CAG-A strain** is a **protective** • Polypoid (5-10%), flat (10-15%), fungating (20-25%), or **infiltrative (40-50%)**^{Q} • **Not as sensitive to chemoradiotherapy** • Treated by a more **aggressive surgical approach**^{Q}.

Pathology
- Esophageal cancer asserts **aggressive biologic behavior**.
- With **only two layers** to the esophageal wall, tumors **rapidly infiltrate through** the muscular wall into surrounding structures^Q.
- The **rich vascular and lymphatic supply facilitates spread to regional lymph nodes**^{Q}.

Clinical Features
- Early-stage cancers: Asymptomatic or mimic symptoms of GERD.

> • **MC symptom: Dysphagia >Weight loss**^{Q}

- **Most patients** with esophageal cancer **present with dysphagia** and **weight loss**, symptoms that usually indicate advanced disease.
- Choking, coughing, and aspiration from a tracheoesophageal fistula (In advanced cases)^Q
- Hoarseness and vocal cord paralysis from direct invasion into the recurrent laryngeal nerve (In advanced cases)^Q
- MC site of metastasis: **Liver**^{Q} >lung >bone
- Paraneoplastic manifestation associated with adenocarcinoma: Motor Neuropathy^Q

Diagnosis
- **Barium swallow: First investigation done**^{Q} in suspected case of **CA esophagus** (classic finding of an **apple core lesion**^{Q})

> • **Endoscopy** with **biopsy: Investigation of choice** for **diagnosis of CA esophagus**^{Q}.
> • **Endoscopic Ultrasound: Investigation of choice** for **staging of CA esophagus**, best for **T staging** and **LN metastasis**^{Q}.

- **CECT (abdomen and chest):** Assess the length of the tumor, thickness of the esophagus and stomach, **regional LN status** and **metastasis to liver** and **lungs**^{Q}.

Treatment of CA Esophagus	
High-grade dysplasia (Tis) or T1a	• Endoscopic Mucosal Resection^Q
Localized Esophageal Cancer	• **T1:** Vagal sparing or transhiatal or **minimal invasive esophagectomy** with limited LN dissection^Q • **T2** and **T3: Neo-adjuvant chemoradiation + Surgery**^{Q} • **Cervical SCC** or **Non-ideal candidate** for resection: **Definitive chemoradiation**^{Q}
Locally Advanced Cancer	• **Chemoradiation**^{Q} (± Surgical resection in T4a)
Metastatic Disease	• **Definitive chemoradiation**^{Q} (for involved distant LN or metastatic disease)
Malignant TEF	• **Coated SEMS**^{Q} (self-expanding metallic stents)

- **Postoperative chemoradiation** is reserved for **GE junction tumors**^{Q}
- **Extent of Resection:** An in-situ **margin of 10 cm**^{Q} should be the goal

Prognosis

Long-term Survival Following Esophagectomy Depends on		
• Depth of tumor invasion (T)^Q	• Number of involved lymph nodes (N)^Q	• Location^Q of the tumor in the esophagus

- **Prognosis is better** for **tumors of** the **cervical esophagus** and tumors **located at GE junction**^Q, in comparison to tumors located in the thoracic esophagus.

TNM CLASSIFICATION OF CARCINOMA OF THE ESOPHAGUS

8th AJCC (2017) TNM Classification of Carcinoma of the Esophagus	
Tis: Carcinoma-in-situ/ High-grade dysplasia	**N1**: Metastasis in **1-2** regional LNs^Q
T1a: Tumor invades **lamina propria or muscularis mucosa**^Q **T1b**: Tumor invades **submucosa**^Q	**N2**: Metastasis in **3-6** regional LNs^Q
T2: Tumor invades **muscularis propria**^Q	**N3**: Metastasis in **7 or more** regional LNs^Q
T3: Tumor invades **adventitia**^Q	**M1**: Distant metastasis^Q
T4a: Tumor invades **pleura, pericardium, azygous vein, diaphragm or peritoneum**^Q **T4b**: Tumor invades other adjacent structures such as **aorta, vertebral body or trachea**^Q	

Stage Grouping — Squamous Cell Carcinoma

Stage	T	N	M	Grade	Location
0	Tis (HGD)	N0	M0	1, X	Any
IA	T1a	N0	M0	1, X	Any
IB	T1a	N0	M0	2-3	Any
	T1b	N0	M0	Any	Any
	T2	N0	M0	1	Any
IIA	T2	N0	M0	2-3, X	Any
	T3	N0	M0	Any	Lower
	T3	N0	M0	1	Upper, middle
IIB	T3	N0	M0	2-3	Upper, middle
	T3	N0	M0	Any	X
	T3	N0	M0	X	Any
	T1	N1	M0	Any	Any
IIIA	T1	N2	M0	Any	Any
	T2	N1	M0	Any	Any
IIIB	T2	N2	M0	Any	Any
	T3	N1-2	M0	Any	Any
	T4a	N0-1	M0	Any	Any
IVA	T4a	N2	M0	Any	Any
	T4b	Any	M0	Any	Any
IVB	Any	Any	M1	Any	Any

Stage Grouping — Adenocarcinoma

Stage	T	N	M	Grade
0	Tis (HGD)	N0	M0	N/A
IA	T1a	N0	M0	1, X
IB	T1a	N0	M0	2
	T1b	N0	M0	1, 2
IC	T1a, T1b	N0	M0	3
	T2	N0	M0	1, 2
IIA	T2	N0	M0	3, X
IIB	T3	N0	M0	Any
	T1	N1	M0	Any
IIIA	T1	N2	M0	Any
	T2	N1	M0	Any
	T3	N0	M0	Any
IIIB	T2	N2	M0	Any
	T3	N1-2	M0	Any
	T4a	N0-1	M0	Any
IVA	T4a	N2	M0	Any
	T4b	Any	M0	Any
	Any	N3	M0	Any
IVB	Any	Any	M1	Any

TYPES OF ESOPHAGECTOMY

Types of Esophagectomy	
Ivor-Lewis	• Transthoracic esophagectomy^Q • **Double incision: Midline laparotomy** followed by **right sided thoracotomy**^Q • Done **for tumors** of **middle 1/3rd** of **esophagus**^Q
Orringer	• Transhiatal esophagectomy^Q • **Double incision: Midline laparotomy** followed by **Cervical incision**^Q • **MC procedure** done for **carcinoma esophagus**^Q

McKeon	• En-bloc esophagectomy^Q • Three incisions: **Right sided thoracotomy**, followed by **midline**^Q **laparotomy**, followed by **cervical incision**^Q • Associated with **maximum morbidity and mortality**^Q

Lymphadenectomy in CA Esophagus	
One-field lymphadenectomy	Removal of the **intra-abdominal nodes** (draining the **proximal stomach** and **distal esophagus**)^Q
Two-field lymphadenectomy	Removal of the **intra-abdominal + Intrathoracic nodes**^Q
Three-field lymphadenectomy	Removal of the **intra-abdominal + Intrathoracic + Cervical LN**^Q

REPLACEMENT CONDUITS AFTER ESOPHAGECTOMY

REPLACEMENT CONDUITS AFTER ESOPHAGECTOMY

- **Best conduit** after esophagectomy (overall): **Stomach**^Q
- **Conduit of choice** after esophagectomy in **CA esophagus: Stomach**^Q
- **Conduit of choice** after esophagectomy in **benign disorders (caustic injuries, acid-peptic disease), unhealthy stomach: Colon**^Q
- **Conduit of choice** for **short segment replacement: Jejunum**^Q

> **Routes of Replacement of Esophagus**
> - **Posterior mediastinum**^Q through the bed of the resected esophagus
> - **Anterior mediastinal** in the **retrosternal**^Q position
> - **Lateral traspleural** placement behind the lung root^Q
> - Antethoracic or presternal **subcutaneous route**^Q

- **Gastric conduit** is based on **right gastric** and **right gastroepiploic vessels**^Q
- **Left colon** is based on **left colic artery** (Branch of IMA), placed in **isoperistaltic** direction.
- **Posterior mediastinal route is preferred (shortest route)**^Q

LEIOMYOMA

LEIOMYOMA

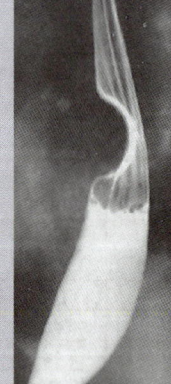

- Leiomyoma is MC benign esophageal tumor^Q.
- The average age **4th-5th** decades, more common in **males**^Q.
- Originate in **smooth muscle**, 90% are located in **lower two thirds** of the esophagus.
- Usually **solitary** and typically **oval**.^Q
- They remain **intramural**, having the bulk of their mass **protruding toward** the **outer wall**
- The **overlying mucosa** is **freely movable** and **normal** in appearance^Q.

Clinical Features
- Many leiomyomas are **asymptomatic. Dysphagia** and **pain** are MC symptoms^Q.
- Location and size tend not to correlate consistently with symptoms

Diagnosis
- **Barium swallow** is IOC for leiomyoma (classical, smooth, contoured, punched-out defect)^Q
- **Endoscopy:** Freely movable mass, which bulges into the lumen,
- **Should not be biopsied** because of an **increased chance** of **mucosal perforation** at the time of surgical enucleation^Q.

Treatment
- **Enucleation** is TOC for leiomyoma^Q.

DYSPHAGIA LUSORIA

DYSPHAGIA LUSORIA

- It is a **disorder of swallowing** caused due to **vascular anomalies**^Q (congenital abnormalities)^Q
- **Vascular rings** and **pulmonary slings** occur as a result of **developmental abnormalities** of the great vessels that cause **compression of the esophagus**^Q.

> - The **MC anomaly** is **right subclavian artery** arising from the **descending aorta** and **travels behind** the **esophagus** to complete its course to the right upper extremity, may cause **significant posterior compression**^Q of the esophagus.

- **Anomalous right aortic arch** with a **left ligamentum arteriosum** and a resultant retroesophageal left subclavian artery will form a **complete ring** that will also cause **posterior esophageal compression**[Q].
- **Pulmonary artery sling** (left pulmonary artery arises from the **right** pulmonary artery instead of from the main pulmonary artery trunk)[Q]

Clinical Features
- Both vascular rings and pulmonary artery slings cause **dysphagia**.
- **Recurrent respiratory infections** and **difficulty in breathing** are also common symptoms.

Diagnosis
- **Barium swallow**: Extrinsic **anterior** or **posterior compression** of the esophagus.
- **Angiography** or **HRCT**: Identify the **anomalous anatomy**[Q].

Treatment
- In **symptomatic patients**, both vascular rings and pulmonary artery slings are **repaired**.
- Results: **Dysphagia resolves** nearly **100% of the time**[Q].

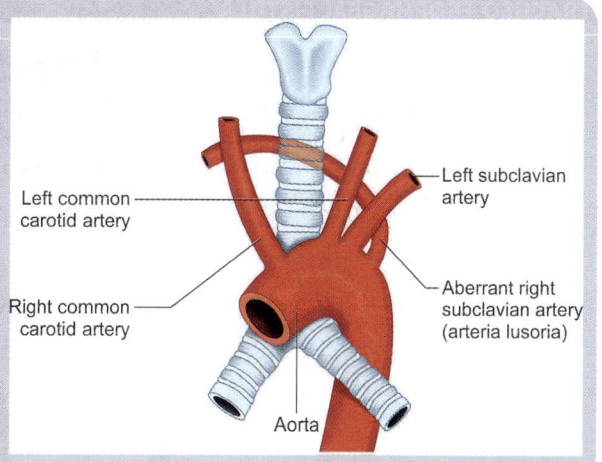

KOMMERELL'S DIVERTICULUM

- An **aberrant right subclavian artery** originating from the proximal descending thoracic aorta can be associated with **aneurysmal change** at the **origin** of the artery, known as **Kommerell's diverticulum**[Q].

BOERHAAVE SYNDROME

BOERHAAVE SYNDROME

- **Spontaneous rupture** usually occurs on **left posterolateral side** of **distal esophagus** into **left pleural cavity** or just above the gastroesophageal junction.
- These patients are typically **male (85%)**, **40 to 60 years** of age, who have a history of **recent emesis**[Q].

Clinical Features

- **Mackler's triad**[Q] of **thoracic pain, vomiting, and cervical subcutaneous emphysema** is seen in spontaneous esophageal perforation.

- Thoracic perforations cause **substernal** and **epigastric pain**[Q].
- **Mediastinal emphysema** & **pleural effusions** are common, but early cervical subcutaneous emphysema is noted in only 20% or less of patients.
- **Fever** & **sepsis** develop with increasing contamination and inflammation of the mediastinum and pleural cavities.
- Patients with an **abdominal perforation** have **epigastric abdominal pain** that is also often referred to the **back** and **left shoulder**[Q].

Diagnosis
- Chest X-ray: **Hydropneumothorax**[Q]
- The **diagnosis** is **confirmed with** a **contrast esophagogram**[Q]. This technique will demonstrate extravasation in 90% of patients.

- **Gastrografin (water soluble)** is **preferred**[Q] to prevent extravasation of barium into the mediastinum or pleura. If **no leak** is seen, a **barium study** should follow.

- **Chest CT**: Mediastinal **air** and **fluid** at the site of perforation.
- **Endoscopy**: If the **esophagogram** is **negative** or if **operative intervention** is planned.

Treatment
- Appropriate **resuscitation**, secured **airway**, **IV fluids** and **broad-spectrum antibiotics** are started immediately, and the patient is monitored in an ICU.

Within 24 Hours	After 24 Hours
• **Golden period** for **primary closure** of an esophageal perforation is within the **first 24 hours**[Q]. • Within 24 hours of perforation, **inflammation** is generally **minimal**, and **primary surgical repair** is recommended[u]. • Mortality rate: **8-20%**	• **Debridement** of devitalized tissue + **Esophageal diversion** or **resection** + Creation of an **esophagostomy** + **Wide drainage** + **feeding jejunostomy**[u] • Mortality rate: **>50%**[Q]

TRACHEO-ESOPHAGEAL FISTULA

TRACHEOESOPHAGEAL FISTULA

- TEF is an **abnormal communication** (fistula) between the **esophagus** and **trachea**[Q].
- TEF is usually **associated with esophageal atresia**, however it **may also exist without atresia**[Q].
- **Prevalence** of TEF is **2.6-3** per **10,000 births**, with a **slight male predominance**[Q].
- **MC anomaly** associated with TEF is **CVS (VSD)**[Q].

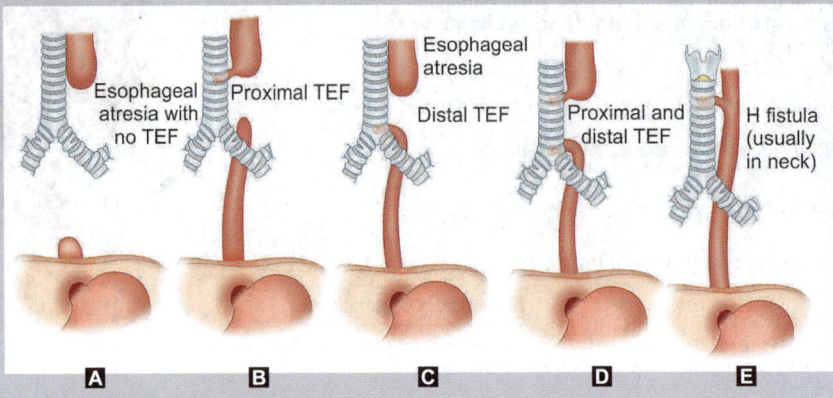

A Esophageal atresia with no TEF **B** Proximal TEF **C** Esophageal atresia, Distal TEF **D** Proximal and distal TEF **E** H fistula (usually in neck)

Classification of TEF
• **Type A:** Atresia only (6%)
• **Type B:** Atresia with proximal TEF (2%)
• **Type C: Atresia with distal TEF (85%): Most common**[Q]
• **Type D:** Atresia with both proximal and distal TEF (rare)
• **Type E:** TEF only (1%)

Clinical Features

- The diagnosis of EA is entertained in an **infant with excessive salivation** along with **coughing** or **choking during** the **first oral feeding**.
- A **maternal history** of **polyhydramnios** is often present.
- The newborn baby with atresia **regurgitates all of its first and subsequent feeds**[Q].
- **Saliva pours continuously** from its mouth[Q].
- Repeated episodes of **coughing, choking** and **cyanosis**[Q] occur on feeding in TEF.

Associated Anomalies
• **MC anomaly** associated with TEF is **CVS (VSD)**.
• Esophageal atresia may occur as part of **VACTERL**[Q] group of anomalies:
– **V**: Vertebral body segmentation defects[Q]
– **A**: Anal atresia[Q]
– **C**: **Cardiovascular** (PDA, **VSD**)[Q]
– **TE**: Tracheoesophageal fistula[Q]
– **R**: Renal (unilateral renal agenesis)[Q]
– **L**: Limb anomalies (radial ray hypoplasia)[Q]

Diagnosis

- The **inability to pass a NG** into the **stomach** is a **cardinal feature** for the **diagnosis of EA**.
- **If gas is present** in the **GIT below** the **diaphragm**, an **associated TEF is confirmed**
- **Inability to pass a NG tube** with **absent radiographic evidence** for gastrointestinal gas is **virtually diagnostic** of an **isolated EA without TEF**.
- **For H-type: Tracheobronchoscopy + Endoscopy** should be performed

Treatment

- **Surgical repair** with **tension free esophageal anastomosis**

Outcome

- The mortality in TEF is **directly related to the associated anomalies**, particularly **cardiac defects** and **chromosomal abnormalities**[Q].

SCHATZKI'S RINGS

Schatzki's Rings

- Consists of a **concentric symmetric narrowing** representing an area of **restricted distensibility** of the **lower esophagus**[Q].

  - **Lying** precisely at the **squamocolumnar mucosal GEJ**, involves **mucosa** and **submucosa**[Q]

- It consists of **esophageal mucosa above** and **gastric mucosa below**.
- It **does not have** a component of **true esophageal muscle**, nor is it **associated with esophagitis**.
- It is **often accompanied** by a **small hiatal hernia**

Clinical Features
- Most patients with Schatzki's rings present with **dysphagia**.
- The **dysphagia** is usually to **solid foods only** and comes on **abruptly** with nearly complete obstruction.

  - **Episodic aphagia: Intermittent obstruction** of the nondistensible ring by **large pieces of meat**[Q].

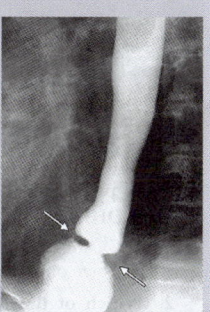

Diagnosis
- Diagnosis of a Schatzki's ring is made with a **barium swallow**[Q].
- Schtazki ring: Type 'B' ring is located at GE junction[Q]

Treatment
- Asymptomatic patients **incidentally found** to have a Schatzki's ring **require no treatment**.
- Best form of treatment of a **symptomatic Schatzki's ring** without reflux: **Esophageal dilation** for relief of the obstructive symptoms.
- Ring with **proven reflux** and mechanically defective sphincter: **Antireflux procedure**
- **Surgical excision** is **not indicated**, can cause **devastating esophageal strictures**.

ANATOMY AND PHYSIOLOGY OF ESOPHAGUS

Anatomy and Physiology of Esophagus

- **Narrowest tube of GIT; Narrowest region of esophagus:** Cricopharynx (15 mm diameter)
- **Extent:** C6-T11[Q]; **Length:** 25-30 cm[Q]
- **Cervical esophagus** begins as a **midline structure** that **deviates slightly** to the **left**[Q] of the trachea as it passes through the neck into the thoracic inlet.
- At the level of the **carina**, it **deviates to the right** to accommodate the arch of the aorta.
- It then winds its way back under the left main-stem bronchus and **remains slightly deviated** to the **left** as it **enters the diaphragm** through the esophageal hiatus[Q].
- Immediately before entering the abdomen, esophagus is pushed anteriorly by **descending thoracic aorta**[Q].

  - Only **Auerbach plexus** is present in **esophagus (Meissner's plexus is absent)**[Q].
  - **Lymphatic channels** in the **lamina propria** are the anatomic features **unique** to the esophagus[Q].

- The **dense submucosal lymphatic plexus** facilitates **early dissemination** of esophageal **malignancies**. In submucosa elastic fibers & collagen combine to make this the **strongest esophageal layer**. Submucosal glands of mixed type are the **characteristic of the esophagus**[Q].

  - **Lacks a serosal layer**[Q]; **Strongest Cayer: submucosa**[Q]
  - **Lining:** Lined by **stratified, non-keratinized squamous epithelium**[Q]

- **Muscles:**
  - **Upper cervical region-** Stratified muscle[Q]
  - **Middle-** Gradual transition from stratified to smooth muscle[Q]
  - **Lower-** Smooth muscle[Q]

Upper Esophageal Sphincter	Lower Esophageal Sphincter
• **Length:** 4-5 cm[Q] • **Pressure:** 60 mm Hg[Q] • Comprises **three skeletal muscle groups:** Distal portion of **inferior** pharyngeal **constrictor**, cricopharyngeus and circular muscle of **proximal esophagus**[Q]	• **Length:** 5 cm[Q] • **Abdominal length:** 2 cm[Q] • **Pressure:** 6-26 mm Hg[Q]

Types of Esophageal Contractions		
Primary Contractions	**Secondary Contractions**	**Tertiary Contractions**
• **Progressive**[Q] contractions • **Triggered by voluntary swallowing**[Q] • **Speed:** 2-4 cm/sec • Reach LES about **9 sec**	• **Progressive**[Q] contractions • **Triggered by distension** or **irritation**[Q] of esophagus (but not by voluntary swallowing)	• **Non progressive, non-peristaltic** contractions[Q] • Occur **spontaneously** and **simultaneously between swallows**[Q]

Multiple Choice Questions

CONGENITAL DIAPHRAGMATIC HERNIA

1. Which of the following is the most important determinant of prognosis in neonatal congenital diaphragmatic hernia (CDH)? *(All India 2011)*
   a. Pulmonary hypertension
   b. Delay in surgery
   c. Size of defect
   d. Gestational age at diagnosis

2. Which of the following is the least important prognostic factor in congenital diaphragmatic hernia? *(All India 2011)*
   a. Pulmonary Hypertension
   b. Delay in emergent surgery
   c. Size of defect
   d. Gestational age at diagnosis

3. All are true about Bochdalek hernia except: *(GB Pant 2011)*
   a. Posterolateral
   b. Left side
   c. Present in second decade
   d. Congenital

4. Most common organ that herniates in Morgagni's hernia:
   a. Spleen
   b. Liver *(MHSSMCET 2009)*
   c. Stomach
   d. Transverse colon

5. Which of the following is contraindication for Bag and mask ventilation? *(AIIMS June 2000)*
   a. Septicemia
   b. Tracheoesophageal fistula
   c. Meconium aspiration
   d. Diaphragmatic hernia

6. False regarding Bochdalek hernia is: *(AIIMS Nov 93)*
   a. Spleen and kidney can herniate
   b. Occurs posterolaterally
   c. Always occurs on right side
   d. Hernia may or may not have sac

7. Not true about Bochdalek hernia:
   a. Seen on right side *(Recent Question 2015, AIIMS Nov 97)*
   b. Associated with hypoplasia of lung
   c. Associated with hiatus hernia
   d. Pericardial cyst is a differential diagnosis

8. The diagnostic feature of congenital diaphragmatic hernia on prenatal ultrasonography is: *(AIIMS June 2001)*
   a. A cyst behind the left atrium
   b. Mediastinal shift with normal heart axis
   c. Peristalsis in the thoracic cavity
   d. Absence of gas bubble under the diaphragm

9. Most common site of Morgagni hernia: *(AIIMS Nov 2006)*
   a. Right anterior
   b. Right posterior
   c. Left anterior
   d. Left posterior

10. In congenital diaphragmatic hernia all are seen except:
    a. Common on left side *(JIPMER 99)*
    b. Abdominal distension
    c. Can be detected antenatally
    d. Heart beat shifted to right

11. Morgagni hernia: *(APPG 98)*
    a. Hernia between the costal and sternal part of the diaphragm
    b. Hernia through the pleuriperitoneal canal
    c. Hernia through the lumbar triangle
    d. Hernia through inguinal canal

12. A neonate with a scaphoid abdomen and respiratory distress has: *(All India 94)*
    a. Congenital pyloric stenosis
    b. Diaphragmatic hernia
    c. Volvulus
    d. Wilms' tumor

13. Most common content of Morgagni foramen: *(Recent Question 2017)*
    a. Stomach
    b. Small intestine
    c. Transverse colon
    d. Spleen

14. Most common diaphragmatic hernia in a newborn infant: *(Recent Question 2017)*
    a. Bochdalek
    b. Morgagni
    c. Paraesophageal type I
    d. Paraesophageal type III

HIATUS HERNIA

15. True about hiatus hernia: *(PGI June 2008)*
    a. Surgery is indicated in all symptomatic cases
    b. Para-esophageal type is more complicated
    c. Para-esophageal type is common type
    d. Common in infants

16. Select the TRUE statement regarding the picture depicted here: *(APPG 2016)*

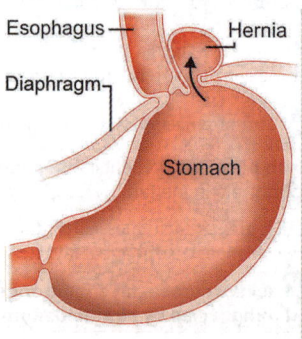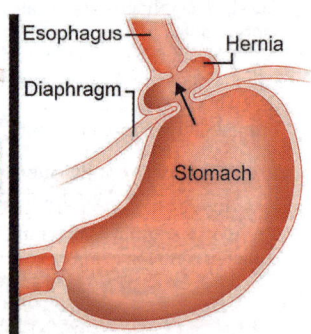

    a. A is known as sliding hernia
    b. Part of upper stomach enters into thorax in both A and B
    c. A is the more common form
    d. A causes symptoms of gastroesophageal reflux

17. The most common complication seen in hiatus hernia is:
    a. Esophagitis *(DNB, 2011, All India 2005)*
    b. Aspiration pneumonitis
    c. Volvulus
    d. Esophageal stricture

18. A 55-year-old male had retrosternal discomfort unrelated to physical exertion. Pain gets worse after lying down there is partial relief with antacids. The most likely diagnosis is: *(UPSC 96)*
    a. Ischemic heart disease
    b. Carcinoma esophagus
    c. Achalasia cardia
    d. Hiatus hernia

19. Most useful investigation in sliding hernia in female: *(UPPG 2008)*
    a. Fluoroscopy   b. Barium meal
    c. Palpation method   d. Ultrasound
20. For hiatal hernia, investigation of choice is:
    a. Barium meal follow through   *(DPG 2006, DPG 2005)*
    b. Barium meal upper GI
    c. Barium meal upper GI in Trendelenburg position
    d. Barium meal double contrast
21. Rossetti modification of Nissen's fundoplication means: *(MHSSMCET 2006)*
    a. Excludes the stomach wall in the wrap
    b. Include only the posterior stomach wall in the wrap
    c. Include only the anterior stomach wall in the wrap
    d. Include both the anterior and the posterior stomach wall in the wrap
22. Fundoplication is used in treatment of: *(DNB 2012, MHPGMCET 2002)*
    a. Hiatus hernia   b. Achalasia cardia
    c. CHPS   d. CA esophagus
23. In Nissen's Fundoplication wrapping is done:
    a. 1/3   b. 1/4   *(MHSSMCET 2009)*
    c. 3/4   d. 1/2
24. Retrocardiac lucency with air fluid level is seen in:
    a. Hiatus hernia   *(Recent Question 2013)*
    b. Distal end esophageal obstruction
    c. Eventration of diaphragm
    d. None
25. What is the most probable diagnosis based on the given barium study image?   *(Recent Question 2016)*
    a. Type I hiatus hernia
    b. Bochdalek hernia
    c. Morgagni hernia
    d. Type II hiatus hernia

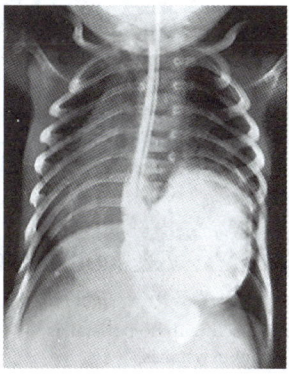
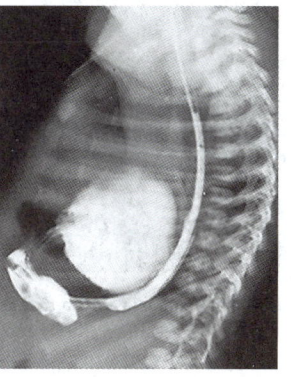

REFLUX ESOPHAGITIS

26. LES pressure is decreased by all except: *(GB Pant 2011)*
    a. Alcohol   b. Protein
    c. Fat   d. Peppermint
27. The lower esophageal sphincter tone (pressure) is increased by: *(COMEDK 2005)*
    a. Glucagon   b. Gastrin
    c. Emptying of the stomach   d. Chocolate

28. The gold standard for diagnosis of gastroesophageal reflux disease (GERD) is: *(Recent Question 2017, MHCET 2016, JIPMER 2014, Orissa 2011, COMEDK 2008, 2007, PGI June 1998)*
    a. Barium swallow
    b. Endoscopy
    c. 24-hours pH monitoring
    d. Esophageal manometry
29. A 35-year-old lady presented with dysphagia, nocturnal asthma and weight loss for 6 years. The most probable diagnosis is: *(COMEDK 2010)*
    a. Achalasia cardia
    b. Lye stricture of esophagus
    c. Gastroesophageal reflux disease
    d. Cancer esophagus
30. Which of the following is the earliest indicator of pathological gastroesophageal reflux in infants (GERD)? *(All India 2011)*
    a. Respiratory symptoms   b. Postprandial regurgitation
    c. Upper GI bleed   d. Stricture esophagus
31. Best test to diagnose gastroesophageal reflux disease and quantify acid output is: *(AIIMS May 2011, Nov 2008)*
    a. Esophagogram   b. Endoscopy
    c. Manometry   d. 24-hours pH monitoring
32. Most important pathophysiological cause of GERD is:
    a. Hiatus hernia   *(AIIMS May 2012)*
    b. Transient LES relaxation
    c. LES hypotension
    d. Inadequate esophageal clearance
33. In GERD, what demonstrates the best anatomical picture? *(MHSSMCET 2007)*
    a. Barium swallow   b. 24-hours pH-monitoring
    c. Endoscopy   d. Manometry
34. Most common complication after Nissen's fundoplication: *(AIIMS GIS Dec 2011, Dec 2006)*
    a. Esophageal injuries   b. Stomach injuries
    c. Liver injuries   d. Pneumothorax
35. All are true about antireflux surgeries except:
    a. Nissen's is 360 degree complete wrap   *(JIPMER GIS 2011)*
    b. Watson is 90 degree posterior
    c. Toupet is 270 degree posterior
    d. Dor is a partial fundoplication
36. Reflux esophagitis is prevented by: *(PGI Dec 2001)*
    a. Long intra-abdominal esophagus
    b. Increased intra-abdominal pressure
    c. Right crus of diaphragm
    d. Increased intra-thoracic pressure
37. Which of the following mechanism can not prevent gastroesophageal reflux? *(AIIMS Nov 98)*
    a. Looping fibers of right crus of diaphragm
    b. Mucosal folds at gastroesophageal junction
    c. Circular muscle fibres of GE sphincter
    d. Angle made by the esophagus with stomach
38. Which one of the following drugs exacerbate reflux esophagitis? *(COMEDK 2004)*
    a. Chlorpropamide
    b. Metoclopramide
    c. Theophylline
    d. Cisapride

39. **The aim of preventing reflux esophagitis by repairing hiatus hernia is achieved by:** *(AIIMS 79, Rohtak 87)*
    a. Bringing the stomach inferior to diaphragm
    b. Reconstitution of the angle of hill
    c. Repair of defect in diaphragm
    d. All of the above

40. **Peptic esophagitis:** *(UPSC 2000)*
    a. Is effectively demonstrated by barium swallow
    b. Is always associated with hiatus hernia
    c. Can be readily confirmed by esophagoscopy
    d. Is associated with the production of higher than normal amounts of gastric acid

41. **Complications of reflux esophagitis:** *(MAHE 2005)*
    a. Stricture   b. Schatzki's ring
    c. Barrett's esophagus   d. All of the above

42. **Most common cause of esophagitis is:** *(AIIMS May 2009)*
    a. Alcohol   b. Smoking
    c. Spicy and hot food   d. Esophageal reflux

43. **What is the name of this fundoplication?**

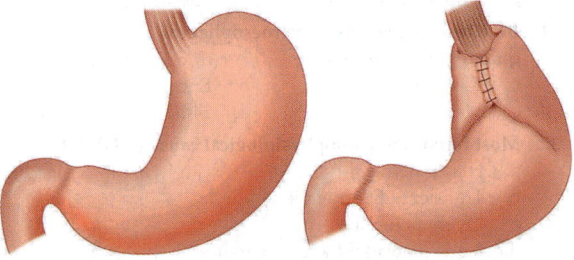

    Normal stomach   After surgery

    a. Nissen's fundoplication   b. Watson fundoplication
    c. Dor fundoplication   d. Toupet fundoplication

ACHALASIA CARDIA

44. **All are true about achalasia except:** *(GB Pant 2011, JIPMER GIS 2011)*
    a. It predisposes to malignancy
    b. Body peristalsis is normal
    c. LES pressure is increased
    d. Dilatation of proximal segment

45. **All of the following are true about achalasia cardia except:** *(Recent Question 2017)*
    a. Achalasia means absence of relaxation
    b. Heller's myotomy is the treatment choice
    c. It is premalignant condition
    d. Caused by selective loss of stimulatory myenteric neurons

46. **All are manometric features of achalasia except:** *(JIPMER GIS 2011)*
    a. High LES pressure
    b. Decreased LES relaxation
    c. Segmental body peristalsis
    d. Manometry helps in diagnosis

47. **A female patient has dysphagia, intermittent epigastric pain. On endoscopy, esophagus was dilated above and narrow at the bottom. Treatment is:** *(AIIMS May 2012)*
    a. PPI
    b. Esophagectomy
    c. Dilatation
    d. Heller's cardiomyotomy

48. **Amyl nitrite inhalation test is used to detect:** *(COMEDK 2005)*
    a. CA esophagus   b. Achalasia cardia
    c. Esophageal diverticulum   d. Tracheoesophageal fistula

49. **Increasing difficulty in swallowing both for solids and liquids in a woman with bird's beak appearance in X-ray seen in:** *(PGI June 2008)*
    a. Achalasia cardia   b. Carcinoma
    c. Reflux esophagitis   d. Barrett's esophagus
    e. Esophagitis

50. **A 30-year-old women comes with dysphagia for both solid and liquids and barium swallow shows parrot beak appearance. On esophageal manometry, LES pressure is increased. Management includes:** *(PGI June 2008)*
    a. Nitrates   b. Ca^{2+} channel blockers
    c. Botulinum toxin   d. Myotomy

51. **Hellers operation is done for:** *(Recent Question 2018, Recent Question 2016, 2014, DNB 2013, 2012)*
    a. Achalasia cardia   b. Hiatus hernia
    c. Diaphragmatic   d. Reflux esophagitis

52. **The defect in achalasia cardia is present in:** *(MAHE 2008)*
    a. Myenteric plexus of Auerbach
    b. Meissner's plexus
    c. Kesselbach's plexus
    d. Mesenteric plexus

53. **What is the diagnosis of barium esophagogram?** *(APPG 2015)*
    a. Achalasia cardia   b. Hiatus hernia
    c. Diffuse esophageal spasm   d. Reflux esophagitis

54. **In achalasia cardia true is:** *(PGI June 2000)*
    a. Pressure at distal end increased with no peristalsis
    b. Low pressure at LES with no peristalsis
    c. Pressure >50mm Hg with peristalsis
    d. Pressure at the distal end increased with normal relaxation

55. **A young patient presents with history of dysphagia more to liquid than solids. The first investigation you will do is:** *(AIIMS June 2003)*
    a. Barium swallow   b. Esophagoscopy
    c. Ultrasound of the chest   d. CT scan of the chest

56. **Treatment for achalasia associated with high rate of recurrence:** *(All India 2002)*
    a. Pneumatic dilatation   b. Laparoscopic myotomy
    c. Open surgical myotomy   d. Botulinum toxin

57. About achalasia cardia all are correct except:
    a. Mostly in women   (APPG 84, Kerala 86, JIPMER 98)
    b. Dilated esophagus narrowing to a point
    c. Heller's operation treatment of choice
    d. Not a premalignant condition

58. All are true of achalasia cardia except: (JIPMER 90)
    a. Dysphagia
    b. Aspiration pneumonitis
    c. Mecholyl test is hyposensitive
    d. X-ray finding of dilated esophagus with a narrow end

59. Following are radiological evidence of Achalasia cardia except: (Karnataka 98)
    a. Smooth narrowing of esophagus
    b. Dilated tortuous esophagus
    c. Absence of air in the fundus
    d. Exaggerated peristalsis

60. Bird's beak appearance is seen in: (Recent Question 2017, Recent Question 2015, J and K 2001)
    a. Volvulus   b. Intussusception
    c. Achalasia   d. Ulcerative colitis

61. This characteristic appearance is seen on barium swallow in: (Recent Question 2016)
    a. Carcinoma esophagus   b. Achalasia cardia
    c. Nutcrackers esophagus   d. Diffuse esophageal spasm

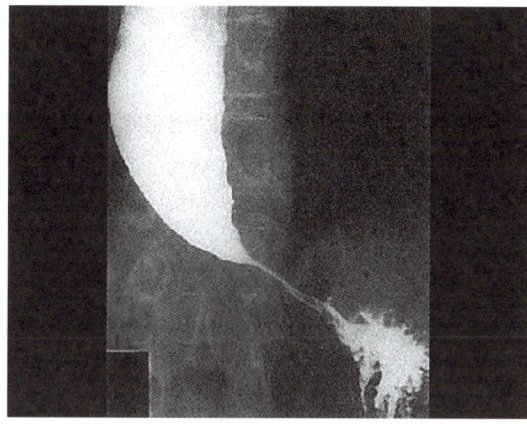

62. Achalasia cardia is characterized by all except: (UPPG 2009)
    a. Most common in women
    b. Dysphagia is most common symptom
    c. Premalignant condition
    d. Parrot beak's appearance

63. True about achalasia cardia is all except: (MHSSMCET 2009)
    a. On repeated Botox injection, recurrence rate increase
    b. More common in young women
    c. Surgery is treatment of choice
    d. Not a premalignant condition

ESOPHAGEAL MOTILITY DISORDERS

64. Corkscrew esophagus is seen in which of the following conditions?   (Recent Question 2017, Recent Question 2015, Bihar PG 2014, NEET 2013, DNB 2008, 2005, 2001)
    a. Carcinoma esophagus   b. Scleroderma
    c. Achalasia cardia   d. Diffuse esophageal spasm

65. This characteristic appearance is seen on barium swallow in: (Recent Question 2016)
    a. Achalasia cardia   b. Nutcrackers esophagus
    c. Diffuse esophageal spasm
    d. Hypertensive LES

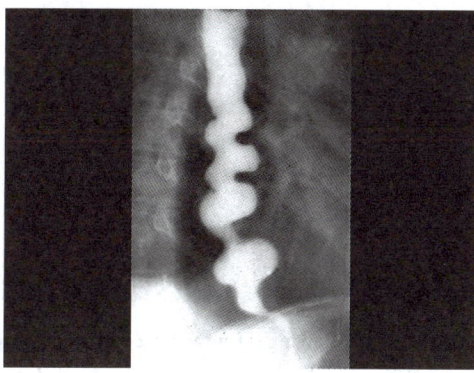

66. Motility in the upper third of the esophagus is decreased in all except:
    a. Pseudo-bulbar palsy   b. Chagas disease
    c. Myasthenia gravis   d. Scleroderma
    e. Cricopharyngeal carcinoma

67. Most common motility disorder leading to dysphagia: (JIPMER 2010)
    a. Nut cracker esophagus   b. Esophageal web
    c. Diffuse esophageal spasm   d. Achalasia cardia

ZENKER'S DIVERTICULUM

68. Best investigation for Zenker's diverticulum is: (Recent Question 2014, AIIMS Nov 2011, AIIMS GIS Dec 2010)
    a. Barium swallow   b. Endoscopy
    c. CECT   d. EUS

69. An elderly male present with history of dysphagia, regurgitation, foul breath and cough. Bilateral lung creps are noted on examination. The most likely diagnosis is: (All India 2012, AIIMS GIS Dec 2010)
    a. Schatzki's ring   b. Zenker's diverticulum
    c. Corkscrew esophagus   d. Plummer-Vinson syndrome

70. True statement about Zenker's diverticulum:
    a. Congenital   (NEET Pattern, GB Pant 2011)
    b. Feeling of obstruction in esophagus
    c. Traction diverticulum
    d. Not present with recurrent aspiration pneumonitis

71. All of the following statements about Zenker's diverticulum are true except: (All India 2009)
    a. Acquired diverticulum
    b. Lateral X-rays on barium swallow are often diagnostic
    c. False diverticulum
    d. Out pouching of the anterior pharyngeal wall just above the cricopharyngeus muscle

72. A 50-year-old male Raju, presents with occasional dysphagia for solids, regurgitation of food and foul smelling breath. Probable diagnosis is: (Recent Question 2016, AIIMS June 99)
    a. Achalasia cardia   b. Zenker's diverticulum
    c. CA esophagus   d. Diabetic gastroparesis

73. A 60-year-old diabetic male patient presented to the OPD with halitosis and dysphagia. Barium swallow was done. What is the diagnosis based on the given findings?
    a. Achalasia cardia   b. Carcinoma esophagus
    c. Zenker's diverticulum d. Leiomyoma

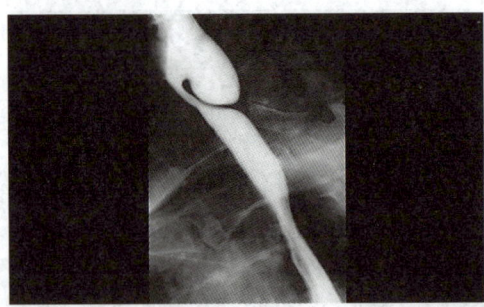

74. Which of the following is true about Zenker's diverticulum? *(PGI Dec 2007)*
    a. It is asymptomatic
    b. Occurs in the mid-esophagus
    c. Treatment is simple excision
    d. It occurs in children

75. Commonest complication of Zenker's diverticulum is: *(AIIMS Nov 96)*
    a. Dysphonia   b. Gastroesophageal reflux
    c. Lung abscess   d. Perforation

76. The pharyngeal diverticulum is a protrusion of mucosa between: *(UPSC 2000)*
    a. The two parts of inferior constrictor muscle of the pharynx
    b. The two parts of middle constrictor muscle of the pharynx
    c. The two parts of the superior constrictor muscle of the pharynx
    d. Cricopharyngeal and posterior part of suprahyoid membrane

77. Dohlman's procedure is used in: *(Recent Question 2013)*
    a. Rectal prolapsed   b. Esophageal achalasia
    c. CA esophagus   d. Zenker's diverticulum

78. Dohlman surgery in Zenker's diverticulum is: *(Recent Question 2019)*
    a. Endoscopic stapling of septum
    b. Endoscopic suturing of pouch
    c. Resection of pouch
    d. Laser excision

ESOPHAGEAL DIVERTICULA

79. Which of the following is a true diverticulum of esophagus? *(AIIMS November 2016)*
    a. Zenker's diverticulum   b. Meckel's diverticulum
    c. Epiphrenic diverticulum d. Parabronchial diverticulum

SCLERODERMA

80. Not a component of POEMS syndrome: *(JIPMER 2010)*
    a. Polyneuropathy   b. Esophageal atresia
    c. Endocrinopathy   d. Multiple myeloma

81. Acronym 'POEMS' stand for: *(PGI May 2011)*
    a. Esophageal dysmotility   b. Polyneuropathy
    c. Endocrinopathy   d. M-protein
    e. Scleroderma

82. Which part of esophagus is mainly affected in scleroderma? *(MHPGMCET 2003)*
    a. Upper third   b. Middle third
    c. Lower third   d. All the above

83. Connective tissue disorder which is associated with gastroesophageal reflux is: *(PGI Dec 99)*
    a. SLE   b. Scleroderma
    c. Behcet's syndrome   d. Dermatomyositis

PLUMMER–VINSON SYNDROME

84. Not true about Plummer-Vinson syndrome is: *(AIIMS 97)*
    a. Occurs in elderly males
    b. Postcricoid webs
    c. Predispose to hypopharynx malignancy
    d. Koilonychia

85. In Plummer-Vinson syndrome, obstruction is due to: *(DPG 2006)*
    a. Esophageal dysmotility   b. Esophageal stenosis
    c. Postcricoid webs   d. None of the above

86. All are features of Plummer-Vinson syndrome except: *(COMEDK 2008)*
    a. Esophageal web   b. Iron deficiency
    c. Achalasia cardia   d. Dysphagia

87. Not a feature of Plummer-Vinson syndrome: *(Punjab 2008)*
    a. Web present in lower part of esophagus
    b. Koilonychia
    c. Premalignant
    d. Common in edentulous females

BARRETT'S ESOPHAGUS

88. True about Barrett's esophagus: *(PGI Dec 2007)*
    a. Long esophageal segment involved
    b. Metaplasia
    c. Peptic ulcer
    d. Para esophageal hernia
    e. Leads to adenocarcinoma

89. All of the following are correct about Barrett's esophagus except: *(Recent Question 2019)*
    a. Predisposes to adenocarcinoma
    b. Columnar to squamous metaplasia
    c. Associated with GERD
    d. Acquired condition

90. A 55 years old patient presented with dysphagia. Identify the diagnosis from upper GI biopsy of esophagus showed in the following picture: *(AIIMS May 2017)*

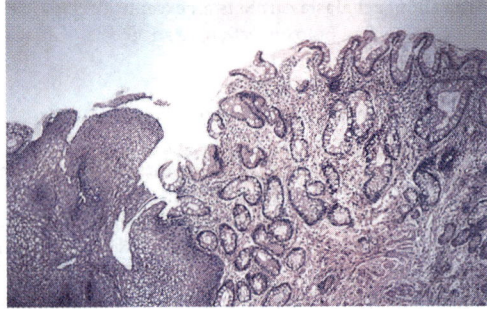

    a. Squamous cell carcinoma   b. Eosinophilic esophagitis
    c. Barrett's esophagus   d. Adenocarcinoma

91. A chronic alcoholic presents with regurgitation and retrosternmal pain. Endoscopic biopsy confirms Barretti's esophagus. What is the most appropriate management in this case? *(JIPMER 2013)*
    a. Endoscopic biopsy every 2 years
    b. PPI
    c. H. pylori treatment
    d. Balloon dilatation

92. Barrett's esophagus is: *(All India 2002, AIIMS June 93)*
    a. Lower esophagus lined by columnar epithelium
    b. Upper esophagus lined by columnar epithelium
    c. Lower esophagus lined by ciliated epithelium
    d. Lower esophagus lined by pseudostratified epithelium

93. Barrett's esophagus is diagnosed by: *(AIIMS May 2012, Nov 2007, DNB 2008)*
    a. Squamous metaplasia   b. Intestinal metaplasia
    c. Squamous dysplasia   d. Intestinal dysplasia

94. Barrett's esophagus can lead to: *(AIIMS June 98)*
    a. Stricture   b. Reflux esophagitis
    c. Peptic ulcer   d. Achalasia

95. True regarding Barrett's esophagus is: *(AIIMS Nov 95)*
    a. Benign course
    b. Premalignant condition
    c. Squamous metaplasia of lower esophagus
    d. Medical treatment is not useful

96. What is the most probable diagnosis on the basis of given endoscopy image? *(Recent Question 2016)*
    a. GAVE   b. Schatzki ring
    c. Barrett's esophagus   d. Esophageal varices

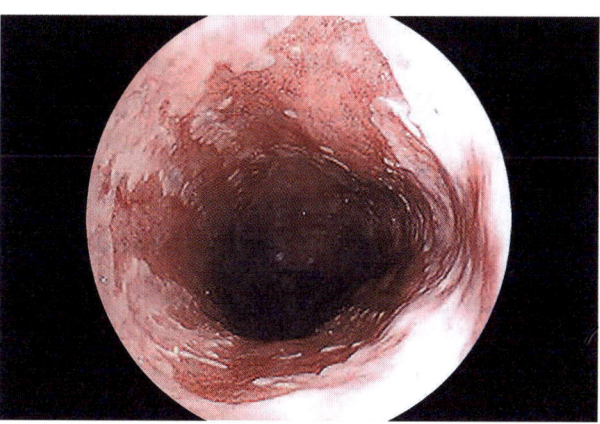

CARCINOMA ESOPHAGUS PREDISPOSING FACTORS

97. All are the predisposing factors for carcinoma esophagus except: *(COMEDK 2011)*
    a. Achalasia
    b. Paterson Brown Kelly Syndrome
    c. Zenker's diverticulum
    d. Ectodermal dysplasia

98. All are risk factors for epidermoid carcinoma except: *(ILBS 2011)*
    a. Achalasia   b. Barrett's esophagus
    c. Nitrosamines   d. Corrosives

99. Premalignant lesion of carcinoma esophagus includes: *(PGI Nov 2011, June 2007)*
    a. Tylosis   b. Plummer-Vinson syndrome
    c. Barrett's esophagus   d. Achalasia cardia
    e. Scleroderma

100. Squamous cell carcinoma of esophagus is caused by: *(MHPGMCET 2009)*
     a. Tobacco/Alcohol   b. Alkalies
     c. GERD   d. All of the above

101. Which is not a predisposing factor for carcinoma esophagus?
     a. Esophageal diverticula   *(Orissa 2011)*
     b. Plummer-Vinson syndrome
     c. Mediastinal fibrosis
     d. Caustic ingestion

102. The adenocarcinoma of esophagus develops in: *(Recent Question 2017, Bihar PG 2014, COMEDK 2014, All India 2002, 98)*
     a. Barrett's esophagus
     b. Long standing achalasia
     c. Corrosive stricture
     d. Alcohol abuse

103. Esophageal carcinoma is not predisposed by: *(PGI June 99, PGI Dec 95)*
     a. Achalasia   b. Scleroderma
     c. Corrosive intake   d. Barrett's esophagus

104. Not a predisposing factor for carcinoma esophagus: *(AIIMS May 2009)*
     a. Diverticula   b. Human papilloma virus
     c. Mediastinal fibrosis   d. Caustic ingestion

105. Risk factor for adenocarcinoma of esophagus: *(KGMC 2011)*
     a. Barrett's esophagus   b. Corrosive injury
     c. Achalasia cardia   d. All of the above

CA ESOPHAGUS CLINICAL FEATURES, DIAGNOSIS AND TREATMENT

106. Which of the following is best indicator of survival in CA esophagus? *(AIIMS GIS May 2008)*
     a. TNM stage
     b. Resection margin
     c. Histology and location
     d. Size of tumor

107. Best prognosis in CA esophagus: *(AIIMS GIS Dec 2010)*
     a. Polypoidal   b. Fungating
     c. Ulcerative   d. Infiltrative

108. Sievert classification is for: *(KGMC 2011)*
     a. Esophageal cancer
     b. Stomach cancer
     c. GE junction tumors
     d. CA pancreas

109. Characteristic features of LN involvement on EUS in CA esophagus are all except: *(AIIMS GIS Dec 2011, May 2008)*
     a. Round contour
     b. Sharp border
     c. Hyperechogenic
     d. Size >1 cm

110. Most commonly used chemotherapy regimen used in CA esophagus: *(AIIMS GIS May 2008)*
     a. 5-FU + Cisplatin   b. Cisplatin + Vinblastine
     c. Cisplatin + Paclitaxel   d. Cisplatin + Epirubicin

111. Which is not used in palliation in CA esophagus?
    (AIIMS GIS May 2008)
    a. EMR
    b. Photodynamic therapy
    c. Laser therapy
    d. Self-expanding stents

112. T-staging of esophagus is best done by:
    (AIIMS GIS Dec 2011, DNB 2002)
    a. EUS
    b. CT
    c. MRI
    d. PET

113. Commonest site of esophagus carcinoma is: (UPPG 2008)
    a. Upper 2/3rd
    b. Middle 1/3rd
    c. Lower 1/3rd
    d. Crico-esophageal junction

114. Barium esophagogram findings in carcinoma esophagus are all except: (UPPG 2009)
    a. Rat-tail deformity
    b. Pencil tip appearance
    c. Apple-core appearance
    d. Filling defect

115. A 60-year-old chronic smoker presented with progressive dysphagia. Barium swallow was done, what is the name of sign? (Recent Question 2017)
    a. Bird beak appearance
    b. Pencil tip appearance
    c. Apple core appearance
    d. Rat tail appearance

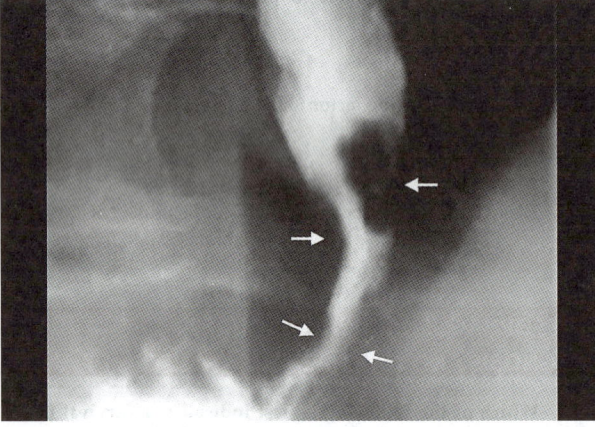

116. MC site of CA esophagus is:
    (MCI Nov 2017, Recent Question 2015, AIIMS Feb 2007)
    a. Middle 1/3rd
    b. Upper 1/3rd
    c. Lower 1/3rd
    d. Lower end of esophagus

117. The commonest site of carcinoma esophagus in India is:
    (AIIMS Nov 2003)
    a. Upper 1/3rd
    b. Middle 1/3rd
    c. Lower 1/3rd
    d. GE junction

118. A patient presents with dysphagia of 4 weeks duration. Now he is able to swallow liquid food only. Which of the following is the one investigation to be done? (DPG 2009 Feb)
    a. Barium studies
    b. Upper GI endoscopy
    c. CT Scan
    d. Esophageal manometry

119. Treatment of choice for CA esophagus: (PGI SS Dec 2009)
    a. Esophagectomy
    b. External radiotherapy
    c. Internal radiotherapy
    d. Chemotherapy

120. Stage of CA esophagus is best decided by:
    (PGI SS June 2009)
    a. Depth of tumor
    b. Size of tumor
    c. Histopathological grade
    d. Age of the patient

121. Esophageal carcinoma is adequately assessed by:
    a. Barium swallow (PGI SS Dec 2009)
    b. Barium swallow + endoscopy
    c. Endoscopy
    d. USG

122. Most common complication of placing stent in CA esophagus: (AIIMS GIS May 2011)
    a. Migration
    b. Chest pain
    c. Perforation
    d. Bleeding

123. What is the diagnosis based on the given findings?

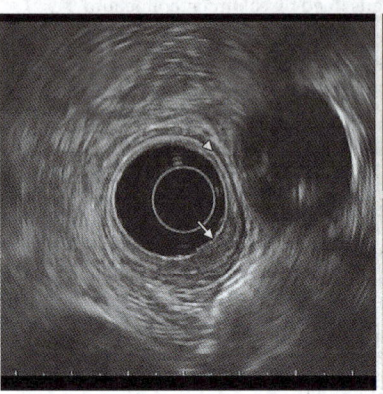
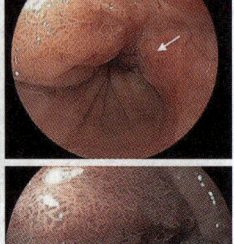
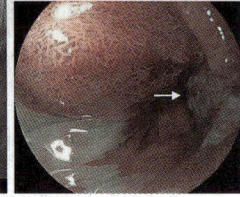

    a. Mallory Weiss syndrome
    b. Carcinoma esophagus
    c. Carcinoma stomach
    d. Esophageal varices

124. Lymph node metastasis in CA esophagus is best detected by: (JIPMER SS 2016, AIIMS GIS May 2011)
    a. PET
    b. EUS
    c. CT
    d. Thoracoscopy + laparoscopy

125. Best palliation in CA esophagus: (GB Pant 2011)
    a. Surgical bypass
    b. Surgical placement of MB tube
    c. Endoprosthesis
    d. Feeding jejunostomy

126. Most common site for squamous cell CA esophagus is:
    (All India 2001)
    a. Upper third
    b. Middle third
    c. Lower third
    d. Gastro-esophageal junction

127. True about CA esophagus: (PGI Dec 2003)
    a. MC in middle 1/3rd
    b. Adenocarcinoma is common variety
    c. Carcinoma develops at the achalasia segment
    d. Smoking is a risk factor
    e. Endoscopy is the investigation of choice

128. Treatment of advanced esophageal cancer is: (DNB 2006)
    a. Chemoradiation only
    b. Curative en-bloc resection
    c. Chemoradiation followed by curative enbloc resection
    d. Chemoradiation followed by palliative enbloc resection

129. Regarding esophagus malignancy-operation all are true except: (MHSSMCET 2009)
    a. Thoracoscopic assisted surgery
    b. Radiotherapy
    c. Chemotherapy + surgery
    d. Transhiatal esophagectomy

130. Transhiatal esophagectomy was planned for adenocarcinoma of lower end of esophagus. The approach would be in the following order: (AIIMS Nov 2007)
    a. Abdomen-Neck
    b. Abdomen-Thorax-Neck
    c. Neck-Thorax-Abdomen
    d. Abdomen-Thorax

131. True about carcinoma esophagus is: (Kerala 94)
    a. Most common site is lower end
    b. Both adeno and squamous cell carcinoma occur
    c. Commonest histology is adenocarcinoma
    d. More common in females

132. Which is the most reliable diagnostic method for staging the esophageal cancer? (UPSC 2006)
    a. MRI
    b. Endoscopic ultrasound
    c. CT scan
    d. Thoracoscopy

133. Early stage of carcinoma esophagus is diagnosed by:
    a. Barium meal (UPPG 2008)
    b. Transesophageal USG
    c. MRI
    d. Endoscopy

134. False statements about carcinoma esophagus are all of the following except: (MCI March 2009)
    a. Most common in lower third
    b. Histologically, adenocarcinoma only
    c. Unrelated to tobacco chewing
    d. It is more common in females

135. Which of the following should never be carried out as a treatment for carcinoma esophagus? (MHPGMCET 2008)
    a. Gastrostomy for palliation
    b. Radiotherapy alone
    c. Radical esophagectomy
    d. Radiotherapy and chemotherapy

136. Treatment of SCC of esophagus: (GB Pant 2011)
    a. Cisplatin
    b. Etoposide
    c. Adriamycin
    d. Bleomycin

137. In Esophageal cancer prognosis is best determined by: (AIIMS May 2015)
    a. Cellular differentiation
    b. Age of patient
    c. T stage
    d. Length of involvement

138. True regarding esophageal squamous cell carcinoma is/are: (PGI May 2018)
    a. Barrett's esophagus is a risk factor
    b. Common in middle third of esophagus
    c. Stomach, jejunum or colon can be used for replacement after surgical removal
    d. Chemoradiation has little role in inoperable patients
    e. Staging is done by CECT

ESOPHAGECTOMY

139. Conduit in gastric pull up is based on: (AIIMS GIS Dec 2011, May 2008)
    a. Right gastric and right gastroepiploic artery
    b. Right gastric and left gastroepiploic artery
    c. Left gastric and right gastroepiploic artery
    d. Left gastric and left gastroepiploic artery

140. Which is the best substitute for esophagus? (MHSSMCET 2005, MP 99, All India 96, PGI Dec 95)
    a. Stomach
    b. Jejunum
    c. Left sided colon
    d. Right sided colon

141. First successful esophagectomy was done by: (AIIMS GIS Dec 2011)
    a. Miculikz
    b. Kaplan
    c. Torek
    d. Orringer

142. Ivor Lewis operation is the treatment of choice for cancer involving .... esophagus: (MHSSMCET 2009)
    a. Upper 1/3rd
    b. Middle 1/3rd
    c. Lower 1/3rd
    d. Entire esophagus

143. Which of the following surgical approach was first described by Orringer for the management of carcinoma esophagus? (J amd K 2005)
    a. Transhiatal
    b. Thoracoscopic
    c. Left thoracoabdominal
    d. Right thoracoabdominal

144. Commonest cause for mortality in Ivor Lewis operations:
    a. Pulmonary atelectasis (AIIMS Nov 98)
    b. Anastomotic leak
    c. Thoracic duct fistula
    d. Sub diaphragmatic collection

145. Which of the following operations was first described by Orringer? (COMEDK 2006)
    a. Enbloc esophagectomy
    b. Transhiatal esophagectomy
    c. Thoracoscopic esophagectomy
    d. Transthoracic esophagectomy

146. The ideal replacement for the esophagus after esophagectomy is: (COMEDK 2010)
    a. Stomach
    b. Jejunum
    c. Colon
    d. Synthetic stent

147. After esophagectomy, stomach tube is based on supply form: (MHSSMCET 2006)
    a. Right gastroepiploic artery
    b. Right gastric artery
    c. Left gastroepiploic artery
    d. Left gastric artery

LEIOMYOMA

148. Commonest benign tumor of the esophagus: (JIPMER 2014, DPG 2009 Feb)
    a. Leiomyoma
    b. Papilloma
    c. Adenoma
    d. Hemangioma

149. This characteristic appearance is seen on barium swallow in: (Recent Question 2017)
    a. Achalasia cardia
    b. Carcinoma esophagus
    c. Leiomyoma
    d. Diffuse esophageal spasm

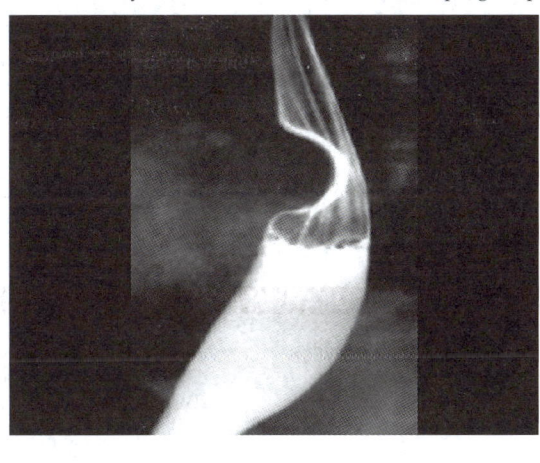

Surgery Essence

150. Endoscopic treatment of leiomyoma of esophagus is contraindicated due to: *(JIPMER GIS 2011)*
   a. Infection
   b. Chances of dissemination
   c. Perforation
   d. Perforation and dissemination

DYSPHAGIA

151. Intermittent dysphagia is caused by: *(PGI June 2004)*
   a. Stricture
   b. Reflux esophagitis
   c. Achalasia cardia
   d. Pharyngeal diverticulum
   e. Diffuse esophageal spasm

152. A 60-year-old patient presenting with dysphagia of 6 weeks duration with solid foods, now can swallow only liquids. Investigation done for diagnosis: *(PGI Dec 2003)*
   a. CXR
   b. Ba swallow
   c. Endoscopy
   d. USG
   e. C.T. Scan

153. Investigation of choice for dysphagia for solids:
   a. Barium swallow
   b. Endoscopy *(PGI Dec 2000)*
   c. X-ray chest
   d. C.T. Scan

154. Odynophagia occurs in: *(AIIMS GIS Dec 2011, PGI June 96)*
   a. Achalasia
   b. Herpes esophagitis
   c. Monilial esophagitis
   d. Barrett's esophagus

155. A 40-year-old female patient presented with dysphagia to both liquids and solids and regurgitation for 3 months. The dysphagia was non-progressive. What is the most likely diagnosis? *(AIIMS May 2006)*
   a. Carcinoma of the esophagus
   b. Lower esophageal mucosal ring
   c. Achalasia cardia
   d. Reflux esophagitis with esophageal stricture

DYSPHAGIA LUSORIA

156. Dysphagia lusoria is caused by: *(Karnataka 2013, PGI SS June 2001)*
   a. Abnormal elongation of arch of aorta
   b. Aneurysm of arch of aorta
   c. Esophageal web
   d. Esophageal diverticula

157. Dysphagia lusoria is due to: *(Recent Question 2016, 2014, AIIMS Nov 2003)*
   a. Esophageal diverticulum
   b. Aneurysm of aorta
   c. Esophageal web
   d. Compression by aberrant blood vessel

158. All are true about dysphagia lusoria except: *(DPG 2008)*
   a. Right aortic arch
   b. Vascular ring
   c. Due to aberrant subclavian artery causing pressure on esophagus
   d. Acquired in later life

ESOPHAGEAL PERFORATION AND INJURY

159. Mackler's triad includes: *(PGI Nov 2009)*
   a. Vomiting
   b. Subcutaneous emphysema
   c. Lower thoracic pain
   d. Peripheral cyanosis
   e. Pleural effusion

160. True about Boerhaave's syndrome: *(PGI Nov 2009)*
   a. MC at lower 1/3rd
   b. Hematemesis is early symptoms
   c. Acute chest pain
   d. Surgically treated
   e. Operation is done after 24 hours

161. True about esophageal injury: *(PGI June 2009)*
   a. Barium swallow is diagnostic
   b. Treatment is primary repair
   c. MC after penetrating injury
   d. Mortality increased if repair after 24 hours

162. Boerhaave's syndrome, true is: *(PGI May 2005)*
   a. Iatrogenic
   b. Silent manifestation
   c. Present with acute chest pain
   d. Treatment is surgical

163. Which is most common site for iatrogenic esophageal perforation? *(Recent Question 2017, Recent Question 2014, DNB 2013, 2012, AIIMS Nov 97)*
   a. Abdominal portion
   b. Cervical portion
   c. Above arch of aorta
   d. Below arch of aorta

164. Commonest cause of esophageal perforation is:
   a. Acid ingestion
   b. Hyperemesis
   c. Instrumentation
   d. Carcinoma infiltrating

165. A 40-year-old female presents with perforation of distal third of esophagus. Best form of management is:
   a. Antibiotics and drainage *(JIPMER GIS 2011)*
   b. Tubal drainage
   c. Primary resection and anastomosis
   d. Esophagectomy with bringing proximal end as fistula in neck

166. In majority of patients with esophageal leaks in thoracic cavity of less than 12 hours duration, the treatment of choice is: *(UPSC 97)*
   a. Primary closure, drainage and antibiotics
   b. Early esophagogastrostomy
   c. Exclusion and diversion of continuity
   d. Total esophagectomy and gastric pull up

167. Best flap for esophagus repair:
   a. Colon
   b. Stomach
   c. Jejunum
   d. Latissimus dorsi

168. In esophageal perforation all are seen except: *(UPPG 2000)*
   a. Pain
   b. Bradycardia
   c. Fever
   d. Hypotension

169. Boerhaave's syndrome is due to: *(Recent Question 2016, DNB 2012, UPPG 2007)*
   a. Drug induced esophagus perforation
   b. Corrosive injury
   c. Spontaneous perforation
   d. Gastroesophageal reflux disease

170. When a 'spontaneous perforation' of the esophagus occurs as a result of severe barotrauma while a person vomits against a closed glottis, the condition is known as: *(UPSC 2008)*
   a. Mallory-Weiss syndrome
   b. Plummer-Vinson syndrome
   c. Kartagener syndrome
   d. Boerhaave's syndrome

171. Longitudinal tear of esophagus is seen in: *(MHPGMCET 2002)*
    a. Boerhaave's syndrome
    b. Mallory-Weiss syndrome
    c. Nutcracker's esophagus
    d. Lye stricture

172. In Boerhaave's syndrome, perforation of esophagus is seen at? *(MHSSMCET 2009)*
    a. Upper anterior
    b. Lower posterior
    c. Upper posterior
    d. Lower anterior

173. Most common site a spontaneous rupture of esophagus is:
    a. Cricopharyngeal junction *(Recent Question 2017, DNB 2009)*
    b. Cardioesophageal junction
    c. Mid esophagus
    d. After the crossing of arch of aorta

174. Investigation of choice for esophageal rupture is? *(DNB 2014)*
    a. Dynamic MRI
    b. Rigid esophagoscopy
    c. Barium contrast swallow
    d. Water soluble low molecular weight contrast swallow

175. Which of the following is true about Boerhaave's syndrome? *(Recent Question 2017)*
    a. May present with peritonitis
    b. Forceful vomiting against open glottis
    c. Upper third esophagus location
    d. Most patients are managed by conservative management

176. Safest contrast in esophageal perforation: *(Recent Question 2018)*
    a. Iohexol   b. Barium sulphate
    c. Gadolinium   d. Hypaque

177. True about esophageal perforation: *(PGI November 2017)*
    a. Morbidity is mainly due to mediastinal infection
    b. Partial tear involving mucosa should be managed conservatively
    c. Simple exploration and end to end anastomosis is done as soon as possible in all cases
    d. Spontaneous perforation most commonly occur in mid thoracic esophagus
    e. Serum amylase levels may be high as a result of absorption of amylase from the pleural cavity

TRACHEOESOPHAGEAL FISTULA

178. Esophageal atresia is most commonly associated with: *(KGMC 2011)*
    a. Respiratory anomalies   b. Anorectal malformations
    c. Genitourinary   d. CVS

179. The most common type of tracheoesophageal fistula is: *(Recent Question 2017, Recent Question 2014, MAHE 2008, 2007)*
    a. Esophageal atresia without tracheoesophageal fistula
    b. Esophageal atresia with proximal tracheoesophageal fistula
    c. Esophageal atresia with distal tracheoesophageal fistula
    d. Esophageal atresia with proximal and distal tracheo-esophageal fistula

180. What is the type of tracheoesophageal fistula (TEF) seen on barium swallow?

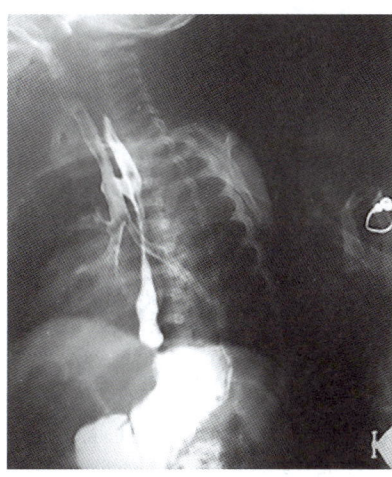

    a. Atresia with proximal TEF
    b. Atresia with distal TEF
    c. Atresia with both proximal and distal TEF
    d. TEF without esophageal atresia

181. Malignant tracheoesophageal fistula best treated with: *(PGI May 2005)*
    a. Radiotherapy
    b. Chemotherapy
    c. Stenting
    d. Tube
    e. Surgical correction

182. Treatment of malignant tracheoesophageal fistula includes: *(PGI June 2007)*
    a. Expandable metal stent
    b. Surgery with graft
    c. Gastrostomy tube
    d. Radiotherapy
    e. Chemotherapy

183. Which one of the following life-threatening congenital anomalies in the newborn presents with polyhydramnios, aspiration pneumonia, excessive salivation and difficulty in passing a nasogastric tube? *(APPG 2016)*
    a. Choanal atresia
    b. Tracheoesophageal fistula
    c. Diaphragmatic hernia
    d. Gastroschisis

184. Which of the following is associated with poor prognosis in tracheo-esophageal fistula in children? *(Recent Question 2016)*
    a. Weight <2000 gms
    b. Major cardiac anomaly
    c. Proximal TE fistula with distal esophageal atresia
    d. Vertebral anomaly

ESOPHAGEAL RINGS AND WEBS

185. Schatzki's ring is: *(PGI Dec 98)*
    a. Mucosal ring at squamocolumnar junction
    b. Muscular ring
    c. Dysphagia is the symptom
    d. Inflammatory stricture

186. What is the diagnosis based on the given barium swallow findings?

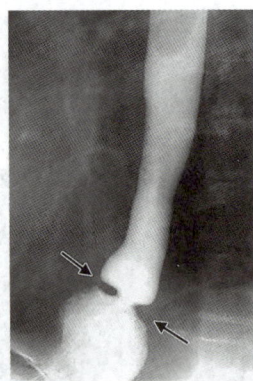

   a. Esophageal web
   b. Carcinoma esophagus
   c. Schatzki ring
   d. Leiomyoma

187. Schatzki ring is seen at: *(UPPG 2009)*
   a. Mid-esophagus
   b. Lower-esophagus
   c. Junction of lower esophagus
   d. None

188. False about Schatzki ring is: *(Punjab 2007)*
   a. Occurs at lower part of esophagus
   b. Involves mucosa and submucosa
   c. Involves mucosa, submucosa and muscularis
   d. Located at squamocolumnar junction

189. True about Schatzki's ring: *(PGI Nov 2010)*
   a. Has skeletal muscle
   b. Located at lower esophagus
   c. Causes dysphagia
   d. Contain all layers of esophagus

190. Schatzki ring: *(DNB 2007, MHSSMCET 2007)*
   a. Can be treated by PPI alone
   b. Occurs at GE junction
   c. Type A ring
   d. Type C ring

191. What is the most probable diagnosis on the basis of given endoscopy image? *(Recent Question 2016)*
   a. GAVE
   b. Schatzki ring
   c. Barrett's esophagus
   d. Esophageal varices

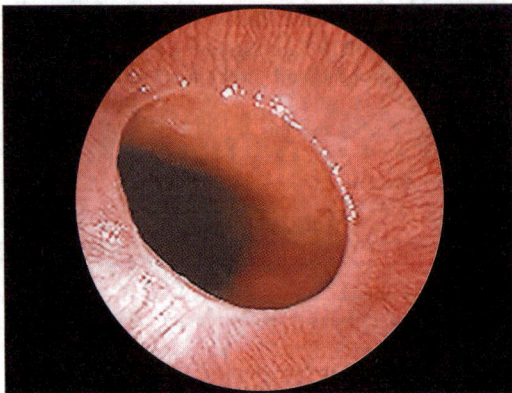

FOREIGN BODY

192. A foreign body usually gets arrested in which part of esophagus? *(DNB 2003)*
   a. Cardiac part of the esophagus
   b. In the middle third of the esophagus
   c. Below the cricopharynx
   d. Above the cricopharynx

193. A child was brought by his mother to the emergency with history of accidental swallowing of coin. Chest X-ray is given below. What is the location of foreign body in this child? *(Recent Question 2016)*
   a. Esophagus
   b. Trachea
   c. Bronchus
   d. None of the above

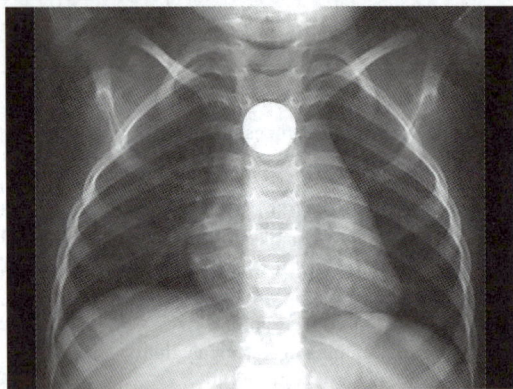

ESOPHAGUS: ANATOMY AND PHYSIOLOGY

194. Which of the following is true about esophageal anatomy? *(JIPMER GIS 2011)*
   a. Cervical esophagus is posterior and little right to trachea
   b. Thoracic esophagus is crossed by aortic arch posteriorly
   c. Thoracic esophagus is crossed by left main bronchus posteriorly
   d. Lower esophagus before entering the diaphragm is anterior and left sided

195. Non-progressive contraction of esophagus are: *(AIIMS May 2011, All India 2009)*
   a. Primary
   b. Secondary
   c. Tertiary
   d. Quaternary

196. Distance between upper incisors and gastroesophageal junction is: *(DPG 97)*
   a. 25 cm
   b. 30 cm
   c. 40 cm
   d. 60 cm

197. Third constriction of the esophagus is at the level of:
   a. Left bronchus crossing the aorta *(CMC 98)*
   b. Where it pierces the diaphragm
   c. Junction of the esophagus and stomach
   d. Cricopharynx

198. Structure not passing through the esophageal hiatus: *(AIIMS Nov 2011)*
   a. Left phrenic nerve
   b. Right vagus nerve
   c. Left vagus nerve
   d. Left gastric artery

199. The normal narrowing in the middle of the esophagus is caused by: *(COMEDK 2007)*
   a. Azygos vein
   b. Hemiazygos vein
   c. Right main stem bronchus
   d. Left main stem bronchus

200. **False statement about esophagus:** *(PGI Nov 2011)*
   a. Thoracic esophagus is supplied directly by aorta
   b. Bleeding from varices occurs from midesophagus
   c. Cervical esophagus drains to deep cervical nodes
   d. It has rich lymphatic network
   e. Abdominal part of esophagus drains to left gastric

201. **Normal LES pressure:** *(Recent Question 2017)*
   a. 6–26 mm Hg   b. 30–50 mm Hg
   c. 50–60 mm Hg   d. 60–70 mm Hg

202. **Dysphagia in esophagus means which invasion?** *(Recent Question 2017)*
   a. Mucosal   b. Submucosal
   c. Transmural   d. Node

DIAPHRAGM

203. **Fluoroscopy is used for diagnosis of:** *(PGI June 98)*
   a. LV function   b. Diaphragmatic palsy
   c. Valvular calcification   d. Pericardial effusion

204. **Diagnosis of traumatic rupture of diaphragm is made by:**
   a. Laparoscopy   *(PGI June 2007)*
   b. Chest X-ray
   c. Diagnostic peritoneal lavage
   d. CT

205. **Diaphragm develops from all of the following structures, except:** *(All India 2011)*
   a. Septum transversum   b. Pleuroperitoneal membrane
   c. Cervical myotomes   d. Dorsal mesocardium

206. **Which of the following incisions is taken for diaphragmatic surgery?** *(AIIMS May 2014)*
   a. Transverse   b. Circumferential
   c. Vertical   d. Radial

MISCELLANEOUS

207. **Pressure of esophagus is .... mm below ambient:** *(PGI Dec 95)*
   a. 3   b. 5
   c. 12   d. 18

208. **'Pencil tip' deformity is seen in:** *(PGI June 95)*
   a. Carcinoma esophagus
   b. Achalasia cardia
   c. Barrett's esophagus
   d. None of the above

209. **Maximum dilatation of esophagus occurs in:** *(Kerala 94)*
   a. Carcinoma at gastroesophageal junction
   b. Achalasia cardia
   c. Stricture at lower end
   d. CREST syndrome

210. **Second swallowing in barium meal studies is found in:** *(JIPMER 95)*
   a. Pharyngeal pouch b. Achalasia cardia
   c. Scleroderma   d. Reflux esophagitis

211. **Hamman's sign is seen with:** *(MHPGMCET 2006)*
   a. Acute pericarditis   b. Aortic dissection
   c. Tracheal compression d. Esophageal perforation

212. **Stricture esophagus is dilated with .... F dilator?**
   a. 30   b. 40   *(MHSSMCET 2009)*
   c. 50   d. 60

213. **Stricture esophagus may be treated by:** *(MHSSMCET 2009)*
   a. Metallic stent   b. Guide wire directed stent
   c. Expandable stents d. Esophagectomy

214. **The Roux loop should be atleast how long to avoid bile reflux esophagitis?** *(MHSSMCET 2010)*
   a. 30 cm   b. 40 cm
   c. 50 cm   d. 60 cm

215. **Feline esophagus is:** *(Recent Question 2018)*
   a. Eosinophilic esophagitis
   b. GERD
   c. Radiation esophagitis
   d. Chemotherapy induced esophagitis

216. **Pharyngo-esophageal reflux is monitored by:** *(Recent Question 2018)*
   a. Esophageal pH monitoring
   b. Dual probe pH monitoring
   c. Barium esophagogram
   d. Radionuclide scintigraphy

217. **Serpiginous ulcers in lower esophagus are seen in:** *(Recent Question 2019)*

   a. CMV esophagitis   b. Candida esophagitis
   c. Corrosive esophagitis d. Pill induced esophagitis

218. **Small punched out lesions on endoscopy in lower esophagus in the immunocompromised patients is seen in:** *(Recent Question 2019)*

   a. CMV esophagitis   b. Candida esophagitis
   c. Corrosive esophagitis d. Herpes simplex esophagitis

Explanations

CONGENITAL DIAPHRAGMATIC HERNIA

1. Ans. a. **Pulmonary hypertension** *(Ref: Sabiston 20/e p1863-1864; Schwartz 10/e p1603-1605; Bailey 27/e p938; Shackelford 7/e p506)*
2. Ans. b. **Delay in emergent surgery** *(Ref: Nelson 20/e p862; Fundamentals of Pediatric Surgery (Springer) 2011/535,536)*

Prognostic Factors in CDH	
Primary Prognostic Factors	**Secondary Prognostic Factors**
Pulmonary hypoplasia (Most important^Q) • **Pulmonary hypoplasia** is the **major determinant** of **survival**^{Q}. • **Degree** of **pulmonary hypoplasia** closely **correlates** with degree of **pulmonary hypertension**^{Q}.	**Antenatal** • **Early gestational age**^{Q} (<24 weeks) • Extradiaphragmatic anomalies^Q • Stomach herniation • Small lung to head circumference ratio • Small fetal abdominal circumference • Polyhydramnios^Q • Size of defect^Q
Pulmonary hypertension (Important)^Q • The **combined effect** of **pulmonary hypoplasia** and **pulmonary hypertension** is believed to be **MC** cause of **mortality** in CDH^Q.	**Postnatal** • **Early presentation**^{Q} (within 6 hours) • PO_2 and PCO_2 unresponsive to ventilation • **Need for** extra-corporeal membrane oxygenation (**ECMO**)^Q
	Side of Defect • **Right sided defects** have **poor prognosis**^{Q}

3. Ans. c. **Present in second decade**
4. Ans. d. **Transverse colon** *(Ref: Sabiston 20/e p1863-1864; Schwartz 9/e p1416-1418; Bailey 27/e p938; Shackelford 7/e p506)*
5. Ans. d. **Diaphragmatic hernia**
6. Ans. c. **Always occurs on right side**
7. Ans. a. **Seen on right side**
8. Ans. c. **Peristalsis in the thoracic cavity**
9. Ans. a. **Right anterior**
10. Ans. b. **Abdominal distension**
11. Ans. a. **Hernia between the costal and sternal part of the diaphragm**
12. Ans. b. **Diaphragmatic hernia**
13. Ans. c. **Transverse colon** *(Ref: Sabiston 20/e p1863; Bailey 27/e p938)*

> *"The foramen of Morgagni: A hernia in the anterior part of the diaphragm with a defect between the sternal and costal attachments. The most commonly involved viscus is the transverse colon."*-Bailey 27/e p938

14. Ans. a. **Bochdalek** *(Ref: Shackelford 7/e p506; Sabiston 20/e p1863; Schwartz 10/e p1604)*

> *"Bochdalek hernias otherwise known as posterolateral hernias, make up 85% of congenital hernias. They occur on the left side 80% of the time."*- Shackelford 7/e p506

HIATUS HERNIA

15. Ans. a. **Surgery is indicated in all symptomatic cases**, b. **Para-esophageal type is more complicated** *(Ref: Sabiston 20/e p1059-1060; Schwartz 10/e p980-984; Bailey 27/e p1083; Shackelford 7/e p494-505)*
16. Ans. b. **Part of upper stomach enters into thorax in both A and B** *(Ref: Sabiston 20/e p1059-1060, Schwartz 10/e p980, Bailey 27/e p1083-1084; Shackelford 7/e p494-505)*
17. Ans. a. **Esophagitis**
18. Ans. d. **Hiatus hernia**
19. Ans. b. **Barium meal** *(Ref: Bailey 27/e p1084)*

Diagnosis of Hiatus Hernia

- The **hernia** may be **visible on** a **plain radiograph** of the **chest** as a **gas bubble**, often with a **fluid level behind** the **heart**[Q].
- A **barium meal** is the **best method of diagnosis**[Q].
- The **endoscopic appearances** may be **confusing**, especially **in large hernias** when it is easy to become disorientated.

20. **Ans. c. Barium meal upper GI in Trendelenburg position** *(Ref: Bailey 27/e p1084)*

Barium Studies in Hiatal Hernia

- To facilitate visualization of the **hernia**, the **patient** may **be placed** in a **Trendelenburg position** during studies of **barium swallowing**[Q].

21. **Ans. c. Include only the anterior stomach wall in the wrap** *(Ref: www.ncbi.nlm.nih.gov/pubmed/8313128)*

Nissen's fundoplication	• **Left crus approach** to a **360-degree wrap** (**Nissen fundoplication**), which is the **procedure of choice** for **GERD**. • **Left crus approach: Direct** and **early view** of the **short gastric vessels** and **spleen**[Q].
Rosetti and **Hell modification** of Nissen's fundoplication	• Include **only anterior stomach wall in** the **wrap**[Q]. • The idea was to reduce dissection in the vicinity of vagus nerve.

22. **Ans. a. Hiatus hernia**
23. **None:** *(Ref: Sabiston 20/e p1051-1053; Schwartz 10/e p980-984; Bailey 27/e p1083; Shackelford 7/e p237-239)*
24. **Ans. a. Hiatus hernia**
25. **Ans. b. Bochdalek hernia** *(Ref: Sabiston 20/e p1579; Schwartz 10/e p1604; Bailey 27/e p938)*

Presence of gastric air bubble or loops of bowel within the chest in newborns are suggestive of congenital diaphragmatic hernia (Bochdalek hernia).

REFLUX ESOPHAGITIS

26. **Ans. b. Protein** *(Ref: Shackelford 7/e p56)* 27. **Ans. b. Gastrin**
28. **Ans. c. 24-hours pH monitoring** *(Ref: Sabiston 20/e p1043-1048; Schwartz 10/e p964-980; Bailey 27/e p1077; Shackelford 7/e p174-180, 215-237)*
29. **Ans. c. Gastroesophageal reflux disease**
30. **Ans. a. Respiratory symptoms** *(Ref: Nelson 20/e p1791)*

Recurrent respiratory symptoms (Wheezing, stridor, chronic cough, apnea, aspiration) are the **earliest indicators** of pathological reflux **among the options provided**.

GERD in Infants

- **Most frequent complications** of **GERD** in **infants** are **failure to thrive** and **recurrent pulmonary symptoms**[Q].
- **Regurgitation alone does not indicate pathological reflux**.
- Presence of **upper GI bleed** is an **uncommon marker** for pathological reflux or esophagitis.
- Presence of **stricture esophagus** is an **uncommon** and **late complication** of untreated pathological GERD.
- **Recurrent pulmonary symptoms** are **frequent** and **early indicators** of **pathological GERD**[Q].

31. **Ans. d. 24-hours pH monitoring**
32. **Ans. b. Transient Les relaxation** *(Ref: Harrison 19/e p1906)*
    - Harrison says "**Transient LES relaxations account for** at least **90%** of **reflux** in **normal subjects** or **GERD patients** without hiatus hernia[Q]."
33. **Ans. a. Barium swallow**

- **IOC** for **anatomical disorders** of esophagus: **Barium swallow**[Q]
- **IOC** for **motility disorders** of esophagus: **Manometry**[Q]

34. **Ans. d. Pneumothorax** *(Ref: Shackelford 7/e p234)*

- **Pneumothorax** (1-5%) is usually **self-limited** but may cause immediate or delayed hemodynamic or respiratory consequences. It is **one of the most common complication** of Nissen's fundoplication.

Complications of Nissen's Fundoplications

Intraoperative
- Pneumothorax (MC)^Q
- Esophageal perforation
- Splenic injury
- Bleeding
- Missed visceral injury

Postoperative
- Slipped or misplaced fundoplication
- Dehiscence
- Transthoracic herniation
- Tight fundoplication

35. Ans. b. Watson is 90 degree posterior
36. Ans. a. Long intra-abdominal esophagus, b. Increased intra-abdominal pressure, c. Right crus of diaphragm
37. Ans. None
38. Ans. c. Theophylline
39. Ans. d. All of the above
40. Ans. None
41. Ans. d. All of the above
42. Ans. d. Esophageal reflux
43. Ans. a. Nissen's fundoplication *(Ref: Sabiston 20/e p1024; Schwartz 10/e p974-976; Bailey 27/e p1079-1080; Shackelford 7/e p237-239)*

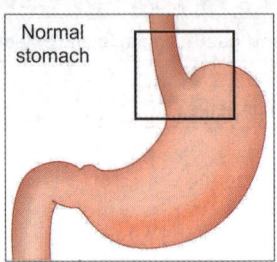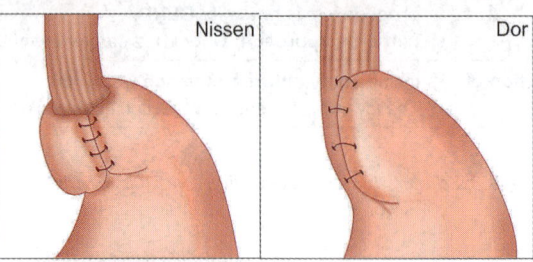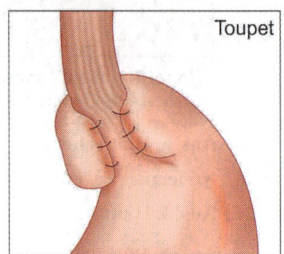

Types of Fundoplication

Type of Fundoplication	Degree of Wrap
Watson	• 90° **anterior** fundoplication^Q
Dor	• 180° **anterior** fundoplication^Q
Toupet	• 180° **posterior** fundoplication subsequently modified to a **270° wrap**^{Q}
Belsey Mark IV	• 270° **anterior** fundoplication^Q
Nissen's	• 360° fundoplication^Q

ACHALASIA CARDIA

44. Ans. b. Body peristalsis is normal *(Ref: Sabiston 20/e p1016-1019; Schwartz 10/e p990-992; Bailey 26/e p1014-1017; Shackelford 7/e p349-352, 354-361)*
45. Ans. d. Caused by selective loss of stimulatory myenteric neurons *(Ref: Sabiston 20/e p1017; Schwartz 10/e p990; Bailey 27/e p1095-1097)*
46. Ans. c. Segmental body peristalsis
47. Ans. d. Heller's cardiomyotomy
48. Ans. b. Achalasia cardia
49. Ans. a. Achalasia cardia
50. Ans. a. Nitrates, b. Ca^{2+} channel blockers, c. Botulinum toxin, d. Myotomy
51. Ans. a. Achalasia cardia
52. Ans. a. Myenteric plexus of Auerbach
53. Ans. a. Achalasia cardia *(Ref: Sabiston 20/e p1016-1019; Schwartz 10/e p1002; Bailey 27/e p1097)*

- Massive esophageal dilation, tortuosity, and a sigmoidal esophagus (megaesophagus) is seen in advanced stage^Q of achalasia cardia

54. Ans. a. Pressure at distal end increased with no peristalsis
55. Ans. a. Barium swallow
56. Ans. d. Botulinum toxin
57. Ans. d. Not a premalignant condition
58. Ans. c. Mecholyl test is hyposensitive *(Ref: www.hon.ch/OESO/free/Vol_4_Prim_Motility/.../ART295.HTML)*

MECHOLYL TEST

- **Mecholyl test** has been used as a means to **demonstrate** the **"denervation supersensitivity"** in patients with **achalasia**^{Q}.
- It has not been reported in patients with the hypertensive LES.

59. Ans. d. Exaggerated peristalsis
60. Ans. a. Volvulus, c. Achalasia

61. **Ans. b. Achalasia cardia** *(Ref: Sabiston 20/e p1016-1019; Schwartz 10/e p1017; Bailey 27/e p1097)*

Achalasia Cardia
Diagnosis
• Barium swallow
• **Dilated esophagus** with a **distal narrowing**^{Q}
• "**Bird's beak**", "**Pencil-tip**" or "**Rat's tail**" **appearance**^{Q}

62. **Ans. a. Most common in women**
63. **Ans. d. Not a premalignant condition**

ESOPHAGEAL MOTILITY DISORDERS

64. **Ans. d. Diffuse esophagus spasm** *(Ref: Sabiston 20/e p1015-1016; Schwartz 10/e p992; Bailey 27/e p1099; Shackelford 7/e p142-143)*

65. **Ans. c. Diffuse esophageal spasm** *(Ref: Sabiston 20/e p1015-1016; Schwartz 10/e p992; Bailey 27/e p1099; Shackelford 7/e p142-143)*

• **Corkscrew** or **rosary-bead** esophagus, **segmental spasm** or **pseudodiverticulosis** appearance^Q **is characteristic of diffuse esophageal spasm.**

66. **Ans. d. Scleroderma, e. Cricopharyngeal carcinoma** *(Ref: Bailey 27/e p1096; Sabiston 20/e p1015)*

Classification of Esophageal Motility Disorders	
Disorders of the **pharyngo-esophageal junction**	• **Neurological: Stroke, motor neuron disease, multiple sclerosis, Parkinson's disease** • **Myogenic: Myasthenia,** muscular dystrophy • Pharyngo-esophageal (**Zenker's**) diverticulum
Disorders of the **body** of the **esophagus**	• Diffuse esophageal spasm • Nutcracker esophagus
Autoimmune disorders- **Systemic sclerosis (CREST)**	• Reflux associated • Idiopathic
Allergic	• Eosinophilic esophagitis • Non-specific esophageal dysmotility
Disorders of the **lower esophageal sphincter**	• Achalasia • Incompetent lower sphincter (i.e. **GERD**)

67. **Ans. d. Achalasia cardia**

ZENKER'S DIVERTICULUM

68. **Ans. a. Barium swallow** *(Ref: Sabiston 20/e p1019-1020; Schwartz 10/e p989; Bailey 27/e p1101; Shackelford 7/e p336-346)*
69. **Ans. b. Zenker's diverticulum**
70. **Ans. b. Feeling of obstruction in esophagus**
71. **Ans. d. Out pouching of the anterior pharyngeal wall just above the cricopharyngeus muscle**
72. **Ans. b. Zenker's diverticulum**
73. **Ans. c. Zenker's diverticulum**
74. **Ans. c. Treatment is simple excision**
75. **Ans. c. Lung abscess**
76. **Ans. a. The two parts of inferior constrictor muscle of the pharynx**
77. **Ans. d. Zenker's diverticulum**
78. **Ans. a. Endoscopic stapling of septum** *(Ref: Sabiston 20/e p1020)*

• *"An alternative to open surgical repair is the endoscopic **Dohlman procedure**, which has become more popular. **Endoscopic division of the common wall between the esophagus and diverticulum** using a laser, electrocautery, or stapler device has been similarly successful. Because of the configuration of the inline stapling device, this approach has been advocated for larger diverticula."*
      —*Sabiston 20/e p1020*

ESOPHAGEAL DIVERTICULA

79. **Ans. d. Parabronchial diverticulum**

SCLERODERMA

80. **Ans. b. Esophageal atresia** *(Ref: Harrison 19/e p718)*

Crow–Fukase Syndrome
• The features of this syndrome are highlighted by an acronym: POEMS^Q • **POEMS**^{Q}: **P**olyneuropathy, **O**rganomegaly, **E**ndocrinopathy, **M**-protein, **S**kin changes.

81. Ans. b. Polyneuropathy, c. Endocrinopathy, d. M-protein
82. Ans. c. Lower third *(Ref: Harrison 19/e p2158; Schwartz 10/e p984-985)*
83. Ans. b. Scleroderma

PLUMMER–VINSON SYNDROME

84. Ans. a. Occurs in elderly males
85. Ans. c. Postcricoid webs
86. Ans. c. Achalasia cardia
87. Ans. a. Web present in lower part of esophagus

BARRETT'S ESOPHAGUS

88. Ans. a. Long esophageal segment involved, b. Metaplasia, c. Peptic ulcer, e. Leads to adenocarcinoma *(Ref: Sabiston 20/e p1050; Schwartz 10/e p967,969,979; Bailey 27/e p1081; Shackelford 7/e p285, 294)*
89. Ans. b. Columnar to squamous metaplasia *(Ref: Schwartz 10/e p967; Sabiston 20/e p1050; Bailey 27/e p1081)*
90. Ans. c. Barrett's esophagus *(Ref: Robbins 9/e p757, 758)*

- The histopathological image of esophagus is showing intestinal type epithelium with goblet cells, typical of Barrett's esophagus.

91. Ans. a. Endoscopic biopsy every 2 years
92. Ans. a. Lower esophagus lined by columnar epithelium
93. Ans. b. Intestinal metaplasia
94. Ans. a. Stricture, c. Peptic ulcer
95. Ans. b. Premalignant condition
96. Ans. c. Barrett's esophagus *(Ref: Sabiston 20/e p1050; Schwartz 10/e p967; Bailey 27/e p1081; Shackelford 7/e p285, 294)*

CARCINOMA ESOPHAGUS PREDISPOSING FACTORS

97. Ans. d. Ectodermal dysplasia *(Ref: Sabiston 20/e p1027-1028; Schwartz 10/e p1003-1014; Bailey 27/e p1085; Shackelford 7/e p375-380)*
98. Ans. b. Barrett's esophagus
99. Ans. a. Tylosis, b. Plummer-Vinson syndrome, c. Barrett's esophagus, d. Achalasia cardia, e. Scleroderma
100. Ans. a. Tobacco/Alcohol, b. Alkalies
101. Ans. c. Mediastinal fibrosis
102. Ans. a. Barrett's esophagus
103. Ans. None
104. Ans. c. Mediastinal fibrosis
105. Ans. a. Barrett's esophagus

CA ESOPHAGUS CLINICAL FEATURES, DIAGNOSIS AND TREATMENT

106. Ans. a. TNM stage *(Ref: Sabiston 20/e p1027-1032; Schwartz 10/e p1003-1014; Bailey 27/e p1088; Shackelford 7/e p416-434)*

Long-term survival following esophagectomy depends on a number of factors such as the **depth of tumor invasion (T)**, the **number of involved lymph nodes (N)**, and on the **location** of the tumor in the esophagus.

107. Ans. a. Polypoidal *(Ref: Sabiston 20/e p1038)*

CARCINOMA ESOPHAGUS

- The **5-year survival rate** varies but can be as **good** as **70% with polypoid lesions** and as poor as 15% with advanced tumors.

108. Ans. c. GE junction tumors *(Ref: Shackelford 7/e p397)*

Siewert Classification GE Junction Tumors	
Type I	Cancer associated with Barrett's esophagus or true esophageal carcinoma **growing down** to the **GE junction**
Type II	Tumor at the **true junction** (within 2 cm of the squamocolumnar junction)
Type III	Tumors of the **subcardial region**

109. Ans. c. Hyperechogenic *(Ref: Shackelford 7/e p420-421)*

Features of Malignant Lymph Nodes on EUS	
Echo-poor (**hypoechoic**) structure	Sharply demarcated borders
Rounded contour	Size >1 cm

110. Ans. a. 5-FU + Cisplatin
111. Ans. a. EMR *(Ref: Shackelford 7/e p438-448)*

Palliation Therapy in Carcinoma Esophagus	
Laser Therapy	Radiation Therapy
Photodynamic Therapy	SEMS

112. **Ans. a. EUS**
113. **Ans. b. Middle 1/3rd** *(Ref: Shackelford 7/e p417)*

   - MC site of SCC of esophagus: **Middle 1/3rd**[Q]
   - MC site of adenocarcinoma of esophagus: **Lower 1/3rd**[Q]
   - MC site of carcinoma esophagus: **Middle 1/3rd (overall)**[Q]

114. **Ans. b. Pencil tip appearance** *(Ref: Surgical radiology Clinical Cases by Prabhakar Fajiah (2007)/113)*

Features of CA Esophagus on Barium Swallow	
• **Mucosal irregularity** and **shouldering**[Q]	• **Annular stricture**[Q]
• **Narrowing**[Q] of the lumen	• **Sharp** and **clear cut edge** of **filling defect**[Q]
• Irregular **"rat-tail" filling defect**[Q] of the distal esophagus with **shouldered edge**[Q]	• **Proximal dilatation**[Q] of the esophagus

   - **"Bird's beak"**, **"Pencil-tip"** or **"Rat's tail" appearance** is seen **in Achalasia**[Q].

115. **Ans. c. Apple core appearance** *(Ref: Sabiston 20/e p1028)*
   - Barium swallow: First investigation done[Q] in suspected case of Carcinoma esophagus (classic finding of an apple core lesion[Q]).

116. **Ans. a. Middle 1/3rd**
117. **Ans. b. Middle 1/3rd**
118. **Ans. a. Barium studies** *(Ref: Sabiston 20/e p1028; Schwartz 10/e p1003-1014; Bailey 27/e p1088; Shackelford 7/e p420)*

   ### Carcinoma Esophagus

   - **Barium swallow** is the **first investigation** for **an esophageal disease**[Q] presenting with dysphagia (it can show irregular filling defect with or without proximal dilatation, annular lesion appear as constricting bands)

Barium Swallow
• A **barium swallow** is **recommended for any patient** presenting **with dysphagia**.
• The **esophagram gives** an **overview of anatomy** and **function**[Q].
• It is **able to differentiate intraluminal from intramural lesions** and to **discriminate between intrinsic** (from a mass protruding into the lumen) **and extrinsic** (from compression of a structures outside the esophagus) **compression**.
• The **classic finding** of an **apple-core lesion** in patients with **esophageal cancer** is recognized easily[Q]

   - **Endoscopy and biopsy** is the **investigation of choice** for **CA esophagus**[Q].
   - For **adequate assessment, both barium swallow** and **endoscopy are required**[Q].

119. **Ans. a. Esophagectomy**
120. **Ans. a. Depth of tumor**
121. **Ans. b. Barium swallow + endoscopy**
122. **Ans. b. Chest pain** *(Ref: Sabiston 20/e p1040; Schwartz 10/e p1008; Bailey 27/e p1094; Shackelford 7/e p439-442)*

   ### Self-Expanding Metallic Stents (SEMS) in Malignant Tracheoesophageal Fistula

   - **SEMS** are relatively easy to insert under fluroscopic guidance with a technical **success rate** of **95%** and **efficacy** of **85-100%** in relieving dysphagia.

     - The **duration of response** is **5-6 months**[Q] and **complications** occur in **10-15%** patients.
     - MC complication of SEMS insertion: Chest pain or odynophagia (13%) > Tumor ingrowth overgrowth (10%) > Stent migration (9%) > Severe reflux (8%)
     - The use of stents coated with **silicone or polyurethane** may prevent or delay tumor ingrowth and subsequent esophageal obstruction.
     - **Coated stents** have been used with good success (>90%) for the treatment of **tracheoesophageal fistula**[Q].

   - Tumor ingrowth may be addressed by insertion of **another stent** or by **tumor ablation.**
   - Placement of stents through proximally located tumors, especially those near the **cricopharyngeus**, is often **not well tolerated.**
   - Stents placed **across GE junction** have a greater tendency to **migrate** and may result in **symptomatic acid reflux**[Q].
   - Fixed diameter **plastic endoluminal prostheses**, associated with **significant morbidity and mortality** and **low rate of dysphagia relief**, have largely been **abandoned**[Q].

123. **Ans. b. Carcinoma esophagus** *(Ref: Sabiston 20/e p1028; Schwartz 10/e p1005; Bailey 27/e p1088)*
124. **Ans. b. EUS** *(Ref: Sabiston 20/e p1028, 1031; Schwartz 10/e p1003-1014; Bailey 27/e p1090; Shackelford 7/e p420-421)*

Carcinoma Esophagus

- EUS is superior to CT or PET for assessment of both T and N stage.
- **Endoscopic ultrasound** (EUS) is the **best diagnostic tool** available to **assess the locoregional extent of disease (T and N Staging)**[Q]
- The **depth of tumor penetration** of the esophageal wall and the **presence of lymph node involvement** can be **assessed with an ultrasound probe** attached to the tip of a flexible endoscope[Q].
- CT is generally **considered** to be **less accurate in determining lymph node involvement than** other modalities such as EUS[Q].

125. Ans. c. Endoprosthesis
126. Ans. b. Middle third
127. Ans. a. MC in middle 1/3rd, b. Adenocarcinoma is common variety, c. Carcinoma develops at the achalasia segment, d. Smoking is a risk factor, e. Endoscopy is the investigation of choice
128. Ans. d. Chemoradiation followed by palliative enbloc resection
129. Ans. b. Radiotherapy
130. Ans. a. Abdomen-Neck *(Ref: Sabiston 20/e p1035; Schwartz 10/e p1009-1012, 1011-1012; Shackelford 7/e p429-430)*

Orringer Transhiatal Esophagectomy

- **Double incision: Midline laparotomy** followed by **cervical incision**[Q]
- **Cervical anastomosis** is done[Q]
- **MC procedure done** for carcinoma esophagus[Q]

131. Ans. b. Both adeno and squamous cell carcinoma occur
132. Ans. b. Endoscopic ultrasound
133. Ans. b. Transesophageal USG
134. Ans. None
135. Ans. a. Gastrostomy for palliation

- A **gastric pull-up in** the **posterior mediastinal position** has the **best functional result,** and every effort is made to **preserve and use this successful combination**.

136. Ans. a. Cisplatin
137. Ans. c. T stage
138. Ans. b. Common in middle third of esophagus, c. Stomach, jejunum or colon can be used for replacement after surgical removal, d. Chemoradiation has little role in inoperable patients

ESOPHAGECTOMY

139. Ans. a. Right gastric and right gastroepiploic artery *(Ref: Sabiston 20/e p1035-1036; Schwartz 10/e p1009; Bailey 27/e p1092; Shackelford 7/e p518-520)*
140. Ans. a. Stomach
141. Ans. c. Torek *(Ref: Shackelford 7/e p416)*

- **First successful esophagectomy** was done **by Torek.**

142. Ans. b. Middle 1/3rd *(Ref: Sabiston 20/e p1035-1036; Schwartz 10/e p1009; Bailey 27/e p1092; Shackelford 7/e p427-430)*

Tumor Margin for Curative Excision

- In GI malignancies (stomach[Q], small intestine[Q], colon[Q] and proximal rectum[Q]), tumor margin for curative excision is 5cm[Q] except:
  - Esophagus: 10 cm[Q]
  - Distal rectum: 2 cm[Q]

143. Ans. a. Transhiatal
144. Ans. b. Anastomotic leak *(Ref: Sabiston 20/e p1035-1036; Schwartz 10/e p1009; Shackelford 7/e p538-545)*

Anastomotic leak following **Ivor Lewis esophagectomy** is a **feared complication** that in the past was associated with a **50% mortality rate**. The **anastomosis is intrathoracic,** leak cause **severe mediastinitis**.

Complications of Esophagectomy	
• Anastomotic Leak (MC)[Q]	• Recurrent laryngeal nerve palsy
• Anastomotic stricture	• Chylothorax
• Pulmonary complications	

Esophagus

ANASTOMOTIC LEAK AFTER ESOPHAGECTOMY

- **Incidence of anastomotic leak** is **higher** following **cervical anastomosis (10-15%)** than intrathoracic anastomosis (5-10%).
- Although **leak** is **more common** following **cervical anastomosis**, it is **rarely life-threatening**[Q].
- **Anastomotic leak** following **Ivor Lewis esophagectomy** is a **feared complication** that in the past was associated with a **50% mortality rate**[Q].
- **Confirmation** is usually possible by **Gastrografin swallow**[Q] or **instillation of contrast** through the nasogastric tube.
- **Immediate intervention** is required, and attempts at **direct repair with muscle flap reinforcement** and **wide drainage** are often successful[Q].
- Patients who are **unstable** or **severely ill** should be **diverted with a spit fistula**, and either excluded at the hiatus, or have the conduit closed and returned to the abdomen[Q].
- **Pulmonary complications** are the **MC cause** of **postoperative morbidity** and **mortality** in **transhiatal esophagectomy**[Q]

145. Ans. b. Transhiatal esophagectomy
146. Ans. a. Stomach
147. Ans. a. Right gastroepiploic artery, b. Right gastric artery

LEIOMYOMA

148. Ans. a. Leiomyoma *(Ref: Sabiston 20/e p1032; Schwartz 10/e p1216; Bailey 27/e p1084; Shackelford 7/e p465-469)*
149. Ans. c. Leiomyoma *(Ref: Sabiston 20/e p1032; Schwartz 10/e p1017; Bailey 27/e p1085)*
    - **Barium swallow** is **IOC** for leiomyoma (**classical, smooth, contoured, punched-out defect**)[Q]
150. Ans. c. Perforation

DYSPHAGIA

151. Ans. b. Reflux esophagitis, d. Pharyngeal diverticulum, e. Diffuse esophageal spasm *(Ref: Sabiston 20/e p1049; Schwartz 10/e p625)*

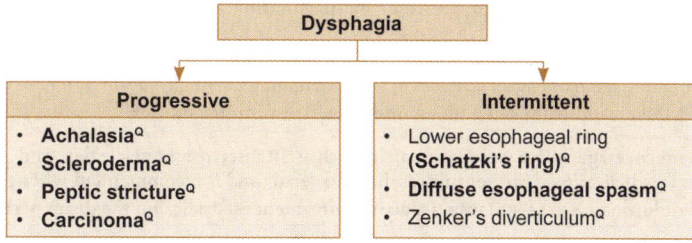

152. Ans. a. CXR, b. Ba swallow, c. Endoscopy, d. USG, e. C.T. Scan
    The clinical history is suggestive of carcinoma esophagus. All of the given investigations are used for the complete work-up.
153. Ans. b. Endoscopy
154. Ans. b. Herpes esophagitis, c. Monilial esophagitis *(Ref: Harrison 19/e p1901, 1909; Bailey 27/e p1103)*
    If **odynophagia** is present, **candidial (monilial)** or **herpes esophagitis** or **pill induced esophagitis** should be suspected.

ODYNOPHAGIA

- Odynophagia means **painful swallowing** seen in **inflammatory lesions** of food passage (i.e. **oral cavity, pharynx** and **esophagus**)
- Causes:
    - **Candidial (monilial)** esophagitis[Q]
    - **Herpes** esophagitis[Q]
    - **Pill induced** esophagitis[Q]

155. Ans. c. Achalasia cardia
    Presence of dysphagia to both solids and liquids suggests the diagnosis of achalasia.

DYSPHAGIA LUSORIA

156. Ans. a. Abnormal elongation of arch of aorta *(Ref: Sabiston 20/e p1610; Bailey 27/e p1105)*

Causes of Dysphagia Lusoria	
• Abnormal right subclavian artery[Q] (MC) • Right aortic arch[Q] • Double aortic arch[Q] • Abnormal innominate artery[Q]	• **Vascular ring (constriction)** formed by a **PDA** or a **ligamentum arteriosum** and the **pulmonary artery** or **aortic arch**[Q].

157. Ans. d. Compression by aberrant blood vessel *(Ref: Sabiston 20/e p1581; Bailey 27/e p1105)*

158. Ans. d. Acquired in later life *(Ref: Sabiston 20/e p1581)*

Dysphagia lusoria is a **disorder of swallowing** caused **due to vascular anomalies**^{Q} (**developmental** or **congenital abnormalities**).

ESOPHAGEAL PERFORATION AND INJURY

159. Ans. a. Vomiting, b. Subcutaneous emphysema, c. Lower thoracic pain *(Ref: Sabiston 20/e p1025-1026; Schwartz 10/e p1018; Bailey 27/e p1073; Shackelford 7/e p478-484)*

160. Ans. a. MC at lower 1/3rd, c. Acute chest pain, d. Surgically treated

161. Ans. a. Barium swallow is diagnostic, b. Treatment is primary repair, c. MC after penetrating injury, d. Mortality increased if repaired after 24 hours

162. Ans. c. Present with acute chest pain, d. Treatment is surgical

163. Ans. b. Cervical portion *(Ref: Sabiston 20/e p1025-1026; Schwartz 10/e p1018; Bailey 27/e p1073; Shackelford 7/e p478-479)*

Esophageal Perforation	
Iatrogenic	**Spontaneous**
• Most common type^Q • Caused by endoscopy^Q • MC site is cervical esophagus (cricopharyngeal area)^Q	• Esophageal rupture after vomiting • MC site: left posterolateral side of the distal esophagus^Q

164. Ans. c. Instrumentation

165. Ans. d. Esophagectomy with bringing proximal end as fistula in neck

166. Ans. a. Primary closure, drainage and antibiotics

167. Ans. b. Stomach *(Ref: Shackelford 7/e p483)*

> **OPERATIVE REPAIR OF ESOPHAGEAL PERFORATION**
>
> - The principles of repair comprise a **clear exposure of** the **perforation** and **debridement** of devitalized tissue, followed by a **primary closure**.
> - Following **debridement** of devitalized tissue, **primary mucosal repair** should then be **performed with interrupted, absorbable suture**, taking care to minimize esophageal stricturing while obtaining adequate suture purchase on vital tissue.
> - The **muscular layer** is then reapproximated with an **interrupted** or **running suture**^{Q}.
>   - Subsequent coverage with a **vascular pedicle**, such as an **intercostal muscle flap**, and **pleural, pericardial,** or **omental pedicle** allows further **buttressing** of a repair and is **recommended whenever feasible**^{Q}.
>   - **Gastric fundus** may also be **suitable tissue reinforcement** especially **for** the distal **perforation**^{Q}.
> - Depending on the site of perforation, any of the antireflux procedures (**Belsey Mark IV, Nissen, Dor, Toupet**) may be used to **buttress the repair**.

168. Ans. b. Bradycardia

169. Ans. c. Spontaneous perforation

170. Ans. d. Boerhaave's syndrome

171. Ans. a. Boerhaave's syndrome

172. Ans. b. Lower posterior

173. Ans. b. Cardioesophageal junction

174. Ans. d. Water soluble low molecular weight contrast swallow

175. Ans. a. May present with peritonitis *(Ref: Sabiston 20/e p1025; Schwartz 10/e p1018; Bailey 27/e p1072)*

176. Ans. d. Hypaque *(Ref: Diseases of the Esophagus By G. Vantrappen, J. Hellemans (2012)/p135)*

> "*Iodinated Contrast* Materials Water-soluble iodinated *contrast* media can be used to visualize the upper gastrointestinal tract. These *contrast* materials are considered *safer* than barium sulfate in patients with *esophageal perforation* or communication between esophagus and airways and when there is a risk of aspiration into the bronchi. *They are also used for the examination of the esophagus in the early postoperative period following esophageal surgery or correction of hiatal hernia. The demonstartion of leak is a contraindication for the withdrawal of the postoperative gastric tube. The most commonly used iodinated water-soluble contrast media are Gastrograffin and Hypaque.*"- *Diseases of the Esophagus By G. Vantrappen, J. Hellemans (2012)/p135*

177. Ans. a. Morbidity is mainly due to mediastinal infection, b. Partial tear involving mucosa should be managed conservatively, e. Serum amylase levels may be high as a result of absorption of amylase from the pleural cavity

TRACHEOESOPHAGEAL FISTULA

178. Ans. d. CVS *(Ref: Sabiston 20/e p1866-1868; Schwartz 10/e p608-609; Bailey 27/e p133; Shackelford 7/e p509-515)*

179. Ans. c. Esophageal atresia with distal tracheoesophageal fistula

180. Ans. d. TEF without esophageal atresia *(Ref: Sabiston 20/e p1867; Schwartz 10/e p1609; Bailey 27/e p133)*

 Type of tracheoesophageal fistula (TEF) seen on barium swallow is H type (TEF without esophageal atresia).

181. Ans. c. Stenting
182. Ans. a. Expandable metal stent, b. Surgery with graft, c. Gastrostomy tube *(Ref: CSDT 11/e p1314; Bailey 27/e p1095)*

MALIGNANT TRACHEOESOPHAGEAL FISTULA

- It is a **sign of incurable esophageal carcinoma**^Q
- Some have advocated **surgical bypass** and **esophageal exclusion**, but this is a major procedure
- **Self expanding metallic stent** is the **best treatment**^Q
- Semi-rigid **prosthetic tubings** may be used (**Gastrostomy tube**)^Q

183. Ans. b. Tracheoesophageal fistula
184. Ans. b. Major cardiac anomaly

ESOPHAGEAL RINGS AND WEBS

185. Ans. a. Mucosal ring at squamocolumnar junction, c. Dysphagia is the symptom *(Ref: Sabiston 20/e p1026-1027; Schwartz 10/e p984; Bailey 27/e p1102; Shackelford 7/e p89-90)*
186. Ans. c. Schatzki ring *(Ref: Sabiston 20/e p1027; Schwartz 10/e p984; Bailey 27/e p1102)*
187. Ans. b. Lower esophagus
188. Ans. c. Involves mucosa, submucosa and muscularis
189. Ans. b. Located at lower esophagus, c. Causes dysphagia
190. Ans. b. Occurs at GE junction *(Ref: Gastroenterol Hepatol (NY); 2010 November 6 (11): 701-704)*

Types of Esophageal Ring on Barium Examination	
Type A	Located **few cm proximal to GE junction**
Type B	**Schatzki's ring: MC esophageal ring** found on esophagogram, **at GE junction**^Q
Type C	Located at **most distal portion of esophagus**, formed by diaphragmatic crural pressure

191. Ans. b. Schatzki ring *(Ref: Sabiston 20/e p1026; Schwartz 10/e p984; Bailey 27/e p1102; Shackelford 7/e p89-90)*

FOREIGN BODY

192. Ans. d. Above the cricopharynx *(Ref: Schwartz 9/e p2378; Dhingra 4/e p64)*

 The first constriction where the esophagus commences is at the **cricopharyngeal sphincter**: This is the **narrowest portion of the esophagus** and is the **most common site of foreign body**.

193. Ans. a. Esophagus

 "Coins in the esophagus are round in appearance on the frontal view whereas coins in the trachea are usually seen on end and are linear in shape."

Foreign Body	
• Coins account for 70% of pediatric ingested foreign bodies	
• Coins will typically become 'stuck' at the level of the cricopharyngeus muscle.	
Coin	**Chest X-ray Anteroposterior (AP) View**
In trachea	• Visualized in the **sagittal plane**^Q (acquired while entering through vocal cords)
In esophagus	• Visualized in **coronal orientation**^Q

ESOPHAGUS: ANATOMY AND PHYSIOLOGY

194. Ans. d. Lower esophagus before entering the diaphragm is anterior and left sided *(Ref: Sabiston 20/e p1067; Schwartz 10/e p941-947; Shackelford 7/e p18-24)*

195. **Ans. c. Tertiary** *(Ref: Sabiston 20/e p1014-1015)*

TERTIARY CONTRACTIONS OF ESOPHAGUS
• Tertiary contractions are **simultaneous, non progressive, non peristaltic waves** that can occur **throughout the esophagus**[Q]
• Tertiary contractions represent **uncoordinated contractions** of the **smooth muscles** that are **responsible for** the **'Cork Screw' appearance** of **esophageal spasm** on Barium swallow
• Tertiary contractions do not have a physiological function and may be **observed in** the **elderly** and in patients with **esophageal motility disorders**[Q]

196. **Ans. c. 40 cm**

Esophageal Constrictions				
No.	Distance from incisor teeth	Bony level	Anatomical Landmark
1	15 cm[Q]	C6	Pharyngoesophageal junction (At beginning[Q])
2	25 cm[Q]		Aortic arch, left bronchus[Q]
3	40 cm[Q]	T10	Pierces diaphragm[Q]

BALD: Beginning, Aortic arch, Left Bronchus, Diaphragm[Q]

197. **Ans. b. Where it pierces the diaphragm**   198. **Ans. a. Left phrenic nerve**
199. **Ans. d. Left main stem bronchus**
200. **Ans. b. Bleeding from varices occurs from midesophagus**
   - **Bleeding from esophageal varices** most commonly occur in the **distal esophagus**[Q].
201. **Ans. a. 6–26 mm Hg** *(Ref: Sabiston 20/e p1016; Bailey 27/e p1068)*

   "The normal LOS is 3–4 cm long and has a pressure of 10–25 mm Hg."-Bailey 27/e p1068

202. **Ans. c. Transmural** *(Ref: Schwartz 10/e p1004)*

DIAPHRAGM

203. **Ans. b. Diaphragmatic palsy**
   - **Fluoroscopy** is used for **diagnosis of diaphragmatic palsy**[Q].
204. **Ans. a. Laparoscopy** *(Ref: Sabiston 20/e p432; Schwartz 10/e p202-203; Bailey 27/e p365)*
205. **Ans. d. Dorsal mesocardium** *(Ref: Langman 11/e p161)*

DEVELOPMENT OF DIAPHRAGM	
• Septum transversum → Central tendon[Q]	• Pleuroperitoneal membranes → Small intermediate muscular portion[Q]
• Mesentery of esophagus → Crura[Q]	• Body wall → Peripheral muscular diaphragm[Q]
• Cervical myotomes (muscular input)[Q]	

206. **Ans. b. Circumferential** *(Ref: Sabiston and Spencer's Surgery of Chest 8/e p chapter 7)*

Circumferential incision is generally taken for diaphragmatic surgery.

DIAPHRAGMATIC INCISIONS
• **Diaphragmatic incisions** can be divided into three groups: **circumferential, central tendon**, and **radial**.
1. **Circumferential incisions:**
– Circumferential incisions in the periphery result in little loss of function.
– Must be at least 5 cm lateral to the edge of the central tendon to avoid the posterolateral and anterolateral branches of the phrenic nerve.
– **Difficult to correctly realign after a long operation.**
– Placement of surgical clips on each side of the muscular incision can greatly facilitate the correct spatial orientation on closing.
2. **Incisions in the central tendon:**
– Do not interrupt any major branch of the nerve itself.
– **Provide excellent visualization of the abdomen from the thorax**, and vice versa.
– **Easy to open and to close.**

3. **Transverse radial incision:**
   - Made from the midaxillary line centrally
   - Relatively safe
   - **May result in segmental diaphragmatic paralysis** if the incision transects the crural or posterolateral branches of the phrenic nerve.

MISCELLANEOUS

207. Ans. b. 5
208. Ans. b. Achalasia cardia
209. Ans. b. Achalasia cardia
210. Ans. a. Pharyngeal pouch

- Second swallow is due to regurgitation of barium from pharyngeal pouch

211. Ans. d. Esophageal perforation *(Ref: Harrison 19/e p1720)*

HAMMAN'S SIGN OR HAMMAN'S CRUNCH

- A **crunching, rasping sound, synchronous with heartbeat, heard over the precordium** and sometimes at a distance from the chest in spontaneous mediastinal emphysema[Q].
- **Hamman's sign** may be present **in acute Mediastinitis** (as in **esophageal perforation**)[Q].

212. Ans. c. 50 *(Ref: Shackelford 7/e p545)*

- To restore **normal swallowing, stricture** should be **dilated** to **at least 16 mm** diameter or **50 French**.[Q]
- **Guidewire directed dilatation** of esophageal strictures is **normal practice** in **most units**[Q].

213. Ans. b. Guide wire directed stent
214. Ans. c. 50 cm *(Ref: Bailey 27/e p1136)*

- The **Roux loop** should be **at least 50 cm** long **to avoid bile reflux esophagitis**[Q]

215. Ans. a. Eosinophilic esophagitis *(Ref: Schwartz 10/e p986)*

"Eosinophilic esophagitis (EE): A barium swallow should be the first test obtained in the patient with dysphagia. EE has a characteristic finding often called the "ringed esophagus" or the "feline esophagus," as the esophageal rings are felt to look like the stripes on a housecat. The endoscopic appearance of EE is also characteristic, and also appears as a series of rings."-Schwartz 10/e p986

216. Ans. b. Dual probe pH monitoring *(Ref: Pediatric Otolaryngology (2014)/p1511)*
217. Ans. a. CMV esophagitis *(Ref: Harrison 20/e p2218)*

"CMV esophagitis occurs primarily in immunocompromised patients, particularly organ transplant recipients. CMV is usually activated from a latent stage. Endoscopically, CMV lesions appear as serpiginous ulcers in an otherwise normal mucosa, particularly in the distal esophagus."-Harrison 20/e p2218

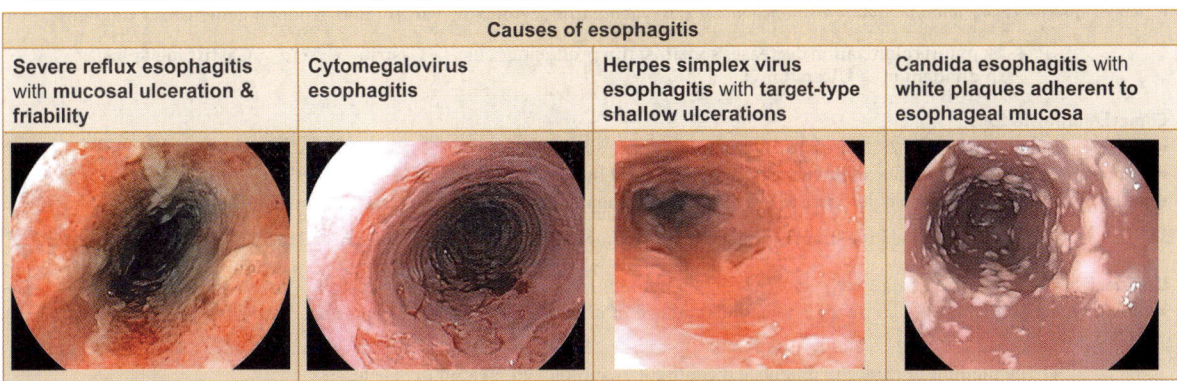

Causes of esophagitis: Severe reflux esophagitis with mucosal ulceration & friability; Cytomegalovirus esophagitis; Herpes simplex virus esophagitis with target-type shallow ulcerations; Candida esophagitis with white plaques adherent to esophageal mucosa

218. Ans. d. Herpes simplex esophagitis *(Ref: Harrison 20/e p2218)*

"Herpes simplex virus type 1 or 2 may cause esophagitis. Vesicles on the nose and lips may coexist and are suggestive of a herpetic etiology. Varicella-zoster virus can also cause esophagitis in children with chickenpox or adults with zoster. The characteristic endoscopic findings are vesicles and small, punched-out ulcerations."-Harrison 20/e p2218

CHAPTER 10

Stomach and Duodenum

HELICOBACTER PYLORI

HELICOBACTER PYLORI

- First successful culture of organism was done by **Marshall and Warren**[Q], who named it Campylobacter pyloridis.

  - Around **90%** of **duodenal ulcers** and **75%** of **gastric ulcer** are associated with **H. pylori infection**[Q].
  - **Gastric antrum** is MC site of colonization[Q].

- It can live only in **gastric epithelium**, because only gastric epithelium expresses specific adherence receptors in vivo that can be recognized by organism.

  - Also found in **heterotopic gastric mucosa** in **proximal esophagus, Barrett's esophagus,** gastric metaplasia in the **duodenum, Meckel's diverticulum,** and heterotopic gastric mucosa in the **rectum**[Q].

- After the person is infected, usually in **childhood,** it is probably for life because **spontaneous remission is rare**[Q].
- There tends to be **inverse relationship** between **infection** and **socioeconomic status**[Q].
- Mechanisms by which **H. pylori** promote ulcer formation include **stimulation** of **gastrin** release, **inhibition** of **somatostatin** release, interruption of inhibitory vagal reflexes and **inhibition** of gastroduodenal **bicarbonate** secretion[Q].
- After eradication of the organism, ulcer **recurrence is rare**[Q].

Characteristic Features

- **Spiral shaped, gram (-)ve rod, motile** with **lophotrichous flagella**[Q]
- The sole source is human gastric mucosa

  - Biochemical reactions: **Catalase, oxidase and urease positive**[Q]

- Grows well when incubated at **37°C in microaerophilic conditions**[Q].
- Media used include **Skirrow's medium, chocolate medium**[Q].

Pathogenesis

- Grows optimally at **pH 6.0-7.0**[Q] and would be killed at pH within the gastric lumen.
- But it survives as it is found deep in mucus layer near epithelial surface, without invading mucosa where physiologic pH is present. It produces **potent urease**, which **provides ammonia** to **buffer acid**[Q].
- Major diseases associated H. pylori virulence factors are **vacuolating cytotoxin (Vac A)**[Q], and group of genes called **CagPal**[Q].

  - H. pylori colonization decreases somatostatin producing cells →↑Gastrin →↑Acid → Gastric metaplasia in duodenum → Ulceration[Q].

Clinical Manifestations

- 90% of duodenal ulcer and **75%** of **gastric ulcer**[Q] are related to H. pylori
- **Increase risk of gastric adenocarcinoma, gastric MALT lymphoma**[Q].
- Extra-gastrointestinal pathologies that are linked include **ischemic heart disease** and **cerebrovascular disease**[Q].

  - **CAG-A positive strain** is **protective for adenocarcinoma** esophagus but **can lead to SCC** of esophagus[Q].

Diagnosis

- **Histologic visualization** of H. pylori is the **gold standard** of **diagnostic test**[Q] (special stains used are **silver, Giemsa, Genta or Warthin starry stain)**[Q].

  - The **method of choice to diagnose** if endoscope is employed is **rapid urease test**[Q].
  - **Serology** is the test of choice for **initial diagnosis** when endoscopy is not required.
  - After treatment, **Urea breath test** is the method of choice but should be performed **after 4 weeks** of therapy[Q].

Accuracy of Diagnostic Methods

- **Chronic inflammation** on a gastric mucosal **biopsy** specimen is **100% sensitive** test[Q].
- **Rapid Urease test** on a gastric mucosal biopsy specimen is **100% specific** test[Q].

PEPTIC ULCER

Gastric Ulcer	Duodenal Ulcer

• **Etiology:**
  – Atrophic gastritis
  – **H. pylori (75%)**[Q]
  – **Smoking, Alcohol**[Q]
  – **Lower socioeconomic status**[Q]
  – Altered mucosal barrier function (**NSAIDs**)[Q]
  – There is either **normochlorhydria** or **achlorhydria**[Q]
  – **Cirrhosis**[Q]
	• **Etiology:**
	  – **Stress, anxiety**: 'hurry, worry, curry'[Q]
	  – **H. pylori (90%)**[Q]
	  – **NSAIDs, steroids**[Q]
	  – Blood group **O+ve**[Q]
	  – **Endocrine: Zollinger-Ellison syndrome, MEN-1, Cushing's syndrome, hyperparathyroidism**[Q]
	  – Alcohol, smoking, vitamin deficiency[Q]
	  – Chronic pancreatitis, Cirrhosis[Q]

• **MC Site:**
  – **Lesser curvature** along the **incisura angularis (Type 1)**[Q]
	• **MC site:**
	  – **1st part** of duodenum (**overall MC site** for peptic ulcer)[Q]

• **Clinical features:**
  – **Equal** in both sexes
  – **Pain** in the **epigastrium after** taking **food**[Q]; relieved by vomiting
  – Pain is uncommon during night
  – **Hematemesis** common
  – Appetite good, but **hesitant to eat** as eating leads to pain that results in **loss of weight**[Q]
	• **Clinical features:**
	  – More common in **males**[Q]
	  – **Pain** in early morning, decreases after food (**hunger pain**[Q])
	  – Pain **common during night**[Q]
	  – **Melena** common
	  – **Appetite good**, eats more frequently and there is **weight gain**[Q]

• **Features on Barium meal:**
  – **Niche** on **lesser curve** with **notch** on **greater curve**[Q]
  – Regular/round margin of ulcer create **spoke wheel pattern**[Q]
  – **Overhanging mucosa** at the margins of a benign gastric ulcer projects inwards, towards the ulcer: **Hampton's line**[Q]
  – Converging mucosal folds at the **base of the ulcer**[Q]
	• **Features on Barium meal:**
	  – **Deformed** or **absent duodenal cap** (because of spasm)[Q]
	  – Appearance of **trifoliate duodenum** due to **secondary duodenal diverticula**[Q]

• **Complications:**
  – **Perforation: MC complication** of gastric ulcer (Into **lesser sac**)[Q]
  – **Hour glass contracture:** Exclusively in women due to **cicatricial contracture** of **lesser curve ulcer**[Q]
  – **Tea pot stomach (hand bag stomach):** Cicatrisation and shortening of the lesser curvature[Q]
  – **Malignant transformation**[Q]
	• **Complications:**
	  – **Bleeding: MC complication**, on **posterior wall**, **gastroduodenal artery**[Q] is most commonly involved
	  – **Perforation:** More on **anterior wall,** if posterior, into pancreas
	  – **Gastric outlet obstruction** due to **pyloric stenosis**- least common[Q]
	  – Duodenal ulcers are **benign (No malignant transformation)**[Q]

TYPES OF GASTRIC ULCER

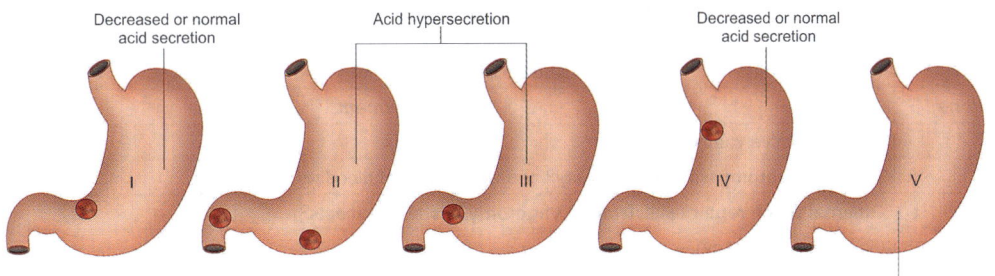

Modified Johnson's Classification of Gastric Ulcer		
Type	Location	Acid Secretion
I	Lesser curvature, near incisura angularis (**MC**)[Q]	Low
II	Body of the **stomach** and **duodenum**[Q]	High[Q]
III	**Prepyloric**[Q] (within 2-3 cm of the pylorus)	High[Q]
IV	High on the **lesser curve**, near **GE junction**[Q]	Low
V	Anywhere, induced by medication (NSAIDs)	Low

Gastric Ulcer	
Benign Ulcer	**Malignant Ulcer**
• Generally at **lesser curvature**[Q] • **Smooth radiating folds**[Q] with **Hampton line and collar**[Q] • **Overhanging margins**[Q] showing regeneration • **Mucosal rugae projects outwards** from the **margins of ulcer**[Q] • **Penetrating sign** (ulcer crater projects into stomach wall rather than into a mass in a stomach wall). • Huge base[Q] • Preserved peristalsis[Q] • Heals within 8-10 weeks[Q]	• At **greater curvature**[Q] • Interrupted **nodular, clubbed folds** with **Lasman Kirklin complex**[Q] (malignant ulcer with no mass) • **Eccentric** with **heaped up** and **everted margins**[Q] • **Mucosal rugae stop far** of the ulcer[Q] • **Carman's meniscus sign** (meniscoid appearance of trapped barium in ulcer bed) • Necrotic base[Q] • No peristalsis[Q] • No healing[Q]

GASTRIC ULCER ON DOUBLE CONTRAST UPPER GI SERIES

Benign Ulcer:
- In benign gastric ulcer, **mucosal folds radiate from crater** in sponge like manner[Q].
- Typically **benign ulcer craters** extend **beyond** the **luminal margin** of the stomach and have **radiating gastric folds**, **ulcer mound** due to mucosal edema, **ulcer collar**[Q] (a lucent ring that separates ulcer crater from gastric mucosa), **Hampton's line** and **Penetrating sign**[Q] (ulcer crater projects into stomach wall rather than into a mass in a stomach wall).

Malignant Ulcer:
- In **malignant ulcers**, **gastric folds** are **amputated** or **clubbed** and do **not reach** the **edge** of ulcer crater have **parallel gastric folds**.
- Malignant ulcers are characterized by **Carman's meniscus sign**[Q] (meniscoid appearance of trapped barium in ulcer bed), **intraluminal crater**[Q] (crater erodes into the mass within the gastric cavity) and **Kirklin complex**[Q] (heaped up margins touching bed causes lucent rim around ulcer on barium meal).

COMPLICATIONS OF PEPTIC ULCER

Complications of Peptic Ulcer
• **Intractability** (Non-healing)
• **Bleeding**: MC complication of peptic ulcer[Q]
• **Perforation**: MC complication of gastric ulcer[Q]
• **Gastric outlet obstruction** (Rare)

Duodenal Ulcer	
Complications	*Treatment*
Intractable	Highly selective vagotomy[Q]
Bleeding	**Truncal vagotomy** with **pyloroplasty**[Q] and oversewing of bleeding vessel
Perforated	**Omental patch repair** (with **Truncal vagotomy** in **stable patients**[Q])
Obstruction	(Rule out malignancy) • **Truncal vagotomy** with **antrectomy** is **ideal procedure**[Q] • **Truncal vagotomy** with **gastrojejunostomy** in cases of **inflammation** and **scarring** of duodenal bulb[Q]

GASTRIC OUTLET OBSTRUCTION

GASTRIC OUTLET OBSTRUCTION

- MC cause of **gastric outlet obstruction**: **CA stomach**[Q]
- **Site of stenosis** or **obstruction** in peptic ulcer disease: **1st** part of the **duodenum**[Q]
- **More common** with **duodenal ulcer** and **type III gastric ulcer** and requires that malignancy should be ruled out.

Stomach and Duodenum

Clinical Features:
- Symptoms of gastric retention, including **early satiety**, **bloating**, indigestion, anorexia, nausea, **vomiting**, epigastric pain, and **weight loss**.
- Patients are frequently **malnourished** and **dehydrated** and have a **metabolic alkalosis**, factors that increase operative risk.

Diagnosis:
- A **saline load test** is helpful, it is performed by emptying the stomach with a nasogastric tube and instilling **750 mL** of saline, the patient is placed in **sitting position**, and **30 minutes** later the nasogastric tube is aspirated, normally **< 400 mL** should remain in the stomach, and 90% of subjects have a residue of less than 200 mL.
- The finding of **> 400 mL** residual saline is consistent with a **diagnosis** of **gastric outlet obstruction**.

Treatment:
- **Surgery** is generally indicated if the obstruction fails to resolve despite **48–72 hours** of adequate **IV fluid replenishment**, **antisecretory therapy** and **nasogastric decompression**[Q].

  - **Truncal vagotomy** and **antrectomy**[Q] is the **ideal procedure**.

- The **inflammation** and **scarring** at **duodenal bulb** or **previous proximal duodenal surgeries** prevents safe performance of an antrectomy, in this setting **truncal vagotomy** with **drainage (Gastrojejunostomy)** is the preferred approach[Q].

TYPES OF VAGOTOMY

Types of Vagotomy		
Highly Selective Vagotomy	**Vagotomy and Drainage**	**Vagotomy and Antrectomy**
• **Procedure of choice** for **chronic** or **intractable** duodenal **ulcers**[Q] • **Nerves of Latarjet** supplying the **antrum** are **preserved**[Q] (and hence gastric motility) • **Drainage procedure** is **not required**[Q] • **Lowest mortality rate** and **side effects**[Q] • **Minimal chances** of **dumping syndrome** and **gastric atony**[Q] • Relatively **high recurrence**[Q]	• **TV** is performed by **division** of **left** and **right vagus nerves above** the **hepatic** and **celiac branches**[Q] just above the GE junction. • **MC operation performed** for **duodenal ulcer**[Q] • **Intermediate morbidity** and **recurrence rate**[Q]	• **Procedure of choice** for **recurrent** duodenal **ulcers**[Q] • **Lowest recurrence rate**[Q] • **High mortality and morbidity**[Q]

OPERATIONS FOR GASTRIC ULCER

Operations for Gastric Ulcer	
Billroth-I Gastrectomy	**Billroth-II Gastrectomy**
• **Gastroduodenostomy**[Q] • Performed when there is a **sufficient portion** of **upper duodenum remaining**[Q] • **Remaining portion of stomach** is **reattached to the duodenum**[Q]	• **Loop gastrojejunostomy**[Q] • Performed if the **stomach cannot be reattached** to **duodenum**[Q] • **Remaining portion of duodenum** is **sealed off**, a **hole is cut into** the **jejunum & stomach is reattached**[Q] at this hole.

Billroth I (Gastroduodenal) anastomosis | Billroth II Gastrectomy (Loop Gastrojejunostomy) | Roux-en-Y Gastrojejunostomy

Polya Gastrectomy

- A type of **posterior gastroenterostomy** which is a **modification of Billroth II operation**.
- **Resection of 2/3** of the **stomach with blind closure** of the **duodenal stump** and **retrocolic anastomosis** of the **full circumference** of the **open stomach to jejunum**^{Q}.

Elective Gastric Ulcer Operations	
Type	**Procedure**
Type I	• **Distal gastrectomy** with Billroth I or II reconstruction^Q
Type II and III	• **Truncal vagotomy** plus **antrectomy**^{Q}
Type IV	• **Schoemaker** procedure^Q • **Pouchet** procedure^Q • **Kelling-Madlener** procedure (For **unstable** patients^Q) • **Csendes** procedure (For **stable** patients^Q)

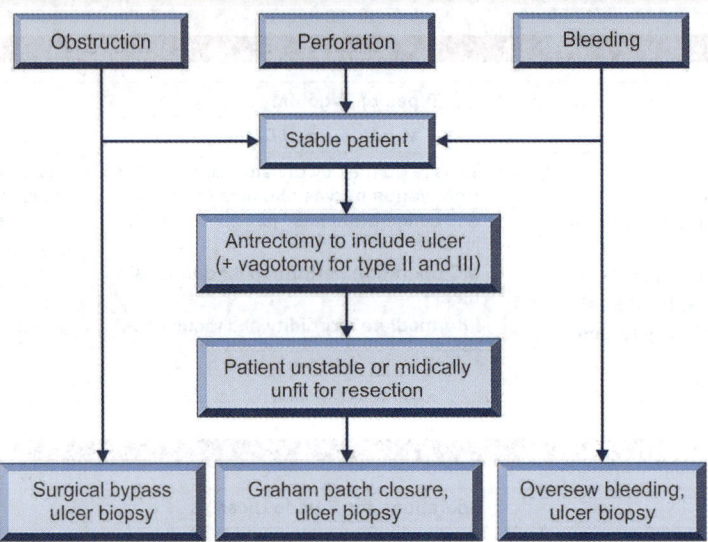

Remember:
- **Benign BPH:** (Benign ulcer- Penetrating sign and Hampton's hump)
- **Malignant CIK:** (Carman's meniscus sign, Intraluminal crater, Kirklin complex)

COMPLICATIONS AFTER GASTRECTOMY

Postgastrectomy/Vagotomy Syndrome

Secondary to Gastric Resection	Secondary to Gastric Reconstruction	Postvagotomy Syndrome
• **Dumping syndrome**^{Q} • Metabolic disturbances^Q	• **Afferent loop** syndrome^Q • **Efferent loop** obstruction^Q • **Alkaline reflux gastritis**^{Q} • **Retained antrum**^{Q} syndrome	• Postvagotomy **diarrhea**^{Q} • Postvagotomy **gastric atony**^{Q} • Incomplete vagal transection^Q

Metabolic Complications after Gastrectomy

- **Metabolic complications** are **more common** and **serious after partial gastrectomy**^{Q} than after vagotomy.
- **More common** in **Billroth II**^{Q} >Billroth I procedure
- **Severity** is directly related to the **extent of gastric resection**^{Q}.
- **MC metabolic defect** appearing **after gastrectomy: Anemia**^{Q}

Anemia

- **MC metabolic defect** appearing **after gastrectomy**: Anemia[Q]
- **Iron deficiency anemia (IDA)** is more common than vitamin B_{12} deficiency anemia[Q].

Iron deficiency anemia:
- More than 30% of **patients** undergoing gastrectomy **suffer from IDA**[Q]
- **Cause:** Combination of **decreased iron intake, impaired iron absorption**, and **chronic blood loss**[Q]
- Addition of **iron supplements** to the patient's diet **corrects IDA**[Q].

Megaloblastic anemia:
- **Megaloblastic anemia** can occur when **>50%**[Q] of the **stomach is removed** such as occurs during **subtotal gastrectomy**[Q].
- **Vitamin B_{12} deficiency** occur **secondary to poor absorption** of the substance owing to **lack of intrinsic factor secretion** in the gastric juice.
- **Treatment: Intramuscular injections** of **cyanocobalamin**[Q] every 3 to 4 months indefinitely because its administration orally is not a reliable route.

Folate deficiency:
- **Folate deficiency** is **rare** after gastric resection
- **May coexist with** either an iron or vitamin B_{12} deficiency.
- Usually be corrected by **dietary supplementation**.

Impaired Absorption

- Common metabolic disturbance after gastric resections is **impaired absorption of fat**.
- **Steatorrhea** may occur as a result of **inadequate mixing of bile salts** and **pancreatic lipase** with ingested fat **because of** the **duodenal bypass**[Q].
- **Deficiency** in uptake **of fat-soluble vitamins** may also occur[Q].
- **Osteoporosis** and **osteomalacia** have also been observed after gastric resection and appear to be **caused by deficiencies** in **calcium**[Q].
- If **fat absorption** is also present, the **calcium malabsorption** is further **aggravated** because **fatty acids bind calcium**[Q].
- **Treatment: Calcium** supplements with **vitamin D**[Q]

DUMPING SYNDROME

Dumping Syndrome

- Dumping syndrome refers to a constellation of **post-prandial symptoms** occurring due to **accelerated emptying** (dumping) of **hyperosmolar stomach contents** into the small bowel.
- It is usually seen in operation which destroys the pyloric sphincter (i.e **gastrectomy, antrectomy** and **drainage procedures**)[Q].
- It also affects a small percentage of patients with highly selective vagotomy due to loss of receptive relaxation of stomach.

Dumping Syndrome	
Early Dumping	**Late Dumping**
It occurs **immediately after meals** (after **15-30 minutes**)[Q]	It is seen **2-3 hrs after meal**[Q]
Dumping of **hyperosmolar contents** into **small bowel**[Q] results in rapid fluid influx from the circulation into gastrointestinal tract. This leads to **acute intestinal distention** and peripheral & splanchnic vasodilatation[Q].	Occurs due to **reactive hypoglycemia**[Q].
This gives rise to **vasomotor & abdominal symptoms**: Epigastric fullness, sweating, light headedness, tachycardia, diarrhea.	Carbohydrate load in small bowel → Increased plasma glucose → Increased insulin secretion → Hypoglycemia
Symptoms can be **ameliorated by lying down & saline infusion**[Q].	Symptoms are **relieved by administration of sugar**[Q].

Management
- **Dietary management:** Diet therapy is done to reduce jejunal osmolality.
  - **Multiple small meals**, food **low in carbohydrate** and **rich in fat** and **proteins** are taken[Q].
  - **Liquids during meals** should be **avoided**[Q].
- **Somatostatin analogues (octreotide):**
  - Diet therapy is usually successful but if it fails, the patient is started on octreotide.

- **Surgery:**
  - Surgery is **rarely required**[Q] as most of the patients improve with time, dietary management and Octreotide.
  - **Surgical procedures** used to treat dumping are:
- Use of an **antiperistaltic loop of jejunum** between the **residual gastric pouch** and **intestine**
- Conversion of **Billroth II to Billroth I** anastomosis
- Conversion to **Roux-en-Y-anastomosis**.

GASTROJEJUNOCOLIC FISTULA

Gastrojejunocolic Fistula

- **Gastrojejunocolic fistula** may **form between transverse colon & upper jejunum** after a **Billroth II surgical procedure**[Q]. (The Billroth procedure attaches the jejunum to the remainder of the stomach).

Clinical Features:
- The **symptoms of GJF** are **diarrhea, epigastric pain** and discomfort, **gastrointestinal bleeding, feculent eructation, fecal vomiting, weight loss** and weakness[Q].
- **Anemia, leukocytosis, electrolyte disturbances** and **hypoalbuminemia** are common laboratory findings[Q].

Diagnosis:

> • **Barium enema** is **diagnostic of GJC fistula**[Q].

- **Investigations used: Barium enema** and **endoscopy**[Q]
- **Success rate** of **barium enema** in **correctly diagnosing** the fistula is **95-100%**[Q]

Treatment:
- The **historical approach** was **2-3-staged operations** even involving a **preliminary diversion colostomy** in order to **ameliorate the nutritional status** of the patient and to **decrease mortality**[Q]
- Three staged operation: (1) colostomy (2) resection of the fistula (3) colostomy closure
- Today, because of the **parenteral & enteral support treatments** and the developments in intensive care conditions, **one-stage resection can be applied**[Q]

UPPER GI BLEED

Risk Stratification Systems for Upper GI Bleeds

- Help to **identify the patients at higher risk of major bleeding or death** (facilitate patient triage)
- Commonly used scoring systems:
  - **Rockall score** (takes account of **endoscopic findings; most useful**[Q])
  - **Blatchford score** (used during **initial assessment, does not require endoscopic data**[Q])

Commonly Used Risk Stratification Systems for Upper GI Bleeds	
Blatchford Score (PUSH + Melena/Syncope + Cardiac/Hepatic Dysfunction)	**Rockall & Baylor Score** (CASDE)
• **P**ulse[Q] • Blood **U**rea nitrogen[Q] • **S**ystolic BP[Q] • **H**emoglobin[Q] • Presence of **M**elena[Q], **S**yncope[Q], **H**epatic[Q] or **C**ardiac dysfunction[Q]	• **C**omorbid disease[Q] (cardiac, hepatic, renal, or disseminated cancer) • **A**ge[Q] (<60 years, 60-79 years, >80 years) • **S**hock[Q] (systolic BP <100 mm Hg, HR >100 beats/min) • **D**iagnosis at the time of endoscopy[Q] (Mallory-Weiss tears, nonmalignant lesions, or malignant lesions) • **E**ndoscopic stigmata of recent bleed[Q]

Bleed Risk Classification
• To **predict risk** of **rebleeding & mortality** in **upper GI bleed** • Predicts **risk on initial presentation** based on **five criteria**: 1. Ongoing **Bleeding**[Q] 2. **Low systolic BP**[Q] (**<100** mm Hg) 3. **Elevated PT**[Q] (**>1.2 times** the control value) 4. **Erratic mental status**[Q] 5. Unstable comorbid **Disease**[Q]

THE FORREST CLASSIFICATION

The Forrest Classification (For Endoscopic Findings and Rebleeding Risk)		
Grade	Description	Rebleeding Risk
Ia	Active, **pulsatile** bleeding^Q	**High**
Ib	**Oozing**^Q, non-pulsatile bleeding	High
IIa	Non-bleeding **visible vessel**^Q	**High**
IIb	Adherent **clot**^Q	Intermediate
IIc	**Black dot**^Q	Low
III	**Clean base**^Q	Low

- High rebleeding risk: I & IIa^Q
- Intermediate risk: IIb^Q
- Low risk: IIc & III^Q

MALLORY WEISS SYNDROME

MALLORY WEISS SYNDROME

- Mallory-Weiss tears are related to **forceful vomiting, retching, coughing,** or **straining**^Q.
- **Forceful contraction** of **abdominal wall** against an **unrelaxed cardia**, resulting in mucosal laceration of **proximal cardia**^Q as a result of the increase in intragastric pressure.

  - Results in **disruption** of gastric mucosa high on the **lesser curve** at **cardia (just below GE junction)**^Q

- Tear is **partial thickness**, extending through the **mucosa and submucosa**^Q

Clinical Features:
- Classically, seen in **alcoholic patients**^Q after a period of **intense retching** and **vomiting** after binge drinking.
- Cause of up to **15% of all severe upper GI bleeds**^Q

  - **Arterial bleeding** (usually from **left gastric artery**^Q), usually **painless** and are **rarely**^Q associated with **massive bleeding**.

- The overall **mortality rate** is **3-4%**, with the **greatest risk** for massive hemorrhage in **alcoholic** patients with **preexisting portal hypertension**^Q.

Diagnosis:
- Usually diagnosed by **history**
- **Endoscopy** is used to **confirm the diagnosis**^Q.

Treatment:
- **Supportive therapy** is often all that is necessary because **90%** of **bleeding episodes** are **self-limited**, and the **mucosa** often **heals within 72 hours**^Q.

  Persistent Bleeding in Mallory Weiss Syndrome is managed by
  - **Endoscopic electrocoagulation**^Q or endoscopic therapy with injection
  - **Angiographic embolization**^Q
  - Surgery consists of laparotomy and **high gastrotomy** with **oversewing of the linear tear**^Q, if above maneuvers fails.

- **Recurrent bleeding** from a Mallory-Weiss tear is **uncommon**^Q.

Remember: A **Sengstaken-Blakemore tube** will **not stop bleeding** in Mallory-Weiss syndrome, as the **bleeding is arterial** and the pressure in the balloon is not sufficient to overcome the arterial pressure and is **contraindicated**^Q.

DIEULAFOY'S GASTRIC LESION

DIEULAFOY'S GASTRIC LESION

- Caused by an **abnormally large (1–3 mm)**^Q, **tortuous artery** coursing through the **submucosa**
- Occurs **6–10 cm** from the **GE junction**, generally in '**fundus**' near the **cardia** along **lesser curvature**^Q.

  - **Erosion** of **superficial mucosa** overlying the artery occur **secondary to pulsations** of **large submucosal vessel**^Q arteriole

- **Artery** is exposed to **gastric contents**, leading to **further erosion & bleeding** occurs^Q.
- **Mucosal defect** is **2–5 mm** in size

Clinical Features:
- More common in **men** (2:1) with **peak incidence** in **5th decade**^Q.
- Associated with **sudden** onset of **massive, painless, recurrent hematemesis** with **hypotension**
- **Recurrent bleeding** with **spontaneous cessation** is common^Q.

Diagnosis:
- **Endoscopy** is the **diagnostic modality of choice**, correctly identifying the lesion in 80% of patients.
  - **Repeated endoscopies** may be needed to correctly identify the lesion because of **intermittent nature** of the **bleeding**^Q.
- **Angiography** showing a **tortous ectatic artery** in the distribution of the **left gastric artery** with accompanied **contrast extravasation** in the setting of acute bleeding.

Treatment:
- **Initial attempts** at **endoscopic control** are **often successful**^Q.
- **Application** of **thermal** or **sclerosant therapy** is **effective** in **80–100% of cases**.^Q
- In cases that fail endoscopic therapy, **angiographic coil embolization** can be **successful**^Q.
- **Gastric wedge resection** to include the offending vessel is reserved **when other modalities have failed**^Q.

WATERMELON STOMACH (GASTRIC ANTRAL VASCULAR ECTASIA)

WATERMELON STOMACH (GASTRIC ANTRAL VASCULAR ECTASIA)

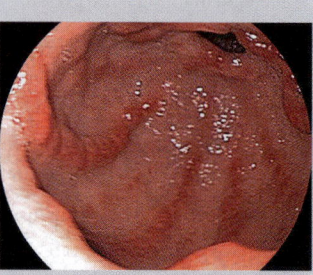

- A rare entity characterized by presence of both **inflammatory** and **vascular components** in **mucosa**^Q.

Pathology:
- **Dilated mucosal blood vessels** in the lamina propria, often containing **thrombi**, with **no evidence of vascular malformation** on angiographic and morphologic examination^Q.
- **Mucosal fibromuscular hyperplasia** and **hyalinization** are often present^Q.
- Predominantly affects the **distal portion (Antrum)**^Q of the stomach

Clinical Features:
- Patients are generally **elderly women** with **chronic bleeding**^Q.
- Most have an **associated autoimmune connective tissue** disorders, and at least **25%** have **chronic liver disease**^Q.
- Patients typically have **iron deficiency anemia** & **chronic blood loss** requiring transfusions^Q.

Diagnosis:
- Diagnosis is based on **typical endoscopic** and **biopsy appearance** of mucosa^Q.
  - Gross endoscopic examination reveals **prominent longitudinal folds** with **parallel striking red stripes** atop the mucosal folds of the **distal stomach**, much like the **rind of a watermelon**^Q.

Treatment:
- Lesions are treated by **endoscopic cautery**^Q.
- In patients with **portal hypertension**, **TIPS** should be considered first^Q.

RISK FACTORS FOR CARCINOMA STOMACH

Factors Associated with Increased Risk of Developing Stomach Cancer	
Nutritional	**Medical**
• **Low fat** or **protein** consumption^Q • **Salted** meat^Q • **High nitrate** consumption^Q • High **complex-carbohydrate** consumption^Q	• **Prior gastric surgery**^Q • **H. pylori**^Q infection • **Epstein-Barr** virus^Q • **Gastric atrophy** and **gastritis**^Q • **Adenomatous polyps**^Q • **Male** gender^Q
Social	**Occupational**
• **Low** social class^Q	• Rubber workers^Q • Coal workers^Q

Environmental	Genetic factors
• Poor food preparation (**smoked, salted**)[Q] • **Lack of refrigeration**[Q] • Poor drinking water (**well water**)[Q] • **Smoking**[Q]	• Blood group '**A**'[Q] • **Pernicious anemia**[Q] • Family history • **Hereditary nonpolyposis colon cancer**[Q] • **Li-Fraumeni syndrome**[Q]

- **Decreased risk of carcinoma stomach:** Aspirin, Diet (high fresh fruit and vegetable intake), Vitamin A and C, calcium, selenium, zinc and iron[Q].
- Alcohol is **not** a risk factor for **CA stomach**[Q].

COX-2 Inhibitors are protective in	
• **Barrett's esophagus**[Q] • **SCC** and **adenocarcinoma** of esophagus[Q]	• **Carcinoma stomach**[Q] • **Desmoid tumors**[Q] • Small duodenal and rectal polyps in FAP[Q]

MÉNÉTRIER'S DISEASE (HYPOPROTEINEMIC HYPERTROPHIC GASTROPATHY)

MÉNÉTRIER'S DISEASE (HYPOPROTEINEMIC HYPERTROPHIC GASTROPATHY)

- A rare, **acquired**[Q], **premalignant**[Q] disease, of unknown cause
- Characterized by **massive gastric folds** in the **fundus**[Q] & **corpus** of the stomach, giving the mucosa a **cobblestone** or **cerebriform appearance**[Q].

- Associated with **CMV infection in children**[Q] & **H. pylori** infection in **adults**[Q].

Pathology:
- **Foveolar hyperplasia** (expansion of surface mucous cells) with **absent parietal cells**[Q].
- **Increased TGF-alpha** has been noted in the **gastric mucosa**[Q]

- Associated with **protein loss** from the stomach, **excessive mucus production**, & **hypochlorhydria** or **achlorhydria**[Q].

Clinical Features:
- Epigastric pain, vomiting, **weight loss, anorexia,** & peripheral **edema**[Q].

Diagnosis:
- **Typical gastric mucosal changes** can be detected by **radiographic** or **endoscopic** examination.
- **Biopsy** should be performed **to rule out gastric carcinoma** or **lymphoma**[Q].
- **Twenty-four-hour pH monitoring** reveals **hypochlorhydria** or **achlorhydria**[Q]
- **Chromium-labeled albumin test** reveals **increased GI protein loss**[Q].

Treatment:
- Medical treatment is limited to **albumin replacement** and maintenance of **adequate nutrition**, acid suppression, octreotide & H. pylori eradication[Q].
- **Total gastrectomy** for **bleeding, severe hypoproteinemia** or **cancer**[Q].

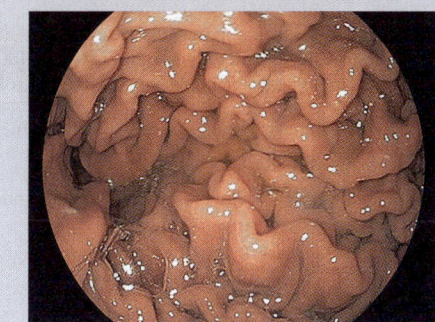

CLASSIFICATION SYSTEM FOR CARCINOMA STOMACH

Lauren Classification System for Carcinoma Stomach

Intestinal	Diffuse
• **Environmental**[Q] • Gastric atrophy, intestinal metaplasia • **Men**[Q] > Women • Increasing incidence with age • **Gland formation**[Q] • **Hematogenous**[Q] spread • **Microsatellite instability**[Q] • **APC gene mutations**[Q] • p53, p16 inactivation[Q] • **Epidemic**[Q] • **Distal** part of the stomach[Q]	• **Familial**[Q] • Blood group '**A**'[Q] • **Women**[Q] > Men • **Younger age group**[Q] • **Poorly differentiated signet ring cells**[Q] • **Transmural/Lymphatic** spread[Q] • **Decreased E-cadherin**[Q] • p53, p16 inactivation[Q] • **Endemic**[Q] • **Proximal** part of the stomach[Q]

Bormann Classification (Based on macroscopic appearance)	
Type I	**Polypoid** or **fungating**^Q cancers
Type II	Fungating & ulcerated with surrounded by **elevated borders**^Q
Type III	Ulcerated lesions **infiltrating** the **gastric wall**^Q
Type IV	Infiltrates diffusely (**Linnitis plastica**)^Q
Type V	Unable to be classified

CARCINOMA STOMACH

Carcinoma Stomach

- Incidence of **gastric cancer**, especially **distal cancer** is **decreasing**^Q; Distribution: **Distal (40%) > Middle (30%) = Proximal (30%)**
- Incidence of **GE junction tumors** are **increasing**^Q
- Approximately **90%** of all tumors of the stomach are **malignant**, the vast majority of which are **gastric adenocarcinoma**^Q.

  - MC genetic abnormalities: **p53** and **COX-2 gene**^Q (SPC: **S**tomach, **p**53 and **C**OX-2 gene)

- Tumor Markers: CEA, CA 19-9, CA-125, CA 72-4 & beta-HCG

Clinical Features

- MC Symptoms: **Abdominal pain (62-91%)**^Q > **weight loss (22-61%)**.
- Typically, pain is constant, nonradiating, & unrelieved by food ingestion.
- **Proximal tumors** involving the gastroesophageal junction often present with **dysphagia**, whereas **distal antral tumors** may present as **gastric outlet obstruction**^Q.

  - **Diffuse mural involvement by tumor**, as occurs in **linnitis plastica**, leads to **decreased distensibility** of the stomach and complaints of **early satiety**^Q.

- **Ascitis, jaundice** or **palpable mass** indicate **incurable disease**^Q.
- **Transverse colon** is a potential site for **malignant fistulization** & **obstruction** from gastric primary tumor.

  - Patients may present with a palpable abdominal mass, a palpable **supraclavicular (Virchow's)** or **periumbilical (Sister Mary Joseph's)** lymph node, **left axilla (Irish nodes)** peritoneal metastasis palpable by rectal examination (**Blummer's shelf**), or a palpable ovarian mass (**Krukenberg's tumor**)^Q via **retrograde lymphatics**^Q most commonly.

- Paraneoplastic syndromes include thrombophlebitis (**Trousseau's syndrome**), neuropathies, nephrotic syndrome, & DIC.

Lymph Node Metastasis

- Relative risk of nodal metastases at a specific nodal location depends on both the **site of origin** of the primary tumor and **width & depth**^Q of invasion of gastric wall.
- **Proximal stomach** & **GE junction tumors**: Higher propensity of spread to nodes in the **mediastinum** & **pericardial region**^Q.
- Tumors in the **body of stomach**: Highest likelihood of spreading to **nodes along** the **greater & lesser curvature, near** the location of **primary tumor** mass^Q.
- Tumors in the **distal stomach**: High likelihood of spread to the **periduodenal, peripancreatic, & porta hepatis** nodes^Q.

Diagnosis

- **Endoscopy with biopsy** is the **best method**^Q to diagnose gastric cancer
- IOC for staging of early gastric cancer: EUS
- Best investigation for preoperative staging: **CECT**^Q

Treatment of Carcinoma Stomach according to site	
Proximal-third	**Extended gastrectomy**, including the **distal esophagus**^Q
Middle-third	**Total gastrectomy** and **D2** LN dissection^Q.
Distal-third	**Intestinal-type**: Subtotal gastrectomy with D2 LN dissection^Q **Diffuse-type**: Total gastrectomy with D2 LN dissection^Q

Recurrence:

- Most recurrences occur **within the first 3 years**^Q.

  - **Loco-regional failure rate is highest** at the **anastomosis or stump (25%)**^Q > **stomach bed (21%)** > regional nodes.

- MC site of metastasis: **Liver**^Q > lung > bone.

Surveillance
- Follow-up should include a **complete history** and **physical examination every 4 months** for **1 year**, then **every 6 months** for **2 years**, and then **annually** thereafter.

Prognosis
- **Prognostic factors** for **CA stomach**: **Depth**^Q of **invasion** and **LN status**^Q

LYMPH NODE STATIONS
1. Right cardiac; **2.** Left cardiac; **3.** Lesser curvature; **4.** Greater curvature; **5.** Suprapyloric; **6.** Infrapyloric **7.** Left gastric; **8.** Common hepatic; **9.** Celiac; **10.** Splenic hilus; **11. Splenic artery;** **12.** Hepatoduodenal ligament; **13.** Retropancreatic; **14.** Mesenteric root; **15.** Transverse mesocolon; **16.** Paraaortic

SISTER MARY JOSEPH NODULE
- **Sister Mary Joseph nodule** or **node**, also called **Sister Mary Joseph sign**, refers to a **palpable nodule bulging into** the **umbilicus** as a result of **metastasis of a malignant cancer** in the **pelvis** or **abdomen**^Q.

    - **Gastrointestinal malignancies** account **for half** of underlying sources (**most commonly gastric cancer, colonic cancer** or **pancreatic cancer**, mostly of the **tail** and **body** of the pancreas), and **men are more likely** to have an **underlying cancer** of the **gastrointestinal tract**^Q.

- **Gynecological cancers** account for about 1 in 4 cases (**primarily ovarian cancer** and also **uterine cancer**)^Q.

Proposed mechanisms for the spread of cancer cells to the umbilicus	
• **Direct transperitoneal spread**^Q • **Via lymphatics**^Q which run alongside the obliterated umbilical vein • **Hematogenous spread**^Q	• **Via remnant structures**: – **Falciform ligament**^Q – **Median umbilical ligament**^Q – **Remnant** of the **vitelline duct**^Q

Prognosis:
- Sister Mary Joseph nodule is **associated** with **multiple peritoneal metastases** and **poor prognosis**^Q.

TNM CLASSIFICATION OF CARCINOMA OF THE STOMACH

8th AJCC (2017) TNM Classification of Carcinoma of the Stomach	
Tis: Carcinoma in situ: intraepithelial tumor without invasion of the lamina propria, high grade dysplasia	**N1:** Metastasis in **1-2** regional LNs^Q
T1a: Tumor invades **lamina propria or muscularis mucosa**^Q	**N2:** Metastasis in **3-6** regional LNs^Q
T1b: Tumor invades **submucosa**^Q	**N3a:** Metastasis in **7-15** regional LNs^Q
T2: Tumor invades **muscularis propria**^Q	**N3b:** Metastasis in **16 or more** regional LNs^Q
T3: Tumor penetrates **subserosal connective tissue** without invasion of visceral peritoneum or adjacent structures^Q	
T4a: Tumor invades **serosa (visceral peritoneum)**^Q	**M1:** Distant metastasis
T4b: Tumor invades **adjacent structures**^Q	

Stage Grouping								
Stage	**IA**	**IB**	**IIA**	**IIB**	**IIIA**	**IIIB**	**IIIC**	**IV**
	T1N0	T1N1 T2N0	T1N2 T2N1 T3N0	T1N3a T2N2 T3N1 T4aN0	T2N3a T3N2 T4aN1-2 T4bN0	T1-2N3b T3-4aN3a T4bN1-2	T3-4aN3b T4bN3a-3b	Any T, Any N, **M1**

GASTRIC STUMP CARCINOMA

GASTRIC STUMP CARCINOMA
- It is defined as **carcinoma** arising in the **gastric remnant > 5 years**^Q following pervious gastric resection **for benign diseases** or **> 15 years**^Q after curative surgery **for malignant disease.**

Etiology
- Thought to be related to **changes in the gastric mucosa** which arise as a result of the **change in the anatomical relationship** between the stomach and the small intestine following surgery.

> • **Enterogastric reflux**^{Q} plays a very **significant role** in the pathogenesis.

- Other important etiological factors include: **Bacterial proliferation** and **hypochlorhydria**^{Q} which increases the mucosal susceptibility to carcinogenesis by N-nitrosamines.

Pathology
- Most of the stump carcinomas are often **near the stoma** but many of these tumors are **quite large at presentation**.
- Equally divided between **intestinal** and **diffuse subtypes**^{Q}.
- **Histologically** they are classified as **Adenocarcinoma**^{Q}, **Adeno-squamous**, Squamous cell carcinoma, Small cell and undifferentiated carcinoma.

Clinical Features
- Usually present **late** and the disease is **advanced**.

Treatment
- **Surgical resection** remains the **only effective** modality of **treatment**.
- Overall average **survival** is **4–6 months**^{Q}.
- **Surgery** whether palliative, has **survival benefit**.

LEATHER BOTTLE STOMACH (LINITIS PLASTICA)

LEATHER BOTTLE STOMACH (LINITIS PLASTICA)

- **Pyloric antrum** is MC site affected in **localized variety**^{Q}
- Stomach is **massively thickened** (feels like **leather**)^Q

Pathology:
- Caused by **proliferation of fibrous tissue** mainly in **submucosa**^{Q}
- Characterized by **Mother of pearl appearance**
- Mucosa appears normal

Clinical Features:
- **Early satiety** due to **reduced stomach capacity**^{Q}
- **LN metastasis** is common^Q

Treatment:
- Treated by **radical gastrectomy**^{Q}

Prognosis:
- Associated with **poor prognosis**^{Q}

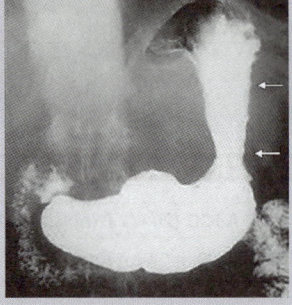
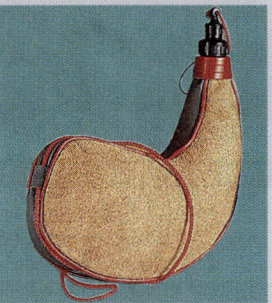

GASTROINTESTINAL STROMAL TUMOR

GASTROINTESTINAL STROMAL TUMOR

- GISTs: **MC mesenchymal tumor** of the GI tract^Q
- MC primary site for GIST: **Stomach (60–70%) > small bowel (20–25%) > colorectum & esophagus (5% each)**^{Q}.

> • **Most GISTs are positive for CD-117 (95%), BCL-2 (80%), CD-34 (70%)**^{Q}.

- **Types: Spindle cell (70%) and Epithelioid (30%)**^{Q}

Pathology:
- Arise from the **muscularis propria** and most likely originate from the **cells of Cajal**^{Q}
- Expression of the receptor tyrosine kinase **KIT (CD 117)**, 5% express platelet derived growth factor receptor alpha (**PDGFRA**)^Q.
- **PDGFRA mutations** in GIST appear to confer a **very favorable prognosis** with **low risk of recurrence**^{Q}.
- New tumor markers of GIST: **DOG-1** (discovered on GIST-1) & **protein kinase C-theta**

Clinical features:
- Patients usually present after the fourth decade, with the mean age of **60 years** at diagnosis.
- MC presentations of gastric GISTs: **GI bleeding** and **pain** or dyspepsia.

Carney triad
Association of **extra-adrenal paragangliomas, pulmonary chondromas & multifocal GIST**^{Q}

Diagnosis:

> - **CT: IOC** for evaluation of **primary tumor** & **accurate staging**[Q]
> - **PET-CT: Gold standard** for **recurrent GIST**[Q]

- **Percutaneous** or **endoscopic biopsy** should only be **performed if the results would obviate the need for surgery**[Q].

Treatment:
- **Bleeding** manifestation is the **MC** indication for **surgery**[Q].
- GIST should be treated with **segmental resection**[Q] (margins of **1cm**)

> - **LN metastasis** are uncommon, regional **lymphadenectomy** is **not recommended**[Q]
> - **Intraoperative incisional biopsy** prior to resection should be **avoided**, because it risks **tumor spillage**[Q]

- **Imatinib**[Q] (selective inhibitor of **type 3** tyrosine kinase KIT), is approved for use in **CD117-positive unresectable** and **metastatic GISTs**.

> - Functional imaging of GIST with **18FDG-PET** scanning represents a useful diagnostic modality for **early-response assessment** with **imatinib therapy**[Q].
> - **Sunitinib**[Q] is used in **imatinib-refractory disease**.
> - **Regorafenib**[Q]: Third line therapy in the **patients failing imatinib & sunitinib therapy**[Q].

Prognosis:
- **Tumor size** is a **predominant factor for survival** in surgical series for primary GIST.
- **MC sites** of **disease failure** after complete resection: **Liver**[Q], **omentum** or **peritoneal cavity**.

> - **Half to two third primaries** will have disease **failure within the liver**[Q] and nearly 40% will have liver as the only site of failure. Generally **hepatic involvement** is **multifocal**.

- **Median time** to **recurrence after resection** of primary GIST is **2 years**[Q].

ABDOMINAL LEIOMYOSARCOMA

ABDOMINAL LEIOMYOSARCOMA

- Leiomyosarcoma describes a **type of soft-tissue cancer** that **occurs within smooth muscle cells**.
- This kind of cancer can be **difficult to detect** as it often causes **no organ dysfunction until** the tumor has gotten to be **large in size**[Q].
- Most common locations: **Uterus & stomach**[Q].

Clinical Features:
- **Asymptomatic** in **initial stage**[Q]
- **Earliest symptom**: **Noticeable lump** or **swelling** within the abdomen.
- The **sign most often cited is bleeding**[Q]. These tumors sometimes **necrose** and **bleed into the bowel**.
- **Leiomyosarcomas** that occur **in the digestive tract** can also cause **gastrointestinal blockage** or **bleeding**[Q], which can manifest as blood in the stool.
- **Uterine leiomyosarcomas** can cause **vaginal bleeding**[Q]

Diagnosis:
- **Endoscopy** can be **used to visualize the tumors**[Q].
- A definitive diagnosis requires a **biopsy**[Q]

Treatment:
- **First-line treatment**: **Surgical removal** of the cancerous tissue.
- **Uterine leiomyosarcoma**: **Total hysterectomy**[Q]
- **Gastric leiomyosarcoma**: **Total gastrectomy**[Q]

GASTRIC LYMPHOMA

GASTRIC LYMPHOMA

- **Stomach** is **MC site** for **lymphoma**[Q] in the GIT
- **MC site** of gastric lymphoma: **Antrum**[Q]

> - **MC gastric lymphoma** is **diffuse large B cell lymphoma**[Q] **(55%)** > extranodal marginal cell lymphoma (**MALT**) (**40%**) > Burkitts lymphoma (3%) > mantle cell and follicular lymphomas.
> - **DLBL** is **MC type of NHL**, **extranodal lymphoma** and **GI lymphoma**.

- **Stomach**, which is devoid of organized lymphoid tissue, is the **MC site** of **MALT lymphoma**^Q.

Clinical Features:
- Lymphomas occur in **older patients** (**sixth** and **seventh** decades)
- More common in **men**
- Vague symptoms, namely **epigastric pain**^Q, early satiety, and fatigue.
- Constitutional **B symptoms** are **very rare**.
- Although overt bleeding is uncommon, **more than half** of patients present with **anemia**^Q.

Diagnosis:
- **Endoscopy**: Nonspecific gastritis or **gastric ulcerations**, with mass lesions being unusual.
- Evidence of distant disease should be sought through upper airway examination, bone marrow biopsy, and CT of the chest and abdomen to detect lymphadenopathy.
- Any **enlarged lymph nodes** should undergo **biopsy**.
- **H. pylori testing** should be performed by histology and, if negative, confirmed by serology.

Staging Systems for Primary Gastrointestinal Non-Hodgkin's Lymphoma		
Ann Arbor	**Description**	**Relative incidence (%)**
IE	Tumor confined to **gastrointestinal tract**	26
IIE	Tumor with spread to **regional lymph nodes**	26
IIE	Tumor with nodal involvement **beyond regional lymph nodes** (para-aortic, iliac)	17
IIIE-IV	Tumor with spread to **other intra-abdominal organs** (liver, spleen) or **beyond abdomen** (chest, bone marrow)	31

Treatment of Gastric Lymphoma	
Low-grade MALT	**High-grade (aggressive)**
• **Confined to gastric wall** and **no t(11;18) translocation**: H.pylori **eradication therapy** and re-evaluate at 12 months	• **Stage I, II, III**: Chemotherapy + RT
• **Lymph node involvement** and **t(11;18) translocation**: H.pylori **eradication therapy** and re-evaluate at 3-6 months; if lymphoma persists: • **Stage I**: XRT • **Stage II**: Chemotherapy + RT	• **Stage IV**: Chemotherapy + RT • **Residual disease**: Further **chemotherapy** or **Surgery**
• **Stage III or IV**: H.pylori **eradication therapy** and Chemotherapy +/- RT	

- **External beam radiotherapy**: 30 Gy with 10 Gy boost
- **Chemotherapy regimens** cyclophosphamide, doxorobucin, vincristine, prednisone (CHOP) +/- rituximab
- **Rituximab** is chimeric monoclonal antibody **against CD-20**, preferred for **high grade MALT** or **DLBL**.

DAWSON'S CRITERIA
(Requirements for the diagnosis of Primary GI lymphoma)

- Absence of **palpable lymphadenopathy**^Q
- **Normal bone marrow biopsy** and **peripheral blood smear**^Q
- Absence of **mediastinal lymphadenopathy**^Q on chest radiographs
- **Disease** grossly **confined to** the affected **viscus**^Q
- **Regional lymphadenopathy only**^Q
- Absence of **hepatic** or **splenic involvement**^Q unless via direct extension of the primary tumor.

PRIMARY GASTRIC HODGKIN'S DISEASE

Primary Gastric Hodgkin's disease

- **Primary gastric Hodgkin's disease** is **extremely rare** (<1% of all gastric lymphomas)
- **Stomach** is the **MC site** of **primary extranodal lymphoma**^Q in adults

Etiology:
- Association of **classic Hodgkin's disease** with **EBV**^Q
- LMP1 (**Latent Membrane Protein 1**) an **essential EBV protein**, commonly expressed and **associated with** the **pathogenesis of Hodgkin's disease**^Q

Diagnosis:
- **Endoscopy: Non-specific gastritis** or **peptic ulcers with mass lesions**^Q
- A full panel of **immunohistochemical markers is essential** to make an **accurate diagnosis** of gastric Hodgkin's disease.

Treatment:
- **Hodgkin's disease** of the **stomach** has been **treated by surgery** while **postoperative chemotherapy** has been employed **for systemic disease**^Q.

Prognosis:
- Prognosis is **poor** with **45–60%** of patients **dying within** the **first year of diagnosis**

BEZOARS

BEZOARS

- Bezoars are **collections** of **nondigestible materials**, usually of vegetable origin (phytobezoar) but also of hair (trichobezoar).
- **Four types of Bezoar:** Phytobezoars, Trichobezoars, Pharmacobezoar and Lactobezoar

Phytobezoar:
- **Most common type**^Q, a high concentration of tannin, exposed to gastric acid form a coagulum leading to bezoar formation
- **Most commonly** found in patients who have undergone **surgery** of the **stomach** and have **impaired gastric emptying**^Q.
- **Diabetics** with **autonomic neuropathy**^Q are also at risk.

> - **Symptoms: Early satiety**, nausea, **pain, vomiting**, and **weight loss** with palpable **large mass**^Q
> - **Diagnosis** confirmed by a **barium examination** or **endoscopy**^Q.

- **Enzymatic therapy** to attempt dissolution of the bezoar. **Papain** and **cellulase** have been used with some success.
- Generally, **enzymatic débridement** is followed by **aggressive Ewald tube lavage** or **endoscopic fragmentation**^Q. Failure of these therapies would necessitate surgical removal.

Trichobezoar:
- Concretions of hair, generally found in **long-haired girls** or **women** who often deny eating their own hair (**trichophagy**)^Q.
- Typically **black** regardless of the color of the hair ingested because of enzymatic oxidation of gastric acid

> - **Most common** type in **Children**^Q
> - **Trichobezoars** are **most likely** to **require surgical management**^Q
> - **Rapunzel Syndrome:** Gastric trichobezoars with a long **extension** of hairs that trails **into the duodenum.**

- **Symptoms:** Pain from **gastric ulceration** and fullness from **gastric outlet obstruction** with occasional **gastric perforation** and **small bowel obstruction**^Q.
- **Larger trichobezoars** require **surgical removal**^Q.
- The trichophagy requires **psychiatric care**^Q because recurrent bezoar formation is common.

Lactobezoar:
- Compact mass of **undigested milk concretions** and have been linked to nearly every **commercially available infant formula** and **breast and cow milk**
- Treated by **withholding oral feedings**

STRESS GASTRITIS (STRESS ULCERATIONS)

STRESS GASTRITIS (STRESS ULCERATIONS/ STRESS EROSIVE GASTRITIS/ HEMORRHAGIC GASTRITIS)

- Characterized by **multiple, superficial** (nonulcerating) **erosions** that **begin in** the **proximal or acid-secreting portion** of the stomach and progress distally^Q.
- **Almost always** seen in the **fundus**^Q & rarely in **distal stomach**.

> - **Cushing's ulcer:** Occur in the setting of central nervous system disease (**Head trauma**)^Q
> - **Curling's ulcer:** as a result of **thermal burn injury** involving **> 35% of BSA**^Q

- **Increased acid secretion** in Cushing's ulcer but **not in Curling's ulcer**^{Q}

Pathophysiology:

- Multifactorial etiology

> - **Impaired mucosal defense** mechanisms against luminal acid such as a **reduction in blood flow**, **mucus**, and **bicarbonate secretion** by mucosal cells, or a **reduction in endogenous prostaglandins**^{Q}.

- In stress (**hypoxia, sepsis,** or **organ failure**), **mucosal ischemia** is the **main factor** responsible for the **breakdown** of these **normal defense mechanisms**^{Q}.

Risk factors or Predisposing clinical conditions		
• ARDS^Q	• Hepatic dysfunction^Q	• Hypotension^Q
• Multiple trauma^Q	• Oliguric renal failure^Q	• Prolonged surgical procedures^Q
• Major burn > 35% of BSA^Q	• Large transfusion^Q requirements	• Sepsis^Q

Clinical Features:

- More than **50%** of patients develop their **stress gastritis within 1–2 days** after a traumatic event.
- Only clinical sign may be **painless upper GI bleeding** that may be delayed at onset.
- **Bleeding** is usually **slow** and **intermittent**^{Q}

Diagnosis:

- **Endoscopy** is required to **confirm the diagnosis**^{Q} and to differentiate stress gastritis from other sources of GI hemorrhage.

Treatment:

- **Definitive fluid resuscitation** with **correction** of any **coagulation abnormalities** and **treatment of the underlying sepsis**^{Q}
- **Intraluminal gastric pH** should be maintained >5.0 with **antisecretory agents**.
- Most of the **superficial erosions** are not actively bleeding **do not require ligature unless** a **blood vessel** is **seen** at its **base**^{Q}.

> - Operation is completed by **closing the anterior gastrotomy** and performing a **truncal vagotomy** & **pyloroplasty**^{Q} to reduce acid secretion.

Prophylaxis:

- **Complete neutralization** of **luminal acid** or **antisecretory therapy** precludes the development of experimental stress gastritis^Q.
- **Sepsis control**, **ventilatory support**, adequate **nutrition** and correction of dyselectrolytemia^Q
- **Drugs** used are: Antacids, H_2-receptor antagonists and sucralfate

GASTRIC VOLVULUS

Gastric Volvulus

- **Organoaxial (two thirds):** Torsion occurs along the stomach's **longitudinal axis**^{Q}
- **Mesenteroaxial (one third):** Torsion occurs along the **vertical axis**^{Q}

Primary Gastric Volvulus	Secondary Gastric Volvulus
• Seen in association with **congenital asplenia** & **wandering spleen**^{Q}	• Occur secondary to some anatomic abnormality, (**Most commonly diaphragmatic hernia**)^Q
• Usually **mesenteroaxial**^{Q}	• Usually **organoaxial**^{Q}
• **Partial** (<180 degree) & **recurrent**^{Q}	• **Paraesophageal hiatal hernia** is the most common cause in **adults** & **congenital diaphragmatic hernia** (Bochdalek hernia) in **children**^{Q}
• Not associated with a diaphragmatic defect	

Clinical Features:

- **Organoaxial gastric volvulus** occurs **acutely** & is associated with a diaphragmatic defect
- **Mesenteroaxial volvulus** is **partial** (< 180 degrees), **recurrent**, and not associated with a diaphragmatic defect.
- Major symptoms at presentation are **abdominal pain** that is acute in onset, distention, vomiting, & **upper GI hemorrhage**^{Q}.

> - **Borchardt's triad: (Epigastric pain + Inability to vomit + Inability to pass a nasogastric tube)** is characteristic feature of gastric volvulus^Q.

Diagnosis:

- **X-ray abdomen: Gas-filled viscus** in the **chest** or upper abdomen^Q.
- **Diagnosis** can be **confirmed** by **barium** contrast study or **endoscopy**^{Q}.

Treatment:
- **Acute volvulus**: It is a **surgical emergency**. Stomach is **reduced** & **uncoiled**. **Diaphragmatic defect** is **repaired** with consideration given to a fundoplication in the setting of a paraesophageal hernia^Q.
- In **strangulation** (5–28%), **compromised segment** of stomach is **resected**^{Q}.
- **Spontaneous volvulus**, without an associated diaphragmatic defect, is treated by **detorsion** & **fixation** of the stomach by gastropexy or tube gastrostomy^Q.

GASTRIC DIVERTICULA

Gastric Diverticula

- Gastric diverticula are **usually solitary** and may be **congenital** or **acquired**^{Q}.
- **Congenital diverticula** are **true diverticula** and contain a full coat of muscularis propria, whereas **acquired diverticula** (perhaps caused by pulsion) usually have a **negligible outer muscle layer**^{Q}.

> - Most gastric diverticula occur in the **posterior cardia** or **fundus**^{Q}.
> - Most of the time gastric diverticula are **asymptomatic**^{Q}.

- However, they **can become inflamed** and may **produce pain** or **bleeding**^{Q}.
- **Perforation** is **rare**.

Treatment:
- **Asymptomatic diverticula do not require treatment**^{Q}
- **Symptomatic lesions** should be **removed**. This can often be done **laparoscopically**^{Q}.

INFANTILE HYPERTROPHIC PYLORIC STENOSIS

Infantile Hypertrophic Pyloric Stenosis

- In HPS, **hypertrophy** of **circular muscle**^{Q} of **pylorus** results in constriction & obstruction of gastric outlet.
- **Acquired condition**
- **Incidence** of **1 in 3000 to 4000**^{Q} live births.
- **Most common between** the ages of **3–6 weeks**^{Q}.
- **Associated anomalies** in **6–20%** cases: Esophageal atresia, Hirschprung's disease, ARM & malrotation

Etiology
- **Ethnic origin** is important because **highest incidence** is found among **whites of Scandinavian**^{Q} decent and **lowest risk** among **African Americans** and **Chinese**.

> - **Males** outnumber females by a ratio of **4:1**^{Q}
> - **First-born males**^{Q} are frequently encountered.

- **Higher risk** for developing HPS in **offspring of parents**^{Q} with **this condition**

Clinical Presentation:
- Infant is **normal at birth, symptomatic between** the ages of **3–6 weeks**^{Q}
- Infants with HPS typically present with **projectile nonbilious vomiting**^{Q}.

> - **Visible gastric peristalsis** may be seen as a wave of contraction **from the left upper quadrant** to the **epigastrium**^{Q}.

- The infants usually **feed vigorously** between episodes of vomiting.
- Typical electrolyte abnormality: **Hypochloremic, hypokalemic, metabolic alkalosis** with **paradoxical aciduria**^{Q}.

Diagnosis:
- **Palpation of the** pyloric tumor or **olive** in the **epigastrium**^{Q} or right upper quadrant by a skilled examiner is **pathognomonic** for the diagnosis of HPS^Q.
- If the olive is palpated, **no additional diagnostic testing** is necessary^Q.

> - When the olive **cannot be palpated**, the diagnosis of HPS can be made with an **ultrasound exam** or fluoroscopic UGI series.
> - Absence of radiation exposure and cost make the **ultrasound** the **usual preferred study**^{Q}.

- **Diagnostic Sonographic measurements:**
  – **Pyloric wall thickness** of at least **4 mm**^{Q} – Transverse diameter **>13 mm** – **Channel length** of at least **17 mm**^{Q}
- **Barium Meal:**
  – **String sign**^{Q}: indicating a narrowed elongated pyloric canal that does not relax is seen (**most specific sign**)
  – **Shoulder sign**^{Q}: caused by hypertrophied muscle indenting the antrum
  – **Double-track sign**^{Q}: caused by redundant mucosa

Treatment:
- Pyloric stenosis is **never a surgical emergency** although dehydration and electrolyte abnormalities may present a **medical emergency**^{Q}
- **Fluid resuscitation** and **correction of electrolyte abnormalities**^{Q} and metabolic alkalosis is essential before surgery.
  - It is important that the underlying metabolic alkalosis is **slowly corrected** with **normal saline**.
  - Treatment of HPS is by a **Ramstedt-Fredet pyloromyotomy** (**cutting across** the **abnormal pyloric musculature**^{Q} while preserving the underlying mucosa).

Postoperative care:
- Postoperatively, infants are usually allowed to resume enteral feedings.
- **Vomiting** after surgery occurs frequently but is **usually self-limited**^{Q}.
- **Complications**: Incomplete myotomy, **mucosal perforation** (usually at the duodenal end), and wound infection.
- If the **mucosa** is **inadvertently opened** then **feeding is delayed for 48 hours**^{Q}.

DUODENAL ATRESIA

Duodenal Atresia

- Occurs as a **result of failure of vacuolization** of the **duodenum** from its solid cord stage.

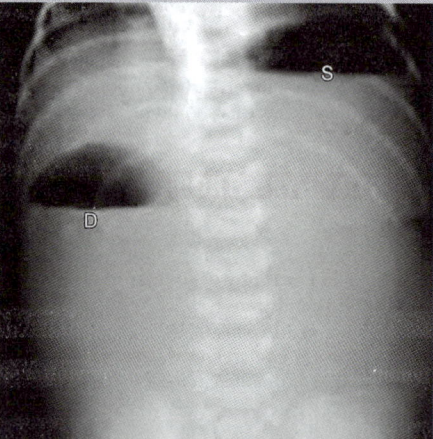

Anatomic variants of Duodenal Atresia
Type I → **Mucosal web** with intact muscular wall (**windsock deformity**)
Type II → Two ends separated by a **fibrous cord**
Type III → **Complete separation with a gap** within the duodenum.

Associated Anomalies
- Prematurity, Down syndrome, polyhydramnios^Q
- Malrotation, annular pancreas, biliary atresia^Q
- Cardiac, renal, esophageal, and anorectal anomalies

Clinical Features
- In most cases, the **duodenal obstruction** is **distal to the ampulla of Vater**, and infants present with **bilious emesis** in the **neonatal period**^{Q}.

Diagnosis
- X-ray abdomen: Double-bubble sign (air-filled stomach and duodenal bulb^Q).

  - **Diagnosis is confirmed**, if there is **no distal air**^{Q}.
  - If **distal air** is present, an **upper GI contrast study** is **performed rapidly**, not only **to confirm the diagnosis** of **duodenal atresia** but also to exclude **midgut volvulus**^{Q}.

Treatment:
- **Diamond-shaped duodenoduodenostomy** is the **treatment of choice**^{Q}.
- 5 'D's of duodenal atresia: **D**A, **D**own's syndrome, **D**istal to ampulla, **D**ouble bubble sign, **D**uodenoduodenostomy

DUODENAL ADENOCARCINOMA

Duodenal Adenocarcinoma

- **Duodenum** is MC site of **small intestinal adenocarcinoma**^{Q}
- 15% in the proximal; 40% in the middle and **45%** in the **distal duodenum (MC)**^{Q}
- **Resectability** and **prognosis** are **better** than other upper GI cancers.

Clinical Features
- Most often presents as **obstruction**, with **nausea, vomiting**, and **abdominal pain** as the most frequent symptoms.
- **Anemia** from bleeding and **biliary** or **pancreatic obstructive symptoms** can also be seen on initial presentation if the tumor is **located within** the **periampullary region**^{Q}.

Diagnosis
- **Endoscopy** is the **diagnostic test of choice** for **duodenal tumors**^{Q}, which allows for direct **visualization** and **biopsy** as needed.

Treatment
- For 1st or 2nd portion: **Whipple procedure**^{Q}
- For 3rd or 4th portion: **Segmental duodenal resection**^{Q}

Multiple Choice Questions

H. PYLORI

1. **H. pylori has been implicated in all, except:** *(Orissa 2011)*
   a. Gastric ulcer
   b. Gastric carcinoma
   c. Gastric lymphoma
   d. Gastric leiomyoma

2. **Which of the following is a common gastric lesion associated with H. pylori and undergoes regression following eradication of the infection?** *(MHPGMCET 2009)*
   a. Inflammatory polyp
   b. Metaplastic polyp
   c. Fundic gland
   d. True adenomas

3. **Eradication of helicobacter pylori has been proved to be beneficial in which of the following disorders of the stomach?** *(COMEDK 2006)*
   a. Low grade MALT lymphoma
   b. Erosive gastritis
   c. Carcinoma stomach
   d. Gastroesophageal disease

4. **A patient of peptic ulcer disease. When investigated endoscopically showed chronic antral gastritis. Which of the following dye will be able to stain the specimen?** *(AIIMS Nov 2000)*
   a. PAS
   b. Zeihl-Neilson stain
   c. Gramstain
   d. Warthin-Starry stain

5. **H. pylori causes:** *(TN 2001)*
   a. Type A Gastritis
   b. Type B gastritis
   c. Autoimmune
   d. Allergic Gastritis

6. **H. pylori infection causes carcinoma by which mechanism:** *(TN 2003)*
   a. Production of nitrosamines
   b. Gastric metaplasia
   c. Increasing acid secretion
   d. Causing mutation

7. **Eradication of H. pylori has been proved to be beneficial in the following condition except:** *(ICS 2005)*
   a. Duodenal ulcer
   b. Gastric ulcer
   c. Low grade MALT lymphoma
   d. Hypertrophic gastritis

8. **H. pylori infection is associated with development of which malignancy:** *(DPG 2011)*
   a. MALTomas
   b. Atherosclerosis
   c. Sarcoma
   d. Gastrointestinal stromal tumor (GIST)

9. **Urease breath test is used to diagnose in which bacteria?** *(Recent Question 2018)*
   a. Streptococci
   b. H. pylori
   c. C. jejuni
   d. Bacteroides

PEPTIC ULCER ETIOLOGY AND CLINICAL FEATURES

10. **Peptic ulcer is associated with all except one:** *(AIIMS Feb 97)*
    a. Cirrhosis
    b. Zollinger Ellison syndrome
    c. Primary hyperparathyroidism
    d. Pernicious anemia

11. **Which one is not associated with peptic ulcer?** *(AIIMS Nov 95)*
    a. Smoking cigarette
    b. Zollinger-Ellison's syndrome
    c. Plummer-Vinson syndrome
    d. Cirrhosis

12. **Which of the following factors contribute to the development of duodenal ulcers?** *(PGI June 2001)*
    a. Lysolecithin
    b. Gastric acid
    c. Alcohol abuse
    d. Prostaglandins
    e. Smoking

13. **Commonest site of peptic ulcer is:** *(All India 99)*
    a. 1st part of duodenum
    b. 2nd part of duodenum
    c. Distal 1/3rd of stomach
    d. Pylorus of the stomach

14. **The most common site of a benign (peptic) gastric ulcer is:** *(AIIMS June 2004)*
    a. Upper third of lesser curvature
    b. Greater curvature
    c. Pyloric antrum
    d. Lesser curvature near incisura angularis

15. **What is correct about duodenal ulcer?** *(Kerala 2003)*
    a. 25% will occur if H. pylori is not eradicated
    b. Magnesium containing drugs may cause constipation
    c. Bismuth is not used for long terms
    d. None of the above

16. **With reference to duodenal ulcers, consider the following statements:** *(UPSC 2007)*
    1. They occur most often in the second part of duodenum
    2. Infection with H. pylori and NSAID - induces injury account for majority of duodenal ulcer
    3. Malignant duodenal ulcers are extremely rare
    4. Eradication of H. pylori has greatly reduced the recurrence rates in duodenal ulcers
    Which of the statements given above are correct?
    a. 1, 2 and 3 only
    b. 2, 3 and 4 only
    c. 1 and 4 only
    d. 1, 2, 3 and 4

17. **Burning epigastric pain is due to:**
    a. Vomiting
    b. Reflux esophagitis
    c. Duodenal ulcer
    d. Gastric ulcer

18. **Increased gastric acid secretion occurs in:** *(AIIMS GIS May 2011)*
    a. Type I gastric ulcer
    b. Type III gastric ulcer
    c. Type IV gastric ulcer
    d. All of the above

19. **Prepyloric or channel ulcer in the stomach is termed as:** *(Recent Question 2016, COMEDK 2008)*
    a. Type 1
    b. Type 2
    c. Type 3
    d. Type 4

20. **Gastric ulcer type III is located at:** *(Recent Question 2017)*
    a. Lesser curvature
    b. Body
    c. Prepyloric region
    d. GE junction

21. **Most common location for chronic gastric ulcer:** *(Recent Question 2018)*
    a. Antrum
    b. Fundus
    c. Greater curve
    d. Lesser curve

22. A 30-year-old male presents to the emergency department with symptoms of epigastric pain radiating to back that wakes him up at night and is relieved by consuming food. He gives history of similar pain in the past which was diagnosed as perforated duodenal ulcer and treated with omental patch surgery on two occasions. Pain before and after surgery has been controlled with proton pump inhibitors and analgesics. The likely diagnosis on this occasion is: *(All India 2011)*
    a. Duodenal Ulcer
    b. Gastric Ulcer
    c. Atrophic Gastritis
    d. Chronic Pancreatitis

PEPTIC ULCER COMPLICATIONS

23. A 30-year-old male presented with massive hematemesis. A 2 × 2 cm ulcer was visualized on upper GI endoscopy on the posterior aspect of first part of duodenum. The bleeding vessel was visualized but bleeding could not be controlled endoscopically. Blood transfusion was done and patient was planned for surgery. His BP was 90/70 and PR = 110/min with Hb = 9 gm% at the time of surgery. Which of the following would be best surgical management? *(All India 2012)*
    a. Antrectomy with ligation of left gastric artery
    b. Duodenotomy with ligation of bleeding vessels with postoperative PPI
    c. Duodenotomy with ligation of bleeding vessels, truncal vagotomy and pyloroplasty
    d. Duodenotomy with ligation of bleeding vessels, highly selective vagotomy

24. Which of the following vessel is most commonly involved in hemorrhage from duodenal ulcer?
    a. IVC *(Recent Question 2016, 2014, All India 2012)*
    b. Gastroduodenal artery
    c. SMA
    d. Inferior pancreatico duodenal artery

25. Most common complication of chronic gastric ulcer is:
    a. Tea pot stomach *(AIIMS June 93)*
    b. Scirrhous carcinoma (Adenocarcinoma)
    c. Perforation
    d. Massive hematemesis

26. In gastric outlet obstruction in a peptic ulcer patient, the site of obstruction is most likely to be:
    (All India 2002, AIIMS June 93)
    a. Antrum
    b. Duodenum
    c. Pylorus
    d. Pyloric canal

27. A Posteriorly perforating ulcer in the pyloric antrum of the stomach is most likely to produce initial localized peritonitis or abscess formation in the following:
    a. Omental bursa (lesser sac) *(PGI June 2009, All India 2003)*
    b. Greater sac
    c. Right subphrenic space
    d. Hepatorenal space (pouch of Morison)

28. A 60-year-old male had a sudden fall in toilet. His BP was 90/50 mm Hg and PR = 100/min. His relatives reported that he is a known case of hypertension and CAD and was regularly taking aspirin, atenolol and sorbitrate. The most likely diagnosis: *(AIIMS May 2012)*
    a. Gastric ulcer with bleeding
    b. Acute MI with cardiogenic shock
    c. Acute CVA
    d. Pulmonary embolism

29. Treatment of perforated peptic ulcer includes: *(PGI Dec 2001)*
    a. IV fluids
    b. Drainage of paracolic gutter
    c. Immediate surgery
    d. Antacids
    e. IV pantoprazole

30. Percentage of patients with perforated peptic ulcer who show free gas under the diaphragm: *(UPPG 2009)*
    a. 100%
    b. 75%
    c. 50%
    d. 90%

31. Commonest cause of death in peptic ulcer patients is:
    (All India 90)
    a. Perforation
    b. Hemorrhage
    c. Pyloric stenosis
    d. Malignancy

32. Investigation of choice in peptic ulcer perforation is:
    (KERALA 94)
    a. USG
    b. X-ray abdomen
    c. Paracentesis
    d. CT scan

33. About 6–8 hours after peptic ulcer perforation the disappearance of abdominal wall rigidity is due to: *(UPSC 95)*
    a. Cessation of acid secretion in the stomach
    b. Revival from initial shock
    c. Dilution of acid in the peritoneal cavity
    d. Fatigue of reflex arc

34. Posterior perforation of peptic ulcer drain into: *(DNB 2009)*
    a. Omental bursa
    b. Greater sac
    c. Foramen of Winslow
    d. Paracolic gutter

35. Prognosis in a case of duodenal perforation is determined by all except: *(PGI 96)*
    a. Age of the patient
    b. Duration of history
    c. Basal pneumonia
    d. Peritonitis

36. The vessel which needs to be ligated in a patient with a bleeding peptic ulcer is: *(APPG 2015)*
    a. Gastroduodenal artery
    b. Superior pancreatico-duodenal artery
    c. Left gastric artery
    d. Left gastroepiploic artery

37. In last decade, duodenal ulcer and its morbidity is reduced due to: *(Recent Question 2015)*
    a. Lifestyle modification
    b. Eradication of H. pylori
    c. Proton pump inhibitors
    d. None of the above

PEPTIC ULCER DIAGNOSIS AND TREATMENT

38. PPI's for peptic ulcer disease should be taken: *(JIPMER 2011)*
    a. Before breakfast
    b. After breakfast
    c. After lunch
    d. After dinner

39. Which of the following acid reducing surgery doesn't require drainage procedure? *(PGI Dec 2007)*
    a. Highly selective vagotomy
    b. Billroth-I operation
    c. Antrectomy
    d. Gastric resection
    e. Truncal vagotomy

40. Highly selective vagotomy preserves: *(MHPGMCET 2002)*
    a. Nerves of Latarjet
    b. Nerve of Kuntz
    c. Nerve of Mayo
    d. All of the above

41. Stump of stomach and duodenum is present in:
    (MHSSMCET 2006)
    a. Billroth-I operation
    b. Billroth-II operation
    c. Whipple's operation
    d. Truncal vagotomy

Stomach and Duodenum

42. **Pyloroplasty of choice when the DU is fibrosed and contracted?** *(MHSSMCET 2009)*
    a. Finney's pyloroplasty
    b. Billroth type I surgery
    c. Billroth type II surgery
    d. Ramsted's operation

43. **H. pylori is associated with ____% of gastric ulcers:**
    a. 5
    b. 20 *(JIPMER 2011)*
    c. 40–60
    d. 80

44. **Barium meal characteristic feature of malignant gastric ulcer is:** *(JIPMER November 2017)*
    a. Hampton line
    b. Carman's meniscus sign
    c. Ulcer cap
    d. Ulcer crater

45. **A patient who has undergone partial gastrectomy presents with neurological symptoms. Most probable diagnosis:** *(JIPMER 2011)*
    a. Folic acid deficiency
    b. Thiamine deficiency
    c. Vitamin B_{12} deficiency
    d. Iron deficiency

46. **Treatment of high lying ulcer near gastroesophageal junction is/are:** *(PGI Nov 2009)*
    a. Pouchet procedure
    b. Kelling-Madlener operation
    c. Csendes procedure
    d. Total gastrectomy
    e. Vagotomy and pyloroplasty

47. **In a highly selective vagotomy, the vagal supply is severed to:** *(COMEDK 2008)*
    a. Proximal two-thirds of stomach
    b. Antrum
    c. Pylorus
    d. Whole of stomach

48. **Incorrect about gastric ulcer:** *(PGI Nov 2009)*
    a. Most common on lesser curvature
    b. 70% H. pylori related
    c. Type IV ulcer most common type
    d. Treatment is primarily medical
    e. 30% GU are associated with malignancy

49. **True statement(s) regarding peptic ulcer disease:**
    a. Anterior ulcer bleeds more commonly *(PGI June 2009)*
    b. Posteriorly perforated ulcer is always management conservatively
    c. Anti-H. pylori drugs must be included in the treatment regime
    d. H. pylori is known to increase incidence of gastric malignancies
    e. Increase acid production in prerequisite for gastric ulcer

50. **All of the following drugs are used in the management of peptic ulcer except:** *(COMEDK 2005)*
    a. Alginic acid
    b. Sucralfate
    d. Misoprostol
    d. Ipratropium

51. **Surgery of choice for chronic duodenal ulcer is:** *(Recent Question 2014, AIIMS June 93)*
    a. Vagotomy + antrectomy
    b. Total gastrectomy
    c. Truncal vagotomy + pyloroplasty
    d. Highly selective vagotomy

52. **Patient presents with recurrent duodenal ulcer of 2.5 cm size, procedure of choice:** *(All India 2001)*
    a. Truncal vagotomy and antrectomy
    b. Truncal vagotomy and gastrojejunostomy
    c. Highly selective vagotomy
    d. Laparoscopic vagotomy and gastrojejunostomy

53. **Lowest recurrence rate in duodenal ulcer treatment is seen with:** *(MHCET 2016, Recent Question 2014, AIIMS Nov 94, All India 2002)*
    a. Highly selective vagotomy
    b. Truncal vagotomy
    c. Truncal vagotomy and antrectomy
    d. Truncal vagotomy and pyloroplasty

54. **Endoscopy is useful in diagnosis of peptic ulcer in following situations except:**
    a. Post bulbar ulcer
    b. Stomal ulcers
    c. Giant duodenal ulcer
    d. Duodenal erosion

55. **All of the following are indications for surgery in a case of duodenal ulcer except:** *(UPCS 96)*
    a. Acute perforation of ulcer
    b. Pyloric stenosis
    c. Massive hemorrhage
    d. Typical periodicity

56. **Maximal reduction in gastric acidity is achieved by:** *(Recent Question 2014, UPCS 97)*
    a. Truncal vagotomy and pyloroplasty
    b. Truncal vagotomy and antrectomy
    c. Partial gastrectomy
    d. Highly selective vagotomy

57. **Perforated peptic ulcer is treated by:** *(SGPGI 2005)*
    a. Vagotomy + Pyloroplasty
    b. Vagotomy + Antrectomy
    c. Vagotomy + repair of perforation
    d. Graham's repair

58. **Lesser curvature anterior seromyotomy is indicated in:**
    a. Gastric ulcer
    b. Gastric CA *(MAHE 2005)*
    c. Duodenal blowout
    d. Duodenal ulcer

59. **The most commonly practiced operative procedure for a perforated duodenal ulcer is:** *(Recent Question 2014, Karnataka 2005)*
    a. Vagotomy and pyloroplasty
    b. Vagotomy and antrectomy
    c. Vagotomy and perforation closure
    d. Graham's omentum patch repair

60. **In a highly selective vagotomy, the vagal supply is severed to:** *(COMEDK 2007)*
    a. Proximal two-thirds of stomach
    b. Antrum
    c. Pylorus
    d. Whole of stomach

61. **Treatment of choice in type III gastric ulcer is:** *(UPPG 2008)*
    a. Vagotomy only
    b. Vagotomy and antrectomy
    c. Vagotomy and pyloroplasty
    d. Highly selective vagotomy

62. **HSV is done in:** *(AIIMS GIS Dec 2006)*
    a. Menetrier's disease
    b. Giant gastric ulcer
    c. Gastric mucosal erosions
    d. Megaesophagus treatment by esophageal mucosal resection

GASTRECTOMY AND COMPLICATIONS

63. **Most common metabolic complication of gastrectomy:** *(AIIMS GIS Dec 2011)*
    a. Iron deficiency anemia
    b. Megaloblastic anemia
    c. Hypocalcemia
    d. Osteoporosis

64. **Most common abnormality after gastric resection and Billroth-II:** *(AIIMS GIS Dec 2009)*
    a. Vitamin B_{12} deficiency
    b. Steatorrhea
    c. Calcium deficiency
    d. Vitamin D deficiency

65. **A patient of partial gastrectomy presents with neurological symptoms. Most probable diagnosis is:** *(JIPMER 2011)*
    a. Folic acid deficiency
    b. Thiamine deficiency
    c. Vitamin B_{12} deficiency
    d. Iron deficiency

66. **Gastric atony occurs in all except:** *(AIIMS GIS Dec 2006)*
    a. Billroth-I
    b. Billroth-II
    c. HSV
    d. Posterior selective vagotomy with anterior seromyotomy

67. **Long-term effects of gastrectomy includes:** *(PGI SS Dec 2009)*
    a. Renal calculi
    b. Vitamin C deficiency
    c. Hypothyroidism
    d. Osteomalacia

68. **Dumping syndrome is due to:** *(Recent Question 2017, Recent Question 2015, All India 99)*
    a. Diarrhea
    b. Presence of hypertonic content in small intestine
    c. Vagotomy
    d. Reduced gastric capacity

69. **Which is not true about dumping syndrome?** *(DNB 2014)*
    a. Post vagotomy
    b. Small frequent meals is beneficial
    c. Starch is beneficial
    d. Clinical features include diarrhea and bloating

70. **All are true regarding early post-cibal syndrome, except:**
    a. Distension of abdomen *(All India 2000)*
    b. Managed conservatively
    c. Hypermotility of intestine is common
    d. Surgery is usually indicated

71. **Duodenal blow out following Billroth gastrectomy most commonly occurs on which day:** *(Recent Question 2015, AIIMS June 93)*
    a. 2nd day
    b. 4th day
    c. 6th day
    d. 12th day

72. **In gastrectomy following occurs except:** *(PGI Dec 97)*
    a. Calcium deficiency
    b. Steatorrhea
    c. Fe^{2+} deficiency
    d. Fluid loss

73. **The earliest manifestation seen after gastrectomy:** *(PGI Dec 2005)*
    a. Incidence of infection
    b. Loss of storage capacity
    c. Loss of HCl
    d. Loss of intrinsic factor

74. **The commonest earliest complication of TV and GJ is:**
    a. Stomal obstruction
    b. Paralytic ileus *(AIIMS 91)*
    c. Gastric leak
    d. Anastomotic hemorrhage

75. **Anemia is greater in which of the following gastric resection:** *(PGI 81, AMU 85)*
    a. Billroth-II
    b. Billroth-I
    c. Both of the above are equal
    d. Neither of the above

76. **A person who had undergone gastrojejunostomy suddenly develops severe diarrhea. Which should be suspected?** *(TN 95)*
    a. Gastric carcinoma
    b. Tuberculosis of abdomen
    c. Gastrojejunocolic fistula
    d. Gastric amoebiasis

77. **The operation where in the stump of the stomach is directly anastomosed to the stump of the duodenum is called:** *(Karnataka 96)*
    a. Polya gastrectomy
    b. Hoffmeister gastrectomy
    c. Billroth-I gastrectomy
    d. Billroth-II gastrectomy

78. **Gastrojejunostomy is an example of:**
    a. Clean contaminated wound *(DNB 2001, JIPMER 2008)*
    b. Clean uncontaminated wound
    c. Unclean uncontaminated wound
    d. Unclean contaminated wound

79. **Which is a clean surgery:** *(Recent Question 2013)*
    a. Hernia surgery
    b. Gastric surgery
    c. Cholecystectomy
    d. Rectal surgery

80. **Duodenal blowout is:** *(APPG 97)*
    a. Perforation of duodenal ulcer
    b. Iatrogenic
    c. Complication of partial gastrectomy
    d. Due to trauma

81. **Postvagotomy diarrhea can be effectively managed by:** *(UPSC 2002)*
    a. Steroids
    b. Thyroxin
    c. Somatostatin analogue
    d. Parathormone

82. **The first gastrectomy was performed in 1881 by:**
    a. Miculikz
    b. Wolfer *(Bihar PG 2016)*
    c. Billroth
    d. Moynihan

83. **All are true about gastric resection except:**
    a. Decreased protein absorption *(DPG 2008)*
    b. Increased intestinal secretion
    c. Calcium deficiency
    d. Increased intestinal motility

UPPER GI BLEED

84. **BLEED risk criteria include all except:** *(AIIMS GIS Dec 2009)*
    a. Ongoing bleeding
    b. Low urine output
    c. BP < 100 mm Hg
    d. Altered mental status

85. **In Forrest classification, high-risk of bleeding is associated with all except:** *(KGMC 2011)*
    a. Visible vessel
    b. Visible pulsatile bleeding
    c. Adherent clot
    d. Visible oozing from vessel

86. **In case of UGI bleeding, all are true about endoscopy except:** *(AIIMS GIS Dec 2009)*
    a. Decreases transfusion requirement
    b. Leads to early discharge of the patient
    c. Can detect causes in all cases
    d. Best tool for localization of bleeding

87. **Investigation of choice for UGI bleed:** *(WBPG 2012, PGI SS 2004, June 97)*
    a. Endoscopy
    b. Angiography
    c. CT
    d. Barium studies

88. **Which of the following is the incorrect statement regarding GI bleeding?** *(AIIMS Nov 2004)*
    a. The sensitivity of angiography for detecting GI bleeding in about 10–20% as compared to nuclear imaging
    b. Angiography can image bleeding at a rate of 0.05–0.1 ml/min or less
    c. 99m Tc-RBC scan will image bleeding at rates as low as 0.05–0.1 ml/min
    d. Angiography will detect bleeding only, if extravasation is occurring during the injection of contrast

89. True about upper GI bleeding: *(PGI DEC 2003)*
    a. Melena is the only symptom
    b. Bleeding occurs beyond the ampula of vater
    c. Endoscopy can best diagnose it
    d. Peptic ulcer is the MC cause
    e. ↑ed BUN

90. A male executive, 50 years of age is seen in seen in casualty with hypotension and hematemesis. There is previous history suggestive of alcohol intake of 100 ml daily. The blood loss is around 2 litres. Most probable diagnosis is: *(AIIMS June 2001)*
    a. Gastritis
    b. Duodenal ulcer
    c. Mallory-Weiss tear
    d. Esophageal varices

91. A 42-year-old company executive presents with sudden upper GI bleed (5 litres) of bright red blood, with no significant previous history. The diagnosis is: *(All India 2000)*
    a. Esophageal varices
    b. Duodenal ulcer
    c. Gastritis
    d. Gastric erosion

92. Which of the following management procedures of acute upper gastrointestinal bleed should possibly be avoided? *(AIIMS Nov 2003)*
    a. Intravenous vasopressin
    b. Intravenous beta-blockers
    c. Endoscopic sclerotherapy
    d. Balloon tamponade

93. Following resuscitation, a patient with bleeding esophageal varices should be treated initially with: *(AIIMS Nov 2004)*
    a. Sclerotherapy
    b. Sengstaken Blackmore tube
    c. Propranolol
    d. Surgery

94. During sclerotherapy (by endoscopy), following are complications except: *(PGI June 98)*
    a. Hepatic encephalopathy
    b. Perforation
    c. Stenosis
    d. Fibrosis

95. A patient presented to emergency ward with massive upper gastrointestinal bleed. On examination, he has mild splenomegaly. In the absence of any other information available, which of the following is the most appropriate therapeutic modality? *(AIIMS Nov 2005)*
    a. Intravenous propranolol
    b. Intravenous vasopressin
    c. Intravenous pantoprazole
    d. Intravenous somatostatin

96. A patient comes with hematemesis and melena. On the upper GI endoscopy there was no significant finding. 2 days later the patient rebleeds. Next line of investigation is:
    a. Emergency angiography *(AIIMS May 2007)*
    b. Repeat upper GI endoscopy
    c. Enteroscopy
    d. Laparotomy

97. The most sensitive test to detect GI bleeding is:
    a. Selective angiography *(Recent Question 2016)*
    b. Radiolabelled erythrocyte scanning
    c. I-131 fibrinogen studies
    d. Stool for occult blood

98. In the Forrest classification for bleeding peptic ulcer with a visible vessel of pigmented protuberance is classified as: *(Recent Question 2016, COMEDK 2006)*
    a. FI
    b. FII a
    c. FII b
    d. FII c

99. A 45-year-old executive suddenly develops hematemesis at home. He is brought to the hospital 4 hours later, there he again has a bout of hematemesis. Total blood loss would be around 2 liters. Most likely diagnosis is: *(AIIMS 2001)*
    a. Gastritis
    b. Esophagitis
    c. Esophageal varices
    d. Duodenal ulcer

100. Most common cause of upper gastrointestinal tract bleeding is: *(Recent Question 2015, 2014, 2013)*
    a. Esophageal varices
    b. Peptic ulcer
    c. Gastritis
    d. Mallory weiss tear

101. Among the following, the least common cause of acute upper GI bleeding is: *(APPG 2015)*
    a. Vascular ectasia
    b. Mallory Weiss tear
    c. Ulcer
    d. Varices

102. Regarding Upper GI bleed, true statement is: *(Recent Question 2018)*
    a. Most common cause is variceal bleeding
    b. It is bleeding upto ampulla of Vater
    c. Most commonly performed management is endoscopic banding
    d. Rockall scoring is used for risk stratification

MALLORY-WEISS TEAR

103. False about Mallory-Weiss syndrome: *(ILBS 2011)*
    a. Massive hemorrhage is MC manifestation
    b. Alcohol is an associated etiology
    c. Conservative treatment is effective in most of the cases
    d. Anti-reflux procedure doesn't have added advantage

104. An old man presenting to the emergency following a bout of prolonged vomiting with excessive hematemesis following alcohol ingestion is likely to suffer from: *(MCI June 2018)*
    a. Mallory-Weiss syndrome
    b. Esophageal varices
    c. Gastric cancer
    d. Bleeding disorder

105. Mallory-Weiss syndrome is partial thickness rupture occurs at: *(Recent Question 2017, Recent Question 2016, WBPG 2014, PGI Dec 97)*
    a. Gastric cardia
    b. Esophagus mucosa
    c. Gastroesophageal junction
    d. Gastroduodenal junction

106. Violent vomiting after forceful retching present with sudden severe hematemesis diagnosis is: *(Recent Question 2018)*
    a. Haemangioma
    b. Carcinoma oesophagus
    c. Mallory-Weiss syndrome
    d. Esophageal varices

107. Bleeding from a Mallory Weiss tear occurs usually from: *(AIIMS May 2015)*
    a. Phrenic vein
    b. Left gastric artery
    c. Short gastric arteries
    d. Coronary vein

DIEULAFOY'S LESION

108. All are true about Dieulafoy's lesion except: *(AIIMS GIS Dec 2011)*
    a. Angiographic embolization is the preferred treatment
    b. Endoscopic treatment can be given
    c. Pulsation of artery causes ulceration
    d. Submucosal artery

109. **Dieulafoy's lesion:** *(PGI SS June 2005)*
    a. Within 6 cm of GE junction
    b. In esophagus
    c. In ileum
    d. In rectum

110. **Dieulafoy's lesion is:** *(Recent Question 2016, MHSSMCET 2006)*
    a. Prolapse gastropathy
    b. Gastric antral vascular ectasia
    c. Gastric hemorrhagic telengectasias
    d. Aberrant vessel in the mucosa that bleeds form a mucosal defect

GASTRIC ANTRAL VASCULAR ECTASIA

111. **All are true about GAVE except:** *(JIPMER GIS 2011)*
    a. Dilated submucosal venous plexus
    b. Bleeding is the most common presentation
    c. Pain is most common clinical symptom
    d. Argon laser treatment is established one

112. **'Watermelon stomach' is:** *(MHSSMCET 2008)*
    a. Prolapse gastropathy
    b. Gastric antral vascular ectasia
    c. Gastric hemorrhagic telengectasias
    d. Aberrant vessel in the mucosa that bleeds form a mucosal defect

113. **What is the most probable diagnosis on the basis of given endoscopy image?** *(Recent Question 2016)*
    a. Dieulafoy's lesion
    b. Gastric antral vascular ectasia
    c. Menetrier's disease
    d. Mallory-Weiss syndrome

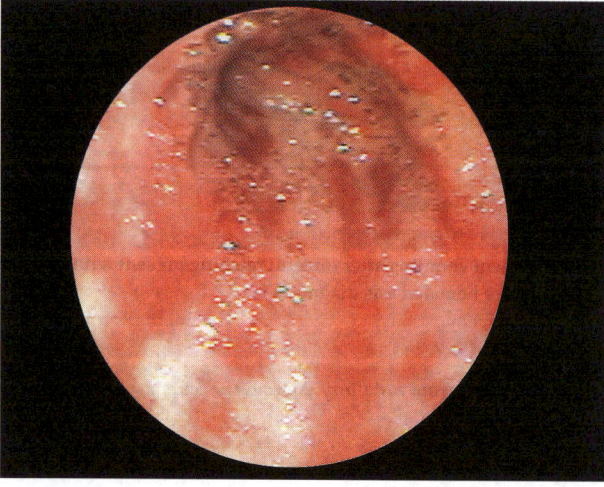

MENETRIER'S DISEASE

114. **Menetrier's disease is characterized by all except:** *(AIIMS GIS Dec 2011)*
    a. Excessive protein loss
    b. Excessive mucus production
    c. Diarrhea
    d. Hyperchlorhydria

115. A 50 years old male presented with the history of epigastric pain, anorexia, weight loss and pedal edema. On laboratory examination, total protein and albumin was low. Endoscopy was performed and the image is given below. What is the most probable diagnosis?

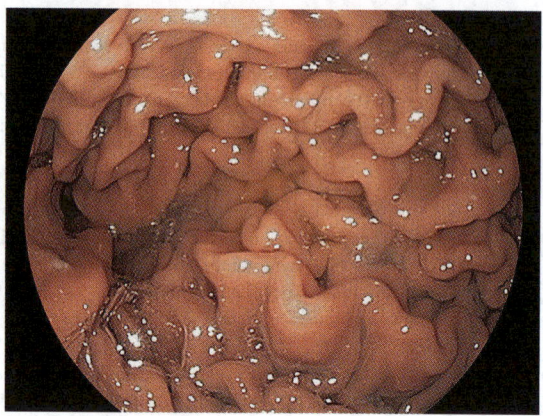

    a. Gastric varices   b. Carcinoma stomach
    c. Hamartomatous polyp   d. Menetrier's disease

116. **All are true about Menetrier's disease except:**
    a. Protein loss *(AIIMS GIS Dec 2006)*
    b. Hyperchlorhydria
    c. Cobblestone appearance of mucosa
    d. Associated with CMV and H. pylori

117. **Thickened gastric folds are found in:** *(PGI June 2003)*
    a. Lymphoma   b. Menetrier's disease
    c. Carcinoma   d. Eosinophilic gastritis
    e. Giardiasis

118. **Menetrier's disease is characterized by all of the following except:** *(COMEDK 2006)*
    a. Giant folds in the pyloric antrum
    b. Foveolar hyperplasia
    c. Hypoalbuminaemia
    d. Hypochlorhydria

GASTRIC POLYPS

119. **Most common benign tumour of the stomach is:**
    a. Adenoma   b. Lipoma
    c. Hamartoma   d. Leiomyoma

120. **The commonest gastric polyp is:** *(COMEDK 2008)*
    a. Hyperplastic polyp   b. Inflammatory polyp
    c. Adenomatous polyp   d. Part of familial polyposis

121. **True regarding hyperplastic gastric polyp is:** *(PGI May 2018)*
    a. Most common gastric polyp
    b. Pre-malignant
    c. Mostly non-Hodgkin's lymphoma
    d. More common in young adults
    e. Surgery is done if they are symptomatic

CARCINOMA STOMACH PREDISPOSING FACTORS

122. **All of the following increases the risk of CA stomach except:** *(PGI SS 2004)*
    a. Benign ulcer   b. Atrophic gastritis
    c. Previous gastric surgery d. Blood group A

123. Due to popularity of refrigeration reducing the need to preserve food, which cancer's incidence has dramatically declined? *(AIIMS May 2013)*
    a. Esophagus
    b. Stomach
    c. Colon
    d. Oropharyngeal malignancies
124. Risk factors for gastric cancer include: *(PGI November 2017)*
    a. Chronic atrophic gastritis
    b. Obesity
    c. Smoking
    d. H. pylori infection
    e. Menetrier's disease
125. Gastric carcinoma is associated with blood group:
    a. A
    b. B *(PGI SS June 2001)*
    c. AB
    d. O
126. E-cadherin is more often mutated in: *(COMEDK 2010)*
    a. Diffuse type of gastric cancer
    b. Intestinal type of gastric cancer
    c. Malignant ulcer of stomach
    d. Erosive gastritis
127. Which of the following anemia is a risk factor for the development of gastric carcinoma? *(DNB 2011, COMEDK 2007)*
    a. Pernicious anemia
    b. Megaloblastic anemia
    c. Aplastic anemia
    d. Hemolytic anemia
128. Risk factor for development of gastric CA: *(All India 2002)*
    a. Blood group 'O'
    b. Duodenal ulcer
    c. Intestinal hyperplasia
    d. Intestinal metaplasia type III
129. Predisposing factor for CA stomach are all except:
    a. Chronic gastric atrophy *(PGI Dec 97)*
    b. Hyperplastic polyp
    c. Metaplasia grade III intestine
    d. Pernicious anemia
130. Predisposing factors for gastric carcinoma are: *(PGI June 2002)*
    a. Atrophic gastritis
    b. Hyperplastic polyp
    c. Adenomatous polyp
    d. Achlorhydria
    e. Animal fat consumption
131. Which of the following is the most significant risk factor for development of gastric carcinoma? *(All India 2006)*
    a. Paneth cell metaplasia
    b. Pyloric metaplasia
    c. Intestinal metaplasia
    d. Ciliated metaplasia
132. All of the following predispose to gastric carcinoma except: *(All India 1990)*
    a. Achlorhydria
    b. 'O' blood group
    c. Pernicious anaemia
    d. Postgastrectomy
133. Precancerous condition of the stomach is: *(Kerala 91)*
    a. Lipoma
    b. Linnitis plastic
    c. Atrophic gastritis
    d. Hyperacidity
134. Malignant transformation is commonly seen in: *(AIIMS 91)*
    a. Stomal ulcer
    b. Gastric ulcer
    c. Chronic duodenal ulcer
    d. Postbulbar ulcer
135. All are true about gastric carcinoma except: *(DNB 2006)*
    a. More in low socioeconomic group
    b. Most common at fundus
    c. H. pylori infection increases risks
    d. Vitamin C protects
136. Gastric malignancy is predisposed with: *(Kerala 2004)*
    a. Blood group O
    b. Intestinal metaplasia
    c. Gastric hyperplasia
    d. Duodenal ulcer
137. AKT-1 amplification is seen in: *(Recent Question 2016)*
    a. CA bladder
    b. CA colon
    c. Breast cancer
    d. Gastric cancer

CA STOMACH CLINICAL FEATURES AND TREATMENT

138. All are true about diffuse carcinoma of stomach except:
    a. Occurs at distal end *(PGI SS June 2001)*
    b. Occurs at cardia
    c. Genetic rather than environmental cause
    d. Occurs in younger patients
139. According to Borrman's classification, Linnitis plastica is: *(AIIMS GIS May 2011)*
    a. Type I
    b. Type II
    c. Type III
    d. Type IV
140. All of the following are true about diffuse gastric cancer according to Lauren's classification except:
    a. Familial *(Recent Question 2017)*
    b. More common in males
    c. Undifferentiated
    d. More common in the proximal part
141. Hereditary diffuse gastric carcinoma is associated with: *(Recent Question 2017)*
    a. Ductal carcinoma NOS subtype
    b. Lobular carcinoma
    c. Ductal carcinoma in-situ
    d. Metaplastic carcinoma
142. Type 1 gastric cancer according to Bormann's classification: *(Recent Question 2017)*
    a. Protruding
    b. Ulcerated
    c. Flat
    d. Excavated
143. GE junction tumor is: *(Recent Question 2017)*
    a. Siewert type I
    b. Siewert type II
    c. Siewert type III
    d. Siewert type IV
144. Not seen in intestinal type of gastric cancer: *(AIIMS GIS Dec 2011, Dec 2009)*
    a. Decreased E-cadherin
    b. APC
    c. Microsatellite instability
    d. p53
145. Not true in case of diffuse carcinoma stomach:
    a. More common *(AIIMS GIS Dec 2009)*
    b. Poorly differentiated with signet ring cells
    c. Transmural or lymphatic spread
    d. Decreased E-cadherin
146. Not seen in intestinal type of gastric cancer: *(AIIMS GIS Dec 2009)*
    a. Decreased E-cadherin
    b. APC
    c. p16
    d. p53
147. All are true about diffuse gastric carcinoma (Lauren's) except: *(JIPMER GIS 2011)*
    a. Blood group 'A'
    b. E-cadherin positive
    c. Hematogenous spread
    d. Common in females
148. Carcinoma stomach which perforates serosa but doesn't involve nearby structures, the stage is: *(KGMC 2011)*
    a. I
    b. II
    c. IIIA
    d. IIIB
149. Diffuse and intestinal variant of CA stomach both have: *(AIIMS GIS Dec 2006)*
    a. E-cadherin
    b. APC
    c. p53
    d. Microsatellite instability

150. **Gastric lymph node station no 5:** *(AIIMS GIS Dec 2009)*
    a. Suprapyloric b. Splenic hilum
    c. Lessar curvature d. Greater curvature

151. **Level 9 lymph node includes:** *(Recent Question 2016, AIIMS GIS Dec 2010)*
    a. Celiac nodes
    b. Splenic hilum
    c. Splenic artery
    d. Hepatoduodenal ligament

152. **Sister Joseph's nodule may indicated cancer of all the following except:** *(COMEDK 2004)*
    a. Somach b. Large bowel
    c. Rectum d. Ovary

153. **Which of the following statements about gastric carcinoma are true?** *(All India 2011)*
    a. Squamous cell carcinoma is the most common histological subtype
    b. Often associated with hypochlorhydria/achlorhydria
    c. Occult blood in stool is not seen
    d. Highly radiosensitive tumor

154. **Most common site of carcinoma of stomach is:** *(JIPMER 2010)*
    a. Proximal stomach b. Gastric antrum
    c. Lesser curvature d. Greater curvature

155. **An ulcero-proliferative lesion in the antrum of the stomach 6 cm in diameter, invading the serosa, with 10 enlarged lymph nodes around and pylorus with no distant metastasis, the TNM staging is:** *(COMEDK 2011)*
    a. T2N1M0 b. T3N2M0
    c. T4N1M0 d. T1N3M0

156. **True about gastric stump carcinoma:** *(PGI Nov 2009)*
    a. Enterogastric reflex is the cause
    b. Prognosis good after surgery
    c. It is always adenocarcinoma in nature
    d. Diffuse type is only variety

157. **All are true about gastric CA except:** *(PGI June 2009)*
    a. H. pylori association is present
    b. D2 gastrectomy include total gastrectomy
    c. Surgical non curative lesion should not be resected
    d. Patient under total gastrectomy should be given vitamin B_{12}
    e. Hematemesis present in majority of patients

158. **Troisier's sign is:** *(MHPGMCET 2008, 2006, APPG 96)*
    a. Metastatic left supraclavicular lymphadenopathy
    b. Carpopedal spasm in hypocalcemia
    c. Migratory thrombophlebitis
    d. Any of the above

159. **Independent risk factor for carcinoma stomach:**
    a. H. pylori *(MHPGMCET 2008)*
    b. Gastrectomy with drainage procedure
    c. Vagotomy with drainage procedure
    d. All of the above

160. **Irish node is most commonly seen in:** *(WB PG 2015)*
    a. Ca stomach b. Ca lung
    c. Ca larynx d. CA endometrium

161. **True about carcinoma stomach include all the following except:** *(MHSSMCET 2007)*
    a. Smoky diet is risk factor
    b. Incidence is now decreasing in Japan and China
    c. Duodenal ulcers are not associated with gastric cancer
    d. Gastric adenocarcinoma is a radioresistant tumor

162. **When carcinoma of stomach develops secondarily to pernicious anemia, it is usually situated in the:**
    a. Pre-pyloric region b. Pylorus *(All India 2006)*
    c. Body d. Fundus

163. **The best prognosis in carcinoma stomach is with:** *(Bihar PG 2014, UPSC 2008, All India 95)*
    a. Superficial spreading type b. Ulcerative type
    c. Linnitis plastica type d. Polypoidal type

164. **All the following indicates early gastric cancer except:** *(Recent Question 2015, DNB 2006, All India 2002, AIIMS Feb 97)*
    a. Involvement of mucosa
    b. Involvement of mucosa and submucosa
    c. Involvement of mucosa, submucosa and muscularis
    d. Involvement of mucosa, submucosa and adjacent lymph nodes

165. **For early diagnosis of CA stomach, which method is used?**
    a. Endoscopy *(AIIMS Feb 97)*
    b. Staining with endoscopic biopsy
    c. Physical examination
    d. Ultrasound abdomen

166. **An adult presented with hematemesis and upper abdominal pain. Endoscopy revealed a growth at the pyloric antrum of the stomach. CT scan showed growth involving the pyloric antrum without infiltration or invasion into surrounding structures and no evidence of distant metastasis. At laparotomy neoplastic growth was observed to involve the posterior wall of stomach and the pancreas extending 6 cm up to tail of pancreas. What will be the most appropriate surgical management?** *(All India 2010)*
    a. Closure of the abdomen
    b. Antrectomy and vagotomy
    c. Partial gastrectomy + distal pancreatectomy
    d. Partial gastrectomy + distal pancreatectomy + splenectomy

167. **Kally, a 60 years old male diagnosed to have carcinoma stomach. CT scan of abdomen showed a mass measuring 4 × 4 cm in the antrum with involvement of celiac nodes and right gastric nodes. Management of choice is:** *(AIIMS June 2001)*
    a. Total gastrectomy b. Subtotal gastrectomy
    c. Palliative d. Chemotherapy

168. **True about early gastric carcinoma:** *(PGI Dec 2002)*
    a. Invasion of mucosa and submucosa with neighboring lymph node
    b. Invasion of mucosa and submucosa irrespective to LN spread
    c. Endoscopic removal of lesions
    d. Conservative gastrectomy

169. **Operability in carcinoma stomach is indicated by all except:**
    a. Involvement of omental nodes
    b. Involvement of lymph nodes at the celiac axis
    c. Lymph node at porta hepatis
    d. Solitary metastatic nodule in the liver
    e. Krukenberg tumor

170. **Linnitis plastica is commonly seen in:** *(Recent Question 2014, DNB 2005, 2001, 2000, All India 91)*
    a. Carcinoma stomach b. Sarcoidosis
    c. Lymphoma d. Leiomyosarcoma

171. **All of the following may be features of a silent carcinoma of the body of the stomach except:**
    a. Obstructive jaundice b. Ascites
    c. Dysphagia d. Krukenberg tumours

172. Presenting symptom of carcinoma stomach is:
    a. Bleeding   b. Obstruction
    c. Perforation   d. Weight loss
173. Gastric carcinoma involving the antrum with lymph node involvements. The pancreas, liver and peritoneal cavity are normal. Most appropriate surgery is:
    a. Total radical gastrectomy   b. Palliative gastrectomy
    c. Gastrojejunostomy   d. None of the above
174. Lymphatic drainage of CA stomach is mostly to: *(DPG 2005)*
    a. Left gastric   b. Pyloric
    c. Celiac   d. None of the above
175. Sister Mary Joseph nodule is most commonly seen with:
    (AIIMS May 2009)
    a. Ovarian cancer   b. Stomach cancer
    c. Colon cancer   d. Pancreatic cancer
176. Which of the following is not associated with this finding given in the image?
    a. Carcinoma pancreas   b. Carcinoma stomach
    c. Testicular tumors   d. Ovarian cancer

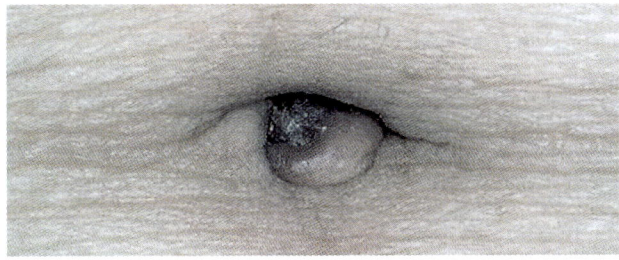

177. Peritoneal dissemination of gastric cancer is best detected by: *(COMEDK 2014)*
    a. USG   b. Laparoscopy
    c. CT   d. MRI
178. Locally invasive gastric carcinoma. Investigation of choice to know depth of cancer invasion: *(Recent Question 2013)*
    a. CECT   b. MRI
    c. Barium   d. EUS
179. Most common cause of Krukenberg's tumor is: *(DNB 2014)*
    a. Ovary   b. Liver
    c. Stomach   d. Kidney

GASTROINTESTINAL STROMAL TUMOR

180. Cell of origin in GIST: *(GB Pant 2011)*
    a. Mesenchymal   b. Argentaffin
    c. Smooth muscle d. Epithelial
181. Which of the following is false about GIST?
    a. More common in female   *(Recent Question 2017)*
    b. >5 cm in size is high-risk
    c. Mesodermal origin
    d. Treatment of choice is segmental resection
182. For high-risk cases of GIST of size >10 cm, imatinib therapy is given for: *(Recent Question 2017)*
    a. 1 year   b. 2 years
    c. 3 years   d. 5 years
183. Treatment of choice for localized GIST:
    (Recent Question 2017)
    a. Segmental resection   b. Total gastrectomy
    c. Distal gastrectomy   d. Imatinib mesylate
184. PDGFRA mutation is seen in: *(Recent Question 2016)*
    a. Aplastic anemia   b. ITP
    c. GIST   d. GI lymphoma
185. Imatinib used in treatment of:
    (Recent Question 2017, Recent Question 2016)
    a. GIST   b. GI lymphoma
    c. CA esophagus   d. CA colon
186. Most common site of GIST: *(Recent Question 2016)*
    a. Esophagus   b. Stomach
    c. Small intestine d. Colon
187. False about GIST: *(KGMC 2011)*
    a. Stomach is most common site
    b. Can present with bleeding
    c. Commonly metastasize to lymph nodes
    d. Can present with peritoneal metastasis
188. Sunitinib is used in: *(KGMC 2011)*
    a. GIST   b. Rectal cancer
    c. Colonic carcinoma d. Pancreatic carcinoma
189. Tyrosine kinase inhibitor imatinib is used for the treatment of: *(JIPMER 2011)*
    a. Fibrosarcoma phylloides   b. GIST
    c. MALT   d. Seminoma
190. A 50 years old male presents with obstructive symptoms. Biopsy of stomach reveals gastrointestinal stromal tumor (GIST). Most appropriate market for GIST is:
    (Recent Question 2017, Recent Question 2016, AIIMS May 2011)
    a. CD-34   b. CD-117
    c. CD-30   d. CD-10
191. Gold standard investigation for recurrent gastrointestinal stromal tumor is: *(AIIMS May 2011)*
    a. MRI   b. MIBG
    c. USG   d. PET-CT
192. True about GIST all except:
    (Recent Question 2015, AIIMS Nov 2010)
    a. Most common in duodenum
    b. Necrosis and ulceration present
    c. PET is used to assess response to therapy
    d. Cell circumscribed
193. Carney triad consists of: *(PGI May 2011)*
    a. Gastric carcinoma   b. Paraganglioma
    c. Pulmonary chordoma   d. Carcinoma bronchus
    e. Chondromatosis
194. GIST (Stromal tumors of GI tract) arise form:
    (MHSSMCET 2008)
    a. Paneth cells   b. Stave cells
    c. Enterocytes   d. Interstitial cells of Cajal
195. Commonest stomach tumour which bleeds:
    a. Adenocarcinoma   b. Squamous carcinoma
    c. Leiomyosarcoma   d. Fibrosarcoma
196. Most common type of gastric sarcoma: *(MCI June 2018)*
    a. Lipoma   b. Glomus tumour
    c. Leiomyosarcoma   d. Leioblastoma
197. Bleeding is seen maximally in which gastric tumors?
    (Punjab 2008)
    a. Adenocarcinoma
    b. Squamous cell carcinoma
    c. Leiomyosarcoma
    d. GIST

198. Which of the following is not true about Gastrointestinal Stromal Tumor (GIST)? *(AIIMS November 2014)*
    a. Originates from interstitial cells of Cajal
    b. Most common mesenchymal tumour of gastrointestinal tract
    c. Prognosis depends on size
    d. ALK gene mutation is seen in most of the cases

GASTRIC LYMPHOMA

199. All are true about stomach lymphoma except:
    a. Most common type is NHL *(GB Pant 2011)*
    b. Large B cell type
    c. Chemosensitive
    d. Most common site is fundus

200. The commonest site of lymphoma in the gastrointestinal system is: *(COMEDK 2007)*
    a. Small bowel   b. Stomach
    c. Large intestine   d. Oesophagus

201. Treatment of gastric lymphoma includes: *(PGI May 2011)*
    a. Chemotherapy   b. Radiotherapy
    c. Surgery   d. Anti-H. pylori treatment
    e. Endoscopic resection

202. Indication of surgery in gastric lymphoma are all except:
    a. Bleeding   *(PGI May 2011, AIIMS Nov 2005, Nov 2002)*
    b. Perforation
    c. Residual disease after chemotherapy
    d. Intractable pain

203. False about gastric lymphoma is: *(AIIMS May 2008)*
    a. Stomach is the most common site
    b. Associated with H. pylori infection
    c. Total gastrectomy with adjuvant chemotherapy is treatment of choice
    d. 5 years survival rate after treatment is 60%

204. The treatment of Hodgkin's disease of stomach is:
    a. Gastric resection   *(Karnataka 89)*
    b. Gastric resection and chemotherapy
    c. Purely medical   d. None of the above

205. The following are true regarding primary gastric lymphoma except: *(APPG 2016)*
    a. More amenable to treatment than gastric adenocarcinoma
    b. H. pylori is implicated especially in MALT type
    c. Mostly of B cell origin
    d. Clinically can be easily differentiated from gastric adenocarcinoma by the presence of early satiety and prominent lymph node metastases

DUODENAL ATRESIA

206. Anomaly associated with duodenal atresia is: *(DNB 2010)*
    a. Down's syndrome   b. Duodenal adenomas
    c. Limb defects   d. Autoimmune disorders

207. Antenatal double bubble appearance on ultrasound is due to: *(Bihar PG 2014, PGI June 97)*
    a. Diaphragmatic hernia   b. Duodenal atresia
    c. Gastric volvulus   d. Intussuception

208. Double Bubble sign is seen with: *(Recent Question 2016, PGI Dec 2006, DNB 2007, 2003, AIIMS May 2009)*
    a. Pyloric stenosis   b. Duodenal atresia
    c. Ileal atresia   d. Esophageal atresia

209. A newborn baby was brought with the history multiple episodes of bilious projectile vomiting. X-ray abdomen was done. What is the diagnosis? *(Recent Question 2016)*
    a. Duodenal atresia
    b. Jejunal atresia
    c. Ileal atresia
    d. Hypertrophic pyloric stenosis

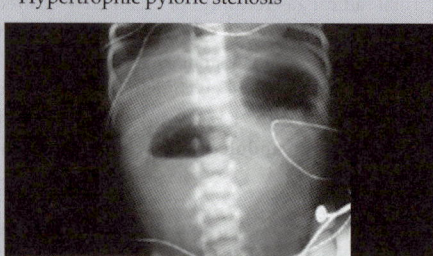

210. Which is the treatment of choice for duodenal atresia? *(DNB, 2011, 2002 MHSSMCET 2005)*
    a. Duodenoduodenostomy   b. Duodenojejunostomy
    c. Bishop-Koop Procedure d. Gastroduodenostomy

211. Duodenal atresia is associated with: *(Recent Question 2017)*
    a. Down's syndrome   b. Patau's syndrome
    c. Turner's syndrome d. Edward's syndrome

HYPERTROPHIC PYLORIC STENOSIS

212. Congenital hypertrophic pyloric stenosis is associated with:
    a. Hypokalemia   *(PGI May 2018, May 2011)*
    b. Hypochloremic metabolic alkalosis
    c. Hypochloremic metabolic acidosis
    d. Hyperchloremic metabolic acidosis
    e. Hyperchloremic metabolic alkalosis

213. A 3 weeks old patient presenting with vomiting and failure to thrive is found to have pyloric stenosis. What should be the next step of management? *(AIIMS May 2011)*
    a. Its emergency so do pyloromyotomy immediately
    b. Fluid resuscitation may be delayed
    c. Correction of electrolyte disturbances
    d. Cardiopulmonary resuscitation

214. Investigation of choice to diagnose hypertrophic pyloric stenosis in infants is: *(Recent Question 2015, 2014, COMEDK 2011)*
    a. Contrast radiology   b. Gastroscopy
    c. Ultrasound abdomen   d. CT abdomen

215. All are seen in hypertrophic pyloric stenosis except: *(NEET Pattern, AIIMS GIS 2003)*
    a. Hyponatremia   b. Hypokalemia
    c. Metabolic acidosis   d. Metabolic alkalosis

216. Hypertrophic pyloric stenosis presents as:
    a. Mass in epigastriumv *(Recent Question 2014, GB Pant 2011)*
    b. More common in girls
    c. Congenital
    d. Present at birth with bilious vomiting

217. Olive shaped mass on feeding is pathognomonic of:
    a. Hypertrophic pyloric stenosis   *(DNB 2005)*
    b. Duodenal atresia
    c. Jejunal atresia
    d. Ileal stenosis

218. An infant after four weeks of birth was brought with the history multiple episodes of nonbilious projectile vomiting. X-ray abdomen was done. What is the diagnosis?

a. Duodenal atresia   b. Jejunal atresia
c. Ileal atresia
d. Hypertrophic pyloric stenosis

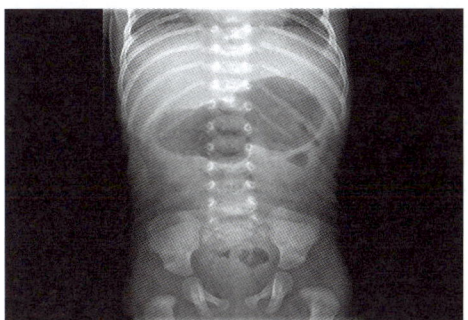

219. **Ramsted's operation is performed for:**
    a. Hirschsprung's disease
    b. CHPS   *(Bihar PG 2014, MHSSMCET 2005, Kerala 94)*
    c. Duodenal atresia
    d. Anorectal malformation

220. **What is the most characteristic of congenital hypertrophic pyloric stenosis?** *(All India 2003)*
    a. Affects the first born female child
    b. The pyloric tumour is best felt during feeding
    c. The patient is commonly marasmic
    d. Loss of appetite occurs early

221. **In a case of hypertrophic pyloric stenosis, the metabolic disturbance is:** *(Recent Question 2017, Recent Question 2016, Bihar PG 2014, JIPMER 2013, All India 2002)*
    a. Respiratory alkalosis
    b. Metabolic acidosis
    c. Metabolic alkalosis with paradoxical aciduria
    d. Metabolic alkalosis with alkaline urine

222. **Metabolic abnormalities associated with infantile pyloric stenosis in early phase include all except:** *(DNB 2012)*
    a. Hypokalemia   b. Aciduria
    c. Hypochloremia   d. None of the above

223. **Make the diagnosis of a 26-day-old infant presenting with recurrent non-bilious vomiting with constipation and loss of weight:** *(AIIMS June 99)*
    a. Esophageal atresia   b. Choledochal cyst
    c. Ileal atresia   d. Pyloric stenosis

224. **If the mucosa was accidentally opened at operation (Ramstedt) it is wise not to feed the child orally for:** *(AMU 90)*
    a. 12 Hours   b. 24 Hours
    c. 48 Hours   d. 1 week

225. **Which of the following is not a feature of ultrasound in CHPS?** *(AIIMS Nov 2011)*
    a. 95% sensitivity by ultrasound
    b. Thickness of pylorus > 4 mm
    c. Channel length > 16 mm
    d. High gastric residue

226. **Hypochloremia, hypokalemia and alkalosis are seen in:** *(DNB 2012, AIIMS June 2003)*
    a. Congenital hypertrophic pyloric stenosis
    b. Hirschsprung's disease
    c. Esophageal atresia
    d. Jejunal atresia

227. **For a patient of gastric outlet obstruction, the OPD fluid management is:** *(PGI June 2003)*
    a. Normal saline   b. Hypertonic saline
    c. Na^+ bicarbonate to counteract aciduria
    d. Hypotonic saline without potassium
    e. Normal saline with potassium

228. **True about hypertrophic pyloric stenosis is all except:** *(DNB 2007)*
    a. Present at 4 weeks
    b. First born male is commonly affected
    c. Ramstedt operation is done
    d. Visible peristalsis is always seen

229. **String sign on barium meal is seen in:**
    a. Duodenal atresia   *(Recent Question 2015)*
    b. Intestinal obstruction
    c. Duodenal ulcer
    d. Congenital hypertrophic pyloric stenosis

230. **The abdominal mass is palpable in .... region in hypertrophic pyloric stenosis.:** *(Recent Question 2018)*
    a. Umbilical   b. Right hypochondrium
    c. Epigastrium   d. Right iliac fossa

GASTRIC OUTLET OBSTRUCTION

231. **Persistent vomiting in G.O.O. causes:** *(PGI Dec 2002)*
    a. Hyponatremic hyperchloremia occur
    b. Hypernatremia without hypochloremic alkalosis
    c. Hypokalemic metabolic alkalosis
    d. Paradoxical aciduria

232. **When peptic ulcer leads to gastric outlet obstruction, the most likely site of obstruction is?** *(Orissa 2011)*
    a. Antrum   b. Pylorus
    c. Lesser curvature   d. First part of duodenum

233. **A patient complains of occasional vomiting of food particles eaten a few days age. His wife reports that his breath smells foul. The most likely diagnosis is:**
    a. Pyloric obstruction   b. Carcinoma stomach
    c. Carcinoma esophagus   d. Achalasia cardia

234. **The most common cause of gastric outlet obstruction in India is:** *(All India 2006)*
    a. Tuberculosis   b. Cancer of stomach
    c. Duodenal lymphoma   d. Peptic ulcer disease

235. **Regarding acute dilation of stomach which is incorrect:**
    a. Occurs with fracture femur
    b. Occurs with plaster
    c. Resolves spontaneously without treatment
    d. Hypophosphatemia is to be avoided

236. **Commonest operation done for peptic ulcer with gastric outlet obstruction is:**
    a. Truncal vagotomy with pyloroplasty
    b. Highly selective vagotomy with pyloroplasty
    c. Truncal vagotomy with gastrojejunostomy
    d. Gastrojejunostomy

237. **A 35 years old male who had chronic duodenal ulcer for the last six years presents with worsening of symptoms loss of periodicity of symptoms, pain on rising in the morning sense of epigastric bloating and postprandial vomiting. The most likely cause of the worsening of his symptoms is the development of:** *(DPG 2010, UPCS 96)*
    a. Posterior penetration   b. Gastric outlet obstruction
    c. Carcinoma   d. Pancreatitis

238. **A patient with antral carcinoma repeatedly vomits. Not seen is:** *(AIIMS 98)*
    a. Acidosis
    b. Hypokalemia
    c. Hyponatremia
    d. Hypochloremia

239. **Most severe degree of alkalosis occurs in obstruction of:**
    a. Cardiac end
    b. Pylorus *(MAHE 98)*
    c. Ileocaecal region
    d. Colon

240. **All of the following are seen in chronic pyloric obstruction except:** *(MCI March 2010)*
    a. Alkaline urine
    b. Acidic urine
    c. Hypochloremia
    d. Hypokalemia

241. **Acute dilatation of stomach is not managed by:**
    a. N/G tube aspiration *(AIIMS June 97)*
    b. Stop oral feeds
    c. Surgery
    d. Fluid and electrolyte balance

242. **Which of the following is true about acute dilatation of stomach?** *(PGI Dec 2005)*
    a. Dilatation of stomach seen on X-ray
    b. Presents with vomiting
    c. Aspiration
    d. Immediately open the abdomen
    e. Atony of stomach

BEZOARS

243. **Bezoar in the stomach present as:** *(Punjab 2009)*
    a. Melena
    b. Perforation
    c. GI obstruction
    d. Diarrhea

244. **The following are the complications of trichobezoars except:**
    a. Hematemesis
    b. Perforation and peritonitis
    c. Obstruction
    d. Malignancy

245. **A female in her twenties presents with complaints of pain abdomen, abdominal distention and vomiting. On examination, she was found to have alopecia and a crepitus in the epigastrium. What is your diagnosis?**
    a. Trichobezoar *(AIIMS November 2014)*
    b. Carcinoma pyloric antrum
    c. Intestinal tuberculosis
    d. Rectus sheath hematoma

246. **True about trichobezoars are all except:** *(MAHE 2006)*
    a. It is caused by Trichuris
    b. It is a psychiatric manifestation
    c. Ball of hairs in the stomach
    d. Pulling the hair and sucking of hair is usually seen

247. **True about gastric bezoar:** *(PGI November 2017)*
    a. After gastrectomy, it does not occur
    b. Caused by ingestion of fruits, vegetable, fibers and hairs
    c. In Rapunzel syndrome, bezoar has a tail-like extension into the small bowel
    d. Surgery is always indicated
    e. It increases chance of gastric ulceration

STRESS GASTRITIS

248. **In case of upper GI bleed associated with stress gastritis all are true except:** *(AIIMS GIS Dec 2009)*
    a. Surgery should be done if transfusion requirements is > 6 units
    b. Vagotomy may be added
    c. Surgery involves anterior gastrotomy with ligation of bleeding ulcers and superficial erosions
    d. Total gastrectomy is rarely indicated

249. **Cushing ulcers are:** *(Recent Question 2019)*
    a. Stress ulcers in burns
    b. Stress ulcers in head injury
    c. Stress ulcers in hiatus hernia
    d. Stress ulcers in analgesic drug abuse

250. **In case of upper GI bleeding due to stress gastritis, all of the following decreases bleeding risk except:**
    a. Treatment of sepsis *(AIIMS GIS Dec 2009)*
    b. Improvement of BP
    c. Elective ventilation
    d. Correction of coagulopathy

251. **All are true about stress gastritis except:** *(GB Pant 2011)*
    a. Backflow H$^+$ uptake by mucosal cells
    b. Decreased HCO$_3$ secretion
    c. Decreased mucosal blood flow
    d. Increased H. pylori infection

252. **Stress-induced ulcers are most commonly found in the:**
    a. Fundus of stomach *(COMEDK 2010)*
    b. Antrum of stomach
    c. Pyloric channel
    d. First part of duodenum

253. **Common sites of for Cushing ulcers include all of the following except:** *(All India 99)*
    a. Esophagus
    b. Stomach
    c. 1st part of duodenum
    d. Distal duodenum

254. **Most common site of Curling's ulcer:** *(Recent Question 2014, AIIMS Nov 2008)*
    a. Ileum
    b. Stomach
    c. Duodenum
    d. Esophagus

255. **Erosive gastritis commonly occurs at:** *(JIPMER 93)*
    a. Body
    b. Fundus
    c. Lesser curvature
    d. Antrum

256. **Curling's ulcer is seen in:** *(NEET 2013, DNB 2008, All India 88)*
    a. Burn patients
    b. Patients with head injuries
    c. Zollinger Ellison syndrome
    d. Analgesic drug abuse

257. **Which of the following is not true of Curling's ulcer?**
    a. Seen in burn patients *(Karnataka 96)*
    b. Are solitary penetrating ulcer
    c. Are shallow multiple erosions
    d. Has also been described in children after head injury or craniotomy

258. **Stress ulcers is caused by all of the following except?** *(APPG 2006)*
    a. Burns
    b. Cortisol therapy
    c. Penicillin therapy
    d. Pulmonary insufficiency

259. **In a burn patient, the doctor is looking for curling ulcer. Which part should be examined?** *(AIIMS Nov 2013)*
    a. 1st part of duodenum
    b. 2nd part of duodenum
    c. 3rd part of duodenum
    d. Junction between 2nd and 3rd part of duodenum

GASTRIC VOLVULUS

260. **All are true about organoaxial gastric volvulus except:**
    a. Borchardt's triad is present (AIIMS GIS Dec 2006)
    b. Usually associated with diaphragmatic defect
    c. Endoscopy usually derotate
    d. Occurs in elderly

261. **Borchardt's triad of acute epigastric pain violent retching and inability to pass a nasogastric tube is seen in patients with:** (J & K 2005)
    a. Achalasia cardia
    b. Acute gastric volvulus
    c. Jejunogastric intussusceptions
    d. Hiatus hernia

262. **Borchardt's triad is characterized by the following except:**
    a. Inability to pass Nasogastric tube (MHSSMCET 2008)
    b. Vomiting
    c. Shock
    d. Diarrhea

STOMACH ANATOMY AND PHYSIOLOGY

263. **Criminal nerve of Grassi:** (ILBS 2011)
    a. Anterior branch of vagus at pylorus
    b. Anterior branch of vagus at cardia
    c. Proximal branch of posterior vagus
    d. Distal branch of posterior vagus

264. **Electrical pacemaker of stomach is situated in:** (Karnataka 2001)
    a. Fundus
    b. Body
    c. Incisura Angularis
    d. Gastroesophageal junction

265. **Function of thick gastric mucosa is:** (All India 97)
    a. Protects epithelium
    b. Neutralizes HCL
    c. Traps foreign particles
    d. None of the above

266. **G-cells are present mostly in:** (TN 91)
    a. Fundus
    b. Cardia
    c. Pyloric antrum
    d. Body

267. **In which of the following organs submucosal glands are present?** (COMEDK 2004)
    a. Colon
    b. Anal canal
    c. Duodenum
    d. Stomach

268. **Ghrelin is responsible for:** (COMEDK 2008)
    a. Stimulation of appetite
    b. Suppression of appetite
    c. Stimulation of sleep
    d. Suppression of sleep

269. **Posterior gastric artery is a branch of:** (JIPMER 2011)
    a. Left gastric artery
    b. Right gastric artery
    c. Splenic artery
    d. Hepatic artery

GASTRIC DIVERTICULUM

270. **Deverticulum of the stomach:** (PGI Nov 2014)
    a. Pain is the main symptom
    b. Usually at cardiac end
    c. Usually on posterior surface
    d. Inversion is the satisfactory treatment
    e. All of the above

271. **The most frequent symptom of gastric diverticulum is:** (Recent Question 2016)
    a. Epigastric lump
    b. Hematemesis
    c. Vomiting
    d. Pain

MISCELLANEOUS

272. **Duodenal stricture is caused by:** (PGI Dec 2002)
    a. Amebiasis
    b. T.B.
    c. CA pancreas
    d. Crohn's disease
    e. Giardiasis

273. **Deficiency of the abdominal muscle is associated with:** (PGI June 99)
    a. Eagle-Barrett syndrome
    b. Christopher syndrome
    c. Megacystitis
    d. Megaureter

274. **Raised gastrin level without associated increase in acid secretion is seen in:** (AIIMS Nov 94)
    a. Carcinoma stomach
    b. Gastrinoma
    c. Pernicious anemia
    d. G-cell hyperplasia

275. **Which is the most common cause of hypergastrinemia?** (MCI November 2017)
    a. Post-vagotomy
    b. After intake of PPI
    c. Resection of small intestine
    d. Atrophic gastritis

276. **Hour glass stomach is seen in:** (AIIMS 92)
    a. Gastric carcinoma
    b. Gastric ulcer
    c. Gastric lymphoma
    d. Corrosive strictures

277. **Highest pickup for gastrojuejunocolic fistula is by:** (J and K 2001)
    a. Ba swallow
    b. Ba meal
    c. Ba enema
    d. Ba meal follow through

278. **Duodenal adenocarcinoma:** (PGI 2004)
    a. Most common small bowel carcinoma
    b. Type of periampullary carcinoma
    c. Jaundice and anemia - most common symptom
    d. Local resection - curative

279. **For gastric lavage in an adult the stomach tube should be passed up to:** (COMEDK 2004)
    a. Up to 20 cm
    b. Up to 30 cm
    c. Up to 40 cm
    d. Up to 50 cm

280. **Thickened gastric folds on barium meal are seen in:** (COMEDK 2010)
    a. Leiomyosarcoma
    b. Scleroderma
    c. Amyloidosis
    d. Linnitis plastica

281. **Duodenal diverticularization is indicated in:** (PGI Nov 2011)
    a. Duodenal fistula
    b. Duodenal polyp
    c. Duodenal ulcer
    d. Pancreatic injury
    e. Duodenal injury

282. **Characteristic features of type A gastritis are all except:** (MHPGMCET 2007)
    a. Gastric antrum is predominantly affected
    b. Chronic hypergastrinemia occurs
    c. Hypochlrhydria occurs
    d. Hypertrophy of gastric enterochromaffin like cells

283. **Finney's stricturoplasty is done when the length of bowel stricture is:** (MHSSMCET 2006)
    a. > 1 cm
    b. > 10 cm
    c. < 10 cm
    d. < 2.5 cm

284. **In Hunt Lawrence pouch reconstruction, the length of pouch is:** (MHSSMCET 2008)
    a. 10 cm
    b. 15 cm
    c. 20 cm
    d. 25 cm

285. **Most common epithelial tumor of stomach:** (Recent Question 2018)
    a. Carcinoid
    b. GIST
    c. Granulosa cell tumor
    d. Sarcoma

Explanations

H. PYLORI

1. **Ans. d. Gastric leiomyoma** *(Ref: Harrison 20/e p2215, 19/e p915)*

Diseases Associated with H. pylori		
Antral Predominant Gastritis	**Corpus Predominant Atrophic Gastritis**	**Non-atrophic Pangastritis (Chronic Superficial gastritis)**
• Duodenal ulcer^Q	• Gastric ulcer^Q • Gastric adenocarcinoma^Q	• MALT lymphoma^Q

2. **Ans. b. Metaplastic polyp**
3. **Ans. a. Low grade MALT lymphoma**
4. **Ans. d. Warthin-Starry stain**
5. **Ans. b. Type B gastritis** *(Ref: Bailey 27/e p1115; Harrison 20/e p2242, 19/e p372e-24t)*

Chronic Gastritis	
Type A	**Type B**
• **Autoimmune** etiology^Q • Circulating antibodies to the parietal cell results in the atrophy of the parietal cell mass, resulting in hypochlorhydria and ultimately achlorhydria^Q. • Associated with pernicious anemia^Q • Primarily involves body and fundus^Q	• Associated with H. pylori infection^Q • Primarily involves antrum^Q

- **Type A:** Autoimmune, Antibodies, Atrophy, Achlorhydria, Anemia
- **Type B:** Bacteria

6. **Ans. b. Gastric metaplasia**   7. **Ans. d. Hypertrophic gastritis**   8. **Ans. a. MALTomas**
9. **Ans. b. H. pylori** *(Ref: Sabiston 20/e p1200; Schwartz 10/e p1053; Bailey 27/e p1114)*

PEPTIC ULCER ETIOLOGY AND CLINICAL FEATURES

10. **Ans. d. Pernicious anemia** *(Ref: Sabiston 20/e p1918; Schwartz 10/e p1053-1073; Bailey 27/e p1116; Shackelford 8/e p673-676, 7/e p701-718)*

Specific Chronic Disorders Associated with PUD	
With strong associations	**With possible associations**
• Systemic mastocytosis^Q • Chronic pulmonary disease^Q • Chronic renal failure^Q • **Cirrhosis**^{Q} • Nephrolithiasis^Q • Alpha1-antitrypsin deficiency^Q	• **Hyperparathyroidism**^{Q} • Coronary artery disease • Polycythemia Vera • Chronic pancreatitis^Q

11. **Ans. c. Plummer-Vinson syndrome**   12. **Ans. b. Gastric acid; c. Alcohol abuse; e. Smoking**
13. **Ans. a. 1st part of duodenum**
14. **Ans. d. Lesser curvature near incisura angularis** *(Ref: Sabiston 20/e p1207)*

GASTRIC ULCERS

- MC type: **Type I gastric ulcer**, is located near **angularis incisura** on the lesser curvature.
- **NSAID ulcers (Type V)** typically occur in the **antrum** but may be located anywhere in the stomach and may be multiple in origin.
- Type II and III: **High acid secretion**^{Q}
- Type I and IV: **Normal** or **low acid secretion**^{Q}
- Association:
  - **Type I:** Blood group 'A'^{Q}
  - **Type II, III, and IV:** Blood group 'O'^{Q}

15. **Ans. d. None of the above** *(Ref: Harrison 20/e p2226, 19/e p1922)*

   - Documented **eradication of H. pylori** in patients with PUD is associated with a dramatic **decrease in ulcer recurrence** to **<10–20%** as compared to **59% in GU patients** and **67% in DU patients** when the **organism is not eliminated**[Q].
   - **Magnesium** containing drugs causes **diarrhea**[Q]
   - **Aluminium**-containing drugs often cause **constipation**[Q]

16. **Ans. b. 2, 3 and 4 only**
17. **Ans. c. Duodenal ulcer; d. Gastric ulcer** *(Ref: Harrison 20/e p2227, 19/e p1918)*

   ### CLINICAL FEATURES OF PEPTIC ULCER

   - **Epigastric pain** described as a **burning** or **gnawing discomfort** can be present in both **DU** and **GU**[Q].
   - The discomfort is also described as an ill-defined, aching sensation or as hunger pain.

     - The **typical pain pattern in DU** occurs **90 minutes to 3 hours after** a meal and is **frequently relieved by antacids** or **food**[Q].
     - Pain that **awakes** the **patient from sleep** (between **midnight** and **3 A.M.**) is the **most discriminating symptom**, with **two-thirds of DU patients** describing this complaint[Q].

   - The **pain pattern** in **GU patients** may be different from that in DU patients, where **discomfort** may actually be **precipitated by food**[Q].
   - **Nausea** and **weight loss** occur **more commonly in GU patients**.

18. **Ans. b. Type III gastric ulcer**
19. **Ans. c. Type 3**
20. **Ans. c. Prepyloric region** *(Ref: Sabiston 20/e p1208; Schwartz 10/e p1057)*
21. **Ans. d. Lesser curve** *(Ref: Sabiston 20/e p1208; Schwartz 10/e p1057)*
22. **Ans. a. Duodenal ulcer**

PEPTIC ULCER COMPLICATIONS

23. **Ans. c. Duodenotomy with ligation of bleeding vessels, truncal vagotomy and pyloroplasty** *(Ref: Sabiston 20/e p1202-1203; Schwartz 10/e p1066; Bailey 27/e p1127; Shackelford 8/e p694-495, 7/e p711-713)*

   ### TREATMENT OF BLEEDING DUODENAL ULCER (SHACKELFORD)

   - The **first priority** during emergency surgery for a **bleeding duodenal ulcer** is **control of** the **bleeding site**[Q].
   - If endoscopy has **failed to precisely identify** the **source** of hemorrhage, a **pyloroduodenotomy** may be **necessary to inspect** the **duodenal bulb** and **gastric antrum**[Q].
   - The **gastroduodenal artery** is the **usual source of bleeding**, which should be **controlled by placement of suture ligatures**[Q].

     - Once the bleeding has been addressed, a **definitive acid-reducing operation** may be **performed**[Q]. With the identification of H. pylori, the utility of a vagotomy has been questioned. **The data**, however, **suggest that, even in the era of H. pylori** and our **ability to eradicate it, a TV perhaps should be performed** in those patients with a **bleeding duodenal ulcer**. There are several **reasons for this recommendation:**
       – Only 40% to 70% of patients with a **bleeding duodenal ulcer** are positive for H. pylori[Q].
       – **H. pylori testing** in the setting of an **acute hemorrhage** is **less reliable**[Q], with the CLO (Campylobacter-like organism) test having a false-negative rate of 18% versus 1% in those not actively bleeding
       – **If an acid-reducing procedure** is **not performed**, up to **50% of patients are at risk of recurrent bleeding**[Q]
       – **Conflicting evidence** that **H. pylori treatment changes** the **risk of recurrent bleeding**[Q].

   - **In contrast to other situations**, the **argument for performing** a **less aggressive operation** in the **face of massive bleeding exposes the patient to a high rebleeding risk post-surgery**[Q].

     - Because it is simple to open the pylorus in a longitudinal fashion, **TV with pyloroplasty** is the **most frequently used operation** for **bleeding duodenal ulcer**[Q].

   - The **pyloric vein of Mayo** is virtually **always present on** the **anterior surface** of the **inferior pylorus**[Q].

24. Ans. b. Gastroduodenal artery *(Ref: Sabiston 20/e p1202-1203; Schwartz 10/e p1053-1073; Bailey 27/e p1127; Shackelford 8/e p694, 7/e p711-714)*

BLEEDING PEPTIC ULCER

- **Bleeding: MC indication** for **operation** and **principal cause** of **death** in PUD patients[Q].
  - The most significant hemorrhage occurs when **duodenal** or **gastric ulcers** penetrate into branches of the **gastroduodenal artery** or **left gastric artery**, respectively[Q].
- **Incidence** of peptic ulcer bleeding **decreased over past decade**, but **mortality** was **stable** for both gastric and duodenal ulcer bleeding, higher in patients of advanced age.
- **Cause of death: Multiple-system organ failure** (not the exsanguinating hemorrhage)

Treatment

- **Irrigation** with **room temperature saline** to lyse red cells in an effort to return clear fluid and to allow for the performance of endoscopy.
- **Figure-of-eight sutures to ligate** the **gastroduodenal artery**[Q]. A 'U' stitch is placed in the ulcer base to **occlude pancreatic branches** of the gastroduodenal artery.
- **Truncal vagotomy** and **pyloroplasty** is the most frequently used operation for **bleeding duodenal ulcer**[Q]

25. Ans. c. Perforation   **26. Ans. b. Duodenum**

27. Ans. a. Omental bursa (lesser sac) *(Ref: Bailey 27/e p1125; Schwartz 9/e p921)*

- **Gastric ulcers perforate into** the **lesser sac**, which can be particularly **difficult to diagnose**[Q].
- A **gastric ulcer perforates into** the **lesser sac**[Q], then no generalized peritonitis can be seen but misleading symptoms may appear.

28. Ans. a. Gastric ulcer with bleeding *(Ref: Harrison 20/e p2227, 19/e p1918)*

- **Hypotension** in an **elderly patient** with history of **aspirin intake** and complaints of **black stool** suggests **GI bleeding** due to **drug induced gastritis**.
- **Bleeding peptic ulcer** due to **NSAIDs** is **more frequent in** individuals **>60 years** of age due to increased use of NSAIDs in this group.

29. Ans. a. IV fluids; c. Immediate surgery; e. IV pantoprazole *(Ref: Sabiston 20/e p1204; Schwartz 10/e p1068; Bailey 27/e p1126; Shackelford 8/e p695, 7/e p713-716)*

MANAGEMENT OF PERFORATED PEPTIC ULCER

- **Perforated peptic ulcer** usually presents as an **acute abdomen.**
- Initially, a **chemical peritonitis** develops from the **gastric and/or duodenal secretions**, but **within hours a bacterial peritonitis supervenes.**
- **Fluid sequestration** into the **third space** of the inflamed peritoneum can be impressive, and **fluid resuscitation is mandatory**[Q].
- The patient is in **obvious distress**, and the abdominal examination shows **peritoneal signs**.
- Usually, **marked involuntary guarding** and **rebound tenderness** is evoked by a gentle examination.

Diagnosis

- **Upright chest x-ray** shows **free air** in about **80%**[Q] of patients.

Treatment

- **Nasogastric aspiration**, **analgesia** and **antibiotics**, resuscitated with isotonic fluid, antisecretary agents (PPI, H_2 receptor antagonist)
- **Surgery** is **almost always indicated**[Q].
- Sometimes, the **perforation has sealed spontaneously** by the time of presentation, and **surgery can be avoided** if the **patient is doing well.**
- Non-operative management in:
  - **Objective evidence** that the **leak has sealed** (i.e., **radiologic contrast study**)[Q]
  - **Absence of clinical peritonitis**[Q].

30. Ans. b. 75% *(Ref: Schwartz 10/e p1061)*

- **Upright chest x-ray** shows **free air** in about **80%** of patients of perforated peptic ulcer.

Stomach and Duodenum

31. Ans. b. Hemorrhage
32. Ans. b. X-ray abdomen
33. Ans. c. Dilution of acid in the peritoneal cavity
34. Ans. a. Omental bursa
35. Ans. c. Basal pneumonia *(Ref: Shackelford 8/e p695, 7/e p714)*
36. Ans. a. Gastroduodenal artery
37. Ans. c. Proton pump inhibitors

PEPTIC ULCER DIAGNOSIS AND TREATMENT

38. Ans. a. Before breakfast *(Ref: Sabiston 20/e p1201; Schwartz 10/e p971,972,979; Bailey 27/e p1119)*
    PPIs are taken before breakfast.
39. Ans. a. Highly selective vagotomy *(Ref: Sabiston 20/e p1205-1206; Schwartz 10/e p1093-1094; Bailey 27/e p1122; Shackelford 8/e p679, 7/e p720-729)*
40. Ans. a. Nerves of Latarjet
41. Ans. a. Billroth-I operation *(Ref: Sabiston 20/e p1208; Schwartz 10/e p1120; Bailey 27/e p1123; Shackelford 8/e p683, 7/e p733-737)*
42. Ans. a. Finney's Pyloroplasty *(Ref: Sabiston 20/e p1206; Schwartz 10/e p1065; Shackelford 8/e p680, 7/e p895)*

    Finney Pyloroplasty is performed in patients with a J-shaped stomach or extensive scarring and narrowing of a significant portion of the duodenal bulb.

    ### DRAINAGE PROCEDURES IN PEPTIC ULCERS

    - **Heineke-Mikulicz Pyloroplasty:** Most commonly performed drainage procedure[Q].
    - **Finney Pyloroplasty:** Performed in patients with a **J-shaped stomach** or **extensive scarring** & **narrowing of a significant portion** of the **duodenal bulb**[Q].
    - **Jaboulay Gastroduodenostomy:** It involves an anastomosis of **distal end** of **stomach to the first** & **second portions of duodenum**, done in **severely scarred** or **deformed pylorus** or **duodenal bulb**[Q].

43. Ans. d. 80 *(Ref: Sabiston 20/e p1197; Schwartz 10/e p1054; Harrison 20/e p2225, 19/e p1039)*

    ### ASSOCIATION OF H PYLORI WITH PEPTIC ULCER

Harrison: **30-60% GUs** and 50-70% of DUs	Sabiston: **75% GUs** and 90% DUs
Schwartz: **70-90% GUs** and 90% DUs	

44. Ans. b. Carman's meniscus sign
45. Ans. c. Vitamin B_{12} deficiency
46. Ans. a. Pouchet procedure; b. Kelling-Madlener operation; c. Csendes procedure *(Ref: Sabiston 20/e p1208; Schwartz 9/e p913-916; Shackelford 8/e p692, 7/e p708-710)*
47. Ans. a. Proximal two-thirds of stomach
48. Ans. c. Type IV ulcer most common type; e. 30% GU are associated with malignancy *(Ref: Harrison 20/e p2226, 19/e p1915; Chandrasoma Taylor 3/e p582, 597)*

    - **MC type** of **gastric ulcer** is **Type I**, is located near **angularis incisura** on the **lesser curvature**[Q].
    - **H. pylori colonization** is seen in **75-80%** of patients with **gastric ulcer**[Q].
    - A **chronic duodenal ulcer never turns malignant**, while **less than 1%** of **chronic gastric ulcer** may **transform into carcinoma**.

49. Ans. c. Anti-H. pylori drugs must be included in the treatment regime; d. H. pylori is known to increase incidence of gastric malignancies
50. Ans. d. Ipratropium *(Ref: Sabiston 20/e p1194-1995, 1200-1201; Schwartz 10/e p1041-1044; Bailey 27/e p1119)*

    ### DRUGS THAT REDUCE GASTRIC ACID SECRETION

    - Proton pump inhibitors[Q]
    - Muscarinic-3 receptors antagonists[Q]
    - Somatostatin[Q]
    - Histamine-2 receptor antagonists[Q]
    - Prostaglandin E-1 receptor agonists[Q] (**Misoprostol**)

    - **Alginates**[Q] are **combined** with **antacids** for use in **reflux esophagitis** because they are believed to **increase adherence to esophageal mucosa**.

51. **Ans. d. Highly selective vagotomy**
52. **Ans. a. Truncal vagotomy and antrectomy**
53. **Ans. c. Truncal vagotomy and antrectomy**
54. **Ans. d. Duodenal erosion** *(Ref: Harrison 20/e p2228, 19/e p1881)*

> ##### ENDOSCOPY
> - **Fiber endoscopy** is especially **useful** in visualizing **postbulbar ulcers, giant duodenal ulcers,** and **stomal ulceration after partial gastrectomy**, all of which can be missed by X-ray.

55. **Ans. d. Typical periodicity**
56. **Ans. b. Truncal vagotomy and antrectomy**
57. **Ans. c. Vagotomy + repair of perforation** *(Ref: Sabiston 20/e p1202-1205; Schwartz 10/e p1068; Bailey 27/e p1123; Shackelford 8/e p691-692, 7/e p701-708)*

Complications	Treatment
Perforated	Type I: • **Distal gastrectomy** in stable patients^Q • Biopsy and patch closure in unstable patients^Q **Type II and III: Patch closure in unstable patients (Truncal vagotomy** with **antrectomy in stable patients)**^Q
Obstruction	**Truncal vagotomy** with **antrectomy**^Q (Rule out malignancy)

58. **Ans. d. Duodenal ulcer** *(Ref: Shackelford 8/e p679, 7/e p704, 708; Schwartz 10/e p1068)*

> ##### OPERATION FOR PEPTIC ULCER
> - **Hill and Baker procedure: Posterior truncal** vagotomy with **anterior HSV**^Q.
> - **Taylor Procedure: Posterior truncal** vagotomy with **anterior lesser curve seromyotomy**^Q. The technique is very suitable for a **laparoscopic** approach.

59. **Ans. d. Graham's omentum patch repair**
60. **Ans. a. Proximal two-thirds of stomach**
61. **Ans. b. Vagotomy and antrectomy**
62. **Ans. d. Megaesophagus treatment by esophageal mucosal resection**

> - **Ménétrier's disease** is associated with **hypochlorhydria (no use of HSV)**.
> - **Giant gastric ulcers** should be treated with **truncal vagotomy + antrectomy**.
> - **Vagotomy**, irrespective if **truncal** or **highly selective**, only has a **temporary effect** in **stress ulceration**, consisting of multiple, punctate, superficial **erosions**, confined initially to the proximal **gastric mucosa**.

GASTRECTOMY AND COMPLICATIONS

63. **Ans. a. Iron deficiency anemia** *(Ref: Sabiston 20/e p1212-1213; Schwartz 10/e p1090-1094; Bailey 27/e p1123; Shackelford 8/e p731, 7/e p757-765)*
    MC metabolic complication after gastrectomy is **iron deficiency anemia**.
64. **Ans. a. Vitamin B$_{12}$ deficiency** *(Ref: Sabiston 20/e p1212; Schwartz 10/e p1094; Bailey 27/e p1124; Shackelford 8/e p731, 7/e p759-760)*
65. **Ans. c. Vitamin B12 deficiency**   66. **Ans. c. HSV**
67. **Ans. d. Osteomalacia**
68. **Ans. b. Presence of hypertonic content in small intestine** *(Ref: Sabiston 20/e p1212; Schwartz 10/e p1090-1092; Bailey 27/e p1123; Shackelford 8/e p719, 7/e p757-759)*
69. **Ans. c. Starch is beneficial**
70. **Ans. d. Surgery is usually indicated**

> - **Surgery** is **rarely required** in **dumping** or **post-cibal syndrome**, as **most of the patients improve with time, dietary management** and **octreotide**^Q.

Stomach and Duodenum

71. **Ans. b. 4th day** *(Ref: Shackelford 7/e p930, 944)*
72. **Ans. d. Fluid loss**
73. **Ans. b. Loss of storage capacity**
74. **Ans. d. Anastomotic hemorrhage**
75. **Ans. a. Billroth-II**
76. **Ans. c. Gastrojejunocolic fistula** *(Ref: Shackelford 6/e p1094, 1110; Bailey 26/e p1039)*
77. **Ans. c. Billroth-I gastrectomy**
78. **Ans. a. Clean contaminated wound** *(Ref: Sabiston 20/e p245; Schwartz 10/e p148)*
79. **Ans. a. Hernia surgery**
80. **Ans. c. Complication of partial gastrectomy**
81. **Ans. c. Somatostatin analogue** *(Ref: Schwartz 10/e p1093; Bailey 26/e p1039; Shackelford 8/e p811, 7/e p760)*

POSTVAGOTOMY DIARRHEA

- About **30%** or more of patients **suffer from diarrhea after gastric surgery**^{Q}.
- For most patients, it is **not severe** and **usually disappears within** the **first 3 to 4 months**^{Q}.
- **Vagotomy** is associated with **alterations in stool frequency**^{Q}.
- **Truncal vagotomy** results in **increased frequency** of **daily bowel movements** in **30-70%** of **patients**^{Q}.

Treatment

- **Postvagotomy diarrhea resolves over time** in most of the patients^Q.
- If symptoms fail to resolve:
  - **Cholestyramine**^{Q} (an anionic exchange resin that absorbs bile salts rendering them unabsorbable and inactive)
  - **Octreotide**^{Q} can be used for **severe postvagotomy diarrhea**

82. **Ans. c. Billroth** *(Ref: Sabiston 20/e p1208; Schwartz 10/e p1120; Bailey 27/e p1120; Shackelford 8/e p683, 7/e p731-742)*
83. **Ans. b. Increased intestinal secretion**

UPPER GI BLEED

84. **Ans. b. Low urine output** *(Ref: Sabiston 20/e p1142; Schwartz 10/e p1060)*
85. **Ans. c. Adherent clot** *(Ref: Sabiston 20/e p1143; Shackelford 8/e p694, 7/e p711)*
86. **Ans. c. Can detect causes in all cases** *(Ref: Sabiston 20/e p1141-1142; Schwartz 10/e p1169; Bailey 27/e p1127)*

ROLE OF ENDOSCOPY IN UPPER GI BLEED

- **Endoscopy: Foundation of diagnosis** and **management** of patients with **an upper GI bleed**^{Q}

Early endoscopy (within 24 hours) results in
- **Reductions** in **blood transfusion requirements**^{Q}
- **Decrease** in the **need for surgery**^{Q}
- **Shorter length** of **hospital stay**^{Q}

- In general, **20–35%** of patients undergoing endoscopy will **require a therapeutic endoscopic intervention**, and **5-10%** will eventually **require surgery**^{Q}.
- **Best tool for localization** of the **bleeding source** is **endoscopy**^{Q}
- In **1–2%** of **patients with upper GI hemorrhage**, the **source cannot be identified** because of **excessive blood impairing visualization** of the mucosal surface.

- **Aggressive lavage** of the stomach with **room temperature normal saline solution before the procedure** can be helpful^Q.

87. **Ans. a. Endoscopy**

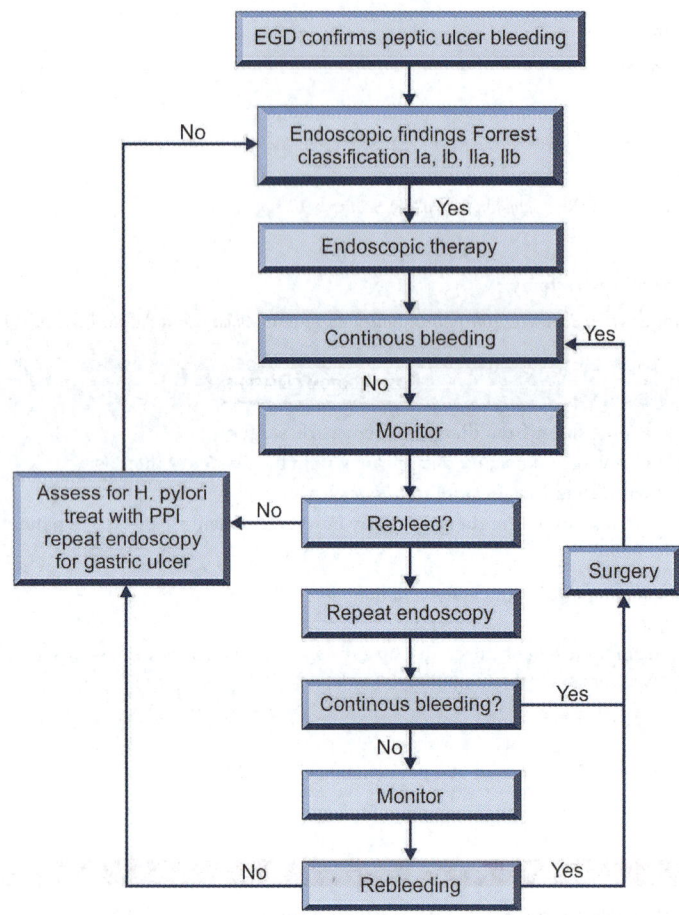

88. **Ans. b. Angiography can image bleeding at a rate of 0.05-0.1 ml/min or less** *(Ref: Sabiston 20/e p1152-1153)*
    Selective angiography, using either the superior or inferior mesenteric arteries, **can detect hemorrhage** in the range of **0.5 to 1.0 mL/min.**

MESENTERIC ANGIOGRAPHY

- **Selective angiography**, using either the superior or inferior mesenteric arteries, **can detect hemorrhage** in the range of **0.5 to 1.0 mL/min**[Q].
- **Only employed** in the **diagnosis of ongoing hemorrhage**[Q].
  - **Particularly useful** in **identifying** the **vascular patterns of angiodysplasias**.
  - It may also be **used for localizing actively bleeding diverticula**[Q].
- **Catheter-directed vasopressin infusion** can provide **temporary control of bleeding**[Q], permitting hemodynamic stabilization, although as many as 50% of patients experience rebleeding when the medication is discontinued.
- It can also be **employed for embolization**[Q].
- **Complications**: Hematomas, arterial thrombosis, contrast reactions, and acute renal failure.

RADIONUCLIDE SCANNING

- **Radionuclide scanning** with **technetium-99m** (^{99m}Tc)-**labeled RBCs** is the **most sensitive** but **least accurate method** for **localization of GI bleeding**[Q].
- With this technique, the **patient's own RBCs** are **labeled** and **reinjected**.
- The **labeled blood** is **extravasated into** the **GI tract lumen**, creating a focus that can be **detected scintigraphically**[Q].
- Initially, images are collected frequently and then at 4 hour intervals for up to 24 hours.

Stomach and Duodenum

- The **tagged RBC scan** can **detect bleeding** as slow as **0.1 mL/min** and is reported to be **more than 90% sensitive**[Q].
- Unfortunately, the **spatial resolution is lacking**, and blood may move retrograde in the colon or distally in the small bowel.
- **Reported accuracy of localization** is **40-60%**, and it is particularly **inaccurate in distinguishing right- from left-sided colonic bleeding**[Q].

89. Ans. c. Endoscopy can best diagnose it; d. Peptic ulcer is the MC cause; e. ↑ed BUN *(Ref: Sabiston 20/e p1202-1203; Schwartz 10/e p1064; Bailey 27/e p1127; Shackelford 8/e p694, 7/e p710-713)*

90. Ans. b. Duodenal ulcer *(Ref: Sabiston 20/e p1143)*

- **Peptic ulcer** is the **most common cause** of **upper GI bleeding**, present in **one-half** to **two-third** of patients with upper GI bleeding. **Bleeding may be** the **initial presenting symptom** in up to 10% of patients with peptic ulcer. **Duodenal ulcer bleeding is more common than gastric ulcer bleeding**.
- Only **10–15%** of **'Heavy'** drinkers develop alcoholic cirrhosis (leading to **esophageal varices**).

91. Ans. b. Duodenal ulcer

92. Ans. b. Intravenous beta-blockers *(RefL Sabiston 20/e p1149; Bailey 27/e p1127; Shackelford 8/e p1582, 7/e p710-713)*

- **Pharmacotherapy** in **variceal bleeding** consists of:
  - **Continuous IV infusion** of somatostatin analogue **octreotide**
  - Infusion of **vasopressin** or vasopressin plus nitroglycerine
- **Beta-blockers** are used in **secondary prevention** of recurrent variceal bleed.
- **Beta-blockers** have **no role in** the **management of acute upper GI bleeding**.

93. Ans. a. Sclerotherapy *(Ref: Sabiston 20/e p1149; Shackelford 8/e p1582, 7/e p1597; Harrison 20/e p2196, 19/e p1890)*

VARICEAL BLEEDING

- In addition to pharmacologic therapy **endoscopy** should be carried out **as soon as possible**
- If varices are found they are treated with either **endoscopic variceal ligation** or **sclerotherapy**[Q].
- **EVL** is the **treatment of choice** for **variceal bleeding**[Q].

94. Ans. a. Hepatic encephalopathy *(Ref: Sabiston 20/e p1150; Schwartz 10/e p1223; Shackelford 8/e p1583, 7/e p1600-1601; Harrison 20/e p2196, 19/e p2064)*

Complications of Injection Sclerotherapy	
• **Esophageal ulcerations**[Q] (May **bleed** or **perforate**)	• Pleural effusion[Q]
• Mediastinitis[Q]	• Pulmonary edema
	• **Late strictures**[Q]

95. Ans. c. Intravenous pantoprazole *(Ref: Sabiston 20/e p1144; Schwartz 10/e p1143)*

96. Ans. b. Repeat upper GI endoscopy *(Ref: Sabiston 20/e p1144)*

- Sabiston says that "The **cause of obscure-overt bleeding** is often a common lesion that is **missed on initial evaluation**. **Repeat upper** and **lower endoscopy** is a **valuable tool** in **identifying missed lesions** because **up to 35% patients** have the **bleeding source identified** on **second look endoscopy**."

97. Ans. b. Radiolabelled erythrocyte scanning *(Ref: Sabiston 20/e p1152)*

- **Radionuclide scanning** with **technetium-99m** (^{99m}Tc)**-labeled RBCs** is the **most sensitive** but **least accurate** method for **localization of GI bleeding**[Q].

98. Ans. b. FII a   99. Ans. d. Duodenal ulcer   100. Ans. b. Peptic ulcer

101. Ans. a. Vascular ectasia

102. Ans. d. Rockall scoring is used for risk stratification *(Ref: Sabiston 20/e p1142; Schwartz 10/e p1060)*

MALLORY-WEISS TEAR

103. Ans. a. Massive hemorrhage is MC manifestation *(Ref: Sabiston 20/e p1145; Schwartz 10/e p1018-1020; Bailey 26/e p994; Shackelford 8/e p656, 7/e p768)*

Massive hemorrhage is **rare in Mallory-Weiss syndrome**.

104. Ans. a. Mallory-Weiss syndrome   105. Ans. a. Gastric cardia   106. Ans. c. Mallory-Weiss syndrome
107. Ans. b. Left gastric artery *(Ref: Harrison 20/e p2199, 19/e p277; Sabiston 20/e p1145; Schwartz 10/e p1145; Shackelford 8/e p656, 7/e p7/768)*

- *"Mallory-Weiss tears are characterized by arterial bleeding.* Most Mallory-Weiss tears stop bleeding spontaneously and supportive treatment is all that is required. If bleeding continues, *infusion of vasoactive substances into the celiac artery or into the left gastric artery often obviates the need for operation."*

DIEULAFOY'S LESION

108. Ans. a. Angiographic embolization is the preferred treatment *(Ref: Sabiston 20/e p1146; Schwartz 10/e p1089; Bailey 27/e p1128; Shackelford 8/e p650, 7/e p769)*

- Initial attempts at **endoscopic control** are often successful. Application of **thermal** or **sclerosant therapy** is **effective in 80–100% of cases. In cases that fail endoscopic therapy, angiographic coil embolization** can be **successful.**

109. Ans. a. Within 6 cm of GE junction   110. Ans. d. Aberrant vessel in the mucosa that bleeds form a mucosal defect

GASTRIC ANTRAL VASCULAR ECTASIA

111. Ans. c. Pain is most common clinical symptom *(Ref: Sabiston 20/e p1146; Schwartz 10/e p1088; Shackelford 8/e p650, 7/e p653-654, 768-769)*
Most common clinical symptom is bleeding, not the pain.
112. Ans. b. Gastric antral vascular ectasia   113. Ans. b. Gastric antral vascular ectasia *(Ref: Sabiston 20 /e p1146; Schwartz 10/e p1088)*

MÉNÉTRIER'S DISEASE

114. Ans. d. Hyperchlorhydria *(Ref: Sabiston 20/e p1231; Schwartz 10/e p1088; Bailey 27/e p1116)*
115. Ans. d. Menetrier's disease *(Ref: Sabiston 20/e p1231; Schwartz 10/e p1088; Bailey 27/e p1116)*

- *History of epigastric pain, anorexia, weight loss and pedal edema and low total protein and albumin levels with massive gastric folds in the stomach giving rise to cobblestone or cerebriform appearance, which is characteristically seen in Menetrier's disease.*

116. Ans. b. Hyperchlorhydria
117. Ans. a. Lymphoma; b. Ménétrier's disease; c. Carcinoma; d. Eosinophilic gastritis *(Ref: Chapman 4th/234; Harrison 19/e p1931)*

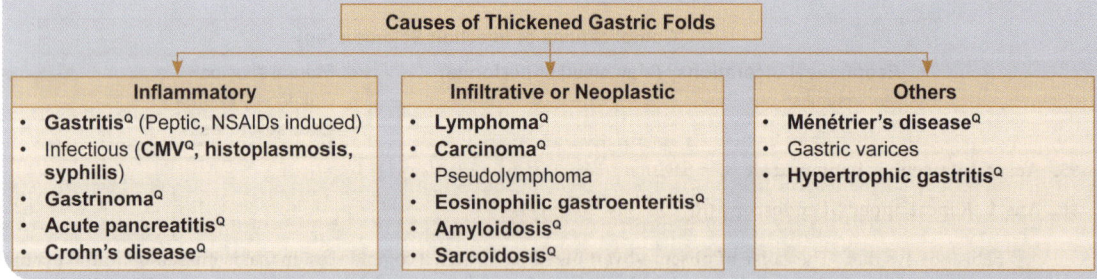

118. Ans. a Giant folds in the pyloric antrum

GASTRIC POLYPS

119. Ans. a. Adenoma *(Ref: Sabiston 20/e p1215; Schwartz 10/e p1076-1077; Bailey 26/e p1045; Shackelford 8/e p764, 7/e p769)*

GASTRIC POLYPS

- There are five types of gastric epithelial polyps inflammatory, hamartomatous, heterotopic, hyperplastic and adenoma. The first three types have negligible malignant potential.

  - MC gastric polyp is the **hyperplastic**[Q] or **regenerative polyp**, which frequently occurs in the setting of gastritis.
  - Polyps that are **symptomatic, > 2 cm** or **adenomatous** should be **removed**.

- Among patients with **FAP, gastric polyps (33–60%)** are **more common** as compared to **gastric adenomas (15%).**
- MC gastric polyp[Q]: Hyperplastic
- MC neplastic gastric polyp: Tubular

120. Ans. a. Hyperplastic polyp
121. Ans. a. Most common gastric polyp, e. Surgery is done if they are symptomatic *(Ref: Schwartz 10/e p1076-1077; Sabiston 20/e p1215)*

CARCINOMA STOMACH PREDISPOSING FACTORS

122. Ans. a. Benign ulcer *(Ref: Sabiston 20/e p1214; Schwartz 10/e p1074-1086; Bailey 27/e p1131; Shackelford 8/e p712, 7/e p774)*
123. Ans. d. Hyperplastic polyps
124. Ans. a. Chronic atrophic gastritis, c. Smoking, d. H. pylori infection, e. Menetrier's disease *(Ref: Schwartz 10/e p1074-1086; Sabiston 20/e p1214; Bailey 27/e p1131)*
125. Ans. a. A
126. Ans. a. Diffuse type of gastric cancer *(Ref: Sabiston 20/e p1216; Schwartz 10/e p1216; Bailey 25/e p1068)*
127. Ans. a. Pernicious anemia
128. Ans. d. Intestinal metaplasia type III
129. Ans. b. Hyperplastic polyp
130. Ans. a. Atrophic gastritis; c. Adenomatous polyp; d. Achlorhydria
131. Ans. c. Intestinal metaplasia
132. Ans. b. 'O' blood group
133. Ans. c. Atrophic gastritis
134. Ans. None of the above
135. Ans. b. Most common at fundus
136. Ans. b. Intestinal metaplasia *(Ref: Shackelford 8/e p712, 7/e p773-774; Schwartz 10/e p1074-1086)*

Precursor lesions of Carcinoma Stomach	
• Adenomatous gastric polyps	• Intestinal metaplasia
• **Chronic atrophic gastritis**	• Ménétrier's disease
• Dysplasia	

INTESTINAL METAPLASIA

- Types: **complete type I** and **incomplete types II** and **III**^{Q}
- The **risk for progression to gastric cancer** is **higher in type III**^{Q} metaplasia than in type I.
- The types differ based on the patterns of **mucin core protein** (MUC) **expression** as well as **cell type composition.**

> - Type I: Presence of **absorptive cells, paneth cells** and **goblet cells** secreting **sialomucins**
> - Incomplete types: Presence of **columnar** and **goblet cells** secreting **sialomucins, sulfomucins** or **both.**

137. Ans. d. Gastric cancer

CA STOMACH CLINICAL FEATURES AND TREATMENT

138. Ans. a. Occurs at distal end *(Sabiston 20/e p1216-1221; Schwartz 10/e p1074-1086; Bailey 27/e p1131; Shackelford 8/e p712, 7/e p774-778)*
139. Ans. d. Type IV *(Ref: Sabiston 19/e p1207; Schwartz 9/e p931; Bailey 27/e p1133)*
140. Ans. b. More common in males *(Ref: Sabiston 20/e p1216; Schwartz 10/e p1079)*
141. Ans. b. Lobular carcinoma *(Ref: Devita 10/e p338)*
142. Ans. a. Protruding *(Ref: Sabiston 20/e p1216; Schwartz 10/e p1079; Bailey 27/e p1133)*
143. Ans. b. Siewert type II *(Ref: Sabiston 20/e p1217)*
144. Ans. a. Decreased E-cadherin
145. Ans. a. More common
146. Ans. a. Decreased E-cadherin
147. Ans. c. Hematogenous spread
148. Ans. b. II

> T4a: Tumor invades **serosa (visceral peritoneum)**   Stage IIB: T1N3, T2N2, T3N1, T4aN0

149. Ans. c. p53
150. Ans. a. Suprapyloric *(Ref: Sabiston 20/e p1219, 19/e p1210; Bailey 27/e p1135)*

LYMPH NODE STATIONS

1. Right cardiac; **2.** Left cardiac; **3.** Lesser curvature; **4.** Greater curvature; **5.** Suprapyloric; **6.** Infrapyloric **7.** Left gastric; **8.** Common hepatic; **9. Celiac**; **10.** Splenic hilus; **11. Splenic artery**; **12. Hepatoduodenal ligament**; **13.** Retropancreatic; **14.** Mesenteric root; **15.** Transverse mesocolon; **16.** Paraaortic

151. **Ans. a. Celiac nodes**   152. **Ans. c. Rectum** *(Ref: Sabiston 20/e p1216; Schwartz 10/e p1069; Bailey 27/e p1135)*

Sister Mary Joseph nodule	
Gastrointestinal malignancies	**Gynecological malignancies**
• Gastric cancer (MC)^Q • Colonic cancer^Q • Pancreatic cancer (mostly **body** and **tail**)^Q	• Ovarian cancer^Q • Uterine cancer^Q

153. **Ans. b. Often associated with hypochlorhydria/achlorhydria**   154. **Ans. b. Gastric antrum**   155. **Ans. None**

T4a: Tumor invades **serosa (visceral peritoneum)**   N3a: Metastasis in **7-15** regional LNs
Stage IIIC: T4aN3, T4bN2, T4bN3

156. **Ans. a. Enterogastric reflex is the cause** *(Ref: Bailey 26/e p1053)*
157. **Ans. b. D2 gastrectomy include total gastrectomty; c. Surgical non curative lesion should not be resected; e. Hematemesis present in majority of patients** *(Ref: Bailey 27/e p1136)*

CARCINOMA STOMACH

- **H. pylori infection** increases risk of gastric cancer by causing **chronic gastritis, loss of gastric acidity** and **bacterial growth** in stomach.
- **Gastrectomy** can be **total** or **subtotal** in **D2 gastrectomy**.
- Patient with **incurable disease** are **not subjected to radical surgery**. Treatment is **palliative systemic chemotherapy**.
- After **gastrectomy**, there is **loss of parietal cell mass** leads to **vitamin B$_{12}$** deficiency and **replacement** should be given **routinely**.
- **MC symptom** of carcinoma stomach is **abdominal pain > weight loss**.
- **Hematemesis** is **very rare** in carcinoma stomach.

158. **Ans. a. Metastatic left supraclavicular lymphadenopathy**   159. **Ans. d. All of the above**   160. **Ans. a. Ca stomach**
161. **Ans. b. Incidence is now decreasing in Japan and China**   162. **Ans. d. Fundus**   163. **Ans. a. Superficial spreading type**

Most Common site of Gastric Malignancies	
CA stomach	Antrum^Q
CA stomach in **pernicious anemia**	Fundus^Q
Diifuse variety	Fundus^Q
Gastric lymphoma	Antrum^Q
Burkitt's lymphoma (by **EBV**)	**Cardia** or **body**^{Q}

164. **Ans. c. Involvement of mucosa, submucosa and muscularis** *(Ref: Sabiston 20/e p1222; Schwartz 10/e p1216; Bailey 27/e p1132)*

EARLY GASTRIC CANCER

- Adenocarcinoma **limited to** the **mucosa** and **submucosa** of the stomach, **regardless of LN status**^{Q}.
- Approx. **10%** of patients will have **LN metastasis**^{Q}.
- Cancer of the lesser curve is more common than cancer of the greater curvature.

Treatment

- Treatment options: **Endoscopic mucosal resection**^{Q}, limited surgical resection or gastrectomy
- **Overall curative rate** with **adequate gastric resection** and **lymphadenectomy is 95%**^{Q}
- **Best prognosis**^{Q}

165. **Ans. b. Staining with endoscopic biopsy** *(Ref: Sabiston 20/e p1218-1221; Schwartz 10/e p1217; Bailey 27/e p1135; Shackelford 8/e p712, 7/e p774-775)*

DIAGNOSIS OF CARCINOMA STOMACH

- **Endoscopy** is the **best method** to **diagnose gastric cancer** as it visualizes the gastric mucosa and allows **biopsy** for a histological diagnosis.

  - **Chromoendoscopy** helps identification of mucosal abnormalities through **topical stains**^{Q}.
  - **Magnification endoscopy** is used to magnify standard endoscopic field by **1.5-150 times**^{Q}.
  - **Narrow band imaging** affords **increased visualization** of the **microvasculature**^{Q}.

- **Confocal laser endomicroscopy** permits in vivo, **three-dimensional microscopy**^{Q} including subsurface structures.
- **EUS** is a tool for **pre-operative staging** and **selection for neoadjuvant therapy**^{Q}.

166. **Ans. c. Partial gastrectomy + distal pancreatectomy** *(Ref: Sabiston 20/e p1221-1225; Schwartz 10/e p1221-1222; Bailey 27/e p1136; Shackelford 8/e p713-715, 7/e p775-778)*

TREATMENT OF CARCINOMA STOMACH

- Maintain **a 5 cm margin proximally** and **distally** to the primary lesion.
- Because of the extensive lymphatic network of the stomach and the propensity for microscopic extension, the traditional surgical approach attempts to maintain **a 5 cm margin proximally** and **distally** to the primary lesion.
- When the general oncologic goal of an **R0 resection** can be achieved by gastric preserving approach in **mid and distal** gastric cancer, **partial gastrectomy** is **preferred** over total gastrectomy.

Treatment of Carcinoma Stomach according to site	
Proximal-third	**Extended gastrectomy**, including the **distal esophagus**[Q]
Middle-third	**Total gastrectomy** and **D2** LN dissection[Q].
Distal-third	**Intestinal-type**: **Subtotal gastrectomy** with **D2** LN dissection[Q] **Diffuse-type**: **Total gastrectomy** with **D2** LN dissection[Q]

- In **subtotal gastrectomy** the luminal extent of the resection comprises about **80%** of the stomach. At the lesser curvature the resection should reach up to about **2 cm below** the anatomic **cardia**. At the greater curvature the resection has to go **beyond** the **right** and **left gastroepiploic arteries**; the small remaining fundus is fed through the short gastric vessels from the splenic hilus.

Indications for Adjuvant Chemoradiation in Carcinoma Stomach
• T3, T4 or **node positive** cancers[Q] • Microscopically positive surgical margins[Q]

- **Spleen preserving D2 resection** is the **recommended** surgical approach for patients with potentially **curable gastric cancer**.
  - **Splenectomy** should be performed only in cases with **intraoperative evidence** of **direct tumor extension** into the **spleen** or when the **primary tumor** is **located in** the **proximal stomach along** the **greater curvature** or **posterior wall of stomach**[Q].
  - **Partial pancreatectomy** should be performed only in cases of **direct tumor extension** to the **pancreas**[Q].

167. **Ans. b. Subtotal gastrectomy**
168. **Ans. b. Invasion of mucosa and submucosa irrespective to L.N. spread; c. Endoscopic removal of lesions; d. Conservative gastrectomy**
169. **Ans. a. Involvement of omental nodes; e. Krukenberg tumor** *(Ref: Schwartz 10/e p1226, 9/e p1068-1074; CSDT 11/e p1175)*

CARCINOMA STOMACH

- Bailey: "**Involvement of other organ per se does not imply incurability**, provided that **it can be removed**."
- Schwartz: "It should be strongly emphasized that **many patients with positive lymph nodes are cured by adequate surgery**. It should also be stressed that often lymph nodes that appear to be grossly involved with tumor turn out to be benign or reactive on pathologic examination. **More than 15 resected lymph nodes** are **required for adequate staging**. Therapeutic nihilism should be avoided and, in the low-risk patient, an aggressive attempt to resect all tumor should be made. The **primary tumor may be resected en bloc with adjacent involved organs** (e.g., **distal pancreas, transverse colon**, or **spleen**) during the course of curative gastrectomy."
- CSDT: "A **solitary metastatic nodule** in **liver** is also **no indication against curable resection**."
- **Periumbilical node**, **Blumer's shelf**, and **Krukenberg's tumor** represent **incurable gastric cancer**.

170. **Ans. a. Carcinoma stomach** *(Ref: Robbins 9/e p772; Sabiston 20/e p1227)*
171. **Ans. c. Dysphagia**
172. **Ans. d. Weight loss**
173. **Ans. d. None of the above**

    Subtotal gastrectomy should be done **for resectable carcinoma stomach** involving **antrum**.
174. **Ans. c. Celiac**
175. **Ans. b. Stomach cancer**
176. **Ans. c. Testicular tumors** *(Ref: Sabiston 20/e p1216; Schwartz 10/e p1079; Bailey 27/e p1135)*
177. **Ans. b. Laparoscopy**

178. **Ans. d. EUS** *(Ref: Schwartz 10/e p1080)*

- The best way to stage the tumor locally is via EUS, which gives fairly accurate (80%) information about the depth of tumor penetration into the gastric wall, and can usually show enlarged (> 5 mm) perigastric and celiac lymph nodes.

179. **Ans. c. Stomach**

GASTROINTESTINAL STROMAL TUMOR

180. **Ans. a Mesenchymal** *(Ref: Sabiston 20/e p1229-1230; Schwartz 10/e p1481-1485; Bailey 26/e p1054; Shackelford 8/e p951, 7/e p1028-1034)*

181. **Ans. a. More common in female** *(Ref: Sabiston 20/e p1229, 1230)*

"Gastric GISTs can manifest at any age, although most typically they manifest in patients older than 50 years. They generally have an equal male-to-female ratio or a slight male predominance." (Sabiston 20/e p1229)

"High-risk GISTs: Defined as >10 cm tumor, mitotic count >10/50 HPF, tumor >5 cm and mitotic count ≥ per 50 HPF, or tumor rupture." (Sabiston 20/e p1230)

182. **Ans. c. 3 years** *(Ref: Sabiston 20/e p1230)*

"The Scandinavian Sarcoma Group (SSG) XVIII trial compared an extended 36-month course of adjuvant imatinib versus a 12-month course after resection for high-risk GISTs (defined as >10 cm tumor, mitotic count >10/50 HPF, tumor >5 cm and mitotic count > per 50 HPF, or tumor rupture). Patients in the extended treatment arm had higher recurrence-free survival (65.6% versus 47.9%) and overall survival (92.0% versus 81.7%) at 5 years after surgery. The results of this trial have established a 3-year course as the standard of care after surgical resection of high-risk GIST." (Sabiston 20/e p1230)

183. **Ans. a. Segmental resection** *(Ref: Sabiston 20/e p1230; Schwartz 10/e p1084; Bailey 27/e p1140)*

"GIST: Wedge resection with clear margins is adequate surgical treatment." (Schwartz 10/e p1084)

184.	Ans. c. GIST	185.	Ans. a. GIST	186.	Ans. b. Stomach
187.	Ans. c. Commonly metastasize to lymph nodes	188.	Ans. a. GIST	189.	Ans. b. GIST
190.	Ans. b. CD-117	191.	Ans. d. PET-CT		
192.	Ans. a. Most common in duodenum	193.	Ans. a. Gastric carcinoma; b. Paraganglioma; c. Pulmonary Chordoma		
194.	Ans. d. Interstitial cells of Cajal				

195. **Ans. c. Leiomyosarcoma** *(Ref: www.ncbi.nlm.nih.gov/pubmed/3771120)*

Leiomyosarcomas that occur **in the digestive tract** can also cause **gastrointestinal blockage** or **bleeding,** which can manifest as blood in the stool.

196. **Ans. c. Leiomyosarcoma**

- Gastrointestinal stromal tumours (**GISTs**) are the **MC mesenchymal tumours** of the **GIT**.
- Formerly **GISTs** were commonly classified histologically as leiomyosarcomas; however, they are now known to **arise from** the **interstitial cells of Cajal.**
- **Majority** of **GISTs** overexpress **KIT** and have characteristic mutations within the gene, which are the targets of **drug treatment with tyrosine kinase inhibitors**.
    - **Leiomyosarcoma** is a **malignant tumour** of **smooth muscle differentiation** and falls into a **group of sarcomas** that show **complex karyotypic changes** with no consistent recurrent genetic abnormality.
- **Upper GI bleeding** is the MC clinical manifestation of **GISTs**[Q], manifesting as hematemesis or melena in **40-65%** of patients. Bleeding occurs because of an ulcer forming in the gastric mucosa overlying the tumor.
- **Bleeding** is **more commonly** seen **in GIST** as compared to **Leiomyosarcoma**[Q].

197. **Ans. d. GIST**

- **Upper GI bleeding** is the **most common clinical manifestation** of **GISTs**, manifesting as hematemesis or melena in **40-65%** of patients.
- **Bleeding occurs because of an ulcer forming** in the **gastric mucosa overlying the tumor**.

198. **Ans. d. ALK gene mutation is seen in most of the cases** *(Ref: Robbins 9/e p775-777; Sabiston 20/e p1229)*

ALK gene mutation is not seen in GIST.

Stomach and Duodenum

ANAPLASTIC LYMPHOMA KINASE (ALK)

- **Anaplastic lymphoma kinase** also known as **ALK tyrosine kinase receptor** or **CD246** (cluster of differentiation 246) is an enzyme that in humans is **encoded by the ALK gene.**
- The **2;5 chromosomal translocation** is associated with approximately **60% anaplastic large-cell lymphomas** (ALCLs). The translocation creates a fusion gene consisting of the ALK (anaplastic lymphoma kinase) gene and the nucleophosmin (NPM) gene: the 3' half of ALK, derived from chromosome 2 and coding for the catalytic domain, is fused to the 5' portion of NPM from chromosome 5.
  - The **EML4-ALK fusion gene** is responsible for approximately 3–5% of **non-small-cell lung cancer** (NSCLC). Also related to **Neuroblastomas**^{Q}.
  - **Germline mutations in the anaplastic lymphoma kinase (ALK) gene** have recently been identified as a **major cause of familial predisposition to neuroblastoma**^{Q}.

GASTRIC LYMPHOMA

199. **Ans. d. Most common site is fundus** *(Ref: Sabiston 20/e p1227-1228; Schwartz 10/e p1074-1084; Bailey 27/e p1140; Shackelford 8/e p960, 7/e p1035-1042)*
   Most common site of gastric lymphoma is fundus is an incorrect statement.

200. **Ans. b. Stomach**

201. **Ans. a. Chemotherapy; b. Radiotherapy; c. Surgery; d. Anti-H. pylori treatment** *(Ref: Sabiston 20/e p1228; Schwartz 10/e p1074, 1084; Bailey 27/e p1140; Shackelford 8/e p966, 7/e p1042)*

Treatment of Gastric Lymphoma	
Low-grade MALT	**High-grade (aggressive)**
• **Confined to gastric wall** and **no t(11:18) translocation**: H.pylori **eradication therapy** and re-evaluate at 12 months	• **Stage I, II, III: Chemotherapy + RT**
• **Lymph node involvement** and **t(11:18) translocation**: H.pylori **eradication therapy** and re-evaluate at 3-6 months; if lymphoma persists: – **Stage I: XRT** – **Stage II: Chemotherapy + RT**	• **Stage IV: Chemotherapy + RT** • **Residual disease**: Further **chemotherapy** or **Surgery**
• **Stage III or IV**: H.pylori **eradication therapy** and **Chemotherapy +/- RT**	

- **External beam radiotherapy**: 30 Gy with 10 Gy boost
- **Chemotherapy regimens** cyclophosphamide, doxorubicin, vincristine, prednisone (CHOP) ± rituximab
- **Rituximab** is chimeric monoclonal antibody **against CD-20**, preferred for **high grade MALT** or **DLBL**.

202. **Ans. d. Intractable pain** *(Ref: Sabiston 20/e p1228; Bailey 26/e p1054; Oxford Surgery 5/e p174)*

Indications of Surgery in Gastric Lymphoma	
• **Failure** of **chemoradiation**^{Q}	• Obstruction^Q
• **Hemorrhage**^{Q}	• Perforation^Q

203. **Ans. c. Total gastrectomy with adjuvant chemotherapy is treatment of choice**
204. **Ans. b. Gastric resection and chemotherapy** *(Ref: http://www.ncbi.nlm.nih.gov/pmc/articles/PMC2117016/)*
205. **Ans. d. Clinically can be easily differentiated from gastric adenocarcinoma by the presence of early satiety and prominent lymph node metastases**

DUODENAL ATRESIA

206. **Ans. a. Down's syndrome** *(Ref: Sabiston 20/e p1870; Schwartz 10/e p1612,1615-1616; Bailey 27/e p1293; Shackelford 8/e p774, 7/e p811-813)*
207. **Ans. b. Duodenal atresia**   208. **Ans. b. Duodenal atresia**
209. **Ans. a. Duodenal atresia**   210. **Ans. a. Duodenoduodenostomy**
211. **Ans. a. Down's syndrome** *(Ref: Sabiston 20/e p1870; Schwartz 10/e p1615; Bailey 27/e p133)*

HYPERTROPHIC PYLORIC STENOSIS

212. **Ans. a. Hypokalemia; b. Hypochloremic metabolic alkalosis** *(Ref: Sabiston 20/e p1869; Schwartz 10/e p1613-1614; Bailey 26/e p113-114; Shackelford 8/e p779, 7/e p813-816)*

Surgery Essence

213. Ans. c. Correction of electrolyte disturbances
214. Ans. c. Ultrasound abdomen
215. Ans. c. Metabolic acidosis
216. Ans. a. Mass in epigastrium
217. Ans. a. Hypertrophic pyloric stenosis
218. Ans. d. Hypertrophic pyloric stenosis *(Ref: Sabiston 20/e p1869)*

Single bubble sign	Congenital Hypertrophic Pyloric Stenosis[Q]
Double bubble sign	Duodenal atresia[Q], Annular pancreas
Triple bubble sign	Jejunal atresia[Q]

219. Ans. b. CHPS
220. Ans. b. The pyloric tumour is best felt during feeding
221. Ans. c. Metabolic alkalosis with paradoxical aciduria
222. Ans. b. Aciduria
223. Ans. d. Pyloric stenosis
224. Ans. c. 48 hours
225. Ans. d. High gastric residue
226. Ans. a. Congenital hypertrophic pyloric stenosis
227. Ans. e. Normal saline with potassium *(Ref: Sabiston 20/e p1205; Schwartz 10/e p1069; Bailey 27/e p1130; Shackelford 8/e p779, 7/e p716-717)*

Fluid resuscitation requires replacement of the chloride and potassium deficiencies.

Gastric Outlet Obstruction

- In cases of **prolonged vomiting**, patients may become **dehydrated** and develop a **hypochloremic hypokalemic metabolic alkalosis** secondary to **loss of gastric juice** rich in **hydrogen, chloride,** and **potassium ions**[Q].
- In this setting, **fluid resuscitation** requires **replacement of** the **chloride** and **potassium deficiencies** in addition to **nasogastric suction for relief of the obstructed stomach**[Q].

228. Ans. d. Visible peristalsis is always seen
229. Ans. d. Congenital hypertrophic pyloric stenosis
230. Ans. c. Epigastrium *(Ref: Sabiston 20/e p1869; Schwartz 10/e p1614; Bailey 27/e p128)*

"Palpation of the pyloric "olive" tumor in the epigastrium by an experienced examiner is pathognomonic for HPS. If the olive is confirmed, no additional diagnostic testing is necessary." (Sabiston 20/e p1869)

GASTRIC OUTLET OBSTRUCTION

231. Ans. c. Hypokalemic metabolic alkalosis; d. Paradoxical aciduria *(Ref: Sabiston 20/e p1205; Schwartz 10/e p1069; Bailey 27/e p1130; Shackelford 8/e p779, 7/e p716-717)*
232. Ans. d. First part of duodenum
233. Ans. a. Pyloric obstruction
234. Ans. b. Cancer of stomach
235. Ans. c. Resolves spontaneously without treatment
236. Ans. c. Truncal vagotomy with gastrojejunostomy
237. Ans. b. Gastric outlet obstruction
238. Ans. a. Acidosis
239. Ans. b. Pylorus *(Ref: http://www.anaesthesiamcq.com/AcidBaseBook/ab7_2.php)*

- **Gastric alkalosis** is **most marked with vomiting** due to **pyloric stenosis** or **obstruction** because the **vomitus is acidic gastric juice only**[Q].
- **Vomiting in other conditions** may involve a **mixture of acid gastric loss** and **alkaline duodenal contents**[Q] and the acid-base situation that results is more variable.
- **Loss of alkaline small intestinal contents** can even **result in an acidosis** if **gastric acid secretion** is **suppressed**[Q].

240. Ans. a. Alkaline urine
241. Ans. c. Surgery *(Ref: Bailey 27/e p1142)*

Acute Gastric Dilatation

- This condition usually occurs in **association with pyloroduodenal disorders** or **after surgery without nasogastric suction**[Q].
- The **stomach**, which may also be **atonic, dilates enormously**[Q].
- Often the **patient is** also **dehydrated** and has **electrolyte disturbances**.
- **Failure to treat** this condition can result in a **sudden massive vomit with aspiration** into the lungs[Q].
- Treatment:
- **Nasogastric suction** with a large-bore tube, **fluid replacement** and **treatment of the underlying condition**[Q].

242. Ans. a. Dilatation of stomach seen on X-ray; b. Presents with vomiting; c. Aspiration; e. Atony of stomach

BEZOARS

243. **Ans. c. GI obstruction** *(Ref: Sabiston 20/e p1233; Schwartz 10/e p1089; Bailey 27/e p1142; Shackelford 8/e p280, 7/e p805)*

    Symptoms of Trichobezoar: Pain from **gastric ulceration** and fullness from **gastric outlet obstruction** with occasional **gastric perforation** and **small bowel obstruction**.

244. **Ans. d. Malignancy**
245. **Ans. a. Trichobezoar**
246. **Ans. a. It is caused by Trichuris**
247. **Ans. b. Caused by ingestion...., c. In Rapunzel syndrome...., e. It increases...** *(Ref: Schwartz 10/e p1089; Sabiston 20/e p1233; Bailey 27/e p1142)*

STRESS GASTRITIS

248. **Ans. c. Surgery involves anterior gastrotomy with ligation of bleeding ulcers and superficial erosions** *(Ref: Sabiston 20/e p1211; Schwartz 10/e p1073-1074)*
249. **Ans. b. Stress ulcers in head injury** *(Ref: Schwartz 10/e p1090; Sabiston 20/e p1211; Bailey 27/e p1142)*
250. **Ans. c. Elective ventilation**
251. **Ans. d. Increased H. pylori infection**
252. **Ans. a. Fundus of stomach**
253. **Ans. d. Distal duodenum**
254. **Ans. b. Stomach**
255. **Ans. b. Fundus**
256. **Ans. a. Burn patients**

- **Cushing ulcer**: Stress gastritis due to **intracranial injury/increased ICP**^{Q}
- **Curling ulcer**: After burn injury (> 35%); in the **body** and **fundus**^{Q}; not in antrum and duodenum
- **Cameron ulcers** or **riding ulcers**: Linear gastric erosions **in hiatal hernias**^{Q}

257. **Ans. b. Are solitary penetrating ulcer; d. Has also been described in children after head injury or craniotomy**
258. **Ans. c. Penicillin therapy**
259. **Ans. a. 1st part of duodenum**

GASTRIC VOLVULUS

260. **Ans. c. Endoscopy usually derotate** *(Ref: Sabiston 20/e p1232; Schwartz 10/e p1090; Shackelford 8/e p280, 7/e p876-878; Bailey 27/e p1142)*
261. **Ans. b. Acute gastric volvulus**
262. **Ans. b. Vomiting**

STOMACH ANATOMY AND PHYSIOLOGY

263. **Ans. c. Proximal branch of posterior vagus** *(Ref: Sabiston 20/e p1188-1189; Schwartz 10/e p1035-1040; Shackelford 8/e p675, 7/e p845)*

STOMACH INNERVATION

- The extrinsic innervation of the stomach is both **parasympathetic through the vagus** and **sympathetic through the celiac plexus**.
- The **vagus nerve originates** in the **vagal nucleus** in the **floor** of the **fourth ventricle** and **traverses** the **neck** in the **carotid sheath** to enter the **mediastinum**, where it **divides into several branches around** the **esophagus**. These branches coalesce above the esophageal hiatus to form the left and right vagus nerves.

- At the **GE junction**, the **left vagus** is **anterior**, and the **right vagus** is **posterior** (**LARP** mnemonic)^Q.

Left vagus	Right vagus
• At the **GE junction**, left vagus is **anterior**^{Q}	• At the **GE junction**, right vagus is **posterior**^{Q}
• Left vagus gives off the **hepatic branch to** the **liver**^{Q} and then continues along the lesser curvature as the **anterior nerve of Latarjet**^{Q}.	• **Criminal nerve of Grassi**^{Q} is the **first branch** of the **right** or **posterior vagus nerve** and is recognized as a **potential etiology of recurrent ulcers** when **left undivided**^{Q}.
	• **Right vagus** also gives a branch off to the **celiac plexus**^{Q} and then continues posteriorly along the lesser curvature.

Truncal vagotomy	• Performed **above** the **celiac** and **hepatic branches of** the **vagi**^{Q}
Selective vagotomy	• Performed **below** the **celiac** and **hepatic branches of** the **vagi**^{u}
Highly selective vagotomy	• Performed by **dividing the crow's feet** to the **proximal stomach** while **preserving** the **innervation of** the **antral** and **pyloric parts** of **stomach**^{Q}.

264. Ans. b. Body *(Ref: Shackelford 8/e p262, 7/e p781)*

Shackelford "The **gastric pacemaker**, which is **located in** the **body along** the **greater curvature**, stimulates both the filling and mixing of food in the body and antrum."

GASTRIC MOTILITY

- **Gastric pacemaker**: Interstitial cells of Cajal (ICCs)^Q
- **Location**: In body^Q along the greater curvature
- **ICCs** are critical for the generation of **sequential contractions**^{Q}

265. Ans. a. Protects epithelium

266. Ans. c. Pyloric antrum *(Ref: Sabiston 20/e p1190)*

Location	Cells
Gastric Body	**MCD PIE** (**M**ucus cells, **C**hief cells, **D** cells, **P**arietal cells, **I**nterneurons and **E**CL cells)^Q
Gastric antrum	**MD GI** (**M**ucus cells, **D** cells, **G** cells and **I**nterneurons)^Q

- **Parietal cells** secrete Ghrelin, Intrinsic factor, Leptin and Acid. (**GILA**)^Q
- **Chief cells** secrete **pepsin** and **leptin**^{Q}

- **Stomach Histology (CMPE)**: Chief cells (44%) > Mucous cells (40%) > Parietal cells (13%) > Endocrine cells (3%)^Q

GASTRIC MORPHOLOGY

- **Muscularis mucosa** is responsible for the **rugae**^{Q} that greatly **increases surface area** and also **marks** the **microscopic boundary** for invasive and non-invasive gastric carcinoma.
- **Submucosa** is the **strongest layer**^{Q} of the gastric wall.
- **Muscularis propria** consists of **three layers**^{Q} of smooth muscle. The **middle layer** is circular and is the **only complete muscle layer** of the stomach wall, this layer becomes **progressively thicker** toward the **pylorus**, where it becomes as a true anatomic sphincter.

EMBRYOLOGY OF STOMACH

- The stomach arises as a **dilatation** in the **tubular embryonic foregut**^{Q}
- Assumes its **normal asymmetric shape** and **position** by the end of the **7th week**^{Q}.
- During the **6th to 10th week** as the stomach enlarges it also **rotates 90 degrees** in a **clockwise direction**^{Q}.

267. Ans. c. Duodenum *(Ref: Sabiston 20/e p1245; Shackelford 8/e p820, 7/e p826)*

- **Brunner's Gland: Submucosal gland** found in the **duodenum**^{Q}

268. Ans. a. Stimulation of appetite *(Ref: Sabiston 20/e p1192; Schwartz 10/e p22,1045,1047,1348; Shackelford 8/e p645, 7/e p645-646)*

GHRELIN

- Secreted by **oxyntic cells** in the **fundus** of the stomach^Q
- First gut peptide found to have **orexigenic (appetite stimulating)** properties^Q.
- **Circulating levels** of ghrelin are **inversely related to BMI, adipose tissue mass** and **plasma insulin** levels^Q.

Primary effects of Ghrelin	
• **Motilin like effects** on gastric motility^Q • **Stimulates release** of **somatostatin** and **PP**^{Q}	• **Stimulates release of growth hormone** from pituitary^Q

269. Ans. c. Splenic artery *(Ref: Sabiston 20/e p1188)*

- **Posterior gastric artery** is a **branch of splenic artery**^{Q}.

GASTRIC DIVERTICULUM

270. **Ans. b. Usually at cardiac end; c. Usually on posterior surface** *(Ref: Schwartz 10/e p1089)*
271. **Ans. d. Pain**

MISCELLANEOUS

272. **Ans. b. T.B., c. CA pancreas, d. Crohn's disease:** *(Ref: Gastrointestinal Radiology 2ed/84)*

Causes of Duodenal Stricture	
• Chronic peptic ulcer^Q disease	• CA head of pancreas^Q
• Crohn's disease^Q	• Annular pancreas^Q
• Tuberculosis^Q	• Pancreatitis^Q
	• Cholecystitis

273. **Ans. a. Eagle-Barrett syndrome** *(Ref: Schwartz 10/e p1634)*

EAGLE-BARRETT SYNDROME OR PRUNE-BELLY SYNDROME

- **Prune-belly syndrome** describes the **wrinkled appearance** of the **anterior abdominal wall** that **characterizes these patients**^{Q}.
- Also known as **Eagle-Barrett syndrome** and the **triad syndrome** because of its **three major manifestations**^{Q}.

Characterized by		
• Extremely lax lower abdominal musculature^Q	• **Dilated urinary tract** including the bladder^Q	• Bilateral undescended testes^Q

- The incidence is **significantly higher** in **males**^{Q}.
- **Most significant comorbidity:** Pulmonary hypoplasia (lead to **death in the most severe cases**)^Q
- **Skeletal abnormalities** include **dislocation** or **dysplasia** of the hip and **pectus excavatum**^{Q}.

Genitourinary Manifestation
• **Major genitourinary manifestation: Ureteral dilatation**^{Q}
• **Ureters** are **typically long** and **tortuous**, and become **more dilated distally**.
• **Ureteric obstruction** is **rarely present**^{Q}.
• The **dilatation is** thought to be **caused by decreased smooth muscle** and **increased collagen** in the ureters^Q.
• Approximately **80%** of affected individuals have **some degree of VUR**, which can **predispose to UTI**^{Q}.

- Most children have adequate renal parenchyma for growth and development^Q.

Treatment:
- **Ureteric surgery** has **no role unless** an area of **obstruction develops**.
- **Bilateral orchidopexy** can be performed in conjunction **with abdominal wall reconstruction at 6-12 months of age**^{Q}.

274. **Ans. c. Pernicious anemia** *(Ref: Sabiston 20/e p1192)*   275. **Ans. d. Atrophic gastritis** *(Ref: Sabiston 20/e p1192)*

Causes of Hypergastrinemia

Ulcerogenic Causes (RAGS)	Non-ulcerogenic Causes (PACH)
• **R**etained excluded antrum^Q	• **P**ernicious anemia^Q
• **A**ntral G-cell hyperplasia or hyperfunction^Q	• **A**ntisecretory agents (PPIs)^Q
• **G**astrinoma^Q	• **A**trophic gastritis^Q
• **G**astric outlet obstruction^Q	• **A**cid-reducing procedure (vagotomy)
• **S**hort-bowel syndrome^Q	• **C**hronic renal failure^Q
	• **H**. pylori infection^Q

276. **Ans. b. Gastric ulcer**

HOUR-GLASS STOMACH

- Hour-glass stomach is caused by **cicatricial contraction** of a **saddle shaped ulcer** at the **lesser curvature**^{Q}

Tea-Pot Stomach (Hand-bag Stomach)

- Tea-pot stomach is caused by **longitudinal shortening** of **gastric ulcer** at the **lesser curvature** of stomach (stomach looks like tea-pot)^Q

277. **Ans. c. Ba enema**
278. **Ans. a. Most common small bowel carcinoma; b. Type of periampullary carcinoma; c. Jaundice and anemia-most common symptom** *(Ref: Sabiston 20/e p1277; Schwartz 10/e p1160; Bailey 25/e p1076; Shackelford 8/e p804-806, 7/e p779)*
279. **Ans. d. Up to 50 cm** *(Ref: Narayan Reddy 20/e p431)*

- In **adults**, **gastric lavage tube** should be passed upto **50 cm mark**^{Q}.

280. **Ans. c. Amyloidosis**
281. **Ans. d. Pancreatic injury; e. Duodenal injury** *(Ref: Sabiston 20/e p1552-1553; Shackelford 8/e p1211, 7/e p688)*

Management of Grade IV and V Pancreatic Injuries

- Due to short of radical resection, other **options designed to divert gastric, pancreatic,** and **biliary secretions away from the duodenum** need to be considered for the management of patients with **grade IV** and **V pancreatic injuries**^{Q}.
- These include **duodenal diverticularization, pyloric exclusion** or **gastrojejunostomy,** and **triple-tube decompression**^{Q}.

  - **Duodenal diverticularization** is accomplished by performing **antrectomy** and **gastrojejunostomy** to achieve gastric diversion, **choledochostomy** to divert bile if the ampulla is injured, **tube duodenostomy** for decompression of the duodenum, **suture repair of any duodenal injuries**, and **extensive periduodenal** and **peripancreatic drainage**^{Q}.

- When **pancreatic injuries** are associated with **major duodenal injuries**. **Drainage** or **resection of the pancreas** can be **combined with suturing** or **stapling** of the **pylorus (pyloric exclusion procedure)** to divert gastric flow from the duodenum^Q.
- Gastrointestinal continuity is then accomplished by **gastrojejunostomy**.
- It is quite remarkable that gastroduodenal continuity is re-established 4 to 6 weeks after pyloric exclusion even when heavy non-absorbable sutures or staples are used.
- The **pyloric exclusion** procedure has **largely replaced** the **duodenal diverticularization** procedure, which entails antrectomy and gastrojejunostomy, as well as drainage and decompression of the duodenal injury and drainage of the pancreatic injury.

282. **Ans. a. Gastric antrum is predominantly affected**

- **Type A gastritis** primarily involves **body** and **fundus**^{Q}

283. **Ans. b. > 10 cm** *(Ref: Shackelford 8/e p875, 7/e p895; Sabiston 19/e p1251)*

- **Finney stricturoplasty** is used for **strictures > 10–15 cm**^{Q}.
- **Heineke-Mikulicz stricturoplasty** is appropriate strictures **< 10 cm**^{Q} in length.

284. **Ans. b. 15 cm** *(Ref: Shackelford 8/e p773, 7/e p810; www.surgery.usc.edu/foregut/demeesterpub/235. Ans.pdf)*

Hunt-Lawrence Pouch

- **Jejunal reservoir (Hunt-Lawrence pouch)** is used for the treatment of **microgastria**.
- Length of pouch: **12–15 cm**^{Q}
- Length of **jejunal limb** used: **35–40 cm**^{Q}

285. **Ans. a. Carcinoid** *(Ref: Schwartz 10/e p1074)*

"Hyperplastic polyps which consist of elongated, branching, dilated glandular structures are the most common epithelial tumors in the stomach (75–90 % of all gastric polyps). They are most likely associated with chronic gastritis and rarely transform into gastric cancer." {Radiology Illustrated: Gastrointestinal Tract edited by Byung Ihn Choi (2014)/p126}

"Carcinoid is the second most common epithelial tumor of the stomach and accounts for 11–41 % of all gastrointestinal carcinoids." {Cytopathology in Oncology edited by Ritu Nayar (2013)/p128}

CHAPTER 11

Peritoneum

RETROPERITONEAL FIBROSIS

Retroperitoneal Fibrosis

- Characterized by **proliferation of fibrous tissue** in the **retroperitoneum**^{Q}
- Fibrosis is usually confined to **central & paravertebral spaces** between the **renal arteries & sacrum** and tends to **encase** the **aorta, IVC & ureters**^{Q}.
- Process usually **begins at the level** of **aortic bifurcation & spreads cephalad**^{Q} upto renal artery generally.

Etiology
- Around **70% cases** are **primary** or **idiopathic (Ormond's disease)**^{Q}

Causes of Secondary (30%)^Q Retroperitoneal Fibrosis
• **Inflammatory conditions: CATH**^{Q} **(Chronic pancreatitis, Actinomycosis, Tuberculosis, Histoplasmosis)** • **Drugs: Methysergide (Most important)**, methyldopa, hydralazine, entacapone, beta-blockers, bromocriptine, phenacetin, amphetamines^Q **(MAHE-BP)** • **Malignancies:** CA prostate, NHL, CA stomach, sarcoma & carcinoid tumor • **Autoimmune disorders:** SLE, PAN & ankylosing spondylitis • **Radiation**

Clinical Features
- More common in **males** of **40-60 years**^{Q}.
- **Early symptoms** are **vague & non-specific**^{Q} (abdominal or flank pain, weight loss, malaise, & hypertension)
- **Obstructive uropathy** (dysuria, frequency, fever due to secondary infection of hydroneprotic kidney) is the **earliest** and **MC specific symptom**^{Q}.

• **Ureters** are **MC involved**, **MC site** is **lower third** of **ureter**. • **Partial or complete obstruction** occurs in **75% patients**^{Q}.

Diagnosis: In absence of uremia, diagnosis is made by IVP.
- **IVP or RGP:**
  - Hydronephrosis with dilated tortuous upper ureter
  - **Medial pulling of ureters** or **pipestem ureters**^{Q}
  - **Extrinsic ureteral compression**^{Q}
- **CT scan is IOC** for retroperitoneal fibrosis^Q.
- **MRI is IOC** in cases of **compromised renal function**, because contrast cannot be given.

Treatment
- **Primary, idiopathic** retroperitoneal fibrosis: **Ureteral stenting** & **immunosuppression** (**TAPS:** Tamoxifen, Azathioprine, Penicillamine, Steroids)^Q
- **Secondary** retroperitoneal fibrosis: **Midline transperitoneal ureterolysis** with **wrapping** the **ureter** with **omental flap** or **lateral retroperitoneal ureteral transposition**^{Q}.

TAPS: Tamoxifen, Azathioprine, Penicillamine, Steroids are used in primary retroperitoneal fibrosis^Q.

SPONTANEOUS BACTERIAL PERITONITIS

Spontaneous Bacterial Peritonitis

- **SBP** is a common and severe complication of ascites characterized by **spontaneous infection of** the **ascitic fluid without an intra-abdominal source**^{Q}.
- **Prevalence** of SBP is **10-30%**^{Q} in patients of ascites, with **20%** in hospital **mortality rate**^{Q}.

• **MC organism** in **adults: E. coli**^{Q} >Klebsiella. • **MC organism** in **children: Group A streptococci**^{Q}

Mechanism

- **Bacterial translocation** with **gut flora traversing** the **intestine into mesenteric lymph nodes**, leading to **bacteremia & seeding of the ascitic fluid**[Q].
- **Predisposing Factors: Bowel preparation**, metabolic **alkalosis**, **dehydration** and **hypoproteinemia**[Q].
- It seen **more commonly in** patients presenting with **GI hemorrhage**[Q].

Clinical Features

- Patients with ascites may present with **fever, altered mental status, elevated WBC count**[Q], and **abdominal pain** or discomfort, or they may present without any of these features.
- **High degree of clinical suspicion** and **peritoneal taps** are important **for** making the **diagnosis.**

Diagnosis

- Presence of **>250**[Q] polymorphonuclear cells of ascitic fluid is consistent with SBP; with ascitic fluid **culture growing single organism**.
- If **more than two organisms** are identified, **secondary bacterial peritonitis** due to a **perforated viscus** should be considered[Q].

> - **Culture negative neutrocytic ascites** is diagnosed, when an ascitic fluid **PMN count of >250 is unaccompanied by a positive ascitic fluid culture**[Q].
> - **Culture negative neutrocytic ascites** carries a **similar prognosis**[Q] **to SBP** and is **managed similarly.**

Treatment

- Treated with **cefotaxime** plus **albumin**[Q]
- **Norfloxacin decreases** the **incidence of SBP**[Q] in patients with variceal bleeding; patients with low-protein ascites and patients with a prior history of SBP.
- **Repeat diagnostic paracentesis** is indicated **after 48 hours** of appropriate antibiotic therapy only if there is a **lack of clinical improvement** or in cases of **secondary bacterial peritonitis**[Q].

Prognosis

- **Occurrence of SBP** is an important **landmark in natural history** of cirrhosis with **1** and **2 year survival** rate of **30%** and **20%,** respectively[Q].

SECONDARY (ACUTE SUPPURATIVE) BACTERIAL PERITONITIS

Secondary (Acute Suppurative) Bacterial Peritonitis

- When **bacteria contaminate** the peritoneum **as a result of spillage** from an intra-abdominal **viscus**[Q].
- Infection in secondary bacterial peritonitis is **polymicrobial**[Q]
- **E. coli & Bacteroides** are **MC organisms**[Q].
- The species of organism isolated vary with the source of the initial process and the normal flora present at the site.

PERITONITIS ASSOCIATED WITH CHRONIC AMBULATORY PERITONEAL DIALYSIS (CAPD)

Peritonitis Associated With Chronic Ambulatory Peritoneal Dialysis (CAPD)

- **Peritonitis** is one of the **MC complications** of **CAPD**[Q], occurring with an incidence of approximately **one episode every 1 to 3 years**[Q].
- **Refractory** or **recurrent peritonitis** is MC cause of **technical failure of CAPD**[Q].

> - **MC organism: Staphylococcus epidermidis**[Q] **(30–50%).**

Clinical Features

- Patients present with **abdominal pain, fever,** and **cloudy peritoneal dialysate** containing **>100 WBC/mm³**, with **>50% of the cells being neutrophils**[Q].
- **Gram staining detects organisms** only in **10–40% of cases**[Q].

Treatment

- CAPD associated peritonitis is treated by the **intraperitoneal administration of antibiotics**, usually a **first generation cephalosporin**[Q].
- Overall, **75% of infections** are **cured by culture-directed antibiotic therapy**[Q].
- **Recurrent** or **persistent peritonitis** requires **removal of** the **dialysis catheter** and resumption of **hemodialysis**[Q].

PNEUMOCOCCAL PERITONITIS

Pneumococcal Peritonitis

- **Primary pneumococcal peritonitis** may **complicate nephrotic syndrome** or **cirrhosis in children**[Q].
- Otherwise **healthy children**, particularly **girls between 3–9 years** of age, **may also be affected**, and it is likely that the **route of infection** is sometimes **via the vagina** and **fallopian tubes**[Q].
- At other times, and **always in males**, the **infection is blood-borne** and **secondary to respiratory tract or middle ear disease**[Q].

Clinical Features
- Onset is sudden, earliest symptom is **pain localized to** the **lower half of the abdomen**.
- Temperature is raised to **39°C or more** and there is usually **frequent vomiting**[Q].
- After **24–48 hours**, **profuse diarrhea** is characteristic and **increased frequency of micturition** (caused by **severe pelvic peritonitis**)[Q]
- On examination, **abdominal rigidity** is **usually bilateral** but is less than in most cases of **acute appendicitis with peritonitis.**[Q]

Diagnosis
- **WBC count ≥ 30 000/μL** with approximately **90% polymorphs** suggests **pneumococcal peritonitis** rather than appendicitis[Q].

Treatment
- Antibiotic therapy + Correcting dehydration and electrolyte imbalance + **Early surgery**[Q]
- **Laparotomy** or **laparoscopy** may be used.

> - If the **exudate** be **odourless** and **sticky**, the **diagnosis of pneumococcal peritonitis** is **practically certain**[Q]

INTRA-ABDOMINAL ABSCESS

Intra-Abdominal Abscess

- **MC site** of intra-peritoneal abscess: **Pelvis**[Q]
- **Right subhepatic space** (lies between inferior surface of liver and hepatic flexure and transverse mesocolon) is the **most dependent portion** of the **abdominal cavity in the recumbent position**[Q].
- **Pelvic cavity** is the **most dependent area** of the **peritoneal cavity** in the **upright position**[Q].

Clinical Features
- **High spiking fevers**, **chills**, **abdominal pain**, **anorexia**, and **delay of return of bowel function**[Q] in the postoperative patient are typical presenting signs and symptoms of intraperitoneal abscess.

Diagnosis
- **CT scan: Investigation of choice** for diagnosis of intra-**abdominal abscess**[Q]

Treatment
- Preferred treatment: CT guided percutaneous drainage[Q]
- **Operative drainage:** If percutaneous drainage is not possible or contraindicated

Pelvic Abscess

- **Pelvis** is the **MC site of an intraperitoneal abscess** because the vermiform **appendix** is **often pelvic in position** and the **fallopian tubes** are **frequent sites of infection**[Q].
- A **pelvic abscess** can also occur as a **sequel to** any case of **diffuse peritonitis** and is **common after anastomotic leakage**[Q] following colorectal surgery

Clinical Features
- Most characteristic symptoms are **diarrhea** & **passage of mucus** in the stools. [Q]
- **Rectal examination** reveals a **bulging** of the **anterior rectal wall**[Q], which, when the abscess is ripe, becomes softly cystic.
- Left to nature, a proportion of these abscesses burst into the rectum, after which the patient nearly always recovers rapidly. If this does not occur, the abscess should be drained deliberately.

Diagnosis
- If any uncertainty exists, the **presence of pus** should be **confirmed by ultrasound** or **CT scanning with needle aspiration** if indicated[Q].

Treatment
> - In women, **vaginal drainage** through the **posterior fornix (Posterior colpotomy)** is often chosen[Q].
> - **In other cases**, when the abscess is definitely pointing into the rectum, **rectal drainage** is employed[Q].

- **Laparotomy** is **almost never necessary**^{Q}.
- **Rectal drainage** of a **pelvic abscess** is far **preferable to suprapubic drainage**, which risks exposing the general peritoneal cavity to infection^Q.
- **Drainage tubes** can also be **inserted percutaneously** or **via the vagina** or **rectum** under ultrasound or CT guidance^Q.

WOUND DEHISCENCE (BURST ABDOMEN)

Wound Dehiscence (Burst Abdomen)

- **Serous** or **serosanguinous discharge** from the wound is the **first sign**^{Q} of dehiscence

> - **Most commonly** observed between **6th** and **8th** post-operative **day**^{Q} (may occur at any time following wound closure)

- Wound dehiscence is **partial** or **total disruption** of any or all layers of the operative wound.
- **Extrusion** of **abdominal viscera** after rupture of all layers is known as **evisceration**^{Q}.

Predisposing Factors for Wound Dehiscence	
Local Risk Factors	**Systemic Risk Factors**

• **Inadequate closure (Most important)**^{Q}
• **Increased** intra-abdominal **pressure**
• **Deficient wound healing** due to:
  – Infections^Q – Seroma^Q
  – **Hematoma**^{Q} – **Presence of drain**^{Q}
	• Old age^Q
	• Obesity^Q
	• Immunosuppression^Q
	• Systemic diseases:
	  – Diabetes^Q – Uremia^Q
	  – Jaundice, Sepsis^Q – Cancer^Q

Management
- Wound dehiscence without evisceration: **Prompt elective closure**^{Q} of the wound
- Wound dehiscence with evisceration:
  - Wound is covered with moist towels
  - Under GA, any exposed bowel or omentum is rinsed with RL containing antibiotics and then returned to abdomen
  - Previous sutures are removed, wound is reclosed (**Tension suturing**^{Q})

DUODENAL STUMP BLOWOUT

Duodenal Stump Blowout

- Duodenal stump blowout is **massive leakage** from **duodenal stump** following **Billroth-II gastrectomy**^{Q}.

Clinical Features
- It usually occurs on **4th to 7th** post-operative **day**^{Q}.
- Usually presents as **sudden intense thoracoabdominal pain, sudden elevation in pulse** and **temperature** or generalized deterioration of condition.

Treatment
- **Adequate drainage** must be instituted **immediately**, which is done by putting a **catheter** through an incision **below the right costal margin**^{Q}.
- **TPN** should be instituted and attention should be directed towards **fluid and electrolyte therapy**^{Q}.
- **Fistula closure** can be anticipated **within 2–3 weeks**^{Q}.

MESENTERIC CYST

Mesenteric Cyst

- Mesenteric cyst is encountered **most frequently** in the **2nd decade of life**
- More common in **women**

Types of Mesenteric cysts	
• **Chylolymphatic (MC)**^{Q} • Simple (**mesothelial**) • **Enterogenous**	• **Urogenital** remnant • **Dermoid** (teratomatous cyst)

Chylolymphatic Cyst	Enterogenous Cyst
• **MC type**, arises in **congenitally misplaced lymphatic tissue** that has **no efferent communication** with **lymphatic system**^Q • Arises most frequently in **mesentery of ileum**^Q. • **Thin wall** of cyst, **filled with clear lymph** or chyle. • Occasionally, the cyst attains a great size. • **Mostly unilocular** and **solitary**^Q • Chylolymphatic cyst **blood supply** is **independent from** that of the **adjacent intestine**^Q • **Enucleation** is possible without the need for resection of gut^Q.	• **Derived** either **from a diverticulum of** the **mesenteric border** of intestine or **from a duplication** of intestine^Q. • **Thicker wall** than a chylolymphatic cyst and it is **lined by mucous membrane**, sometimes ciliated^Q. • **Content** is **mucinous** and is either **colorless** or **yellowish brown** as a result of past hemorrhage. • **Muscle in** the **wall** of an **enteric duplication cyst** and **adjacent bowel** has a **common blood supply**^Q • **Removal of the cyst** always entails **resection** of the **related portion of intestine**^Q.

Clinical Features

- A painless abdominal swelling^Q
- **Recurrent attacks** of **abdominal pain**^Q with or without vomiting (temporary impaction of a food bolus in a segment of bowel narrowed by the cyst or possibly from torsion of the mesentery)
- **Acute abdominal pain** may arises as a result of: **Torsion, rupture, hemorrhage, infection**.

> • **Tillaux triad:** Fluctuant swelling near the umbilicus + moves freely in a plane perpendicular to the attachment of the mesentery + zone of resonance around the cyst^Q.

Diagnosis

- **CT scan: Investigation of choice** for **diagnosis of mesenteric cyst**^Q
- **USG:** Helpful in diagnosis

Treatment

- **Chylolymphatic cysts: Enucleation** is **treatment of choice**^Q
- **Enterogenous cyst: Resection & anastomosis** is the **treatment of choice**^Q
- **Aspiration alone** has a **high rate of cyst recurrence**^Q.

PSEUDOMYXOMA PERITONEI

Pseudomyxoma Peritonei

- Pseudomyxoma peritonei describes **mucinous ascites** arising from a **ruptured appendiceal** or **ovarian adenocarcinoma**^Q.
- **MC site** of primary: **Appendix**^Q
- **Peritoneum** becomes **coated with a mucus-secreting tumor** that **fills the peritoneal cavity** with **tenacious semisolid mucus** and **large, loculated cystic masses**^Q.
- Occurs **most commonly** in **40–50 years** of age
- Occurs with **equal frequency** in **men** and **women**^Q.

Clinical Features

- Patients are **often asymptomatic**^Q until late in the course of their disease.
- **On presentation**, **global deterioration in health** long before the diagnosis is made
- **Abdominal pain & distention** and **nonspecific complaints** are common.
- **Physical examination:** A new **hernia**, **ascites**, **distended abdomen** with **nonshifting dullness**^Q and, occasionally, a palpable abdominal mass.

Diagnosis

- **CT (chest, abdomen & pelvis):** Information regarding the **diagnosis** and the **ability to resect the tumor completely** or **perform an adequate cytoreduction**^Q.
- **Preoperative colonoscopy: Differentiate a mucinous neoplasm of** the **appendix from** that **arising from the colon**^Q.
- Often, the **diagnosis is made at laparotomy** (peritoneal cavity containing **tenacious semisolid mucus** and **large, loculated cystic masses**)

Treatment

- **Cytoreduction** (Resection of as much of the tumor as possible) + **Intraperitoneal hyperthermic chemotherapy (IPHC)**^Q.

> • **Operative management:** Omentectomy, stripping of involved peritoneum, resection of involved organs and appendectomy with right hemicolectomy^Q

Prognosis

- **Adenomucinosis** (Adenocarcinoma of appendix): **Best survival rate** (75% at 5 years)
- **Peritoneal mucinous carcinomatosis**: **Worst** (14% at 5 years)

ACUTE MESENTERIC LYMPHADENITIS

Acute Mesenteric Lymphadenitis

- Syndrome of **acute right lower quadrant abdominal pain** associated with **mesenteric lymph node enlargement** and a **normal appendix**^{Q}.
- Diagnosis is made upon **exploration** of the abdomen of a **patient suspected of having acute appendicitis** at which time a **normal appendix** and **enlarged mesenteric lymph nodes**^{Q} are discovered.
- Occurs **most commonly** in **children** and **young adults**^{Q}
- Equal frequency in males and females.
- **Etiology often remains unknown**, although **some cases** are associated with **Yersinia infection of the ileum.**
- **Yersinia enterocolitica** has been **associated with** this **syndrome** in **children**^{Q}.

MALIGNANT PERITONEAL MESOTHELIOMA

Malignant Peritoneal Mesothelioma

- MC primary malignant peritoneal neoplasm: **Malignant mesothelioma**^{Q}
- Results from malignant transformation of the simple squamoid epithelium covering the peritoneal cavity.
- **More common** in **males**, **median age** of presentation is **50 years**.
- Most patients had **exposure to asbestos**^{Q}.

Clinical Features

- Most patients present with **abdominal pain** and **weight loss.**
- **Ascites** is common and often **intractable.**
- **Omentum** may become **diffusely involved with tumor**, present as an **epigastric mass.**
- In contrast to pseudomyxoma peritonei, **local invasion of intra-abdominal organs**, such as the liver, intestine, bladder, and abdominal wall, **can occur.**
- **Encasement of bowel** can create a **malignant bowel obstruction**.

Diagnosis

- **CT scan**: Mesenteric thickening, peritoneal studding, hemorrhage within the tumor, and **ascites**^{Q}.

Treatment

- **Complete surgical resection** is usually **not possible** because of the extent of disease.

Prognosis

- Median survival is 30–60 months

Multiple Choice Questions

RETROPERITONEAL FIBROSIS

1. **Ormond's disease is:** *(MHPGMCET 2009, 2007)*
   a. Retractile testis
   b. Idiopathic retroperitoneal lymphadenopathy
   c. Idiopathic retroperitoneal fibrosis
   d. Idiopathic mediastinitis

2. **Retroperitoneal fibrosis most commonly presents with:**
   a. Pedal edema   b. Ascites   *(JIPMER 2011)*
   c. Ureteric obstruction   d. Back pain

3. **Most common organ involved in retroperitoneal fibrosis is:**
   (Recent Question 2014, AIIMS Nov 93)
   a. Aorta   b. Ureter
   c. Inferior vena cava   d. Sympathetic nerve plexus

4. **Localized idiopathic fibrosis is seen in all of the following except:** *(UPSC 2001)*
   a. Riedel's struma   b. Hypertrophic scar
   c. Sclerosing cholangitis   d. Panniculitis

5. **False about retroperitoneal fibrosis is:** *(Recent Question 2015)*
   a. Ureter is most commonly involved
   b. More common in females
   c. Primary idiopathic form is called Ormond's disease
   d. Corticosteroids are mainstay of treatment

PERITONITIS

6. **All are true about SBP except:** *(ILBS 2012)*
   a. In hospital mortality rate is 20%
   b. Neutrocytic ascites has better prognosis
   c. Norfloxacin is useful for prevention
   d. Cefotaxime is used for treatment

7. **Emergency operation done in cases of:** *(PGI Nov 2010)*
   a. Volvulus   b. Obstructed hernia
   c. Appendicular perforation with paralytic ileus
   d. Toxic megacolon   e. Colonic perforation

8. **Investigation for acute abdomen includes:** *(PGI May 2010)*
   a. USG   b. Multidetector CT
   c. Contrast enhanced CT   d. X-ray abdomen
   e. Echocardiography

9. **A post-op patient presents with peritonitis and massive contamination because of duodenal leak. Management of choice is:** *(AIIMS June 2001)*
   a. Four quadrant peritoneal lavage
   b. Duodenostomy + Feeding jejunostomy + Peritoneal lavage
   c. Total parenteral nutrition
   d. Duodenojejunostomy

10. **In which of the following condition, air under both sides of diaphragm is visualized?** *(PGI Dec 2001, June 2001)*
    a. Perforated Meckel's diverticulum
    b. Uterine rupture following illegal abortion
    c. Perforation of duodenal ulcer
    d. Liver abscess
    e. Appendicular perforation

11. **Which of the following causes least irritation of the peritoneal cavity?** *(All India 99)*
    a. Bile   b. Blood
    c. Gastric enzyme   d. Pancreatic enzyme

12. **A 30-year-old a male patient presented with abdominal pain, fever, nausea, vomiting and respiratory distress. His BP was found to be 80/40 mm Hg and pulse rate of 115/min. The following chest X-ray was recorded in emergency. What is the immediate management?** *(AIIMS May 2016)*
    a. IV fluids and antibiotics followed by laparotomy
    b. Immediate laparotomy
    c. Intravenous fluids
    d. Intravenous potassium

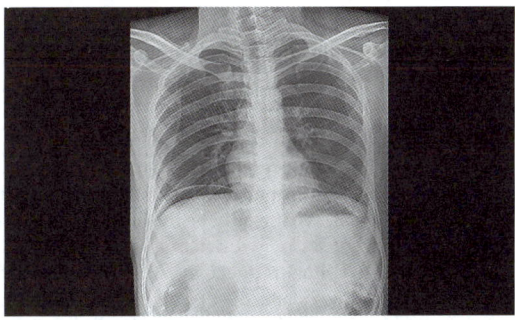

13. **A 40 years old male was brought to emergency with severe abdominal pain. On examination, pulse rate was 112/minute and systolic BP was 80 mm Hg. Chest X-ray is given below. What is the most appropriate management?**
    (Recent Question 2019)
    a. Exploratory laparotomy   b. Saline wash of stomach
    c. Intercostal tube drainage   d. IV antibiotics

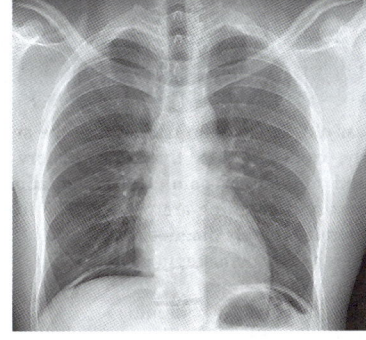

14. **Most common cause of peritonitis in adult male is:**
    (Recent Question 2014, All India 93)
    a. Duodenal ulcer perforation   b. Abdominal tuberculosis
    c. Enteric perforation   d. Perforated appendix

15. **Apart from Escherichia coli, the other most common organism implicated in acute suppurative bacterial peritonitis is:** *(Recent Question 2014, All India 2006)*
    a. Bacteroides   b. Klebsiella
    c. Peptostreptococcus   d. Pseudomonas

16. Primary peritonitis with pneumococcus is associated with:
    a. Lymphomas   b. Nephrotic syndrome
    c. Carcinoids   d. None of the above

17. Generalized diffuse peritonitis has been compared to second and third degree burns of:
    a. 13%   b. 30%
    c. 45%   d. 60%

18. Early surgery is indicated in:
    a. Amoebiasis peritonitis   b. Biliary peritonitis
    c. Typhoid peritonitis   d. All

19. Most common cause of generalized peritonitis in a 40-year-old adult male is: *(AIIMS 92)*
    a. Enteric perforation
    b. Ruptured liver abscess
    c. Duodenal ulcer perforation
    d. Perforated CA stomach

20. The commonest organism seen in peritonitis is: *(TN 2001)*
    a. Escherichia coli   b. Clostridium welchii
    c. Staphylococci   d. Klebsiella

21. Which of the following complications is not seen with peritonitis? *(MAHE 2006)*
    a. Renal failure   b. Residual abscess
    c. Endotoxic shock   d. Bone marrow suppression

22. A 25-year-old female presents with pyrexia for ten days, develops acute pain in periumbilical region spreading all over the abdomen. What would be the most likely cause? *(Recent Question 2014, UPSC 2007)*
    a. Perforation peritonitis due to intestinal tuberculosis
    b. Generalized peritonitis due to appendicular perforation
    c. Typhoid enteric perforation and peritonitis
    d. Acute salpingo-oophoritis with peritonitis

23. Spontaneous peritonitis in cirrhosis patients; the polymorphonuclear cells are: *(NEET 2013, UPPG 2008)*
    a. More than 200 cells/cumm   b. More than 300 cells/cumm
    c. More than 400 cells/cumm   d. More than 500 cells/cumm

24. Which of the following is true regarding classical spontaneous bacterial peritonitis? *(NEET 2013, COMEDK 2010)*
    a. Ascitic fluid neutrophil count is 250/cumm
    b. Bowel perforation should be present
    c. Multiple organisms are isolated from ascetic fluid
    d. Board-like rigidity is present in abdomen

25. A 10-year-old female who used to use the swimming pool regularly, comes with a three day history of vomiting, fever and abdominal pain. On examination, abdominal tenderness and guarding are present. The liver dullness is not obliterated. Likely diagnosis is: *(AIIMS 99)*
    a. Gangrenous intussusceptions
    b. Perforation
    c. Spontaneous biliary peritonitis
    d. Primary peritonitis

26. Sonu, a 15-year-old girl, a regular swimmer presents with sudden onset of pain in abdomen, abdominal distension and fever of 39°C and obliteration of the liver dullness. Most probable diagnosis is: *(Recent Question 2014, AIIMS June 2001, Nov 99)*
    a. Ruptured typhoid ulcer
    b. Primary bacterial peritonitis
    c. Ruptured ectopic pregnancy
    d. UTI with PID

27. All of the following regarding diagnosis of acute peritonitis are correct except: *(MCI March 2007)*
    a. Raised WBC count in peritoneal aspirate
    b. Moderately raised amylase levels are diagnostic of peritonitis
    c. CT scan may aid in diagnosis
    d. Upright films shows free air under the diaphragm

MESENTERIC CYST

28. Most common type of mesenteric cyst is: *(MHSSMCET 2005)*
    a. Enterogenous   b. Chylolymphatic
    c. Urogenital   d. Teratomatous

29. True about mesenteric cyst: *(PGI Dec 2005)*
    a. Moves perpendicular to the line of attachment
    b. Teratomatous is most common
    c. Chylolymphatic cyst has separate blood supply
    d. Surgical removal of bowel along cyst is treatment of choice in all the cyst

30. Mesenteric cyst whose removal entrails removals of part of gut: *(TN 95)*
    a. Chylolymphatic cyst b. Enterogenous cyst
    c. Dermoid   d. All

31. All are mesenteric cyst except: *(DNB 2007)*
    a. Dermoid cyst   b. Chylolymphatic cyst
    c. Gartner's cyst   d. Enterogenous cyst

32. A part of adjacent intestine will be removed in: *(JIPMER 2012)*
    a. Enterogenous cyst   b. Chylolymphatic cyst
    c. Dermoid cyst   d. Mesothelial cyst

ASCITES

33. Transudative ascites is/are associated with: *(PGI May 2011)*
    a. Myxedema   b. Budd-Chiari syndrome
    c. Acute pancreatitis d. Portal vein thrombosis
    e. Congestive heart failure

34. Serum-ascites albumin gradient >1.1 g/dL is seen in: *(COMEDK 2005)*
    a. Nephrosis   b. Cirrhosis
    c. Pancreatic ascites d. Neoplasm

35. Mucinous ascites is seen in: *(PGI June 2000)*
    a. Stomach CA   b. TB
    c. Nephrotic syndrome d. Cirrhosis

36. The following are true regarding ascites except:
    a. Only when the amount of fluid present exceeds 1500 ml. It can be recognized clinically *(Kerala 2000)*
    b. Shifting dullness is absent when there is a very large accumulation of fluid
    c. In cirrhosis there is obstruction to the venous outflow of the liver due to obliterative fibrosis of the intra hepatic venous bed
    d. A transudate has a protein content of greater than 30 gms of protein per litre
    e. In Meig's syndrome it is associated with pleural effusion and solid fibroma of ovary

37. Pseudochylous ascites occurs in:
    a. Cirrhosis   b. Hyperlipidemia
    c. Filariasis   d. Malignant ascites

38. A patient came with ascites. Ascitic fluid analysis was done and found to have SAAG more >1.1. All of the following can be the cause except: *(AIIMS November 2017)*
    a. Cirrhosis   b. Liver failure
    c. Metastasis to liver d. Tubercular peritonitis

39. True statement regarding tubercular peritonitis and ascites:
    (PGI November 2017)
    a. SAAG <1.1 gm/dL in ascitic fluid
    b. Elevated adenosine deaminase level
    c. Protein <25–30 gm/L
    d. The diagnosis can be made up by laparoscopy with directed biopsy of the peritoneum

PSEUDOMYXOMA PERITONEI

40. In pseudomyxoma peritonei, mucinous cyst-adenocarcinoma of which following organ is involved: *(Orissa 2011)*
    a. Pancreas   b. Ovary
    c. Kidney   d. Abdominal testis

41. Pseudomyxoma peritonei arises from: *(PGI Dec 2008)*
    a. Carcinoma ovary   b. Ovarian cyst
    c. Ovarian dermoid   d. Adenocarcinoma colon
    e. Mucocele of appendix

42. True about pseudomyxoma peritonei: *(PGI June 2004)*
    a. Seen in male only
    b. Cytoreductive surgery needed
    c. Always appendectomy needed
    d. Radiation therapy given
    e. Locally malignant tumor

43. All are true about pseudomyxoma peritonei except:
    a. Common in male   *(UPPG 2007)*
    b. Associated with ovary tumors
    c. Yellow jelly collection of fluid
    d. Appendiceal adenocarcinoma

44. All are true about pseudomyxoma peritonei except:
    a. Associated with ovarian tumors   *(DPG 2008)*
    b. Appendix is most common site of origin
    c. Yellow jelly collection of fluid
    d. Common in male

45. False about pseudomyxoma peritonei is: *(JIPMER May 2018)*
    a. Recurrence after surgery
    b. Refractory to drugs
    c. Hyperthermic intraperitoneal chemotherapy is treatment option
    d. Most commonly associated with appendiceal tumor

ABDOMINAL ABSCESS

46. Commonest site of intraperitoneal abscess is: *(Orissa 2011)*
    a. Lesser sac   b. Greater sac
    c. Pelvis   d. Paracolic gutter

47. The part of peritoneal cavity that is most dependent in supine position: *(MHSSMCET 2009)*
    a. Right subphrenic space   b. Lesser sac
    c. Supra mesocolic space   d. Right subhepatic space

48. Most common site of intra-abdominal abscess:
    (MHPGMCET 2006)
    a. Pelvic   b. Subphrenic space
    c. Mesenteric   d. Paracolic gutters

49. Most common cause of infection and collection of fluid in the left subhepatic space: *(MHPGMCET 2009)*
    a. Perforation at the lesser curvature of stomach
    b. Complicated acute pancreatitis
    c. Ruptured abscess of the left lobe of the liver
    d. Perforation of posterior duodenal wall ulcer

50. Posterior perforated ulcer on pyloric antrum cause abscess formation in: *(PGI June 2009)*
    a. Greater sac   b. Lesser sac
    c. Pouch of Morrison   d. Omental bursa
    e. Right subphrenic

51. In a patient recovering from peritonitis, which of the following would be the most characteristic sign of pelvic abscess:
    a. Fever and abdominal pain   *(MHPGMCET 2008)*
    b. Tachycardia
    c. Mucus in the stool for first time
    d. All of the above

52. Treatment of pouch of Douglas abscess is:
    (Recent Question 2016)
    a. Laparotomy   b. Posterior colpotomy
    c. Antibiotics   d. Extraperitoneal drainage

53. Most common site for intra abdominal abscess following laparotomy is: *(AIIMS 92)*
    a. Sub hepatic   b. Subphrenic
    c. Pelvic   d. Paracolic

54. Correct about subphrenic abscess is:
    a. Rarely chest symptoms   b. Toxemia
    c. Rarely toxaemia   d. No sign and symptoms

55. The most favored treatment for a pelvic abscess in cul-de-sac is: *(DPG 96)*
    a. Laparotomy   b. Colpotomy
    c. External I and D   d. Antibiotics

56. Colopotomy is done to treat: *(APPG 98)*
    a. Ischeorectal abscess   b. Pelvic abscess
    c. Appendicular abscess   d. Perianal abscess

57. Most pathognomic in pelvic abscess is: *(UPPG 2007)*
    a. Constipation   b. Mucopurulent discharge
    c. Loose stool   d. Bleeding

58. Most common site of intraperitoneal abscess is: *(DPG 2008)*
    a. Right superior intraperitoneal space
    b. Right inferior intraperitoneal space
    c. Left superior intraperitoneal space
    d. Left superior intraperitoneal space

59. Most common site of intra-peritoneal abscess: *(APPG 2008)*
    a. Morrison's pouch   b. Omental bursa
    c. Pelvic region   d. Left subhepatic pouch

60. A posteriorly perforating ulcer in the pyloric antrum of the stomach is likely to produce initial localized peritonitis or abscess formation in the: *(AIIMS Nov 2004)*
    a. Greater sac
    b. Left subhepatic and hepatorenal spaces (Pouch of Morrison)
    c. Right subphrenic space   d. Lesser sac

61. A patient developed wound infection post laparotomy for pyoperitoneum, was treated conservatively. Now, granulation tissue is seen in the wound. Next step in management is: *(Recent Question 2015)*
    a. Daily dressing   b. Mesh repair
    c. Incision and drainage
    d. Re-suturing with interrupted stitches

PNEUMOPERITONEUM

62. Treatment of pneumoperitoneum, as a result of colonoscopic perforation in a young patient is: *(PGI June 98)*
    a. Temporary colostomy   b. Closure + lavage
    c. Permanent colostomy   d. Symptomatic

63. Best investigation for air in peritoneal cavity is: *(CMC 98)*
    a. USG   b. Laparotomy
    c. Laparoscopy   d. X-ray abdomen-erect view

64. In pneumoperitoneum following are seen except: (PGI 97)
    a. Hypertension   b. Bradycardia
    c. Tachycardia   d. Hypercapnia
65. In which one of the following conditions is gas under diaphragm not seen? (UPSC 2005)
    a. Perforated duodenal ulcer b. Typhoid perforation
    c. After laparotomy
    d. Spontaneous rupture of esophagus
66. Rigler's sign is seen in: (COMEDK 2008)
    a. Ulcerative colitis   b. Crohn's disease
    c. Megacolon   d. Pneumoperitoneum
67. The best view to visualized minimal pneumo-peritoneum:
    a. AP view abdomen   (All India 2012)
    b. Erect view abdomen
    c. Right lateral decubitus with horizontal beam
    d. Left lateral decubitus with horizontal beam
68. Advantage of carbon dioxide in laparoscopy are all except: (Rohtak 97)
    a. Non-irritant   b. Non-inflammable
    c. Minimally absorbed d. No tissue reaction
    e. None
69. The given finding of X-ray is rarely seen in which of the following? (Recent Question 2016)
    a. Gastric perforation   b. Duodenal perforation
    c. Ileal perforation   d. Appendicular perforation

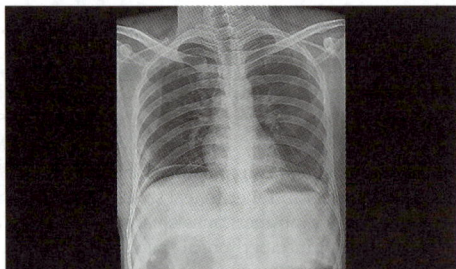

PERITONEUM ANATOMY

70. True about boundaries of lesser sac: (PGI 2000)
    a. Posteriorly stomach   b. Crus of diaphragm
    c. Spleen   d. Greater omentum
71. Lesser sac of stomach is bounded by: (PGI 2000)
    a. Posterior wall of stomach b. Visceral surface of spleen
    c. Under surface of liver   d. Greater omentum
72. Lesser omentum has following contents except: (PGI 97)
    a. Hepatic vein   b. Hepatic artery
    c. Portal vein   d. Bile duct
73. True about relation of epipolic foramen is: (AIIMS 97)
    a. Portal vein posteriorly   b. IVC inferiorly
    c. Hepatic art superiorly   d. Bile duct anteriorly
74. Root of mesentery is crossed by: (AIIMS May 2011)
    a. Horizontal part of duodenum
    b. Left gonadal vessels   c. Left ureter
    d. Superior mesenteric artery

WOUND DEHISCENCE

75. Burst abdomen most commonly occurs on the: (Recent Question 2014)
    a. 2nd day   b. 3rd day
    c. 7th day   d. 9th day
    e. 5th day

76. On 7th post operative day, abdominal wound shows pink serosanguinous discharge. It suggests: (DNB 2001)
    a. Impending wound dehiscence
    b. Infection in the abdomen
    c. Stitch abscess   d. Healing wound

MESENTERIC LYMPHADENITIS

77. Acute mesenteric lymphadenitis is caused by: (All India 94)
    a. E. coli   b. α-hemolytic streptococci
    c. Hemophilus   d. Yersinia
78. The commonest cause of acute mesenteric adenitis is: (Recent Question 2016)
    a. Tuberculosis   b. Brucellosis
    c. Pneumococcal infection d. Idiopathic

MISCELLANEOUS

79. Which of the following is not characteristic of visceral pain?
    a. Poor localization   b. Diffuse in nature
    c. High threshold   d. Very rapid adaptation
80. Odorless peritoneal fluid is noticed in:
    a. Perforated peptic ulcer b. Perforated ileum
    c. Perforated appendix   d. T.B. peritonitis
81. "Peritoneal mice" is: (Kerala PG 2015, APPG 97)
    a. Pseudomyxoma peritonei b. Appendices epiploicae
    c. Peritoneal seedings of tumour
    d. Endometriosis
82. Malignant change in lipoma is most common in: (Rohtak 2000)
    a. Thigh   b. Nape of neck
    c. Retroperitoneum   d. Back
83. Retractile mesenteris may be seen in: (NIMHANS 86)
    a. Ormond's disease   b. Gardner's syndrome
    c. Turner's syndrome d. Down's syndrome
84. 'Gas' in the tissue should be differentiated with:
    a. Pseudomyxoma peritonei   (UPPG 2007)
    b. Pseudomonas infection c. Clostridium nouyi infection
    d. Non clostridial infection
85. The mesentery of small intestine, along its attachment to the posterior abdominal wall, crosses all of the following structures except: (AIIMS Nov 2004)
    a. Left gonadal vessels   b. Third part of duodenum
    c. Aorta   d. Right ureter
86. Which is the baseline investigation in the case of an acute abdomen in this high-tech era? (Kerala 2003)
    a. Abdomen CT   b. Abdomen X-ray
    c. USG   d. Colonoscopy
87. Which of the following abdominal structure will be responsible for sharp pain while doing abdominal surgery?
    a. Parietal peritoneum   (AIIMS Nov 2000)
    b. Liver parenchyma   c. Small intestine
    d. Colon
88. 'Peritoneal mice' come from: (MHPGMET 2005)
    a. Appendices epiploicae b. Pseudomyxoma peritonei
    c. Metastases   d. All
89. Median survival in malignant peritoneal mesothelioma: (MHPGMET 2005)
    a. 6–10 months   b. 4–12 months
    c. 4–6 months   d. 12–20 months
90. Most common primary malignant peritoneal tumour: (Recent Question 2017)
    a. Mesothelioma   b. Desmoid tumor
    c. Lipoma   d. Fibroma

Explanations

RETROPERITONEAL FIBROSIS

1. **Ans. c. Idiopathic retroperitoneal fibrosis** *(Ref: Sabiston 20/e p1087, Campbell 11/e p1143, 10/e p1008-112)*
2. **Ans. d. Back pain**
3. **Ans. b. Ureter**
4. **Ans. b. Hypertrophic scar** *(Ref: Bailey 27/e p31, 1064, 25/e p598)*

   Hypertrophic scar is not an idiopathic fibrosis, fibrosis occurs after incision.
5. **Ans. b. More common in females**

PERITONITIS

6. **Ans. b. Neutrocytic ascites has better prognosis** *(Ref: Sabiston 20/e p1078; Schwartz 10/e p149-150; Bailey 27/e p1048)*

   Culture negative neutrocytic ascites carries a **similar prognosis to SBP** and is **managed similarly.**

7. **Ans. a. Volvulus, b. Obstructed hernia, c. Appendicular perforation with paralytic ileus, d. Toxic megacolon, e. Colonic perforation** *(Ref: Sabiston 20/e p1252; Schwartz 10/e p1149)*

Indications of Immediate Surgery in Intestinal Obstruction	
• **Obstructed** or **strangulated hernia**[Q]	• **Volvulus**[Q] of gut
• **Operative decompression**[Q] needed (in **Toxic megacolon**)	• **Acute obstruction**[Q]
	• **Colonic perforation**[Q]

8. **Ans. a. USG, b. Multidetector CT, c. Contrast enhanced CT, d. X-ray abdomen** *(Ref: Sabiston 20/e p1126-1129; Schwartz 10/e p1147)*

INVESTIGATIONS IN ACUTE ABDOMEN
• **Plain X-ray**: Important role in imaging of patients with acute abdominal pain (useful for **intestinal obstruction** and **perforation**)[Q].
• **USG**: Extremely accurate in detecting **gallstones** and **GB pathology**[Q]
• **CECT** and **MDCT**: Improvement in imaging techniques, especially MDCT has **revolutionized** the **diagnosis of acute abdomen**[Q].

9. **Ans. c. Total parenteral nutrition** *(Ref: Schackelford 7/e p930, 944)*

   This is a case of **duodenal stump blowout**. Best treatment is **adequate drainage immediately** by putting a **catheter** through an incision **below the right costal margin**[Q]. **TPN** should be instituted and attention should be directed towards **fluid and electrolyte therapy**[Q].

   Since drainage by putting a **catheter** through an incision **below the right costal margin**[Q] option is not there, best option will be TPN.

10. **Ans. a. Perforated Meckel's diverticulum, b. Uterine rupture following illegal abortion, c. Perforation of duodenal ulcer, e. Appendicular perforation** *(Ref: Chapman 4/e p212)*

Causes of Pneumoperitoneum	
1. Perforation of GI Tract: • Peptic ulcer[Q] • Inflammation (**Diverticulitis, appendicitis, toxic megacolon, necrotizing enterocolitis**)[Q] • Infarction • Malignant neoplasm • Pneumatosis cystoides rupture[Q] • Iatrogenic (**Endoscopy**)[Q] 2. **Penetrating abdominal injury**[Q]	3. **Iatrogenic**: • Surgery, peritoneal dialysis, • Drainage catheter, biopsy 4. **Through female genital tract**: • Spontaneous • Iatrogenic (perforation, culdocentesis, tubal patency test)[Q] 5. **Gas forming peritonitis**[Q] 6. **Pneumothorax with pleuroperitoneal fistula**

11. **Ans. b. Blood** *(Ref: Harrison 20/e p954, 19/e p1989)*

    - **Gastric juice, pancreatic juice, bile, urine** and **meconium irritate peritoneal cavity** and lead to **aseptic** or **chemical peritonitis**[Q].
    - **Chemical irritation** of the peritoneum is **greatest for acidic gastric juice** and **pancreatic enzymes**[Q].
    - The chemical irritation caused by stomach acid & activated pancreatic enzymes is extreme and secondary bacterial infection may occur.

12. **Ans. a. IV fluids and antibiotics followed by laparotomy** *(Ref: Sabiston 20/e p1134; Bailey 27/e p1051)*

    Chest X-ray is showing air under the right dome of diaphragm, which is seen in perforation peritonitis. In cases of perforation peritonitis, laparotomy is the treatment of choice after fluid resuscitation of the patient and IV antibiotics.

13. **Ans. a. Exploratory laparotomy** *(Ref: Schwartz 10/e p1061; Sabiston 20/e p1134; Bailey 27/e p1051)*

14. **Ans. a. Duodenal ulcer perforation** *(Ref: Sabiston 20/e p1121)*

    MC cause of peritonitis in **adult male**: **Peptic** ulcer **perforation**

    ### PERITONITIS

    - The **most common cause is** a **perforation of** the **abdominal viscus-most commonly**, **a perforated ulcer**^{Q}, may occur as a result of perforation of any part of the bowel; other causes include a benign ulcer, a tumor, or trauma.
    - MC cause of peritonitis in **adult male**: **Peptic** ulcer **perforation**^{Q}

15. **Ans. a. Bacteroides** *(Ref: Sabiston 20/e p1078; Bailey 27/e p1049)*
16. **Ans. b. Nephrotic syndrome** *(Ref: Bailey 27/e p1053)*
17. **Ans. c. 45%**
18. **Ans. d. All**
19. **Ans. c. Duodenal ulcer perforation**
20. **Ans. a. Escherichia coli**
21. **Ans. None or d. Bone marrow suppression** *(Ref: Bailey 27/e p1052)*

Complications of Peritonitis	
Abdominal Complications	Systemic Complications
• Adhesive small bowel obstruction^Q • Paralytic ileus^Q • Residual or recurrent abscess^Q • Portal pyemia (liver abscess)^Q	• Bacteraemic/endotoxic shock^Q • Bronchopneumonia/respiratory failure^Q • Renal failure^Q • Bone marrow suppression^Q • Multisystem failure

22. **Ans. c. Typhoid enteric perforation and peritonitis** *(Ref: Sabiston 20/e p1266-1267; Schwartz 10/e p1154; Bailey 27/e p1248; Harrison 20/e p1176, 19/e p1050-1051)*

23. **Ans. a. More than 200 cells/cumm**
24. **Ans. a. Ascitic fluid neutrophil count is 250/cumm**
25. **Ans. d. Primary peritonitis** *(Ref: Sabiston 20/e p1125; Bailey 27/e p1050)*

Primary (Pneumococcal) peritonitis	• Liver dullness is **not obliterated**^{Q}
Perforation (Secondary) peritonitis	• Liver dullness is **obliterated**^{Q}

    ### LIVER DULLNESS

    - Right mid-axillary line is percussed from above downwards. The percussion note will be resonant in the upper part of the mid-axillary line. At the **upper border of** the **liver**, the **resonant note** is **replaced by dull note**.
    - If the **liver dullness** is **replaced by a resonant note**, it indicates **presence of free gas under diaphragm** as occurs in the **perforation of gastrointestinal tract**^{Q}.

26. **Ans. a. Ruptured typhoid ulcer**
27. **Ans. b. Moderately raised amylase levels are diagnostic of peritonitis**

MESENTERIC CYST

28. **Ans. b. Chylolymphatic** *(Ref: Sabiston 20/e p1082; Schwartz 10/e p1459-1460; Bailey 27/e p1063)*
29. **Ans. a. Moves perpendicular to the line of attachment, c. Chylolymphatic cyst has separate blood supply**
30. **Ans. b. Enterogenous cyst**
31. **Ans. c. Gartner's cyst**
32. **Ans. a. Enterogenous cyst**

ASCITES

33. **Ans. a. Myxedema, b. Budd-Chiari syndrome, d. Portal vein thrombosis, e. Congestive heart failure** *(Ref: Sabiston 20/e p1077)*

Classification of Ascites by Serum-Ascites Albumin Gradient

High Gradient (>1.1 g/dL) or Transudate First PSM CAB		Low Gradient (<1.1 g/dL) or Exudate BT in PNS	
• **F**ulminant hepatic failure^Q • **F**atty liver of pregnancy • **P**ortal vein thrombosis^Q • **S**inusoidal obstruction syndrome • **M**yxedema^Q	• **M**ixed ascites • **M**assive liver metastases • **C**irrhosis (MC)^Q • **C**ardiac ascites^Q • **A**lcoholic hepatitis^Q • **B**udd-Chiari syndrome^Q	• **B**iliary ascites • **B**owel obstruction or infarction^Q • **T**ubercular peritonitis^Q • **P**eritoneal carcinomatosis (MC)^Q	• **P**ost-operative lymphatic leak • **P**ancreatic ascites • **N**ephrotic syndrome^Q • **S**erositis in connective tissue disease

- MC cause of **low-albumin gradient ascites**: Peritoneal carcinomatosis^Q
- MC cause of **high-albumin gradient ascites**: Cirrhosis^Q

34. **Ans. b. Cirrhosis**

35. **Ans. a. Stomach CA** *(Ref: Harrison 16/e p245)*

CAUSES OF MUCINOUS ASCITES

- Pseudomyxoma peritonei^Q
- Colloid carcinoma of stomach^Q or colon^Q with peritoneal implants

36. **Ans. a. Only when the amount of fluid present exceeds 1500 ml. It can be recognized clinically, d. A transudate has a protein content of greater than 30 gms of protein per litre** *(Ref: Bailey 26/e p979)*

CLINICAL FEATURES OF ASCITES

- **Ascites** can be **recognized clinically** when the amount of **fluid exceeds 150 ml**^{Q}.
- **Abdomen** is **distended evenly with fullness of** the **flanks**, which are dull to percussion.
- Usually, **shifting dullness is present**^{Q} but **when there is a very large accumulation of fluid this sign is absent**^{Q}. In such cases, on flicking the abdominal wall, a characteristic fluid thrill is transmitted from one side to the other.
- In **cirrhosis**, there is **obstruction to** the **portal venous system**, which is caused by **obliterative fibrosis** of the **intrahepatic venous bed**^{Q}. Lymph flow may be increased.
- **Meig's syndrome**: Ascites and **pleural effusion** are associated with **solid fibroma** of the **ovary**^{Q}. The effusion disappear when the tumour is excised.

37. **Ans. d. Malignant ascites** *(Ref: Bailey 27/e p1059)*

PSEUDOCHYLOUS ASCITES

- **Abnormal accumulation** in the peritoneal cavity **of a milky fluid that resembles chyle**.
- The **turbidity of the fluid** is **caused by cellular debris** in the fluid^Q.
- Pseudochylous ascites is **indicative of** an **abdominal tumor** or **infection**^{Q}.

CHYLOUS ASCITES

- In some patients the **ascitic fluid appears milky** because of an **excess of chylomicrons (triglycerides)**^{Q}.

Causes of Chylous Ascites	
• Malignancy (**Lymphomas-MC**^{Q}) • **Cirrhosis**^{Q} • **Tuberculosis** • **Filariasis**^{Q} • **Nephrotic syndrome**^{Q}	• Sarcoidosis • Abdominal trauma (including surgery) • Constrictive pericarditis • Congenital lymphatic abnormality^Q

- The **prognosis is poor** unless the underlying condition can be cured.
- In addition to other measures used to treat ascites, patients should be placed on a **fat-free diet** with **medium-chain triglyceride**^{Q} supplements.

38. **Ans. d. Tubercular peritonitis** *(Ref: Harrison 20/e p1245, 19/e p287)*

39. **Ans. a. SAAG...., b. Elevated adenosine....., d. The diagnosis can.....** *(Ref: Sabiston 20/e p1077)*

PSEUDOMYXOMA PERITONEI

40. **Ans. b. Ovary** *(Ref: Sabiston 20/e p1080; Schwartz 10/e p1258-1259; Bailey 27/e p1059)*
41. **Ans. a. Carcinoma ovary, d. Adenocarcinoma colon, e. Mucocele of appendix** *(Ref: Recent Advances in Surgery, Irving Taylor/83)*

    - "In addition to the **association of PMP** with **appendiceal** and **ovarian tumors**, there are cases reports suggesting occasional origin from other intra-abdominal organs such as the colon, rectum, stomach, GB, bile duct, small intestine, urinary bladder, lung, breast fallopian tube and pancreas. With the exception of **colorectal mucinous adenocarcinoma**, which **often simulate PMP**, these are rare and only account for less than 5% of total cases."

42. **Ans. b. Cytoreductive surgery needed, c. Always appendectomy needed, e. Locally malignant tumor**
43. **Ans. a. Common in male**   44. **Ans. d. Common in male**
45. **Ans. b. Refractory to drugs** *(Ref: Schwartz 10/e p1258-1259; Sabiston 20/e p1080; Bailey 27/e p1059)*

ABDOMINAL ABSCESS

46. **Ans. c. Pelvis** *(Ref: Maingot 11/e p179-184; Bailey 27/e p1055)*
47. **Ans. d. Right subhepatic space**   48. **Ans. a. Pelvic**
49. **Ans. b. Complicated acute pancreatitis** *(Ref: Bailey 27/e p1056)*

> **LEFT SUBHEPATIC SPACE (LESSER SAC)**
>
> - The **commonest cause** of **infection** here is **complicated acute pancreatitis**^{Q}.
> - In practice, a **perforated gastric ulcer rarely causes a collection** here because the **potential space is obliterated by adhesions**.

50. **Ans. b. Lesser sac, d. Omental bursa** *(Ref: Bailey 27/e p1056; Schwartz 10/e p1068)*
    - **Gastric ulcers perforate into** the **lesser sac**, which can be particularly **difficult to diagnose**.^{Q}
    - A **gastric ulcer perforates into** the **lesser sac**^{Q}, then no generalized peritonitis can be seen but misleading symptoms may appear.
51. **Ans. d. All of the above** *(Ref: Bailey 27/e p1055)*
52. **Ans. b. Posterior colpotomy**   53. **Ans. c. Pelvic**   54. **Ans. b. Toxemia**
55. **Ans. b. Colpotomy**   56. **Ans. b. Pelvic abscess**   57. **Ans. b. Mucopurulent discharge**
58. **Ans. b. Right inferior intraperitoneal space** *(Ref: Bailey 27/e p1055)*

    Most common site of intra-peritoneal abscess is pelvis. Best option among the options provided is **inferior space,** right inferior intraperitoneal space.

59. **Ans. c. Pelvic region**   60. **Ans. d. Lesser sac**   61. **Ans. d. Re-suturing with interrupted stitches**

PNEUMOPERITONEUM

62. **Ans. b. Closure + lavage** *(Ref: Schackelford 8/e p1694, 7/e p1747-1748; Schwartz 10/e p1180)*

> **RISKS ASSOCIATED WITH COLONOSCOPY**
>
> - **Risks of colonoscopy: Perforation** and **hemorrhage**^{Q}
>
>   > - MC site of **bleeding after colonoscopy: Stalk** after polypectomy.
>   > - MC site of **perforation** during colonoscopy: **Sigmoid colon**^{Q}
>
> - **Perforation** can be caused by **excessive air pressure**, **tearing** of the antimesenteric border of the colon **from excessive pressure** on colonic loops, and at the sites of **electrosurgical applications**^{Q}
>
> **Management**
>
> - Patients with **perforation** but **no peritoneal signs** can be **safely managed with careful monitoring** (Bowel rest + Broad spectrum antibiotics + Close observation^Q)
> - A **large perforation** recognized during the procedure **requires surgical exploration**. Because the **bowel has almost always been prepared** prior to the colonoscopy, there is usually **little contamination** associated with these injuries and **most can be repaired primarily**^{Q}.

63. **Ans. d. X-ray abdomen-erect view** *(Ref: Bailey 27/e p1051)*

    - Bailey says "**A radiograph of** the **abdomen may confirm** the **presence of dilated gas-filled loops of bowel** (consistent with a paralytic ileus) or **show free gas**, although the **latter is best shown on an erect chest radiograph**. If the patient is too ill for an 'erect' film to demonstrate free air under the diaphragm, a **lateral decubitus film is just as useful**, showing gas beneath the abdominal wall."

Peritoneum

64. **Ans. b. Bradycardia**
65. **Ans. d. Spontaneous rupture of esophagus**
66. **Ans. d. Pneumoperitoneum** *(Ref: Sabiston 20/e p1127; Bailey 27/e p190-191)*

PNEUMOPERITONEUM

- **Best projection** to demonstrate **pneumoperitoneum**: Chest X-ray[Q]
- If the **patient cannot get into** an **erect position** then **left lateral decubitus** projection is required[Q].
- Patient should be in that position for **10 min**[Q] at least for **air to rise up**.
- By careful technique even **1 ml of air can be detected**

Supine Film Signs of Pneumoperitoneum	
Football sign	Collection of **air in** the **centre of abdomen over a fluid collection**[Q]
Rigler's sign	Visualization of **both aspects of bowel** wall being **outlined by air** on either side[Q]
Cupola sign	**Large amount of gas under** the **diaphragm**[Q]
Triangle sign	Air between bowel loop[Q]

- **Chilladiti syndrome** or **interposition of colon between liver** and **diaphragm** can mimic pneumoperitoneum[Q]

67. **Ans. d. Left lateral decubitus with horizontal beam**   68. **Ans. c. Minimally absorbed**

- **Carbon dioxide** has the **advantage of being noncombustible** and **rapidly absorbed from the peritoneal cavity**; however, it **may lead to hypercarbia in** patients with **significant cardiopulmonary disease**[Q].

69. **Ans. d. Appendicular perforation** *(Ref: Chapman 4/e p212)*

    Gas below right dome of diaphragm is rarely seen in appendicular perforation due to little amount of gas.

PERITONEUM ANATOMY

70. **Ans. d. Greater omentum** *(Ref: BDC 4/e vol II p/232, 240)*

LESSER SAC (OMENTAL BURSA)

- A **large recess of peritoneal cavity behind stomach, lesser omentum** and **caudate lobe of liver**, which separates stomach bed from stomach.
- It is **closed all around** except in upper part of its right border where it **communicates with the greater sac through** the **epiploic foramen**[Q].
- Level of epiploic foramen: T12 vertebra[Q]

Boundaries of Lesser Sac	
Anterior	**Posterior**

• **Caudate lobe** of liver[Q]
• **Stomach**[Q]
• **Lesser omentum**[Q]
• **Greater omentum**[Q] (anterior 2 layers)
	• **Greater omentum**[Q] (posterior 2 layers)
	• **Structures forming stomach bed:**
	  – **Diaphragm**[Q] – **Left kidney** and **suprarenal** gland
	  – **Pancreas**[Q] – **Transverse mesocolon**[Q]
	  – **Splenic flexure** of colon – **Splenic artery**[Q]
	  – Spleen (sometimes)

71. **Ans. a. Posterior wall of stomach, d. Greater omentum**   72. **Ans. a. Hepatic vein**
73. **Ans. d. Bile duct anteriorly**   74. **Ans. a. Horizontal part of duodenum** *(Ref: BDC 4/e vol II p/227)*

MESENTERY

- Mesentery is a **fan shaped fold** of peritoneum that **attaches** the **jejunum** and **ileum** to **posterior abdominal wall**[Q].
- **Root** of mesentery is **15 cm long**[Q].
- It is **directed obliquely downwards** and **to the right**, extending from:
  - Duodenojejunal flexure on the left side of L2 vertebra[Q]
  - Upper part of right sacroiliac joint[Q]

Root of Mesentery Crosses Following Structures in Order	
1. **4th (ascending) and 3rd (horizontal) part of duodenum**[Q] 2. **Abdominal aorta**[Q] 3. **IVC**[Q]	4. **Right ureter**[Q] 5. **Right psoas major**[Q] 6. **Right testicular** or **ovarian vessels**[Q]

WOUND DEHISCENCE

75. **Ans. c. 7th day** *(Ref: CSDT 11/e p24; Bailey 27/e p299)*
76. **Ans. a. Impending wound dehiscence**

MESENTERIC LYMPHADENITIS

77. **Ans. d. Yersinia** *(Ref: Sabiston 20/e p1082-1083; Bailey 27/e p1062)*
78. **Ans. d. Idiopathic**

MISCELLANEOUS

79. **Ans. d. Very rapid adaptation** *(Ref: Guyton 13/e p626; Ganong 25/e p167)*

> **CHARACTERISTIC FEATURES VISCERAL PAIN**
>
> - **Visceral pain** is **poorly localized**, often the pain is **referred** or **radiating**^{Q}
> - **Pain of hollow viscus** is often **felt as a colic**^{Q} (it comes and goes to reappear again).
>   - **Highly localized** types of **damage** to the viscera **seldom cause severe pain**
>   - Often accompanied by **vomiting** and **hypotension**^{Q}

80. **Ans. a. Perforated peptic ulcer**
81. **Ans. b. Appendices epiploicae** *(Ref: Bailey 27/e p1060)*

> **PERITONEAL LOOSE BODIES (PERITONEAL MICE)**
>
> - Peritoneal loose bodies **almost never cause symptoms**^{Q}.
> - One or more may be **found in** a **hernial sac** or in the **pouch of Douglas**^{Q}.
> - The loose body may **come from an appendix epiploica**^{Q} that has undergone axial rotation followed by necrosis of its pedicle and detachment but they are **also found in** those who suffer from **subacute attacks of pancreatitis**^{Q}.
> - These hyaline bodies attain the **size of a pea** or **bean** and **contain saponified fat surrounded by fibrin**.

82. **Ans. c. Retroperitoneum** *(Ref: Bailey 27/e p1065)*

A **retroperitoneal lipoma is often malignant** (liposarcoma) and **may increase rapidly in size**.

> **RETROPERITONEAL LIPOMA**
>
> - The patient may seek advice on account of a swelling or because of **indefinite abdominal pain**.
> - **Women** are more often affected. These swellings **sometimes reach** an **immense size**.
> - **Diagnosis** is usually by **ultrasound** and **CT scanning**^{Q}.
> - A **retroperitoneal lipoma** sometimes **undergoes myxomatous degeneration**, a complication that **does not occur in a lipoma in any other part of** the **body**^{Q}.
> - Moreover, a **retroperitoneal lipoma is often malignant (liposarcoma)** and may **increase rapidly in size**^{Q}.

83. **Ans. a. Ormond's disease** *(Ref: Schwartz 10/e p1458)*

> **RETRACTILE MESENTERITIS**
>
> - **Retroperitoneal fibrosis** has been **associated with** a variety of sclerosing diseases, among these is a variant known as **retractile mesenteritis**
> - Involve predominantly the **mesentery of small intestine** and **associated vessels**, involvement of mesocolon and colon is less frequent.

84. **Ans. c. Clostridium nouyi infection**
85. **Ans. a. Left gonadal vessels**
86. **Ans. b. Abdomen X-ray**
87. **Ans. a. Parietal peritoneum**
88. **Ans. a. Appendices epiploicae**
89. **Ans. b. 4–12 months** *(Ref: Sabiston 20/e p1081, 19/e p1103)*
90. **Ans. a. Mesothelioma** *(Ref: Sabiston 20/e p1080)*

"The most common primary malignant peritoneal neoplasm is malignant mesothelioma, which results from malignant transformation of the simple squamoid epithelium covering the peritoneal cavity."-Sabiston 20/e p1080

CHAPTER 12

Intestinal Obstruction

SMALL BOWEL OBSTRUCTION

SMALL BOWEL OBSTRUCTION

- **Adhesions** secondary to previous surgery are the **MC cause of SBO**^{Q}.
- Causes: **Adhesions (60%) > Malignant tumors (20%) >Hernia (10%) > Crohn's disease (5%)**^{Q}
  - **Metastatic** or **peritoneal carcinomatosis** are the **MC malignancies** leading to **SBO**^{Q}.
- Primary **colonic cancers** (particularly those arising from the **cecum** & **ascending colon**) may present as a **SBO**^{Q}.

Pathophysiology
- **Early in the course** of an obstruction, **intestinal motility & contractile activity increase** in an effort to **propel luminal contents**^{Q} past the obstructing point.
- **Increase in peristalsis** early in the course of bowel obstruction is present **both above** and **below the point of obstruction**^{Q} (diarrhea in partial or even complete small bowel obstruction **in the early period)**
- **Later in the course** of obstruction, the **intestine becomes fatigued & dilates**^{Q}, with contractions becoming less frequent & less intense.
- As the **bowel dilates, water & electrolytes accumulate** both **intraluminally** & in the **bowel wall**^{Q} itself.
  - This **massive third-space fluid** loss accounts for the **dehydration & hypovolemia**^{Q}.
  - **Metabolic effects** of **fluid loss** depend on the **site & duration** of the obstruction.
- As the **intraluminal pressure increases** in the **bowel**, a **decrease in mucosal blood flow** can occur.

Clinical Features
- **Cardinal symptoms** of intestinal obstruction: **Colicky abdominal pain (1st symptom)**^{Q}, nausea, vomiting, **abdominal distention,** and a **failure to pass flatus** & **feces** (i.e., **obstipation)**^{Q}.
- **Typical crampy abdominal pain** occurs **in paroxysms** at **4- to 5-minute intervals** & occurs **less frequently with distal obstruction**^{Q}.
  - Nausea & **vomiting** are **more common** with **proximal obstruction.**
  - **Cramping abdominal pain** is the **initial** and **most prominent symptom** in **distal obstruction**^{Q}
  - **Abdominal distention** is **more common** in **distal obstruction**^{Q}
- **Abdominal distention** occurs as the obstruction progresses, and the **proximal intestine becomes increasingly dilated**^{Q}.
  - As the **obstruction** becomes **more complete** with **bacterial overgrowth**, the **vomitus becomes more feculent,** indicating a **late** and **established intestinal obstruction**^{Q}.
- Patient may present with **tachycardia** & **hypotension**^{Q}, demonstrating the severe dehydration that is present.
- **Fever suggests** the possibility of **strangulation**^{Q}.
- **Abdominal distention** is dependent **on the level of obstruction**^{Q}.

- **Early in the course** of bowel obstruction, **peristaltic waves** can be observed, particularly **in thin patients,** and auscultation of the abdomen may demonstrate **hyperactive bowel sounds** with **audible rushes** associated with **vigorous peristalsis**^{Q} (i.e., borborygmi).
- **Late** in the obstructive course, **minimal** or **no bowel sounds** are noted.

- **Localized tenderness, rebound,** & **guarding** suggest **peritonitis** and the likelihood of **strangulation**^{Q}.
- **Rectal examination:** To assess for **intraluminal masses** and to **examine the stool** for **occult blood**^{Q} (an indication of malignancy, intussusception, or infarction)

Diagnosis
- **X-ray Abdomen: Confirm** the **clinical suspicion** and **define** more accurately the **site of obstruction (60%** diagnostic **accuracy)**^{Q}
  - **Supine radiographs: Dilated loops** of **small intestine**^{Q} without evidence of colonic distention, **diagnose site & level of obstruction**^{Q}
  - **Erect radiographs: Multiple air-fluid levels,** which often layer in a **stepwise pattern**^{Q} (up to 3-5 air fluid levels <2.5 cm in length is **normal)**
  - **Supine films** are **better than erect** for **diagnosis of intestinal obstruction**^{Q}

CT Scan

- Used in **complex patients,** in whom the **diagnosis** is **not readily apparent**[Q]
- **Highly sensitive** for **diagnosing complete** or **high-grade obstruction** of **the small bowel and for determining the location** and **cause of obstruction.**
- **Less sensitive** for **partial small bowel obstruction**[Q]
- Useful for **extrinsic cause** of bowel obstruction (e.g. abdominal tumors, inflammatory disease, or abscess) and **determining bowel strangulation**

- Enteroclysis is investigation of choice in **low-grade, intermittent** SBO[Q]
- **Barium studies: Precisely demonstrate** the **level of** the **obstruction** and **cause** in certain cases[Q]
- **Ultrasound:** Useful in **pregnant patients**[Q]

> - **Leukocytosis may** be found in patients with **strangulation,** but **does not necessarily denote strangulation**[Q].
> - Absence of leukocytosis does not eliminate strangulation as a possibility

TREATMENT OF ACUTE INTESTINAL OBSTRUCTION

TREATMENT OF ACUTE INTESTINAL OBSTRUCTION

- **Fluid Resuscitation & Antibiotics**[Q]: Aggressive intravenous (IV) replacement with an isotonic saline solution such as lactated Ringer's.
- **Urine output** should be monitored by the placement of a Foley catheter.
- **Elderly patients** may require **central venous assessment**[Q]
- **Tube Decompression**[Q]: Nasogastric suction **reduces** the **risk of pulmonary aspiration** of vomitus and minimizing further **intestinal distention** from preoperatively swallowed air.

> - Patients with a **partial intestinal obstruction** may be **treated conservatively** with **resuscitation** and **tube decompression** alone[Q].
> - **Resolution of symptoms** and discharge **without** the need for **surgery** has been reported in **60–85%** of patients with a **partial obstruction**[Q].

- **Clinical deterioration** of the patient or **increasing small bowel distention** on abdominal radiographs **during tube decompression** warrants **prompt operative intervention**[Q].

Operative Management

- **Complete SBO** requires **operative intervention**[Q].
- **Adhesiolysis:** In cases of intestinal obstruction secondary to an **adhesive band**[Q]
- **Incarcerated hernias** can be managed by **manual reduction** of the herniated segment of bowel and **closure of the defect**[Q].

Consideration of laparoscopic management in patients with	
• **Mild abdominal distention**[Q] allowing adequate visualization	• **Partial** obstruction[Q]
• **Proximal** obstruction[Q]	• Anticipated **single-band** obstruction[Q]

Simple Obstruction	Strangulating Obstruction
• Simple obstructions that involve **mechanical blockage** of the flow of **luminal contents**[Q] • **Vascular supply** is **not compromised**[Q]	• Usually involves a **closed-loop obstruction**[Q] • **Vascular supply** to a segment of intestine is **compromised**[Q], can lead to intestinal infarction. • Associated with an **increased morbidity** and **mortality risk**[Q] • **Classic signs:** Tachycardia, fever, leukocytosis, and a constant, noncramping abdominal pain[Q]. • **CT scan:** Useful only in **detecting** the **late stages** of **irreversible ischemia** (e.g. **pneumatosis intestinalis, portal venous gas**)[Q].

PARALYTIC ILEUS

PARALYTIC ILEUS

- Caused by **impaired intestinal motility**
- **Paralytic ileus** is a state in which there is **failure of transmission of peristaltic waves** secondary to **neuromuscular failure**[Q].

Pathophysiology

- The most frequently encountered factors are **abdominal operations, infection and inflammation, electrolyte abnormalities,** and **drugs**.
- Characteristic sequence of return of normal motility: **Small intestinal motility returning to normal** within the **first 24 hours, gastric motility within 48 hours & colonic motility returning to normal 3 to 5 days**[Q].

Paralytic Ileus: Common Etiologies	

• Abdominal **surgery**[Q]
• **Uremia**[Q]
• Infection:
  – Sepsis
  – Intra-abdominal abscess
  – **Peritonitis**[Q]
  – **Pneumonia**[Q]
	• **Medications:**
	  – **Anticholinergics**[Q]
	  – **Opiates**[Q]
	  – **Phenothiazines**[Q]
	  – **Calcium channel blockers**[Q]
	  – Tricyclic antidepressants

• **Electrolyte abnormalities:**
  – **Hypokalemia**[Q]
  – **Hypomagnesemia**[Q]
  – **Hypermagnesemia**[Q]
  – **Hyponatremia**[Q]
	• **Hypothyroidism**[Q]
	• Ureteral colic
	• **Retroperitoneal hemorrhage**[Q]
	• **Spinal cord injury**[Q]
	• Myocardial infarction
	• **Mesenteric ischemia**[Q]

Clinical Features
- Paralytic ileus is a state in which there is **failure of transmission of peristaltic waves secondary to neuromuscular failure**.
- The resultant stasis leads to **accumulation of fluid & gas within the bowel with associated distention, vomiting, absent or diminished bowel sounds** and **absolute constipation**[Q].

> • Pain is colicky in mechanical obstruction, **pain is not a feature of paralytic ileus** and if present a steady, diffuse discomfort[Q]

Diagnosis
- **Abdominal X-ray: Dilated bowel loops** with **multiple air fluid levels**[Q]

> • Radiological picture is similar to small bowel obstruction, the **only differentiating point** is presence of gas in colon & rectum in paralytic ileus[Q].

Paralytic Ileus	Mechanical Obstruction
• **Pain** is **not a feature of paralytic ileus** and if present a steady, diffuse discomfort[Q]. • **Bowel sounds** are **hypoactive or absent**[Q] • **Presence of gas in colon & rectum**[Q] in paralytic ileus on abdominal X-ray	• Pain is **colicky**[Q] in mechanical obstruction • **Hyperactive bowel sounds**[Q] in mechanical obstruction • **Absence of gas** in **colon & rectum** in mechanical (complete)[Q] small bowel obstruction

POST-OPERATIVE ILEUS

Post-operative Ileus

- Following most abdominal operations or injuries, the motility of the GI tract is transiently impaired.
- **Proposed mechanisms** responsible for this dysmotility are **surgical stress-induced sympathetic reflexes, inflammatory response** mediator release, and **anesthetic/analgesic effects**[Q]; each of which can inhibit intestinal motility.

> • **Return of normal motility: Small intestine**[Q] (within 24 hours) >Gastric (48 hours)[Q] > Colonic (3–5 days)[Q]
> • **Post-operative ileus** is most pronounced in **colon**[Q]

- **Characteristic sequence** of return of normal motility: **Small intestinal motility** returning to normal **within the first 24 hours, gastric motility** within **48 hours** and **colonic motility** returning to normal **3 to 5 days**[Q].
- Because **small bowel motility is returned before colonic** and gastric motility, listening for **bowel sounds** is **not a reliable indicator** that ileus has fully resolved[Q].

Management of Post-operative Ileus
- The **essence of treatment** is **prevention**, with the **use of nasogastric suction** and **restriction of oral intake until bowel sounds** and the **passage of flatus return**[Q].
- **Following general principles** should be applied:
  - The **primary cause** must be **removed**[Q].
  - **Gastrointestinal distension** must be **relieved by decompression**[Q].
  - Close attention to **fluid** and **electrolyte balance**[Q] is essential.
  - There is no place for the routine use of peristaltic stimulants.

- Rarely, in resistant cases, medical therapy with an **adrenergic blocking agent** in association with **cholinergic stimulation**, e.g. **neostigmine (Catchpole regimen)**Q, may be used, provided that an intraperitoneal cause has been excluded.

> - If **paralytic ileus** is **prolonged** and **threatens life**, a **laparotomy** should be considered to exclude a hidden cause and facilitate bowel decompressionQ

INTUSSUSCEPTION

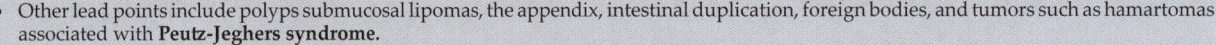

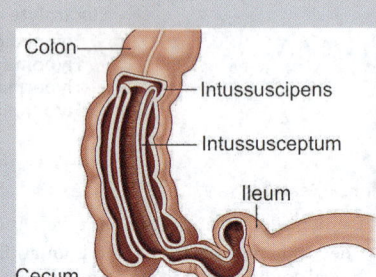

- **Telescoping** of one portion of the intestine into the other.
- **Middle layer** is **isolated between two sharp bends** and **first to become gangrenous**Q.

> - **Apex is most prone to gangrene**
> - **Highest incidence** between 4 and **10 months**Q of age
> - Approx **80–90%** of cases occur **between 3 and 36 months**Q

- **Mostly idiopathic** in **infants** and **toddlers**Q (no clear etiology).
- **MC type: Ileocolic**Q > Ileo-ileocolic > Ileo-ileal > Colocolic

Etiology and Predisposing Factors

- **Upper respiratory tract infections** or **gastroenteritis**Q (adenovirus and rotavirus have been implicated) have been **thought to be contributory** to the development of "idiopathic" intussusception. **Hypertrophy** of **Peyer's patches**Q can be seen at surgery, but no single etiologic factor predominates.

> - Approximately **5–10%** of cases have a true **pathologic lead point**. The **older the toddler**, the **more likely** there will be a **lead point**Q
> - **MC lead point is Meckel's diverticulum**Q > **Polyp**Q

- Other lead points include polyps submucosal lipomas, the appendix, intestinal duplication, foreign bodies, and tumors such as hamartomas associated with **Peutz-Jeghers syndrome**.

> - **Henoch-Schönlein purpura:** Submucosal hemorrhage acts as a **lead point**Q
> - **Cystic fibrosis:** Risk for **recurrent intussusception**Q

Clinical Features

- **Typical history:** Sudden, short-duration, cyclic crampy abdominal painQ.
- **During** these **episodes** the infant cries inconsolably with the **knees drawn up**Q.
- **Between episodes** the infant is **asymptomatic**Q.

> - **Vomiting** is almost **universal**Q
> - **Initially the passage of stools may be normal** while later on blood mixed with mucus is evacuated - red currant jelly stool

- An abdominal mass may be palpated - a **sausage shaped abdominal mass**Q (increase in size & firmness during the paroxysm of pain)
- There may be an **associated feeling of emptiness** in the **right iliac fossa (Sign of Dance)**Q
- **Occult** or **gross blood in 60–90%** of cases on rectal examinationQ
- **Apex** may be **palpable** or even **protrude from anus** in extensive **ileocolic** or **colocolic intussusception**Q

Diagnosis

- **USG: Kidney-shaped mass** in the longitudinal view or a **target sign** in the transverse view

> - **Hydrostatic reduction** by **contrast agent** or **air enema (preferred)** is the **diagnostic** & **therapeutic procedure of choice**Q
> - **Successful reduction** is confirmed by **reflux of air**Q (or barium) into the small bowel

Treatment

- **Hydrostatic reduction** by **contrast agent** or **air enema** is the **diagnostic** & **therapeutic procedure of choice**Q.
- The success rate with air or barium reduction should exceed 70%Q.

> - **Failure of reduction** or the **presence of peritonitis** mandates **operative intervention**Q, which can be performed laparoscopically or by a standard approach
> - **Definitive surgical procedure: Ileocolectomy with primary anastomosis**Q

Recurrence

- **Recurrence** after **successful hydrostatic reduction** is **5–10%**, recurrence rate after operative reduction is 1–4%.
- **Recurrence** is usually **managed by hydrostatic reduction**Q.
- **Third recurrence**Q is an **indication for operative intervention** to look for a **lead point**.

Radiological Investigations in Intussusception

Plain X-ray Film	Barium Enema	Ultrasound
• Features of **small intestinal obstruction**[Q] • **Abdominal soft tissue density** in some cases which may show: • **Target sign**[Q]: Soft tissue mass with concentric area of lucency due to mesenteric fat. • **Meniscus sign**[Q]: Crescent of gas within colonic lumen that outlines the apex of intussusception	• **Claw sign**[Q]: Rounded apex of intussusception protrudes into the contrast column • **Coiled spring sign**[Q]: Edematous mucosal folds of returning limb of intussusception outlined by contrast material.	• **Target sign** or **Bull's eye sign** on **transverse scan**[Q] • **Pseudokidney sign** on **longitudinal scan**[Q]

MECONIUM SYNDROME

Meconium Syndrome

- The meconium syndromes of infancy represent a complex **group of gastrointestinal conditions associated with cystic fibrosis** (CF), with considerable overlap in clinical presentation and management.
    - The **abnormal chloride transport** in **patients with CF** results in **tenacious, viscous secretions** affecting a wide variety of organs, including **the intestine, pancreas, lungs, salivary glands, reproductive organs,** and **biliary tract**[Q]
- The **clinical presentation** of the meconium syndromes ranges from a **meconium plug** to **simple** and **complicated meconium ileus**[Q].

Meconium Plug
- Meconium plug syndrome is a frequent **cause** of **neonatal intestinal obstruction**
- **Associated with**
    - **Hirschsprung's disease**[Q], **Maternal diabetes**[Q]
    - **Hypothyroidism**[Q], **Cystic Fibrosis**[Q]

Clinical Features
- **Affected infants** are often **preterm**[Q]
- Present with signs and symptoms of **distal intestinal obstruction**[Q]
- **Abdominal distention** is a **prominent feature**[Q]

Diagnosis
- Abdominal X-ray: Multiple dilated loops[Q] of intestine.
- **Diagnostic** and **therapeutic procedure** of **choice** is a **water-soluble contrast enema**[Q].

Treatment
- **Diagnostic** and **therapeutic procedure** of **choice** is a **water-soluble contrast enema**[Q]. This often **results** in the **passage of a plug** of **meconium** and **relief of the obstruction**[Q]

MECONIUM ILEUS

Meconium Ileus

Simple Meconium Ileus
- **Meconium ileus** in the newborn represents the **earliest clinical manifestation of CF** and **affects roughly 15% of patients** with this inherited disease.
- In simple meconium ileus, the **terminal ileum** is **dilated** and filled with thick, tarlike, inspissated meconium[Q].
- **Smaller pellets** of **meconium** are found in the **more distal ileum**, leading into a **relatively small colon**[Q].

Clinical Features
- Present with signs and symptoms of **distal intestinal obstruction**[Q].

Diagnosis

Abdominal X-ray in Meconium Ileus
- **Dilated, gas-filled loops** of **small bowel**[Q]
- **Absence of air-fluid levels**[Q]
- Mass of meconium within the right side of the abdomen mixed with gas to give a **ground-glass** or **soap bubble appearance**[Q].

- Investigation of choice: Water-soluble (Gastrografin) contrast enema^Q.

Treatment
- **Water-soluble (Gastrografin) contrast enema** is successful in **relieving the obstruction** in up to **75%** of cases^Q, with a bowel perforation rate of less than 3%.
  - **Contrast agents** are **hypertonic** relative to serum, so **infants** should be **well hydrated** and electrolytes and vital signs carefully monitored following the procedure
- **Operative management** is required when the **obstruction cannot** be **relieved** with **contrast enema**^Q.
- **Simple evacuation** of the **luminal meconium** without the need to create a stoma is all that is necessary in most cases.
- **Irrigate** the **proximal** and **distal bowel with** either **warmed saline solution** or **4% N-acetylcysteine**^Q.
- **Bishop-Koop operation** with irrigation stoma is **rarely used in meconium ileus**.

COMPLICATED MECONIUM ILEUS

COMPLICATED MECONIUM ILEUS

- Meconium ileus is considered complicated when **perforation** of the **intestine** has taken place.
  - This may occur **in utero**^Q or the **early neonatal period**^Q
  - Meconium peritonitis is an **aseptic chemical peritonitis**^Q caused by **spillage of meconium**
- **Meconium within** the **peritoneal cavity** results in **severe peritonitis** with a **dense inflammatory response** and **calcification (Snow-storm sign on USG**^Q**)**.
- The presentation of complicated meconium ileus is variable and includes formation of a **meconium pseudocyst, adhesive peritonitis** with or without **secondary bacterial infection**, or **ascites**^Q.
- **Treatment**: Most patients are **managed non-operatively** with **enema** or **oral polyethylene glycol solution**.

ACUTE MESENTERIC ISCHEMIA

Acute Mesenteric Ischemia	
Emboli (50%)^Q:	
– **Arrhythmia, Valvular disease**^Q**,** Myocardial infarction	– Hypokinetic ventricular wall
– Cardiac aneurysm, Aortic atherosclerotic disease	
Thrombosis (25%): Atherosclerotic disease	
Nonocclusive (5–15%):	
– **Pancreatitis, Heart failure, Sepsis**^Q	– Cardiac bypass, **Burns, Renal failure**^Q
Venous occlusion:	
– Hypercoagulable state	– Sepsis Compression, Pregnancy, Portal hypertension

ACUTE MESENTERIC ISCHEMIA

Clinical Features
- Early diagnosis is the **key to successful management** of AMI^Q.
- Most patients have **nonspecific symptoms** of abdominal pain^Q.
- **Abdominal pain out of proportion** to the findings on physical examination and persisting **beyond 2 to 3 hours** is the classic picture.
- Diarrhea, nausea, vomiting, and anorexia can also be part of the initial symptom complex.
- **Melena** or **hematochezia in 15%**, and **occult fecal blood** is found in **half** of the patients.
- Leukocytosis is common.

Diagnosis

- **IOC in AMI is mesenteric arteriography**^Q

- **CT scan: Wall hyperdensity**, absence of **wall enhancement**, wall thickening, bowel dilation, **pneumatosis, gas** in **mesenteric vein branches** and in **portal vein** branches.
- **Hemoconcentration, leukocytosis** and **metabolic acidosis** is present.
- **Hyperkalemia** and **hyperphosphatemia** in bowel infarction should be suspected.

Treatment

- Effective management: **Early diagnosis**, **aggressive resuscitation**, **early revascularization**, and ongoing supportive care.
- **Mucosal layer** is the **most sensitive to ischemia**, **bacterial translocation** should be anticipated and **intravenous antibiotics**[Q] used to treat the associated bacteremia.

> - **Catheter-directed papaverine** to **reverse** the **severe mesenteric vasospasm**[Q] is initiated early after arteriography
> - **Anticoagulation** is given **to prevent propagation**[Q] of mesenteric thrombus

- In addition to aggressively correcting the low cardiac output, terminating vasoconstrictor use, and discontinuing digitalis preparations, **intra-arterial papaverine infusion** is the **treatment of choice**[Q].
- In the **absence of peritonitis**, supportive care with **anticoagulation** and **continued papaverine** infusion is recommended.
- **Evidence of peritonitis**: Exploratory laparotomy, with conservative resection of necrotic bowel.

Investigation of Choice	
Acute mesenteric ischemia[Q]	**Angiography**[Q]
Mesenteric venous thrombosis[Q]	**CECT**[Q]
Chronic mesenteric ischemia[Q]	**Aortography**[Q]

NON-OCCLUSIVE MESENTERIC ISCHEMIA

Non-occlusive Mesenteric Ischemia

- Accounts for **20%** of all cases of AMI
- Has manifestations similar to those of mesenteric arterial thrombosis, but it occurs with **patent mesenteric arteries.**
- **Splanchnic vasoconstriction** is the underlying pathophysiologic process and is **precipitated by hypoperfusion** from **medications, depressed cardiac output**, or renal or **hepatic disease**[Q].
- BP in the bowel **falls below 40 mm Hg, ischemia** develops leading to **infarction** and bowel necrosis

Increased Risk of Non-occlusive mesenteric ischemia[Q]	
• **Acute myocardial infarction**[Q]	• **Hemodialysis patients**[Q]
• **CHF, dysrhythmia**[Q]	• **Recent history of cardiopulmonary bypass**
• **Sepsis, hypovolemia**	• **Major abdominal surgery**[Q]
• Use of **splanchnic vasoconstrictors**[Q]	• **Pancreatitis, aortic dissection, or burns**[Q]

- Nonocclusive mesenteric ischemia is typified by **diffuse spasm** of the **SMA branches** with **intermittent areas** of **narrowing and dilation.**

> - **Arteriogram**: **Diffuse vasospasm** with **marked narrowing** of the major branches of the SMA, often with the **"string of sausages" appearance**[Q] with **reflux of contrast** into the aorta

- **Perfusion** is **markedly compromised** because the **intense distal vasospasm** causes high peripheral resistance, with frequent reflux of contrast into the aorta.

EMBOLIC OCCLUSION IN ACUTE MESENTERIC ISCHEMIA

Embolic Occlusion in Acute Mesenteric Ischemia

- Accounts for **40–50%** of cases of AMI.
- **Most emboli** originate in the **heart** and are **secondary to myocardial infarction**[Q], **cardiac arrhythmia**, endocarditis, cardiomyopathy, ventricular aneurysm, valvular disorders, or depressed left ventricular function as a result of ischemic heart disease.

> - Most mesenteric emboli lodge in the **SMA** (branches from the aorta at **an oblique angle**)[Q]
> - More than 50% of emboli lodge in the **mid to distal segment** of the **SMA**[Q]

- Key to successful management: **High index of suspicion** leading to early diagnosis, **aggressive resuscitation**, and **early mesenteric revascularization**.
- **Acute SMA embolism**: **Sudden** and **dramatic symptoms** because of the absence of collateral circulation.
- **Severe abdominal pain** contrast markedly with the **absence of physical findings**[Q].
- **Rectal examination** is **not helpful** because the presence of occult blood is typically a late occurrence.

MESENTERIC VENOUS THROMBOSIS

MESENTERIC VENOUS THROMBOSIS

- MVT accounts for 5–15% of patients with mesenteric ischemia.
- SMV is MC involved, frequently with **extension of thrombus into portal vein**[Q].

- **IMV** is most often **spared**[Q]

Clinical Features
- Most commonly, patients complain of **midabdominal colicky pain**[Q]
- Nausea, vomiting, diarrhea, and anorexia frequently accompany their abdominal discomfort.
- Occult blood in the stool in half of the patients, gross bleeding such as hematemesis, hematochezia, or melena occurs in approximately 15%.
- Family history of venous thromboembolism[Q] in half of the patients
- **Bowel infarction** ultimately develops in **30–60%**[Q].

Diagnosis
- Elevation of the WBC count in 50–65% of patients.
- Serum amylase is usually normal, and serum lactate is elevated only in patients with advanced bowel ischemia and suggests necrosis[Q].

- **CECT** with IV contrast is the **diagnostic test of choice**[Q] for patients with suspected **acute MVT**

Treatment
- Rapid initiation of **systemic anticoagulation**[Q] is important.
- Exploratory laparotomy in localized or diffuse peritoneal irritation,
- Acute thrombus in large veins: Thrombectomy followed by recombinant tissue plasminogen activator solution.
- The patient is treated with heparin intraoperatively and anticoagulation is continued postoperatively[Q].

Prognosis
- MVT have a **high risk of recurrence (35–70%)**[Q], most frequently within 30 days, thus emphasizing the need for early and persistent anticoagulation.
- **Mortality rate** is high, **up to 50%**.

CHRONIC MESENTERIC ISCHEMIA

CHRONIC MESENTERIC ISCHEMIA

- CMI is **most commonly** the result of **advanced atherosclerotic disease** of **multiple mesenteric arteries**[Q].
- **Symptomatic CMI is rare** because of the **good collateral circulatory network** that exists between the mesenteric vessels
- **Symptomatic disease** is more common in **females**[Q]
- **Risk factors**: Positive **family history**, **smoking**, **hypertension**, and **hypercholesterolemia**[Q].

Causes of Chronic Mesenteric Ischemia
• Atherosclerotic disease[Q] • Arterial hyperplasia/dysplasia • Inflammatory disease[Q]

Clinical Features
- **Classical picture: Postprandial abdominal pain (intestinal angina** or **intestinal claudication)** leading to an **aversion to food** and **weight loss**[Q].
- Pain is characteristically **diffuse**, midabdominal, midepigastric, and **crampy** in nature.
- Pain develops **within 15–45 minutes** after eating (severity related to the **size of the meal** ingested)

Diagnosis
- **Evaluation** of the mesenteric arteries frequently **begins with a duplex scan**.
- **Aortography** with AP and lateral views is **diagnostic technique of choice**[Q].

Treatment
- **Revascularization** by **balloon angioplasty** or **stent placement** for **elderly patients** (poor candidates for surgery). **Restenosis** and **reintervention** rates may be **high (30–50%)**

- **Definitive therapy:** Surgery with **transaortic endarterectomy** or **bypass grafting**
- **Results of surgery** are generally **highly gratifying** in properly selected patients, with **rapid resolution of symptoms** and **return of weight**

- **Long-term patency** of the grafts is excellent, **exceeding 90%**.

COLONIC PSEUDO-OBSTRUCTION

Colonic Pseudo-obstruction

- **Pseudo-obstruction** of the colon describes the condition of **distention of the colon,** with signs and symptoms of **colonic obstruction,** in the **absence of** an actual **physical cause** of the obstruction[Q]
- Acute colonic pseudo-obstruction is also known as **Ogilvie's syndrome**[Q]
- Two types: Primary and secondary
- **Secondary pseudo-obstruction is more common**[Q]

Pathophysiology

- **Mechanism** thought to play: **Sympathetic overactivity overriding the parasympathetic system**[Q]
- Indirect support for this theory has been derived from the **success in treating** the syndrome with **neostigmine,** a **parasympathomimetic agent**[Q]
- **Further support** comes from reports of **immediate resolution of** the syndrome after administration of an **epidural anesthetic** that provides sympathetic blockade

Primary Pseudo-obstruction

- It is a motility disorder:
  - A **familial visceral myopathy** (hollow visceral myopathy syndrome) or
  - A **diffuse motility disorder involving** the **autonomic innervation** of the intestinal wall.

Causes of secondary Pseudo-obstruction

Neuroleptic medications[Q]	Uremia[Q]
Opiates[Q]	Lupus, scleroderma, dermatomyositis[Q]
Severe metabolic illness	Parkinson's disease[Q]
Myxedema (Hypothyroidism[Q])	Traumatic retroperitoneal hematomas[Q]
Hyperparathyroidism[Q]	Diabetes mellitus[Q]

Clinical Features

- **Acute form:** Most commonly affects patients with **chronic renal, respiratory, cerebral, or cardiovascular disease, involves only** the colon[Q].
- **Chronic form:** Affects other parts of the gastrointestinal tract, usually presents as bouts of **subacute** and **partial intestinal obstruction,** and tends to **recur periodically.**

- **Acute colonic pseudo-obstruction** should be suspected when a **medically ill patient** suddenly **develops abdominal distention**[Q]
- **The abdomen is** tympanitic, **usually** nontender, **and bowel sounds** are **usually present**

Diagnosis

- **Abdominal X-ray: Distended colon,** with the **right** and **transverse segments**[Q] tending to be **most dramatically affected** (radiologic appearance of large bowel obstruction). **Transition point** is frequently present, usually at or near the **splenic flexure**[Q].

- Most useful investigation: Water-soluble contrast enema[Q]
- Contrast enema differentiate mechanical obstruction and pseudo-obstruction

Treatment

- **Initial treatment:** Nasogastric decompression, replacement of extracellular fluid deficits, and correction of electrolyte abnormalities[Q].
- **All medications** that **inhibit bowel motility,** such as opiates, **should be discontinued.**
- Most patients improve with this regimen[Q].

- Treat this condition with **neostigmine**[Q]
- **Mechanical obstruction should be excluded** (either by water-soluble contrast enema or colonoscopy) **before the administration of neostigmine**[Q]
- **Resolution** is indicated by the **passage of stool** and **flatus** by the patient, **within ten minutes** of drug administration

LARGE BOWEL OBSTRUCTION

Large Bowel Obstruction

- Classified as **dynamic (mechanical)** or **adynamic (pseudo-obstruction).**
- **Mechanical obstruction** is characterized by **blockage** of the **large bowel** (luminal, mural, or extramural), resulting in **increased intestinal contractility**[Q]
- **Pseudo-obstruction** is characterized by the **absence of intestinal contractility,** often associated with **decreased** or **absent motility** of the **small bowel** and **stomach**[Q]

- MC cause of LBO: Colorectal cancer[Q] (CA Rectum > sigmoid)
- Adhesions (MC cause of small bowel obstruction) are rarely a cause of colonic obstruction.

Pathophysiology
- Colon becomes distended as gas (about **two thirds is swallowed air**, the remainder includes the products of bacterial fermentation), **stool**, and **liquid accumulate** proximal to the site of blockage.
- In **obstructed hernia** or **volvulus**, the **blood supply** can become **compromised**, or **strangulated**; initially, the **venous return** is **blocked**[Q]
- **Vascular compromise** of the **obstructed colon** can occur due to **excessive distention**[Q]
- **Closed-loop obstruction**: When **both** the **proximal** and **distal** parts of the bowel are **occluded**[Q] (strangulated hernia or volvulus)
- **Closed-loop obstruction** is seen when a **cancer occludes** the **lumen of the colon** in the **presence of a competent ileocecal valve**[Q]
- **Increasing colonic distention causes** the pressure in the **cecum** to become so **high** that the vessels in the bowel wall are occluded, and **necrosis** and **perforation**[Q] can occur

Clinical Features
- Cancers of **rectum** or **left colon** are **more likely to obstruct**[Q] than those arising in the more capacious proximal colon.
- **Failure to pass stool** and **flatus** associated with **increasing abdominal distention** and **cramping abdominal pain**[Q].

Diagnosis
- Abdominal X-ray: Distended colon[Q]
- CT scan: Helpful in revealing an **inflammatory process** such as **diverticulitis**.
- Water-soluble contrast enema: For the **diagnosis of** suspected case of **volvulus** or **distal sigmoid cancer**[Q]

Treatment
- Virtually **all patients with complete acute large bowel obstruction** require **prompt surgical intervention**[Q] and should not undergo a trial of non-operative management.
- Acute large bowel obstruction in patients **with competent ileocecal valve** is a **true surgical emergency** because of **high chances of perforation (MC site: Cecum)**[Q].
- Once diagnosis has been made, **surgical exploration** should be undertaken **as soon as possible after appropriate resuscitation**[Q]

Treatment of Large Bowel Obstruction	
Site of Obstruction	**Procedure**
Right-sided colonic obstruction (cancer or volvulus)	Resection with **ileo-transverse anastomosis**[Q]
Cancer of sigmoid colon	• **Hartmann's operation**[Q] (sigmoidectomy with descending colostomy & closure of the rectal stump), • **Sigmoidectomy** with **primary colorectal anastomosis**[Q] • **Abdominal colectomy** with **ileorectal anastomosis**[Q]
Cancer of **distal** or **mid rectum**	**Loop colostomy** or **defunctioning colostomy**[Q] (to relieve obstruction) followed by **neoadjuvant chemoradiation**[Q], (with the plan to resect the primary lesion at a later time)

	Small Bowel Obstruction	Large Bowel Obstruction
Valvulae conniventes	Thin complete lines[Q] Seen in jejunum[Q]	Absent
Haustra	Absent	Thick incomplete bands[Q]
No of loops	Many[Q]	Few
Distribution of loops	Central[Q]	Peripheral[Q]
Diameter of loops	3–5 cm[Q]	>5 cm[Q]
Radius of curvature	Small[Q]	Large[Q]
Solid feces	Absent	Present[Q]

SIGMOID VOLVULUS

Sigmoid Volvulus

- Volvulus can occur in any segment of **large bowel attached to a long & floppy mesentery**[Q] or fixed to the retroperitoneum by a narrow base of origin[Q]
  - **MC site** of volvulus: **Sigmoid colon**
  - **More commonly anticlockwise** (can be both clockwise or anticlockwise)
- Equal frequency in both sexes[Q]

Associated Predisposing Factors

- Age: **60–70 years**^Q.
- **Chronic constipation**^Q
- **Institutionalized** or **neurologically impaired or psychiatric patients**^Q (their medication may decrease intestinal motility, or they may fail to pass stool regularly, leading to fecal loaded large bowel predisposing to volvulus)
- **Diet high in fibre** and **vegetables**^Q (as in **third world countries**)

Clinical Features

- Present as **acute** or **subacute intestinal obstruction**
- **Sudden onset** of **severe abdominal pain, vomiting, & obstipation.**
- **Abdomen is markedly distended** and **tympanitic,** with the **distention** often **more dramatic**^Q than would be associated with other causes of obstruction.
- Severe abdominal pain, **rebound tenderness,** & **tachycardia** are **ominous signs**^Q.

Radiological (X-ray) Characteristics

- **Markedly dilated sigmoid colon** with the **appearance of a bent inner tube** or **coffee bean appearance**^Q.
- **Inferior convergence** of the dilated loop **points towards left side** of pelvis. Whorl sign on CT scan.

> - Contrast enema demonstrates the point of obstruction with the pathognomic **'birds beak'** or **'bird of prey'** or **'ace of spades' sign**^Q

Management of Sigmoid Volvulus

- **Initial management: Resuscitation**^Q followed by **endoscopic decompression** and **detorsion**^Q.
- **Decompression/detorsion**^Q can be achieved by placement of **rectal tube** through a **proctoscope** or the use of a **colonoscope.**
- If detorsion/decompression cannot be achieved with either the rectal tube or colonoscope, **laparotomy with resections of the sigmoid colon**^Q is done.

> - Even if **detorsion** of the sigmoid volvulus is successful, **risk of recurrence is high** (50%)^Q
> - **Sigmoid colectomy** is indicated after the patient has stabilized

- Any evidence of **bowel gangrene** or **perforation contraindicates non-operative decompression** and an **immediate surgical exploration**^Q is done.
- **Paul-Mikulicz operation:** In cases of **suspicion of impending gangrene**

CECAL VOLVULUS

CECAL VOLVULUS

- Cecal volvulus is **actually** a **cecocolic volvulus**^Q
- Consists of an **axial rotation** of the **terminal ileum, cecum,** and **ascending colon**^Q with concomitant twisting of the associated mesentery.
- Cause: Lack of fixation of the cecum to the retroperitoneum.^Q

> - Cecal volvulus occurs in **clockwise direction**^Q
> - **More common** in **women**^Q
> - Affects a **younger age group** as compared to sigmoid volvulus, in **5th decade**^Q

Predisposing Factors for Cecal volvulus	
• **Previous surgery**^Q	• **Malrotation**^Q
• **Pregnancy**^Q	• **Obstructing lesions of the left colon**^Q

Clinical Features

- Sudden onset of **abdominal pain & distention.**
- Presents with **features of small bowel obstruction.**
- **Asymmetric distention** of the abdomen, with a **tympanitic mass palpable** in either **the left upper quadrant** or **midabdomen**^Q.

Diagnosis

- Abdominal X-ray: Dilated cecum, displaced to the left side of the abdomen.
- **Distended cecum** assumes a **gas-filled comma shape** or **kidney bean shape**^Q, the **concavity** of which faces **inferiorly** and to the **right**.
- **Haustral markings** in the **distended loop** indicate that the dilated bowel is colon.
- **Torsion results in small bowel obstruction**^Q (radiographic pattern of SBO)

- Contrast enema is used to confirm the diagnosis and to exclude a carcinoma of the distal bowel as a precipitating cause of the volvulus[Q]

Treatment
- Most cases require **operation to correct** the **volvulus & prevent ischemia**[Q].
- If **ischemia** has already occurred, **immediate operation** is obviously required.

> - **Right colectomy** with **primary anastomosis** is the **procedure of choice**[Q]
> - In **frankly gangrenous bowel, resection** of the gangrenous bowel **with ileostomy** is a safer approach

- **Recurrence rates are high with ceropxy**, and **right colectomy** remains the **procedure of choice for cecal volvulus.**

Cecal bascule
- A condition in which **cecum folds** in **a cephalad direction anteriorly** over a **fixed ascending colon**[Q]
- Cecal bascule **commonly causes intermittent bouts** of abdominal pain
- Mobile cecum permits **intermittent episodes** of **isolated cecal obstruction** that are **spontaneously relieved**[Q] as the cecum falls back into its normal position

> - **Sigmoid volvulus** is **more commonly anticlockwise** (can be **both clockwise** or **anticlockwise**)[Q]
> - **Cecal volvulus** and **small intestine volvulus** are mostly **clockwise**[Q]

MALROTATION: EMBRYOLOGY

Malrotation: Embryology

- **Rapid growth** plus **elongation** of the **midgut** starting in the **fifth week** leads to **herniation** of midgut with **superior mesenteric vessels** as its **stalk**[Q].
- The midgut undergoes **270-degree counterclockwise rotation**[Q] around the superior mesenteric vessels.
- This **initial rotation** results in the **normal position** of the DJ flexure in the **left upper quadrant** at the level of the gastric antrum[Q].
- The **DJ flexure** becomes **fixed** to the **posterior abdominal wall** by the **ligament of Treitz**. As a result of this rotation and fixation, the **third portion** of the **duodenum** lies **posterior** to the **SMA**[Q].

> - In the **10th week** the **herniated intestinal loop** begins to **return**[Q] to the abdominal cavity.
> - The **cecocolic loop** undergoes another **270-degree counterclockwise rotation**[Q] around the **SMA**, which leads to the **normal position** of the **cecum** in the **right lower quadrant**.

- Subsequently, the ascending colon and descending colon become fixed to the posterior abdominal wall.
- During the **fourth** and **fifth weeks** of gestation, the **small intestine mesentery attaches** itself to the **posterior abdominal wall** in a broad base **extending** diagonally from the **DJ flexure** to the **cecum**[Q].

> - MC rotational abnormality: Non-rotation[Q]
> - MC type of malrotation: Incomplete rotation[Q]

TYPES OF MALROTATION

Types of Malrotation

Nonrotation
- MC rotational abnormality
- **Failure of counterclockwise rotation**[Q] after return of the midgut to the abdominal cavity.
- Duodenal 'C' loop, ligament of Treitz and **small intestine** is on **right side** of abdomen.
- Cecum is on the **left side** of abdomen[Q]
- **Proximal jejunum** & **ascending colon** are **fused** as **one pedicle**, through which **blood supply** to the **entire midgut (SMA)**[Q] is located.

Incomplete Rotation
- **Counterclockwise rotation** is **arrested** at around **180 degrees**[Q].
- **Most common**[Q] **forms** of malrotation.

> - The **small intestine** lies on the **right side** with the **DJ flexure** to the **right** of the **vertebral column**, and the **duodenum** has a **corkscrew configuration**[Q].
> - The **large intestine** lies on the **left side** with the **cecum** at **abnormal locations**, usually in the **midline**[Q].

- Other forms of fixation anomalies may be due to **failure of fixation** of the **ascending colon** in the **right hypochondrium**. Associated with this abnormal fixation is a **narrow intestinal mesentery** and **Ladd's bands**.
- **Ladd's bands** represent the **retroperitoneal attachments** that normally **fix** the **cecum** and **ascending colon** to the **posterior abdominal wall**. Because the right colon is more medial, the **bands extend across** the **duodenum** from the right upper quadrant **to** the **cecum** and **ascending colon**^{Q}.

Reverse Rotation

- In **reverse rotation**, part of the **rotation** occurs in a **clockwise direction** around the SMA.
- **Duodenum** assumes an **anterior position** and the **colon lies posterior** to the duodenum and the SMA.

Hyperrotation

- If the **counterclockwise rotation** extends **beyond 270 degrees**, the **cecum** comes to rest in the **left hypochondrium position.**

MALROTATION

MALROTATION

- Patients have a **30–62% risk** of **having associated anomalies**, and **most involve GIT**^{Q}.
- Incidence of clinically symptomatic malrotation is **1 in 6000 live births**^{Q}.
- Malrotation may initially be recognized at any age

  - Approximately in **90% of patients symptoms develop before 1 year of age**, with **50% to 75%** appearing **within the first month**^{Q} of life.

Clinical Features

- Malrotation can be totally asymptomatic and discovered only during work-up for an unrelated condition or during an autopsy examination.
- **Malrotation without volvulus** may be manifested as **chronic, vague abdominal pain**, with **or without intermittent bilious emesis**, & **failure to thrive**^{Q}.

  - **Neonates** typically have **bilious emesis,** which may be the **only initial symptom of midgut volvulus**^{Q}.
  - **Systemic signs** such as increasing lethargy with poor perfusion, temperature instability, cardiopulmonary compromise, and low urine output in cases of **delayed diagnosis**^{Q}.

- Hematologic studies may show metabolic acidosis, thrombocytopenia, & leukopenia.
- **Acute onset of bilious vomiting** in a **neonate** is a **sign of malrotation** until proved otherwise. It demands **immediate radiologic evaluation**^{Q}.

Diagnosis

Upper Gastrointestinal Contrast Study

- **Gold standard test** for **diagnosis** is an **upper gastrointestinal contrast study**^{Q}.
- Malrotation is diagnosed by an **abnormal position** of the **ligament of Treitz**^{Q}.
- **Normal location** is typically to the **left of vertebral column** & posterior to stomach^Q

- **Volvulus** can be diagnosed by **contrast-enhanced upper gastrointestinal series** showing a **corkscrew configuration** of upper portion of small intestine or a **"bird's beak" appearance** at **third portion**^{Q} of duodenum.

Treatment

Acutely ill child with **peritonitis**	**Emergency surgery**^{Q} without radiologic studies
Symptomatic from volvulus	Nasogastric decompression, intravenous fluid, and broad-spectrum antibiotics followed by urgent surgery^Q
Chronic symptoms or **symptom-free**	**Elective correction**^{Q}

In Malrotation

- **Plain abdominal radiographs** are **not helpful** in **ruling in** or **out** midgut **volvulus**^{Q}.
- A **contrast enema** study is **not part** of the **work-up** for malrotation. The presence of a **normally located** cecum in the right lower quadrant **does not rule out malrotation**^{Q}

Operative Treatment of Malrotation

- The standard approach via a **right upper quadrant transverse incision**^{Q}.
- **If volvulus** is present, it should be **reduced by counterclockwise rotation**^{Q} as necessary because volvulus usually occurs in a clockwise direction

- Bowel with **uncertain viability** should be wrapped with **warm moist gauze** sponges for at least 15 minutes
  - **Frankly gangrenous bowel** should be resected and a stoma or stomas fashioned.
  - **Ladd's bands,** which represent the posterior peritoneal attachments of the right colon that cross over the duodenum, **should be divided** on the **lateral aspect** of the duodenum^Q.
- **Widening of the mesenteric base** is necessary, & **duodenum** is **mobilized & straightened** by dividing the abnormal ligament of Treitz and Ladd's bands.
- **Incidental appendectomy** should be performed to **avoid diagnostic confusion** in the future **because** the cecum will be **placed in** the **left lower quadrant**^{Q}.
  - **Duodenum** and **proximal jejunum** are placed on the **right side**^{Q}
  - **Terminal ileum** and **cecum** are placed in the **left hypochondrium**^{Q}

Multiple Choice Questions

ACUTE INTESTINAL OBSTRUCTION

1. True about strangulation of intestine is: *(MHPGMCET 2001)*
   a. Arterial blood flow affected first
   b. Usually venous blood flow affected first
   c. Blood flow normal
   d. No gangrene

2. Most common cause of hyponatremia in surgical practice:
   a. Small intestinal obstruction *(MHPGMCET 2008)*
   b. Duodenal fistula
   c. Pancreatic fistula
   d. Intussusception

3. Best investigation for acute intestinal obstruction is: *(Recent Question 2014)*
   a. Barium studies
   b. X-ray
   c. USG
   d. ERCP

4. Early sign of intestinal strangulation: *(PGI SS June 2001)*
   a. Continuous pain
   b. Abdominal rigidity and shock
   c. Abdominal fluid
   d. Dilated bowel loops on USG

5. The most common cause of small intestinal obstruction is: *(Recent Question 2014)*
   a. Intussusception
   b. Iatrogenic adhesions
   c. Trauma
   d. Carcinoma

6. Commonest cause of acute intestinal obstruction is: *(Recent Question 2016)*
   a. Adhesions
   b. Volvulus
   c. Inguinal hernias
   d. Internal hernias

7. A 40 years old male was brought to the emergency with the history of multiple episodes of colicky pain, bilious vomiting with no passage of feces and flatus. X-ray abdomen was done. On the basis of findings, what is the diagnosis? *(Recent Question 2016)*
   a. Duodenal obstruction
   b. Jejunal obstruction
   c. Ileal obstruction
   d. Colonic obstruction

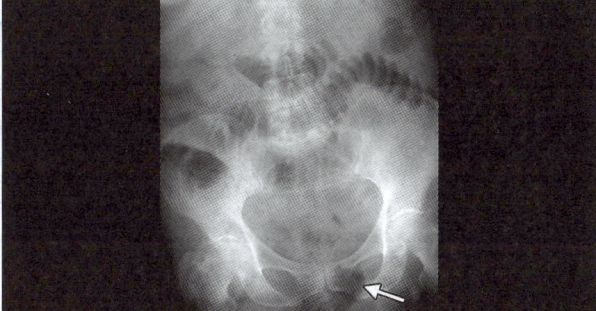

8. While doing emergency laparotomy for an intestinal obstruction, which organ would you first visualize to say whether it is small bowel or large bowel obstruction? *(AIIMS November 2018)*
   a. Ileum
   b. Sigmoid colon
   c. Cecum
   d. Rectum

9. The commonest cause of intestinal obstruction in a 30 years old Indian female: *(All India 93)*
   a. TB stricture
   b. Crohn's disease
   c. Postoperative adhesions
   d. Adenocarcinoma

10. Acute intestinal obstruction is characterized by: *(PGI Dec 2003)*
    a. Vomiting is common in duodenal obstruction
    b. Pain after each attack of vomiting is characteristic of ileal obstruction
    c. In colonic obstruction distension is common than vomiting
    d. X-ray erect posture is diagnostic
    e. Colicky pain to steady pain indicates strangulation

11. Features of intestinal obstruction: clinically/investigation by: *(PGI June 2006)*
    a. Abdominal distension
    b. Vomiting
    c. Fluid level in X-ray >4
    d. Localized tenderness
    e. Diarrhea

12. In intestinal obstruction, investigations needed are: *(PGI Dec 2001)*
    a. Barium swallow
    b. Intestinal barium meal
    c. Stomach barium meal
    d. Erect X-ray abdomen
    e. Supine X-ray abdomen

13. A 30-years old lady presented with acute pain abdomen, constipation and vomiting suspecting acute intestinal obstruction. The investigation of choice for the patient is:
    a. X-ray abdomen erect posture *(PGI June 2003)*
    b. Ba enema
    c. USG
    d. CT scan

14. A women of 35-years, comes to emergency department with symptoms of pain in abdomen and bilious vomiting but no distension of bowel. Abdominal X-ray showed no air fluid level. Diagnosis is: *(Recent Question 2014; AIIMS June 2009)*
    a. CA rectum
    b. Duodenal obstruction
    c. Adynamic ileus
    d. Pseudo-obstruction

15. One of the following will always present with bilious vomiting: *(All India 94)*
    a. Pyloric stenosis
    b. Esophageal atresia
    c. Atresia of the 3rd part of the duodenum
    d. Malrotation of the gut

16. Distended abdomen in intestinal obstruction is mainly due to: *(All India 95, PGI Dec 98)*
    a. Diffusion of gas from blood
    b. Fermentation of residual food
    c. Bacterial action
    d. Swallowed air

17. In case of new born, the commonest cause of intestinal obstruction is: *(AIIMS Nov 95)*
    a. Annular pancreas
    b. Duodenal atresia
    c. Jejunal atresia
    d. Esophageal atresia

18. Regarding adhesive intestinal obstruction, true is:
    (AIIMS Nov 94)
    a. Avoid surgery for initial 48–72 hours
    b. Never operate
    c. Operate after minimum 10 days of conservative treatment
    d. Immediate operation

19. Water loss is severe if intestinal obstruction occurs at:
    (JIPMER 90)
    a. First part of duodenum   b. Third part of duodenum
    c. Mid-jejunum   d. Ileum

20. The first to appear in a cause of acute intestinal obstruction is:
    (Recent Quetions 2016)
    a. Constipation   b. Colicky pain
    c. Vomiting   d. Distension

21. Primary feature of small intestinal obstruction: *(APPG 96)*
    a. Fever   b. High peristalsis with colic
    c. Abdominal distension   d. Empty rectum

22. Best way to diagnose lower small intestinal obstruction:
    a. Pain abdomen   *(PGI 96)*
    b. Abdominal distension
    c. Profuse vomiting
    d. Multiple air gas shadows on X-ray

23. For intestinal obstruction immediate operation should not be done in case of: *(Kolkata 2000)*
    a. Postop adhesion   b. Appendix perforation
    c. Volvulus   d. Obstructed hernia

24. Which of the following is most suggestive of neonatal small bowel obstruction?   *(All India 2003)*
    a. Generalized abdominal distension
    b. Failure to pass meconium in the first 24 hours
    c. Bilious vomiting
    d. Refusal of feeds

25. What is the sure sign of intestinal obstruction?
    (Recent Question 2013)
    a. Vomiting and distension   b. Jelly like stool
    c. Diarrhoea   d. Localized tenderness

26. Ileal obstruction due to round worm obstruction treatment is: *(Recent Question 2013)*
    a. Resection with end to end anastomosis
    b. Resection with side to side anastomosis
    c. Enterotomy, removal of worms and primary closure
    d. Diversion

27. Investigation of choice for intermittent GI obstruction:
    (Recent Question 2017)
    a. X-ray   b. USG
    c. Enteroclysis   d. Barium meal follow-through

28. Step ladder pattern of gas shadow is seen in:
    (Recent Question 2017)
    a. Duodenal obstruction   b. Intestinal obstruction
    c. Gastric outlet obstruction d. Sigmoid volvulus

INTUSSUSCEPTION

29. A neonate presents with colicky pain and vomiting with sausage-shaped lump in the abdomen, diagnosis is:
    (UPPG 2009)
    a. Enterocolitis   b. Perforation of the abdomen
    c. Intussusception   d. Acute appendicitis

30. All statement about adult intussusception are true except:
    (PGI Nov 2009)
    a. Idiopathic and more enteric rather than colonic
    b. Lead point present in majority of cases
    c. Resection of bowel is adequate for large bowel intussusception
    d. Hydrostatic reduction with barium or air are done if bowel is not gangrenous

31. A previously healthy infant presents with recurrent episode of abdominal pain. The mother says that the child has been passing altered stool after episodes of pain, but gives no history of vomiting or bleeding per rectum. Which of the following is the most likely diagnosis?   *(All India 2011)*
    a. Rectal polyps   b. Intussusception
    c. Meckel's diverticulum d. Necrotizing enterocolitis

32. True about Intussusceptions in children: *(PGI Nov 2010)*
    a. Most common variety is ileocolic
    b. Associated with pathological lead point
    c. May be seen after viral infection
    d. Can be relieved by barium enema
    e. Surgery is always indicated

33. True statement about treatment of intussusception:
    a. Air enema   *(PGI Nov 2010)*
    b. Saline enema
    c. Ba enema
    d. Hydrostatic reduction
    e. Colonoscopy is always done to confirm diagnosis

34. A 10-month-old child was brought to your hospital having recurrent attacks of pain abdomen. On examination, sausage shaped mass was palpable in the right lumbar region. Barium enema was done. What is the diagnosis on the basis of barium enema findings?
    a. Colorectal polyp   b. Rectal prolapse
    c. Intussusception   d. Carcinoma colon

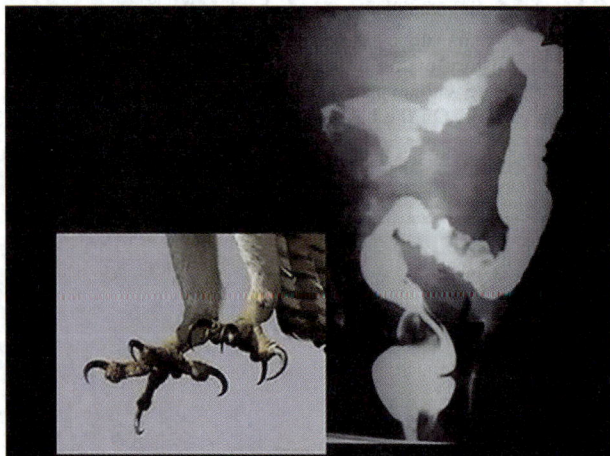

35. Intussusception usually begins from: *(DNB 2007)*
    a. Jejunum   b. Terminal ileum
    c. Colon   d. Rectum

36. The most common type of intussusception:
    (MCI June 2018, DNB 2009, 2005, 2001, 2000, MHPGMCET 2009)
    a. Ileocolic   b. Colocolic
    c. Ileoileal   d. Retrograde

37. All are true about intussusception except:
    (AIIMS GIS May 2011)
    a. Barium must be used in children after 48 hours
    b. X-ray shows paucity of colonic gas
    c. X-ray shows lump shadow
    d. USG show pseudo-kidney sign

38. A child was operated for small intestine mass with intussusception and after the operation the tumor was diagnosed in histological section. Which is the most likely tumor associated? (AIIMS Nov 2012)
    a. Carcinoid
    b. Villous adenoma
    c. Lymphoma
    d. Smooth muscle tumor

39. What is intussuscipiens? (Recent Question 2014)
    a. The entire complex of intussusception
    b. The entering layer
    c. The outer layer
    d. The process of reducing the intussusception

40. What is the name of sign in this barium enema done in the patient of intussusception?
    a. Meniscus sign
    b. Claw sign
    c. Coiled spring sign
    d. Target sign

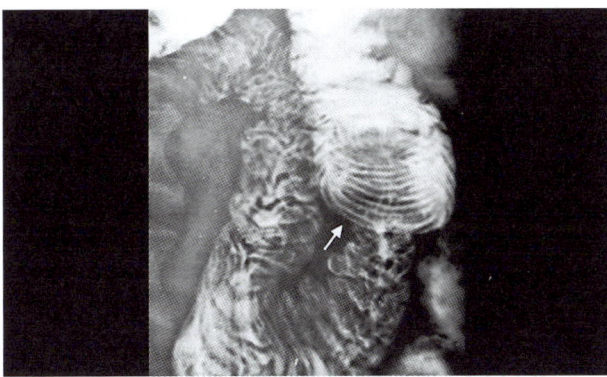

41. A 10-months old infant presents with acute intestinal obstruction. Contrast enema X-ray shows the intussusceptions. Likely cause is: (All India 2002)
    a. Payers patch hypertrophy
    b. Meckel's diverticulum
    c. Mucosal polyp
    d. Duplication cyst

42. Features of intussusceptions are: (PGI June 2001)
    a. Pincer sign
    b. Target sign
    c. Dove sign
    d. Coiled spring sign
    e. Dance sign

43. Recurrent pain abdomen with intestinal obstruction and mass passes per rectum goes in favor of: (PGI Dec 99)
    a. Internal herniation
    b. Stricture
    c. Strangulated hernia
    d. Intussusception

44. Recurrent obstruction, mass per rectum and diarrhea in child: (Recent Question 2014)
    a. Intussusception
    b. Rectal prolapsed
    c. Internal hernia
    d. Hemorrhoids

45. Commonest cause of intussusception is: (WBPG 2015)
    a. Submucous lipoma
    b. Meckel's diverticulum
    c. Hypertrophy of submucous Peyer's patches
    d. Polyp

46. Intussusception is frequently associated with:
    (JIPMER 2014, 2012)
    a. Submucosal lipoma
    b. Intramural lipoma
    c. Subserusal lipoma
    d. Subfascial lipoma

47. Which of the following is true about intussusception?
    a. Common in neonates (DPG 2005)
    b. Fever always present
    c. Not associated with tumors of intestine
    d. Usually relieved by barium enema

48. The least common type of intussusception is:
    (Recent Question 2016)
    a. Multiple
    b. Colocolic
    c. Ileoileal
    d. Ileoilecolic

49. Henoch-Schnolein purpura may rarely cause:
    a. Intussusception
    b. Volvulus
    c. Atrial fibrillation
    d. Hernia

50. Claw sign seen in: (APPG 2008)
    a. Intussusception
    b. Volvulus
    c. Both
    d. None

51. A young patient was brought to the emergency with colicky abdominal pain, bilious vomiting. CT findings are given below. What is the name of this sign?
    a. Claw sign
    b. Coiled spring sign
    c. Meniscus sign
    d. Target sign

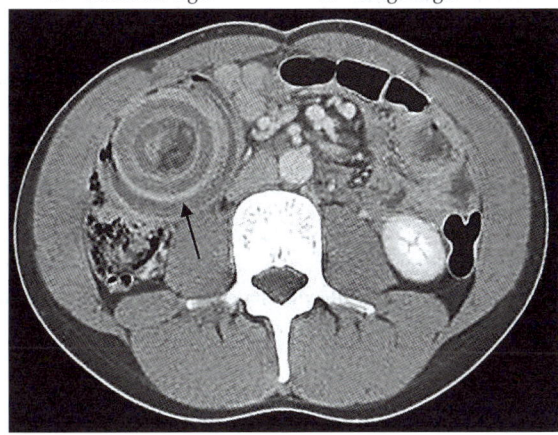

52. Complete treatment of intussusception is indicated by:
    (APPG 2008)
    a. Free passage of barium in the terminal ileum
    b. Passage of feces and flatus along with barium
    c. Improvement of clinical condition
    d. None

53. A 12-months old male child suddenly draws up his legs and screams with pain. This is repeated periodically throughout the night interspersed with periods of quiet sleep. When seen after 12 hours the child looks pale, has just vomited and passed thin blood-stained stool; there is a mass around umbilicus. What is the most likely diagnosis? (UPSC 97)
    a. Appendicitis
    b. Intussusception
    c. Gastroenteritis
    d. Roundworm obstruction

54. Sign of Dance is: (MAHE 2005)
    a. Empty right iliac fossa in intussusception
    b. Pincer shaped appearance in barium enema in intussusception
    c. Tenderness at the McBurney's point
    d. Passing of large quantities of urine in hydronephrosis

55. Which of the following is true about intussusception in children? *(Recent Question 2017)*
    a. Most common type is ileocecocolic
    b. Most common type is colocolic
    c. Entering tube is intussuscipiens
    d. Contrast enema is not useful in the management

56. A patient has acute abdominal pain with blood and mucus in stool with palpable mass per abdomen is due to: *(Recent Question 2014; AIIMS June 2000)*
    a. Meckel's diverticulum   b. Volvulus
    c. Intussusception
    d. Hypertrophic pyloric stenosis

57. A 6 months old child woke up in night, crying with abdominal pain, which got relieved on passing red stool. What is the most likely diagnosis? *(AIIMS November 2014)*
    a. Meckel's diverticulum   b. Intussusception
    c. Malrotation   d. Intestinal obstruction

MECONIUM SYNDROME

58. A new born child has not passed meconium for 48 hours. What is the diagnostic procedure of choice? *(All India 2008)*
    a. USG   b. Contrast enema
    c. CT   d. MRI

59. Snow storm ascites is seen in: *(APPG 2005)*
    a. Meconium ileus   b. Hirschsprung's disease
    c. Ileocaecal tuberculosis   d. Pseudomyxoma peritonei

60. Extraluminal abdominal calcifications in the newborn may be seen in: *(COMEDK 2010)*
    a. Meconium aspiration   b. Hirschsprung's disease
    c. Meconium peritonitis   d. Meconium plug syndrome

61. Intra-abdominal calcification in a plane X-ray abdomen is most often seen in: *(Karnataka 95)*
    a. Meconium ileus   b. Meconium peritonitis
    c. Meconium plug syndrome   d. Necrotising enterocolitis

62. Which one of the following statements regarding meconium peritonitis is not correct? *(UPSC 2000)*
    a. It is a septic peritonitis
    b. It develops in later intra-uterine life or during or just after delivery
    c. This condition should always be considered when a baby is born with tense abdomen
    d. Plain X-ray abdomen of this condition reveals calcification on liver and spleen

63. Meconium ileus is associated with: *(All India 2000, 98, 96)*
    a. Fibrocystic disease of pancreas
    b. Liver aplasia
    c. Cirrhosis of liver   d. Malnutrition

64. Which of the following statement is correct about the surgical management of meconium ileus?

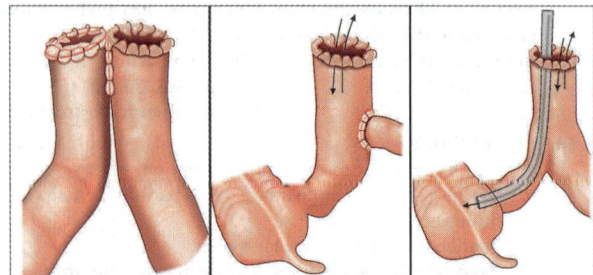

    a. 1-Paul Mikulicz, 2-Bishop-Koop, 3-Santulli
    b. 1-Paul Mikulicz, 2- Santulli, 3- Bishop-Koop
    c. 1- Santulli, 2-Bishop-Koop, 3- Paul Mikulicz
    d. 1- Bishop-Koop, 2- Paul Mikulicz, 3-Santulli

65. Fluid levels are not visible in: *(PGI June 98)*
    a. Meconium ileus   b. Intussusception
    c. Colon pouch   d. Duodenal obstruction

66. A new born girl not passed meconium for 48 hours, has abdominal distention and vomiting. Initial investigation of choice would be: *(AIIMS Nov 2007)*
    a. Manometry
    b. Genotyping for cystic fibrosis
    c. Lower GI contrast study
    d. Serum trypsin immunoblot

67. Meconium peritonitis occurs: *(PGI June 99)*
    a. Just before birth   b. Just after birth
    c. Before and after birth   d. Due to birth trauma

MESENTERIC ISCHEMIA

68. Occlusion to superior mesenteric artery affects jejunum and:
    a. Pyloric antrum   *(UPPG 2010)*
    b. Fundus of stomach
    c. Duodenum distal to the opening of CBD
    d. Greater curvature
    e. Descending colon

69. Most common cause of acute mesenteric ischemia is: *(AIIMS May 2011, Nov 2008)*
    a. Arterial thrombosis   b. Venous thrombosis
    c. Embolism   d. Non occlusive disease

70. All are causes of dynamic intestinal obstruction except:
    a. Gallstones   b. Bands   *(JIPMER 2010)*
    c. Intussusception
    d. Mesenteric vascular occlusion

71. A young female complains of pain in umbilical region since few days, which is more especially after taking meals. What is the likely diagnosis? *(MHSSMCET 2005)*
    a. Peptic ulcer disease   b. Meckel's diverticulum
    c. Typhlitis   d. Abdominal angina

72. If patient with superior mesenteric artery thrombosis doesn't develop collateral circulation, then what is the best treatment? *(MHSSMCET 2005)*
    a. Resection anastomosis   b. Endarterectomy
    c. Arterial reconstruction   d. Papaverine injection

73. Which of the following is a common cause of abdominal angina? *(MHSSMCET 2006)*
    a. SMA thrombosis   b. SMA embolism
    c. SMA aneurysm   d. SMA rupture

74. Ischemia of which of the vessel would cause least damage?
    a. Renal artery   b. SMA   *(AIIMS Nov 2011)*
    c. IMA   d. Celiac trunk

75. All are true about non-obstructive mesenteric ischemia except: *(AIIMS GIS Dec 2006)*
    a. Vasopressor treatment   b. Cardiac shock
    c. Burns   d. Hypercoagulable state

76. String of lakes appearance on angiography is seen in:
    a. Chronic mesenteric ischaemia   *(Recent Question 2016)*
    b. Non-occlusive mesenteric ischemia
    c. Mesenteric venous thrombosis
    d. Mesenteric arterial thrombosis

77. All are true about acute mesenteric ischemia except:
    a. Branch point of middle colic artery is most common location for embolism *(AIIMS GIS 2003)*
    b. Acute venous thrombosis is best judged on CT
    c. Non-obstructive mesenteric ischemia has very good prognosis
    d. Gold standard investigation is angiography

78. All are true about mesenteric ischemia except:
    a. Due to embolism to SMA *(AIIMS GIS 2003)*
    b. Most common cause is AF
    c. Embolus gets lodged most commonly at branching of SMA from aorta
    d. Most common cause of small bowel syndrome in adults

79. Type of mesenteric ischemia best visualized by CECT: *(AIIMS GIS Dec 2006)*
    a. Mesenteric ischemia by embolic occlusion
    b. Acute mesenteric artery thrombosis
    c. Non-occlusive mesenteric ischemia
    d. Acute mesenteric venous thrombosis

80. A 65-years old Ramdeen presents with abdominal pain and distension of abdomen. His stools were maroon colored and he gives a past history of cerebrovascular accident and myocardial infarction. What will be the probable diagnosis? *(AIIMS Nov 2000, Nov 97)*
    a. Ulcerative colitis
    b. Acute mesenteric ischemia
    c. Irritable bowel syndrome
    d. Crohn's disease

81. A man aged 60 years has history of IHD and atherosclerosis. He presents with abdominal pain and maroon stools. Most likely diagnosis: *(All India 2001)*
    a. Acute intestinal obstruction
    b. Acute mesenteric ischemia
    c. Peritonitis
    d. Appendicitis

82. True about mesenteric vein thrombosis: *(PGI Dec 2003)*
    a. Peritoneal signs always present
    b. Thrombectomy is always done
    c. Heparin is given
    d. Surgery can lead to short bowel syndrome

83. Identify the following vessel in this arteriography: *(Recent Question 2018)*
    a. Superior mesenteric artery
    b. Inferior mesenteric artery
    c. Splenic artery
    d. Common hepatic artery

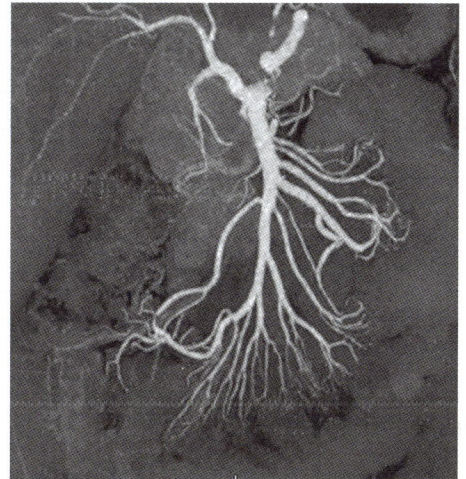

PARALYTIC ILEUS

84. Post-operative ileus is most pronounced in: *(AIIMS Nov 2011, AIIMS GIS Dec 2010)*
    a. Colon
    b. Stomach
    c. Ileum
    d. Duodenum

85. Paralytic ileus is seen in: *(PGI June 99)*
    a. Spinal cord injury
    b. Hypocalcemia
    c. Hypermagnesemia
    d. Uremia

86. Prolonged postoperative ileus is best treated by: *(PGI Dec 98)*
    a. Long tube insertion
    b. Calcium pentonthenate
    c. Laparotomy and exploration
    d. Peristaltic stimulants

87. First to recover from post-operative ileus: *(Recent Question 2016, DNB 2014, 2008)*
    a. Small intestine
    b. Stomach
    c. Colon
    d. None

88. Paralytic ileus is characterized by all except: *(SGPGI 2005)*
    a. No bowel sound on auscultation
    b. No passage of flatus
    c. Gas filled loops of intestine with multiple fluid levels
    d. Loops of intestine are not seen due to loss of peristalsis

89. Routine management of paralytic ileus includes all of the following except: *(MCI March 2005)*
    a. Electrolyte correction
    b. Nasogastric aspiration
    c. Parasympathomimetics
    d. IV fluids

90. First to recover from paralytic ileus: *(Recent Question 2017)*
    a. Stomach
    b. Small intestine
    c. Rectum
    d. Colon

91. True about postoperative ileus is: *(MHPGMCET 2003)*
    a. No intestinal sounds heard
    b. Intestinal peristalsis never becomes normal again
    c. Is due to hypernatremia
    d. Begins 2-3 days postoperatively

92. Most common electrolyte imbalance that causes paralytic ileus is: *(DNB 2014)*
    a. Hyponatremia
    b. Hypernatremia
    c. Hypokalemia
    d. Hyperkalemia

LARGE BOWEL OBSTRUCTION

93. A patient has presented with left sided colonic malignancy with obstruction in emergency. What is the treatment of choice? *(MHSSMCET 2005)*
    a. Hartman's Procedure
    b. Total colectomy
    c. Left hemi-colectomy
    d. Defunctioning colostomy

94. Treatment of obstructing, resectable right colonic cancer: *(AIIMS GIS Dec 2010)*
    a. Ileotransverse anastomosis after right hemicolectomy
    b. Diverting ileostomy
    c. Subtotal colectomy with ileorectal anastomosis
    d. Subtotal colectomy with exteriorization of the both ends

95. A patient of CA rectum presents with obstruction. Treatment: *(PGI SS June 2006)*
    a. Defunctioning colostomy
    b. Hartmann's procedure
    c. Anterior resection
    d. Abdomino-perineal resection

96. What are the features of colonic obstruction? *(PGI Dec 2000)*
    a. No passage of gas absolutely (Obstipation)
    b. No passage of stools absolutely
    c. Distention of abdomen
    d. Mild fever initially
    e. Fecal vomitus

97. Most common cause of colonic obstruction is:
    (Recent Question 2016)
    a. Volvulus   b. Hernia
    c. Adhesions   d. Neoplasm

98. In obstruction of the large gut rupture occurs at the:
    a. Cecum   b. Ascending colon
    c. Transverse colon   d. Descending colon

99. Commonest cause of colonic obstruction in neonates is:
    a. Meconium ileus   b. Aganglionic colon
    c. Ileal atresia   d. Volvulus

100. Acute mechanical large bowel obstruction should be operated early because: *(UPSC 95)*
    a. Electrolyte imbalance due to third space loss
    b. Septicemia from absorption of bowel contents
    c. Early gangrene and perforation
    d. Respiratory embarrassment to massive abdominal distension

101. Acute mechanical large bowel obstruction should be operated early because of the risk of: *(UPSC 97)*
    a. Respiratory embarrassment due to abdominal distension
    b. Electrolyte imbalance from vomiting
    c. Septicemia from bowel contents
    d. Closed-loop obstruction and cecal perforation

PSEUDO-OBSTRUCTION

102. Ogilvie's syndrome results from the denervation of the colon distal to the: *(COMEDK 2006)*
    a. Hepatic flexure   b. Mid-transverse colon
    c. Splenic flexure   d. Descending colon

103. True about Ogilvie's syndrome are all except:
    (Recent Question 2016, 2015; AIIMS Nov 2007)
    a. It is caused by mechanical obstruction of the colon
    b. It involves entire/part of the large colon
    c. It occurs after previous surgery
    d. It occurs commonly after narcotic use

104. Investigation of choice for pseudo-obstruction:
    a. Water soluble contrast enema *(AIIMS GIS Dec 2006)*
    b. Barium enema
    c. CECT   d. Colonoscopy

105. Colonic Pseudo-obstruction occurs in all, except:
    (AIIMS June 94)
    a. Diabetes mellitus   b. Dermatomyositis
    c. Scleroderma   d. Hyperthyroidism

106. Ogilvie's syndrome: *(Recent Question 2017)*
    a. Acute colonic pseudo-obstruction
    b. Chronic colonic pseudo-obstruction
    c. Fecal obstruction
    d. Intussusception

107. Most common cause of Ogilvie's syndrome:
    (Recent Question 2017)
    a. Head injury   b. Electrolyte abnormalities
    c. Carcinoma   d. Drugs

108. A 56-year-old woman has not passed stools for the last 14 days. X-ray shows no air fluid levels, Probable diagnosis is:
    a. Paralytic ileus *(Recent Question 2014; All India 2001)*
    b. Aganglionosis of the colon
    c. Intestinal pseudo-obstruction
    d. Duodenal obstruction

109. Acute pseudo-obstruction of the colon known as:
    (DNB 2012, UPPG 2007)
    a. Sjogren's syndrome b. Gardener's syndrome
    c. Ogilvie's syndrome d. Peutz-Jegher's syndrome

VOLVULUS

110. Sigmoid volvulus: *(PGI SS Dec 2009)*
    a. Clockwise
    b. CECT is diagnostic
    c. Rigid sigmoidoscopy is the initial treatment
    d. Sigmoidectomy is contraindicated

111. Most common site of volvulus: *(DNB 2012, GB Pant 2011)*
    a. Sigmoid colon   b. Caecum
    c. Transverse colon   d. Stomach

112. False about volvulus: *(AIIMS GIS May 2008)*
    a. Sigmoid volvulus is most common
    b. In absence of ischemia, mesocolopexy is done
    c. Ogilvie's syndrome refers to cecal volvulus
    d. Elective sigmoid resection after detorsion

113. False regarding cecal volvulus: *(ILBS 2011)*
    a. Present with small bowel obstruction
    b. Present with air fluid levels in right upper quadrant and convexity towards left
    c. Endoscopic derotation is not effective like sigmoid volvulus
    d. Cecopexy can be a form of treatment

114. This characteristic appearance is seen in:
    a. Gastric volvulus   b. Small intestinal volvulus
    c. Cecal volvulus   d. Sigmoid volvulus

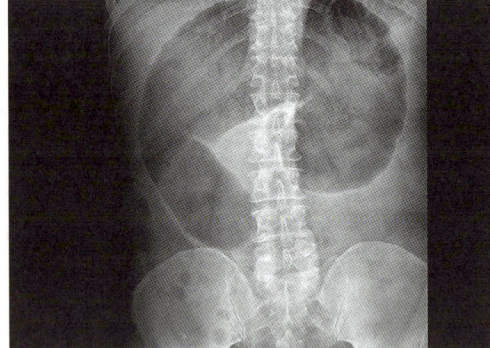

115. In cecal volvulus: *(AIIMS GIS Dec 2006)*
    a. Resolves with endoscopic treatment as frequently as sigmoid volvulus
    b. Right hemicolectomy is the treatment of choice
    c. Conservative management
    d. Colonoscopic decompression

116. Obstruction with multiple air fluid levels in a newborn, suggest diagnosis of: *(MHSSMCET 2010)*
    a. Duodenal atresia   b. Ileal atresia
    c. Ladd's band   d. Midgut volvulus

117. **'Bird of prey' sign is seen in the radiographic barium examination of:** *(COMEDK 2008)*
    a. Gastric volvulus
    b. Intussusception
    c. Sigmoid volvulus
    d. Cecal volvulus
118. **True about colonic volvulus:** *(PGI Nov 2010)*
    a. Most common in caecum
    b. Common in psychiatric patient
    c. Bird's beak sign
    d. May present as intestinal obstruction
119. **False about cecal volvulus:** *(AIIMS GIS 2003)*
    a. Mostly resolve with colonoscopic reduction
    b. More common than cecal basecule
    c. Right hemicolectomy is TOC
    d. Truly is cecocolic volvulus
120. **Which of the following statement about volvulus is false?**
    a. More common in psychiatric patients *(All India 2008)*
    b. Sigmoid volvulus is more common than caecal volvulus
    c. Lower GI scopy is contraindicated in sigmoid volvulus
    d. Volvulus of caecum is managed by conservative methods
121. **Coffee bean sign is usually seen in:** *(J and K 96)*
    a. Volvulus
    b. Pyloric obstruction
    c. Intussusception
    d. Intestinal obstruction
122. **This characteristic appearance is seen in:** *(Recent Question 2017)*
    a. Gastric volvulus
    b. Small intestinal volvulus
    c. Cecal volvulus
    d. Sigmoid volvulus

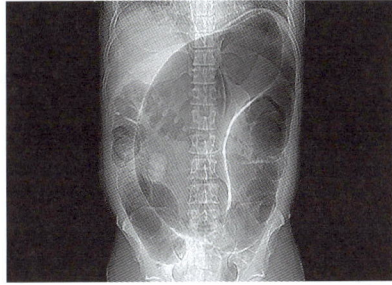

123. **Definitive treatment of sigmoid volvulus is:** *(PGI June 97)*
    a. Surgical correction
    b. Colectomy
    c. Enema
    d. Endoscopic correction
124. **Predisposing factors for sigmoid volvulus are:** *(Kerala 97)*
    a. Band of adhesion
    b. Long pelvic mesocolon
    c. Narrow attachment of pelvic mesocolon
    d. Loaded pelvic colon
    e. All of the above
125. **Rotation of sigmoid volvulus occurs:** *(AMU 2005)*
    a. Clockwise
    b. Anticlockwise
    c. Initially clockwise later anticlockwise
    d. Either clockwise or anticlockwise
126. **Sigmoid volvulus rotation occurs:** *(UPPG 2007, 2005)*
    a. Clockwise
    b. Anticlockwise
    c. Both clockwise and anti clockwise
    d. Axial in direction
127. **Which of the following statements abut sigmoid volvulus is incorrect?** *(DPG 2009 March)*
    a. More common with laxative abuse
    b. Non-operative treatment has no role
    c. Recurrence rate around 40%
    d. Sigmoid resection is definitive treatment
128. **All are predisposing factors for sigmoid volvulus except:** *(DNB 2007)*
    a. Hirschprung's diseases
    b. Chagas diseases
    c. Chronic constipation
    d. Tuberculosis
129. **Least common volvulus site in neonate is:** *(JIPMER 2013)*
    a. Ilioileal
    b. Large bowel volvulus
    c. Small bowel volvulus
    d. Gastric volvulus
130. **Midgut volvulus symptoms appear at:** *(Recent Question 2017)*
    a. 1st week
    b. 2nd week
    c. 3rd week
    d. 4th week

MALROTATION

131. **Child presents with recurrent abdominal pain and bilious vomiting. Condition was diagnosed by barium follow through. Surgery was done, mesenteric widening, appendectomy, cutting the Ladd's band. What is the diagnosis?**
    a. Recurrent cecal volvulus *(AIIMS Nov 2010)*
    b. Malrotation
    c. Recurrent appendicitis
    d. Stricture TB
132. **The cecum is found to be placed below the stomach and in the midline. Which of the following abnormality must have taken place while rotation of the gut?** *(AIIMS Nov 2010)*
    a. Non-rotation
    b. Malrotation
    c. Reversed rotation
    d. Mixed rotation
133. **Malrotation presents as:** *(PGI Dec 2002)*
    a. Mass abdomen
    b. Bleeding PR
    c. Bilious vomiting
    d. Hematemesis

MISCELLANEOUS

134. **Bowel can get strangulated in all of the following space except:** *(AIIMS Nov 2000)*
    a. Rectouterine pouch
    b. Ileocolic recess
    c. Paraduodenal recess
    d. Omental recess
135. **Spastic ileus is seen in:** *(PGI Dec 99)*
    a. Porphyria
    b. Retroperitoneal abscess
    c. Hypokalemia
    d. MI
136. **True about visceral pain:** *(PGI Nov 2011)*
    a. It is poorly localized
    b. Resembles "fast pain" produced by noxious stimulation of the skin
    c. Mediated by B fibers in the dorsal roots of the spinal nerves
    d. Causes relaxation of nearby skeletal muscles
    e. Shows relatively rapid adaptation
137. **A young healthy male patient presented with abdominal pain and history of altered bowel habits from the last 6 months. On CT examination, there was dilated distal part of ileum, thickened ileocecal junction with thickened cecum with presence of sacculations on the antimesenteric border. The vascularity of adjoining mesentery is also increased and there is surrounding mesentery fat. Which of the following is not a differential diagnosis?** *(AIIMS Nov 2013)*
    a. Ulcerative colitis
    b. Crohn's disease
    c. Tuberculosis
    d. Ischemic bowel disease

Explanations

ACUTE INTESTINAL OBSTRUCTION

1. **Ans. b. Usually venous blood flow affected first** *(Ref: Sabiston 20/e p1252; Schwartz 10/e p1147; Bailey 27/e p1281)*
   - Venous return is compromised before arterial supply in strangulated intestinal obstruction^Q.
2. **Ans. a. Small intestinal obstruction** *(Ref: Bailey 24/e p56)*

Hyponatremia
• The **most frequent cause** of **sodium depletion** in **surgical practice** is **obstruction** of the **small intestine**^{Q}, with its rapid loss of gastric, biliary, pancreatic and intestinal secretions by antiperistalsis and ejection, whether by vomiting or aspiration.
• **Duodenal, total biliary, pancreatic and high intestinal external fistulae** are all notorious for bringing about **early and profound hyponatremia**^{Q}.

3. **Ans. b. X-ray**
4. **Ans. a. Continuous pain** *(Ref: Sabiston 20/e p1252; Schwartz 10/e p1147; Bailey 27/e p1281)*
5. **Ans. b. Iatrogenic adhesions**
6. **Ans. a. Adhesions**
7. **Ans. b. Jejunal obstruction**
8. **Ans. c. Cecum** *(Ref: Bailey 27/e p1294)*

"After full resuscitation, the abdomen should be opened through a midline incision. Care should be taken to ensure that the loss of tamponade of the abdominal wall does not lead to increased caecal distension and rupture (this starts with splitting along the line of the taenia coli on the antimesenteric border). Distension of the caecum will confirm large bowel involvement. Identification of a collapsed distal segment of the large bowel and its sequential proximal assessment will readily lead to identification of the cause." –Bailey 27/e p1294

9. **Ans. c. Postoperative adhesions**
10. **Ans. a. Vomiting is common in duodenal obstruction, c. In colonic obstruction distension is common than vomiting, d. X-ray erect posture is diagnostic, e. Colicky pain to steady pain indicates strangulation** *(Ref: Sabiston 20/e p1249-1252; Schwartz 10/e p1147-1149; Bailey 27/e p1281)*
11. **Ans. a. Abdominal distension, b. Vomiting**
12. **Ans. d. Erect X-ray abdomen, e. Supine X-ray abdomen**
13. **Ans. a. X-ray abdomen erect posture**
14. **Ans. b. Duodenal obstruction** *(Ref: Sabiston 20/e p1249; Schwartz 10/e p1147; Bailey 27/e p1285-1286)*
    - Abdominal pain, bilious vomiting without abdominal distention is suggestive of proximal small intestinal obstruction, distal to ampulla of Vater (Duodenal obstruction).

    - Nausea and **vomiting** are **more common** with **proximal obstruction**^{Q}
    - **Abdominal distention** is **more common in distal obstruction**^{Q}

15. **Ans. c. Atresia of the 3rd part of the duodenum**
16. **Ans. d. Swallowed air** *(Ref: Sabiston 20/e p1250; Schwartz 10/e p1147; Bailey 26/e p1186)*

Consideration of Laparoscopic Management in Patients with	
Gas	**Fluid**
• **Swallowed air**^{Q} is the major source (**Nitrogen**^{Q} is not well Absorbed by intestinal mucosa)	• Enormous quantities of fluid from the extracellular Space are lost into gut (third space loss)
• Gases produced by **bacterial fermentation** (H_2, CO_2, CH_4)	• Net **GI secretion** is enhanced in obstruction

17. **Ans. b. Duodenal atresia** *(Ref: Bailey 27/e p133, 1293)*

    - MC site of intestinal atresia: Duodenum^Q
    - MC cause of neonatal intestinal obstruction: Duodenal atresia^Q

18. **Ans. a. Avoid surgery for initial 48–72 hours** *(Ref: Sabiston 20/e p1252; Schwartz 10/e p1149; Bailey 27/e p1293)*

    TREATMENT OF ADHESIVE OBSTRUCTION

    - **Initial management** is based on **intravenous rehydration and nasogastric decompression; occasionally, this treatment is curative**^{Q}.
    - Although an initial conservative regimen is considered appropriate, **regular assessment is mandatory to ensure that strangulation does not occur**^{Q}.

- **Conservative treatment should not be prolonged beyond 72 hours**^Q
- When, as is usual, laparotomy is required, although multiple adhesions may be found, **only one may be causative. This should be divided** and the **remaining adhesions left in situ**^Q unless severe angulation is present. Division of these adhesions will only cause further adhesion formation.
  - When obstruction is caused by an area of **multiple adhesions**, the adhesions should be **freed by sharp dissection**^Q
- **To prevent recurrence,** the bare area should be **covered with Omental grafts**^Q.
- **Laparoscopic adhesiolysis** may be considered in **highly selected cases** of **chronic subacute obstruction**^Q

19. Ans. a. First part of duodenum
20. Ans. b. Colicky pain *(Ref: Bailey 27/e p1285)*

Symptoms of Intestinal Obstruction

- Symptoms of intestinal obstruction: **Pain, vomiting, distention** and **constipation**
- **Pain** is the **first symptom encountered**^Q; it occurs **suddenly** and is usually **severe**.

Pain in Intestinal Obstruction
- It is **colicky in nature** and is usually **centred on the umbilicus (small bowel)** or **lower abdomen (large bowel)**^Q
- The pain coincides with **increased peristaltic activity**^Q
- With increasing distension, the colicky pain is replaced by a mild constant diffuse pain
- The development of **severe pain** is indicative of the **presence of strangulation**^Q
- **Pain may not be a significant feature** in **postoperative simple mechanical obstruction** and **does not** usually occur in paralytic ileus^Q

21. Ans. b. High peristalsis with colic
22. Ans. d. Multiple air gas shadows on X-ray
23. Ans. a. Postop adhesion
24. Ans. c. Bilious vomiting
25. Ans. a. Vomiting and distension
26. Ans. c. Enterotomy, removal of worms and primary closure *(Ref: Schwartz 10/e p1149; Farquharson's 8/e p470; Sabiston 20/e p1253)*

- Resection of small bowel is done when the affected bowel segment is of questionable viability.
- Diversion is the first step in case of colonic obstruction, followed by resection and anastomosis of affected segment and then closure of diversion colostomy at a later date.
- Intestinal luminal obstruction such as due to Bezoars or fecoliths of worm intestations are dealt with by enterotomy and removal followed by primary closure.

27. Ans. c. Enteroclysis
28. Ans. b. Intestinal obstruction *(Ref: Sabiston 20/e p1242)*

"Characteristic findings of small bowel obstruction on supine radiographs are dilated loops of small intestine, without evidence of colonic distention. Upright radiographs demonstrate multiple air-fluid levels, which often layer in a stepwise fashion."
—Sabiston 20/e p1242

INTUSSUSCEPTION

29. Ans. c. Intussusception *(Ref: Sabiston 20/e p1879; Schwartz 10/e p1622; Bailey 27/e p1287; Shackelford 8/e p986, 7/e p1059-1061)*
30. Ans. a. Idiopathic and more enteric rather than colonic *(Ref: Bailey 27/e p1287)*

Intussusception in Adults
- Bailey says **"Adult** cases of **intussusceptions** are **invariably associated with** a **lead point,** which is usually a **polyp** (e.g. Peutz-Jegher's syndrome), a **submucosal lipoma** or other **tumor**^Q."
- "In adults, **colocolic**^Q intussusception is **common** but in **children, ileocolic** is the **commonest** variety (77%)."

31. Ans. b. Intussusception
32. Ans. a. Most common variety is ileocolic, b. Associated with pathological lead point, c. May be seen after viral infection, d. Can be relieved by barium enema
33. Ans. a. Air enema, b. Saline enema, c. Ba enema, d. Hydrostatic reduction
34. Ans. c. Intussusception *(Ref: Sabiston 20/e p1879; Schwartz 10/e p1622; Bailey 27/e p1289; Shackelford 8/e p986, 7/e p1060-1061)*

Radiological Investigations in Intussusception

Plain X-ray Film	Barium Enema	Ultrasound
• Features of **small intestinal obstruction**[Q] • **Abdominal soft tissue density** in some cases which may show: – **Target sign**[Q]: Soft tissue mass with concentric area of lucency due to mesenteric fat. – **Meniscus sign**[Q]: Crescent of gas within colonic lumen that outlines the apex of intussusception.	• **Claw sign**[Q]: Rounded apex of intussusception protrudes into the contrast column • **Coiled spring sign**[Q]: Edematous mucosal folds of returning limb of intussusception outlined by contrast material.	• **Target sign** or **Bull's eye sign** on **transverse scan**[Q] • **Pseudokidney sign** on **longitudinal scan**[Q]

35. Ans. b. Terminal ileum
36. Ans. a. Ileocolic
37. Ans. a. Barium must be used in children after 48 hours *(Ref: Sabiston 20/e p1879; Schwartz 10/e p1622; Bailey 27/e p1293; Shackelford 8/e p986, 7/e p1060-1061)*
38. Ans. c. Lymphoma *(Ref: Sabiston 20/e p1879; Schwartz 10/e p1622; Bailey 27/e p1284; Shackelford 8/e p986, 7/e p771)*
39. Ans. c. The outer layer
40. Ans. c. Coiled spring sign
41. Ans. a. Payers patch hypertrophy
42. Ans. b. Target sign, d. Coiled spring sign, e. Dance sign
43. Ans. d. Intussusception
44. Ans. a. Intussusception
45. Ans. c. Hypertrophy of submucous Peyer's patches
46. Ans. a. Submucosal lipoma
47. Ans. d. Usually relieved by barium enema
48. Ans. a. Multiple *(Ref: Bailey 27/e p1284)*

Types of Intussusception (in decreasing order)

1. **Ileocolic (77%)**[Q]	4. Colocolic (2%): **MC in adults**
2. Ileo-ileo-colic (12%)	5. Multiple (1%)
3. Ilioileal (5%)	6. Retrograde (0.2%)

49. Ans. a. Intussusception
50. Ans. a. Intussusception
51. Ans. d. Target sign *(Ref: Sabiston 20/e p1879; Schwartz 10/e p1622; Bailey 27/e p1284)*

• The given sign is target sign, seen in intussusception.

52. Ans. a. Free passage of barium in the terminal ileum

• In intussusception, **successful reduction** is **confirmed** by **reflux of air (or barium)**[Q] into the small bowel

53. Ans. b. Intussusception
54. Ans. a. Empty right iliac fossa in intussusceptions
55. Ans. a. Most common type is ileocecocolic *(Ref: Sabiston 20/e p1879; Schwartz 10/e p1622; Bailey 27/e p1283)*
56. Ans. c. Intussusception
57. Ans. b. Intussusception

MECONIUM SYNDROME

58. Ans. b. Contrast enema *(Ref: Sabiston 20/e p1876; Schwartz 10/e p1617-1619; Shackelford 8/e p979, 7/e p1053-1054)*

• Failure to pass meconium **in the first 2 days** of life (48 hours) is typically **suggestive of a lower GI tract obstruction** such as Hirschprung's disease, meconium plug syndrome or anorectal malformation. A **contrast enema** is the **most suitable primary investigation to make the diagnosis**, amongst the options provided.

59. Ans. a. Meconium ileus *(Ref: Sabiston 20/e p1875; Schwartz 10/e p1617-1619; Bailey 27/e p1294, 134; Shackelford 8/e p978, 7/e p1053-1054)*
60. Ans. c. Meconium peritonitis *(Ref: Sabiston 20/e p1876; Schwartz 10/e p1617-1619; Bailey 27/e p134; Shackelford 8/e p979, 7/e p1054)*
61. Ans. b. Meconium peritonitis
62. Ans. a. It is a septic peritonitis

• Meconium peritonitis is an aseptic chemical peritonitis caused by spillage of meconium

63. Ans. a. Fibrocystic disease of pancreas *(Ref: Sabiston 20/e p1875; Schwartz 10/e p1617; Shackelford 8/e p978, 7/e p1053-1054)*

• Meconium ileus in the newborn represents the earliest clinical manifestation of CF and affects roughly 15% of patients with this inherited disease

Cystic Fibrosis

Diagnosis

• The **diagnosis of CF is usually confirmed in** the **postoperative period**[Q].

  • The **pilocarpine iontophoresis sweat test** revealing a **chloride concentration >60 mEq/L** is the **most reliable** and **definitive method to confirm the diagnosis of CF**[Q]. This test may not be reliable in infants and is usually performed later

• A **more immediate test** includes **detection of the mutated CFTR gene**[Q]. This test, coupled **with a careful family history** and **clinical presentation, permits confirmation** of the **diagnosis in most infants**[Q].

64. **Ans. a. 1-Paul Mikulicz, 2-Bishop-Koop, 3-Santulli** *(Ref: Sabiston 20/e p; Schwartz 10/e p1619; Bailey 27/e p1294)*

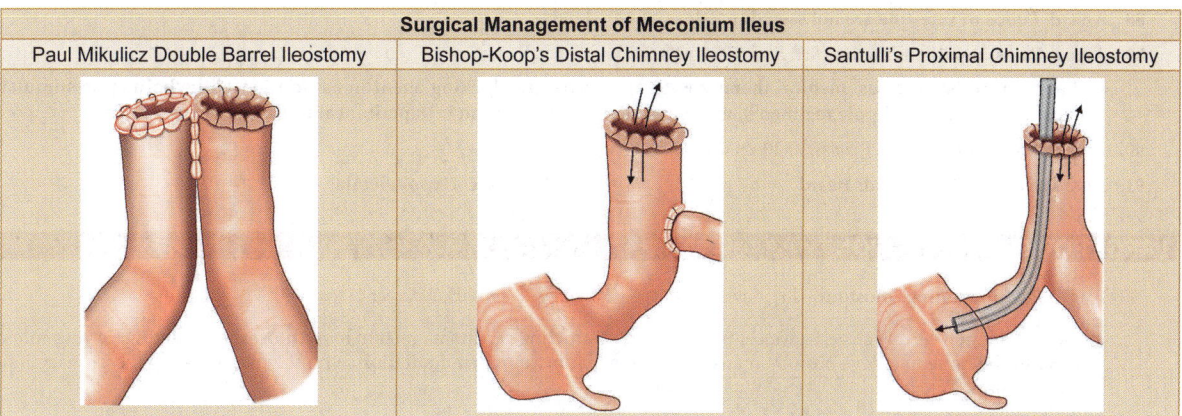

Surgical Management of Meconium Ileus		
Paul Mikulicz Double Barrel Ileostomy	Bishop-Koop's Distal Chimney Ileostomy	Santulli's Proximal Chimney Ileostomy

65. **Ans. a. Meconium ileus**
66. **Ans. c. Lower GI contrast study**
67. **Ans. a. Before and after birth**
    - Meconium peritonitis may occur in utero or the early neonatal period.

MESENTERIC ISCHEMIA

68. **Ans. c. Duodenum distal to the opening of CBD** *(Ref: Bailey 27/e p1253)*

> **SUPERIOR MESENTERIC ARTERY**
> - SMA supplies the **midgut**, from **distal part of duodenum** to **proximal 2/3rd of transverse colon**^{Q}.

69. **Ans. c. Embolism** *(Ref: Sabiston 20/e p1155; Schwartz 10/e p859-866; Bailey 27/e p1253; Shackelford 8/e p1028, 7/e p1075-1077)*
70. **Ans. d. Mesenteric vascular occlusion**
71. **Ans. d. Abdominal angina** *(Ref: Sabiston 20/e p1155; Schwartz 10/e p859-866; Bailey 27/e p1253; Shackelford 8/e p1033, 7/e p1084-1092)*
72. **Ans. a. Resection anastomosis**   73. **Ans. a. SMA thrombosis**   74. **Ans. c. IMA** *(Ref: Grays 40/e p1141)*

> - Grays Anatomy: **Occlusion of IMA does not always result in irreversible ischemia** of the **descending** and **sigmoid colon**, because the **marginal artery of colon** usually **receives an adequate supply** from the **left branch of the middle colic artery**^{Q}

75. **Ans. d. Hypercoagulable state** *(Ref: Sabiston 20/e p1155; Schwartz 10/e p859-866; Bailey 27/e p1253; Shackelford 8/e p1031, 7/e p1081-1082)*
76. **b. Non-occlusive mesenteric ischemia**   77. **Ans. c. Non-obstructive mesenteric ischemia has very good prognosis**
78. **Ans c. Embolus gets lodged most commonly at branching of SMA from aorta** *(Ref: Sabiston 20/e p1155; Schwartz 10/e p859-866; Bailey 27/e p1253; Shackelford 8/e p1028, 7/e p1077-1078)*
    - More than 50% of emboli lodge in the mid to distal segment of the SMA.
79. **Ans. d. Acute mesenteric venous thrombosis** *(Ref: Sabiston 20/e p1155; Schwartz 10/e p918-927; Bailey 27/e p1253; Shackelford 8/e p1031, 7/e p1082-1084)*
80. **Ans. b. Acute mesenteric ischemia** *(Ref: Sabiston 20/e p1155; Schwartz 10/e p859-866; Bailey 27/e p1253; Shackelford 8/e p1028, 7/e p1077-1082)*
81. **Ans. b. Acute mesenteric ischemia**   82. **Ans. c. Heparin is given, d. Surgery can lead to short bowel syndrome**
83. **Ans. a. Superior mesenteric artery** *(Ref: Sabiston 20/e p1239; Schwartz 10/e p863)*

> - Coronal maximum intensity projection of the superior mesenteric artery and its branches. This image was created on a workstation with CT data from a state-of-the-art 16-slice multidetector CT scanner. Note the fine detail that is visible of the end-organ arteries of the jejunum and ileum.

PARALYTIC ILEUS

84. **Ans. a. Colon** *(Ref: Sabiston 20/e p306; Schwartz 10/e p1151-1152; Bailey 27/e p1297)*
85. **Ans. a. Spinal cord injury, c. Hypermagnesemia, d. Uremia** *(Ref: Sabiston 20/e p306; Schwartz 10/e p1151-1152; Bailey 27/e p1297)*
86. **Ans. c. Laparotomy and exploration** *(Ref: Bailey 27/e p1297)*
    - If paralytic ileus is prolonged and threatens life, a laparotomy should be considered to exclude a hidden cause and facilitate bowel decompression.

87. Ans. a. Small intestine
88. Ans. d. Loops of intestine are not seen due to loss of peristalsis
89. Ans. c. Parasympathomimetics *(Ref: Bailey 25/e p1202)*
    - Rarely, in resistant cases, medical therapy with an adrenergic blocking agent in association with cholinergic stimulation, e.g. neostigmine (the Catchpole regimen^Q), may be used, provided that an intraperitoneal cause has been excluded.
90. Ans. b. Small intestine *(Ref: Sabiston 20/e p306; Bailey 27/e p1296)*
91. Ans. a. No intestinal sounds heard   92. Ans. c. Hypokalemia

LARGE BOWEL OBSTRUCTION

93. Ans. d. Defunctioning colostomy *(Ref: Sabiston 20/e p1337; Bailey 27/e p1265, Naingot 11/e p501)*
    - Most common site of colorectal cancer is rectum, in obstructing carcinoma rectum **loop colostomy or defunctioning colostomy should be done** to relieve obstruction followed by **neoadjuvant chemoradiation**, with the plan to resect the primary lesion at a later time.
94. Ans. a. Ileotransverse anastomosis after right hemicolectomy   95. Ans. a. Defunctioning colostomy
96. Ans. a. No passage of gas absolutely (Obstipation), b. No passage of stools absolutely, c. Distention of abdomen
97. Ans. d. Neoplasm   98. Ans. a. Cecum   99. Ans. b. Aganglionic colon
100. Ans. c. Early gangrene and perforation   101. Ans. d. Closed-loop obstruction and cecal perforation

    - Virtually **all patients with complete acute large bowel obstruction** require **prompt surgical intervention** and should not undergo a trial of non-operative management
    - **Acute large bowel obstruction** in patients **with competent ileocecal valve** is **a true surgical emergency** because of **high chances of perforation (MC site: Cecum)**^Q
    - Once diagnosis has been made, **surgical exploration** should be undertaken **as soon as possible after appropriate resuscitation**^Q

PSEUDO-OBSTRUCTION

102. Ans. c. Splenic flexure *(Ref: Sabiston 20/e p1336; Bailey 27/e p1297)*
    - **Ogilvie's syndrome: Distended colon,** with the **right** and **transverse segments** tending to **be most dramatically affected. Transition point** is frequently present, usually **at or near** the **splenic flexure.**
103. Ans. a. It is caused by mechanical obstruction of the colon   104. Ans. a. Water soluble contrast enema
105. Ans. d. Hyperthyroidism
106. Ans. a. Acute colonic pseudo-obstruction *(Ref: Sabiston 20/e p1337; Schwartz 10/e p1221; Bailey 27/e p1297)*

    "*Colonic pseudo-obstruction: This may occur in an acute or a chronic form. The former, also known as Ogilvie's syndrome, presents as acute large bowel obstruction."-Bailey 27/e p1297*

107. Ans. b. Electrolyte abnormalities *(Ref: Sleisenger 10/e p1877; Sabiston 20/e p1337; Schwartz 10/e p1221; Bailey 27/e p1297)*
108. Ans. c. Intestinal pseudo-obstruction   109. Ans. c. Ogilvie's syndrome

VOLVULUS

110. Ans. c. Rigid sigmoidoscopy is the initial treatment *(Ref: Sabiston 20/e p1335; Schwartz 10/e p1219-1220; Bailey 27/e p1295; Shackelford 8/e p1809, 7/e p1850-1853)*
111. Ans. a. Sigmoid colon
112. Ans. c. Ogilvie's syndrome refers to cecal volvulus *(Ref: Sabiston 20/e p1335; Schwartz 10/e p1219; Bailey 27/e p1297; Shackelford 8/e p1684, 7/e p1853-1854)*
113. Ans. d. Cecopexy can be a form of treatment
114. Ans. c. Cecal volvulus *(Ref: Sabiston 20/e p1335; Schwartz 10/e p1220; Bailey 27/e p1289)*
    - **Cecal volvulus: Distended cecum** assumes a **gas filled comma shape or kidney bean shape**^Q, the concavity of which faces **inferiorly and to the right.**
115. Ans. b. Right hemicolectomy is the treatment of choice
116. Ans. d. Midgut volvulus

Intestinal Obstruction

117. Ans. c. Sigmoid volvulus
118. Ans. b. Common in psychiatric patients, c. Bird's beak sign, d. May present as intestinal obstruction
119. Ans. a. Mostly resolve with colonoscopic reduction
120. Ans. c. Lower GI scopy is contraindicated in sigmoid d. Volvulus of cecum is managed by conservative methods
121. Ans. a. Volvulus
122. Ans. d. Sigmoid volvulus *(Ref: Sabiston 20/e p1335; Schwartz 10/e p1219; Bailey 27/e p1284)*
    - **Sigmoid volvulus: Markedly dilated sigmoid colon** with the **appearance of a bent inner tube** or **coffee bean appearance**^{Q}.
123. Ans. b. Colectomy
124. Ans. d. Loaded pelvic colon
125. Ans. d. Either clockwise or anticlockwise
126. Ans. c. Both clockwise and anti-clockwise

- **Sigmoid volvulus** is **more commonly anticlockwise** (can be **both clockwise** or **anticlockwise**)^Q
- **Cecal volvulus** and **small intestine volvulus** are mostly **clockwise**^{Q}

127. Ans. b. Non-operative treatment has no role
128. Ans. d. Tuberculosis *(Ref: Schwartz 10/e p1221, 9/e p1055)*
    - Hirschsprung's disease and Chagas disease can lead to megacolon, a risk factor for sigmoid volvulus.
129. Ans. b. Large bowel volvulus
    - Small bowel volvulus is most common form of volvulus in neonates. Colonic volvulus is very rare.
130. Ans. a. 1st week *(Ref: Bailey 25/e p85)*

"Midgut volvulus can occur at any age, although it is seen most often in the first few weeks of life."

MALROTATION

131. Ans. b. Malrotation *(Ref: Sabiston 20/e p1871; Schwartz 10/e p1616-1617; Shackelford 8/e p970, 7/e p1046-1048; Bailey 27/e p134-135)*
132. Ans. d. Mixed rotation *(Ref: Sabiston 20/e p1871; Schwartz 10/e p1616)*

    Mixed rotation of gut:
    - The intestine doesn't rotate as it re-enters the abdomen after physiological hernia.
    - **Caecum lies just inferior to the pylorus of the stomach.** It may result in volvulus (twisting) of intestine, which leads to obstruction further

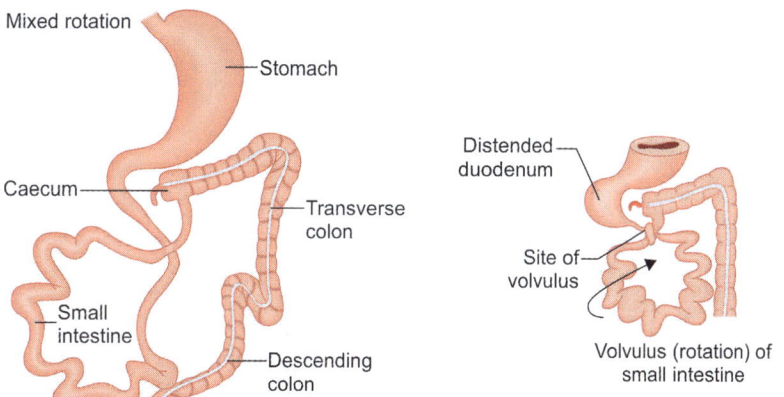

133. Ans. b. Bleeding PR, c. Bilious vomiting

MISCELLANEOUS

134. Ans. a. Rectouterine pouch
135. Ans. a. Porphyria *(Ref: Harrison 19/e p1982)*

SPASTIC ILEUS

- Spastic ileus or dynamic ileus is rare, results from extreme and prolonged contraction of the intestine.

Spastic ileus is seen in	
• Heavy metal poisoning^Q	• Porphyria^Q
• Uremia^Q	• Extensive intestinal ulceration^Q

136. **Ans. a. It is poorly localized** *(Ref: Guyton 13/e p627; Ganong 25/e p167)*

CHARACTERISTIC FEATURES VISCERAL PAIN

- **Visceral pain** is **poorly localized,** often the pain is **referred or radiating**[Q]
  - **Highly localized** types of **damage** to the viscera **seldom cause severe pain**
  - Often accompanied by **vomiting** and **hypotension**[Q]
- **Pain of hollow viscus** is often **felt as a colic**[Q] (it comes and goes to reappear again).
- There are **no proprioceptors in viscera** and few temperature and touch sense organs. Pain receptors are present, although they are more sparsely distributed than in somatic structures.
  - **Afferent fibers** from visceral structures **reach the CNS via sympathetic** and **parasympathetic pathways.**
  - Their **cell bodies** are located **in the dorsal roots** and the **homologous cranial nerve ganglia.**
  - Specifically, there are **visceral afferents in the facial, glossopharyngeal**, and **vagus nerves**; in the thoracic and upper lumbar dorsal roots; and in the sacral roots.
- Essentially **all visceral pain** that originates **in the thoracic** and **abdominal cavities** is transmitted through **small type C pain fibers** and, therefore, can transmit only the chronic-aching-suffering type of pain.

137. **Ans. d. Ischemic bowel disease** *(Ref: Sabiston 20/e p1155; Schwartz 10/e p1167; Bailey 27/e p1253; Schackelford 8/e p1023, 7/e p1077-1082)*

- **In ischemic bowel disease or mesenteric ischemia, vascularity of adjoining mesentery is decreased.**
- History of **abdominal pain** and **altered bowel habits** with **thickened cecum and ileocecal junction** and **increased vascularity of surrounding mesentery** can be observed in Ulcerative colitis, Crohn's disease and tuberculosis.

Mesenteric Ischemia

- Findings on **CT scans associated with bowel ischemia** include **dilation of the bowel lumen, bowel wall thickening, abnormal bowel wall enhancement, arterial occlusion, venous thrombosis, and intramural or portal venous gas**[Q].
- **Dilation of an ischemic bowel segment** suggests **interruption of normal peristaltic activity**[Q].
- **Symmetrical bowel wall thickening greater than 3 mm** in a **distended segment**[Q] of bowel suggests ischemia.
- Greater degrees of bowel wall thickening should raise suspicion of mesenteric venous thrombosis (MVT).
- **Intravenous contrast** is useful in demonstrating the heterogeneity of the ischemic bowel wall **(lack of bowel wall enhancement)** and may show **occlusion of mesenteric arteries if given by rapid bolus administration**[Q].

CHAPTER 13

Small Intestine

MECKEL'S DIVERTICULUM

MECKEL'S DIVERTICULUM

- Most commonly encountered congenital anomaly of the small intestine[Q]
- Occur 2% of the population[Q].

Rule of two in Meckel's diverticulum	
• 2% prevalence[Q]	• Half of these who are symptomatic are <2 years[Q] of age
• 2 inch in length[Q]	• 2 feet proximal to ileocecal valve[Q]

- True[Q] diverticulum as it has all the 3 layers of the intestine[Q].
- Located on the antimesenteric border of the ileum 45 to 60 cm proximal to the ileocecal valve
- Results from incomplete closure of omphalomesenteric or vitellointestinal duct.
- An equal incidence among men & women[Q].

  - MC heterotopic tissue: Gastric mucosa (50%)[Q] >Pancreatic mucosa (5%) >colonic mucosa (rarely)

Clinical Features
- Most are entirely benign & incidentally discovered during autopsy, laparotomy, or barium studies

  - MC clinical presentation is GI bleeding (25-50%)[Q]
  - Hemorrhage: MC symptomatic presentation in children ≤2 years[Q]

- Hemorrhage is manifested as painless bright red blood from the rectum, with intermittent episodes[Q] persisting without treatment.
- Source of the bleeding is a chronic acid-induced ulcer in the ileum adjacent to a Meckel's diverticulum that contains gastric mucosa.
- Intestinal obstruction (31%): Due to volvulus, intussusception, or, rarely, incarceration of the diverticulum in an inguinal hernia (Littre's hernia)[Q].

Complications of Meckel's Diverticulum

• MC complication in children & young adults: Bleeding[Q]	• MC complication in adults: Intestinal obstruction[Q]

- Diverticulitis (10-20%) is more common in adult patients.
- Progression of the diverticulitis may lead to perforation and peritonitis.

  - When the appendix is found to be normal during exploration for suspected appendicitis, the distal ileum should be inspected for the presence of an inflamed Meckel's diverticulum[Q].

Diagnosis
- Most accurate diagnostic test in children: Scintigraphy with sodium 99mTc-pertechnetate[Q].

  - 99mTc-pertechnetate is preferentially taken up by the mucus-secreting cells of gastric mucosa & ectopic gastric tissue in the diverticulum[Q]. (Sensitivity-85%, specificity-95% and an accuracy-90% in the pediatric age group)
  - Less accurate in adults because of the reduced prevalence of ectopic gastric mucosa[Q]
  - Sensitivity & specificity can be improved by pentagastrin and glucagon or H2-receptor antagonists (cimetidine)[Q].

- In adults with normal nuclear medicine findings, barium studies should be performed.

Treatment
- Symptomatic Meckel's diverticulum: Diverticulectomy or resection of the segment of ileum[Q] bearing the diverticulum.
- Segmental intestinal resection is required for bleeding because the bleeding site usually is in the ileum adjacent to the diverticulum[Q].
- Asymptomatic diverticula found in children during laparotomy should be resected[Q].

  - Incidentally found Meckel's diverticulum should be removed at any age up to 80 years as long as no additional conditions (e.g., peritonitis) made removal hazardous[Q].

INTESTINAL ATRESIA

Intestinal Atresia

- **MC site** of **intestinal atresia: Duodenum**[Q]
- **MC cause** of **neonatal intestinal obstruction: Duodenal atresia**[Q]

Jejunoileal Atresia

- **Atresia & stenosis** are among the **MC causes** of **neonatal intestinal obstruction**[Q].
- Incidence of jejunoileal atresia is **1 in 300 to 1500**[Q] live births.
- **Gender ratio** is **equal**.
- **Jejunal atresia** is slightly **more common** than ileal atresia.
- In 80-90% of cases the atresia is **isolated**. However, in up to **20%** of cases **atresias are multiple**.

> - **Cystic fibrosis** is an important comorbid condition with **reported incidence** is **10-20%**. **White infants** with **jejunoileal atresia** have **more than 210 times** the **risk for cystic fibrosis**[Q].

Clinical Features

- Infants with atresia or stenosis usually have **bilious vomiting** on the **first day of life**.
- The **higher the obstruction**, the **earlier the vomiting**.
- **Abdominal distention** is more pronounced with **distal obstruction**.
- More than 60% of these **infants fail** to **pass meconium** in the **first day** of life, may have **grayish mucoid contents** in the rectal vault[Q].

Diagnosis

- Can be diagnosed by **prenatal ultrasonography**[Q].
- Associated with **maternal polyhydramnios**[Q].
- **Abdominal radiographs** show **gas-** and **fluid-filled bowel loops** with **absence of gas distally**[Q].

Treatment

- Management includes **intravenous fluid**, **decompression** of the stomach, withholding of enteral feeding, and **antibiotics**.
- **After resuscitation** the infant is taken to the operating room for **exploratory laparotomy**.
- The goals of the operation are to **restore intestinal continuity after resection** of the **atretic segment** while preserving intestinal length.

Prognosis

- The prognosis in these patients is **excellent**, with **survival rates of 90%**[Q].
- Risk of **adhesive bowel obstruction** & **necrotizing enterocolitis (NEC)**[Q]

SMALL INTESTINAL DUPLICATION

Small Intestinal Duplication

- Intestinal duplications are **mucosa-lined structures** that are **in continuity** with the GI tract.
- **MC site** of **duplication: Ileum** (within the **leaves of mesentery**)[Q]
- Located **along mesenteric border**, contain **all** the **three layers** of **bowel**[Q]
- **Share a common wall** & **blood supply** with **adjacent bowel**[Q]

Types of Small Intestinal Duplication	
Cystic	Tubular
- **More common (75%)**[Q] - **Do not have communication** with **the lumen**[Q] of normal small intestine - Manifested as **partial small bowel obstruction**[Q]	- Less common (25%) - Parallel to the **normal bowel lumen**[Q] - **Higher incidence of communication**[Q] with the existing lumen of small intestine - Significant incidence of **ectopic gastric mucosa**[Q]. - **Bleeding**[Q] is a common manifestation

Clinical Features

- **Recurrent abdominal pain**, emesis from **intestinal obstruction**, & **hematochezia**[Q].
- **Bleeding** from **ulceration in the duplication** or in the **adjacent intestine** if the duplication contains **ectopic gastric mucosa**[Q].

Diagnosis
- CT, ultrasonography, and **technetium pertechnetate** scanning can be very helpful.
- **USG:** Classical **triple layer effect**[Q]

Treatment
- **Short duplications:** Resection of the cyst and adjacent intestine with **end-to-end anastomosis**[Q]
- **Long duplications:**
  - Multiple enterotomies and **mucosal stripping**[Q] in the duplicated segment, which will allow the walls to collapse and become adherent.
  - Divide the common wall using a **linear cutting stapler**[Q] to form a common lumen.
- **Excellent prognosis** in duplications who undergo **complete excision**[Q] without compromise of the length of remaining intestine

SMALL INTESTINAL DIVERTICULA

DUODENAL DIVERTICULA
- **Relatively common**, representing the **second MC site** for diverticulum formation **after the colon**.
- More common in **women** (rare in patients <40 years)
- **Two thirds to three fourths** are found in **periampullary region**[Q] (within a **2 cm of ampulla**) and project from medial wall of duodenum.

Clinical Features
- **Mostly asymptomatic**, usually **noted incidentally** by an upper GI studies for an unrelated problem
- **Less than 5%** of duodenal diverticula will **require surgery** because of a **complication** of the diverticulum itself.
- Major complications are **obstruction** of **biliary** or **pancreatic ducts** that may contribute to **cholangitis & pancreatitis**, respectively; **hemorrhage; perforation**; and rarely, blind loop syndrome.

> - Only those **diverticula associated with ampulla of Vater** are significantly related to **complications of cholangitis & pancreatitis**[Q].

- In these patients, the **ampulla** most often **enters** the duodenum **at superior margin of diverticulum** rather than through the diverticulum itself.

Diagnosis
- Diagnosis by **endoscopy** or by **plain abdominal films** showing an **atypical gas bubble**[Q]

Treatment
- **Asymptomatic**, found incidentally: **No treatment**
- **MC** and **most effective treatment** for **symptoms** or **complications**: **Diverticulectomy**[Q]

SMALL INTESTINAL (JEJUNO-ILEAL) DIVERTICULA
- **Less common** than duodenal diverticula, occur **more commonly along** the **mesentery**
- **False diverticula**, occurring mainly in an **older age group** (after sixth decade).
- With an increased frequency in the **proximal jejunum** and **distal ileum**
- **Jejunal diverticula** are **more common** and are **larger** than those in the ileum.

> - **Jejunal diverticula** are **multiple**, usually protrudes from mesenteric border of the bowel and may be **overlooked at surgery** because they are **embedded within** the **small bowel mesentery**[Q]

Clinical Features
- **Mostly asymptomatic**, discovered incidentally
- **Vague chronic abdominal pain, malabsorption**, functional pseudo-obstruction, & chronic low-grade GI hemorrhage.
- **Acute complications** are **diverticulitis**, with or without abscess or perforation; **GI hemorrhage**; & **intestinal obstruction.**
- Stasis of intestinal flow with **bacterial overgrowth** resulting in **steatorrhea** & **megaloblastic anemia**, with or without neuropathy.
- **Perforation** is the MC complication of jejunoileal diverticular disease and is a sequel of **diverticulitis**[Q]

Treatment
- **No treatment** for incidentally noted, **asymptomatic jejunoileal diverticula**[Q]
- In case of **obstruction, bleeding, & perforation**: Intestinal resection & end-to-end anastomosis.
- In **malabsorption** secondary **bacterial overgrowth**: **Antibiotics**[Q]

PNEUMATOSIS INTESTINALIS

PNEUMATOSIS INTESTINALIS

- An uncommon condition presenting as **multiple gas-filled cysts** of gastrointestinal tract.
- Located in the **subserosa**, **submucosa**, and, rarely, muscularis layer

> - **MC site: Jejunum**^{Q} > ileocecal region > colon (Can occur anywhere)

- **Equal incidence** among **males** and **females**^{Q}
- Most commonly occurs in the **4th-7th decades**^{Q} of life.
- Pneumatosis **in neonates** is usually associated with **necrotizing enterocolitis**^{Q}.

Pathology
- On histologic section, **honeycomb appearance**^{Q}.
- Cysts are **thin walled** & break easily.
- **Spontaneous rupture** gives rise to **pneumoperitoneum**.

Predisposing Factors
- **COPD**^{Q}
- **Immunocompromised state**^{Q}.
- **Diabetes**^{Q}
- **Inflammatory, obstructive**, or **infectious conditions** of the intestine^Q.
- **Endoscopy** and **jejunostomy** placement; **ischemia**^{Q}

Clinical Features
- Symptoms are **nonspecific**, most commonly **diarrhea, abdominal pain, abdominal distention**, nausea, vomiting, weight loss, and **mucus in stools**^{Q}.
- **Pneumoperitoneum** occurs usually in association with **small bowel** rather than large bowel **pneumatosis**^{Q}.

> - **Pneumatosis intestinalis** represents one of the few cases of **sterile pneumoperitoneum** and should be considered in the patient with **free abdominal air** but **no evidence of peritonitis**^{Q}.

Diagnosis
- On **plain films**, **radiolucent areas** within the **bowel wall** (appear as **grapelike clusters** or **tiny bubbles**)^Q
- Alternatively, **barium contrast** or **CT studies** can be used to **confirm the diagnosis**^{Q}.

Treatment
- Management of the **uncomplicated primary disease** is **conservative**.

> - When **symptoms demand treatment**, the **first line** is **intermittent high flow oxygen therapy**^{Q}, providing a concentration of 70% continuously for 5 days by nasal specula.
> - Cysts may resolve with antibiotics, particularly **metronidazole**^{Q}.
> - In **resistant cases**, maintenance treatment with **sulfasalazine**^{Q} may be helpful.

RADIATION ENTERITIS

RADIATION ENTERITIS

- Radiation therapy affect rapidly dividing cells in small intestine
- Rapidly dividing cells in small intestinal epithelium **may sustain severe, acute**, and **chronic deleterious effects**.

> - **Serious late complications** are **unusual** if the **total radiation dosage** is <4000 cGy^Q
> - **Morbidity risk increases** with dosages >5000 cGy^Q.

Pathology
- **Radiation damage** tends to be **acute** and **self-limiting**^{Q}.
- Late effects of radiation injury:
  - Damage to small submucosal blood vessels^Q
  - Progressive obliterative arteritis & submucosal fibrosis^Q
  - Thrombosis & vascular insufficiency^Q

Predisposing Factors
- Previous **abdominal operations**^{Q}
- Preexisting **vascular disease, hypertension, diabetes**^{Q}
- Adjuvant treatment: **5-FU, doxorubicin, dactinomycin** and **methotrexate**^{Q}

Clinical Features
- **Radiation damage** tends to be **acute** & **self-limiting**, with symptoms consisting mainly of **diarrhea, abdominal pain**, & **malabsorption**^{Q}.

- **Late effects** of radiation injury resulting eventually in **thrombosis** & **vascular insufficiency** leading to **necrosis** & **perforation** of the involved intestine, but **more commonly stricture formation** with symptoms of **obstruction** or **small bowel fistulas**[Q].

Prevention
- By **adjusting ports** & **dosages of radiation** to deliver optimal treatment specifically to the tumor and not to surrounding tissues.
- **Exclude the small bowel** from the irradiated field by **reperitonealization, omental transposition**, & placement of **absorbable mesh slings**.
- **Sucralfate** is used to **prevent diarrhea** associated with abdominal radiation.
- **Superoxide dismutase** reduces complications.

- Most effective radioprotectant: **Amifostine**[Q] (WR-2721)

Treatment
- **Acute radiation enteritis:** Control symptoms with **antispasmodics, analgesics antidiarrheal agents**[Q].

- **Operative intervention:** Obstruction (MC), **fistula** formation, **perforation** & **bleeding**[Q]
- **Operative procedures:** Bypass or resection with reanastomosis.

GASTROINTESTINAL TUBERCULOSIS

GASTROINTESTINAL TUBERCULOSIS

- **Mycobacterium tuberculosis**[Q] is responsible for **all the cases** of GI tuberculosis
- M. bovis has largely been eliminated by public health measures
- More common in **poor socioeconomic status**[Q]

Pathogenesis

Primary Intestinal Tuberculosis	Secondary Intestinal Tuberculosis
• Ingestion of **contaminated food**[Q] may cause primary tuberculosis (this route of infection has decreased in recent years)	• Arises from **swallowed sputum**[Q] containing tuberculous bacilli • Influenced by **virulence** & **quantity of bacilli** and host resistance of infection[Q]

- When the intestines become infected by **lymphatic spread** from the mesenteric nodes, **nodal disease** is considered as the **primary site** & intestinal involvement is secondary.
- **Earliest intestinal lesions** are found in **submucosa**[Q], while the overlying mucosa is normal.

Sites of Intestinal Involvement
- MC site is **terminal ileum** & **ileocecal junction**[Q]
- Other regions in decreasing frequency are: colon, jejunum, rectum, anal canal, duodenum, stomach & esophagus
- **Site of predilection** is dictated by the factors: abundance of **lymphoid tissue**, rate of **absorption** of intestinal contents, **prolonged stasis** & **digestive activity** of intestinal contents[Q]

Pathology

Ulcerative Tuberculosis (60%)	Hyperplastic Tuberculosis (10%)	Sclerotic or Fibrotic Tuberculosis (30%)
• **Tuberculous** intestinal **ulcers** are usually **deep** & **transversely placed**[Q] in the direction of lymphatics • **Multiple ulcers** may be seen, most often in **terminal ileum**[Q] • Disease progression is associated with the appearance of **inflammatory mass** around the bowel. • **Diseased** part of the **GIT** becomes **thickened** and **serosal surface** is studded with **tubercles**. • Marked **increase** in **mesenteric fat** with **fat wrapping** around the bowel loops • **Regional lymph nodes** become **enlarged** and may **caseate**, leading to **mesenteric abscess** formation • Bowel perforation is **rare** and is usually confined by perilesional inflammatory mass	• A **fibroblastic reaction** occurs in submucosa and subserosa resulting in **marked thickening** of the **bowel wall**[Q] • Involvement of adjacent mesentery, lymph nodes and omentum, results in **formation** of a **mass lesion** • Hyperplastic lesions are due to **reduced bacterial virulence** & **increased host resistance**	• Associated with **strictures** of intestine, typically described as "**napkin-ring strictures**" which may be **single** or **multiple** • When multiple, strictures may occur in **short segment** of bowel or over the **entire length** of intestine.

Clinical Features

- **Initial symptoms** are vague & **non-specific**[Q]
- As the diseases progress, individual may develop **fever** (in **two third**), **night sweats**, malaise, weakness, **anorexia** & **weight loss**[Q].
- **MC symptom** of GI tuberculosis is **abdominal pain**[Q].
- **Diarrhea** is another common symptom.
- Abdominal distention suggests presence of ascites or subacute intestinal obstruction

Primary Small Bowel Disease	Colonic Tuberculosis
• **Stools** are large in amount, **foul smelling** and resemble those seen in patients with **malabsorption**[Q].	• **Stools** may be **watery, small** in amount and mixed with **blood** when disease affects predominantly the **colon**[Q].

Complications

- Intestinal obstruction & malabsorption are MC complications[Q]
- Bowel perforation & GI hemorrhage are less common

Diagnosis

- **Laboratory tests**: MC abnormality is raised ESR (90% cases)[Q]

Ascitic Fluid Showing	
• **Lymphocytosis**[Q] (WBC >500/mm³)	• **SAAG <1.1**[Q]
• **High protein**[Q] content (>2.5 gm/dL)	• **Adenosine deaminase** is **raised**, (sensitivity & specificity of 95%[Q])

RADIOLOGICAL IMAGING

Ultrasound

- **Club-sandwich appearance**[Q] (presence of alternating echogenic & echofree layers produce by bowel wall, serosa & adjacent bowel loops with interloop fluid collection)

CT Scan

- **High density appearance** of ascitic fluid due to **elevated protein content**[Q]
- **Thickening** of bowel wall and ileocecal valve

BARIUM STUDIES IN GI TUBERCULOSIS

- **Earliest feature** is **spasm** & **hypermotility** with **edema of valve**[Q]
- **Thickening of valve lips** with **narrowing** of terminal ileum (Fleishner or umbrella sign[Q]) is characteristic of TB.
- In advance disease, characteristic deformity includes **symmetric, annular, napkin ring stenosis**[Q] and obstruction or shortening and pouch formation.
- **Cecum** become **shrunken** & **retracted** out of the iliac fossa due to **contraction of mesocolon (pulled up cecum**[Q])
- **Loss of ileocecal angle** with **dilated terminal ileum** imparting **goose neck deformity**[Q]
- **Narrowing of terminal ileum** due to irritability, along with shortened rigid cecum called as **"Sterlein sign"**[Q]
- **Persistent narrow stream** of **barium** in the bowel indicates stenosis known as **String sign**[Q]

Remember: **String sign** & **Sterlein sign** are also seen in **Crohn's disease** and are **not specific for TB**[Q].

Treatment

- Treatment of GI tuberculosis is **ATT**.
- **Fever, malaise** & **weight loss subside** in a **few weeks**[Q].
- **Majority of patients** (70%) with **symptoms** of **subacute intestinal obstruction** and evidence of intestinal **strictures** show **complete resolution** of the **radiological abnormality**[Q]

Indications of Surgery in GI Tuberculosis	
• Intestinal obstruction secondary to stricture (MC)[Q]	• Severe GI hemorrhage[Q]
• Free perforation[Q]	• Intra-abdominal abscess[Q]
	• Internal or external fistula[Q]

ENTERIC FEVER OR TYPHOID

ENTERIC FEVER OR TYPHOID

- Enteric fever is a potentially life-threatening systemic disease characterized by **fever** and **abdominal pain**[Q]
- It is caused by **Salmonella typhi** or **paratyphi**[Q]
- **Typhoid** is the **MC cause of ileal perforation** in **tropical countries (India)**[Q].

Pathology

- Ulceration & necrosis of ileocecal Peyer's patches^Q
- Ulcer is **parallel to the long axis** of gut and is usually situated in the **lower ileum (longitudinal ulcers)**^{Q}
- **Perforation** of a typhoid ulcer usually occurs during the **third week**^{Q} and is occasionally the first sign of the disease.

Clinical Features

- **Fever & abdominal pain** are hallmark symptoms^Q
- Non-specific symptoms: Headache, cough, sweating, myalgia, arthralgia, fatigue
- **Paralytic ileus** is the MC complication^Q of typhoid.
- **Intestinal hemorrhage (2nd MC)**^{Q} may be the leading symptom.

Complications of Enteric Fever	
• **Paralytic ileus (MC)**^{Q}	• Phlebitis
• Intestinal **hemorrhage (2nd MC)**^{Q}	• Genitourinary inflammation
• **Perforation**^{Q}	• Arthritis
• **Cholecystitis**^{Q}	• Osteomyelitis

Characteristic Signs

- **Rose spots, splenomegaly, leucopenia** with **shift to left**^{Q}
- **Lipopolysaccharide endotoxin** is responsible for **leucopenia** and **splenomegaly**^{Q}
- **Relative bradycardia** despite of **high fever**^{Q}

ENTEROCUTANEOUS FISTULA

ENTEROCUTANEOUS FISTULA

- Enterocutaneous fistulas are **most commonly iatrogenic**, usually the result of a **surgical misadventure**^{Q}

Surgical Misadventure Leading to Enterocutaneous Fistula

- **Anastomotic leakage**^{Q}
- **Injury** of the **bowel or blood supply**^{Q}
- **Laceration** of the bowel by **wire mesh** or **retention suture**^{Q}

Etiology of Enterocutaneous fistula	
• **Iatrogenic (MC)**^{Q}	• Inflammatory bowel disease
• **Erosion** by **suction catheters adjacent abscesses**, or **trauma**^{Q}	• Mesenteric vascular disease
• **Previous radiation therapy**^{Q}	• Intra-abdominal sepsis
• **Intestinal obstruction**^{Q}	• **Crohn's disease**^{Q} leading to spontaneous fistula in 2% cases

Clinical Features

Typical Clinical Presentation
• **Typical clinical presentation** is that of a **febrile, postoperative patient** with an **erythematous wound**^{Q}.
• When a **few skin sutures** are **removed**, a **purulent** or **bloody discharge** is noted; leakage of enteric **contents** then occurs, sometimes immediately, but **often within 1 or 2 days**^{Q}.

- If the **diagnosis is in doubt**, **confirmation** can be obtained by **oral administration** of a **nonabsorbable marker**, such as **charcoal** or **Congo red**, or by **injection of water-soluble contrast medium** into the fistula^Q.

  - In general, the **more proximal the fistula** in the intestine, the **more serious the problem**, with **greater fluid and electrolyte loss**^{Q}.
  - The **drainage** has a greater digestive capacity, and the **distal segment** is **not available** for **absorption of nutrients**^{Q}.

Diagnosis

- **Fistulogram**^{Q} to determine:
  - **Presence** and **extent** of any **abscess cavities**
  - **Extent** of **bowel wall disruption**
  - Whether a **distal obstruction** is present
  - **Length** of the tract
  - **Location** of the fistula
- **CT** is helpful in determining whether **underlying collections** of **fluid** or **pus** are present.

Treatment

- Successful management requires establishment of **controlled drainage**, usually using a **sump suction apparatus**; **management of sepsis**; **prevention of fluid** and **electrolyte depletion**; **protection of the skin**; and **provision of adequate nutrition**^{Q}.
- When **sepsis** has been **controlled** and **nutritional therapy** has been instituted, a course of **conservative management**^{Q} should be followed.

- > • Most of these fistulas heal spontaneously within 4-6 weeks of conservative management^Q. If closure is not accomplished after this time, surgery is indicated.
- This **period of conservative management** not only allows those **fistulas to heal spontaneously** but also **allows for optimization of nutritional status** and **control of the wound** and **fistula sites**^{Q}.
- Also, a **reasonable delay permits** the **peritoneal reaction** and **inflammation to subside**, thus **making** a **second operation easier** and **safer**^{Q}.

> • **Preferred operation**: Fistula tract excision and segmental resection of the involved segment of intestine and reanastomosis^Q.

- **Simple closure** of the fistula after removing the fistula tract **almost always results in** a **recurrence** of the fistula.
- If an **unexpected abscess** is encountered or if the **bowel wall is rigid** and **distended** over a **long distance**, thus making primary anastomosis unsafe, **exteriorization of both ends** of the **intestine** should be accomplished.

Complications
- **Sepsis**, **fluid** and **electrolyte depletion**, **necrosis** of the **skin** at the site of external drainage, and **malnutrition**^{Q}.
- **Mortality rates** for patients with enterocutaneous fistulas remain high (**15-20%**)

Factors Preventing Spontaneous Fistula Closure

• **High output (>500 mL/day)**^{Q}	• **Radiation enteritis**^{Q}
• **Severe disruption** of intestinal continuity^Q (**>50%** of bowel circumference)	• **Distal obstruction**^{Q}
	• **Undrained abscess cavity**^{Q}
• **Active inflammatory bowel disease**^{Q} of bowel segment	• **Foreign body**^{Q} in the fistula tract
• **Cancer**^{Q}	• **Fistula tract <2.5 cm** long^Q
	• **Epithelialization** of fistula tract^Q

SUPERIOR MESENTERIC ARTERY SYNDROME

Superior Mesenteric Artery Syndrome

- Vascular compression of **third portion**^{Q} of duodenum by **superior mesenteric artery** as it passes over this portion of duodenum.
- Also known as **Wilkie's syndrome**, **cast syndrome**, and **arteriomesenteric duodenal ileus** or **compression**^{Q}

Three Mechanical Factors Must be Present
- An abnormally **narrow, aortomesenteric angle**^{Q}
- An abnormally **highly fixed transverse duodenum**^{Q}
- An **abnormal course** of the **mesenteric artery**^{Q} continuing inferiorly, anterior to the unyielding vertebral column

- **Most commonly** seen in **young asthenic individuals**, with **women** being more commonly affected than men^Q.
- **SMA** normally **leaves aorta** at an **acute angle (50-60°)**
- Normally a **mass of fat** and **lymphatics** near **origin of SMA** is believed to **protect duodenum from compression.**

Predisposing Factors
• Rapid weight loss^Q	• Scoliosis^Q
• Supine immobilization^Q	• Placement of a body cast^Q
• Rapid growth of height^Q	

Clinical Features
- Symptoms include profound nausea and vomiting, **abdominal distention, weight loss, & postprandial epigastric pain**^{Q}, which varies from intermittent to constant depending on the severity of the duodenal obstruction.
- **Weight loss** usually occurs **before** the **onset of symptoms** and contributes to the syndrome.

Diagnosis
- **Barium** upper gastrointestinal series or **hypotonic duodenography**^{Q}, which demonstrates abrupt or near-total cessation of flow of barium from the duodenum to the jejunum.
- CT has been useful in certain instances.

Treatment
- **Conservative measures** are tried initially and have been **increasingly successful** as **definitive treatment.**
- **Operative treatment of choice** is **duodenojejunostomy**^{Q}.

SMALL-BOWEL NEOPLASM

Small-Bowel Neoplasm

- MC tumor of small bowel: **Stromal tumor**^{Q} >**Adenoma**^{Q}
- MC tumor of small bowel in children: **Lymphoma**^{Q}
- MC malignant tumor of small bowel: **Adenocarcinoma**^{Q} > **Carcinoid**
- MC site of small bowel malignancy, carcinoids, lymphoma: **Ileum**^{Q}

Small-Bowel Malignancies

- **MC malignant neoplasms** of the **small bowel**: Adenocarcinoma^Q >Carcinoid >malignant GISTs >lymphomas.
- **Adenocarcinomas** are **more numerous** in the **proximal small bowel**, whereas the **other malignant lesions** are **more common** in the **distal intestine (ileum)**^{Q}.

Clinical Features
- In contrast to benign lesions, malignant neoplasms **almost always produce symptoms**^{Q}

> - **MC symptom**: Abdominal pain >weight loss^Q

- **Obstruction** develops in **15-35%** of patients and, in contrast to the intussusception produced by benign lesions, is usually the **result of tumor infiltration** and **adhesions**.
- **Diarrhea** with tenesmus and **passage of large amounts** of mucus may occur.
- Adenocarcinomas may produce the typical constricting apple-core lesions similar to those observed in the colon.

> - **Gastrointestinal bleeding** is more common with leiomyosarcomas^Q.

- A **palpable mass** may be felt in **10-20%** of patients, and **perforations** develop in about **10%**, usually secondary to lymphomas and sarcomas.

Diagnosis
- Barium meal follow through (BMFT): Accurate diagnosis in 50–70% of patients with malignant neoplasms of the small intestine
- **Enteroclysis (small bowel enema)**: Diagnostic accuracy of about **90%**^{Q}

Treatment
- **Wide resection** including **regional lymph nodes**^{Q}.

> - Often, **surgical resection for cure** is **not possible**. Therefore, **palliative resection should be performed to prevent** further complications of **bleeding, obstruction**, and **perforation**^{Q}.

- Preferred chemotherapy regimen: **FOLFOX**^{Q}

Prognosis
- **Only half** of the patients operated on for malignant tumors of the small intestine **have lesions amenable to curative resection**.
- **One third** have a **distant metastasis** at the time of initial surgery
- Overall **5-year survival rate after surgical treatment** of malignant tumors is only **25%**
- **Adenocarcinoma** has the **poorest prognosis**, with an overall **survival rate** of **15-20%**.

GASTROINTESTINAL LYMPHOMA

Gastrointestinal Lymphoma

- Any segment of the gastrointestinal tract may be secondarily involved by systemic dissemination of non-Hodgkin lymphomas.
- However, **up to 40%** of **lymphomas arise** in sites **other than lymph nodes**, and the **gut is the most common location**^{Q}.

> - **Intestinal lymphoma** involves the **ileum (MC)**^{Q}, jejunum, and duodenum, in decreasing frequency, a pattern that mirrors the **relative amount of normal lymphoid cells** in these anatomic areas.

- **Primary GI lymphomas** usually arise as **sporadic neoplasms**^{Q}
- Intestinal tract lymphomas can be classified into **B-Cell** and **T-Cell lymphomas**^{Q}.
- **Intestinal T-cell lymphoma** is usually **associated with** a **long-standing malabsorption syndrome** (such as **celiac disease**)^Q.
- **MC splenic neoplasm** is **NHL**^{Q}.

- Stomach is the MC site for extranodal lymphoma^Q.
- Typical presentation of small bowel lymphoma: Thick walled infiltrating mass with aneurysm dilatation without obstruction^Q.

Primary GI Lymphomas Occur More Frequently in	
Chronic gastritis caused by H. pylori^Q	Congenital immunodeficiency states^Q
Chronic sprue^Q like syndromes	HIV infection^Q
Natives of the Mediterranean region^Q	Following organ transplantation with immunosuppression^Q

Pathology
- All the gut lymphoid tissue is mucosal & submucosal, early lesions appear as plaque-like expansions of the mucosa and submucosa.
- Diffusely infiltrating lesions may produce full-thickness mural thickening, with effacement of the overlying mucosal folds and focal ulceration.
- Diffuse infiltrating type is more common than polypoidal^Q.

CARCINOID TUMORS

CARCINOID TUMORS

- Distribution (BIRACS)^Q: Bronchus> Ileum > Rectum > Appendix > Colon > Stomach
- Combined incidence of carcinoid tumor in duodenum + jejunum + ileum (small intestine) > Bronchus^Q
- MC site of carcinoid tumor: GI tract >Respiratory tract^Q
- Arise from enterochromaffin cells^Q at the base of the crypts of Lieberkuhn in the GI tract.

Foregut carcinoids	Mostly argyrophilic^Q (silver staining only with the addition of a reducing agent)
Midgut carcinoids	Argentaffinic^Q (silver staining)
Hindgut carcinoids	Mixed (60-70% argyrophilic & 8-16% argentaffinic)^Q

- MC foregut location for carcinoid tumors: Stomach^Q
- Colonic carcinoids occur more commonly on the right side, in the ascending or proximal transverse colon^Q.
- Small bowel carcinoids are multiple in 25% of cases^Q.
- Appendiceal carcinoids are typically solitary lesion^Q.

> - Highest percentage of non-localized disease (PCS): Pancreatic^Q (91%) >colonic (77%) >small intestinal carcinoid tumors (75%)
> - Highest percentage localized disease (LOAR)^Q: Laryngeal carcinoid tumors (100%) >Ovary, appendix >rectum

Pathology
- GIT carcinoids produce a variety of peptide hormones, the most common is serotonin^Q.
- Foregut carcinoids produce low levels of serotonin^Q (5-hydroxytryptamine) but may secrete 5-hydroxytryptophan or adrenocorticotrophic hormone.
- Hindgut carcinoids rarely produce serotonin^Q but may produce other hormones such as somatostatin and peptide YY.
- Gastric carcinoid patients are deficient in the enzyme dopa-decarboxylase, the enzyme responsible for conversion of 5-hydroxytryptophan to serotonin (5-hydroxy tryptamine).

Malignant potential in Carcinoids depends on (LSD Growth)			
Location^Q	**S**ize^Q	**D**epth of invasion^Q	**G**rowth pattern^Q

- In small bowel carcinoid (SBC), frequent coexistence of a second primary malignant neoplasm of a different histological type, this usually is a synchronous adenocarcinoma, most commonly in the colon & breast^Q.
- Associated with MEN-I in 10% of cases^Q.

Clinical Features
- MC symptom of SBC: Intermittent intestinal obstruction^Q

MALIGNANT CARCINOID SYNDROME

- Occur in fewer than 10% of patients with carcinoid tumors.
- Midgut carcinoids are the MC source^Q of carcinoid syndrome.
- Attacks may be spontaneous or precipitated by stress, alcohol, a large meal or sexual intercourse.
- Common symptoms and signs include cutaneous flush (80%)^Q; diarrhea (76%); hepatomegaly (71%); cardiac lesions (70%); asthma (25%).

> - Bright-red patchy flushing which is typically seen with gastric carcinoids^Q

- **Diarrhea** is directly **related to serum serotonin level** (serotonin stimulates secretin release), **episodic** usually occurring **after meals**, **watery** and often **explosive**; and serotonin antagonist **methylsergide** effectively **controls** the symptoms (**Ondansetron** is particularly **effective in** treating **diarrhea** apparently through the **restoration of normal colonic motility**)[Q].
- MC cardiac lesions: TR > PR > TS > PS

> **Atypical or Variant Carcinoid Syndrome**
> - Occur in patients with **gastric carcinoid tumors**[Q].
> - These patients experience **cutaneous flushes** that are **patchy** and **highly pruritic**.
> - **Diarrhea, bronchospasm**, and **cardiac lesions** are **rare**.
> - The syndrome is due to large release of **histamine** from the tumor rather than serotonin.

Diagnosis
- Elevated urinary levels of **5-HIAA**[Q] (5-hydroxyindoleacetic acid) measured **over 24 hours** with high-performance liquid chromatography are **highly specific**[Q].

> - Plasma concentration of **chromogranin A** is **100% specific**[Q]

- Provocative tests using **pentagastrin, calcium**, or **epinephrine** are used to reproduce the symptoms of carcinoid tumors. The administration of **pentagastrin** is the **safest** and **most reliable** and the **most frequently used**[Q].
- Radiographic imaging is difficult because of the **small size** of **most tumors** and their common **submucosal location**[Q].
- The submucosal location lends to **more accurate localization with contrast studies** especially **enteroclysis**[Q], than with conventional sectional imaging such as CT scan.

> - Initial imaging procedure to **localize** & **stage** the carcinoid tumors: **SRS**[Q]
> - Best investigation for localization: **DOPA-PET**[Q]

Treatment

> **SURGERY**
> - Carcinoid tumors of the **jejunum** & **ileum: segmental resection** and **en-bloc lymphadenectomy**[Q].
> - **Resection** of primary tumor **regardless of metastasis**, to avoid complications from growth of primary tumor in terms of **bleeding, obstruction** & **abdominal pain** especially with **midgut carcinoids** because of their propensity to cause **intense fibrosing reaction**[Q].

> **MEDICAL THERAPY**
> - It includes chemotherapy and biological agents such as **somatostatin analogs** and **interferon alpha**[Q].
> - Chemotherapy: Dacarbazine, epirubicin & 5-FU (DEF)[Q].
> - **Octreotide** administration leads to reduction of symptoms, including flushing and diarrhea.
> - Newer treatment includes **In111-Octreotide** and **I124-labeled MIBG (metaiodobenzylguanide)**[Q].

> **TARGETED RADIOTHERAPY**
> - **Smart bombs**[Q]- **Radiolabeled somatostatin analogues** that deliver radiation specifically to carcinoids cells. Indium-111-labeled pentetreotide demonstrate an enhanced tumor regression response.

Prognosis
- Carcinoid tumors have the **best prognosis** of all **small bowel tumors**, whether the disease is **localized** or **metastatic**[Q].

> - Most useful prognostic marker is an elevated level of **chromogranin A**[Q].
> - **Midgut carcinoid** has the **best prognosis**[Q].

- **Female gender** and **younger age**[Q] is associated with **better prognosis**
- One of the main determinants of survival is the **presence of liver metastases**[Q].

BLIND LOOP SYNDROME

> **BLIND LOOP SYNDROME**

- A rare condition manifested by **diarrhea, steatorrhea, megaloblastic anemia**, weight loss, abdominal pain[Q].
- **Deficiencies** of the fat-soluble vitamins (**A, D, E, & K**) and **neurologic disorders**[Q].

Etiopathogenesis
- **Underlying cause: Bacterial overgrowth** in **stagnant areas** of the small bowel produced by **stricture, stenosis, fistulas**, or **diverticula**[Q] (e.g., jejunoileal or Meckel's diverticulum).
- **Bacterial overgrowth** competes for **vitamin B_{12}**, producing systemic deficiency of vitamin B_{12} & **megaloblastic anemia**[Q].

Clinical Features
- Manifested by **diarrhea, steatorrhea, megaloblastic anemia,** weight loss, abdominal pain
- Deficiencies of the fat-soluble vitamins (A, D, E, and K), as well as **neurologic disorders**[Q].

Diagnosis
- Diagnosed with **cultures obtained** through an **intestinal tube (gold standard** diagnostic test)
- By **indirect tests** such as the ^{14}C-xylose or ^{14}C-cholylglycine breath tests. Excessive bacterial use of ^{14}C substrate leads to an **increase in** $^{14}CO_2$.

> - In **Schilling test**, vitamin B_{12} excretion is not altered by the addition of intrinsic factor, but a course of a **broad-spectrum antibiotic** (e.g., tetracycline) should **return vitamin B_{12} absorption to normal**[Q].

Treatment
- **Parenteral vitamin B_{12} therapy + Broad-spectrum antibiotic** (tetracycline or amoxicillin-clavulanate)[Q].
- For most patients, a **single course of therapy (7-10 days)** is sufficient, and the patient may remain symptom-free for months.
- **Surgical correction** of the condition producing stagnation and blind loop syndrome **produces a permanent cure** and is indicated in those patients who **require multiple rounds of antibiotics** or are on **continuous therapy**[Q].

SHORT BOWEL SYNDROME

Short Bowel Syndrome

- **Malabsorptive condition** that arises secondary to **removal of significant segments of the small intestine**[Q].
- Most common causes are **Mesenteric infarction**[Q], **Crohn's disease**[Q], **Trauma**[Q], **Volvulus**[Q].
- Normal length of small intestine: 600 cm[Q].
- Length <200 cm leads to short bowel syndrome[Q].

Changes Seen in Terminal Ileal Resection	
- **Malabsorption** of **bile salts** and **vitamin B_{12}** (which are normally absorbed in this region) - Vitamin B_{12} Malabsorption → **Megaloblastic anemia**[Q] - **Bile salts Malabsorption** → **Unabsorbed bile salts** escape into **colon** and **stimulate fluid secretion** from the colon → **watery diarrhea**[Q]. - Decreased bile salts in the bile → **Cholesterol gall stones**[Q]	- **Reduction in bile salt pool** → **steatorrhea**[Q] and **Malabsorption** of **fat soluble vitamins** (due to fat malabsorption) - **Unabsorbed fatty acids** bind with **calcium** → Increased concentration of **free oxalates** (oxalates bind with calcium normally and therefore escape without intestinal absorption) → Free oxalates are absorbed → **Oxalate kidney stones**[Q].

Removal of Ileocecal Valve
- **Bacterial overgrowth**[Q] from the **colon** → **diarrhea & malabsorption**[Q]
- Decrease in **intestinal transit time**[Q]

Adaptive Response
- Resection of up to 70% of **small bowel** usually can be **tolerated** if the terminal ileum & ileocecal valve are preserved.
- **Length alone**, however, is **not the only determining factor of complications** related to small bowel resection.

> - **Proximal bowel resection** is **tolerated** much **better than distal resection**[Q]
> - Because the **ileum can adapt** and **increase its absorptive capacity more efficiently than the jejunum**[Q].

Treatment
- **Early phase:** Control diarrhea, **replacement** of **fluid and electrolytes**, and **TPN**[Q]
- H2-receptor antagonists or **PPI** for **acid hypersecretion**[Q]
- **Cholestyramine**[Q] for **cathartic effects** of **unabsorbed bile salts** in the colon.

> - **Hypergastrinemia** and **gastric hypersecretion** occur after massive small bowel resection and **greatly contribute to diarrhea after a massive small bowel resection**[Q].

Intestinal Lengthening Operation
- **Bianchi Procedure**[Q]: Longitudinal intestinal lengthening and tailoring
- **STEP:** Serial transverse enteroplasty procedure[Q]

BOWEL ANASTOMOSIS

Bowel Anastomosis

- **Good surgical technique** is **more important than** the choice of suture material:
  - Gentle handling[Q] of the bowel
  - Adequate hemostasis[Q]
  - Meticulous approximation[Q] of well-vascularized bowel
  - Tension-free anastomosis[Q]

Two-layer Anastomoses	One-layer Anastomoses
• **Inner layer** is an **absorbable** 3-0 or 4-0 running **full-thickness stitch**[Q] • **Outer layer** is an **inverting**, usually 3-0, **seromuscular stitch**, which may be running or interrupted **nonabsorbable**[Q].	• A **full-thickness technique**, interrupted or running with **nonabsorbable suture**[Q]

- For **multiple strictures** involving **long segment** of **small intestine, stricturoplasty** is preferred to **prevent short bowel syndrome**[Q].

Multiple Choice Questions

MECKEL'S DIVERTICULUM

1. All are true statement about Meckel's diverticulum except:
   (Recent Question 2014; PGI Nov 2010)
   a. Occurs in 2% of population
   b. Perforation occurs
   c. Common on anti-mesenteric border
   d. Contains ectopic gastric tissue
   e. Diarrhea very common

2. Meckel's diverticulum follows the rule of 2. Which of the following is false? *(Recent Question 2018)*
   a. Occurs in approximately 2% of population
   b. Approximately 2 inches in length
   c. Generally present 2 feet proximal to ileocecal valve
   d. 2% are symptomatic

3. Ectopic mucosa of Meckel's diverticulum is diagnosed by:
   (AIIMS GIS Dec 2011, Dec 2010)
   a. Tc-99 radionuclide scan   b. Angiography
   c. CT   d. Endoscopy

4. All are true about Meckel's diverticulum except:
   a. Congenital   *(GB Pant 2011)*
   b. True diverticula
   c. Develop from omphalomesenteric duct
   d. All incidentally detected Meckel's diverticulum should be resected

5. Most common presenting complication of Meckel's diverticulum: *(Orissa 2011)*
   a. Hemorrhage   b. Intussusception
   c. Meckel's diverticulitis   d. Intestinal obstruction

6. What does the intraoperative photograph above depicts?
   (APPG 2015)
   a. Transverse colon   b. Fallopian tube
   c. Meckel's diverticulum   d. Intussusception

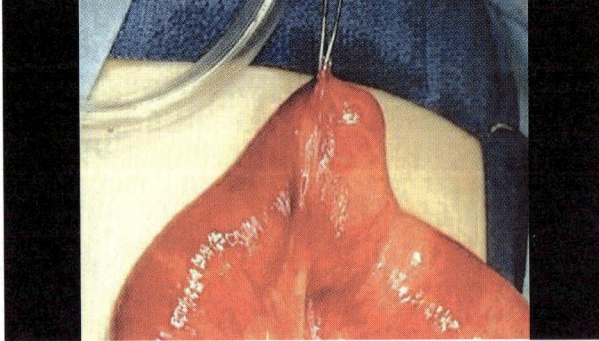

7. Meckel's diverticulum is a derivative of:
   (All India 94, AIIMS May 2005)
   a. Allantoic diverticulum   b. Vitellointestinal duct
   c. Ventral mesogastrium   d. Ductus arteriosus

8. The most frequent congenital anomaly of the GI tract is:
   a. Imperforate anus   b. Meckel's diverticulum
   c. Malrotation   d. Duodenal atresia

9. All of the following are true about Meckel's diverticulum except: *(All India 96)*
   a. Bleeding   b. Intussusception
   c. Arises at the mesenteric border
   d. Located 60 cm from the cecal valve

10. Which one of the following statements is incorrect regarding Meckel's diverticulum?   *(Recent Question 2015)*
    a. Is found on the antimesenteric border of the small intestine
    b. Consists of mucosa without a muscle coat
    c. Heterotopic gastric mucosa can ulcerate and cause a brisk gastrointestinal bleed
    d. A fibrous band between the apex and umbilicus can cause intestinal obstruction

11. Best investigation for diagnosis of ectopic gastric mucosa in Meckel's diverticulum: *(AIIMS June 99)*
    a. Fluoroscopy   b. Occult blood test in stool
    c. Ultrasound abdomen   d. Radionuclide scan

12. A wide mouthed Meckel's diverticulum is found accidently on laparotomy. What will be the treatment of choice?
    a. Resection of diverticulum
    b. Leave as such
    c. Ligate at base
    d. Resection with part of ileum

13. Complications of Meckel's diverticulum include: *(Kerala 86)*
    a. Hemorrhage   b. Intussusception
    c. Strangulation   d. All are correct

14. Which one of the following conditions is diagnosed by Tc^{99}-Pertechnate scintigraphy?   *(UPSC 2004)*
    a. Pharyngeal diverticulum   b. Duodenal diverticulum
    c. Meckel's diverticulum   d. Colonic diverticulum

15. The Meckel's diverticulum is situated within about ____ cm from the ileocecal valve: *(COMEDK 2008, 2007)*
    a. 25   b. 60
    c. 75   d. 100

16. Which of the following statement is not true about Meckel's diverticulum?   *(DPG 2007)*
    a. Most common congenital anomaly of small intestine
    b. Most common is ectopic gastric mucosa
    c. Bleeding may occur from the wall
    d. Wide mouth stapling at the base for non bleeding cases

17. Uncommon complication of Meckel's diverticulum:
    (MCI Sept 2005)
    a. Intussusception   b. Diverticulitis
    c. Malignancy   d. Increased bleeding

18. Common congenital anomaly of midgut is: *(COMEDK 2008)*
    a. Hirschsprung's disease   b. Omphalocele
    c. Duodenal atresia   d. Meckel's diverticulum

19. Efficacy of Tc-Pertechnate scan is increased by all except:
    (AIIMS GIS Dec 2006)
    a. Glucagon   b. Pentagastrin
    c. Cimetidine   d. Metoclopramide

20. What is false about Meckel's diverticulitis?
    a. Present in 3% of the population   *(AIIMS November 2015)*
    b. Presents with periumbilical pain
    c. Remnant of proximal part of vitellointestinal duct
    d. Lies on the anti-mesenteric border

Small Intestine

21. Which of the following is true about Meckel's diverticula?
    (Recent Question 2017)
    a. Most common congenital anomaly of the intestine
    b. Always contain heterotopic mucosa
    c. Pseudodiverticula
    d. Located on mesenteric border

SMALL INTESTINAL DIVERTICULA

22. True about small bowel diverticula: *(PGI June 2005)*
    a. Contains all the layers of bowel wall
    b. Common in terminal ileum
    c. Surgical treatment is not required
    d. Seen on the mesenteric border

23. All are true about duodenal diverticula except:
    (AIIMS GIS May 2011)
    a. Whenever found, should be treated due to increased risk of complications
    b. Most common site is periampullary region
    c. Can cause acute pancreatitis
    d. Most are asymptomatic

24. Feature(s) of Jejunal diverticula is/are: *(PGI Nov 2010)*
    a. ↑ Folate absorption   b. ↓ Ferritin absorption
    c. ↓ B12 absorption   d. Urea breath test
    e. Steatorrhea

GASTROINTESTINAL TUBERCULOSIS

25. Which one is not true regarding hyperplastic ileocecal tuberculosis? *(AIIMS June 97, All India 2001)*
    a. Mass in right iliac fossa
    b. Common site ileocecal region
    c. X-ray shows indrawing of caecum from ileum
    d. Conservative management is treatment of choice

26. Which is true about intestinal tuberculosis?
    a. Common site is appendix *(PGI Dec 99, PGI June 96)*
    b. Causes intestinal perforation
    c. Commonly associated with pulmonary TB
    d. Caused by M. tuberculosis

27. Small intestinal tuberculosis can cause:
    a. Diarrhea   b. Constipation
    c. Structure   d. Malabsorption

28. Most common indication for laparotomy in intestine TB is:
    (PGI 93)
    a. Peritonitis   b. Intestine obstruction
    c. Doubtful diagnosis   d. Lower GI bleeding

29. Not true about hyperplastic tuberculosis: *(UPPG 2000)*
    a. Most common site is ileo-cecal region
    b. Presents as mass in right iliac fossa
    c. Surgery is the treatment of choice
    d. Barium studies are characteristic

30. Kalu, 35-year-old male presented with the history of recurrent attacks of colicky abdominal pain. Barium meal follow through was done. What is the name of this radiological sign? *(Recent Question 2016)*
    a. String sign of Kantor   b. Goose neck appearance
    c. Fleischner sign   d. Umbrella sign

31. Most common indication for operation in tuberculosis of intestine is: *(Kerala 2001)*
    a. Obstruction   b. Perforation
    c. Mass abdomen   d. GI symptoms

32. Commonest site of tuberculosis of the intestines:
    a. Stomach   b. Ileum   *(All India 89)*
    c. Jejunum   d. Colon

33. Commonest site involved in Ileocecal TB:
    a. Intestinal wall   b. Lymph node
    c. Mesentery   d. Intestinal mucosa

34. True regarding barium study of ileocecal tuberculosis:
    (PGI June 2009)
    a. String sign   b. Goose neck sign
    c. Right sided obstruction   d. Pulled up caecum
    e. Sterlein sign

35. The most common cause of perforation of the distal ileum in India is: *(UPSC 2005)*
    a. Tuberculosis   b. Typhoid
    c. Amoebiasis   d. Regional enteritis

36. Pulled up cecum is seen in: *(Recent Question 2014, 2013)*
    a. CA colon   b. Carcinoid
    c. Ileocecal tuberculosis   d. Crohn's disease

37. Fleischner sign on barium study is seen in? *(DNB 2014)*
    a. Ileocecal TB   b. Crohn's disease
    c. Small bowel carcinoid
    d. Typhoid

SUPERIOR MESENTERIC ARTERY SYNDROME

38. All are true regarding superior mesenteric artery syndrome, except: *(All India 2000)*
    a. Caused by compression of distended duodenum
    b. Common in young females
    c. Does not occur in obese individuals
    d. Most common in 6th-7th decade

39. What is probable diagnosis of a patient with spinal POP cast presenting with bilious vomiting?
    a. Acute dilation of stomach
    b. Duodenal obstruction
    c. Peritonitis
    d. Acute pancreatitis

40. All of the following is true regarding superior mesenteric artery syndrome, except: *(MHSSMCET 2008)*
    a. Common in young females
    b. Caused by compression of third part of duodenum
    c. Vomiting and post-prandial abdominal pain are typical symptoms
    d. Gastrojejunostomy is treatment of choice in chronic cases

41. Which of the following is wrong regarding superior mesenteric artery syndrome? *(AIIMS May 2018)*
    a. Superior mesenteric artery is compressed by third part of duodenum at the ligament of Treitz attachment
    b. Superior mesenteric artery has a normal angle between 38-65 degree in relation to duodenum
    c. Strong procedure is corrective surgery in which ligament of Treitz is divided
    d. Superior mesenteric artery syndrome is characterized by an angle less than 25 degree due to loss of intervening mesenteric pad of fat

PNEUMATOSIS INTESTINALIS

42. A young, apparently healthy patient presented with air under bilateral domes of diaphragm, which is because of:
    a. Pneumatosis cystoides intestinalis *(GB Pant 2011)*
    b. Diverticulitis
    c. Perforated peptic ulcer
    d. Band with Meckel's diverticulum

43. Treatment of choice for pneumatosis intestinalis, which is uncomplicated: *(MHPGMCET 2007)*
    a. High flow oxygen therapy
    b. Steroids and antibiotics
    c. Surgical resection
    d. Sulfasalazine therapy

44. Pneumatosis intestinalis in plain abdominal Roentgenogram is seen in: *(Orissa 2011)*
    a. Meconium ileus
    b. Neonatal necrotizing enterocolitis
    c. Duodenal atresia
    d. Intestinal obstruction

45. All are correct regarding pneumatosis cystoides except one:
    a. Spontaneous regression is seen *(AIIMS June 95)*
    b. Surgical resection indicated
    c. May cause tension pneumoperitoneum
    d. May cause severe bleeding

46. When the gas filled cysts are found in subserosa or submucosa of small intestine or colon, it is called:
    a. Pneumatosis cystoides intestinalis *(AMU 2005)*
    b. Colonoscopy
    c. Double contrast barium enema
    d. Mesenteric cyst

47. Pneumatosis intestinalis is diagnostic of: *(COMEDK 2009)*
    a. Ileal perforation
    b. Necrotizing enterocolitis
    c. Meconium ileus
    d. Colonic aganglionosis

SHORT BOWEL SYNDROME

48. Which one of the following gastrointestinal disorders predisposes to urolithiasis? *(UPSC 2007)*
    a. Peutz-Jegher's syndrome
    b. Short bowel syndrome
    c. Familial polyposis coli
    d. Ulcerative colitis

49. True about small bowel resection: *(PGI November 2017)*
    a. If jejunum is cut, ileum can compensate jejunal function
    b. If ileum is cut, jejunum can compensate ileum function
    c. Ileum resection is generally better tolerated, as jejunal shows better capacity to compensate
    d. Bile acid malabsorption leads to diarrhea

50. Which is not seen in massive resection of small bowel? *(AIIMS June 95, All India 98, PGI June 99, DPG 2008)*
    a. Hypogastrinemia
    b. Vitamin B_{12} deficiency
    c. Malabsorption
    d. Oxalate stone

51. In a patient with ileal resection, ileocecal valves were spared. Which of the following can develop? *(PGI May 2018)*
    a. Bacterial over growth
    b. Malabsorption
    c. Steatorrhea
    d. Cholelithiasis
    e. Renal oxalate stones

52. Complications of short bowel syndrome: *(GB Pant 2011)*
    a. Gall stones
    b. Oxalate renal stones
    c. Cirrhosis
    d. All of the above

53. Deficiency of which of the following vitamin is most commonly seen in short bowel syndrome with ileal resection? *(DNB 2012, All India 2012)*
    a. Vitamin B_{12}
    b. Vitamin B_1
    c. Folic acid
    d. Vitamin K

54. Renal calculus is seen in massive bowel resection due to:
    a. Reduced renal calcium excretion *(AIIMS Nov 94)*
    b. More calcium absorption in gut
    c. More oxalate absorption in gut
    d. None of the above

55. Resection of 90% of the ileum and jejunum causes all the following except: *(All India 94)*
    a. Hypogastrinemia
    b. Steatorrhea
    c. Anemia
    d. Extracellular volume depletion

56. Mechanism of action of teduglutide in short bowel syndrome: *(Recent Question 2019)*
    a. GLP-2 analogue
    b. HT1a inhibitor
    c. GLP-1 analogue
    d. C-peptide analogs

RADIATION ENTERITIS

57. Multiple strictures in intestine are found in: *(All India 2000)*
    a. Radiation enteritis
    b. Duodenal ulcer
    c. Ulcerative colitis
    d. Gastric erosion

58. Dose of radiation causing small intestinal radiation enteritis: *(AIIMS GIS Dec 2006)*
    a. 2300 rad
    b. 5000 rad
    c. 5500 rad
    d. 6000 rad

59. Intestine can tolerate a maximum dose of radiation upto:
    a. 3000 rad
    b. 4000 rad *(ILBS 2011)*
    c. 5000 rad
    d. 6000 rad

ENTERIC FEVER

60. Typhoid perforation occurs during: *(MHSSMCET 2005, MHPGMCET 2006, UPPG 2009, AIIMS 89)*
    a. 1st week
    b. 2nd week
    c. 3rd week
    d. 4th week

61. A 14-year-old girl with history of prolonged fever and abdominal discomfort is observed to have splenomegaly and leucopenia. In the course of disease she developed acute abdominal event and died. Which of the following is the likely finding on autopsy? *(All India 2012)*
    a. Transverse ulcers
    b. Longitudinal ulcers
    c. Pin point ulcers
    d. Pseudopolyps

62. Typhoid perforation is diagnosed by:
    a. Plain X-ray of abdomen in erect posture
    b. Rectal examination
    c. Gastric aspiration
    d. Barium enema

63. A 24-year-old male, who has been having fever for 15 days starts having acute pain and distension of abdomen. Abdominal examination reveals generalized tenderness with guarding. The most likely diagnosis is: *(Recent Question 2015)*
    a. Acute appendicitis
    b. Acute pancreatitis
    c. Enteric perforation
    d. Duodenal ulcer perforation

Small Intestine

64. Which of the following statement is correct about the given ulcers?

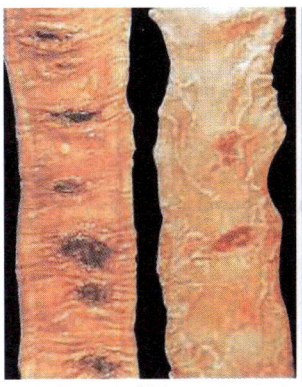 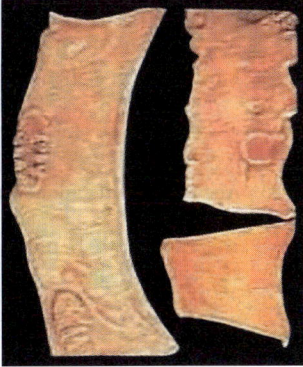

   a. 1-Crohn's disease & 2-Ulcerative colitis
   b. 1- Ulcerative colitis & 2- Crohn's disease
   c. 1- Typhoid & 2- Tuberculosis
   d. 1-Tuberculosis & 2-Typhoid

SMALL BOWEL RESECTION AND ANASTOMOSIS

65. Anastomosis of small bowel is done by: *(J and K 95)*
   a. Suture in 1 layer by non-absorbable suture
   b. Suture in 2 layers by non-absorbable suture
   c. Suture in 2 layers by absorbable sutures
   d. Suture in layers by absorbable suture

66. Treatment of choice in multiple intestinal strictures of segment of Jejunum is: *(AIIMS 92)*
   a. Resection and end to end anastomosis
   b. Nobles procedure
   c. Stricturoplasty
   d. End to side anastomosis

ENTERIC FISTULA

67. All are associated with non-healing of fistula except: *(GB Pant 2011)*
   a. Contained abscess   b. Distal obstruction
   c. Non-epithelialization   d. Radiating enteritis

68. Causes of non-healing of enterocutaneous fistula are all except: *(AIIMS GIS May 2011)*
   a. Epithelialization of track
   b. Radiation enteritis
   c. Acute inflammatory disease
   d. Track length >3 cm

69. Favorable features for closure of enterocutaneous fistula are all except: *(AIIMS GIS Dec 2011)*
   a. Tract <1 cm
   b. No sepsis
   c. No underlying bowel disease
   d. No distal obstruction

70. All of the following delay healing of enterocutaneous fistula except: *(JIPMER GIS 2011)*
   a. Radiation   b. Foreign body
   c. >2 cm fistulous tract   d. High output

71. Fistula leading to highest electrolyte in balance is:
   a. Gastric   b. Duodenal *(DNB 2009)*
   c. Sigmoid   d. Rectal

INTESTINAL ATRESIA AND DUPLICATION

72. A neonate presented with bilious vomiting and X-ray showing disproportionate size of bowel loops with no air-fluid levels. Most likely diagnosis is: *(KGMC 2011)*
   a. Intestinal atresia   b. Midgut volvulus
   c. Meconium ileus   d. Meconium plug syndrome

73. Most common site of intestinal duplication:
   a. Duodenum   b. Jejunum
   c. Ileum   d. Colon *(PGI SS June 2001)*

74. Commonest cause of intestinal obstruction in neonate is: *(MHPGMCET 2001)*
   a. Meconium ileus   b. Intestinal atresia
   c. Hirschsprung's disease   d. Volvulus

75. True about duplication of intestine is: *(PGI June 98)*
   a. Spherical type is MC
   b. Tubular type is attached longitudinally with bowel
   c. Spherical cyst communicates with lumen
   d. All of the above

76. Commonest site of intestinal atresia is in the: *(KGMC 2011)*
   a. Duodenum   b. Jejunum
   c. Ileum   d. Colon

77. The treatment of choice in duodenal atresia: *(All India 89)*
   a. Gastrojejunostomy   b. Duodenojejunostomy
   c. Bishop koop procedure   d. Duodenoduodenostomy

78. What is the type of given intestinal atresia?

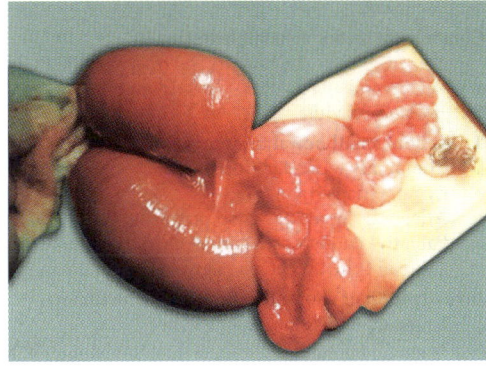

   a. Type I   b. Type II
   c. Type III   d. Type IV

79. "Apple peel bowel with loss of dorsal mesentery is feature of which type of ileal atresia"? *(APG 2015)*
   a. Type 1   b. Type 2
   c. Type 3   d. Type 4

80. Duplication of the small intestine is associated with:
   a. Heterotopic mucosa *(Recent Question 2017)*
   b. Smooth muscle component
   c. Spinal /vertebral defects
   d. All are correct

81. A newborn baby was brought with the history multiple episodes of bilious projectile vomiting. X-ray abdomen was done. What is the diagnosis? *(Recent Question 2017)*
   a. Duodenal atresia
   b. Jejunal atresia
   c. Ileal atresia
   d. Hypertrophic pyloric stenosis

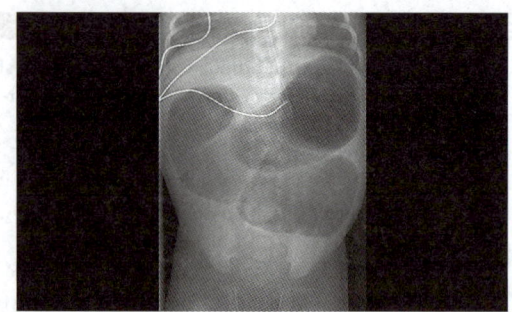

NEOPLASMS OF SMALL INTESTINE

82. **Most common tumor of small bowel in children:**
    (GB Pant 2011)
    a. Lymphoma b. Carcinoma
    c. Leiomyosarcoma d. Adenocarcinoma

83. **In small intestinal malignancy:** (PGI SS June 2009, June 2006)
    a. Most common site is jejunum
    b. Most common site is ileum
    c. Most common type is adenocarcinoma
    d. Less common due to decreased intestinal transit and increased enzymatic action

84. **Most common malignancy of small bowel:** (PGI SS 2004)
    a. Adenocarcinoma
    b. Carcinoid tumors
    c. Lymphoma
    d. Papilloma

85. **Commonest tumor of small intestine is:**
    (All India 96, AIIMS Feb 97, PGI June 95)
    a. Leiomyoma b. Lymphoma
    c. Adenocarcinoma d. Hemangioma

86. **True about small bowel tumour:** (PGI June 2003)
    a. Commonly located in duodenum
    b. Lymphoma is common
    c. Adenocarcinoma has good prognosis
    d. Palliative surgeries are done even in presence of metastasis
    e. Adjuvant chemotherapy is given

87. **Investigation of choice for small intestine tumor:**
    a. Ba meal follow through
    b. Echo (JIPMER 98)
    c. X-ray abdomen
    d. CT scan with contrast

88. **True about duodenal adenocarcinoma:** (PGI 2004)
    a. Commonest small intestinal tumor
    b. Arises from periampullary region
    c. Jaundice and anaemia found
    d. 5-year survival is 5%
    e. Surgery is only curative

89. **True about abdominal lymphoma:** (PGI Nov 2011)
    a. GIT lymphoma-most commonly has polypoid appearance
    b. Primary small-intestinal lymphomas are most commonly located in the ileum
    c. Lymphoma is most common primary malignant neoplasm of spleen
    d. Stomach is most common site for extranodal lymphoma
    e. MALT lymphoma is associated with H. pylori infection

90. **Most common primary for small bowel metastasis:**
    (AIIMS GIS May 2011)
    a. Lungs b. Melanoma
    c. Breast d. Kidney

91. **False statement regarding benign small bowel tumour is:**
    a. Accidentally discovered during surgeries (JIPMER 2013)
    b. Most commonly asymptomatic
    c. Cause hemorrhage
    d. Causes malabsorption

92. **Most common malignancy of small bowel:**
    (Recent Question 2017)
    a. Adenocarcinoma b. Carcinoid tumor
    c. Leiomyosarcoma d. Lymphoma

93. **Aneurysmal dilatation of small bowel is seen in:**
    (Recent Question 2017)
    a. Small bowel lymphoma
    b. Gallstone ileus
    c. Duodenal atresia
    d. Sjogren syndrome

CARCINOID TUMORS

94. **All are true about carcinoid tumors except:** (GB Pant 2011)
    a. Small bowel is the least common site
    b. Multifocal in 30% cases
    c. Associated with synchronous adenocarcinoma
    d. Associated with MEN-1 in 10% cases

95. **All of the following statements about carcinoid tumors are true except:** (All India 2012)
    a. It is the most common malignant tumor of the small intestine
    b. Extensive involvement of small intestine is associated with higher probability of lung metastasis
    c. Five year survival for carcinoids tumors is > 60%
    d. Appendiceal carcinoids are more common in females

96. **Least common volvular disease in carcinoids is:**
    a. TS b. TR (JIPMER GIS 2011)
    c. PR d. PS

97. **All are seen in carcinoid syndrome except:** (HPU 2005)
    a. Diarrhea b. Constipation
    c. Liver metastasis d. 5-HT secretion

98. **The metabolite excreted in the urine carcinoid syndrome is:**
    (MHCET 2016)
    a. VMA b. 17-Ketosteroid
    c. Histamine d. 5-HIAA

99. **All of the following are associated with carcinoid syndrome except:** (MCI Sept 2005)
    a. Cyanosis b. Diarrhea
    c. Flushing d. Acute appendicitis

100. **All of the following about gastrointestinal carcinoid tumors are true, except:** (All India 2010)
    a. Small intestine and appendix account for almost 60% of all gastrointestinal carcinoid
    b. Rectum is spared
    c. 5-years survival for carcinoid tumors is >60%
    d. Appendiceal carcinoids are more common in females than males

101. **True about carcinoid syndrome:** (PGI Nov 2011)
    a. Associated with MEN-1
    b. Serum chromagranin-A is elevated
    c. Urinary excretion of 5-HIAA in increased
    d. Urinary excretion of 5-HIAA is decreased
    e. Octretoide is used for treatment

Small Intestine

102. **False about carcinoid syndrome:** *(PGI May 2011)*
    a. Foregut carcinoid-↑serotonin in blood
    b. Midgut carcinoid-↑serotonin in blood
    c. Foregut carcinoid-↑serotonin in blood
    d. Midgut carcinoid-normal urinary 5-HIAA

103. **Which of the following is true of small bowel carcinoids?**
    a. Most common site is duodenum *(AIIMS Nov 2006)*
    b. It does not cause endocardial fibroelastosis
    c. Increased risk of CA lung
    d. It is the most common malignancy of small intestine

104. **Increased level of 5 HIAA is seen in which disease?**
    (Recent Question 2018)
    a. Carcinoid tumor   b. Phenylketonuria
    c. Pheochromocytoma   d. Adenocarcinoma

105. **Most common site for carcinoid tumor is:**
    (Recent Question 2013)
    a. Esophagus   b. Lung
    c. Appendix   d. Ileum

SMALL INTESTINE TRANSPLANTATION

106. **All are true about intestinal transplant except:**
    a. Principal barrier to widespread application is vigorous rejection reactions *(JIPMER GIS 2011)*
    b. Severe form of GVHD occurs when T cells of graft respond to foreign HLA cells
    c. Uniquely dangerous complication is loss of protective mucosal barrier, bacterial translocation and severe sepsis
    d. Majority of intestinal grafts are multi-visceral grafts

MISCELLANEOUS

107. **Gangrene of intestine is seen in all the following conditions, except:** *(All India 2000)*
    a. Tricuspid valve endocarditis
    b. Shock
    c. Mesenteric artery thrombosis
    d. Volvulus

108. **What is the investigation for small intestine abnormalities except?** *(PGI Dec 2005)*
    a. Enteroclysis   b. Radionuclide
    c. CT enteroclysis   d. MR enteroclysis
    e. USG enteroclysis

109. **Small intestinal biopsy is diagnostic in:** *(PGI June 2006)*
    a. Whipple's disease   b. Abetalipoproteinemia
    c. Celiac disease   d. Agammaglobulinemia

110. **In intestine, lipoma is commonest in:**
    a. Rectum   b. Sigmoid colon
    c. Caecum   d. Ileum

111. **Mass in right iliac fossa can be:** *(Kerala 94)*
    a. Ileocecal Tb   b. Ileocecal neoplasm
    c. Ameboma   d. All of the above

112. **Intestine get strangulated most commonly in which space?**
    (SGPGI 2005)
    a. Omental bursa   b. Paraduodenal space
    c. Rectouterine space d. Subphrenic

113. **Regarding abdominal cocoon all statements are true except:**
    a. Common in young girl   *(PGI Nov 2009)*
    b. Associated with liver fibrosis
    c. Fibrosis of small bowel and stomach
    d. Chronic peritonitis is seen
    e. Seen in tropical and subtropical region

114. **Maximum water reabsorption in the gastrointestinal tract occurs in:** *(All India 2011)*
    a. Stomach   b. Jejunum
    c. Ileum   d. Colon

115. **On contrast radiography which among the following is false?** *(AIIMS May 2011)*
    a. Ileum is featureless
    b. Colon has haustrations
    c. Jejunum is feathery
    d. Distal part of duodenum has a cap

116. **Pain in hypogastric region may arise from:** *(PGI May 2010)*
    a. Uterus   b. Left colon
    c. Urinary bladder   d. Gallbladder

117. **Vitellointestinal duct closure is usually done at what age?**
    (MHSSMCET 2007)
    a. At birth   b. 9 months
    c. 6 weeks   d. 12 months

118. **Which of the following is most prominent feature of immunoproliferative small intestine disease (IPSID)?**
    (AIIMS May 2012)
    a. Malabsorption   b. Obstruction
    c. Bleeding   d. Abdominal pain

Explanations

MECKEL'S DIVERTICULUM

1. Ans. e. Diarrhea very common *(Ref: Sabiston 20/e p1284; Schwartz 10/e p1163-1165; Bailey 27/e p1252; Shackelford 8/e p911, 7/e p695-698)*
2. Ans. d. 2% are symptomatic *(Ref: Schwartz 10/e p1163; Sabiston 20/e p1284; Bailey 27/e p1252)*
3. Ans. a. Tc-99 radionuclide scan
4. Ans. d. All incidentally detected Meckel's diverticulum should be resected
5. Ans. a. Hemorrhage
6. Ans. c. Meckel's diverticulum *(Ref: Sabiston 20/e p1284; Schwartz 10/e p1164; Bailey 27/e p131)*
7. Ans. b. Vitellointestinal duct
8. Ans. b. Meckel's diverticulum
9. Ans. c. Arises at the mesenteric border
10. Ans. b. Consists of mucosa without a muscle coat
11. Ans. d. Radionuclide scan
12. Ans. a. Resection of diverticulum *(Ref: Sabiston 20/e p1286; Shackelford 8/e p912, 7/e p698, 1065)*

> **Incidentally Detected Meckel's Diverticulum**
> - Epidemiologic studies suggest that resection of asymptomatic Meckel's diverticulum is indicated in most patients because of **6.4% life time risk of complications** from a Meckel's diverticulum that persist over increasing age groups; a cumulative incidence of early **(12%)** and late **(7%)** post-operative morbidity and mortality after resection of symptomatic Meckel's diverticula and the 2% life time risk of developing complications after incidental diverticulectomy. Authors concluded that **barring any strong contraindications, incidentally discovered Meckel's diverticula should be removed.**

13. Ans. d. All are correct
14. Ans. c. Meckel's diverticulum
15. Ans. b. 60
16. Ans. d. Wide mouth stapling at the base for non bleeding cases *(Ref: Bailey 27/e p1252)*

Wide mouth stapling at the base for non bleeding ulcer is not done in Meckel's diverticulum.

> **MECKEL'S DIVERTICULECTOMY**
> - A Meckel's diverticulum that is broad based should **not be amputated at its base** and invaginated in the same way as a vermiform appendix, because of **risk of stricture**.
> - Furthermore, this does not remove hetrotopic epithelium where it is present.

17. Ans. c. Malignancy
18. Ans. d. Meckel's diverticulum
19. Ans. d. Metoclopramide
20. Ans. a. Present in 3% of the population
21. Ans. a. Most common congenital anomaly of the intestine *(Ref: Sabiston 20/e p1284; Schwartz 10/e p1164; Bailey 27/e p131)*

SMALL INTESTINAL DIVERTICULA

22. Ans. d. Seen on the mesenteric border *(Ref: Sabiston 20/e p1280; Schwartz 10/e p1165; Bailey 27/e p1251; Shackelford 8/e p909-9/0, 7/e p691-700)*

> - MC acquired diverticula of the **small bowel: Duodenal diverticula**[Q]
> - MC true congenital diverticulum of the small bowel: Meckel's diverticulum[Q]
> - Most small intestinal diverticula are false diverticula except Meckel's diverticulum[Q]
> - Most small intestinal diverticula arises from mesenteric aspect except Meckel's diverticulum[Q]

23. Ans. a. Whenever found, should be treated due to increased risk of complications *(Ref: Sabiston 20/e p1281; Schwartz 10/e p1165; Bailey 27/e p1251; Shackelford 8/e p910, 7/e p691-695)*
24. Ans. c. ↓ B12 absorption, e. Steatorrhoea *(Ref: Sabiston 20/e p1282; Schwartz 10/e p1167; Bailey 27/e p1252; Shackelford 8/e p909, 7/e p698-700)*

GASTROINTESTINAL TUBERCULOSIS

25. Ans. d. Conservative management is treatment of choice *(Ref: Sabiston 20/e p1079-1268; Bailey 27/e p1249)*
26. Ans. b. Causes intestinal perforation, c. Commonly associated with pulmonary TB, d. Caused by mycobacterium TB

- MC site of GI tuberculosis: **Ileocecal region**^Q
- MC type of Abdominal tuberculosis: **Peritoneal tuberculosis**^Q

27. Ans. a. Diarrhea, c. Stricture, d. Malabsorption   28. Ans. b. Intestine obstruction
29. Ans. c. Surgery is the treatment of choice
30. Ans. a. String sign of Kantor   *(Ref: Sabiston 20/e p1263; Bailey 27/e p1248)*
31. Ans. a. Obstruction
32. Ans. b. Ileum   33. Ans. d. Intestinal mucosa
34. Ans. a. String sign, b. Goose neck sign, c. Right sided obstruction, d. Pulled up cecum, e. Sterlein sign
35. Ans. b. Typhoid   *(Ref: J Indian Med Assoc 199; 89:255-6)*

- **Ileal perforation** is a common problem seen in **tropical countries**. The **commonest cause being typhoid fever**^Q.
- In **western countries** the causes are **malignancy, trauma** and **mechanical etiology**, in the order of frequency^Q.

36. Ans. c. Ileocecal tuberculosis   37. Ans. a. Ileocecal TB

SUPERIOR MESENTERIC ARTERY SYNDROME

38. Ans. d. Most common in 6th-7th decade *(Ref: Sabiston 20/e p1292; Shackelford 8/e p782, 7/e p866)*
39. Ans. b. Duodenal obstruction
40. Ans. d. Gastrojejunostomy is treatment of choice in chronic cases *(Ref: Sabiston 20/e p1292)*

- TOC in annular pancreas: **Duodenoduodenostomy**^Q
- TOC in duodenal atresia: Diamond shaped **Duodenoduodenostomy**^Q
- TOC in SMA syndrome: **Duodenojejunostomy**^Q

41. Ans. a. Superior mesenteric artery is compressed by....... *(Ref: Sabiston 20/e p1292)*

PNEUMATOSIS INTESTINALIS

42. Ans. a. Pneumatosis cystoides intestinalis *(Ref: Sabiston 20/e p1289; Schwartz 10/e p1170-1171; Shackelford 8/e p768, 7/e p1057-1058)*
43. Ans. a. High flow oxygen therapy   44. Ans. b. Neonatal necrotizing enterocolitis
45. Ans. b. Surgical resection indicated   46. Ans. a. Pneumatosis cystoides intestinalis
47. Ans. b. Necrotizing enterocolitis

SHORT BOWEL SYNDROME

48. Ans. b. Short bowel syndrome *(Ref: Sabiston 20/e p1291; Schwartz 10/e p1171-1173; Bailey 27/e p1256; Shackelford 8/e p921, 7/e p998-1014)*
49. Ans. a. If jejunum is cut...., d. Bile acid malabsorption *(Ref: Schwartz 10/e p1171-1173; Sabiston 20/e p1291; Bailey 27/e p1256)*
50. Ans. a. Hypogastrinemia
51. Ans. b. Malabsorption, c. Steatorrhea, d. Cholelithiasis, e. Renal oxalate stones *(Ref: Schwartz 10/e p1171-1173; Sabiston 20/e p1291; Bailey 27/e p1256)*
52. Ans. d. All of the above   53. Ans. a. Vitamin B_{12}
54. Ans. c. More oxalate absorption in gut   55. Ans. a. Hypogastrinemia *(Ref: Harrison 20/e p2255, 19/e p1443)*

- Harrison says "**Gastric hypersecretion** of **acid** occurs in many patients **following large resection** of the **small intestine**. The etiology is unclear but may be **related to reduced hormonal inhibition** of acid secretion or **increased gastrin levels** due to **reduced small intestinal catabolism** of circulating gastrin."

56. Ans. a. GLP-2 analogue *(Ref: Sabiston 20/e p1292)*

- "Randomized controlled trials have shown that *teduglutide, a GLP-2 analogue* that is *resistant to degradation by the proteolytic enzyme dipeptidyl peptidase 4 and therefore has a longer half-life than GLP-2, is well tolerated and has led to the restoration of intestinal functional and structural integrity through significant intestinotrophic and proabsorptive effects. It is the first targeted therapeutic agent to gain approval for use in adult short bowel syndrome with intestinal failure.*"
  Sabiston 20/e p1292

RADIATION ENTERITIS

57. Ans. a. Radiation enteritis *(Ref: Sabiston 20/e p1290; Schwartz 10/e p1162-1163; Shackelford 8/e p915, 7/e p986-997)*
58. Ans. b. 5000 rad   59. Ans. b. 4000 rad

ENTERIC FEVER

60. **Ans. c. 3rd week** *(Ref: Sabiston 20/e p1266; Bailey 27/e p1248; Harrison 20/e p1175)*
61. **Ans. b. Longitudinal ulcers**
62. **Ans. a. Plain X-ray of abdomen in erect posture**
63. **Ans. c. Enteric perforation**
64. **Ans. d. 1-Tuberculosis & 2-Typhoid** *(Ref: Sabiston 20/e p1266; Schwartz 10/e p1154; Bailey 27/e p82)*

Tuberculosis	Typhoid
Transverse ulcers in ileum	Longitudinal ulcers in ileum

SMALL BOWEL RESECTION AND ANASTOMOSIS

65. **Ans. a. Suture in 1 layer by non-absorbable suture** *(Ref: Shackelford 8/e p1008, 7/e p920-928)*
66. **Ans. c. Stricturoplasty**

- For **multiple strictures** involving **long segment** of **small intestine, stricturoplasty** is preferred to **prevent short bowel syndrome**[Q].

ENTERIC FISTULA

67. **Ans. c. Non-epithelialization** *(Ref: Sabiston 20/e p1287; Schwartz 10/e p1158; Bailey 27/e p1256; Shackelford 8/e p888, 7/e p944-946)*
68. **Ans. d. Track length >3 cm**
69. **Ans. a. Tract < 1 cm**
70. **Ans. c. > 2 cm fistulous tract**
71. **Ans. b. Duodenal** *(Ref: Sabiston 20/e p1287)*

- In general, the **more proximal the fistula** in the intestine, the **more serious the problem**, with **greater fluid** and **electrolyte loss**[Q].
- The **drainage** has a **greater digestive capacity**, and the **distal segment** is **not available** for **absorption** of **nutrients**[Q].

INTESTINAL ATRESIA AND DUPLICATION

72. **Ans. a. Intestinal atresia** *(Ref: Sabiston 20/e p1870-1871; Schwartz 10/e p1615-1616; Bailey 27/e p133; Shackelford 8/e p973, 7/e p1049-1051)*
73. **Ans. c. Ileum** *(Ref: Shackelford 8/e p978, 7/e p1051-1053)*
74. **Ans. b. Intestinal atresia**
75. **Ans. a. Spherical type is MC, b. Tubular type is attached longitudinally with bowel**
76. **Ans. a. Duodenum**
77. **Ans. d. Duodenoduodenostomy**
78. **Ans. c. Type III** *(Ref: Sabiston 20/e p1871; Schwartz 10/e p1616; Bailey 27/e p133-134)*

- **"Apple** peel" atresia or "Christmas tree" atresia is type IIIb of intestinal atresia.

Small Intestine

Classification of Intestinal Atresia	
Type I	**Membranous atresia** with **intact bowel & mesentery**
Type II	**Blind ends** separated by a **fibrous cord**
Type IIIa	**Blind ends** separated by a **V-shaped mesenteric defect**
Type IIIb	**"Apple peel"** atresia^Q or **"Christmas tree"** ^Q atresia
Type IV	**Multiple atresias ("string of sausages")**^Q

79. Ans. c. Type 3 *(Ref: Sabiston 20/e p1871; Shackelford 7/e p1050)*
80. Ans. d. All are correct *(Ref: Schwartz 10/e p1624; Bailey 27/e p136)*   81. Ans. b. Jejunal atresia

NEOPLASMS OF SMALL INTESTINE

82. Ans. a. Lymphoma *(Ref: Schwartz 10/e p1159; Bailey 27/e p1250; Shackelford 8/e p 965, 7/e p771)*
83. Ans. b. Most common site is ileum *(Ref: Sabiston 20/e p1277; Schwartz 10/e p1159; Shackelford 8/e p965, 7/e p771)*

- **Duodenum** is **MC site** of **Atresia** and **Adenocarcinoma**^Q.
- **Jejunum** is **MC site** of (**PIA**): **P**neumatosis Intestinalis, **A**ngiodysplasia^Q
- **Ileum** is **MC site** of (**DAL-3**): **D**uplication, **A**denoma (tubular), **L**ipoma, **L**ymphoma, **L**eiomyoma^Q.

84. Ans. b. Carcinoid tumors   85. Ans. a. Leiomyoma *(Ref: Shackelford 7/e p771)*
86. Ans. d. Palliative surgeries are done even in presence of metastasis *(Ref: Sabiston 20/e p1271; Schwartz 9/e p999-1001; Bailey 27/e p1251)*
87. Ans. a. Ba meal follow through, d. CT scan with contrast
88. Ans. b. Arises from periampullary region, c. Jaundice and anemia found, e. Surgery is only curative
89. Ans. b. Primary small-intestinal lymphomas are most commonly located in the ileum, c. Lymphoma is most common primary malignant neoplasm of Spleen, d. Stomach is most common site for extranodal lymphoma and e. MALT lymphoma is associated with H. pylori infection *(Ref: Harrison 20/e p571, 19/e p537; Sabiston 20/e p1278)*
90. Ans. b. Melanoma *(Ref: Sabiston 20/e p1280)*

- **Cutaneous melanoma**^Q is the **MC extra-abdominal source** to **involve the small intestine**; others include adenocarcinoma of the **breast** and **carcinoma** of the **lung**.

91. Ans. d. Causes malabsorption
92. Ans. a. Adenocarcinoma *(Ref: Sabiston 20/e p1276; Schwartz 10/e p1159)*

"Adenocarcinomas constitute approximately 50% of the malignant tumors of the small bowel."-Sabiston 20/e p1276

93. Ans. a. Small bowel lymphoma *(Ref: Clinical Imaging of Small Intestine 2/e p415)*

"The typical presentation of a small bowel lymphoma is a thick walled infiltrating mass with aneurysmal dilatation without obstruction. Aneurysmal dilatation is based on destruction of small bowel wall and myenteric nerve plexus."
(Ref: Clinical Imaging of Small Intestine 2/e p415)

CARCINOID TUMORS

94. Ans. a. Small bowel is the least common site *(Ref: Sabiston 20/e p1272; Schwartz 10/e p1161; Bailey 27/e p1250; Harrison 20/e p598, 19/e p563)*
95. Ans. b. Extensive involvement of small intestine is associated with higher probability of lung metastasis *(Ref: Sabiston 20/e p1276; Schwartz 10/e p1162; Bailey 27/e p1250)*

Extensive involvement of **small intestine by carcinoid tumor** is associated with **higher probability** of liver (not the lung) metastasis.

- **MC malignant tumor** of **small intestine: Adenocarcinoma**^Q > **Carcinoid**
- **Carcinoid tumors** have the **best prognosis** of **all small bowel tumors**, whether the disease is localized or metastatic.
- **Resection of a carcinoid tumor localized** to **its primary site** approaches a **100% survival rate**^Q.
- **Five-year survival rates** are about **65%** among patients **with regional disease** and 25% to 35% among those with distant metastasis.
- **Appendiceal carcinoids** are **more common in females**^Q.
- **Extensive involvement** of **small intestine** is associated with **higher probability** of **liver metastasis**^Q

96. Ans. d. PS   97. Ans. b. Constipation   98. Ans. d. 5-HIAA
99. Ans. d. Acute appendicitis   100. Ans. b. Rectum is spared

101. Ans. a. Associated with MEN-I, b. Serum chromogranin A is elevated, c. Urinary excretion of 5-HIAA in increased, e. Octreotide is used for treatment
102. Ans. a. Foregut carcinoid-↑serotonin in blood, d. Midgut carcinoid-normal urinary 5-HIAA
103. Ans. d. It is the most common malignancy of small intestine
104. Ans. a. Carcinoid tumor *(Ref: Sabiston 20/e p1273; Schwartz 10/e p1161; Bailey 27/e p1251)*
105. Ans. b. Lung

SMALL INTESTINE TRANSPLANTATION

106. Ans. d. Majority of intestinal grafts are multivisceral grafts *(Ref: Sabiston 20/e p668; Schwartz 10/e p352-354; Bailey 27/e p1555; Shackelford 8/e p934, 7/e p1008-1012)*

MISCELLANEOUS

107. Ans. a. Tricuspid valve endocarditis
    Shock, mesenteric artery thrombosis and volvulus can lead to gangrene of intestine.
108. Ans. e. USG enteroclysis *(Ref: Schwartz 10/e p1161,1163,1164; Shackelford 8/e p868, 7/e p868, 884, 993)*

ENTEROCLYSIS (SMALL BOWEL ENEMA)

- **Contrast** in injected directly through **Frekas tube directly into distal duodenum**, filling the small bowel loops[Q].
- The opacified small bowel loops can be **imaged** then **using X-rays** (Barium enteroclysis), **CT** (CT enteroclysis) or **MRI** (MRI enteroclysis).[Q]

Enteroclysis is Investigation of Choice in
- Partial, intermittent small intestinal obstruction[Q]
- Small intestinal diverticula[Q]
- Crohn's disease[Q]

109. Ans. a. Whipple's disease, b. Abetalipoproteinemia, d. Agammaglobulinemia *(Ref: Harrison 20/e p2251, 19/e p1940)*

Disease that can be Diagnosed by Small-intestinal Mucosal Biopsies	
Lesions	**Pathologic Findings**
Diffuse, Specific	
• Whipple's disease[Q]	• **Lamina propria** contains **macrophages containing PAS +** material
• Agammaglobulinemia[Q]	• No plasma cells; either **normal or absent villi ("flat mucosa")**
• Abetalipoproteinemia[Q]	• Normal villi; **epithelial cells vacuolated with fat postprandially**
Patchy, Specific	
• Intestinal lymphoma	• Malignant cells in lamina propria and submucosa
• Intestinal lymphangiectasia	• Dilated lymphatics; clubbed villi
• Eosinophilic gastroenteritis	• Eosinophil infiltration of lamina propria and mucosa
• Amyloidosis	• Amyloid deposits
• Crohn's disease	• **Noncaseating granulomas**
• Infections	• Specific organisms
• Mastocytosis	• **Mast cell infiltration of lamina propria**
Diffuse, Nonspecific	
• Celiac disease	• **Short** or **absent villi**; mononuclear infiltrate; epithelial cell damage; hypertrophy of crypts
• Tropical sprue	• Similar to celiac disease
• Bacterial overgrowth	• Patchy damage to villi; lymphocyte infiltration
• Folate deficiency	• **Short villi; decreased mitosis in crypts; megalocytosis**
• Vitamin B_{12} deficiency	• Similar to folate deficiency
• Radiation enteritis	• Similar to folate deficiency
• Zollinger-Ellison syndrome	• **Mucosal ulceration** and **erosion** from acid
• Protein-calorie malnutrition	• **Villous atrophy; secondary bacterial overgrowth**
• Drug-Induced enteritis	• Variable histology

110. Ans. d. Ileum
111. Ans. d. All of the above
112. Ans. a. Omental bursa

113. **Ans. b. Associated with liver fibrosis** *(Ref: www.emedicine_hlml/cocoon)*

IDIOPATHIC SCLEROSING ENCAPSULATING PERITONITIS (ABDOMINAL COCOON)

- It is a rare condition of **unknown cause** in which **intestinal obstruction** results from the **encasement of variable lengths** of bowel by a **dense fibrocollagenous membrane** that gives the **appearance of a cocoon**[Q].

Causes of Secondary Cocoon	
• **Previous abdominal surgery or peritonitis**[Q]	• Use of **providone iodine** for abdominal wash out
• Chronic ambulatory peritoneal dialysis (**CAPD**)[Q]	• Placement of **Lee Veen shunt** for **refractory ascites**[Q]
• **Prolonged use** of beta blocker propranolol[Q]	• **SLE**[Q]

Clinical Features
- Occurrence of **intestinal obstruction** in a relatively **young girl without** an **obvious cause**[Q]
- History of similar episodes that **resolved spontaneously**[Q]
- Abdominal pain and **vomiting**[Q]
- Presence of a **non tender soft mass** on abdominal palpation
- Features of **increasing abdominal distension**, **jaundice** and features suggestive of liver pathology

Diagnosis
- Barium meal follow through: Serpentine configuration of **dilated small bowel**[Q]
- CT scan is helpful

Treatment
- Laparotomy with **removal of the membrane**, after which recovery is usually complete

114. **Ans. b. Jejunum** *(Ref: Ganong 25/e p464)*

- **Maximum water absorption** from **GIT** occurs in **jejunum**[Q] (5500 mL) >**Ileum** (2000 mL) >**Colon** (1300 mL).

SMALL INTESTINE (ANATOMY AND PHYSIOLOGY)

- Average length: 600 cm
- **Duodenum: 20 cm; Jejunum: 250 cm; Ileum: 350 cm**[Q]
- **Largest endocrine organ** of the body: **Small bowel**[Q]
- **Strongest component** of small intestine: **Submucosa**[Q] (used for manufacturing **catgut sutures**)
- **Pacemaker** of **small bowel** is located in: **Duodenum**[Q]
- Proximal bowel (**jejunum**) absorbs: Calcium, iron, folate and **fats**[Q]
- Distal bowel (**ileum**) absorbs: Bile salts, vitamin B12[Q]

115. **Ans. d. Distal part of duodenum has a cap** *(Ref: BDC 4/e vol II/p251)*

The first part of duodenum has duodenal cap or bulb, not the distal part.

SMALL INTESTINE RADIOGRAPHY

- The **first part of duodenum** is visible as a **triangular shadow** on barium studies known as **duodenal cap**[Q].
- The **small intestine** contains **mucosal folds** known as **plicae ciculares** or **valvulae conniventes**[Q] that are visible of barium studies and help in the distinction between small intestine and colon.
- **Colon** can be identified by the presence of **haustrations**[Q].
- **Valvulae conniventes** are **more prominent** in jejunum giving the **'feathery'**[Q] **appearance** on barium. These **mucosal folds** are **gradually reduced distally** giving **'featureless'** appearance of distal **ileum**[Q].

116. **Ans. a. Uterus, b. Left colon, c. Urinary bladder** *(Ref: BDC 4/e vol II/p221)*

PAIN IN HYPOGASTRIUM AND PELVIS

- Common causes of pain in this area include **rectal disease** (rectal cancer, proctitis), **bladder diseases** (stones, cystitis, carcinoma), and **uterus** (salpingo-oophoritis, uterine cancer) in females.

117. **Ans. c. 6 weeks** *(Ref: Bailey 27/e p131)*

- **Spontaneous obliteration** of **omphalomesenteric** or **vitallointestinal duct** occurs **before** the **6th week** of **intrauterine life**[Q].

118. **Ans. a. Malabsorption** *(Ref: Harrison 19/e p537, 719)*

IMMUNOPROLIFERATIVE SMALL-INTESTINAL DISEASE (IPSID)

- **IPSID** is recognized as an **infectious pathogen–associated human lymphoma** that has **association with Campylobacter jejuni**[Q].
- It **involves mainly** the **proximal small intestine** resulting in **malabsorption, diarrhea,** and **abdominal pain**[Q].
- IPSID is associated with **excessive plasma cell differentiation** and **produces truncated alpha heavy chain proteins lacking the light chains** as well as the **first constant domain**[Q].

Treatment

- **Early-stage IPSID** responds to **antibiotics (30–70% complete remission)**[Q].
- **Most untreated IPSID** patients progress to **lymphoplasmacytic** and **immunoblastic lymphoma**[Q].
- **Patients not responding to antibiotic therapy** are considered for treatment with **combination chemotherapy** used to treat low-grade lymphoma[Q].

CHAPTER 14

Large Intestine

HIRSCHSPRUNG'S DISEASE

Hirschsprung's Disease

- Occurs in **1** out of every **5000 live births**^Q

  - **MC affected site**: **Rectosigmoid (75%)**^Q > splenic flexure or transverse colon (17%) > **Entire colon** with **variable extension into** the **small bowel**^Q (8%)

- **Increased Risk**: Positive family history^Q & **Down syndrome**^Q

Pathogenesis
- One type of **neurocristopathies**^Q; Consequence of **defective migration of neural crest cell to colonic mucosa**^Q
- Characterized pathologically by **absent ganglion cells** in the **myenteric (Auerbach's)** & **submucosal (Meissner's) plexus** with **hypertrophy of nerve trunks**^Q in the plexus
- Associated with **muscular spasm** of the **distal colon** & **internal anal sphincter** resulting in a **functional obstruction**^Q
- **Abnormal bowel** is the **contracted distal segment**, whereas the **normal bowel** is the **proximal, dilated portion**^Q.

Clinical Presentation		
Neonates	**First few weeks of life**	**Otherwise healthy children and adults**
• **Suspected in** all neonates presenting with: – **Delayed passage** of **meconium beyond** the **first 24 hours of life**^Q – **Abdominal distension following feeds**^Q	• **Suspected in** any child presenting in first few weeks of life with: – **Gross** abdominal **distension**^Q – **Chronic constipation**^Q – **Failure to thrive**^Q	• **Short segment Hirschsprung disease** should be suspected in **otherwise healthy children** and **adults**^Q presenting with: – **Severe constipation without fecal soiling**^Q – **Faecal soiling** is usually **not a feature** of this **condition**.

Digital Examination
- **Rectum** is **empty** on digital examination^Q;   **Rapid expulsion of feces** often follows examination^Q
- **Contracted rectal wall** can sometimes be appreciated by examining finger

Diagnosis		
Rectal biopsy	**Anorectal manometry**	**Radiology**
• **Gold standard for** the **diagnosis of** Hirschsprung's disease • Confirms the diagnosis on demonstration of: – Aganglionosis^Q – Hypertrophic nerve trunks^Q – Increased acetylcholine esterase staining^Q	• Useful as a **screening test**^Q • Rectoanal inhibitory **reflex is absent**^Q	• **Water soluble contrast enema** indicates the **length** and **site** of **involved intestine**. • Important positive findings include: – **Coning down** of **transition zone** – Irregularity in mucosa – **Abnormal contraction** of intestine

- **Repeated tube decompression** and gentle **rectal washouts** with 30-50 ml of **normal saline** have a positive and significant clinical impact on these patients.

Treatment of Hirschsprung's Disease	
Short segment disease	**Long segment disease**
• **Extended myectomy**^Q removing a **strip of rectal wall** up to the area where normal ganglion cells start may be sufficient	• **Temporary colostomy**^Q for a few months to allow proximal intestine to return to its normal caliber followed by **definitive procedures**: – Swenson^Q – Duhamel^Q – Soave^Q

Prognosis
- **Excellent** overall survival
- MC post-operative problems: Constipation (MC)[Q] >soiling >incontinence >enterocolitis.

COLONIC DIVERTICULA

Colonic Diverticula

- A **diverticulum** is an **abnormal sac or pouch protruding from the wall of a hollow organ**
- **True diverticulum** is composed of **all layers of the intestinal wall**[Q]
- **False diverticulum (pseudodiverticulum) lacks a portion** of the **normal bowel wall**[Q].

> - **Acquired diverticula** are the **MC type**[Q] and are mainly **false**[Q] diverticula
> - **MC site**[Q] of **colonic diverticula: Sigmoid colon**

Pathogenesis
- Diverticula are **herniation of mucosa through** the **muscularis propria**

> - **Protrusion** occurs **at the point** where the **nutrient artery penetrates** through **the muscularis propria**[Q], resulting in a break of the colonic wall, **mainly on mesenteric side**

- In some cases, the **arteriole** penetrating the wall can be **displaced over** the **dome** of **diverticulum** which results in **massive hemorrhage**[Q]

> - Another factor is **increased intraluminal pressure**[Q], **diets low in fiber** reduce the stool bulk which in turn leads to **increased peristaltic activity**, particularly in the **sigmoid colon**. This increases the intraluminal pressure.

- Diverticulosis is **more common in the western world**[Q], its **rare** in the **underdeveloped & developing countries**, where **diets include** more **fibre** and **roughage**[Q].

> - There is often a striking hypertrophy of the muscular layers of the colonic wall[Q] associated with diverticulosis.
> - This thickening of the colonic wall, most commonly affecting the sigmoid colon, may precede the appearance of diverticula[Q].

Diagnosis
- **Barium enema** is **investigation of choice** for **colonic diverticulosis**[Q].
- **Thickening** of the **circular muscle fibres** develops a **concertina** or **saw-tooth appearance** on **barium enema**[Q].
- **Investigation of choice** for **colonic diverticulosis: Barium enema**[Q]
- **Investigation of choice** for **diverticulitis: CT scan**[Q]

COLORECTAL POLYPS

Histological Classification of Colorectal Polyps	
Neoplastic Polyps	**Non-neoplastic polyps**

Adenomatous polyps or Adenomas:
- Tubular
- Tubulovillous
- Villous
	1. Hyperplastic polyps
	2. Hamartomatous polyps:
	   – Juvenile polyps
	   – PJS
	3. Inflammatory polyps

NON-NEOPLASTIC POLYPS

Non-neoplastic Polyps

- **Hyperplastic Polyps**
  - **MC colorectal polyp**[Q]
  - Account for **>90% of all colorectal polyps**, mostly found in the **rectosigmoid**[Q].
  - Histologic appearance of these polyps is serrated (**saw-toothed appearance**)[Q]
  - **No malignant potential**[Q]

Large Intestine

- **Hamartomatous Polyps**
  - A hamartomatous polyp is a localized overgrowth of normal, mature intestinal epithelial cells.
  - Usually lined with normal epithelium over a submucosal core.
  - Juvenile polyps are the MC type of colorectal hamartomas^Q

  > **Juvenile polyps**
  > - Juvenile polyps are the **MC type of colorectal hamartomas**^{Q}
  > - Occur most commonly in children **<5 years of age**^{Q}.
  > - Up to 80% of juvenile polyps occur as a **single lesion of the rectum**^{Q}
  > - Typical symptoms are **rectal bleeding**, **mucus discharge**, **diarrhea**, & **abdominal pain**^{Q}.
  > - Also called **retention polyps** due to the inflammatory obstruction of the crypt necks that leads to cystic dilation of the mucus-filled glands.
  > - **No increased risk of cancer**^{Q}

  > **Peutz-Jegher's Syndrome (AD)**
  > - PJS is also characterized by **hamartomatous polyps**^{Q}.
  > - Histological characteristics: **Arborization** & **Pseudoinvasion**^{Q}

- **Inflammatory Polyps**
  - Inflammatory polyps occur more frequently in **chronic ulcerative colitis**^{Q}, but are also seen in **Crohn's disease**^{Q}.
  - Inflammatory polyps have **no malignant potential**^{Q} and **require no treatment**^{Q} other than that of underlying colitis.

ADENOMATOUS POLYPS

Adenomatous Polyps

- **MC neoplastic polyp** is adenomatous, which harbors malignant potential^Q.
- Most colon cancers arise from adenomatous polyps (adenoma)^Q.
- Conditions associated with adenomatous polyps: Strong association with ureterosigmoidostomies^Q, acromegaly^Q and streptococcus bovis bactermia^Q

Probability of development of malignancy depends upon		
Gross Appearance of lesion	**Histology**	**Size**
• Pedunculated • **Sessile (Increased risk)**^{Q}	• **Tubular (MC)**^{Q} • Tubulovillous • **Villous (Highest risk)**^{Q}	• <1 cm • 1-2 cm • **>2 cm (Increased risk)**^{Q}

Adenomatous Polyps			
Types	**Incidence**	**Villous tissue**	**Risk of Malignancy**
Tubular	65-80%^{Q}	<25%	5%
Tubulovillous	10-25%	25-75%	20%
Villous	5-10%	>75%^{Q}	40%^{Q}

PEUTZ-JEGHER'S SYNDROME (AD)

Peutz-Jegher's Syndrome (AD)

- **Hamartomatous polyps** (usually <100) throughout the GIT, **most common in jejunum**^{Q}
- Associated with **hypermelanotic macule** in the **perioral region, buccal mucosa**^{Q}.
- Mucocutaneous pigmentation usually occurs during infancy and most commonly noted in perioral & buccal region.

  > - Pigment spots usually appear in first few years of life, reach a maximum level in early adolescence and can fade in adulthood^Q. However, pigmentation on the buccal mucosa remains throughout the life^Q.
  > - **Pigmented macules** of PJS have **no malignant potential**^{Q}.

- Polyposis develops by age 20, occur most commonly in the jejunum (**jejunum**^{Q} >colon >stomach).

Histology
- Smooth muscle extends into the superficial epithelial layer in a tree like manner known as **arborization**[Q].
- **Pseudoinvasion (epithelial cell trapping)**[Q] is noted in up to 10% of polyps >3 cm.

Genetics
- It exhibits **autosomal dominant** inheritance[Q]
- Chromosome **19p13.3** encodes the serine threonine kinase **LKB1/STK11**[Q].

Extraintestinal Features
- **Increased risk** for **extraintestinal cancer** of the **pancreas**, **thyroid**, **breast** (may be bilateral), **lung**, **gallbladder**, **biliary tract (cholangiocarcinoma)**[Q].
- **Increased risk of gynecologic malignancies of the ovary** (bilateral sex cord tumors with annular features) & **uterus** (well-differentiated adenocarcinoma of the cervix, known as **adenoma malignum**)[Q]
- In men there is **increased risk** of **feminizing Sertoli cell tumors** of the testis[Q].

COWDEN'S DISEASE

COWDEN'S DISEASE

- Characterized by **multiple hamartomatous tumors** arising from all three embryonal cell layers (ectoderm, mesoderm & endoderm), **mucocutaneous lesions**, **developmental anomalies**[Q] and a predilection to develop **breast & thyroid neoplasia**.
- Polyps arise more commonly from **ectodermal**[Q] rather than endodermal elements.
- MC feature: **Multiple trichilemmomas**[Q] (type of benign hair shaft tumor)
- 2nd MC system involved: CNS
- Associated with megalencephaly, ataxia, epilepsy, dysplastic gangliocytoma of the cerebellum known as **Lhermitte Duclos syndrome**[Q].
- Polyps are typically small & occur from mouth to anus, but are observed **most commonly in the colon**[Q].
- Developmental disorders include **high arched palate** & **adenoid facies, prominent forehead, hypoplastic mandible.**[Q]
- Gene: PTEN gene (10q23.3)[Q]

Associations
- Estimated lifetime risk of thyroid cancer (mainly FCT): **10%**
- Estimated lifetime risk of **breast cancer: 30-50%**.
- **No increased risk** of **invasive gastrointestinal malignancy**[Q]

CRONKHITE-CANADA SYNDROME

CRONKHITE-CANADA SYNDROME

- It is an **acquired**[Q], nonhereditary, non-familial gastrointestinal polyposis disorder associated with **skin pigmentary changes, hair loss, & nail atrophy (onychodystrophy).**[Q]
- **No evidence of colorectal malignancy**[Q]

Characteristic Features
- MC symptom is **diarrhea**[Q].
- **Hair loss** occur in **all part of body**[Q] and hair regrowth during spontaneous remission and after therapy.
- Polyps are found throughout the gastrointestinal tract with **characteristic esophageal sparing**[Q].
- MC site of polyp: **Stomach**[Q]

> - **Mortality** associated with this syndrome is up to 60% due to associated non-malignant complications (**diarrhea, dehydration, hypoproteinemia**)[Q].

Management
- Supportive care, with management of fluids, electrolytes, nutrition and anemia is important consideration.
- Medical management is usually required for 6-12 months, and corticosteroids have been used with success for disease recurrence[Q]

RUVALCABA-MYHRE-SMITH SYNDROME

RUVALCABA-MYHRE-SMITH SYNDROME

- Also referred to as **Bannayan-Zonana syndrome**[Q], **Ruvalcaba-Riley Smith syndrome**, and Bannayan-Riley-Ruvalcaba syndrome
- Characterized by **hamartomatous polyposis** and **OLD HM-2**

Large Intestine

OLD HM-2
• Ocular abnormalities, Lipomas, Developmental abnormalities • Hashimoto's thyroiditis, Hyperpigmentation of penis. • Macrocephaly, Mental retardation

- **No increased risk of colorectal carcinoma**, other **gastrointestinal** or **extraintestinal malignancy**^{Q}

FAMILIAL ADENOMATOUS POLYPOSIS (AD)

Familial Adenomatous Polyposis (AD)

- FAP is an **autosomal dominant**^{Q} inherited syndrome
- Results in the development of **>100 adenomatous polyps**^{Q}.
- Location of APC gene: **Long arm of chromosome 5q21.**
- Increased number of polyps predisposes patients to a greater risk of cancer^Q.
- Accounts for **<1%**^{Q} of all cases of CRC
- **Earliest phenotypic change** present is known as **aberrant crypt formation**^{Q}

  - **Average age of adenoma development** in FAP is **15 years**^{Q}, with approximately 15% manifesting polyps by 10 years, 75% by 20 years, and 90% by 30 years of age.
  - If left untreated, colorectal cancer develops in nearly **100%**^{Q} of these patients **by age 40 years**^{Q}

Extra-Intestinal Features		
• **Osteomas (mandible & skull)**^{Q} • **Desmoid tumors**^{Q}	• Thyroid papillary tumors • **Medulloblastomas**^{Q} • Hypertrophic gastric fundic polyps^Q	• **CHRPE**^{Q} • Benign dental abnormalities • Epidermoid cyst

- Congenital hypertrophy of the retinal epithelium (CHRPEs) are asymptomatic and have no malignant potential; and are significantly larger, multiple, bilateral and with mixed pigment than sporadic CHRPE.

  - After CRC, **MC malignancy** diagnosed in patients with FAP is **periampullary adenocarcinoma of duodenum**^{Q}.
  - After the CRC is eliminated by surgery, **periampullary tumors**^{Q} are **MC cause of death** among individuals with FAP.

- Others are tumors of the brain, hepatoblastoma, adrenal gland, thyroid, pancreas, biliary tree, stomach, & small intestine.

Diagnosis

  - MC method used to screen for APC mutations is the **APC gene testing** by protein truncation test^Q

- **Protein truncation test** detects 80% of disease causing mutations but does not detect missense mutation^Q.
- Combination of **protein truncation test** & **strand gel electrophoresis** has upto 90% mutation detection rate^Q.

  - **Direct DNA sequencing** is the **most accurate method of detecting APC mutations**, with 95% detection rate^Q.
  - If a disease causing mutation is documented in a family, the accuracy of the test for other at risk family members is almost 100%^{Q}.

- A **positive screening test** should be **confirmed with a diagnostic modality**
- Confirmatory tests include direct DNA sequencing, allele-specific oligonucleotide hybridization (ASO-hybridization), ASO amplification (ASO PCR), RFLP, and ligase chain reaction^Q.

Management

- After the colorectal cancer is eliminated by surgery, **periampullary tumors** are the **MC cause of death**^{Q} among individuals with FAP.

  - **Prophylactic proctocolectomy** is recommended for patients with FAP, given the near 100% risk of early-onset CRC^Q.
  - **Treatment of choice: Total proctocolectomy with ileal pouch-anal anastomosis (IPAA)**^{Q}.

GARDNER'S SYNDROME (AD)

Gardner's Syndrome (AD)

The combination of FAP with:
- Bony lesions (**osteomas**^{Q}, cortical thickening of long bones & ribs)
- Benign lymphoid polyposis of ileum^Q

- **CHRPE**[Q]
- **Dental anomalies**[Q] (impacted tooth, supernumerary tooth, dental cyst)
- **Desmoid tumors** & **sebaceous cyst**[Q]

TURCOT'S SYNDROME (AR)

Turcot's Syndrome (AR)

- **MC brain tumors** are **medulloblastoma** & particularly **glioblastoma**.
- It is a phenotypic variant of FAP and is transmitted by an **autosomal recessive** gene.
- Turcot's syndrome kindreds fall into two groups based on their types of brain tumor and particularly genetic alteration.
- **Medulloblastoma in FAP**[Q]
- **Glioblastoma multiforme** in **HNPCC**[Q]

HEREDITARY NONPOLYPOSIS COLORECTAL CANCER (AD)

Hereditary Nonpolyposis Colorectal Cancer (AD)

- HNPCC is an **autosomal dominant**[Q] inherited syndrome
- **Defective mismatch repair genes** are located on chromosomes **2, 3 & 7**[Q].
- HNPCC is responsible for **3-5%**[Q] of **all cases of CRC**.

> - Incidence of adenomas in HNPCC and CRC is similar to that of the general population with sporadic CRC.
> - Adenomas in patients with HNPCC have higher incidence of high-grade dysplasia & villous architecture[Q].
> - Polyps in patients with HNPCC develop at a younger age, larger than general population & **distributed equally**[Q] **throughout colon**.

- CRC are mostly **poorly differentiated** & **mucinous** and have **signet ring histology** and **"Crohn's like" pattern** of tumor infiltrating lymphocytes[Q].
- Patients with HNPCC have survival that is equivalent, if not better than patients with sporadic CRC of similar stage.
- Predominance of **right sided colon cancer** & **increased incidence of synchronous** & **metachronous CRC**.

> - Lynch syndrome I: CRC only[Q]
> - Lynch syndrome II: CRC & associated malignancies[Q]

Diagnosis
- **Gold standard for diagnosis** of HNPCC is the **detection of a germline mutation in MMR gene**[Q].
- Mismatch repair genes associated with HNPCC: (hMLH1, hMLH3, hPMS1, hPMS2) and (hMSH2, hMSH3, hMSH6)[Q].

> - More than 90% of cases are due to mutation in **hMLH1** or **hMSH2**[Q].

- **Revised Amsterdam criteria**: Used to **select at risk patients** for HNPCC[Q]
- **Bethesda guidelines**: To direct patient selection **for MSI testing**[Q]

Extraintestinal Features
- **Endometrial** (39-60%)[Q], **gastric** (13-19%)[Q], **ovarian** (6-12%)[Q], small intestine, pancreatic, thyroid, transitional cell epithelium of the urinary tract (renal pelvic, ureter, bladder); brain cancers.
- MC extraintestinal feature: **Endometrial cancer**[Q].
- HNPCC associated tumor of the CNS: Glioblastoma

> - Association with **benign & malignant tumors of sebaceous glands & keratocanthomas** is called **Muir-Torre syndrome**[Q]

Management:
- **Surveillance colonoscopy** should begin **at 20 years of age**[Q] & repeated every 2 years until 35 years the age of & **then annually** thereafter[Q].
- In women: Periodic vacuum curettage is **begun at age 25 years**[Q], as are **pelvic USG** & **CA-125** levels.
- **Annual tests for occult blood in urine** because of risk for ureteral & renal pelvic cancer.
- Procedure of choice: **Abdominal colectomy with ileorectal anastomosis**[Q] (when colon cancer is detected)
- **Annual proctoscopy** is mandatory after abdominal colectomy **to detect carcinoma rectum**[Q]
- **In females** with no further plans for childbearing, a **prophylactic total abdominal hysterectomy & bilateral salpingo-oophorectomy** are recommended[Q].

SCREENING FOR COLORECTAL CANCER

Screening for Colorectal Cancer

- **American Cancer Society** suggests **fecal Hemoccult screening annually** & **flexible sigmoidoscopy every 5 years beginning at age 50 for asymptomatic individuals**[Q] having no colorectal cancer risk factors.
  - The American Cancer Society has also endorsed a **"total colon examination"** (i.e., **colonoscopy** or **double-contrast barium enema**) **every 10 years as an alternative**[Q] to Hemoccult testing with periodic flexible sigmoidoscopy.
- **Colonoscopy** has been shown to be **superior to double-contrast barium enema** and also to have a **higher sensitivity** for detecting villous or dysplastic adenomas or cancers[Q] than the strategy employing occult fecal blood testing & flexible sigmoidoscopy.
  - **Double-contrast barium enema** is done when **colonoscopy is contraindicated**[Q]

Colorectal cancer is an ideal candidate for screening
• It is a common and serious problem[Q]
• Precursor lesions exist[Q]
• It is slow growing[Q]
• Testing is available[Q]

RISK FACTORS FOR COLORECTAL CANCER

Risk Factors for the Development of Colorectal Cancer	
1. Dietary Factors: – High animal fat diet[Q] – Low fiber diet[Q] – Alcohol[Q] 2. Hereditary syndromes: – FAP[Q] – HNPCC[Q]	3. Inflammatory bowel disease (Both UC & Crohn's disease)[Q] 4. Streptococcus bovis bacteremia[Q] 5. Ureterosigmoidostomy[Q] 6. Smoking[Q] 7. Acromegaly[Q] 8. Pelvic irradiation[Q]

CHEMOPREVENTION

Chemoprevention

- There is significant chemopreventive role of **NSAIDs, Calcium** carbonate, **Selenium** and **Hormone replacement therapy** in colorectal neoplasia[Q].
- **High fiber diet** has been found to have **protective effect** by increasing the **stool bulk**, diluting the **toxins**, and reducing the **colonic transit time** and thus **reducing exposure time to fecal carcinogens**[Q]

CARCINOMA COLON

Carcinoma Colon

- Most common form of colon cancer is **sporadic**[Q] in nature, without an associated strong family history.
- MC site of colon cancer: **Sigmoid**[Q]; Least common site: **Hepatic flexure**[Q]
- MC site of metastasis: **Liver >Lung**[Q]
- **Mucin production worsens** the prognosis since mucin aids tumor extension[Q]

> - **Incidence** of metastasis is related to **depth of invasion**[Q]
> - **Chemotherapy regimen: FOLFOX-IV (5-FU, Leucovorin, Oxaliplatin)**[Q]

Clinical Features

- **Symptoms** of colonic carcinoma are **non-specific** and generally **develop** when the **cancer is locally advanced**[Q].

Symptoms associated with colon cancer	
• **Abdominal pain (44%): MC**[Q]	• Hematochezia or melena (40%)
• Change in bowel habit (43%)	• Weakness or malaise (20%)

Right Colon	Left Colon

• **Fungating** or **cauliflower**[Q] type growth
• **Cancer** may become quiet **large without** any **obstructing symptoms** due to relative **liquid** stool consistency[Q]
• **Lesions ulcerate** leading to **chronic insidious blood loss**[Q]
• Patients present with:
  – **Melena, anemia, fatigue**[Q]
  – **Abdominal pain**[Q]
  – **Mass** in **right iliac fossa**[Q]
• **Good prognosis**[Q] as compared to left
	• **Annular, constricting** or **stenosing** growth[Q]
	• **Symptoms** of **obstruction** is **more common**[Q]
	• Patients present with:
	  – **Decrease** in **stool caliber**[Q]
	  – **Alteration** of **bowel habbits** (increasing **constipation**)[Q]
	  – **Palpable lump**[Q]
	• **Poor prognosis** (more **infiltrative**)[Q]

- **Lesions of transverse colon** are having **mixed symptoms** of bleeding and obstruction[Q].

Diagnosis

- **Barium enema:** "**Apple core**" or "**napkin ring**" lesion, caused by a **constricting carcinoma**[Q]

Colonoscopy
• **Gold standard for diagnosis** of **colon cancer**[Q].
• **Permits biopsy** of the tumor **to verify the diagnosis**[Q]
• Inspect entire colon to **exclude metachronous polyps** or **cancers**[Q]
• **Incidence** of a **synchronous cancer** is about 3%[Q]

- **Tumors causing complete obstruction:** Water-soluble contrast enema is useful in to **establish the anatomic level** of the **obstruction**[Q].
- **IOC for staging of carcinoma colon: CECT**[Q]

8th AJCC (2017) TNM Classification of Colorectal carcinoma	
Tis: Carcinoma in situ: intraepithelial or invasion of lamina propria	**N1:** Metastasis in **1-3** regional LNs
	N1a: Metastasis in **1** regional LN
T1: Tumor invades **submucosa**[Q]	**N1b:** Metastasis in **2-3** regional LN
T2: Tumor invades **muscularis propria**[Q]	**N1c: Tumor deposits** in in the **subserosa, mesentery**, or **nonperitonealized pericolic** or **perirectal tissues without regional LN metastasis**[Q]
T3: Tumor **invades subserosa** or **into non-peritonealized pericolic or perirectal tissues**[Q]	
T4a: Tumor **penetrates** the surface of **visceral peritoneum**[Q]	**N2a:** Metastasis in **4-6** regional LN[Q]
	N2b: Metastasis in **7 or more** regional LN[Q]
T4b: Tumor directly **invades** or is **adherent** to other **organs** or **structures**[Q]	**M1a:** Metastasis confined to **one organ or site** (e.g. Liver, lung, ovary, non-regional node) without peritoneal metastases[Q]
	M1b: Metastasis to **more than one organ**[Q]
	M1c: Metastasis to **peritoneum with or without other organ involvement**[Q]

Stage Grouping					
I	II	IIIA	IIIB	IIIC	IV
T1N0 T2N0	IIA: T3N0 IIB: T4aN0 IIC: T4bN0	T1-T2, N1 T1, N2a	T1-T2, N2b T2-T3, N2a T3-T4a, N1	T3-T4a, N2b T4a, N2a T4b, N1-N2	IVa: Tany Nany M1a IVb: Tany Nany M1b IVC: Tany Nany M1c

Modified Duke's (Modified Astler-Collar) Classification	
Stage	**Description**
A	Confined to the mucosa
B1	**Partially penetrated** the **muscularis propria**[Q]
B2	**Fully penetrated**[Q] the muscularis propria
C1	**Lymph node invasion without penetration** of the entire bowel wall[Q]
C2	**Lymph node invasion with penetration**[Q] of the entire bowel wall
D	**Distant metastasis**[Q]

Treatment of Colon Cancer According to Stage	
Stage 0: (Tis, N0, M0)	• **Endoscopic polypectomy for** polyps containing **carcinoma in situ**
Stage I: (T1, N0, M0) **Malignant Polyp**	• Segmental colectomy^Q
Stages I and II: (T1–3, N0, M0) **Localized Colon Carcinoma**	• Surgical resection^Q
Stage III: (Tany, N1, M0) **Lymph Node Metastasis**	• **Surgical resection + Adjuvant chemotherapy**^Q (routinely) • **Reference regimen: FOLFOX-IV**^Q (5-FU, Leucovorin, Oxaliplatin)
Stage IV: (Tany, Nany, M1) **Distant Metastasis**	• **MC site of metastasis: Liver > Lung**^Q • **Resection (metastasectomy)** for **isolated, resectable metastasis + adjuvant chemotherapy**^Q • **Palliation** for unresectable disease

Indications of adjuvant chemotherapy in Stage II
1. Insufficient lymph node sampling^Q (<12 nodes resected with the specimen)
2. Perivascular invasion^Q
3. Poorly differentiated histology^Q
4. Bowel obstruction or perforation^Q

CHEMOTHERAPY IN CA COLON

CHEMOTHERAPY IN CA COLON

- **FOLFOX-IV**^Q **(5-FU, Leucovorin, Oxaliplatin)** is the **reference regimen** with **infusional 5-FU**
- **Irinotecan** based regimen should **not be used in the adjuvant setting,** as randomized data have shown increased toxicity and no long term benefit.
- **Bevacizumab, cetuximab** and **panitumumab** should also **not be used** in the **adjuvant setting,** as they add toxicity and expense, and do not add benefit.
- **Irinotecan, bevacizumab and cetuximab** are used for **systemic metastatic disease** or **stage IV**^Q.

POST-RESECTION FOLLOW-UP

POST-RESECTION FOLLOW-UP

- In candidates for resection of recurrent disease (e.x. hepatic resection) serum **CEA** testing should be performed **every 3 to 4 months** for 2 to 3 years after resection of the primary tumor. (**Half-life** of **CEA** is **7-14 days**^Q.)
- **CEA** is **most sensitive** for detection of **retroperitoneal** & **hepatic metastases**^Q.
- Rationale for **colonoscopy** is **not to define recurrent cancer;** major rationale is to **define synchronous** or **metachronous bowel tumors,** usually polyps.
- **Colonoscopy** is recommended at **1 year after resection**^Q, and every **3 years** thereafter.

PROGNOSTIC FACTORS IN COLORECTAL CARCINOMA

PROGNOSTIC FACTORS IN COLORECTAL CARCINOMA

- **Most important prognostic factor** for **colorectal carcinoma: Stage of the disease**^Q
- Single **most important independent prognostic factor** for colorectal carcinoma: **LN status**^Q
- **Stage of disease** gives **information related to depth of penetration** into bowel wall & **extent of regional node spread,** both of which are the two most important independent prognostic factors^Q.

NO EFFECT ON PROGNOSIS

NO EFFECT ON PROGNOSIS

- **No effect on Prognosis: Tumor size** and **duration** of **symptoms**^Q
- **Tumor size** and **configuration** (endophytic, exophytic, annular) **do not carry any prognostic significance**^Q in colorectal carcinoma

- **Left sided colon cancers** are **more infiltrative** at the time of **diagnosis than right lesions,** associated with **poor prognosis**^Q.

COLONIC ISCHEMIA

COLONIC ISCHEMIA

- **Intestinal ischemia** occurs **most commonly** in the **colon**[Q].
- Unlike small bowel ischemia, **colonic ischemia is rarely associated with major arterial** or **venous occlusion**[Q].
- **Most colonic ischemia** appears to **result from low flow** and/or **small vessel occlusion**[Q].

> - MC site of ischemic colitis: Splenic flexure[Q]

- **Ligation** of the **IMA during aortic surgery** predisposes **to colonic ischemia**[Q].
- **Splenic flexure** is the **MC site**[Q] of ischemic colitis (any segment of the colon may be affected)
- **Rectum** is **relatively spared** because of its **rich collateral circulation**[Q].

Risk factors for Colonic Ischemia	
• Vascular disease[Q]	• Vasculitis[Q]
• Diabetes mellitus[Q]	• Hypotension[Q]

Clinical Features
- Diagnosis of ischemic colitis is often based upon the **clinical history** and **physical examination**[Q].
- **Mild ischemia:** Diarrhea (usually bloody) **without abdominal pain**[Q].
- **Severe ischemia:** Intense abdominal pain (often out of proportion to the clinical examination), **tenderness, fever,** and **leukocytosis**[Q]
- **Peritonitis** and/or **systemic toxicity** are signs of **full-thickness necrosis** and **perforation.**

Diagnosis
- **Abdominal X-ray: Thumb printing**[Q] (due to **mucosal edema** and **submucosal hemorrhage**)[Q].
- **CT scan:** Nonspecific **colonic wall thickening** and **pericolic fat stranding**[Q].
- **Angiography** is usually not **helpful**[Q] because major arterial occlusion is rare.

> - **Sigmoidoscopy:** Characteristic **dark, hemorrhagic mucosa**[Q]
> - **Risk of precipitating perforation** is **high**, so **sigmoidoscopy** is **relatively contraindicated**[Q] in ischemic colitis.

Treatment
- **Majority** of patients with ischemic colitis **can be treated medically**[Q].
- **Bowel rest** and **broad-spectrum antibiotics** are the mainstay of therapy (**80% of patients recover**[Q] with this regimen)

Indications of Surgery
• Failure to improve after 2 to 3 days of medical management[Q]
• Progression[Q] of symptoms
• Deterioration in clinical condition[Q]

Complications
- **Stricture (10-15%): MC site of stricture is sigmoid colon**[Q]
- **Chronic segmental ischemia** (15-20%).

PSEUDOMEMBRANOUS COLITIS

PSEUDOMEMBRANOUS COLITIS

- **PMC** is caused by **C. difficile**, a **gram-positive**[Q] bacillus.
- **C. difficile colitis** is the **leading cause of nosocomially acquired diarrhea**[Q].

Pathogenesis
- Colitis is thought to result from **overgrowth** of this **organism** after depletion of the **normal commensal flora** of the gut **with the use of antibiotics**[Q].

> - **Clindamycin**[Q] was the first **antimicrobial** agent associated with **C. difficile colitis**, almost any antibiotic may cause this disease.
> - Toxins produced: **Toxin A** (an **enterotoxin**) and **toxin B** (a **cytotoxin**)[Q].

- **Immunosuppression, medical comorbidities, prolonged hospitalization** or **nursing home residence,** and **bowel surgery** increase the risk[Q].

Clinical Features
- The **spectrum of disease** ranges from **watery diarrhea** to **fulminant, life-threatening** colitis

Diagnosis
- Diagnosis is made after **detection of one** or both toxins by:
  - Stool cytotoxin assay[Q] ELISA[Q]
- **Colonoscopy:** Characteristic **ulcers, plaques,** and **pseudomembranes**[Q]
- **CECT: Accordion sign**[Q] is seen

Treatment
- **Immediate cessation** of **offending antimicrobial agent**[Q].
- **Mild disease:**
  - **Oral metronidazole** (10-day course): **Drug of choice**[Q]
  - **Oral vancomycin:** Second-line agent, used in **metronidazole allergy** or in **recurrent disease**[Q]
- **Severe disease:** Bowel rest, IV hydration, and IV metronidazole or oral vancomycin[Q].

> - **Recurrent colitis** occurs in up to **20%** of patients and may be **treated by a longer course** of oral metronidazole or **vancomycin** (up to 1 month).
> - **Fulminant colitis,** characterized by septicemia and/or evidence of perforation, **requires emergent laparotomy**[Q].

HEYDE'S SYNDROME

Heyde's syndrome

- Heyde's syndrome is a **triad of aortic stenosis,** an **acquired coagulopathy** and **anemia due to bleeding from intestinal angiodysplasia**[Q].
- It is due to the induction of von-Willebrand disease type IIA by the valvular stenosis[Q].

Clinical Features:
- **Gastrointestinal hemorrhage** may present as **hematemesis, melena,** or **hematochezia.**
- **It is not necessary for the aortic stenosis to lead to any other symptoms,** but **evidence of heart failure, syncope,** or **chest pain may be present** if the stenosis is severe.

Diagnosis:
- **Endoscopy** or **colonoscopy** shows **angiodysplasia**[Q] (Dilated mucosal and submucosal veins).
- **Colonoscopy** is the **mainstay of diagnosis** because it allows both visualization of the pathology and therapeutic intervention in colonic, rectal, and distal ileal sources of bleeding[Q].

LOWER GI BLEEDING

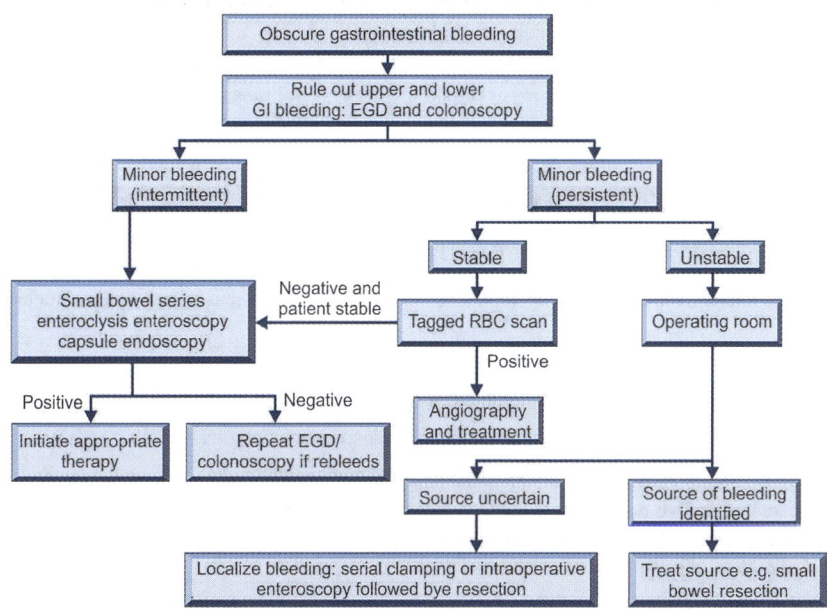

Lower Gastrointestinal Bleeding

Colonic Bleeding (95%)	%	Small Bowel Bleeding (5%)
Diverticular disease[Q]	30-40	**Angiodysplasias**
Anorectal disease[Q]	5-15	Erosions or ulcers (potassium, NSAIDs)
Ischemia	5-10	Crohn's disease
Neoplasia	5-10	Radiation
Infectious colitis	3-8	Meckel's diverticulum
Postpolypectomy	3-7	Neoplasia
Inflammatory bowel disease	3-4	Aortoenteric fistula
Angiodysplasia	3	
Radiation colitis/proctitis	1-3	
Other	1-5	
Unknown	10-25	

LOWER GASTROINTESTINAL BLEED

- Lower gastrointestinal bleed is defined as a bleeding from a site distal to the ligament of Treitz[Q].
- MC site of lower GI bleed: colon (95%)[Q]
- MC cause of lower GI bleed in India: Hemorrhoids[Q] (Rarely massive bleeding)

> - **MC cause of significant lower GI bleed: Diverticular disease (overall)**[Q]
> - **MC cause** of significant small bowel bleed: angiodysplasia[Q]
> - **MC cause** of recurrent, obscure lower GI bleed: Vascular ectasia[Q] (angiodysplasia)

VASCULAR ECTASIA (ANGIODYSPLASIA)

Vascular Ectasia (Angiodysplasia)

- **MC vascular lesions** found in the **colon: Vascular ectasia**[Q]
- **MC cause** of recurrent lower intestinal bleeding after 60 years of age: Vascular ectasia[Q]
- Arise from **age-related degeneration of previously normal colonic blood vessels**[Q].
- Acquired condition[Q]

> - Almost **always occur in** the **cecum** or the **proximal ascending colon**[Q]
> - Usually multiple, are **<5 mm**[Q] in diameter
> - **Rarely identified** with **gross inspection** or **routine pathologic examination**
> - **Diagnosed with colonoscopy** or **angiography**
> - **Angiography: Slow emptying** of **vein**[Q] and dilation of **submucosal vessels**[Q]

- Not associated with synchronous angiomatous lesions of the skin, mucous membranes, or other viscera[Q].
- API: "Hemorrhoids and anal fissure are the most common cause of lower GI bleeding, however the bleeding is rarely **massive**[Q]."

BOWEL PREPARATION

Bowel Preparation

- Normal microbial organisms in the colon compose up to 90% of the dry weight of feces, reaching concentrations up to 109 organism/ml of feces[Q].

> - **Bacteroides: MC colonic microbe**[Q] (anaerobe)
> - **Escherichia coli: MC aerobic colonic microbe**[Q]

- Colon is generally cleansed in preparation for colonic operations and adequate colonoscopy or contrast enema.

Bowel Preparation Consists of
1. **Special diet: Two days prior** to surgery, patient is put on **clear fluids**
2. **Purging** the fecal contents **(mechanical preparation)** by using cathartic, night before surgery
3. **Antibiotics** effective against colonic bacteria

- **Complete bowel obstruction** and **free perforation** are **absolute contraindications** to bowel preparation^Q.

Agents Used for Purging
• **Polyethylene glycol solution** (PEG)^Q
• **Sodium phosphate solution**^Q

- Sodium phosphate has been linked to rare, but serious, electrolyte imbalances in patients with impaired renal function^Q.
- PEG is the recommended bowel preparation in patients with renal insufficiency, cirrhosis, ascites, or congestive heart failure^Q.
- Benefit from routine single-dose administration of parenteral antibiotics 30 minutes before incision^Q is well-established.
- Antibiotics active against both aerobes and anaerobes are ideal:
  - Second- or third-generation cephalosporins^Q
  - Fluoroquinolone + metronidazole^Q
  - Clindamycin^Q

> • A preparation often used consists of **erythromycin base** (1g) and neomycin (1g) given in **three preoperative doses** the **day before surgery**^Q

COLONIC INJURIES

COLONIC INJURIES

- Colon injuries are generally the result of penetrating trauma^Q.
- The incidence of infectious complications after a colonic injury is related to inadequate treatment or delay in diagnosis^Q.

Diagnosis
- Physical examination is particularly useful to establish that laparotomy is necessary after a stab wound to the abdomen, if peritoneal signs are present^Q

> • A negative physical examination does not rule out the presence of a colonic injury, particularly in patients with stab wounds to the back and flanks^Q.

- An objective evaluation of the abdomen is warranted after stab wounds and may include DPL or a triple-contrast (oral, IV, and rectal) CT scan^Q.

> • Gunshot wounds to the abdomen usually indicate the necessity for laparotomy, and with few exceptions, no further workup is necessary^Q and the colonic injury will be diagnosed during abdominal exploration.

- Presence of blood on rectal examination is strong evidence of colon or rectal injury^Q.

Treatment
- Primary repair can be selected when known associated complicating factors have been excluded^Q.

Indications of Primary Repair
• **Early diagnosis** (within **4-6 hours**)^Q
• **Absence of prolonged shock or hypotension**^Q
• **Absence of gross contamination**^Q of the peritoneal cavity
• **Absence** of **associated** colonic **vascular injury**^Q
• **Less than 6 units** of **blood transfused**^Q
• **No requirement** for the use of **mesh**^Q to permanently close the abdominal wall

- Low-risk penetrating colonic injuries: **Primary closure** or **resection and primary anastomosis**^Q
- High-risk colon injuries or those associated with **severe injuries**: **Resection** and **colostomy**^Q.

Complications
- **Abscess** formation, anastomotic **leak** and **peristomal hernia**

Multiple Choice Questions

HIRSCHSPRUNG'S DISEASE

1. **True about Hirschsprung's disease:** *(PGI May 2010, Dec 2008)*
   a. Aganglionic segment is contracted not dilated
   b. Descending colon is most common site of aganglionosis
   c. Barium enema is diagnostic
   d. It is seen in infants and children only
   e. Barium enema show calcification

2. **Duhamel's operation is done for:** *(MHSSMCET 2005)*
   a. Hirschsprung's disease   b. Meconium ileus
   c. Annular pancreas   d. Imperforate anus

3. **Hirschsprung's disease is best diagnosed by:**
   (All India 2012, AIIMS GIS Dec 2011)
   a. Rectal biopsy   b. Anal manometry
   c. CT   d. MRI

4. **Not true regarding Hirschsprung's disease is:**
   (Recent Question 2015; AIIMS Nov 97)
   a. Autosomal dominant
   b. Absent ganglionic cells in myenteric plexus
   c. Absent ganglionic cell in submucous plexus
   d. Rectal biopsy is diagnostic

5. **Aganglionic segment is encountered in which part of colon in case of Hirschsprung's disease?**
   (Recent Question 2014; AIIMS Nov 99)
   a. Distal to dilated segment
   b. In whole colon
   c. Proximal to dilated segment
   d. In dilated segment

6. **Hirschsprung's disease involves which region of intestine?**
   (MCI March 2008)
   a. Colon   b. Rectum
   c. Rectosigmoid part   d. Terminal ileum

7. **Treatment of choice in a child with short segment Hirschsprung's disease with minimal symptoms:**
   a. Conservative treatment   b. Extended myectomy
   c. Swenson operation   d. Duhamel's operation

8. **Investigation of choice in Hirschsprung's disease is:**
   (Recent Question 2017, AIIMS Nov 2005, DNB 2005, 2000, PGI Dec 98)
   a. Rectal manometry   b. Rectal examination
   c. Rectal biopsy   d. Ba enema

9. **True statements about congenital megacolon include all of the following except:** *(All India 97)*
   a. Dilatation and hypertrophy of pelvic colon
   b. Loud borborygmi
   c. Symptoms appear within 3 days following birth
   d. Large stool

10. **In Hirschsprung's disease, aganglionic segment is:**
    (DNB 2010)
    a. Normal or dilated   b. Normal or contracted
    c. Dilated or contracted   d. Always dilated

11. **Fecal soiling in children is most commonly due to:**
    (PGI June 99)
    a. Hirschsprung's disease   b. Chronic constipation
    c. Rectal atresia   d. None of the above

12. **Absence of ganglion in myenteric plexus is seen in:**
    (PGI June 97)
    a. Crohn's disease   b. Ulcerative colitis
    c. Hirschsprung's disease   d. Intussusception

13. **A newborn presented with bloated abdomen shortly after birth with passing of less meconium. A full thickness biopsy of the rectum was carried out. Which one of the following rectal biopsy findings is most likely to be present?**
    a. Fibrosis of submucosa   *(All India 2005)*
    b. Hyalinisation of the muscular coat
    c. Thickened muscularis propria
    d. Lack of ganglion cells

14. **Following procedures (except one) are done for correction of Hirschsprung's disease:** *(Recent Question 2016)*
    a. Duhamel's   b. Soave's
    c. Swenson's   d. Bayar's

15. **When rectal washouts are given to Hirschsprung's disease, the following fluid is used:** *(Karnataka 95)*
    a. 5% dextrose   b. Normal saline
    c. Soap solution   d. Tap water

16. **All are features of congenital megacolon except:** *(All India 97)*
    a. Large bulky stools   b. Tight anal ring
    c. Pseudodiarrhoea   d. Failure to thrive

17. **Hirschsprung's disease is treated by:** *(APPG 98)*
    a. Colostomy
    b. Excision of aganglinonic segment
    c. Colectomy
    d. Sodium chloride wash

18. **A 3 years old male child presents with history of constipation and abdominal distension for the last two years. The plain radiograph of abdomen reveals fecal matter containing distended bowel loops. A barium enema study done subsequently shows a transition zone at the recto-sigmoid junction with reversal of recto-sigmoid ratio. The most probable diagnosis is:** *(AIIMS Nov 2003)*
    a. Anal atresia   b. Malrotation of the gut
    c. Hirschsprung's disease   d. Congenital megacolon

19. **Most common presentation of Hirschsprung's disease:**
    (Recent Question 2017)
    a. Abdominal distention   b. Vomiting
    c. Failure to pass meconium   d. Failure to thrive

COLONIC DIVERTICULA

20. **Acquired diverticula are most commonly in seen in:**
    (Recent Question 2015; MHSSMCET 2007)
    a. Jejunum/ileum   b. Transverse colon
    c. Sigmoid colon   d. Ascending colon

21. **True regarding colovesical fistula is:** *(JIPMER 2013)*
    a. Commonly presents with pneumaturia
    b. Barium enema is diagnostic
    c. Common in Females
    d. May be a surgical complication

22. Most common fistula in diverticulosis of colon"
    (MHSSMCET 2010, 2006)
    a. Colocutaneous   b. Colovaginal
    c. Vesicovaginal   d. Colovesical

23. A 40 years old male patient presented with mild abdominal pain, mild constipation with a feeling of incomplete evacuation and mucus in stools for the past four years. On examination, tenderness is presenting left iliac fossa. The most likely diagnosis is: (AIIMS May 2012)
    a. Ulcerative colitis
    b. Diverticular disease of colon
    c. Irritable bowel syndrome
    d. Carcinoma colon

24. Colonic diverticulosis is best diagnosed by:
    (Recent Question 2015; AIIMS May 2007)
    a. Colonoscopy   b. Nuclear scan
    c. Barium enema   d. CT scan

25. This characteristic appearance is seen on barium enema in:
    (Recent Question 2018)
    a. Colonic polyps   b. Colonic diverticula
    c. Carcinoma colon d. Ischemic colitis

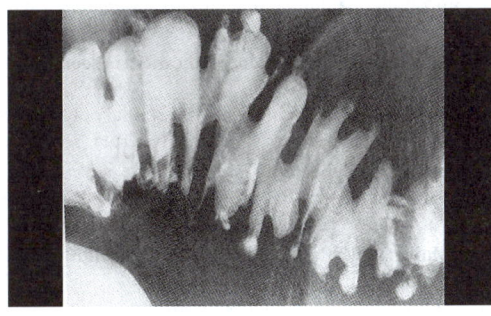

26. Massive colonic bleeding in a patient of diverticulosis is from: (All India 2000)
    a. Inferior mesenteric artery
    b. Superior mesenteric artery
    c. Celiac artery
    d. Gastro-duodenal artery

27. In acute diverticulitis of the colon, the sigmoidoscopic finding is: (Kerala 87)
    a. Mucosa is inflamed
    b. Minute diverticuli seen
    c. Saw toothed appearance
    d. Sigmoidoscope cannot be passed beyond 15 cm

28. Diverticular disease is not common in: (Karnataka 94)
    a. Colon   b. Jejunum
    c. Duodenum   d. Stomach

29. Which of the following about acute diverticulitis is incorrect? (DPG 2009 March)
    a. Sigmoid is the commonest site
    b. Peri-colic abscess can occur
    c. Fistulization is an emergency
    d. Conservative treatment may be successful in severe attack

30. The most common site of bleeding diverticula is: (DPG 2008)
    a. Sigmoid colon   b. Descending colon
    c. Rectum   d. Ascending colon

31. The term "Left sided appendicitis" as popularly called is nothing but:
    a. Diverticulitis   b. Ascending colitis
    c. Descending colitis d. Typhilitis

32. A obese old patient with diverticular disease if presents with perforation, what will the treatment of choice?
    a. Primary resection and anastomosis (MHSSMCET 2005)
    b. Hartman's procedure
    c. Conservative approach
    d. Left Hemicolectomy

33. Best investigation to diagnose colonic diverticulitis:
    (Recent Question 2017)
    a. Barium enema   b. CECT
    c. Ultrasound   d. MRI

34. Hinchey classification is used in cases of: (MHCET 2016)
    a. Complicated diverticulitis
    b. Complicated pancreatitis
    c. Complicated hepatitis
    d. Complicated meningitis

COLORECTAL POLYPS

35. According to Hagitt's classification, a polyp invading neck in between head and stalk is level:
    a. 1   b. 2
    c. 3   d. 4

36. All are predisposing factor for colorectal carcinoma except:
    (AIIMS GIS 2003)
    a. Turcot's syndrome   b. Muir-Torre syndrome
    c. Cowden's syndrome   d. Juvenile polyposis coli

37. Intestinal polyps that can potentially grow into cancer:
    (DNB 2005, 2001, MHPGMCET 2007)
    a. Adenomatous polyp   b. Hyperplastic polyp
    c. Juvenile polyp   d. Hamartomatous polyp

38. Cowden's disease is characterized by the following except:
    (MHPGMCET 2007)
    a. Fibrocystic disease of breast and breast cancer
    b. Facial trichilemmomas
    c. Potentially malignant intestinal polyps
    d. Acral keratosis

39. Not associated with GI malignancy: (GB Pant 2011)
    a. Cowden's syndrome   b. Peutz-Jegher's syndrome
    c. Juvenile polyposis   d. Gardner's syndrome

40. All are true about risk factor for malignancy in polyp except:
    a. Pedunculated polyp   b. > 2 cm (GB Pant 2011)
    c. Villous polyp   d. Cellular atypia

41. A 17-year-old patient develops intussusception for which he was operated and a segment of intestine showing multiple polyps was resected. Microscopy showed the following pathology. What is the likely diagnosis? (AIIMS November 2015)
    a. Tubulovillous polyps   b. Hamartomatous polyps
    c. Inflammatory polyps   d. Adenocarcinoma

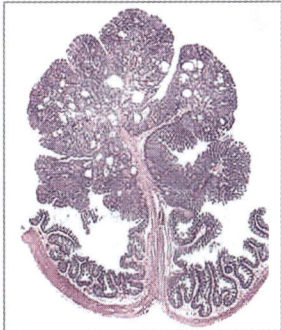

42. **Carcinoma of the colon develops in all patients with:**
    a. Juvenile polyposis (COMEDK 2005)
    b. Hamartomatous polyps
    c. Inflammatory polyps
    d. Familial adenomatous polyposis

43. **Diagnosis of colonic polyps is best done radiologically using:** (COMEDK 2010)
    a. Barium meal series
    b. Double-contrast barium enema
    c. Instant enema
    d. Water-soluble contrast enema

44. **Which polyp has maximum malignant potential?**
    (Recent Question 2015; AIIMS June 93)
    a. Sessile b. Pedunculated
    c. Superficial spreading d. Any of the above

45. **Incidence of malignancy is maximum in:** (AIIMS Feb 97)
    a. Villous adenoma b. Juvenile polyps
    c. Hyperplastic polyps d. Tubular adenoma

46. **All the following statements regarding malignant potential of colorectal polyps are true except:** (AIIMS Nov 2002)
    a. Polyps of the familial polyposis coli could invariably undergo malignant change
    b. Pseudopolyps of ulcerative colitis has high risk of malignancy
    c. Villous adenoma is associated with high risk of malignancy
    d. Juvenile polyps have little or no risk

47. **True about neoplastic colorectal polyps:** (PGI June 2003)
    a. Sessile polyps > 1 cm is malignant
    b. MC site is colon and rectum
    c. Adenomatous polyp is premalignant
    d. Tubular adenoma is malignant
    e. Pseudpolyps are premalignant

48. **Which of the following polyps is not premalignant?**
    a. Juvenile polyposis syndrome (PGI June 2003)
    b. Peutz-Jegher's syndrome
    c. Ulcerative colitis
    d. Familial polyposis coli
    e. Cronkhite Canada syndrome

49. **All of the following are pre-malignant except:**
    (AIIMS November 2014)
    a. Crohn's disease b. Ulcerative colitis
    c. Peutz-Jegher's syndrome d. Barrett's esophagus

50. **Polyp associated with highest risk of malignant transformation is:** (MHCET 2016)
    a. Juvenile b. Villous adenoma
    c. Tubular adenoma
    d. Polyp of Peutz-Jegher's syndrome

51. **Which of the following colonic polyps is not premalignant?**
    a. Juvenile polyps (All India 2006, AIIMS Nov 2006)
    b. Hamartomatous polyps associated with Peutz-Jegher's syndrome
    c. Villous adenoma d. Tubular adenomas

52. **All the following polyps are premalignant except:**
    a. Juvenile polyposis syndrome (All India 2007)
    b. Familial polyposis syndrome
    c. Juvenile polyp
    d. Peutz-Jegher's syndrome

53. **In children MC type of polyp is:** (PGI Dec 98)
    a. Juvenile polyp b. Solitary polyp
    c. Familial polyposis
    d. Multiple adenomatous polyp

54. **Metabolic abnormality seen in large colorectal villous adenoma:** (AIIMS May 2008)
    a. Hypokalemic metabolic alkalosis
    b. Hypokalemic metabolic acidosis
    c. Chlorine sensitive metabolic acidosis
    d. Chlorine resistant metabolic alkalosis

55. **Lalita, a female patient presents with pigmentation of the lips and oral mucosa and intestinal polyps. Her sister also gives the same history. Most probable diagnosis is:**
    (DNB 2011, AIIMS June 2001, All India 2000)
    a. Carcinoid tumor b. Melanoma
    c. Villous adenoma d. Peutz-Jegher's syndrome

56. **A 25 years old man has pigmented macules over the palms, soles and oral mucosa. He also has anemia and abdominal pain. Which one of the following is the most likely diagnosis?** (WBPG 2015; APPG 2015)
    a. Incontinentia pigmenti b. Peutz-Jegher's syndrome
    c. Cushing's syndrome d. Albright's syndrome

57. **Strong correlation with colorectal cancer is seen in:**
    (All India 2003)
    a. Peutz-Jegher's polyp b. Familial polyposis coli
    c. Juvenile polyposis d. Hyperplastic polyp

58. **Prophylactic polypectomy is done is:**
    a. Peutz-Jegher's syndrome b. Gardner's syndrome
    c. Familial polyposis d. None of the above

59. **On colonoscopy which of the following is highly malignant?**
    a. Single pedunculated polyp (JIPMER 98)
    b. Multiple flat polyps about hundreds
    c. Multiple pedunculated polyp
    d. Solitary flat polyp

60. **A 25-year-old male presented to your OPD with recurrent abdominal pain. On the basis of the image of the patient, what is the most probable diagnosis?**
    a. Cowden's disease b. HNPCC
    c. Peutz-Jegher's syndrome
    d. Cronkhite Canada syndrome

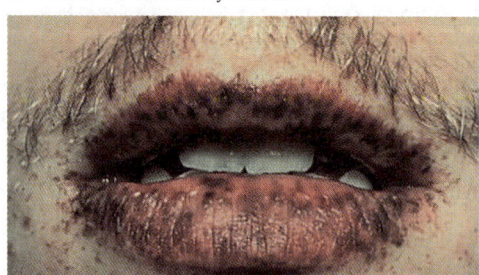

FAMILIAL ADENOMATOUS POLYPOSIS

61. **Which of the following is not true about FAP?**
    a. AR inheritance
    (JIPMER Nov 2017, JIPMER SS 2016, AIIMS May 2011)
    b. Screening done by sigmoidoscopy
    c. Polyps develop in late adulthood
    d. Epidermal cysts and osteomas may occur

62. **All are true about FAP except:** *(JIPMER GIS 2011)*
    a. Gastric and duodenal polyps are most common
    b. Most of the gastric polyps represents fundal gland hyperplasia
    c. Increased risk of ampullary carcinoma
    d. CHRPE can be detected by ophthalmoscopy in 25% patients

63. **Recommended treatment of FAP involving sigmoid colon:** *(AIIMS GIS Dec 2006)*
    a. Total colectomy with ileorectal anastomosis
    b. Total colectomy with IPAA
    c. Segmental resection
    d. Total proctocolectomy with IPAA

64. **Are true about FAP except:** *(AIIMS GIS Dec 2006)*
    a. > 100 polyps for diagnosis
    b. Mutation in APC gene
    c. Budesonide prevent CA colon
    d. Endometrial carcinoma is a prominent association

65. **Which is not true about familial polyposis?** *(AIIMS GIS May 2008)*
    a. FAP: 100% risk of CRC cancer
    b. Juvenile polyposis: 20% risk of CRC cancer
    c. HNPCC: 30-60% risk of endometrium cancer
    d. Cowden's syndrome: 30% risk of CRC cancer

66. **Most common associated cancer in FAP:** *(AIIMS GIS Dec 2009)*
    a. CA pancreas
    b. Periampullary carcinoma
    c. CA thyroid
    d. Stomach

67. **Which of the following is true about FAP?** *(GB Pant 2011)*
    a. In stomach, most common are gastric adenomas
    b. Gastric carcinoma is common
    c. Duodenal carcinoma in 50% patients
    d. Duodenal adenoma in 60-90% patients

68. **Gardner's syndrome is associated with all except:** *(PGI SS Dec 2009)*
    a. Brain tumor
    b. Desmoid tumor
    c. Osteoma
    d. Abnormal dentition

69. **"Gardner's syndrome" has all the following except:** *(COMEDK 2005)*
    a. Colonic polyp
    b. Multiple epidermal cyst
    c. Bony exostosis
    d. Giant gastric folds

70. **True about familial polyposis colon cancer syndrome except:**
    a. Autosomal recessive *(JIPMER 2011)*
    b. Associated with fibroma and osteomas
    c. Associated with brain tumors
    d. 100% incidence of colon carcinoma

71. **Turcot's syndrome is associated with:** *(PGI June 2002)*
    a. Duodenal polyps
    b. Familial adenomatous polyposis
    c. Brain tumors
    d. Villous adenoma
    e. Hyperplastic polyps

72. **The most common facial abnormality in Gardner's syndrome:** *(AIIMS Nov 2005)*
    a. Ectodermal dysplasia
    b. Odontome
    c. Multiple osteomas
    d. Dental cysts

73. **Following genetic counseling in a family for Familial polyposis coli, next screening test is:** *(MCI June 2018, AIIMS Nov 2006)*
    a. Flexible sigmoidoscopy
    b. Colonoscopy
    c. Occult blood in stools
    d. APC gene

74. **Desmoid tumor is associated with:** *(JIPMER 2014, 2013)*
    a. Colonic polyps
    b. Pancreatic cancer
    c. Ovarian cancer
    d. Gastric cancer

75. **Which of the following is associated with FAP?** *(Recent Question 2017)*
    a. Gardner's syndrome
    b. Peutz-Jegher's syndrome
    c. Juvenile polyps
    d. Hamartomatous polyp

76. **All the following are True regarding Familial Adenomatous Polyposis except:** *(APPG 2015)*
    a. It is due to a mutation of APC gene in chromosome 15
    b. > 100 colorectal polyps are present
    c. It is an autosomal dominant disorder
    d. Congenital Hypertrophy of Retinal Pigment Epithelium is seen in upto 50% patients

HEREDITARY NON-POLYPOSIS COLON CANCER

77. **Lynch syndrome is also known as:** *(KGMC 2011)*
    a. FAP
    b. PJS
    c. HNPCC
    d. Cowden's syndrome

78. **Multiple cutaneous sebaceous adenomas are seen in:** *(All India 2011)*
    a. Gardner's syndrome
    b. Turcot's syndrome
    c. Muir-Torre syndrome
    d. Cowden syndrome

79. **Patient with proximal CA colon with endometrial and ovarian carcinoma has:** *(Recent Question 2018, AIIMS GIS Dec 2006)*
    a. Lynch syndrome
    b. Gardener's syndrome
    c. Cowden's disease
    d. Cronkhite-Canada syndrome

80. **Amsterdam criteria includes all except:** *(AIIMS GIS Dec 2009)*
    a. At least three relatives should be affected
    b. All the three should be first degree relative
    c. Two successive generations affected
    d. FAP excluded

81. **Most common extra-intestinal malignancy in HNPCC:** *(AIIMS GIS May 2011)*
    a. Pancreatic carcinoma
    b. CA stomach
    c. Small bowel carcinoma
    d. Transitional cell carcinoma

82. **Most common mismatch repair gene mutation in HNPCC:**
    a. MSH-2 and hMLH-1
    b. PMS-1 *(GB Pant 2011)*
    c. MSH-6
    d. PMS-2

83. **Microsatellite instability is most common in:**
    a. FAP *(PGI SS June 2005)*
    b. HNPCC
    c. Sporadic colonic carcinoma
    d. Juvenile polyposis

COLORECTAL CANCER: RISK FACTORS

84. **Premalignant conditions is/are:** *(PGI Dec 2006)*
    a. Ulcerative colitis
    b. Amoebic colitis
    c. Familial polyposis coli
    d. Juvenile polyp
    e. Peutz-Jegher's syndrome

85. **Based on epidemiological studies, which of the following has been found to be most protective against carcinoma colon?** *(DNB 2011, AIIMS May 2011, All India 2009)*
    a. High fiber diet
    b. Low fat diet
    c. Low selenium diet
    d. Low protein diet

86. **Genetic abnormality in case of late adenoma to carcinoma in CA colon:** *(AIIMS GIS Dec 2009)*
    a. APC
    b. K-ras
    c. DCC
    d. p53

87. All of the following genes may be involved in development of carcinoma of colon except: *(All India 2009)*
    a. APC
    b. Beta-Catenin
    c. K-ras
    d. Mismatch repair genes

88. Cholecystectomy may lead to increased risk of: *(COMEDK 2004)*
    a. Proximal colon cancer
    b. CA. pancreas
    c. Hepatic cancer
    d. Cholangiocarcinoma

89. Commonly undergoing malignant transformation is/are: *(PGI June 2006)*
    a. FAP
    b. Crohn's disease
    c. Ulcerative colitis
    d. Enteric colitis
    e. Juvenile polyp

CARCINOMA COLON CLINICAL FEATURES AND DIAGNOSIS

90. Most common site of colonic carcinoma: *(GB Pant 2010, UPPG 2009; NEET 2013)*
    a. Sigmoid
    b. Transverse
    c. Descending
    d. Ascending

91. Constricting type of colonic carcinoma is seen in: *(MHPGMCET 2001)*
    a. Left colon
    b. Right colon
    c. Transverse colon
    d. Caecum

92. Patient having diarrhea and colic on and of with mass in right iliac fossa. Most probable diagnosis is: *(DNB 2009)*
    a. Carcinoma rectum
    b. Carcinoma cecum
    c. Carcinoma sigmoid
    d. Carcinoma transverse colon

93. Carcinoma right colon is most commonly of which type? *(AIIMS Nov 94, UPPG 2008)*
    a. Stenosing
    b. Ulcerative
    c. Tubular
    d. Fungating

94. True regarding carcinoma colon is: *(AIIMS Nov 2000)*
    a. Lesion on left side of the colon presents with features of anemia
    b. Mucinous carcinoma has a good prognosis
    c. Duke's A stage should receive adjuvant chemotherapy
    d. Solitary liver metastasis is not a contraindication for surgery

95. On barium enema, this appearance is seen in:
    a. Ischemic colitis
    b. Carcinoma colon
    c. Colonic diverticula
    d. Colonic polyposis

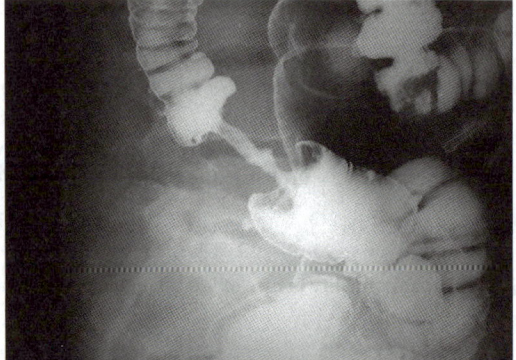

96. True about virtual colonscopy: *(PGI June 2009)*
    a. Have better image than conventional colonoscopy
    b. VC is performed by CT and MRI
    c. Take more time than conventional colonscopy
    d. Easy to take tissue sample
    e. Helpful in pathology outside colon

97. Colonic disease can be diagnosed by all except: *(PGI May 2010)*
    a. Virtual colonoscopy
    b. Ba enema
    c. Ba swallow
    d. Ba follow through
    e. Enteroclysis

98. Colonic metastases are related with:
    a. Pre-op CEA level *(AIIMS GIS Dec 2010, 2011)*
    b. Depth of invasion
    c. Size of tumor
    d. Circumferential involvement

99. Which of the following is true about colon carcinoma?
    a. Inherited in 30% cases *(PGI SS Dec 2009)*
    b. Synchronous lesion is seen in 1% cases
    c. Metachronous lesion is seen in up to 12% cases
    d. Carcinoma is inevitable in untreated cases of FAP

100. What is an acceptable screening technique for detecting recurrent colon cancer? *(COMEDK 2004)*
    a. Screening sigmoidoscopy
    b. Screening the stool for occult blood
    c. Stool cytology
    d. Measurement of CEA levels

101. Most important prognostic factor for colorectal carcinoma is:
    a. Site of lesion *(AIIMS May 2011)*
    b. Tumour size and characteristics
    c. Age of patient
    d. Lymph node status

102. The tendency of colonic carcinoma to metastasize is best assessed by: *(Recent Question 2014; AIIMS Nov 2003)*
    a. Size of tumor
    b. Carcinoembryonic antigen (CEA) levels
    c. Depth of penetration of bowel wall
    d. Proportion of bowel circumference involved

103. Which of the following is true about colon carcinoma?
    a. Right sided colon carcinoma associated with young individuals *(PGI Dec 2005)*
    b. Most common site is sigmoid colon
    c. Right sided colon carcinoma present as chronic anemia
    d. Not resectable in case of metastasis
    e. Right sided colon has better prognosis than left sided colon

104. The incidence of carcinoma of the caecum in relation to colonic adenocarcinoma is:
    a. 2%
    b. 4.5%
    c. 20%
    d. 44%
    e. 62%

105. The best investigation for colorectal carcinoma: *(Kerala 97)*
    a. Exfoliative cytology
    b. Air contrast barium enema
    c. Ultrasound
    d. Colonoscopy and biopsy

106. Tenesmus occurs in lesions of:
    a. Ileum
    b. Right side of colon
    c. Descending colon
    d. Sigmoid colon

107. The area of the colon which is least visualized by barium studies:
    a. Sigmoid
    b. Hepatic flexure
    c. Splenic flexure
    d. Caecum

108. The commonest site of perforation during colonoscopy is: *(UPSC 2000)*
    a. Caecum
    b. Hepatic flexure
    c. Splenic flexure
    d. Sigmoid colon

109. A 58-year-old female complains of dull aching pain in right iliac fossa. On examination, gross pallor was found and a mass was palpable in right iliac fossa. What is the most likely diagnosis? *(AIIMS November 2014)*
    a. Appendicular mass
    b. Ileocecal tuberculosis
    c. Diverticulitis
    d. Carcinoma ascending colon

CARCINOMA COLON STAGING

110. Three lymph nodes in CA colon represents: *(KGMC 2011)*
    a. IB
    b. IA
    c. II
    d. III

111. Stage IIIC in colorectal cancer: *(GB Pant 2011)*
    a. T2N0M0
    b. T2N2M0
    c. T2N1M0
    d. T4N1M0

CARCINOMA COLON TREATMENT

112. Management of carcinoma rectosigmoid with obstructive carcinoma in elderly frail: *(PGI Nov 2009)*
    a. Colostomy
    b. Abdomino-perineal resection (APR)
    c. Resection and primary anastomosis
    d. Hartmann procedure
    e. Laser recanalisation

113. Treatment of carcinoma left colon with acute obstruction includes: *(PGI June 2008)*
    a. Hartman's procedure
    b. Left colectomy with anastomosis
    c. Proximal colostomy
    d. Extended right colectomy with ileoanal anastomosis
    e. Primary anastomosis should never be attempted

114. Treatment included in management of unresectable colorectal cancer liver metastases: *(PGI May 2011)*
    a. Portal vein embolization
    b. Radiotherapy
    c. Resection
    d. Staged operation
    e. Chemotherapy

115. In case of elective surgery of carcinoma sigmoid colon, which of the following should be done? *(PGI June 2004)*
    a. Mechanical bowel wash
    b. Broad spectrum antibiotic given 48 hours before operation
    c. Broad spectrum antibiotic at the time of operation
    d. None

116. After undergoing surgery, for carcinoma of colon a patient developed single liver metastasis of 2 cm. What you do next? *(BIHAR PG 2014; All India 2002, All India 98)*
    a. Resection
    b. Chemoradiation
    c. Acetic acid injection
    d. Radiofrequency ablation

117. A 60 years old man suffering from left colon carcinoma presented with acute left colonic obstruction the treatment is: *(PGI June 2003)*
    a. Primary resection and Hartman's procedure
    b. Defunctioning colostomy
    c. Right hemicolectomy
    d. Resection of whole left bowel and end to end anastomosis
    e. Conservative treatment

118. True about treatment of carcinoma left colon with acute obstruction: *(PGI June 2008)*
    a. Hartman's procedure
    b. Left colectomy with anastomosis
    c. Proximal colostomy
    d. Extended right colectomy with ileoanal anastomosis
    e. Primary anastomosis should never be attempt

119. Ramu is 60 years old male with CA descending colon presents with acute intestinal obstruction. In emergency department treatment of choice is: *(AIIMS Nov 99, Nov 98, Feb 97)*
    a. Defunctioning colostomy
    b. Hartman's procedure
    c. Total colectomy
    d. Left hemicolectomy

120. All the following are true regarding colorectal cancers except: *(APPG 2016)*
    a. Macroscopic variants are annular, tubular or cauliflower
    b. Left hemicolectomy is the treatment of choice for splenic flexure tumors
    c. Duke's classification was originally described for rectal tumors
    d. Arise from adenomatous polyp after genetic mutations influenced by environmental factors

COLONIC ISCHEMIA

121. Thumb printing appearance of colon on barium enema is seen in: *(COMEDK 2004)*
    a. Diverticulitis
    b. Ischemic colitis
    c. Ulcerative colitis
    d. Carcinoma colon

122. This characteristic appearance is seen on barium enema in:
    a. Colonic polyps
    b. Colonic diverticula
    c. Ischemic colitis
    d. Carcinoma colon

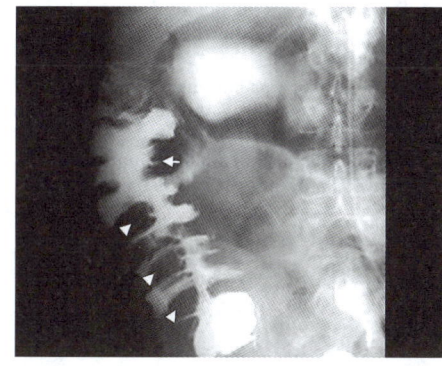

123. Are true about ischemic colitis except: *(JIPMER GIS 2011)*
    a. IMA is commonly occluded in cases needing aortic surgeries
    b. Ischemia is more common in small bowel as compared to large bowel
    c. Most common site of post ischemic stricture is sigmoid
    d. Transection of IMA doesn't need reimplantation if aortic surgery is attempted

124. Most common site of post ischemic stricture is: *(JIPMER GIS 2011, GB Pant 2011, MHSSMCET 2010)*
    a. Ascending colon
    b. Hepatic flexure
    c. Splenic flexure
    d. Sigmoid colon

125. Commonest site for ischemic colitis is:
    (AIIMS June 95, PGI Dec 97)
    a. Hepatic flexure   b. Splenic flexure
    c. Descending colon   d. Ascending colon

126. A 60 years old man presents with acute onset of pain in lower abdomen followed by repeated rectal bleeding. Examination revealed pulse rate of 100/minute, BP 160/96 mm of Hg and a localized tenderness in the left hypochondrium. Stools examination reveals only a few pus cells and sigmoidoscopy was normal. Which one of the following is the most likely diagnosis?   (UPSC 96)
    a. Idiopathic ulcerative colitis
    b. Bacillary dysentery
    c. Ischemic colitis   d. Amoebic colitis

127. True about acute ischemic colitis: (PGI November 2017)
    a. Most common site involved are sigmoid colon and splenic flexure
    b. Most commonly occur in young female
    c. Abdominal radiographs show thumb print sign
    d. Commonly present as pain in abdomen with bloody diarrhea
    e. Acute thrombotic mesenteric occlusion is also known as intestinal angina

PSEUDOMEMBRANOUS COLITIS

128. Pseudomembranous colitis is associated with:
    (COMEDK 2005)
    a. Campylobacter   b. Clostridium difficile
    c. Clostridium retgari   d. Salmonella typhi

129. Which among the following is the drug of choice for clostridium difficile-induced colitis?   (COMEDK 2009)
    a. Gentamicin   b. Ciprofloxacin
    c. Metronidazole   d. Linezolid

130. A patient on antibiotics for treatment for peritonitis presents with mucus diarrhea. Most probable cause could be:
    a. Ulcerative colitis   (MCI Sept 2009)
    b. Activation of latent tuberculosis
    c. Antibiotic associated diarrhea
    d. Gastritis

131. In a patient of pseudomembranous colitis, CECT was done. What is the name of sign seen on CECT?
    (Recent Question 2017)
    a. Accordion sign   b. Whorl sign
    c. Central stellate scar   d. Honeycombing

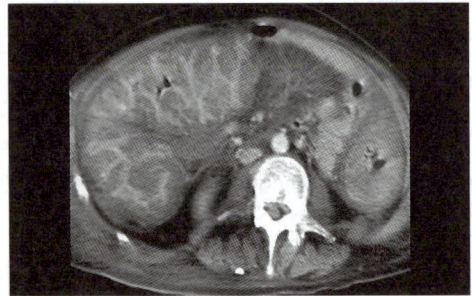

COLONIC RESECTION AND ANASTOMOSIS

132. After hemicolectomy, on the 6th post operative day patient developed serous discharge from the wound, following are to be done: (PGI Dec 2003)
    a. Dressing of the wound only
    b. Start IVF
    c. Do urgent laparotomy
    d. Do Ba-enema to see for anastomotic leak

133. On the 4th postoperative day of laparotomy a patient presents with bleeding and oozing from the wound. Management is:
    a. Dressing of wound and observe for dehiscence
    b. IV fluids   c. Send for USG abdomen
    d. Start treatments for peritonitis
    e. Urgent surgery   (PGI June 2006)

134. Cattel's maneuver is mobilization of: (MHSSMCET 2005)
    a. Sigmoid colon
    b. Descending colon
    c. Small bowel
    d. Caecum and ascending colon

135. Dunking maneuver is used in: (MHSSMCET 2009)
    a. Left hemicolectomy
    b. Right Hemicolectomy
    c. Right extended hemicolectomy
    d. Anterior resection

ENTERIC FISTULA

136. True about enterocutaneous fistula: (PGI Dec 2000)
    a. High output fistula drains 500 mL/day
    b. Malignancy is most common cause
    c. Fluid and electrolyte loss can occur
    d. No skin damage

137. Most common cause of colonic fistula in India at age of 27 years: (UPPG 2008)
    a. Crohn's disease   b. Ulcerative colitis
    c. Tuberculosis   d. Carcinoma rectum

LOWER GI BLEED

138. A 65-year-old man presented with an episode of syncope. He said he felt dizzy during defecation and noticed gross bleeding in the pan. Fecal occult blood test done 3 months ago as a part of routine screening for colon cancer was negative. There is no history of recent weight loss. What is the likely colonoscopic finding?   (AIIMS November 2014)
    a. Early stage carcinoma colon
    b. Sigmoid diverticulitis
    c. Microscopic colitis
    d. Dilated mucosal and submucosal veins in the colon

139. Heyde's syndrome is: (COMEDK 2010)
    a. Mitral stenosis, arthritis and biliary cirrhosis
    b. Mitral regurgitation, hiatus hernia and cirrhosis
    c. Aortic stenosis, gastrointestinal bleeding and angiodysplasia of colon
    d. Pulmonary arterial hypertension, tricuspid regurgitation and cirrhosis

140. First investigation to be done in a patient with recurrent fecal occult blood loss: (MHSSMCET 2006)
    a. Esophagogastroscopy   b. Colonoscopy
    c. Barium enema   d. Close Observation

141. Most common cause of heavy bleeding in 70 years old male:
    (Recent Question 2014; KGMC 2011)
    a. Colorectal carcinoma   b. Colonic diverticulosis
    c. Polyp   d. Angiodysplasia

142. False about vascular ectasia: (AIIMS GIS 2003)
    a. Associated with cutaneous lesions
    b. The bleed is usually small and recurrent and never massive
    c. The treatment may involve subtotal colectomy in some cases
    d. Associated with aortic stenosis

143. Which of the following is the least common possibility about angiodysplasia of colon? *(Recent Question 2015)*
    a. Involvement of cecum
    b. Involvement of rectum in 50% of cases
    c. Affecting age group > 40 years
    d. Cause of troublesome lower GI haemorrhage

144. Most common cause of lower GI bleed in India is: *(AIIMS Nov 94)*
    a. Benign tumour
    b. Non specific ulcer
    c. Cancer rectosigmoid
    d. Hemorrhoids

145. Painless lower GI bleed is seen in child with: *(PGI Dec 2000)*
    a. Meckel's diverticulum
    b. Rectal polyp
    c. Anal fissure
    d. Acute Appendicitis

146. A patient presents with lower gastrointestinal bleed. Sigmoidoscopy shows ulcers in the sigmoid. Biopsy from this area shows flask-shaped ulcers. Which of the following is the most appropriate treatment? *(AIIMS Nov 2005)*
    a. Intravenous ceftriaxone
    b. Intravenous metronidazole
    c. Intravenous steroids sulphasalazine
    d. Hydrocortisone enemas

147. Following is least common about angiodysplasia of colon:
    a. Involvement of cecum *(All India 96)*
    b. Involvement of rectum in 50% of cases
    c. Affecting age group > 40 years
    d. Cause of troublesome lower G.I. hemorrhage

148. The most useful investigation for profuse lower gastrointestinal bleeding is: *(UPSC 2005)*
    a. Proctosigmoidoscopy
    b. Colonoscopy
    c. Double contrast barium enema
    d. Selective arteriography

149. Most common cause of lower gastro intestinal bleeding is: *(UPPG 2007)*
    a. Diverticulosis
    b. Colorectal carcinoma
    c. Angiodysplasia
    d. Anal fissure

150. The commonest cause of significant lower gastrointestinal bleed in a middle aged person with unknown reason is: *(DPG 2009 March)*
    a. Sigmoid diverticula
    b. Angiodysplasia
    c. Ischemic colitis
    d. Ulcerative colitis

151. Most common site of angio dysplasia is: *(DNB 2007)*
    a. Sigmoid colon
    b. Transverse colon
    c. Ascending colon
    d. Descending colon

152. All of the following are cause of blood in stools in children except:
    a. Meckel's diverticulum
    b. Carcinoma
    c. Intussusception
    d. Juvenile polyp

153. The commonest cause of significantly lower gastrointestinal bleed in a middle aged person without any known precipitating factor may be due to: *(MCI March 2008, Sept 2010)*
    a. Ulcerative colitis
    b. Ischemic colitis
    c. Angiodysplasia
    d. Diverticulum of sigmoid colon

154. Massive bleeding per rectum in a 70 years old patient is due to: *(DNB 2005, 2000, All India 2000)*
    a. Diverticulosis
    b. Carcinoma colon
    c. Colitis
    d. Polyps

155. Guaiac test is used for: *(PGI 82)*
    a. Pentosuria
    b. Fructosuria
    c. For occult blood in stool
    d. Pancreatitis

BOWEL PREPARATION

156. Full bowel preparation is avoided in all, except: *(AIIMS June 94)*
    a. Carcinoma colon
    b. Hirschsprung's disease
    c. Ulcerative colitis
    d. Irritable bowel syndrome

157. Complete bowel preparation is done in a case of: *(AIIMS Nov 99)*
    a. Colonic carcinoma
    b. Hirschsprung's disease
    c. Irritable bowel disease
    d. Ulcerative colitis

158. Agent not used for bowel preparation: *(AIIMS GIS May 2011)*
    a. Metronidazole
    b. Polymyxin
    c. Erythromycin
    d. Neomycin

LARGE INTESTINE ANATOMY AND PHYSIOLOGY

159. What is epicolic node? *(Recent Question 20216, APPG 2008)*
    a. Node draining colon
    b. Adjacent to aorta
    c. Epitracheal node
    d. None

160. True about colonic organisms is: *(PGI Dec 98)*
    a. Distal ileum 103–105 organisms
    b. Colon 1010–1011 organisms
    c. First organism in new born is coliforms and streptococcus
    d. Chyme in jejunum contains many bacteria

161. Antiperistalsis is seen in: *(AIIMS 91)*
    a. Distal colon
    b. Jejunum
    c. Proximal colon
    d. Ileum

162. Mass movement of the colon would be abolished by:
    a. Extrinsic denervation *(COMEDK 2005)*
    b. Distension of the colon
    c. Gastrocolic reflex
    d. Destruction of Auerbach's plexus

163. Which of the following is the terminal group of lymph node for colon? *(AIIMS May 2011)*
    a. Paracolic
    b. Epicolic
    c. Preaortic
    d. Ileocolic

164. Which of the following is not degraded by colonic flora? *(AIIMS May 2011)*
    a. Pectin
    b. Lignin
    c. Starch
    d. Glucose

MISCELLANEOUS

165. A patient suffered bullet injury to left side of the colon and presented in the causality department after 12 hours. What will be the management? *(AIIMS Nov 2000)*
    a. Proximal defunctioning colostomy
    b. Primary closure
    c. Proximal colostomy and bringing out the distal end as mucus fistula
    d. Resection and primary anastomosis

166. Functional GI disorders can be differentiated from organic GI disorders by: *(SGPGI 2005)*
    a. Abdominal pain
    b. Diarrhea
    c. Tenesmus
    d. Bleeding PR

167. All are true about colonic lipoma except: *(PGI SS June 2001)*
    a. Squeeze sign on radiology
    b. Most common site is cecum
    c. Most commonly subserosal
    d. Most commonly submucosal

Explanations

HIRSCHSPRUNG'S DISEASE

1. Ans. a. Aganglionic segment is contracted not dilated *(Ref: Sabiston 20/e p1866; Schwartz 10/e p1624-1626; Bailey 27/e p1096)*
2. Ans. a. Hirschsprung's disease
3. Ans. a. Rectal biopsy
4. Ans. a. Autosomal dominant
5. Ans. a. Distal to dilated segment
6. Ans. c. Rectosigmoid part
7. Ans. b. Extended myectomy
8. Ans. c. Rectal biopsy
9. Ans. d. Large stool
10. Ans. b. Normal or contracted
11. Ans. b. Chronic constipation
12. Ans. c. Hirschsprung's disease
13. Ans. d. Lack of ganglion cells
14. Ans. d. Bayar's
15. Ans. b. Normal saline

> - **Repeated tube decompression** and gentle **rectal washouts** with 30-50 ml of **normal saline**^{Q} have a positive and significant clinical impact on these patients

16. Ans. a. Large bulky stools
17. Ans. b. Excision of aganglionic segment
18. Ans. c. Hirschsprung's disease
19. Ans. a. Abdominal distention *(Sabiston 19/e p1848; Schwartz 10/e p1625)*

COLONIC DIVERTICULA

20. Ans. c. Sigmoid colon *(Ref: Sabiston 20/e p1330; Schwartz 10/e p1201; Bailey 27/e p1273; Shackelford 8/e p1827, 7/e p1879-1895)*
21. Ans. a. Commonly presents with pneumaturia
22. Ans. d. Colovesical
23. Ans. b. Diverticular disease of colon
24. Ans. c. Barium enema

> - **Investigation of choice** for **colonic diverticulosis: Barium enema**^{Q}
> - **Investigation of choice** for **diverticulitis: CT scan**^{Q}

25. Ans. b. Colonic diverticula *(Ref: Sabiston 20/e p1331; Schwartz 10/e p1201; Bailey 27/e p1274)*
26. Ans. b. Superior mesenteric artery *(Ref: Sabiston 20/e p1330; Schwartz 10/e p1201; Bailey 27/e p1273; Shackelford 8/e p1830, 7/e p1883-1884)*
    Although diverticular disease is much more common on the left side, right-sided disease is responsible for more than half episodes of bleeding (from SMA).

COLONIC DIVERTICULA

- MC cause of **significant lower GI bleeding: Diverticula**^{Q}
- **Bleeding occurs** in **3-15%** of individuals with diverticulosis
- **Bleeding** occurs at the **neck of** the **diverticulum** and is believed to be secondary to bleeding from the vasa recti as they penetrate through the submucosa.

  > - Of those that bleed, **more than 75% stop spontaneously**^{Q}, although about **10% rebleed within 1 year** and almost **50% within 10 years**.
  > - Although **diverticular disease** is **much more common** on the **left side**, **right-sided disease** is **responsible for more than half episodes of bleeding**^{Q}.

- **Best method** of **diagnosis** and **treatment: Colonoscopy**^{Q}
- **Epinephrine injection, electrocautery, endoscopic clips** have been successfully applied **to control the hemorrhage**^{Q}.
- If none of these maneuvers is successful or if hemorrhage recurs, **colonic resection** is indicated.
- **Blind hemicolectomy** is associated with **rebleeding in more than half** of patients,
- **Subtotal colectomy does not eliminate the risk** for recurrent hemorrhage^Q
- **Mortality rate** of **emergent subtotal colectomy** for bleeding: **30%**^{Q}

27. Ans. a. Mucosa is inflamed
28. Ans. b. Jejunum *(Ref: Shackelford 8/e p1826, 7/e p1879)*

INCIDENCE OF DIVERTICULA

- **Most common** sites of diverticula: **CMD PES JAI** (Colon > Meckel's > Duodenum > Pharynx > Esophagus > Stomach > Jejunum > Appendix > Ileum)^Q

29. **Ans. c. Fistulization is an emergency** *(Ref: Sabiston 20/e p1333)*

- Sabiston says "In diverticulitis, fistula between colon and bladder: **a fistula arising from the colon is rarely a cause for emergency surgery**[Q]; infact, the **patient general condition** is **often improved** when the abscess fistulizes and drains. **Antibiotics** should be administered to reduce the adjacent cellulitis, and the **diagnostic steps** should be taken to confirm the cause of the fistula **before a definitive operation** is undertaken."

30. **Ans. d. Ascending colon**   31. **Ans. a. Diverticulitis**
32. **Ans. b. Hartman's procedure** *(Ref: Sabiston 20/e p1333)*

GENERALIZED PERITONITIS AFTER DIVERTICULAR PERFORATION

- **Generalized peritonitis** resulting from diverticulitis can have two causes:
  - **Diverticular perforation into the peritoneal cavity (perforation is not sealed by the body's normal defenses)**
  - **Abscess bursts** into the unprotected peritoneal cavity
- In either situation, the result is an **overwhelming infection** that requires **immediate operative intervention**[Q].

Clinical Features
- **Diffuse abdominal tenderness**, with voluntary and involuntary guarding over the entire abdomen.
- **Elevated white blood count, fever, tachycardia**, and **hypotension**[Q].

Diagnosis
- **Abdominal X-ray** or **CT scans** may **reveal intraperitoneal free air**[Q]
- **Absence of extra-intestinal air does not exclude** the **diagnosis**[Q].

Treatment
- **Immediate laparotomy** is **mandatory**[Q] to identify and excise the segment of colon containing the perforation.

  - The **proper operation** in this situation is to **resect** the **diseased sigmoid colon, construct** a **colostomy** using noninflamed descending colon, and **suture** the **divided end** of the **rectum closed.** This procedure is called **Hartmann's operation**[Q].

- **Hartmann's operation** is the **most common technique** for **emergency operations** required for **control of infection secondary to diverticulitis**[Q].
- **Anastomosis** between the **descending colon** and **rectum** to restore intestinal continuity is done **after a period of at least 10 weeks**[Q]

33. **Ans. b. CECT** *(Ref: Sabiston 20/e p1331; Schwartz 10/e p1201; Bailey 27/e p1274)*   34. **Ans. a. Complicated diverticulitis**

COLORECTAL POLYPS

35. **Ans. b. 2** *(Ref: Sabiston 20/e p1366; Shackelford 8/e p1998, 7/e p2030-2032)*

HAGGIT'S CLASSIFICATION FOR POLYPS

- **Haggit's classification**[Q] for polyps containing cancer according to the depth of invasion
- By definition, all sessile polyps with invasive carcinoma are level 4 by Haggitt criteria

Level	Depth of Invasion by Carcinoma
0	**Does not invade muscularis mucosa** (carcinoma-in-situ or Intramucosal carcinoma)[Q]
1	**Invades** through the **muscularis mucosa into submucosa** but is limited to head of the polyp.
2	**Invades** the level of **neck** of polyp (junction between head & stalk)[Q]
3	**Invades** any **part of the stalk**[Q]
4	**Invades into submucosa** of bowel wall **below the stalk of polyp** but **above the muscularis propria**[Q].

36. **Ans. c. Cowden's syndrome** *(Ref: Sabiston 20/e p1368; Schwartz 10/e p1205-1206; Bailey 27/e p1418; Shackelford 8/e p1973, 7/e p2047)*

- No increased risk of invasive gastrointestinal malignancy is seen in Cowden's syndrome[Q].

37. **Ans. a. Adenomatous polyp** *(Ref: Sabiston 20/e p1368; Schwartz 10/e p1205-1206; Bailey 27/e p1259; Shackelford 8/e p 1963, 7/e p2030-2032)*
38. **Ans. c. Potentially malignant intestinal polyps** *(Ref: Sabiston 20/e p1368; Schwartz 10/e p292,1206; Bailey 27/e p1418; Shackelford 8/e p 1973, 7/e p2047)*
39. **Ans. a. Cowden's syndrome**   40. **Ans. a. Pedunculated polyp**
41. **Ans. b. Hamartomatous polyps** *(Ref: Sabiston 20/e p1364; Schwartz 10/e p1206; Bailey 27/e p1327)*

42. **Ans. d. Familial adenomatous polyposis**
43. **Ans. b. Double contrast barium enema** *(Ref: Harrison 20/e p 574, 19/e p541; Bailey 27/e p1260)*

> - Best investigation for diagnosis of colorectal polyps: Colonoscopy >Double-contrast barium enema^Q

44. **Ans. a. Sessile** 45. **Ans. a. Villous adenoma**
46. **Ans. b. Pseudopolyps of ulcerative colitis has high risk of malignancy**
47. **Ans. a. Sessile polyps >1 cm is malignant, b. MC site is colon and rectum, c. Adenomatous polyp is premalignant**
48. **Ans. a. Juvenile polyposis syndrome, b. Peutz-Jegher's syndrome, c. Ulcerative colitis, e. Cronkhite Canada syndrome** *(Ref: Schwartz 10/e p1206)*
49. **Ans. c. Peutz-Jegher's syndrome** 50. **Ans. b. Villous adenoma**
51. **Ans. a. Juvenile polyps** 52. **Ans. c. Juvenile polyp** 53. **Ans. b. Solitary polyp**
54. **Ans. b. Hypokalemic metabolic acidosis** *(Ref: Harrison 19/e p269)*

> #### MCKITTRICK-WHEELOCK SYNDROME
> - Villous adenoma causing profuse watery diarrhea and hypokalemia, hyponatremia, hypochloremia and metabolic acidosis^Q.
> - Severe volume loss can lead to acute renal failure and cardiovascular collapse^Q.
> - Treatment is resuscitation followed by resection^Q.

55. **Ans. d. Peutz-Jegher's syndrome** *(Ref: Sabiston 20/e p 1372; Schwartz 10/e p1202; Bailey 27/e p1250; Shackelford 8/e p 1972 8/e p 1972, 7/e p2045-2046)*
56. **Ans. b. Peutz-Jegher's syndrome** 57. **Ans. b. Familial polyposis coli**
58. **Ans. d. None of the above**
59. **Ans. b. Multiple flat polyps about hundreds** *(Ref: Sabiston 20/e p1368; Shackelford 8/e p2047)*
60. **Ans. c. Peutz-Jegher's syndrome**

FAMILIAL ADENOMATOUS POLYPOSIS

61. **Ans. a. AR inheritance** *(Ref: Sabiston 20/e p1360; Schwartz 10/e p1206-1207; Bailey 27/e p1259; Shackelford 8/e p 1963 7/e p2033-2041)*

> #### SPIGELMAN'S CRITERIA
> - Spigelman's criteria predict the malignant risk of duodenal polyposis^Q in patients with FAP and guide surveillance and management.
> - Spigelman's criteria are determined by duodenal polyp number, size, histology and dysplasia (score: 0-12).

62. **Ans. d. CHRPE can be detected by ophthalmoscopy in 25% patients** 63. **Ans. d. Total proctocolectomy with IPAA**
64. **Ans. d. Endometrial carcinoma is a prominent association** *(Ref: Shackelford 8/e p 1968, 7/e p2038)*

Endometrial carcinoma is a prominent association in HNPCC, not the FAP.

> - Management of duodenal polyps in patients with FAP includes medical intervention (with NSAIDs such as sulindac), endoscopic polyp ablation, and surgical resection^Q.
> - Sulindac has been used because of its potential to stabilize, and in some cases reverse, the development of gastrointestinal neoplasia, especially colorectal adenomas^Q.
> - Sulindac is most successful in the treatment of small (<1 cm) duodenal polyps^Q

65. **Ans. d. Cowden's syndrome: 30% risk of CRC cancer** 66. **Ans. b. Periampullary carcinoma**
67. **Ans. d. Duodenal adenoma in 60-90% patients** *(Ref: Shackelford 8/e p 1968, 7/e p2037)*

> - Incidence of duodenal polyps in the patients with FAP: 90-100%^{Q}
> - Incidence of duodenal carcinoma in the patients with FAP: 0-5%^{Q}

68. **Ans. a. Brain tumor** *(Ref: Sabiston 20/e p1368; Schwartz 10/e p666,1207,1485; Bailey 27/e p1259; Shackelford 8/e p 1968 7/e p2035, 2055)*
69. **Ans. d. Giant gastric folds**
70. **Ans. a. Autosomal recessive**
71. **Ans. b. Familial adenomatous polyposis, c. Brain tumors** *(Ref: Sabiston 20/e p1368)*
72. **Ans. c. Multiple osteomas** *(Ref: Sabiston 20/e p1361)*

Large Intestine 459

Gardner's Syndrome (AD)

- Skeletal abnormalities, the most common of which are osteomas, are an essential component of Gardner syndrome.
- The osteomas are characterized by slow, continuous growth, and occur most frequently in the mandible[Q], the outer cortex of the skull and the paranasal sinuses.
- The angle of the mandible is a particularly diagnostic site[Q].

73. Ans. d. APC gene

- Most common method used to screen for APC mutations is the APC gene testing by protein truncation test[Q]

74. Ans. a. Colonic polyps
75. Ans. a. Gardner's syndrome *(Ref: Sabiston 20/e p1361; Schwartz 10/e p1207; Bailey 27/e p1259)*
76. Ans. a. It is due to a mutation of APC gene in chromosome 15

HEREDITARY NON-POLYPOSIS COLON CANCER

77. Ans. c. HNPCC *(Ref: Sabiston 20/e p1370; Schwartz 10/e p291-292,1183,1207; Bailey 27/e p1260; Shackelford 8/e p 1974, 7/e p1753-1754)*
78. Ans. c. Muir-Torre syndrome
79. Ans. a. Lynch syndrome
80. Ans. b. All the three should be first degree relative *(Ref: Sabiston 20/e p1370; Schwartz 10/e p292; Shackelford 8/e p 1974, 7/e p2041-2042)*

Revised Amsterdam Criteria

- The Revised Amsterdam criteria are used to select at-risk patients[Q] (all criteria must apply).

Criteria

- Three or more relatives who are diagnosed with an HNPCC-associated cancer (colorectal, endometrium, small bowel, ureter, or renal pelvis) in which one affected person is a first-degree relative of the other two[Q]
- At least two successive generations are affected[Q]
- One or more cases of cancer are diagnosed before age 50 years[Q]
- FAP has been excluded[Q], and tumors have undergone pathology review

  - The Bethesda guidelines are established to direct patient selection for MSI testing[Q]

81. Ans. b. CA stomach *(Ref: Sabiston 20/e p1371; Schwartz 10/e p291-292; Shackelford 8/e p 1976, 7/e p2043)*

Extra-intestinal malignancies in HNPCC

- Endometrial (39-60%)[Q] >gastric (13-19%)[Q] >ovarian (6-12%)[Q]
- Rare Malignancies: Small intestine, pancreatic, thyroid, transitional cell epithelium of the urinary tract (renal pelvic, ureter, bladder); brain cancers.

82. Ans. a. MSH-2 and hMLH-1
83. Ans. b. HNPCC

RISK FACTORS COLORECTAL CANCER

84. Ans. a. Ulcerative colitis, c. Familial polyposis coli *(Ref: Schwartz 10/e p291-292)*
85. Ans. a. High fiber diet *(Ref: Maingot 11/e p626-627; Schwartz 10/e p1204)*

- **High fiber diet** has been found to have **protective effect** by **increasing** the **stool bulk, diluting** the **toxins,** and **reducing** the **colonic transit time** and thus **reducing exposure time to fecal carcinogens**[Q]

86. Ans. d. p53 *(Ref: Sabiston 20/e p1360; Schwartz 10/e p1204)*

- The most frequently mutated tumor suppressor gene in human neoplasia is p53 (TP53), located on **chromosome 17p**[Q]
- **Mutations in p53** are present in **75% of colorectal cancers** and occur, rather late[Q] in the adenoma-carcinoma sequence.

FEARON-VOGELSTEIN ADENOMA CARCINOMA MULTISTEP MODEL

- **Earliest mutations** in adenoma-carcinoma sequence occur in **APC gene**[Q]. **Earliest phenotype change** present is known as **aberrant crypt formation**[Q] & **most consistent genetic aberrations** within these cells are abnormally short proteins known as **APC truncations.**
- Most APC truncation mutations occur in mutational cluster region of the gene, an area **responsible** for **beta-catenin binding**[Q].
- **Mutations in p53** are present in **75% of colorectal cancers** and **occur rather late**[Q] in the adenoma-carcinoma sequence.

87. **Ans. b. Beta-Catenin** *(Ref: Sabiston 20/e p1360)*

Gene Mutations that Cause Colon Cancer	
Mutation type	**Genes Involved**
Germline	• **APC** and **MMR**[Q]
Somatic	• **Oncogenes:** Myc, Ras, Src, erbB2[Q] • **Tumor suppressor genes:** p53, DCC, APC[Q] • **MMR genes:** bMSH2, bMLH1, bPMS1, bPMS2, bMSH6, bMSH3[Q]
Genetic polymorphism	• APC[Q]

ADENOMATOUS POLYPOSIS COLI (APC) GENE

- APC gene is a tumor suppressor gene located on chromosome 5q21[Q].
- Its product is 2843 amino acids in length and forms a cytoplasmic complex with GSK-3β (a serine-threonine kinase), β-catenin, and axin[Q].

- **APC** participates in cell cycle control by regulating the intracytoplasmic pool of β-catenin[Q].
- **APC** influences cell cycle proliferation by regulating Wnt expression[Q].

- The **Wnt signaling proteins** are closely associated with the **APC-β-catenin pathway.**
- Under normal conditions, **reduced intracytoplasmic β-catenin levels inhibit Wnt expression.**
- When **APC** is **mutated** however, β-catenin levels rise, and **Wnt is activated.**

88. **Ans. a. Proximal colon cancer** *(Ref: Maingot 11/e p628)*

- Bile acids can induce hyperproliferation of the intestinal mucosa[Q] via a number of intracellular mechanisms.
    - **Cholecystectomy**, which alters the enterohepatic cycle of bile acids, has been associated with a **moderately increased risk** of proximal colon cancers[Q].
- It cannot be ruled out, however, that it is less the effect of the cholecystectomy than the impact of other, not yet identified factors in the lithogenic bile of such patients.
- A number of cofactors have been identified that **may enhance** or **neutralize the carcinogenic effects of bile acids,** e.g., the amount of **dietary fat, fiber, or calcium**[Q].
- **Calcium**, in fact, **binds bile acids** and thus may **reduce their negative impact**[Q].

89. **Ans. a. FAP, b. Crohn's disease, c. Ulcerative colitis**

CARCINOMA COLON CLINICAL FEATURES AND DIAGNOSIS

90. **Ans. a. Sigmoid** *(Ref: Bailey 27/e p1262)*

Site of Carcinoma	Frequency
• **Rectum (MC)**[Q]	• 38%
• **Sigmoid colon (2nd MC)**[Q]	• 21%
• **Cecum**	• 12%
• Transverse colon	• 5.5%
• Ascending colon	• 5%
• Descending colon	• 4%
• Splenic flexure	• 3%
• Hepatic flexure (LC)[Q]	• 2%

91. **Ans. a. Left colon** *(Ref: Sabiston 20/e p1372; Bailey 27/e p1262)*
92. **Ans. b. Carcinoma cecum**
93. **Ans. d. Fungating**
94. **Ans. d. Solitary liver metastasis is not a contraindication for surgery** *(Ref: Sabiston 20/e p 1377; Schwartz 10/e p1293-1294; Bailey 27/e p1264)*

95. **Ans. b. Carcinoma colon** *(Ref: Sabiston 20/e p1371; Bailey 27/e p1262)*

- **Barium enema**: "**Apple core**" or "**napkin ring**" **lesion**, caused by a **constricting carcinoma**[Q]

96. **Ans. a. Have better image than conventional colonoscopy, b. VC is performed by CT and MRI, e. Helpful in pathology outside colon** *(Ref: Harrison 20/e p 2205, 19/e p1898-1899)*

VIRTUAL COLONOSCOPY

- VC is **a medical imaging procedure** which **uses x-rays** and **computers** to produce **two-**and **three-dimensional images** of the **colon** and **rectum** and display them on a screen
- VC is **performed via CT** or with **MRI**[Q]
- After the examination, the **images produced** by the scanner must be **processed into a 3D image**[Q] (a cine program allows the user move through the bowel as if performing a normal colonoscopy).

  - VC is used to **diagnose colonic polyps, diverticulosis and cancer**[Q].
  - VC provides a **secondary benefit** of **revealing diseases** or **abnormalities outside** the **colon**[Q]

- VC provides **clearer, more detailed images than** a **barium enema**[Q]
- Takes **less time** than either a conventional **colonoscopy** or **barium enema**[Q]

Disadvantages of Virtual Colonoscopy

- Radiologist **cannot take tissue samples (biopsy)** or **remove polyps**[Q] during VC (conventional colonoscopy must be performed if abnormalities are found)
- **VC** performed **with CT exposes** the patient to **ionizing radiation**[Q]

97. **Ans. c. Ba swallow, d. Ba follow through, e. Enteroclysis**

- **Barium swallow** is used for anatomical disorders of **esophagus**[Q].
- **Barium meal** is used for anatomical disorders of **stomach**[Q].
- **Barium meal follow through** is used for anatomical disorders of **small intestine**[Q].
- **Barium enema** is used for anatomical disorders of **large intestine**[Q].
- **Enteroclysis** is also known as **small bowel enema**, used for small intestine[Q].

98. **Ans. b. Depth of invasion** *(Ref: Schwartz 10/e p1209; Shackelford 7/e p2133)*

- **Incidence** of **metastasis** (hence **prognosis**) is **related** to **depth of invasion**[Q]
- **No effect on Prognosis: Tumor size** and **duration** of symptoms[Q]
- **Tumor size** and **configuration** (endophytic, exophytic, annular) **do not carry** any **prognostic significance**[Q] in colorectal carcinoma.

99. **Ans. d. Carcinoma is inevitable in untreated cases of FAP**   100. **Ans. a. Screening sigmoidoscopy**
101. **Ans. d. Lymph node status** *(Ref: Schwartz 10/e p1203-1216)*
102. **Ans. c. Depth of penetration of bowel wall**
103. **Ans. b. Most common site is sigmoid colon, c. Right sided colon carcinoma present as chronic anemia, e. Right sided colon has better prognosis than left sided colon** *(Ref: Robbins 8/e p863)*

- **Left sided colon cancers** are **more infiltrative at** the time of **diagnosis than right lesions**, associated with **poor prognosis**[Q].

104. **Ans. None: Incidence of carcinoma in cecum is 12%**[Q].
105. **Ans. d. Colonoscopy and biopsy**   106. **Ans. d. Sigmoid colon**   107. **Ans. a. Sigmoid**
108. **Ans. d. Sigmoid colon** *(Ref: Shackelford 8/e p1694, 7/e p1747-1748; Harrison 19/e p1881)*

RISKS ASSOCIATED WITH COLONOSCOPY

- **Risks of colonoscopy: Perforation** and **hemorrhage**[Q]
- **MC site** of **bleeding after colonoscopy: Stalk** after polypectomy.
- **MC site** of **perforation** during colonoscopy: **Sigmoid colon**[Q]
- **Perforation** can be caused by excessive air **pressure**, **tearing** of the antimesenteric border of the colon **from excessive pressure** on colonic loops, and at the sites of **electrosurgical applications**[Q]

109. **Ans. d. Carcinoma ascending colon**

CARCINOMA COLON STAGING

110. **Ans. d. III** *(Ref: Sabiston 20/e p1374)*   111. **Ans. d. T4N1M0**

CARCINOMA COLON TREATMENT

112. **Ans. a. Colostomy, d. Hartmann procedure, e. Laser recanalisation** *(Ref: Sabiston 20/e p1376; Schwartz 10/e p1212-12133; Bailey 27/e p1264)*

- Maingot: "Hartmann's operation is an **excellent palliative procedure** done in **elderly people** who are **not fit for major surgery** like APR and also **in locally advanced tumors**[Q]."
- **Unresectable rectal cancer** can be palliated by fulgration (electrocoagulation) or laser photocoagulation[Q].
- **Diverting colostomy** is performed **for obstructing rectal cancer that cannot be resected**[Q].

Treatment of Large Bowel Obstruction	
Right-sided colonic obstruction (cancer or volvulus)	**Resection** with ileo-**transverse anastomosis**[Q]
Cancer of sigmoid colon	**Hartmann's operation**[Q] (sigmoidectomy with descending colostomy and closure of the rectal stump), **Sigmoidectomy** with **primary colorectal anastomosis**[Q] **Abdominal colectomy** with **ileorectal anastomosis**[Q].
Cancer of **distal or mid rectum**	**Loop colostomy** or **defunctioning colostomy** (to relieve obstruction) followed by **neoadjuvant chemoradiation**[Q], (with the plan to resect the primary lesion at a later time)

113. **Ans. a. Hartman's procedure, b. Left colectomy with anastomosis, c. Proximal colostomy, d. Extended right colectomy with ileoanal anastomosis**

114. **Ans. d. Staged operation, e. Chemotherapy** *(Ref: Sabiston 20/e p1377)*

COLORECTAL LIVER METASTASES

- With **improved response rates to modern chemotherapy** and advances in hepatic surgery, however, **more patients** are **now candidates for hepatectomy**[Q] than in the past.
  - For patients with **unresectable disease, preoperative chemotherapy** has been shown to **convert some patients** to **complete resection**[Q].
  - **Combinations of chemotherapy** and **complete resection** of **hepatic metastases** are **associated with long-term survival** in **up to 50%** of patients in modern series.
- **Complete resection** of hepatic metastases **appears to be a critically important treatment modality** that is **necessary for long-term survival**[Q].

METASTATIC COLORECTAL CARCINOMA

- At present, only patients who have recurrence of colorectal carcinoma with defined **isolated liver, lung, ovarian, or anastomotic metastasis should undergo surgery**[Q].

Pulmonary Metastasis
- Prognostic factors include the **number** of metastases, **size** of the lesion, lymph node involvement, presence of additional metastatic sites and in some series pre-thoracotomy CEA levels.
- Neither primary disease free survival nor primary colorectal cancer stage significantly affect survival rates after thoracotomy.

Prophylactic Bilateral Oophorectomy
- Incidence of **ovarian cancer** with a history of colorectal cancer is **five times,** so the prevention of primary ovarian cancer in postmenopausal women is considered to be the main benefit.

115. **Ans. a. Mechanical bowel wash, c. Broad spectrum antibiotic at the time of operation**
116. **Ans. a. Resection**
117. **Ans. a. Primary resection and Hartman's procedure, b. Defunctioning colostomy, d. Resection of whole left bowel and end to end anastomosis**
118. **Ans. a. Hartman's procedure, b. Left colectomy with anastomosis, c. Proximal colostomy, d. Extended right colectomy with ileoanal anastomosis**
119. **Ans. b. Hartman's procedure**
120. **Ans. b. Left hemicolectomy is the treatment of choice for splenic flexure tumors**

COLONIC ISCHEMIA

121. Ans. b. Ischemic colitis *(Ref: Sabiston 20/e p1356; Schwartz 10/e p1221; Bailey 27/e p1276; Shackelford 8/e p 1820, 7/e p1866-1877)*
122. Ans. c. Ischemic colitis *(Ref: Sabiston 20/e p1356; Schwartz 10/e p1222; Bailey 27/e p1277)*
    - **Thumb printing**[Q] (due to **mucosal edema** and **submucosal hemorrhage**)[Q] is characteristic feature of ischemic colitis.
123. Ans. b. Ischemia is more common in small bowel as compared to large bowel

   - Indeed, the **IMA is frequently occluded** in **conditions requiring aortic surgery**, and **in such circumstances, transection of the IMA does not require reimplantation**[Q]. However, **in this situation**, the **left colon is dependent** on **collateral blood supply**, and transient hypotension at the time of the vascular procedure or immediately after surgery may result in ischemic injury to the vulnerable colonic mucosa.
   - In **aortic surgeries, the IMA is assessed for backbleeding.** If there is **strong backbleeding** (stump pressure >40 mm Hg), the **IMA is ligated close to the aorta** or oversewn from within the sac. **Poor backbleeding from the IMA is a sign of insufficient collateral circulation** to the **sigmoid colon,** and **reimplantation of the IMA with a patch of the aorta into** the **aortic limb is warranted**[Q].

124. Ans. d. Sigmoid colon
125. Ans. b. Splenic flexure
126. Ans. c. Ischemic colitis
127. Ans. a, c, d, e. Most common site..., Abdominal radiographs..., Commonly present..., Acute thrombotic... *(Ref: Schwartz 10/e p1221; Sabiston 20/e p1356; Bailey 27/e p1276)*

PSEUDOMEMBRANOUS COLITIS

128. Ans. b. Clostridium difficile *(Ref: Sabiston 20/e p1133; Schwartz 10/e p1222; Bailey 27/e p1273)*
129. Ans. c. Metronidazole
130. Ans. c. Antibiotic associated diarrhea
131. Ans. a. Accordion sign

COLONIC RESECTION AND ANASTOMOSIS

132. Ans. b. Start IVF, c. Do urgent laparotomy *(Ref: CSDT 11/e p24)*

WOUND DEHISCENCE (BURST ABDOMEN)

- **Serous** or **serosanguinous discharge** from the wound is the **first sign**[Q] of dehiscence
  - **Most commonly** observed between 5th and 8th post-operative **day**[Q] (may occur at any time following wound closure)
- Wound dehiscence is **partial** or **total disruption** of any or all layers of the operative wound.
- **Extrusion** of **abdominal viscera** after rupture of all layers is known as evisceration[Q].

Predisposing Factors for Wound Dehiscence	
Local Risk Factors	**Systemic Risk Factors**

• **Inadequate closure (Most important)**[Q]
• **Increased** intra-abdominal **pressure**
• **Deficient wound healing** due to:
  – Infections[Q]
  – Seroma[Q]
  – Hematoma[Q]
  – Presence of drain[Q]
	• Old age[Q]
	• Obesity[Q]
	• Immunosuppression[Q]
	• Systemic diseases:
	  – Diabetes[Q]
	  – Uremia[Q]
	  – Jaundice, Sepsis[Q]
	  – Cancer[Q]

Management
- **Wound dehiscence** without evisceration: **Prompt elective closure**[Q] of the wound
- **Wound dehiscence** with evisceration:
  - Wound is **covered with moist towels**
  - Under GA, **any exposed bowel or omentum** is rinsed with RL containing **antibiotics** and then **returned to abdomen**
  - Previous sutures are removed, wound is reclosed **(Tension suturing**[Q])

133. Ans. b. IV fluids, e. Urgent surgery
134. Ans. d. Cecum and ascending colon *(Ref: Sabiston 20/e p443)*

Maneuvers for Retroperitoneal Exposure			
Kocher's Maneuver	**Extended Kocher's Maneuver**	**Mattox Maneuver**	**Cattel-Braasch Maneuver**
• Surgical maneuver to **expose structures** in the **retroperitoneum**[Q] **behind** the **duodenum** and **pancreas**[Q] • Used for **mobilization of duodenum**[Q]	• **Right sided medial visceral rotation**[Q] • **Right colon** and **duodenum is reflected medially**[Q] • **Exposes IVC, Infrarenal aorta, right renal artery** and **iliac vessels**[Q] • Recommended for **drainage of inframesocolic hematoma**[Q]	• **Left sided medial visceral rotation**[Q] • Left sided viscera (**Left kidney, left colon, spleen and pancreas**) are brought to midline[Q] • **Exposes** entire length of **abdominal aorta, celiac axis, proximal part** of **mesenteric arteries** and **proximal left renal artery**[Q] • Recommended for **drainage** of **central supra-mesocolic hematoma**[Q]	• For **extensive retroperitoneal exposure**[Q] • **Right colon** is **fully mobilized** and **reflected medially**[Q] • Good option for **exposure of the infrapancreatic segment**[Q]

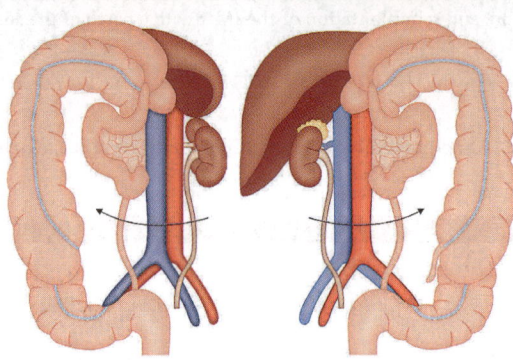

Left medial visceral rotation to expose the abdominal-aorta   Right medial visceral rotation to expose the infrahepatic vena cava

135. **Ans. b. Right hemicolectomy**

ENTERIC FISTULA

136. **Ans. a. High output fistula drains 500 mL/day, c. Fluid and electrolyte loss can occur**   137. **Ans. a. Crohn's disease**

LOWER GI BLEED

138. **Ans. d. Dilated mucosal and submucosal veins in the colon** *(Ref: Harrison 19/e p731; Bailey 27/e p1276)*

    Diagnosis in a 65-year-old patient of bleeding per rectum with syncope and negative fecal occult blood test and no history of recent weight loss is Heyde's syndrome. The colonoscopic finding in Heyde's syndrome is dilated mucosal and submucosal veins in the colon.

139. **Ans. c. Aortic stenosis, gastrointestinal bleeding and angiodysplasia of colon** *(Ref: Harrison 20/e p 829, 19/e p731; Bailey 27/e p1276)*
140. **Ans. b. Colonoscopy** *(Ref: Sabiston 20/e p1151)*

    • Colonoscopy is the mainstay of diagnosis because it allows both visualization of the pathology and therapeutic intervention in colonic, rectal, and distal ileal sources of bleeding[Q].

141. **Ans. b. Colonic diverticulosis** *(Ref: Sabiston 20/e p1151)*
142. **Ans. a. Associated with cutaneous lesions** *(Ref: Sabiston 20/e p1153; Shackelford 8/e p 1815, 7/e p1856-1863; Bailey 27/e p1276)*
143. **Ans. b. Involvement of rectum in 50% of cases**
144. **Ans. d. Hemorrhoids** *(Ref: API Medicine 6/e p509, 511)*

    • API: "Hemorrhoids and anal fissure are the most common cause of lower GI bleeding, however the bleeding is rarely **massive**[Q]."

145. **Ans. a. Meckel's diverticulum, b. Rectal polyp**
146. **Ans. b. Intravenous metronidazole** *(Ref: Harrison 20/e p 1572, 19/e p1365; Bailey 27/e p1272)*

AMEBIC COLITIS

• MC site of **amebic colitis: Cecum and ascending colon**[Q]
• **Flask shaped ulcers** on **colonoscopy** confirms the **diagnosis of amebic colitis**[Q]

Drug Therapy for Amebiasis

- **Asymptomatic carrier:** Luminal agents **(Iodoquinol, paromomycin)**^{Q}
- **Acute colitis: Metronidazole** and **luminal agents**^{Q}
- **Amebic liver abscess: Metronidazole, tinidazole** and **luminal agents**^{Q}

147. Ans. b. Involvement of rectum in 50% cases
148. Ans. b. Colonoscopy
149. Ans. a. Diverticulosis
150. Ans. a. Sigmoid diverticula
151. Ans. c. Ascending colon
152. Ans. None > b. Carcinoma
153. Ans. d. Diverticulum of sigmoid colon
154. Ans. a. Diverticulosis
155. Ans. c. For occult blood in stool *(Ref: Harrison 20/e p 574, 19/e p540)*

BOWEL PREPARATION

156. Ans. a. Carcinoma colon *(Ref: Sabiston 20/e p252; Schwartz 10/e p1194-1195)*
157. Ans. a. Colonic carcinoma
158. Ans. b. Polymyxin

LARGE INTESTINE ANATOMY AND PHYSIOLOGY

159. Ans. a. Node draining colon *(Ref: Grays 40/e p1077)*

Lymphatic drainage of Large Intestine

- Lymphatic drainage also **follows** the **arterial anatomy.**
- **Lymphatics from** the **colon** and **proximal two thirds** of the **rectum** ultimately **drain into** the **para-aortic nodal chain,** which empties into the **cisterna chyli**^{Q}.
- **Superior** and **inferior mesenteric nodes** are part of **Pre-aortic group** of lymph nodes^Q.
- **Lymphatics draining** the **distal rectum** and **anal canal** may **drain either** to the para-aortic nodes or laterally, through the internal iliac system, to the superficial inguinal nodal basin (dentate line roughly marks the level where lymphatic drainage diverges)
- Lymph nodes are commonly grouped into levels depending on their location.

Epicolic	Located **along** the **bowel wall** and in the **epiploicae**^{Q}
Paracolic	Located **adjacent to** the **marginal artery**^{Q}
Intermediate	Located **along** the **main branches**^{Q} of the large blood vessels
Primary or terminal	Located on the **superior** or **inferior mesenteric artery**^{Q}

160. Ans. b. Colon 1010-1011 organisms *(Ref: Jawetz Microbiology 23rd/1154; Sabiston 20/e p1320; Schwartz 10/e p1179)*

Normal Microbial Flora of Intestinal Tract

- **At birth,** the **intestine is sterile,** but organisms are soon introduced with food.
- In the **breastfed children,** the organisms present in the intestine: **Lactic acid streptococci** and **Lactobacilli**^{Q}
- In **normal adults,** the **stomach acidity** keeps the number of **microorganism** at **minimum,** unless obstruction at the pylorus favors the proliferation of gram positive cocci and bacilli.
- As the **pH of intestinal contents** becomes **alkaline,** the resident **flora gradually increases**^{Q}.
- In **diarrhea, bacterial count decreases,** whereas count **increases in intestinal obstruction**^{Q}.

Part of GIT	No. of Microorganisms
Stomach	10^3-10^5/gm of contents
Duodenum	10^3-10^6/gm of contents
Jejunum and Ileum	10^5-10^8/gm of contents
Cecum and Transverse colon	10^8-10^{11}/gm of contents
Sigmoid and Rectum	10^{11}/gm of contents^Q

466 Surgery Essence

161. **Ans. c. Proximal colon** *(Ref: Sabiston 20/e p1324, 19/e p1307)*

MOTILITY PATTERN OF COLON

- **Right colon** is the **fermentation chamber** of the **human GI tract**[Q]
- **Bacteria** are **most metabolically active** in **cecum**[Q]
- **Left colon** is a site **of storage** and **dehydration of stool**[Q].

Site	Motility Pattern
Right colon	**Antiperistaltic**, or **retropulsive waves**[Q] generate retrograde flow of colonic contents back to the cecum.
Left colon	Antegrade tonic contractions[Q]

- **Mass peristalsis** is interspersed with the propulsive and retropulsive contractions and occurs at varying intervals, **more frequently after meals**[Q].
- **Mass peristaltic contraction** advances a **column of colonic contents** through **one third of** the **colonic length**[Q].
- **Increased postprandial contractility** is **greater in** the **sigmoid**[Q] **than** in the transverse colon.
- **Gastrocolic reflex:** Effects of a meal on colonic motility[Q]

162. **Ans. d. Destruction of auerbach plexus** *(Ref: Ganong 25/e p472)*

Auerbach Plexus	Meissner's Plexus
• Situated **between** and innervates **outer longitudinal** and **inner circular layers**[Q] • Primarily concerned with **peristalsis**[Q]	• Situated between **middle circular layer** and **mucosa**[Q] • Also known **as submucosal plexus**[Q] • Primarily concerned with **intestinal secretion**[Q]

163. **Ans. c. Preaortic**

164. **Ans. b. Lignin** *(Ref: Sabiston 20/e p1321)*

FERMENTATION IN COLON

- Both microbiota and host obtain clear benefits from this association.
- Bacteria supply the host with butyrate[Q] (main fuel for colonic epithelial cells)
- Bacterial fermentation products are absorbed and used as a source of energy.
- Main sources of energy for intestinal bacteria are complex carbohydrates: starches & nonstarch polysaccharides (NSPs), also known as dietary fiber[Q].

  - **Lignin** is **not fermented** by **human colonic flora** and **attracts water**[Q], thus producing bulk.
  - **Celluloses** are **only partially fermented**[Q].
  - **Fruit pectins** are **completely fermented**[Q].

- **Highly fermentable NSPs** provide **minimal bulk** and **slow transit time**[Q].
- **Constipation, diverticulosis,** and **colon cancer** are **uncommon in** populations with a **high intake of roughage** (i.e., **waterinsoluble NSPs**)[Q].

Water-insoluble fibers (Lignin)	• Used for the treatment of constipation[Q]
Water-soluble NSPs (Pectin)	• Used to treat diarrhea[Q]

MISCELLANEOUS

165. **Ans. c. Proximal colostomy and bringing out the distal end as mucus fistula** *(Ref: Sabiston 20/e p443)*

166. **Ans. d. Bleeding PR**

167. **Ans. c. Most commonly subserosal** *(Ref: Maingot 11/e p838)*

SHORT CHAIN FATTY ACIDS (SCFA)

- **Short chain fatty acids** are produced **in** the **colon** and **absorbed from it**[Q].
- **SCFAs: Acetate (60%), Propionate (25%), Butyrate**[Q] **(15%)**
- Formed by action of colonic bacteria on complex carbohydrates, resistant starches, and other component of dietary fibers.

Anatomy of Colon

- The **meandering artery** or **Arc of Riolan**[Q] is a collateral branch that **connects** the **proximal MCA to the LCA** and runs in the transverse mesocolon parallel to the left branch of the MCA.
- **Griffith's point**[Q]: **splenic flexure**, where the vascular arcades connecting the MCA and LCA are often absent
- **Sudek's point**[Q]: inconsistent marginal artery at the junction of the **lowest sigmoid branch** and the **superior hemorrhoidal artery**

  - **Jackson Membrane**[Q]: Adhesion from the **right abdominal wall** to the **anterior taenia** of the ascending colon.
  - **Gerlach valves**[Q]: A mucosal fold **covering** the **appendiceal orifice**.
  - **Fold of Treves**[Q]: **Inferior ileocecal fold (does not contain any vessel**, referred as the **bloodless fold of Treves)**

- **Fold of Treves** is the **only antimesenteric epiploic appendage** normally found on the **small intestine** and **marks** the **junction** of the ileum and cecum[Q]

  - **Widest portion** of colon: **Cecum**[Q]
  - **Narrowest portion** of colon: **Sigmoid**[Q]
  - **MC site** of **colonic rupture** caused **by distal obstruction: Cecum**[Q]
  - Colon absorbs water, NaCl[Q]; secretes K+, HCO3 and mucus[Q]
  - MC site of ischemic colitis: Splenic flexure

Large Intestine

- Length of **cecum**: 7.5 cm (x=7.5 cm)
- Length of **Transverse colon**: 45 cm (6x)
- Length of **Sigmoid colon**: 30 cm (4x)
- Length of **Ascending colon**: 15 cm (2x)
- Length of **Descending colon**: 22.5 cm (3x)

CHAPTER 15

Ileostomy and Colostomy

STOMA

STOMAS

- May be **colostomy** or **ileostomy**
- May be **temporary** or **permanent**
- **Temporary** or **defunctioning stomas** are usually fashioned as **loop stomas**
- An **ileostomy is spouted**; a **colostomy is flush**[Q]
- **Ileostomy effluent** is usually **liquid** whereas **colostomy effluent** is usually **solid**[Q]
- **Ileostomy patients** are more likely to develop **fluid & electrolyte problems**
- An **ileostomy** is usually sited in the **right iliac fossa**[Q]
- A **temporary colostomy** may be **transverse** and sited in the **right upper quadrant**[Q]
- **End-colostomy** is usually sited in the **left iliac fossa**[Q]
- All patients should be counseled by a stoma care nurse before operation

STOMA FORMATION

STOMA FORMATION

- A **colostomy** is a **connection** of the **colon to** the **skin** of the abdominal wall.
- An **ileostomy** involves **exteriorization** of the **ileum on** the abdominal **skin**.
- **MC indications** of **stoma formation**: Colorectal cancer, chronic ulcerative colitis and Crohn's disease[Q]
- **Ileostomy revisions** are most commonly performed **for Crohn's disease**[Q].

  - **Appearance of a fistula** adjacent to a stoma usually **indicates recurrence of Crohn's disease**[Q].
  - A special complication in portal hypertension: **Varices** can form **in** the **peristomal skin**[Q].

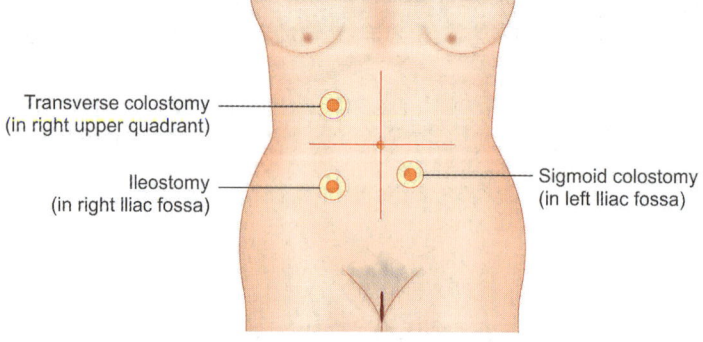

Sites of Stoma Formation

ILEOSTOMY

ILEOSTOMY

- **Opening** constructed **between** the **small intestine** and the **abdominal wall**, usually by **using distal ileum**.

  - **Indications** of **Permanent ileostomy**: For patients who require **removal of the entire colon** and **rectum** (Crohn's disease or ulcerative colitis[Q])
  - **Indications** of **loop ileostomy**: Cases where **multiple** and **complex anastomoses** must be **performed distally** (Crohn's disease or CA rectum[Q]).

- **Loop ileostomy use** is becoming **more frequent** (because of the complex sphincter-preserving operations being performed for **UC** and **FAP**)

Types of ileostomies	
• End ileostomy (Brooke) • Loop ileostomy • Loop-end ileostomy	• Continent ileostomy (Kock pouch) • Urinary conduit

Continent Ileostomy

- Continent ileostomy, or **Kock pouch**, has been used as an **alternative to** a **conventional ileostomy** for **selected patients** with **UC** or **FAP**ᵠ.

> • Contraindicated in Crohn's diseaseᵠ (risk of **recurrent disease**)
> • Not recommended for well-functioning end ileostomyᵠ.

- It involves construction of an **internal pouch with** a **continent nipple valve**.
- The **complication rate** for construction of this **continent ileostomy** has been **high** because of the difficulty in maintaining continence of the nipple valve and position of the pouch so that intubation can be easily accomplished.

Continent Ileostomy	
Advantages	**Disadvantages**
• Patient **need not wear** an **appliance**ᵠ • Patient is **continent between intubations**ᵠ • **Better quality of life**ᵠ	• **Not all patients** are **continent** • Require **multiple intubations** during the day • **Difficulty in intubation** • Prolonged surgery with substantial risk of complications.

COLOSTOMY

COLOSTOMY

- **MC indication** for **fashioning a colostomy: CA rectum**ᵠ
- Colostomies are also constructed as **treatment for obstructing lesions** of the **distal large intestine** and for **actual or potential perforations**ᵠ.

Type by Anatomic Location	
• End-sigmoid colostomy (MC)ᵠ • End-descending colostomyᵠ	• Transverse colostomy • Cecostomy

> • However, **if** the **IMA** is **transected** during an operation for **CA rectum**, the **blood supply** to the **sigmoid colon** is **no longer dependable**, and it **should not be used** for stoma construction. Therefore, an **"end-descending"** colostomy is usually **preferable** to an end-sigmoid colostomyᵠ.

- **Location of** the **colostomy** should **avoid any deep folds of fat**, **scars**, and **bony prominences** of the abdominal wallᵠ.

Type by Function
• To **provide decompression of** the **large intestine**ᵠ • To **provide diversion of** the **feces**ᵠ

Decompressing Colostomy	Diverting Colostomy
Indications • **Distal obstructing lesions** causing **massive dilation** of the **proximal colon** without **ischemic necrosis**ᵠ • **Severe sigmoid diverticulitis** with **phlegmon**ᵠ • **Selected patients** with **toxic megacolon**ᵠ	**Indications** • When **distal segment** of **bowel** has been **completely resected** (as during **APR**)ᵠ • **Known** or **suspected perforation** or **obstruction** of the **distal bowel** (e.g., **obstructing carcinoma**, **diverticulitis**, **leaking anastomosis**, or **trauma**ᵠ) • **Destruction** or **infection of** the **distal colon**, **rectum**, or **anus** (e.g., Crohn's **disease** or failed anal sphincter reconstruction)ᵠ
Types of Decompressing Stomas • **Blow-hole cecostomy** • **Blow hole transverse** colostomy • **Tube type** of **cecostomy** • **Loop-transverse** colostomy	**Types of Diverting Stomas** • **Loop-transverse** colostomy • **Loop sigmoid colostomy**

STOMAL COMPLICATIONS

- MC complication of both end & loop colostomy: Parastomal hernia[Q]
- Parastomal hernia is more common in end colostomy[Q] as compared to loop colostomy.
- Prolapse is more common in loop colostomy
- MC complication of ileostomy: Skin irritation[Q]
- MC early complication of ileostomy: Ischemic necrosis[Q]

STOMAL COMPLICATIONS

- Stomas are widely used in the treatment of colorectal, intestinal, and urologic diseases.
- An intestinal stoma can be an ileostomy, colostomy, or urostomy, end, loop, or end-loop, temporary or permanent, diverting or decompressing, or continent or incontinent.
  - A tube cecostomy and a blowhole are considered temporary decompressing colostomies performed in emergencies[Q].
- Technical factors are most important in minimizing the complication rate of stoma construction and are largely preventable.
- Early complications are considered those that occur within 30 days[Q] after surgery.

Clinical Presentation and Diagnosis	
Ischemic necrosis[Q]	From impaired perfusion to the terminal portion of the bowel as a result of a tight aperture, overzealous trimming of mesentery, or mesenteric tension.
Stomal retraction[Q]	Occurs early as a result of tension on the bowel or ischemic necrosis of the stoma.
Late retraction[Q]	Caused by increased thickness of the abdominal wall with weight gain.
Stenosis[Q]	As a result of a small aperture (natural maturation), ischemia, recurrence of Crohn's disease, or development of carcinoma.
Mucocutaneous separation	As a result of ischemia, inadequate approximation of mucosa to the dermal layer of skin, excessive bowel tension, or peristomal infection.
Stomal prolapse[Q]	Most alarming to the patient and can result in incomplete diversion of stool, interfere with the stoma appliance, lead to leakage of stool, or become associated with obstructive symptoms and incarceration.
Parastomal hernia[Q]	Occurs to some degree in most patients.
Peristomal fistula	Sign of Crohn's disease, may result from a deep suture used to mature the stoma, or may be caused by trauma from an appliance.
Chemical dermatitis[Q]	Caused by contact of the stoma effluent with peristomal skin[Q]. Manifested as erythema, ulceration (ileostomy effluent), encrustation (urostomy effluent), or pseudoepitheliomatous hyperplasia.
Traumatic dermatitis	Occurs during change of the stomal device, from stripping of adhesive, or as a result of friction or pressure from the stomal device or supportive belt. Manifested as erythema, erosion and ulceration.
Diarrhea and dehydration[Q]	Commonly occurs in older patients, in hot weather, during strenuous exercise, and in association with short bowel syndrome.
Cutaneous manifestations of the disease[Q]	Damaged peristomal skin in psoriasis[Q]. Pyoderma gangrenosa in IBD[Q]. Parastomal varices in portal hypertension[Q].

Stomal Complications				
	Early (RAPID-O)		**Late (SPF-GO)**	
Stoma	• Poor location • Retraction* • Ischemic necrosis[Q]	• Detachment • Abscess formation • Opening wrong end	• Prolapse[Q] • Stenosis[Q] • Parastomal hernia[Q]	• Fistula formation[Q] • Gas • Odor
Peristomal skin	• Excoriation[Q] • Dermatitis*		• Parastomal varices • Dermatoses	• Cancer • Skin manifestations of IBD
Systemic	• High output*		• Bowel obstruction[Q] • Nonclosure	

- *May also develop as a late complication

Multiple Choice Questions

ILEOSTOMY AND COLOSTOMY

1. **Most common complication of end colostomy:** *(JIPMER 2011)*
   a. Parastomal hernia
   b. Prolapse
   c. Perforation
   d. Bleeding

2. **Known complication of stoma (e.g., Colostomy stoma):** *(MHPGMCET 2009)*
   a. Prolapse
   b. Stenosis
   c. Retraction
   d. All of the above

3. **Continent ileostomy is done in all the following except:**
   a. Ulcerative colitis with poor anal tone *(MHSSMCET 2005)*
   b. Crohn's disease
   c. Redo Hirschsprung's disease
   d. All

4. **Mercedes procedure is used in:** *(MHSSMCET 2008)*
   a. Discrepancy in size of ileum and stoma
   b. Ileostomy stenosis
   c. Ileostomy prolapse
   d. Ileostomy leak

5. **Early postoperative complication of ileostomy:** *(AIIMS Nov 2006)*
   a. Obstruction
   b. Prolapse
   c. Diarrhea
   d. Necrosis

6. **Guyrope's technique is related to:** *(MHSSMCET 2009)*
   a. Ileal resection and anastomosis
   b. Ileostomy
   c. Colostomy
   d. All of the above

7. **Which of the following in a not a recognized complication of colostomy?** *(MHSSMCET 2011)*
   a. Prolapse
   b. Necrosis
   c. Stenosis
   d. Constipation

8. **Early postoperative complication of ileostomy:** *(JIPMER 2014, AIIMS May 2012)*
   a. Obstruction
   b. Prolapse
   c. Diarrhea
   d. Necrosis

9. **The following regarding colostomy are true except:** *(Kerala 2000)*
   a. A colostomy is an artificial opening made in large bowel to divert the faeces to the exterior
   b. Temporary colostomy is established to defunction and anastomosis
   c. Permanent colostomy is formed after the resection of rectum by the abdominoperineal technique
   d. Double barreled colostomy is commonly done now a days
   e. Colostomy hernia is common complication

10. **Parastomal hernia is most frequently seen with:** *(All India 2009)*
    a. End colostomy
    b. Loop colostomy
    c. End ileostomy
    d. Loop ileostomy

11. **Early complications of ileostomy are all except:**
    a. High output
    b. Ischemic necrosis
    c. Retraction
    d. Stenosis *(GB Pant 2011)*

12. **Parastomal hernia is most frequently seen with:** *(Bihar PG 2016)*
    a. End colostomy
    b. Loop colostomy
    c. End ileostomy
    d. Loop ileostomy

13. **Prolapse is more frequently associated with:** *(Recent Question 2016)*
    a. End colostomy
    b. Loop colostomy
    c. End ileostomy
    d. Loop ileostomy

14. **Most common complication of ileostomy is:** *(Recent Question 2016)*
    a. Ischemic necrosis
    b. Skin irritation
    c. Prolapse
    d. Parastomal hernia

15. **Which of the following stoma is formed in Hartman's procedure?** *(Recent Question 2017)*
    a. End colostomy
    b. End ileostomy
    c. Loop ileostomy
    d. Cecostomy

16. **This complication is most commonly seen in which type of stoma?**

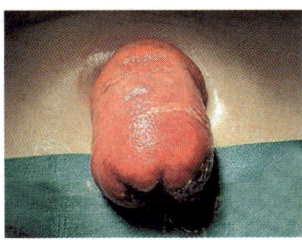

   a. End ileostomy
   b. Loop ileostomy
   c. End colostomy
   d. Loop colostomy

Explanations

ILEOSTOMY AND COLOSTOMY

1. **Ans. a. Parastomal hernia** *(Ref: Sabiston 20/e p1326-1330; Schwartz 10/e p1192-1193; Bailey 27/e p1278; Shackelford 8/e p2159, 7/e p2248-2260; Maingot 11/e p141-148)*
2. **Ans. d. All of the above** *(Ref: Sabiston 20/e p1326-1330; Schwartz 10/e p1192-1193; Bailey 27/e p1278; Shackelford 8/e p2157, 7/e p2256-2260; Maingot 11/e p153-154)*
3. **Ans. b. Crohn's disease** *(Ref: Sabiston 20/e p1327-1328; Schwartz 10/e p1192-1193; Bailey 27/e p1254-1255; Maingot 11/e p154-166)*
4. **Ans. a. Discrepancy is size of ileum and stoma**

Mercedes Procedure^Q	Used when there is **discrepancy between** the **size of** the **ileal loop** and the **ileostomy stoma**.
Mercedes benz or seagull sign^Q	Rarely the **centre of gallstone** may contain **radioluscent gas** in a **triradiate** or **biradiate fissure**. This gives **characteristic dark shapes** on **radiograph**
Mercedes sign incision^Q	**Excision of xiphoid** process and **downward traction on** the **liver** provides **excellent exposure of** the **hepatic veins** and **suprahepatic IVC**

5. **Ans. d. Necrosis** *(Ref: Sabiston 20/e p1328-1329; Schwartz 10/e p1193; Bailey 27/e p1255; Maingot 11/e p164-165)*
   - Schwartz says "**Stoma necrosis** may occur in the **early post-operative period** and usually is **caused by skeletonizing** the **distal small bowel** and / **creating an overly tight fascial defect**.
6. **Ans. b. Ileostomy** *(Ref: www.ncbi.nlm.nih.gov/pubmed/2658641)*
   - **Guy rope principle** is **used to evert** the **necessary length** of **bowel in** creation of **ileostomy**.

GUY ROPE PRINCIPLE
- In the creation of a **permanent ileostomy**, a fully everted nipple ensures a good fit of the stomal appliance.
- In normal bowel segment this may not pose a problem, but **forceful attempts at eversion in diseased, thickened**, and **friable bowel** may **result in damage to** the **bowel segment**.
- In order to prevent this, **guy rope principle** is **used to evert** the **necessary length** of **bowel**^Q.

7. **Ans. d. Constipation**
8. **Ans. d. Necrosis**
9. **Ans. d. Double barreled colostomy is commonly done now a days** *(Ref: Bailey 27/e p1277)*
   - Bailey says "**Double-barrelled colostomy** was designed so that it **could be closed by crushing the intervening 'spur'** using an **enterotome** or **a stapling device**. It is **rarely used now**, but occasionally the colon is divided so that both ends can be brought to the surface separately, ensuring that the distal segment is completely defunctioned."

10. **Ans. a. End colostomy**
11. **Ans. d. Stenosis**
12. **Ans. a. End colostomy**
13. **Ans. b. Loop colostomy**
14. **Ans. b. Skin irritation**
15. **Ans. a. End colostomy**
16. **Ans. d. Loop colostomy** *(Ref: Sabiston 20/e p310-311; Schwartz 10/e p1193; Bailey 27/e p1277; Shackelford, 8/e p2160, 7/e p2248-2260; Maingot 11/e p141-148)*

- MC complication of **both end & loop colostomy: Parastomal hernia**^Q
- **Parastomal hernia** is **more common in end colostomy**^Q as compared to loop colostomy.
- Prolapse is **more common in** loop colostomy.
- **MC complication** of **ileostomy: Skin irritation**^Q
- **MC early complication** of ileostomy: **Ischemic necrosis**^Q

CHAPTER 16

Inflammatory Bowel Disease

CROHN'S DISEASE

CROHN'S DISEASE

- Chronic, transmural inflammatory disease of GIT for which the cause is unknown[Q].
- Can involve any part of alimentary tract from mouth to anus but most commonly affects small intestine & colon[Q].

  - Involvement of both large & small intestine: 55%[Q]
  - Involvement of only small intestine: 30%[Q]
  - Involvement of only large intestine: 15%[Q]

- Crohn's disease primarily attacks young adults[Q] in 2nd & 3rd decades of life.
- More common in smokers & urban dwellers[Q] & females taking OCPs
- Strong familial association[Q]

  - Upper GI Crohn's disease is most frequently found in gastric antrum & duodenum[Q].
  - In patients with colonic disease, rectal sparing is characteristic[Q].

Etiology: Unknown

- Infectious agents proposed as potential causes: Mycobacterium paratuberculosis & measles virus[Q].
- The identification of CARD-15/NOD2 mutation[Q] (on chromosome 16q, also known as IBD-1 locus) provided the first definitive genetic link to the condition and is relatively specific for Crohn's disease.

IBD-1 (chromosome 16q)	Relatively specific for Crohn's disease[Q]
IBD-2 (chromosome 12q)	More common in Ulcerative colitis[Q]

Pathology

- Diseased bowel separated by areas of grossly appearing normal bowel (skip areas)[Q].
- Extensive fat wrapping caused by circumferential growth of mesenteric fat[Q] around the bowel wall (creeping fat).
- Thickened, firm, rubbery, & almost incompressible bowel wall[Q].
- Involved segments are adherent to adjacent intestinal loops or other viscera, with internal fistulas[Q].
- Mesentery of the involved segment is thickened, with enlarged lymph nodes[Q].

  - Earliest gross pathologic lesion is a superficial aphthous ulcer[Q] noted in the mucosa.

- Linear ulcers may coalesce to produce transverse sinuses with islands of normal mucosa in between (cobblestone appearance[Q])
- Inflammatory reaction is characterized by extensive edema, hyperemia[Q] lymphangiectasia, an intense infiltration of mononuclear cells, and lymphoid hyperplasia[Q].

  - Characteristic histologic lesions of Crohn's disease are noncaseating granulomas with Langerhans' giant cells[Q].
  - Granulomas are found in the wall of bowel or in regional lymph nodes[Q] in 60-70% of patients

Clinical Features

- MC symptom is intermittent & colicky abdominal pain, most commonly noted in lower abdomen[Q].
- Diarrhea is the next most frequent symptom and is present, at least intermittently, in about 85% of patients.
- In contrast to ulcerative colitis, patients with Crohn's disease typically have fewer bowel movements, & stools rarely contain mucus, pus, or blood[Q].

  - Main intestinal complications of Crohn's disease include obstruction & perforation[Q].
  - Fistulas occur between the sites of perforation & adjacent organs, usually at the site of a previous laparotomy[Q].

- Long-standing Crohn's disease predisposes to cancer of small intestine & colon[Q].
- Perianal disease (fissure, fistula, stricture, or abscess[Q]) is common

- In **Crohn's disease, ileum** is **MC site** of **fistula (enterocutaneous & enterovesical)**, MC site of **perforation** and MC site of **carcinoma**[Q].

Diagnosis
- IOC for **diagnosis** of **Crohn's disease**: **CT Enteroclysis**[Q]
- **Serology**: Anti-Saccharomyces cerevisiae **(ASCA**[Q]**)** autoantibodies have **specificity of 92%** for **Crohn's disease**.

Radiological Findings of Crohn's Disease	
• **Aphthous ulceration**: Earliest radiographic findings in enteroclysis[Q] • **Deep ulcers**[Q] • **Cobble stone appearance**[Q] • **Fat halo sign**[Q] on CT: Low attenuation of submucosal fat around bowel • **Creeping fat sign**[Q]	• **Hose-pipe like appearance**[Q]: Long stricture extending up to ileocecal valve with thickened wall; corresponds to "**String sign of Kantor**"[Q] • **Raspberry thorn** or **rosethorn appearance**[Q]: Linear fissures throughout the bowel • **Comb sign**[Q]: Vascular jejunization of ileum

CROHN'S DISEASE OF THE ANORECTUM

Crohn's Disease of the Anorectum

- **Anal manifestations** of Crohn's disease can be **most devastating** because of their **painful nature** and their **threat to** the **patient's continence**[Q]
- Occur in nearly **20% of patients** with Crohn's disease.

> - Typically presents in three ways: Ulceration (MC[Q]), fistula and stricture.
> - Fistulas tend to be chronic, indurated, and cyanotic and are often painless[Q].

Clinical Features
- Patients may suffer from **fissures, fistulas**, and **abscesses**[Q].
- Symptoms and signs of **anal Crohn's disease** may include **pain, swelling, bleeding, soilage** or **frank incontinence**, and **fever**.

> - Edematous, purplish tags are characteristic of the disease.

Evaluation
- **Anorectal examination** should include **inspection, digital examination, anoscopy**, and **proctosigmoidoscopy**[Q].

Treatment
- Although **conservatism is paramount in importance**, patients should not be undertreated if treatment is indicated.
- **Surgery** is usually warranted for **pain** resulting from a **poorly draining** or **undrained abscess**[Q].

> - Fissures caused by Crohn's disease are often multiple and located off the midline; they usually respond to conservative measures[Q], such as sitz baths, stool softeners, and oral analgesics.
> - Sphincterotomy and fissurectomy should be avoided in perianal Crohn's disease[Q].

- **Infliximab**[Q] has been **very successful** in the treatment of **fistulizing perianal Crohn's** disease with **closure rates** between 25% and 67%.

> - Most successful strategy is **a staged approach** to perianal disease.
> - **Control of local sepsis** is an **essential first step**[Q].
> - **Abscesses** need to be **drained** and **fistula tracts** require **chronic drainage with non-cutting setons**[Q].
> - Once the perianal sepsis is controlled, **infliximab** treatment is initiated.
> - After two to three infliximab infusions, **setons are removed to permit closure of the fistulas**[Q].

- If the **fistulas do not close** and the **local sepsis has resolved, definitive surgical therapy** may be undertaken[Q].

EXTRAINTESTINAL MANIFESTATIONS OF CROHN'S DISEASE

Extraintestinal Manifestations of Crohn's Disease	
• **Skin**: Erythema multiforme, **Erythema nodosum**, Pyoderma gangrenosum • **Eyes**: Iritis, Uveitis, Conjunctivitis • **Blood**: Anemia, **Thrombocytosis, Phlebothrombosis, Arterial thrombosis**	• **Joints**: Peripheral arthritis, Ankylosing spondylitis • **Liver**: Nonspecific triaditis, **Sclerosing cholangitis** • **Kidney**: Nephrotic syndrome • **Pancreas**: Pancreatitis • **General**: Amyloidosis

ULCERATIVE COLITIS

ULCERATIVE COLITIS

- UC occurs **more commonly** in **developed countries**^Q
- More commonly affects patients **< 30 years**; More common in females taking OCPs
- **More common** in **whites, Jews,** and persons of **northern European ancestry**^Q

Etiology
- Infectious agents, including **C. difficile** & **Campylobacter jejuni**^Q, have been implicated as playing a causative role in the pathogenesis, but such a role has not been confirmed.
- A **family history of IBD** is a **significant risk factor**^Q.

> - **Smoking** appears to confer a **protective effect**^Q
> - Both **UC** and **Crohn's disease** are **more common in women** who **use OCPs**^Q
> - Patients who have had an **appendectomy** appear to be at **decreased risk for developing UC**^Q.

Pathology
- Major **pathologic process involves mucosa** & **submucosa** of colon, with **sparing** of the **muscularis**^Q.
- **Typical gross appearance: Hyperemic mucosa**^Q
- **Rectal involvement** (**proctitis**) is the **hallmark of disease**^Q, & diagnosis should be seriously questioned if the rectal mucosa is not affected.
- **Pseudopolyps**, or **inflammatory polyps** are seen in UC.
- **Diagnostic characteristic** of UC: **Continuous uninterrupted inflammation** of mucosa, **beginning in distal rectum** & **extending proximally**^Q to a variable distance.

> - **Most characteristic lesion of UC: Crypt abscess**^Q (collections of neutrophils fill & expand the lumina of individual crypts of Lieberkühn)
> - **Crypt abscesses** are **not specific for UC**^Q and can be seen in Crohn's disease and infectious colitis.

- **Crypt branching** may be seen in **chronic UC** and is an **important characteristic**^Q.
- **Number of goblet cells** in the crypts **is diminished**, as is mucus production.

Clinical Features
- **Diarrhea** with **passage of mucus**^Q
- **More urgency** than with Crohn's disease, because of **distal proctitis**^Q.
- **Rectal bleeding** is common in UC

> - **Rectal involvement** is present in almost **100%** of patients with UC, whereas anal involvement is rare.
> - **Crohn's disease** may have **normal rectal mucosa** (so-called **rectal sparing**^Q), although **anal disease** (e.g. **fissures, fistulas, abscesses**) is **common**^Q.

Laboratory Investigations
- Increased CRP, ESR & platelet count; Decreased hemoglobin
- **Fecal lactoferrin**^Q: **Highly sensitive & specific marker** for detecting **intestinal inflammation**^Q
- **Fecal calprotectin**^Q levels **correlate well** with histologic **inflammation, predict relapses & detect pouchitis**
- Both **fecal lactoferrin & calprotectin**^Q are integral part of management & to **rule out active inflammation versus symptoms of irritable bowel or bacterial overgrowth**^Q
- **p-ANCA** is having **92% specificity** for **UC**^Q.

Diagnosis
- In the **acute phase** of UC, **proctosigmoidoscopy** is sufficient because the rectum is invariably inflamed.
- **Colonoscopy**: If patient is **not having acute flare**, colonoscopy is used **to assess** the disease **extent & severity**^Q
- **Earliest colonoscopic finding: Decreased vascularity** with **erythematous & edematous mucosa**^Q
- **Disease severity** of UC can be graded by **Modified Truelove and Witts Classification**^Q

Radiology
- **Earliest radiological change: Fine mucosal granularity**^Q
- **Deep ulceration** appear as **"collar-button" ulcers**^Q indicating that ulceration has penetrated the mucosa
- **Double contrast barium enema**: Primary radiologic tool **for confirming** the **diagnosis** & assessing the **extent** and **severity** of UC^Q.

End stage or Burned out UC is Characterized Radiographically by

- Shortening of colon[Q]
- Loss of normal redundancy in sigmoid region, at splenic & hepatic flexures[Q]
- Featureless mucosa[Q]
- Absence of discrete ulceration
- Narrow caliber of bowel[Q]
- Disappearance of haustral pattern[Q]/Ahaustral colon[Q]/Pipestem colon[Q]/Lead pipe sign[Q]/Garden hose appearance[Q]/Stove pipe appearance[Q]

- Approximately **15–20%** of patients with **severe UC** have an associated **backwash ileitis**, characterized by a **fixed, patulous ileocecal valve** and a **dilated, granular terminal ileum** on **double contrast barium studies**[Q].

EXTRAINTESTINAL MANIFESTATIONS OF ULCERATIVE COLITIS

Extraintestinal Manifestations of Ulcerative Colitis

- Arthritis
- Ankylosing spondylitis
- Erythema nodosum
- Pyoderma gangrenosum
- Primary sclerosing cholangitis (PSC)

MANAGEMENT PROTOCOL OF IBD

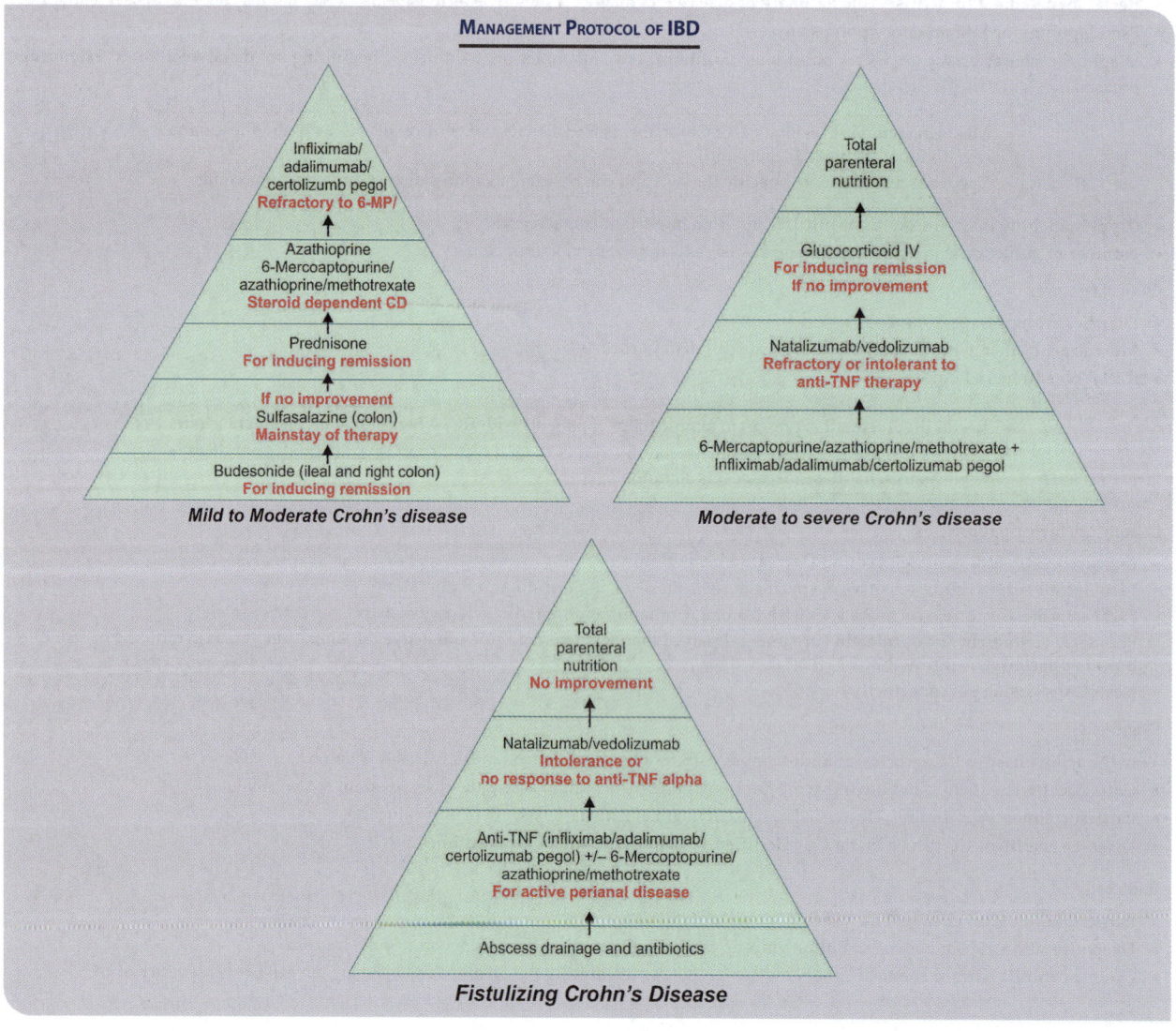

Inflammatory Bowel Disease

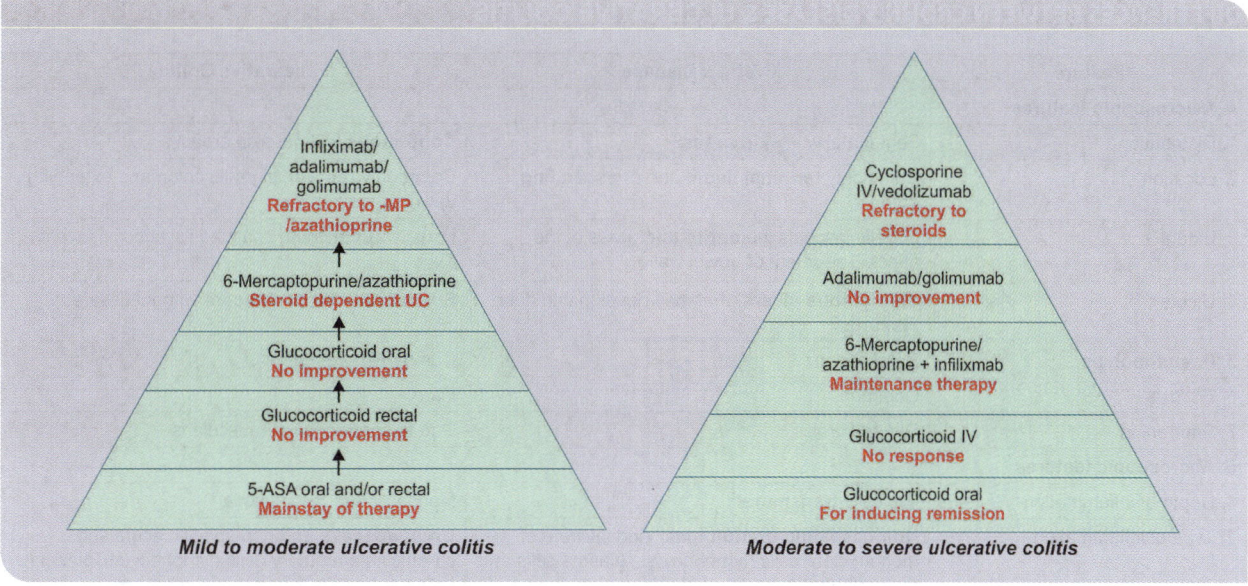

Mild to moderate ulcerative colitis | **Moderate to severe ulcerative colitis**

SURGICAL OPTIONS FOR ULCERATIVE COLITIS

Indications of Surgery in Ulcerative Colitis	
• Intractability^Q	• Massive colonic bleeding^Q
• Dysplasia, **carcinoma**^Q	• Toxic megacolon^Q

Surgical Options for Ulcerative Colitis	
• Total proctocolectomy with ileostomy	• Total abdominal colectomy with end-ileostomy
• Restorative proctocolectomy with IPAA^Q	
• Total proctocolectomy with a continent ileal reservoir (Kock pouch)^Q	

Indications of Surgical Options in Ulcerative Colitis

Total Proctocolectomy with End Ileostomy
- Total proctocolectomy has the advantage of removing all diseased mucosa, thereby preventing further inflammation and the potential for progression to dysplasia or carcinoma^Q.
- **Major disadvantage:** Need for a **permanent ileostomy**
- **Older patients**, those with **poor sphincter function**, and patients with **carcinomas in the distal rectum** may be candidates for this procedure^Q.

Total Proctocolectomy with Continent Ileostomy
- **Major problem with the Kock pouch** is the **high complication rate** necessitating **reoperation** in up to **50%** of patients^Q.
- **MC problem** is a **slipped valve**, which occurs when the intussuscepted limb everts and the continent nipple is lost.
- **Other complications:** Inflammation of the ileal pouch mucosa (so-called **pouchitis**) in 15% to 30% of cases, fistula formation (10%), and stoma stricture (10%).
- **Kock procedure should not be performed** in **obese patients, debilitated patients**, or **any patient with** a **physical** or **mental handicap**^Q that would prohibit safe catheterization of the reservoir.
- Procedure is **contraindicated in** patients with **Crohn's disease** because of **high incidence of its recurrence**, causing failure of pouch.

Total Proctocolectomy with Ileal Pouch-Anal Anastomosis (IPAA)
- Restorative proctocolectomy with IPAA has become the most common definitive operation for the surgical treatment of UC.

Complications of Total Proctocolectomy With IPAA	
• **Pouchitis** (7–33%)^Q	• Anastomotic and pouch suture line **leaks**
• **Small bowel obstruction** (up to 27%)	• **Pouch-vaginal fistula**
• Pelvic sepsis	

DIFFERENCES BETWEEN CROHN'S DISEASE & ULCERATIVE COLITIS

Feature	Crohn's Disease	Ulcerative Colitis
A. Macroscopic features		
1. Distribution	Segmental with **skip areas**[Q]	**Continuous** without skip areas[Q]
2. Location	Commonly **terminal ileum** and/or **ascending colon**	Commonly **rectum,** sigmoid colon and extending upwards
3. Extent	Usually involves the **entire thickness** of the affected segment of bowel wall	Usually **superficial,** confined to mucosal layers
4. Ulcers	**Serpiginous ulcers,** that may develop into deep **Fissures**[Q]	**Superficial mucosal ulcers** without fissures
5. **Pseudopolyps**	Rarely seen	Commonly present[Q]
6. Fibrosis	Common	Rare
7. Shortening	Due to fibrosis	Due to contraction of muscularis
B. Microscopic features		
1. Depth of inflammation	Typically **transmural**[Q]	Mucosal[Q] and Submucosal
2. Type of inflammation	**Non-caseating granulomas**[Q] and infiltrate of mononuclear cells (lymphocytes, plasma cells and macrophage)	**Crypt abscess** and non-specific acute and chronic inflammatory cells (lymphocytes, plasma cells neutrophils, eosinophils, mast cells)
3. Mucosa	Patchy ulceration	Hemorrhagic mucosa with ulceration
4. Submucosa	Widened due to edema and lymphoid aggregates	Normal or reduced in width
5. Muscularis	Infiltrated by inflammatory cells	Usually spared, except in cases of **Toxic Megacolon**[Q]
6. Fibrosis	Present	Usually absent
C. Complications		
1. **Fistula formation**	**Internal** and **external fistulae** in 10% case	Extremely **rare**[Q]
2. Malignant changes	Less common but present	May occur in disease of more than 10 years duration (**more common**[Q])
3. **Fibrous strictures**	Common[Q]	Never[Q]
4. **Toxic megacolon**	–	Risk present[Q]
5. Named Features	**String Has CRF** • **String** sign of Kantor[Q] • **H**ose pipe appearance[Q] • **C**reeping fat sign[Q] • **C**omb sign[Q] • **R**aspberry thorn appearance[Q] or **R**osethorn appearance[Q] • **F**at halo sign on CT[Q]	**GPL Stove Collar Button** • **G**arden hose appearance[Q] • **P**ipestem colon[Q] • **L**ead pipe sign[Q] • **S**tove pipe appearance[Q] • **C**ollar button ulcer[Q]

Remember
- Earliest change in **Crohn's disease** is **Apthoid ulceration**[Q].
- Earliest Change in Ulcerative colitis is Blurring of mucosal stripe and granular appearance[Q].
- **Surgery** is palliative in **Crohn's disease**[Q] whereas **curative in ulcerative colitis**[Q].
- Risk of **carcinoma colon: UC = CD**[Q]
- Risk of **small intestinal malignancies: CD > UC**[Q]
- Risk of **cholangiocarcinoma: UC > CD**[Q]

Multiple Choice Questions

INFLAMMATORY BOWEL DISEASE

1. **Crohn's disease can be seen in:** *(COMEDK 2007)*
   a. Jejunum only
   b. Colon only
   c. Terminal ileum and right side
   d. Mouth to anus

2. **Cobble stone appearance is seen in:**
   (Kerala PG 2015, COMEDK 2008, 2007)
   a. Ulcerative colitis   b. Crohn's disease
   c. Appendicitis   d. Carcinoma rectum

3. **String sign of Kantor seen in:** *(APPG 2008)*
   a. Crohn's disease   b. Ulcerative colitis
   c. Both of the above   d. None of the above

4. **Which of the following statements about Crohn's disease is incorrect?** *(DPG 2009 March)*
   a. Granuloma present frequently
   b. It is separate and distinct form ulcerative colitis
   c. Cigarette smoking is a risk factor
   d. Rectum spared in 50% patients with large bowel involvement

5. **True statement regarding anorectal Crohn's disease:**
   a. Ulceration, fistula is common
   b. Fistulas are painless and indurated
   c. Non-cutting setons are used in management
   d. All of the above

6. **A middle-aged female presented with recurrent bloody diarrhea. Colonoscopy reveals multiple geographic ulcers and histopathological examination is shown below. What is the likely diagnosis?** *(AIIMS May 2017)*
   a. Crohn's disease
   b. Adenocarcinoma colon
   c. Pseudomembranous colitis
   d. Ulcerative colitis

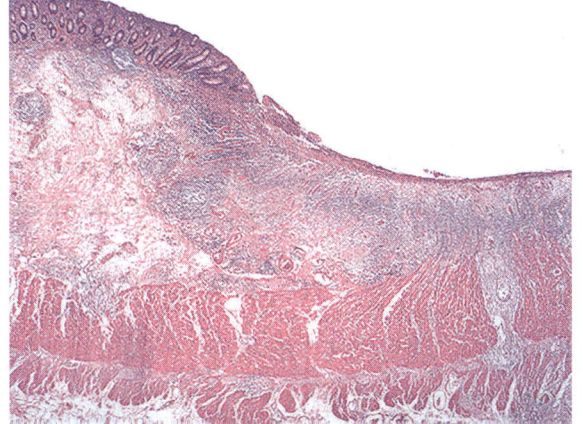

7. **Ulcerative colitis starts from:** *(GB Pant 2011)*
   a. Rectum   b. Sigmoid colon
   c. Ascending colon   d. Any part

8. **Crohn's disease is best diagnosed by** *(GB Pant 2011)*
   a. Upper GI series   b. Enteroclysis
   c. Capsule endoscopy   d. CECT

9. **Characteristic of Crohn's disease:** *(GB Pant 2011)*
   a. Transmural involvement with skip lesions
   b. Large bowel involvement
   c. Pseudopolyps
   d. Involvement of mucosa only

10. **All are true about ulcerative colitis except:** *(PGI SS June 2007)*
    a. Terminal ileum may be involved
    b. Stricture formation is present
    c. Malignancy after 10 years
    d. Crypt abscess is pathognomonic

11. **Skip lesions are seen in:**
    (Recent Question 2016, AIIMS May 2009)
    a. Ulcerative colitis   b. Typhoid
    c. Crohn's disease   d. Tuberculosis

12. **A patient gives chronic history of diarrhea and blood in stool presents with multiple fistulae in the perineum and multiple stricture in small intestine. The diagnosis is:** *(AIIMS June 2000)*
    a. In Crohn's disease   b. Radiation enteritis
    c. Ulcerative colitis   d. Ischemic bowel disease

13. **Crohn's disease is associated with following:** *(DPG 96)*
    a. Stomach not involved
    b. No granulomatous + Transmucosal fissures
    c. Continuous involvement
    d. Through and through involvement of thickness of bowel wall

14. **On barium study, these findings are seen in:**
    (Recent Question 2016)
    a. Ulcerative colitis
    b. Ischemic colitis
    c. Tuberculosis
    d. Crohn's disease

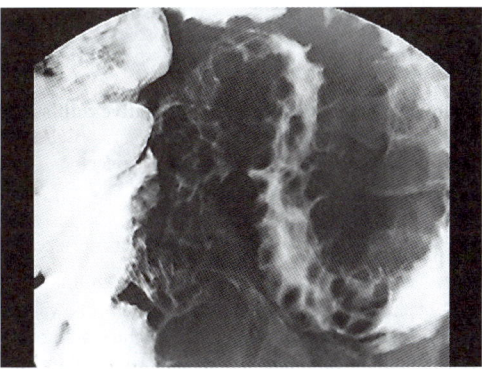

15. **Skip lesions with tuberculoid granulomas is characteristic of:**
    a. Hodgkin's lymphoma   b. Sarcoidosis
    c. Crohn's disease   d. Ulcerative colitis

16. False regarding involvement in Crohn's disease: *(AIIMS 94)*
    a. Anorectal area
    b. Rectum
    c. Small intestine with right colon
    d. Large alone without involvement of small intestine

17. UC can be differentiated from Crohn's disease by all except: *(DNB 2005, AIIMS GIS May 2011)*
    a. Pseudopolyps
    b. Rectal sparing
    c. Discontinuous lesions
    d. Deep longitudinal ulcers

18. Histological difference between Ulcerative colitis and Crohn's disease is presence of: *(Recent Question 2019)*
    a. Crypt abscess
    b. Diffuse distribution of pseudopolyps
    c. Mucosal edema
    d. Lymphoid aggregates in the mucosa

19. Inflammatory bowel disease found in children: *(PGI June 2006)*
    a. Ulcerative colitis
    b. Tropical sprue
    c. Crohn's disease
    d. Celiac disease
    e. Cystic fibrosis

20. About ulcerative colitis, true statement is/are: *(PGI May 2018)*
    a. No skip lesion
    b. Almost always includes rectum
    c. Can present with pain and bloody diarrhea
    d. More common in smokers
    e. Transmural involvement

21. In a 27 years old male, most common cause of a colovesical fistula would be: *(All India 2001, 99)*
    a. Crohn's disease
    b. Ulcerative colitis
    c. TB
    d. Cancer colon

22. The commonest site of involvement in the Crohn's disease is: *(COMEDK 2005)*
    a. Jejunum
    b. Transverse colon
    c. Terminal ileum
    d. Rectum

23. The indications of colonoscopy in a patient with ulcerative colitis are all of the following except: *(COMEDK 2010)*
    a. Diagnosis of the extent of inflammation
    b. Differentiating if from Crohn's disease
    c. Diagnosis of toxic megacolon
    d. Monitoring the response to treatment

24. Crohn's disease is associated with: *(COMEDK 2011)*
    a. NOD2/CARD-15 gene
    b. P53 suppressor gene
    c. Philadelphia chromosomes
    d. BRAC-1 gene

25. Following statements regarding ulcerative colitis is true:
    a. Smoking has a protecting effect *(COMEDK 2011)*
    b. Smoking does not have a protective effect
    c. There is no relation to smoking
    d. Smoking causes relapses

26. Skip lesions are characteristic of *(Recent Question 2016, JIPMER 2010)*
    a. Typhoid
    b. Ischemic bowel disease
    c. Ulcerative colitis
    d. Crohn's disease

27. Which one is commonly associated with Crohn's disease? *(PGI Nov 2009)*
    a. Cologastric
    b. Coloureteric
    c. Colovesical
    d. Coloduodenal
    e. Colovaginal

28. All are true about Ulcerative colitis except: *(PGI Nov 2009)*
    a. All layers are involved
    b. Malabsorption
    c. Backwash ileitis in 10–15%
    d. Mesalazine maintains the disease in remission
    e. Rarely recurs after surgery

29. On barium study, these findings are seen in: *(Recent Question 2016)*
    a. Ulcerative colitis
    b. Ischemic colitis
    c. Tuberculosis
    d. Crohn's disease

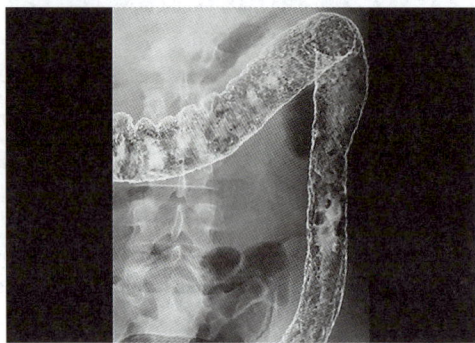

30. Which of the following is true about ulcerative colitis? *(JIPMER SS 2016, DNB 2011, MHPGMCET 2005, 2002)*
    a. Premalignant condition
    b. Cobblestone mucosa is characteristic
    c. Almost always leads to toxic megacolon
    d. Rarely affects rectum

31. Pathognomonic of Crohn's disease *(MHSSMCET 2009)*
    a. Transmural inflammation
    b. Stricture of small bowel
    c. Contiguous involvement
    d. Lead pipe colon

32. Hose pipe appearance of intestine is a feature of: *(Recent Question 2013)*
    a. Crohn's disease
    b. Malabsorption syndrome
    c. Ulcerative colitis
    d. Hirschsprung's disease

33. Earliest gross pathologic lesion seen in Crohn's Disease: *(Recent Question 2018)*
    a. Apthous ulcer
    b. Creeping fat
    c. Enlarged lymph nodes
    d. Strictures

34. Which of the following is true about ulcerative colitis? *(Recent Question 2018)*
    a. 20% end up in surgery in 1 year of diagnosis
    b. Extra intestinal problems are managed medically
    c. Steroid dependent cases need surgery
    d. Surgery is palliative in ulcerative colitis

35. Which of the following statement is not true regarding Crohn's disease? *(Recent Question 2018)*
    a. Rectum is not involved
    b. Continuous lesion visualized in endoscopy
    c. Noncaseating granulomas
    d. Cobblestone appearance

IBD EXTRAINTESTINAL MANIFESTATIONS

36. In ulcerative colitis, after colectomy least likely to resolve is:
    a. Ankylosing spondylitis
    b. PSC *(AIIMS GIS 2003)*
    c. Pyoderma gangrenosum
    d. Erythema nodosum

37. Non-correctable lesion after colectomy for UC:
    (AIIMS GIS May 2008)
    a. Skin lesions
    b. Arthritis
    c. PSC
    d. Iritis

38. Pyoderma-gangrenosum is most commonly associated with:
    (All India 99)
    a. Ulcerative colitis
    b. Crohn's disease
    c. Amoebic colitis
    d. Ischemic colitis

39. All are true associations of ulcerative colitis except:
    (PGI Dec 99)
    a. Erythema nodosum
    b. Circinate balanitis
    c. Sclerosing cholangitis
    d. Aphthous stomatitis

40. All of the following extraintestinal manifestations of ulcerative colitis respond to colectomy except:
    a. Primary sclerosing cholangitis
    b. Pyoderma gangrenosum
    c. Episcleritis
    d. Peripheral arthralgia

41. The following are complications of ulcerative colitis except:
    a. Peptic ulceration
    b. Arthritis *(All India 90)*
    c. Sclerosing cholangitis
    d. Toxic megacolon

42. Type of renal stone formed in a patient with regional enteritis:
    (JIPMER 2011)
    a. Calcium oxalate
    b. Cysteine
    c. Struvite
    d. Urate

43. Most common stones in ulcerative colitis: *(DPG 2007)*
    a. Oxalate
    b. Cysteine
    c. Uric acid
    d. Phosphate

IBD TREATMENT

44. Treatment of choice in case of chronic ulcerative colitis is:
    (AIIMS June 95)
    a. Colectomy with ileostomy
    b. Colectomy + manual proctectomy + ileoanal pouch anastomosis
    c. Proctocolectomy with ileoanal anastomosis
    d. Ileorectal anastomosis

45. Surgical treatment of ulcerative colitis: *(PGI June 2005)*
    a. Done in late cases only
    b. Done in cases where medical treatment fails
    c. Pouch surgery done
    d. Restorative proctocolectomy done in emergency cases

46. Which sulphonamide is used for the treatment of ulcerative colitis?
    (All India 88)
    a. Sulphamethiazole
    b. Sulphathalazole
    c. Sulphaguanidine
    d. Salazopyrin

47. Sulfasalazine exerts its primary action in ulcerative colitis by inhibition of:
    (COMEDK 2004)
    a. Folic acid synthesis
    b. Formation of prostaglandins (PG)
    c. Phospholipase C
    d. Formation of interleukins

48. Procedure of choice in ulcerative colitis with acute perforation is:
    (Recent Question 2016)
    a. Defunctioning ileostomy
    b. Closure of perforation
    c. Proximal diversion colostomy
    d. Total colectomy and ileostomy

49. Sulfonamide useful in treating ulcerative colitis is:
    (All India 91)
    a. Sulfadiazine
    b. Sulfasalazine
    c. Sulfamethoxazole
    d. Sulfadimidine

50. Best treatment for remission of acute ulcerative colitis is:
    (AIIMS 97)
    a. Sulphasalazine
    b. Prednisolone
    c. Aminosalicyclic acid
    d. NSAIDS

51. Indication of emergency surgery in ulcerative colitis is/are:
    a. Toxic megacolon *(PGI Nov 2011)*
    b. Massive colonic hemorrhage
    c. Extraintestinal manifestation
    d. Colonic perforation
    e. Colonic dysplasia

52. After subtotal colectomy for toxic megacolon in CD, lowest recurrence is with: *(AIIMS GIS 2003)*
    a. Complete proctectomy with Brooke ileostomy
    b. Ileorectal anastomosis
    c. Koch's pouch
    d. IPAA

53. Treatment of choice in ulcerative colitis: *(GB Pant 2011)*
    a. Total proctocolectomy with IPAA
    b. Total colectomy with IRA
    c. Total colectomy with ileostomy
    d. Total proctocolectomy with ileostomy

54. Not an indication for surgery in ulcerative colitis:
    a. Presence of dysplasia on colonic biopsy *(PGI SS Dec 2009)*
    b. Pancolitis
    c. Toxic megacolon
    d. Failure of response to medical therapy of acute colitis

55. True statement regarding management of ileocaecal Crohn's disease is: *(JIPMER, 2014, 2007)*
    a. Avoid antibiotics
    b. Avoid steroids in first week
    c. 5-ASA reduces small bowel obstruction
    d. Cholestyramine improves diarrhea, worsens steatorrhea

COLITIS ASSOCIATED CARCINOMA

56. Risk of carcinoma in ulcerative colitis: *(GB Pant 2011)*
    a. 20% after 20 years
    b. 20% after 30 years
    c. 30% after 30 years
    d. 50% after 30 years

57. Risk of malignancy in ulcerative colitis is more in:
    a. Onset in childhood *(PGI Dec 2001)*
    b. Extensive involvement of colon
    c. Disrupted architecture with crypt abscesses
    d. Pseudopolyps
    e. Recurrence after treatment

58. Not true about malignancy arising from ulcerative colitis is:
    a. Takes at least 10 years to develop *(PGI June 99)*
    b. Left sided is more common
    c. Associated with dysplasia of the rest of the colon
    d. Younger age of onset is associated with increased chance of carcinoma

59. In ulcerative colitis, carcinoma arises from: *(PGI Dec 98)*
    a. Pseudopolyps
    b. Dysplastic sites
    c. Familial polyps
    d. Multiple adenomatous polyp

60. Ulcerative colitis progressing to malignancy is characterized by following except: *(PGI 97)*
    a. Risk increases with the time
    b. Prognosis worsens
    c. Prognosis depends on period
    d. Arise from pseudo polyps

61. False about malignancy in ulcerative colitis:
    a. Poorly differentiated with higher stage *(AIIMS GIS 2003)*
    b. Related to extent of disease
    c. Poor prognosis as compared to sporadic
    d. Evenly distributed

62. All are true about colonic cancer in UC except:
    a. In younger patients *(AIIMS GIS Dec 2010)*
    b. Depends upon duration of disease
    c. Depends on extent of UC in colon
    d. Risk of cancer irrespective of grade of dysplasia

IBD COMPLICATIONS

63. Toxic megacolon is seen in: *(COMEDK 2009)*
    a. Carcinoma colon   b. Gastrocolic fistula
    c. Ulcerative colitis   d. Amoebic colitis

64. A middle aged male patient presents with fever and diarrhea for 1 week and acute onset pain abdomen for 6 hours. An erect abdominal X-ray was taken as shown. What is the likely diagnosis? *(AIIMS May 2017)*
    a. Pseudomembranous colitis
    b. Adenocarcinoma colon
    c. Pneumatosis intestinalis
    d. Toxic megacolon

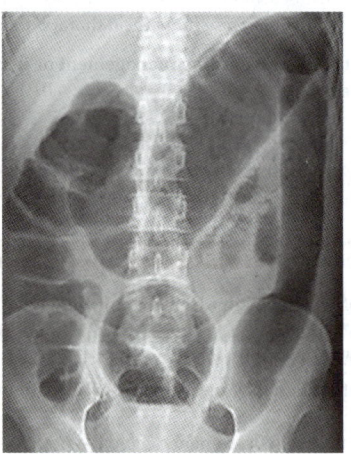

65. Treatment of choice in toxic megacolon: *(MHSSMCET 2005)*
    a. Total colectomy
    b. Segmental resection
    c. Colostomy
    d. Clindamycin, Metronidazole, Steroids

66. Toxic megacolon is seen in: *(Orissa 2011)*
    a. Crohn's disease   b. Ulcerative colitis
    c. Diverticulosis   d. All of the above

67. In which of the following conditions acquired secondary megacolon is seen?
    a. Fissure in-ano
    b. Complete absence of parasympathetic ganglion cells
    c. Absence of sympathetic ganglion cells
    d. Rectal malignancy

68. All of the following are known complications of ulcerative colitis except: *(PGI June 95)*
    a. Stricture   b. Perforation
    c. Toxic megacolon   d. Carcinoma

69. Most common cause of death in Crohn's disease is due to:
    a. Sepsis *(AIIMS May 2009)*
    b. Thromboembolic complication
    c. Electrolyte disturbance
    d. Malignancy

70. Incidence of pouchitis in patients treated for ulcerative colitis with IPAA is: *(JIPMER GIS 2011)*
    a. 7–33%   b. 7–15%
    c. 18–56%   d. 6–8%

71. All are true about pouchitis except: *(JIPMER GIS 2011)*
    a. Probiotics have shown promising response
    b. Cause may be related to mucosal ischemia
    c. Most commonly seen in ulcerative colitis surgeries
    d. Episodes of pouchitis will not respond to antibiotics

72. Most common complication of UC with IPAA: *(AIIMS GIS Dec 2010)*
    a. Small bowel obstruction   b. Pouchitis
    c. Pelvic sepsis   d. Leak

73. Most common cause of death in Crohn's disease is due to:
    a. Sepsis *(AIIMS GIS Dec 2010)*
    b. Thromboembolic complication
    c. Electrolyte disturbance
    d. Malignancy

74. Most common postoperative complication of IPAA in ulcerative colitis is: *(AIIMS Nov 2011)*
    a. Pouchitis   b. Pelvic abscess
    c. Small bowel obstruction   d. Perianal complications

75. A patient of Crohn's disease underwent resection anastomosis. Now present on 7th post-op day with anastomotic leak from a fistula. Every day leakage volume adds up to 150–200 ml. There is no intra-abdominal collection and the patient is stable without any complaints. What will be next line of management? *(AIIMS May 2012)*
    a. Conservative treatment and leave him and hope for the spontaneous resolution
    b. Perform laparotomy and check for leakage site and healthy margins
    c. Perform laparotomy and completely exteriorize the fistula
    d. Perform laparotomy and place drain and leave

Explanations

INFLAMMATORY BOWEL DISEASE

1. **Ans. d. Mouth to anus:** *(Ref: Sabiston 20/e p1254; Schwartz 10/e p1153-1157; Bailey 27/e p1242-1243; Shackelford 8/e p865, 7/e p1966-1969)*
2. **Ans. b. Crohn's disease**
3. **Ans. a. Crohn's disease**
4. **Ans. d. Rectum spared in 50% patients with large bowel involvement**
5. **Ans. d. All of the above** *(Ref: Sabiston 20/e p1411; Schwartz 10/e p1153-1157; Bailey 27/e p1242-1243; Shackelford 8/e p865, 7/e p1968)*
6. **Ans. a. Crohn's disease** *(Ref: Robbins 9/e p798-799; Sabiston 20/e p1258; Bailey 27/e p1242)*
7. **Ans. a. Rectum**
8. **Ans. b. Enteroclysis**
9. **Ans. a. Transmural involvement with skip lesions**
10. **Ans. b. Stricture formation is present** *(Ref: Sabiston 20/e p1339; Schwartz 10/e p1197-1198; Bailey 27/e p1243; Shackelford 8/e p865, 7/e p1961-1966)*
11. **Ans. c. Crohn's disease**
12. **Ans. a. In Crohn's disease**
13. **Ans. d. Through and through involvement of thickness of bowel wall**
14. **Ans. d. Crohn's disease** *(Ref: Sabiston 20/e p1257; Schwartz 10/e p1155; Bailey 27/e p1244)*

    Radiograph of a small bowel follow-through demonstrates scattered islands of normal intestinal mucosa adjacent to multiple ulcerations resulting in cobblestone appearance of the distal ileum. Cobblestone appearance is seen in Crohn's disease.

15. **Ans. c. Crohn's disease**
16. **Ans. b. Rectum**
17. **Ans. a. Pseudopolyps**
18. **Ans. a. Crypt abscess** *(Ref: Schwartz 10/e p; Sabiston 20/e p1340; Bailey 27/e p)*

    > "The typical microscopic finding in ulcerative colitis is inflammation of the mucosa and submucosa. The most characteristic lesion is the crypt abscess, in which collections of neutrophils fill and expand the lumina of individual crypts of Lieberkühn."
    > – Sabiston 20/e p1340

19. **Ans. a. Ulcerative colitis, c. Crohn's disease**
20. **Ans. a. No skip lesion, b. Almost always includes rectum, c. Can present with pain & bloody diarrhea**
21. **Ans. a. Crohn's disease** *(Ref: Sabiston 20/e p1350; Smith 17/e p581)*

    ### COMMON CAUSES OF COLOVESICAL FISTULA
    - **Diverticulitis (50–60%** More common in patients **> 40 years**^{Q}
    - **CA colon (20–25%** More common in patients **> 50 years**^{Q}
    - **Crohn's disease 10%** Seen in **2nd to 3rd decade**^{Q}

22. **Ans. c. Terminal ileum**
23. **Ans. c. Diagnosis of toxic megacolon** *(Ref: Bailey 27/e p1268)*

    Colonoscopy is not done in toxic colon for the fear of aggravating the disease or perforation.

    ### INDICATIONS OF COLONOSCOPY AND BIOPSY IN ULCERATIVE COLITIS
    - To establish the **extent of inflammation**^{Q}
    - To **monitor** the **response of treatment**^{Q}.
    - To distinguish **between UC and Crohn's disease**^{Q}
    - To assess long standing cases for **malignant change**^{Q}

24. **Ans. a. NOD2/CARD-15 gene**
25. **Ans. a. Smoking has a protecting effect**
26. **Ans. d. Crohn's disease**
27. **Ans. a. Cologastric, c. Colovesical, d. Coloduodenal, e. Colovaginal** *(Ref: Sabiston 20/e p1350)*

    - Sabiston says "Fistula may develop between intestine and any other intra-abdominal organ, including bladder, bowel, uterus, vagina and stomach."
    - Harrison says "Fistula involving stomach or duodenum arise from the small or large bowel and do not necessarily signify the presence of upper GI tract involvement."

28. **Ans. a. All layer are involved, b. Malabsorption**
    - Both are the features of Crohn's disease.

29. **Ans. a. Ulcerative colitis** *(Ref: Sabiston 20/e p1341; Schwartz 10/e p1198; Bailey 27/e p1268)*

    Given radiograph demonstrates an ahaustral, pipe-like appearance of colon (pipestem colon or lead pipe sign).

30. **Ans. a. Premalignant condition**   31. **Ans. a. Transmural inflammation**   32. **Ans. a. Crohn's disease**
33. **Ans. a. Apthous ulcer** *(Ref: Sabiston 20/e p1350; Schwartz 10/e p1153; Bailey 27/e p1243)*

    - *"The earliest lesion characteristic of Crohn's disease is the aphthous ulcer."* - Schwartz 10/e p1153

34. **Ans. b. Extra intestinal problems are managed medically** *(Ref: Sabiston 20/e p1341; Schwartz 10/e p1196; Bailey 27/e p1267)*
35. **Ans. b. Continuous lesion visualized in endoscopy**

IBD EXTRAINTESTINAL MANIFESTATIONS

36. **Ans. b. PSC.** *Ref: Sabiston 20/e p1341; Schwartz 10/e p1197-1198; Bailey 27/e p1267; Shackelford 8/e p1889, 7/e p1962)*

Extraintestinal Manifestations of Ulcerative Colitis	
• Arthritis	• Pyoderma gangrenosum
• Ankylosing spondylitis	• Primary sclerosing cholangitis (PSC)
• Erythema nodosum	

    - **Colectomy** has **no effect** on the **course of PSC in UC**[Q].
    - **Pyoderma gangrenosum** is **more common in UC**[Q].
    - **EPASU** is **more common in Crohn's disease**[Q].
    - **EPASU:** Erythema nodosum, Peripheral arthritis, Ankylosing spondylitis, Stones **(Cholilithiasis** and **oxalate stones)**, Ureteral obstruction[Q].
    - **MC cutaneous manifestation of IBD: Erythema nodosum**[Q]
    - **Erythema nodosum** is the **most responsive to treatment** of the bowel and persistence of the lesion indicates inadequate control of IBD[Q].

37. **Ans. c. PSC**   38. **Ans. a. Ulcerative colitis**
39. **Ans. b. Circinate balanitis**

    - Circinate balanitis is seen in Reiter's syndrome, not in ulcerative colitis.

40. **Ans. a. Primary sclerosing cholangitis**   41. **Ans. a. Peptic ulceration**
42. **Ans. a. Calcium oxalate**   43. **Ans. a. Oxalate** *(Ref: Harrison 20/e p2269, 19/e p1958)*

Urologic Manifestations of IBD
• The **most frequent genitourinary complications** are **calculi, ureteral obstruction,** and **ileal bladder fistulas**[Q].
• **Calcium oxalate stones** develop **secondary to hyperoxaluria,** which results from **increased absorption of dietary oxalate**[Q].
• Normally, dietary calcium combines with luminal oxalate to form insoluble calcium oxalate, which is eliminated in the stool.
• In patients with **ileal dysfunction, nonabsorbed fatty acids bind calcium** and **leave oxalate unbound**[Q].
• The **unbound oxalate** is then **delivered to the colon,** where it is **readily absorbed,** especially **in the presence of inflammation**[Q].

IBD TREATMENT

44. **Ans. c. Proctocolectomy with ileonal anastomosis** *(Ref: Sabiston 20/e p1344; Schwartz 10/e p1187-1188; Bailey 27/e p1269; Shackelford 8/e p1919, 7/e p1974)*

Indications of Surgery in Ulcerative Colitis	
• Intractability[Q]	• Massive colonic bleeding[Q]
• Dysplasia, carcinoma[Q]	• Toxic megacolon[Q]

    - Older patients or those with fecal incontinence should undergo a total proctocolectomy with an end ileostomy.
    - Younger patients with no evidence of rectal dysplasia should undergo restorative proctocolectomy and IPAA with a double-stapled anastomosis and diverting loop ileostomy.
    - Patients with confirmed rectal dysplasia should be treated with mucosectomy and a hand-sewn IPAA.
    - Patients with significant debility who are poor operative candidates should undergo a total abdominal colectomy with a very low Hartmann closure and an end ileostomy.

45. Ans. b. Done in cases where medical treatment fails, c. Pouch surgery done
46. Ans. d. Salazopyrin *(Ref: Sabiston 20/e p1343; Bailey 27/e p1269)*
    - Salazopyrin is brand name of sulfasalazine.
47. Ans. b. Formation of prostaglandins (PG) *(Ref: Harrison 20/e p2270, 19/e p1959; Shackelford 8/e p1896, 7/e p1970)*

    - **5-ASA** compounds exert its local anti-inflammatory effect by **inhibiting leukotriene production (PG synthesis)** by **inhibition of 5-lipooxygenase activity;** also inhibits the **production of IL-1** and **TNF**[Q].

Commonly Used 5-ASA Formulations in IBD
• **Sulfasalazine**
• Oral **mesalamine** agents
• Azo compounds: **Balsalazide, Olsalazine**

48. Ans. d. Total colectomy and ileostomy
49. Ans. b. Sulfasalazine
50. Ans. b. Prednisolone
51. Ans. a. Toxic megacolon, b. Massive colonic hemorrhage, d. Colonic perforation
52. Ans. a. Complete proctectomy with Brooke ileostomy
53. Ans. a. Total proctocolectomy with IPAA
54. Ans. b. Pancolitis
55. Ans. c. 5-ASA reduces small bowel obstruction

COLITIS ASSOCIATED CARCINOMA

56. Ans. b. 20% after 30 years *(Ref: Schwartz 10/e p1195,1197-1198; Bailey 27/e p1268; Shackelford 8/e p1919, 7/e p1964)*

    - The **risk of malignancy** in Crohn's pancolitis is similar to UC pancolitis, i.e. **2% after 10 years, 8% after 20** years and **18% after 30** years approximately[Q].

57. Ans. a. Onset in childhood, b. Extensive involvement of colon *(Ref: Sabiston 20/e p1342; Schwartz 10/e p1195,1197-1198; Bailey 27/e p1268)*

Risk Factors for Cancer in Ulcerative Colitis patient
• The **duration** of colitis[Q]
• The **extent** of colonic involvement[Q]
• The presence of concomitant **PSC and family history of CRC**[Q] (regardless of the family history of IBD)
• **Pancolitis** (disease extending proximal to the splenic flexure) and disease diagnosed at a **young age**[Q]

    - **UC-related CRC** tends to be **multicentric** and **evenly distributed** throughout the colon. Tumour tend to be **infiltrative, highly aggressive** and **poorly differentiated**[Q].
    - No significant difference between sporadic and **UC-related CRC** with respect to **prognosis**[Q].
    - Cumulative risk of cancer increases with duration of ulcerative colitis, reaching **25% at 25 years**[Q], **35% at 30 years**[Q], **45% at 35 years**[Q] and **65% at 40 years**[Q]

58. Ans. b. Left sided is more common *(Ref: Sabiston 20/e p1342; Schwartz 10/e p1197-1198; Bailey 27/e p1268; Shackelford 8/e p1824, 7/e p1963-1965)*

Colitis Associated Colon Cancer (CAC)	Sporadic Colon Cancer (SCC)
• **Arise from flat dysplasia** or **dysplasia associated lesion or mass**[Q]	• Arise from **adenomatous polyps**[Q]
• **Multiple synchronous colon cancer** in **12%**[Q]	• **Multiple synchronous colon cancer** in **3–5%**[Q]
• Mean age: **30 years**[Q]	• Mean age: **60 years**[Q]
• **Distributed uniformly**[Q] throughout the colon	• **Left side predominance**[Q]
• **Mucinous** or **anaplastic cancers** are more common[Q]	• Mucinous or anaplastic cancers are **less common**[Q]

59. Ans. b. Dysplastic sites
60. Ans. d. Arise from pseudo polyps
61. Ans. c. Poor prognosis as compared to sporadic
62. Ans. d. Risk of cancer irrespective of grade of dysplasia

IBD COMPLICATIONS

63. Ans. c. Ulcerative colitis *(Ref: Sabiston 20/e p1344; Schwartz 10/e p1195,1198,1199; Bailey 27/e p1267; Shackelford 8/e p1919, 7/e p1965-1966)*

Toxic Megacolon

- Toxic megacolon is a **serious life-threatening condition** that can occur in patients with **ulcerative colitis, Crohn's colitis**, and **infectious colitides** such as **pseudomembranous colitis**[Q]
- This **decompensation** results in a **necrotic thin-walled bowel** in which **pneumatosis**[Q] can often be seen radiographically.

Management
- **Medical treatment** is associated with a **high rate of recurrence** with subsequent **urgent operation**[Q] has been reported.
- **Aggressive preoperative stabilization** is required, using **volume resuscitation** with **crystalloid solutions** to prevent dehydration secondary to third-space fluid losses, stress-dose steroids for patients previously on steroid therapy, **and broad-spectrum antibiotics**[Q].

  - **Total abdominal colectomy** with **ileostomy** and preservation of the rectum is **treatment of choice** for **toxic megacolon**[Q].
  - It serves the **main purpose of removing the diseased colon** and **avoiding a difficult** and **morbid pelvic dissection**[Q].

64. **Ans. d. Toxic megacolon** *(Ref: Sabiston 20/e p313, 1289; Essentials of Radiology By Fred A. Mettler 3/e p149)*

- *History of diarrhea for long duration (suggestive of ulcerative colitis) with acute history of abdominal pain and dilated transverse and descending colon is suggestive of toxic megacolon. Ulcerative colitis is a predisposing factor for toxic megacolon.*

Organ	Diameter in Megacolon
Cecum	>12 cm[Q]
Ascending colon	>8 cm
Transverse colon	>6 cm[Q]
Rectosigmoid or descending colon	>6.5 cm

65. **Ans. a. Total colectomy**
66. **Ans. b. Ulcerative colitis a. Crohn's disease**
67. **Ans. d. Rectal malignancy**
68. **Ans. a. Stricture** *(Ref: Sabiston 20/e p1341; Schwartz 10/e p1195,1198,1199; Bailey 27/e p1267)*

- **Inflammation** is **purely mucosal** in **ulcerative colitis**, **strictures** are **highly uncommon**. Any **stricture diagnosed** in a patient with **ulcerative colitis** is presumed to be **malignant** until proven otherwise.

69. **Ans. d. Malignancy** *(Ref: Sabiston 20/e p1265, 1352)*

- Long-term survival studies have suggested that patients with **Crohn's disease** have a **death rate** that is about **two to three times higher** than that in the general population.
- **Gastrointestinal cancer**[Q] remains the **leading cause of disease-related death** in patients with **Crohn's disease;** other causes of disease-related deaths include **sepsis, thromboembolic complications,** and **electrolyte disorders.**

70. **Ans. a. 7–33%** *(Ref: Sabiston 20/e p1348; Schwartz 10/e p1194; Shackelford 8/e p1932-1935, 7/e p1995-1997)*

Pouchitis

- **Inflammation** of the **mucosa** of the **ileal pouch**, or **pouchitis**, occurs in **7-33%** of patients with UC **treated by IPAA**[Q].
- The **cause** is **unknown** but may be related to **bacterial overgrowth, mucosal ischemia,** or **other local factors**[Q].

Clinical features:
- Pouchitis typically presents with **increased stool frequency, fever, bleeding, cramps,** and **dehydration**[Q].

Treatment:
- Episodes usually respond to **rehydration** and **oral antibiotics**, usually **metronidazole** or **ciprofloxacin**[Q].
- **Probiotics** have been reported to **provide dramatic resolution** in **some cases** of **pouchitis resistant to antibiotic therapy**[Q].

  - The diagnosis of **Crohn's disease** must also be entertained in patients with **significant pouchitis** that does not **respond to medical treatment**[Q].

71. **Ans. d. Episodes of pouchitis will not respond to antibiotics**
72. **Ans. b. Pouchitis**
73. **Ans. d. Malignancy**
74. **Ans. a. Pouchitis**

75. **Ans. a. Conservative treatment and leave him and hope for the spontaneous resolution** *(Ref: Sabiston 20/e p1287; Schwartz 10/e p1158; Bailey 27/e p1256)*

> **TREATMENT OF ENTEROCUTANEOUS FISTULA**
>
> - Successful management requires establishment of **controlled drainage**, usually using a **sump suction apparatus; management of sepsis; prevention of fluid** and **electrolyte depletion; protection of the skin;** and **provision of adequate nutrition**[Q].
> - When **sepsis** has been **controlled** and **nutritional therapy** has been instituted, a course of **conservative management**[Q] should be followed.
>   - **Most of these fistulas heal spontaneously** within **4–6 weeks** of **conservative management**[Q]. If closure is not accomplished after this time, surgery is indicated.
> - This **period of conservative management** not only allows those **fistulas to heal spontaneously** but also **allows for optimization of nutritional status** and **control of the wound and fistula sites**[Q].
> - Also, a **reasonable delay permits** the **peritoneal reaction** and **inflammation to subside,** thus **making** a **second operation easier** and **safer**[Q].
>   - **Preferred operation: Fistula tract excision** and **segmental resection** of the **involved segment of intestine** and **reanastomosis**[Q].
> - **Simple closure** of the fistula after removing the fistula **tract almost always results in** a **recurrence** of the fistula.
> - If an **unexpected abscess** is encountered or if the **bowel wall is rigid** and **distended** over a **long distance,** thus making primary anastomosis unsafe, **exteriorization of both ends** of the **intestine** should be accomplished.

CHAPTER 17

Vermiform Appendix

ACUTE APPENDICITIS

ACUTE APPENDICITIS

- Acute appendicitis is the MC general surgical emergency^Q
- Worldwide, **perforated appendicitis** is the **leading general surgical cause** of **death**^Q.

Pathophysiology
- **Obstruction of the lumen**^Q is believed to be the **major cause** of **acute appendicitis**^Q.
- **Obstruction of the lumen** may be **caused by inspissated stool** (fecalith^Q or appendicolith^Q), **lymphoid hyperplasia**^Q, **vegetable matter** or **seeds**^Q, **parasites**, or a **neoplasm**^Q.

  - Obstruction of appendiceal lumen contributes to **bacterial overgrowth & continued secretion of mucus** leads **to intraluminal distention & increased wall pressure**. Luminal distention produces the **visceral pain** sensation experienced by the patient as **periumbilical pain**.

- Subsequent impairment of lymphatic & venous drainage leads to mucosal ischemia.

Bacteriology
- **MC bacteria isolated** in perforated appendicitis: Bacteroides fragilis (80%) > E. coli (77%)^Q.

Clinical Features
- **Diagnosis** can be **made primarily** on the basis of the **history & physical examination** in **most cases**.
- **Typical presentation**: Periumbilical pain followed by **anorexia & nausea**.

  - The **pain** then **localizes to** the **right lower quadrant** as the inflammatory process progresses to involve the parietal peritoneum overlying the appendix.
  - This **classic pattern of migratory pain** is the **most reliable symptom** of **acute appendicitis**.
  - A **bout of vomiting** may occur. **Fever ensues, followed by** the development of **leukocytosis**.
  - **Occasional patients** have **urinary symptoms** or **microscopic hematuria**

- **Tenderness** is **directly over** the **appendix**, at **McBurney's point**.
- **Rectal & pelvic examinations** are **most likely** to be **negative** (Tenderness on examination in pelvic appendix)

Dunphy's sign^Q	Pain on coughing^Q	
Rovsing's sign^Q	Pain in the **right lower quadrant** during **palpation of** the **left lower quadrant**^Q	
Ten Horn sign	Pain on gentle traction of right testis	
Obturator sign^Q	Pain on **internal rotation of** the **hip**^Q	Suggestive of **pelvic appendix**^Q
Iliopsoas sign^Q	Pain on **extension** of the **right hip**^Q	Suggestive of **retrocecal appendix**^Q

Diagnosis
- IOC for diagnosis of acute appendicitis in children: USG^Q
- Gold standard for diagnosis of acute appendicitis: CECT^Q

Laboratory Studies
- **WBC count** is **elevated**, with **more than 75% neutrophils** in most patients^Q.
- **Normal WBC count** and **differential** is found in **10% of patients** with acute appendicitis^Q.
- **High WBC count** (>20,000/mL) suggests **complicated appendicitis** with **gangrene** or **perforation**^Q.
- **Microscopic hematuria** is **common in appendicitis** (**gross hematuria** may **indicate** the presence of a **kidney stone**)^Q

Ultrasound

- USG has a **sensitivity of 85%** and a **specificity >90%** for the diagnosis of acute appendicitis in patients of abdominal pain.
- **Characteristic findings**: Appendix ≥ 7 mm diameter, a **thick-walled, noncompressible luminal structure** seen in cross section (**target lesion**), or the **presence of an appendicolith**[Q].
- Commonly used in **children** and **pregnant patients**[Q] with equivocal clinical findings suggestive of acute appendicitis.

Plain X-ray

- A **calcified appendicolith** is **visible** in only **10–15%** of patients with acute appendicitis.
- **Failure of the appendix to fill during** a **barium enema** has been **associated with appendicitis**[Q] (this finding lacks sensitivity & specificity because up to 20% of normal appendices do not fill).

CT Scan

- **CT scan**: **Sensitivity of 90%** and a **specificity of 80-90%** for the diagnosis of **acute appendicitis** in patients with abdominal pain[Q].
- **Classic findings** on CT: **Distended appendix > 7 mm** in diameter and **circumferential wall thickening & enhancement** (appearance of a **halo** or **target**)[Q]
- **CT detects appendicoliths** in **50%** of patients with appendicitis.
- **Most valuable for older patients** and in patients with atypical symptoms

Treatment

- Most patients are managed by prompt **appendectomy**[Q].

ALVARADO (MANTRELS) SCORES

Alvarado (MANTRELS) scores

	Manifestations	Score
Symptoms	• **M**igratory RIF pain • **A**norexia • **N**ausea and vomiting	1 1 1
Signs	• **T**enderness (RIF) • **R**ebound tenderness • **E**levated temperature	2 1 1
Laboratory	• **L**eucocytosis • **S**hift to left	2 1
	Total	10

Scores	Prediction
9–10	**Appendicitis is certain**
7–8	**High likelihood** of appendicitis
5–6	**Equivocal**
1–4	Appendicitis can be **ruled out**

- **CT scanning** is **appropriate for making diagnosis in** patients with **Alvarado scores** of **5 and 6 (in equivocal cases)**[Q].

MANAGEMENT OF ACUTE APPENDICITIS

Management of Acute Appendicitis

- Most patients are managed by **prompt surgical removal of** the **appendix**[Q].
- A **brief period of resuscitation**[Q] is usually sufficient to ensure the safe induction of general anesthesia.
- **Preoperative antibiotics**[Q] cover aerobic and anaerobic colonic flora.
- **Single** preoperative **dose of antibiotics** in **nonperforated appendicitis** reduces postoperative **wound infections** and **intra-abdominal abscess** formation[Q].
- **Perforated** or **gangrenous appendicitis**: Continue **postoperative IV antibiotics until** the **patient is afebrile**[Q].

  - **Appendectomies** are performed **laparoscopically**, particularly **in fertile women, obese patients**, and cases of **diagnostic uncertainty**[Q].
  - **Open appendectomy** is usually performed through a **transverse right lower quadrant incision (Davis-Rockey)** or an **oblique incision (McArthur McBurney)**[Q].
  - For **uncomplicated cases**, a **transverse, muscle-splitting incision** lateral to the rectus abdominis muscle **over McBurney's point is preferred**[Q].

OCHSNER-SHERREN REGIME

MANAGEMENT OF APPENDICULAR MASS

- If an **appendix mass** is present and the **condition of the patient** is **satisfactory**, standard treatment is the **conservative Ochsner-Sherren regimen**^{Q}.
- This strategy is based on the premise that **inflammatory process** is **already localized** and that **inadvertent surgery is difficult**^{Q} and **may be dangerous**. It may be impossible to find the appendix and, a **fecal fistula** may form.
- For these reasons, it is wise to observe a non-operative programme but to be prepared to operate should clinical deterioration occur.

> - **CECT abdomen** should be performed & **antibiotic therapy** (Metronidazole + 3rd generation cephalosporin or **single dose of ertapenem**) should be given^Q.
> - An **abscess**, if present, should be **drained radiologically**^{Q}.

- **Temperature** & **pulse rate** should be recorded **4-hourly** and a **fluid balance** record maintained.
- **Clinical deterioration** or **evidence of peritonitis** is an indication for early laparotomy^Q.

> - **Clinical improvement** is usually evident **within 24-48 hours**^{Q}.
> - **Failure of the mass to resolve** should raise **suspicion of a carcinoma** or **Crohn's disease**^{Q}.

- Using this regimen, approximately **90% of cases resolve without incident**.
- The **great majority of patients will not develop recurrence**, and it is **no longer considered advisable to remove** the **appendix** after an interval of 6–8 weeks^Q.

Criteria for stopping conservative treatment of an appendix mass		
• A rising pulse rate^Q	• Increasing or spreading abdominal pain^Q	• Increasing size of the mass^Q

APPENDICITIS IN PREGNANCY

APPENDICITIS IN PREGNANCY

- Appendicitis is the **MC nonobstetric surgical disease of abdomen during pregnancy**^{Q}.
- Risk during pregnancy is the **same as** it is **in nonpregnant women** of the same age
- Incidence is **1 in 2000** pregnancies.
- Can occur in any trimester, with a **slight increase**^{Q} in frequency during the **2nd trimester.**
- **Perforation** is **more common in the 3rd trimester**^{Q}
- Fetal mortality can rise up to **35–50%** in cases of **perforation**^{Q}.

Clinical Features
- Diagnosis may be difficult because symptoms of **nausea, vomiting, & anorexia**, as well as elevated **WBC count**, are common during pregnancy^Q.
- **Location of tenderness varies with gestation**^{Q}.
- After the fifth month of gestation, appendix is shifted superiorly above the iliac crest & appendiceal tip is rotated medially into right upper quadrant by gravid uterus.

Diagnosis
- **Ultrasound**^{Q} is helpful for establishing the diagnosis & **location** of inflamed appendix.

Treatment
- **Early appendectomy**^{Q} is the appropriate therapy in suspected appendicitis **during all stages** of pregnancy.
- **Laparoscopic appendectomy is safe**^{Q}

APPENDICULAR PERFORATION

APPENDICULAR PERFORATION

- **Immediate appendectomy** has long been the **recommended treatment** for acute appendicitis because of the presumed **risk of progression to rupture**^{Q}.
- The overall rate of perforated appendicitis is **25.8%**.
- **Children <5 years**^{Q} of age and **patients > 65 years**^{Q} of age have the **highest rates of perforation** (45 & 51%, respectively).

Risk Factors for Appendicular Perforation (Fecolith DIE in Pelvic Surgery)	
• **Fecalith**^{Q}	• **Extremes of ages**^{Q}
• **Diabetes mellitus**^{Q}	• **Pelvic** appendix^Q
• **Immunosuppression**^{Q}	• Previous abdominal **surgery**^{Q}

- It has been suggested that **delays in presentation** are **responsible for the majority of perforated appendices**^{Q}.
- **Appendiceal rupture** occurs **most frequently distal** to the **point of luminal obstruction along the antimesenteric border** of the appendix^Q.

> - **Rupture should be suspected** in the presence of **fever** with a **temperature of > 39°C** (102°F) and a **WBC count of > 18,000 cells/mm³**.
> - **MC bacteria isolated** in perforated appendicitis: Bacteroides fragilis (80%) > E. coli (77%)^Q.

APPENDICEAL CARCINOID

APPENDICEAL CARCINOID

- Appearance: **Firm, yellow, bulbar mass** in the **appendix**^{Q}
- **Majority of carcinoids** are **located in the tip**^{Q} of the appendix.
- **Mean tumor size** for carcinoids is **2.5 cm**^{Q}.
- Carcinoid tumors **usually present with localized disease** (64%)^Q.

Clinical Features

- **Carcinoid syndrome** is **rarely associated**^{Q} with appendiceal carcinoid unless widespread metastases are present.
- **Symptoms attributable directly to** the **carcinoid are rare**^{Q}, although the tumor can occasionally obstruct the appendiceal lumen much like a fecalith and result in acute appendicitis
- **Malignant potential** is **related to size**, with **tumors < 1 cm rarely resulting in extension outside of** the **appendix**^{Q} or adjacent to the mass.

Treatment of Appendiceal Carcinoid	
Size	Treatment option
Up to 1 cm	• Appendectomy^Q
> 1–2 cm	• **Appendectomy if located at tip or mid-appendix** • **Right hemicolectomy** if: – **Located at base**^{Q} – **Invading mesoappendix**^{Q} – **LN involvement**^{Q}
> 2 cm	• **Right hemicolectomy**^{Q}

Prognosis

- Patients with **carcinoid tumors** have the **best 5-year survival** (83%)^Q.

MUCOCELE OF APPENDIX

MUCOCELE OF APPENDIX

- A mucocele of the appendix is an **obstructive dilatation** by **intraluminal accumulation** of **mucoid material**^{Q}.
- Caused by one of four processes: **retention cysts, mucosal hyperplasia, cystadenomas,** and **cystadenocarcinomas**^{Q}.
- **Intact mucoceles < 2 cm** are **almost always benign**^{Q}.
- Larger mucoceles are more likely to be neoplastic.

Clinical Features

- **Clinical presentation** is **nonspecific** (an **incidental finding** at **operation**)
- An **intact mucocele** presents **no future risk** for the patient; however, the **opposite is true** if the **mucocele has ruptured** and **epithelial cells have escaped into** the **peritoneal cavity**^{Q}.

Treatment

- **Every effort** is **made to keep the mucocele intact during extraction**, including **placing** the **specimen in a bag** or **converting** a laparoscopic procedure **to an open procedure**^{Q}, if necessary.
- **Presence of a mucocele does not mandate** performance of a **right hemicolectomy**^{Q}.

> - Surgery include: **Appendectomy + Wide resection of** the **mesoappendix** to include all the appendiceal lymph nodes + **Collection** and **cytologic examination** of all **intraperitoneal mucus** + **Inspection of** the **base** of the appendix^Q.

- **Right hemicolectomy** is **reserved for** patients with a **positive margin at** the **base** of the appendix or **positive periappendiceal lymph nodes**^{Q}.

APPENDICEAL ADENOCARCINOMA

APPENDICEAL ADENOCARCINOMA

- Appendiceal adenocarcinomas found in < 1% of **appendectomy specimens**.
- Most are **discovered incidentally**[Q].
- **Typical patient** is **older** and the **duration of symptoms** is **usually longer**.
- **Mucinous adenocarcinoma cell type** is **most common** and has a **better prognosis**[Q] after resection than the colon or signet ring cell type, with 5-year survival rates approaching 50%.
- **Right hemicolectomy** is **recommended**[Q].

APPENDICULAR LYMPHOMA

APPENDICULAR LYMPHOMA

- **MC site of extranodal lymphoma: GIT**[Q] (**Stomach**[Q] > **small intestine**[Q] > pharynx > colon > esophagus).
- Appendicular lymphoma is rare
- More common in **males**[Q]

Pathology
- **MC type of extranodal lymphoma: DLBL**[Q]
- Lymphoma of the appendix is almost exclusively **non-Hodgkin's B-cell lymphoma**[Q]

Clinical Features
- **MC manifestation: Acute appendicitis**[Q] from luminal obstruction
- Other symptoms: Insidious onset of **pain in RIF**[Q] & an associated **palpable mass**[Q]

Diagnosis
- **USG: Diffuse hypoechoic thickening**[Q] with cystic dilation of the lumen (relative **maintenance of vermiform appearance**[Q])
- **CECT:** Diameter ≥ 3 cm (**Aneurysmal dilatation of lumen**[Q] is seen)

Treatment
- **Surgery (right hemicolectomy) + chemotherapy** is the **best treatment option**[Q] for appendiceal lymphoma.
- **Chemotherapy regimen: CHOP**[Q] (**C**yclophosphamide, **H**ydroxydaunorubicin or doxorubicin, **O**ncovin or vincristine, **P**rednisone)
- Addition of **Rituximab**[Q] (monoclonal antibody **against CD20**) improves overall survival.

APPENDECTOMY

CONVENTIONAL APPENDECTOMY

- When the preoperative diagnosis is considered reasonably certain, the incision that is widely used for appendectomy is the so called **gridiron incision** (gridiron: a **frame of cross-beams** to **support a ship** during repairs)[Q].

  - **Gridiron incision (described first by McArthur**[Q]) is **made at right angles** to a **line joining** the **anterior superior iliac spine to** the **umbilicus**, its **centre being along** the line at **McBurney's point**[Q].

- If **better access** is required, it is possible to **convert** the **gridiron to a Rutherford Morison incision**[Q] by **cutting** the **internal oblique** and **transversus muscles** in the line of the incision.

  - In recent years, a **transverse skin crease (Lanz**[Q]) **incision** has become **more popular**, as the **exposure is better** and **extension**, when needed, **is easier**.
  - **Lanz incision** is also known as: **Modified McBurney incision/ Rocky Davis incision/ Bikini incision.**
  - The **incision**, appropriate in length to the size and obesity of the patient, is made approximately **2 cm below** the **umbilicus centred on** the **mid-clavicular-midinguinal line**.
  - It is a **muscle splitting incision**[Q] along the **direction of fibers**.

- When the **diagnosis is in doubt**, particularly in the **presence of intestinal obstruction**, a **lower midline abdominal incision**[Q] is to be **preferred** over a right lower paramedian incision.

  - **Rutherford Morison's incision** is useful if the **appendix is para** or **retrocaecal & fixed**[Q].
  - It is **essentially an oblique muscle-cutting incision** with its **lower end over McBurney's point** & extending **obliquely upwards** and **laterally** as necessary. All layers are divided in the line of the incision[Q].

STEPS OF APPENDECTOMY

Steps of Appendectomy

- **Cecum** is identified by the **presence of taeniae coli**, a turgid **appendix** may be **felt at the base** of the cecum^Q.
- **Base of** the mesoappendix is **clamped in artery forceps, divided** and **ligated**^{Q}.
- **Appendix** is **crushed near its junction** with the **cecum** in artery forceps, which is removed and reapplied just distal to the crushed portion^Q.
- An **absorbable ligature** is **tied around** the **crushed portion** close to the cecum^Q.
- **Appendix** is **amputated** between the artery forceps and the ligature.
- An **absorbable purse-string** or **'Z' suture** may then be **inserted into** the **cecum** about 1.25 cm from the base^Q.
- **Stump** of the appendix **is invaginated while** the **purse-string** or **'Z' suture is tied**, thus burying the appendix stump^Q.
- Many surgeons believe **invagination** of the appendiceal stump **is unnecessary**^{Q}.

Methods to be adopted in special circumstances	
Edematous and **inflamed cecal wall**	• **Purse string suture** is **not applied**^{Q} • **Stump** is **not invaginated**^{Q}
Inflamed base of appendix	• **Base** is **not crushed** for the fear of spread of infection by way of lymphatics and blood stream^Q. • **Base** is **ligated close to the cecal wall**^{Q}, after which the appendix is amputated and the stump invaginated.
Gangrenous base of appendix	• **Neither crushing nor ligation**^{Q} • Two **stitches** are **placed through** the **cecal wall close to the base** of the gangrenous appendix, which is **amputated flush with** the **cecal wall**^{Q}, after which these stitches are tied. **Further closure** is effected by means of a **second layer** of **interrupted seromuscular sutures**^{Q}.

COMPLICATIONS OF APPENDECTOMY

Complications of Appendectomy

- **Wound infection: MC postoperative complication**^{Q} (in 5-10% of all patients).
- **Intra-abdominal abscess**^{Q}
- **Ileus**^{Q}
- **Respiratory** complications (rare)^Q
- **Venous thrombosis** and **embolism**
- **Portal pyaemia** (pylephlebitis)
- **Adhesive intestinal obstruction:**
  - **MC late complication** of appendectomy^Q.
  - At operation, a **single band adhesion** is often **found to be responsible**^{Q}.
- **Fecal fistula**^{Q}
  - **Leakage from** the **appendicular stump** occurs **rarely**, but may follow if the **encircling stitch** has been **put in too deeply** or if the **cecal wall was involved by edema** or **inflammation**^{Q}.
  - Occasionally, a **fistula may result following appendicectomy in Crohn's disease**^{Q}.
  - **Conservative management** with low-residue enteral nutrition will usually **result in closure**^{Q}.

ANATOMY OF APPENDIX

Anatomy of Appendix

- **Appendix, ileum,** and **ascending colon** are all **derived from** the **midgut**^{Q}.
- **Appendiceal artery (end artery),** a **branch of** the **ileocolic artery,** supplies the appendix^Q.
- **Length: 2–20 cm** (average length is 9 cm in adults)^Q.
- **Base of the appendix** is **located at the convergence of** the **taeniae along the inferior aspect of** the **cecum**^{Q}
- **MC location: Retrocecal**^{Q}
- **Least common location: Post-ileal**^{Q}

Multiple Choice Questions

ACUTE APPENDICITIS

1. **Most common initiating factor in acute appendicitis is:** *(JIPMER GIS 2011)*
   a. Luminal obstruction b. Bacterial infection
   c. Lymphoid hyperplasia d. Perforation

2. **When acute appendicitis is suspected, it can be confirmed by:** *(PGI June 2007, June 2002)*
   a. Clinical examination b. USG
   c. CT scan d. Blood counts
   e. Upper GI endoscopy

3. **True about appendicular rupture is all except:** *(PGI Dec 99)*
   a. Common in extremes of age
   b. Common in people with fecolith obstruction
   c. Early antibiotics prevent rupture
   d. Appendectomy is done always in presence of rupture

4. **Most dangerous position of appendix is:** *(Recent Question 2015)*
   a. Retrocecal b. Paracolic
   c. Pelvic d. Retroperitoneal

5. **A young boy presented to the casualty with history of fever, pain abdomen and vomiting. On examination, he was febrile with a pulse rate of 104/min. The resident was eliciting the sign shown below. Identify the sign.** *(AIIMS May 2017)*

   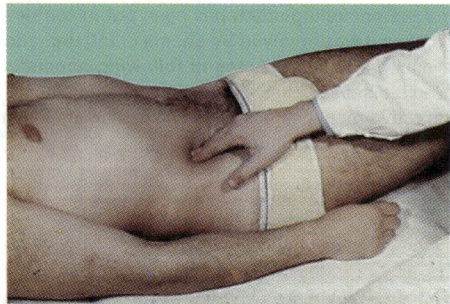

   a. Rovsing's sign b. Ballance sign
   c. McBurney's point tenderness
   d. Psoas sign

6. **In a case of retrocecal appendicitis which movement aggravates pain?** *(AIIMS Nov 2007)*
   a. Flexion b. Extension
   c. Medial rotation d. Lateral rotation

7. **Earliest symptoms in acute appendicitis is:** *(DNB 2003)*
   a. Pain b. Fever
   c. Vomiting d. Rise of pulse rate

8. **A patient with Crohn's disease was opened and an inflamed appendix found. The treatment of choice is:**
   a. Appendectomy *(Recent Question 2016)*
   b. Ileocolic resection and anastomosis
   c. Close the abdomen and start medical treatment
   d. None of the above

9. **When the rectum is inflated with air through a rectal tube, pain and tenderness occur in the right iliac fossa in case of appendicitis? This is known as:** *(Recent Question 2014)*
   a. Aaron's sign b. Battle's sign
   c. Bastedo sign d. MC Burney's sign

10. **The frequent mechanism in perforation of appendix is:**
    a. Impacted faecolith *(DNB 89, 91)*
    b. Tension gangrene due to the accumulating secretions
    c. Necrosis of lymphoid patch
    d. Retrocaecal infection

11. **Acute appendicitis is due to:** *(AIIMS 90, AMU 90)*
    a. Faecolith b. Worms of ileo-caecal region
    c. Streptococcal infections d. Abuse of purgatives
    e. None of the above

12. **All are useful in acute appendicitis except:** *(Kerala 94)*
    a. Antibiotics b. Analgesics
    c. IV Fluids d. Purgation

13. **Most common organism isolated from perforated appendicitis:** *(AIIMS GIS May 2008)*
    a. E. coli b. Pseudomonas
    c. Klebsiella d. Enterococcus

14. **Diffuse peritonitis following appendicitis is usually seen:** *(Recent Question 2013, ICS 2000)*
    a. When appendicular perforation occurs early (within 24 hours)
    b. When perforation occurs late (after 24 hours)
    c. Particularly in non-obstructive appendicitis
    d. When antibiotics are withheld

15. **All of the following signs are not seen in acute appendicitis except:** *(TN 2001)*
    a. Rovsing's b. Murphy's
    c. Boa's sign d. Mack wen's sign

16. **All are to be done in case of 20-years old female coming to casualty with right iliac fossa pain, with local guarding and tenderness, except:** *(AIIMS Nov 99)*
    a. IV glucose b. Pethidine 100 mg IM
    c. Nil orally d. X-ray abdomen

17. **Aaron's sign is seen in:**
    a. Achalasia cardia b. Hiatus hernia
    c. Mediastinum emphysema d. Acute appendicitis

18. **Rovsing sign is seen in:** *(PGI 95)*
    a. Acute appendicitis b. Acute cholecystitis
    c. Pancreatitis d. None

19. **A 15-year-old boy is admitted with a history and physical finding consistent with appendicitis. Which of the following findings is most likely to be positive?** *(COMEDK 2004)*
    a. Pelvic crepts b. Iliopsoas sign
    c. Murphy's Sign d. Flank ecchymosis

20. **False about appendicitis in children:** *(JIPMER 2011)*
    a. Localized pain is the single most important symptom
    b. Vomiting precedes abdominal pain
    c. Perforation occurs in 80% of cases <5 years
    d. 60% perforation occurs within 48 hours

21. Most common occurrence before appendicitis:
    a. Blockage of lumen   b. Ileitis   *(PGI Nov 2011)*
    c. Gastroenteritis   d. Perforation
22. In appendicitis, the initial periumbilical pain is eventually localized to right iliac fossa because of:
    a. Peritoneum   b. Iliopsoas
    c. Colon   d. Caecum
23. Which of the following clinical signs is not associated with acute appendicitis?   *(MHPGMCET 2009)*
    a. Pointing sign   b. Rovsing's sign
    c. Cullen's sign   d. Obturator sign
24. "Ten horn" sign is a feature of: *(MHSSMCET 2011)*
    a. Rectus muscle hematoma   b. Acute pancreatitis
    c. Choledocholithiasis   d. Acute appendicitis
25. Alvarado scale is for:
    (Recent Question 2017, DNB 2012, MHSSMCET 2011)
    a. Diverticulitis
    b. Mesenteric lymphadenitis
    c. Acute appendicitis
    d. Pelvic abscess
26. Which of the following organisms produces signs and symptoms that mimic acute appendicitis?   *(Recent Question 2015)*
    a. Enteropathic Escherichia coli
    b. Enterobius vermicularis
    c. Trichomonas hominis
    d. Yersinia enterocolitica
27. From the surgery done below, name the scoring used to diagnose this condition: *(Recent Question 2018)*

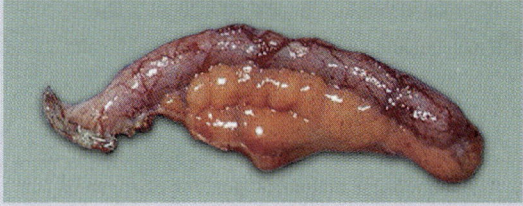

    a. Alvarado   b. Ranson
    c. Apache-II   d. BISAP
28. Alvarado score consists of: *(Recent Question 2013)*
    a. Leucopenia   b. Anorexia
    c. Diarrhea   d. Periumbilical pain
29. Most common differential diagnosis for appendicitis:
    a. Gastroenteritis   *(Recent Question 2013)*
    b. Mesenteric lymphadenopathy
    c. Intussusception
    d. Meckel's diverticulitis
30. Investigation of choice for acute appendicitis in children:
    (AIIMS May 2015, November 2014, May 2013)
    a. CT scan   b. Ultrasound
    c. MRI   d. X-ray

APPENDICITIS IN PREGNANCY

31. Regarding appendicitis in pregnancy, false is: *(ILBS 2011)*
    a. MC cause of acute abdomen in first trimester
    b. Pregnancy doesn't increase the risk
    c. Conservative management by antibiotics should be tried
    d. After rupture, fetal mortality is around 30–40%
32. A pregnant female presents with pain in abdomen on examination, tenderness is found in right lumbar region. TLC is 12,000/cmm, and urine examination is normal, for diagnosis further test done is: *(AIIMS June 99)*
    a. Chest X-ray with abdominal shield
    b. Ultrasound abdomen
    c. Non contrast CT abdomen
    d. Laparoscopy
33. Which is the best test for diagnosis of acute appendicitis in a pregnant female?   *(MHSSMCET 2008)*
    a. Alder's test   b. Aaron's test
    c. Angell's test   d. Mc Burney's test

OCHSNER-SHERREN REGIME

34. Ochsner-Sherren regimen is used for treatment of:
    (DNB 2012, 2000, MHPGMET 2005)
    a. Appendicular abscess   b. Appendicular mass
    c. Acute appendicitis   d. Appendicular mucocele
35. A 26-years old male presented with 4 day history of pain in the right sided lower abdomen with frequent vomiting. Patients general condition is fair and clinically a tender lump was felt in the right iliac fossa. Most appropriate management for this case would be: *(Recent Question 2014)*
    a. Exploratory laparotomy
    b. Immediate appendectomy
    c. Ochsner-Sherren regimen
    d. External drainage
36. True about appendicular mass is all except: *(DPG 2006)*
    a. Ochsner-Sherren regime followed
    b. Develops after 72 hours
    c. Fever is present
    d. Operation is to be done immediately
37. A 25-years old man presents with 3 days history of pain in the right lower abdomen and vomiting. Patient's general condition is satisfactory and clinical examination reveals a tender lump in right iliac fossa. The most appropriate management in this case would be: *(Recent Question 2015)*
    a. Immediate appendectomy   b. Exploratory laparotomy
    c. Ochsner-Sherren regimen   d. External drainage

NEOPLASM OF APPENDIX

38. Most common neoplasm of appendix is:
    (Recent Question 2015, AIIMS Nov 93)
    a. Lymphoma   b. Adenocarcinoma
    c. Leiomyosarcoma   d. Argentaffinoma
39. A 25-year-old patient presented with mass in right iliac fossa, which after laparotomy was found to be carcinoid of 2.5 cm in diameter. What will be next step in management?
    (Recent Question 2013, AIIMS Nov 2000)
    a. Segmental resection   b. Appendectomy
    c. Right hemicolectomy   d. Do yearly 5-HIAA assay
40. What is the treatment of patient with carcinoid tumor of appendix of size more than 2 cm?   *(AIIMS June 99)*
    a. Right hemicolectomy   b. Appendectomy
    c. Appendectomy + abdominal CT scan
    d. Appendectomy + 24 hours urinary HIAA
41. Mucocele of the appendix is: *(All India 89)*
    a. Benign tumour   b. Low grade malignancy
    c. Retention cyst   d. Infective process

Surgery Essence

42. Treatment of an incidentally detected appendicular carcinoid measuring 2.5 cm is: *(MCI March 2009)*
    a. Right hemicolectomy
    b. Limits resection of the right colon
    c. Total colectomy
    d. Appendectomy

43. Most common tumor occurring in appendix: *(JIPMER 2010)*
    a. Melanoma
    b. Carcinoid tumor
    c. Adenocarcinoma
    d. Mucinous carcinoma

44. Treatment of choice for mucinous adenocarcinoma of appendix: *(MHSSMCET 2009)*
    a. Right hemicolectomy
    b. Appendectomy
    c. Percutaneous aspiration
    d. Total colectomy

APPENDICULAR LYMPHOMA

45. Best treatment option for appendicular lymphoma:
    a. Right hemicolectomy *(Recent Question 2016)*
    b. Chemotherapy
    c. Right hemicolectomy + chemotherapy
    d. None

APPENDECTOMY

46. Grid-iron incision was first described by: *(MHSSMCET 2005)*
    a. McArthur
    b. Rutherford Morrison
    c. Hamilton Bailey
    d. Lanz

47. Stump size in appendectomy should not be more than:
    a. 1 mm
    b. 2 mm *(MHSSMCET 2010)*
    c. 3 mm
    d. 4 mm

48. During appendectomy if it is noticed that base of appendix is inflamed then further line of treatment is: *(DPG 2011, PGI 96)*
    a. No appendectomy
    b. No burying of stump
    c. Hemicolectomy
    d. Cecal resection

49. The nerve commonly damaged during McBurney's incision is: *(Recent Question 2013, Bihar PG 2014, All India 2003)*
    a. Subcostal
    b. Iliohypogastric
    c. 11th thoracic
    d. 10th thoracic

50. Which of the following statements is not true of McBurney's incision? *(Karnataka 94)*
    a. Most suitable if the diagnosis of appendicitis is definite
    b. If it is converted into a muscle cutting incision it is called Rutherford Morison's incision
    c. Inguinal hernia is a sequele of the incision
    d. The incision can be extended upwards or downwards

51. A Gridiron incision becomes a Rutherford Morison's incision is extended by: *(Karnataka 94)*
    a. Splitting the muscles laterally
    b. Cutting the muscles laterally
    c. Cutting the muscles medially into the rectus sheath
    d. Incising vertically along the rectus muscle

52. Which one of the following is a muscle-splitting incision? *(ICS 2005)*
    a. Kocher's
    b. Rutherford-Morrison
    c. Pfannenstiel
    d. Lanz

53. An appendicular fistula is least likely to heal if: *(Kerala 98)*
    a. The stump was sutured with vicryl
    b. There is stenosis/narrowing of the sigmoid colon
    c. Superadded infection
    d. None

54. All of the following are early complications arising after appendectomy for acute appendicitis except:
    a. Ileus
    b. Sterility
    c. Intestinal obstruction
    d. Pulmonary complications

55. Fecal fistula after appendectomy may occur due to:
    a. Adhesions *(MHPGMCET 2003)*
    b. Gangrenous appendicitis
    c. Undiagnosed ileo-cecal disease
    d. Postoperative infection

56. Which of the following is a muscle splitting incision?
    a. Kocher's incision *(AIIMS November 2016)*
    b. Lanz incision
    c. Rutherford-Morrison incision
    d. Pfannenstiel incision

57. Incision at McBurney's point corresponds to: *(Recent Question 2017)*
    a. Tip of appendix
    b. Base of appendix
    c. Midpoint of appendix
    d. Base of cecum

APPENDIX ANATOMY AND PHYSIOLOGY

58. All are true about appendicular artery except: *(DPG 97)*
    a. Supplies only appendix
    b. Supplies terminal ileum also
    c. Is an end artery
    d. Branch of lower division of ileocolic artery

59. True statement about appendix: *(PGI June 2006)*
    a. Does not have mesentery
    b. Has taenia coli
    c. Develops from midgut
    d. Supplied by appendicular branch of ileocolic artery

60. The commonest anatomical position of appendix is: *(Karnataka 2013, DNB 2012, MHPGMCET 2007, 2001)*
    a. Retrocaecal
    b. Pelvic
    c. Paracecal
    d. Preileal

61. The fold of Treves is: *(MAHE 2005)*
    a. The fold of mucous membrane projecting into the lumen of the rectum
    b. The ilio-appendicular fold of peritoneum
    c. The fold of mucous membrane around the papilla of water
    d. The fold of peritoneum over the inferior mesenteric vein

MISCELLANEOUS

62. Malone procedure is used in: *(KGMC 2011)*
    a. Anorectal incontinence
    b. Urinary incontinence
    c. Neurogenic bladder
    d. GERD

63. Which of the following present as acute abdomen?
    a. Acute intermittent porphyria *(Karnataka 89)*
    b. Tabes
    c. Pneumonitis of lower lobe
    d. All

Explanations

ACUTE APPENDICITIS

1. **Ans. a. Luminal obstruction** *(Ref: Sabiston 20th/e p1297; Schwartz 10/e p1243-1251; Bailey 27/e p1302; Shackelford 8/e p1951, 7/e p2019-2023)*
2. **Ans. a. Clinical examination, b. USG, c. CT scan, d. Blood counts**
3. **Ans. c. Early antibiotics prevent rupture** *(Ref: Sabiston 20/e p1302; Schwartz 10/e p1250-1251; Shackelford 8/e p1953, 7/e p2027)*

    Early antibiotic doesn't prevent rupture, most patients are managed by **prompt surgical removal of** the **appendix**.
4. **Ans. c. Pelvic**
5. **Ans. c. McBurney's point tenderness** *(Ref: Sabiston 20/e p1299; Schwartz 10/e p1244; Bailey 27/e p1303)*

    - The given clinical picture is suggestive of acute appendicitis. In the image, resident is eliciting McBurney's point tenderness in the patient of acute appendicitis.
    - *"Abdominal examination typically reveals a quiet abdomen with tenderness and guarding on palpation of the right lower quadrant. The location of the tenderness is classically over McBurney point, which is located one-third the distance between the anterior superior iliac spine and the umbilicus."-Sabiston 20/e p1299*
6. **Ans. b. Extension** *(Ref: Sabiston 20th/e p1299; Schwartz 10/e p, 1259; Bailey 27/e p1304; Shackelford 8/e p1952, 7/e p2020)*
7. **Ans. a. Pain**
8. **Ans. a. Appendectomy**
9. **Ans. c. Bastedo sign** *(Ref: www.medilexicon.com)*

Bastedo Sign
• An **obsolete sign** in **chronic appendicitis**^{Q}
• **Pain** and **tenderness** in **right iliac fossa** on **inflation of** the **colon with air**^{Q}

10. **Ans. b. Tension gangrene due to the accumulating secretions**
11. **Ans. a. Faecolith, b. Worms of ileo-caecal region**
12. **Ans. d. Purgation** *(Ref: Sabiston 20/e p1300; Schwartz 10/e p1243-1251; Bailey 27/e p1308; Shackelford 8/e p1953, 7/e p2022-2024)*
13. **Ans. a. E. coli**
14. **Ans. a. When appendicular perforation occurs early (within 24 hours)** *(Ref: Bailey 27/e p1303)*

    - In **late stages**, **greater omentum** and **small bowel** becomes **adherent to inflamed appendix**, walling off the spread of **peritoneal contamination**^{Q}.
15. **Ans. a. Rovsing's**
16. **Ans. None** *(Ref: Harrison 16/e p84)*

    - Harrison 14 says "Narcotics or analgesics should be withheld until a definitive diagnosis or a definitive plan has been formulated, because these agents often make it more difficult to secure and to interpret the history and physical findings."
    - Harrison 16 says "**Narcotics** or **analgesics should not be withheld** until a definitive diagnosis or a definitive plan has been formulated; **obfuscation of diagnosis by adequate analgesia is unlikely**^{Q}."
17. **Ans. d. Acute appendicitis** *(Ref: Sabiston 20/e p1126)*
18. **Ans. a. Acute appendicitis**
19. **Ans. b. Iliopsoas sign**
20. **Ans. b. Vomiting precedes abdominal pain** *(Ref: Sabiston 20/e p1297; Bailey 27/e p1303)*

    - **Typical presentation**: **Periumbilical pain** followed by **anorexia** and **nausea**^{Q}.
    - **Localized pain** is the **most important symptom**^{Q}
    - **Perforation** occurs in **80% of cases < 5-years**
    - Approximately **60% perforation** occurs **within 48 hours**

21. **Ans. a. Blockage of lumen**
22. **Ans. a. Peritoneum**
23. **Ans. c. Cullen's sign**
24. **Ans. d. Acute appendicitis**
25. **Ans. c. Acute appendicitis**
26. **Ans. d. Yersinia enterocolitica** *(Ref: Sabiston 20/e p1082, 19/e p1105)*

27. Ans. a. Alvarado *(Ref: Schwartz 10/e p1245; Sabiston 20/e p1132; Bailey 27/e p1307)*
28. Ans. b. Anorexia
29. Ans. b. Mesenteric lymphadenopathy
30. Ans. b. Ultrasound

APPENDICITIS IN PREGNANCY

31. Ans. c. Conservative management by antibiotics should be tried *(Ref: Sabiston 20/e p2048, 1306; Schwartz 10/e p1256-1257; Bailey 27/e p1304)*
    Surgery should be **performed during pregnancy** when **appendicitis is suspected**, just as it would be in a nonpregnant woman.
32. Ans. b. Ultrasound abdomen
33. Ans. a. Alder's test *(Ref: www.ncbi.nlm.nlh.gov/.../PMC3398111)*

ALDER'S TEST

- **Localizing the area** of **maximal abdominal tenderness** and **maintaining constant pressure** on that point while the **patient is being turned to left**^{Q}.
- If the **pain is constant**, pain is of **extra-uterine origin**; if **pain disappears** it is more likely to be **uterine** or **tubal origin**^{Q}.
- This is a **very useful** and **important clinical test** which may be **employed in all cases** of an **acute abdomen in pregnancy**^{Q}.

OCHSNER-SHERREN REGIME

34. Ans. b. Appendicular mass
35. Ans. c. Ochsner-Sherren regimen
36. Ans. d. Operation is to be done immediately
37. Ans. c. Ochsner-Sherren regimen

NEOPLASM OF APPENDIX

38. Ans. d. Argentaffinoma *(Ref: Sabiston 20/e p1308; Schwartz 10/e p1258; Bailey 27/e p1315; Shackelford 8/e p1956, 7/e p2028)*

- MC neoplasm of appendix: Carcinoid tumor
    - **MC malignant neoplasm of appendix (MAC):** Mucinous adenocarcinoma^Q (**38%**) > **A**denocarcinoma (**26%**) > **C**arcinoid (**17%**).

39. Ans. c. Right hemicolectomy *(Ref: Sabiston 20/e p1308; Schwartz 10/e p1258; Bailey 27/e p1315; Shackelford 8/e p1956, 7/e p2028)*
40. Ans. a. Right hemicolectomy
41. Ans. a. Benign tumour, b. Low grade malignancy, c. Retention cyst *(Ref: Sabiston 20/e p1308; Schwartz 10/e p1258; Bailey 27/e p1315; Shackelford 8/e p1956, 7/e p2028)*
42. Ans. a. Right hemicolectomy
43. Ans. b. Carcinoid tumor
44. Ans. a. Right hemicolectomy *(Ref: Sabiston 20/e p1308)*

APPENDICEAL ADENOCARCINOMA

- Appendiceal adenocarcinomas found in **< 1%** of **appendectomy specimens**.
- Most are **discovered incidentally**^{Q}.
- **Typical patient** is **older** and the **duration of symptoms** is **usually longer**.
- **Mucinous adenocarcinoma cell type** is **most common** and has a **better prognosis**^{Q} after resection than the colon or signet ring cell type, with 5-year survival rates approaching 50%.
- **Right hemicolectomy** is **recommended**^{Q}.

APPENDICULAR LYMPHOMA

45. Ans. c. Right hemicolectomy + chemotherapy

APPENDECTOMY

46. Ans. a. McArthur *(Ref: Bailey 27/e p1309)*
47. Ans. c. 3 mm *(Ref: Maingot 11/e p602)*

No matter how the appendix is divided, the **residual appendiceal stump should be no longer than 3 mm to minimize** the **possibility of stump appendicitis** in the future.

STUMP APPENDICITIS

- Appendicitis in the remaining appendiceal stump after appendectomy
- The residual appendiceal **stump should not be more than 3 mm**^{Q} to minimize the possibility of stump appendicitis.

48. **Ans. b. No burying of stump** *(Ref: Sabiston 20/e p1300; Schwartz 10/e p1251-1256; Bailey 27/e p1309; Shackelford 8/e p1955, 7/e p2023-2024)*
49. **Ans. b. Iliohypogastric** *(Ref: Bailey 25/e p1213)*

    - **Right inguinal hernia** is **more common** following a **gridiron incision** for appendectomy, and is **due to injury** to the **iliohypogastric nerve**[Q].
    - IH → IH (IlioHypogastric nerve → Inguinal Hernia)

50. **Ans. d. The incision can be extended upwards or downwards** *(Ref: Bailey 27/e p1309)*

    - In **McBurney's incision**, incision is **extended upwards** and **laterally**, not downwards.

51. **Ans. b. Cutting the muscles laterally**   52. **Ans. d. Lanz**
53. **Ans. b. There is stenosis/narrowing of the sigmoid colon** *(Ref: Sabiston 20/e p1287)*

    - **Unrelieved obstruction** of the tube **distal to fistula** is a **cause of persistence** of fistula.

54. **Ans. b. Sterility**
55. **Ans. c. Undiagnosed ileo-cecal disease** *(Ref: Bailey 27/e p1314)*
    - **Leakage from** the **appendicular stump** occurs rarely, but may follow **if the encircling stitch** has been **put in too deeply** or if the **cecal wall** was **involved by edema** or **inflammation**. Occasionally, a fistula may result **following appendectomy in Crohn's disease**.
56. **Ans. b. Lanz incision**
57. **Ans. b. Base of appendix** *(Ref: Netter's Surgical Anatomy and Approaches E-Book By Conor P Delaney (2013)/p240)*

    "An open incision is made at McBurney's point, located one-third the distance between the anterior superior iliac spine and the umbilicus. This area generally corresponds to the location of the base of the appendix."-Netter's Surgical Anatomy and Approaches E-Book By Conor P Delaney (2013)/p240

APPENDIX ANATOMY AND PHYSIOLOGY

58. **Ans. b. Supplies terminal ileum also** *(Ref: Sabiston 20/e p1296)*
59. **Ans. c. Develops from midgut, d. Supplied by appendicular branch of ileocolic artery**
60. **Ans. a. Retrocaecal**
61. **Ans. b. The ilio-appendicular fold of peritoneum** *(Ref: Sabiston 20/e p1296)*

    - **Jackson Membrane**[Q]: Adhesion from the **right abdominal wall** to the **anterior taenia** of the ascending colon.
    - **Gerlach valves**[Q]: A mucosal fold **covering** the **appendiceal orifice.**
    - **Fold of Treves**[Q]: Inferior ileocecal fold (**does not contain any vessel**, referred as the **bloodless fold of Treves**)

MISCELLANEOUS

62. **Ans. a. Anorectal incontinence** *(Ref: Bailey 27/e p137; Shackelford 7/e p2292)*

    APPENDICOSTOMY

    - Use in urologic reconstruction as an **appedicovesicostomy** in patients requiring chronic catheterization for bladder emptying (**Mitrofanoff procedure**)[Q]
    - An **appendicolostomy** for patients in whom the bladder is absent or too small is created by implanting the appendix under the taeniae of a detubularized patch of cecum or sigmoid colon.
    - **Conduit for decompression** after colon surgery or for the **chronic administration** of medications or **enema** (**Malone Procedure**)[Q]

63. **Ans. d. All** *(Ref: Bailey 27/e p1305)*

Rare Differential Diagnoses of Acute Appendicitis	
- **Preherpetic pain**[Q] of the right 10th and 11th dorsal nerves	- **Diabetes mellitus**[Q]
- **Tabetic crises** (**Tabes**[Q])	- **Typhlitis** or **leukemic ileocecal syndrome**[Q]
- **Acute intermittent porphyria**[Q]	

CHAPTER 18

Rectum and Anal Canal

HEMORRHOID

HEMORRHOID

- Recent theories regard hemorrhoids as **normal anatomical structures**[Q].
- These are **cushions of submucosal tissue** containing **venules, arterioles, smooth muscle fibres & elastic connective tissue (VASE)**.
- Three hemorrhoidal cushions are found in the **left lateral, right anterior & right posterior position (3, 7 & 11 O' Clock)**[Q]
- Hemorrhoids or **piles** are **symptomatic anal cushions**.

- **More common** when intra-abdominal pressure is raised, e.g. in obesity, constipation & pregnancy[Q]
- **Symptoms:** bright-red, painless bleeding, mucus discharge & prolapse
- Hemorrhoids cannot be palpated, **best diagnosed by proctoscopy**[Q].

Internal Hemorrhoids	External Hemorrhoids
• Located **proximal to** the **dentate line**[Q] • **Painless**, can be **ligated**[Q] • **Banding** is **preferred**[Q]	• Located **distal to dentate line**[Q] • Also known as **5-days painful self curing lesion**[Q] • **Painful, not ligated**[Q] • **Excision is done**[Q] • Repeated thrombosis leads to **semi-ripe black currant appearance**

Classification of Internal Hemorrhoids	
1st degree	**Painless bleeding**[Q], no prolapse
2nd degree	**Prolapse** through the anus, on straining but **reduce spontaneously**[Q]
3rd degree	Prolapse through the anal canal and **require manual reduction**[Q]
4th degree	Permanently prolapsed and **cannot be manually reduced**.[Q]

Treatment
- Mere presence of hemorrhoids is not necessarily an indication of treatment.
- Treatment is **only indicated** if they are symptomatic. **Best treatment** is the **least invasive** one which is **possible to alleviate** the **symptoms**[Q].

Treatment of Hemorrhoids	
Medical therapy	• Bleeding from **1st & 2nd degree** hemorrhoids often improve with the addition of **dietary fibre, stool softeners** and other **diet regulation**[Q].
Rubber band ligation	• Done for **1st, 2nd & selected 3rd degree** hemorrhoids[Q]
Infrared photocoagulation	• Done for **1st & 2nd degree** hemorrhoids
Sclerotherapy	• Done for **1st, 2nd & selected 3rd degree** hemorrhoids[Q] • Most commonly used sclerosant is **5% phenol in almond** or **arachis oil**.
Operative hemorrhoidectomy[Q]	• **3rd & 4th degree** hemorrhoid[Q] • **2nd degree not cured by non-operative methods**[Q] • **Mixed** (combine internal/external hemorrhoids)[Q] • **Fibrosed hemorrhoids**

Operative Hemorrhoidectomy
• **Milligan-Morgan open** hemorrhoidectomy[Q]   • **Ferguson closed** hemorrhoidectomy[Q] • **Whitefield submucosal** hemorrhoidectomy[Q]   • **Longo's stapler** hemorrhoidectomy[Q]

RECTAL PROLAPSE

RECTAL PROLAPSE

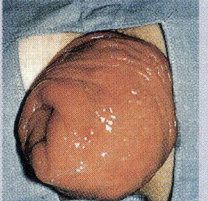

- **Mucous membrane** & **submucosa** of the rectum **protrude outside** the anus for approximately **1–4 cm**[Q].
- It may be **mucosal** or **full thickness** (whole wall of the rectum is included)
- Commences as a **rectal intussusception**[Q]
- In **children**, the prolapse is usually mucosal and should be **treated conservatively**
- In the **adult**, the prolapse is **often full thickness** and is frequently **associated with incontinence**[Q]
- **Surgery** is **necessary** for **full-thickness rectal prolapse**[Q]

Clinical Features

Children	• **Mucosal prolapse** often commences **after an attack of diarrhea**, or from **loss of weight** & **consequent loss of fat** in the **ischiorectal fossae**[Q]. • It may also be **associated with fibrocystic disease, neurological causes** & **maldevelopment of** the **pelvis**[Q].
Adults	• Often associated with **third-degree hemorrhoids**[Q]. • In the **female a torn perineum**, and in the **male straining from urethral obstruction, predisposes to mucosal prolapse**[Q]. • In **old age**, both **mucosal & full-thickness prolapse** are associated with **atony of** the **sphincter mechanism**[Q].

- **Prolapsed mucous membrane** is **pink** (prolapsed internal hemorrhoids are **plum colored, trifoliate** & **more pedunculated**)[Q]

Diagnosis

- Before operative intervention, a careful **history, physical examination**, & **colonoscopy** should be performed.
- **Manometry** should be done **in cases** associated **with incontinence**[Q].

Abdominal Procedures	Perineal Procedures

• Considered the **surgical procedures of choice** for **young & fit individuals**[Q]
• **Not suitable for elderly & infirm patients**[Q]
• Are most likely **to improve continence**[Q]
• Have **least recurrence rates**[Q]
• **Postoperative constipation** is the **MC side effect**[Q]
• **Abdominal Procedures**
• Abdominal rectopexy
  – **Suture Rectopexy**
  – **Mesh Rectopexy**
    – Posterior (**Well's Ivalon's**)[Q]
    – Anterior (**Ripstein's**)[Q]
    – Lateral (**Orr-Loygue**)
    – Ventral
  – **Resection Rectopexy** (Frykman and Goldberg)
• Anterior resection[Q]
	• **Relatively minor procedures** that may be performed under local or regional anaesthesia
	• **Well tolerated by elderly, frail & unfit patients**[Q]
	• Less likely to improve continence
	• **Recurrence rates** varying from **5–35% higher than** following **abdominal rectopexy**[Q]
	• **Postoperative constipation** is **infrequent**[Q]
	
	Perineal Procedure
	• Delorme's muscosectomy[Q]
	• Thiersh and encirclement[Q]
	• Altemeier rectosigmoidectomy[Q]

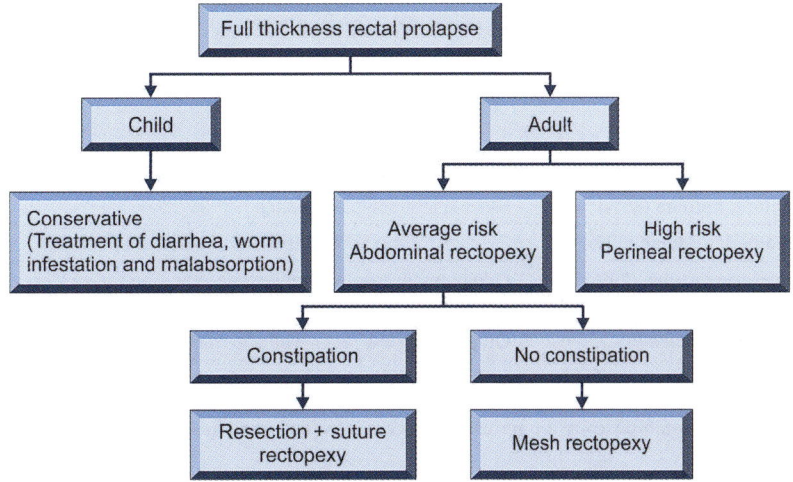

ANO-RECTAL ABSCESS

Ano-Rectal Abscess

- Acute sepsis in the region of the anus is common.
- More common in men^Q
- Subdivided into: Perianal (MC)^Q, Ischiorectal (2nd MC)^Q, submucous & pelvirectal
- Underlying conditions: Fistula-in-ano (MC), Crohn's disease, diabetes, immunosuppression^Q

> **Cryptoglandular Theory of Intersphincteric Anal Gland Infection**
> - Upon **infection of a gland, pus,** which **travels along** the **path of least resistance,** may **spread caudally** to **present as** a **perianal abscess** or **ischiorectal abscess**^{Q}

- MC organism responsible: E. coli^Q > Bacteroides^Q

Clinical Features

- Usually produces a **painful, throbbing swelling in** the **anal region** with **swinging pyrexia**
- Patients with infection in the larger **fatty-filled ischiorectal space,** in which **tissue tension is much lower,** usually **present later,** with **less well localized symptoms** but more constitutional upset & fever.

> - Increased incidence of infection in ischiorectal fossa is due to **poor blood supply**^{Q}.

Treatment

- Drainage of pus + Antibiotics^Q
- Always look for a **potential underlying problem**^{Q}

> - For **perianal & ischiorectal sepsis** (with an **incidence of 60% & 30%** respectively), **drainage** is **through the perineal skin,** usually through a **cruciate incision** over the **most fluctuant point**, with excision of the skin edges to de-roof the abscess.

- **Modified Hanley's technique:** Used for drainage of horseshoe ischiorectal abscess^Q

FISTULA-IN-ANO

Fistula-in-ano

- **Fistula-in-ano** is a **chronic abnormal communication, runs outwards** from the **anorectal lumen** to an **external opening** on the skin of the **perineum** or **buttock**
- Usually **results from anorectal abscess (cryptoglandular abscess**^{Q}**)**
- **Other causes:** Crohn's disease, tuberculosis, lymphogranuloma venereum, actinomycosis, rectal duplication, foreign body and malignancy
- **Types: High** or **Low** (according to whether **internal opening** is **below** or **above** the **anorectal ring**^{Q})

Clinical Presentation

- Non-specific anal fistulae are **more common in men** than women.
- Most commonly affect patients in **3rd-5th decade**
- Patients usually complain of **intermittent purulent discharge & pain**^{Q} (which increases until temporary relief occurs when the pus discharges).
- There is a **previous episode of acute anorectal sepsis** that settled (**incompletely**) spontaneously or with antibiotics, or which was surgically drained.

> - **Passage of flatus or feces through** the **external opening** is suggestive of a **rectal** rather than an anal **internal opening**^{Q}.

Parks Classification of Fistula-in-ano (ITS-E)	
Intersphincteric fistulae (45%): MC^Q	Runs in interspinteric space
Trans-sphincteric fistulae (30%)	Extends through both internal and external sphincters
Suprasphincteric fistulae (20%)	Originates in the Intersphincteric plane and tracks up and around the entire external sphincter
Extrasphincteric fistulae (5%)	Originates in the rectal wall and tracks lateral to both sphincters

Clinical Assessment

- A full **medical history** & **proctosigmoidoscopy** are **necessary** to gain information about **sphincter strength** and to **exclude associated conditions**.

Key Points to Determine	
• Site of the internal opening^Q • Site of the external opening^Q • Course of the primary track^Q	• Presence of secondary extensions^Q • Presence of other conditions complicating the fistula^Q

- Full examination under anesthesia should be repeated before surgical intervention.
- Dilute hydrogen peroxide, instilled via the external opening, is a very useful way of demonstrating the site of the internal opening

> - MRI is the 'gold standard' for fistula imaging^Q
> - Usually reserved for difficult recurrent cases^Q
> - Advantage of MRI: Its ability to demonstrate secondary extensions, which may be missed at surgery and which are the cause of persistence^Q.

- Fistulography and CT: Useful techniques if an extrasphincteric fistula is suspected.

Treatment
- Treatment options: Fistulotomy, fistulectomy, setons, advancement flaps and glues, VAAFT
- Laying open is the surest method of eradication, but sphincter division may result in incontinence^Q

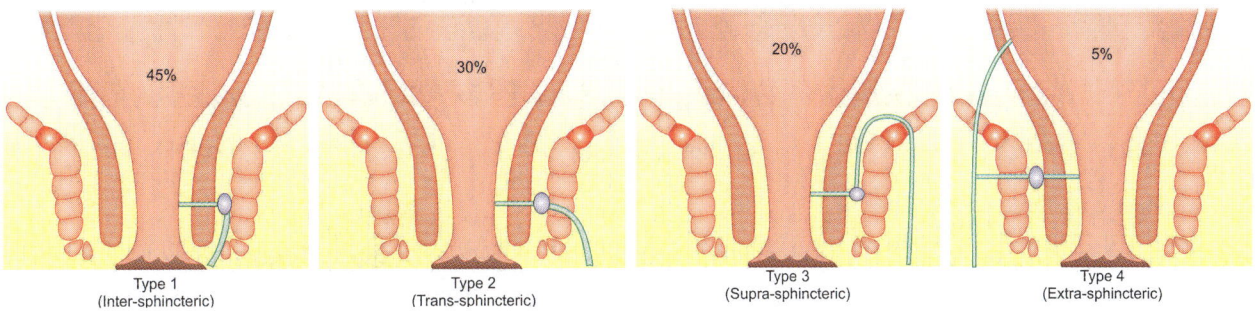

Type 1 (Inter-sphincteric) 45% • Type 2 (Trans-sphincteric) 30% • Type 3 (Supra-sphincteric) 20% • Type 4 (Extra-sphincteric) 5%

Goodsall's rule

- Used to indicate the likely position of the internal opening according to the position of the external opening(s)

> **According to Goodsall's rule**
> - Fistulas with external openings anterior to horizontal imaginary line drawn across the mid-point of anus connect to the internal opening by short straight track^Q.
> - Fistulas with external openings posterior to horizontal line run a curvilinear course and open internally into posterior midline^Q (at 6 o'clock position^Q).

- **Exceptions** of Goodsall's rule:
  - If an anterior external opening is > 3 cm from the anal margin. Such fistula track to the posterior midline.
  - When there is an anterior and also a posterior opening of the same fistula, the rule of posterior opening applies.

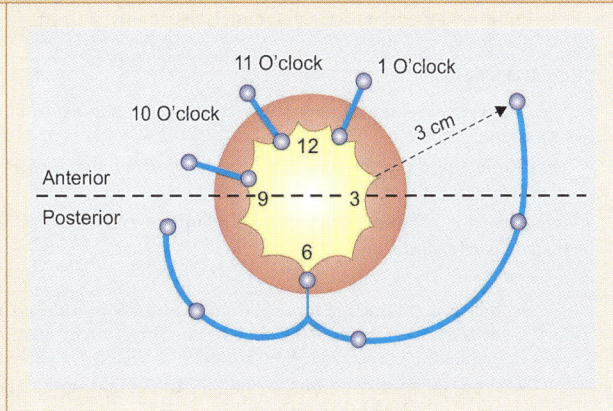

ANAL FISSURE (FISSURE-IN-ANO)

ANAL FISSURE (FISSURE-IN-ANO)

- An anal fissure is a longitudinal split in the anoderm, extending from anal verge to dentate line^Q.
- MC site: Mid-line posteriorly^Q (6'O Clock Position)^Q
- MC symptom: Pain^Q

Etiology
- **Trauma caused by** the **strained evacuation** of a **hard stool** or from the **repeated** passage of **diarrhea**[Q].
- **Anterior anal fissure:** More common in women, arise **following vaginal delivery**.

Clinical Features
- **Acute fissure:** Characterized by **severe anal pain** associated **with defecation** with passage of fresh blood, normally noticed on the tissue after wiping.

> - **Chronic fissures:** Characterized by a **hypertrophied anal papilla + Sentinel tag + Deep canoe shaped ulcer**[Q]

- Mostly seen in **young adults**, **men** & **women are affected equally**[Q].

Treatment
- **Conservative initially**, consisting of **sitz bath** (in a basin containing **warm antiseptic lotion**), **stool-bulking agents** & **softeners**, **nitrates** and **calcium channel blockers** to relax the **anal sphincter** and **improve blood flow**[Q]
- **Surgery** if above fails, consisting of **lateral internal sphincterotomy** or **anal advancement flap**[Q]

Treatment of Anal Fissure
• **Chemical sphincterotomy: Nitroglycerine (0.2%**[Q]**)** or **diltiazem (2%**[Q]**)** for relaxation of anal sphincter
• **Lord's procedure: Dilatation** of **sphincter** under GA, not practiced due to **high rate of incontinence**[Q]
• **Notara's lateral sphincterotomy: Surgical procedure of choice** for anal fissure[Q]
• **Anal advancement flap:** An **inverted house-shaped flap** of **perianal skin** is carefully mobilized on its blood supply and **advanced without tension to cover** the **fissure**, and then sutured with interrupted absorbable sutures.

PILONIDAL SINUS

PILONIDAL SINUS

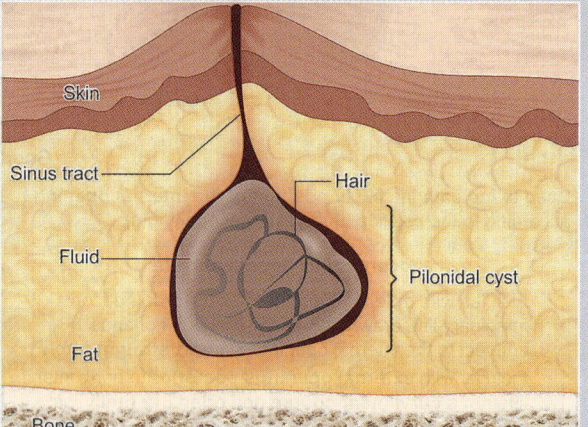

- **Acquired** disease, seen in **hairy males**[Q]
- **Seen in** age group of **20–29 years**
- **Found in** the **natal cleft overlying** the **coccyx**[Q]

> - Consisting of **noninfected, midline openings communicating with** a **fibrous track** lined by granulation tissue and containing hair lying loosely within the lumen.
> - **Common** among **military personnel**, also known as **'jeep disease'**[Q].

Etiopathogenesis
- **Hair follicles** have almost **never been demonstrated** in the walls of the sinus.
- **Hair Projecting** from the sinus **are dead hair**, with their pointed ends directed towards the blind end of the sinus.
- **Recurrence** is **common, even though adequate excision** of the **track is carried out**[Q].

> - It is thought that the **combination of buttock friction** & **shearing forces** in that area **allows shed hair** or **broken hairs to drill through** the **midline skin**, or that **infection in relation** to a **hair follicle** allows **hair to enter the skin** by the **suction** created by movement of the buttocks, so creating a **subcutaneous, chronically infected, midline track**[Q].
> - From this primary sinus, **secondary tracks may spread laterally**, which may emerge at the skin as **granulation tissue-lined, discharging openings**[Q].

Clinical Features
- Characteristically seen in **dark-haired individuals** rather than those with softer blond hair
- Patients complain of **intermittent pain, swelling** & **discharge** at the base of the spine
- History of repeated abscesses that have **burst spontaneously** or which have been incised, **usually away from** the **midline**[Q].

> - **Primary sinus** may have **one or many openings**, all of which are **strictly in** the **midline between** the level of **sacrococcygeal joint** and **tip of coccyx**[Q].
> - **Interdigital pilonidal sinus** is an **occupational disease of hairdressers**[Q]
> - Also seen in **axilla** & **umbilicus**[Q]

Treatment
- **Conservative treatment:** For minor symptoms, **simple cleaning out** of tracks & **removal of all hair**, with **regular shaving** of the area and **strict hygiene**, may be recommended[Q].
- Treatment of an **acute exacerbation (abscess):** Abscess drainage with **thorough curettage** of **granulation tissue** and **hair**[Q].

Surgical Treatment of Chronic Pilonidal Disease
- **Laying open of all tracks** with or without **marsupialisation**[Q]
- **Excision of all tracks** with or without primary closure[Q]
- **Excision of all tracks** & **closure by Limberg's flap**[Q], Karydakis flap or rhomboid flap[Q]
- **Bascom's procedure**[Q]: Incision lateral to the midline to gain access to the sinus cavity, which is rid of hair & granulation tissue and excision & closure of the midline pits. The lateral wound is left open.

SOLITARY RECTAL ULCER SYNDROME

Solitary Rectal Ulcer Syndrome
- SRUS is located on **anterior** or **anterolateral**[Q] rectal wall, **7–10 cm** from **anal verge**[Q]
- May involve bowel anywhere from sigmoid to anorectal junction
- **More common** in **women**, age **20-40 years**
- **Multiple ulcers** may be present within a single patch of diseased mucosa in **10–15%** cases
- Endoscopically, **only half** of the patients with SRUS **have an actual ulcer**. The **remaining** patients have an area of **mucosal erythema, mucosal nodules** or **frank polyps**, which may or may not have surface ulcerations.

Etiology
- Internal intussusception[Q]
- Anterior rectal wall prolapse[Q]
- Increased intrarectal pressure[Q]

Histopathology
- **Mucosal hyperplasia, crypt distortion** or **elongation**[Q]
- **Hypocellular lamina propria**[Q]
- **Subepithelial fibrosis, thickened muscularis mucosa**[Q]
- **Tongues** of muscle extending to the mucosa[Q]

Clinical Features
- Patients are **typically young** and **female**, with an **average age of 25 years** and a **history of straining** and **difficult evacuation**[Q].
- Commonly presents with **rectal bleeding** in the **setting of straining** or **constipation, pain, mucus discharge**[Q].

Diagnosis
- **Defecography:** Radiologic procedure of choice and usually **reveals the underlying disorder**[Q].
- **Full-thickness rectal prolapse, internal prolapse, paradoxical Puborectalis syndrome** (failure of relaxation of the pelvic floor musculature on straining) and **thickened rectal folds are common findings**[Q].

Treatment
- **Non-operative therapy** (high fiber diet, defecation training to avoid straining, laxatives or enema) is **effective in majority of the patients**[Q].
- **Surgery** (either **abdominal** or **perineal repair of prolapse**) is reserved for highly symptomatic patients, who have **failed all medical intervention**[Q].
- **Rectopexy** corrects **anterior rectal wall prolapse**[Q].

CARCINOMA RECTUM

Carcinoma Rectum
- MC site of colorectal cancer: Rectum[Q]
- MC type: Adenocarcinoma[Q]
- Multiple in 5% cases[Q]
- Usually **present as an ulcer**, but polypoid and infiltrating types are also common.

> - **MC site of metastasis: Liver**[Q] (34%) >Lungs (22%) >Adrenals (11%)
> - With **improved response rates** to **modern chemotherapy** and advances in hepatic surgery, however, **more patients are now candidates for hepatectomy**[Q] than in the past.
> - **Dose of radiotherpay** given in CA rectum: **60 Gray**[Q]

Clinical Features
- Age of presentation in CA rectum: Above 55 years
- **Bleeding** is the **earliest** and **MC symptom**[Q].
- Sense of incomplete defecation[Q]

Sense of Incomplete Defecation
- Sensation that there are more feces to be passed (**tenesmus**, a distressing **straining to empty** the **bowels without resultant evacuation**[Q]).
- This is a very important **early symptom** and is almost invariably present in tumours of the **lower half of the rectum**[Q].
- The patient may endeavor to **empty the rectum several times a day** (**spurious diarrhea**), often with the **passage of flatus** and **a little blood-stained mucus** ('bloody slime')[Q].

- **Alteration in bowel habit:** Patient has to **get up early in order to defecate**[Q], or one who **passes blood & mucus** in addition to feces (**'early-morning bloody diarrhea'**[Q]).
- Patient with an **annular carcinoma** at the rectosigmoid junction suffers with **increasing constipation**, and the one with a **growth in the ampulla** of the rectum who has **early-morning diarrhea**[Q].

> - **Pain in the back**, or **sciatica**, occurs when the **cancer invades the sacral plexus**[Q].
> - **Weight loss** is suggestive of **hepatic metastases**[Q].

Diagnosis

- **Sigmoidoscopy** (**rigid,** not flexible) and **Biopsy:** Investigation of choice for **diagnosis of CA rectum**[Q]
- **TRUS** (Transrectal ultrasound): Best for **'T' staging**[Q]
- **Endorectal coil MRI:** Best for predicting **LN invasion** and **overall staging**[Q]
- **CECT:** Evaluation of **metastasis**

Treatment of Carcinoma Rectum	
Stage 0 (Tis, N0, M0)	- **Local excision**[Q]
Stage I: Localized Rectal Carcinoma (T1–2, N0, M0)	- **Polypectomy** with clear margins[Q] - **Radical resection** in good-risk patients with **unfavorable histologic characteristics** and located in the **distal third** of the rectum[Q]
Stage II: Localized Rectal Carcinoma (T3–4, N0, M0)	- **Preoperative chemoradiation + radical resection**[Q]
Stage III: Lymph Node Metastasis (Tany, N1, M0)	- **Preoperative chemoradiation + radical resection**[Q]
Stage IV: Distant Metastasis (Tany, Nany, M1)	- **Palliative procedures**[Q] - Resection to control pain, bleeding, or tenesmus

Treatment Options for Carcinoma Rectum	
Low Anterior Resection	- **Sphincter saving operation**[Q] - Performed for the **cancers** of **proximal third** to **two third** of the **rectum** (Located **> 5 cm above**[Q] the **anal verge**) - Descending colon is anastomosed with the distal rectum
Abdominoperineal Resection (APR or Miles Procedure)	- **Complete excision** of **rectum** and **anus**, by concomitant dissection through the abdomen and perineum with **creation of permanent colostomy**[Q] - Performed for carcinoma of **lower rectum** (at or **below 5 cm** from **anal verge**)
Hartmann's Procedure	- When there is **too much destruction** or **sepsis** to allow a safe anastomosis[Q] - For **elderly** or **severely unstable patients**[Q] who would not stand a lengthy anterior resection or APR procedure

CARCINOMA ANAL CANAL

Carcinoma Anal Canal

- **MC type** of CA anal canal: **SCC >BCC >Melanoma**[Q]
- **Median age** at diagnosis: **60 years**[Q]

> - **MC symptom: Bleeding PR**[Q]
> - **MC site of metastasis: Lung**[Q]
> - **MC site of LN metastasis: Inguinal LNs**[Q]

Risk Factors for Carcinoma Anal Canal	
- **HPV infection (16, 18, 31, 33)**[Q] - **HIV** or **immunosuppression**[Q] - **Smoking**[Q] - **Anal receptive intercourse**[Q]	- **Sexual promiscuity**[Q] - **Chronic inflammation**[Q] - **Anal intra-epithelial neoplasia**[Q] - History of **vulvar** or **cervical cancer**[Q]

Clinical Features

- **Most patients** present with **rectal bleeding & pain**[Q].
- Patients are **frequently misdiagnosed** as having a benign anorectal condition such as **hemorrhoids**[Q].

> - Additional symptoms: **Incontinence, change in bowel habits, pelvic pain,** and **rectovaginal** or **rectovesical fistulas** are **ominous**[Q] suggest **advanced malignancy** with **infiltration into the sphincters** or **penetration into the rectal wall**[Q].

Diagnosis
- **Proctoscopy** with **biopsy: Investigation of choice** for diagnosis of **CA anal canal**[Q].
- **CT abdomen & pelvis: Mandatory** because **all of the draining lymph nodes** are **not palpable**[Q].
- **CT scan:** Evaluate distant metastasis

Treatment
- **Nigro regimen: Chemoradiation** is the **treatment of choice**[Q].
- More than **80%** are **cured by chemoradiation**. If any **residual tumor** is **left** behind after chemoradiation, **APR** is performed[Q].

> - **Chemotherapy regimen: 5-FU + Mitomycin C/Cisplatin**[Q]
> - First **chemotherapy** is given **followed by radiotherapy**[Q].

Prognosis
- Overall **5-year survival: 66%**

8th AJCC (2017) TNM Classification of Carcinoma of the Anal Canal & Anal Margin

Tis: Carcinoma in situ (Bowen disease, high-grade squamous intraepithelial lesions (HSIL), anal intraepithelial neoplasia II-III (AIN II-III)	**N1a:** Metastases to **inguinal, mesorectal, and/or internal iliac LNs**[Q]
T1: Tumor ≤2 cm in greatest dimension[Q]	**N1b:** Metastases to **external iliac LNs**[Q]
T2: >2 cm but <5 cm in greatest dimension[Q]	**N1c:** Metastases to **external iliac and in inguinal, mesorectal, and/or internal iliac LNs**[Q]
T3: >5 cm in greatest dimension[Q]	**M1:** Distant metastasis
T4: Invading adjacent structures: **vagina, urethra, or bladder**[Q] (involvement of the sphincter muscle alone, rectal wall, or perirectal subcutaneous tissue or skin is not classified as T4)	

Stage Grouping

0	I	IIA	IIB	IIIA	IIIB	IIIC	IV
Tis N0M0	T1 N0M0	T2 N0M0	T3 N0M0	T1-2 N1 M0	T4 N0M0	T3-4 N1M0	Any T Any N M1

PAGET'S DISEASE OF ANAL CANAL

Paget's Disease of Anal Canal
- **MC site of extra-mammary Paget's disease: Anogenital region** >Axilla >eyelid
- **MC site in females: Vulva**[Q]
- More common in females, median age of **65 years**.
- It can be associated with the **presence of rectal adenocarcinoma**[Q]

> - **Perianal Paget's** is associated with an **underlying visceral malignancy** in **20–86%** of cases[Q].
> - MC synchronous tumor: Colorectal adenocarcinoma[Q]

Pathology
- Found in both the **anal canal** and **margin**.

> - **Perianal Paget's cells** are **foamy** and **vacuolar in appearance**[Q]
> - **Positive for PAS, mucicarmine, Alcian blue,** and **cytokeratin 7**[Q].

Clinical Features
- Occurs in **apocrine, hair-bearing areas**[Q].
- **Erythematous, pruritic, scaling plaques** with **well-defined serpiginous borders** are a **typical feature** of the disease[Q].
- Lesions may also **appear ulcerated** and **crusty with a serous discharge**.

Diagnosis
- **Diagnosis** is made **on biopsy**[Q].

Treatment
- **Wide local excision** is **treatment of choice**[Q].
- **Recurrence rates** as high as **61%** have been reported **following excision** of perianal Paget's disease[Q].
- **Re-excision** is the **usual recommendation**[Q]

ANAL CANAL MELANOMA

ANAL CANAL MELANOMA

- MC site of melanoma: **Skin >Eye >Anorectum**[Q]
- **More common** in **females**[Q]
- The tumor can appear **small** and **polypoid**, or **large and ulcerating**.

Clinical Features
- Most common symptoms include **bleeding, itching**, the presence of a **mass, pain, tenesmus**, or **changes in bowel habits**[Q].
- Like anal squamous cell carcinoma, **misidentification of the tumor as a hemorrhoid**[Q] is a common mistake.
- **Mesorectal lymph node metastases** are found in **40–60%** of patients at initial presentation and **inguinal adenopathy** is present in at **least 20%**.
- **Distant spread** occurs to the **bone, lung**, and **liver**.

Diagnosis
- Diagnosis is frequently made **following hemorrhoidectomy** or **local excision** of the perianal mass.
- Like melanoma of the skin, **anorectal melanoma** is **staged by depth** or **thickness** of the lesion.

Treatment
- **Wide local excision** has **replaced APR** for the **treatment of anal melanoma**[Q].
- **Wide local excision with negative margins** for those patients **without anal sphincter involvement**[Q].
- **Palliative APR**: Large tumor **invading sphincter**s[Q]

Prognosis
- Regardless of stage, 5-year survival rates for anorectal melanoma is **very poor**, averaging about **6%**.
- The **median survival time** following diagnosis is **12–18 months**[Q].

MANAGEMENT OF PATIENTS WITH ANORECTAL MALFORMATIONS

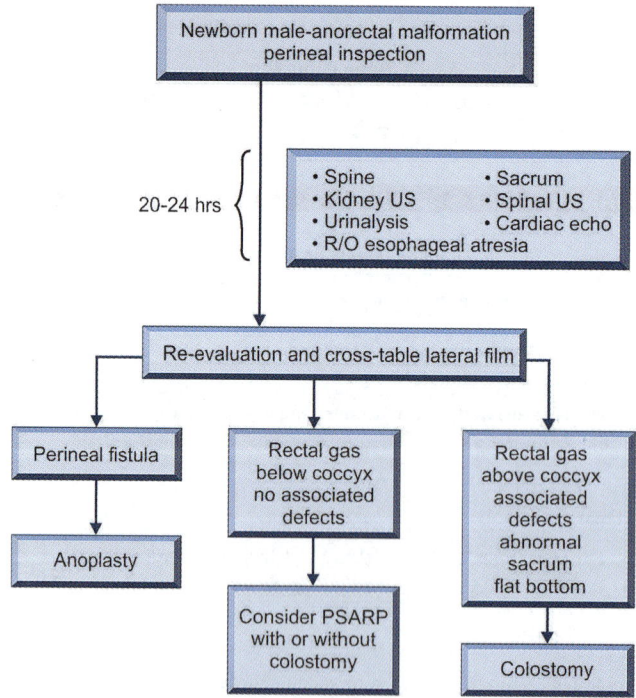

MANAGEMENT OF PATIENTS WITH ANORECTAL MALFORMATIONS

- The principles of management centre around **diagnosing** the **type of defect** present, **Low** or **High**, depending on the **site of termination of rectum** in **relation to pelvic floor**[Q].
- Wangensteen-Rice (**Invertogram**) is performed **6–12 hours after birth**[Q].

High Lesions	Low Lesions
• **Rectum ends above** the level of the **level-ani complex**[Q]	• **Rectum ends below** the level of **levator ani complex**[Q]

Clinical Clues Suggesting Low Lesion	Clinical Clues Suggesting High Lesion

• **Bucket Handle**[Q]:
  – Presence of a **prominent midline skin tag stem tap,** below which one can pass an instrument.
	• **Flat bottom**[Q]:
	  – This usually reflects **poor muscle structures** and is always associated with **very high defects**.

• **Midline Raphe Fistula:**
  – A subepethelial meconial fistula which looks like a black ribbon, placed in the midline in the perineum.
	• **Meconuria (Meconium in urine**[Q]**):**
	  – The presence of meconium in urine means that some form of **communication exists** between the **urinary tract** and **rectum**.
	  – It suggests a **high lesion**.

• **Perineal Fistula (meconial)**[Q]**:** – The presence of meconium coming out through a small orifice located usually anteriorly to the centre of anal dimple	
• **Anal Stenosis:** – Very narrow anal canal	
• **Anal membrane:** – Very thin epithelial membrane through which one can see meconium	

Management

- **High lesions:** Patients with **high lesions** are **difficult to manage** and **require** an **initial protective colostomy. Posterior Saggital Anorectoplasty (PSARP)** is performed **after 4-8 weeks**.
- **Low lesions:** Can be **treated** with a **perennial anoplasty** (without the need of a protective colostomy).

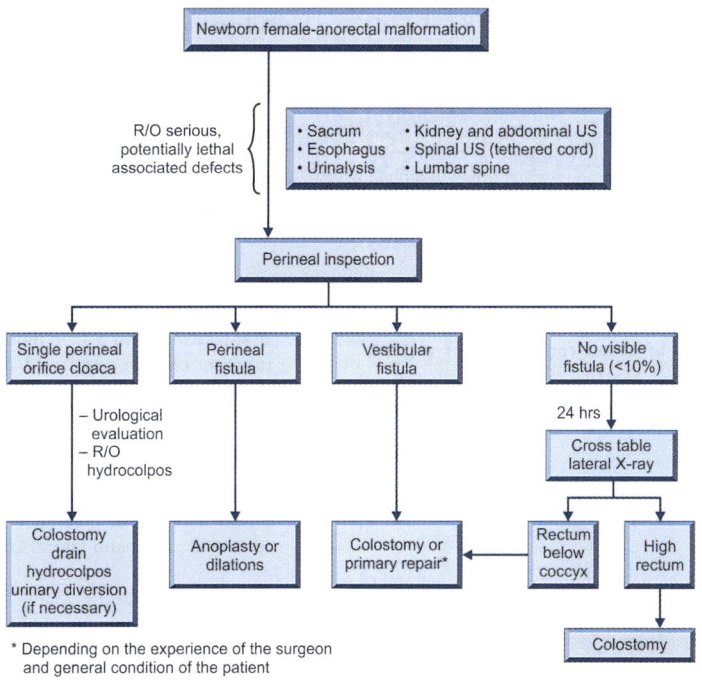

Multiple Choice Questions

VILLOUS ADENOMA

1. **Villous polyp of rectum manifest:** *(Recent Question 2016)*
   a. Bleeding PR
   b. Mucus diarrhea with hypokalemia
   c. Prolapse rectum
   d. Obstruction

2. **In villous papillomas of the rectum which is lost:** *(DNB 2007, 2003)*
   a. Na$^+$
   b. Mg^{2+}
   c. K$^+$
   d. All

3. **The best surgical management for villous adenoma of the rectum is:** *(Recent Question 2016)*
   a. Local resection of lesion
   b. Repeated sigmoidoscopy
   c. Abdomino perineal resection
   d. Electrolyte infusion and chemotherapy

4. **Rectal adenoma is associated with:** *(JIPMER 2003)*
   a. Familial polyposis coli
   b. Hypokalemia
   c. Intussusception
   d. Hemorrhoids

5. **Regarding villous adenoma all are true *except*:** *(WBPG 2014)*
   a. Dysentery
   b. Watery diarrhea
   c. Hypokalemia
   d. Constipation

RECTAL POLYP

6. **Rectal polyps usually present with:** *(SGPGI 2005, UPPG 97)*
   a. Obstruction
   b. Perforation
   c. Bleeding
   d. Malignant change

7. **A toddler has few drops of blood coming out of rectum. Probable diagnosis is:** *(AIIMS May 2013, AIIMS May 2012)*
   a. Juvenile rectal polyp
   b. Adenomatous polyposis coli
   c. Rectal ulcer
   d. Piles

8. **Most common cause of fresh bleeding per rectum in a 5-years old child is:** *(WBPG 2012, AIIMS June 93)*
   a. Volvulus
   b. Trauma
   c. Worm infestation
   d. Rectal polyp

CARCINOMA RECTUM

9. **All are true about TME for CA rectum except:**
   a. Decreases local recurrence *(AIIMS GIS Dec 2009)*
   b. Decreases incidence of impotence
   c. Decreases incidence of bladder dysfunction
   d. Decreases survival

10. **Local excision in CA rectum is done in all except:**
    a. Within 6 cm of anal verge *(AIIMS GIS Dec 2009)*
    b. Lesion < 4 cm
    c. Involvement of < 40% circumference
    d. T1 and T2 cancer with or without lymph node involvement

11. **In CA rectum, preoperatively:** *(AIIMS GIS Dec 2009)*
    a. Only RT is given
    b. Only chemotherapy is given
    c. Chemoradiation is given
    d. Chemoradiation is given postoperatively only

12. **In rectal carcinoma, distal margin should be at least:**
    a. 2 cm
    b. 3 cm *(PGI SS June 2001)*
    c. 4 cm
    d. 5 cm

13. **True about surgical treatment of rectal cancer:**
    a. Irrigation of divided bowel ends with cytotoxic solution may reduce local true recurrence *(PGI SS Dec 2009)*
    b. Intramural spread is commonly > 4 cm
    c. Minimum of 5 cm distal resection margin is required
    d. Mesorectum is devoid of lymph nodes

14. **Dukes A stage of rectal carcinoma is managed by:**
    a. Surgical resection only *(DNB 2008)*
    b. Surgical resection + selective adjuvant chemotherapy
    c. Surgical resection + routine adjuvant chemotherapy
    d. Chemotherapy primarily

15. **All are true about rectal cancer except:** *(JIPMER GIS 2011)*
    a. Most common symptom is hematochezia
    b. Precise location of tumor is done with rigid proctosigmoidoscopy
    c. Dissection lateral to endopelvic fascia investing the mesorectum causes local recurrence
    d. Radiation dose is 60 Gray

16. **False about indications of local resection in CA rectum:**
    a. T2N0, T1N1 *(AIIMS GIS 2003)*
    b. < 10 cm from anal verge
    c. < 4 cm or < 40% of circumference involved
    d. Well differentiated with no LN involvement

17. **Best treatment for a 4 cm moderate grade rectal cancer at the junction of lower and mid one thirds, with less than one third circumference of the rectum being involved?**
    a. Radiotherapy *(MHSSMCET 2008, 2006)*
    b. Anterior resection
    c. Transanal resection
    d. Abdomino-perineal resection

18. **Distal margins of clearance required for treatment of CA rectum is .... and lateral and proximal margins ....** *(MHSSMCET 2010)*
    a. 2 cm and 5 cm
    b. 3 cm and 5 cm
    c. 5 cm and 2 cm
    d. 5 cm and 3 cm

19. **A patient with carcinoma of rectum which is 5 cm form anal verge, which procedure you will prefer to perform:**
    a. Anterior resection *(MHSSMCET 2005)*
    b. Abdominoperineal resection
    c. Hartman's procedure
    d. Defunctioning colostomy

20. **Which of the following is the investigation of choice for assessment of depth of penetration and perirectal nodes in rectal cancer?** *(AIIMS Nov 2004)*
    a. Transrectal ultrasound
    b. CT scan pelvis
    c. MRI Scan
    d. Double contrast barium enema

21. Vimal, a 70-years old male presents with a history of lower GI bleed for last 6 months. Sigmoido-scopic examination shows a mass, of 4 cm about 3.5 cm above the anal verge. The treatment of choice is: (AIIMS June 2001)
    a. Colostomy
    b. Anterior resection
    c. Abdominoperineal resection
    d. Defunctioning anastomosis

22. A patient comes with rectal carcinoma situated 6 cm above dentate line with no nodal metastasis. Treatment of choice will be: (AIIMS Nov 97)
    a. Anterior resection   b. APR
    c. Radiotherapy   d. Hartman's procedure

23. For a rectal carcinoma at 5 cm from the anal verge, the best acceptable operation is: (All India 2004)
    a. Anterior resection
    b. Abdominoperineal resection
    c. Posterior resection
    d. APR done in lesion of upper zone

24. Commonest presentation of CA rectum is:
    a. Diarrhea   (JIMPER 2012, DPG 95)
    b. Constipation
    c. Bleeding P/R
    d. Feeling of incomplete defecation

25. Sphincter saving surgery for rectal malignancy is not done in: (PGI Dec 2001)
    a. Age over 50 years
    b. Lymph node involvement
    c. Infiltration of lamina propria
    d. More than 4 cm from anal verge
    e. High grade tumor

26. In which case anterior resection is the method of treatment? (AIIMS Feb 97)
    a. CA sigmoid colon   b. CA rectum
    c. CA colon   d. CA anal canal

27. Prognosis for carcinoma rectum is best assessed by:
    a. Site of tumour   (AIIMS 87, Karnataka 89)
    b. Histological grading
    c. Size of tumors
    d. Duration of the symptoms

28. Best procedure in mid rectal carcinoma is: (AIIMS 92)
    a. Abdomino perineal resection
    b. Anterior resection
    c. Perineal loop
    d. Transverse colostomy

29. Treatment of carcinoma rectum 5 cm from anal verge without nodal metastasis is: (Kerala 94)
    a. Abdominoperineal resection
    b. Radiotherapy
    c. Endoscopic resection
    d. Chemotherapy

30. Which of the following is more aggressive rectal carcinoma?
    a. Adenocarcinoma   (MAHE 2006)
    b. Secondary mucoid carcinoma
    c. Signet ring carcinoma
    d. Squamous cell carcinoma

31. A punch biopsy shows carcinoma rectum with fixed mass and X-ray chest normal. Which of the following is least useful investigation? (UPPG 2008)
    a. Rigid proctoscope   b. Barium enema
    c. CT chest   d. MRI-abdomen and pelvis

32. Ideal management in an old and frail patient presenting with a mass situated 15 cm away from anal orifice:
    a. Abdomino-perineal resection (MCI March 2005)
    b. Colonoscopic removal
    c. Hartman's operation
    d. Anterior resection

33. Aim of surgery in carcinoma rectum is: (MCI March 2010)
    a. Limited excision of the rectum
    b. Sacrificing gastrointestinal continuity
    c. Preserving the anal sphincter
    d. Preserving mesorectum

34. Anterior resection is contraindicated in the following:
    a. Age more than 60 years   (PGI 90)
    b. Undifferentiated carcinoma
    c. Melanin in liver
    d. Cancer is less than 5 cm from anorectal margin

35. Which one of the following statements is false regarding carcinoma rectum? (APPG 2015)
    a. Hartmann's operation is done in old debilitated patients
    b. Per rectal examination can diagnose only 10% of cases
    c. Early morning spurious diarrhea and tenesmus can occur
    d. Growth confined to rectal wall is stage A of Modified Duke staging

HEMORRHOIDS

36. Not true about hemorrhoids: (AIIMS GIS May 2008)
    a. First degree- no prolapse
    b. Excision for externo-internal piles
    c. Third degree- no surgery
    d. Conservative treatment in first degree

37. Hemorrhoids managed by manual reduction: (AIIMS GIS May 2011)
    a. I degree   b. II degree
    c. III degree   d. IV degree

38. Which of the following is not true about hemorrhoids?
    a. Pruritus is not common   (PGI SS June 2007)
    b. Can be palpated on DRE in absence of complications
    c. Band ligation is most commonly done office procedure
    d. Stapled hemorrhoidectomy causes less postoperative pain

39. True about treatment of hemorrhoids: (PGI Nov 2010)
    a. Band ligation
    b. 5% phenol in almond oil is used as sclerosant
    c. May be resolved by diet modification
    d. Hemorrhoidectomy is TOC

40. External hemorrhoids below the dentate line are:
    a. Painful (AIIMS May 2012, All India 2007, AIIMS Nov 2006)
    b. Ligation is done as management
    c. Skin tag is not seen in these cases
    d. May turn malignant

41. Injection sclerotherapy is ideal for the following: (All India 2004)
    a. External hemorrhoids   b. Internal hemorrhoids
    c. Posterior resection   d. Local resection

42. Commonest complication following haemorrhoidectomy is: (MHSSCET 2005, AIIMS 92)
    a. Hemorrhage   b. Infection
    c. Fecal impaction   d. Urinary retention

43. Treatment of choice in 2nd degree piles is: (AIIMS 92)
    a. Cryosurgery   b. Sclerotherapy
    c. Banding   d. Surgery

44. Treatment of primary piles is: *(Kerala 94)*
    a. Surgery b. Sclerotherapy
    c. No treatment d. Analgesics
45. Best investigation to diagnose piles is: *(Kerala 94)*
    a. Proctosigmoidoscopy b. Barium enema
    c. Ultrasound d. Proctoscopy
46. Five-day self subsiding pain is diagnostic of: *(APPG 97)*
    a. Anal fissure
    b. Fistula-in-ano
    c. Thrombosed external hemorrhoids
    d. Thrombosed internal hemorrhoids
47. The following are true of hemorrhoids except:
    a. They are arteriolar dilatations *(JIPMER 2001)*
    b. They are common causes of painless bleeding
    c. They cannot be per rectally palpated
    d. They can be banded
48. All of the following are true in management of hemorrhoids except: *(DPG 2009 March)*
    a. Excisional surgery is cornerstone
    b. Fiber supplementation is effective
    c. Improvement in bowel function is helpful
    d. Ligation with rubber bands effective
49. Most important disadvantage of cryosurgery for hemorrhoid is: *(DPG 2005)*
    a. Pain b. Infection
    c. Profuse watery discharge d. Hemorrhage
50. Which of the following is true about hemorrhoids? *(DNB 2008)*
    a. More common with portal hypertension
    b. External hemorrhoids are proximal to dentate line
    c. Internal hemorrhoids bleed profusely and painless
    d. Internal hemorrhoids are covered by anoderm
51. A patient with external hemorrhoids develops pain while passing stools. The nerve mediating this pain is: *(Recent Question 2015)*
    a. Hypogastric nerve b. Sympathetic plexus
    c. Splanchnic visceral nerve d. Pudendal nerve
52. What is the grade of hemorrhoid based on the image given below?
    a. Grade I b. Grade II
    c. Grade III d. Grade IV

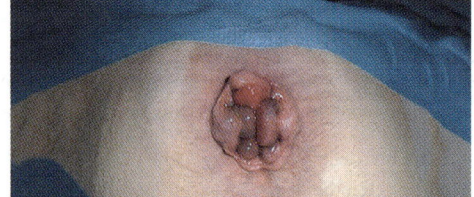

53. Indications of hemorrhoidectomy include: *(PGI May 2018)*
    a. Large first & second degree hemorrhoids
    b. Third & fourth degree hemorrhoids
    c. If not able to differentiate prolapsed hemorrhoids & lower rectal prolapse
    d. Complicated by strangulations
    e. Failure of conservative therapy

SOLITARY RECTAL ULCER SYNDROME

54. All are true regarding solitary rectal ulcer syndrome except:
    a. Usually in anterior wall *(DNB 2002)*
    b. Associated with rectal prolapse
    c. Usually malignant d. Bowel training helps alot
55. Colitis cystica profunda is seen in case of: *(AIIMS GIS Dec 2009)*
    a. SRUS b. Rectal carcinoma
    c. Rectocele d. Fissure
56. Most common site of SRUS: *(GB Pant 2011)*
    a. Posterior, 7–10 cm from anal verge
    b. Anterior, 7–10 cm from anal verge
    c. Posterior, 2–3 cm from anal verge
    d. Anterior, 2–3 cm from anal verge
57. True about solitary rectal ulcer syndrome is all/except:
    a. Increased muscle layer proliferation *(AIIMS May 2007)*
    b. Crypt distortion
    c. Lamina propria infiltration with lymphocyte
    d. Subepithelial fibrosis
58. Not true regarding solitary rectal ulcer: *(AIIMS Nov 97)*
    a. 20% are multiple
    b. Recurrent rectal prolapsed is a cause
    c. Involves posterior wall
    d. Managed by digital reposition
59. Treatment of solitary rectal ulcer are all except:
    a. Laxatives b. Rectopexy *(PGI Dec 2007)*
    c. Banding d. Sclerosant injection
    e. Enema

RECTAL PROLAPSE

60. A 40-years old male presented with reducible rectal prolapse with history of constipation from the last 10 years, redundant sigmoid with fecal matter, best form of management for this patient: *(ILBS 2011)*
    a. Delorme procedure b. Anterior resection
    c. Rectopexy d. Mesh fixation
61. Rectal prolapse is common in: *(WBPG 2014)*
    a. 1–3 months b. 3–5 months
    c. 5–8 months d. 8–12 months
62. Treatment of rectal prolapse in childhood is:
    a. Lahaut's operation *(AIIMS June 94)*
    b. Incision of prolapsed mucosa
    c. Thiersch wiring d. Ripstein operation
63. Recurrent prolapse of the rectum in children is treated by: *(Recent Question 2015)*
    a. Thiersch wiring b. Digital reposition
    c. Excision d. Ripstein's operation
64. Delorme's procedure is used for: *(WBPG 2012, MHPGMCET 2007, SGPGI 2004)*
    a. Rectal prolapse b. Solitary rectal ulcer
    c. Rectal bilharziasis d. Proctalgia fugax
65. A 30-years old male present with complete rectal prolapse. Which of the following procedure is associated with lowest risk of recurrence? *(All India 2012)*
    a. Delorme's procedure b. Thiersch procedure
    c. Abdominal rectopexy d. Altmeir's procedure
66. A young male patient presents with compete rectal prolapse. The surgery of choice is: *(All India 2010)*
    a. Abdominal rectopexy b. Delormes procedure
    c. Anterior resection d. Goodsall's procedure

Rectum and Anal Canal

67. In old age for rectal prolapse palliative surgery in a patient unfit for surgery is: *(Recent Question 2013)*
    a. Delorme's procedure
    b. Well's procedure
    c. Thiersch's operation
    d. Low anterior resection

68. Which of the following is a perineal procedure for rectal prolapse? *(Recent Question 2017)*
    a. Delorme
    b. Ripstein
    c. Resection rectopexy
    d. Frykman Goldberg procedure

69. A 60-year-old male presented to your OPD with this problem. What is the preferred treatment? *(Recent Question 2017)*
    a. Frykman-Goldberg procedure
    b. Well's procedure
    c. Delorme procedure
    d. Ripstein procedure

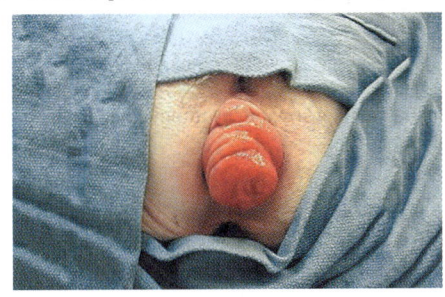

ANORECTAL ABSCESS

70. Commonest type of anorectal abscess is: *(DNB 2012)*
    a. Ischio rectal
    b. Submucous
    c. Pelvi-rectal
    d. Perianal

71. The increased incidence of infection in the ischiorectal fossa is due to: *(All India 89)*
    a. Absence of deep fascia
    b. Proximity to anus
    c. Poor blood supply
    d. Presence of fibrofatty tissue

72. Most common cause of anorectal abscess is:
    a. Inflammation of anal gland *(MAHE 2007, 2008)*
    b. Folliculitis
    c. Inflammation of rectal mucosa
    d. Rectum

FISTULA-IN-ANO

73. Most common anorectal fistula: *(AIIMS GIS Dec 2009)*
    a. Intersphincteric
    b. Transsphincteric
    c. Suprasphincteric
    d. Extrasphincteric

74. An AIDS patient presents with fistula in ano. His CD_4 count is below 50. Treatment of choice is: *(Punjab 2008, MAHE 2001)*
    a. Seton
    b. Fistulectomy
    c. Both
    d. Medical

75. Which type of malignancy is found in anorectal fistula?
    a. Squamous cell carcinoma *(PGI June 2005)*
    b. Transitional cell carcinoma
    c. Adenocarcinoma
    d. Columnar carcinoma

76. True statement regarding 'Fistula in ano' is:
    a. Posterior fistulae have straight tracks *(All India 2001)*
    b. High fistulae can be operated with no fear of incontinence
    c. High and low divisions are made in relation to the pelvic floor
    d. Intersphincteric is the most common type

77. The treatment of choice in fistula in ano: *(JIPMER 93)*
    a. Anal dilatation
    b. Fissurotomy
    c. Fistulectomy
    d. Fistulotomy

78. High or low fistula in ano is termed according to its internal opening present with reference to: *(UPSC 2008)*
    a. Anal canal
    b. Dentate line
    c. Anorectal ring
    d. Sacral promontory

79. Ideal investigation for fistula-in-ano is: *(Recent Question 2014, MCI March 2008)*
    a. Endoanal ultrasound
    b. MRI
    c. Fistulography
    d. CT scan

80. Seton used in fistula in ano surgery is draining seton and: *(Recent Question 2014, 2013)*
    a. Cutting seton
    b. Dissolving seton
    c. Dissecting seton
    d. Fibrosing seton

81. Name of this seton used for converting high lying fistula to low lying fistula:

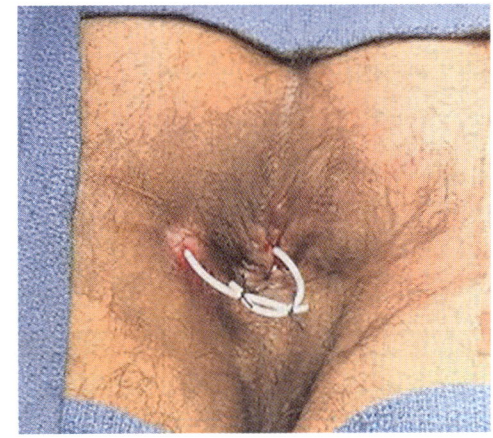

    a. Cutting seton
    b. Draining seton
    c. Marking seton
    d. Staging seton

ANAL FISSURE

82. Most common site of chronic fissure in ano: *(GB Pant 2011)*
    a. Anterior
    b. Posterior
    c. Lateral
    d. Anterolateral

83. Percentage of GTN used in fissure: *(GB Pant 2011)*
    a. 2%
    b. 0.2%
    c. 0.02%
    d. 20%

84. All are treatment of acute fissure in ano except:
    a. Conservative *(AIIMS Sept 96)*
    b. Dilatation under GA
    c. Lateral sphincterotomy
    d. External sphincterotomy

85. Sitz Bath consists of which of the following? *(Karnataka 96)*
    a. Patient bathed in normal saline
    b. Bathed in molten wax
    c. Sitz in a basin containing warm antiseptic lotion
    d. Sitz in a basin containing molten wax

86. Rectal examination should not be done in: *(JIPMER 90)*
    a. Anal fissure
    b. Fistula in ano
    c. Prolapsed piles with bleeding
    d. Anal stenosis

87. Internal sphincterotomy is the treatment of choice for:
 (Recent Question 2016)
    a. Piles
    b. Fistula
    c. Fissure-in-ano
    d. Carcinoma

88. Anal fissure best diagnosed by:
    a. Anoscopy *(Recent Question 2014, All India 2008)*
    b. History and superficial clinical examination
    c. PR examination
    d. USG

89. Lateral internal sphincterotomy is useful for:
 (Recebt Question 2014)
    a. Anal fistula
    b. Anal canal strictures
    c. Hemorrhoids
    d. Anal fissure

90. A sentinel pile indicatess: *(MHPGMCET 2008, 2007)*
    a. Internal hemorrhoids
    b. Pilonidal sinus
    c. Fissure-in-ano
    d. Fistula-in-ano

91. Most common site for anal fissure is:
 (Recent Question 2013)
    a. 3 o'clock
    b. 6 o'clock
    c. 2 o'clock
    d. 10 o'clock

92. Which of the following is not indicated in fissure-in-ano?
 (Recent Question 2017)
    a. Botox injection
    b. Topical steroids
    c. Topical calcium channel blockers
    d. Topical nitroglycerine

PILONIDAL SINUS

93. Which is not a feature of pilonidal sinus? *(PGI June 95)*
    a. Branching tracts are common
    b. Recurrence is uncommon
    c. Bony involvement is uncommon
    d. Seen in drivers

94. The following statement about pilonidal sinus is true:
    a. More common in females *(All India 2007)*
    b. Mostly congenital
    c. Prognosis after surgery is poor
    d. Treatment of choice is surgical excision of sinus tract

95. Jeep's disease is also known as:
 (Recent Question 2017 MCI March 2008)
    a. Anal incontinence
    b. Hemorrhoids
    c. Pilonidal sinus
    d. Anal fissure

96. All of the following are true regarding pilonidal sinus except: *(MCI Sept 2009)*
    a. Seen predominantly in women
    b. Occurs only in sacrococcygeal region
    c. Tendency for recurrence
    d. Obesity is a risk factor

97. All are true about pilonidal sinus except:
 (PGI November 2017)
    a. More common in young female
    b. It may occur due to combination of buttock friction and shearing forces in affect area
    c. Direction of the sinuses are cephaloid
    d. May lead to recurrent abscess formation
    e. Recurrence is common even after surgery

98. Position for the treatment of pilonidal sinus:
 (Recent Question 2015)
    a. Jack knife
    b. Sim's position
    c. Prone
    d. Supine

99. Which of the following flap based procedure is used for pilonidal sinus surgery? **(AIIMS November 2018)**
    a. Rhomboid flap
    b. Rotational flap
    c. Free flap
    d. Circular flap

CARCINOMA ANAL CANAL

100. Treatment of choice for squamous cell carcinoma of anal canal: *(Recent Question 2013, DNB 2012, JIPMER 2011)*
    a. Abdominoperineal resection
    b. Chemoradiation
    c. Wide local excision
    d. CO_2 laser

101. Not included in treatment of squamous cell carcinoma of anal margin: *(PGI May 2011)*
    a. Radiotherapy f/b chemotherapy
    b. Chemotherapy f/b radiotherapy
    c. Local excision
    d. Radical surgery
    e. Abdominoperineal resection

102. Most common surgical complication of condyloma acuminata? *(MHSSMCET 2008)*
    a. Infection
    b. Recurrence
    c. Hemorrhage
    d. Malignant change

103. Virus that has increased association with anal warts:
    a. HPV
    b. HIV *(MHPGMCET 2009)*
    c. LMV
    d. EBV

104. Quadrivalent vaccine available for HPV protects against:
 (JIPMER 2010)
    a. HPV 6, 11, 31, 32
    b. HPV 11, 16, 30, 33
    c. HPV 6, 11, 16, 18
    d. HPV 16, 18, 31, 35

105. Commonest type of carcinoma anal canal is:
 (Recent Question 2014, AIIMS June 97)
    a. Squamous cell carcinoma
    b. Adenocarcinoma
    c. Adenocanthoma
    d. Papillary type

106. Anal carcinoma is most commonly: *(PGI June 97)*
    a. Adenocarcinoma
    b. Epidermoid
    c. Mixed
    d. None of the above

107. Treatment of squamous cell carcinoma of anal canal is:
 (Karnataka 2012, AIIMS Nov 2002)
    a. Cisplatin based chemotherapy followed by radical radiotherapy
    b. Abdominoperineal resection
    c. Radical radiotherapy
    d. Radical radiotherapy followed by mitomycin-C based chemotherapy

108. Which of the following statements is true for Nigro's regimen? *(All India 2008)*
    a. It is a regimen for anal canal neoplasm
    b. It incorporates chemotherapy with radiation as an alternative to surgery
    c. Has the advantage of preserving continence
    d. All of the above

109. A 50-years old male, working as a hotel cook, has four dependent family members. He has been diagnosed with an early stage squamous cell cancer of anal canal. He has more than 60% chances of cure. The best treatment option is:
 (All India 2003)
 a. Abdomino-perineal resection
 b. Combined surgery and radiotherapy
 c. Combined chemotherapy and radiotherapy
 d. Chemotherapy alone

110. For CA Anal canal, treatment of choice is: *(DNB 2012, GB Pant 2011, AIIMS Feb 97, Nov 97, June 98, All India 2006)*
 a. Surgery
 b. Surgery + Radiotherapy
 c. Chemoradiation
 d. Chemotherapy

111. In carcinoma of anus distal margin of clearance of anal canal of at least: *(Recent Question 2014, CMC 2001)*
 a. 2 cm
 b. 5 cm
 c. 4 cm
 d. 7 cm

112. Anal margin carcinoma is mostly: *(PGI SS June 2005)*
 a. SCC
 b. BCC
 c. Bowen's disease
 d. Melanoma

PAGET'S DISEASE OF ANAL CANAL

113. Paget's disease of anal canal is: *(JIPMER GIS 2011)*
 a. Squamous cell carcinoma in situ
 b. Squamous cell adenoma
 c. Intra-epithelial adenocarcinoma
 d. Marginal anal cell carcinoma

114. Which of the following is true about extra-mammary Paget's disease? *(JIPMER 2011)*
 a. MC site is vulva
 b. MC site is penis
 c. MC site is vagina
 d. MC site is perianal region

ANAL CANAL MELANOMA

115. True about melanoma of the anal canal is: *(PGI June 99)*
 a. Present usually as anal bleeding
 b. AP resection gives better result than local excision
 c. Local recurrence at the same site after resection
 d. Radiosensitive

ANORECTAL MALFORMATIONS

116. A newborn baby presents with absent anal orifice and meconuria. What is the most appropriate management: *(MHCET 2016, All India 2008)*
 a. Transverse colostomy
 b. Conservative
 c. Posterior saggital anorectoplasty
 d. Perineal V-Y plasty

117. Invertogram is taken after:
 a. 2 hours after birth
 b. 4 hours after birth
 c. 6 hours after birth
 d. 8 hours after birth

118. A 45-year-old female presented to your OPD with this lesion in the left breast. What is the most probable diagnosis?
 a. DCIS
 b. LCIS
 c. Peau-d'orange
 d. Paget's disease of nipple

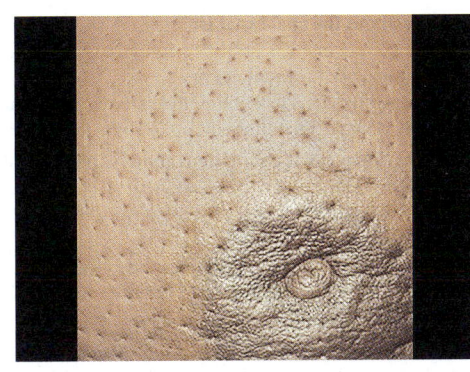

119. Anorectal anomalies are commonly associated with: *(JIPMER 2011)*
 a. Cardiac anomalies
 b. Duodenal atresia
 c. CNS malformations
 d. Abdominal

120. A neonate is brought with history of not having passed meconium on examination there is no anal opening but a dimple. Investigation of choice is: *(JIPMER 90)*
 a. X-ray erect posture
 b. X-ray supine posture
 c. Gastrograffin study
 d. Invertogram

RECTUM AND ANAL CANAL ANATOMY AND PHYSIOLOGY

121. Resting tone of rectum is decreased in all except:
 a. Micturition *(All India 91)*
 b. Retained feces in the rectum
 c. Prolapse rectum
 d. Trauma involving the perineum

122. The length of a standard proctoscope is: *(TN 2004)*
 a. 4 inches
 b. 6 inches
 c. 8 inches
 d. 3 inches

123. Length of flexible sigmoidoscope: *(Recent Question 2015)*
 a. 30 cm
 b. 40 cm
 c. 60 cm
 d. 70 cm

124. Muscle which is primarily responsible for rectal continence: *(Recent Question 2016)*
 a. External sphincter
 b. Internal sphincter
 c. Puborectalis
 d. Sacrococcygeus

125. Below the pectineal line the lymphatic spread is to ..... nodes: *(Recent Question 2016)*
 a. Superficial inguinal
 b. Internal iliac
 c. External iliac
 d. Para aortic

126. Internal sphincter of rectum is formed by:
 a. Levator ani *(DPG 96)*
 b. Puborectalis
 c. Longitudinal muscle fibers condensation
 d. Circular muscles fibers condensation

127. What is false regarding dentate line? *(AIIMS 98)*
 a. Glands of Morgagni open below the line
 b. Anal glands open at the line
 c. Dentate line lies 2 cms above the anal verge
 d. Transitional epithelium lies above the dentate line

128. True statement about upper half of anal canal is:
 a. Insensitive to pain
 b. Drained by superficial inguinal lymph node
 c. Lined by squamous epithelium
 d. Supplied by superior mesenteric artery

129. **Not true about the anal canal is:** *(PGI 99)*
    a. Completely lined by stratified squamous epithelium
    b. Supplied by pudendal nerve
    c. Drained by veins forming portosystemic anastomosis
    d. Part below pectinate line is supplied by inferior rectal artery

130. **Which of the following statement about valves of Houston is true?** *(All India 2012, AIIMS GIS Dec 2011)*
    a. The middle valve corresponds to middle convex fold to right
    b. The upper valve corresponds to peritoneal reflection
    c. The valve contain all the three layer of muscle wall
    d. Valves disappear after mobilization of rectum

131. **A patient with external hemorrhoids develops pain while passing stools. The nerve mediating this pain is:** *(Bihar PG 2014, DNB 2011, All India 2002)*
    a. Hypogastric nerve
    b. Pudendal nerve
    c. Splanchnic visceral nerve
    d. Sympathetic plexus

132. **In an adult male, on per rectal examination, the following structures can be felt anteriorly except:** *(All India 2005)*
    a. Internal iliac lymph nodes
    b. Bulb of the penis
    c. Prostate
    d. Seminal vesicle when enlarged

133. **The following are important in maintenance of normal fecal continence except:** *(All India 95)*
    a. Anorectal angulation
    b. Rectal innervations
    c. Internal sphincter
    d. Haustral valve

134. **Which of the following is not a component of anorectal ring?** *(AIIMS May 2013)*
    a. External anal sphincter
    b. Puborectalis
    c. Anococcygeal raphe
    d. Internal anal sphincter

135. **External anal sphincter is innervated by:** *(AIIMS Nov 2013)*
    a. S2, S3, S4
    b. S2, S3
    c. L5, S1
    d. L2, L3

136. **Dentate line measurement from anal margin:** *(WBPG 2014)*
    a. 1 cm
    b. 1.5 cm
    c. 2 cm
    d. 2.5 cm

MISCELLANEOUS

137. **Hemangioma of the rectum:** *(PGI June 2007)*
    a. Common tumor
    b. Fatal hemorrhage seen
    c. Ulcerative colitis like symptoms seen
    d. None

138. **Bleeding per rectum is present in all, except:** *(AIIMS June 94)*
    a. Meckel's diverticulum
    b. Sigmoid volvulus
    c. Carcinoma rectum
    d. Ulcerative colitis

139. **A young office executive, on tout, presents with bright red painless bleed since 7 days and abdominal pain. External and per-rectal examinations are normal. As attending general practitioner what will be your next step:** *(AIIMS Nov 2010)*
    a. Proctoscopy
    b. Do a barium enema
    c. Refer to surgeon for sigmoidoscopy
    d. Refer to gastroenterologist for colonoscopy

140. **Not a cause of acute anal pain:** *(AIIMS Nov 2012)*
    a. Thrombosed hemorrhoids
    b. Acute anal fissure
    c. Fistula-in-ano
    d. Perianal abscess

Explanations

VILLOUS ADENOMA

1. **Ans. a. Bleeding PR, b. Mucus diarrhea with hypokalemia** *(Ref: Sabiston 20/e p1363; Schwartz 10/e p1205-1206; Bailey 27/e p1326; Harrison 20/e p264, 19/e p254, 305)*
   - Villous adenoma causes **profuse watery diarrhea** and **hypokalemia, hyponatremia, hypochloremia** and **metabolic acidosis**[Q].
   - **Best treatment: Submucosal resection** endoscopically or surgically (Provided cancerous change has been excluded)

2. Ans. a. Na^+, c. K^+
3. Ans. a. Local resection of lesion
4. Ans. b. Hypokalemia
5. Ans. a. Dysentery

RECTAL POLYP

6. Ans. c. Bleeding
7. Ans. a. Juvenile rectal polyp
8. Ans. d. Rectal polyp

Rectal Polyps

- Occur most commonly in **children < 5 years** of age[Q].
- Occur as a **single lesion** of the **rectum**[Q]
- Typical symptoms are **rectal bleeding, mucus discharge, diarrhea**, and **abdominal pain**[Q].

CARCINOMA RECTUM

9. **Ans. d. Decreases survival** *(Ref: Sabiston 20/e p1379; Schwartz 10/e p1203-1216; Bailey 27/e p1335; Schackelford 8/e p1986, 7/e p2123-2124)*

Total Mesorectal Excision	
Advantages	**Disadvantages**
• Significant **increase in 5-year survival rates**[Q]	• **TME is a more complex operation**[Q]
• **Decrease in local recurrence** rate[Q]	• Associated with a **longer operating time**, more **blood loss, longer hospital stay**[Q]
• **Decrease** in the incidence of **impotence** and **bladder dysfunction**[Q].	• **Higher leakage rate, higher stoma rate**[Q].

10. **Ans. b. Lesion <4 cm, c. Involvement of <40% circumference. d. T1 & T2 cancer with or without lymph node involvement** *(Ref: Sabiston 20/e p1379)*

    "Local excision does not allow complete removal of lymph nodes in the mesorectum, so operative staging is limited. *In addition, definitive treatment of early-stage rectal cancers by local excision has been shown to be associated with a threefold to five-fold higher recurrence rate compared with similar stage cancers treated by radical surgical resection before guidelines for specific selection criteria. Over time, the selection criteria have been refined to select only patients for this procedure who will have acceptable long-term outcomes.* **The operation is indicated for mobile tumors smaller than 3 cm in diameter that involve less than 30% of the rectal wall circumference and that are located in the distal rectum. These tumors should be stage T1 (limited to the submucosa), be well or moderately differentiated histologically, and have no vascular or lymphatic invasion. There should be no evidence of nodal disease on preoperative ultrasound or MRI.** *Adherence to these principles results in acceptable local recurrence rates compared with treatment by abdominal perineal resection.*"

Carcinoma Rectum Amenable to Local Excision for Curative Intent	
Physical Features	**Endorectal Ultrasound**
• Tumor **<3 cm** in **diameter**[Q]	• **T1, T2 lesions**[Q]
• Tumor **<30%** of bowel **circumference**[Q]	• No regional LN involvement
• Tumor located in distal rectum[Q]	
• Tumor **freely mobile**[Q] on digital rectal examination	

11. **Ans. c. Chemoradiation is given** *(Ref: Sabiston 20/e p1377-1381; Schwartz 10/e p1203-1216; Bailey 27/e p1337)*

12. **Ans. a. 2 cm** *(Ref: Sabiston 20/e p1378; Schwartz 9/e p1050; Bailey 27/e p1326)*

Tumor Margin for Curative Excision

- In GI malignancies (**stomach**[Q], **small intestine**[Q], **colon**[Q] and **proximal rectum**[Q]), tumor margin for curative excision is **5 cm**[Q] except:
  – **Esophagus: 10 cm**[Q]
  – **Distal rectum: 2 cm**[Q]

13. **Ans. a. Irrigation of divided bowel ends with cytotoxic solution may reduce local true recurrence** *(Ref: Bailey 25/e p1236)*

    - Bailey says "In each of the procedures, it is essential to ensure that **any free tumour cells released by mobilisation of** the **rectum are destroyed by irrigation of** the **rectal lumen with a cancercidal solution** such as **1% cetrimide**[Q]. By so doing, the implantation of such cells and subsequent local recurrence is prevented. However, it should be realised that, although a **small percentage of local recurrences** are **due to implantation of shed cells**, the **majority result from inadequate removal of** the **tumour** at the time of the **initial operation**[Q]."

14. **Ans. a. Surgical resection only**
15. **Ans. c. Dissection lateral to endopelvic fascia investing the mesorectum causes local recurrence**

    Dissection **medial to endopelvic fascia** investing the mesorectum **causes local recurrence.**

16. **Ans. a. T2N0, T1N1**
17. **Ans. c. Transanal resection**

    Best treatment for this patient is **local resection**, as the **tumor** is **involving less than one third circumference of** the **rectum. Transanal resection** is the best among the provided options.

18. **Ans. a. 2 cm and 5 cm** *(Ref: Bailey 27/e p1332)*

    - Bailey says "Provided a **minimum distal margin of clearance** of **2 cm**[Q] can be secured, it is safe to restore gastrointestinal continuity (Williams). The **principles of the operation** involve **radical excision** of the **neoplasm, removal of the mesorectum** and **high proximal ligation of the inferior mesenteric lymphovascular pedicle**[Q]."
    - The **proximal** and **radial margin** should be **at least 5 cm**[Q].

19. **Ans. b. Abdominoperineal resection** *(Ref: Sabiston 20/e p1378-1380; Schwartz 10/e p1189; Bailey 27/e p1336)*
20. **Ans. c. MRI Scan** *(Ref: Sabiston 20/e p1378; Schwartz 10/e p1214; Bailey 27/e p1330; Maingot 11/e p701)*

    #### ENDORECTAL-COIL MRI

    - **Endorectal-Coil MRI** can **identify involved perirectal nodes** on the basis of characteristics other than size. It can **identify foci** not only **within** the **mesorectum** but also **outside the mesorectal fascia** such as **pelvic side walls**[Q].
    - **Best for** predicting **LN invasion** and **overall staging**[Q]

21. **Ans. c. Abdominoperineal resection**
22. **Ans. a. Anterior resection**
23. **Ans. b. Abdominoperineal resection**
24. **Ans. c. Bleeding P/R**
25. **Ans. d. More than 4 cm from anal verge**
26. **Ans. b. CA rectum**
27. **Ans. b. Histological grading** *(Ref: Sabiston 20/e p1377)*

    #### NO EFFECT ON PROGNOSIS

    - **No effect on Prognosis: Tumor size** and **duration** of symptoms[Q]
    - **Tumor size** and **configuration** (endophytic, exophytic, annular) **do not carry** any **prognostic significance**[Q] in colorectal carcinoma.

28. **Ans. b. Anterior resection**
29. **Ans. a. Abdominoperineal resection**
30. **Ans. c. Signet ring carcinoma**
31. **Ans. b. Barium enema**
32. **Ans. c. Hartmann's operation**
33. **Ans. c. Preserving the anal sphincter**
34. **Ans. d. Cancer is less than 5 cm from anorectal margin**
35. **Ans. b. Per rectal examination can diagnose only 10% of cases**

HEMORRHOIDS

36. **Ans. c. Third degree no surgery** *(Ref: Sabiston 20/e p1400-1402; Schwartz 10/e p1222-1225; Bailey 27/e p1355; Schackelford 8/e p1852, 7/e p1896-1906)*

    Surgery can be done for 3rd degree not controlled by other measures.

37. **Ans. c. III degree**
38. **Ans. b. Can be palpated on DRE in absence of complications**

    - Hemorrhoids cannot be palpated, **best diagnosed by proctoscopy**[Q].

39. **Ans. a. Band ligation, b. 5% phenol in almond oil is used as sclerosant, c. May be resolved by diet modification, d. Hemorrhoidectomy is TOC**
40. **Ans. a. Painful**
41. **Ans. b. Internal hemorrhoids**

Rectum and Anal Canal

42. Ans. d. Urinary retention *(Ref: Bailey 27/e p1360, 26/e p1256, 25/e p1259; Sabiston 20/e p1401, 19/e p1389-1391; Schwartz 10/e p1223-1224, 9/e p1059)*

Complications of Hemorrhoidectomy	
Early Complications	**Late Complications**
• **Pain (MC)**^Q • **Acute retention** of **urine (2nd MC)**^Q • Reactionary hemorrhage	• Secondary hemorrhage • Anal stricture • Anal fissure • Incontinence

43. Ans. c. Banding
44. Ans. a. Surgery, b. Sclerotherapy
45. Ans. d. Proctoscopy
46. Ans. c. Thrombosed external hemorrhoids
47. Ans. a. They are arteriolar dilatations
48. Ans. a. Excisional surgery is cornerstone *(Ref: Bailey 27/e p1357)*

Mere presence of hemorrhoids is not necessarily an indication of treatment. Treatment is **only indicated** if they are **symptomatic**. **Best treatment** is the **least invasive one which is possible** to **alleviate** the **symptoms.**

49. Ans. a. Pain *(Ref: Bailey 24/e p1259)*

Most important disadvantage of cryosurgery for hemorrhoid is pain.

CRYOSURGERY

- The extreme cold (**-196°C**) of **liquid nitrogen** application causes **coagulation necrosis of the piles,** which subsequently separated and dropped off.
- **Cryosurgery for hemorrhoids cause:**
  – Pain^Q
  – Mucous discharge^Q (Not the watery discharge)

50. Ans. c. Internal hemorrhoids bleed profusely and painless
51. Ans. d. Pudendal nerve
52. Ans. d. Grade IV *(Ref: Sabiston 20/e p1401; Schwartz 10/e p1223; Bailey 27/e p1355)*
53. Ans. b. Third & fourth degree hemorrhoids, d. Complicated by strangulations, e. Failure of conservative therapy

SOLITARY RECTAL ULCER SYNDROME

54. Ans. c. Usually malignant
55. Ans. a. SRUS *(Ref: Sabiston 20/e p1387-1388; Schwartz 10/e p1219, 9/e p1054; Bailey 27/e p1324)*
56. Ans. b Anterior, 7–10 cm from anal verge
57. Ans. c. Lamina propria infiltration with lymphocyte
58. Ans. c. Involves posterior wall
59. Ans. c. Banding, d. Sclerosant injection

RECTAL PROLAPSE

60. Ans. b. Anterior resection *(Ref: Sabiston 20/e p1382; Schwartz 10/e p1218-1219; Bailey 27/e p1323; Schackelford 8/e p1783, 7/e p1824-1832)*

Abdominal rectopexy is the **procedure of choice** for **complete rectal prolapse** in **young** and **fit patients.**
Perineal procedures (Delorme's procedure) are reserved for elderly and frail patients.
Abdominal rectopexy has the **least recurrence rates** and is **most likely to improve continence.**
Perineal procedures are reserved for elderly, frail and infirm patients, who are unlikely to tolerate major 'abdominal' procedures.

61. Ans. d. 8–12 months
62. Ans. c. Thiersch wiring *(Ref: Bailey 27/e p1323)*

TREATMENT OF RECTAL PROLAPSE IN CHILDHOOD

- Prolapse during childhood is **best managed conservatively,** the **only exception** is **persistence of prolapse despite effective treatment of diarrhea,** worm infestation and malabsorption^Q. These cases are **managed by surgery.**

Conservative Treatment	Operative Treatment
• Effective **control of diarrhea, worm infestation** and **correction of malnutrition**^Q • **Sclerotherapy:** • Usually **reserved for prolapse of** the **redundant mucosa after** an **anoplasty** or **rectoplasty** for an **imperforate anus**^Q • **5% phenol** in **olive oil** is **injected submucosally**^Q	• **Thiersch operation**^Q: – **Anal encirclement**^Q • Ideally suited for prolapse in **myelomeningocele** and **sacral agenesis**^Q • **Lockhart Mummery Rectopexy**^Q: • **Simplest** and **safest** operation in childhood complete rectal prolapse^Q • **Posterior rectal wall stiffening**

63. Ans. a. Thiersch wiring
64. Ans. a. Rectal prolapse

65. Ans. c. Abdominal rectopexy   66. Ans. a. Abdominal rectopexy

| WAR | Wells Abdominal Ripstein |
| PAD | Perineal Altmier's Delorme |

67. Ans. c. Thiersch's operation
68. Ans. a. Delorme *(Ref: Sabiston 20/e p1397; Schwartz 10/e p1219; Bailey 27/e p1323)*   69. Ans. c. Delorme procedure

ANORECTAL ABSCESS

70. Ans. d. Perianal *(Ref: Sabiston 20/e p1406; Schwartz 10/e p1227; Bailey 27/e p1362; Schackelford 8/e p1871, 7/e p1914)*
71. Ans. c. Poor blood supply   72. Ans. a. Inflammation of anal gland

FISTULA-IN-ANO

73. Ans. a. Intersphincteric *(Ref: Sabiston 20/e p1407-1408; Schwartz 10/e p1229-1231; Bailey 27/e p1363; Schackelford 8/e p1874, 7/e p1767, 1914-1924)*
74. Ans. a. Seton *(Ref: Sabiston 20/e p1408; Schwartz 10/e p1231; Bailey 27/e p1366; Schackelford 8/e p1881, 7/e p1923-1924)*

SETONS
- A **seton** is a **ligature of silk, nylon, silastic or linen**^{Q}.
- Used for **marking, draining, cutting or staging**^{Q}.
- A **high fistula** may be **converted into a low fistula by setons**^{Q}

Setons are Useful in the Management of
- **Complex anorectal fistulas** with **risk of incontinence** or **poor healing**^{Q}
- Patients with **Crohn's disease**^{Q}
- **Immunocompromised (HIV)** and **incontinent** patients^Q
- Patients with **chronic diarrheal states**^{Q}
- **Anterior fistula in women**^{Q}

75. Ans. a. Squamous cell carcinoma, b. Transitional cell carcinoma *(Ref: Schackelford 7/e p1926)*

CARCINOMA ASSOCIATED WITH FISTULA-IN-ANO
- MC type of carcinoma to arise in fistula-in-ano: **Colloid carcinoma**^{Q} (44%) > **Squamous cell carcinoma** (34%) > **Adenocarcinoma** (22%)
- **Clue to early diagnosis** is the appearance of **mucin globules**^{Q} in Fistulotomy or fistulectomy specimens

76. Ans. d. Intersphincteric is the most common type   77. Ans. d. Fistulotomy
78. Ans. c. Anorectal ring   79. Ans. b. MRI
80. Ans. a. Cutting seton
81. Ans. a. Cutting seton *(Ref: Sabiston 20/e p1408; Schwartz 10/e p1231; Bailey 27/e p1366-1367; Schackelford 8/e p1881, 7/e p1923-1924)*

ANAL FISSURE

82. Ans. b. Posterior *(Ref: Sabiston 20/e p1402-1404; Schwartz 10/e p1225; Bailey 27/e p1352; Schackelford 8/e p1865, 7/e p1906-1912)*
83. Ans. b. 0.2%   84. Ans. d. External sphincterotomy
85. Ans. c. Sitz in a basin containing warm antiseptic lotion   86. Ans. a. Anal fissure
87. Ans. c. Fissure-in-ano   88. Ans. b. History and superficial clinical examination
89. Ans. d. Anal fissure   90. Ans. c. Fissure-in-ano

ATYPICAL FISSURES
- A **fissure sited elsewhere** around the anal circumference or **with atypical features** should raise the **suspicion of a specific etiology**^{Q}
- **Early examination** under anesthesia, **with biopsy** and **culture to exclude:**
  - **Crohn's disease, tuberculosis**^{Q}
  - **STD** (syphilis, Chlamydia, chancroid, lymphogranuloma venereum, HSV, CMV, Kaposi's sarcoma, B-cell lymphoma)
  - **HIV-related ulcers**^{Q}
  - **Squamous cell carcinoma**^{Q}

91. Ans. b. 6 o'clock   92. Ans. b. Topical steroids *(Ref: Sabiston 20/e p1405; Schwartz 10/e p1226; Bailey 27/e p1352)*

PILONIDAL SINUS

93. **Ans. b. Recurrence is uncommon** *(Ref: Sabiston 20/e p1408-1409; Schwartz 10/e p1233; Bailey 27/e p1347; Schackelford 8/e p1790, 7/e p1833-1840)*
    Recurrence is **common**, even though **adequate excision** of the **track is carried out**.
94. **Ans. d. Treatment of choice is surgical excision of sinus tract**
95. **Ans. c. Pilonidal sinus**   96. **Ans. a. Seen predominantly in women**
97. **Ans. a. More common in young female** *(Ref: Schwartz 10/e p1233; Sabiston 20/e p1408-1409; Bailey 27/e p1347)*
98. **Ans. a. Jack knife**   99. **Ans. a. Rhomboid flap** *(Ref: Sabiston 20/e p1409)*

> "In patients with recurrent disease who have undergone multiple prior surgical interventions, flap-based procedures, such as a V-Y advancement flap, rhomboid flap, Z-plasty, Bascom repair, or Karydakis flap, may be beneficial. Limited comparative studies of the various flap-based procedures exist. A rhomboid fasciocutaneous flap that serves to flatten the gluteal cleft has been shown to have lower recurrence rates compared with a V-Y advancement flap. A Karydakis flap and rhomboid flap are essentially equivalent in published series. In most practices, the complex flap closures are reserved for patients with refractory disease for whom previous simple measures have failed." -*Sabiston 20/e p1409*

CARCINOMA ANAL CANAL

100. **Ans. b. Chemoradiation** *(Ref: Sabiston 20/e p1412-1413; Schwartz 10/e p1218; Bailey 27/e p1371; Schackelford 8/e p2095, 7/e p2166-2170)*
101. **Ans. a. Radiotherapy f/b chemotherapy, d. Radical surgery** *(Ref: Sabiston 20/e p1412; Schwartz 10/e p1218; Bailey 27/e p1371; Schackelford 8/e p2100, 7/e p2173)*

ANAL MARGIN TUMORS

- These tumors **arise on the perianal skin**[Q] beyond the anal verge.
- **Squamous cell carcinoma** of the **anal margin** is treated by **primary surgical excision** similarly to skin cancers[Q].
- **Metastases** are **late** and **rare**, and recurrences are **typically locoregional**.
- **Symptoms** include **pain, bleeding, itching**, and **palpable mass**.
- **Diagnosis** is often suspected by the experienced clinician on inspection, but **biopsy prior to definitive treatment** is imperative.

  - **Small lesion: Wide-local excision**[Q]
  - **Large lesion** or **sphincter involvement: Chemoradiation**[Q]

102. **Ans. b. Recurrence**
103. **Ans. a. HPV** *(Ref: Sabiston 20/e p1412; Schwartz 10/e p485,1232,1233,1678,1680; Bailey 27/e p1368; Schackelford 8/e p2101, 7/e p2172)*

ANAL WARTS OR CONDYLOMATA ACCUMINATA

- HPV forms the **etiological basis of: Anal** and **perianal warts**, **AIN**, and **SCC of the anus**[Q].
- Subtypes (**16, 18, 31, 33**) are **associated with a greater risk of progression** to **dysplasia** and **malignancy**[Q].
- **Condylomata accuminata** is the **MC STD encountered by colorectal surgeons**[Q]
- Most frequently observed in **homosexual men**[Q].

Clinical Presentation
- Many are **asymptomatic** but **pruritus, discharge, bleeding** and **pain** are **usual presenting complaints**[Q].
- Rarely, **relentless growth** results in giant condylomata (**Buschke- Löwenstein tumour**), which may obliterate the anal orifice[Q].
- **Diagnosis** is **confirmed by biopsy**[Q]

Treatment
- Application of **25% podophyllin**[Q]
- **Surgical excision**[Q]
- **Recurrence is common**[Q]

104. **Ans. c. HPV 6, 11, 16, 18** *(Ref: Maingot 11/e p732)*

HPV VACCINES

- **Gardisil** is a **recombinant vaccine** against HPV **types 6, 11, 16, 18**[Q].
- It is **currently approved** for use in **females age 9–26 years** of age and requires a series of **three injections over a 6 month** period[Q].

  - Nearly **100% prevention rate** in **genital warts, vulvar, vaginal**, and **cervical precancerous lesions** caused by the **serotypes against** which the **vaccine is directed**[Q].

- Vaccine is **only effective** in patients **not previously exposed** to the **viruses included in** the **vaccine**, and it **confers no protection against viruses not covered** by the vaccine[Q]

105. Ans. a. Squamous cell carcinoma
106. Ans. b. Epidermoid

EPIDERMOID CARCINOMA OF ANUS

- **Epidermoid carcinoma** of the **anus** includes **SCC, cloacogenic** carcinoma, **transitional carcinoma** and **basaloid carcinoma**[Q].
- The **clinical behavior** and **natural history** of these tumors **are similar**[Q].

107. Ans. a. Cisplatin based chemotherapy followed by radical radiotherapy
108. Ans. d. All of the above
109. Ans. c. Combined chemotherapy and radiotherapy
110. Ans. c. Chemoradiation
111. Ans. a. 2 cm
112. Ans. a. SCC

PAGET'S DISEASE OF ANAL CANAL

113. Ans. c. Intra-epithelial adenocarcinoma *(Ref: Sabiston 20/e p1413-1414; Bailey 27/e p1372; Schackelford 8/e p 2101, 7/e p2174-2175; Maingot 11/e p743-744)*
114. Ans. a. MC site is vulva

ANAL CANAL MELANOMA

115. Ans. a. Present usually as anal bleeding *(Ref: Sabiston 20/e p1415; Schwartz 10/e p1218; Bailey 27/e p1371; Schackelford 8/e p2100, 7/e p2173; Maingot 11/e p742)*

ANORECTAL MALFORMATIONS

116. Ans. a. Transverse colostomy *(Ref: Sabiston 20/e p1877-1879; Schwartz 10/e p1626-1628; Bailey 27/e p1345-1347)*

- The presence of **meconium in urine reflects** some form of **communication between** the **urinary tract** and **rectum**, and suggests a **high type of anorectal malformation**[Q].
- Such **patients require** a **diverting colostomy**. The **colostomy decompresses** the **bowel** and **provides protection during** the **healing of subsequent repair**[Q].
- **Posterior Saggital Anorectoplasty (PSARP)** is performed **after 4–8 weeks**.
- The presence of **meconium in urine** and a **flat bottom** are considered **indications of a protective colostomy**[Q].

117. Ans. c. 6 hours after birth
118. Ans. c. Peau-d'orange
119. Ans. a. Cardiac anomalies
120. Ans. d. Invertogram

- Anorectal malformations are associated with VACTERL abnormalities.

RECTUM AND ANAL CANAL ANATOMY AND PHYSIOLOGY

121. Ans. b. Retained feces in the rectum
122. Ans. a. 4 inches *(Ref: Bailey 27/e p1320)*

Proctoscope	10–12 cm[Q]
Rigid sigmoidoscope	25 cm[Q]
Flexible sigmoidoscope	60 cm[Q]
Colonoscope	160 cm[Q]

123. Ans. c. 60 cm
124. Ans. c. Puborectalis *(Ref: Maingot 11/e p663)*
125. Ans. a. Superficial inguinal
126. Ans. d. Circular muscles fibers condensation
127. Ans. d. Transitional epithelium lies above the dentate line
128. Ans. a. Insensitive to pain

Anal Canal		
Upper (Mucous) Zone	Middle (Transitional) Zone	Lower (cutaneous) Zone
• Length: **15 mm**[Q] • Lined by **simple columnar mucous membrane** showing **anal columns** of **Morgagni, anal valves, anal sinus, anal papilla**[Q]. • **Pain insensitive**[Q]	• Length: **15 mm**[Q] • Lined by **non-keratinized stratified squamous epithelium** without sweat and sebaceous gland[Q] • **Pain sensitive**[Q]	• Length: **8 mm**[Q] • Lined by non-keratinized stratified squamous epithelium **with sweat and sebaceous gland**[Q] • **Pain sensitive**[Q]

- **Dentate/ Pectinate line** lies **between upper** and **middle part**^Q
- **White line** of **Hilton** lies **at lower limit of middle**^Q (transitional) part
- **Anal glands** open at the **dentate line**^Q

129. **Ans. a. Completely lined by stratified squamous epithelium**
130. **Ans. d. Valves disappear after mobilization of rectum** *(Ref: Sabiston 20/e p1394; Schwartz 10/e p1178; Bailey 27/e p1318; Schackelford 8/e p1670, 7/e p1703)*

VALVES OF HOUSTON

- The **middle valve** folds to the **left**^Q (corresponds to the anterior peritoneal reflection) and the proximal and distal to the right.
- These valves are more properly called **folds**, for they have **no specific function** as impediments to flow.
- They are lost following **full surgical mobilization**^Q of the rectum, a maneuver that may provide approx. **5 cm** of **additional length** to the rectum^Q.

131. **Ans. b. Pudendal nerve** *(Ref: Gray's 40/e p1098)*

	Pudendal Nerve	
Root Value	**Course**	**Branches and Supply**
• S2, S3, S4^Q	• **Leaves pelvis** through **greater sciatic foramen**^Q • **Enter perineum** through **lesser sciatic foramen**^Q	• **Main** sensory motor **nerve of perineum**^Q and **sensory nerve** of **external genitalia** • **Dorsal nerve** of **penis/clitoris** • **Inferior rectal nerve**^Q supply **anal mucosa** (lower ½), **perineal skin** and **external anal sphincter** • **Perineal nerve**

132. **Ans. a. Internal iliac lymph nodes**
133. **Ans. d. Haustral valve** *(Ref: Sabiston 20/e p1394; Bailey 27/e p1339)*

FECAL CONTINENCE

- Normal fecal continence requires:
  - **Adequate rectal wall compliance** to accommodate the fecal bolus^Q
  - **Appropriate neurogenic control** of the **pelvic floor** and **sphincter** mechanism^Q
  - **Functional internal and external sphincter muscles**^Q

ANAL CANAL PHYSIOLOGY

- **Resting pressure** or **tone**: Due to **Internal sphincter** (90 cm H$_2$O)^Q
- **Squeeze pressure**: Contraction of the **external anal sphincter** and **puborectalis muscle**^Q
- **Principal mechanism that provides continence**: Pressure differential between the **rectum** (6 cm H$_2$O) and **anal canal** (90 cm H$_2$O)^Q.
- **Anorectal angle** is produced by the **anterior pull of** the **puborectalis muscle** as it encircles the rectum at the anorectal ring and contributes to fecal continence. **This angle** may act as a **flap valve** or have a **sphincter-like function**^Q.

134. **Ans. c. Anococcygeal raphe** *(Ref: BDC 5/e pVol-III/e p428; Maingot 11/e p663)*

Anorectal ring is a muscular ring present at the anorectal junction. It is formed by the **fusion of** the **Puborectalis, uppermost fibers of external sphincter** and the **internal sphincter**.

- BDC says "**Anorectal ring** is a **muscular ring** present at the anorectal junction. It is formed by the **fusion of** the **Puborectalis, uppermost fibers of external sphincter** and the **internal sphincter**. It is easily felt by a finger in anal canal. **Surgical division** of this ring results in **rectal incontinence**. The ring is **less marked anteriorly** where the fibers of Puborectalis are absent."

ANORECTAL RING

- Rectal continence depends solely on the **anorectal ring**^Q and any damage to this ring results in rectal incontinence.
- The anorectal ring is **muscular ring** present at the **anorectal junction**^Q.

Anorectal Ring is formed by Fusion of		
• Puborectalis^Q	• Deep external anal sphincter^Q	• Internal anal sphincter^Q

- The **Puborectalis muscle** appears to be **most important muscle for maintaining fecal continence**^Q.

135. **Ans. a. S2, S3, S4** *(Ref: Gray's 40/e p1158-1159)*

External anal sphincter is innervated by **inferior rectal branch of pudendal nerve** (**anterior divisions** of S2, S3, S4[Q] sacral spinal nerves) **mainly** and by **perineal branch of S4**.

Anal Sphincter

External Anal Sphincter
- **Voluntary**[Q]
- Sphincter complex of **striated muscles**, composed mainly of **type 1 (slow twitch) skeletal muscle fibers**[Q] suited for prolonged contraction
- Contributed by fibers from **Puborectalis part of levator ani muscle**[Q] (in **upper most** part); **superficial transverse perineal muscles anteriorly**[Q] and **anococcygeal raphe posteriorly** (in **upper third**); and **anococcygeal ligament**[Q] (in middle third).
- It is **innervated by inferior rectal branch of pudendal nerve (anterior divisions** of S2, S3, S4[Q] sacral spinal nerves) **mainly** and by **perineal branch of S4**.
- It also receives **nerve to levator ani (Puborectalis)**, with which it contracts in unison to maintain continence when internal sphincter is relaxed (except during defecation).

Internal Anal Sphincter
- **Involuntary**[Q]
- Formed by **thickening of inner circular smooth muscle layer**[Q] of upper end of anal canal.
- This sphincter remains in **state of tonic contraction most of the time to maintain resting tone or pressure**[Q] (90 cm H_2O) and to prevent leakage of fluid and flatus.
- Its **contraction is maintained by sympathetic fibers** from **superior rectal** (periarterial) and **hypogastric plexuses**; and inhibited (relaxed) by parasympathetic pelvic splanchnic nerves

136. **Ans. c. 2 cm**

- The dentate line lies abut 2 cm proximal to the anal margin and roughly corresponds to the level where the distal squamous mucosa meets the more proximal columnar mucosa

MISCELLANEOUS

137. **Ans. b. Fatal hemorrhage seen, c. Ulcerative colitis like symptoms seen** *(Ref: Bailey 27/e p1327)*

HEMANGIOMA OF RECTUM
- Hemangioma of the rectum is an **uncommon cause** of **serious hemorrhage**[Q].
- When localized in the **lower part** of the **rectum** or **anal canal**, a hemangioma can be **excised**[Q].
- When the **lesion is diffuse**, or lying in the **upper part** of the rectum, the **symptoms simulate ulcerative colitis**[Q].
- Diagnosis is often missed for a long period, or it is mistakenly thought to be a carcinoma.
- **Selective angiography** and **embolization** may be **helpful**, but **excision of** the **rectum** is sometimes **required**[Q].

138. **Ans. b. Sigmoid volvulus**

139. **Ans. a. Proctoscopy** *(Ref: Bailey 27/e p1356)*

- Hemorrhoids are most likely cause of fresh, painless bleed in this young patient. Next step would be to check for hemorrhoids by proctoscopy before going for more invasive procedures like sigmoidoscopy or colonoscopy to diagnose other conditions.

140. **Ans. c. Fistula in-ano** *(Ref: Bailey 27/e p1364; Sabiston 20/e p1407; Schwartz 10/e p1229-1231)*

Fistula-in-ano is not a cause of acute anal pain (Patients usually complain of **intermittent purulent discharge** and **pain**).

CHAPTER 19

Hernia and Abdominal Wall

HERNIA

Hernia

- **Hernia** is derived from the Latin word for **rupture**.
- A hernia is defined as an **abnormal protrusion** of an organ or tissue **through a defect**^Q in its surrounding walls.

Nyhus Classification System	
Type I	• **Indirect hernia**; **internal ring normal**; typically **in infants, children, young adults**^Q
Type II	• **Indirect hernia**; **internal ring enlarged**^Q without impingement on the floor of the inguinal canal; does not extend to the scrotum
Type IIIA	• **Direct hernia**^Q (size is not taken into account)
Type IIIB	• **Indirect hernia** enlarged enough to **encroach upon** the **posterior** inguinal **wall**; **indirect sliding** or **scrotal hernias** and **pantaloon hernias**^Q
Type IIIC	• **Femoral hernia**^Q
Type IV A B C D	• Recurrent hernia • **Direct**^Q • Indirect • Femoral • Combined

Gilbert Classification System			
Type 1	**Small, indirect**	Type 5	**Diverticular**, direct
Type 2	**Medium**, indirect	Type 6	**Combined (pantaloon)**
Type 3	**Large**, indirect	Type 7	**Femoral**^Q
Type 4	**Entire floor, direct**^Q		

SCHUMPELICK CLASSIFICATION SYSTEM

- The major feature is the **addition of orifice sizing** to traditional systems.
- The **defects** are then **graded according to size**.

• **L**: **Lateral indirect** site • **M**: **Medial direct** • **F**: **Femoral**	• **Type I**: Defect size **<1.5 cm** in diameter • **Type II**: Defect size **1.5-3 cm** • **Type III**: Defect size **>3 cm**

RISK FACTORS FOR HERNIA

Risk Factors for Hernia	
Weakness of Abdominal Muscles	**Increased Intra-abdominal Pressure**
• **Patent processus vaginalis**^Q • Patent canal of nuck causing indirect inguinal hernia in females • **Connective tissue disorders**^Q like Ehlers Danlos syndrome • Congenital conditions like **Extrophy of bladder**, **Prune Belly syndrome**^Q • **Advancing age**^Q • **Chronic debilitating disease**^Q • **Defective collagen synthesis**^Q • Previous **right lower quadrant incision**^Q • **Cigarette smoking**^Q	• **Chronic cough**^Q (Bronchitis, tuberculosis) • **Chronic obstructive pulmonary disease**^Q • **Obesity**^Q • Chronic **constipation** with **straining** at stool • **Enlarged prostate** with **straining** at micturition • **Pregnancy**^Q • **Cirrhosis** with **ascites**^Q • **Heavy weight lifting**^Q • Chronic ambulatory peritoneal dialysis • Intra-abdominal tumors • Chronically enlarged pelvic organs

Other Risk Factors	
• Birth weight <1500 gm (Pre-term)^Q • Family history of a hernia	• Arterial aneurysms^Q • Sex: Indirect inguinal hernia is more common in boys^Q
• MC type of hernia in males: Indirect inguinal hernia^Q • MC type of hernia in females: Indirect inguinal hernia^Q	• Femoral hernia is more common in females^Q. • Direct inguinal hernia is more common in the elderly^Q

INDIRECT INGUINAL HERNIA

Types of Indirect Inguinal Hernia

- **Bubonocele**: Hernia is **limited to inguinal canal**
- **Funicular: Processus vaginalis is closed just above** the **epididymis**, contents of sac can be felt separately from testis
- **Complete (Vaginal)**: Hernial sac is continuous with tunica vaginalis of testis. Testis appear to **lie within** the **lower part of hernia**

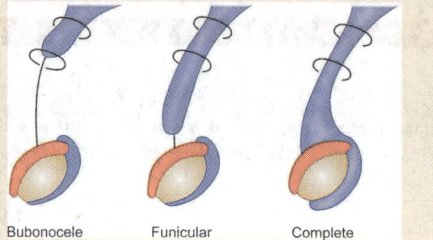
Bubonocele   Funicular   Complete

DIRECT INGUINAL HERNIA

Direct Inguinal Hernia

- In **adult males, 35%** of inguinal hernias **are direct**^{Q}
- At presentation, **12%** of patients will have a **contralateral hernia**^{Q}
- **Fourfold increased risk** of future **development of** a **contralateral hernia** if one is not present at the original presentation.
- **Always acquired**^{Q}
- **Sac passes through** a **weakness** or **defect of transversalis fascia** in the **posterior wall** of the inguinal canal.
- Patient has **poor lower abdominal musculature**, presence of elongated bulgings (**Malgaigne's bulges**).

  • **Women** practically **never develop** a **direct inguinal hernia**^{Q}.

Predisposing Factors
- Smoking^Q
- Occupations that involve **straining** and **heavy weight lifting**^{Q}

  • **Damage** to the **iliohypogastric nerve (previous appendectomy)** is another cause, because of the resulting **weakness of** the **conjoined tendon**^{Q}.
  • **IH → IH** (Ilio**H**ypogastric nerve → **I**nguinal **H**ernia^Q)

Clinical Features
- Direct hernias **do not attain a large size** or descend into the scrotum.
- In contrast to an indirect inguinal hernia, a **direct inguinal hernia lies behind** the **spermatic cord**.
- Sac is often **smaller than hernial mass would indicate**, the protruding mass mainly consisting of **extraperitoneal fat**^{Q}.

  • As the **neck of the sac is wide, direct inguinal hernias do not often strangulate**^{Q}

Management of Inguinal Hernia

- **Objectives** of treatment:
  – **Treatment of hernia sac**
  – **Inguinal floor reconstruction**

Treatment of Hernia Sac	Inguinal Floor Reconstruction
• Basic operation is **inguinal herniotomy**, which entails **dissecting out** & **opening** the **hernial sac, reducing any contents** and then **transfixing the neck** of the sac & **removing the remainder**^{Q}. • **Direct sacs** are usually too broad for ligation and should not be opened but instead are simply **inverted into peritoneal cavity**^{Q}.	• **Management of** the **hernia sac is sufficient for children & young adults**^{Q} • **Reconstruction** (repair or strengthening) of the inguinal floor is **necessary in all adult hernias to prevent recurrence**^{Q}. • **Types of repair**: – **Primary tissue repair**^{Q} – **Anterior tension-free mesh repair**^{Q} – **Preperitoneal repairs**: **Open** & **laparoscopic** approach^Q

Hernia and Abdominal Wall

Inguinal Floor Reconstruction

Primary Tissue Repair	Anterior Tension-free Mesh Repair	Laparoscopic and Preperitoneal Repairs
• **Posterior wall** of inguinal wall is **strengthened by approximation of tissues with sutures**[Q]. • There is **no use of prosthetic material**[Q]. • **Advantages**: **Simplicity** of repair & **absence** of any **foreign body** in groin • **Disadvantage**: Higher recurrence rates due to **tension** on the repair & **slower return to unrestricted physical activity**[Q]. **Types:** – **Bassini repair**[Q] – Halsted repair – **McVay**[Q] (Cooper ligament) repair – **Shouldice repair**[Q] – Darn repair	• Current practice in hernia management employ **synthetic mesh** to **bridge the defect** • **Recurrence** is **very low** • **Types:** – **Lichtenstein repair**[Q]: Mesh is used to reconstruct the inguinal floor. – **Patch & plug repair**[Q]: **Plug** of mesh is **inserted into** the hernia **defect** and sutured in place. Then another piece of **mesh** is **placed over** the **inguinal floor**.	• Preperitoneal space is reached by either transabdominal laparoscopy (**TAPP**) or by totally extraperitoneal repair (**TEP**). • **Both techniques** are **similar in actual repair** but **differ in the manner** by which the **preperitoneal space is accessed**. • **TAPP (Transabdominal PrePeritoneal)** [Q]: – Peritoneal space is reached by conventional laparoscopy and pre-peritoneum overlying the inguinal floor is dissected away as a flap. • **TEP (Totally ExtraPeritoneal)** [Q]: – Preperitoneal space is accessed without entering the peritoneal cavity

Landmarks in Laparoscopic Repair

Triangle of Doom	Triangle of Pain	Corona Mortis
• Bounded **laterally** by **gonadal vessels**[Q] • **Medially** by **vas deferens**[Q] • **Apex** oriented superiorly at the **internal ring**[Q] • Contain **external iliac vessels**[Q], deep circumflex iliac vein, femoral nerve & genital branch of genitofemoral nerve.	• Also known as **Electrical hazard zone**[Q] • Bounded **medially** by **gonadal vessels**[Q] • **Superiorly** by **iliopubic tract**[Q] • **Laterally** by **peritoneum**[Q] • This triangle **contains** from lateral to medial: – Lateral femoral cutaneous nerve[Q] (MC injured nerve in laparoscopic hernia repair) – Anterior femoral cutaneous[Q] – Femoral branch of the genitofemoral nerve[Q] – Femoral nerve[Q]	• Also known as **Crown of death**[Q] – Vascular connections between the obturator and external iliac systems[Q] • **Aberrant obturator artery** arises from **inferior epigastric artery**, **arches over** the **Coopers ligament** and **joins** the **normal obturator artery**[Q] to complete a vascular ring • **Significant hemorrhage**[Q] may occur **if accidentally cut** and it is **difficult to achieve** subsequent **hemostasis**

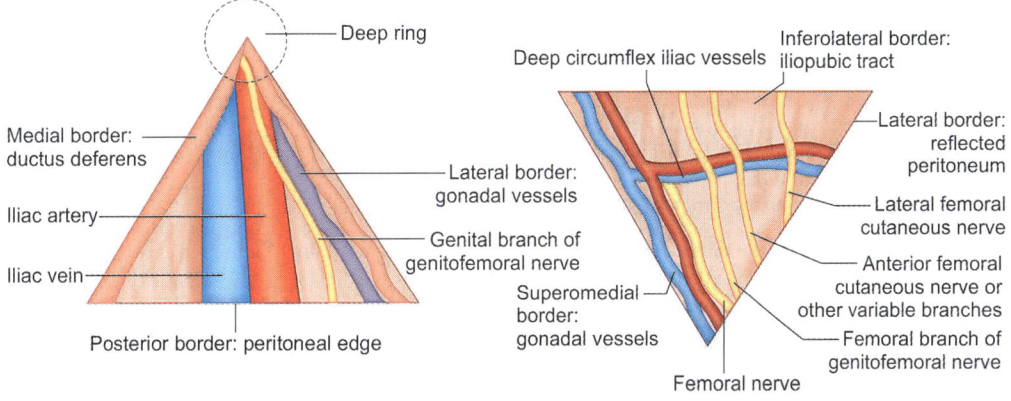

Space of Retzius (Retropubic space)	• Extra-peritoneal space between pubic symphysis & urinary bladder[Q]
Space of Bogros (Retroinguinal space)	• Extra-peritoneal space situated deep to inguinal ligament[Q] • Situated laterally & cranially to Retzius space

Complications of Groin Hernia Repairs	
• Recurrence	• Bladder injury
• Chronic groin pain	• Wound infection
• **Seroma**	• **Osteitis pubis**
• Hematoma	• Prosthetic complications (Contraction, Erosion, Infection)
• **Ischemic orchitis**	
• **Testicular atrophy**	

- MC injured nerve in laparoscopic hernia repair: Lateral cutaneous nerve of thigh^Q > Genitofemoral nerve (GFN)^Q
- MC injured nerve in open hernia repair: **I**lioinguinal nerve^Q > Ilio**H**ypogastric nerve^Q > **G**enital branch of GFN^Q (GHI in reverse sequence)

STRANGULATED INGUINAL HERNIA

Strangulated Inguinal Hernia

- **Indirect inguinal hernias strangulate more commonly**, the direct variety not so often because of wide neck of the sac.
- Strangulation occurs **more often in patients** who have **worn a truss for a long time** and in those with a partially reducible or an irreducible hernia.

> - MC constricting agent: Neck of the sac^Q > External inguinal ring in children > Adhesions within the sac (rarely).
> - MC contents: Small intestine^Q > Omentum

- It is **rare for** the **large intestine to become strangulated in** an **inguinal hernia**, even when the hernia is of the sliding variety.

Strangulation During Infancy
• Incidence of strangulation in infancy is 4% and the **ratio of girls to boys is 5:1.**
• **More frequently**, the **hernia is irreducible** but not strangulated.
• **In most cases** of **strangulated inguinal hernia** occurring **in female infants**, the **content of the sac is an ovary** or an **ovary plus its fallopian tube**^{Q}.

Diagnosis
- Diagnosis of strangulation is made **on clinical grounds.**

Clinical Features of Strangulated Inguinal Hernia
• In addition to patient having developed an **irreducible hernia** and an **intestinal obstruction**, patient develops **sudden pain**, at **first situated over hernia**, followed by **generalized abdominal pain**.
• Hernia is **tense & extremely tender**^{Q}.
• **Overlying skin** may be **discolored** with a **reddish** or **bluish tinge**^{Q}.
• There is **no expansile cough impulse**^{Q}.

Treatment
- **Vigorous resuscitation** with IV fluids, **nasogastric aspiration & antibiotics is essential** followed by **emergency operation**^{Q}.
- Inguinal herniotomy for strangulation:
  - An **incision** is made **over the most prominent part** of the swelling.

> - Each layer covering the anterior surface of the body of the sac "near fundus"^{Q} is incised and, if possible, stripped off the sac.
> - The sac is then incised and any fluid, which may be highly infective, drained effectively^Q.

- **Devitalised omentum is excised** after being securely ligated.
- **Viable intestine is returned to** the **peritoneal cavity**^{Q}.
- **Doubtfully viable** and **gangrenous intestine is excised**^{Q}.

> - If the **incision** has been **soiled** or **gangrenous bowel resected**^{Q}, prosthetic mesh should not be used^Q.
> - **Biosynthetic meshes** made **from collagen** or **dermis** are totally absorbed, are more suited to use in a contaminated environment^Q.

FEMORAL HERNIA

FEMORAL HERNIA

- Femoral hernia is the **3rd MC type of primary hernia**.
- Accounts for **20% of hernias in women**[Q] and **5% in men**.
- More common in **multipara**[Q]
- More common on **right side**; Bilateral in **20%**[Q]

> - It **cannot be controlled by a truss**[Q]
> - Of all hernias it is the **most liable to become strangulated**[Q] because of:
>   – **Narrowness of the neck** of sac[Q]   – **Rigidity of femoral ring**[Q]
> - Strangulation is the **initial presentation** of **40%** of femoral hernias[Q]
> - Should be **operated on as soon as possible**[Q]

Anatomy
- **Femoral canal** occupies the **most medial compartment** of the **femoral sheath** and extends from femoral ring to **saphenous opening**[Q].
- Femoral canal is **1.25 cm long & 1.25 cm wide at its base**[Q], which is directed upwards.
- Femoral canal **contains fat, lymphatic vessels & lymph node of Cloquet**[Q].

> **Boundaries of Femoral Ring**
> - **Anteriorly** by the **inguinal ligament**[Q]
> - **Posteriorly** by Astley **Cooper's** (iliopectineal) **ligament, pubic bone & pectineus fascia**[Q]
> - **Medially** by **Gimbernat's** (lacunar) **ligament**[Q], which is also prolonged along the iliopectineal line, as Astley Cooper's ligament
> - **Laterally** by a **thin septum separating** it from the **femoral vein**[Q]

Clinical Features
- Rare before puberty
- Prevalence rises between **20-40 years**[Q] of age and this continues to old age.
- A small femoral hernia may be unnoticed by the patient or disregarded for years, perhaps **until the day it strangulates**[Q].
- **Mass** or **bulge below & lateral to pubic tubercle**[Q]

Treatment
- **Low inguinal** operation (**Lockwood**[Q])
- **Inguinal** operation (**Lotheissen**[Q])
- **High inguinal** operation (**McEvedy**[Q])
- Midline Abdominal Extraperitoneal Femoral Hernioplasty (**Henry Procedure**[Q]): This is now considered as the **procedure of choice**; does not damage the transversalis fascial floor; reducing the risk of a subsequent inguinal hernia.

Variants of Femoral Hernia	
Laugier's femoral hernia[Q]	• Hernia through a **gap in** the **lacunar** (Gimbernats) **ligament** • Diagnosis is based on **unusual medial position** of a **small femoral hernia sac** • **Always strangulated**
Narath's femoral hernia[Q]	• Occurs in patients with **congenital dislocation of hip** • Due to **lateral displacement of** the **psoas muscle** • Hernia lies hidden **behind** the **femoral vessels**
Cloquet's hernia[Q]	• **Sac lies under** the **pectineus** fascia

SPIGELIAN HERNIA

SPIGELIAN HERNIA

- Spigelian hernia **occurs through** the **spigelian fascia**[Q]
- **Spigelian fascia** is composed of **aponeurotic layer** between **rectus muscle** medially & **semilunar line** laterally[Q].

> - Nearly **all spigelian hernias occur at** or **below the arcuate line**[Q].
> - **Absence of posterior rectus fascia** may **contribute to** an **inherent weakness** in this area[Q].
> - These hernias are **often interparietal**, with the **hernia sac dissecting posterior to external oblique aponeurosis**[Q].
> - **Spigelian hernia** sac **always penetrates** the **spigelian aponeurosis** & **usually penetrates** the **internal oblique** musculature[Q].

Clinical Features
- Most **spigelian hernias** are **small (1-2 cm** in diameter)
- Develop during **4 to 7 decades** of life.
- Patients often present with **localized pain** in the area **without a bulge** because the **hernia lies beneath** the intact **external oblique aponeurosis**[Q].

Diagnosis
- **Ultrasound** or **CT** of the abdomen can be **useful to establish** the **diagnosis**[Q].

Treatment
- A spigelian hernia is **repaired** because of the **risk for incarceration**[Q] associated with its **relatively narrow neck**.
- Defect is **closed transversely by simple suture repair**[Q] of the transversus abdominis and internal oblique muscles, followed by closure of the external oblique aponeurosis.
- **Larger defects** are repaired using a **mesh prosthesis**[Q].
- **Recurrence** is **uncommon**[Q].

SLIDING HERNIA (HERNIA EN GLISSADE)

Sliding Hernia (Hernia en Glissade)

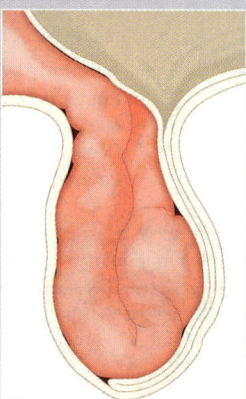

- Hernias in which **posterior wall of** the **sac is formed by a viscus**[Q]
- Viscera is **liable to be injured,** if the **hernia sac is resected during surgery**[Q]
- **More common** on **left side**[Q]

Most Common Content	
• Left side: **Sigmoid colon**[Q] & its mesentery (**MC**)	• Right side: **Cecum**[Q]

- **Other contents**: Appendix, urinary bladder, uterus, fallopian tube, ovary or ureter
- **Primary danger**: Failure to recognize the **visceral component** of hernia sac **before injury to the bowel or bladder**[Q].

Clinical Features
- Occurs almost exclusively in **men**[Q].
- **More common** on the **left side**[Q]; rarely bilateral
- Patient is **nearly always over 40 years of age**, the incidence rising with age[Q].

> • Occasionally, **large intestine is strangulated** in a **sliding hernia**; more often, **non-strangulated large intestine is present behind the sac containing strangulated small intestine**[Q].

Treatment
- **Operation** is indicated
- **Sliding hernia contents** are reduced into the peritoneal cavity, and **any excess hernia sac is ligated & divided**[Q].

> • Sliding hernia is a cause of considerable discomfort, **impossible to control with a truss**[Q].

LUMBAR HERNIA

Lumbar Hernia

- Lumbar hernias can be either **congenital (20%)** or **acquired (80%)**[Q]
- Occur in the **lumbar region** of the **posterior abdominal wall**[Q].
- **More common** on **left side, in men**[Q]

> • Hernias through the **superior lumbar triangle (Grynfeltt's triangle)** are **more common**[Q].
> • **Grynfeltt's triangle** is bounded by the **12th rib, paraspinal muscles & internal oblique muscle**[Q].

- **Less common** are hernias through the **inferior lumbar triangle (Petit's triangle)**[Q]
- **Petit's triangle** is bounded by **iliac crest, latissimus dorsi muscle, & external oblique muscle**[Q].
- **Weakness of lumbodorsal fascia** through either of these areas results in **progressive protrusion of extraperitoneal fat** and a **hernia sac**[Q].

Clinical Features
- **MC presentation**: Unilateral bulge in the flank[Q].
- Lumbar hernias are **not prone to incarceration**[Q].

Treatment
- Lumbar hernia be repaired at the **time of discovery**; the exception is in **newborns** and be undertaken after a child is **6 months of age**^{Q}.
- **Dowd's operation** is done for **lumbar hernia**^{Q}.
- **Repair** is **best done by placement of prosthetic mesh**, which can be sutured to the margins of the hernia^Q.

OBTURATOR HERNIA

Obturator Hernia

- Also known as **skinny old lady hernia** or **French hernia**^{Q}.
- **Thin, elderly, & debilitated women** are at greatest risk
- More common in **female** secondary to the **larger & more oblique** design of the **obturator canal**^{Q}.
- Occur more frequently on the **right** in **female** patients and on the **left** in **male** patients^Q.
- **Bilateral** in **6%** cases.

Predisposing Factors	
• Women with **wider pelvis & more triangular obturator canal**^{Q} • **Malnutrition**^{Q}	• Chronic constipation, COPD, ascites, kyphoscoliosis^Q • **Multiparity**^{Q} • Age **70-79 years**^{Q}

Clinical Features
- Patients present **most commonly with intestinal obstruction**^{Q} (jejunum or ileum within the hernial sac).

Howship-Romberg Sign^Q	• **Pain radiating down** the **medial thigh** to the **knee** due to compression of obturator nerve (anterior division) by the hernial sac • **Pathognomonic for** an **incarcerated hernia** • Present in **25-50%** cases
Hannington Kiff sign^Q	• Absence of the **obturator reflex** in the thigh **due to compression of obturator nerve.**

Treatment
- **Operation** is **indicated**
- **Posterior approach** (either open or laparoscopic) **is preferred**^{Q}.

PARADUODENAL HERNIA

Paraduodenal Hernia

- It is the **MC** variety of **congenital internal hernia**^{Q}
- Nearly **75%** are **left-sided, more common** in **male**s

> • Herniation into the **left Paraduodenal fossa (Fossa of Landzert**^{Q}**)** occurs more frequently than herniation into the **right fossa (Fossa of Kolb**^{Q}**)**.

- **Small bowel herniate** through the **vascular arch of Treitz** formed by the **inferior mesenteric vein** and the **ascending branch of left colic artery**^{Q}
- **Herniated bowel** is **posterior** to the **mesocolon**; with the **afferent limb** being the **4 part of** the **duodenum** and **efferent limb** being the **terminal ileum**^{Q}.

Clinical Features
- Occur between **4 to 5 decade**

> • **Postprandial pain with postural variation** is a **characteristic symptom**^{Q}

- Commonly PDH manifest as **acute intestinal obstruction.** Life time risk of **incarceration** is **50%**.

Diagnosis
- On barium study the **small bowel** is **clustered** to the **left of the midline** with a well-circumscribed edge that corresponds to the hernial sac.
- However **all radiologic studies may be normal** especially in **chronic intermittent cases**, because hernia may **reduce spontaneously**. These investigations are **most often diagnostic** during an **acute episode**^{Q}.

Treatment
- **Reduction of hernia sac** and **closure of the defect**^{Q} or incision of the hernia sac

UMBILICAL HERNIA

Umbilical Hernia

- Umbilical hernias **in infants** are **congenital**^Q and are quite common.
- **Strong predisposition** in individuals of **African descent**.
- **Close spontaneously** in most cases by the **age of 2 years**^Q.
- **Complications** are **unusual**^Q.
- Those that **persist after the age of 5 years** are frequently **repaired surgically**^Q

Indications of Surgery in Umbilical Hernia	
• Persisting **beyond 5 years**^Q • **Symptomatic**^Q • **Strangulated**^Q	• Defect **size >2 cm**^Q • **Progressive enlarging**^Q hernia after the age 1-2 years

Treatment
- **Small defects: Closed primarily**^Q
- **Defects >3 cm: Closed using prosthetic mesh**^Q.

Mayo's Repair
- **Vest-over-pants repair** proposed by Mayo employs **imbrication of superior** and **inferior fascial edges**^Q.
- Because of **increased tension on** the **repair** and **recurrence rates** of 30%, it is **rarely performed today**^Q.

Abdominal Wall Defects

Omphalocele	Gastroschisis
• **Intestine fails to return**, abdominal **contents protruding** directly **through** the **umbilical ring** with a **sac covering** the **bowel**^Q • **Abdominal contents** are **covered with peritoneum** on the **inside & amnion on the outside**^Q. • **Size of defect** is **variable**, ranging from a small opening through which a **small portion of intestine** is herniated to a **large one** in which **entire bowel & liver** are **included**^Q. • **Chromosomal abnormalities**^Q are present in roughly **30%** of infants, including **trisomies 13, 18 & 21**^Q. • **More than half** of infants have other **major** or **minor malformations**, with **cardiac being** the **most common**^Q, followed by musculoskeletal, gastrointestinal & genitourinary. • Close association with **Beckwith-Wiedemann syndrome**^Q (omphalocele, hyperinsulinemia, and macroglossia). • **Poor prognosis**^Q due to **associated abnormalities**.	• **Fetal gut** is **extruded** through a defect in abdominal wall • **Defect** is **always on** the **right side of umbilical ring** with an **intact umbilical cord**^Q • **Covering sac is absent**^Q. • **Risk for associated anomalies** is **low**^Q. • **Association with intestinal atresia** in up to 15%. • Atresias may involve the **small and large intestine**^Q. • Babies are more often **small for gestational age** and **born to mothers with** a history of **cigarette, alcohol, and recreational drug use** and intake of **aspirin, ibuprofen, and pseudoephedrine** during the first trimester^Q • **Increased risk in mothers younger than 20 years**^Q. • In patients with gastroschisis, the **intestine** is often **thickened, edematous, matted together,** and **foreshortened**^Q. • **Good prognosis**^Q

EPIGASTRIC HERNIA (FATTY HERNIA OF THE LINEA ALBA, EPIGASTRIC LIPOMA)

Epigastric Hernia (Fatty Hernia of the Linea Alba, Epigastric Lipoma)

- About 3% to 5% of the population has epigastric hernias.
- **More common** in **men**^Q.
- **Located between** the **xiphoid process & umbilicus**^Q

> • **Multiple in** up to 20% of patients, and **about 80% are just off**^Q the midline.

- Usually **within 5 to 6 cm of** the **umbilicus**.
- **Defects** are **small** and often **produce pain out of proportion** to their size owing to **incarceration of preperitoneal fat**^Q.

Clinical Features
- **Majority** of these hernias are **asymptomatic**
- Sometimes such a hernia gives rise to **attacks of local pain**. This may be because the **fatty contents become nipped sufficiently** to produce **partial strangulation**^Q.

> • **Referred pain**: It is not uncommon to find that the patient, who may not have noticed the hernia, complains of **pain suggestive of a peptic ulcer**^Q.

Treatment
- Repair usually consists of **excision of** the **incarcerated preperitoneal tissue & simple closure of the fascial defect**^Q.

INCISIONAL HERNIA

Incisional Hernia

- Postoperative ventral abdominal wall hernia or incisional hernia is the result of a **failure of fascial tissues to heal** & **close** following laparotomy[Q].
- As the approximated **fascial tissue separates**, bowel & omentum herniates through the opening, **covered by a peritoneal sac**[Q].

> - **Highest incidence** is seen with **large, midline, vertical, lower abdominal incisions**[Q].
> - **Incidence** seems to be **lower in smaller incisions**

- Modern rates of incisional hernia range from **2-11%**.
- **One-third** of these hernias will present **5-10 years postoperatively**.

Risk Factors for Incisional Hernia		
Surgery Related	**Surgeon Related**	**Patient Related**
• Emergency surgery[Q] • Wound infection[Q] • Midline vertical incisions[Q]	• Wounds closed under **excessive tension**[Q] • Poor technique[Q] • Use of **absorbable sutures**[Q]	• Advanced age, malnutrition[Q] • Ascites, Steroid use[Q] • Diabetes, obesity[Q] • Smoking, coughing[Q] • Vomiting & distension[Q]

Clinical Features
- **Bulge** in the abdominal wall originating deep to the skin scar.
- Symptoms aggravated by **coughing** or **straining** as the hernia contents protrude through the abdominal wall defect.
- In **large ventral hernias**, the **skin** may present with **ischemic** or **pressure necrosis** leading to **frank ulceration**[Q].

Treatment
- **Operative repair**: Primary **suture repair** of the hernia, **open repair** with prosthetic mesh, and **laparoscopic incisional hernia repair**[Q].

> • Laparoscopic incisional hernia repair (**IPOM**- Intraperitoneal onlay mesh repair) has the **lowest rate of recurrence**[Q]

- Major complication from **open, nonmesh incisional hernia repair**: Recurrence[Q]
- **Recurrence rates** vary between **10-50%**, typically reduced by **>50%** with the use of prosthetic mesh
- Risk of recurrence is likely **related to the tension** placed on the repair in large hernias
- Incisional hernias with a **diameter >4 cm** should be **repaired with mesh**[Q].

UMBILICAL ADENOMA OR RASPBERRY TUMOUR

Umbilical adenoma or Raspberry tumour

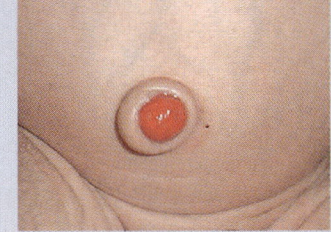

- **Commonly seen in infants** but only occasionally later in life[Q].
- Due to a **partially** (occasionally a completely) **unobliterated vitellointestinal duct**[Q].
- **Mucosa prolapsing through** the umbilicus gives rise to a **raspberry-like tumour**[Q]
- **Moist** and **tends to bleed**

Treatment
- **Pedunculated tumour**: A **ligature is tied around**[Q] it, in a few days, the polypus drops off.
- If tumour reappears after this procedure: **Umbilectomy**[Q]

DESMOID TUMOR

Desmoid Tumor

- MC primary malignant neoplasm of the mesentery: Desmoid tumor
- Arises from **musculoaponeurotic structures** of abdominal wall, especially **below** the level of umbilicus[Q].
- It is a **completely unencapsulated fibroma**[Q] and is **so hard** that it **creaks when it is cut**[Q].
- Distribution: Extra-abdominal (60%), abdominal wall (25%), intra-abdominal (15%).
- About **80% of cases** occur **in women**[Q], many of whom have borne children

> • Occurs **occasionally in scars**[Q] of old hernial or other abdominal **operation wounds**.
> • **Surgical trauma**[Q]: Important etiological factor
> • **Estrogens stimulate**[Q] desmoid growth
> • Occur in cases of **FAP**[Q] **(Gardener's syndrome)**

Pathology
- Tumour is composed of **fibrous tissue** containing **multinucleated plasmodial masses** resembling **foreign body giant cells**[Q].
- Usually of **very slow growth**, it **tends to infiltrate muscle** in the **immediate area**[Q].
- Eventually it **undergoes a myxomatous change** and it then **increases in size more rapidly**.
- **Metastasis does not occur**[Q], no sarcomatous change

Clinical Features
- **Desmoids classically arise in pregnancy** as an **abdominal mass independent of uterus**.
- **MC presentation: Abdominal mass**
- Affected patients may present with a **painful versus asymptomatic firm mass, bowel obstruction, or bowel ischemia**.

Diagnosis
- **MRI** is **investigation of choice** for extremity & abdominal wall desmoids[Q].
- **Biopsy** is required to **establish the diagnosis**.

Treatment
- **Wide local excision** (with **2 cm margin**) is **treatment of choice**[Q].
- **Surgery + Radiotherapy:** For **recurrent desmoid tumors**[Q]
- Doxorubicin, dacarbazine, or carboplatin can produce remission in up to 50% of patients.

Prognosis
- Involvement of margins is associated with **recurrence rates** as high as **80%**.

Multiple Choice Questions

CLASSIFICATION OF HERNIA

1. Type IIIA in Nyhus classification of hernia:
   (MCI November 2017, DNB 2011)
   a. Direct inguinal hernia   b. Indirect inguinal hernia
   c. Femoral hernia   d. Umbilical hernia

2. Type 7 Gilbert hernia is:
   a. Direct inguinal hernia   b. Indirect inguinal hernia
   c. Femoral hernia   d. Umbilical hernia

3. Femoral hernia in Nyhus classification: *(WBPG 2014)*
   a. IIIA   b. II
   c. IIIC   d. IV

RISK FACTORS FOR HERNIA

4. The following are the risk factors for inguinal hernia:
   a. Family history of inguinal hernia *(PGI Dec 2007)*
   b. Weight lifter   c. COPD
   d. Female   e. Obesity

INGUINAL HERNIA

5. Most common type of hernia in females is:
   (AIIMS Feb 97, DPG 2005, JIPMER GIS 2011)
   a. Direct inguinal hernia   b. Indirect inguinal hernia
   c. Femoral hernia   d. Umbilical hernia

6. For differentiating inguinal hernia and femoral hernia the landmark will be: *(AIIMS Nov 98)*
   a. Public symphysis   b. Femoral artery
   c. Inferior epigastric level d. Public tubercle

INDIRECT INGUINAL HERNIA

7. True about inguinal hernia: *(PGI June 2003)*
   a. It is more common in female
   b. Right sided is more common than left side
   c. Direct hernia is less likely to undergo strangulation
   d. Femoral hernia is more common in female

8. All of the following statements are true about repair of groin hernias except: *(AIIMS Nov 2004)*
   a. Lichtenstein tension free repair has a low recurrence rate
   b. TEP repair is an extraperitoneal approach to laparoscopic repair of groin hernia
   c. In Shouldice repair, non-absorbable mesh is used
   d. The surgery can be done under local anesthesia in selected cases

9. Most important step in the repair of an indirect inguinal hernia is:
   a. Herniotomy
   b. Narrowing of the internal ring
   c. Bassini's repair
   d. Transfixation of the neck of the sac

10. The treatment of choice for inguinal hernia in infants is:
    (MCI June 2018)
    a. Herniotomy   b. Herniorrhaphy
    c. Truss   d. Hernioplasty

11. On examination of the patient for a hernia, it is useful to realize that:
    a. An impulse is often much better seen than felt
    b. The internal abdominal ring lies 1.25 cm above the midpoint of poupart's ligament
    c. The external abdominal ring lies 1.25 cm above and medial to ASIS
    d. None of the above

12. A patient is advised to avoid strenuous activity following herniorrhaphy for a period of:
    a. One day   b. One week
    c. 3 weeks   d. 6 weeks

13. Which one of the following is not performed in Lichtenstein tension free hernioplasty? *(Karnataka 2006)*
    a. High ligation of indirect hernia sac
    b. Mesh sutured to the conjoint tendon and inguinal ligament
    c. Conjoint tendon sutured to inguinal ligament
    d. Spermatic cord is placed in two tails of the internal ring

14. True statement regarding direct inguinal hernia: *(UPPG 2008)*
    a. Most common inguinal hernia in women is direct
    b. Direct hernia is medial to inferior epigastric artery
    c. Repair of the transversalis fascia and the internal ring
    d. Descends downwards and inwards towards the scrotum

15. Content of epilocele is: *(DNB 2011)*
    a. Omentum   b. Intestine
    c. Colon   d. Urinary bladder

16. Triangle of Doom is bounded by all of the following except:
    (AIIMS Nov 2008)
    a. Cooper's ligament   b. Vas deferens
    c. Gonadal vessels   d. Peritoneal reflection

17. Which of the following is correct regarding the boundaries of triangle of Doom? *(AIIMS May 2018)*
    a. Medially vas deferens, laterally gonadal vessels, inferiorly peritoneum
    b. Laterally vas deferens, medially gonadal vessels, inferiorly peritoneum
    c. Laterally medial umbilical ligament, medially gonadal vessels, inferiorly peritoneum
    d. Laterally gonadal vessels, medially lateral umbilical ligament, inferiorly peritoneum

18. What is the name of this triangle?
    a. Triangle of doom   b. Triangle of pain
    c. Triangle of death   d. Corona mortis

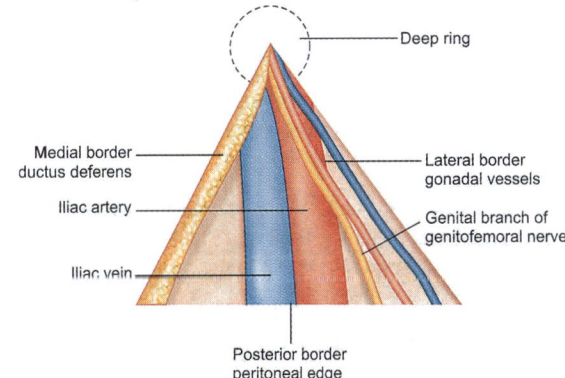

19. True regarding indirect inguinal hernia are all except:
    a. Most common type of hernia   (MCI March 2008)
    b. Always unilateral
    c. Inguinal herniotomy is the basic operation
    d. Transillumination distinguishes it from hydocele

20. Most common type of hernia in the young age group:
                                             (MCI Sept 2006)
    a. Femoral hernia   b. Direct inguinal hernia
    c. Indirect inguinal hernia   d. Umbilical hernia

21. Least recurrence rate in incisional hernia repair is following:
                                             (JIPMER 2010)
    a. On lay mesh repair   b. Intraperitoneal mesh repair
    c. Inlay mesh repair   d. Shouldice repair

22. Inguinal herniotomy includes all of the following except:
    a. Dissection and opening of the hernial sac   (Orissa 2011)
    b. Reduction of contents
    c. Transfixation of the neck and excision of redundant sac
    d. Repair of stretched inguinal ring and fascia transversalis

23. Hesselbach's triangle is bounded by the following, except:
    a. Rectus abdominis muscle   (Orissa 2011)
    b. Transversus abdominis muscle
    c. Inferior epigastric artery
    d. Inguinal ligament

24. Ilioinguinal nerve is damaged while incising:
    a. External oblique aponeurosis   (MHSSMCET 2006)
    b. Internal oblique muscle
    c. Transverse abdominis
    d. Linea alba

25. Shouldice repair is: (PGI SS June 2007)
    a. Multilayered repair of inguinal canal
    b. Conjoint tendon is sutured to inguinal ligament
    c. Conjoint tendon is sutured to Cooper's ligament
    d. Transabdominal repair

26. Are true about hernia repair except: (JIPMER GIS 2011)
    a. Bassini's repair is between inguinal ligament and conjoint tendon
    b. Shouldice repair is involvement of the posterior wall strengthening
    c. Mcvay's repair is for femoral hernia
    d. Lichtenstein is a tension free-mesh repair

27. Funicular hernia is type of: (DNB 2007)
    a. Direct inguinal hernia   b. Indirect inguinal hernia
    c. Femoral Hernia   d. Umbilical hernia

28. A child presented with a swelling in the right groin region. When the swelling was reduced, a gurgling sound was heard. Which of the following is an incorrect statement?
                                             (AIIMS November 2015)
    a. The sac contains omentum only
    b. The hernia lies above and medial to pubic tubercle
    c. Patent processus vaginalis
    d. This type of hernia is most common in children

29. A 3-year-old child comes with hydrocele of the hernia sac. Management will include: (AIIMS May 2015)
    a. Herniotomy   b. Herniorrhapy
    c. Observation only   d. Operate after 5 years of age

30. Triangle of doom is related to: (Recent Question 2014)
    a. Laparoscopic Nissen's fundoplication
    b. Laparoscopic hernia surgery
    c. Endoscopic thyroidectomy
    d. Thoracoscopic thymectomy

31. Inguinal hernia in a child is associated with:
                                             (Recent Question 2017)
    a. Patent processus vaginalis   b. Ectopia vesicae
    c. Undescended testis   d. All are correct

32. Triangle of doom is seen during which type of hernia surgery: (Recent Question 2017)
    a. Laparoscopic   b. Open
    c. Both   d. None

COMPLICATIONS OF HERNIA

33. Which of these would you like to do for a case of strangulated hernia?   (PGI June 2002)
    a. X-ray   b. USG abdomen
    c. Aspiration of contents of sac
    d. Correction of hypovolemia
    e. Prepare OT for urgent surgery

34. In a case of strangulated hernia management is:
                                             (PGI June 2006, Dec 2006)
    a. USG-abdomen   b. X-ray abdomen
    c. Aspirate contents   d. Immediate surgery
    e. IV fluids

35. Which of the following is not done in case of obstructed inguinal hernia?   (PGI June 2003, PGI Dec 2001)
    a. Aspiration of the sac for diagnosis
    b. X-ray abdomen
    c. USG abdomen
    d. Do early surgery

36. During surgery of hernia, the sac of a strangulated inguinal hernia should be opened at the:
                                             (AIIMS Nov 96, AIIMS June 2004)
    a. Neck   b. Body
    c. Fundus   d. Deep ring

37. Treatment of strangulated hernia is: (Kerala 94)
    a. Observation   b. Immediate surgery
    c. Manual reduction   d. Analgesics

38. Which is the 1st sign of strangulation of inguinal hernia?
    a. Tense   b. Tenderness   (UPPG 96)
    c. Irreducible   d. Redness

39. During laparoscopic inguinal hernia repair a tacker was accidently placed below and lateral to the iliopubic tract. Postoperatively the patient complained of pain and soreness in the thigh. This is due to the involvement of:
                                             (AIIMS November 2015, May 2015)
    a. Lateral cutaneous nerve of thigh
    b. Ilioinguinal nerve
    c. Genital branch of genitofemoral nerve
    d. Obturator nerve

40. Most common nerve injured during hernia surgery:
                                             (Recent Question 2017, 2014)
    a. Ilioinguinal nerve   b. Iliohypogastric nerve
    c. Genitofemoral nerve d. None of the above

FEMORAL HERNIA

41. True about femoral hernia is: (PGI Dec 98)
    a. Occurs exclusively in females
    b. Pregnancy is common cause
    c. Doesn't strangulate
    d. In males associated with cryptorchidism

42. What is the type of hernia?
    a. Direct inguinal hernia   b. Indirect inguinal hernia
    c. Femoral hernia   d. Obturator hernia

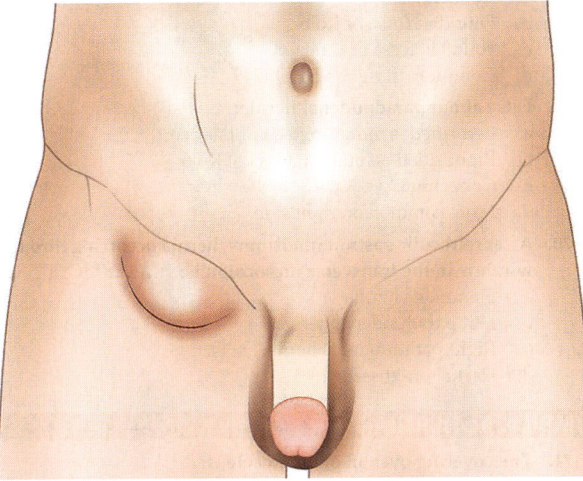

43. Which structures live immediately lateral to femoral hernia? *(AIIMS Nov 2011)*
    a. Lateral cutaneous nerve of thigh
    b. Femoral nerve
    c. Femoral artery
    d. Femoral vein

44. Femoral hernia is characteristically ..... the public tubercle. *(MHPGMCET 2007, TN 89)*
    a. Lateral and below   b. Medial and above
    c. Lateral and above   d. Medial and below

45. In the treatment of femoral hernia, Lockwood's operation refers to: *(Karnataka 2006)*
    a. Low inguinal operation   b. High inguinal operation
    c. Inguinal operation   d. Laparoscopic surgery

46. Strangulation most commonly occurs in: *(DNB 2012, MCI Sept 2005)*
    a. Femoral hernia
    b. Direct inguinal hernia
    c. Indirect inguinal hernia
    d. Lumbar hernia

47. Medial boundary of femoral ring is formed by: *(JIPMER 2011)*
    a. Inguinal ligament
    b. Pectineal ligament
    c. Lacunar ligament
    d. Septum separating it from femoral vein

48. A patient with femoral hernia can be managed by:
    a. Bassini repair   b. Hunters repair
    c. Shouldice repair   d. McVay repair

49. Hernia that lies under the fascia of pectineus muscle is: *(MHSSMCET 2006)*
    a. Cloquet's hernia   b. Laugier's hernia
    c. Narath's hernia   d. Obturator hernia

50. In Laugier's hernia opening is in the: *(WBPG 2014)*
    a. Lacunar ligament   b. Conjoint tendon
    c. External oblique   d. Peritoneum

51. Neck of sac of femoral hernia lies: *(Recent Question 2013)*
    a. Below and lateral to pubic tubercle
    b. Above and lateral
    c. Above and medial
    d. Below and medial

SPIGELIAN HERNIA

52. All are true about Spigelian hernia except:
    a. Usually occurs above arcuate line   *(JIPMER GIS 2011)*
    b. Picked up by USG or CT
    c. Hernia sac will be posterior to the external oblique aponeurosis
    d. Usually small and asymptomatic

53. Spigelian hernia is seen in: *(All India 99)*
    a. Lumbar triangle   b. Subumbilical region
    c. Paraumbilical region   d. Supraumbilical region

54. Spigelian hernia is a type of hernia occurring at:
    (Recent Question 2013 PGI June 95, PGI June 2000)
    a. Medial border of rectus abdominis
    b. Lateral border of rectus abdominis
    c. Lumbar region
    d. Femoral canal

55. Spigelian hernia is: *(MCI March 2005)*
    a. Passes through the obturator canal
    b. Hernia occurring through the linea alba
    c. Hernia through the triangle of Petit
    d. Hernia occurring at the level of arcuate line

56. Spigelian hernia is a defect within the following muscle:
    (COMEDK 2004)
    a. Rectus abdominis   b. Internal oblique
    c. Transversalis abdominis   d. External oblique

57. True statement regarding Spigelian hernia is: *(PGI May 2018)*
    a. Protrudes through linea alba
    b. Occurs at the termination of transverse abdominis muscle
    c. Occurs at the lateral edge of rectus abdominis muscle
    d. Content of hernia mostly include small intestine
    e. Surgery is the treatment of choice

SLIDING HERNIA

58. Most common content in 'Hernia en glissade' is:
    (PGI June 96, All India 95)
    a. Omentum   b. Urinary bladder
    c. Caecum   d. Sigmoid colon

59. What is the name of this hernia?
    a. Ogilvie's hernia   b. Hernia-en-Glissade
    c. Pantaloon's hernia   d. Spigelian hernia

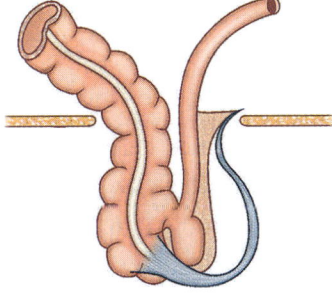

60. Viscera forms wall of which hernia? *(PGI Dec 95)*
    a. Lumbar hernia
    b. Sliding hernia
    c. Epigastric hernia
    d. Femoral hernia
61. Sliding constituent of a large direct hernia is: *(All India 88)*
    a. Bladder
    b. Sigmoid colon
    c. Caecum
    d. Appendix
62. Most useful investigation in sliding hernia in female: *(UPPG 2008)*
    a. Fluroscopy
    b. Barium-meal
    c. Palpation method
    d. Ultrasound
63. If caecum is involved as a part of the wall of hernia sac and is not its content, then it will be known as: *(Recent Question 2014, 2008)*
    a. Richter's hernia
    b. Spigelian hernia
    c. Sliding hernia
    d. Interstitial hernia

LUMBAR HERNIA

64. About lumbar hernia, false statements:
    a. Superior triangle is Grynfeltt's triangle
    b. Inferior triangle is Petit's triangle
    c. Mostly acquired
    d. More common on right side
65. Which of the following statement is incorrect about this hernia?

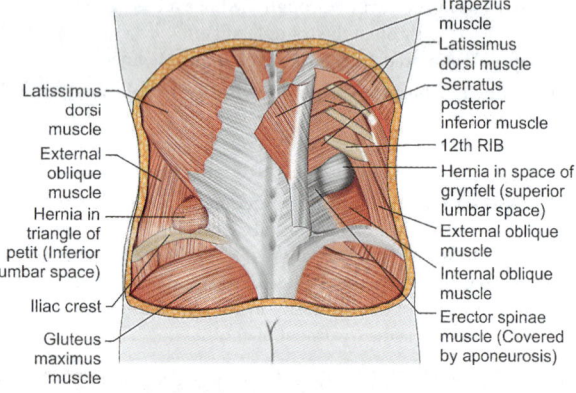

    a. More commonly congenital
    b. Hernia through Grynfeltt's triangle is more common
    c. Petit's triangle is bounded by the iliac crest, latissimus dorsi and external oblique muscle
    d. Grynfeltt's triangle is bounded by 12th rib, paraspinal and internal oblique muscle

OBTURATOR HERNIA

66. True about obturator hernia in adults: *(PGI Nov 2009)*
    a. More common in space of Lorentz
    b. Common in female
    c. Chronic constipation risk factor
    d. Surgical treatment should be done
    e. May present with intestinal obstruction
67. Howship-Romberg sign is seen in: *(JIPMER SS 2016, Recent Question 2016)*
    a. Sliding hernia
    b. Obturator hernia
    c. Lumbar hernia
    d. Paraduodenal hernia

PARADUODENAL HERNIA

68. False about paraduodenal hernia: *(PGI Nov 2009)*
    a. Congenital
    b. Found in fossa of Kolb
    c. Found in fossa of Landzert
    d. Common on right side
69. False about paraduodenal hernia: *(AIIMS GIS 2003)*
    a. Left sided is found in fossa of Landzert
    b. Right sided is found in fossa of Kolb
    c. Congenital
    d. More common on right side
70. After retrocolic gastrojejunostomy, hernia occurring through window in the transverse mesocolon is: *(MHSSMCET 2008)*
    a. Stammer's hernia
    b. Left paraduodenal hernia
    c. Right paraduodenal hernia
    d. Hernia-en-glissede

UMBILICAL HERNIA

71. The covering over an omphalocele is:
    a. Skin
    b. Amniotic membrane
    c. Chorionic membrane
    d. None of the above
72. Omphalocele is caused by: *(DNB 2010)*
    a. Duplication of intestinal loops
    b. Abnormal rotation of the intestinal loop
    c. Failure of gut to return to the body cavity from its physiological herniation
    d. Reversed rotation of the intestinal loop
73. In Moore's classification of omphalocele (exomphalos), type I umbilical defect is less than .. cm:
    a. 0.5
    b. 2.5
    c. 3.5
    d. 4.5
74. Exomphalos major should be operated at: *(DNB 91)*
    a. Birth
    b. 3 months of age
    c. 1 year
    d. 3 years
75. Mayo's operation is done for: *(Recent Question 2016)*
    a. Spigelian hernia
    b. Femoral hernia
    c. Richter's hernia
    d. Umbilical hernia
76. What is the most probable diagnosis based on the given image? *(Recent Question 2017)*

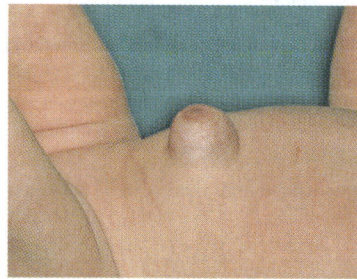

    a. Omphalocele
    b. Gastroschisis
    c. Umbilical hernia
    d. Ectopia vesicae
77. Umbilical hernia in a child - indication for surgery is/are: *(MAHE 2007)*
    a. Failure to disappear by 3 years
    b. >2 cm size
    c. Symptomatic
    d. All of the above

78. What is false regarding gastroschisis and omphalocele? *(DNB 2012, AIIMS 2000)*
    a. Intestinal obstruction is common in gastroschisis
    b. Gastroschisis is associated with multiple anomalies
    c. Umbilical cord is attached in normal position in gastroschisis
    d. Liver is the content of omphalocele

79. Hernia that is least likely to strangulate is: *(AIIMS Nov 93)*
    a. Femoral hernia
    b. Direct inguinal hernia
    c. Indirect inguinal hernia
    d. Umbilical hernia

80. Incidence of exomphalos: *(MHPGMCET 2006)*
    a. 1 in 1000
    b. 1 in 3000
    c. 1 in 5000
    d. 1 in 10,000

81. True regarding gastroschisis is: *(DNB 2003)*
    a. An omphalocele
    b. An anterior abdominal wall tumor
    c. A variant of gastric carcinoma
    d. Herniation of abdominal contents through body wall

82. What is the diagnosis based on the given image?
    a. Gastroschisis
    b. Omphalocele
    c. Umbilical hernia
    d. Ectopia vesicae

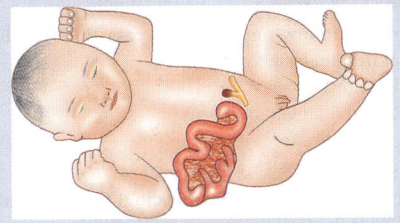

83. What is the diagnosis based on the given image? *(Recent Question 2017)*
    a. Gastroschisis
    b. Omphalocele
    c. Umbilical hernia
    d. Epigastric hernia

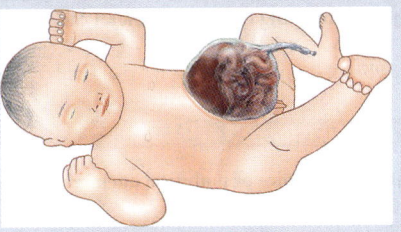

84. In omphalocele abdominal wall defect is more than:
    a. 0.5 cm
    b. 2.5 cm *(WBPG 2014)*
    c. 4 cm
    d. 6 cm

85. Omphalocele is caused by: *(Recent Question 2019)*
    a. Duplication of intestinal loops
    b. Abnormal rotation of intestinal loops
    c. Failure of gut to return to body cavity after its physiological herniation
    d. Reversed rotation of intestinal loops

EPIGASTRIC HERNIA

86. The hernia which often simulates a peptic ulcer is: *(WB PG 2015, MCI March 2007, Karnataka 94)*
    a. Umbilical hernia
    b. Fatty hernia of the linea alba
    c. Incisional hernia
    d. Inguinal hernia

87. True about epigastric hernia is: *(AIIMS May 2012)*
    a. Located below the umbilicus and always in the midline
    b. Located above the umbilicus and always in the midline
    c. Located above the umbilicus and on either side
    d. Can be seen anywhere on abdomen

RICHTER'S HERNIA

88. The sac contains only a portion of the circumference of the intestine: *(UPPG 2007, 2005)*
    a. Richter's hernia
    b. Littre's hernia
    c. Spigelian hernia
    d. Lumbar hernia

89. Strangulation without obstruction is seen in: *(DNB 2005)*
    a. Inguinal hernia
    b. Femoral hernia
    c. Richter's hernia
    d. Littres hernia

90. Richter hernia is most common in: *(Recent Question 2014)*
    a. Hiatus hernia
    b. Femoral hernia
    c. Lumbar hernia
    d. Direct inguinal hernia

LITTRE'S HERNIA

91. Which of the following is content of Littre's hernia? *(DNB 2012, MHPGMET 2005)*
    a. Urinary bladder
    b. Meckel's diverticulum
    c. Circumference of intestinal wall
    d. Appendix

92. Hernia containing Meckel's diverticulum is: *(MHSSMCET 2005)*
    a. Richter's hernia
    b. Pantaloon hernia
    c. Littre's hernia
    d. Mydel's hernia

MISCELLANEOUS HERNIA

93. About hernia, false statements: *(PGI Dec 2003)*
    a. In children, indirect inguinal hernia is treated medically
    b. In Richter's hernia, absolute constipation seen
    c. Indirect inguinal hernia is the MC type
    d. Deep inguinal ring is lateral and above the public tubercle

94. True about hernia: *(PGI Dec 2003)*
    a. External abdominal hernia is common
    b. Direct hernia usually acquired
    c. Strangulation is common in femoral hernia
    d. Direct hernia is acquired in old age
    e. TOC for indirect inguinal hernia is surgery

95. True about hernia: *(PGI Dec 2000)*
    a. Direct hernias are usually acquired
    b. Femoral is most common hernia to strangulate
    c. External abdominal hernia are most common
    d. 50% old people suffer from direct type of hernia with strangulation
    e. Treatment of choice for indirect inguinal hernia is surgery

96. Causes of recurrent hernia:
    a. Absorbable sutures
    b. Sliding hernia
    c. Missed sac
    d. Infection

97. Hernia with hydrocele is .... hernia. *(Recent Question 2016)*
    a. Gibbon's
    b. Fruber's
    c. Dobson's
    d. Leobel's

98. Hernia into pouch of Douglas is ...... hernia.
    a. Beclard's
    b. Bochdaleks
    c. Blandin's
    d. Berger's

99. The person whose work on the radical cure of hernia immortalised his name was: *(Karnataka 96)*
    a. William Halsted
    b. Eduardo Bassini
    c. Mc Vay
    d. Koontz
100. Truss cannot prevent progression of which type of inguinal hernia? *(UPPG 99)*
    a. Sliding
    b. Littre's
    c. Indirect
    d. Direct
101. What is the name of this hernia?
    a. Pantaloons' hernia
    b. Sliding hernia
    c. Maydl's hernia
    d. Spigelian hernia

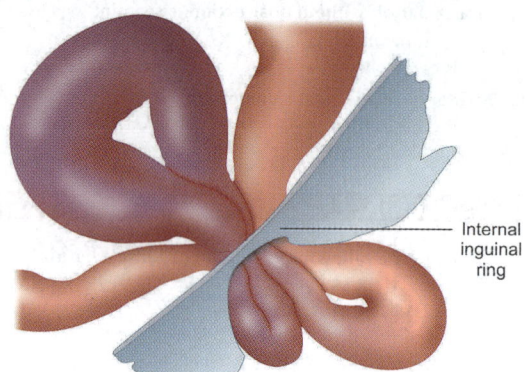

INCISIONAL HERNIA

102. Which of the following does not predispose to abdominal wall dehiscence? *(JIPMER 92)*
    a. Faulty technique
    b. Malignancy
    c. Raised intra-abdominal pressure
    d. Old age
103. Ventral hernia is a/an: *(AMC 99)*
    a. Incisional hernia
    b. Umbilical hernia
    c. Femoral hernia
    d. Inguinal hernia
104. Incisional hernia, not true is: *(DPG 2006)*
    a. Faulty operative technique
    b. There is distension of abdomen
    c. Associated with infection of the wound
    d. Caused by use of local anesthesia
105. Hernia prone to re-occur apter primary repair: *(JIPMER 2013)*
    a. Femoral
    b. Epigastric
    c. Spigelian
    d. Incisional
106. Point A in the given image represents which type of repair for ventral hernia? *(Recent Question 2016)*
    a. Onlay
    b. Inlay
    c. Retromuscular
    d. Preperitoneal

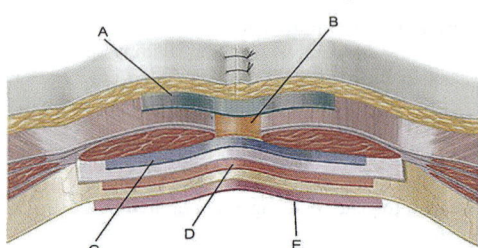

HERNIA AND ABDOMINAL WALL ANATOMY

107. A patient operated for direct inguinal hernia developed anesthesia at the root of the penis and adjacent part of the scrotum, the nerve likely to be injured is: *(AIIMS Nov 2001)*
    a. Genital branch of genitofemoral nerve (supply dartos muscle)
    b. Femoral branch of genitofemoral nerve
    c. Iliohypogastric nerve
    d. Ilioinguinal nerve
108. During repair of indirect inguinal hernia, while releasing the constriction at the deep inguinal ring, the surgeon takes care not to damage one of the following structures:
    a. Falx inguinalis (conjoint tendon) *(AIIMS Nov 2003)*
    b. Interfovelar ligament
    c. Inferior epigastric artery
    d. Spermatic cord
109. Preservation of ilioinguinal nerve is an important step in inguinal hernia operation while: *(UPSC 97)*
    a. Incising the subcutaneous tissue
    b. Incising the external oblique aponeurosis
    c. Incising the cremasteric fascia
    d. Isolating the sac
110. All of the following structures pass through the inguinal cannal in females except: *(All India 2012)*
    a. Ilioinguinal nerve
    b. Round ligament of uterus
    c. Lymphatics from uterus
    d. Inferior epigastric artery
111. Which of the following is true about deep inguinal ring?
    a. Defect in fascia transversalis *(DPG 97)*
    b. Transmits deep inferior epigastric artery
    c. Lies just above and lateral to public tubercle
    d. Opening in external oblique aponeurosis
112. On an average, the distance between femoral ring and saphenous opening (length of femoral canal) is:
    a. 1.25 cm
    b. 2.50 cm
    c. 3.75 cm
    d. 5.00 cm

UMBILICAL ADENOMA

113. Treatment of choice of umbilical adenoma in a new born is:
    a. Occlusion with a coin
    b. Strapping
    c. Surgery
    d. Masterly inactivity
114. "Raspberry tumour" is another name for: *(Recent Question 2013)*
    a. Umbilical fistula
    b. Umbilical granuloma
    c. Umbilical adenoma
    d. Meckel's diverticulum
115. Raspberry tumour is: *(JIPMER 98)*
    a. Neoplastic
    b. Inflammatory
    c. Traumatic
    d. Congenital

DESMOID TUMOR

116. Treatment of desmoid tumor is: *(AIIMS Nov 93)*
    a. Conservative
    b. Radiotherapy
    c. Surgery
    d. Radiotherapy following chemotherapy

117. Regarding desmoid tumour which is not correct?
    a. Often seen below the umbilicus *(DNB 2002)*
    b. Unencapsulated
    c. More common in women
    d. Metastasis does not occur
    e. Highly radiosensitive

118. Recurrent fibroma refers to desmoid tumor arising in:
    a. Uterus
    b. Scar tissue
    c. Ovary
    d. Muscle

119. Treatment of choice of desmoid tumour is: *(AIIMS June 94)*
    a. Surgery
    b. Chemotherapy
    c. Radiotherapy
    d. Surgery + Radiotherapy

120. What is the treatment of choice in desmoid tumors?
    a. Irradiation *(DNB 2009, UPSC 2008)*
    b. Wide excision
    c. Local excision
    d. Local excision following radiation

121. Regarding desmoid tumour, true is: *(MHSSMCET 2011)*
    a. Mostly females are affected
    b. Well-capsulated tumor
    c. Common above the level of umbilicus
    d. Radiotherapy is treatment of choice

122. Most common presentation of abdominal desmoid tumor is: *(AIIMS November 2017)*
    a. Abdominal pain
    b. Abdominal mass
    c. Fever
    d. Rectal prolapse

PATENT VITELLO-INTESTINAL DUCT

123. Patent vitello-intestinal duct should preferably be operated at:
    a. Birth
    b. 6 months of age
    c. 12 months of age
    d. 3 years of age

124. The patent vitello-intestinal duct most often discharges:
    a. Mucus
    b. Pus
    c. Urine
    d. Faeces

PATENT URACHUS

125. A new born presents with discharge of urine from the umbilicus for 3 days. Diagnosis is: *(UPPG 2008)*
    a. Meckel's diverticulum
    b. Mesenteric cysts
    c. Urachal fistula
    d. Umbilical hernia

126. A child complains of fluid coming out of umbilicus on straining. What is the diagnosis? *(AIIMS November 2014)*
    a. Urachal fistula
    b. Gastroschisis
    c. Patent vitellointestinal duct
    d. Congenital umbilical hernia

MISCELLANEOUS

127. Which age group most often present with jaundice due to omphalitis in infants is?
    a. At birth
    b. 24-72 hours
    c. 1-3 weeks
    d. 3-6 weeks

128. Congenital hydrocele is best treated by: *(PGI 2001)*
    a. Eversion of sac
    b. Excision of sac
    c. Lords procedure
    d. Herniotomy

129. Bleeding from the umbilicus in an adult female during menstruation is suggestive of: *(All India 94)*
    a. Bleeding diathesis
    b. Vicarious menstruation
    c. Persistent urachus
    d. Purpura

130. A new born presents with mid anterior abdominal wall defect with characteristic spontaneous disappearance at age 4 years: *(UPPG 2008)*
    a. Patent urachus
    b. Omphalocele
    c. Ectopia vesicae
    d. Umbilical hernia

131. Most common cause of umbilicus not separated at age of 2 years: *(UPPG 2008)*
    a. Raspberry tumour
    b. Leukocyte adhesion deficiency
    c. Patent urachus
    d. Umbilical granuloma

132. Pascal's law is used in which technique of hernia repair?
    a. Lichtenstein mesh repair *(DNB 2010)*
    b. Stoppa's preperitoneal repair
    c. Bassini's repair
    d. Darning repair

133. All of the following are true about hernia surgery except: *(AIIMS Nov 2012)*
    a. Surgery should not be done unless patient becomes symptomatic
    b. Hernia in children is treated with herniotomy
    c. Absorbable mesh should not be used for surgery
    d. Surgery can be done using laparoscopy

134. Method of reduction of inguinal hernia: *(Recent Question 2013)*
    a. Kugel maneuver
    b. Taxis
    c. McVay procedure
    d. Stoppa technique

Explanations

CLASSIFICATION OF HERNIA

1. **Ans. a. Direct inguinal hernia** *(Ref: Sabiston 20/e p1098; Schwartz 10/e p1634-1635)*
2. **Ans. c. Femoral hernia** *(Ref: Schwartz 10/e p1496, 9/e p1316; Schackelford 7/e p567-568)*
3. **Ans. c. IIIC**

RISK FACTORS FOR HERNIA

4. **Ans. a. Family history of inguinal hernia, b. Weight lifter, c. COPD, e. Obesity** *(Ref: Sabiston 20/e p1092; Schwartz 10/e p1500; Bailey 27/e p1023-1024)*

INGUINAL HERNIA

5. **Ans. b. Indirect inguinal hernia** *(Ref: Sabiston 20/e p1092; Schwartz 10/e p1634-1635; Bailey 27/e p1029; Schackelford 8/e p573, 7/e p558)*

   - **MC type** of hernia **in males: Indirect inguinal hernia**^{Q}
   - **MC type** of hernia **in females: Indirect inguinal hernia**^{Q}
   - **Femoral hernia** is **more common in females**^{Q}.
   - **Direct inguinal hernia** is **more common in** the **elderly**^{Q}

6. **Ans. d. Public tubercle** *(Ref: Sabiston 20/e p1092, 19/e p1114, 1126; Schwartz 10/e p1634-1635, 9/e p1308; Bailey 27/e p1029, 26/e p954-960; Schackelford 7/e p561)*

Inguinal Hernia	Femoral Hernia
Neck of sac lies **above** and **medial** to the **pubic tubercle**^{Q}	**Neck of sac** lies **below** and **lateral** to the **pubic tubercle**^{Q}

INDIRECT INGUINAL HERNIA

7. **Ans. b. Right sided is more common than left side, c. Direct hernia is less likely to undergo strangulation, d. Femoral hernia is more common in female** *(Ref: Sabiston 20/e p1092-1093; Schwartz 10/e p1634-1635; Bailey 27/e p1029)*

8. **Ans. c. In Shouldice repair, non-absorbable mesh is used** *(Ref: Sabiston 20/e p1097-1102; Schwartz 10/e p1634-1635; Bailey 27/e p1032; Schackelford 8/e p603, 7/e p568-579)*

   In **Shouldice repair**, inguinal floor is strengthened by approximation of tissues using non-absorbable sutures, **mesh is not used**.

9. **Ans. b. Narrowing of the internal ring**

   Most important step of hernia repair is narrowing of internal ring.

10. **Ans. a. Herniotomy**
11. **Ans. a. An impulse is often much better seen than felt**
12. **Ans. None**

    After herniorrhapy, avoid strenuous activity for 6 months.

13. **Ans. c. Conjoint tendon sutured to inguinal ligament** *(Ref: Sabiston 20/e p1100; Schwartz 10/e p1508; Bailey 27/e p1032; Schackelford 8/e p602, 7/e p576)*

    #### LICHTENSTEIN TENSION-FREE REPAIR

    - Initial **exposure** and **mobilization of cord structures** is identical to other open approaches.
    - Lichtenstein repair **does not include routine division of** the **transversalis fascia**^{Q}.
    - **Internal inguinal ring is not reconstructed** using canal structures.
    - **Floor** and **internal ring** are **reinforced through** the application of the **mesh.** ^{Q}
    - **Mesh** is **split to accommodate** the **spermatic cord**^{Q}.
    - **Rounded edge** is **attached** to the **anterior rectus sheath**^{Q} just medial to the pubic tubercle
    - **Inferior margin** of the mesh is then **sutured to the shelving edge** of the **inguinal ligament**^{Q}

14. **Ans. b. Direct hernia is medial to inferior epigastric artery** *(Ref: Sabiston 20/e p1092-1093; Schwartz 10/e p1503; Bailey 27/e p1029)*

Hernia and Abdominal Wall

	Indirect Hernia	Direct Hernia
Age	• Any age	• Common in **elderly**^Q
Herniation	• **Protrusion** through **deep inguinal ring**; Herniation occurs latter^Q	• **Herniation** through **posterior wall** of inguinal canal
Shape	• **Pyriform/oval** in shape^Q	• **Globular/round** shape
Descent	• **Obliquely** and **downwards**	• **Directly forwards**
Descent to scrotum	• **Descent to** the **bottom of scrotum** and becomes **complete**^Q	• **Rarely** descent to the bottom of the scrotum
Neck	• Narrow^Q	• Wide^Q
Sac	• **Lateral** to **inferior epigastric artery**	• **Medial** to **inferior epigastric artery**
Zieman's test	• **Cough impulse** on **index finger**^Q	• **Cough impulse** on **middle finger**
Invagination test	• **Tip** of finger	• **Pulp** of finger
Ring occlusion test	• **Does not bulge**	• **Bulge medial to occluding finger**
Coverings (from inside out)	• Extraperitoneal tissue • **Internal spermatic fascia**^Q • **Cremasteric fascia**^Q • External spermatic fascia • Skin	• Extraperitoneal tissue • **Fascia transversalis** • **Conjoint tendon** • External spermatic fascia • Skin
	• Commonly **unilateral**	• Commonly **bilateral**^Q
Obstruction/strangulation	• **Common**	• **Rare**
Sac	• Should be **opened during surgery**	• **Not necessary**, unless obstruction is present

15. **Ans. a. Omentum** *(Ref: Bailey 27/e p1031)*
16. **Ans. a. Cooper's ligament** *(Ref: Sabiston 20/e p1101-1102; Schwartz 10/e p1496)*
17. **Ans. a. Medially vas deferens, laterally gonadal vessels, inferiorly peritoneum** *(Ref: Schwartz 10/e p1496; Sabiston 20/e p1101-1102)*
18. **Ans. a. Triangle of Doom**
19. **Ans. b. Always unilateral**
20. **Ans. c. Indirect inguinal hernia**
21. **Ans. b. Intraperitoneal mesh repair**
22. **Ans. d. Repair of stretched inguinal ring and fascia transversalis**
23. **Ans. b. Transversus abdominis muscle** *(Ref: Sabiston 20/e p1096; Bailey 27/e p1033; Schackelford 8/e p599, 7/e p560)*

Hesselbach's Triangle		
Lateral Border	**Medial Border**	**Base**
• Epigastric artery^Q	• **Lateral border** of **rectus abdominis**^Q where it is attached to pubic crest	• **Inguinal ligament**

- **Indirect inguinal hernia** comes out of abdominal cavity **through deep inguinal ring**^Q, travel inguinal canal and becomes superficial through superficial inguinal ring.
- **Direct inguinal hernia** enters inguinal canal through **medial half** of **weak posterior wall** (**Hesselbach's triangle**^Q) and becomes superficial through superficial inguinal ring.

24. **Ans. a. External oblique aponeurosis** *(Ref: Sabiston 20/e p1096; Schwartz 10/e p1495-1517, 1974; Bailey 27/e p1029)*

External oblique aponeurosis is in close relation to ilioinguinal nerve and hence during operation for inguinal hernia, prevention of injury to ilioinguinal nerve to avoid later development of incisional hernia is very important.

Nerves in Relation to Inguinal Hernia

Ilioinguinal Nerve	Iliohypogastric Nerve	Genitofemoral Nerve
• **Pierces transversus abdominis** and **internal oblique** above the iliac crest and **inters inguinal canal**^Q. • It emerges from superficial inguinal **ring** to supply skin of: – **Proximomedial skin** of **thigh**^Q – **Skin** over **penile root**^Q – **Upper part** of **scrotum**^Q	• **Pierces transversus abdominis**, travels **between transversus abdominis** and **internal oblique** until it **pierces** the aponeurosis of **both obliques**^Q just above the external ring • It divides into two branches. – **Lateral cutaneous** supplies **posterolateral gluteal skin**^u – **Anterior cutaneous** supplies **suprapubic skin**^Q	• Divides into two branches – **Genital branch** of genitofemoral nerve **enters** the **inguinal canal** at **deep ring** and **supplies**^Q **cremaster** and **scrotal skin** – **Femoral branch** of genitofemoral nerve **passes behind** the **inguinal ligament**, enters femoral sheath lateral to femoral artery, pierces the anterior layer of femoral sheath and fascia lata and **supplies** the **skin anterior** to **upper part of femoral triangle**^Q.

25. **Ans. a Multilayered repair of inguinal canal** *(Ref: Sabiston 20/e p1099; Schwartz 10/e p1495, 1506-1507; Bailey 27/e p1032; Schackelford 8/e p603, 7/e p575)*

SHOULDICE REPAIR

- Primary tenets of the procedure involve **extensive dissection** and **reconstruction of inguinal canal anatomy**[Q].
- The use of a **continuous suture in multiple layers** resulted in the **dual advantage of distributing tension** over several layers and **preventing subsequent herniation** between interrupted sutures[Q].
- Consists of division and **double breasting** of the **transversalis fascia**[Q]

26. **Ans. None** *(Ref: Sabiston 20/e p1099; Schwartz 10/e p1506, 9/e p1320-1322; Bailey 27/e p1032; Schackelford 8/e p603, 7/e p573-576)*

- **Bassini's repair:** A **triple-layer repair** is then performed to restore integrity to the floor. The **medial tissues**, including the **internal oblique, transversus abdominis** muscle and **transversalis fascia**, are fixed to the shelving edge of the inguinal ligament and **pubic periosteum** with interrupted sutures (Inguinal ligament is **sutured to conjoint tendon**[Q]).
- **Shouldice repair** leads to **posterior wall strengthening**[Q]
- The **advantage of the McVay** (Cooper's ligament) **repair** is the ability to **address both inguinal** and **femoral canal defects**[Q].

27. **Ans. b. Indirect inguinal hernia**
28. **Ans. a. The sac contains omentum only** *(Ref. Sabiston 20/e p1097; Schwartz 10/e p1503; Bailey 27/e p1031)*

Content of Hernia	Name	Reduction
Omentum	Omentocele[Q]	• Omentum is doughy[Q] • The last portion is more difficult to reduce than the first[Q].
Intestine	Enterocele[Q]	• Gurgles on reduction[Q] • First portion is more difficult to reduce than the last[Q].

29. **Ans a. Herniotomy** *(Ref: Sabiston 20/e p1884; Schwartz 10/e p1634; Bailey 27/e p1503)*
30. **Ans. b. Laparoscopic hernia surgery**
31. **Ans. d. All are correct** *(Ref: Campbell 11/e p3182)*
32. **Ans. a. Laparoscopic** *(Ref: Sabiston 20/e p1103; Schwartz 10/e p1499)*

COMPLICATIONS OF HERNIA

33. **Ans. d. Correction of hypovolemia, e. Prepare OT for urgent surgery** *(Ref: Sabiston 20/e p1104; Schwartz 10/e p1634-1635; Bailey 27/e p1034)*
34. **Ans. d. Immediate surgery, e. IV fluids**
35. **Ans. a. Aspiration of the sac for diagnosis, b. X-ray abdomen, c. USG abdomen**
36. **Ans. c. Fundus**
37. **Ans. b. Immediate surgery**
38. **Ans. b. Tenderness**
39. **And. a. Lateral cutaneous nerve of thigh** *(Ref: Sabiston 20/e p1105; Schwartz 10/e p1514)*

> "**Neuropathic groin pain** is *caused by damage to a nerve in the groin region and may be due to partial or complete division, stretching, contusion, crushing, suturing, or electrocautery. The nerves that are usually involved are the **ilioinguinal nerve, iliohypogastric nerve**, both the genital and femoral branches of the **genitofemoral nerve**, and the **lateral femoral cutaneous nerve of the thigh**. The first two are especially prone to injury during an open herniorrhaphy, while the latter (i.e. Lateral cutaneous nerve of thigh) are more likely damaged during laparoscopy. The genital and femoral branches of the genitofemoral nerve and the lateral cutaneous nerve of the thigh are most at risk when the surgeon staples below the iliopubic tract when lateral to the internal spermatic vessels. A burning, tingling pain along the lateral aspect of the thigh in the distribution of the lateral femoral cutaneous nerve is known as **meralgia paresthetica**, and is due to entrapment of that nerve; the affected skin area may be hyperaesthetic and/or pruritic, and patients may complain of the tactile hallucination of a sensation of small insects creeping under the skin (formication)." (Schwartz 10/e p1514)*

40. **Ans. a. Ilioinguinal nerve**

FEMORAL HERNIA

41. **Ans. b. Pregnancy is common cause** *(Ref: Sabiston 20/e p1104; Schwartz 10/e p1504; Bailey 27/e p1035; Schackelford 8/e p606, 7/e p547-554)*
42. **Ans. c. Femoral hernia**
43. **Ans. d. Femoral vein**
44. **Ans. a. Lateral and below**
45. **Ans. a. Low inguinal operation**
46. **Ans. a. Femoral hernia**
47. **Ans. c. Lacunar ligament**
48. **Ans. d. McVay repair** *(Ref: Schwartz 9/e p2514)*

McVay repair closes the femoral space, is effective for femoral hernia.

49. **Ans. a. Cloquet's hernia** *(Ref: Bailey 25/e p978-979)*
50. **Ans. a. Lacunar ligament**
51. **Ans. a. Below and lateral to pubic tubercle**

Hernia and Abdominal Wall

SPIGELIAN HERNIA

52. Ans. a. Usually occurs above arcuate line *(Ref: Sabiston 20/e p1113; Bailey 27/e p1041; Schackelford 8/e p580, 7/e p609-610)*
53. Ans. b. Subumbilical region
54. Ans. b. Lateral border of rectus abdominis
55. Ans. d. Hernia occurring at the level of arcuate line
56. Ans. b. Internal oblique
57. Ans. c. Occurs at the…., d. Content of hernia…, e. Surgery is the…..

SLIDING HERNIA

58. Ans. d. Sigmoid colon *(Ref: Sabiston 20/e p1104; Bailey 27/e p1029)*
59. Ans. b. Hernia-en-Glissade *(Ref: Sabiston 20/e p1104; Bailey 25/e p977)*
60. Ans. b. Sliding hernia
61. Ans. b. Sigmoid colon
62. Ans. b. Barium-meal *(Ref: CSDT 12/e p771)*

> An **upper GI barium series (Barium meal)** is the preferred examination in the **investigation of sliding hiatus hernia**. In this question, sliding hernia means sliding hiatus hernia.
> By the way, CSDT says "Finding a **segment of colon in** the **scrotum on barium enema** strongly suggests a **sliding hernia.**"

63. Ans. c. Sliding hernia

LUMBAR HERNIA

64. Ans. d. More common on right side *(Ref: Sabiston 20/e p1115; Schwartz 10/e p1742; Bailey 27/e p1042; Schackelford 8/e p606, 7/e p613-616)*
65. Ans. a. More commonly congenital *(Ref: Sabiston 20/e p1115; Bailey 27/e p1042)*

> **Lumbar hernias can be either congenital (20%) or acquired (80%).**

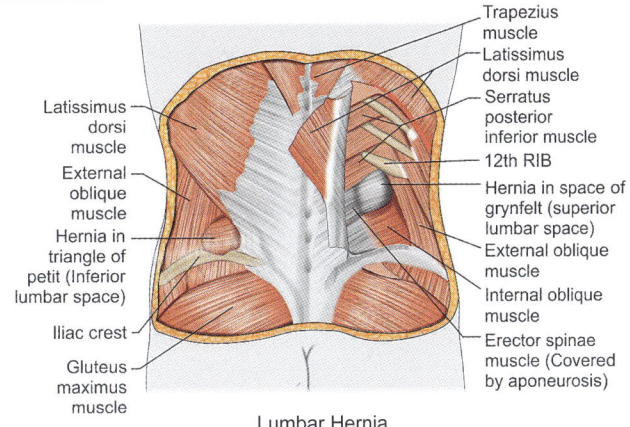

Lumbar Hernia

OBTURATOR HERNIA

66. Ans. b. Common in female, c. Chronic constipation risk factor, d. Surgical treatment should be done, e. May present with intestinal obstruction *(Ref: Sabiston 20/e p1113; Bailey 27/e p1029; Schackelford 8/e p611, 7/e p616-618)*
67. Ans. b. Obturator hernia

PARADUODENAL HERNIA

68. Ans. d. Common on right side *(Ref: Sabiston 20/e p1083; Schackelford 8/e p861, 7/e p954-955)*
69. Ans. d. More common on right side
70. Ans. a. Stammer's hernia *(Ref: www.ncbi.nlm.nih.gov› Ann Surg › v.177(5); May 1973)*

> **STAMMER'S HERNIA**
>
> - **Internal hernia** occurring **through window in** the **transverse mesocolon after** retrocolic **gastrojejunostomy** is known as Stammer's hernia[Q].
> - Stammer's Hernia **can lead to colonic ischemia**

UMBILICAL HERNIA

71. Ans. b. Amniotic membrane *(Ref: Sabiston 20/e p1883; Schwartz 10/e p1455,1631; Bailey 27/e p1037)*
72. Ans. c. Failure of gut to return to the body cavity from the physiological herniation
73. Ans. b. 2.5 *(Ref: pubmedcentralcanada.ca/e ppmcc/articles/.../annrcse01490-0010.pdf)*

Moore's Classification of Omphalocele	
Type	Diameter of Defect
Type 1	<2.5 cm^Q
Type 2	2.5 to 5 cm
Type 3	>5 cm

74. Ans. a. Birth *(Ref: Sabiston 20/e p1883; Schwartz 10/e p1453,1631,1632; Bailey 27/e p135)*
75. Ans. d. Umbilical hernia *(Ref: Sabiston 20/e p1107; Schwartz 10/e p1455,1631; Bailey 27/e p1037; Schackelford 8/e p579, 7/e p599-600)*
76. Ans. c. Umbilical hernia *(Ref: Sabiston 20/e p1107; Schwartz 10/e p1631; Bailey 27/e p1037)*
77. Ans. d. All of the above
78. Ans. b. Gastroschisis is associated with multiple anomalies
79. Ans. b. Direct inguinal hernia
80. Ans. c. 1 in 5000
81. Ans. d. Herniation of abdominal contents through the body wall
82. Ans. b. Gastroschisis
83. Ans. b. Omphalocele
84. Ans. c. 4 cm

Omphalocele/exomphalos: Congenital herniation of abdominal contents at the umbilicus (i.e. into the umbilical cord). Occasionally divided into:
- < 4 cm—Umbilical cord hernia
- > 4 cm—Omphalocele

85. Ans. c. Failure of gut to return to body cavity after its physiological herniation *(Ref: Schwartz 10/e p1455; Sabiston 20/e p1883; Bailey 27/e p1037)*

EPIGASTRIC HERNIA

86. Ans. b. Fatty hernia of the linea alba *(Ref: Sabiston 20/e p1108; Schwartz 10/e p1455; Bailey 27/e p1039; Schackelford 8/e p573, 7/e p597)*
87. Ans. c. Located above the umbilicus and on either side

- Epigastric hernias are multiple in up to **20%** of patients, and **about 80%** are **just off the midline**^{Q}.

RICHTER'S HERNIA

88. Ans. a. Richter's hernia *(Ref: Bailey 27/e p1024)*

Richter's Hernia

- Richter's hernia is a hernia in which the **sac contains only a portion of** the **circumference** of the **intestine**^{Q} (usually small intestine).
- It usually **complicates femoral** and, rarely, obturator hernias.

Strangulated Richter's Hernia
- **Operation** is frequently **delayed** because the **clinical features mimic gastroenteritis**^{Q}.
- The **local signs of strangulation** are often **not obvious**^{Q}.
- Patient may not vomit and, although colicky pain is present
- **Bowels** are often **opened normally** or there **may be diarrhea**^{Q}.
- **Absolute constipation** is **delayed** until paralytic ileus supervenes.
- For these reasons, **gangrene of the knuckle of bowel** and **perforation** have often **occurred before operation** is undertaken^Q.

89. Ans. c. Richter's hernia
90. Ans. b. Femoral hernia

LITTRE'S HERNIA

91. **Ans. b. Meckel's diverticulum** *(Ref: Bailey 27/e p1252)*
92. **Ans. c. Littre's hernia**

> **LITTRE'S HERNIA**
>
> - **Littre's hernia** is the **protrusion of a Meckel's diverticulum**^{Q} through a potential abdominal opening.

MISCELLANEOUS HERNIA

93. **Ans. a. In children, indirect inguinal hernia is treated medically, b. In Richter's hernia, absolute constipation seen, d. Deep inguinal ring is lateral and above the public tubercle** *(Ref: BDC 4/e pvol II/e p208)*

- **Surgery** is the **only treatment option for hernia in any age group**, there is no role of medical treatment.
- **Deep ring** is **situated 1.25 cm above** the **inguinal ligament**, **midway between** the **symphysis pubis** and **ASIS**^{Q}.
- **Deep ring** is an **opening in** the **fascia transversalis**^{Q}.
- **Superficial ring** lies **immediately above the pubic tubercle**, as a **triangular gap in** the **external oblique aponeurosis**^{Q}.
- **Clinical features** mimic **gastroenteritis** in **strangulated Richter's hernia**^{Q}.

94. **Ans. a. External abdominal hernia is common, b. Direct hernia usually acquired, c. Strangulation is common in femoral hernia, d. Direct hernia is acquired in old age, e. TOC for indirect inguinal hernia is surgery**

95. **Ans. a. Direct hernias are usually acquired, b. Femoral is most common hernia to strangulate, c. External abdominal hernia are most common, e. Treatment of choice for indirect inguinal hernia is surgery**

96. **Ans. a. Absorbable sutures, c. Missed sac, d. Infection** *(Ref: Bailey 27/e p1034)*

> **RECURRENT HERNIAS**
>
> - **Reported recurrence rates** vary between **0.2% and 15%** depending on the technique employed.
> - Only **50% of recurrences** will become apparent **within 2 years**^{Q}.
> - Causes of **recurrent inguinal hernias**, especially those that appear in the **first postoperative year**, are usually due to **errors of observation, judgment, or surgical technique**^{Q}.
>
> | Causes of Recurrence | |
> |---|---|
> | • **Failure to perform high ligation** or **reduce the peritoneal sac** with an **indirect hernia**^{Q} | • **Metabolic problems** of the tissues in the groin^Q |
> | • **Inadequate closure** of the **internal ring**^{Q} | • **Infection**^{Q} that destroys the repair |
> | • **Missed sac**^{Q} | • **Continuing failure** of the floor of the canal^Q |

> **DUAL (SADDLE-BAG or PANTALOON) HERNIA**
>
> - This type of hernia **consists of two sacs** that **straddle the inferior epigastric artery**, **one sac being medial** and the **other lateral** to this vessel.
> - The condition is not rare and is a **cause of recurrence**, one of the sacs having been overlooked at the time of operation.

97. **Ans. a. Gibbon's**

Gibbon's hernia	• **Hernia with hydrocele**^{Q}
Berger's hernia	• **Hernia into pouch of Douglas**^{Q}
Beclard's hernia	• **Femoral hernia through opening of saphenous vein**^{Q}
Amyand's hernia	• Inguinal hernia **containing appendix**^{Q}
Ogilve's hernia	• Hernia through the **defect in conjoint tendon** just lateral to where it inserts with the rectus sheath^Q
Stammer's hernia	• **Internal hernia** occurring **through window in** the **transverse mesocolon after** retrocolic **gastrojejunostomy**^{Q}
Peterson hernia	• Hernia **under Roux limb** after **Roux-en-Y gastric bypass**^{Q}
Velpeau hernia	• Hernia **in front of** femoral vessels
Holthouse hernia	• Inguinal hernia with **extension of the loop of intestine along inguinal ligament**.

98. Ans. d. Berger's
99. Ans. b. Eduardo Bassini
100. Ans. a. Sliding
101. Ans. c. Maydl's hernia *(Ref: Abdominal Wall Hernias: Principles and Management by Robert Bendavid (2012)/p563)*

Maydl's hernia (Hernia-in-W)

- In **Maydl's hernia**, a loop of bowel in the form of **'W'** lies in the hernial sac & central portion of the **'W' loop is strangulated** and **lies within the abdominal cavity**.
- Maydl's hernia is a **complication of large hernial sacs**

INCISIONAL HERNIA

102. **Ans. d. Old age** *(Ref: Sabiston 20/e p1109; Schwartz 10/e p1454-1455; Bailey 27/e p1039; Schackelford 8/e p574, 7/e p602-608)*
     Old age is a risk factor for incisional hernia, but not for wound dehiscence.

103. Ans. a. Incisional hernia

104. Ans. d. Caused by use of local anesthesia

105. Ans. d. Incisional

106. **Ans. a. Onlay** *(Ref: Sabiston 20/e p1111)*

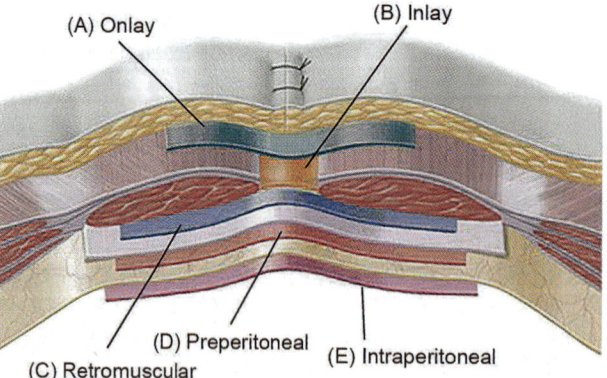

Mesh Placement in Abdominal Wall Reconstruction		
Onlay (Overlay)	**Underlay (Sublay)**	**Inlay**
• Placement of **mesh over anterior fascia** after closure of the fascial defect[Q] • Mesh is **placed outside the abdominal cavity** avoiding direct contact with abdominal viscera[Q]	• Placement of **mesh below the fascial components**[Q] (retrorectus, preperitoneal, or intraperitoneal position) • **Intra-abdominal pressure** acts to **hold the mesh** and **prevent migration** due to wide overlap of mesh and fascia[Q].	• **Mesh is sutured to the fascial edge without overlap**[Q] • Associated with **high recurrence rate**[Q] because high intra-abdominal pressure pulls away the mesh from fascial edges

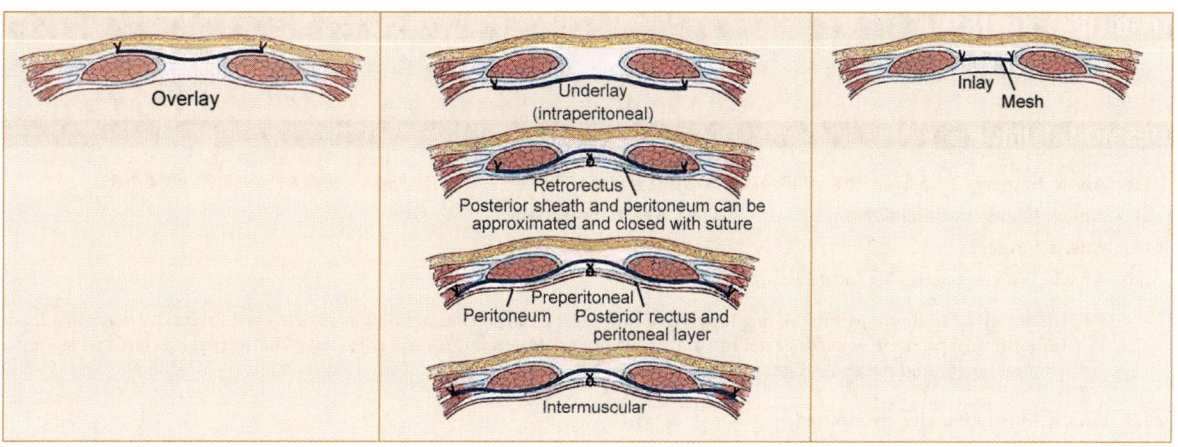

HERNIA AND ABDOMINAL WALL ANATOMY

107. **Ans. d. Ilioinguinal nerve**

108. **Ans. c. Inferior epigastric artery** *(Ref: BDC 4/e pvol II/e p208)*

    Deep ring lies immediately lateral to inferior epigastric artery, so artery is being in danger of getting damaged while releasing the constriction at the deep ring.

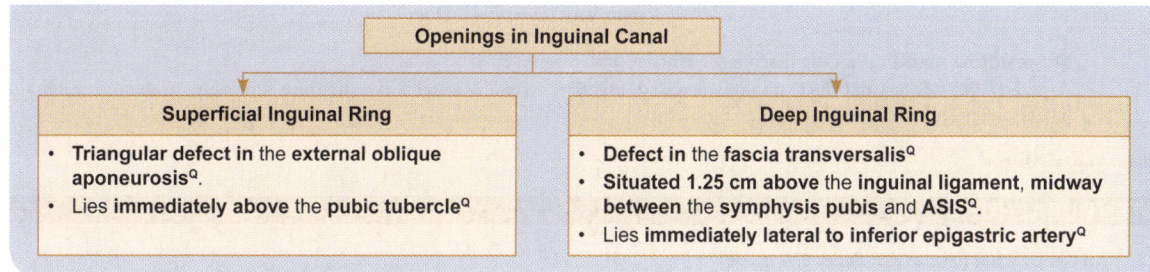

109. **Ans. b. Incising the external oblique aponeurosis**

110. **Ans. d. Inferior epigastric artery** *(Ref: BDC 5/e pvol II/e p224)*

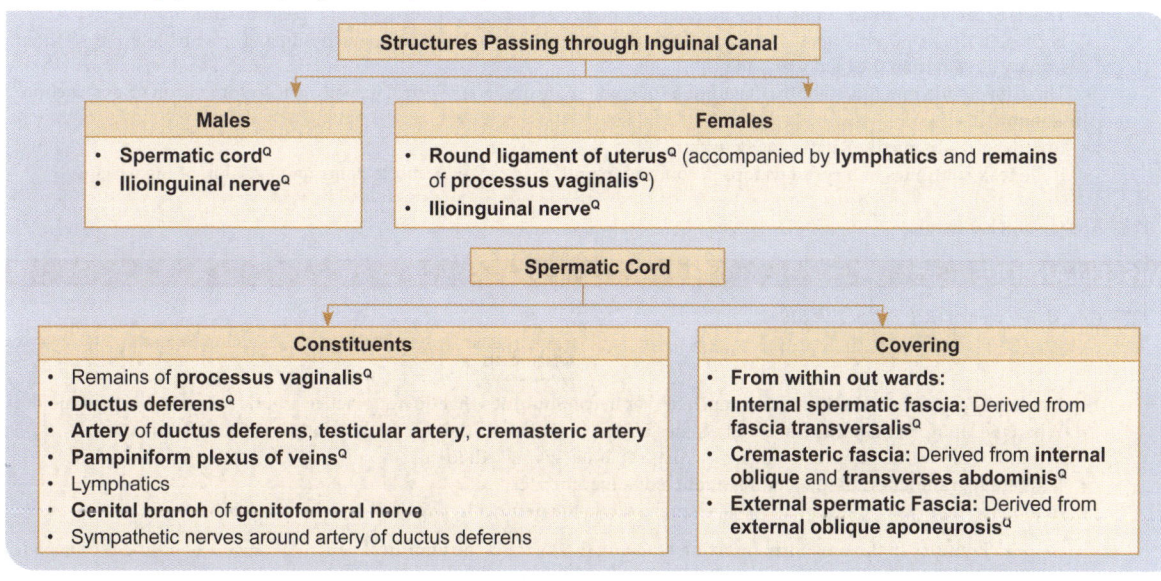

111. **Ans. a. Defect in fascia transversalis**   112. **Ans. a. 1.25 cm**

UMBILICAL ADENOMA

113. Ans. None *(Ref: Bailey 26/e p968)*
114. Ans. c. Umbilical adenoma
115. Ans. d. Congenital

DESMOID TUMOR

116. Ans. c. Surgery *(Ref: Sabiston 20/e p1072-1074; Schwartz 10/e p1485; Bailey 27/e p1045; Schackelford 8/e p1967, 7/e p974, 2035)*
117. Ans. e. Highly radiosensitive
118. Ans. b. Scar tissue
119. Ans. a. Surgery
120. Ans. b. Wide excision *(Ref: Devita 9/e p1573)*

- Devita says "In desmoid tumors, **postoperative radiation** is **not recommended** in patients **with negative margins**. **Residual tumor** from a primary lesion **does not invariably lead to treatment failure** and **adjuvant radiation may be omitted** as long as local progression would not cause significant morbidity."

121. Ans. a. Mostly females are affected
122. Ans. b. Abdominal mass *(Ref: Sabiston 20/e p765, 1073, 1085; Schwartz 10/e p1454; Bailey 27/e p1045)*

- "Patients with a desmoid tumor present with an asymptomatic mass or with symptoms related to mass effect from the tumor." *(Sabiston 20/e p1073)*

PATENT VITELLO-INTESTINAL DUCT

123. Ans. b. 6 months of age *(Ref: Bailey 27/e p1044)*

PATENT VITELLOINTESTINAL DUCT

- The **resulting umbilical fistula discharges mucus**^{Q} and, rarely, feces.
- A **patent vitellointestinal duct** should be **excised, together with** a **Meckel's diverticulum** if present, preferably when the child is about **6 months**^{Q} old.

124. Ans. a. Mucus

PATENT URACHUS

125. Ans. c. Urachal fistula *(Ref: Bailey 27/e p1044)*

PATENT URACHUS

- A **patent urachus seldom reveals** itself **until maturity** or **even old age**^{Q}.
- This is because the **contractions of** the **bladder commence at the apex** of the organ and **pass towards the base**^{Q}.
- Because it opens into the apex of the bladder a **patent urachus is closed temporarily during micturition** and so the potential urinary stream from the bladder is cut off.
- Thus, the **fistula remains unobtrusive until a time when** the **organ is overfull**, usually due to **some form of obstruction**^{Q}.

Treatment
- Remove the obstruction^Q in the lower urinary tract.
- If the **leak continues** or a **cyst develops** in connection with the urachus: **Umbilectomy** and **excision of the urachus**^{Q}

126. Ans. a. Urachal fistula

MISCELLANEOUS

127. Ans. d. 3-6 weeks *(Ref: Bailey 27/e p1044)*

OMPHALITIS

- Incidence of an **infected umbilicus** is much higher in **communities that do not practice aseptic severance** of the umbilical cord.
- When the stump of the umbilical cord becomes inflamed, **antibiotic therapy** usually **localizes the inflammation.**
- By employing warm, moist dressings, the crusts separate, giving exit to pus.
- **Exuberant granulation tissue** requires a **touch of silver nitrate**.
- In more serious cases, infection is liable to spread along the **defunct hypogastric arteries** or **umbilical vein**.

  - **Jaundice in the newborn:** Infection reaching the **liver via** the **umbilical vein** may cause a stenosing intrahepatic cholangiolitis, appearing some **3-6 weeks after birth**^{Q}.

128. **Ans. d. Herniotomy**
129. **Ans. b. Vicarious menstruation**
130. **Ans. d. Umbilical hernia**
131. **Ans. b. Leukocyte adhesion deficiency**

- **Leukocyte adhesion deficiency** is associated with **recurrent bacterial infection** and **impaired wound healing**[Q].

132. **Ans. b. Stoppa's preperitoneal repair** *(Ref: Recent advances in surgery 10/e p166)*

STOPPA'S PREPERITONEAL REPAIR

- In **Stoppa's preperitoneal repair**, the expanding intra-abdominal pressure holds the mesh in place without suture fixation.
- According to **Pascal's law,** any additional pressure exerted upon an enclosed fluid mass is transmitted equally in all directions.
- Use of large mesh extending 3-5 cm beyond the edge of defect in all sides **utilizes Pascal's law.**

133. **Ans. a. Surgery should not be done unless patient becomes symptomatic** *(Ref: Sabiston 20/e p1097; Schwartz 10/e p1509; Bailey 27/e p1026)*

- Sabiston says "**Most surgeons recommend operation on discovery of an inguinal hernia** because the natural history of a groin hernia is that of **progressive enlargement** and **weakening**, with the **potential for incarceration** and **strangulation."**
- Bailey says " The **basic operation** is **inguinal herniotomy**, which entails dissectiong out and opening the hernial sac, reducing any content and then transfixing the neck of the sac and removing the remainder. It is employed either by itself or as the first step in a repair procedure (herniorrhaphy). By itself, it is **sufficient for** the **treatment of hernia in infants, adolescents** and **young adults."**
- **Non-absorbable mesh** is **used in hernia surgery**.
- **Surgery can be done using laparoscopy (TEP or TAPP)**

134. **Ans. b. Taxis** *(Ref: Schwartz 10/e p1505)*

CHAPTER 20

Spleen

IDIOPATHIC THROMBOCYTOPENIC PURPURA

Idiopathic Thrombocytopenic Purpura (ITP)

- ITP is characterized by a **low platelet count** despite **normal bone marrow** & **absence of other causes of thrombocytopenia**[Q].
- ITP is predominantly a **disease of young women**[Q].
- ITP manifests differently in **children**: Both genders are **affected equally**[Q], onset is **sudden**, thrombocytopenia is **severe**, and **complete spontaneous remissions** are seen in **80% of affected children**[Q].
- **Girls >10 years** with **more chronic purpura** are those in whom the **disease seems to persist**[Q].

Pathology
- **Autoantibodies are responsible** for the **disordered platelet destruction** mediated by **overactivated platelet phagocytosis within** the **reticuloendothelial system**[Q].
- **Relative bone marrow failure**[Q] (production cannot match destruction of thrombocytes to compensate sufficiently).

Clinical Features
- Typical presentation: **Purpura, epistaxis, & gingival bleeding**[Q].
- Less commonly, gastrointestinal bleeding & hematuria are noted.

  - Despite the destruction of platelets by splenic macrophages, **spleen** is normally **not enlarged in ITP**[Q].

Diagnosis
- **Diagnosis of ITP involves exclusion** of other relatively common causes of thrombocytopenia: **pregnancy**, drug-induced thrombocytopenia (e.g., **heparin, quinidine, quinine, sulfonamides**), **viral infections**, & **hypersplenism**[Q]

Treatment of ITP	
Asymptomatic patients with platelet counts **>50,000/mm³**	**Observation**[Q]
Platelet counts **30,000-50,000/mm³**	**Observation** with more routine follow-up[Q]
Symptomatic patients with **platelets counts <50,000/mm³** or **platelet counts <30,000/mm³**	**Glucocorticoid** (prednisone, 1 mg/kg body weight/day)[Q]
Platelets counts <20,000/mm³ with **significant mucous membrane bleeding** or **life-threatening hemorrhage**	**Hospitalization**[Q]

- **Platelet transfusion** is indicated only for those who experience **severe hemorrhage**.
- **IV immunoglobulin** is important for the **treatment of acute bleeding, in pregnancy,** or for **patients being prepared for operation,** including **splenectomy**.
- Other treatment options: Long-term **glucocorticoid therapy, azathioprine** or **cyclophosphamide**.

  - **Indications of splenectomy in ITP:**
    - **Failure of medical therapy**[Q]
    - **Prolonged use of steroids** with **undesirable effects**[Q]
    - Most cases of **first relapse**[Q]
- **Splenectomy** provides a **permanent response** without subsequent need for steroids in **75-85% of patients**[Q].
- **Laparoscopic splenectomy**[Q] has become the **gold standard for ITP** patients.
- **Responses** usually occur **within the first postoperative week**.
- For patients with **extremely low platelet counts (<10,000/mm³)** platelets should be available for surgery but should **not be given preoperatively**.
- Once the **splenic artery is ligated**[Q], **platelets are given** to those who continue to bleed.

INDICATIONS OF SPLENECTOMY

- MC indication for splenectomy: Trauma[Q]
- MC indication for elective splenectomy: ITP[Q]

Indications for Splenectomy

Splenectomy always indicated:	Splenectomy rarely indicated:
• **Primary splenic tumor**[Q] • **Hereditary spherocytosis**[Q] **Splenectomy usually indicated:** • **Primary hypersplenism**[Q] • **Chronic ITP**[Q] • **Splenic vein thrombosis** causing **gastric varices**[Q] • **Splenic abscess**[Q]	• Chronic leukemia • Splenic lymphoma • Macroglobulinemia • Thalassemia major • Sickle cell disease • Congestive splenomegaly and hypersplenism due to PHT • Felty's syndrome • Hairy cell leukemia • Chediak-Higashi syndrome • Sarcoidosis
Splenectomy sometimes indicated:	**Splenectomy not indicated:**
• **Splenic injury**[Q] • **Autoimmune hemolytic disease**[Q] • Elliptocytosis with hemolysis • Nonspherocytic hemolytic anemia • **Hodgkin's disease (for staging**[Q]) • **Thrombotic thrombocytopenic purpura**[Q] • **Idiopathic myelofibrosis**[Q] • **Splenic artery aneurysm**[Q] • Wiskott-Aldrich syndrome • Gaucher's disease • Mastocytosis (aggressive disease)	• Asymptomatic hypersplenism • Splenomegaly with infection • Splenomegaly associated with elevated IgM • Hereditary hemolytic anemia of moderate degree • Acute leukemia • Agranulocytosis

HEREDITARY SPHEROCYTOSIS

Hereditary Spherocytosis

- **Autosomal dominant** disease **affecting** the production of **spectrin**, a RBC **cytoskeletal protein**[Q].

Pathology

> **Loss** of **spectrin**[Q] → RBCs lack biconcave shape[Q] → Affects RBCs deformability[Q] → Increased osmotic fragility[Q] → More **susceptible to trapping** and **destruction** by the **spleen**[Q].

Clinical Features
- **Anemia**, occasionally with **jaundice**, and **splenomegaly**[Q].

Diagnosis
- Diagnosis is made by examination of a **peripheral blood smear, increased reticulocyte count, increased osmotic fragility**, and a **negative Coombs' test**[Q].

Treatment
- **Anemia** can be **successfully treated with splenectomy**[Q]
- **Splenectomy** should be **delayed until the age of 5 years to preserve immunologic function** of the **spleen** and **reduce the risk of OPSI**[Q].
- Presence of **pigmented gallstones: Cholecystectomy**[Q]

SPLENECTOMY

Splenectomy

- Most serious sequela is **overwhelming postsplenectomy infection (OPSI)**, with meningitis, pneumonia, or bacteremia.
- OPSI is **typically caused by polysaccharide-encapsulated organisms**, such as **Streptococcus pneumoniae, Neisseria meningitidis, & Hemophilus influenzae**[Q].

> - When elective splenectomy is planned, **vaccination against encapsulated bacteria** should be given **at least 2 weeks before surgery**[Q].
> - If spleen is removed in **emergency, vaccination** should be given **as soon as possible**[Q] following surgery.

- **Vaccines** should be given for **Streptococcus pneumoniae, Hemophilus influenzae type b & Meningococcus**[Q].
- In addition to above given 3 vaccines, **annual influenza immunization**[Q] is also advised as influenza has been implicated as a risk factor for secondary bacterial infections.
- **Booster injection** of **pneumococcal vaccine** should be given **every 5-6 years**[Q].
- Harrison says that "**Routine chemoprophylaxis** with oral **penicillin** can result in the **emergence of drug-resistant strains** and is **not recommended.**"

Splenectomy Outcomes

Increased risk of Infections	Hematologic Outcomes

• Life threatening infection in asplenic patients is attributable to **loss of splenic macrophages, diminished tuftsin production, & loss of** spleen's **reticuloendothelial screening function.**
• After splenectomy, **ability to filter & phagocytose bacteria**, particularly **encapsulated bacteria (Streptococcus pneumoniae, Hemophilus influenzae, Neisseria meningitides) & parasitized blood cells is lost**[Q].
• **MC infection after splenectomy**: Streptococcus pneumoniae[Q] (50–90% cases)
	• **Immediately after splenectomy:**
	  – Leucocytosis[Q]
	  – **Thrombocytosis** (these levels **returns to normal** within 2–3 weeks)[Q]
	• **Chronic manifestations:**
	  – Anisocytosis & poikilocytosis[Q]
	  – **Howell Jolly bodies**[Q] (nuclear remnants)
	  – **Heinz bodies**[Q] (denatured hemoglobin)
	  – **Basophilic stippling**[Q] & occasional nucleated erythrocytes

Other common bacterial infections
- **Hemophilus influenzae type b**[Q]
- **Meningococcus**[Q]
- **Group A** and **B streptococcus**[Q]
- Capnocytophaga canimorsus
- Enterococcus species
- Bacteroides • Salmonella • Bartonella

Protozoal that invade the RBCs
- Babesia, Ehrlichia, Plasmodium (BEP)[Q]

COMPLICATIONS OF SPLENECTOMY

Complications of Splenectomy

Pulmonary Complications:
- **Left lower lobe atelectasis**: MC complication[Q]
- Pleural effusion
- Pneumonia

Hemorrhagic Complications:
- Subphrenic hematoma

Infectious Complications:
- Subphrenic abscess
- Wound infection

Pancreatic Complications:
- Pancreatitis
- Pseudocyst
- Pancreatic fistula

Thromboembolic Complications:
- DVT
- Portal vein thrombosis

- **DVT prophylaxis** is **routinely recommended**[Q].
- In patients with **hemolytic anemia** or **myeloproliferative disorders & splenomegaly**, **thrombotic risk** is **heightened**, particularly the risk of **portal vein thrombosis**[Q].
- Patients undergoing splenectomy for **malignancy** or **myeloproliferative disorders** should be strongly considered for **perioperative pharmacoprophylaxis**, either **LMWH** or **unfractionated heparin**[Q].

OVERWHELMING POSTSPLENECTOMY INFECTION

Overwhelming Postsplenectomy Infection (OPSI)

- OPSI is **MC fatal late complication** of **splenectomy**.

  - Mortality associated with OPSI: 40-50%[Q]
  - Infection may occur at any time after splenectomy[Q], Life long risk remains[Q]
  - Most infections occurr more than 2 years after splenectomy usually after 5 years of splenectomy.
  - Risk is greatest in thalassemia major & sickle cell anemia[Q]

Clinical Features

- OPSI **typically begins with** a **prodromal phase** characterized by **fever, rigors** & **chills** and other **nonspecific symptoms**, including sore throat, malaise, myalgias, diarrhea, & vomiting.

  > - **Progression of** the **illness is rapid**, with the **development of hypotension, DIC, respiratory distress, coma,** & **death within hours of presentation**[Q].
  > - **Despite antibiotics** and **intensive care**, the **mortality rate** is between **50-70% for florid OPSI**[Q].

- **Most frequently involved organism** in OPSI is **S. pneumoniae**[Q] (50-90% of cases)
- Other organisms involved in OPSI: **H. influenzae, N. meningitidis, Streptococcus** and **Salmonella spp**[Q].

  > - **Risk for OPSI** is **greater** in **splenectomy for malignancy** or **hematologic conditions** than for those who underwent splenectomy for trauma[Q].
  > - **Risk is greater for young children**[Q] (<4 years of age).

SPLENIC TUMORS

- MC neoplasm of spleen: **Lymphoma**[Q] (Non-Hodgkin's lymphoma)
- MC primary tumor of spleen: **Hemangioma**[Q]
- MC primary malignant tumor of spleen: **Angiosarcoma**[Q] (Hemangiosarcoma)

HEMANGIOMA SPLEEN

Hemangioma Spleen

- **Hemangioma: MC benign tumor** of the **spleen**[Q].
- **Primarily asymptomatic**, **incidentally found** at autopsy[Q]
- May be **singular, multiple,** or **even involve** the **entire spleen**[Q].

Clinical Features

- **Symptoms result** when the **tumor enlarges** to **encroach on adjacent organs**.
- **Spontaneous rupture**[Q] can occur in up to **25% of cases**.
- A **consumptive coagulopathy** may be present due to the **platelet trapping** in the **cavernous spaces** of the lesion[Q].

Diagnosis

- **CT scan** demonstrates **splenomegaly**[Q].
- **Angiography** demonstrates a **"laking" effect** similar to that seen with hepatic hemangiomas

Treatment

- **Nonsurgical treatment** is employed for **small, asymptomatic, incidentally detected hemangiomas**[Q].
- **Splenectomy** is **the treatment of choice** for **larger** and **symptomatic hemangiomas**[Q].

SPLENIC CYST

- MC true splenic cyst: **Parasitic** or **hydatid cyst** (Echinococcus)[Q] (10%)
- MC non-parasitic splenic cyst: **Pseudocyst** (secondary to **trauma**)[Q] (70–80%)
- MC congenital nonparasitic splenic cyst: **Epidermoid cysts**[Q]

SPLENIC ABSCESS

Splenic Abscess

- **Unusual but potentially life threatening illness**[Q]
- **Mortality rate** of **15–20%** in previously **healthy patients**, with **single unilocular lesions**, to **80%** for **multiple abscesses** in **immunocompromised patients**[Q].

Predisposing Factors for Splenic Abscess	
• Malignancies^Q	• Hemoglobinopathies^Q
• Polycythemia vera^Q	• Urinary tract infections
• Endocarditis^Q	• IV drug use^Q
• Prior trauma^Q	• AIDS^Q

- Approximately **70%** of **splenic abscesses result from hematogenous spread** of the **infective organism** from another location, as in **endocarditis, osteomyelitis,** and **IV drug use**^Q.
- **Gram-positive cocci** (*Staphylococcus-MC*^Q, *Streptococcus*, or *Enterococcus* spp.) and **gram-negative enteric organisms** are typically involved.

> • **Salmonella** and **Enterobacter spp**. and other enteric organisms are commonly seen in splenic abscess in patients of sickle cell anemia.

- **Fungal abscesses** (e.g., *Candida* spp.) also occur, **typically in immunosuppressed patients**^Q.

Clinical Features
- Splenic abscesses present with **nonspecific symptoms**: Vague **abdominal pain, fever, peritonitis,** and **pleuritic chest pain**^Q.
- Splenomegaly is not typical.

Diagnosis
- **CT: Investigation of choice** for diagnosis of **splenic abscess**^Q.
- **USG**: Diagnosis can also be made with ultrasound.

Treatment
- **Unilocular abscesses: Percutaneous drainage + antibiotics** (success rates 75–90%)^Q
- **Multilocular lesions: Splenectomy + Drainage** of the left upper quadrant + **Antibiotics**^Q

SPLENIC ARTERY ANEURYSM

SPLENIC ARTERY ANEURYSMS

- MC site of intra-abdominal aneurysm: Aorta >Splenic artery^Q

> • MC site of splanchnic artery aneurysm: Splenic artery^Q
> • MC causes: Arteriosclerosis^Q
> • Usually **saccular**, multiple aneurysm is **20%**^Q

- **Calcification** is present in **one-third**, and **mostly situated** in the **distal third**^Q of the splenic artery.
- Four times **more common in women** (possible factors include **multiparity, portal hypertension, arterial fibrodysplasia, pancreatitis**, and, less commonly, trauma, arteritis, and septic emboli)^Q
- Aneurysmal **rupture** in **pregnancy** usually occurs during the **third trimester**^Q.

Factors Increasing the Risk of Rupture	
• Young age^Q	• Presence of **hypertension**^Q
• **Absence of** aneurysmal **calcification**^Q	• Aneurysm diameter **>1.5 cm**^Q

Management
- Documented **aneurysmal enlargement** and **symptoms** caused by aneurysm are **indications of operation**^Q.
- An aneurysm detected in a **female** who anticipate pregnancy should be removed and one **detected during pregnancy** should be **removed before** the **third trimester**^Q.

> - **Proximal aneurysms** are **excised** after proximal and distal ligations.
> - **Mid-splenic aneurysms** are **excluded** by proximal and distal ligations of the splenic artery and all collateral vessels.
> - **Distal** or **hilar aneurysm** is the **most common** and is treated with **aneurysmectomy** and **splenectomy**^Q.

Multiple Choice Questions

IDIOPATHIC THROMBOCYTOPENIC PURPURA

1. **Best time to give platelets in ITP, 48,000/μL:** *(ILBS 2011)*
   a. After ligation of splenic artery
   b. Preoperatively
   c. Postoperatively
   d. After ligation of splenic vein

2. **False about ITP:** *(PGI SS Dec 2005)*
   a. More common in females
   b. Splenomegaly
   c. Altered peripheral platelet count
   d. Increased bone marrow megakaryocytes

3. **All are true about ITP except:** *(JIPMER GIS 2011)*
   a. Low platelet count, normal bone marrow seen
   b. In adults, most common in young women
   c. Chronicity if occurs in children, common in girls
   d. Remission occurs in 70% of cases of adult ITP

4. **In the diagnosis of idiopathic thrombocytopenic purpura, one of the statements is true:** *(COMEDK 2006)*
   a. In the bone marrow smear, there is decreased number of megakaryocytes
   b. In the bone marrow smear, there is increased number of megakaryocytes
   c. Prothrombin time is prolonged
   d. Partial thromboplastin time is prolonged

5. **An evidence that splenectomy might benefit a patient with idiopathic thrombocytopenic purpura includes which of the following?** *(UPSC 2007)*
   a. A significant enlargement of the spleen
   b. A high reticulocyte count
   c. Patients age less than five years
   d. An increase in platelet count on corticosteroid therapy

6. **A patient with ITP is being planned for splenectomy. What is the best time for platelet infusion in this patient:**
   a. 2 hours before surgery *(All India 2010, 2008)*
   b. At the time of skin incision
   c. After ligating the splenic artery
   d. Immediately after removal of spleen

7. **During splenectomy in ITP, platelet infusion is given:**
   a. Immediately after ligating splenic artery *(DPG 2008)*
   b. Immediately after removal of spleen
   c. After incision
   d. Next day of surgery

8. **Which of the following is the best treatment for ITP?** *(Recent Question 2019)*
   a. Prednisolone   b. Azathioprine
   c. Splenectomy   d. Platelet transfusion

HYPERSPLENISM

9. **All are seen in hypersplenism except:** *(AIIMS GIS Dec 2011)*
   a. Anemia   b. Thrombocytopenia
   c. Splenomegaly   d. Hypocellular bone marrow

10. **Which of the following doesn't fit into definition of hypersplenism?** *(JIPMER GIS 2011)*
    a. Bone marrow hypoplasia b. Splenomegaly
    c. Pancytopenia   d. Antiplatelet antibodies

11. **Hypersplenism is associated with:** *(PGI Dec 97)*
    a. Pancytopenia   b. Thrombocytopenia
    c. Leucopenia   d. Polycythemia

SPLENECTOMY

12. **Most common complication of splenectomy:**
    a. OPSI   *(AIIMS GIS Dec 2011)*
    b. Avascular necrosis of greater curvature of stomach
    c. Pancreatitis
    d. Atelectasis

13. **In contemporary world, most common indication for splenectomy is:** *(DNB 2005, 2000 JIPMER GIS 2011)*
    a. Trauma   b. Hemolytic anemia
    c. ITP   d. Infections

14. **Splenectomy can be curative in all of the following except:**
    a. Thalassemia *(DNB 2007, 2005, 2003, MHSSMCET 2005)*
    b. Sickle cell disease
    c. Hereditary spherocytosis
    d. ITP

15. **Splenectomy is indicated in:** *(MHPGMET 2005)*
    a. Spherocytosis   b. Pyropoikilocytosis
    c. Elliptocytosis d. All

16. **Splenectomy is done to tide over the acute crises of uncontrollable:** *(MHPGMCET 2006)*
    a. ITP   b. TTP
    c. HUS   d. All of the above

17. **Auto splenectomy is seen in one of the following hemolytic anemias:** *(MHCET 2016, COMEDK 2006)*
    a. Hereditary spherocytosis
    b. Sickle cell anaemia
    c. Thalassemia
    d. Immunohemolytic anemia

18. **Vaccine for post splenectomy infection is given against all except:** *(MCI Sept 2009, Punjab 2007)*
    a. Streptococcus pneumonia b. Haemophilus influenza
    c. Neisseria meningitides   d. E. coli

19. **All of the followings are true about OPSI except:**
    a. Develops 1-5 years after splenectomy *(PGI June 2009)*
    b. Maximum risk is within 1 year of splenectomy
    c. Begin with headache, myalgia and fever
    d. May present with severe septic shock
    e. Usually not respond with antibiotic treatment

20. **Which of the following is not an absolute indication of splenectomy?** *(All India 2000)*
    a. Splenic abscess
    b. Hereditary spherocytosis
    c. Fibrosarcoma
    d. Autoimmune hemolytic anemia

21. **Splenectomy is most useful in:** *(All India 96)*
    a. Sickle cell anemia
    b. Thalassemia
    c. Hereditary spherocytosis
    d. Acquired autoimmune hemolytic anemia

22. **Splenectomy is not done in:** *(AIIMS June 2001)*
    a. Myelofibrosis
    b. Sickle cell anemia
    c. Hereditary spherocytosis
    d. Splenic abscess

23. **Most common infection after splenectomy is:**
    (Recent Question 2016, PGI May 2005, June 97, AIIMS Nov 93)
    a. Anaerobic
    b. Staphylococcal
    c. Streptococcal
    d. Pneumococcal

24. **Most common complication of splenectomy is:** *(AIIMS Nov 93)*
    a. Hematemesis
    b. Left lower lobe atelectasis
    c. Peritoneal effusion
    d. Acute dilatation of stomach

25. **In which case pneumococcal vaccine is most effective?**
    a. When given preoperatively *(AIIMS Nov 97)*
    b. When given post operatively
    c. Against all strains of bacteria
    d. Against gram negative bacteria

26. **Postsplenectomy sepsis is common in:** *(PGI June 2000)*
    a. ITP
    b. Thalassemia
    c. Hereditary spherocytosis
    d. Trauma

27. **Which is the commonest postsplenectomy infection?**
    (DNB 2003, 2002, 2001, All India 2000, AIIMS Nov 99; Recent Question 2013)
    a. Streptococcus pyogenes
    b. Staphylococcus aureus
    c. Streptococcus pneumoniae
    d. Pseudomonas aeruginosa

28. **Most common complication of splenectomy is:** *(AIIMS 92)*
    a. Pancreatic leak
    b. Pulmonary complications
    c. Pneumococcal peritonitis
    d. Hemorrhage

29. **Splenectomy is least useful in:** *(All India 89)*
    a. Congenital elliptocytosis
    b. Thalassemia major
    c. Congenital spherocytic anaemia
    d. Hereditary nonspherocytic hemolytic anaemia

30. **Most common infections after splenectomy are:** *(DPG 2010)*
    a. Capsulated bacteria
    b. Uncapsulated bacteria
    c. Gram-positive sepsis
    d. Gram-negative bacteria

31. **Splenectomy can lead to:** *(DNB 2012, MCI Sept 2005)*
    a. Leucopenia
    b. Thrombocytosis
    c. Thrombocytopenia
    d. Thrombocytopenia and leucopenia

32. **In a female who had Steroid Resistant ITP it was decided to perform splenectomy. On day 3 post laparoscopic surgery patient had fever. Which of the following scenarios is most likely?** *(AIIMS May 2015)*
    a. Left lower lobe consolidation
    b. Port site infection
    c. Intra-abdominal collection
    d. Urine for pus should be sent

SPLENIC TRAUMA

33. **The innovative method for treatment of moderate splenic injury:** *(Recent Question 2014, MHSSMCET 2006)*
    a. Conservative management
    b. Mesh repair
    c. Splenorrhaphy
    d. Splenectomy

34. **Kehr sign is seen in:**
    (Recent Question 2014, MHSSMCET 2009, AIIMS June 94)
    a. Splenic injury
    b. Liver injury
    c. Renal injury
    d. Mesenteric hematoma

35. **Management of grade 3 splenic trauma in a stable child:** *(PGI Nov 2010)*
    a. Embolization
    b. Partial splenectomy
    c. Total splenectomy
    d. Conservative

36. **True about blunt abdominal trauma with splenic rupture:** *(PGI June 2008)*
    a. Kehr's sign-discoloration around umbilicus
    b. Spleen is most common organ to be involved
    c. Splenectomy is treatment of choice for splenic rupture
    d. Cullen's sign seen

37. **Kehr's sign seen in splenic rupture is:**
    (AIIMS Nov 93, All India 95)
    a. Pain over left shoulder
    b. Pain over right scapula
    c. Periumbilical pain
    d. Pain over renal angle

38. **In splenic injury, conservative management is done in:**
    a. Hemodynamically unstable *(AIIMS June 99)*
    b. Young patient
    c. Shattered spleen
    d. Extreme pallor and hypotension

39. **The most important radiological sign of splenic rupture is:**
    a. Obliteration of psoas shadow *(Bihar PG 2014)*
    b. Obliteration of splenic shadow
    c. Indentation of the left side air bubble
    d. Fracture of one or more lower ribs on left side

40. **Accidental small splenic rupture is treated with:**
    a. Catgut sutures
    b. Silk sutures
    c. Omental patch
    d. Catgut suturing with omental patch
    e. Splenectomy

41. **In a patient presenting with abdominal trauma, fracture rib and bruise over left hypochondrium probable diagnosis is:** *(PGI 96)*
    a. Rupture left lobe of liver
    b. Rupture right lobe of liver
    c. Splenic rupture
    d. Rupture stomach

42. **All of the following are true regarding splenic-rupture except:** *(MCI Sept 2009)*
    a. Elevation of the left dome of diaphragm
    b. Obliterated psoas shadow
    c. Obliterated colonic gas shadow
    d. Obliterated splenic outline

43. **A 27-year-old patient presented with left sided abdominal pain to the emergency room; 6 hours after an RTA. He was hemodynamically stable and FAST positive. A CECT (contrast enhanced CT) scan showed grade III splenic laceration. What will be the most appropriate treatment?** *(All India 2010)*
    a. Splenectomy
    b. Splenorrhaphy
    c. Splenic artery embolization
    d. Conservative management

SPLENIC TUMORS

44. **Most common tumor of spleen is:** *(All India 2000)*
    a. Lymphoma
    b. Sarcoma
    c. Hemangioma
    d. Metastasis

45. **Most common malignancy affecting spleen is:**
    (UPSC 2008, PGI June 97)
    a. Angiosarcoma
    b. Hamartoma
    c. Secondaries
    d. Lymphoma

46. **Most common cause of isolated splenic metastasis is:**
    (All India 2012)
    a. Carcinoma pancreas
    b. Carcinoma stomach
    c. Carcinoma ovary
    d. Carcinoma cervix

47. **True regarding hemangioma of the spleen:** *(MCI March 2005)*
    a. Least common benign tumour of the spleen
    b. May transforms into a haemangiosarcoma
    c. Malignant transformation may be managed conservatively
    d. None of the above

SPLENIC ABSCESS

48. A patient presents with fever for 3 weeks. On examination he is observed to have splenomegaly. Ultrasonography reveals a hypoechoic shadow in spleen near the hilum. Gram-negative bacilli are isolated on blood culture. Which of the following is the most likely causative organism?
    (All India 2010)
    a. Cytomegalovirus
    b. Toxoplasmosis
    c. Salmonella
    d. Lymphoma virus

SPLENIC CYST

49. **Most common cysts of the spleen are:** *(All India 2010)*
    a. Hydatid cyst
    b. Dermatoid cyst
    c. Pseudocyst
    d. Lymphangioma

ACCESSORY SPLEEN

50. **Commonest site of accessory spleen is:**
    (Recent Questions 2017, DNB 2012, AIIMS Nov 93)
    a. Lienorenal ligament
    b. Hilum of spleen
    c. Gastro splenic ligament
    d. Around tail of pancreas

51. **Spleniculi are seen in:** *(PGI June 95)*
    a. Colon
    b. Hilum
    c. Liver
    d. Lungs

52. **Accessory spleen in is found at all sites, except:**
    a. Hilum *(AIIMS 1994)*
    b. Presacral area
    c. Tail of pancreas
    d. Greater omentum, small bowel mesentery

53. **Spleniculi are most commonly found in:**
    (UPPG 2009, Orissa 2011)
    a. Splenic hilum
    b. Tail of pancreas
    c. Greater omentum
    d. Gastrocolic ligament

54. **True about splenunculi:** *(JIPMER May 2018)*
    a. It is encapsulated
    b. Most common site is tail of pancreas
    c. Often single
    d. Have more red pulp than spleen

MISCELLANEOUS

55. **Splenic vein thrombosis is best treated by:** *(USPC 97)*
    a. Splenectomy
    b. Porto-caval shunt
    c. Spleno-renal shunt
    d. Mesenterico-caval shunt

56. **The spleen contains about .... % of the total blood volume:**
    a. 1
    b. 2
    c. 5
    d. 7

57. **Splenosis means:**
    a. Infection of spleen
    b. Presence of accessory spleens
    c. Rupture of spleen and distribution of its tissue on peritoneum
    d. Non-functioning spleen

58. **True statement about splenosis:** *(PGI Nov 2017)*
    a. Occur after traumatic rupture of the spleen
    b. Function as normal spleen
    c. Multiple small implants of splenic tissue on the peritoneal surfaces
    d. Peritoneal nodules of metastatic carcinoma
    e. Benign tumor of spleen

59. **One of the following does not cause increase in the size of spleen in later stages:** *(MAHE 2001)*
    a. Sickle cell anemia
    b. Cirrhosis
    c. Infectious mononucleosis
    d. Hairy cell leukemia

60. **Removal of senescent RBC from circulation by spleen is called:**
    a. Culling
    b. Pitting
    c. Filtering
    d. Phagocytosis

61. **Downward displacement of enlarged spleen is prevented by:** *(All India 98)*
    a. Lienorenal ligament
    b. Phrenicocolic ligament
    c. Upper pole of right kidney
    d. Sigmoid colon

62. **Regarding spleen, true is:** *(AIIMS 91)*
    a. Arises from ventral mesogastrium
    b. Inferior border is notched
    c. Axis of spleen lies along 9th rib
    d. Derives its nerve supply from celiac plexus

63. **Right sided isomerism is associated with:** *(All India 2011)*
    a. Asplenia
    b. One spleen
    c. Two spleens
    d. Polysplenia

64. **Splenic vein thrombosis is most commonly caused by:**
    a. Chronic pancreatitis *(MHPGMCET 2001)*
    b. Carcinoma pancreas
    c. Spleen trauma
    d. Perforation of duodenum

65. **Tropical splenomegaly is caused by:** *(MHPGMCET 2009)*
    a. Malaria
    b. Kala-azar
    c. Schistosoma
    d. All of the above

66. **Most common splanchnic aneurysm:** *(AIIMS GIS 2003)*
    a. Splenic artery
    b. Hepatic artery
    c. Gastroduodenal artery
    d. Superior mesenteric artery

Explanations

IDIOPATHIC THROMBOCYTOPENIC PURPURA

1. **Ans. a. After ligation of splenic artery** *(Ref: Sabiston 20/e p1559-1560; Schwartz 10/e p90; Bailey 27/e p1182; Shackelford 8/e p1635, 7/e p1659-1661)*
2. **Ans. b. Splenomegaly**
3. **Ans. d. Remission occurs in 70% cases of adult ITP**
4. **Ans. b. In the bone marrow smear, there is increased number of megakaryocytes** *(Ref: Sabiston 20/e p1560)*
5. **Ans. d. An increase in platelet count on corticosteroid therapy**
6. **Ans. c. After ligating the splenic artery**
7. **Ans. a. Immediately after ligating splenic artery**
8. **Ans. c. Splenectomy** *(Ref: Sabiston 20/e p1560; Bailey 27/e p1182)*

HYPERSPLENISM

9. **Ans. d. Hypocellular bone marrow** *(Ref: Sabiston 20/e p1562; Schwartz 10/e p1427; Bailey 27/e p1184)*

HYPERSPLENISM

- Characterized by **splenic enlargement,** any combination of **anemia, leucopenia** or **thrombocytopenia, compensatory bone marrow hyperplasia** & **improvement after splenectomy**[Q].
- Careful clinical judgment is required to balance the long- and short-term risks of splenectomy against continued conservative management.

10. **Ans. a. Bone marrow hypoplasia**
11. **Ans. a. Pancytopenia, b. Thrombocytopenia, c. Leucopenia**

SPLENECTOMY

12. **Ans. d. Atelectasis** *(Ref: Sabiston 20/e p1567; Schwartz 10/e p1429-1445; Bailey 27/e p1185; Shackelford 8/e p1649, 7/e p1674-1676)*
13. **Ans. a. Trauma** *(Ref: Sabiston 20/e p1564; Schwartz 10/e p206-207; Bailey 27/e p1185)*

    Overall, the **most common indication for splenectomy** is **trauma** to the **spleen**, whether external trauma (blunt or penetrating) or iatrogenic injury (e.g. during operative procedures for other reasons).

14. **Ans. b. Sickle cell disease**

    Splenectomy is not curative in sickle cell disease.

15. **Ans. d. All**
16. **Ans. a. ITP**
17. **Ans. b. Sickle cell anemia**

Autosplenectomy	Sickle cell anemia[Q]
Autonephrectomy	Renal TB[Q]

18. **Ans. d. E. coli** *(Ref: Sabiston 20/e p1564; Schwartz 10/e p1429-1445; Bailey 27/e p1186; Shackelford 8/e p1649, 7/e p1674-1676)*
19. **Ans. b. Maximum risk is within 1 year of splenectomy** *(Ref: Sabiston 20/e p1567; Schwartz 10/e p1444, 9/e p1262; Bailey 27/e p1187; Shackelford 8/e p1649, 7/e p1674-1676)*

    Infection may occur at any time after splenectomy; in one recent series, **most infections occurred more than 2 years after splenectomy** and **42% occurred more than 5 years after splenectomy**.

20. **Ans. d. Autoimmune hemolytic anemia**
21. **Ans. c. Hereditary spherocytosis** *(Ref: Sabiston 20/e p1561; Schwartz 10/e p1429,1431; Bailey 27/e p1183; Shackelford 8/e p1638, 7/e p1662)*
22. **Ans. None**
23. **Ans. d. Pneumococcal**
24. **Ans. b. Left lower lobe atelectasis**
25. **Ans. a. When given preoperatively** *(Ref: Sabiston 20/e p1567, 19/e p1567)*

    - When elective splenectomy is planned, **vaccination against encapsulated bacteria** should be given **at least 2 weeks before surgery**.
    - If spleen is removed in **emergency, vaccination** should be given **as soon as possible** following surgery.

26. Ans. a. ITP, b. Thalassemia, c. Hereditary spherocytosis
27. Ans. c. Streptococcus pneumoniae
28. Ans. b. Pulmonary complications
29. Ans. b. Thalassemia major
30. Ans. a. Capsulated bacteria
31. Ans. b. Thrombocytosis
32. Ans. a. Left lower lobe consolidation *(Ref: Sabiston 20/e p1567; Schwartz 10/e p1444; Bailey 27/e p1186; Shackelford 8/e p1649, 7/e p1674-1676)*
    Fever on post-operative day 3 after laparoscopic splenectomy suggests left lower lobe consolidation.

    > "Left lower lobe atelectasis is the most common complication after OS; pleural effusion and pneumonia also can occur. Hemorrhage can occur intra-operatively or postoperatively, presenting as subphrenic hematoma. Transfusions have become less common since the advent of LS, although the indication for operation influences the likelihood of transfusion as well. Subphrenic abscess and wound infection are among the perioperative infectious complications."- *Schwartz 10/e p1444*

SPLENIC TRAUMA

33. Ans. a. Conservative management *(Ref: Sabiston 20/e p435-437; Schwartz 10/e p206; Shackelford 8/e p1624, 7/e p1638)*

    The innovative method for treatment of moderate splenic injury is conservative management.

    SPLENORRHAPHY

    - **Splenorrhaphy** represents a variety of **"spleen-sparing"** techniques aimed at **controlling the hemorrhage from a splenic injury**[Q] while sparing the patient the long-term immunologic consequences of splenectomy.
        - **Splenorrhaphy** is most appropriately considered in cases of **less severe splenic injury** (e.g., grades I and II, and occasionally grade III)[Q].
        - Splenorrhaphy **should not be attempted to** repair **extensive** or **complex shatter** or **crush-type injuries** of the spleen, **nor** is it well-**advised** to undertake splenorrhaphy **in** the face of **multiple concomitant traumatic injuries** or **associated hypotension**[Q].
    - The placement of a **simple monofilament suture** through the **splenic parenchyma** (often in a mattress technique and incorporating a **piece of Gelfoam** or an **omental patch** placed at the site of bleeding) will often **bring** about **satisfactory hemostasis**[Q].
    - **Wrapping** the **entire spleen** with **either absorbable** or **nonabsorbable mesh**[Q] has been described as a means of **effecting external tamponade** and **controlling bleeding** and has not been associated with significantly increased risk of infectious complications.

34. Ans. a. Splenic injury *(Ref: Sabiston 20/e p436; Shackelford 8/e p1593, 7/e p1636)*

Kehr's sign[Q]	• **Pain** may **be referred to tip** of **left shoulder** in **splenic rupture** (Kehr's sign)[Q] • Due to **irritation of undersurface of diaphragm** with **blood** and pain is referred to the shoulder through the affected fibers of phrenic nerve (**C4** & **C5**[Q]) • Kehr's sign can be **elicited by bimanual compression** of the **left upper quadrant**[Q] after the patient has been in Trendelenberg's position for about 10 minutes prior to maneuver.
Ballance's sign[Q]	• A fixed area of **percussible dullness** in the **left upper quadrant** due to **coagulation of blood from** the **injured spleen**[Q].

35. Ans. d. Conservative *(Ref: Sabiston 20/e p435-437; Schwartz 10/e p206; Bailey 27/e p1180; Shackelford 8/e p1604, 7/e p1636-1639)*
36. Ans. b. Spleen is most common organ to be involved
37. Ans. a. Pain over left shoulder
38. Ans. b. Young patients
39. Ans. b. Obliteration of splenic shadow
40. Ans. d. Catgut suturing with omental patch *(Ref: Shackelford 7/e p1638)*

    - The placement of a **simple monofilament suture** through the **splenic parenchyma** (often in a mattress technique and incorporating a **piece of Gelfoam** or an **omental patch** placed at the site of bleeding) will often **bring** about **satisfactory hemostasis**.

41. Ans. c. Splenic rupture
42. Ans. c. Obliterated colonic gas shadow *(Ref: emedicine.medscape.com/article/373694-overview)*

Signs of Splenic Injury in X-ray Abdomen	
• **Obliteration** of **spleen outline**[Q] • **Intendation of gastric air bubble** on the **left side**[Q] • Some of the **left lower ribs** may be **fractured**[Q]	• **Obliteration** of **psoas shadow**[Q] • **Elevation** of **left hemidiaphragm**[Q] • **Increased free fluid** in **between air filled intestinal coils**[Q]

43. Ans. d. Conservative management

SPLENIC TUMORS

44. **Ans. a. Lymphoma** *(Ref: Maingot 11/e p1085; Bailey 26/e p1094)*
45. **Ans. d. Lymphoma**
46. **Ans. c. Carcinoma ovary** *(Ref: Oncological Imaging by Paul Silvermann 2012/chapter 31/The spleen)*

    In case of **"isolated"** splenic metastasis, **ovarian** and **colorectal carcinomas** are the most common causes.

    - Causes of **isolated splenic metastasis**: **Carcinoma Ovary**^{Q} (27%) >**Colorectal carcinoma** (26%) >**Uterine cancer** (17%)
    - **MC primary** for **metastasis to spleen**: **Malignant melanoma**^{Q} (30-50%) > **CA Breast** (21%) > **CA Lung** (18%).

47. **Ans. d. None of the above** *(Ref: Shackelford 8/e p1643, 7/e p1651)*

SPLENIC ABSCESS

48. **Ans. c. Salmonella** *(Ref: Sabiston 20/e p1564; Schwartz 10/e p1436, 9/e p1255; Bailey 26/e p1090; Shackelford 8/e p1644, 7/e p1655-1658)*

SPLENIC CYST

49. **Ans. c. Pseudocyst** *(Ref: Sabiston 20/e p1563-1564; Schwartz 10/e p1436; Bailey 27/e p1178; Shackelford 8/e p1643, 7/e p1650-1651)*

ACCESSORY SPLEEN

50. **Ans. b. Hilum of spleen**
51. **Ans. b. Hilum**
52. **Ans. b. Presacral areas**
53. **Ans. a. Splenic hilum**
54. **Ans. a. It is encapsulated** *(Ref: Schwartz 10/e p1425; Sabiston 20/e p1561; Bailey 27/e p1178)*

MISCELLANEOUS

55. **Ans. a. Splenectomy** *(Ref: Sabiston 20/e p1531; Schwartz 10/e p1280-1281)*
56. **Ans. b. 2** *(Ref: Sabiston 20/e p1556; Schwartz 10/e p1423-1445)*

   ### SPLEEN

   - **Normal weight:** 75-100 gm^Q
   - **Average blood flow:** 300 ml/min^Q
   - Functions as the **primary filter** of the **reticuloendothelial system**^{Q}, sequestering and removing antigens, bacteria, senescent or damaged cellular elements
   - **Important role** in humoral immunity, producing IgM, opsonins, tuftsin & properdin^Q
   - **Important component** of the **complement activation system**^{Q}
   - **Source** of extramedullary hematopoiesis^Q.
   - **Contains 2%** of **total blood volume** (known as **blood bank** of **body**)^Q
   - **Normally spleen cannot be palpated; spleen** can be **palpable** when it is **enlarged 2.5 times**^{Q}.

57. **Ans. c. Rupture of spleen and distribution of its tissue on peritoneum** *(Ref: Shackelford 7/e p1616)*

   ### SPLENOSIS

   - **Splenosis** or regeneration of miniscule splenic remnants in the **peritoneal cavity**^{Q}
   - May be **encountered in cases** of **traumatic rupture** where **splenic tissue disseminates** throughout the **peritoneal cavity**^{Q}.

58. **Ans. a. Occur after....., b. Function as...., c. Multiple small implants.....**
59. **Ans. a. Sickle cell anemia**
60. **Ans. a. Culling**
61. **Ans. b. Phrenicocolic ligament** *(Ref: Grays 40/e p1107-1108, 1214, 1228, 1191)*

SPLENIC ANATOMY

- Spleen is **largest lymphatic organ**[Q]
- Related to **9th, 10th** and **11th ribs**; **Long axis** is along **10th rib**[Q]
- **Develops from** cephalic part of **dorsal mesogastrium**
- **Superior border** is **notched** at **anterior margin**[Q]
- Nerve supply from celiac plexus[Q]

Ligaments Related to Spleen
• **Phrenicocolic ligament** prevents downward displacement[Q]
• **Linorenal ligament** contain **tail of pancreas** and **splenic vessels**[Q]
• **Gastrosplenic ligament** contain **short gastric vessels**[Q]

62. **Ans. d. Derives its nerve supply from celiac plexus**
63. **Ans. a. Asplenia** *(Ref: Nelson 20/e p2233)*

Right Isomerism (Asplenia)	Left Isomerism (Polysplenia)
• **Spleen** is **absent**, **either side** of midline **resembles right side**[Q]	• **Multiple small spleens** placed on either side of midline, **either side** of midline **resembles left side**[Q]
• Also known as **bilateral right sidedness**	• Also known as **bilateral left sidedness**
• Asplenia is associated with **severe cardiac abnormalities**	• Associated with **less severe cardiac abnormalities**
• Relatively **poor prognosis**	• Relatively **better prognosis**

64. **Ans. a. Chronic pancreatitis**
65. **Ans. d. All of the above** *(Ref: Bailey 27/e p1182, 26/e p1091)*

TROPICAL SPLENOMEGALY

- **Massive splenic enlargement** frequently occurs **in** the **tropics from malaria**, **kala-azar** and **schistosomiasis**[Q].
- Occasionally, splenomegaly cannot be fully attributed to these diseases.
- It may result from **occult infection** or be **related to malnutrition**.
- The **massive splenomegaly** observed in this condition **may require removal** for those patients **disabled by anemia** or **local symptoms**[Q].
- **Lifelong antimalarial therapy** is indicated **in malaria endemic areas**[Q].

66. **Ans. a. Splenic artery** *(Ref: Sabiston 20/e p1788; Schwartz 10/e p1438; Bailey 27/e p1179; Shackelford 8/e p1045, 7/e p1098-1100)*

SECTION 4

Urology

CHAPTERS

- ☐ Kidney and Ureter
- ☐ Urinary Bladder
- ☐ Prostate and Seminal Vesicles
- ☐ Urethra and Penis
- ☐ Testis and Scrotum

CHAPTER 21

Kidney and Ureter

RENAL CALCULI

Renal Calculi

- Peak incidence 20–40 years, more common in **males**^Q
- **Infectious stones** are more common in **females**^Q
- For formation of stones, a period of **abnormal crystalluria** is required. Urine must be supersaturated with salt of the stone forming crystal (**Supersaturation & crystallization**)^Q

Clinical Features
- MC symptom is **pain**^Q.
- Severity of pain is **not related** to **size of stone**^Q

> - Stone in **upper ureter** or **renal pelvis** → pain referred to **testis**^Q in males, labia majora in females^Q
> - Stone in **mid ureter** → referred along **iliohypogastric**^Q nerve to **iliac fossa**, mimicking appendicitis
> - Stone in **lower ureter** → referred along **ilioinguinal**^Q nerve to **thigh, scrotum and perineum**^Q.

- Stone approaching **bladder** → bladder symptoms (frequency, urgency & dysuria)
- Stone in the **intramural ureter** → **strangury**^Q.
- **Drug of choice** for **ureteric colic** is diclofenac (voveran).

TYPES OF RENAL CALCULI

Types of Renal Calculi

- **Calcium oxalate**
  - **MC** type of **kidney stone (85%)**^Q
  - Risk factors are **hypercalciuria, hypercalcemia, hyperoxaluria**
  - Have **hard, small** and **jagged surface**
  - On section-wavy concentric laminae
- **Uric acid stones**
  - About **5–10 %** of all kidney stones, **MC radiolucent urinary calculi**^Q, formed in **acidic urine**
  - Patients with uric acid stones may have **gout, myeloproliferative disorders** or Lesch-Nyhan syndrome (hyperuricemia)

> **Uric Acid Stones Management**
> - Cornerstone of treatment: **Low purine diet, hydration** and **alkalization of urine**^Q
> - **Allopurinol**^Q (Inhibits conversion of hypoxanthine & xanthine to uric acid)
> - **Acetazolamide**^Q (may be added if urine pH is <6.5)

- **Struvite stones (Infection stones)**
  - Composed of **calcium, ammonium, magnesium phosphate (Triple phosphate stones)**^Q
  - Tend to grow in **alkaline urine**^Q, especially with **Proteus infection** and **fill whole of the PCS**, forming **staghorn calculi**^Q
  - Formed in **high urinary concentration** of **ammonia**
  - More common in **women**^Q (increased susceptibility for UTI)
  - Most of the **stag horn calculi** are **silent**^Q and cause **progressive destruction** of **renal parenchyma**^Q.
  - Increased tendency to form struvite calculi is seen in: **Foreign body** in the urinary tract (**Foley's catheter**) and **Neurogenic bladder**^Q/Bladder dysfunction/Bladder outlet obstruction.

> **Struvite Stones Management**
> - Complete stone removal + Treatment of a metabolic abnormality + Correction of any anatomic abnormalities contributing to stasis
> - **PCNL + ESWL (best treatment option)**^Q
> - **Antibiotics** to prevent stone recurrences or growth after operative procedure
> - **Acetohydroxamic acid (irreversible inhibitor of urease)**^Q decreases likelihood of precipitation
> - **Low calcium, low phosphorus diet**

- **Cystine**
  - **Extremely hard stone**, formed in **acidic urine**; Radio-opaque due to double sulphur bonds[Q]
  - Relatively **resistant** to fragmentation by **ESWL**
  - Occur in cystinuria with typical **"ground glass" appearance** with a **round smooth outline**[Q]
  - Typical **benzene** or **hexagonal cystine crystals**[Q] in urine.

Cystine Stones Management
• Stone removal
• To lower cystine concentration in urine (**Low methionine diet** and **alkalization**)[Q]
• **Cystine complexing agents**: D-Penicillamine[Q] and Alpha-mercaptopropionylglycine (MPG)[Q]
• **Alpha-MPG is better tolerated than d-penicillamine**

- **Xanthine**
  - Seen in **xanthinuria, radioluscent**[Q]
  - Stones are **smooth, brick red colored, round** and show **lamination on cross section**[Q]
  - Management: High fluid intake (most effective therapy) and **Allopurinol**[Q]
- **Indinavir**
  - A **protease inhibitor** used in **AIDS patients**, resulting in **radioluscent calculi**[Q] in 6% patients.
- **Silicate**: Associated with **long term use of antacids** containing **silica**[Q]
- **Triamterene**: Antihypertensive medication, leading to **radioluscent**[Q] stones

RENAL CALCULI: INVESTIGATIONS

RENAL CALCULI

Laboratory Investigations

- **Urine:** pH, microscopic examination (RBCs, pus cells and crystalluria) and culture for splitting organisms

• **Acidic urine**: CCU (**C**alcium oxalate, **C**ystine, **U**ric acid)[Q]
• **Alkaline urine**: Calcium **Phosphate**, **Struvite**[Q]

Crystalluria: To Determine the Stone Composition	
Crystal	Appearance
Calcium oxalate monohydrate	**Dumbbell** or hourglass[Q]
Calcium oxalate dehydrate	**Enveloped or bipyramidal**[Q]
Calcium phosphate (apatite)	**Amorphous**[Q], Flat shaped plates or wedge-shaped prisms
Brushite	**Needle shaped**[Q]
Struvite	**Coffin lid**[Q]
Uric acid	Multifaceted, irregular plates or rosettes[Q]
Cystine	**Hexagonal** or benzene ring[Q]

Radiographic Investigations

- **X-ray KUB:**
  - Ninety percent are **radiopaque**[Q]
  - Radiolucent stones (TIXU): Triamterene, indinavir, xanthine & uric acid[Q]
- **USG:** A screening tool for hydronephrosis or stone within collecting system.
- **IVP:**
  - Early films (At 1 and 5 min for promptness of contrast excretion and Any obstruction along urinary tract)
  - Delayed films (Identifies cause of delayed contrast excretion)

• **Non-contrast spiral CT**[Q] is the **most sensitive investigation** for **renal/ureteric calculus**[Q].

- **Retrograde pyelogram (RGP):**
  - Better delineation of anatomy. Especially useful **if distal ureter not visualized**[Q] well.
  - **Excludes unsuspected** additional **ureteric calculi** and allows **assessment of coexistent ureteric disease** such as **stricture**[Q], which may complicate the operative and post operative course.

Radionuclide Evaluation

- **DMSA** (Dimercaptosuccinic acid): Renal **morphology**[Q] (scar)
- **DTPA** (Diethylene Triamine Pentacetic Acid): To assess **perfusion** (Effective renal plasma flow) & **function**[Q] (Total and differential GFR), less effective than MAG-3 for decreased renal function

- MAG-3 (Mercapto-acetyl glycine): Best for **renal perfusion**^{Q} (Assess renal plasma flow).

> - **Metabolic workup** should be done **in young** patients, with **recurrent** calculi, **multiple** calculi and in **nephrocalcinosis**^{Q}, struvite stones, uric acid stones and cystine stones.

MANAGEMENT OF RENAL AND URETERIC CALCULI

Management of Renal and Ureteric Calculi

Indications of Conservative Treatment (for 4-6 weeks)

(Feature of stone likely to pass spontaneously)
- **Single** stone ≤ 5 mm^Q
- Stone in **lower third** of ureter^Q
- Ureter is **undilated**^{Q}
- Evidence of **downward movement**^{Q}

Surgical Intervention
- ESWL (Extracorporeal shock wave lithotripsy)
- PCNL (percutaneous nephrolithotomy)
- URS (Ureteroscopy)
- Laparoscopic stone surgery
- OSS (Open stone surgery)

- The majority (80-85%) of **simple renal calculi** are treated satisfactorily with **ESWL**^{Q}.
- Rests are managed by **PCNL/URS**
- OSS is the least common treatment modality now days.

INDICATIONS OF OPEN STONE SURGERY

Indications of Open Stone Surgery

- **Anatomic abnormality** requiring open operative intervention (e.g. PUJO)^Q
- **Nonfunctioning kidney** with stone (nephrectomy)^Q

TREATMENT DECISIONS BY STONE BURDEN

Treatment Decisions by Stone Burden

- Stone ≤ 2 cm: ESWL^Q
- Unless factors of stone composition, location, or renal anatomy shift the balance towards more invasive modalities (PCNL/URS).
- Stone > 2 cm: PCNL^Q
- Stag horn calculi: (PCNL + ESWL) is TOC^Q
- Initial approach is **PCNL, followed by ESWL,** as an adjunct to minimize the number of repeat PCNL accesses.

ESWL (EXTRACORPOREAL SHOCK WAVE LITHOTRIPSY)

ESWL (Extracorporeal Shock Wave Lithotripsy)

- **High energy shock waves**^{Q} are produced outside the patient's body, which are focused on stones with help of fluoroscopy or ultrasound.
- The **change in density** between the **soft renal tissue** and **hard stone** causes **release of energy** at the stone surface which causes "**compression induced tensile cracking** of stones"^{Q}
- Incoming shock wave result in fragmentation of stones from **erosion & shattering**^{Q}
- The stone fragments into small pieces and may pass down the ureter.
- **Strongest** or **Gold standard lithotripter** for ESWL is **Dornier unmodified HM-3.**^{Q}

> - **Difficult (hard) stones** for ESWL: Brushite, Hydroxyapatite, Cystine, Calcium oxalate monohydrate (BHC-2)^Q

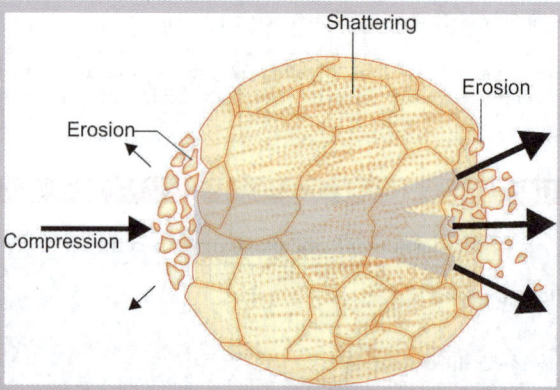

Factors Responsible for Decreasing the Chances of Stone Free Status
- **Stone burden:** Multiple stones, > 2 cm and **staghorn calculi**[Q]
- (ESWL is best suited for stone < 2 cm in renal pelvis or calyces with no distal obstruction)
- **Reduced clearance:** Lower calyceal location, marked **hydronephrosis or scarring**, **calyceal diverticulum** or **horseshoe kidney**[Q].
- **Stone composition:**
    - **Difficult:** Brushite, Hydroxyapatite, Cystine, Calcium oxalate monohydrate **(BHC-2)**[Q]
    - **Breakable:** Uric acid, struvite, Calcium oxalate dihydrate.

Contraindications of ESWL		
Absolute	**Relative**	
• **Pregnancy**[Q] • **Bleeding disorder**[Q]	• **UTI**[Q] • Unrelieved **distal obstruction**[Q] • Cardiac **pacemaker**[Q] • **Uncontrolled hypertension**[Q] • Severe **orthopaedic deformity**	• Weight **> 300 pounds** • Severe **renal failure**[Q] • **Aneurysm**

Complications of ESWL
- **Acute injury** to the **renal parenchyma** leading to **hematuria** & **edema**[Q] around the kidney.
- **Chronic renal injury** leading to accelerated **rise** in the systemic **blood pressure**, **decrease** in **renal function** and increase in rate of **stone recurrence**[Q].
- **Lung parenchymal injury** (if exposed)
- **Extrasystoles**
- **Infection** due to release of bacteria in fragment
- **Steinstrasse** (street of stones or columnation of stone gravel in ureter)[Q]

PCNL (PERCUTANEOUS NEPHROLITHOTOMY)

PCNL (Percutaneous Nephrolithotomy)

- Removal of kidney stone via a **'track'** developed **between** the **surface of skin** & **collecting system** of kidney.
- **Posterior approach**[Q] is most commonly used, **through the posterior calyx** rather than into the renal pelvis, as it **avoids damage** to **posterior branches of renal artery**[Q], which are closely associated with renal pelvis.

Indications of PCNL
- **Obstructive uropathy**[Q] (contraindication for ESWL)
- **Large volume stone (>2 cm)**, **stag horn calculi**[Q]
- Other modalities failure (**Ureteroscopic failure or ESWL failure**)[Q]
- **Lower pole calyceal stone**[Q]
- **Difficult (hard) stones for ESWL:** Brushite, Hydroxyapatite, Cystine, Calcium oxalate monohydrate (BHC-2)[Q]

Complications
- Bleeding, (MC complication)
- Urinary extravasation
- Sepsis
- Injury to other viscera like **pleura (MC)**[Q], colon, spleen
- Retained fragments

URETEROSCOPY

Ureteroscopy

- Ureteroscopic stone extraction is **highly efficacious** for **lower ureteric calculi**[Q].
- The use of small-caliber ureteroscopes and the advent of balloon dilatation or ureteral access sheaths have increased **stone-free rates (66–100%)** dramatically.

Indications
- **Lower ureteric calculi**[Q]
- **Upper ureteric calculi** of **ESWL failure**[Q]
- Suspicion of **urothelial tumor**[Q] (filling defect, Brush cytology)
- **Ureteric dilatations** or **DJ stents**[Q]
- Retrieval of **foreign body**[Q]

Complications
- Iatrogenic injuries or **ureteric perforations**[Q]

URETERIC CALCULI

Ureteric Calculi

Proximal and Mid-ureteral Stones
- Stone ≤ 1 cm: **ESWL**[Q] is primary approach. **Ureteroscopy** is preferred in **failed ESWL, distal obstruction** or **impacted stones**.
- Stone > 1 cm: **Ureteroscopy**[Q] is primary approach. PCNL for large proximal stones or impacted calculi.

Distal ureteral stones
- Stone ≤ 1 cm: ESWL and Ureteroscopy equally successful. **Ureteroscopy**[Q] is the primary approach
- Stone > 1 cm: **Ureteroscopy**[Q]

Remember: For **all ureteric stones, ureteroscopy** is the **primary approach except ≤ 1 cm proximal** and **mid-ureteral stones**Q.

INTRACORPOREAL LITHOTRIPSY

Intracorporeal Lithotripsy

Techniques
- **Electro hydrolytic lithotripter (EHL)**
  - **Narrow safety margin**, may damage ureteral mucosa but **least expensive**
  - **Suitable** for **bladder calculi**[Q].
  - **Successfully fragments 90% of calculi**[Q]
- Ultrasonic lithotripter
- Ballistic lithotripter
- **Laser lithotripter (Holmium-YAG lager)**
  - Ho-YAG is the **best laser source** for **intracorporeal lithotripsy**[Q], primarily through a **photothermal mechanism** that causes **stone vaporization**[Q].
  - **Most effective** and **versatile** with good safety margin
  - **Fragments all stones** regardless of composition. It **can cut through the metal**. So, caution must be exercised while using a basket.
  - **Potential side effect** is **production of cyanide**[Q] when **uric acid stones** are **treated**. This has been reported in vitro. The clinical experience has suggested **no significant cyanide toxicity**[Q].
  - Major disadvantage is **initial high cost** of the device and the laser fibers.

EMPHYSEMATOUS PYELONEPHRITIS

Emphysematous Pyelonephritis

- **Necrotizing infection** characterized by the **presence of gas** within the **renal parenchyma** or **perinephric tissue**[Q].
- About **80–90%** of patients have **diabetes**[Q], rest are associated with urinary tract obstruction from calculi or papillary necrosis, more common in **females**
- Bacteria most frequently cultured from the urine include **E. coli**[Q] (MC), **Klebsiella pneumoniae**, and **Enterobacter cloacae**.
- **Decreased host immunity**[Q] is **most important factor**.

Clinical Features
- Triad "**Fever, flank pain,** and **vomiting**^{Q}" almost always present and fails initial management with parenteral antibiotics
- **Pneumaturia** may be present.
- The **mortality** rate is **19–43%**^{Q}.

Diagnosis
- **Plain X-ray**: **Gas**^{Q} overlying the affected kidney
- **CT scan**^{Q} is **more sensitive** than USG in **detecting** the **presence of gas**^{Q} in the renal parenchyma

Management
- Fluid resuscitation, **prompt control of blood glucose** and **relief of urinary obstruction**^{Q} is essential with **parenteral antibiotics (3-4 weeks)**^{Q}.
- In addition, **percutaneous drainage**^{Q} is helpful in accelerating resolution of the infection and minimizing the morbidity and mortality of the infection.
- Most cases require **nephrectomy**^{Q}.

Prognosis
- Poor prognostic factors: High creatinine, low platelet, presence of **renal/perirenal fluid** with a **bubbly/loculated gas** pattern or **gas** in the collecting system.

XANTHOGRANULOMATOUS PYELONEPHRITIS

Xanthogranulomatous Pyelonephritis
- XGP is a form of **chronic bacterial infection**^{Q} of the kidney
- **Most commonly caused** by **Proteus** >E. coli
- The **affected kidney** is almost always **hydronephrotic** and **obstructed**^{Q}.

Pathology
- In most cases, XGP occurs **unilaterally**. Severe inflammation and necrosis obliterate the kidney parenchyma. Usually **pelvis** is **not dilated** due to peripelvic fibrosis.

> - It is **difficult to distinguish** XGP **from clear cell RCC** pre-operatively.
> - Even **frozen section** has **difficulties to distinguish** XGP **from clear cell RCC**.

- Characteristically, **foamy lipid-laden histiocytes (xanthoma cells)**^{Q} are present and may be mistaken for renal clear cell carcinoma.

Clinical Features
- Flank pain, fever, chills, and persistent bacteriuria with palpable flank mass.
- A history of **urolithiasis**^{Q} is present in **50%** of the patients, **staghorn calculi**^{Q} in **80%** cases.
- Primarily occurs **unilaterally**, azotemia or renal failure is **not seen**.

Diagnosis
- **Urinalysis**: Demonstrates **WBCs** and **protein**.
- **Proteus species (MC)**^{Q} or **E. coli** are commonly cultured from the urine, **one third** of patients have **no growth**, most likely because they have recently received antibiotic therapy.
- **Serum blood analysis**: Anemia and **hepatic dysfunction**^{Q} in approximately **50%** of patients.
- **CT scan is IOC for XGP**.
- **USG**: Enlarged kidney with a large central echogenic area and **anechoic parenchyma**^{Q}.

Management
- Kidney-sparing surgery (**partial nephrectomy**) is indicated XGP.
- **Nephrectomy** in cases of **extensive infection**.

PYONEPHROSIS

Pyonephrosis
- Bacterial infection of a **hydronephrotic, obstructed kidney**^{Q}, which leads to **suppurative destruction** of the renal parenchyma and potential loss of renal function.
- Kidney is a **bag of pus**^{Q}.
- **MC cause: Renal stones**^{Q}. Others are infected hydronephrosis, acute pyelonephritis.

Clinical Features
- Mostly **unilateral**^{Q}, characterized by triad of **anemia, fever** and **swelling in loin**^{Q}.

Diagnosis
- **USG** diagnose pyonephrosis.

Management
- Immediate institution of **antibiotic therapy** and **drainage**^{Q} of the infected collecting system.
- Antibiotics should be started before manipulation of the urinary tract.
- In the **ill patient**, drainage of the collecting system with a **percutaneous nephrostomy**^{Q} tube
- **Nephrectomy** in **destroyed** or **non-functioning kidney**

PERINEPHRIC ABSCESS

PERINEPHRIC ABSCESS

- Sources of perinephric abscesses are mainly **extension** of **cortical abscesses** or **hematogenous**^{Q}.
- Generally caused by **E. coli** or **Proteus**^{Q} species.

Clinical Features
- **High grade swinging fever**^{Q}, abdominal tenderness and flank mass

Diagnosis
- **Urine cultures** (positive only if communication with collecting system is present, so most are usually negative) identify causative organisms in **one-third**^{Q} and **blood cultures** in **half**^{Q} of cases
- Accurately detected on **USG** or **CT scans**.

Management
- Appropriate **antibiotic therapy**^{Q}. If the patient **does not respond within 48 hours** of treatment, **percutaneous drainage**^{Q} under CT or ultrasound guidance is indicated.
- If the abscess still does not resolve, then **open surgical drainage** or **nephrectomy**^{Q} may be necessary.
- Follow-up imaging is needed to confirm the resolution of the abscesses.

GENITOURINARY TUBERCULOSIS

GENITOURINARY TUBERCULOSIS

- Tubercle bacilli (**M. tuberculosis**) may invade one or more organs of genitourinary tract and cause **chronic granulomatous infection**^{Q}.
- More common in **males**^{Q} (young adults of age **20-40** years)

Etiology
- M. tuberculosis reaches the genitourinary organs by **hematogenous route** from **lungs**^{Q}.
- The **primary site** is often **not symptomatic** or **apparent**^{Q}.

> - Tubercle bacilli lodge in **periglomerular capillaries** and form **cortical granulomas**^{Q} after hematogenous spread from a distant focus.
> - These contain **dormant bacilli** that may remain stable, but have the potential to multiply, years later producing the disease.
> - **Spontaneous healing** is the **usual response**^{Q}.

- Development of **disease** depends on the **interaction between pathogen & immune response of host**^{Q}.
- In whole of genitourinary tract, **Kidney & prostate** is the **primary site of infection**^{Q} (hematogenous). Rest organs are involved by ascent or descent.
- Generally **testis** is **not involved**^{Q}.

Pathogenesis
- **Granulomas** at renal pyramid → Enlarge (**tubercular abscess**) → Burst into **PC system** & **pus discharge** in urine (sterile pyuria^Q).
- **Vesical irritability** is an **early clinical manifestation**^{Q}.

Complications

> **Stenosis** of calyceal neck or pelvic ureteric junction → **Hydronephrosis & pyonephrosis** → **Perinephric abscess** → Kidney replaced by caseous material (**putty kidney**) → **Calcification (Cement Kidney)** → **Autonephrectomy** (a calcified non-functioning kidney, representing end-stage disease)^Q.

- **Autonephrectomy** is the final result of marked parenchymal fibrosis & obstructive uropathy.
- **Scarring** with **stricture formation**[Q] is one of the most typical lesions of tuberculosis and most commonly affects **juxtavesical portion** of **ureter**.
- **Inflammation** of **bladder mucosa** in early stages → **tubercle formation** (seen endoscopically as **white** or **yellow raised nodules**[Q] surrounded by halo of hyperemia) → Mural fibrosis (**Thimble bladder**)[Q]
- **Large calcifications** in the **prostate** & **beaded appearance** of **vas deferens**[Q]

Clinical Features

> - Earliest symptom is urinary frequency[Q]

- **Active tuberculosis** elsewhere in the **body** is found in **less than half** of patients with **genitourinary tuberculosis**[Q].
- In tuberculosis of epididymis, an abscess may drain spontaneously through the scrotal wall. A **chronic draining sinus** should be regarded as **tubercular** until proved otherwise.

> **Tuberculosis of genital tract should be considered in the presence of following situations**
> - **Chronic cystitis**[Q] that refuses to respond to adequate treatment
> - **Sterile pyuria**, **gross** or **microscopic hematuria**[Q]
> - Non-tender enlarged epididymis with **beaded** or thickened **vas**[Q]
> - **Chronic draining scrotal sinus**[Q]
> - **Induration** or **nodulation** of **prostate** and **thickening** of one or both **seminal vesicle**[Q]

Diagnosis
- Diagnosis rest on **demonstration** of **tubercle bacilli** in the **urine** by **culture** or **PCR**[Q].

> **Urine:** Pyuria with **acid urine**, **sterile** on ordinary culture (**Persistent pyuria without organisms** on culture means **tuberculosis** until proved otherwise), culture for tubercle bacilli from the **first morning urine sample** is positive in high percentage of patients.

- **Plain X-ray:** May show **calcified lesions** or **punctate calcifications**[Q] in renal parenchyma
- **IVP: IOC for diagnosis of early renal TB**[Q]

> **IVP in Tuberculosis**
> - Earliest sign is **"moth-eaten" calyx**[Q] (Obliteration of clear cut outline of renal papilla) due to erosion.
> - **Obliteration** of one or more **calyces** (calectasis, hydronephrosis)
> - SOL in pelvis (**TB abscess**) seen as **splaying of calyces**[Q]
> - **Ureteric strictures**[Q] (single or multiple)
> - **Shrunken bladder** with irregular wall (**Thimble bladder**)[Q]
> - Absence of function of kidney due to complete ureteral occlusion and renal destruction (**autonephrectomy**)[Q]

- **RGP:** Extensive calcification or thickness of the ureter (**Pipe-stem ureter**)[Q], are usually associated with **pyonephrosis**.

> **Cystoscopy in Tuberculosis**
> - Earliest sign is **pallor**[Q] around ureteric orifice.
> - Other features are **tubercular ulcer** and **golf hole ureteric orifice**[Q].

- **CECT is IOC** for **genitourinary tuberculosis**[Q].
- **MRI:** Diffuse, radiating streaky areas of low signal intensity in the prostate (watermelon skin sign)

Treatment
- **ATT** and **Surgery (for complications)**[Q]

> **Surgery in Genitourinary Tuberculosis**
> Optimal time of surgery is **3-6 weeks**[Q] after ATT is started.
> **Procedures**
> - **Ureteral dilatations** offer >50% chances of cure in **ureteric strictures**[Q]
> - **Pyeloplasty** for PUJ obstruction
> - **Boari operation** or bowel interposition for **ureteral strictures**[Q]
> - **Augmentation** or substitution **cystoplasty** for **bladder contracture**[Q]
> - **Nephroureterectomy** for **nonfunctioning kidney** (as the ureters are usually refluxing)
> - **Partial nephrectomy** for **polar lesions** not responding to ATT

> **Indications of Surgery in Genitourinary TB**
> - Associated **RCC/malignancy**[Q]
> - **Non-functioning** kidney with **hypertension**[Q]
> - **Non-functioning** kidney with **totally destroyed parenchyma** or **deranged function**[Q]

HYDRONEPHROSIS

HYDRONEPHROSIS

- Hydronephrosis is an **aseptic dilatation** of the kidney caused by **obstruction to the outflow of urine**.

Unilateral Hydronephrosis		
Extramural Obstruction	**Intramural Obstruction**	**Intraluminal Obstruction**
• **Tumour** from **adjacent structures**[Q], e.g. carcinoma of the **cervix, prostate**, rectum, colon or cecum • **Idiopathic retroperitoneal fibrosis**[Q] • **Retrocaval ureter**[Q]	• **Congenital stenosis** (PUJ obstruction)[Q] • **Ureterocele** and congenital small ureteric orifice • **Inflammatory stricture**[Q] • **Neoplasm** of the **ureter** or **bladder** cancer involving the **ureteric orifice**[Q]	• **Calculus** in the **pelvis** or **ureter**[Q] • **Sloughed papilla** in papillary **necrosis**[Q] (especially in **diabetics**[Q], **analgesic abusers**[Q] and those with **sickle cell disease**[Q]) may obstruct the ureter

Bilateral Hydronephrosis	
Congenital	**Acquired**
• **Posterior urethral valves**[Q] • **Urethral atresia**[Q]	• **BPH** or **CA prostate**[Q] • Postoperative **bladder neck scarring**[Q] • **Urethral stricture**[Q] • **Phimosis**[Q]

Pathology
- There is **calyceal dilatation** & **renal parenchyma** is **destroyed by pressure atrophy**[Q].
- A **kidney** destroyed by longstanding hydronephrosis is a **thin-walled, lobulated, fluid-filled sac**.
- **Urethral obstruction** tends to lead to **detrusor hypertrophy**, which can lead to **obstruction of** the **ureters** in their **intramural course**[Q].

Clinical Features

Unilateral Hydronephrosis
- Unilateral hydronephrosis is more common in women and on the right.
- **Presenting features** include the following:
  - **Mild pain** or **dull aching** in the **loin**, often with a sensation of dragging heaviness made worse by excessive fluid intake. The **kidney may be palpable**[Q].
  - **Attacks of acute renal colic** may occur with no palpable swelling.
  - **Intermittent hydronephrosis** (Dietl's crisis)[Q]. A **swelling in the loin** is associated with **acute renal pain**. Some hours later the **pain is relieved** and the **swelling disappears** when a **large volume of urine is passed**[Q].

Bilateral Hydronephrosis
- From lower urinary obstruction symptoms of **bladder outflow obstruction**[Q] predominate.
- The kidneys are unlikely to be **palpable**[Q] because renal failure intervenes before the kidneys become sufficiently large.

Diagnosis
- **Ultrasound**[Q] is the least invasive means of detecting hydronephrosis and is regularly used to diagnose **PUJ obstruction** in utero.
- **Excretion urography** is only helpful if there is **significant function** in the **obstructed kidney**.
- **Isotope renography (DTPA scan)**[Q] is the **best test** to establish that dilatation of the **renal collecting system** is **caused by obstruction**.
- Very occasionally, a **Whitaker test** is indicated.

Treatment
- The **indications for operation** are **bouts of renal pain, increasing hydronephrosis, evidence of parenchymal damage** and **infection**[Q].
- **Conservation of renal tissue**[Q] is the aim; nephrectomy should be considered only when the renal parenchyma has been largely destroyed.
- **Mild cases** should be **followed by serial USG** and **operated upon if dilation is increasing**[Q].

PERCUTANEOUS NEPHROSTOMY

PERCUTANEOUS NEPHROSTOMY

- Percutaneous nephrostomy is occasionally essential, if not life saving, in the treatment of **acute** or **chronic upper urinary tract obstruction**[Q].
- It is the **first step** in **obtaining antegrade access to the kidney**[Q] for various procedures.

Indications of Percutaneous Nephrostomy
• **Acute** or **chronic upper urinary tract obstruction**[Q] in which access to the kidney is impossible from the lower urinary tract • **Creatinine** level is **rising above the reference range**[Q] and the urine cannot be drained through the ureter • **Renal pelvis disorders** (UPJ obstruction, horseshoe kidneys, ureter duplex, ureter fissures, double renal collecting systems)[Q] • **Hydronephrosis in renal transplant allografts**[Q] • **Treatment of staghorn calculi** and **large** or **lower-pole kidney stones**[Q]	• **Contraindications to ESWL**[Q] • **Stones** or **tumors associated with distal obstruction** or a **foreign body**[Q] that cannot be removed through the ureter • When **rapid dilation of the nephrostomy tract** is **required**[Q] • To diagnose ureteral obstruction, filling defects, and anomalies via antegrade radiography • Tumors, such as sarcomas, ovarian tumors, and other retroperitoneal tumors

ANGIOMYOLIPOMA

ANGIOMYOLIPOMA

- AML is a **benign** clonal neoplasm consisting of varying amounts of **mature adipose tissue, smooth muscle & thick-walled vessels**[Q]

  - Approximately **20–30%** are found in patients with **tuberous sclerosis (TS)**[Q]
  - **AML in TS** is more likely to be **bilateral & multicentric**, presents with **accelerated growth rates & symptomatic presentation**[Q]

- Who do not have TS (**70-80%**), pronounced **female predominance**, present **later** during **5th** or **6th decade**[Q]
- **Massive retroperitoneal hemorrhage** from AML (**Wunderlich's syndrome**)[Q] is seen in **10%** of patients. It's the most significant and feared complication.
- **Pregnancy** appears to **increase the risk of hemorrhage**[Q] from AML

Diagnosis

- **CT scan: Presence of fat**[Q] within a renal lesion virtually **excludes the diagnosis of RCC** and is considered **diagnostic of AML**.
- **Lack of calcification**[Q]

- **USG:** Well circumscribed, **highly echogenic lesion**, often associated with **shadowing**.
- **Angiography: Aneurysmal dilation**[Q] is found in **50% of AMLs**
- Positive immunoreactivity for **HMB-45**[Q], is **characteristic** for **AML** (used to differentiate AML from sarcoma)

Treatment

- **Asymptomatic** AML upto **4 cm: Follow up** with imaging at 6-12 months.
- **Symptomatic** or **> 4 cm:** Intervention is required.
  - **Nephron sparing approach** for small symptomatic AML by selective **embolization**[Q] (most preferred) or **partial nephrectomy**
  - **Total nephrectomy** for larger lesions or **life threatening hemorrhage**[Q]

ONCOCYTOMA

ONCOCYTOMA

- Represents **3–7%** of all solid renal masses; Arise from **oncocytes, rich in mitochondria**[Q]
- Most renal oncocytomas **cannot be differentiated** from **eosinophilic variant of chromophobe RCC**[Q] by clinical or radiographic means

Pathology

- In grossly, tumors are light brown or tan, **homogeneous**, and **well circumscribed**, not truly encapsulated
- A **central scar** without prominent necrosis or hypervascularity.
- Ultrastructurally, **packed** with **numerous large mitochondria**, which contributes to their **distinctive staining characteristics**[Q]

Diagnosis

- **CT scan: Central stellate scar**[Q]
- **Angiography: Spoke-wheel pattern**[Q] of feeding arteries
- **MRI:** well-defined capsule, central stellate scar, and distinctive intensities on T1 and T2 images

Treatment

- A **nephron-sparing approach**[Q] is preferred.

Central Stellate Scar is seen in	
• FNH[Q] • Fibrolamellar HCC[Q]	• Serous cystadenoma[Q] (pancreas) • Renal oncocytoma[Q]

CLASSIFICATION OF RCC

CLASSIFICATION OF RCC

- **Clear cell carcinoma:**
  - **MC type** of RCC, **mainly sporadic**^{Q}.

  > - Both sporadic & familial cases are associated with **loss of sequence** on **chromosome 3** either by **translocation (3:6, 3:8, 3:11)** or **deletion**^{Q}.
  > - This region harbors the **VHL gene**^{Q}

  - Arise from **proximal convoluted tubule (PCT)** particularly of **cortex**^{Q}.
  - Occurs as **solitary unilateral lesion**^{Q}, often a pseudocapsule is formed around tumor by compression of surrounding tissue.
  - Tumor cells are **clear** and contain **glycogen & lipids**^{Q}.
  - Most are **well differentiated**^{Q}.
- **Papillary carcinoma:**
  - Characterized by **papillary growth pattern**^{Q}.

  > - MC cytogenetic abnormalities are **trisomies 7, 16, & 17**^{Q}.
  > - Loss of 18 in sporadic form, trisomy 7 in familial form.
  > - This is due to **mutated MET gene** on chromosome **7**^{Q}.

  - **Arise from proximal convoluted tubule (PCT)**^{Q}, can be **multifocal & bilateral**^{Q}
  - Typically **hemorrhagic & cystic**.
  - Papillary carcinoma is the **MC type** of RCC in patients with **dialysis associated cystic disease**^{Q}.
  - Composed of **cuboidal & low columnar cells**^{Q}.
  - **Psammoma bodies** may be present.
- **Chromophobe renal carcinoma:**
  - Represent 5% of RCC, composed of cells with **prominent cell membrane & eosinophilic cytoplasm** with a **halo around nucleus**.
  - Relative **transparent cytoplasm** with a **fine reticular pattern** described as 'Plant cell' appearance.
  - Associated with **best prognosis**

  > - These tumors exhibit **multiple chromosome loss & extreme hypodiploidy**^{Q}.
  > - Loss of multiple chromosomes 1^Q, 2^Q, 6, 10, 13, 17, 21 & Y^Q.

  - Arises from **intercalated cells** of **collecting duct**^{Q}.
  - Composed of **pale eosinophilic cells** often with a **perinuclear halo**^{Q}.
- **Collecting duct (bellini duct) carcinoma:**
  - **Rarest type** of RCC^Q, composed of malignant cells enmeshed within a prominent fibrotic stroma typically in medullary location.
  - Arise from **collecting duct cells** in the **medulla**^{Q}.
  - **Hobnail pattern** on histology^Q
  - Has got **very aggressive course**^{Q}.
  - Associated with **desmoplastic reaction**^{Q}
- **Remember:** **Medullary cell carcinoma** is seen **almost exclusively** in association with **sickle cell trait**.

RENAL CELL CARCINOMA

- MC type of RCC: **Clear cell carcinoma**^{Q}
- MC type seen with **dialysis associated cystic disease: Papillary carcinoma**^{Q}
- **Exclusively** associated with **sickle cell trait: Medullary cell carcinoma**^{Q}
- Best prognosis: **Chromophobe carcinoma**^{Q}

RENAL CELL CARCINOMA

RENAL CELL CARCINOMA (GRAVITZ TUMOR, HYPERNEPHROMA, INTERNIST'S TUMOR, RADIOLOGIST'S TUMOR)^Q

- **MC malignant tumor** of adult kidney and **most lethal**^{Q} of all malignancies
- More common in **males**, in 6th & 7th decade
- Majority are **sporadic**
- Hereditary variants are **VHL syndrome, Hereditary clear cell carcinoma** and **Hereditary papillary carcinoma**^{Q}
- Tumor usually involve **upper pole**^{Q}

Risk Factors
- Most significant risk factors are **smoking & tobacco chewing**[Q]
- Other risk factors are obesity, hypertension, exposure to **Asbestos**, petroleum products and **cadmium**, chronic renal failure (specially due to **analgesic nephropathy**)[Q]

Spread
- Characteristic feature of RCC is tendency to **invade renal vein**. Further extension produces a **continuous cord of tumor** in IVC and even in **right side of heart**[Q].
- **MC route** is **hematogenous**[Q]

> - MC sites of distant metastasis are **lungs (cannon ball deposits & pulsating secondaries)**[Q] > bone> liver> brain.

- **Lymphatic spread** occurs when tumor extends beyond renal capsule.

Notable Features of RCC
- Encapsulated in spite of being malignant (**pseudocapsule**)
- **Spontaneous regression**[Q]
- **Refractoriness** to **cytotoxic agents**[Q]
- **Response** to **biological response modifiers (IL-2 & IFN-alpha)**[Q]
- **Prolonged** period of **stable disease**[Q]

Clinical Features
- Classical triad of **gross hematuria, abdominal mass & pain** is seen in **10% cases**[Q] (**Too late triad**)
- MC and **consistent presentation** is **hematuria**[Q].
- Other symptoms are fever, weight loss, malaise, **acute & non-reducing varicocele, lower limb edema** due to IVC obstruction.

RCC: Paraneoplastic Syndromes (20%)
- **Raised ESR: MC** paraneoplastic manifestation[Q]
- **Hypercalcemia:**
  - Due to production of **PTH-rp**[Q]
  - **Only paraneoplastic syndrome** in which **medical therapies** are proven **useful**.
- **Hypertension**[Q] (**Renin** production from tumor)
- **Polycythemia**[Q] (**Erythropoietin** production from tumor)
- **Stauffer's syndrome:**
  - **Non-metastatic hepatic dysfunction**[Q] due to raised **IL-6**[Q] leading to **increased ALP, PT** and **bilirubin**
  - Hepatic function **normalizes after nephrectomy**[Q]
- Others are: **Cushing syndrome**, hypoglycemia, anemia, gynecomastia, amenorrhea

Diagnosis

- **Diagnostic IOC: CT** (95% accurate)[Q]
- **MRI** is **most accurate** non-invasive investigation for detecting **tumor thrombus** in **renal vein** or **IVC**. Distinguishes **tumor thrombus** from **bland thrombus**[Q]
- **Inferior venocavogram**[Q] is **most sensitive & specific** but **invasive** means to detect involvement of **IVC**.

- **Renal arteriography** is done before **renal sparing surgery** (partial nephrectomy), but 3-D helical CT is also sufficient.
- Specific **plain X-ray** finding is **central calcification**[Q].

FNAC is not Routinely done in RCC, Indications are
• Suspected **secondaries**[Q]	• Clinical suspicion of **renal abscess**[Q]
• Suspected **lymphoma**[Q]	• To prove pathological diagnosis in **disseminated** or **unresectable disease**[Q]

Treatment

Localized RCC
- **TOC** is **open radical nephrectomy**[Q]
- Chemotherapy & radiotherapy is not effective

- Patient with **Stauffer's syndrome** are also candidate for **radical nephrectomy**[Q].
- **Radical nephrectomy** or **debulking** is done **for cytoreduction** in both **locally advanced** and **metastatic RCC**[Q].

Indications of Nephron Sparing Surgery

- **Bilateral RCC** or **VHL syndrome**[Q]
- RCC involving a **solitary functioning kidney**[Q]
- Unilateral carcinoma and a functioning opposite kidney affected by a condition that might threaten its future function (e.g. RAS)
- Low stage or ≤ **4 cm RCC**[Q] at any location

Locally Advanced and Metastatic RCC

- **Sunitinib** is the **first line treatment** for **metastatic RCC** (response rate: **31%**)[Q]
- Combined **IL-2** & **IFN-alpha** is the **2nd line** treatment for **metastatic RCC** (response rate: **15%**)[Q]
- Chemotherapy with **vinblastine**[Q], as it is single most effective agent
- **Removal of thrombus** should be considered in **renal or IVC extension**[Q]
- **Radiotherapy** for **symptomatic bone metastasis**[Q]

Prognostic Factors

- **Pathologic stage**[Q] is single **most important** prognostic factor
- **Lymph node involvement** is a **poor** prognostic factor

Staging and Grading

- TNM (preferred) and **Robson's**[Q] staging are used for RCC.
- **Fuhrman**[Q] histological system is used for **grading**.
- **Leibovich prognostic score** (0–11) **for RCC**: Based on **tumor stage, grade, size, involvement of LN & tumor necrosis** histologically[Q].

8th AJCC (2017) TNM Staging for Renal Cell Carcinoma

T: Primary tumor	N: Regional lymph nodes
T1a: Tumor ≤**4 cm** and confined to the kidney[Q] **T1b**: Tumor >**4 cm** and ≤**7.0 cm** and confined to the kidney[Q]	N0: No regional lymph nodes metastasis N1: Metastasis in regional lymph node
T2a: Tumor >**7 cm** but ≤**10 cm** and confined to the kidney[Q] **T2b**: Tumor >**10 cm** and confined to the kidney[Q]	
T3a: Tumor grossly extends into **renal veins** or its **segmental (muscle containing) branches**, or tumor invades perirenal and/or renal sinus fat but **not beyond Gerota's fascia**[Q]	M: Distant metastases M0: No distant metastasis M1: Distant metastasis present
T3b: Tumor grossly extents into **vena cava below diaphragm**[Q]	
T3c: Tumor extends into the **vena cava above** the **diaphragm** or **invades** the **wall of vena cava**[Q]	
T4: Tumor invades **beyond Gerota's fascia**[Q] (including contiguous extension into ipsilateral adrenal gland)	

Stage I	Stage II	Stage III	Stage IV
T1N0M0	T2N0M0	T1-3 N1 M0 T3 N0 M0	T4 anyN M0 AnyT anyN **M1**

Pediatric Tumors

- MC **malignant** tumor of infancy - MC **extracranial solid** tumor in children - MC **abdominal** malignancy in children	- **Neuroblastoma**[Q]
- MC **primary malignant renal** tumor of **childhood**	- **Wilms' tumor**[Q]
- MC **renal tumor** of **infancy**	- **Congenital mesoblastic nephroma**[Q]
- MC **soft tissue** tumor in **infants & children**	- **Rhabdomyosarcoma**[Q]
- MC **solid tumor** of **childhood**	- **Brain tumor**[Q]
- MC **cancer of childhood**	- **Leukemia**[Q] (30%) >**Brain tumors**[Q] (22%)

WILMS' TUMOR

WILMS' TUMOR

- Wilms' tumor: **MC primary renal tumor** of childhood (2-5 years)[Q].
- Wilms' tumor: **2nd MC malignant abdominal tumor** in children (MC is **neuroblastoma**).
- Arise from kidney, composed of **three elements- Blastema, Epithelium & Stroma**[Q]. (BESt)
- MC presenting feature is **asymptomatic abdominal mass or swelling**[Q].
- Mostly **unilateral**.

> - Characterized by **triad of abdominal mass, fever & microscopic hematuria**[Q].

- Fever typically resolve after tumor resection

Associated Malformations

- **WAGR Syndrome**[Q]: It consists of **aniridia, genital anomalies & mental retardation**. The risk of **Wilms' tumor is increased** by **33%** in this syndrome[Q]. Associated with **WT-1 gene deletion** located on chromose[Q] **11p 13**
- **Denys-Drash Syndrome**[Q]: It consists of **gonadal dysgenesis** (Male pseudohermaphroditism), **nephropathy** leading to **renal failure**. Majority of patients with this syndrome **have renal failure**.
- **Beckwith-Wiedmann Syndrome**[Q]: It consists of **enlargement of body organs**, **hemi-hypertrophy**, **renal medullary cysts** and **abnormal large cells** in **adrenal cortex**, macroglossia, omphalocele, hepatoblastoma. Associated with **WT-2 gene deletion** located on chromosome **11p 15.5**.

Diagnosis

- **USG (first investigation)**[Q] or CT abdomen for staging.
- **MRI** is **superior** to other imaging modalities in **delineating nephroblastomatosis elements**.
- **Calcification** tends to be more **crescent shaped, discrete & peripheral**[Q] in comparison of finely stippled calcification of neuroblastoma.

Treatment

- **Surgical excision (transperitoneal radical nephrectomy)** is treatment of choice.
- **Routine exploration** of **contralateral kidney** is **not necessary** if imaging is satisfactory and doesn't suggest bilateral process.

> - In unfavorable histology, **Radiation therapy** should be **started within 10 days**[Q] after nephrectomy, **Chemotherapy** should be **started 5 days after surgery**[Q].

- **Chemotherapy:** *VCD* (Vincristine + Cyclophosphamide + Doxorubicin or dactinomycin)
- **Whole lung irradiation** is recommended for **pulmonary metastasis**.

Preoperative Treatment should be Considered	
• **Solitary kidney**[Q] • **Bilateral**[Q] renal tumors • Tumor in **horse shoe kidney**[Q]	• Tumor **thrombus in IVC above** the level of **hepatic veins**[Q] • **Respiratory distress** due to **metastatic**[Q] disease

Prognosis

- **Histology**[Q] of Wilms' tumor & **tumor stage** is identified as most important **determinant of prognosis**[Q] (Histology > Stage).

The **postchemotherapy based staging system** is the **'SIOP' staging** system developed by the **International society of oncology**.
Two Staging Systems are currently being used for the staging of Wilms' Tumor.

Prechemotherapy Staging System	Postchemotherapy Staging System
• Developed by the **National Wilms' Tumor staging Group (NWTSG** - Staging system) • This staging system is widely used in **North America** and **Canada** • 'NWTSG' approach involves **employment of 'primary surgery'**. • **Chemotherapy** with or without **Radiation therapy** is given **after surgery** • **Staging** is done **at time of surgery (Prechemotherapy)**	• Developed by the **International Society of Pediatric Oncology (SIOP** - Staging system) • This staging system is widely used in Europe • 'SIOP' approach involves employment of **preoperative chemotherapy without histological confirmation** of Wilms' tumor. • **Primary chemotherapy** for **all patients** regardless of extent • **Staging** is done **at time of surgery (Postchemotherapy)**

CARCINOMA RENAL PELVIS

Carcinoma Renal Pelvis

- Transitional cell carcinoma accounts for **90%** of **upper urinary tract cancers**[Q].
- Urothelial cancer often presents as a **widespread urothelial abnormality**: Patients with a single upper-tract carcinoma are at **risk** for developing **bladder carcinoma (30-50%)**[Q] and **contralateral upper urinary tract carcinoma (2-4%)**.
- More common in **males**

Etiology
- Smoking[Q]
- Excessive analgesic (Phenacetin) intake[Q]
- Industrial dyes or solvents[Q]
- Balkan's nephropathy[Q]

Clinical Features
- **Painless gross hematuria (MC)**[Q], flank pain, irritative voiding symptoms

Diagnosis
- **Ureteroscopic brush cytology for malignant cells**[Q]
- **IVP** showing **radioluscent intraluminal filling defects**[Q]

> - **CT urography** is **IOC** for evaluation of **upper urinary tract**[Q]
> - Ureteral tumors are often characterized by **ureteral dilation below** the **site** of the **lesion**, creating the appearance of a **"goblet"** (better **appreciated** on **RGP**)[Q]
> - **Bergman sign**[Q]: A ureteral catheter passed upto ureter may coil distal to the ureter

Treatment
- **Nephroureterectomy** with a cuff of bladder[Q].
- Periodic follow up with cystourethroscopy as **risk** for developing **bladder carcinoma (30-50%)** and **contralateral upper urinary tract carcinoma (2–4%)**[Q].

RENAL INJURIES

Renal Injuries

- Kidney is the **most commonly injured** part of **urinary tract**[Q]
- MC cause of blunt renal injury is **motor vehicle accident**[Q].
- **Hematuria** is the **best indicator**[Q] of traumatic urinary system injury.
- More than 80% of patients sustaining **penetrating renal injuries** have **other intra-abdominal injuries**[Q].
- Blunt renal injuries are generally divided into minor and major injuries.
- **Minor injuries** account for approximately **85%**[Q] of cases.

> **Penetrating wounds** causing **small parenchymal injuries** are generally treated by **débridement, primary repair,** and **drainage**[Q].

- **Injuries involving the hilum** are **seldom repaired primarily**[Q], and in most circumstances total nephrectomy is necessary.

Imaging Studies

> **Contrast enhanced CT is the IOC for Renal Injuries**[Q]
>
> **Indications**
> - Gross hematuria[Q]
> - Microscopic hematuria with hypotension[Q] anytime during initial resuscitation

- **IVP** should be done to see the **function of the opposite kidney**[Q]
- **Arteriography** is used to **define arterial injuries** suspected on CT or to **localize arterial bleeding** that can be controlled by **embolization**[Q].

Grade	Type	Description
I	Contusion	Microscopic (**>3 RBCs/HPF**)[Q] or gross hematuria, urological studies normal
	Hematoma	**Subcapsular,** nonexpanding without parenchymal laceration.
II	Hematoma	Nonexpanding **perirenal** hematoma, confined to renal retroperitoneum
	Laceration	**<1 cm** parenchymal depth of renal cortex **without urine extravasation**[Q].
	Laceration	**>1 cm** parenchymal depth of renal cortex **without collection system rupture or urinary extravasation**[Q]

Grade	Type	Description
IV	Laceration	Parenchymal laceration **extending through collecting system**[Q]
	Vascular	**Main renal artery** or **vein injury** with contained hemorrhage
V	Laceration	Completely **"Shattered kidney"**[Q]
	Vascular	**Avulsion of renal hilum**, devascularising the kidney.

Note: Advance one grade for bilateral injuries upto grade III.

Management

Nonoperative

- **Most (>95%)** of **renal injuries** can be **managed non-operatively**[Q].
- Significant renal injuries (Grade II–V) are found only in **5%** of renal trauma.
- A **hemodynamically stable patient** with an **injury well staged by a CT scan** can usually be **managed without renal exploration**[Q]. Hospital admission, bed rest, vital monitoring and repeated CT scan is required.

Renal Exploration in Injuries

- Renal exploration should be done by transabdominal approach in order to have a control on the renal vessels first[Q].

Absolute Indications	Relative Indications
• Persistent renal bleeding[Q] • Expanding or pulsatile perirenal hematoma[Q]	• Urinary extravasation • Non viable tissue (>20% necrosis) • Segmental arterial injury

Indications of Nephrectomy

- Hemodynamically **unstable patient**, with **low body temperature** and **poor coagulation**, with a **normal contralateral kidney**[Q].
- **Extensive renal injuries**[Q] when the patient's life would be threatened by an attempt at renal repair.
- Already **poorly functioning hydronephrotic kidney**[Q] with continuous bleeding

COMPLICATIONS AFTER RENAL TRAUMA

Complications after Renal Trauma

- **Complication rate** after renal trauma is **3–10%**[Q]
- **Urinoma** is the **MC complication**[Q] after renal trauma
- **Delayed bleeding** usually occurs **within 1–2 weeks**[Q] after injury

Early Complications	Late Complications
• Urinoma, delayed bleeding • Urinary fistula, abscess • Hypertension	• Hydronephrosis, pyonephrosis • Stone formation, AV fistula • Delayed hypertension

RUPTURE OF THE URETER

Rupture of the Ureter

Ureteric Injury during Operation

- **MC cause** of injury to the ureters is **surgical trauma** during **hysterectomy** or other **pelvic surgery**[Q]
- **Preoperative catheterization** of ureters makes them easier to **protect** during surgery[Q]
- **Injuries discovered** at the time of surgery should be **repaired immediately**[Q]

Clinical Features

- Unilateral Injuries
- **No symptoms**[Q]: Secure ligation of a ureter may simply lead to silent atrophy of kidney.
- **Loin pain** and **fever**[Q]: Possibly with **pyonephrosis**, occur with infection of the obstructed system. **Urography** shows **no function**, which will be permanent unless steps are taken quickly to **relieve the obstruction** by inserting a **percutaneous nephrostomy**.
- A **urinary fistula**[Q] develops through the **abdominal** or **vaginal wound**. **Nephrostomies**[Q] may be inserted and **repair postponed** until edema and inflammation have subsided.

Diagnosis
- The diagnosis is rarely made until there is swelling in the loin or iliac fossa associated with a reduction of urine output.
- **Excretion urogram** or **CECT: Extravasation** of **contrast** from the injured ureter[Q].

Treatment
- Early repair is safe provided that the patient is fit for surgery

Injury Recognized at the time of Operation
• **Ureterovesical continuity** should be restored unless the patient's condition is poor[Q].
• **Deliberate ligation** of the proximal ureter and **temporary percutaneous nephrostomy** is then the best course **until the patient is well enough** for a repair[Q].

Methods for Repairing a Damaged Ureter	
• **No loss** of length	• **Spatulation** and **end-to-end anastomosis** without tension[Q]
• **Little loss** of length	• Mobilise kidney • **Psoas hitch**[Q] of bladder • **Boari operation**[Q]
• **Marked loss** of length	• **Transureteroureterostomy** • **Interposition** of isolated **bowel loop** or mobilised **appendix**[Q] • Nephrectomy[Q]

Bilateral Ureteral Injury
• Ligation of both ureters leads to **anuria**[Q].
• Ureteric catheters will not pass and urgent relief of obstruction by **nephrostomy** or **immediate surgery**[Q] is essential.

Boari Operation
- A **strip of bladder** wall is fashioned into a **tube** to **bridge the gap**[Q] between the cut ureter and the bladder[Q].

ADULT POLYCYSTIC KIDNEY DISEASE (AD)

Adult Polycystic Kidney Disease (AD)

- Inheritance is **autosomal dominant**[Q] with 100% gene penetrance, 50% offsprings are affected.
- **Chromosome** affected: **16 & 4**[Q]; Protein abnormality: **Polycystin**[Q]
- Usually **bilateral**[Q]
- An important cause of **renal failure**, accounting for **10-15%** of patients **who receive hemodialysis**.

Pathology
- Kidneys are **grossly enlarged**[Q] with multiple cysts
- Cyst are distributed **uniformly**[Q] throughout cortex & medulla
- Cysts contain straw colored fluid that may become hemorrhagic
- **Renal arteriolar thickening** is a prominent finding in **adults**

Presentation
- Usually occurs in 3rd or 4th decade
- MC clinical feature is **hypertension (75% adults & 25% children)**[Q] due to activation of rennin angiotensin system[Q].
- **Pain** due to infection (pyelonephritis)/obstruction/sudden hemorrhage.
- **Hematuria**[Q], **nocturia** (due to impaired concentrating ability), **nephrolithiasis** (15–20%)[Q]
- Progressive decline in renal function leading CRF
- MC cause of death: Cardiovascular disorders[Q]

ADPKD Extra-renal manifestations	
• Cysts: **Liver (MC)**[Q], spleen, **pancreas** and **ovaries** • **Berry aneurysms** (10–40%)[Q] • Cyst in seminal vesicles (40%), Arachnoid membrane (8%)	• **Colonic diverticulosis**[Q] • **Mitral valve prolapse**[Q]

Diagnosis
- **USG:** Enlarged kidney with uniformly increased medullary echogenecity

IVP in ADPKD
• Stretching of the calyces by the cysts (**spider leg** or **bell like deformity**)^Q • **Bubble appearance**^{Q} (calyceal distortion) • **Swiss cheese appearance**^{Q}

- CT scan is **IOC**^{Q} in ADPKD

Management
- Treatment is mainly aimed to control UTI, hypertension, calculi & general measures for uremia (low protein diet)
- Pain relief by percutaneous aspiration with instillation of sclerosing agent or **Rovsing's operation (deroofing of the cyst)**^{Q}
- Dialysis or **renal transplantation** (only definitive treatment) for renal failure^Q.

INFANTILE POLYCYSTIC KIDNEY DISEASE (AR)

INFANTILE POLYCYSTIC KIDNEY DISEASE (AR)

- Rare, **autosomal recessive**^{Q}, usually bilateral
- Always become apparent during childhood, rarely upto 20 years, **most severe forms** are seen **earliest in life**^{Q}.
- If diagnosed at **birth**, **child dies** in 2 months due to **uremia** and **pulmonary hypoplasia**^{Q}
- Associated with **hepatic fibrosis**, leading to portal hypertension and hepatic failure; **pulmonary fibrosis**^{Q}

Diagnosis
- **IVP:** Delayed function with characteristic radial or medullary streaking (**sunburst pattern**)^Q

Treatment
- No cure, only **palliative support**^{Q} (respiratory care, surgery for esophageal varices, hemodialysis and renal transplantation)

PELVIURETERIC JUNCTION (PUJ) OBSTRUCTION

PELVIURETERIC JUNCTION (PUJ) OBSTRUCTION

- A blockage of the ureter at the junction with the renal pelvis resulting in restriction of urine flow
- MC cause of **fetal hydronephrosis**^{Q}
- More common in **boys**^{Q}, mainly **left sided**, **bilateral** in **10–15%** cases

Causes of PUJ Obstruction	
Congenital	**Acquired**
• **Aperistaltic segment**^{Q} due to disorganization of smooth muscle or collagen deposition • Crossing **aberrant renal vessel**^{Q}	• **Calculus**^{Q} • **Instrumentation**^{Q} • **Infection**^{Q}

Associated Abnormalities
- **PUJ Obstruction** of **opposite kidney (MC)**^{Q} in 40%
- **VUR**^{Q}
- **VATER defects**^{Q} (Vertebral anomalies, anorectal malformations, TE fistula, Radial and renal dysplasia)

Clinical Presentation
- Most infants are **asymptomatic**^{Q}
- Most infants are discovered by **palpable abdominal mass** or **prenatal USG**^{Q}.

Diagnosis
- **USG:** Diagnoses **hydronephrosis**, but does not diagnose whether it is obstructive.
- **IVP:** It was the primary radiological study to define PUJO but now **replaced by DTPA scan**^{Q}.

DTPA Scan
• **Investigation of choice for PUJO** to establish that hydronephrosis is due to obstruction.

- Pressure flow studies (**Whitaker test**)^Q
  - **Invasive test**, used only in cases of **equivocal result** of renal scan^Q.
  - Measures **differential pressure between kidney** and **bladder**
  - A percutaneous puncture of kidney is made; **contrast fluid** is infused at a constant rate with monitoring of intra-pelvic pressure. An **abnormal rise** confirms obstruction.
- **Retrograde Pyelogram:** Anatomic delineation more clear. Show the **distal end of obstruction**^{Q}.

Treatment
- **Conservative** in children with **good renal function without any complication**
- Pyeloplasty or nephrectomy

Types of Pyeloplasty	
Open	**Endoscopic**

A. **Anderson Hynes (Dismembered) pyeloplasty**:
• **Gold standard for PUJ obstruction**[Q]
• For large **redundant pelvis** with **high insertion of ureter**[Q].
• Advantages: Broad applicability, including **preservation of anomalous vessels**[Q] and **excision of** the **pathological UPJ and appropriate repositioning**[Q] successful reduction pyeloplasty
B. **Foley V-Y pyeloplasty**: Best applied for **high insertion** of the ureter
C. **Flaps (Spiral and vertical)**
	• For **small pelvis**[Q] with PUJ dependent for good funnel drainage and **intrarenal pelvis**[Q].
	• More than **2 cm** long area of **stricture** is a **contraindication**[Q].
	• Endoscopic procedures are:
	  – a. **Endopyelotomy** (percutaneous or retrograde) advised for associated renal stone
	  – b. **Balloon dilatations** or **Lasers**

Indications for Nephrectomy in PUJO
• **Permanent severe loss** of renal function (< 10% function)[Q] • **Unmanageable complication** in hydronephrotic kidney (**Severe recalcitrant infection, Intractable pain, Hypertension**)[Q]

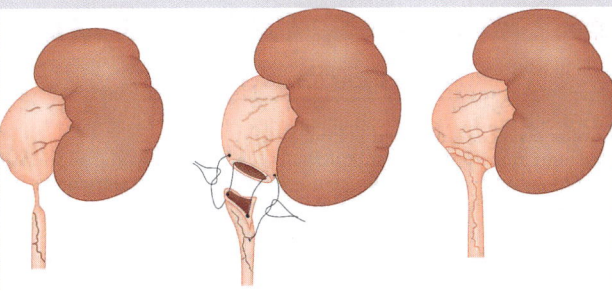

Anderson-Hynes dismembered pyeloplasty

RENAL AGENESIS

RENAL AGENESIS

- Incidence of **unilateral**[Q] renal agenesis is **1 in 1000**[Q], more common in **males**[Q] and on **left side**[Q] in unilateral renal agenesis.
- Ureter is **absent** on the side of the unformed kidney in **50%**[Q] cases, in rest blind ureter is found.
- Bilateral is incompatible with life and rare.
- Associated anomalies: **Oligohydramnios**[Q], **pulmonary hypoplasia**[Q] (due to **defective proline synthesis**), **amnion nodosum**[Q], **Potter's facies**[Q] (seen in bilateral RA).
- Unilateral renal agenesis is associated with **unicornuate** or **bicornuate uterus** and **septate vagina** in females.
- **Colonic shadow** is placed **more laterally**[Q] on X-ray KUB due to **unilateral renal agenesis.**

POTTER'S FACIES

- Hypertelorism, prominent inner canthal fold[Q]
- Blunted nose, recessive chin, broad and low set ears, limb deformities[Q]
- Seen in **bilateral renal agenesis**[Q]

MEDULLARY SPONGE KIDNEY (AR)

MEDULLARY SPONGE KIDNEY (AR)

- Dilatation of **distal portion of** the **collecting duct** with **numerous associated cysts** giving kidneys an **appearance of sponge**
- **Autosomal recessive** defect, **usually bilateral**[Q], affecting all of the papillae, but it may be unilateral
- **Infection** & **calculi** are occasionally seen as a result of urinary stasis in the tubules.

Associated with
- **Hemihypertrophy**[Q] of the body
- **Hypercalcemia**[Q]
- **Stone formation**[Q] (Calcium oxalate or calcium phosphate)
- **Nephrocalcinosis**[Q] (Calcium deposition in renal parenchyma)

Clinical Features
- Symptoms are due to **infection** & **stone formation**[Q].
- MC symptom: Renal colic > UTI > gross hematuria.

Diagnosis
- Made on the basis of excretory urogram or contrast-enhanced CT scan.

IVP (Excretory urogram): IOC to diagnose medullary sponge kidney[Q]
• "Bristles on brush"[Q] appearance due to dilated ducts • "Bouquet of flowers"[Q] appearance due to calcification in the ectatic ducts

Treatment
- There is **no treatment** for medullary sponge kidney.
- Therapy is directed toward the complications (e.g. pyelonephritis and renal calculi).

RETROCAVAL URETER

Retrocaval Ureter (Circumcaval Ureter)

- An **embryologically normal ureter** becomes **entrapped behind IVC**[Q]
- Because of **abnormal persistence of right posterior subcardinal**[Q] (as opposed to the supracardinal) **vein**. This forces the right ureter to encircle the vena cava from behind (**Altered development of IVC**)[Q]
- **Right ureter** typically **deviates medially behind** the **IVC**[Q], winding about and crossing in front of it from medial to lateral direction, to resume a normal course to the bladder.
- More common in **males**[Q]

Clinical Features
- Signs & Symptoms of **ureteric obstruction**[Q]

Diagnosis
- MRI is **IOC** to delineate **anatomy** clearly and **non-invasively**[Q]
- IVP: "Reverse J", "Fish Hook" or "Shepherd crook"[Q] deformity.
- Retrograde ureterography

Surgical Management
- Ureteral division with **relocation ureteroureterostomy** in cases of obstruction.

HORSESHOE KIDNEY

Horseshoe Kidney

- MC renal fusion abnormality[Q] with incidence of **1:400**[Q], more common in **males**[Q]
- Fusion at the **lower poles**[Q] by a parenchymatous or fibrous isthmus

Etiopathogenesis
- Fusion occurs before kidneys have rotated at their long axes
- The axes of these masses are **vertical**[Q] whereas axes of normal kidneys are oblique to spine, because they lie along the edges of the psoas muscle
- **Pelvis and ureters** are usually **anteriorly placed**[Q] or anteromedial, crossing anteriorly to isthmus
- **Calyces** point **posteriorly**[Q]. Lowermost calyx extends **caudally** or even **medially**[Q]
- **Migration** is incomplete. Inferior mesenteric artery (**IMA**) **prevents full ascent**[Q]
- **Isthmus** usually located adjacent to **L3-L4** vertebra, just below the origin of IMA from aorta
- **Ureteral compression** can occurs due to **anteriorly displaced ureter**[Q] or from obstruction by **aberrant vessels** leading to hydronephrosis and infection.

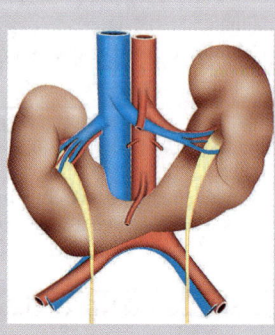

Associated Abnormalities (Present in one-third[Q] cases)	
• CVS (VSD) and CNS involvement • Anorectal malformations[Q] • Unicornuate or bicornuate uterus[Q]	• Renal: VUR and PUJ obstruction in one third[Q] cases • Hypospadias, undescended testis[Q]

Clinical Features
- Most are **asymptomatic**[Q], mostly it is an autopsy finding
- MC symptom: **vague abdominal pain**[Q]
- Rovsing syndrome: abdominal pain, nausea and **vomiting**[Q] on hyperextension of spine

Diagnosis is usually made on IVP showing
• **Low lying kidneys**[Q], closed to vertebral column
• **Vertical axes**[Q] through kidneys point towards the LS spine
• Characteristic orientation of the calyces, directed posterior to each renal pelvis, with the **lowermost calyx** pointing **caudally** or **even medially** (**Hand joining sign**)[Q]
• High insertion of the ureter appears to drape over a midline mass (**Flower vase-like curves of ureters**)[Q]

> • Angiography is done before surgery as **blood supply is unpredictable**[Q] but not needed usually as helical CT is useful.

Complications
- Prone to **ureteral obstruction** due to high incidence of **aberrant renal vessels**[Q] and the necessity for ureters to arch over the renal tissues
- Hydronephrosis, stone, **infection**[Q]
- Large fused kidney occupying the concavity of sacrum may cause **dystocia**[Q]

Treatment
- **Pyeloplasty** is done only in symptomatic cases, **isthmus is not divided**[Q].

AORTIC ANEURYSM WITH HORSESHOE KIDNEY
- **Preoperative angiography is essential**[Q] for the proper evaluation of the renal arteries, as there are multiple aberrant renal arteries arising from aorta
- Isthmus rarely needs to be divided
- **Left retroperitoneal approach**[Q] is preferred.

BENIGN RENAL CYST

Benign Renal Cyst
- MC **benign renal lesions**[Q], represent > 70% of all **asymptomatic**[Q] renal masses.
- More common in **men**, and can be **solitary** or **multiple**[Q]
- Prevalence **increases with age**, can be found in > 50% of patients > **50 years**[Q]
- Treatment: Percutaneous **drainage and sclerosis**[Q] with 95% alcohol.

Bosniak's Classification of Simple and Complex Cyst	
Category I	Simple benign cyst[Q] with good through-transmission, no echoes within the cyst, sharply, marginated smooth wall; requires **no surgery**
Category II	Looks benign with **septation, minimal calcification**, and **high density**; requires **no surgery**[Q]
Category II F	**Calcification** in wall **thicker** and more **nodular**[Q] than in category II, septa have **minimal enhancement**; requires **no surgery**
Category III	**Complicated lesion** cannot confidently be distinguished from malignancy, **more calcification**, more **prominent septation**; more likely to be **benign** than malignant; requires **surgical exploration**[Q] and/or removal
Category IV	**Malignant lesion**[Q] with large cystic components, **irregular margins; solid vascular elements**; requires **surgical removal**[Q]

URETEROCELE

Ureterocele
- Cystic dilation of terminal ureter
- More common in **females**[Q]

Types
- **Intravesical (20%)**: Most often with **single ureter**[Q]
- **Ectopic (80%)**: Nearly always involve the **upper pole** of **duplicated ureters**[Q].

Clinical Features
- MC presentation is **UTI or urosepsis**[Q]
- Palpable abdominal mass (due to **hydronephrosis**)

- **Prolapse** through female urethra as a cyst
- **Calculi** due to urinary stasis, mostly in distal ureter

Diagnosis
- **USG:** Hydroureteronephrosis, cyst in bladder
- **IVP:** Typical **Adder head** or **Cobra head** or **Spring onion appearance**[Q] is diagnostic of ureterocele
- **MCU:** A **smooth filling defect**[Q] in the trigonal area
- **Cystoscopy:** Enlarging & collapsing cysts[Q] as urine flows

Treatment
- Significant upper pole function: **Endoscopic incision** or **cyst excision & reimplantation**[Q]
- Poor upper pole function: Upper pole nephrectomy and partial ureterectomy.

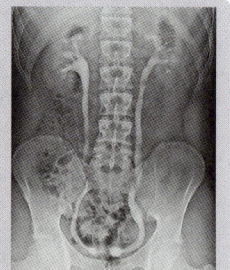

DUPLICATION OF URETER (AD)

DUPLICATION OF URETER (AD)

- MC congenital anomaly of **upper urinary tract**[Q]
- Mode of inheritance is **autosomal dominant**[Q]
- More common in **females** and often **bilateral**[Q]
- "Yo-Yo" effect[Q] in **fused ureter** (incomplete duplication) is seen.

Types
- **Incomplete duplication:** Both ureters join together and a single ureteric opening
- **Complete duplication:** Both ureters open separately
  - **Weigert-Meyer's rule**[Q]: In cases of complete duplication, the upper pole ureter and the lower pole ureter rotate on their long axes so that the **upper pole ureteric orifice** is **medial & caudal** to the **lower pole orifice**[Q].
  - **Upper pole ureter** becomes **ectopic & obstructed**[Q], whereas the **lower pole ureter** end laterally and have a **short intravesical tunnel** leading to VUR[Q].

Clinical Features
- Many patients are **asymptomatic**[Q]
- A common presentation is **persistent** or **recurrent infections**[Q].

> - In **females**, the **upper pole ureter** may be **ectopic**, with an **opening distal** to the **external sphincter**[Q] or even **outside the urinary tract**.
> - Such patients have **classic symptoms: incontinence** characterized by **constant dribbling** with a **normal pattern of voiding**[Q].

- In **males**, because the mesonephric duct becomes the vas and seminal vesicles, the **ectopic ureter** is **always proximal** to the **external sphincter**[Q], and associated **incontinence does not occur**[Q].

Diagnosis
- **IVP:** Shows **duplication** in most of cases
- **MCU** discloses **VUR** (in lower pole ureter) and demonstrate presence of **ureterocele** (in upper pole ureter).

Treatment
- Treatment of reflux alone is not influenced by duplication in most of the cases.
- Lower grade reflux is treated medically and higher grade surgically
- **Surgery** is reserved for **upper pole obstruction** or **ectopy**[Q]. If renal function in one segment is very poor, **heminephrectomy** is the most appropriate treatment.

> - MC congenital anomaly of **upper urinary tract: Duplication** of ureter[Q]
> - MC congenital anomaly of **genitourinary tract: VUR**[Q]

ECTOPIC URETERAL ORIFICE

ECTOPIC URETERAL ORIFICE

- Around 80% is associated with a **duplication collecting system**[Q].
- More common in **females**[Q]

Location
- **Males: Prostatic**[Q] or **posterior urethra (MC)**[Q], lateral in bladder
- **Females: Anterior urethra (MC)**[Q], vestibule, vagina

Clinical Features
- **Females: Continuous incontinence** with an otherwise **normal voiding**[Q], **persistent vaginal discharge** (Ureter opening in **vagina**)[Q]
- **Males:** MC presentation is **UTI, no urinary incontinence**[Q], recurrent epididymo-orchitis (Epididymitis in a prepubertal boy, ectopic ureter should be ruled out).

Complications
- Ectopic ureter may be severely obstructed, causing massive **hydronephrosis**

Diagnosis
- **IVP: Drooping lily sign**[Q] (Non visualized upper pole of a duplex system displaces the lower pole down, looking like a drooped down lily flower on IVP)

Treatment
- **Mainly expectant,** if there are no symptoms.
- **Ureteric reimplantation** or **upper pole nephrectomy**[Q] depending on moiety function.

VESICOURETERIC REFLUX (VUR)

Vesicoureteric Reflux (VUR)
- VUR is the **most common inheritable disease**[Q] of the genitourinary tract.
- **Autosomal dominant** mode of transmission.
- Overall incidence is **>10%**[Q] and in children with UTI is 30%
- **Majority** of cases (75%) are **asymptomatic**[Q].
- Major cause of VUR is **attenuation of trigone**[Q] and its contiguous **intravesical ureteric musculature**[Q].

Types

Primary	Secondary
• The length of **submucosal ureter** may be **short** • **Deficiency** of the **longitudinal muscle**[Q] of the intravesical ureter resulting in an inadequate valvular mechanism	• Caused by **elevated pressures** in the bladder • **MC anatomical cause**: Posterior urethral valves (**50%** have **VUR**)[Q] • Other causes: **Neurogenic bladder** or bladder dysfunction

Investigations
- **MCU is IOC for VUR**[Q]
- **DMSA scan: IOC for pyelonephritis** and **cortical renal scarring**[Q]
- Urine culture

MCU Grading of VUR (International classification)	
Grade I	Reflux into **non dilated ureter**[Q]
Grade II	Reflux into **pelvis & calyces**[Q] without dilation
Grade III	**Mild to moderate dilation** of the **ureter, renal pelvis & calyces**[Q] with minimal blunting of the fornices
Grade IV	**Dilation** of the **pelvis & calyces** with **blunting**[Q].
Grade V	**Gross dilation** of the **ureter, pelvis & calyces**; loss of papillary impression and **ureteral tortuosity**[Q].

Natural History
- With bladder growth and **maturation**, most low-grade reflux **resolves spontaneously**[Q].
- **Severe grades** of reflux are **less likely to resolve**[Q].
- **Mean age** of reflux resolution is **6-7 years**[Q].

• Resolution rates: Grades I & II: 80–84%, Grade III: 50%, Grade IV: 20-30%, Grade V: 0-5%[Q]

- Younger children, especially the **neonates**, are more likely to have spontaneous **resolution**[Q]
- Reflux of **infected urine** cause **pyelonephritis**. Repeated such episodes lead to **renal scarring** and **nephropathy** resulting in **hypertension** and **azotemia**[Q].
- If urine is kept sterile, significant nephropathy rarely occurs.

Management
- **Medical management**: Keep the **urine sterile**[Q] and wait for spontaneous resolution

Medical Management Recommended as the Initial Management for
• All prepubertal children with **grade I-III reflux**[Q] as most of the cases usually resolve. • **Unilateral grade IV reflux**, especially in **young children**[Q].

Drugs used in VUR
• **Age up to 6 weeks**: Amoxicillin or **Ampicillin**[Q]. • **Age after 6 weeks**: The biliary system is mature enough to handle **TMP-SMX** (**DOC** for **prophylaxis**)[Q]. Usually **nighttime doses** are given. Other option is **nitrofurantoin**.

- Periodic cultures every **3 months**^{Q} for evaluation of breakthrough infections.
- **DMSA scan** if recurrent bouts of **pyelonephritis**^{Q} are suspected. Yearly radiographic studies for resolution.
- **Surgical management:** Ureterovesicoplasty or **ureteric reimplantation**^{Q} and **STING**^{Q} (Suburethral transurethral injection of teflon paste) are the treatment options.

Methods of Ureteric Implantation
- **Lich-Gregoir technique**^{Q} by direct implantation of ureter
- **Leadbetter-Politano technique**^{Q} involves creation of a submucosal anti-reflux tunnel.

Indications of Surgical Management in VUR
- **Breakthrough UTIs**^{Q} despite prophylactic antibiotics
- Severe grades of reflux- **grade V** or **bilateral grade IV**^{Q}
- **New renal scars** or **deterioration of renal function**^{Q} as on serial USG of DMSA scan.
- Reflux that **persist in girls** at full linear growth (**at puberty**)^Q
- Reflux **associated with** congenital abnormalities (**Bladder diverticula**)^Q.
- **All secondary reflux**, which **persist**^{Q} after correction of the primary cause e.g. fulguration of posterior urethral valves or management of uninhibited detrusor.

RENAL ARTERY ANEURYSMS

Renal Artery Aneurysms

- Most are **saccular**^{Q}, and **75%** occur at the **bifurcation** of the **primary** or **secondary branches**^{Q}.
- **Medial fibroplasia**^{Q} is the **MC cause** of **true renal aneurysms**, followed by degenerative atherosclerosis and polyarteritis nodosa. **Spontaneous** or **traumatic dissection** is the MC cause of false renal aneurysms^Q.

Clinical Features
- Usually **asymptomatic**^{Q} or have associated renal artery occlusive disease and renovascular hypertension or ischemic nephropathy.
- **Rupture** occurs in **< 3%**^{Q} **of cases**, but when the aneurysm ruptures in a **pregnant woman**, the **fetal mortality rate** is 75%, and the **maternal mortality rate** is **50%**^{Q}.

Diagnosis
- Around 50% are **diagnosed incidentally**^{Q}, when renal arteriogram is performed for another reason or during workup for hypertension.
- Plain film of abdomen may show intra-renal or extra-renal **ring like calcification**^{Q}.

Treatment
- Surgical repair

Indications of Surgery
- Any aneurysm **>2 cm**^{Q}
- Woman of **childbearing age**^{Q}
- **Enlarging**^{Q} on serial X-rays
- **Poorly calcified** or **poor access** to **healthcare**^{Q}

- Patients who are followed for renal artery aneurysms at regular intervals should have thorough medical control of their blood pressure.

HEPATORENAL SYNDROME

Hepatorenal Syndrome

- HRS is a state of **functional renal failure** (reduced GFR) **without renal pathology** in patients with **severe liver disease**^{Q}.
- **Low cardiac output** and **high** plasma rennin predicts development of HRS^Q
- Occurs in about **10%** of patients with **advanced cirrhosis** or **acute liver failure**^{Q}.

Pathophysiology of HRS
- **Marked disturbances** in the **arterial renal circulation**: Increase in renal vascular resistance accompanied by a **reduction in systemic vascular resistance**^{Q}.
- The reason for **renal vasoconstriction** is most likely **multifactorial** and is poorly understood.
- **Structurally** or **histologically kidneys** are **normal** and **recover function after** successful **liver transplantation**^{Q}.
- **Pathogenic hallmark** of HRS is **intense renal vasoconstriction** with **co-existent vasodilatation**^{Q}.

- In HRS, **urine sodium** is typically **< 10 mEq/L** with **hyperosmolar urine**, oliguria (< 400 mL/24 hr), fractional excretion of sodium < 1; and urine creatinine-to-plasma creatinine ratio > 30:1.

Type 1 HRS	Type 2 HRS
• Characterized by a **progressive impairment**^{Q} in **renal function** and a **significant reduction** in **creatinine clearance** within **1–2 weeks** of presentation^Q. • **Poor outcome**^{Q}	• Characterized by a **reduction in glomerular filtration rate**^{Q} with an **elevation of serum creatinine** level, but it is **fairly stable**^{Q} • Associated with a **better outcome**

Clinical Features
- HRS is often seen in patients with refractory ascites and requires exclusion of other causes of acute renal failure.

Diagnosis
- The diagnosis is made usually in the presence of a **large amount of ascites** in patients who have a **stepwise progressive increase** in creatinine^Q.

International Ascitic Club Criteria for HRS	
• Serum **creatinine > 1.5 mg/dL**^{Q} • **Absence of shock, bacterial infection, nephrotoxic drugs, diarrhea** or **renal fluid losses**^{Q} • **Absence** of significant **proteinuria** (< 500 mg/day)^Q • **No evidence** of **obstructive uropathy**^{Q}	• **Low urine volume** (< 500 mL/day) and **low urine sodium** (< 10 mEq/L)^Q • **No sustained improvement** in renal function **after diuretic withdrawal** and expansion of plasma volume with **1.5 L** of **isotonic saline**^{Q}

Treatment
- **Drug of choice** is **terlipressin**^{Q} (**albumin** improves the therapeutic response)
- **Midodrine + octreotide + IV albumin** may **reverse renal failure**^{Q} in some patients with HRS
- **Best therapy for HRS:** Liver transplantation (recovery of renal function is typical in this setting)^Q
- In patients with either **type 1** or **type 2 HRS**, the **prognosis is poor** unless transplant can be achieved within a short period of time.

URINARY ASCITES

Urinary Ascites

- **Forty percent** of neonatal ascites is caused **by urinary conditions**^{Q}.
- **Urinary ascites** occurs when **high intraluminal pressure forces urine to extravasate from the kidney**^{Q}, usually across a renal fornix.
- Urine then **enters the retroperitoneum** and **travels across the peritoneum as a transudate**.
- If aspirated from the peritoneal cavity, **ascites** or **extravasated urine** contains **electrolyte & creatinine levels similar to serum**^{Q}.
- The **urine within the peritoneum** is subject to the **large absorptive mesothelial surface that quickly normalizes these values**, masking the identity of ascitic fluid as urine.
- **Diagnosis** of urinary ascites may be difficult and **may require definitive upper tract drainage** in the form of **nephrostomy tubes** in order to establish the etiology of the ascites and allow its resolution.
- **Urinary ascites** in the case of **distal obstruction** may **serve to lower urinary pressures** and offer **some protection to the developing kidneys**^{Q}.

Causes of Urinary Ascites	
• **Posterior urethral valves**^{Q} • **Urethral stricture**^{Q} • **Urethral atresia**^{Q} • **Bladder outlet obstruction**^{Q} • **Ectopic ureterocele**^{Q} • **Neurogenic bladder**^{Q}	• **Hydrocolpos** • **Sacrococcygeal teratoma**^{Q} • **Bladder perforation**^{Q} during delivery • **Urachal lacerations** secondary to umbilical artery catheterization

PATENT URACHUS

Patent Urachus

- A patent urachus is suspected in the **neonatal period** by **continuous** or **intermittent drainage of fluid from umbilicus**^{Q}
- **Most common organisms** cultured from the umbilical drainage include **Staphylococcus aureus, Escherichia coli**^{Q}
- **Additional presentations** include an **enlarged** or **edematous umbilicus & delayed healing of cord stump**^{QW}

Diagnosis
- **Diagnosis is confirmed by** demonstration of the **fluid-filled canal** on **longitudinal ultrasound** or **contrast filling on retrograde fistulogram** or **voiding cystourethrogram (VCUG)**^{Q}

Management
- Management of an **infected urachus with abscess formation** includes **initial drainage under antibiotic coverage**^{Q}
- Once the infection has subsided, **complete excision** of the **patent urachus including a bladder cuff** is required
- **Removing all anomalous tissue avoids:**
  - **Recurrences** or **stone formation**^{Q}
  - Prevents the rare event of later transformation into a **malignant adenocarcinoma**^{Q}.

Multiple Choice Questions

RENAL AND URETERIC CALCULI

1. Renal calculi associated with proteus infection:
 (All India 2011, 2009)
 a. Uric acid b. Triple phosphate
 c. Calcium oxalate d. Xanthine

2. Nephrolithiasis occurs with the toxicity of: *(COMEDK 2005)*
 a. Ritonavir b. Saquinavir
 c. Indinavir d. Nelfinavir

3. Not true about 'Struvite Stones' is: *(AIIMS Nov 2001)*
 a. Better known as staghorn calculus
 b. These are triple phosphate stones
 c. Common in infected urine
 d. Usually seen in acidic urine

4. Randall's plaques causes: *(TN 98)*
 a. Bile stones b. Urinary stones
 c. Premalignant lesions d. Bacterial infections

5. Commonest stone in case of UTI: *(AIIMS Nov 97)*
 a. Phosphate b. Urate
 c. Cysteine d. Calcium oxalate

6. Oxalate stones are found in: *(PGI June 2006)*
 a. Ethylene glycol b. Ethanol
 c. Diethyl glycol d. Methyl alcohol

7. Staghorn calculus is made of:
 (Recent Question 2017, DNB 2012, UPSC 97)
 a. Oxalate b. Phosphate
 c. Uric acid d. Cystine

8. Renal stones which are laminated and irregular in outline are: *(Recent Question 2013)*
 a. Uric acid b. Calcium oxalate
 c. Struvite d. Cystine

9. Most common renal stone: *(Recent Question 2017)*
 a. Calcium oxalate stone b. Uric acid stone
 c. Staghorn calculi d. Cystine stone

10. Stone formed in alkaline urine is: *(Recent Question 2017)*
 a. Calcium oxalate b. Calcium phosphate
 c. Cysteine d. Uric acid

11. Chronic laxative abuse can result in the formation of which type of stone? *(Recent Question 2018)*
 a. Xanthine b. Cysteine
 c. Ammonium urate d. Struvite

12. Potent producer of urease is: *(Recent Question 2017)*
 a. E. coli b. Proteus
 c. Klebsiella d. Pseudomonas

13. Struvite stone is caused by which metal? *(Recent Question 2018)*
 a. Magnesium b. Calcium
 c. Sodium and potassium d. Both a and b

RENAL AND URETERIC CALCULI CLINICAL FEATURES

14. Locate the renal stone with pain radiating to medial side of thigh and perineum due to slipping of stone in males:
 a. At pelvic brim *(AIIMS June 2010, All India 96)*
 b. Intramural opening of ureter
 c. Junction of ureter and renal pelvis
 d. At crossing of gonadal vessels and ureter

15. A patient was admitted with complaints of ureteric stone. He was on treatment with IV fluids and analgesics. Suddenly he developed radiating pain to the pubic area and medial aspect of the thigh. The stone is coming down. What is the most probable site of lodgment of the stone? *(DPG 2011)*
 a. At renal pelvis b. At pelvic brim
 c. At the level of gonadal vessels
 d. Intramural portion of the ureter

16. Triad of renal colic, swelling in loin which disappears after passing urine is called: *(All India '96)*
 a. Kocher's triad b. Saint's triad
 c. Dietl's crisis d. Charcot's triad

17. Ureteric colic due to stone is caused by:
 (UPPG 2010, All India 2008)
 a. Stretching of renal capsule due to back pressure
 b. Increased peristalsis of ureter to overcome the obstruction
 c. Irritation of intramural ureter
 d. Extravasation of urine

18. A patient with alkaline urine which is cloudy with plenty of pus cells is suffering from infection with: *(Kerala 89)*
 a. E. coli b. Proteus
 c. TB d. None

19. Referred pain from ureteric colic is felt in the groin due to involvement of the following nerve: *(All India 2003)*
 a. Subcostal b. Iliohypogastric
 c. Ilioinguinal d. Genitofemoral

20. Commonest presentation of bilateral ureteric stones:
 a. CRF b. UTI *(AIIMS 91)*
 c. Pain d. Hematuria

21. Most severe pain in ureteric stone is seen in cases of:
 a. Oxalate stones *(UPPG 99)*
 b. Triple phosphate
 c. Cystine stone d. Uric acid stone

22. Ureteric colic characterized by all except: *(UPPG 2007)*
 a. Acute onset
 b. Stillness of the patient
 c. Responds to antispasmodics
 d. Radiates to the groin

23. Treatment of choice of ureteric colic is: *(GB Pant 2010)*
 a. Nitrites b. Pethidine
 c. Adrenaline d. Diclofenac

RENAL AND URETERIC CALCULI DIAGNOSIS AND TREATMENT

24. A petient present with pain and tenderness in the left iliac fossa. USG shows a 3 cm stone in the renal pelvis without any hydro-nephrosis. Most appropriate management:
 a. PCNL *(AIIMS May 2012)*
 b. ESWL
 c. Diuretics
 d. Medical dissolution threapy with KCl

25. All are radioopaque except one: *(AIIMS June 2000)*
    a. Oxalate
    b. Uric acid
    c. Cystine
    d. Mixed
26. What is the name of this intervention performed frequently for renal stone removal?
    a. ESWL
    b. PCNL
    c. Ureteroscopy
    d. Laparoscopic stone surgery

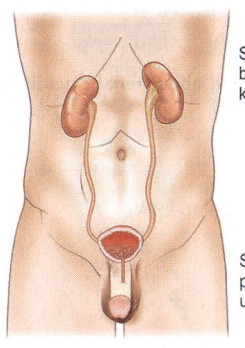
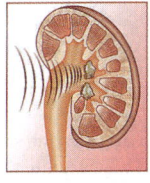
Shock waves break up kidney stones
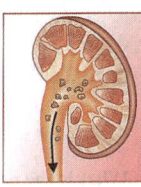
Small pieces pass through urinary tract

27. What is the name of this intervention performed frequently for renal stone removal?
    a. ESWL
    b. PCNL
    c. Ureteroscopy
    d. Laparoscopic stone surgery

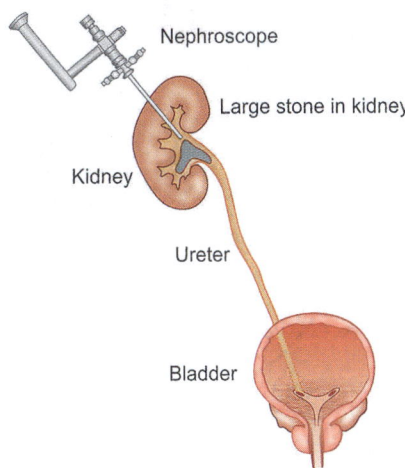

28. A child presents with complaints of abdominal colic and hematuria USG showed a renal stone 2.5 cm in diameter in renal pelvis the next step in management of this case:
    (AIIMS Nov 2000)
    a. ESWL
    b. Pyelolithotomy
    c. Nephroureterostomy
    d. Conservative
29. Which of the following stones is hard to break by ESWL?
    (All India 2010)
    a. Calcium oxalate monohydrate
    b. Calcium oxalate dehydrate
    c. Uric acid
    d. Struvite
30. Ramesh, 30-year-old male presented with repeated attacks of renal colics. X-ray KUB was done. Findings are suggestive of:
    a. Calcium oxalate stone
    b. Uric acid stone
    c. Struvite stone
    d. Cystine stone

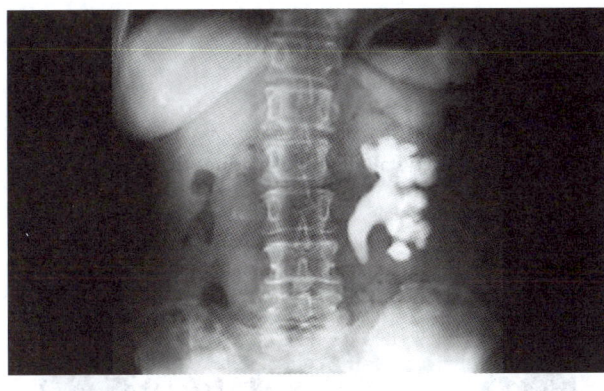

31. A 50 years old female is admitted with abdominal pain and anuria. Radiological studies revealed: bilateral impacted ureteric stones with hydronephrosis. Urine analysis showed RBCs with pus cells in urine. Serum creatinine level was 16 mg/dl and urea level was 200 mmol/l. Which of the following should be the immediate treatment? *(All India 2010)*
    a. Hemodialysis
    b. 'j' stent drainage
    c. Lithotripsy
    d. Ureteroscopic removal of stones
32. What complication should one expect when PCNL is done through 11th intercostals space? *(All India 2010)*
    a. Hydrothorax
    b. Hematuria
    c. Damage
    d. Remnants fragments
33. Which of the following is not a contraindication for extra corporeal shockwave lithotripsy (ESWL) for renal calculi?
    a. Uncorrected bleeding diathesis *(AIIMS June 2003)*
    b. Pregnancy
    c. Ureteric stricture
    d. Stone in a calyceal diverticulum
34. A 10 mm calculus in the right lower ureter associated with proximal hydroureterone-phrosis is best treated with:
    a. ESWL *(All India 2003)*
    b. Antegrade percutaneous access
    c. Open ureterolithotomy
    d. Ureteroscopic retrieval
35. Treatment used for lower ureteric stone is: *(AIIMS June 98)*
    a. Endoscopic removal
    b. Diuretics
    c. Drug dissolution
    d. Laser
36. Correct order of stones on the basis of images of crystals:
    a. Calcium oxalate, struvite, uric acid, cystine
    b. Calcium oxalate, uric acid, struvite, cystine
    c. Uric acid, calcium oxalate, struvite, cystine
    d. Struvite, uric acid, calcium oxalate cystine

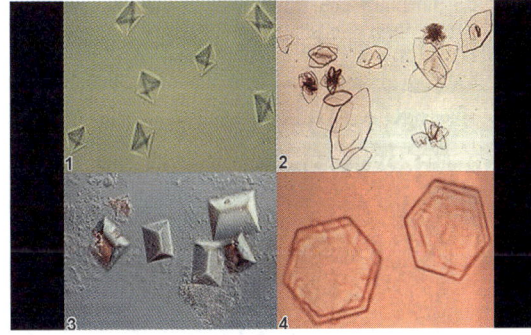

37. **Steinstrasse is:** *(Recent Questions 2017, HPU 2001)*
    a. Staining of stones
    b. Stones
    c. Failure of ESWL
    d. Ureteric obstruction due to fragments in ureter

38. **Identify the crystals depicted in urine microscopy.**
    (APPG 2015)
    a. Oxalate crystals b. Cystine crystals
    c. Struvite crystals d. Uric acid crystals

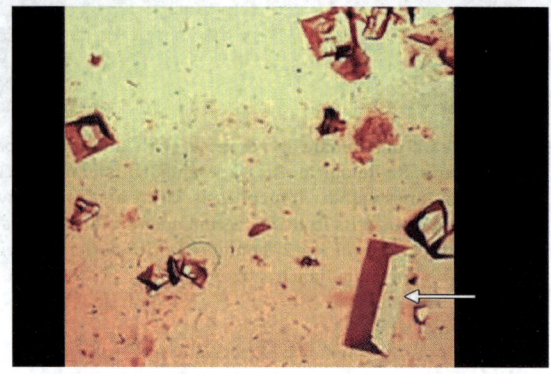

39. **Which of the following statements about the Holmium: YAG laser is incorrect?** *(AIIMS June 2004)*
    a. It has a wavelength of 2100 nm
    b. Its use for uric acid stones has caused deaths due to generation of cyanide
    c. It is effective against the hardest urinary stones
    d. It can even cut the wire of stone baskets

40. **All are indicated in a patient with cystinuria with multiple renal stones except:** *(AIIMS Nov 2012)*
    a. Cysteamine b. Increase fluid intake
    c. Alkalinization of urine d. Penicillamine

41. **Percentage of renal stones which are radio opaque:**
    a. 10% b. 25
    c. 37% d. 75%
    e. 90%

42. **Dormia basket is used for removal of renal calculi in the:**
    a. Pelvic ureteric junction b. Upper 1/3rd of ureter
    c. Middle 1/3rd of ureter d. Lower 1/3rd of ureter

43. **Which is false regarding ureteric stones?** *(AIIMS 92)*
    a. Urine is always infected
    b. Should be removed immediately
    c. Source is always the kidneys
    d. Pain in referred to tip of penis in intramural stones

44. **Identify this crystal found in urine analysis.**
    a. Calcium carbonate stone *(AIIMS November 2015)*
    b. Ammonium phosphate stone
    c. Uric acid
    d. Calcium oxalate stone

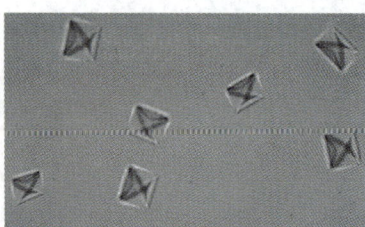

45. **Which one of the following is radiolucent stone?**
    (Recent Question 2017, 2015, GB Pant 2010, MCI Sept 2007)
    a. Calcium oxalate b. Cystine
    c. Uric acid d. Phosphate

46. **Treatment of choice for 0.5 mm renal calyx stone is:**
    a. ESWL b. PCNL *(DNB 2007)*
    c. Ureteroscopy d. Cystoscopy

47. **All are risk factors for nephrolithiasis except:** *(DNB 2007)*
    a. Renal tubular acidosis b. High protein intake
    c. High calcium intake d. Hypercalciuria

48. **All of the following statement about renal calculi are true, except:** *(All India 93)*
    a. Cystine stones form in acidic urine
    b. Struvite stones form in alkaline urine
    c. Oxalate stones are radiopaque
    d. Uric acid stones are resistant to ESWL

49. **Staghorn calculus is made of:** *(DNB 2000)*
    a. Oxalate b. Phosphate
    c. Uric acid d. Cystine

50. **What is the name of this intervention?**

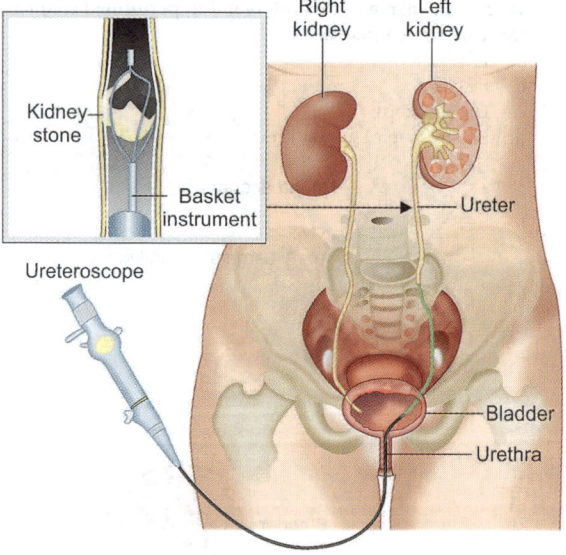

    a. ESWL
    b. PCNL
    c. URS
    d. Electrohydraulic lithotripsy

51. **Treatment used for lower ureteric stone is:** *(AIIMS June 98)*
    a. Endoscopic removal b. Diuretics
    c. Drug dissolution d. Laser

52. **Chandu, 45-year-old male shows calcification on the right side of his abdomen in an AP view. In lateral view the calcification is seen to overlie the spine. Most likely diagnosis is:** *(All India 2001)*
    a. Gallstones b. Calcified mesenteric nodes
    c. Renal stones d. Calcified rib

53. **Which of the following advises is not given to a 35 years old female patient with recurrent renal stone?** *(AIIMS Nov 2012)*
    a. Increase water b. Restrict protein
    c. Restrict salt d. Restricted calcium intake

54. Which of the following are radiolucent renal stones?
    (MHPGMCET 2002, JIPMER 2012)
    a. Uric acid stones   b. Cystine stones
    c. Mixed stones   d. Calcium oxalate stones

55. Which of the following statement is true about the given image? *(Recent Question 2018)*

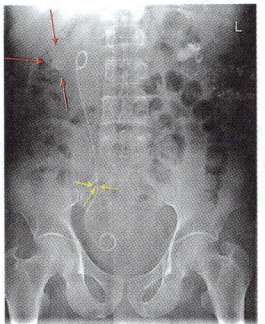

    a. Stent for bile duct obstruction caused by malignancy
    b. DJ stent after ESWL
    c. Stent for pancreatic duct obstruction caused by malignancy
    d. PCNL

56. Which of the following is not true regarding ureteric calculus? *(MHPGMCET 2008)*
    a. Severity of pain increases with size of the calculus
    b. Hematuria is invariably seen in all cases
    c. Pain may radiate to the anterior aspect of thigh
    d. Pain may radiate to tip of the penis

57. Commonest cause of ureteric obstruction: *(MHSSMCET 2006)*
    a. Stone   b. Clot
    c. Cast   d. Carcinoma

58. LASER used in treatment of ureteric calculi:
    (MHSSMCET 2008, 2006, All India 2003)
    a. Holmium b. Nd-Yag
    c. Argon   d. CO_2

59. Following is true about PCNL except: *(MHSSMCET 2009)*
    a. Bleeding is least concerned complication
    b. Involves the placement of a hollow needle into the renal colleting system through the soft tissue of the loin and the renal parenchyma
    c. Perforation of the colon or pleural cavity during placement of the percutaneous track
    d. Perforation of the collecting system may occur

60. A patient is passing stones recurrently in urine for past few years. All are to be restricted in diet except: *(AIIMS Nov 2010)*
    a. Protein restriction
    b. Calcium restriction
    c. Salt restricted
    d. Phosphate restriction

61. Management of 4 cm size renal staghorn calculus:
    (AIIMS November 2017)
    a. ESWL   b. PCNL
    c. Intra renal repair surgery d. Open pyelolithotomy

RENAL INFECTIONS

62. Most common cause of emphysematous pyelonephritis:
    (GB Pant 2011, COMEDK 2008)
    a. E. coli   b. Proteus
    c. Klebsiella   d. Pseudomonas

63. Sheela, a middle aged diabetic female presented with flank pain and fever. On U/S the kidney was irregular and showed fat density lesion with calculi. The diagnosis is most probably: *(AIIMS Nov 2001)*
    a. TB kidney
    b. Xanthogranulomatous kidney
    c. Chronic pyelonephritis
    d. Renal abscess

64. Following is true of pyonephrosis except: *(AIIMS 92)*
    a. Commonly associated with renal calculi
    b. Always unilateral
    c. Is a complication of hydronephrosis
    d. Follows acute pyelonephritis

65. Subcapsular nephrectomy is indicated is: *(PGI 93)*
    a. Perinephric abscess   b. Hydronephrosis
    c. Pyonephrosis   d. Solitary adenocarcinoma

66. A boy is suffering from acute pyelonephritis. Most specific urinary finding will be: *(AIIMS May 2012)*
    a. WBC cast   b. Leucocyte esterase test
    c. Nitrite test   d. Bacteria in Gram stain

67. Xanthogranulomatous pyelonephritis is often associated with infection by: *(DNB 2010, COMEDK 2009)*
    a. Proteus   b. E. coli
    c. H. influenza   d. Klebsiella

68. Most common predisposing factor for chronic pyelonephritis is: *(DNB 2004, 2000)*
    a. Diabetes mellitus   b. Renal stone
    c. Posterior urethral valve d. Vesicoureteric reflux

GENITOURINARY TUBERCULOSIS

69. Most common route of infection in kidney tuberculosis:
    (Recent Question 2015, All India 93)
    a. Ascending spread
    b. Hematogenous
    c. Lymphatic spread
    d. Direct invasion

70. The most sensitive imaging modality to detect early renal tuberculosis is: *(Recent Questions 2017)*
    a. Intravenous urography
    b. Computed tomography
    c. Ultrasound
    d. Magnetic resonance imaging

71. Earliest sign of renal tuberculosis on IVP:
    a. Caliectasis
    b. Moth eaten calyx
    c. Splaying of calyces
    d. Hydronephrosis

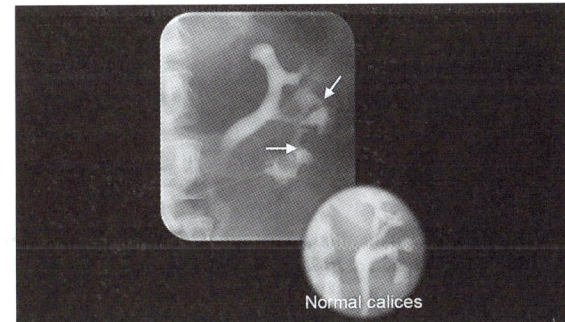

72. **In genitourinary TB, true is:** *(PGI Dec 98)*
    a. Sterile pyuria is consistent finding
    b. AFB in early morning sample is always positive
    c. MC site is pelvis
    d. Commonest cause of pyelonephritis

73. **Renal tuberculosis originates in the:** *(Recent Questions 2017)*
    a. Renal papilla
    b. Renal medulla
    c. Afferent tubules
    d. Efferent arteriole of glomerulus

74. **"Golf-hole" ureter is seen in:** *(WBPG 2015, 2014; Karnataka 94)*
    a. Ureteric calculus
    b. Ureteral polyp
    c. Tuberculosis of ureter
    d. Retroperitoneal fibrosis

75. **Earliest and often the only presentation of TB kidney is:** *(DNB 2005, 2001)*
    a. Increased frequency
    b. Pain
    c. Hematuria
    d. Renal calculi

76. **In a patient who was has acid-fast bacilli in the urine:**
    a. Calcification of the bladder is common
    b. Bladder disease is associated with extensive renal disease
    c. Ureteric involvement causes shortening of the ureters
    d. Renal disease can produce changes identical to reflux nephropathy
    e. Ureteric calculi are commonly present

77. **A 35 years old male came to hospital with dysuria and pus cells on examination. Urine culture came negative (sterile pyuria). After few hours patient deteriorated suddenly and died due to renal failure. Gross autopsy pictures of kidneys shown. Family history of renal disease was present. What is the diagnosis?** *(JIPMER November 2017)*

    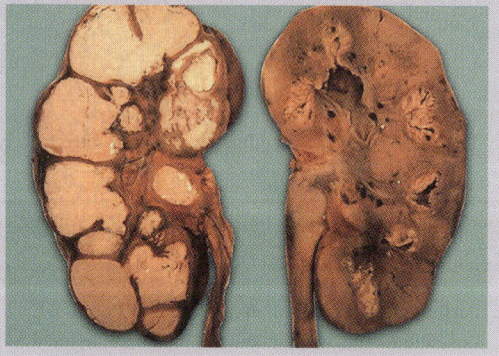

    a. Renal cell cancer
    b. Renal tuberculosis
    c. Cystic renal disease
    d. Metastasis

78. **Genitourinary TB in a male patient presents with:**
    a. Painful and tender epididymis *(JIPMER 2011)*
    b. Bacteriuria without pyuria
    c. Renal cysts (unilateral)
    d. Microscopic hematuria

79. **Sterile pyuria is characteristically seen in:** *(All India 2011)*
    a. Renal tuberculosis
    b. Chronic Hydronephrosis
    c. Wilms' Tumor
    d. Neuroblastoma

80. **In a patient of genitourinary tuberculosis, IVP was done. What is the name of the sign seen in the image?**
    a. Moth eaten calyx
    b. Pipe stem ureter
    c. Bladder calcification
    d. Thimble bladder

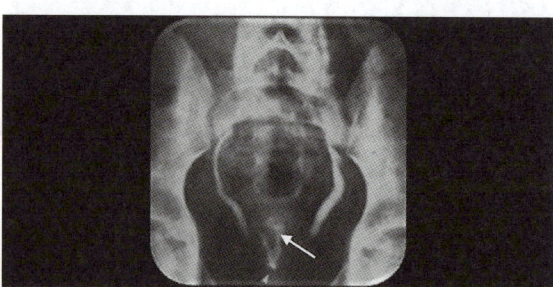

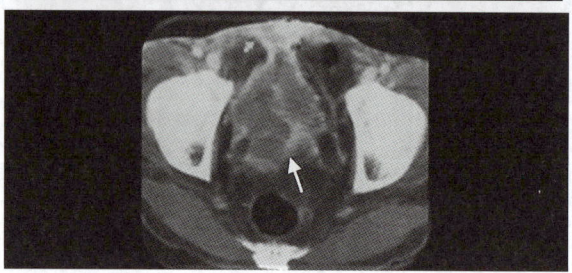

HYDRONEPHROSIS

81. **A lady present with unilateral hydronephrosis on USG. She is asymptomatic. Ureteropelvic drainage is normal. What is/are treatment modality for her?** *(PGI Dec 2008)*
    a. Pyloroplasty
    b. Analgesia SOS
    c. Under observation
    d. Follow up by USG

82. **Unilateral hydronephrosis is due to:** *(AMC 99)*
    a. Bladder neck contracture
    b. Stricture urethra
    c. Carcinoma of prostate
    d. Ureterocele

83. **A 60 years old male with poor stream of urine, post void residual urine is 400 mL, bilateral hydronephrosis and prostate weighing 70g. His urea is 120 and creatinine 3.5. Ideal "next immediate" step:** *(AIIMS Nov 2010)*
    a. Catheterize with Foley catheter
    b. Bilateral PC nephrostomies
    c. CT to rule out carcinoma
    d. MRI pelvis

84. **Hydronephrosis due to obstruction of ureter is best diagnosed by:** *(MHPGMCET 2008)*
    a. IVU
    b. Radioisotope scan
    c. Retrograde pyelography
    d. Whitaker test

85. **What is the name of radiological sign seen in a patient with history of renal stones?**
    a. Cup sign
    b. Honeycombing
    c. Egg in cup appearance
    d. Rim sign

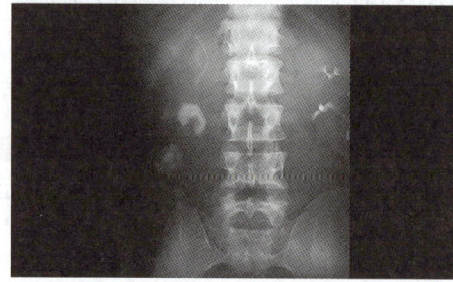

DIAGNOSTIC AND LABORATORY INVESTIGATIONS

86. DTPA scan of hypertensive young lady is normal, USG shows small kidney on left side. Next investigation will be:
    a. CT Scan abdomen   *(AIIMS Nov 2000)*
    b. Retrograde pyelogram
    c. Digital subtraction angiography
    d. DMSA

87. After a single episode of painless gross hematuria in a boy. Doctor performed an excretory urogram showing a filling defect towards the lower renal infundibulum 1.5 cm in size. What will be the next investigation to be done?
    (Karnataka 2003, AIIMS Nov 2000)
    a. Cystoscopy   b. Urine cytology
    c. USG   d. Retrograde pyelography

88. An absolute contraindication for IVP is: *(All India 96)*
    a. Allergy to the drug   b. Multiple myeloma
    c. Blood urea > 200 mg   d. Renal tumor

89. During investigation of hydronephrosis, isotope renogram is useful mainly in: *(UPSC 2000)*
    a. Detecting vesicoureteric reflux
    b. Anatomical definition
    c. Distinguishing between non-obstructed system
    d. Identifying ectopic kidney tissue

90. Pseudo kidney is: *(J and K 2001)*
    a. Thickened bowel loop on USG
    b. Hydronephrosis
    c. Unascended kidney
    d. Undescended testes

91. The investigation of choice for renal scarring defect in kidney: *(Recent Question 2016, All India 2012)*
    a. DMSA scan
    b. DTPA scan
    c. Dexa scan
    d. MCU

92. The substance present in the gallbladder stones or the kidney stones can be best identified by the following techniques:
    a. Fluorescence spectroscopy   *(All India 2003)*
    b. Electron microscopy
    c. Nuclear magnetic resonance
    d. X-ray diffraction

93. Reflux nephropathy is diagnosed mainly by: *(MCI Sept 2005)*
    a. X-ray KUB
    b. Micturating cystourethrogram
    c. CT scan   d. MRI

94. A patient presents with hematuria of several days and dysmorphic RBC casts in urine. The site of origin is:
    a. Kidney   b. Ureter   *(AIIMS Nov 2001)*
    c. Bladder   d. Urethra

95. Isotope Renogram: *(Karnataka 94)*
    a. Study of rennin mechanism
    b. Contrast study of kidneys, ureter and bladder
    c. Utilized in mapping the anatomy of kidneys
    d. Graphic representation of radioactivity of kidneys

96. 'Rim' and 'ball' nephrograms in intravenous urography are seen in: *(COMEDK 2009)*
    a. Normal kidneys
    b. Acute obstructive nephropathy
    c. Chronic obstructive nephropathy
    d. Chronic renal failure

97. Radiation exposure is the least in the following procedure:
    a. Micturating cystourethrogram   *(AIIMS Nov 2010)*
    b. IVP
    c. Bilateral nephrostogram   d. Spiral CT for stones

98. Indications of percutaneous nephrostomy: *(PGI Nov 2010)*
    a. Stone removal
    b. Ureteral obstruction
    c. Anterograde renography
    d. Renal tumor resection
    e. Ischemic renal failure

99. One of the following is characterized by RIM sign:
    (AIIMS Nov 98)
    a. Hydronephrosis
    b. Hypernephroma
    c. Chronic pyelonephritis
    d. Polycystic kidney

100. Percutaneous nephrostomy is indicated in: *(DNB 2001)*
    a. Polycystic kidney disease
    b. Solitary adenocarcinoma
    c. Simple hydronephrosis   d. Pyonephrosis

101. Most useful investigation in a child, who recovered from the bout of pyelonephritis: *(Recent Question 2017)*
    a. DTPA scan   b. DMSA scan
    c. MCU   d. IVP

BENIGN RENAL TUMORS

102. Regarding angiomyolipoma of kidney, what is incorrect?
    a. Pain in the loin   *(AIIMS Nov 94)*
    b. Presents with hypertension
    c. Bleeding is self limited
    d. Nephrectomy is the treatment of choice

103. A complex renal cyst was incidentally detected on ultrasound in a patient following which he underwent a CT for an insurance workup. What is the likely diagnosis?
    (AIIMS May 2017)

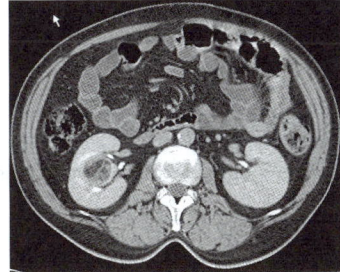

    a. Oncocytoma   b. Angiomyolipoma
    c. Perinephric cyst   d. Renal cell carcinoma

104. Central stellate scar on CT scans are seen in:
    (COMEDK 2008)
    a. Renal hemangioma   b. Renal oncocytoma
    c. Wilms' tumour   d. Papillomas

RENAL CELL CARCINOMA TYPES

105. Renal cell carcinoma histopathologicaly showing 'perinuclear halo' and "Plant like" structure in malignant cells is seen in:
    a. Clear cell tumor   *(PGI Dec 2000)*
    b. Papillary carcinoma
    c. Collecting duct carcinoma
    d. Chromophobe cell carcinoma

106. **Which of the following statements is true regarding kidney tumors?** *(PGI Dec 2001)*
    a. Mutated VHL gene is associated with clear cell carcinoma
    b. Extreme hyperdiploidy occurs
    c. Extreme hypodiploidy occurs
    d. Renal papillary carcinoma has defect in chromosome 8
    e. Oncocytoma has defect in chromosome 11

107. **The most common histological variant of renal cell carcinoma is:** *(Bihar PG 2016)*
    a. Clear cell type   b. Chromophobe type
    c. Papillary type   d. Tubular type

108. **Chromophobe variant to renal cell carcinoma is associated with:** *(All India 2010)*
    a. VHL gene mutations
    b. Trisomy of 7 and 17 (+7, +17)
    c. 3 p deletions (3 p-)
    d. Monosomy of 1 and Y (-1, -Y)

109. **Bilateral renal cell carcinoma is seen in:** *(COMEDK 2008)*
    a. Eagle-Barett's syndrome
    b. Beckwith-Weidman syndrome
    c. von-Hippel Lindau (VHL) syndrome
    d. Bilateral angiomyolipoma

110. **Most common site of origin of RCC:** *(MHSSMCET 2008)*
    a. PCT   b. DCT
    c. Collecting ducts d. Loop of Henle

111. **Sickle cell anemia is associated with which type of renal cell carcinoma?** *(JIPMER November 2017)*
    a. Medullary   b. Papillary
    c. Chromophobe d. Colloid

RENAL CELL CARCINOMA CLINICAL FEATURES, PARANEOPLASTIC SYNDROMES

112. **All can be seen in hypernephroma, except:** *(AIIMS Nov 93)*
    a. Polycythemia   b. Renal vein thrombosis
    c. Hypertension   d. Hematuria

113. **Not correct regarding renal cell carcinoma:**
    a. May be associated with varicocele
    b. May invade renal vein *(AIIMS Nov 94, June 95)*
    c. More common in female
    d. Arises from proximal convoluted tubule

114. **Most common site for secondary metastasis in a case of hypernephroma:** *(AIIMS Feb 97)*
    a. Adrenal   b. Lungs
    c. Brain   d. Bones

115. **Painless gross hematuria occurs in:** *(All India 94)*
    a. Renal cell carcinoma b. Polycystic kidney
    c. Stricture of urethra d. Wilms' tumor

116. **In renal cell carcinoma, which is true?** *(JIPMER 95)*
    a. Hypercalcemia   b. Polycythemia
    c. Cushing syndrome d. All

117. **Cannon ball deposits seen in the lungs are characteristic of:**
    a. Seminoma testis b. Carcinoid *(DNB 2003)*
    c. Hypernephroma   d. Pheochromocytoma

118. **Bilateral RCC may be seen in:** *(DNB 2002)*
    a. Tuberous sclerosis
    b. von-Willebrand's disease
    c. von-Hippel Lindau disease
    d. von-Recklinghausen disease

119. **All are features of hypernephroma except:** *(HPU 2005)*
    a. Persistent pyrexia   b. Hematuria
    c. Polycythemia   d. Lower pole involvement

120. **All are true about renal cell carcinoma except:** *(DPG 2006)*
    a. Invasion of renal vein means inoperability
    b. Presents with abdominal pain, hematuria
    c. Arises from tubular epithelium
    d. More common in males

121. **Regarding RCC all are true except:** *(DPG 2005)*
    a. Renal lump, pain abdomen, hematuria
    b. Associated with anemia and low ESR
    c. Propensity to invade IVC
    d. Invasion of renal vein is contraindication for surgery

122. **Not correct regarding renal cell carcinoma:** *(Recent Questions 2017)*
    a. May be associated with varicocele
    b. May invade renal vein
    c. More common in female
    d. Arises from proximal convoluted tubule

123. **A 55-year-old male with 35 pack years presented with painless mass in left scrotal sac and microscopic hematuria. On laboratory investigation, Alpha-fetoprotein and lactate dehydrogenase was negative. What is the diagnosis?** *(AIIMS May 2013)*
    a. Epididymitis   b. Seminoma
    c. Renal cell carcinoma d. Carcinoma lung

124. **All can be seen in hypernephroma, except:** *(AIIMS Nov 93)*
    a. Polycythemia   b. Renal vein thrombosis
    c. Hypertension   d. Hematuria

125. **Paraneoplastic syndrome associated with RCC are all of the following except:**
    a. Polycythemia   b. Hypercalcemia
    c. Malignant hypertension d. Cushing syndrome

126. **Most common presentation of renal adenocarcinoma:** *(COMEDK 2005)*
    a. Hematuria   b. Local pain
    c. Mass   d. Fever

127. **Commonest manifestation of Grawitz's tumor in male:**
    a. Secondary deposits *(MHPGMCET 2009)*
    b. Pathological fracture c. Hematuria
    d. Rapidly developing varicocele

RENAL CELL CARCINOMA DIAGNOSIS AND TREATMENT

128. **A patient presented with renal cell carcinoma invading IVC and renal vein. False statement is:** *(AIIMS Nov 2001, June 2001)*
    a. Pre operative biopsy is not necessary
    b. IVC involvement indicates inoperability
    c. Pre-op radiotherapy is not essential
    d. Chest X-ray should be done to rule out pulmonary metastasis

129. **Most important prognostic indicator for renal cell carcinoma:** *(AIIMS May 2009)*
    a. Nuclear grade   b. Histological type
    c. Size   d. Pathological staging

130. **A 60 years old male, who is a chronic smoker, presented with 'too late' triad. Chest X-ray film image is given below. What is the most probable diagnosis?** *(Recent Question 2016)*
    a. Carcinoma bladder   b. Carcinoma renal pelvis
    c. Choriocarcinoma   d. Renal cell carcinoma

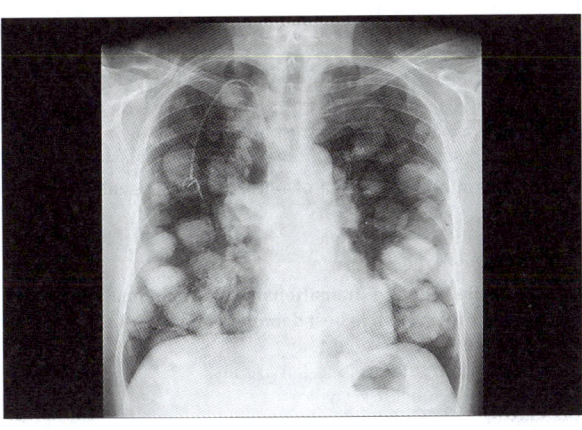

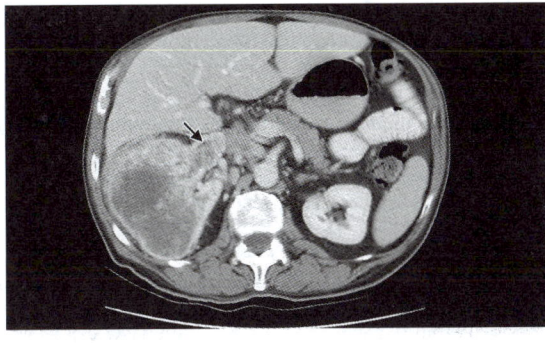

131. The treatment of choice in renal cell carcinoma with the tumor if less than 4 cm in size is: *(AIIMS Nov 2004)*
    a. Partial nephrectomy
    b. Radical nephrectomy
    c. Radical nephrectomy + post operative radiotherapy
    d. Radical nephrectomy + chemotherapy

132. False regarding hypernephroma is:
    (Recent Question 2014, AIIMS Nov 93)
    a. Radiosensitive
    b. Arise from cortex usually from pre existing adenoma
    c. May present with rapidly developing varicocele
    d. Usually adenocarcinoma

133. A 30 years old male presents with pain on the right flank and hematuria. CECT abdomen reveals a large 8 x 8 cm sized solid mass in the right kidney and 3 x 3 cm solid mass occupying the upper pole of left kidney. The most appropriate surgical treatment for this patient is: *(AIIMS Nov 2002)*
    a. Bilateral radical nephrectomy
    b. Right radical nephrectomy and biopsy of the mass from opposite kidney
    c. Right radical nephrectomy and left partial nephrectomy
    d. Right radical nephrectomy only

134. Ideal approach for renal malignancy is:
    a. Transperitoneal
    b. Retroperitoneal
    c. Lumbar incision
    d. Abdominothoracic incision

135. Renal collar to prevent spread of malignancy from kidney is put around: *(JIPMER 93)*
    a. Aorta   b. IVC
    c. Renal vein   d. Renal artery

136. A 40 years old man presented with painless hematuria Bimanual examination revealed a ballotable mass over the right flank. Subsequently right nephrectomy was done and mass was seen to be composed of cells with clear cytoplasm. Areas of hemorrhage and necrosis were frequent. Cytogenic analysis of this mass is likely to reveal an abnormality of:
    (All India 2004)
    a. Chromosome 1   b. Chromosome 3
    c. Chromosome 11   d. Chromosome 5

137. A 65 years old male banker came for an ultrasound to renew his medical insurance. In right kidney, a complex cyst was found and the picture of CT scan is given below. Most likely diagnosis is: *(AIIMS May 2017)*
    a. Oncocytoma   b. Angiomyolipoma
    c. Perinephric cyst d. Renal cell carcinoma

138. A patient with a suspected renal tumor/mass is diagnosed by exfoliative urinary cytology. Which of the following histological types is most likely to be diagnosed on urinary exfoliative cytology? *(All India 2012)*
    a. Transitional cell carcinoma
    b. Adenocarcinoma
    c. Well differentiated carcinoma (Low grade)
    d. All three type can be easily detected on exfoliative cytology

139. The commonest systemic abnormality associated with renal cell carcinoma is: *(COMEDK 2009)*
    a. Hypertension   b. Polycythemia
    c. Elevated ESR   d. Pyrexia

140. A 40 years old patient with a single kidney presents with a solitary exophytic mass of 4 cm localized at its lower pole. Which amongst the following is the best recommended management option?
    a. Partial nephrectomy   b. Radical nephrectomy
    c. Radical nephrectomy with dialysis
    d. Radical nephrectomy with immediate renal transplantation

141. Radical Nephrectomy include all of the following except:
    a. Early ligation of vessels   *(MHSSMCET 2008)*
    b. Lymphadenectomy
    c. Keeping fascia back in place
    d. Removal of kidney including the Gerota's fascia

142. In radical nephrectomy, following structures are removed except: *(Recent Question 2017)*
    a. Gerota's fascia   b. Ipsilateral adrenal gland
    c. Surrounding hilar nodes d. Para-aortic nodes

143. Best investigation for diagnosis and extension of IVC thrombus in renal cell carcinoma: *(Recent Question 2016)*
    a. MRI   b. CT
    c. Venacavography   d. USG

144. Stage T3 renal cell carcinoma: *(Recent Question 2017)*
    a. Tumor invades beyond Gerota's fascia
    b. Contiguous extension into the ipsilateral adrenal gland
    c. Tumor grossly extends into the inferior vena cava
    d. Confined to the kidney

WILMS' TUMOR

145. Commonest presentation of Wilms' tumour is:
    (Recent Questions 2017)
    a. Hematuria   b. Abdominal lump
    c. Hydronephrosis   d. Pain in abdomen

146. **True regarding Wilms' tumour is:** *(AIIMS Nov 94)*
    a. Bone metastasis
    b. Always unilateral
    c. Very commonly metastasize to liver
    d. Worst prognosis among infants

147. **The most important determinant of prognosis in Wilms' tumor is:** *(All India 2006)*
    a. Stage of disease
    b. Loss of heterozygosity of chromosome 1p
    c. Histology
    d. Age less than 1 year at presentation

148. **The ideal timing of radiotherapy for Wilms' tumor after surgery is:** *(All India 2006)*
    a. Within 10 days
    b. Within 2 weeks
    c. Within 2 months
    d. Anytime after surgery

149. **Neuroblastoma differs from Wilms' tumor radiologically by all except:** *(AIIMS June 2001)*
    a. Calcification
    b. Aorta and IVC are not eroded but pushed aside
    c. Same location
    d. Intraspinal extension of tumor

150. **Earliest symptom of Wilms' tumour:** *(Recent Questions 2017)*
    a. Hematuria
    b. Pyrexia
    c. Abdominal mass
    d. Metastases

151. **The triad of Wilms' tumour is:**
    a. Hematuria
    b. Mass abdomen
    c. Pain
    d. Fever
    e. Weight loss

152. **All are true about Wilms' tumour except:** *(All India 97)*
    a. Fever and weakness are clinical features
    b. Arises from primitive cells
    c. Hematuria almost always present
    d. It presents as abdominal mass

153. **Good prognosis in Wilms' tumour is seen in:** *(Punjab 2008, Kerala 91)*
    a. 2-5 years
    b. Less than 1 year
    c. Male child
    d. Female child

154. **All are true regarding Wilms' tumour except:** *(AIIMS 92)*
    a. Preoperative use of Actinomycin D
    b. Postoperative radiotherapy
    c. Good prognosis in infants
    d. Neuroblastoma is the commonest differential diagnosis

155. **Commonest site of metastasis of Wilms' tumour is:** *(AIIMS 94)*
    a. Bones
    b. Lungs
    c. Liver
    d. Brain

156. **Which of the following is the postchemotherapy based staging system in Wilms' tumor?** *(All India 2009)*
    a. National Wilms' tumor staging system (NWTSG)
    b. International society of Pediatric Oncology (SIOP)
    c. AJCC TNM
    d. Chadwick

157. **All are associated with Wilms' tumor except:** *(AIIMS Feb 97)*
    a. Aniridia
    b. Male pseudo hermaphrodite
    c. Arthogryposis multiplex congenita
    d. Hemihypertrophy

158. **Which of the following is the treatment of choice for stage I Wilms' tumor?** *(All India 2012)*
    a. Laparoscopic nephrectomy
    b. Open nephroureterectomy
    c. Chemotherapy
    d. Observation

159. **Wilms' tumor chromosome is:** *(JIPMER 2012)*
    a. 13 q
    b. 13 p 14
    c. 11 p 13
    d. 17

TUMORS OF RENAL PELVIS

160. **Commonest type of cancer of the renal pelvis and upper ureter is:** *(Recent Questions 2017)*
    a. Transitional cell carcinoma
    b. Adenocarcinoma
    c. Squamous cell carcinoma
    d. Nephroblastoma

161. **Epidermoid carcinoma of renal pelvis is usually associated with:** *(Karnataka 94)*
    a. Multiple papillomas
    b. Pelvic calculus
    c. Tuberculosis of kidney
    d. Filariasis

162. **'Stipple sign' in transitional cell carcinoma of the renal collecting system is best demonstrated by:** *(COMEDK 2009)*
    a. Intravenous urography
    b. Retrograde pyeloureterography
    c. Radionuclide scan
    d. Ultrasound scan

163. **Nephroureterectomy is indicated in:** *(DNB 2011)*
    a. Renal cell carcinoma
    b. Chronic pyelonephritis
    c. Polycystic kidney disease
    d. Transitional carcinoma of the pelvis extending till ureter

164. **Gold standard treatment of TCC involving renal pelvis:** *(Recent Question 2016)*
    a. Radical nephroureterectomy
    b. Pelviureterectomy
    c. Radical nephrectomy
    d. Conservative Nephrectomy

165. **In a chronic smoker, who presented with hematuria, RGP was performed as patient was having carcinoma renal pelvis. What is the name of sign seen on this film?**
    a. Bergman sign
    b. Stipple sign
    c. Goblet sign
    d. Both b and c

RENAL TRAUMA

166. **Which of the following is true about renal trauma?**
    a. Urgent IVP is indicated *(All India 95)*
    b. Exploration of the kidney to be done in all cases
    c. Lumbar approach to kidney is preferred
    d. Renal artery aneurysm is common

167. **All except one are correct regarding renal trauma:**
    a. Observation is best *(AIIMS June 95)*
    b. IVP is indicated
    c. Exploration indicated in all cases
    d. Hematuria is a cardinal sign

168. **Which does not happen in unilateral renal trauma?**
    a. Hypertension
    b. Uremia *(AIIMS 92)*
    c. Clot formation
    d. Perinephric hematoma

169. After RTA, a young male presented with non-pulsatile retroperitoneal hematoma. On table IVU was done. Right kidney was not visualized. Left kidney showed immediate excretion of dye. What is next step in the management?
    a. Nephrectomy *(AIIMS Nov 2011)*
    b. Open Gerotas fascia and explore proximal renal vessels
    c. Perform retrograde pyelography
    d. Perform on table angiography

170. Renal trauma is best treated by: *(UPSC 98)*
    a. Observation and supportive measures
    b. Early drainage of perirenal hematoma
    c. Heminephrectomy
    d. Nephrostomy

171. Forty eight after sustaining a blunt abdominal injury, a 15-year-old by presents with hematuria and pain in the left side of abdomen. On examination, he has a pulse rate of 96/minute with a BP of 110/70 mm Hg. His Hb is 10.8 gm% with a PCV of 31%. Abdominal examination revealed tenderness in left lumbar region but no palpable mass. The most appropriate investigation to diagnose and find the extent of renal injury would be: *(UPSC 2005)*
    a. Sonographic evaluation of abdomen
    b. Intravenous pyelography
    c. Contrast enhanced computed tomography
    d. MR urography

172. What percent of cases with injury to kidney require surgical exploration? *(MAHE 2008)*
    a. 20%   b. 90%
    c. 50%   d. 70%

173. During renal rupture the nephrectomy is not attempted until: *(UPPG 2010)*
    a. Fluid replacement
    b. Antibiotics covers
    c. Contralateral renal function is ascertained
    d. Renal angiogram

174. In renal trauma, which statement is not correct?
    a. Exploration is indicated in 90% of cases *(Orissa 2011)*
    b. Hematuria is a cardinal sign
    c. Transperitoneal approach is preferred
    d. IVP is urgently indicated

175. Number of grades of blunt trauma kidney by C.T. scan are:
    a. 3   b. 4   *(Orissa 2011)*
    c. 5   d. 6

176. Absolute indication for surgical exploration after renal trauma? *(MHSSMCET 2008)*
    a. Hematuria
    b. Pulsatile hematoma
    c. Cortical renal contusion
    d. Delayed arterial injury

177. A 25-year-old male presents to emergency with history of road traffic accident two hours ago. The patient is hemodynamically stable. Abdomen is soft. On catheterization of the bladder, hematuria is noticed. The next step in the management should be: *(Recdent Question 2016, AIIMS Nov 2004)*
    a. Immediate laparotomy
    b. Retrograde cystourethrography (RGU)
    c. Diagnostic peritoneal lavage (DPL)
    d. Contrast enhanced computed tomography (CECT) of abdomen

178. Following a blunt trauma abdomen, a patient had renal laceration and urinoma. Even after 12 days, urinoma persisted, but patient was stable and there was no fever. Next step in management would be: *(AIIMS November 2017)*
    a. Percutaneous exploration and repair
    b. Wait and watch
    c. J-shaped urinary stent
    d. Percutaneous nephrostomy

URETERIC INJURY

179. Inadvertent surgical injury of the ureter leads to:
    a. Complete renal atrophy   b. Hematuria
    c. Renal failure   d. Hydronephrosis
    e. Hypertension

180. Commonest cause of ureteric injury during surgical operation is: *(UPPG 2007, 2006)*
    a. Abdominoperineal resection
    b. Hysterectomy
    c. Prostatectomy
    d. Colectomy

POLYCYSTIC KIDNEY DISEASE

181. All of the following are features of adult polycystic kidney disease except: *(COMEDK 2005)*
    a. Autosomal recessive trait   b. Present as renal mass
    c. Haematuria   d. Renal failure

182. Polycystic kidney disease is associated with all of the following except: *(COMEDK 2010)*
    a. Cerebral aneurysms
    b. Mitral valve prolapsed
    c. Renal cell carcinoma
    d. Hepatic cysts

183. Not true about polycystic kidney disease is: *(AIIMS Nov 97)*
    a. Autosomal dominant
    b. Proteinuria < 2 gm/day
    c. Leads to CRF
    d. Decompression of cyst leads to normal renal function

184. Image of kidney in a patient having polycystin 2 mutation is given below. What is the inheritance mode in this disease? *(Recent Question 2016)*
    a. Autosomal dominant   b. Autosomal recessive
    c. X-linked dominant   d. X-linked recessive

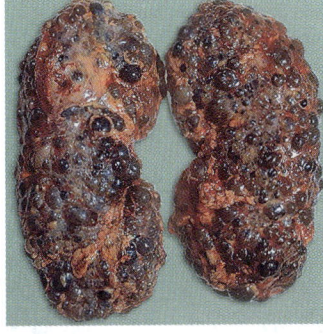

185. In adult polycystic kidney, all are true except:
    a. Hypertension is rare *(AIIMS June 2001)*
    b. Hematuria is a common symptom
    c. Cysts are seen in liver spleen and pancreas
    d. Autosomal dominant transmission is seen

186. **True of autosomal dominant polycystic kidney disease I and II respectively:** *(PGI June 2002)*
    a. Chromosomes 16 and 5
    b. 16 and 4
    c. 11 and 5
    d. 11 and 4
    e. 4 and 5
187. **Polycystic kidneys can be associated with:**
    a. Cysts in liver
    b. Coarctation of aorta
    c. Berry aneurysms
    d. All
188. **Polycystic kidney may be associated with cyst in all the sites except:** *(Bihar PG 2014, All India 91)*
    a. Lung
    b. Liver
    c. Pancreas
    d. Brain
189. **Treatment of choice in polycystic kidney is:** *(Kerala 91)*
    a. Removal of cyst
    b. Nephrectomy
    c. Dialysis
    d. Renal transplant
190. **The incidence of liver cysts in childhood polycystic kidney disease is:** *(All India 92)*
    a. 5%
    b. 10%
    c. 18%
    d. 50%
191. **What is the diagnosis on the basis of CECT findings?**
    a. ADPKD
    b. Bilateral RCC with multiple liver metastasis
    c. Multiple secondaries with unknown primary
    d. HCC with multiple metastasis to kidneys

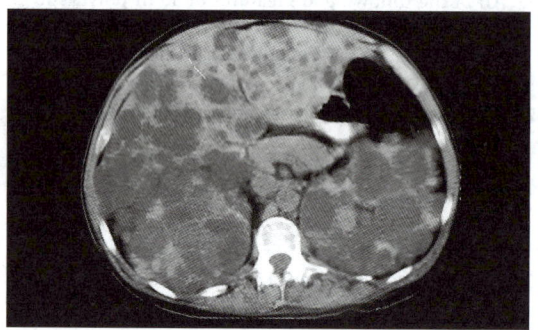

192. **Polycystic disease of the kidney may have cysts in all the following organs except:** *(All India 2004)*
    a. Lungs
    b. Liver
    c. Pancreas
    d. Spleen
193. **IVP was done in the patient of ADPKD. What is the name of this sign?** *(Recent Question 2016)*
    a. Spider leg appearance
    b. Swiss cheese appearance
    c. Bubble appearance
    d. Bristles of brush appearance

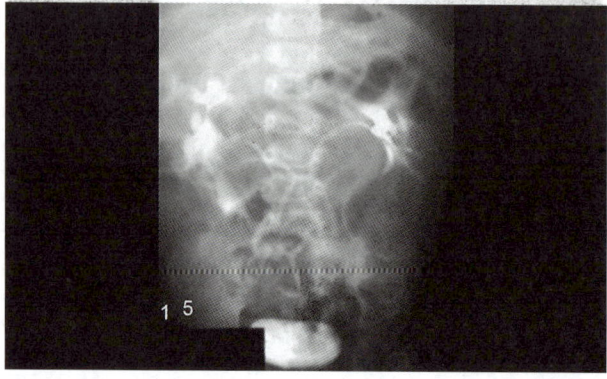

194. **The typical appearance of "spider leg" on excretory urography is seen in:** *(Recent Question 2016, UPSC 2008)*
    a. Hydronephrosis
    b. Polycystic kidney
    c. Medullary sponge kidney
    d. Renal cell carcinoma
195. **All are true about polycystic kidney except:** *(UPPG 2009)*
    a. Inherited as autosomal recessive
    b. Hypertension and hematuria are common symptoms
    c. Spider leg deformity
    d. Associated with cysts in the liver and spleen
196. **True about adult polycystic kidney disease is all except:**
    a. Autosomal dominant inheritance *(AIIMS 2001)*
    b. Hypertension is rare
    c. Can be associated with cysts in liver, lungs and pancreas
    d. Pyelonephritis is common
197. **Which of the following is the common extrarenal involvement in autosomal dominant polycystic kidney disease?**
    a. Mitral valve prolapse *(AIIMS Nov 2004)*
    b. Hepatic cysts
    c. Splenic cysts
    d. Colonic diverticulosis
198. **Which one of the following statements is wrong regarding adult polycystic kidney disease?** *(AIIMS May 2004)*
    a. Kidneys are enlarged in size
    b. The presentation is unilateral
    c. Intracranial aneurysms may be associated
    d. Typically manifests in the 3rd decade
199. **All of the following are true about childhood polycystic kidney disease, except:**
    a. Autosomal dominant
    b. Pulmonary hypoplasia may be seen
    c. Renal cysts are present at birth
    d. Congenital hepatic fibrosis may be seen
200. **All the following are features of polycystic disease of kidneys except:** *(MCI June 2018)*
    a. Hematuria
    b. Hypertension
    c. Renal failure
    d. Erythrocytosis

PUJ OBSTRUCTION

201. **Not true about congenital PUJ obstruction is:**
    a. Can be associated with renal agenesis *(AIIMS Nov 2001)*
    b. Can be diagnosed antenatally
    c. Bilateral in 10–15% of cases
    d. Aberrant vessel is the most common cause
202. **All are true in PUJO except:**
    a. Commoner in boys
    b. Bilateral lesions occur in 10-40%
    c. Right sided lesions predominate
    d. Intrinsic lesions predominate
203. **Most infants and children with PUJO present with:**
    a. Pain *(GB Pant 2008)*
    b. Hematuria
    c. Painless abdominal mass
    d. Renal failure
204. **Best management for a symptomatic 6 years male with PUJ obstruction:** *(GB Pant 2010)*
    a. Endopyelotomy
    b. Foley V-Y pyeloplasty
    c. Dismembered pyeloplasty
    d. Wait and watch

205. Anderson-Hynes operation is performed for:
    a. Achalasia cardia   (MCI June 2018)
    b. Pyloric stenosis   c. Pseudopancreatic cyst
    d. Pelviureteric junction obstruction

206. This surgery is performed for which of the following condition?
    a. Carcinoma renal pelvis   b. PUJ obstruction
    c. Ureteric strictures   d. VUR

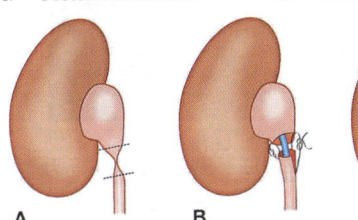
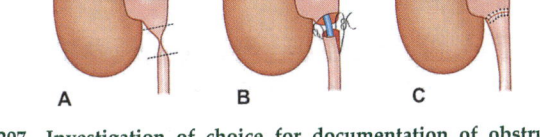

207. Investigation of choice for documentation of obstructive nature of pelvicalyceal system dilatation:
                                 (Recent Questions 2017)
    a. IVP   b. DTPA scan
    c. Whittaker test   d. Ultrasound

208. Not true about PUJ obstruction is: (AIIMS Nov 2001)
    a. Retrograde pyelography is useful to locate the site of obstruction
    b. Endoscopic pyelotomy is contraindicated
    c. Whittakar test is of clinical significance
    d. Dismembered pyeloplasty is the procedure of choice

209. Distention of abdomen with passage of large amount of urine is known as: (MHPGMCET 2001)
    a. Dietl's crisis   b. Anderson-Hynes crises
    c. Meteriorism   d. Strangury

CONGENITAL ANOMALIES OF KIDNEY

210. Potter facies and oligohydramnios are pathognomic of:
    a. Bilateral renal agenesis   b. Unilateral renal agenesis
    c. bilateral renal disease   d. Unilateral cystic disease

211. Potter's facies is characterized by:
    a. Hyperteleorism   b. Prominet inner canthus
    c. Recessive chin   d. Low set ears
    e. All are true

212. A symptom of medullary sponge kidney disease is:
    a. Nocturia   b. Anemia   (All India 95)
    c. Azotemia   d. UTI

213. IVP was done in a patient having hypercalcemia and nephrolithiasis. What is the diagnosis based on IVP findings?
    a. ADPKD   b. ARPKD
    c. Medullary sponge kidney
    d. Congenital cystic nephroma

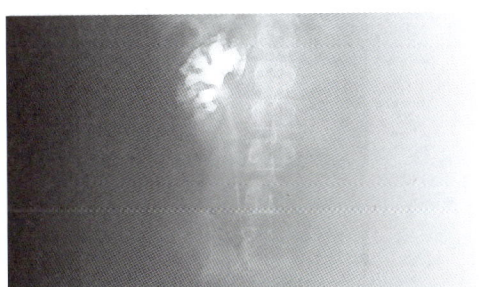

214. Which of the following is the most common renal vascular anomaly?   (All India 2010)
    a. Supernumerary renal arteries
    b. Supernumerary renal veins
    c. Double renal arteries   d. Double renal veins

215. Renal collar which surrounds the aorta has its two limbs split by: (All India 99)
    a. Left renal vein   b. Left renal artery
    c. Isthmus of horseshoe kidney
    d. All of the above

216. Persistent fetal lobulation of adult kidney is due to:
    a. Congenital renal defect   (AIIMS Nov 2007)
    b. Obstructive uropathy
    c. Intrauterine infections and scar
    d. Is a normal variant

217. Incidence of Renal ectopia is: (All India 92)
    a. 1:100000   b. 1:75000
    c. 1:10,000   d. 1:1000

218. An absent kidney is found in: (AMU 2005)
    a. 1:200 individuals   b. 1:700 individuals
    c. 1:1400 individuals   d. 1:5000 individuals

219. Medullary cystic disease of the kidney is best diagnosed by:
    a. Ultrasound   b. Nuclear scan
    c. Urography   d. Biopsy

ABERRANT RENAL ARTERY

220. Aberrant renal artery, all true except:
    a. More common in women
    b. Usually towards left
    c. May cause hydronephrosis
    d. Usually divided to gain access to renal pelvis

221. All are true of aberrant renal artery except: (PGI 93)
    a. Bilateral   b. Leads to hydronephrosis
    c. Common in females d. More common on left side

RETROCAVAL URETER

222. 'Reverse J' deformity on IVP is seen in:
    a. Congenital megaureter   b. Ureterocele
    c. Retrocaval ureter   d. VUR

223. Given radiological sign is seen in:
    a. PUJ obstruction
    b. Aberrant left renal artery
    c. Retrocaval ureter
    d. Retroperitoneal fibrosis

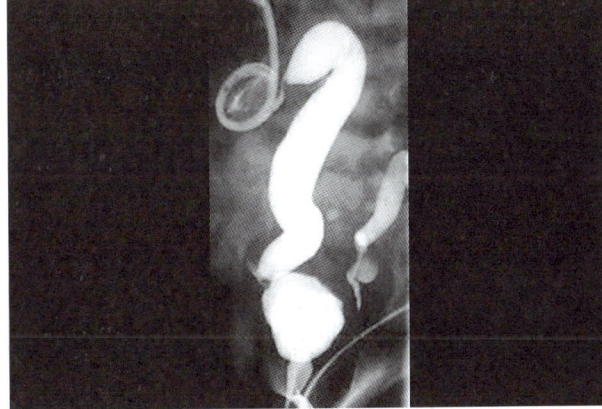

224. Retrocaval ureter occurs due to persistence of:
    a. Azygous vein   *(Recent Question 2016)*
    b. Hemiazygous
    c. Anterior cardinal vein
    d. Posterior cardinal vein

HORSESHOE KIDNEY

225. Which is false of Horseshoe kidney?   *(AIIMS 92)*
    a. Spider like appearance in IVP
    b. Ureteral obstruction common
    c. Lower calyx is reversed
    d. Heminephrectomy improves function

226. Isthmus of horses is located at what level?
    (Recent Questions 2017)
    a. L1-L2 vertebra   b. L3-L4 vertebra
    c. L4-L5 vertebra   d. L2-L3 vertebra

227. "Hand joining sign" and 'Flower vase' pattern of uteters is characteristic of: *(Recent Questions 2017)*
    a. Sigmoid kidney   b. Horseshoe kidney
    c. Crossed ectopia   d. L-shaped kidney

228. With regard to horse-shoe kidneys, true is:
    a. Usually symptomatic
    b. Most cases require surgery
    c. Division of isthmus is usually required to ensure adequate dependent drainage
    d. Isthmus may contain aberrant vessels

229. Horseshoe kidney ascent is prevented by:
    a. Superior mesenteric artery   *(Recent Question 2017)*
    b. Superior mesenteric vein
    c. Inferior mesenteric artery
    d. Inferior mesenteric vein

RENAL CYST

230. Spider leg appearance in IVP is suggestive of:
    a. Renal cyst   b. Renal carcinoma
    c. Renal Tb   d. Hydronephrosis
    e. Chronic renal failure

231. Which of the following is the most common renal cystic disease in infants is?
    a. Polycystic kidney   b. Simple renal cyst
    c. Unilateral renal dysplasia d. Calyceal cyst

URETEROCELE

232. Cobra head appearance on excretory urography is suggestive of: *(MCI March 2010)*
    a. Horseshoe kidney   b. Duplication of renal pelvis
    c. Simple cyst of kidney   d. Ureterocele

233. Treatment of choice for ureterocele?   *(MHSSMCET 2009)*
    a. DJ stent   b. Laparoscopic repair
    c. LASER ablation   d. Endoscopic diathermy

234. Adder head appearance on IVP is/are seen in: *(PGI Nov 2011)*
    a. Polycystic kidney   b. Ureterocele
    c. Horseshoe kidney   d. Hydronephrosis
    e. Ectopic ureter

235. A 3-year-old girl presents with recurrent UTI. On USG shows hydronephrosis with filling defect and negative shadow of bladder with no ectopic orifice: *(UPPG 2004)*
    a. Vesicoureteric reflux   b. Hydronephrosis
    c. Ureterocele   d. Sacrococcygeal teratoma

236. This characteristic appearance is seen on IVP in:
    (Recent Question 2019, 2017)
    a. Tuberculosis   b. VUR
    c. Ureterocele   d. Ureteric stone

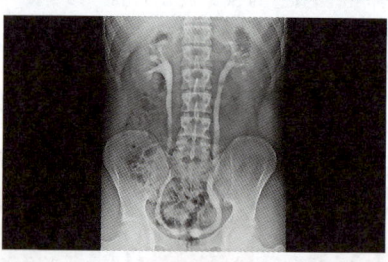

URETERIC ABNORMALITIES

237. Ectopic ureter opening is not located in:
    (MAHE 2005, AIIMS Nov 98)
    a. Bulbar urethra   b. Prostatic urethra
    c. Seminal vesicle   d. Bladder neck

238. What is the diagnosis based on IVP findings?
    a. VUR   b. ADPKD
    c. Ectopic ureteric orifice   d. Ureterocele

239. Most common congenital anomaly of the upper renal tract is: *(Recent Questions 2017)*
    a. Duplication of renal pelvis b. Duplication of ureter
    c. Ectopic ureteric orifice   d. Congenital megaureter

240. On the basis of given IVP image, what is the most probable diagnosis?   *(Recent Question 2016)*
    a. Bilateral duplication of ureter
    b. Right bifid and left complete duplication of ureter
    c. Right bifid and left incomplete duplication of ureter
    d. Left bifid and right complete duplication of ureter

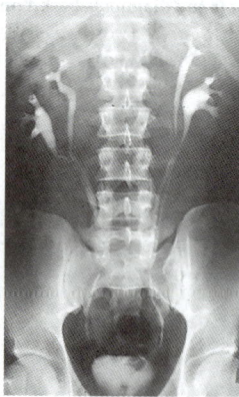

241. A 9 years old boy presented with abdominal pain and recurrent UTI, IVP reveals duplication of left ureter. The most likely site of ectopic opening would be: *(All India 99)*
    a. Prostatic urethra
    b. Ejaculatory duct
    c. Seminal vesicle
    d. Vas deference

242. Ectopic ureter may be frequently associated with:
    a. Oliguria
    b. Dysuria
    c. Bilateral hydroureter
    d. Paradoxical incontinence

243. True statement about duplex draining system of urinary tract are all except: *(Recent Question 2015, Punjab 2007)*
    a. It is most common anomaly of the upper urinary tract
    b. Upper moiety drains lower in the bladder
    c. Lower pole moiety is more prone to obstruction and upper pole more prone to reflux
    d. Yo-Yo Reflux may occur if ureters get fused

244. Yo-Yo reflux is seen in: *(Recent Question 2017)*
    a. Duplication of ureter
    b. Polycystic kidney disease
    c. Medullary sponge kidney
    d. Ureterocele

245. Given diagram represent which rule?
    a. Weigert-Meyer's rule
    b. Pascal's rule
    c. Lambert's rule
    d. Beer's rule

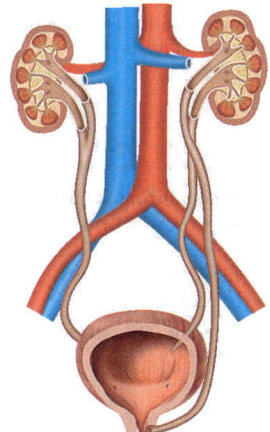

246. Weigert-Meyer's rule applies to:
    a. Fusional anomalies
    b. Renal dysplasia
    c. Polycystic kidney disease
    d. Ureteral duplications

247. In a patient with complete ureteral duplication, the opening of ureter draining the upper pole of the kidney is:
    a. Above and medial to the lower pole ureter
    b. Above and lateral to the lower pole ureter
    c. Below and medial to the lower pole ureter
    d. Below and lateral to the lower pole ureter
    e. Always lateral to lower pole ureter

248. According to Weigert-Meyer's rule of duplication of ureter, the lower pole ureter in urinary bladder is: *(JIPMER November 2017)*
    a. Lateral and cephalad to the upper pole ureter
    b. Lateral and caudal to the upper pole ureter
    c. Medial and cephalad to the upper pole ureter
    d. Medial and caudal to the upper pole ureter

249. In the male, the most common site of termination of the ectopic ureter is the:
    a. Posterior urethra
    b. Anterior urethra
    c. Seminal vesicles
    d. Vas deference

250. In the female, the most common site of termination of the ectopic ureter is the: *(Recent Question 2016)*
    a. Vestibule
    b. Fallopian tube
    c. Ovary
    d. Uterus

251. Presentation and evaluation of ectopic ureter, all are true except:
    a. In males there is duplication in 80% of cases
    b. Can present as abdominal mass or HDN on antenatal USG
    c. IVP will usually show a functioning but dilated upper pole segment and identify the site of ureteral opening
    d. The lower pole is seen as the classic 'drooping lily' sign

252. Classic symptom of ectopic ureter in females:
    a. Painful defecation *(Recent Question 2016)*
    b. Urinary frequency
    c. Ureteral incontinence with otherwise normal voiding
    d. Labial swelling

253. MC presentation of ectopic ureter in males:
    a. Recurrent UTI
    b. Epididymitis
    c. Pelvic pain
    d. Seminal vesicle infections

VESICOURETERIC REFLUX

254. In case of vesicoureteric reflux which will be investigation of choice: *(AIIMS Nov 98)*
    a. Micturating cystourethrogram
    b. IVP
    c. Cystography
    d. Radionuclide study

255. In a patient suspected to be suffering from vesicoureteric reflex, which one of the following radiological investigations may confirm the diagnosis? *(UPSC 2007)*
    a. Intravenous urography
    b. Micturating cystourethrography
    c. Pelvic ultrasound
    d. Antegrade pyelography

256. Reflux into pelvis and calyces without dilatation:
    a. I
    b. II
    c. IV
    d. IV

257. A 5-year-old child was brought with history of recurrent UTI, fever and abdominal pain. MCU was done. What is the diagnosis based on the given image?
    a. Grade II VUR
    b. Grade III VUR
    c. Grade IV VUR
    d. Grade V VUR

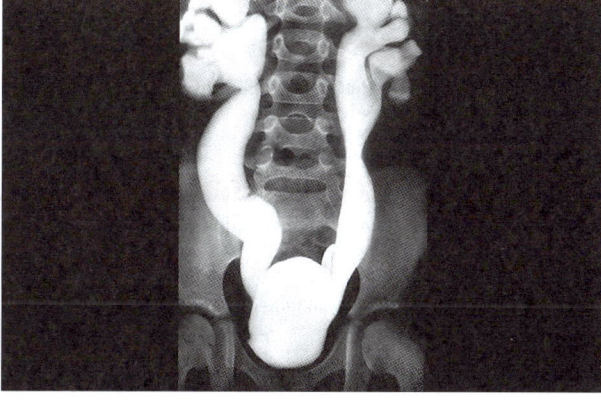

Urology

258. Treatment of choice for grade IV vesicoureteric reflux with recurrent UTI: *(AIIMS June 2000)*
    a. Cotrimoxazole
    b. Bilateral reimplantation of ureter
    c. Injection of collagen in the ureter
    d. Endoscopic resection of ureter

259. Which of the following statements is true of primary grade IV-V vesicoureteric reflux in young children? *(AIIMS May 2006)*
    a. Renal scarring usually begins in the midpolar regions
    b. Postnatal scarring may occur even in the absence of urinary tract infections
    c. Long-term outcome is comparable in patients treated with either antibiotic prophylaxis or surgery
    d. Oral amoxicillin is the choice antibiotic for prophylaxis

260. The most common cause of renal scarring in a 3 years old child is:
    a. Trauma
    b. Tuberculosis
    c. VUR induced pyelonephritis
    d. Interstitial nephritis

RENAL ARTERY ANEURYSM

261. The risk of rupture in renal artery aneurysms is:
    a. Less than 1%   b. 5%
    c. 20%   d. 75%
    e. None of the above

HEPATORENAL SYNDROME

262. Features of hepatorenal syndrome are: *(PGI June 2006)*
    a. Urine sodium < 10 meq/L
    b. Normal renal histology
    c. Renal functional abnormal even after liver become normal
    d. Proteinuria

263. Which of the following statements are incorrect with regard to hepatorenal syndrome in a patient with cirrhosis?
    a. Creatinine clearance 40 ml/min   *(All India 2003)*
    b. Urinary sodium < 10 mEq/L
    c. Urine osmolality lower than plasma osmolality
    d. No sustained improvement in renal function after volume expansion

264. Which of the following statement is incorrect with regard to hepatorenal syndrome in a patient with cirrhosis?
    a. The creatinine clearance is > 40 ml/min
    b. The urinary sodium is < 10 mmol/L
    c. The urine osmolality is lower than the plasma osmolality
    d. There is poor response to volume expansion

DIALYSIS

265. The following are the complications of hemodialysis except:
    a. Hypotension   b. Peritonitis
    c. Hypertension   d. Bleeding tendency

RENAL TRANSPLANT

266. First autologous renal transplantation was done:
    a. Hardy   b. Kavosis   *(All India 2010)*
    c. Higgins   d. Studor

267. All of the following statements are correct about renal transplantation except: *(AIIMS Nov 2004)*
    a. Renal transplantation is heterotopic
    b. Cyclosporine is the mainstay of immuno-suppression
    c. In India, organ harvesting from brain dead patients is not permitted by law
    d. Kidney after removal is flushed with cold perfusion solution

268. After renal transplant, the commonest malignancy is: *(AIIMS June 97)*
    a. Lymphoma   b. Renal cell carcinoma
    c. Skin cancer   d. Adrenal cancer

269. Not true about right kidney is: *(DNB 2003, AIIMS June 2001)*
    a. Right kidney is preferred over the left for transplantation
    b. It is lower than the left kidney
    c. Right renal vein is shorter than the left
    d. Right kidney is related to the duodenum

270. After renal transplantation, which drug is given? *(PGI June 96)*
    a. Cyclophosphamide b. Corticosteroids
    c. Interferon   d. Cyclosporine

271. Urinary ascites is due to: *(PGI Dec 98)*
    a. Injury to bladder during birth
    b. Ureteric obstruction
    c. Congenital urethral atresia
    d. Urethral valves

272. A newborn presents with discharge of urine from the umbilicus for 3 days. Diagnosis is:
    a. Meckel's diverticulum   b. Mesenteric cysts
    c. Urachal fistula   d. Omphalocele

KIDNEY AND URETER ANATOMY AND PHYSIOLOGY

273. Ureters are identified during surgery by: *(AIIMS 96)*
    a. Peristalsis due to flow of urine
    b. Rich arterial plexus
    c. Relation to renal vein and artery
    d. Relation to lumbar plexus

274. All of the following structures cross the right ureter anatomically except: *(All India 2012)*
    a. Terminal ileum
    b. Vas deferens
    c. Genitofemoral nerve
    d. Right colic and ileocolic vessels

275. Ureteric construction is seen at all the following positions, except: *(All India 2002)*
    a. Ureteropelvic junction
    b. Ureterovesicle junction
    c. Crossing of iliac artery
    d. Ischial spine

276. The narrowest part of the ureter is at the: *(AIIMS Nov 2005)*
    a. Ureteropelvic junction   b. Iliac vessel crossing
    c. Pelvic ureter   d. Ureterovesicle junction

277. All the following are true regarding blood supply to the kidney, except: *(All India 2002)*
    a. Stellate veins drain superficial zone
    b. It is a type of portal-circulation
    c. The renal artery divides into five segmental arteries before entering the hilum
    d. Its segmental arteries are end-arteries

278. The commonest site of surgical ureterovaginal fistula is:
    a. Below infudibulopelvic ligament   *(PGI 99)*
    b. Below uterine artery in the Mackenrodts ligament
    c. Vaginal angle
    d. Above uterine artery

279. **True about ureter is:** *(AIIMS 91)*
    a. Gonadal vessels lie anterior to it
    b. It lies in front of great vessels
    c. About 50 cm long   d. Nerve supply from T8-T10
    e. Internal iliac artery

280. **What is column of Bertini in kidney?** *(APPG 2008)*
    a. Renal tumour
    b. Tongue like papillary projection
    c. Calculus   d. None

281. **Ureter is diagnosed during operation by:** *(All India 98)*
    a. Venous plexus   b. High arterial supply
    c. Peristaltic movements   d. Circumference

282. **The resting ureteric pressure:** *(PGI June 99)*
    a. 5–7 cm of H_2O b. 15–30 cm of H_2O
    c. 7–10 cm of H_2O d. 0–5 cm of H_2O

283. **Left loin nephrectomy, structure not cut is:** *(PGI Dec 98)*
    a. Trapezius   b. Serratus inferior posterior
    c. Latissimus Dorsi   d. Internal oblique

284. **Unilateral small smooth kidney is seen in:** *(Karnataka 2003)*
    a. Reflux nephropathy   b. Lobar infarction
    c. Renal artery stenosis
    d. Chronic glomerulonephritis

285. **The neonatal kidney achieves concentrating ability equivalent to adult's kidney by:**
    a. One year of age   b. Eighteen months of age
    c. Three to six months of age   d. Just before puberty

MISCELLANEOUS

286. **A 60 years old male presents with hematuria at onset of micturition, cause is:** *(AIIMS June 99)*
    a. Urethral stone   b. Bladder tumor
    c. Ureteric stone   d. Prostatitis

287. **A 23 years old male who is otherwise normal complains of mild pain in his right iliac fossa in a waveform pattern which increases during the right and he becomes exhausted and is admitted in the hospital. On examination there is mild hematuria. Urine examination reveals plenty of RBCs, 50WBCs/hpf. Urine pH is 5.5. Most likely diagnosis is:**
    a. Glomerulonephritis   b. CA urinary bladder
    c. Ureteral calculus   d. Cystitis

288. **What is oliguria?** *(MCI June 2018, Recent Question 2015)*
    a. Excretion of less than 300 mL in 24 hours
    b. Excretion of less than 500 mL in 24 hours
    c. Excretion of less than 300 mL in 12 hours
    d. Excretion of less than 100 mL in 24 hours

289. **Normal capacity of the renal pelvis is:**
    a. 7 mL   b. 10 mL
    c. 15 mL   d. 20 mL

290. **Low and fixed specific gravity of urine is seen in:**
    a. Diabetes mellitus   *(SGPGI 2005)*
    b. Diabetes insipidus
    c. Chronic renal failure
    d. Acute glomerulonephritis

291. **Auto nephrectomy is seen in:** *(JIPMER 95)*
    a. Sickle cell anemia
    b. Renal TB
    c. Sarcoidosis
    d. Lymphoma

292. **Urine incontinence is seen in all except:**
    a. Ureterovaginal fistula   *(MHPGMCET 2003)*
    b. Vesicovaginal fistula
    c. Ectopic ureter
    d. Urerthrovaginal fistula

293. **If due to a certain pathology there is marked loss of ureter, then what is best therapeutic options?** *(MHSSMCET 2005)*
    a. Transureterostomy
    b. Psoas Hitch operation
    c. Intestinal segment substitute
    d. Boari's flap operation

294. **According to American Urology Association, definition of microscopic hematuria:** *(Recent Question 2016)*
    a. >3 RBCs/hpf   b. >20 RBCs/hpf
    c. >50 RBCs/hpf   d. >100 RBCs/hpf

295. **Sickle cell trait is associated with which type of RCC?** *(JIPMER November 2017)*
    a. Medullary   b. Papillary
    c. Chromophobe   d. Clear cell

Explanations

RENAL AND URETERIC CALCULI

1. **Ans. b. Triple phosphate** *(Ref: Smith 18/e p255; Campbell 11/e p1182-1196; Bailey 27/e p1406)*
2. **Ans. c. Indinavir**
3. **Ans. d. Usually seen in acidic urine**
4. **Ans. b. Urinary stones** *(Ref: Campbell 11/e p1175)*

RANDALL'S PLAQUES

- **Randall's plaques** are **soft tissue calcifications**[Q] found in the **deep renal medulla** skirting the surface of the epithelium of the papilla, where they **act as nucleating elements** for **renal calculi** or **stones**[Q].

5. **Ans. a. Phosphate**
6. **Ans. a. Ethylene glycol** *(Ref: Smith 18/e p254)*

CALCIUM OXALATE CRYSTALS

- **Calcium oxalate crystals** in the urine are the **most common constituent** of human **kidney stones**, and **calcium oxalate crystal formation** is also one of the **toxic effects of ethylene glycol poisoning**[Q].
- **Excessive oxalate** may occur **secondary to the accidental** or **deliberate ingestion of ethylene glycol** (partial oxidation to oxalate[Q]. This may result in diffuse and massive deposition of calcium oxalate crystals and may occasionally lead to renal failure.

7. **Ans. b. Phosphate**
8. **Ans. b. Calcium oxalate**
9. **Ans. a. Calcium oxalate stone** *(Ref: Campbell 11/e p1209; Smith 18/e p252; Bailey 27/e p1406)*
10. **Ans. a. Calcium phosphate** *(Ref: Campbell 11/e p1237; Smith 18/e p251)*
11. **Ans. c. Ammonium urate** *(Ref: Campbell 11/e p1195, 1196)*

"Conditions associated with ammonium acid urate crystallization include laxative abuse, recurrent urinary tract infection, recurrent uric acid stone formation, and inflammatory bowel disease."-Campbell 11/e p1195

"The underlying pathophysiologic mechanism of ammonium acid urate stone formation due to laxative abuse has been postulated to be the result of dehydration due to gastro-intestinal fluid loss causing intracellular acidosis and enhanced ammonia excretion. Because urinary sodium is low in the setting of laxative use, urate complexes with abundant ammonia, thereby leading to urinary supersaturation of ammonium acid urate."- Campbell 11/e p1196

12. **Ans. b. Proteus** *(Ref: Campbell 11/e p1194; Smith 18/e p255; Bailey 27/e p1406)*
13. **Ans. d. Both a and b** *(Ref: Campbell 11/e p1213; Smith 18/e p255; Bailey 27/e p1406)*

RENAL AND URETERIC CALCULI CLINICAL FEATURES

14. **Ans. a. At pelvic brim** *(Ref: Smith 18/e p257; Campbell 1/e p1-2; Bailey 27/e p1407)*
15. **Ans. b. At pelvic brim**
16. **Ans. c. Dietl's crisis** *(Ref: Bailey 27/e p1411)*

DIETL'S CRISIS

- **Intermittent hydronephrosis (Dietl's crisis):** A swelling in the **loin** is associated with **acute renal pain**. Some hours later the **pain is relieved** and the **swelling disappears** when a **large volume of urine is passed**[Q].

17. **Ans. b. Increased peristalsis of ureter to overcome the obstruction** *(Ref: Smiths 18/e p257)*
    - The **severity** and **colicky nature** of **ureteric colic pain** are **caused by** the **hyperperistalsis** and **spasm** of **smooth muscles** of the **ureter** as it attempts to **rid** itself of a **foreign body** or to **overcome obstruction**.

PAIN FROM ACUTE OBSTRUCTION OF URETER (STONE OR BLOOD CLOT)

- **Ureteral pain** is typically **stimulated by acute obstruction** (passage of a **stone** or a **blood clot**)[Q].
- **Back pain** from **renal capsular distention**[Q] combined with **severe colicky pain** (due to **renal pelvic and ureteral muscle spasm**[Q] that radiates from the costovertebral angle down toward the lower anterior abdominal quadrant, along the course of the ureter.
- The **severity** and **colicky nature** of this pain are caused by the **hyperperistalsis**[Q] and **spasm**[Q] of this **smooth muscle organ** as it attempts to **rid itself of a foreign body** or to **overcome obstruction**.

18. Ans. b. Proteus
19. Ans. b. Iliohypogastric
20. Ans. c. Pain
21. Ans. a. Oxalate stones *(Ref: Bailey 27/e p1406)*

OXALATE STONES

- **Oxalate stones** are **irregular** in shape and **covered with sharp projections,** which tend to **cause bleeding**[Q].
- The **surface** of the calculus is **discolored** by **altered blood**[Q].
- A **calcium oxalate monohydrate** stone is **hard** and **radiodense**[Q].

22. Ans. b. Stillness of the patient
23. Ans. d. Diclofenac

RENAL AND URETERIC CALCULI DIAGNOSIS AND TREATMENT

24. Ans. a. PCNL *(Ref: Smith 18/e p272; Campbell 11/e p1236; Bailey 27/e p1409)*
25. Ans. b. Uric acid
26. Ans. a. ESWL
27. Ans. b. PCNL
28. Ans. a. ESWL *(Ref: Campbell 11/e p1236, 1247, 1251; Bailey 27/e p1408)*

The best treatment in this situation is PCNL. Since PCNL is not mentioned in the option, the best option is ESWL despite of size 2.5 cm, as it is preferred over other three for the management of renal stones.

29. Ans. a. Calcium oxalate monohydrate *(Ref: Smith 18/e p268; Campbell 11/e p1268; Bailey 27/e p1408)*

- "Calculi composed of cystine, callium oxalate monohydrate are known to be resistant to fragmentation (ESWL)"

30. Ans. c. Struvite stone *(Ref: Smith 18/e p255; Campbell 11/e p1182-1196; Bailey 25/e p1295-1300)*
31. Ans. b. 'j' stent drainage *(Ref: 'Acute Care Surgery: Principles and Practice' (Springer) 2007/571)*

- **Prompt drainage** of **hydronephrosis** by **'J' stent drainage** is the single **best option to manage uremia** in this patient **with bilateral renal calculi, to allow recovery of renal function** at the **earliest**[Q].
- **Hemodialysis** may be **used afterwards** if **renal recovery** is **prolonged necessitating removal of waste products**[Q]
- **Prompt drainage** of hydronephrosis **by 'J' stent placement** is the **procedure of choice for hydronephrosis** complicated with **renal failure** in the **setting of urinary obstruction**[Q].
- Prompt drainage of hydronephrosis is indicated of renal function is compromised or urinary infection (UTI) is suspected, to preserve/salvage renal function.
- **Prompt drainage** can be achieved **by placement** of a **ureteral sent** or through **percutaneous nephrostomy**[Q].

  - The **drainage procedure of choice** in **emergent situations** is **cystoscopy with placement of internalized double 'J' ureteral stent**. This procedure has the advantage of being a **completely internal drainage system**[Q].
  - **Percutaneous nephrostomy** may be used to allow urinary drainage if the **stone is too impacted to allow passage** of a **guide wire for sent placement**[Q]

32. Ans. a. Hydrothorax *(Ref: Smith 18/e p272; Campbell 11/e p1282; Bailey 27/e p1409)*

- **PCNL** done through the **11th intercostals space** traverses the **lower aspect of pleura** and can **result in significant hydrothorax** from **large amount of irrigative fluid.**

33. Ans. d. Stone in a calyceal diverticulum *(Ref: Smith 17/e p264-268; Campbell 11/e p1278, 10/e p1380-1381)*
34. Ans. d. Ureteroscopic retrieval *(Ref: Smith 18/e p272; Campbell 11e p1283; Bailey 27/e p1408)*
35. Ans. a. Endoscopic removal *(Ref: Campbell 11/e p1283; Bailey 27/e p1408)*
36. Ans. b. Calcium oxalate, uric acid, struvite, cystine *(Ref: Smith 18/e p 255; Campbell 11/e p1182-1196; Bailey 27/e p1406)*
37. Ans. d. Ureteric obstruction due to fragments in ureter
38. Ans. c. Struvite crystals
39. Ans. b. Its use for uric acid stones has caused deaths due to generation of cyanide *(Ref: Smith 18/e p167; Campbell 11/e p1262)*
40. Ans. a. Cysteamine *(Ref: Harrison 19/e p1871; Smith 18/e p256; Campbell 11/e p1229)*

- **Patient with cystinuria with multiple renal stones** should be **treated with increase urine volume** (high fluid intake), **alkalinization of urine, Penicillamine** and **tiopronin.** (α-Mercaptopropionyl glycine).

41. **Ans. e. 90%** *(Ref: Smith 18/e p265)*

> **IMAGING OF URETERIC COLIC (CALCULUS)**
>
> - **Spiral CT (Non-contrast CT)**[Q] has become the **study of choice** in **emergent situations,** as the **entire urinary tract** can be **scanned rapidly** and **without contrast injection**[Q].
> - **Calculi** can be **readily identified** and **distinguished** from **clot** or **tumor**[Q].

- **A plain film** of the abdomen and **renal ultrasound** examination will **diagnose most stones**[Q].
- About of **90%** of **calculi** are **radiopaque**[Q] (calcium, cystine).
- **Excretory urography** is necessary to **verify their location** within the urinary tract and also affords a **qualitative measure** of **renal function**.
- An **acutely obstructed kidney** may show only **increasing density** of **renal shadow** without significant radiopaque material in calices.
- A **non-opaque stone** (uric acid) will be seen as a **radiolucent defect** in the opaque contrast media.

42. **Ans. d. Lower 1/3rd of ureter**
43. **Ans. a. Urine is always infected, b. Should be removed immediately**
44. **Ans. d. Calcium oxalate stone** *(Ref: Smith 18/e p255; Campbell 11/e p1182-1196, 10/e p1296-1302; Bailey 25/e p1295-1300)*

In the given image, which shows enveloped or bipyramidal crystals are seen in calcium oxalate (dihydrate) stones.

Calcium Oxalate	Calcium Oxalate Monohydrate	Brushite
Enveloped or bipyramidal[Q]	Dumbbell or hourglass[Q]	Needle shaped[Q]

Struvite	Uric Acid	Cystine
Coffin lid[Q]	Multifaceted, irregular plates or rosettes[Q]	Hexagonal or benzene ring[Q]

45. **Ans. c. Uric acid**
46. **Ans. a. ESWL**
47. **Ans. c. High calcium intake**
48. **Ans. d. Uric acid stones are resistant to ESWL**
49. **Ans. b. Phosphate**
50. **Ans. c. URS** *(Ref: Sabiston 20/e p2071, Schwartz 10/e p1666, Bailey 27/e p1408-1409)*
51. **Ans. a. Endoscopic removal**
52. **Ans. c. Renal stones** *(Ref: Bailey 27/e p1388)*

X-Ray KUB

- **Kidney stones** should be looked **opposite** to **second lumbar vertebra**^{Q}.
- In a **lateral X-ray** of abdomen **gallstones** are **anterior** and **renal** and **ureteric stones** overlie the **lumbar spine**^{Q}.

Opacities on a plain X-ray that may be confused with renal calculus	
• Calcified mesenteric LN	• **Phleboliths**: calcification in the walls of **veins**, especially in the **pelvis**
• **Gallstones** or concretion in the **appendix**	• **Calcified tuberculous lesion** in the **kidney**
• **Tablets** or **foreign bodies** in the alimentary canal (e.g. cyclopenthiazide)	• **Calcified adrenal gland**
• **Ossified tip** of the **12th rib**	

53. **Ans. d. Restricted calcium intake** *(Ref: Harrison 19/e p1870; Smith 18/e p253)*

- A **source of calcium** at each meal may **actually help prevent oxalate stones from forming** as the **calcium binds with oxalate** in **food** and thus **prevents the oxalate from being absorbed** into the body^Q.

Dietary Modification in Stone Disease

Increase Intake of	Decrease Intake of
• Fluid^Q	• Oxalate^Q
• Dietary calcium^Q	• Animal protein^Q
• Potassium and phytates^Q	• Sucrose
• Vitamin C^Q	• Fructose
	• Sodium

54. **Ans. a. Uric acid stones**
55. **Ans. b. DJ stent after ESWL** *(Ref: Sabiston 20/e p2114; Schwartz 10/e p1666; Bailey 27/e p1408)*
56. **Ans. a. Severity of pain increases with size of the calculus** *(Ref: Bailey 27/e p1407)*
    - The **severity of pain** is **not related to the size** of the **stone.**

Ureteric Colic

- There is a pattern of severe exacerbation on a background of continuing pain
- Radiates to the groin, penis, scrotum or labium as the stone progresses down the ureter
- The **severity of pain** is **not related** to the **size** of the **stone**^{Q}
- The pain is **almost invariably associated with haematuria**^{Q}
- There may be few physical signs

57. **a. Stone**
    - MC cause of **ureteric obstruction: Stone**^{Q}
    - MC cause of **ureteric colic** in **hematuria: Clot**^{Q}

58. **Ans. a. Holmium**
59. **Ans. a. Bleeding is least concerned complication**
60. **Ans. b. Calcium restriction** *(Ref: Smith 18/e p253)*
61. **Ans. b. PCNL** *(Ref: Campbell 11/e p1240; Smith 18/e p272; Bailey 27/e p1409)*

RENAL INFECTIONS

62. **Ans. a. E. coli** *(Ref: Smith 18/e p206; Campbell 11/e p279-280)*
63. **Ans. b. Xanthogranulomatous kidney** *(Ref: Smith 18/e p208; Campbell 11/e p287)*
64. **Ans. b. Always unilateral** *(Ref: Smith 18/e p209; Campbell 11/e p283; Bailey 27/e p1412)*

- For **HDN, DJ stenting** and **percutaneous nephrostomy**, both are having **same results** but **DJ stenting is less invasive**.
- For **pyonephrosis, percutaneous nephrostomy** is **better** than DJ stenting.

65. **Ans. c. Pyonephrosis** *(Ref: P Modi, G Kadam, R Goel - Journal of Endourology, 2007)*

- A **subcapsular nephrectomy** (SN) is sometimes needed to successfully **remove** the **kidney** because of the **dense perinephric adhesions** in **pyonephrosis**.

66. **Ans. c. Nitrite test** *(Ref: Smith 18/e p200)*

Sensitivity and Specificity of Urinalysis in UTI		
Tests	Sensitivity (%)	Specificity (%)
Esterase	83 (67–94)	**78** (64–92)
Nitrite	53 (15–82)	**98 (90–100)**[Q]
Esterase or Nitrite	**93** (90–100)	72 (58–91)
White blood cells	73 (32–100)	81 (45–98)
Bacteria	81 (16–99)	**83** (11–100)
Any above	99.8 (99–100)	70 (60–92)

67. **Ans. a. Proteus**
68. **Ans. d. Vesicoureteric reflux** *(Ref: Bailey 27/e p1404)*

- **Chronic pyelonephritis** is so often **associated with vesicoureteric reflux** that some feel that it is **better named "Reflux nephropathy"**. It is important cause of renal damage and death from end-stage renal failure.

GENITOURINARY TUBERCULOSIS

69. **Ans. b. Hematogenous** *(Ref: Smith 18/e p223-225; Campbell 11/e p422; Bailey 27/e p1405)*
70. **Ans. a. intravenous urography** *(Campbell 11/e p425)*
    - IVU is the gold standard for imaging early renal TB.

Intravenous urography: The majority of cases will show positive findings on excretary urography, **the most common findings being hydrocalycosis, hydronephrosis or Hydroureter due to stricture formation. Early signs include the moth-eaten appearance of calyceal erosion and papillary irregularity.** These signs are best seen on early excretary **films because they are often masked by increasing density of the contrast on later films of the IVU**. Cavitory lesions communicating with the collecting system are characteristic of TB.

71. **Ans. b. Moth eaten calyx** *(Ref: Smith 18/e p224; Campbell 11/e p425; Bailey 27/e p1405)*
72. **Ans. a. Sterile pyuria is consistent finding**
73. **Ans. a. Renal papilla** *(Ref: Smith 18/e p223; Campbell 11/e p422; Bailey 27/e p1405)*

PATHOGENESIS OF GENITO-URINARY TUBERCULOSIS

- **Granulomas** at **renal pyramid** → Enlarge (**tubercular abscess**) → **Burst** into **PC system** and **pus discharge** in urine (sterile pyuria[Q]).
- **Vesical irritability** is an **early clinical manifestation**[Q].

74. **Ans. c. Tuberculosis of ureter**

CYSTOSCOPY IN TUBERCULOSIS

- **Earliest sign** is **pallor**[Q] around ureteric orifice.
- Other features are **tubercular ulcer** and **golf hole ureteric orifice**[Q].

75. **Ans. a. Increased frequency**
76. **Ans. b. Bladder disease is associated with extensive renal disease, c. Ureteric involvement causes shortening of the ureters, d. Renal disease can produce changes identical to reflux nephropathy**
77. **Ans. b. Renal tuberculosis** *(Ref: Campbell 11/e p425; Smith 18/e p224; Bailey 27/e p1405)*
78. **Ans. d. Microscopic hematuria**
79. **Ans. a. Renal tuberculosis**
80. **Ans. d. Thimble bladder**

HYDRONEPHROSIS

81. **Ans. b. Analgesia SOS, c. Under observation, d. Follow up by USG** *(Ref: Bailey 27/e p1411)*
82. **Ans. d. Ureterocele**
83. **Ans. a. Catheterize with Foley catheter** *(Ref: Bailey 27/e p1412, 1349; CSDT 13/e p922)*

   - **Catheterization** is **mandatory for acute urinary retention**^{Q}. Spontaneous voiding may return, but a **catheter** should be **left indwelling for 3 days** while detrusor tone returns.

84. **Ans. b. Radioisotope scan**
85. **Ans. d. Rim sign**

   ### Chronic Hydronephrosis
   - **Rim sign:** On IVP, rim sign is seen due to **chronic hydronephrosis** (**Atrophic changes in kidney** with the **dilatation of pelvicalyceal system**). The **inner margin of hydronephrotic rim in concave towards the renal hilum**.

DIAGNOSTIC AND LABORATORY INVESTIGATIONS

86. **Ans. c. Digital subtraction angiography** *(Ref: Bailey 27/e p1389)*
   - **Hypertension** in a **young female** is most likely due to **renal artery stenosis**, caused by **fibromuscular dysplasia**. **DSA** will show the stenosis.

   ### Renal Artery Stenosis
   - **Satisfactory imaging** of the **renal vessels** can even be achieved by **digital subtraction angiography**^{Q} after intravenous injection of contrast medium.
   - **Intra-arterial angiography** is considered **"gold standard"** for **diagnosis of large vessel disease**^{Q}, usually performed simultaneous with planned intervention.

87. **Ans. c. USG**
   - Causes of **filling defect** on **IVP: Stone, mass, cyst**^{Q}.
   - After excretory urogram, **next best investigation** will be **USG** for **lesion characterization**^{Q}.

88. **Ans. a. Allergy to the drug** *(Bailey 27/e p1389)*

   ### Intravenous Urography (IVU)
   - Although **IVU** gives **excellent images** of the **urinary tract**, its **use should be restricted** because in a **few patients** the **iodine** in the **contrast medium** may **provoke** a **potentially life-threatening anaphylactic reaction**^{Q}.
   - Patients with a **history of allergy, atopy** and **eczema** are **particularly vulnerable**^{Q}, but severe reactions may occur without warning.

89. **Ans. c. Distinguishing between non-obstructed system** *(Ref: Bailey 27/e p1392)*
   - A **99mTc-DTPA scan** is particularly **useful to prove** that **collecting system dilatation** is **caused by obstruction**.

   ### Radioisotope Scanning
   - **Radioisotope scanning** is used in particular to obtain **information about function** in **individual renal units**^{Q}.
   - Diethyltriaminepentaacetic acid (**DTPA**) **behaves** in the kidney **like inulin**: it is **filtered by the glomeruli** and **not absorbed by the tubules**. Using a gamma camera, DTPA labelled with technetium-99m can be followed during its transit through individual kidneys to give a **dynamic representation of renal function**.
   - A **99mTc-DTPA scan** is particularly **useful to prove** that **collecting system dilatation** is **caused by obstruction**. In **obstruction**, **radioactivity** will **remain in the kidney** even if urine flow is stimulated by administration of a diuretic like furosemide^Q.
   - Other substances [dimercaptosuccinic acid (**DMSA**), mercaptoacetylglycine (**MAG-3**) and **sodium orthoiodohippurate (Hippuran)**] labelled with suitable radioactive isotopes have similarly been used to investigate renal function^Q.
   - **Isotope bone scanning** is fundamental to the staging of kidney and prostate cancers, which typically **metastasise to the skeleton**^{Q}.

90. **Ans. a. Thickened bowel loop on USG** *(Ref: Sutton 7/e p873)*

   - **Pseudokidney sign** or **target sign** is **USG finding** of **intussusception**^{Q}.

91. **Ans. a. DMSA scan** *(Ref: Bailey 27/e p1392)*
    - **Renal scarring** or **structure of kidney** is best demonstrated by a **DMSA scan**.

Investigation of Choice	
ADPKD (Retroperitoneal Fibrosis)	CT scan[Q]
Medullary Sponge Kidney	IVP[Q]
VUR	MCU[Q]
Retrocaval ureter	MRI[Q]
PUJ Obstruction	DTPA scan[Q]
Renal structure or surface	DMSA scan[Q]

92. **Ans. d. X-ray diffraction** *(Ref: www.imaging.robarts.ca/.../2005pmb50)*

    ### X-ray Diffraction
    - The **X-ray diffraction** is dedicated to **materials identification** and characterize through single crystal and power X-ray diffraction analysis.
    - Monoenergetic **X-ray diffraction (XRD) analysis** is an **established standard** for the assessment of **urinary stone composition**[Q].
    - For the **precise determination** of true **stone composition, x-ray diffraction analysis** has often been the **method of first choice**[Q].

93. **Ans. b. Micturating cystourethrogram**

94. **Ans. a. Kidney** *(Ref: Smith 18/e p528; Campbell 11/e p23)*

Clinical Significance of Different Casts	
1. **Hyaline casts**	• A **normal constituent**[Q] of urine and has no attached significance[Q] • **Tom Horsfall protein**[Q] is protein secreted by **epithelial cells** of **loop of henle**. This protein may be excreted as Hyaline cast[Q]
2. **RBC cast**	• Are suggestive of **glomerular injury**[Q] or **acute glomerulonephritis**
3. **WBC casts**	• Are suggestive of **interstitial injury** and may be seen in **interstitial nephritis**[Q] • **WBC cast** with **bacteria** indicate **pyelonephritis**[Q]
4. **Brood granular casts**	• Are seen in **CRF**[Q] and suggests interstitial fibrosis and dilatation of tubules.
5. **Pigmented muddy brown granular casts**	• Are suggestive of ischemic or nephrotoxic injury[Q] **(Tubular Necrosis)**

95. **Ans. d. Graphic representation of radioactivity of kidneys**

96. **Ans. c. Chronic obstructive nephropathy** *(Ref: Wolfgang 2/e p550)*

Cortical Rim Nephrogram is seen in	
• Acute total main renal artery occlusion[Q] • Renal vein thrombosis[Q]	• Acute tubular necrosis[Q] • Severe chronic urinary obstruction[Q]

    - **Rim and ball nephrogram** on IVP is seen in **chronic obstructive nephropathy**[Q].
    - **Rim sign** is seen in **chronic hydronephrosis**[Q].

97. **Ans. a. Micturating cystourethrogram**

Procedure	Mean Effective Dose (mSv) Value
X-ray abdomen	0.7
Intravenous urogram (6 films)	2.5[Q]
MCU	1.2[Q]
Cystography	1.8
Lithotripsy	1.3
Nephrostomy	3.4[Q]
PCNL	4.5
Ureteric stenting	4.7
CECT abdomen	10[Q]
Renal angiogram	2 to 30
Kidney stent insertion	12.7

Kidney and Ureter

98. **Ans. a. Stone removal, b. Ureteral obstruction, c. Anterograde renography, d. Renal tumor resection** *(Ref: Bailey 27/e p1412; Campbell 11/e p153)*

> "Percutaneous nephrostomy is indicated to drain the upper urinary tract collecting system in cases of obstruction at an intrarenal location, at the ureteropelvic junction, or anywhere in the ureter".

- For **HDN**, **DJ stenting** and **percutaneous nephrostomy**, both are having **same results** but **DJ stenting** is **less invasive**^{Q}.
- For **pyonephrosis, percutaneous nephrostomy** is **better** than DJ stenting^Q.

99. **Ans. a. Hydronephrosis**
100. **Ans. d. Pyonephrosis**
101. **Ans. b. DMSA scan** *(Ref: Campbell 11/e p285, 2940; Smith 18/e p206; Bailey 27/e p1404)*

BENIGN RENAL TUMORS

102. **Ans. c. Bleeding is self limited, d. Nephrectomy is the treatment of choice,** *(Ref: Smith 18/e p331; Campbell 11/e p1309; Bailey 27/e p1416)*

103. **Ans. b. Angiomyolipoma** *(Ref: Campbell 11/e p1306, 10/e p1499; Bailey 27/e p1416)*

> *In the given CT image, the renal mass is containing fat content, which is suggestive of angiomyolipoma, which is a fat containing benign renal neoplasm.*

> "Angiomyolipoma is the only benign renal tumor that is confidently diagnosed on cross-sectional imaging. The presence of fat (confirmed on non-enhanced thin-cut CT by a value of −20 Hounsfield Units [HU] or less) within a renal lesion is considered the diagnostic hallmark. Findings of more than 20 pixels with attenuation less than −20 HU and of more than 5 pixels with attenuation less than −30 HU have been shown to have a positive predictive value of 100%. Ultrasonography shows a well-circumscribed, highly echogenic lesion with shadowing. On angiography (or CT-angiography) aneurysmal dilation is found in 50% of angiomyolipomas. The size of the aneurysms has been reported to correlate with the risk of rupture. MRI can be used in difficult cases or in lieu of CT, with findings on fat-suppressed images being highly suggestive of the diagnosis."-Campbell 11/e p1306

104. **Ans. b. Renal oncocytoma** *(Ref: Smith 18/e p330; Campbell 11/e p1305)*

Central Stellate Scar is seen in	
• FNH^Q	• Serous cystadenoma^Q (pancreas)
• Fibrolamellar HCC^Q	• Renal oncocytoma^Q

RENAL CELL CARCINOMA: TYPES

105. **Ans. d. Chromophobe cell carcinoma** *(Ref: Smith 18/e p333; Campbell 11/e p1329; Bailey 27/e p1417)*
106. **Ans. a. Mutated VHL gene is associated with clear cell carcinoma, c. Extreme hypodiploidy occurs**
107. **Ans. a. Clear cell type**
108. **Ans. d. Monosomy of 1 and Y (-1, -Y)** *(Ref: Smith 18/e p333; Campbell 11/e p1329; Bailey 27/e p1417)*

- These tumors exhibit **multiple chromosome loss** and **extreme hypodiploidy**^{Q}.
- Loss of multiple chromosomes **1^Q, 2^Q**, 6, 10, 13, 17, 21 and **Y^Q**.

109. **Ans. c. von-Hippel Lindau (VHL) syndrome**
110. **Ans. a. PCT** *(Ref: Smith 18/e p333; Campbell 11/e p1329; Bailey 27/e p1417)*
111. **Ans. a. Medullary** *(Ref: Campbell 11/e p1333)*

- "Renal medullary carcinoma is a subtype of RCC that occurs almost exclusively in patients with the sickle cell trait. It is typically diagnosed in young African-Americans, often in the third decade of life, and many cases are both locally advanced and metastatic at the time of diagnosis."-Campbell 11/e p1333

RENAL CELL CARCINOMA CLINICAL FEATURES, PARANEOPLASTIC SYNDROMES

112. **Ans. None** *(Ref: Smith 18/e p355; Campbell 11/e p1334; Bailey 27/e p1417)*

Incidence of Systemic Syndromes Associated with RCC	
Syndrome	%
↑ ESR	55.6
Hpertension	37.5
Anemia	36.3
Calhexia, weight loss	34.5
Pyrexia	17.2
Abnormal liver function	14.4
Hypercalcemia	4.9
Polycythemia	3.5
Neuromyopathy	3.2
Amyloidosis	2.0

113. Ans. c. More common in female
114. Ans. b. Lungs
115. Ans. a. Renal cell carcinoma
116. Ans. d. All
117. Ans. a. Seminoma testis, c. Hypernephroma *(Ref: Smith 18/e p333)*

- **Cannon-Ball pulmonary metastases** are **characteristic feature of RCC and testicular carcinoma**. As a rule, RCC produces spherical or round cannon-ball metastases.

118. Ans. c. von-Hippel Lindau disease
119. Ans. d. Lower pole involvement
120. Ans. a. Invasion of renal vein means inoperability
121. Ans. d. Invasion of renal vein is contraindication for surgery, b. Associated with anemia and low ESR
122. Ans. c. More common in female
123. Ans. c. Renal cell carcinoma
124. Ans. None
125. Ans. None > d. Cushing syndrome
   - Cushing syndrome is the least common among the given options.
126. Ans. a. Hematuria
127. Ans. c. Hematuria

RENAL CELL CARCINOMA DIAGNOSIS AND TREATMENT

128. Ans. b. IVC involvement indicates inoperability *(Ref: Smith 18/e p340; Campbell 11/e p1355; Bailey 27/e p1419)*

- 45–70% of patients with RCC and IVC thrombus can be cured with an aggressive surgical approach including radical nephrectomy and IVC thrombectomy.

129. Ans. d. Pathological staging
130. Ans. d. Renal cell carcinoma *(Ref: Campbell 11/e p1340; Harrison 19/e p578)*

Renal Cell Carcinoma
- **Cannon Ball pulmonary metastases** are **characteristic feature of RCC**[Q].
- As a rule, **RCC produces spherical or round cannon-ball metastases**[Q].

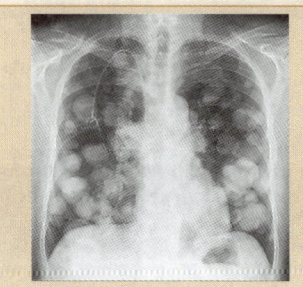 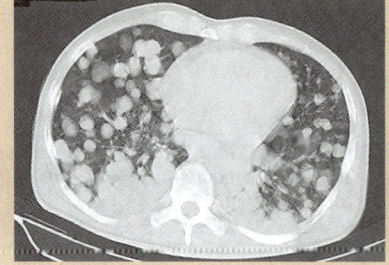 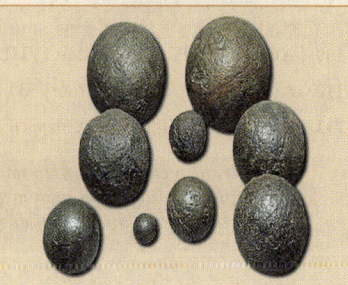

131. Ans. a. Partial nephrectomy
132. Ans. a. Radiosensitive
133. Ans. c. Right radical nephrectomy and left partial nephrectomy
134. Ans. a. Transperitoneal

Kidney and Ureter

135. Ans. c. Renal vein
136. Ans. b. Chromosome 3
137. Ans. d. Renal cell carcinoma *(Ref: Smith 18/e p336; Campbell 11/e p1338; Bailey 27/e p1419)*

Most likely diagnosis for an asymptomatic complex cyst in a 65 years old male as given in CT image, which appears as exophytic mass is renal cell carcinoma.

> "CT scanning is more sensitive than US or IVU for detection of renal masses. A typical finding of RCC on CT is a mass that becomes enhanced with the use of intravenous contrast media. In general, RCC exhibits an overall decreased density in Hounsfield units compared with nor- mal renal parenchyma but shows a heterogeneous pattern of enhancement or increased attenuation (slightly decreased from the surrounding parenchyma) when contrast is used. In addition to defining the primary lesion, CT scanning is also the method of choice in staging the patient by visualizing the renal hilum, perinephric space, renal vein and vena cava, adrenals, regional lymphatics, and adjacent organs."-Smith 18/e p336

138. Ans. a. Transitional cell carcinoma
139. Ans. c. Elevated ESR
140. Ans. a. Partial nephrectomy
141. Ans. c. Keeping fascia back in place *(Ref: Smith 18/e p339; Campbell 11/e p1345)*

- The prototypical concept of **Radical nephrectomy** encompasses the basic principles of **early ligation of the renal artery and vein**, **removal of the kidney** with primary **dissection external to the Gerota's fascia**, **excision of the ipsilateral adrenal gland**, and **performance of a complete regional lymphadenectomy** from the **crus of the diaphragm** to the **aortic bifurcation**^{Q}.
- It has been well demonstrated that **removal of the ipsilateral adrenal gland** is **not routinely necessary** in the absence of radiographic adrenal enlargement **unless the malignant lesion extensively involves the kidney, is locally advanced**, or is **located in the upper portion** of the kidney **immediately adjacent to the adrenal gland**^{Q}.

RADICAL NEPHRECTOMY

- Radical nephrectomy is the **primary treatment for localized RCC**.
- Its goal is to achieve the **removal of tumor** and to take a **wide margin of normal tissue**.
- **Radical nephrectomy** encompasses:
  - Basic principles of **early ligation of** the **renal artery** and **vein**^{Q} (Artery followed by vein) First vein is incircled then artry is ligated.
  - **Removal of the kidney** with primary **dissection external to the Gerota's fascia**^{Q}
  - **Excision of the ipsilateral adrenal gland**^{Q}
  - Performance of a **complete regional lymphadenectomy** from the **crus of the** diaphragm to the **aortic bifurcation**^{Q}.

142. Ans. d. Para-aortic nodes *(Ref: Campbell 11/e p1345)*
143. Ans. c. Venacavagraphy
144. Ans. c. Tumor grossly extends into the inferior vena cava *(Ref: Campbell 11/e p1337; Smith 18/e p334)*

WILMS' TUMOR

145. Ans. b. Abdominal lump *(Ref: Smith 18/e p342; Campbell 11/e p3572; Bailey 27/e p1421)*
146. Ans. a. Bone metastasis
147. Ans. c. Histology
148. Ans. a. Within 10 days
149. Ans. c. Same location
150. Ans. c. Abdominal mass
151. Ans. a. Hematuria, b. Mass abdomen, d. Fever
152. Ans. c. Hematuria almost always present
153. Ans. b. Less than 1 year
154. Ans. a. Preoperative use of actinomycin D
155. Ans. b. Lungs
156. Ans. b. International society of Pediatric Oncology (SIOP) *(Ref: Campbell 11/e p3575-3576, , Schwartz 10/e p1638-1639)*

The postchemotherapy based staging system is the 'SIOP' staging system developed by the International society of oncology.

157. Ans. c. Arthrogryposis multiplex congenita
158. Ans. b. Open nephroureterectomy *(Ref: Campbell 11/e p3574)*

- The **treatment of choice** for **satge I Wilms' tumor** is **transperitoneal radical nephrectomy (radical nephroureterectomy)**^{Q} followed by **chemotherapy with or without radiotherapy** depending upon tumor histology.

159. Ans. c. 11 p13

TUMORS OF RENAL PELVIS

160. Ans. a. Transitional cell carcinoma *(Ref: Smith 18/e p322; Campbell 11/e p1370)*

- **Urothelial (transitional cell) carcinoma make up > 90% of upper urinary tract tumors**

161. **Ans. b. Pelvic calculus**
162. **Ans. b. Retrograde pyeloureterography** *(Ref: Smith 18/e p324; Campbell 11/e p1371)*

- **Goblet sign** and **Stipple sign** describe the **appearance of ureteral dilation below** the **site** of an **intraluminal ureteral filling defect**, **best seen at** retrograde pyelography (**RGP**)^Q.
- The **Stipple sign** refers to the **pointillistic end-on appearance**^{Q} on IVP or RGP of **contrast material tracking into** the **interstices** of a papillary lesion.
- Because maturity of TCC have a papillary configuration, **presence of this sign** should **raise** the **suspicion of TCC**, while the **Stipple sign** is **best seen** in **large papillary bladder tumors**^{Q}, it can occur anywhere in urothelial tumor, which expresses papillary architecture.

163. **Ans. d. Transitional carcinoma of pelvis extending till ureter**
164. **Ans. a. Radical nephroureterectomy**
165. **Ans. d. Both b and c** *(Ref: Smith 18/e p322; Campbell 11/e p1370; Bailey 27/e p1421)*

RENAL TRAUMA

166. **Ans. a. Urgent IVP is indicated** *(Ref: Smith 18/e p286; Campbell 11/e p1151; Bailey 27/e p1413)*
167. **Ans. c. Exploration indicated in all cases**   168. **Ans. b. Uremia**
169. **Ans. b. Open Gerota's fascia and explore proximal renal vessels** *(Ref: Smith 18/e p286; Campbell 11/e p1151)*

- The correct option should be "take the control or explore proximal renal vessels before opening Gerota's fascia", to avoid excessive intra-operative bleeding.

Excretory Urography (IVU or IVP)- Campbell 11/e p1151

- Historically, **excretory urography** was the most commonly used modality to evaluate genitourinary injuries. Largely replaced by CT, a limited role includes the intraoperative "single-shot" IVP. The **indications are uncommon**, but when the surgeon encounters an unexpected **retroperitoneal hematoma surrounding a kidney during abdominal exploration**, the study can provide essential information^Q.
- The **main purpose** of the **one-shot IVP** is to **assess the presence of a functioning contralateral kidney** and to **radiographically stage the injured side**^{Q}.
- If **findings are not normal** or **near normal**, the **kidney should be explored to complete the staging** of the injury and **reconstruct any abnormality found**^{Q}.

- In the given problem, patient is having a **non-pulsatile hematoma**, which is **not an indication** for **surgical exploration**.
- **On table IVU** was done **to see** the **function of contralateral kidney**, the function of opposite kidney should be ascertained before planning nephrectomy in any trauma patient.
- **Angiography** is **largely used to define arterial injuries suspected on CT** or to **localize and control arterial bleeding**. Renal **embolization** has proved useful in the **primary setting with persistent bleeding** in a **hemodynamically stable patient**.
- **Take the control** or **explore proximal renal vessels before opening Gerota's fascia**", to avoid excessive intra-operative bleeding.

170. **Ans. a. Observation and supportive measures**   171. **Ans. c. Contrast enhanced computed tomography**
172. **Ans. a. 20%** *(Ref: Smith 18/e p287)*

- **Minor renal injuries** from **blunt trauma** account for **85% of cases** and **do not usually require operation**^{Q}.
- **Bleeding stops spontaneously** with **bed rest** and **hydration**^{Q}.
- Cases in which **operation is indicated** include those associated with **persistent retroperitoneal bleeding, urinary extravasation,** evidence of **nonviable renal parenchyma,** and **renal pedicle injuries** (less than 5% of all renal injuries)^Q.

173. **Ans. c. Contralateral renal function is ascertained**   174. **Ans. a. Exploration is indicated in 90% of cases**
175. **Ans. c. 5**   176. **Ans. b. Pulsatile hematoma**
177. **Ans. d. CECT of abdomen**
178. **Ans. c. J-shaped urinary stent** *(Ref: Campbell 11/e p3736)*

Management of urinoma is by endoscopic intervention, with cystoscopy, retrograde pyelography, placement of a ureteral stent, urethral catheter drainage, and intravenous antibiotics.

Kidney and Ureter

URETERIC INJURY

179. Ans. a. Complete renal atrophy, d. Hydronephrosis *(Ref: Smith 18/e p288; Bailey 27/e p1414)*
180. Ans. b. Hysterectomy

POLYCYSTIC KIDNEY DISEASE

181. Ans. a. Autosomal recessive trait *(Ref: Smith 18/e p537; Campbell 11/e p3017; Bailey 27/e p1402)*
182. Ans. c. Renal cell carcinoma
183. Ans. d. Decompression of cyst leads to normal renal function
184. Ans. a. Autosomal dominant *(Ref: Campbell 11/e p3017; Smith 18/e p537)*
185. Ans. a. Hypertension is rare
186. Ans. b. 16 and 4
187. Ans. a. Cysts in liver, c. Berry aneurysms
188. Ans. a. Lung
189. Ans. d. Renal transplant
190. Ans. d. 50%
191. Ans. a. ADPKD
192. Ans. a. Lungs
193. Ans. a. Spider leg appearance *(Ref: Smith 18/e p537; Campbell 11/e p3017; Bailey 27/e p1402)*

IVP in ADPKD	
• Stretching of the calyces by the cysts (**spider leg** or **bell like deformity**)^Q	• **Bubble appearance**^{Q} (calyceal distortion) • **Swiss cheese appearance**^{Q}

194. Ans. b. Polycystic kidney
195. Ans. a. Inherited as autosomal recessive
196. Ans. b. Hypertension is rare
197. Ans. b. Hepatic cyst
198. Ans. b. The presentation is unilateral
199. Ans. a. Autosomal dominant *(Ref: Campbell 11/e p3017; Bailey 27/e p1402)*
200. Ans. d. Erythrocytosis *(Ref: Campbell 11/e p3017; Smith 18/e p537; Bailey 27/e p1402)*

PUJ OBSTRUCTION

201. Ans. d. Aberrant vessel is the most common cause *(Ref: Smith 18/;e p575; Campbell 11/e p1105; Bailey 26/e p1290-1292)*
202. Ans. c. Right sided lesions predominate
203. Ans. c. Painless abdominal mass
204. Ans. c. Dismembered pyeloplasty
205. Ans. d. Pelviureteric junction obstruction *(Ref: Campbell 11/e p1105; Smith 18/e p575)*
206. Ans. b. PUJ obstruction
207. Ans. b. DTPA scan
208. Ans. b. Endoscopic pyelotomy is contraindicated
209. Ans. a. Dietl's crisis

CONGENITAL ANOMALIES OF KIDNEY

210. Ans. a. Bilateral renal agenesis *(Ref: Smith 18/e p513; Campbell 11/ep3007, 2975; Bailey 27/e p1410)*
211. Ans. e. All are true
212. Ans. d. UTI *(Ref: Smith 18e p522; Campbell 11/e p3037)*

   • MSK is usually a benign process, and it may remain asymptomatic and undetected for life. Clinical presentation usually occurs after age 20 years with most common presentation being renal colic (50-60%), followed by urinary tract infection (20-30%) and gross hematuria (10-18%)

213. Ans. c. Medullary sponge kidney *(Ref: Smith 18/e p522; Campbell 11/e p3037)*

IVP (Excretory urogram): IOC to diagnose medullary sponge kidney^Q
• **"Bristles on brush"**^{Q} appearance due to dilated ducts • **"Bouquet of flowers"**^{Q} appearance due to calcification in the ectatic ducts

214. Ans. a. Supernumerary renal arteries *(Ref: Campbell's 10/e p26; Smith 18/e p522)*

- Vascular anomalies involving the kidney are very common being present in 25% to 40% of kidneys.
- **Supernumerary renal arteries** with two or more renal arteries supplying each kidney are the **most common renal vascular anomaly**.

ABNORMALITIES OF RENAL VASCULATURE

- **MC renal vascular anomaly** is the presence of **supernumerary renal arteries**[Q].
- **Variations** of the **main renal artery** and **vein** are common, present in **25% to 40%** of kidneys.
- **MC variation** is occurrence of **supernumerary renal arteries (two or more arteries to a single kidney**[Q])
- **MC sub-group** of **supernumerary renal arteries** is a **duplicated renal artery (double renal artery)**[Q] involving a second diminutive renal artery supplying each kidney
- Supernumerary renal veins are also common, but occur about half as commonly as supernumerary renal arteries.

215. **Ans. a. Left renal vein** *(Ref: Smith 18/e p522)*

RENAL COLLAR

- The **main renal vein** divides and sends **one limb anterior** and **another limb posterior** to **aorta** to reach the **IVC**[Q].
- Formed on the **left side**[Q] and represents **persistence of the embryonic state**.

216. **Ans. d. Is a normal variant** *(Ref: www.ajronline.org/content/188/5/1380.full)*

PERSISTENT FETAL LOBULATION

- **Persistent fetal lobulation** is a **normal variant** seen occasionally **in adult kidneys**.
- It occurs when there is **incomplete fusion** of the **developing renal lobules**[Q].
- Embryologically, the kidneys originate as distinct lobules that fuse as they develop and grow.
- It is often seen on **ultrasound, CT** or **MRI** as **smooth indentations of the renal outline in between renal pyramids**[Q].
- They should be **distinguished from renal cortical scarring**, which **generally overlie the pyramids**[Q].

217. **Ans. d. 1:1000** *(Ref: Campbell 10/e p3136, Smith 18/e p522)*

ECTOPIC KIDNEY

- The **actual incidence** among **autopsy series** varies from **1 in 500** to **1 in 1200** but the **average occurrence** is about **1 in 900**[Q].

218. **Ans. c. 1:1400 individuals** *(Ref: Campbell 11/e p3007, 10/e p3128; Smith 18/e p513)*

- Most autopsy series suggest that **unilateral renal agenesis** occurs **once in 1100 births**[Q].
- In an historical survey of excretory urograms, the incidence ranged between **1 in 1500**[Q].

219. **Ans. d. Biopsy** *(Ref: Campbell 11/e p3021; Smith 18/e p537)*

MEDULLARY CYSTIC DISEASE

- **Excretory urography** and **ultrasonography** frequently **fail to detect cysts** because they are **small**[Q].
- Cysts may be seen on **imaging studies** if they are large enough, but, **early in the disease, cysts are rarely visible**[Q].
- It is **best diagnosed by biopsy**[Q].
- Histologically, there is a **characteristic triad**:
  - **Irregular thickening** and **disintegration** of the **tubular basement membrane**
  - **Marked tubular atrophy** with cyst development
  - **Interstitial cell infiltration with fibrosis**

ABERRANT RENAL ARTERY

220. **Ans. d. Usually divided to gain access to renal pelvis** *(Ref: Smith 18/e p522)*

ABERRANT RENAL ARTERY

- Arteries that originate from vessels other than aorta or the main renal artery
- **Unilateral**[Q], more common on **left side**[Q], involving **lower pole**[Q] of kidney
- May cause **hydronephrosis** due to **extrinsic compression**[Q]
- These are **end arteries**[Q], therefore any injury or division may lead to lower pole infarction.

> - The **renal arteries** are **end-arteries**, **division** leads to **infarction** of parenchyma[Q].
> - **Renal veins** have **extensive collaterals** and an aberrant vein **can be divided** with impunity[Q].

221. **Ans. a. Bilateral**

Kidney and Ureter

RETROCAVAL URETER

222. Ans. c. Retrocaval ureter *(Ref: Smith 18/e p575; Campbell 11/e p1125; Bailey 27/e p1402)*
223. Ans. c. Retrocaval ureter *(Ref: Smith 18/e p575; Campbell 11/e p1125; Bailey 27/e p1402)*

> **Retrocaval Ureter** (Circumcaval ureter)
> **Diagnosis**
> - **MRI** is **IOC** to delineate **anatomy** clearly & **non-invasively**[Q]
> - **IVP**: "Reverse J", "Fish Hook" or "Shepherd crook"[Q] deformity.

224. Ans. d. Posterior cardinal vein

HORSESHOE KIDNEY

225. Ans. a. Spider like appearance in IVP, d. Heminephrectomy improves function *(Ref: Smith 18/e p520; Campbell 11/e p2996; Bailey 27/e p1399)*
226. Ans. b. L3-L4 vertebra   227. Ans. b. Horseshoe kidney   228. Ans. d. Isthmus may contain aberrant vessels
229. Ans. c. Inferior mesenteric artery *(Ref: Campbell 11/e p2293; Smith 18/e p520; Bailey 27/e p1399)*

RENAL CYST

230. Ans. a. Renal cyst *(Ref: Smith 18/e p515; Campbell 11/e p1300; Bailey 27/e p1402)*
231. Ans. a. Polycystic kidney *(Ref: Smith 18/e p514; Campbell 11/e p3017)*

> - Incidence of polycystic kidney: **1 in 400**[Q] (0.25%)
> - **Simple renal cyst** is **MC cystic disease** in **human kidney** (incidence is **0.22% from birth to 18 years**)[Q]

URETEROCELE

232. Ans. d. Ureterocele *(Ref: Smith 18/e p571; Campbell 11/e p3076; Bailey 27/e p1401)*
233. Ans. d. Endoscopic diathermy   234. Ans. b. Ureterocele   235. Ans. c. Ureterocele
236. Ans. c. Ureterocele *(Ref: Smith 18/e p571; Campbell 11/e p3076; Bailey 26/e p1286)*
   - **IVP**: Typical **Adder head** or **Cobra head** or **Spring onion appearance**[Q] is diagnostic of ureterocele

URETERIC ABNORMALITIES

237. Ans. a. Bulbar urethra *(Ref: Smith 18/e p570; Campbell 11/e p3098; Bailey 27/e p1400)*
238. Ans. c. Ectopic ureteric orifice   239. Ans. b. Duplication of ureter

> - MC congenital anomaly of **upper urinary tract**: **Duplication** of **ureter**[Q]
> - MC congenital anomaly of **genitourinary tract**: **VUR**[Q]

240. Ans. b. Right bifid and left complete duplication of ureter   *(Ref: Campbell 11/e p3075; Smith 18/e p578)*
    Right Incomplete (bifid) with Left Complete Duplication of Ureter

Normal system

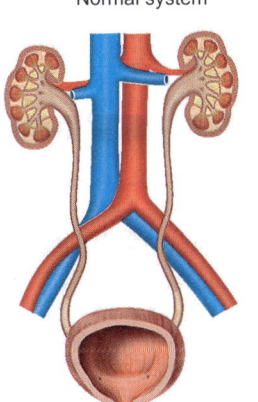

Duplex kidney

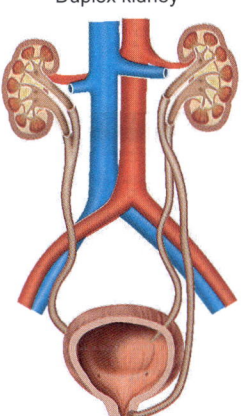

241. Ans. a. Prostatic urethra *(Ref: Smith 18/e p573; Campbell 11/e p3075; Bailey 27/e p1400)* 242. Ans. d. Paradoxical incontinence
243. Ans. c. Lower pole moiety is more prone to obstruction and upper pole more prone to reflux
244. Ans. a. Weigert-Meyer's rule *(Ref: Smith 18/e p570; Campbell 11/e p3098; Bailey 27/e p1400)*
245. Ans. a. Duplication of ureter *(Ref: Campbell 11/e p3075)* 246. Ans. d. Ureteral duplications
247. Ans. c. Below and medial to the lower pole ureter
248. Ans. a. Lateral and cephalad to the upper pole ureter *(Ref: Campbell 11/e p3098; Smith 18/e p570; Bailey 27/e p1400)*
249. Ans. a. Posterior urethra 250. Ans. a. Vestibule
251. Ans. a. In males, there is duplication in 80% cases
    - **Ectopic ureteral orifice** is associated with a **duplication collecting system**^{Q} in **80%**, in **females**^{Q}, not in males.
252. Ans. c. Ureteral incontinence with otherwise normal voiding 253. Ans. a. Recurrent UTI

VESICOURETERIC REFLUX

254. Ans. a. Micturating cystourethrogram *(Ref: Smith 18/e p191; Campbell 11/e p3141)*
255. Ans. b. Micturating cystourethrography 256. Ans. a. I
257. Ans. d. Grade V VUR *(Ref: Smith 18/e p191; Campbell 11/e p3141)*

International classification of vesicoureteral reflux

Grade I	Grade II	Grade III	Grade IV	Grade V
Contrast appears in the nondilated ureter	Contrast appears in the renal pelvis and calyces without dilation	Mild to moderate dilation of the ureter, renal pelvis, and calyces, with minimal blunting of the fornices	Moderate ureteral tortuosity and dilation of the renal pelvis and calyces	Gross dilation of the ureter, renal pelvis, and calyces; loss of papillary impressions; and ureteral tortuosity

258. Ans. a. Cotrimoxazole
259. Ans. b. Postnatal scarring may occur even in the absence of urinary tract infections
    - Although **UTI** is the **most important cause** for **scarring** and **nephropathy** in patients with **VUR**, scarring can occur even **in the absence of UTI** due to **pressure effect of reflux**^{Q} on the **renal tissue**.
260. Ans. c. VUR induced pyelonephritis

RENAL ARTERY ANEURYSM

261. Ans. b. 5% *(Ref: Smith 18/e p523; Campbell 11/e p2999)*

HEPATORENAL SYNDROME

262. Ans. a. Urine sodium < 10 mEq/L, b. Normal renal histology *(Ref: Sabiston 20/e p1043; Blumgart 5/e p389; Schackelford 7/e p1449, 1527; Harrison 19/e p2066)*
263. Ans. c. Urine osmolality lower than plasma osmolality
    - **Hepatorenal syndrome** is associated with **urine osmolality greater than plasma osmolality**^{Q}.
264. Ans. a. The creatinine clearance is > 40 mL/min, c. The urine osmolality is lower than the plasma osmolality

DIALYSIS

265. Ans. b. Peritonitis, c. Hypertension *(Ref: Harrison 19/e p1824)*

COMPLICATIONS DURING HEMODIALYSIS

- **Hypotension** is the **MC acute complication** of **hemodialysis**, particularly among patients with diabetes mellitus.
- **Muscle cramps** during dialysis are also a common complication of the procedure.
- **Anaphylactoid reactions** to the dialyzer, particularly on its first use, have been reported most frequently with the **bioincompatible cellulosic-containing membranes**.
- **Cardiovascular disease** constitutes the **major cause of death in patients with ESRD**. **Cardiovascular mortality** and **event rates are higher in dialysis patien**ts than in patients post-transplantation, although rates are extraordinarily high in both populations.

RENAL TRANSPLANT

266. Ans. a. Hardy *(Ref: Campbell 11/e p1087)*

First autologous renal transplantation was performed by 'Hardy' in 1963Q
'In 1963, Hardy performed the first renal autotransplantation to resolve on extensive ureteral lesion'.

267. Ans. c. In India, organ harvesting from brain dead patients is not permitted by law *(Ref: Bailey 27/e p1546-1547)*

RENAL TRANSPLANTATION

- **Most** of the **organs** used for transplantation are **obtained from brainstem-dead, heart-beating deceased donors**[Q] and in the majority of cases multiple organs are procured.
- **In India**, for **organ harvesting from brain dead patients**[Q], the relatives are formally asked to sign a prescribed form, in contrast to U.K., where the transplant co-ordinators and nurse just write and sign in the file about the consent given.
- **After removal from the donor**, the **kidney is flushed with chilled organ preservation solution** and, **if necessary**, **stored briefly on ice**[Q] until transplanted into the recipient.
- **Calcineurin blockers** are especially useful in renal transplant patients. These include **cyclosporine** and **tacrolimus**[Q].

268. Ans. c. Skin cancer *(Ref: Bailey 27/e p1542)*

MALIGNANCY AFTER TRANSPLANTATION

- After transplantation there is an increased risk of developing most types of malignancy but the **risk is particularly high for** those types of **tumour in which viral infection plays an etiological role**.
- The risk is particularly high for **skin cancer**[Q] and a condition called post-transplant lymphoproliferative disorder (**PTLD**)[Q].
- The **risk of skin cancer after transplantation rises with age** and with exposure to sunlight, and it has been predicted that **50% of transplant patients** will **develop a skin malignancy within 20 years** of **transplantation**[Q].
- **Transplant patients** also have a **300-fold increased risk of developing Kaposi's sarcoma**[Q], although this malignancy is still very uncommon after transplantation.

269. Ans. a. Right kidney is preferred over the left for transplantation *(Ref: Bailey 27/e p1549)*

If the left kidney has a single renal artery (10% of kidneys have two or more renal arteries) it is usually chosen for transplantation because it has a longer renal vein, which simplifies the transplant operation[Q].

RENAL TRANSPLANTATION

- **Before the donation** it is essential to **perform imaging** (usually **MR angiography** or **CT angiography**) to **delineate the anatomy** of the **arterial supply to the kidneys**[Q].
- If the **left kidney** has a **single renal artery** (10% of kidneys have two or more renal arteries) it is **usually chosen for transplantation** because it has a **longer renal vein**, which **simplifies the transplant operation**[Q].
- The presence of **multiple arteries does not necessarily preclude donation** although implantation of living donor kidneys with multiple arteries may **increase the chances of vascular complications** developing **after implantation**[Q].

270. Ans. b. Corticosteroids, d. Cyclosporine *(Ref: Bailey 27/e p1540)*

IMMUNOSUPPRESSIVE DRUG REGIMEN IN RENAL TRANSPLANTATION

- Combination of **glucocorticoid** with **cyclosporine** or **tacrolimus**, **azathioprine** or **mycophenolate mofetil** and sometimes **antilymphocyte antibody preparation**[Q].

271. **Ans. d. Urethral valves** *(Ref: Campbell's 11/e p2891)*   272. **Ans. c. Urachal fistula** *(Ref: Campbell's 11/e p3176)*

KIDNEY AND URETER ANATOMY AND PHYSIOLOGY

273. **Ans. a. Peristalsis due to flow of urine** *(Ref: Oxford Urology 6/e p2123)*

- **Ureters** are situated retroperitoneally, and are **identified by peristalsis**^{Q}.

KIDNEY AND URETER: ANATOMY AND PHYSIOLOGY

- **Kidney** receives **20%** of **cardiac output**
- Renal **vein** is **anterior**, renal **artery** in **middle**, renal **pelvis** is **posterior (VAP)**
- Main renal artery divides into **4–5 segmental arteries. First and most consistent division** is **posterior** branch.
- There are 2 or more LNs at the renal hilum **(first site of metastasis)**^{Q}.
- From the **left kidney**, lymphatic trunk then **drain into para-aortic nodes.**
- From the **right kidney**, lymphatics drain **into hilar lymph node, inter-aortocaval** and **paracaval nodes.**

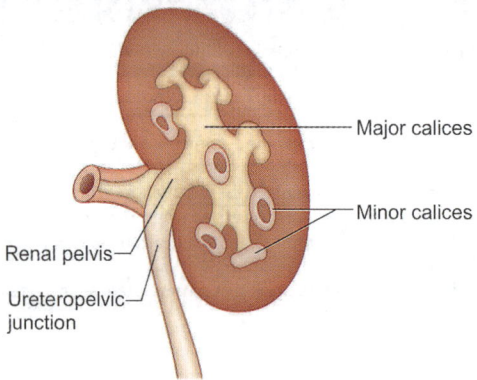

274. **Ans. c. Genitofemoral nerve** *(Ref: BDC 5/e p325, 326)*
- The **genitofemoral nerve lies posterior to** the **ureter**^{Q}. The ureter lies on the genitofemoral nerve, which is posterior.

275. **Ans. d. Ischial spine** *(Ref: Snell's 7/e p284, 382)*

- At the **level of ischial spine ureter changes its direction** from **down-backward to forward - medially** but there is **no constriction**.
- The normal **anatomical narrowing of ureter** are the **potential sites of obstruction by ureteric (kidney) stone.**

NORMAL ANATOMICAL NARROWING OF URETER

- **Uretero-pelvic junction**^{Q}
- Where ureter **cross the brim** of pelvic inlet^Q (at site of **crossing of iliac artery**^{Q})
- Juxtaposition of **vas deferens** or **broad ligament**
- **Uretero-vesicle junction**^{Q}
- **Ureteric orifice**

276. **Ans. d. Ureterovesicle junction**   277. **Ans. b. It is a type of portal-circulation** *(Ref: Snell's 7/e p283)*

Renal Circulation	
Artery	**Vein**
• **Right renal artery** is **longer than left**^{Q}.	• **Left renal vein** is **longer than right**^{Q}
• Close to hilum, renal artery divides into **5 segmental arteries**, that are **end-arteries**^{Q}	• **Stellate veins** drain most superficial zone of renal cortex^Q
• Renal artery → 5 segmental arteries → Arcuate artery → Interlobular artery → Afferent glomerular arteriole^Q	• **Left kidney is preferred for transplantation** due to **longer renal vein**^{Q}

278. **Ans. b. Below uterine artery in the Mackenrodt's ligament** *(Ref: Keith and Moore 4/e p374, 384)*

- **Maximum chance** of **ureteric injury** is **in hysterectomy**, while **ligating uterine vessels in** the **Mackenrodt's ligament**^{Q}.
- Ureter is also vulnerable to injury when ovarian vessels are being ligated during oophorectomy.

279. Ans. a. Gonadal vessels lie anterior to it *(Ref: Keith and Moore 4/e p281)*

- **Gonadal vessels** and **colic vessels** lie **anterior to ureter**; **IVC** is **medial**; **gonadal vein** and **inferior mesenteric vein** is **on left side**^{Q}.

280. Ans. b. Tongue like papillary projection   281. Ans. c. Peristaltic movements   282. Ans. d. 0–5 cm of H_2O

- **Resting ureteric pressure** is **~0–5 cm H_2O**^{Q}
- **Ureteric contraction pressures** range from **20–80 cm H_2O**^{Q}.

283. Ans. a. Trapezius *(Ref: Smith 18/e p339)*

NEPHRECTOMY

- Two common approaches:
  – **Transperitoneal abdominal**^{Q} approach   – **Retroperitoneal loin**^{Q} approach
- **Retroperitoneal loin approach** is **preferred** method **except in malignant tumors** and **renal injuries** (to exclude other injuries)^Q

NEPHRECTOMY (LOIN APPROACH)

- Following muscles are cut in loin approach:
  – **Lattisimus dorsi**^{Q} – **Serratus posterior-inferior**^{Q} – **External and internal oblique, transversus abdominis**^{Q}

284. Ans. c. Renal artery stenosis   285. Ans. a. One year of age

- The **neonatal kidney achieves concentrating ability** equivalent to **adult's kidney** by **one year** of age^Q
- The **neonatal kidney achieves adult's GFR** by **two years of age**^{Q}.

MISCELLANEOUS

286. Ans. a. Urethral stone

Relation of hematuria to micturition	Site of bleeding
Blood appears **at the beginning**	Urethra^Q
Blood appears **at the end**	Vesical^Q
Blood is **intimately mixed** throughout the process	**Prerenal, renal** or **vesical**^{Q}

287. Ans. c. Ureteral calculus
- Clinical picture is suggestive of ureteric colic.

288. Ans. a. Excretion of less than 300 mL in 24 hours   289. Ans. a. 7 mL

- The average capacity of the renal pelvis is 4–8 mL^Q.

290. Ans. c. Chronic renal failure *(Ref: Smith 18/e p49)*
- Low and fixed specific gravity of urine is seen in chronic renal failure.

291. Ans. b. Renal TB

Autosplenectomy	Sickle cell anemia^Q
Autonephrectomy	Renal TB^Q

292. Ans. d. Urerthrovaginal fistula *(Ref: Bailey 27/e p1429-1430, 25/e p1320)*   293. Ans. a. Transureterostomy
294. Ans. a. >3 RBCs/hpf
295. Ans. a. Medullary *(Ref: Campbell 11/e p1333)*

"Renal medullary carcinoma is a subtype of RCC that occurs almost exclusively in patients with the sickle cell trait. It is typically diagnosed in young African-Americans, often in the third decade of life, and many cases are both locally advanced and metastatic at the time of diagnosis."-*Campbell 11/e p1333*

CHAPTER 22

Urinary Bladder

EXSTROPHY OF BLADDER (ECTOPIA VESICAE)

EXSTROPHY OF BLADDER (ECTOPIA VESICAE)

- Extrophy of bladder is **complete ventral defect** of **Urogenital sinus** and the **overlying skeletal system**^{Q}.
- **Defect in the infraumbilical part** of **anterior abdominal wall**, associated with **incomplete development of anterior wall of the bladder**^{Q}.

Embryology
- Basic defect is abnormal overdevelopment of the **cloacal membrane** and **its rupture**.
- Timing of this rupture of this **defective cloacal membrane determines the variant** of the extrophy-epispadias complex that results.

Clinical Features
- **Posterior wall of the bladder protrudes through the defect** with mucosal edges fused with skin and **urine spurts** onto the abdominal wall from the **ureteral orifices**^{Q}.
- **Rectus muscles** which are inserted on the pubic rami are also **widely separated**^{Q}.
- An **umbilical hernia**^{Q} though usually small is present along with extrophic bladder.

  - In males, **complete epispadias** with a **wide & shallow scrotum**. Undescended testis & **inguinal hernias**^{Q} are common.
  - **Females** also have **epispadias** with **bifid clitoris** and **wide separation** of the **labia**^{Q}.

- **Anus** is **dislocated anteriorly** in both sexes and there may be **rectal prolapse**^{Q}.

Complications
- Consequences of untreated bladder exstrophy are **total urinary incontinence**^{Q} and an increased incidence of bladder cancer, usually **adenocarcinoma**.
- Many untreated exstrophy of bladder reveal fibrosis, derangement of muscularis mucosa and chronic infection leading to **hydronephrosis**^{Q}.

Treatment
- **Enterocystoplasty**^{Q} is the method of choice to augment bladder capacity and aid in reservoir function.
- **Urinary diversion with cystectomy**^{Q} is treatment of choice for small, fibrotic or inelastic bladder.
- **Complete reconstruction** is achieved by:
  - Bladder closure with **sacral osteotomy** and **lengthening of penis**^{Q} (Posterior iliac osteotomy^Q is done in ectopia vesicae)
  - Antiureteral reflux procedure with **bladder neck reconstruction**^{Q}
  - Repair of epispadiac penis^Q

BLADDER STONE

Vesical Calculus	
Primary Bladder Calculi	**Secondary Bladder Calculi**
Develop in **absence of** any **known functional, anatomic or infectious factors**^{Q}	Develop in concert with **bladder outlet obstruction**^{Q}, infection, **impaired bladder emptying** or a **foreign body**.

MIGRANT BLADDER CALCULI

- Found in **upper urinary tract, passed into bladder** and **retained**
- Most stones migrate out of ureter into bladder are < 1 cm and easily passed into urethra
- Calculi that are **retained**, are associated with **small bladder outlet** or **bladder outlet obstruction**
- Retained upper tract stones may grow to large size in bladder

BLADDER STONE

- Most renal stones that are small enough to pass through the ureters are also small enough to pass through a normally functioning bladder and an unobstructed urethra[Q].
- In older men with bladder stones composed of uric acid, the stone most likely formed in the bladder[Q].
- Stones composed of calcium oxalate are usually initially formed in the kidney[Q].
- In adults, MC type of vesical stone (seen in >50% of cases) is composed of uric acid[Q].
- Less frequently, bladder calculi are composed of calcium oxalate, calcium phosphate, ammonium urate, cystine, or magnesium ammonium phosphate (when associated with infection).

Endemic Bladder Calculi
- In children, stones are composed mainly of **ammonium acid urate**[Q], **calcium oxalate**, or an impure mixture of ammonium acid urate and calcium oxalate with calcium phosphate.
- The common link among endemic areas relates to **feeding infants human breast milk** and **polished rice**[Q].
- These foods are **low in phosphorus**, ultimately leading to **high ammonia excretion**[Q].
- These children also usually have a **high intake of oxalate-rich vegetables** (increased oxalate crystalluria) and **animal protein (low dietary citrate)**[Q].

- Vesical calculi may be single or multiple, especially in the presence of bladder diverticula, and can be small or large enough to occupy the entire bladder. They **range from soft to extremely hard**, with **surfaces** ranging from **smooth** and **faceted** to **jagged** and **spiculated** ("jack" stones)[Q].
- Jack stones are composed of **calcium oxalate dihydrate**[Q]

PRIMARY BLADDER CALCULI (ENDEMIC BLADDER CALCULI)

Primary Bladder Calculi (Endemic Bladder Calculi)
- Mainly seen in **underdeveloped countries**[Q] (North Africa, Thailand, Myanmar, Indonesia), in **pediatric age** group.
- Most common in children <10 years, with a peak incidence at 2 to 4 years of age.
- More common in boys than in girls.
- Common in **Rajasthan, Andhra Pradesh**[Q] and some north-eastern states of **India.**
- Related to **chronic dehydration** and **low protein, low phosphate, exclusive milk & high carbohydrate diet**[Q].
- Low phosphate diet increases urinary ammonium excretion leading to **ammonium urate stones**[Q].

Diagnosis
- **USG bladder**: Identifies the stone with its **characteristic shadowing** and **stone moves** with **changing body position.**

Treatment
- **Small stones**: Removed or crushed transurethrally **(Cystolitholapexy)**[Q]
- **Larger stones**: Disintegrated by **transurethral electrohydraulic lithotripsy** or **Cystolithotomy**[Q]

- Primary bladder calculi **rarely recur after treatment**[Q].

SECONDARY BLADDER CALCULI

Secondary Bladder Calculi
- **Most** bladder stones are secondary, more common in **older males**[Q] (>50 years), usually because of **bladder outlet obstruction**[Q].
- **MC type: Uric acid** (sterile urine) > **Struvite stones**[Q] (Infected urine)
- Bladder stones are **usually solitary**[Q], multiple in 25% patients.

Etiology
- Bladder outlet obstruction (MC cause)[Q]
- Neurogenic bladder[Q]
- Foreign body (**Foley's catheter**, forgotten DJ stents)[Q]
- Bladder **diverticula**[Q]

Clinical Features
- Typical symptoms are **intermittent, painful voiding** and **terminal hematuria** with **severe pain at the end of micturition**[Q].
- **Pain** may be referred to the **tip of the penis** or to the **labia majora**[Q].

Diagnosis
- A large percentage of bladder stones are **radiolucent (uric acid)**[Q].
- **USG bladder**: Identifies the stone with its **characteristic shadowing** and **stone moves** with **changing body position**[Q].

Treatment
- **Small stones**: Removed or crushed transurethrally **(Cystolitholapexy)**[Q]
- **Larger stones**: Disintegrated by **transurethral electrohydraulic lithotripsy** or **Cystolithotomy**[Q]

Stones of Genitourinary Tract	
MC renal stone: Calcium oxalate[Q]	MC primary bladder stone: Ammonium urate[Q]
MC bladder stone: Uric acid[Q] > Struvite	MC prostate stone: Calcium phosphate[Q]

MALACOPLAKIA

Malacoplakia
- Inflammatory disease of the bladder that can also affect ureters & kidneys
- In the bladder, it manifests as plaques or nodules made of **large histiocytes (von Hansemann cells)**[Q] with laminar **inclusion bodies (Michaelis-Gutmann bodies)**[Q] form around bacterial fragments (E. coli) which acts as nidus.
- Believed to result from the **inadequate killing** of **bacteria** by macrophages or monocytes that exhibit **defective phagolysosomal activity**[Q].

Risk Factors
- **Immunosuppression** (Steroids, Transplantation)[Q]
- Diabetes, Lymphoma, Rheumatoid arthritis[Q]

Clinical Features
- More commonly affects **women** and associated with a history of **UTI**.
- Patients with malacoplakia often have **chronic illness** or are **immunosuppressed**.[Q]
- Irritative voiding symptoms (**urgency** and **frequency**) and **hematuria** are common.

Diagnosis
- **USG or CT** may demonstrate a **mass in the bladder** and **evidence of obstruction** if the disease extends to the ureter.
- **Culture** of the lesion can yield bacteria, most commonly **E. coli**.

Management
- **TMP-SMX** and **fluoroquinolones**[Q] are recommended in the treatment of malacoplakia.
- In **malacoplakia limited** to the **lower urinary tract**, **antibiotic therapy** alone is usually sufficient.
- Best chance of **cure: Antibiotics + Surgery**[Q]
- The **prognosis is poor** and **mortality rate is high** in patients having **bilateral renal involvement**, regardless of treatment.

SCHISTOSOMIASIS (BILHARZIASIS)

Schistosomiasis (Bilharziasis)
- Schistosomiasis is an infection with **Schistosoma haematobium**[Q].
- Endemic in **Africa, Egypt & Middle East**
- More common in **Males**[Q]

S. hematobium	Affects bladder[Q]
S. japonicum	Affects liver & small intestine[Q]
S. mansoni	Affects large intestine[Q]

Lifecycle
- **Man**[Q] is the **only definitive host** & **intermediate host** is **snail**[Q].
- Life cycle begins with the passage of **eggs** into **freshwater** regions through **urine**[Q].
- When the **eggs are hatched**, **miracidia** are produced. These **penetrate** the **snail** and eventually form into **cercariae**.

  - Eggs → **Miracidium**[Q] (penetrate the snail) → **Cercaria**[Q] (penetrate skin of man) → Migrate to **vesical venous plexus**[Q] for reproduction → Eggs in urine[Q]

- Fluke embryos (**cercariae**) **penetrate** the **skin** of man from infected water and migrate to the **vesical venous plexus**, where **sexual reproduction** takes place[Q].
- **Eggs** are laid in the **submucosal veins** & **penetrate** the **bladder wall** to enter **urine**[Q].

Pathology

- Schistosoma **eggs** are **highly antigenic** and induce **intense granulomatous reaction** in bladder resulting in **bladder fibrosis** with **ureteric or urethral strictures**[Q].
- **Calcification** of **dead eggs** within bladder can produce a **calcified bladder** or **bladder stones**[Q].

Complications

- **Bladder calcification:** Schistosomiasis is the **MC cause**[Q] of bladder calcification worldwide.
- Urolithiasis, ascending urinary tract infection, urethral & ureteric stricture with subsequent hydronephrosis, & renal failure.
- **Squamous cell carcinoma**[Q] (Most serious complication)

Symptoms

- **MC symptom** of urinary schistosomiasis is **urinary frequency**[Q].

> - **Swimmer's itch** is the **first clinical sign** due to local inflammatory response from **cercarial penetration (<24 hours)**[Q]
> - **Katayama fever (Acute schistosomiasis)**[Q]: Generalized allergic reaction associated with onset of egg laying, which includes fever, urticaria, lymphadenopathy, hepatosplenomegaly & eosinophilia (**3 weeks to 4 months**)

- Acute inflammation phase when eggs are deposited, penetrate tissues and excreted (**hematurea, frequency & terminal dysurea**)
- Fever, rigor, toxemia & uremia are manifestations of renal involvement
- Signs:
  - In early uncomplicated cases, there are essentially no clinical findings.
  - In **advanced cases**, rectal examination may reveal a **fibrosed prostate, enlarged seminal vesicle** or **thickened bladder base**[Q].

Diagnosis

- Demonstration of schistosomal **eggs** in **early morning urine sample**[Q]
- **Sandy patches** (eggs in trigone) on **cystoscopy**[Q]
- IVU, RGU or cystography may show **mucosal irregularity**, inflammatory pseudo polyps, ureterits cystica, **ureteral dilation & stricture, reduced bladder capacity**[Q]

> - **Calcification** in the **wall of the bladder** or distal ureters on **plain radiographs (Fetal head appearance)**[Q]
> - **Calcifications** of the **distal ureters** have a characteristic pattern of **linear or parallel calcifications**[Q] on plain radiographs

Treatment

- **Praziquantel**[Q] **(DOC), metrifonate**[Q] or **oxaminiquine**[Q] are the drugs used in schistosomiasis.
- Surgery to treat the bladder contraction or for resection of the bladder cancer.

BLADDER DIVERTICULA

BLADDER DIVERTICULA

- The **normal intravesical pressure** during **voiding** is about **35–50 cm H$_2$O**[Q]; however, pressures as great as 150 cm H$_2$O may be reached by a **hypertrophied bladder** endeavoring to **force urine past an obstruction**[Q].
- This **pressure causes** the lining between the inner layer of **hypertrophied muscle to protrude**, forming **multiple saccules**.
- If one or more, but usually one, **saccule** is **forced through the bladder wall**, it becomes a **diverticulum**[Q].

Types

Congenital diverticula

- As a result of a **developmental defect**[Q].
- These are **situated in the midline anterosuperiorly** and represent the **unobliterated vesical end** of the **urachus**[Q].

Pulsion diverticula

- The usual cause is **bladder outflow obstruction**[Q].

Pathology

- Diverticula are **lined by bladder mucosa** and the **wall is composed of fibrous tissue only**[Q]

Clinical Features

- An **uninfected diverticulum** of the bladder usually causes **no symptoms**[Q].
- The patient is nearly **always male (95%)** and **over 50 years of age**[Q].
- **Symptoms** are those of associated **urinary tract obstruction**, recurrent infection and **pyelonephritis**[Q].
- **Hematuria** (due to infection, stone or tumour) is a symptom in about **30%**.
- In a few patients **micturition occurs twice in rapid succession**[Q] (the second act may follow a change of posture)

Diagnosis
- Diverticula are usually **discovered incidentally** on **cystoscopy** or **ultrasound**^{Q}.

Treatment
- **Operation** is necessary **only for the treatment of complications**^{Q}.
- If the **diverticulum is small** and **associated outflow obstruction** has been **dealt with by prostate resection**, there is **no reason to resect the diverticulum**^{Q}.
- Even a large diverticulum may not require treatment in the absence of infection or other complications.

Complications of Bladder Diverticula	
• Recurrent urinary infection • Squamous cell metaplasia and leucoplakia	• Bladder stone • Hydronephrosis and hydroureter • Neoplasm

INTERSTITIAL CYSTITIS (HUNNER'S ULCER)

INTERSTITIAL CYSTITIS (HUNNER'S ULCER)

- **Confined to women; Etiology obscure**
- **Chronic pancystitis**, often with marked infiltration with lymphocytes & macrophages.
- **Ulceration of the mucosa** occurs in the **fundus of bladder**.
- In severe cases the **bladder capacity is reduced to 30–60 mL**.
- **Characteristic linear bleeding ulcer** is caused by **splitting of the mucosa** when the bladder is distended under anaesthesia.

Clinical Features
- **First symptom** is **increased frequency**
- Pain, relieved by micturition and aggravated by jarring and over-distension of the bladder, is another characteristic symptom. Haematuria also occurs.
- In most patients **pyuria & urinary infection are absent**.

Diagnosis
- **Cystoscopy: Characteristic ulcer in the fundus**, but it may be absent.
- It is important to **check urinary cytology** and to **biopsy the mucosa to exclude underlying neoplastic disease**.

Treatment
- Treatment is difficult & unsatisfactory.
- **Hydrostatic dilatation** under anaesthesia may give relief for some months.
- **Instillation of dimethylsulphoxide** results in improvement in some patients.

BLADDER RUPTURE

BLADDER RUPTURE

- Bladder injuries occur most often from **external force** to **full bladder** and often associated with **pelvic fractures**^{Q}.
- **Pelvic fracture** accompanies bladder rupture in **90%**^{Q} cases.
- Classic triad suggestive of bladder rupture: **Suprapubic pain and tenderness + Difficulty in ability to pass urine + Hematuria**^{Q}

Extraperitoneal (80%)
- MC cause is **pelvic fracture**^{Q}.
- Diagnosed by **cystogram** or **CT cystography**^{Q}

  - **Flame sign** or **pear sign**^{Q} (pattern of contrast extravasation) or **tear drop bladder**^{Q} is seen
  - Treated by **simple catheter drainage**^{Q} (Typically **10 days** of catheter drainage will provide adequate healing time)

- **Surgical repair** is indicated in cases of **repeated blockade** of catheter due to bleeding, **projecting bone fragment** or **tear extending** to the **bladder neck**^{Q}.

Intraperitoneal (20%)
- **Blow, kick or fall** on **fully distended bladder**^{Q} leads to intraperitoneal rupture
- Usually seen in **males**, MC site of rent is **dome**^{Q} of bladder.

> Apart from classic triad suggestive of bladder rupture (Suprapubic pain and tenderness + Difficulty in ability to pass urine + Hematuria) patients develop **peritonism** and **abdominal distention**[Q].

- Diagnosis is made by **retrograde cystography** or **CT cystography**.
- X-ray abdomen shows **ground glass appearance**[Q] (due to fluid in abdomen).
- **Laparotomy** with **peritoneal lavage** and **bladder repair** with **SPC**[Q] should be done.
- **Cystography (gold standard)**[Q] reveals **distorted bladder** with **extravasation** of **contrast** in **perivesical space** and **streaks of contrast** into **fascial planes** giving rise to typical **"sun-burst" appearance**[Q].
- USG shows **bladder in bladder appearance**[Q] due to **perivesical collection** and rent may be detected.

Risk Factors for Carcinoma Urinary Bladder

Transitional Cell Carcinoma	Squamous Cell Carcinoma
• **Cigarette smoking**[Q]: main etiological factor, account for about 50% bladder cancer • Occupational exposure to chemicals: **Naphthylamine, benzidine, acrolein, aniline dyes, hydrocarbons**[Q] • **Schistosoma hematobium**[Q]: Risk factor **for both TCC and SCC, more for SCC** • Drugs: **Phenacetin and Chlornaphazine**[Q] • **Cyclophosphamide**[Q] • **Pelvic irradiation**[Q] • Occupations associated with increased risk: **Chemical, dye, rubber, petroleum, leather and printing industry workers**[Q]	• **Schistosoma hematobium**[Q]: Risk factor for both TCC and SCC, more for SCC • **Chronic irritation**: Urinary calculi, long term indwelling catheters, chronic urinary tract infections[Q] • **Bladder diverticula**[Q]

Types of Carcinoma Urinary Bladder

Transitional Cell Carcinoma	Squamous Cell Carcinoma (Bilharzial carcinoma)[Q]	Adenocarcinoma Urinary Bladder
• More than **90%** of bladder cancer are **TCC**[Q] • Most commonly appear as **papillary or exophytic lesions**[Q]	• Account for **5–10%**, arise from **lateral bladder wall and dome**[Q] • Often **nodular and invasive**[Q] at the time of diagnosis • Do not respond to TURBT, partial cystectomy or chemotherapy • Treatment is **Radical cystectomy**[Q] • Stage to stage and grade to grade prognosis is same as TCC	• Account for **< 2%** bladder cancer • **Urachal remnants** and **ectopia vesicae** are **risk factors**[Q] • Three types: **primary vesical, urachal and metastatic**[Q] • Adenocarcinoma also occur in **intestinal urinary conduits, augmentations, pouches** and **ureterosigmoidostomies**[Q] • **Primary adenocarcinoma** arise along the **floor** whereas adenocarcinoma arising from **urachus** occur at the **dome** • Treatment: Radical cystectomy with **pelvic lymphadenectomy**[Q] • Poor response to chemotherapy and radiotherapy

- MC benign mesenchymal tumor of urinary bladder: **Leiomyoma**[Q]
- MC malignant mesenchymal tumor of urinary bladder: **Leiomyosarcoma**[Q]
- MC malignant mesenchymal tumor of urinary bladder in **children**: **Embryonal rhabdomyosarcoma**[Q]

CARCINOMA URINARY BLADDER

Carcinoma Urinary Bladder

- More common in **whites**, **higher socio-economic status** and in **males**[Q], in **6th & 7th** decade
- 75% are **localized** to bladder and 25% have **spread to regional nodes** or **distant sites** at the time of presentation
- Most tumors develop at **trigone & adjacent posterolateral wall**[Q] with ureteral involvement
- Tumors tend to be **multifocal**[Q] in bladder

Pathology
- MC type grossly is papillary & histologically, TCC.[Q]

Precursor Lesions of Invasive Urothelial Cancer
- **Non-invasive papillary tumor (Kiss ulcer)**[Q] causes painless, profuse paroxysmal hematuria
- Carcinoma in situ (Malignant cystitis)[Q]

> **Carcinoma in situ (Malignant cystitis)**
> - Typically presents as **irritative**^{Q} lower urinary symptoms
> - Common in **high grade**^{Q} tumors
> - **Urinary cytology** is **IOC**^{Q}
> - Urine cytology is **positive** in **80–90%** cases because of **poor cohesiveness** of cells
> - Associated with increased chances of **recurrence** and **poor prognosis**
> - Treatment: **Two cycles of BCG**^{Q}, radical cystectomy in cases recurrence

Clinical Features
- MC symptom: **Painless hematurea**^{Q} (85% cases)
- Hematuria is **gross** or microscopic, **intermittent**^{Q} rather than constant
- **Vesical irritability**^{Q}: Frequency, urgency and dysurea
- Bone pain & abdominal pain in advanced disease
- MC site of **lymphatic metastases**: Pelvic lymph nodes (obturator is MC)^Q
- MC site of **hematogenous spread**: **Liver**^{Q} > lung

Diagnosis

Cystoscopy
- Diagnosis and initial staging is made by **cystoscopy and transurethral resection (TUR)**^{Q}
- **Urinary Cytology**
- Cytologic examination of exfoliated cells are useful in **detecting cancer in symptomatic patients** and **assessing response to treatment**^{Q}
- Most useful for **early diagnosis of recurrence in TCC**^{Q}

> **Exfoliated Markers for Detection of Bladder Cancer**
> - Newer urinary tumor markers like **BTA test, urinary nuclear matrix protein (NMP22)** can detect cancer **specific proteins in urine (BTA/NMP22)**^{Q}
> - **Hyaluronidase, Lewis-X antigen** on exfoliated urothelial cells
> - Determination of **telomerase activity** in exfoliated cells
> - Have been used to **detect new index tumors** and **recurrent tumors**^{Q}
> - Expected to play important role in near future

- CT and MRI: used for **staging**^{Q}

Management
- **Cystoscopy** and **TUR** or **biopsy**; **further management** is based on **stage, grade, size, multiplicity** and **recurrence pattern**^{Q}
- Systemic chemotherapy: MVAC (**M**ethotrexate + **V**inblastine + **A**driamycin + **C**isplatin)
- **Drugs used for Intravesical chemotherapy**: BCG, mitomycin-c, epirubicin, thiotepa

Prognosis
- There is strong correlation between **tumor grade and stage** and tumor recurrence, progression and survival
- In patients with **organ confined disease**, presence of **lymph node metastases** appears to be the **most important prognostic factor**
- Presence of **lymphovascular invasion** is associated with **poor prognosis**^{Q}

8th AJCC (2017) TNM Staging for CA Bladder	
T: Primary tumor	**N: Regional lymph nodes**
Ta: Non-invasive papillary carcinoma^Q **Tis**: Carcinoma in situ "Flat tumor"^{Q}	**N1**: **Single** regional **LN** in true **pelvis** (hypogastric, obturator, external iliac or presacral LN)^Q
T1: Tumor invades **subepithelial connective tissue**^{Q}	**N2**: **Multiple** regional **LN** in true **pelvis** (hypogastric, obturator, external iliac or presacral LN)^Q
T2a: **Superficial** muscularis propria **invasion (inner half)**^{Q} **T2b**: **Deep** muscularis propria **invasion (outer half)**^{Q}	**N3**: LN metastasis to **common iliac LNs**^{Q}
T3a: **Microscopic extension** into perivesical fat^Q **T3b**: **Macroscopic extension** into perivesical fat^Q	**M: Distant metastases**
T4a: Cancer invading **pelvic viscera** (e.g., prostatic stroma, vaginal wall, rectum, uterus)^Q **T4b**: Extension to **pelvic sidewalls**, **abdominal walls**, or **bony pelvis**^{Q}	**M0**: No distant metastasis **M1**: Distant metastasis present

Treatment of CA Bladder	
Tis	Intravesical BCG[Q]
Ta (single, low to moderate grade, not recurrent)	Complete TUR[Q]
Ta (large, multiple, high grade or recurrent) and T1	Complete TUR followed by intravesical chemo or immunotherapy[Q]
T2-T4	• Radical cystectomy[Q] • Neoadjuvant chemotherapy followed by radical cystectomy[Q] • Radical cystectomy followed by adjuvant chemotherapy • Neoadjuvant chemotherapy followed by concomitant chemotherapy and irradiation
Any T, N+, M+	Systemic chemotherapy followed by selective surgery or irradiation

BCG

BCG

- BCG is attenuated strain of **Mycobacterium bovis**[Q]
- **Mechanism of action**: Immunologically mediated
  - Exact mechanism is not known[Q]
  - Binds to fibronectin on bladder cells and **elicits T_{H1} response**[Q]
- **Most effective**[Q] intravesical chemotherapy

Contraindications of BCG	
Absolute	Relative
• **Immunosupressed**[Q] patients • **Gross hematurea**[Q] • **Immediately after TURBT**[Q] • **Traumatic catheterization**[Q] • Total **urinary incontinence**[Q] • **History** of **BCG sepsis**[Q]	• Deranged LFT • Previous history of Koch's • UTI • Poor performance status

Side Effects

- MC is **frequency, urgency and dysuria**[Q]
- Patients with **severe BCG sepsis** (high fever, chills confusion, hypotension, jaundice) should be treated with **ATT**[Q].

URINARY DIVERSION

Urinary Diversion

- Urinary diversion can lead to **stricture** at anastomosis, **reflux of urine**, reabsorption of solutes leading to **dyselectrolytemia**[Q].
- **Gold standard conduit** for urinary diversion: **Ileal conduit**[Q]
- Ileal conduit is best for urinary diversion as it is **simplest to perform**[Q] and associated with minimal intra-operative and immediate post-operative complications.
- **Ileal or colonic conduits** (Ureterosigmoidostomy):
  - Hyperchloremic, hypokalemic metabolic acidosis[Q]
  (DK Raised HCl in ureterosigmoidostomy: Decreased K^+, raised H^+ and Cl^-)
- **Jejunal conduits**:
  - Hypochloremic, hyponatremic, hyperkalemic, metabolic acidosis[Q]
  (RH Khurana Decreases NaCl in jejunal conduit: Raised H^+, K^+; Decreased Na^+, Cl^-)
- **Stomach conduit**:
  - Hypochloremic, hypokalemic, metabolic alkalosis[Q]
  (Everything decreases in stomach conduit: Decreased H^+, K^+, Cl^-)

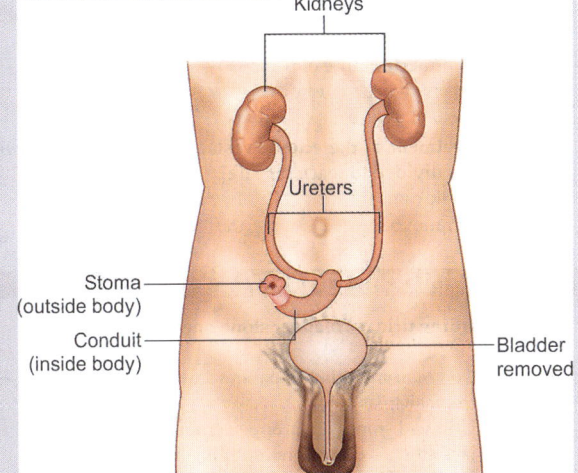

Multiple Choice Questions

ECTOPIA VESICAE

1. In ectopia vesicae, bone divided is: *(MHSSMCET 2011)*
   a. Pubic bone
   b. Sacrum
   c. Coccyx
   d. Iliac bone

2. Ectopic vesicae includes all except: *(COMEDK 2005)*
   a. Hypospadias
   b. Extrophy of bladder
   c. Defective abdominal wall
   d. Bifid clitoris

3. What is the diagnosis based on the given image? *(JIPMER November 2017)*
   a. Gastroschisis
   b. Omphalocele
   c. Umbilical hernia
   d. Ectopia vesicae

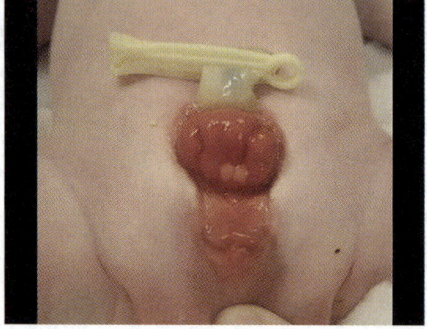

4. All of the following are features of exstrophy of the bladder except: *(All India 97)*
   a. Epispadias
   b. Cloacal membrane is present
   c. Posterior bladder wall protrudes through the defects
   d. Umbilical and inguinal hernia

5. Which is not seen in complete ectopic vesicae:
   a. Umbilical hernia *(Recent Quetsion 2016)*
   b. Visible uretero vesical efflux
   c. Hypospadias
   d. Waddling gate

6. About ectopia vesicae, following is true except: *(PGI June 98)*
   a. CA bladder may occur
   b. Ventral curvature of penis
   c. Incontinence of urine
   d. Visible ureterovesical efflux

7. For treatment of the ectopic-vesiae, which of the following bone is divided to reach the site? *(UPPG 2004)*
   a. Pubic rami
   b. Iliac bone
   c. Ischium bone
   d. Symphysis

URINARY BLADDER STONES

8. Regarding urinary bladder stone one is not true: *(AIIMS June 98)*
   a. Common in pediatric patient in tropics than that of non tropical areas
   b. Uric acid stones are dropped from above
   c. Jack stone is due to urea splitting bacteria
   d. Commonly distal passage obstruction cause stone

9. Secondary vesical calculus refers to stones formed due to:
   a. Hypercalciuria *(Karnataka 2006)*
   b. Injury
   c. Infection
   d. Migrating from above

10. A 60 years old man presented with intermittent painful voiding of urine. What is the diagnosis based on clinical picture and the given image? *(Recent Question 2018)*

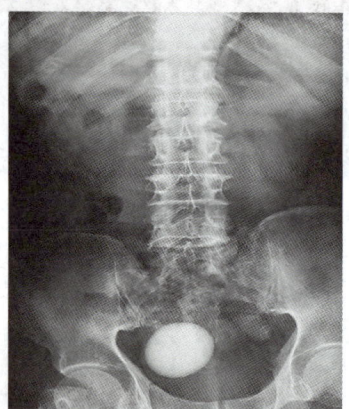

   a. Bladder stone
   b. Ureteric stone
   c. Prostate calcification
   d. Schistosomiasis

11. Not true about bladder stones is: *(AIIMS Nov 2001)*
    a. Rare in Indian children
    b. Primary stones are rare
    c. Small stones can be removed per urethra
    d. Maximum stones are radioopaque

12. The commonest bladder stone is: *(Recent Question 2016)*
    a. Triple phosphate
    b. Xanthine
    c. Uric acid
    d. Cysteine

13. What is the composition of this stone?

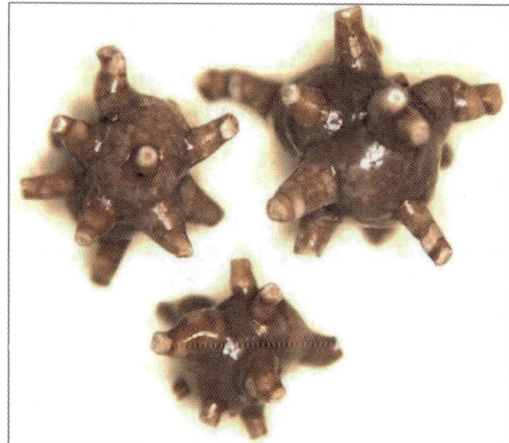

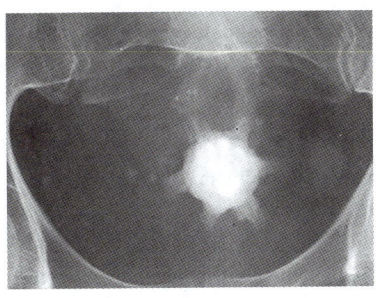

a. Calcium oxalate monohydrate
b. Calcium oxalate dihydrate
c. Calcium phosphate
d. Calcium carbonate

14. **The following is true about bladder stones:**
    a. Girls more than boys
    b. Treatment is litholapexy
    c. Always forms in kidneys and passes down to bladder
    d. Usually asymptomatic

15. **Jack stone calculi is seen in which anatomic part:**
    a. Prostate   b. Kidney   *(MAHE 2006)*
    c. Ureter   d. Bladder

16. **Which of the following is false regarding endemic bladder stones?**   *(AIIMS Nov 2013)*
    a. Always associated with recurrence
    b. High incidence in cereal based diet
    c. Peak incidence in 3 years old children in India
    d. Most common type is ammonium urate or calcium oxalate

URINARY BLADDER: MALAKOPLAKIA

17. **Malakoplakia of the urinary bladder is considered to be associated with:**   *(COMEDK 2005)*
    a. TB   b. Urothelial carcinoma
    c. Schistosomiasis d. Defect in phagocytosis

18. **True about malakoplakia is:**   *(MHPGMCET 2002)*
    a. Benign lesion of urinary bladder
    b. May turn into malignancy
    c. Michaelis-Gutmann bodies are characteristic feature
    d. May cause sever hematuria and lead to death

URINARY BLADDER: TUBERCULOSIS

19. **Cystoscopic findings in TB bladder are all except:**
    a. Cobblestone mucosa   *(PGI Dec 97)*
    b. Thimble bladder
    c. Golf hole ureter
    d. Whitish efflux from the ureteric holes

20. **Thimble bladder is seen in:**
    (Recent Question 2015, All India 91)
    a. Acute tuberculosis
    b. Chronic tuberculosis
    c. Neurogenic bladder
    d. Schistosomiasis

21. **Treatment of 'Thimble bladder' is:**   *(Recent Question 2015)*
    a. Anti-tubercular treatment
    b. Corticosteroids
    c. Ileocystoplasty
    d. Anti-tubercular drugs + steroids

SCHISTOSOMIASIS

22. **A patient, Ramu presents with hematuria for many days. On investigations he is found to have renal calculi, calcifications in the wall of urinary bladder and small contracted bladder; most probable cause is:**   *(AIIMS Nov 2001)*
    a. Schistosomiasis   b. Amyloidosis
    c. Tuberculosis   d. CA urinary bladder

23. **One of the following disease will show urinary bladder calcification radiologicaly which resemble fetal head in pelvis:**   *(AIIMS June 2000)*
    a. Tuberculosis   b. Schistosomiasis
    c. Chronic cystitis   d. Malignancy

24. **Metrifonate is effective against:**   *(COMEDK 2008)*
    a. Amebiasis   b. Leishmaniasis
    c. Schistosomiasis   d. Giardiasis

25. **In a patient of schistosomiasis, X-ray pelvis was done. What is the name of this sign?**

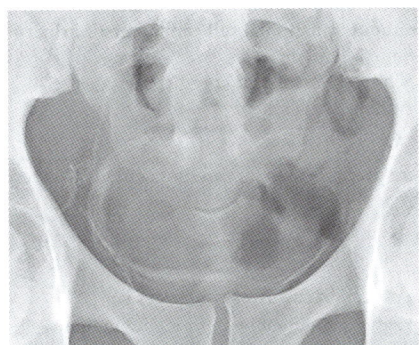

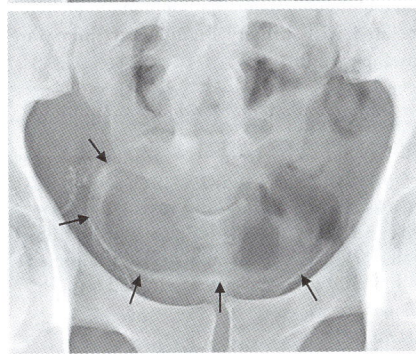

a. Fetal head appearance   b. Rim sign
c. Linear calcification   d. Goblet sign

CARCINOMA URINARY BLADDER: RISK FACTORS

26. **Carcinoma common in dye industry workers:**
    (MHPGMCET 2001)
    a. Skin   b. Scrotum
    c. Urinary bladder   d. Maxilla

27. **Transitional cell carcinoma can be seen in:**
    (MHSSMCET 2006)
    a. Analgesic nephropathy
    b. Urate nephropathy
    c. Pulmonary infections
    d. Myocardial infarction

28. **Transitional cell carcinoma of bladder is associated with:**
    (PGI June 2001)
    a. Schistosomiasis   b. Naphthylamine
    c. Smoking   d. Tuberculosis of bladder

29. **Squamous cell tumor of urinary bladder is due to:** *(PGI June 97)*
    a. Stone   b. Schistosomiasis
    c. Chronic cystitis d. Diabetes mellitus

30. **Squamous cell carcinoma of urinary bladder is predisposed to by:** *(PGI June 2002)*
    a. Urolithiasis   b. Persistent urachus
    c. Schistosomiasis   d. Polyp
    e. Smoking

31. **In a survey, many children are examined and were found to have urogenital abnormalities. Which congenital anomaly is associated with increased risk of bladder carcinoma?**
    a. Medullary sponge kidney   *(AIIMS Nov 97)*
    b. Bladder exstrophy
    c. Unilateral renal agenesis
    d. Doubler ureter

32. **True about transitional cell carcinoma of urinary bladder:**
    a. Smoking predisposes   *(PGI Dec 2003)*
    b. Schistosoma infection predisposes
    c. Aniline dye workers
    d. Radiation

33. **All are precancerous for carcinoma bladder except:**
    (Recent Question 2015, All India 91)
    a. Tuberculosis bladder   b. Aniline dyes
    c. Schistosomiasis   d. Chronic ulcer

34. **'Kiss cancer' of the urinary bladder is:**
    a. Highly malignant   b. Malignant
    c. Benign   d. Pre-malignant

35. **Associated with urinary bladder carcinoma are all of the following except:** *(MCI Sept 2009)*
    a. Smoking   b. HPV infection
    c. Schistosomiasis   d. Cyclophosphamide

36. **A 63-year-old male from the middle east presented with hematuria. The urine showed RBCs but no RBC casts. BUN level was normal. cystoscopy revealed an irregular growth on the mucus of the bladder. A biopsy from this growth revealed features of squamous cell carcinoma. The etiology of this cogidition is most likely linked to:** *(COMEDK 2014)*
    a. Cigarette smoking
    b. HPV infection
    c. Parasitic infection
    d. Chronic alcohol abuse

37. **Which of the following drug causes carcinoma bladder?**
    (Recent Question 2017)
    a. Cyclophosphamide   b. Cisplatin
    c. Taxane   d. Tamoxifen

CARCINOMA URINARY BLADDER: TYPES

38. **SCC of bladder is best treated by:** *(GB Pant 2011)*
    a. Chemotherapy   b. Radical cystectomy
    c. Radiotherapy   d. TUR

39. **Most common bladder tumor:** *(GB Pant 2011)*
    a. TCC   b. SCC
    c. Rhabdomyosarcoma d. Sarcoma

40. **Most common tumor of urinary bladder is:**
    a. Squamous cell carcinoma   *(DNB 2008, PGI June 97)*
    b. Adenocarcinoma
    c. Transitional carcinoma
    d. Stratified squamous carcinoma

41. **Most malignant carcinoma of the bladder is:**
    a. Malignant villous tumor   b. Solid tumor
    c. Carcinomatous ulcer   d. Adenocarcinoma

42. **It is true of carcinoma of the urinary bladder that:**
    a. It usually occurs in childhood
    b. Occurs more often in aniline dye workers
    c. It is located most frequently in the trigone
    d. Papillary formation is rare

43. **Bladder tumors mostly arises from:** *(All India 91)*
    a. Mucosa   b. Submucosa
    c. Muscularis mucosa   d. Serosa

44. **About transitional cell carcinoma of bladder following is correct:**
    a. Most common site is fundus
    b. Prognosis is excellent if muscle layer is invaded
    c. Exposure to industrial carcinogens predisposes
    d. Most of carcinomas are flat, solid and deeply infiltrating

CARCINOMA URINARY BLADDER: CLINICAL FEATURES AND DIAGNOSIS

45. **A 55-year-old smoker presents with history of five episodes of macroscopic hematuria each lasting for about 4–5 days in the past five years. Which of the following investigations should be performed to evaluate the suspected diagnosis?**
    a. Urine microscopy and cytology   *(All India 2011)*
    b. X-ray KUB
    c. Ultrasound KUB
    d. DTPA scan

46. **CA urinary bladder commonly presents as:** *(PGI Dec 2003)*
    a. Hematuria   b. Frequency
    c. Dysuria   d. Abdominal lump

47. **Most constant and persistent feature of CA bladder is:**
    a. Increased frequency   *(PGI Dec 95)*
    b. Hematuria
    c. Recurrent UTI
    d. Pain abdomen

48. **What is true about carcinoma bladder?** *(AIIMS June 94)*
    a. Common in smokers
    b. Commoner in females than that in males
    c. Mostly adenocarcinoma
    d. Pain in suprapubic region is the first symptom

49. **A 67 years old chronic heavy smoker presents with 2 weeks history of frank hematuria. Ultrasound pelvis shows a filling defect. Most probable diagnosis:** *(JIPMER May 2018)*
    a. Bladder diverticula
    b. Adenocarcinoma of bladder
    c. Squamous cell carcinoma of bladder
    d. Transitional cell carcinoma of bladder

50. **A 60-year-old smoker came with a history of painless gross hematuria for one day. Most logical investigation would be:**
    a. Urine routine   *(All India 2007)*
    b. Plain X-ray KUB
    c. USG KUB
    d. Urine microscopy for malignant cytology

51. A 60-year-old smoker came with the history of painless gross hematuria for one day. The investigation of choice would be: *(AIIMS Nov 2006)*
    a. Urine routine and microscopy
    b. Plain X-ray KUB
    c. USB KUB
    d. Urine for malignant cytology

52. False statement regarding urothelial bladder tumor is: *(PGI May 2018)*
    a. Most common variety
    b. Schistosomiasis is not a risk factor
    c. Strongly related to smoking
    d. Pain is the most common presenting feature
    e. Most common site is trigone

53. An elderly male presents with one episode of gross heematuria. All of the following investigations are recommended for this patient except: *(All India 2007)*
    a. Cystoscopy
    b. Urine microscopy for malignant cells
    c. Urine tumor markers
    d. Intravenous pyelogram

54. Urinary cytology is a useful screening test for the diagnosis of: *(Recent Question 2016)*
    a. Renal cell carcinoma
    b. Wilms' tumour
    c. Urothelial carcinoma
    d. Carcinoma prostate

55. Which of the following is a tumor marker for bladder cancer? *(Recent Question 2017)*
    a. AFP
    b. CEA
    c. Bladder surface protein
    d. NMP-22

56. A 60 years old smoker male patient presents with painless gross hematuria for 1 day. IVU shows 1.2 cm filling defect at the lower pole of infundibulum. Which is the next best investigation to be done? *(MCI November 2017)*
    a. Cystoscopy
    b. Urine cytology
    c. USG abdomen
    d. DMSA scan

CARCINOMA URINARY BLADDER: TREATMENT

57. Treatment of choice for low grade superficial bladder carcinoma: *(JIPMER 2011)*
    a. Local excision
    b. Radical cystectomy
    c. Intravesical BCG
    d. Chemotherapy

58. A lady who presented with hematuria was found to have Stage II Transitional Cell Carcinoma of bladder. Which of the following statements about management of her condition is true?
    a. Cystoscopic fulguration is the standard treatment
    b. 70% chance of requiring cystectomy in 5 years after TURP
    c. History of smoking is not a risk factor
    d. There is no role of chemotherapy

59. BCG is used in the treatment of: *(MHPGMCET 2006)*
    a. Carcinoma cervix
    b. Carcinoma colon
    c. Carcinoma of urinary bladder
    d. All

60. pT2, pT3 or CIS carcinoma bladder not responding to BCG is best treated by: *(MHSSMCET 2008)*
    a. Intravesical mitomycin-C and interferon
    b. Systemic chemotherapy
    c. Cystoscopic
    d. Radical cystectomy

61. Treatment of choice for bladder pTa: *(MHSSMCET 2010)*
    a. Endoscopic tumor resection
    b. Endoscopic tumor resection and intravesical chemotherapy
    c. Partial cystectomy with intravesical
    d. Radical cystectomy with or without radical radiotherapy BCG

62. Which of the following is the most effective intravesical therapy for superficial bladder cancer? *(AIIMS Nov 2005)*
    a. Mitomycin
    b. Adriamycin
    c. Thiotepa
    d. BCG

63. Which of the following is not an intravesical chemotherapeutic agent? *(UPSC 2005)*
    a. Mitomycin C
    b. BCG
    c. Epirubicin
    d. Thiotepa

64. A 65-year-old male smoker presents with gross total painless hematuria. The most likely diagnosis is: *(All India 2003)*
    a. Carcinoma of urinary bladder
    b. Benign prostatic hyperplasia
    c. Carcinoma prostate
    d. Cystolithiasis

65. BCG is used in tumour therapy: *(JIPMER 98)*
    a. Bladder
    b. Stomach
    c. Esophagus
    d. Colon

66. A 60-year-old female presented with hematuria and diagnosed transitional cell carcinoma of bladder stage T1N1M0. Best treatment modalities is: *(UPPG 2008)*
    a. Transurethral resection
    b. Transurethral resection and intravesical chemo-immunotherapy
    c. Total cystectomy and pelvic lymphadenectomy
    d. Systemic chemotherapy

67. Identify the false statement regarding urothelial cell carcinoma of the bladder. *(APPG 2016)*
    a. Ileal conduit diversion is required after cystectomy
    b. Intravesical chemotherapy and immunotherapy are not found to be beneficial in Non Muscular Invasive Bladder Cancer (NMIBC)
    c. Radical cystectomy following chemotherapy has been shown to be of benefit in Muscle Invasive Bladder Cancer
    d. Strongly associated with smoking & Schistosoma hematobium

68. Laser used in carcinoma bladder: *(Recent Question 2017)*
    a. Carbon dioxide laser
    b. Nd-YAG laser
    c. Ho-YAG laser
    d. Argon laser

69. Chemotherapy used for metastatic bladder cancer:
    a. AC (Adriamycin and Cisplatin) *(Recent Question 2016)*
    b. Interferon
    c. MVAC (Methotrexate, Vinblastine, Adriamycin and Cisplatin)
    d. Cisplatin alone

URINARY BLADDER INJURY

70. A person after pelvic fracture could not pass urine. On examination bladder is not palpable. What is probable diagnosis? *(PGI Dec 2008)*
    a. Posterior urethra rupture, with retention of urine
    b. Rectourethral injury
    c. Intraperitoneal rupture of bladder
    d. Extraperitoneal rupture of bladder

71. **True about extraperitoneal urinary bladder rupture is all except:**
    a. Associated with fracture   (MHPGMCET 2002)
    b. More common than intraperitoneal bladder rupture pelvis in about 70% cases
    c. Commonly associated with anterior urethral rupture
    d. Can be managed conservatively without surgical intervention

72. **Urine gests collected in which place in case of extraperitoneal rupture of bladder:**   (AIIMS Nov 95)
    a. Groin
    b. Below urogenital diaphragm
    c. Above urogenital diaphragm
    d. Perineal space

73. **In extraperitoneal rupture of bladder, urine extravasates in:**
    a. Groin   (AIIMS Nov 94, All India 93)
    b. Intraperitoneal region
    c. Extraperitoneal region
    d. Perivesical space

74. **Tear-drop bladder is seen in:**   (PGI June 99)
    a. Tuberculosis
    b. Hunner's ulcer
    c. Perivescial hemorrhage with rupture
    d. Perivesical hemorrhage without rupture

75. **A 40-year-old male was brought to the casualty with history RTA. Cystography was done. What is the name of sign seen in the image?**
    a. Pear sign   b. Flame sign
    c. Tear drop bladder   d. Rim sign

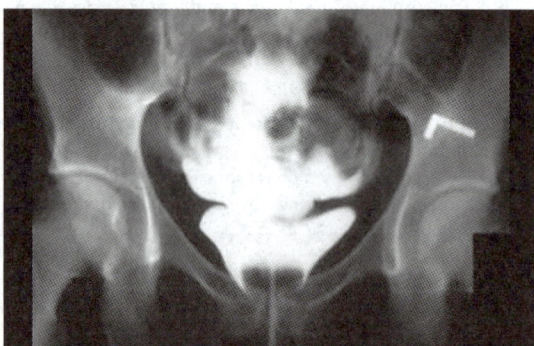

76. **A 40-year-old male was brought to the casualty with history RTa. Cystography was done. What is the name of sign seen in the image?**
    a. Pear sign   b. Flame sign
    c. Tear drop bladder   d. Rim sign

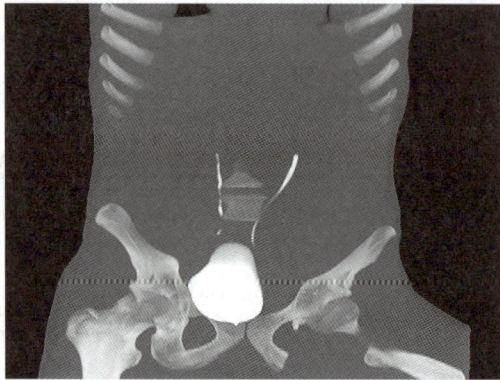

77. **A 40-year-old male was brought to the casualty with history RTa. Cystography was done. What is the name of sign seen in the image?**
    a. Pear sign   b. Flame sign
    c. Tear drop bladder   d. Rim sign

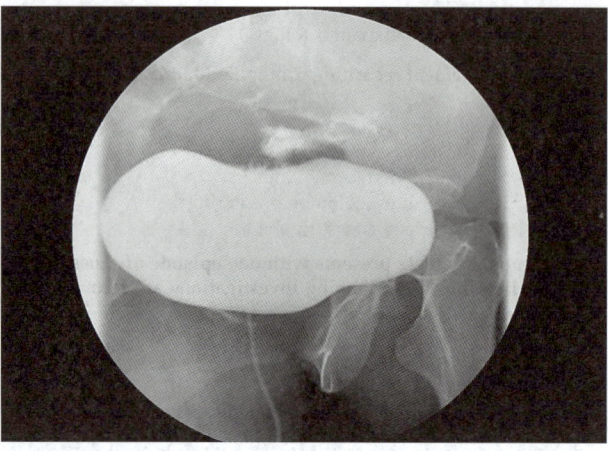

78. **Intraperitoneal bladder rupture management:**
    a. Requires laparotomy   (Recent Question 2017)
    b. Antegrade cystogram is needed
    c. Simple catheter drainage is the treatment
    d. Conservative management

79. **Most reliable investigation in bladder rupture is:**
    a. IVP
    b. Cystoscopy
    c. Retrograde cystogram
    d. Catheterization

URINARY DIVERSION

80. **In ureterosigmoidostomy all occur except:**   (JIPMER 98)
    a. Hyponatremia
    b. Hyperkalemia
    c. Hyperchloremia
    d. Acidosis

81. **Urinary diversion is indicated in the following except?**   (MHSSMCET 2008)
    a. Ectopia vesicae
    b. Carcinoma bladder
    c. Neurogenic bladder
    d. Bladder hematoma

82. **Which among the following will complicate as hyperchloremic acidosis?**   (AIIMS June 98)
    a. Ureterosigmoidostomy
    b. Diarrhea
    c. Vomiting
    d. Ileoplasty

URINARY INCONTINENCE

83. **Urinary incontinence results from all except:**
    a. Neurogenic bladder
    b. Vesico vaginal fistula
    c. Ectopic ureter
    d. Rectovesical fistula

84. Postmicturition dribbling is due to: (AMU 2005)
    a. Detrusor
    b. Dribbling decreased in case of urethral stricture
    c. Collection of urine in 'U' shaped curve of bulb of penis
    d. Neurogenic bladder
85. To differentiate between stress incontinence and detrusor instability investigation done is: (AIIMS June 97)
    a. Cystosurethroscopy
    b. Urodynamic study
    c. MCU
    d. Retrograde urethroscopy
86. In which case cystometric study is indicated? (AIIMS Nov 98)
    a. Neurogenic bladder
    b. Stress incontinence
    c. Fistula
    d. Urge incontinence

MISCELLANEOUS

87. Which is a normal finding in cystometry? (PGI 97)
    a. Absence of systolic detrussor contraction
    b. Residual volume of 75 ml
    c. Leakage on coughing
    d. First sensation of urination at 300 ml
88. Commonest cause for pulsion diverticulum of the urinary bladder is:
    a. Benign enlargement of prostate
    b. Fibrous prostate
    c. Contracture of bladder neck
    d. Stricture urethra
89. Catheterization of bladder done in: (PGI Dec 2006)
    a. CA prostate
    b. Postoperative retention
    c. Preoperative before taking the patient for appendicitis
    d. Stricture
    e. Rupture
90. A young lady presents with symptoms of urinary tract infection. All of the following findings on a midstream urine sample support the diagnosis of uncomplicated acute cystitis, except: (All India 2011)
    a. Positive nitrite test
    b. CFU count < 1000/ml
    c. Detection of one bacteria/field on Gramstain
    d. > 10 WBC/HPF
91. Normal intravesical pressure during voiding: (MHPGMCET 2007)
    a. 20–35 cm H_2O b. 35–50 cm H_2O
    c. 50–65 cm H_2O d. 65–80 cm H_2O
92. What is Marion's disease? (MHSSMCET 2005)
    a. Benign prostatic hypertrophy
    b. Superficial thrombophlebitis of breast
    c. Bladder outlet obstruction
    d. Interstitial cystitis
93. Marion's disease is due to: (DNB 90)
    a. Muscular hypertrophy of internal sphincter of urinary bladder
    b. Fibrosis of the neck of bladder
    c. Vesicular diverticula
    d. Vesicular calculi
94. What is the name of this operation? (Recent Question 2016)
    a. Lich-Gregoir operation
    b. Anderson Hynes operation
    c. Boari's operation
    d. Leadbetter-Politano operation

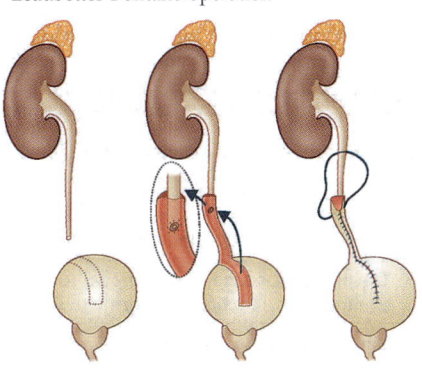

95. What is Boari's FLAP surgery? (MHSSMCET 2005)
    a. Ureterostomy   b. DJ stent in situ
    c. Bowel interposition
    d. Flap of the bladder wall fashioned into a tube replace lower ureter
96. In Boari operation: (GB Pant 2011)
    a. Ureteric retransplant
    b. Lower ureteric reconstruction
    c. Diversion   d. Bowel interposition
97. Interstitial cystitis is also known as: (DNB 2012)
    a. Eosinophilic cystitis   b. Radiation cystitis
    c. Hunner's cystitis   d. Tubercular cystitis
98. All are seen in cystitis except: (DNB 2014)
    a. Fever   b. Hematuria
    c. Dysuria   d. Nocturia
99. After a surgery, the surgeon asked the intern to remove the Foley's catheter but he could not do it. The surgeon himself tried to remove the Foley's catheter but he was unsuccessful. What should be done next? (AIIMS May 2016)
    a. CT guided rupture of bulb of Foley's
    b. Inject ether to dissolve the balloon and pull it out
    c. Inject water to over distend the balloon until it bursts and Foley's can be removed
    d. Use ultrasound guidance to locate and prick the balloon and then remove the catheter

Explanations

ECTOPIA VESICAE

1. **Ans. d. Iliac bone** *(Ref: Smith 18/e p583; Campbell's 11/e p3194; Bailey 27/e p1424-1425)*
   Posterior iliac osteotomy is done in ectopia vesicae.
2. Ans. a. Hypospadias
3. Ans. d. Ectopia vesicae
4. Ans. b. Cloacal membrane is present
5. Ans. c. Hypospadias
6. Ans. b. Ventral curvature of penis
7. Ans. b. Iliac bone

URINARY BLADDER STONES

8. **Ans. b. Uric acid stones are dropped from above** *(Ref: Smith 18/e p275; Campbell 11/e 1291; Bailey 27/e p1434)*

Vesical Calculus	
Primary Bladder Calculi	**Secondary Bladder Calculi**
• Develop in **absence of** any **known functional, anatomic** or **infectious factors**[Q]	• Develop in concert with **bladder outlet obstruction**[Q], infection, impaired bladder emptying or a **foreign body**.

9. **Ans. c. Infection** *(Ref: Smith 18/e p275; Campbell 11/e p1292; Bailey 27/e p1434)*
10. **Ans. a. Bladder stone** *(Ref: Bailey 27/e p1435; Smith 18/e p276; Campbell 11/e p1291-1292)*
11. **Ans. d. Maximum stones are radio-opaque** *(Ref: Smith 18/e p275; Campbell 11/e p1292; Bailey 27/e p1435)*
12. **Ans. c. Uric acid**
13. **Ans. b. Calcium oxalate dihydrate** *(Ref: Radiology Review Manual By Wolfgang Dähnert 7/e p1006)*

Spiculated stone or Jackstone (Child's toy jack) are composed of calcium oxalate dihydrate and more common in bladder.

Radiographic Shape of Stone	
Spiculated stone or Jackstone (Child's toy jack)	Composition: Calcium oxalate dihydrate Location: Urinary bladder >Kidney
Mulberry stone	Mamillated contour Composition: Calcium oxalate dihydrate
Seed calculi	**Small stones of similar size with lapidary effect** (like cut gems) Formed in **small cavity (calyceal diverticulum, cyst, hydronephrosis)**

14. Ans. b. Treatment is litholapexy
15. Ans. d. Bladder
16. **Ans. a. Always associated with recurrence** *(Smith 18/e p275; Campbell 11/e p1292; Bailey 27/e p1434)*

URINARY BLADDER: MALACOPLAKIA

17. **Ans. d. Defect in phagocytosis** *(Ref: Smith 18/e p212; Campbell 11/e p289)*
18. **Ans. c. Michaelis-Gutmann bodies are characteristic feature**

URINARY BLADDER: TUBERCULOSIS

19. **Ans. d. Whitish efflux from the ureteric holes** *(Ref: Smith 18/e p227; Campbell 11/e p427; Bailey 27/e p1442)*
20. Ans. b. Chronic tuberculosis
21. Ans. c. Ileocystoplasty

SCHISTOSOMIASIS

22. **Ans. a. Schistosomiasis** *(Ref: Smith 18/e p230; Campbell 11/e p437; Bailey 27/e p1442)*
23. Ans. b. Schistosomiasis
24. Ans. c. Schistosomiasis
25. **Ans. a. Fetal head appearance** *(Ref: Schwartz 10/e p1286; Bailey 27/e p1444)*

Urinary Bladder

Schistosomiasis
• **Calcification** in the **wall of the bladder (Fetal head appearance)**[Q]
• **Calcifications** of the **distal ureters** have a characteristic pattern of **linear or parallel calcifications**[Q] on plain radiographs

CARCINOMA URINARY BLADDER: RISK FACTORS

26. Ans. c. Urinary bladder *(Ref: Smith 18/e p312; Campbell 11/e p2187-2188; Bailey 27/e p1446)*
27. Ans. a. Analgesic nephropathy
28. Ans. a. Schistosomiasis; b. Naphthylamine; c. Smoking
29. Ans. a. Stone; b. Schistosomiasis; c. Chronic cystitis
30. Ans. a. Urolithiasis; c. Schistosomiasis
31. Ans. b. Bladder exstrophy
32. Ans. a. Smoking predisposes; b. Schistosoma infection predisposes; c. Aniline dye workers; d. Radiation
33. Ans. a. Tuberculosis bladder; d. Chronic ulcer
34. Ans. c. Benign *(Ref: Bailey 27/e p1445, 26/e p1330)*

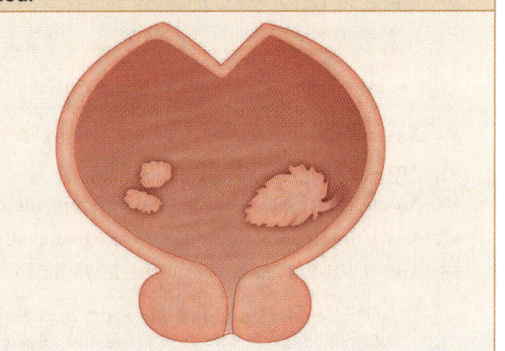

Benign Papillary Tumour
• **'Kiss' cancer**: **Papillary tumour** with **daughter implantation**
• The papilloma consists of a **single frond** with a **central vascular core** with **villi**; it looks like a **red sea anemone**
• Inverted papilloma is a condition in which the proliferative cells penetrate under normal mucosa so that the lesion is covered with smooth urothelium.
• It is **benign**.

35. Ans. b. HPV infection
36. Ans. c. Parasitic infection
37. Ans. a. Cyclophosphamide *(Ref: Campbell 11/e p2188; Smith 18/e p310; Bailey 27/e p1446)*

CARCINOMA URINARY BLADDER: TYPES

38. Ans. b. Radical cystectomy *(Ref: Smith 18/e p313; Campbell 11/e p2225; Bailey 27/e p1451)*
39. Ans. a. TCC
40. Ans. c. Transitional carcinoma
41. Ans. b. Solid tumour *(Ref: Bailey 27/e p1448)*

> • **Muscle-invasive tumours** are **nearly always solid** although there may be a low tufted surface.
> • These tumours are **often large** and **broad based**[Q], having an irregular, ulcerated, appearance within the bladder.
> • The **incidence of metastases**, whether from lymphatic invasion in the pelvis or blood-borne to the lung, liver or bones, is **much more common** and will cause the **death of 30–50% of patients**[Q].

SQUAMOUS CELL TUMOURS

> • **Squamous cell tumours** tend to be **solid** and are **nearly always associated with muscle invasion**[Q].
> • This is the **most prevalent form of bladder cancer** in areas where **bilharzia is endemic**.
> • Squamous cell tumours may be **associated with chronic irritation** caused by **stone disease** in the bladder **as a result of metaplasia**[Q].

42. Ans. b. Occurs more often in aniline dye workers, c. It is located most frequently in the trigone
43. Ans. a. Mucosa
44. Ans. c. Exposure to industrial carcinogens predisposes

CARCINOMA URINARY BLADDER: CLINICAL FEATURES AND DIAGNOSIS

45. Ans. a. Urine microscopy and cytology *(Ref: Smith 18/e p313; Campbell 11/e p2197; Bailey 27/e p1447)*
46. Ans. a. Hematuria
47. Ans. b. Hematuria
48. Ans. a. Common in smokers
49. Ans. d. Transitional cell carcinoma of bladder
50. Ans. d. Urine microscopy for malignant cytology
51. Ans. d. Urine for malignant cytology
52. Ans. b. Schistosomiasis is not a risk factor, d. Pain is the most common presenting feature

53. Ans. c. Urine tumor markers
54. Ans. c. Urothelial carcinoma
55. Ans. d. NMP-22
56. Ans. a. Cystoscopy

CARCINOMA URINARY BLADDER: TREATMENT

57. Ans. a. Local excision *(Ref: Smith 18/e p316; Campbell 11/e p2207; Bailey 27/e p1450-1451)*
58. Ans. b. 70% chance of requiring cystectomy in 5 years after TURP

- Treatment of stage II bladder cancer is **radical cystectomy** or **neoadjuvant chemotherapy** followed by **radical cystectomy**.
- Rests of the three options are wrong.

59. Ans. c. Carcinoma of urinary bladder
60. Ans. d. Radical cystectomy
61. Ans. a. Endoscopic tumor resection
62. Ans. d. BCG *(Ref: Smith 18/e p318, 17/e p316; Campbell 11/e p2212-2216; Bailey 27/e p1450, 26/e p1334)*

Drugs used in Intravesical Chemotherapy			
• Mitomycin C^Q	• Epirubicin^Q	• Thiotepa^Q	• BCG (most effective)^Q

63. Ans. b. BCG *(Ref: Smith 17/e p316-317; Campbell 10/e p2343-2345; Bailey 27/e p1450)*
64. Ans. a. Carcinoma of urinary bladder
65. Ans. a. Bladder
66. Ans. c. Total cystectomy and pelvic lymphadenectomy
67. Ans. b. Intravesical chemotherapy and immunotherapy are not found to be beneficial in Non Muscular Invasive Bladder Cancer (NMIBC)
68. Ans. b. Nd-YAG laser *(Ref: Campbell 11/e p2210)*

"Laser coagulation allows minimally invasive ablation of tumors up to 2.5 cm in size. The neodymium : yttrium-aluminum-garnet (Nd : YAG) laser has the best properties for use in bladder cancer."-Campbell 11/e p2210

69. Ans. c. MVAC (Methotrexate, Vinblastine, Adriamycin and Cisplatin)

URINARY BLADDER INJURY

70. Ans. d. Extraperitoneal rupture of bladder *(Ref: Smith 18/e p290; Campbell 11/e p2386; Bailey 27/e p1428)*
71. Ans. c. Commonly associated with anterior urethral rupture *(Ref: Smith 18/e p290; Campbell 11/e p2368; Bailey 27/e p1425)*

Bladder Rupture	
Extraperitoneal (80%)	**Intraperitoneal (20%)**
• MC cause is **pelvic fracture**^Q. • Classic triad: **Suprapubic pain and tenderness + Difficulty** in ability **to pass urine + Hematuria** • Diagnosed by **cystogram** or **CT cystography**^Q • **Flame sign** or **pear sign**^Q (pattern of contrast extravasation) is seen • Treated by **simple catheter drainage** (Typically **10 days** of catheter drainage will provide adequate healing time)^Q • **Surgical repair** is indicated in cases of **repeated blockade** of catheter due to bleeding, **projecting bone fragment** or **tear extending** to the **bladder neck**^Q.	• **Cause: Blow, kick** or **fall on fully distended bladder**^Q • Usually seen in **males**, **MC site of rent** is **dome** of **bladder**^Q. • Apart from classic triad suggestive of bladder rupture (Suprapubic pain and tenderness + Difficulty in ability to pass urine + Hematuria) patients develop **peritonism** and **abdominal distention**^Q. • Diagnosis is made by **retrograde cystography** or **CT cystography**^Q. • **X-ray** abdomen shows **ground glass appearance**^Q (due to fluid in abdomen) • **Laparotomy** with **peritoneal lavage** and **bladder repair** with **SPC** should be done^Q.

72. Ans. c. Above urogenital diaphragm
73. Ans. d. Perivesical space
74. Ans. c. Perivesical hemorrhage with rupture
75. Ans. b. Flame sign *(Ref: Smith 18/e p290; Campbell 11/e p2386; Bailey 27/e p1425)*
76. Ans. a. Pear sign
77. Ans. c. Tear drop bladder
78. Ans. a. Requires laparotomy *(Ref: Campbell 11/e p2387; Smith 18/e p291; Bailey 27/e p1425)*
79. Ans. c. Retrograde cystogram

Urinary Bladder

URINARY DIVERSION

80. **Ans. b. Hyperkalemia** *(Ref: Smith 18/e p394, 401; Campbell 11/e p2344-2345; Bailey 27/e p1452-1453)*
81. **Ans. d. Bladder hematoma** *(Ref: Bailey 27/e p1452)*

INDICATIONS OF EXTERNAL URINARY DIVERSION
- To **relieve distal obstruction**[Q]
- When the **bladder has been removed** or has **lost normal neurological control**[Q]
- **Incurable fistula**[Q]
- **Irremovable obstruction**[Q]

82. **Ans. a. Ureterosigmoidostomy**

URINARY INCONTINENCE

83. **Ans. d. Rectovesical fistula** *(Ref: Bailey 27/e p1430)*

Rectovesical fistula doesn't cause urinary incontinence, as the level of fistula is above the sphincter mechanism.

Causes of Incontinence	
Problems of social control	• **Uninhibited detrusor hyperreflexia** and **impaired social perception** in **dementia**[Q]
Storage problems	• **Small bladder capacity owing to fibrosis** (tuberculosis, radiotherapy or interstitial cystitis)[Q] • **Small functional capacity**[Q] owing to severe detrusor instability, neurogenic dysfunction or infection
Impairment of emptying	• **Chronic retention**[Q] or **neurogenic bladder dysfunction**[Q] have **small functional bladder capacities** with **detrusor overactivity** causing incontinence, despite having large residual volumes of urine.
Weak sphincter	• This leads to **genuine stress incontinence**[Q]
Fistulae	• **Leakage from fistulae** (vesicovaginal)[Q] or **upper tract duplication** with an **ectopic ureter**[Q].

84. **Ans. c. Collection of urine in 'U' shaped curve of bulb of penis**
85. **Ans. b. Urodynamic study** *(Ref: Bailey 27/e p1432)*

DETRUSOR INSTABILITY
- **Phasic increases in pressure** give rise to **urgency** and **urge incontinence (detrusor instability)**[Q].
- This abnormality is found in **patients with neurogenic bladder dysfunction**, such as in **multiple sclerosis (MS)** or **Parkinson's disease** or **following a stroke** or **spinal injury**, when it is known as **detrusor hyperreflexia**[Q].
- About **50% of men with bladder outflow obstruction** have **detrusor instability**, and in **about half of them the instability resolves after prostatectomy**[Q].
- **Idiopathic detrusor instability** is common and must be distinguished from genuine stress incontinence (GSI) in women before performing bladder neck suspension procedures.

GENUINE STRESS INCONTINENCE
- This is defined as **urinary leakage occurring during increased bladder pressure** when this is **solely due to increased abdominal pressure**[Q] and not to increased true detrusor pressure.
- It is **caused by sphincter weakness**[Q].

USES OF URODYNAMIC TESTING
- To **distinguish GSI** (due to sphincter weakness) **from detrusor instability** in **women**[Q]
- For the **classification of neurogenic bladder dysfunction**[Q]
- To **distinguish bladder outflow obstruction** from **idiopathic detrusor instability** in **men**[Q]
- To **investigate incontinence** or **other lower urinary tract symptoms**[Q]

86. **Ans. a. Neurogenic bladder** *(Ref: Bailey 27/e p1429)*

CYSTOMETRY

- **Cystometric studies** are **urodynamic studies** in which the **pressure changes** in the **bladder** is simultaneously **measured** with **bladder filling** and **during micturition**[Q].
- It **helps in accurate assessment** of **detrusor** and **sphincter activity** especially if a **neurogenic abnormality** is suspected[Q].

MISCELLANEOUS

87. **Ans. a. Absence of systolic detrusor contraction**
    Rest three options are false.

88. **Ans. c. Contracture of bladder neck** *(Ref: Bailey 27/e p1437)*
    Pulsion diverticula: The usual cause is **bladder outflow obstruction**.

89. **Ans. a. CA prostate; b. Postoperative retention** *(Ref: Bailey 27/e p1437)*

    - **Retention of urine** can occur **after major** and **lengthy operations** of the **anal canal** and **perineal region**[Q]. So, in these types of operations, it is usual to forestall a **catheter before** or **at the conclusion of the operation**.
    - **Appendicitis** is **not a major operation**, so catheterization is usually not recommended.
    - **Prostatic cancer** presents with **bladder outlet obstruction**. This is **relieved by catheterization**[Q].
    - If the catheter will not pass, it is usually due to poor technique, lack of anesthesia, traumatization of urethra or a urethral stricture.
    - If the catheter cannot be passed, suprapubic puncture and urethral instrumentation should be done.

90. **Ans. a. Positive nitrite test** *(Ref: Smith 18/e p200)*

Sensitivity and Specificity of Urinalysis in UTI		
Tests	**Sensitivity (%)**	**Specificity (%)**
Esterase	83 (67–94)	**78** (64–92)
Nitrite	53 (15–82)	**98** (90–100)[Q]
Esterase or Nitrite	**93** (90–100)	72 (58–91)
White blood cells	73 (32–100)	81 (45–98)
Bacteria	81 (16–99)	**83** (11–100)
Any above	99.8 (99–100)	70 (60–92)

91. **Ans. b. 35–50 cm H_2O** *(Ref: Bailey 27/e p1431)*
    - The **normal voiding pressure** should not exceed **60 cm H_2O in men** and about **40 cm H_2O in women**, with a **flow rate** of between **20 and 25 mL/sec.**

    ### URODYNAMIC TESTING

    - The principle is to **artificially simulate bladder filling** and emptying while **obtaining pressure measurements**[Q].
    - The patient attends with a **full bladder** and is **allowed to void** in private to **measure the maximum urinary flow rate**[Q].
    - After voiding, the **residual urine** is measured **by ultrasound**[Q].
    - **Radiographic screening** may be carried out **to assess bladder neck closure** and **urinary leakage during movement** or **coughing** (stress incontinence) or **during bouts of phasic detrusor pressure** (detrusor instability)[Q].
    - The **normal bladder** will accept approximately **400–550 ml** when filled at room temperature at a rate of < 50 ml/min.
    - The **pressure increase** in the **bladder** should be **< 15 cm H_2O**[Q]. In addition, phasic pressure increases should not be seen.
    - The **normal voiding pressure** should not exceed **60 cm H_2O in men**[Q] and about **40 cm H_2O in women**, with a **flow rate** of between **20 and 25 ml/sec**[Q].

92. **Ans. c. Bladder outlet obstruction** *(Ref: Bailey 27/e p1467)*

    ### MARION'S DISEASE

    - **Congenital obstruction** of the **posterior urethra** due to **muscular hypertrophy** and **stenosis of the bladder neck**

93. **Ans. a. Muscular hypertrophy of internal sphincter of urinary bladder**
94. **Ans. c. Boari's operation** *(Ref: Bailey 27/e p1415)*

Boari operation
• A **strip of bladder** wall is fashioned into a **tube** to **bridge the gap**^{Q} between the cut ureter and the bladder. • Used for **lower ureteric reconstruction** • **Boari flap** provides the **needed length** to create a **tension-free anastomosis** between the **ureter and the bladder**^{Q}

95. **Ans. d. Flap of the bladder wall fashioned into a tube replace lower ureter** *(Ref: Bailey 27/e p1415)*
96. **Ans. b. Lower ureteric reconstruction**
97. **Ans. c. Hunner's cystitis** *(Ref: Bailey 27/e p1443; Smith 18/e p585)*
98. **Ans. a. Fever** *(Ref: Smith 17/e p206)*
99. **Ans. d. Use ultrasound guidance to locate and prick the balloon and then remove the catheter** *(Ref: http://www.aafp.org/afp/2000/0915/p1397.html)*

Best technique in this situation is ultrasound-guided rupture of balloon.

CHAPTER 23

Prostate and Seminal Vesicles

BENIGN PROSTATIC HYPERPLASIA (BPH)

BENIGN PROSTATIC HYPERPLASIA (BPH)

Incidence and Epidemiology
- BPH originates in the **transition zone**^{Q}, incidence is **age related**^{Q}
- The prevalence of BPH is **20%** in **41–50** years, **50%** in **51–60** years, **> 90%** older than **80** years.

Etiology
- Seems to be **multifactorial** and **endocrine controlled**^{Q}.
- Prostate is composed of **stromal & epithelial elements**^{Q}, and each, either alone or in combination, can give rise to **hyperplastic nodules**^{Q} and symptoms associated with BPH.

Pathology
- BPH develops in the **transition zone**. It is truly a **hyperplastic process**^{Q}.
- Nodular growth pattern is composed of varying amounts of **stroma & epithelium**.
- **Stroma** is composed of **collagen & smooth muscle**^{Q}.

  - **Alpha-blocker** therapy result in **excellent responses**^{Q} in patients with BPH having significant component of **smooth muscle**, while those with BPH predominantly composed of **epithelium** might respond better to **5-alpha-reductase inhibitors**^{Q}.
  - **Effects starts early** with **alpha-blockers** whereas **effect starts after 1 month** and may **take 6 months for maximum effect** with **5-alpha-reductase inhibitors**^{Q}.

- Patients with significant components of **collagen** in the stroma **may not respond** to **either form** of medical therapy.
- As **BPH nodules** in the transition zone enlarge, **compress** the outer zones of the prostate, resulting in the formation of a **surgical capsule** separating the transition zone from the peripheral zone, and serves as a **cleavage plane** for **open enucleation**^{Q} of the prostate.

Pathophysiology
- **Prostatic size** on DRE **correlates poorly with symptoms** because the **median lobe** is **not** readily **palpable**^{Q}.

  - **Prostatic stroma**, composed of **smooth muscle & collagen**, is rich in **adrenergic nerve supply**. The level of autonomic stimulation thus sets a tone to the prostatic urethra. Use of **alpha-blocker therapy decreases this tone**, resulting in a decrease in outlet resistance^Q.
  - **Irritative voiding complaints** of BPH result from the **secondary response** of bladder to the **increased outlet resistance**^{Q}.

- Bladder outlet obstruction leads to **detrusor muscle hypertrophy, hyperplasia & collagen deposition**^{Q} (collagen deposition is most likely responsible for a decrease in bladder compliance).

Symptoms
- **Obstructive symptoms** include **hesitancy, decreased force** & caliber of stream, sensation of incomplete bladder emptying, **double voiding** (urinating a second time within 2 hours of the previous void), **straining to urinate & post-void dribbling**^{Q}.
- **Irritative symptoms** include **frequency, urgency & nocturia (FUN)**^{Q}
- **IPSS (International Prostatic Symptom Score)**: score can range from 0–35. **Mild: 0–7, moderate: 8–19, severe: 20–35**.

Signs
- **Size & consistency** of the prostate is noted.
- BPH usually results in a **smooth, firm, elastic enlargement** of the prostate.
- **Induration** is suggestive of **cancer** and the need for further evaluation (**PSA, TRUS and biopsy**)^Q.

Imaging
- **IVP or ultrasound** is recommended only in the **presence of concomitant urinary tract disease** or **complications** from BPH (hematuria, urinary tract infection, renal insufficiency, history of stone disease).
- **Uroflowmetry.** (Q_{max} **>15 mL/sec is normal**, 10–15 ml/sec is equivocal and **< 10 mL/sec** is suggestive of **obstruction**)^Q
- **Cystometrograms** and **urodynamic profiles** are reserved to differentiate outflow obstruction from neurogenic bladder (**voiding pressure > 80 cm H_2O** signifies **outlet obstruction**)^Q

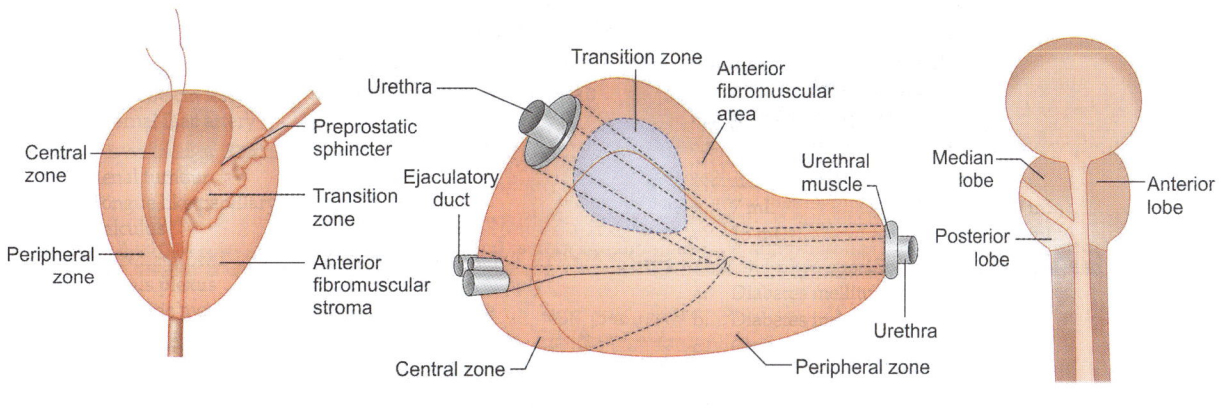

Anatomy of the prostate gland

MEDICAL THERAPY IN BPH

MEDICAL THERAPY IN BPH

- **Alpha-blockers:** (Prazosin, terazosin, doxazosin, tamsulosin, alfuzosin, **silodosin**^{Q})
  - **Relaxes smooth muscle & decreases urethral resistance**^{Q}.
  - **Side effects**: orthostatic hypotension, dizziness, tiredness, retrograde ejaculation, rhinitis & headache^Q.
- **5-Alpha-reductase inhibitors:** (Finasteride, dutasteride, triptorelin pamoate)
  - **Blocks** the conversion of **testosterone** to **dihydrotestosterone**, affecting the **epithelial component**^{Q} of the prostate, resulting in a **reduction in the size of gland**^{Q} and improvement in symptoms.

  > - **Six months of therapy** are **required** to see the **maximum effects** on prostate size (**20% reduction**)^Q and symptomatic improvement. However, **symptomatic improvement** is seen **only in** men with **enlarged prostates (> 40 cm^3)**^{Q}.

  - **Side effects**: decreased libido, decreased ejaculate volume and impotence^Q.
- **Combination therapy**
  - The **reduction in risk** associated with **combination therapy** (66% risk reduction) is **greater than** that associated with **doxazosin or finasteride alone**^{Q}.
  - Patients most likely to benefit from combination therapy: whom **baseline risk of progression** is **very high**, generally patients with **larger glands** and **higher PSA values**^{Q}.

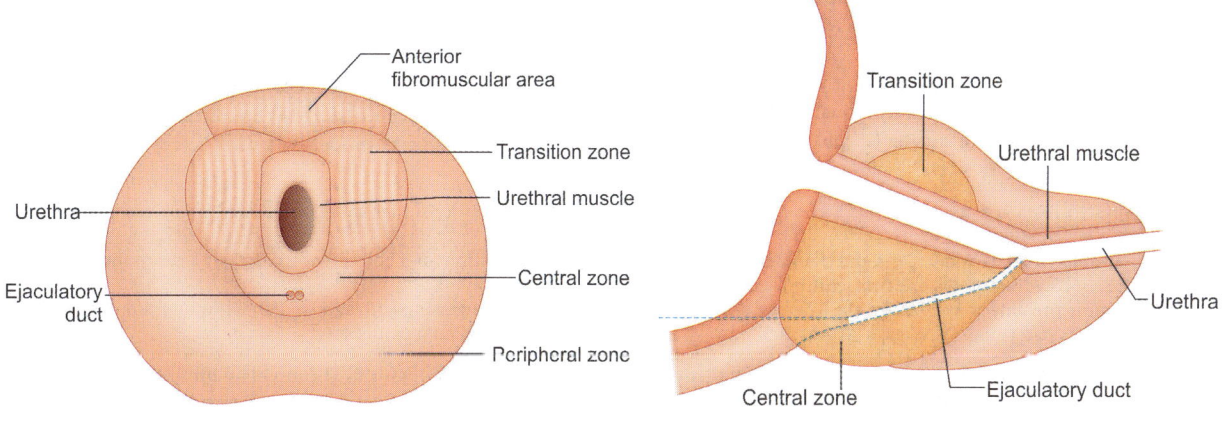

Absolute Indications for Surgery in BPH
1. **Refractory urinary retention**^{Q} (failing at least one attempt at catheter removal) 2. **Recurrent UTI**^{Q} 3. **Recurrent gross hematuria**^{Q} 4. Bladder **stones**^{Q} 5. **Renal insufficiency**^{Q} 6. Minimal improvement on medical treatment^Q

TREATMENT OF BPH

TREATMENT OF BPH

- **MC indication** for surgery is **symptoms interfering** with **quality of life**^{Q} (bothersome symptoms & symptoms of BOO).

CONVENTIONAL SURGICAL THERAPY

- **TURP (Gold standard)**^{Q}:
  - Cystoscopic removal of strips of prostatic tissue using diathermy loop.
  - **Two techniques: NESBIT technique** (preferred) & Mauer Mayer technique
  - Best irrigant fluid is **1.5% glycine**^{Q} (**Electrolyte solutions** like NaCl are **not compatible** with **electrocautery**, so **not used**).
  - **Glycine** is composed of **glycolic acid** and **ammonium**, which can **cause CNS (visual) toxicity.**^{Q}
  - **TURIS: TUR in saline using bipolar cautery**^{Q}
  - **Chips of prostate are removed by Ellik's evacuator.**

  > - **Verumontanum** is the single most important anatomical **landmark in TURP**^{Q}.
  > - **Verumontanum** lies immediately **proximal to external sphincter** and serve as the **distal landmark for prostate resection** to prevent injury to the external sphincter.
  > - **Verumontanum: Distal landmark** for **prostate resection**^{Q}.
  > - **Verumontanum:** Landmark for **proximal limit** of **external sphincter**^{Q}.

  - **Resection** proceeds at **1 gm/minute** for **an hour**.
  - **Risks of TURP:** Retrograde ejaculation (**75%**)^Q, impotence (5–10%)^Q & incontinence (< 1%)^Q.
  - **Complications:** Bleeding, **urethral stricture** or **bladder neck contracture**^{Q}, perforation of the prostate capsule with extravasation, and if severe, TUR syndrome.

TUR syndrome (Dilutional hyponatremia or water intoxication)
• **TUR syndrome (Dilutional hyponatremia** or **water intoxication**)^Q resulting from a hypervolemic, hyponatremic state due to **absorption of** the **hypotonic irrigating solution**. • **Clinical Features**: Nausea, vomiting, confusion, hypertension, bradycardia, & **visual disturbances**^{Q}. • The risk increases with **resection times > 90 minutes** or **gland size > 75 gm**. • **Treatment** includes **diuresis** (furosemide) and in **severe cases**, **hypertonic saline (3%)** administration.

Late Complications of TURP
• **Bladder neck stenosis (4%) > Urethral stricture (3.6%)** • **Bladder neck stenosis** is seen more often with **small (< 30 gm) fibrotic prostates.**

- **Transurethral incision of the prostate (TUIP):**
  - For **posterior commissure hyperplasia** (elevated bladder neck), involves **two incisions** using the **Collins knife** at the **5- and 7-O'clock** positions.
  - The **incisions** are started **just distal** to the **ureteral orifices** and are extended **outward** to the **verumontanum**.

  > - **TUIP lowers** the **incidence of bladder neck contracture** when **compared to TURP**, so **TUIP** should be strongly **considered** in patients with **smaller gland** in place of TURP.
  > - **TUIP** is used for **smaller (20 gm) prostate, young patients.**
  > - **Decreased incidence** of **retrograde ejaculation** as compared to TURP.

- **Open simple prostatectomy: Glands > 75 gm**, concomitant bladder **diverticulum** or a bladder **stone** or if **dorsal lithotomy** positioning is **not possible**.
  - **Suprapubic prostatectomy:** Performed **transvesically (Frayer's)**^{Q} and **operation of choice** in dealing with concomitant bladder pathology **(Bladder stones** or **diverticulum)**^{Q}.
  - **Retropubic prostatectomy (Millin's)**^{Q}: Transverse incision is made in surgical capsule of prostate and enucleation is done.
  - **Perineal prostatectomy (Youngs)**^{Q}: Abandoned now

  > • **Carcinoma prostate** originates in **peripheral zone** of prostate, so prostatectomy for **BPH confers no protection** for subsequent cancer^Q.

Minimally Invasive Therapy in BPH
1. **Laser therapy**: Two main energy sources of lasers have been utilized- **holmium:YAG (best)**[Q], **Nd:YAG**. 2. Transurethral electrovaporization 3. Hyperthermia 4. Transurethral needle ablation 5. High intensity focused ultrasound 6. Intraurethral stents

ACUTE BACTERIAL PROSTATITIS

Acute Bacterial Prostatitis

- Acute inflammation of prostate associated with UTI
- Caused by **ascending urethral infection** or **reflux** of **infected urine**[Q] into prostatic ducts
- MC organism: **E. coli**[Q]
- Patients present with sudden onset **high grade fever** with **chills** and **rigors**, severe **irritative symptoms** and **enlarged, tender** and **boggy prostate**[Q]
- **Catheterization** and **prostatic massage** is **contraindicated**[Q]
- MC used antibiotics are: **TMP-SMX** and **Ciprofloxacin** (Both are having better **concentration in prostatic tissue**)[Q]
- Around **4-6 weeks**[Q] of antibiotic therapy is used to avert chronic bacterial prostatitis.

CHRONIC BACTERIAL PROSTATITIS

Chronic Bacterial Prostatitis

- Due to **persistent bacterial infection**[Q] of prostate
- Insidious in onset, characterized by **relapsing or recurrent UTI**[Q] caused by persistence of pathogen in prostatic fluid despite of antibiotic therapy
- **Diagnosis** is made by **microscopic examination** and **culture** of prostatic expressate and culture of urine obtained before and after prostatic massage[Q]
- **Treated** by chronic antibiotic suppression (3–4 months).[Q]

PROSTATIC ABSCESS

Prostatic Abscess

- Most cases result from **complications** of **acute bacterial prostatitis**[Q]
- **Fluctuation** is a **very late sign**[Q]
- Predisposing factors: Diabetes, renal insufficiency, immunosuppression, urethral instrumentation, chronic indwelling catheter[Q]
- Diagnosis: **TRUS** or **pelvic CT scan** is crucial for diagnosis and treatment
- Treated by **transurethral drainage** and **antibiotics**[Q]

PROSTATIC CALCULI

Prostatic Calculi

- Thought to represent **calcified corpora amylacea**[Q], which is composed of **calcium phosphate**[Q]
- Usually **phosphate**, seen on **TRUS** in **nearly all elderly males**[Q]
- Lie at the **periphery** of **transition zone** (posterior and posterolateral zones of prostate)
- Usually **asymptomatic** due to peripheral location, tend to **occur in clusters**[Q]
- **Calculi do not predispose** to **infections**[Q]
- But if **infections** occurs **in the presence of calculi**, it is almost **impossible to eradicate**[Q] the as the calculi may get infected and serve as a source of bacterial persistence and recurrent UTI.

PROSTATE CANCER

Prostate Cancer

- MC cancer of males, MC cause of bone secondaries[Q]
- African-American men have highest incidence, less common in Asians[Q]
- Best screening protocol for CA prostate: PSA + DRE[Q]

Risk Factors
- Advancing age & increased fat intake[Q] increase the risk
- Lycopene, Vitamin A & E and selenium decrease the risk[Q]
- MC genetic alteration in CA prostate is hypermethylation of glutathione transferase (GSTP-1)[Q] gene promoter located on chromosome 11[Q].

Pathology
- MC type is adenocarcinoma[Q] >TCC
- Prostatic adenocarcinoma are often multifocal & heterogenous[Q]
- It is often accompanied by premalignant lesion PIN (prostatic intraepithelial neoplasia)

> - Neoplastic glands are smaller, more crowded and lack branching & papillary infoldings.
> - Diagnosis of CA prostate based on absence of basal cell layer[Q].

- Basal cell layer is present in normal glands, BPH glands and the precursor lesions of CA prostate[Q].
- Site: Peripheral zone- 75%[Q], Transition zone- 15%, Central zone- 10%

Spread
- Spread occurs by direct local invasion and through hematogenous and lymphatics
- Local invasion most commonly involves seminal vesicles & base of bladder[Q]

> - Hematogenous spread occurs mostly to bone (axial skeleton is MC site with lumbar spine[Q] being most frequently implicated) forming osteoblastic secondaries[Q]
> - Visceral metastasis most commonly involve lungs[Q] > liver > adrenal glands
> - Lymphatic metastasis are most often identified in obturator nodes[Q]

- CNS involvement is usually a result of direct extension from skull metastasis[Q]

Clinical Features
- Most patients with early-stage CA prostate are asymptomatic, being peripheral[Q].
- Presence of symptoms suggest locally advanced or metastatic disease
- DRE: Hard, irregular, nodular prostate with median sulcus obliteration[Q]

Laboratory Findings
- Azotemia (bilateral ureteral obstruction), anemia in metastatic disease, raised ALP in bony metastasis
- PSA velocity >0.75 ng/ml/yr indicates carcinoma[Q]

Prostate Biopsy
- TRUS guided biopsy is done in patients with abnormal DRE or elevated PSA or both[Q].
- Differentiation of tumor is graded by Gleason score[Q]. A sum of 7 or more suggests an aggressive cancer.

Imaging
- TRUS is used for staging, most lesions are hypoechoic[Q].

Endorectal MRI in CA Prostate

- **Most optimal imaging** to appreciate the **prostate anatomy**[Q]
- Prostate cancer is associated with **lower levels of citrate** & **higher levels of choline** and **creatine**[Q] compared to BPH or normal tissues.
- The combined information provided by **MRI & MR spectroscopy** (for detection of citrate) may allow for a **more accurate assessment** of cancer **location & stage**[QQ]

Axial imaging in CA Prostate

- **CT scan** is mainly used to detect **LN metastasis**
- Intravenous administration of **superparamagnetic nanoparticles**, which gain access to lymph nodes by means of interstitial-lymphatic fluid transport, at the time of high resolution MRI, appears to **improve visualization** of **small nodal metastasis**[Q]

Bone Scan
- Patients with PSA ≥ 15 ng/ml or greater, locally advanced disease (T3b, T4) are at higher risk for bone metastasis, and should be considered for bone scan[Q].

Prostascint (Antibody imaging for prostate cancer)
- **Indium-111 capromab pendetide** is used in Prostascint
- **Radiolabeled monoclonal antibody** directed against **prostate specific membrane antigen**
- Helpful in **detecting soft tissue metastasis including LN metastasis** in biopsy proven prostate cancer which appear to be localized

Capsules of Prostate
- **True capsule:** Formed by **condensation** of the **peripheral part** of the gland^Q
- **False capsule:** Fomed by **visceral layer** of the **pelvic fasica**^{Q}.

Batson Periprostatic Venous Plexus
- Located **between two (true & false) capsule**
- In front this plexus **recieves deep dorsal vein of plexus & ends in internal iliac vein**^{Q}
- Has **valveless communication with vertebral plexus**, leading to **early metastasis to lumbar vertebra**^{Q}
- Via **hematogenous spread**, prostate cancer **first involve Batson periprostatic venous plexus** & then into **vertbral plexus** of veins^Q

GLEASON SCORE AND GRADING SYSTEM

GLEASON SCORE AND GRADING SYSTEM

- **Gleason score** is the MC used histological grading system for **prostate cancer**^{Q}.
- The **two most predominant histological patterns** of the prostate cancer are assigned a **Gleason grade** ranging from **1–5**^{Q}.

   - **Primary grade** is assigned to the **pattern of cancer** that is **most commonly observed** in the histological slides of the specimen^Q.
   - **Secondary grade** is assigned to the **second most commonly observed pattern** in the specimen.
   - **Gleason score** is the **sum of the two grades**. Thus it is also known as **Gleason sum**^{Q}.

- If the entire specimen has only one pattern present, then both the primary and secondary grades are reported as the same grade.

   - The **Gleason grade** ranges from **1 to 5**, with 5 having the **worst prognosis**^{Q}.
   - The **Gleason score** ranges from **2 to 10**^{Q}.

- The **Gleason score** is used to help **evaluate the prognosis** of men with prostate cancer. Together with other parameters, the Gleason score is incorporated into a strategy of prostate cancer staging which predicts prognosis and help guide therapy.

   - A point of importance is that the **primary Gleason grade** is **most important**^{Q} with respect to placing patients in prognostic groups.
   - For example in patients with a **Gleason score 7**, a **Gleason 4+3** is a **more aggressive cancer** than a **Gleason 3+4**.

TUMOR MARKERS OF CA PROSTATE (APART FROM PSA)

TUMOR MARKERS OF CA PROSTATE (APART FROM PSA)

- **Prostatic acid phosphatase:**
  - PAP activity is **1000 fold greater** in the **prostate**^{Q} than any other tissue
  - PAP is **not prostate specific**^{Q} and detectable levels are noted after prostatectomy
  - **Increased in renal, liver** and **bony malignancies**^{Q}
- **Alkaline phosphatase:**
  - **Raised in liver involvement** or **bony metastasis**^{Q}
- **Alpha-methyl co-A racemase**^{Q}
- **Hepsin**^{Q}
- **DD3**^{Q}

PROSTATE SPECIFIC ANTIGEN (PSA)

PROSTATE SPECIFIC ANTIGEN (PSA)

- It is a **glycoprotein**, serine protease.^{Q}
- **Free: 10–40%;**^{Q} **Complexed** to antiprotease: **60–90%**^{Q}
- **Formed in prostate**^{Q}, secreted in seminal fluid
- Causes **liquefaction** of **seminal coagulum**^{Q}

- Normal value: ≤ 4 ng/ml^Q (in > 50 years); Value > 20 ng/ml is **diagnostic of CA prostate**^{Q}
- **PSA** is the single test with **highest positive predictive value** for **CA prostate**^{Q}.
- **PSA** is **prostate specific, not** the **cancer specific**^{Q}
- **Level of PSA** is directly related to **tumor burden**^{Q}

- Its use without DRE is not recommended as 25% of men with CA prostate have PSA levels <4 ng/ml.
- **Best use of PSA** is **monitoring** after **radical prostatectomy**^{Q}

PSA related Investigations

PSA Density	PSA Velocity	Free PSA
• PSA/Prostate volume • If ≥ 0.15, biopsy^Q recommended	• Rate of change of PSA per year^Q • ≥ 0.75 ng/ml/year indicates carcinoma^Q • Assessment at every 18 months	• Free PSA (in %) appears to be most useful in distinguishing between those with and without CA prostate when total PSA levels fall in the range of 4–10 ng/ml^Q

Prostate Specific Antigen (PSA)

Increased PSA	Decreased PSA
• CA prostate^Q, BPH^Q • Acute prostatitis, Chronic prostatitis^Q • Prostatic abscess^Q • Catheterization, Cystoscopy^Q • Prostatic biopsy^Q (TRUS) • DRE^Q, Sexual intercourse	• Castration^Q • Anti-androgen therapy^Q • Radiotherapy or chemotherapy^Q for CA prostate • Radical prostatectomy^Q

8th AJCC (2017) TNM Staging for CA Prostate

T: Primary tumor	N: Regional lymph nodes
Tis: Carcinoma in situ (**PIN**)	**N0**: No regional LN metastasis
T1a: ≤5% of tissue in resection for benign disease has cancer, normal DRE^Q **T1b**: >5% of tissue in resection for benign disease has cancer, normal DRE^Q **T1c**: Tumor identified by **needle biopsy** (e.g., because of elevated PSA)^Q	**N1**: Metastasis in a regional LNs^Q (**obturator, internal iliac, external iliac, presacral LNs**)
T2a: Tumor involves **one half of one lobe** but not both lobes^Q **T2b**: Tumor involves **more than one half of one lobe** or less **T2c**: Tumor involves **both lobes**^{Q}	**M: Distant metastases**
T3a: **Extracapsular extension** on one or both sides including bladder neck involvement^Q **T3b**: **Seminal vesicle** involvement^Q	**M1a**: Distant metastasis in **non-regional** lymph nodes^Q **M1b**: Distant metastasis to **bone**^{Q} **M1c**: Distant metastasis to **other sites**^{Q}
T4: Tumor is fixed or invades adjacent structures other than seminal vesicles: **external sphincter, rectum, levator muscles and/or pelvic wall**^{Q}	

Treatment of CA Prostate

T1a	• **Incidentally found tumors** at TURP, by definition **low volume (≤5%)**, usually **well-differentiated** associated with **very slow growth rate**^{Q}. • Managed by **watchful waiting** (Regular follow up with **DRE & PSA**)^Q
T1b, T1c and T2	• Management depends on patient's age, life expectancy, performance status and patient's preference. • In **younger, fitter men (<70 years)**: **Radical prostatectomy**^{Q} or **radiotherapy**^{Q}, if surgery is contraindicated • **Elderly (>70 years)** with **life expectancy <10 years**: **Watchful waiting**^{Q} (Progress rate is very slow, 10% at 10 years)
Advanced disease (T3, T4 or any metastasis)	• Palliative treatment, androgen ablation or palliative radiotherapy • **Androgen ablation** (Hormone therapy) is **first line of treatment**: **Orchiectomy + Flutamide** or **LHRH + Flutamide** • **Palliative radiotherapy**^{Q}

New Drugs in metastatic, castration resistant CA Prostate
- **Cabazitaxel** and **Sipuleucel-T**^{Q}

SEMEN ANALYSIS

Semen Analysis

- **Fresh semen** is a coagulum that **liquefies 15-30 minutes** after ejaculation^Q.
- **Ejaculate volume** should be at least **1.5 mL**^{Q}, as smaller volumes may not sufficiently buffer against vaginal acidity.
- **Sperm concentration** should be > 20 million sperm/mL^Q.
- **Sperm motility** and **sperm cytology** or **morphology**^{Q} is another measure of semen quality.
- **Sperm morphology** is a **sensitive indicator** of **overall testicular health**^{Q}, because these characteristics are determined during spermatogenesis.

Abnormalities

• **Low ejaculate volume** may indicate:
  – **Retrograde ejaculation**^{Q} — **Ejaculatory duct obstruction**^{Q}
  – **Incomplete collection**^{Q} — **Androgen deficiency**^{Q}
• Azoospermia:
  – **Testicular failure**^{Q} — Obstruction of **vas deferens**^{Q}
• Absence of fructose:
  – **Seminal vesicle agenesis** or **obstruction**^{Q}

Semen Analysis-Minimal Standards of Adequacy
Ejaculate volume: 1.5–5.5 mL^Q
Sperm concentration: >20 × 10^6 sperm/mL^Q
Motility: >50%^{Q}
Forward progression: 2 (scale 1–4)^Q
Morphology: >30% WHO normal forms (> 4% **Kruger** normal forms)
No agglutination (clumping), **white cells**, or **increased viscosity**^{Q}.

Transrectal Ultrasound
• High-frequency (5–7) mHz **transrectal ultrasound** (TRUS) offers **super imaging** of the **prostate, seminal vesicles**, and **ejaculatory ducts**^{Q}. • Due to both accuracy and convenience, **TRUS** has **replaced surgical vasography** in the **diagnosis of obstructive lesions** that **cause infertility**^{Q}.

SPERM ASPIRATION

Sperm Aspiration

- **Sperm aspiration techniques** are indicated for men in whom the **transport of sperm is not possible** because the **ductal system is absent** or **surgically unreconstructable**^{Q}.
- An example of this is **vasal agenesis**. **Acquired forms of obstruction** may also exist, the most common of which is **failed vasectomy reversal**^{Q}.
- **Aspiration procedures** can involve **microsurgery** to **collect sperm** from the sperm reservoirs within the genital tract^Q.
- At present, **sperm** are routinely **aspirated** from the **vas deferens, epididymis**, or **testicle**^{Q}.

  - In cases of **sperm aspiration** from the **testicle** and **epididymis**, IVF along with intracytoplasmic sperm injection **(ICSI)** is required^Q.
  - An **obvious prerequisite** for these procedures is **ongoing sperm production**^{Q}.
  - Although **evaluated indirectly** by **hormone levels** and **testis volume**, the **most direct way to verify sperm production** is with a **testis biopsy**^{Q}.

Vasal Aspiration	Epididymal Aspiration	Testis Sperm Retrieval
• Vasal aspiration provides the **most mature** or **fertilizable sperm**^{Q}, as they have **already passed** through the **epididymis**^{Q}, where **sperm maturation is completed**.	• Epididymal sperm aspiration is performed when the **vas is not present** or is **scarred** and **unusable**^{Q}. • **Epididymal sperm** are **not as mature as vasal sperm**^{Q}; as a consequence, **epididymal sperm require ICSI to fertilize the egg**^{Q}.	• The **most recently developed aspiration technique**^{Q} • Indicated for patients in whom there is an **unreconstructable blockage** in the **epididymis**, or in cases of **severe testis failure**^{Q}, in which so few sperm are produced that they cannot reach the ejaculate.

Multiple Choice Questions

BENIGN PROSTATIC HYPERPLASIA

1. Benign prostatic hyperplasia first develops in the:
   a. Periurethral transition zone *(COMEDK 2011)*
   b. Peripheral zone
   c. Central zone
   d. Anterior fibromuscular stroma

2. In BPH most common lobe involved is:
   (Recent Question 2016, WBPG 2015, AIIMS June 2000)
   a. Lateral   b. Posterior
   c. Median   d. Anterior

3. Most common site of BPH: *(Recent Question 2017)*
   a. Peripheral zone   b. Middle zone
   c. Transition zone   d. Central zone

4. Which is the earliest symptom of benign hypertrophy of prostate? *(Karnataka 94, 96)*
   a. Frequency   b. Hematuria
   c. Incontinence   d. Strangury

5. Which of the following is an absolute indication for surgery in cases of benign prostatic hyperplasia? *(All India 2003)*
   a. Bilateral hydroureteronephrosis
   b. Nocturnal frequency
   c. Recurrent urinary tract infection
   d. Voiding bladder pressures > 50 cm of water

6. Which of the following lasers is used for treatment of benign prostatic hyperplasia as well as urinary calculi?
   (All India 2003)
   a. CO_2 laser   b. Excimer laser
   c. Ho: YAG laser   d. Nd-YAG laser

7. A 60-years old diabetic and hypertensive with second grade prostatism admitted for prostatectomy developed myocardial infarction. Treatment now would be: *(All India 99)*
   a. Finasteride   b. Terazocin
   c. Finasteride and terazocin d. Diethyl stilbestrol

8. The following statements regarding finasteride are true except: *(All India 2005)*
   a. It is used in the medical treatment of benign prostatic hypertrophy
   b. Impotence is well documented after its use
   c. It blocks the conversion of dihydrotestosterone to testosterone
   d. It is a 5-α reductase inhibitor

9. Indication for surgery in benign prostatic hypertrophy are all except: *(Recent Question 2016)*
   a. Prostatism   b. Chronic retention
   c. Hemorrhage   d. Enlarged prostate

10. Grade I benign prostate with outflow obstruction is best treated with:
    a. Retropubic prostatectomy b. Transurethral resection
    c. Transvesicle prostatectomy d. Androgen therapy

11. Assessment of patient with prostatism include all except:
    a. Rectal examination *(APPG 2013, DPG 2009 March)*
    b. Serum prostate specific antigen
    c. Pressure flow urodynamic studies
    d. Transrectal ultrasound scanning

12. In follow up of BPH, most important indication of surgery is:
    a. Prostate size > 75 gm *(AIIMS Nov 2010)*
    b. Single episode of UTI requiring 3 days of antibiotics
    c. Cannot use medication due to hypertension
    d. Bilateral hydronephrosis

13. What of the following is an absolute indication for surgery in cases of benign prostatic hyperplasia?
    (MHSSMCET 2005, All India 2003)
    a. Bilateral hydroureteronephrosis
    b. Nocturnal frequency
    c. Recurrent urinary tract infection
    d. Voiding bladder pressures > 50 cm of H_2O

14. The drug that has the fastest onset of action in benign prostatic hyperplasia is: *(COMEDK 2008)*
    a. Finasteride   b. Tamsulosin
    c. Dutasteride   d. Flutamide

15. In the management of symptomatic benign prostatic hyperplasia with finasteride the period of trial required for determining a satisfactory response is: *(COMEDK 2009)*
    a. 1 month   b. 2 months
    c. 4 months   d. 6 months

16. Mechanism of action of Silodosin: *(Recent Question 2016)*
    a. Alpha antagonist   b. Beta antagonist
    c. Anticholinergic   d. PDE5 inhibitor

17. Which of the following drug can decrease the size of prostate? *(AIIMS November 2017)*
    a. Tamsulosin   b. Sildenafil
    c. Finasteride   d. Prazosin

TURP AND COMPLICATIONS

18. The most important use of transrectal ultrasonography (TRUS) is for: *(COMEDK 2007)*
    a. Screening for CA prostate
    b. Distinguishing prostate cancer from BPH
    c. Systematic prostate biopsy in suspected prostate cancer
    d. Guiding transurethral resection of prostate cancer

19. The most common complication of transurethral resection of prostate (TURP): *(COMEDK 2007, 2008, 2009)*
    a. Erectile dysfunction
    b. Retrograde ejaculation
    c. Urinary incontinence
    d. Impotence

20. Delirium, mental confusion and nausea in patients who had undergone transurethral resection of prostate suggests:
    (MCI Nov 2017, Sept 2009)
    a. Hypernatremia   b. Sepsis
    c. Hepatic coma   d. Water retention

21. Which of the following is the most common cause of delayed urinary tract obstructive symptoms after TURP?
    a. Stricture of the navicular fossa *(All India 2011)*
    b. Stricture of the membranous urethra
    c. Stricture of the bulb of urethra
    d. Bladder neck stenosis

22. During TURP, surgeon takes care to dissect above the verumontanum to prevent injury to: *(All India 2011)*
    a. External urethral sphincter
    b. Urethral crest
    c. Prostatic utricle
    d. Trigone of bladder

23. What is the reason for following set of symptoms after prostatic surgery- restlessness, vomiting and change in sensorium? *(AIIMS June 99)*
    a. Electrolyte imbalance
    b. Bladder neck obstruction
    c. Acute pyelonephritis
    d. Ureter stenosis

24. TURP was done in an old patient of BHP, after which he developed altered sensorium cause is?
    (MCI June 2018, AIIMS June 2001, AIIMS June 99)
    a. Hypernatremia
    b. Hypokalemia
    c. Hyponatremia
    d. Hypomagnesemia

25. Commonest cause of periumbilical pain after 30 min. of TURP done under spinal anesthesia with Bupivacaine:
    a. Meteorism *(AIIMS June 2000)*
    b. Perforation of bladder
    c. Recovery from bupivacaine anaesthesia
    d. Mesentery artery ischemia

26. Which of the following substances is not used as an irrigant during transurethral resection of the prostate?
    (AIIMS Nov 2003)
    a. Normal saline   b. 1.5% glycine
    c. 5% dextrose   d. Distilled water

27. A 70 years old patient benign prostatic hyperplasia underwent transurethral resection of prostate under spinal anaesthesia. One hour later, he developed vomiting and altered sensorium. The most probable cause is:
    (MHSSMCET 2008, AIIMS June 2001, All India 2003)
    a. Over dosage of spinal anesthetic agent
    b. Rupture of bladder
    c. Hyperkalemia
    d. Water intoxication

28. All of the following can be seen after transurethral resection of prostate except: *(AIIMS Nov 2000)*
    a. Congestive cardiac failure
    b. Transient blindness
    c. Convulsions
    d. Hypernatremia

29. TUR (Transurethral resection) syndrome is due to:
    a. Hyponatremia   b. Hypokalemia *(UPSC 95)*
    c. Hypovolemia   d. Hypoxia

30. Consider the following conditions:
    1. Urinary flow rate < 10 cc/second
    2. Residual volume of urine > 100 cc
    3. Serum level of prostatic specific antigen > 10 mmol/litre
    4. Trabeculated urinary bladder
    Which of the above are indications of TURP for BHP?
    a. 1, 2 and 3   b. 2, 3 and 4
    c. 1, 2 and 4   d. 1, 3 and 4

31. Which one of the following is used as an irrigation solution during transurethral resection of the prostate?
    a. 1.5% glycine *(COMEDK 2014)*
    b. Physiological Saline
    c. Ringer's lactate
    d. 5% dextrose

32. True about transurethral resection of the prostate:
    (PGI November 2017)
    a. More morbidity than retropubic prostatectomy
    b. Can cause retrograde ejaculation
    c. Open prostatectomy is preferred in larger obstructive mass
    d. Less risk of bleeding in transurethral laser vaporization than in TURP
    e. Resectoscope is passed through the urethra and prostate resected into multiple pieces and removed

CARCINOMA PROSTATE

33. Most common site of development of carcinoma of prostate is: *(Recent Question 2015, DNB 2012, Orissa 2011, MHPGMCET 2002, 2001)*
    a. Peripheral zone   b. Central zone
    c. Transitional zone   d. Fibromuscular stroma

34. On MRI, origin of carcinoma prostate is seen in:
    (Recent Question 2017)
    a. Peripheral zone   b. Central zone
    c. Transition zone   d. Periurethral zone

35. A 49-years old man suffering from carcinoma of prostate was x-rayed. He showed areas of sclerosis and collapse of T10 and T11 vertebrae in x-ray. The spread of this cancer to the above vertebrae in X-ray. The spread of this cancer to the above vertebrae was through: *(AIIMS Nov 2002)*
    a. Sacral canal
    b. Lymphatic vessels
    c. Internal vertebral plexus of veins
    d. Superior rectal vein

36. Mr. Chaturvedi, a 70 years old man comes to casualty with urinary retention and back pain. Which investigation should be performed? *(AIIMS Nov 2000, Nov 99)*
    a. Serum acid phosphatase   b. Serum calcium
    c. Serum alkaline phosphates d. Serum electrophoresis

37. A 65 years old male was diagnosed with prostate cancer three years back and was treated by surgery and hormone therapy. Presently he has developed urinary symptoms and progressive backache. What is the tumor marker, which can be indicative of disease relapse? *(AIIMS Nov 2003)*
    a. CA-125   b. Beta-HCG
    c. CEA   d. PSA

38. Specific marker for prostatic cancer is: *(PGI Dec 99)*
    a. Alkaline phosphatase   b. Prostate specific antigen
    c. Acid phosphatase   d. CA-125

39. Screening of prostate CA commonly done by:
    (PGI Nov 2010, May 2005)
    a. DRE (digital rectal exam)
    b. USG
    c. MRI
    d. PSA
    e. CT scan

40. A 50 years old male with positive family history of prostate cancer has come to you for a screening test. The most sensitive screening test to pickup prostate cancer is:
    a. DRE *(All India 2007)*
    b. PSA
    c. DRE+ PSA
    d. Endorectal coil MRI with T1W and T2W images

41. Transrectal ultrasonogram in evaluation of carcinoma prostate is most useful for: *(All India 2008)*
    a. Taking guided biopsy
    b. Identifying seminal vesicle invasion
    c. Nodal sampling
    d. Measuring the extent of invasion

42. In prostatic metastasis, the site most commonly involved is: *(PGI June 99)*
    a. Obturator nodes
    b. Perivesical nodes
    c. Pre-sacral nodes
    d. Para aortic nodes

43. CA prostate commonly metastasizes to the vertebrae: *(All India 2001)*
    a. Because valveless communication exist with Batson's periprostatic plexus
    b. Via drainage to sacral lymph node
    c. Of direct spread
    d. None of above

44. Secondary deposits form prostatic carcinoma is commonest in: *(Recent Question 2015)*
    a. Bone
    b. Kidney
    c. Liver
    d. Brain

45. In carcinoma prostate with metastasis which is raised? *(Recent Question 2016)*
    a. ESR
    b. Alkaline phosphatase
    c. Acid phosphatase
    d. Bilirubin

46. A patient presents with complains of sciatica. On radiological examination there was sclerotic lesions on his skull. Which of the following is most likely to be elevated in this patient? *(AIIMS 2000)*
    a. CEA
    b. Prostate specific antigen
    c. Alkaline phosphatase
    d. Alpha-1 antitrypsin

47. Serum acid phosphatase is raised in: *(MCI June 2018)*
    a. Osteosarcoma
    b. Prostatic carcinoma
    c. Paget's disease
    d. Hyperparathyroidism

48. Normal level of PSA in males is: *(DNB 2011)*
    a. < 4 ng/ml
    b. 4–10 ng/ml
    c. > 10 ng/ml
    d. PSA is not produced by normal males

49. Gleason scoring is done for: *(Recent Question 2017, DNB 2009)*
    a. Prostatic cancer
    b. Lung cancer
    c. Bladder cancer
    d. Hodgkins lymphoma

50. Which of the following is true about prostate cancer screening? *(APPG 2008)*
    a. Digital screening along with PSA is additive
    b. Prostate cancer is common among young males
    c. Tumor markers are diagnostic
    d. Bleeding per rectum is earliest manifestation of disease

51. True about prostate CA is: *(DPG 2008)*
    a. Arises in the periurethral zone
    b. Extremely radio sensitive
    c. Obturator nodes are most commonly involved
    d. PSA is not used in workup

52. Gleason score: all are true except: *(AIIMS May 2011, Nov 2008)*
    a. Used for grading prostate cancer
    b. Scores range from 1–10
    c. Higher the score, poorer the prognosis
    d. Helps in planning management

53. Osteoblastic metastasis commonly arise from: *(JIPMER 2014, 2013, AIIMS May 2013)*
    a. Breasts
    b. Prostate
    c. Lung
    d. RCC

54. Best screening marker of prostate cancer is: *(UPPG 2009)*
    a. AFP
    b. Prostate specific antigen
    c. CA 19-20
    d. CA 125 to 26

55. The most important use of transrectal ultrasonography (TRUS) is for: *(COMEDK 2007)*
    a. Screening for CA prostate
    b. Distinguishing prostate cancer from BPH
    c. Systematic prostate biopsy in suspected prostate cancer
    d. Guiding transurethral resection of prostate cancer

56. Treatment for metastatic CA Prostate: *(JIPMER 2011)*
    a. GnRH analogue
    b. Estrogen therapy
    c. Radiotherapy with chemotherapy
    d. Radiotherapy

CARCINOMA PROSTATE TREATMENT

57. Which is not used in carcinoma prostate? *(PGI Dec 97)*
    a. Estrogen
    b. Progesterone
    c. Cyproterone acetate
    d. Flutamide

58. An 85-years old man underwent transurethral resection of prostate. A histological examination of his specimen showed foci of adenocarcinoma management will be: *(AIIMS Nov 2000)*
    a. Endocrine therapy
    b. Radical surgery
    c. Hormone therapy
    d. No further treatment

59. A 75-years old frail elderly man underwent TURP. The biopsy revealed adenocarcinoma. What is the next line of management? *(All India 94)*
    a. Radiotherapy
    b. Surgery followed by hormonal replacement therapy
    c. Conservative treatment
    d. Surgery followed by radiotherapy

60. Which of the following is the most troublesome source of bleeding during a radical retropubic prostatectomy? *(All India 2005)*
    a. Dorsal venous complex
    b. Inferior vesical pedicle
    c. Superior vesical pedicle
    d. Seminal vesicular artery

61. A 70-years old man with CA prostate with osteoblastic secondaries in pelvis and lumbar vertebra showed well differentiated Adeno Carcinoma prostate on needle biopsy. He is ideally treated by:
    a. Radical prostatectomy
    b. TURP
    c. Radiation
    d. Hormonal manipulation

62. Management of Carcinoma prostate in a 50-years old man revealed after TURP: *(MHSSMCET 2006)*
    a. No treatment required
    b. Hormonal therapy
    c. Bilateral subcapsular orchidectomy
    d. Radical prostatectomy

63. A 70-year-old man with prostate cancer was given radiotherapy. The recurrence of the cancer is monitored biochemically by: *(AIIMS Nov 2012)*
    a. Androgens only
    b. Prostate specific antigen and carcinoembryonic antigen
    c. Prostate specific antigen only
    d. ALP and CEA

64. Treatment of metastatic prostate carcinoma is: *(JIPMER 2011)*
    a. Radiotherapy
    b. Estrogen only
    c. GnRH analogs
    d. Radiotherapy with chemotherapy

65. Which of the following drugs is useful for treatment of advanced prostate cancer? *(AIIMS November, May 2014)*
    a. Goserelin
    b. Ganirelix
    c. Cetrorelix
    d. Abarelix

66. Regarding prostatectomy which one of the statements is false: *(APPG 2015)*
    a. Water intoxication and hyponatremia can give rise to CHF
    b. Perineal prostatectomy (Young) is a commonly done surgical procedure
    c. Retrograde ejaculation occurs in about 65% of men
    d. Intraurethral stents are helpful in the management of men who are grossly unfit (ASA grade 4)

67. Sipuleucel-T is a vaccine for: *(Recent Question 2017)*
    a. RCC
    b. Testicular tumor
    c. Carcinoma prostate
    d. Carcinoma bladder

68. Ketoconazole action in prostate carcinoma is: *(Recent Question 2017)*
    a. Pituitary inhibition
    b. Adrenal ablation
    c. Inhibits DHT formation
    d. Androgen antagonist

PROSTATITIS

69. Complication which commonly accompanies acute prostatitis: *(Recent Question 2016)*
    a. Epididymitis
    b. Orchitis
    c. Seminal vesiculitis
    d. Sterility

70. A 60 years old male presented with fever, chills and dysuria. Patient was hospitalized in emergency for 5 days. PSA level was 7.4. Next best step in this patient: *(AIIMS Nov 2013)*
    a. Repeat PSA
    b. TURP
    c. TRUS guided biopsy
    d. Antibiotics and admit

71. Most common organism responsible for acute bacterial prostatitis: *(Recent Question 2018)*
    a. E. coli
    b. Peptostreptococci
    c. Enterococci
    d. Streptococci agalactiae

INFERTILITY

72. Semen analysis of a young man who presented with primary infertility revealed low volume, fructose negative ejaculate with azoospermia. Which of the following is the most useful imaging modality to evaluate the cause of his infertility? *(All India 2003)*
    a. Colour duplex ultrasonography of the scrotum
    b. Transrectal ultrasonography
    c. Retrograde urethrography
    d. Spermatic venography

73. Absence of fructose in semen indicates: *(PGI Dec 2008)*
    a. Obstruction to seminal vesicles
    b. Obstruction at prostatic urethra
    c. Vas deferens obstruction
    d. Testicular failure

74. A 25 years old married male presents with infertility. He had undergone retroperitoneal lymph node dissection at age of 15 years for embryonal carcinoma of right testis. Semen analysis shows-quantity-0.5 mL, no. sperm, no fructose. Biopsy of testis shows normal spermatogenesis. Best treatment here would be:
    a. Artificial insemination of donor *(All India 99)*
    b. Penile-prosthesis
    c. Microtesticular aspiration and intracytoplasmic injection
    d. None of the above

75. A 55-year-old diabetic patient presented with impotence with history of failure to get erection after papaverine intracavernous injection. Color Doppler shows no abnormality of arteries but shows mild venous run-off. Treatment of choice: *(All India 99)*
    a. Intracavernous injection of papaverine
    b. Penile prosthetic implants
    c. Vacuum constriction device
    d. Psychotherapy

76. The most important in assessing fertility potential is:
    a. Sperm count
    b. Sperm motility
    c. Sperm morphology
    d. Quantity of ejaculated semen
    e. None of the above

77. Which of the following is true about obstructive azoospermia?
    a. ↑FSH and ↑LH *(All India 2011)*
    b. Normal FSH and normal LH
    c. ↑LH, normal FSH
    d. ↑FSH, normal LH

78. In a couple for treatment of infertility from the last four years, female partner is normal. Male partner has 0.8 ml semen volume per ejaculate on two repeated samples and absent fructose, with no sperms on examination under microscope. What is the next line of management? *(AIIMS Nov 2013)*
    a. Per-rectal examination to check ejaculatory duct obstruction
    b. Give antioxidants
    c. Testicular biopsy
    d. Transrectal ultrasound to detect duct obstruction

79. Fructose absence in semen analysis suggests: *(Recent Question 2017)*
    a. Bilateral vas deferens obstruction
    b. Ejaculatory duct obstruction
    c. Testicular failure
    d. Prostatic urethral obstruction

PROSTATE ANATOMY AND PHYSIOLOGY

80. Corpora amylaciae is seen in: *(Kerala 94)*
    a. Thymus
    b. Lymph node
    c. Spleen
    d. Prostate

81. Hot flush is not associated with: *(PGI Dec 2008)*
    a. Medical castration
    b. Surgical castration
    c. Ketoconazole therapy
    d. Androgen receptor blockade
    e. Radical prostatectomy

82. Medical castration is effected by: *(Kerala 90)*
    a. Deithylstilbesterol
    b. LHRH analogues
    c. Gossypol
    d. Hanovan

83. Complimentary operation done at the time of prostatectomy is:
    a. Vasectomy
    b. Circumcision
    c. Hernia repair
    d. All of the above

84. Prostate calculi are usually composed of:
    a. Calcium oxalate
    b. Calcium phosphate
    c. Struvite
    d. Uric acid

Explanations

BENIGN PROSTATIC HYPERPLASIA

1. Ans. a. Periurethral transition zone *(Ref: Smith 18/e p350; Campbell 11/e p2433; Bailey 27/e p1458)*
2. Ans. c. Median
3. Ans. c. Transition zone *(Ref: Campbell 11/e p2433; Smith 18/e p350; Bailey 27/e p1458)*   4.   Ans. a. Frequency
5. Ans. a. Bilateral hydroureteronephrosis, c. Recurrent urinary tract infection *(Ref: Campbell 11/e p2509; Bailey 27/e p1463)*
6. Ans. c. Ho: YAG laser *(Ref: Smith 18/e p356; Campbell 11/e p2526)*
7. Ans. b. Terazocin *(Ref: Smith 18/e p354; Campbell 11/e p2473; Bailey 27/e p1464)*
8. Ans. c. It blocks the conversion of dihydrotestosterone to testosterone   9.   Ans. d. Enlarged prostate
10. Ans. b. Transurethral resection *(Ref: Smith 18/e p356; Campbell 11/e p2510; Bailey 27/e p1464)*
11. Ans. d. Transrectal ultrasound scanning *(Ref: Bailey 27/e p1462; Smith 18/e p218)*

    In prostatitis, DRE examination reveals **tender, enlarged glands** that are **irregular** and **warm**. PSA levels are often **elevated**. TRUS is only **indicated in** patients who **do not respond to conventional therapy**.

    ### LET US CONSIDER EVERY OPTION

    - In prostatitis, DRE examination reveals **tender, enlarged glands** that are **irregular** and **warm**^{Q}.
    - PSA levels are often **elevated**^{Q}.
    - TRUS is only **indicated in** patients who **do not respond to conventional therapy**^{Q}.

12. Ans. d. Bilateral hydronephrosis   13.   Ans. a. Bilateral hydroureteronephrosis, c. Recurrent urinary tract infection
14. Ans. b. Tamsulosin   15.   Ans. d. 6 months   16.   Ans. a. Alpha antagonist
17. Ans. c. Finasteride *(Ref: Goodman Gilman 12/e p308, 1205; Katzung 13/e p720)*

    "Finasteride has been reported to be moderately effective in reducing prostate size in men with benign prostatic hyperplasia and is approved for this use in the USA."-Katzung 13/e p720

TURP AND COMPLICATIONS

18. Ans. c. Systematic prostate biopsy in suspected prostate cancer *(Ref: Rumack's Diagnostic Ultrasound 3/e p411)*

Uses of TRUS in CA prostate	
• To guide biopsy	• To guide therapy

19. Ans. b. Retrograde ejaculation *(Ref: Smith 18/e p354; Campbell 11/e p2515; Bailey 27/e p1466)*
20. Ans. d. Water retention   21.   Ans. d. Bladder neck stenosis   22.   Ans. a. External urethral sphincter
23. Ans. a. Electrolyte imbalance   24.   Ans. c. Hyponatremia
25. Ans. b. Perforation of bladder *(Ref: Bailey 27/e p1466)*

    ### COMPLICATIONS OF TURP

    - **Perforation of the bladder** or the **prostatic capsule** can occur at the time of transurethral surgery.
    - This usually occurs from a **combination of inexperience** in association with a **large prostate** or **heavy blood loss**.
    - A **large perforation with marked extravasation** may require the **insertion of a small suprapubic drain**.
    - If not detected, it may **present postoperatively** after the effect of spinal anesthesia, as **suprapubic pain**.

26. Ans. a. Normal saline *(Ref: Campbell 11/e p2510)*

    The use of an ionic solution (i.e., normal saline) leads to dissipation of the cutting current and poor cutting efficacy

27. Ans. d. Water intoxication   28.   Ans. d. Hypernatremia
29. Ans. a. Hyponatremia   30.   Ans. c. 1, 2 and 4
31. Ans. a. 1.5% glycine *(Ref: Campbell 11/e p2510)*
32. Ans. b. Can cause......, c. Open prostatectomy..., d. Less risk of bleeding..., e. Resectoscope is passed...

CARCINOMA PROSTATE

33. Ans. a. Peripheral zone *(Ref: Smith 18/e p357; Campbell 11/e p2594; Bailey 27/e p1469)*
34. Ans. a. Peripheral zone *(Ref: Campbell 11/e p2396; Smith 18/e p357; Bailey 27/e p1469)*
35. Ans. c. Internal vertebral plexus of veins
36. Ans. a. Serum acid phosphatase *(Ref: Smith 18/e p360; Campbell 11/e p2602-2605; Bailey 27/e p1469)*
37. Ans. d. PSA *(Ref: Smith 18/e p360; Campbell 11/e p2602; Bailey 27/e p1471)*
38. Ans. b. Prostate specific antigen
39. Ans. a. DRE (Digital rectal exam), d. PSA
40. Ans. c. DRE+ PSA
41. Ans. a. Taking guided biopsy
42. Ans. a. Obturator nodes
43. Ans. a. Because valveless communication exist with Batson's periprostatic plexus *(Ref: Campbell 11/e p2594)*
44. Ans. a. Bone
45. Ans. c. Acid phosphatase
46. Ans. b. Prostate specific antigen
47. Ans. b. Prostatic carcinoma
48. Ans. a. < 4 ng/ml
49. Ans. a. Prostate cancer
50. Ans. a. Digital screening along with PSA is additive
51. Ans. c. Obturator nodes are most commonly involved
52. Ans. b. Scores range from 1 to 10 *(Ref: Smith 18/e p362; Bailey 27/e p1472; Campbell 11/e p2595)*

    Gleason score ranges from 2 to 10.

53. Ans. b. Prostate *(Ref: Harrison 19/e p580; Devita 9/e p2512-2513; CSDT 12/e p1202)*

    Osteoblastic metastasis commonly arises from carcinoma prostate.

    - MC site of primary for **bone metastasis: CA Breast**[Q]
    - MC cause of **osteoblastic secondaries** in males: **CA Prostate**[Q]
    - MC cause of **osteoblastic secondaries** in females: **CA Breast**[Q]
    - MC tumor metastasize to bone in females: **CA Breast**[Q]

54. Ans. b. Prostate specific antigen
55. Ans. c. Systematic prostate biopsy in suspected prostate cancer
56. Ans. a. GnRH analogue *(Ref: Smith 18/e p372)*

    - In metastatic CA prostate, Androgen ablation (Hormone therapy) is **first line of treatment: Orchiectomy + Flutamide** or **LHRH + Flutamide**[Q].
    - **Leuprolide** and **goserelin** are **GnRH analogues**, which are **used primarily** for the treatment of **hormone-responsive prostate cancer**[Q].

CARCINOMA PROSTATE TREATMENT

57. Ans. b. Progesterone *(Ref: Smith 18/e p371; Campbell 11/e p2789; Bailey 27/e p1474)*
58. Ans. d. No further treatment
59. Ans. c. Conservative treatment
60. Ans. a. Dorsal venous complex
61. Ans. d. Hormonal manipulation
62. Ans. d. Radical prostatectomy
63. Ans. c. Prostate specific antigen only *(Ref: Smith 18/e p371; Campbell 11/e p2617; Bailey 27/e p1473; Harrison 19/e p581)*

    Cancer control (in CA Prostate) after radiotherapy has been defined by various criterias including: *(Ref: Harrison 19/ep581)*
    - A decline in PSA to less than 0.5 or 1 ng/ml
    - "Non-rising" PSA values
    - **Negative biopsy** of the prostate 2 years after completion of the treatment
        The current standard definition of biochemical failure (the Phoenix definition) is a rise in PSA by ≥ 2 ng/ml higher than the lowest PSA achieved

64. **Ans. c. GnRH analogs**
65. **Ans. a. Goserelin** *(Ref: Katzung12/e p972; Goodman and Gilman 12/e p1763-1764; Smith 18/e p372; Campbell 11/e p291)*

    Goserelin is useful for the treatment of advanced prostate cancer.

    > "The **treatment of choice** for patients with **advanced prostate cancer** is **elimination of testosterone production** by the testes through either **surgical** or **chemical castration**. Bilateral orchiectomy or estrogen therapy in the form of diethylstilbestrol was previously used as first-line therapy. Presently, the use of **GnRH agonists**-including **leuprolide** and **goserelin**, alone or in combination with anti-androgen (e.g. **flutamide, bicalutamide** or **nilutamide**) is **the preferred approach.**"- *Katzung12/e p972*

66. **Ans. b. Perineal prostatectomy (Young) is a commonly done surgical procedure**
67. **Ans. c. Carcinoma prostate** *(Ref: Campbell 11/e p2813; Smith 18/e p373)*

    > "In prostate cancer, several immunologic strategies have been under clinical development. The most important of these include the **sipuleucel-T (Provenge)** autologous prostatic acid phosphatase (PAP)-loaded dendritic cell vaccine, the **GVAX** allogeneic recombinant whole cell vaccine, and **CTLA-4** inhibitory approaches."- *Campbell 11/e p2813*

68. **Ans. b. Adrenal ablation** *(Ref: Campbell 11/e p2787; Smith 18/e p372; Bailey 27/e p1474)*

PROSTATITIS

69. **Ans. c. Seminal vesiculitis** *(Ref: Smith 18/e p218; Campbell 11/e p310, 313; Bailey 27/e p1474)*
70. **Ans. d. Antibiotics and admit** *(Ref: Smith 18/e p218; Campbell 11/e p310, 313; Bailey 27/e p1475)*

    - A **60 years old male** presented with **fever, chills and dysuria**. Patient was hospitalized in emergency for 5 days. **PSA level was 7.4**. This patient is most probably suffering from **acute bacterial prostatitis** and **treated by antibiotics**.

71. **Ans. a. E. coli** *(Ref: Campbell 11/e p305; Smith 18/e p218; Bailey 27/e p1474)*

    > "The most common cause of bacterial prostatitis is the Enterobacteriaceae family of gram- negative bacteria, which originate in the gastrointestinal flora. The most common organisms are strains of Escherichia coli, which are identified in 65% to 80% of infections."- *Campbell 11/e p305*

INFERTILITY

72. **Ans. b. Transrectal ultrasonography** *(Ref: Smith 18/e p699)*

    - **Sperms** are produced in **seminiferous tubules** and then **stored** and **matured within** the **epididymis**^{Q}.
    - **Vas deferens carries** the **sperms** from epididymis **to the urethra** where they open by separate openings into prostatic urethra^Q.
    - **Just before opening**, each vas deferens is **joined by ducts of seminal vesicles**^{Q}.
    - **Vas deferens** and **seminal vesicle ducts** join to **form** the **ejaculatory duct**^{Q}

73. **Ans. a. Obstruction to seminal vesicles** *(Ref: Smith 18/e p696)*

    - **Absence of fructose** in the semen indicates **seminal vesicle agenesis** or **obstruction of its duct** or the **ejaculatory duct**^{Q}.

74. **Ans. c. Microtesticular aspiration and intracytoplasmic injection** *(Ref: Smith 18/e p713)*
75. **Ans. c. Vacuum constriction device** *(Ref: Campbell 11/e p738)*

    ### Vacuum Erection Device Therapy

    - In **patients who do not respond** to or **decline oral** or **local vasoactive pharmacotherapeutic options**^{Q}, vacuum erection device therapy may be alternatively explored.

      > - The **principle** of **vacuum erection device therapy** is to **mechanically create negative pressure surrounding** the **penis** in order to **engorge it with blood** and then **restrain blood egress from** the **organ** to **maintain** the **erection-like effect**^{Q}.

    - **Efficacy rates** in achieving **satisfactory erections** of **67–90%**, but **satisfaction rates** with the device are lower, ranging from **34 to 68%**.
    - The device is **more acceptable to older men** in a **steady relationship** compared with young, single men.

> - Success is limited in patients with severe vascular abnormalities such as proximal venous leakage or arterial insufficiency or fibrosis secondary to priapism or prosthesis infection[Q].
- Further, it may offer a means to preserve the elasticity of penile tissues after priapism or penile prosthesis explantation or after surgical correction of Peyronie's disease[Q].
- It has been suggested to facilitate erection recovery after treatments for prostate cancer[Q].

76. **Ans. b. Sperm motility**
77. **Ans. b. Normal FSH and normal LH** *(Ref: Shaw's 13/e p203; Oxford textbook of Medicine 4/e p283)*

    Obstructive azoospermia is associated with **normal levels** of **FSH** and **LH.**

Azoospermia		
Obstructive Azoospermia	**Hypogonadotrophic Azoospermia**	**Hypergonadotrophic Azoospermia**
Azoospermia due to obstruction: • Normal FSH and LH[Q] • Normal testosterone[Q] • Testicular volume is usually normal[Q]	Azoospermia due to **hypothalamic** or **pituitary failure:** • Low FSH and LH[Q] • Low testosterone[Q] • Testicular volume is usually reduced[Q]	Azoospermia due to **testicular (end organ) failure:** • Persistently elevated FSH[Q] • Testicular volume is usually reduced[Q]

78. **Ans. d. Transrectal ultrasound to detect duct obstruction** *(Ref: Smith 18/e p713)*

    > - *Absent fructose with no sperms in ejaculate is suggestive of obstruction of vas deferens with seminal vesicle agenesis or obstruction. Next line of management in this patient would be transrectal ultrasound to detect duct obstruction.*
    > - *"High-frequency (5-7) mHz transrectal ultrasound (TRUS) offers superb imaging of the prostate, seminal vesicles, and ejaculatory ducts[Q].*
    > - *Due to both accuracy and convenience, TRUS has replaced surgical vasography in the diagnosis of obstructive lesions that cause infertility[Q]."*

79. **Ans. b. Ejaculatory duct obstruction** *(Ref: Campbell 11/e p599; Smith 18/e p709)*

PROSTATE ANATOMY AND PHYSIOLOGY

80. **Ans. d. Prostate** *(Ref: Smith 18/e p369; Campbell 11/e p305; Bailey 27/e p1456-1457)*
81. **Ans. e. Radical prostatectomy** *(Ref: Bailey 27/e p1473; Campbell 11/e p2794)*

    HOT FLASHES

    - **Hot flashes** (also called **hot flushes**, **vasomotor symptoms**) have been recognized as a **side effect of androgen ablation (medical or surgical)**[Q]
    - Described as a **subjective feeling** of **warmth** in the **upper torso** and **head** followed by **objective perspiration**
    - Are among the **most common side effects of androgen ablation**[Q], affecting between **50%** and **80%** of patients
    - **Treatment** of hot flashes should be **reserved for** those who find them **bothersome**[Q].
    - **Drugs used** for treatment: **DES, oral progestogens, cyproterone acetate**, clonidine, sertraline, venlafaxine[Q]

82. **Ans. a. Diethylstilbestrol, b. LHRH analogues** *(Ref: Smith 18/e p372)*

Androgen Ablation Therapy for Prostate Cancer	
Level	**Agent**
Pituitary	• Diethylstilbestrol[Q] • Goserelin[Q] • Leuprolide[Q]
Adrenal	• Ketoconazole[Q] • Aminoglutethimide[Q]
Testicle	• Orchiectomy[Q]
Prostate cell	• **Bicalutamide**[Q] • **Flutamide**[Q] • **Nilutamide**[Q]

83. **Ans. None**
84. **Ans. b. Calcium phosphate** *(Ref: Smith 18/e p277; Campbell 11/e p305; Bailey 27/e p1468)*

CHAPTER 24

Urethra and Penis

HYPOSPADIAS

HYPOSPADIAS

- Hypospadias results when **fusion of urethral folds is incomplete**, and urethral **meatus opens** on the **underside of penis** or **perineum (ventral surface of penis)**[Q].

  - Occurs in **1:250 male births** and **multifactorial**[Q] in inheritance.
  - Hypospadias is MC congenital malformation of urethra[Q].

- Estrogens & progestins given during pregnancy increase the risk.
- **Anterior forms** are **more** common[Q] then posterior because fusion of urethral folds is from posterior to anterior.
- **70% cases** are **distal penile** or **coronal**[Q].
- **Circumcision is not done** in patients with hypospadias, as the prepuce can later be **used in surgical repair**[Q].

Types of Hypospadias		
• Glanular	• Penile	• Scrotal
• Coronal	• Penoscrotal	• Perineal
• Subcoronal		

- **Surgical pathology** in addition to ventrally placed ectopic meatus, hypospadias has:
- **Chordee** ventral curvature of penis due to contracture of fibrous cord which has replaced the distal urethra and corpus spongiosum. **Severity of chordee** is proportional to **degree of hypospadias**[Q].
- **Hooded prepuce** deficient on ventral aspect and excess **on dorsal aspect**[Q].
- **Stenosis of ectopic meatus**[Q]
- Multiple urethral orifices
- **Flattening of glans**[Q]
- Microphallus

Associated Abnormalities
- **Undescended testis**[Q] (10%) with or without sexual ambiguity
- **Inguinal hernia**[Q] (10%)
- Urinary tract abnormality (upper and lower)

Associated Problems
- Abnormal stream, **painful erection** (chordee) & **infertility** (in proximal or posterior types)[Q]

Management
- Treatment is not required in anterior variety. (repair is done for cosmetic reasons only)
- **Optimal time** of repair is **6–12 months**[Q].
- **Meatal advancement** or **local skin flap advancement**[Q] is the surgical procedure done along with removal of chordee.

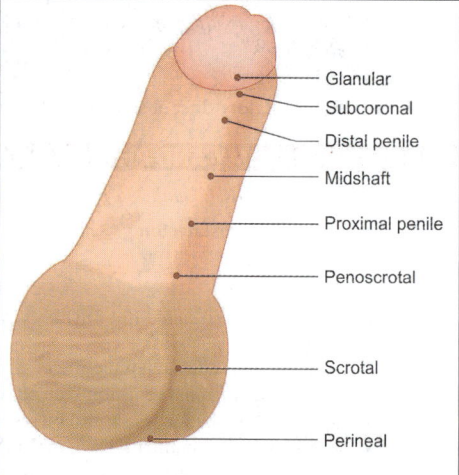

Named Procedures in Hypospadias
• **Dennis-Brown** technique (Two stage)[Q]
• **MAGPI**[Q] (Meatal advancement and glanuloplasty integrated) for coronal or subcoronal
• **Mathiew procedure**[Q] (Perimeatal based flap, one stage) for distal penile
• **Asopa** or **Duckett**[Q] technique using vascularized preputial island (one stage)
• **Thiersch-Duplay** or **Bracka**[Q] technique for proximal penile

Complications of Surgery
- MC complications is **urethral fistula**^{Q} (10%)
- **Meatal stenosis**^{Q} due to devascularisation of distal neourethra
- **Urethral stricture and stenosis** due to poor vascularity of flap, **persistent chordee**^{Q}

- Incidence of **hypospadias: 1 in 250**^{Q}
- Incidence of **horse-shoe kidney: 1 in 400** (0.25%)^Q
- Incidence of **renal agenesis: 1 in 1000**^{Q}

EPISPADIAS

EPISPADIAS

- Urethra opens on the **dorsum (upper aspect)** of the penis in males, in females there is a **fissure in the wall**^{Q} of the urethra which opens above the clitoris

Associated Anomalies
- **Extrophy of bladder**^{Q} (ectopia vesicae) with pubic diastasis and waddling gait
- **Dorsal Chordee**^{Q}
- VUR in 40% cases^Q

Clinical Features
- **Females:** Bifid clitoris & separation of the labia. Most are **incontinent**^{Q} because of maldevelopment of the urinary sphincters.
- **Males:** Patients with **glandular epispadias** seldom have urinary incontinence. However, incontinence in **penopubic is 95%** and **penile epispadias is 75%**^{Q}.
- Epispadias is a mild form of bladder exstrophy, and in severe cases, exstrophy and epispadias coexist.

Management
- **Surgery** is required to **correct the incontinence**, **remove the chordee** to straighten the penis, and **extend the urethra** out onto the glans penis^Q.
- **Bladder augmentation** combined with the **artificial sphincter** may be required in patients in whom incontinence cannot be corrected.

POSTERIOR URETHRAL VALVE

POSTERIOR URETHRAL VALVE

- **Symmetrical folds of urothelium** extending **distally from prostatic urethra to external urinary sphincter**^{Q}.

  - **Exclusively** an anomaly of **male urethra**^{Q}.
  - Four types, **Type 1 is MC** (lies just **distal to the verumontanum** or **at the verumontanum**)^Q

- Acts as a **flap valve**^{Q} (one way valve)- allows catheter, but balloons out during micturition and obstructs stream.

Clinical Features
- **Newborns** may present with **palpable abdominal masses** (distended bladder, hydronephrotic kidneys & ascites)^Q
- Infants with **urinary infection & sepsis**^{Q}.
- Sometimes, the valves are **incomplete**^{Q} and the patient remains **without symptoms** until adolescence or adulthood.
- Approximately **30%** of patients experience **end stage renal disease.**^{Q}
- **Vesicoureteral reflux** occurs in **50% of patients**^{Q}.

Associated with
- **Oligohydramnios**^{Q}
- Renal parenchymal dysplasia (**most important factor** in overall **prognosis**)^Q
- Abnormal bladder function (25%)^Q
- Pulmonary hypoplasia (**MC cause of death**)^Q

Investigations

- **Investigation of choice: MCU**^{Q} (shows proximal urethral dilatation with distal stricture)

- **Cystoscopy:** Shows dilation of urethra above valve.
- **Prenatal diagnosis by ultrasound**, showing **bilateral hydroureteronephrosis with enlarged thickened bladder** as early as **28 weeks**^{Q} of gestation (**Keyhole sign** on **prenatal** USG).

Management

- First a small polyethylene **feeding tube** is **inserted** in the bladder and left for several days. Then further management is done according to serum creatinine level.
  - **Normal serum creatinine** - transurethral ablation (**endoscopic fulgration**)[Q] of the valves
  - **Increased serum creatinine** and the worsening of condition – **vesicostomy (Blockson's technique is best)** to bypass the obstruction and **when normal creatinine levels** are achieved, transurethral ablation (**endoscopic fulgration**)[Q] is done.

Prognosis

- **Bladder dysfunction** and **renal hypoplasia** is associated with **poor prognosis** and is major cause of progressive renal failure[Q].
- **Pulmonary hypoplasia** is MC cause of **death**[Q].

PHIMOSIS

Phimosis

- Phimosis is a condition in which the **contracted foreskin cannot be retracted over the glans**[Q].
- **Chronic infection** from **poor local hygiene** is its **most common cause**[Q].
- Most cases occur in **uncircumcised males**, although excessive skin left after circumcision can become stenotic and cause phimosis.

Types

- Congenital
- **Acquired:** Usually presents late in life and associated with **inflammation, balanitis xerotica obliterans, trauma** or **cancer**[Q].

Clinical Features

- **Difficulty in micturition**[Q] is the main symptom.
- **Ballooning of prepuce during micturition**[Q] is suggestive of phimosis.
- Edema, erythema, and tenderness of the prepuce and the presence of purulent discharge usually cause the patient to seek medical attention.
- Inability to retract the foreskin is a less common complaint.

Complications

- Balanoposthitis, Hydronephrosis or hydroureter
- **Prepucial calculi, carcinoma under foreskin**[Q]

Treatment

- **Local steroid** cream for **4–6 weeks**[Q].

  > **Circumcision** should be done if **no response to steroids, recurrent balanitis** or **balanoposthitis, age > 16–18 years**[Q].

- If phimosis is associated with considerable **infection**, it should be treated with **broad-spectrum antimicrobial drugs**. The **dorsal slit of foreskin**[Q], if improved drainage is necessary.
- **Circumcision** for phimosis should be **avoided in children requiring general anesthesia; except** in cases with **recurrent infections**[Q].
- The procedure should be **postponed until** the child reaches an age when **local anesthesia** can be used.

PARAPHIMOSIS

Paraphimosis

- **Acquired** condition in which the **foreskin**, once retracted over the glans, **cannot be replaced** in its normal position.
- It is uncommon for the urethra to be compressed, so the **micturition** is normally **not affected**[Q].

Pathology

- **Chronic inflammation** under the redundant foreskin leads to **contracture** of **preputial opening** (phimosis) and formation of a **tight ring of skin** when the foreskin is retracted behind the glans.
- The **skin ring** causes **venous congestion** leading to **edema** and **enlargement** of the **glans**[Q].
- As the condition progresses, **arterial occlusion & necrosis of the glans**[Q] may occur.

Treatment

- **Ice bags, gentle manual compression**[Q] and injection of a solution of **hyaluronidase** in normal saline may help to reduce swelling.
- **Circumcision:** If conservative method fails

PRIAPISM

Priapism

- **Painful, persistent erection**^{Q} not normally associated with sexual excitement or desire, which does not subside after sexual excitement or desire.
- Most patients present with an **erection** of **at least 24 hours**^{Q} duration.
- **Priapism is an emergency**, if therapy is delayed for 36–48 hours, then marked tissue damage (due to ischemia) is likely to occur with **cavernosal fibrosis** and **impotence**^{Q}.

Types
- **High flow (non-ischemic) priapism**^{Q}: Occurs secondary to **penile or perineal trauma**, arterial sinusoidal shunt within corpus cavernosum.
- **Low flow (ischemic) priapism**^{Q}: Painful priapism, can lead to **compartment syndrome**, **more common** than high flow Priapism, caused by **Sickle cell anemia**, leukemia, spinal cord lesions, fat emboli, **malignant penile inflammation**^{Q}, autonomic neuropathy, drugs (**Trazadone**)^Q
- Majority due to **vasoactive intracorporeal injections**^{Q}

Clinical Presentation: Two peak ages
- **Children 5–10 years old**: Most common due to **sickle cell disease**^{Q}, attacks are usually nocturnal and the patient awakens with painful erection.
- **Adults 20–50 years**: Mostly **iatrogenic**^{Q}, priapism involves only corpora cavernosa. The spongiosum and glans are flaccid.

Diagnosis
- Diagnosis is **mainly clinical**^{Q}, only investigation useful to supplement clinical examination is **doppler**.

Treatment
- If present early, **within 4–6 hours**: **Ketamine**^{Q} (dissociative anesthesia) causes 50% detumescence.

> - **Aspiration** and **saline irrigation** till the aspirate is bright red, followed by injection of diluted **phenylephrine**^{Q}.
> - **Active treatment** in high flow priapism as it represents a **compartment syndrome**^{Q}.

- **Selective internal pudendal arteriography** and **selective embolization of** the **artery** feeding the shunt for **high flow non-ischemic priapism**^{Q}
- **Operative intervention:**
- **Winter's procedure** (percutaneous **cavernoglandular** shunt)^Q
  - Corpora spongiosa shunt
  - Corpora saphenous shunt

Surgical Management of Ischemic Priapism
(surgical creation of shunt to allow blood to drain from the corpora cavernosa)

Corporo-glanular shunt	Corporo-spongiosal shunt	Corporo-saphenous shunts	Corporo-dorsal vein shunt
• Shunts created between **glans penis** and **corpora cavernosa**^{Q}. • These are **distal shunts** and represent the **first line** surgical therapy. **Examples:** • Winter shunt^Q • Al-Ghorab shunt^Q • Ebbehoj and T shunt	• Shunts created between **corpora cavernosa** and **corpora spongiosa**^{Q} • These are **proximal shunts** and are performed in rare circumstances **Examples:** • **Quackel** or **Sacher shunt**^{Q}	• **Shunts** created between **corpora cavernosa** and **saphenous vein**^{Q} • Rarely performed **Examples:** • **Grayhack shunt**^{Q}	• Shunt between **corpora cavernosa** and superficial or deep **dorsal vein** of **penis**^{Q} • Rarely performed **Examples:** • **Barry shunt**^{Q}

PEYRONIE'S DISEASE

Peyronie's Disease

- Peyronie's disease (**plastic induration of penis/ penile fibromatosis**^{Q}) usually seen **over 40 years** of age.

> It is due to **fibrous plaques** in one or both corpus cavernosum of varying sizes **involving tunica albuginea**^{Q} which may later calcify or ossify.

- Cause remains obscure, the dense fibrous plaque is microscopically consistent with **findings of severe vasculitis**.
- Palmar fibromatosis (**Dupuytren's contracture**), plantar fibromatosis and penile fibromatosis (**Peyronie's disease**) are components of the same pathological process called **superficial fibromatosis**^{Q}.
- **Galezia's Triad: (DPR)** Dupuytren's contracture + Peyronie's disease + Retroperitoneal fibrosis^Q

Clinical Features
- **Painful erection**, **curvature of penis** and **poor erection distal to involved area**[Q].
- No pain when the penis is in nonerect state.
- **Palpable induration** or **mass** appears usually on the **dorsolateral aspect**[Q] of the penis.

Treatment
- **Spontaneous remission** occurs in about **50% cases**[Q], so observation & emotional support advised initially.
- If the penile deformity is distressing, **Nesbitt's operation**[Q] can be performed to straighten the penis.
- **Nesbitt operation**: Straightening of penis by **placing non-absorbable sutures** in **corpus cavernosum opposite** to the **plaque**.

URETHRAL INJURY

Urethral Injury
- Urethral injuries occur most often in **men**, usually associated with **pelvic fractures** or **straddle type falls**.
- Urethra is separated in two anatomic divisions:
  - **Posterior urethra: Prostatic urethra + Membranous urethra**[Q]
  - **Anterior urethra: Bulbous urethra + Penile urethra**[Q]

INJURIES TO POSTERIOR URETHRA

Injuries to Posterior Urethra

Etiology
- The part of urethra **most likely injured** in **pelvic fracture** is **membranous urethra**[Q].
- Membranous urethra is **sheared** at the bulbomembranous or **prostatomembranous junction**[Q].
- **Bulbomembranous junction** is **more prone than prostato membranous junction** during pelvic fracture (posterior urethra is densely adhered to pubis via urogenital diaphragm & puboprostatic ligaments)

Clinical Features
- **Retention of urine + Blood at urethral meatus + Pelvic hematoma and High lying prostate**[Q]
- Presence of blood at external urethral meatus indicates that **immediate urethrography**[Q] is necessary to establish the diagnosis.
- Associated with **deep extravasation** of **urine** in **pelvis** & **retroperitoneal tissues**[Q].
- **Pie in sky appearance**[Q] on **IVP** in **membranous urethral injury**.
- **Superior displacement** of **prostate does not occur** if the **puboprostatic ligaments** remain **intact**.

Instrumental Examination
- The only instrumentation involved should be for **urethrography**[Q].

> - **Catheterization or urethroscopy** should **not** be **done in every case** (as its associated with an **increased risk** of **hematoma, infection, and conversion of partial urethral tear** into **complete transection** of **urethra**)[Q].
> - In suspected **partial injury, gentle single attempt** to **catheterize** the patient **acts as** a **stent** over which **urethra heals**[Q].

Complications
- **Bladder rupture** may be associated with posterior urethral injuries in **20% of cases**[Q].
- **Stricture, impotence,** and **incontinence**[Q] are complications of prostatomembranous disruption.

> - **Stricture** following **primary repair** and **anastomosis** occurs in about **50% of cases**, with **delayed repair** incidence of stricture can be reduced to about **5%**[Q].

- The incidence of **impotence after primary repair** is 30–80%, can be **reduced to 30–35%** by **delayed urethral reconstruction**[Q].

Diagnosis
- When blood is noticed at meatus, **immediate RGU** should be done to rule out urethral injury.

Treatment

Immediate Management
- **No urethral instrumentation** or **manipulation** and **suprapubic cystostomy**

> - In suspected **partial injury, gentle single attempt** to **catheterize** the patient **acts as** a **stent** over which **urethra heals**.

- **Incomplete laceration** of the posterior urethra **heals spontaneously**, and the **suprapubic cystostomy** can be **removed within 2–3 weeks**[Q].
- **SPC** remains the **gold standard** for **initial management**, endoscopic alignment can be done **over guidewire** if patient presents **within 7–10 days**[Q].

Delayed Urethral Reconstruction
- **Reconstruction** of the urethra after prostatic disruption can be undertaken **within 3 months**[Q].

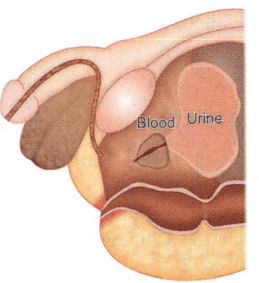
Injury to the posterior (membranous) urethra

INJURIES TO ANTERIOR URETHRA

INJURIES TO ANTERIOR URETHRA

Etiology
- **Direct blow to the perineum**^{Q} is the mechanism of injury.
- **Straddle injury**^{Q} may cause laceration or contusion of the urethra.
- **Self-instrumentation** or **iatrogenic instrumentation** may cause **partial disruption**^{Q}.

Pathology and pathogenesis: MC site is bulbar urethra.

A. Contusion
- Is a sign of crush injury without urethral disruption. Perineal hematoma usually resolves without complications.

B. Laceration
- A **severe straddle injury**^{Q} may result in laceration of part of the urethral wall, allowing extravasation of urine.
- If the **extravasation** is unrecognized, it may **extend into the scrotum, along the penile shaft, and up to the abdominal wall and limited only by Colles' fascia** and often results in **sepsis, infection,** and **serious morbidity**^{Q}.

Clinical Features
- Retention of urine + Blood at urethral meatus + Perineal hematoma and Normal prostate on P/R^Q
  - **Superficial extravasation** of urine, urine collects in **scrotum, anterior perineum,** beneath **superficial fascia** of **penis** and spreads **under fascia scarpa**^{Q}.
- **Massive urinary extravasation** and **infection** in the perineum and scrotum in delayed presentation

Complications
- **Heavy bleeding** from **corpus spongiosum** injury and urethral **meatus**^{Q}.
- **Sepsis and infection**^{Q} due to **urinary extravasation** (Aggressive debridement and drainage for infection)
- **Stricture** at the **site of injury**^{Q}

Treatment
- **Urethral contusion:**
  - After urethrography, if the voiding occurs normally, without pain or bleeding, no additional treatment.
- **Urethral lacerations:**
  - **Suprapubic cystostomy**^{Q} for complete urinary diversion while the urethral laceration heals.
- **Urethral laceration with extensive urinary extravasation:**
  - Suprapubic cystostomy for urinary diversion and antibiotic therapy for Infection and abscess formation

Prognosis
- **Urethral stricture** is a major complication but in **most cases** do **not require surgical reconstruction**^{Q}.

STRICTURE URETHRA

STRICTURE URETHRA

- Area of narrowing in the caliber of urethra due to formation of scar in the tissues surrounding the urethra
- Male urethra is **more prone** to **trauma** & **stricture**^{Q} formation.
- **Large catheters** and **instruments** are more likely than small ones to cause **ischemia, internal trauma** leading to **stricture**^{Q}.

Etiology
- **Traumatic (MC)**^{Q}, straddle injuries for anterior and pelvic fracture for posterior urethra

- Inflammatory or infectious (Infection from **long-term catheter use**^Q is a major cause, gonococcal urethritis is seldom a cause of strictures today)
- Ischemia
- Malignant
- Congenital (**Fossa navicularis** and **membranous urethra** is **MC site**^Q of congenital urethral stricture)

Pathophysiology
- Healing occurs by scar formation after injury to urothelium
- Process of **scar formation** occurs in **spongy erectile tissues**^Q (corpus spongiosa) of the penis that surrounds urethra (**spongiofibrosis**^Q)
- Scar tissue contracts, reduces the caliber of urethral lumen, causing **resistance** to **antegrade flow** of urine.

Clinical Features
Obstructive voiding symptoms
- **Decreased force** of urinary stream, improving with pressure (**MC**)^Q
- **Spraying** or **double stream**^Q
- **Incomplete emptying** of the bladder, **terminal dribbling** and urinary **intermittency**^Q
- Urinary retention, dilation of proximal urethra and prostatic ducts, urinary tract infections

Complications
- Prostatitis, cystitis, urinary diverticula and chronic UTI
- **Severe prolonged obstruction** result in decompensation of UV junction resulting in **reflux, hydronephrosis** and **renal failure**^Q
- **Urethral fistula** and **periurethral abscess**^Q commonly develop in association with chronic severe strictures

Diagnosis
- **Location, length, depth** and **density** of stricture should be evaluated for appropriate treatment.
- **Retrograde urethrogram** or **MCU**^Q to demonstrate location and extent of stricture

RGU
- MCU and RGU, both are required for adequate assessment
- MCU for posterior urethra, RGU for anterior urethra
- **Cystourethroscopy** for visualization of stricture
- **High frequency ultrasound** for **short bulbar strictures** (more accurate in measuring stricture length than RGU and is helpful in determining whether to excise or graft)
- **MRI** for defining the **distorted pelvic anatomy** associated with **posterior urethral strictures**^Q resulting from trauma.

Management
- **Periodic urethral dilations** to stretch the scar without producing additional scarring.
- **Internal urethrotomy**: Incising the stricture transurethrally using endoscopic equipment to release scar tissue. The incision is made under direct vision at **12 O'clock** position with urethrotome, with curative success rate of **20–35%** (**Good** success in **short strictures without spongiofibrosis**^Q)

Open Reconstruction
- **Excision & re-anastomosis** for strictures ≤ **2 cm**^Q: Complete excision of the fibrotic segment with a widely spatulated **tension-free re-anastomosis**, most dependable technique
- **Excision & tissue transfer** for strictures > **2 cm**^Q: Full-thickness skin graft tissue is harvested from the desired non-hair bearing location, **penile skin, bladder epithelium**, or **buccal mucosa** (**MC** and **best results**)^Q.
- **Urethral stents**: Endoscopically placed, designed to be incorporated into wall of urethra and provide a patent lumen.

CARCINOMA PENIS

Carcinoma Penis

- Most commonly occur in **6th decade**^Q of life, but "40% patients are less than 40 years"
- Most commonly associated etiologic factor is **poor hygiene**^Q
- **Phimosis**^Q is commonly associated (50%)

> - **Neonatal circumcision** confers **immunity**^Q against **CA penis, HIV** or **STDs**, but **not if done later.**

- Most important **carcinogens** are **smegma** and **HPV infection (16, 18, 31, 33)**^Q.

Premalignant Lesions
- **Buschke-Lowenstein tumour**^Q (Verrucous carcinoma): Tumour destroy adjacent tissue by compression, no metastasis usually. (Locally Malignant)
- **Balanitis Xerotica Obliterans**^Q: Whitish patch on glans, meatus and urethra, meatal stenosis.
- **Leukoplakia**^Q (more common in **diabetics**)
- Cutaneous horn
- Long standing genital warts

Carcinoma in Situ
- **Bowen's disease**^{Q}: Intraepithelial skin neoplasm (solitary thickened, grey white plaque with ulceration and scabbing) with HPV association in 80% cases. Converts into infiltrating **SCC in 10%**. **No high incidence of visceral malignancy**. When it involves **glans** and **prepuce**, it is called **Erythroplasia of Queyrat**^{Q}
- **Erythroplasia of Queyrat**^{Q}: **Red velvety plaques** over **glans** or **prepuce**, treated by **5% 5-FU cream** or ND YAG laser.

Clinical Features
- **Squamous cell carcinoma (80%)**^{Q} is the **MC type**, most commonly originates from glans^Q>prepuce>sulcus>shaft (GPS).
- Others are **transitional cell carcinoma (15%)**, basal cell carcinoma, malignant melanoma, sarcoma.
- **MC symptom** is **lesion itself** associated with foul smelling discharge.
- **Phimosis** is associated in **50%**.
- There is **little or no pain**.
- Lesions are typically confined to penis at the time of presentation.

> - **More than 50% patients** of CA Penis presents with **enlarged inguinal lymph nodes**^{Q}.
> - 50% of patients presenting with **enlarged inguinal lymph inguinal lymph nodes are reactive** (non-metastatic), used to **subside after 4-6 weeks of antibiotics**^{Q}.
> - **Priapism** is the MC and earliest symptom of metastatic CA penis^Q.
> - **MC cause of death** is bleeding caused by **erosion of femoral artery** by **metastatic inguinal lymph nodes**^{Q}.
> - **2nd MC** cause of death is **sepsis**.

- **Hypercalcemia**^{Q} is seen **in absence** of **osseous metastasis** in **20%** of patients, appears to **correlate with volume of disease**^{Q}.

Patterns of Spread
- **Buck's fascia**^{Q} and **tunica albuginea** represents a **barrier to corporal invasion** and **hematogenous spread**.
- Primary dissemination is to **inguinal**, **femoral** and **iliac** LNs.

> - **Prepuce** and **shaft skin** drain into the **superficial inguinal LNs**^{Q} (Superficial to tensor fascia lata).
> - **Glans** and **corporal bodies** drain to **both superficial** and **deep inguinal LNs**^{Q} (deep to tensor fascia lata).
> - **Anterior urethra** to **inguinal LN** and **posterior urethra** to **internal iliac LNs**.
> - **Penile drainage** is **bilateral** because of **multiple croos-connections**^{Q}.

- Penetration of buck's fascia and tunica albiginea leads to invasion of vascular corpora and vascular dissemination (rare).
- **Distant metastases** in **< 10% cases**, may involve **lung**, liver bone or brain.

Diagnosis
- **Good incisional biopsy**^{Q} from the periphery of the lesion from its junction with the normal tissue for grade and depth of invasion is **mandatory for diagnosis**.

> - **Sentinel lymph node biopsy (CABANA procedure)** is done for inguinal LN status.

Radiological Investigations
- Assessment of depth by **USG** or **MRI**^{Q} (CT is not effective)

> - **MRI is IOC for staging in CA penis**.

Treatment
- Without any treatment of invasive carcinoma, **death within 2 years**.
- Small non-invasive lesion involving prepuce: **5-FU cream, Nd-YAG laser, radiotherapy + close follow-up** is mandatory/ Wide excision or circumcision

> - Lesions involving **glans or distal shaft**: **Partial penectomy** with **2 cm margin**^{Q}
> - Lesions involving **proximal shaft** or 2 cm margins are not achieved: **Total penectomy** with **perineal urethrostomy**^{Q}.
> - **Bilateral Ilioinguinal LN dissection**^{Q} for metastatic lymph nodes.

- Chemotherapy used are **Bleomycin**, 5-FU, **Cisplatin**, methotrexate.
- **Radiotherapy** for selected **superficial small lesions**.

Prognosis
- Survival correlates with **presence** or **absence of nodal disease**^{Q}.

Jackson (Extent of spread)^Q Staging for CA Penis	
Stage I	Confined to **glans** or **prepuce**
Stage II	Extension to **shaft**
Stage III	**Operable inguinal LN metastasis**
Stage IV	**Inoperable** inguinal LN metastasis or **local** or **advanced spread**

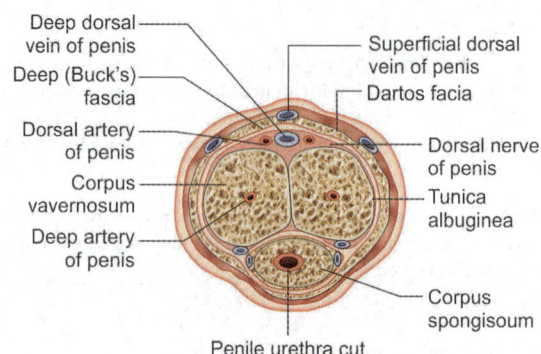

8th AJCC (2017) TNM Staging for CA Penis	
T: Primary tumor	**N: Regional lymph nodes**
Tis: Carcinoma in-situ^Q **Ta**: **Noninvasive verrucous carcinoma**^Q	**N1**: Palpable mobile **unilateral inguinal LN**^Q
T1a: Invades **subepithelial connective tissue** without lymphovascular invasion and is not poorly differentiated^Q	**N2**: Palpable mobile **multiple** or **bilateral inguinal LNs**^Q
T1b: Invades subepithelial connective tissue **with lymphovascular invasion** or **poorly differentiated**^Q	**N3**: **Fixed inguinal nodal masses** or **pelvic lymphadenopathy unilateral or bilateral**^Q
T2: Invades **corpus spongiosum** with or without invasion of urethra^Q	**M: Distant metastases**
T3: Invades **corpus cavernosum** with or without invasion of urethra^Q	
T4: Invades **other adjacent structures**^Q	M0: No distant metastasis M1: Distant metastasis present

Stage 0	Stage I	Stage IIA	Stage IIB	Stage IIIA	Stage IIIB	Stage IV
Tis N0M0 Ta N0M0	T1a N0M0	T1b N0M0 T2 N0M0	T3 N0M0	T1-3 N1 M0	T1-3 N2 M0	T4 anyN M0 Any T **N3** M0 Any T any N **M1**

CARCINOMA MALE URETHRA

Carcinoma of Male Urethra

- **Chronic irritation** and **infection**^Q are the strongest risk factors
- Incidence of **urethral stricture** in men with development of urethral cancer: 24–76%^Q
- **HPV-16**^Q has a causative role in SCC of urethra
- **MC presenting symptom: Palpable mass** associated with **obstructive voiding symptoms**^Q

Pathology
- **MC site** is **bulbomembranous urethra**^Q > penile urethra > prostatic urethra

> - Overall, **MC type is SCC**^Q > TCC > adenocarcinoma.
> - **MC type** of carcinoma **prostatic urethra** are **TCC**^Q > SCC.
> - **MC type** of carcinoma **penile urethra** are **SCC**^Q > TCC.

- Lymphatics of the **anterior urethra** drain into the **superficial** and **deep inguinal LNs**^Q
- Lymphatics of the **posterior urethra** drain into **external iliac, obturator** and **hypogastric LNs**^Q.

Diagnosis
- **MRI with gadolinium** is **IOC** for evaluating **local soft tissue, LNs metastasis**^Q

Treatment
- Surgery is **mainstay of treatment**^Q. Radiotherapy is also used.
- **Ilioinguinal node dissection** only in presence of palpable adenopathy.

Multiple Choice Questions

HYPOSPADIAS

1. **True about hypospadias:** *(JIPMER 2011)*
   a. Associated with chordee
   b. 50% associated with undescended testis
   c. Due to failure of fusion of posterior wall of urethra
   d. Circumcision done immediately

2. **True about hypospadias:** *(PGI May 2010)*
   a. Defect seen in ventral penis
   b. Always associated with chordee
   c. Associated with hooded prepuce
   d. Circumcision should be avoided

3. **Circumcision is contraindicated in:**
   (NEET 2013; WBPG 2012; GB Pant 2010)
   a. Paraphimosis   b. Meatal stenosis
   c. Hypospadias   d. Phimosis

4. **True about hypospadias is all except:** *(MHPGMCET 2003)*
   a. Sex determination is not possible
   b. Prepuce is hooded
   c. Incidence is 1 in 3000 male births
   d. May not require surgical treatment

5. **Most common congenital anomaly of urethra:**
   (MHSSMCET 2008)
   a. Hypospadias   b. Epispadias
   c. Meatal stenosis   d. PU valve

6. **Commonest hypospadias is:** *(DNB 2011, 2001, AIIMS Dec 95)*
   a. Penile   b. Glandular
   c. Scrotal   d. A or C

7. **All are true about hypospadias, except:** *(AIIMS June 93)*
   a. Circumcision in infancy is contraindicated
   b. Avoid surgery till puberty
   c. No treatment required in glandular variety
   d. If associated chordee is present, 2 stage operation is done

8. **The best time for surgery of hypospadias is:** *(All India 2003)*
   a. 1–4 months of age
   b. 6–10 months of age
   c. 12–18 months of age
   d. 2–4 years of age

9. **Features of hypospadias are all except:**
   a. Chordee   *(WBPG 2014, All India 98)*
   b. Hooded prepuce
   c. No-treatment required with glandular variety
   d. Cryptorchidism

10. **In hypospadias all are seen except:** *(BIHAR 2014; PGI Dec 99)*
    a. Hooded penis   b. Dorsal chordee
    c. Spatulated glans   d. Meatal stenosis

11. **Which is not true of hypospadias?** *(AIIMS 92)*
    a. Chordee is reversed after 5 years
    b. Glandular type needs no treatment
    c. Circumcision should not be done
    d. Surgical correction has good results in infancy

12. **Penis is curved in downward direction in all types of hypospadias except:** *(Recent Question 2016)*
    a. Glandular   b. Coronal
    c. Penile   d. Perineal

13. **In severe hypospadias the possibility of an intersex problem is settled by:**
    a. Careful inspection of genitals
    b. Biopsy for gonadal tissue
    c. Karyotyping   d. Hormone assay

14. **All of the following are seen in hypospadias except:**
    (All India 96)
    a. Ectopia vesicae   b. Hooded prepuce
    c. Chordee   d. Infertility

15. **Which of the following urethral anomaly is the most common?** *(TN 99)*
    a. Hypospadias   b. Pin hole meatus
    c. Epispadias   d. Stricture urethra

16. **Which of the following is true regarding hypospadias?**
    (APPG 2015)
    a. It is attributed to failure of complete urethral tubularisation in the fetus
    b. Urethral opening is most commonly in the perineum
    c. Urethra opens proximally and dorsally
    d. It is seen in 1 in 1500 boys

17. **Read the following statements and choose the appropriate answer:**
    Statement A (Assertion) - Ritual circumcision is contraindicated in infants with hypospadias
    Statement R (Reasoning) - In hypospadias, foreskin is deficient dorsally and there is a variable degree of chordee *(APPG 2016)*
    a. Statements A & R are both Correct but R is not the Reasoning for A
    b. Statement A is wrong but Statement R is Correct
    c. Statements A & R are both Correct and R is the reasoning for A
    d. Statement A is Correct but Statement R is wrong

18. **Which of the following developmental defects of the urogenital sinuses never occurs in the female?** *(APPG 2016)*
    a. All these defects can occur
    b. Hypospadias
    c. Ectopia vesicae
    d. Epispadias

19. **Best age for hypospadias repair:** *(Recent Question 2017)*
    a. Before 1 year   b. 2 years
    c. 4 years   d. 5 years

20. **Name of surgery in hypospadias:** *(Recent Question 2017)*
    a. Dennis-Brown   b. Ombridann's
    c. Ladd and Gross   d. Keetley-Torek

21. **Order of correction of hypospadias:** *(JIPMER November 2017)*
    a. Straightening of penis – Balanoplasty – Urethroplasty
    b. Urethroplasty – Balanoplasty – Straightening
    c. Straightening – Urethroplasty – Balanoplasty
    d. Balanoplasty – Urethroplasty – Straightening

EPISPADIAS

22. Epispadias is associated with: *(All India 2008)*
    a. Bifid pubic symphysis
    b. Chordee
    c. Anal atresia
    d. Intestinal obstruction

23. Epispadias in relation to hypospadias:
    a. Is more common
    b. Less common
    c. Occurs with the same frequency
    d. Is difficult to treat

POSTERIOR URETHRAL VALVE

24. All are true about posterior urethral valve except:
    a. Most common in boys *(GB Pant 2011)*
    b. Can be detected by prenatal USG
    c. Early catheterization should be done
    d. Diagnosed by early urethroscopy

25. A three years old boy presents with poor urinary stream. Most likely cause is: *(AIIMS June 2003)*
    a. Stricture urethra
    b. Neurogenic bladder
    c. Urethral calculus
    d. Posterior urethral valve

26. A male child with recurrent UTI with dribbling of urine most likely cause is: *(Punjab 2011)*
    a. VUR
    b. Posterior urethral valves
    c. Stricture urethra
    d. Neurogenic bladder

27. For posterior urethral valve-investigation of choice is: *(BIHAR PG 2014; AIIMS June 97, PGI Dec 2002, Dec 2003, June 2003)*
    a. Cystoscopy
    b. MCU
    c. Cystourethroscopy
    d. Retrograde urethroscopy

28. Posterior urethral valve are commonly observed in:
    a. Boys
    b. Girls
    c. Adult males
    d. Adult females

29. Most common uropathic obstruction in children is:
    a. Stricture *(UPPG 2009)*
    b. Stones
    c. Posterior urethral valve
    d. Anterior urethral valve

30. Most common location of posterior urethral valve: *(PGI SS 2004, MHPGMCET 2008)*
    a. Proximal to verumontanum
    b. Distal to verumontanum
    c. At the level of verumontanum
    d. At the bladder neck

31. Posterior urethral valve is usually seen:
    a. Above verumontanum *(MHSSMCET 2005, 2006, 2008)*
    b. Below verumontanum
    c. At the level of bladder neck
    d. At the level of verumontanum

PHIMOSIS

32. The recommended treatment for preputial adhesions producing ballooning of prepuce during micturition in a 2 years old boy is: *(AIIMS June 2003)*
    a. Wait and watch policy
    b. Circumcision
    c. Dorsal slit
    d. Preputial adhesions release and dilatation

33. A five years old child presents with ballooning of prepuce after micturition. Examination of penis reveals prepucial adhesions. Which of the following the best treatment:
    a. Adhesiolysis and dilatation *(All India 2011)*
    b. Circumcision
    c. Dorsal slit
    d. Conservative management

34. Which of the following statement is false about the given conditions?

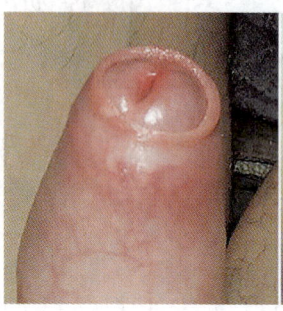 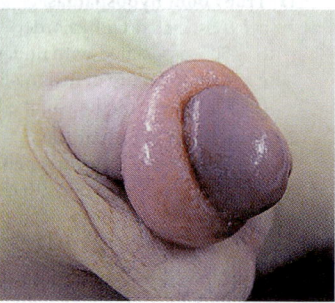

   a. Both 1 & 2 can be congenital
   b. Both 1 & 2 can be acquired
   c. Both 1 & 2 can be treated by circumcision
   d. None of the above

PARAPHIMOSIS

35. Not true about paraphimosis is: *(AIIMS June 98)*
    a. Iatrogenic
    b. Seen in diabetes mellitus
    c. Gangrene of glans
    d. Circumcision is the treatment

36. Which of the following are TRUE regarding the picture depicted here of a patient who underwent Foley's catheterization? *(APPG 2016)*
    (P) Obstruction of venous and lymphatic return from glans
    (Q) Commonly due to sickle cell anemia
    (R) The condition occurred due to the doctor forgetting to replace the retracted prepuce
    (S) Previous circumcision is the cause of this condition here

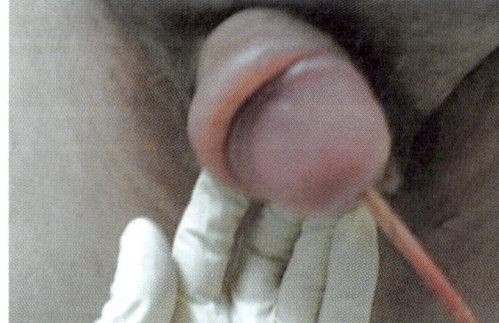

   a. PQRS are all true
   b. Only R and S are true
   c. Only P and R are true
   d. Only P and S are true

37. About paraphimosis true is: *(PGI June 96)*
    a. Catheter induced
    b. Circumcision is treatment
    c. Hyaluronidase injection
    d. All of the above

CIRCUMCISION

38. Circumcision is done in a child in which of the following conditions: *(TN 91)*
   a. Phimosis
   b. Recurrent balanitis
   c. Paraphimosis
   d. All of the above

39. Indications of circumcision are all except: *(MHPGMCET 2002)*
   a. Chronic balanoposthitis
   b. Jew religion
   c. Carcinoma penis
   d. Paraphimosis

40. All are true regarding circumcision except: *(JIPMER November 2017)*
   a. Hemorrhage due to bleeding from frenular artery
   b. Increases sexual drive
   c. Avoid correction of congenital anomaly
   d. Reduces sexually transmitted infections

PRIAPISM

41. The Grayhack shunt is established between: *(All India 2010)*
   a. Corpora cavernosa and corpora spongiosa
   b. Corpora cavernosa and saphenous vein
   c. Corpora cavernosa and dorsal vein
   d. Corpora cavernosa and glans

42. Persistent priapism is rarely seen as a consequence of: *(COMEDK 2010)*
   a. Sickle cell disease
   b. Leukemia
   c. Spinal cord disease
   d. Prolonged sexual activity

43. In Priapism, cavernous blood study will reveal:
   a. $PO_2 < 30\%$, $PCO_2 > 60\%$ *(MHSSMCET 2009)*
   b. $PCO_2 > 60\%$
   c. $PCO_2 > 60\%$
   d. $PO_2 < 60\%$

44. In children persistent priapism may result due to:
   a. Thrombosis of venous plexus
   b. Leukemia
   c. Wilms' tumour
   d. Trauma

45. Priapism in a polytrauma patient signify:
   a. Penile injury *(Recent Question 2017)*
   b. Spinal cord injury
   c. Significant head injury
   d. Pelvic injury

PEYRONIE'S DISEASE

46. Palpable fibrous plaque on dorsal penile shaft indicates: *(DPG 2005, Karnataka 95)*
   a. Paget's disease
   b. Potter's syndrome
   c. Prehn's sign
   d. Peyronie's disease

47. This condition is associated with which of the following?

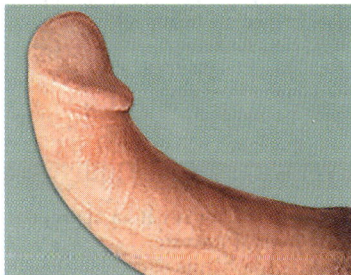

   a. Retroperitoneal fibrosis
   b. Dupuytren's contracture
   c. Both of the above
   d. None of the above

48. The following statements are true about Peyronie's disease except: *(AIIMS Nov 2002)*
   a. Patient presents with complaints of painful erection
   b. Condition affects adolescent males
   c. The condition can be associated with Dupuytren's contracture of the tendon of the hand
   d. Spontaneous regression occurs in 50% of the cases

49. All are true about Peyronie's disease except:
   a. Self limiting *(UPPG 2007, 2006)*
   b. Medical treatment is effective
   c. Association with Dupuytren's contracture
   d. Calcified plaques

50. Peyronie's disease is: *(MHPGMCET 2007)*
   a. Browning of penis
   b. Ectopic opening of urethra
   c. Curved deformity of penis due to fibrous plaque
   d. Absent glans penis

51. Nesbitt's operation is done for: *(MHPGMCET 2009, 2005)*
   a. Ectopic testis
   b. Hypospadias
   c. Peyronie's disease
   d. Any of the above

52. Peyronie's contracture is seen in: *(Recent Question 2014; 2013)*
   a. Dupuytren's disease
   b. Hypospadias
   c. Epispadias
   d. Exstrophy

URINARY TRACT INFECTION

53. What will be next investigation to be done in case of a 2 years old female child with 1st episode of UTI? *(AIIMS June 98)*
   a. Abdominal ultrasound
   b. DMSA scan
   c. 6 monthly urine culture
   d. Nothing actively needed

54. A child with recurrent urinary tract infection is most likely to show: *(All India 2005)*
   a. Posterior urethral valves
   b. Vesicoureteric reflux
   c. Neurogenic bladder
   d. Renal and ureteric calculi

55. Which fruit juice helps in preventing UTI? *(AIIMS Nov 2011, Nov 2006)*
   a. Grape
   b. Raspberry
   c. Cranberry
   d. Orange

56. Commonest organism giving rise to urinary tract infection: *(Recent Question, 2017)*
   a. E. coli
   b. Proteus
   c. Staphylococcus
   d. Streptococcus

57. Urinary tract infection exists when the bacterial count in 1 ml. midstream specimen of urine is: *(Recent Question, 2016)*
   a. 100
   b. 1000
   c. 10^4
   d. 10^5 or over

58. The most reliable urine specimen is obtained by: *(UPSC 2005)*
   a. Urethral catheterization
   b. Catheter aspiration
   c. Midstream voiding
   d. Suprapubic aspiration

URINARY RETENTION

59. Acute urinary retention in a male child may be due to: *(Recent Question 2016)*
   a. Prostatic radiotherapy
   b. Urethral stricture
   c. Hysteria
   d. Meatal ulcer with scabbing

60. Acute onset of anuria in elderly men:
   a. Bilateral infraction of kidneys
   b. Obstructive urinary disease
   c. Acute tubular necrosis
   d. Acute cortical

61. Most frequent causes of acute retention of urine include all except: *(DPG 2009 March)*
    a. Meatal ulcer with scabbing in children
    b. Haemorrhoidectomy
    c. Herniorrhaphy
    d. Fecal impaction

62. Urinary retention in child is most commonly caused by:
    a. Metal scab with ulceration *(PGI Dec 2003)*
    b. Posterior urethral valve
    c. Urethral stricture
    d. Epispadias
    e. Congenital short penis

URETHRAL INJURY

63. A 25 years old male presents to emergency department following a road traffic accident. On examination there is pelvic fracture and blood at urethral meatus. Following are true about patient except: *(AIIMS Nov 2002)*
    a. Anterior urethra is the most likely site of injury
    b. Retrograde urethrography should be done after the patient is stabilized
    c. Foley catheter may be carefully passed if the RGU is normal
    d. Rectal examination may reveal a large pelvic

64. Not true about urethral injuries is: *(AIIMS Nov 2001)*
    a. Catheterize the patient immediately
    b. Can be associated with fracture pelvis
    c. Bladder injury is associated with post urethral injuries
    d. Blood at the external urethral meatus is an imp feature

65. All of the following can be done in a case of pelvic fracture with pelvic hematoma and had not passed urine since trauma except: *(AIIMS Nov 99)*
    a. Pass indwelling urethral catheter
    b. IV fluid infusion
    c. IV pyelography
    d. Digital per rectal examination

66. Membranous urethral rupture causes collection of blood in:
    a. Ischiorectal fossa *(Recent Question, 2014; AIIMS Nov 93)*
    b. Deep perineal pouch
    c. Superficial inguinal region
    d. Pelvic diaphragm

67. All are true about bulbar urethral rupture, except:
    a. Perineal hematoma *(DNB 2011, AIIMS June 93)*
    b. Floating prostate on per rectal examination
    c. Collection of urine in perineum
    d. Bleeding per urethra

68. Following trauma, a patient presents with a drop of blood at the trip of urinary meatus. He complains of inability to pass urine. Next step should be: *(All India 2001)*
    a. IVP should be done
    b. MCU should be done
    c. Catheterize, drain bladder, and remove the catheter thereafter
    d. Catheterize, drain bladder and retain in catheter thereafter

69. In case of pelvic fracture with urethral injury, the most important first step in management is:
    a. Repair in injured urethra
    b. Fixation of pelvic fracture
    c. Treatment of shock and hemorrhage
    d. Splinting urethra with catheters

70. Commonest late complication of traumatic rupture of urethra is: *(JIPMER 92)*
    a. Diverticulum   b. Retrograde ejaculation
    c. Stricture   d. Chordee

71. Rupture of membranous urethra occurs more commonly due to: *(AIIMS 92)*
    a. Thin unsupported wall b. Fixity of urethra
    c. Angulation   d. Proximity to bladder

72. Treatment of fracture pelvis with rupture urethra is:
    a. Suprapubic cystostomy *(Kerala 95)*
    b. Explore and correct the fracture, repair urethra
    c. Catheterization
    d. Urethrogram to assess injury

73. Urine extravasation occurs in the following in case of penile urethral rupture, except: *(JIPMER 2003)*
    a. Ischiorectal fossa   b. Scrotum
    c. Abdomiadias
    d. Below superficial fascia of penis

74. A young man gets into a fight after taking beer and is kicked by the lower abdomen. There was pelvic fracture. Blood at meatus. Most likely cause is: *(MCI Nov 2017)*
    a. Rupture of membranous urethra
    b. Bulbar urethral injury
    c. Kidney laceration
    d. Ureteric injury

75. All the features of membranous urethral injury except:
    a. Blood of meatus   b. Retention of urine
    c. Pelvic fracture   d. None *(MAHE 2007, 2008)*

76. A patient was brought to the hospital with a history of RTA eight hours back. A few drops of blood were noted at the external urethral meatus. He had not passed urine and his bladder palpable per abdomen. The probable diagnosis is:
    a. Urethral injury *(AIIMS Nov 2006)*
    b. Rupture bladder
    c. Urethral injury with extravasation of urine in the retroperitoneum
    d. Anuria due to hypovolemia

77. With the knowledge of anatomy of the pelvis and perineum, which of the following is true regarding collection of urine in urethral rupture above deep perineal pouch? *(AIIMS Nov 2012)*
    a. Medial aspect of thigh b. Scrotum
    c. True pelvis only   d. Anterior abdominal wall

78. Following urethral rupture, immediate procedure to be done is: *(MCI Sept 2008, March 2009)*
    a. Urinary catheterization b. Suprapubic cystostomy
    c. Referral to a urologist d. Observation

79. A 32-year-old man with pelvic fracture is in urinary retention with blood at the external urinary means. Retrograde urethrogram shows prostatomembrane disruption. The most appropriate immediate treatment is: *(COMEDK 2014)*
    a. Urethral catheterization
    b. Exploration and repair of urethra
    c. Suprapubic cystostomy
    d. Perineal urethrostomy

URETHRAL STRICTURE

80. Which of the following is not an appropriate investigation for anterior urethral stricture? *(AIIMS June 97)*
    a. Magnetic resonance imaging
    b. Retrograde urethrogram
    c. Micturating cystourethrogram
    d. High frequency ultrasound

81. The commonest cause of an obliterative stricture of the membranous urethra is: *(All India 2003)*
    a. Fall-astride injury
    b. Road-traffic accident with fracture pelvis and rupture urethra
    c. Prolonged catheterization
    d. Gonococcal infection

82. What is the location of stricture in the given RGU?

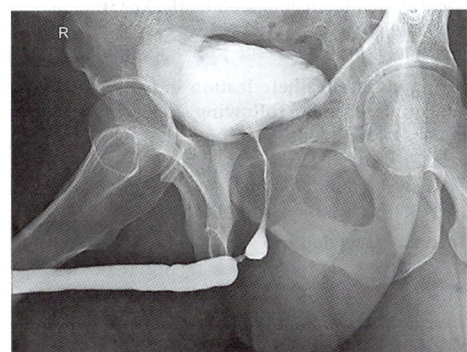

    a. Membranous urethra
    b. Bulbar urethra
    c. Penile urethra
    d. Prostatic urethra

83. The following are complications of stricture urethra except: *(Karnataka 96)*
    a. Periurethral abscess
    b. Inguinal hernia
    c. Hydronephrosis
    d. Papilloma of bladder

84. Commonest cause of urethral stricture in a young person is:
    a. Trauma
    b. Gonococcal *(Karnataka 96)*
    c. Syphilis
    d. Tuberculosis

85. The recent treatment of short bridle passable stricture of urethra in the penile and bulbous urethra is:
    a. Internal urethrotomy with Thompson-Walker's urethrotome *(MAHE 2005)*
    b. Optical internal urethrotomy
    c. Syme's operation
    d. Wheelhouse operation

86. Optical urethroplasty is done in: *(UPPG 2007)*
    a. Congenital stricture of urethra
    b. Hypospadias
    c. Epispadias
    d. Testicular tumors

87. On exertion urine stream increased in: *(APPG 96)*
    a. Prostate enlargement
    b. Marion's disease
    c. Posterior urethral valves
    d. Urethral stricture

88. Post gonococcal stricture urethra is most commonly situated in the: *(Recent Questions 2015)*
    a. Bulbar urethra
    b. Penoscrotal junction
    c. Distal part of spongy urethra
    d. Just distal to external meatus

89. Most common cause of urethral stricture is: *(Recent Questions 2013)*
    a. Trauma
    b. Infection
    c. Congenital
    d. Post endoscopy

90. A 40 years old patient of pelvic injury presents with stricture of bulbar urethra of 1.5 cm length. Best management:
    a. Urethral dilatation *(Recent Question 2017)*
    b. Excision with end-to-end urethroplasty
    c. Partial graft urethroplasty
    d. Urethrotomy

CARCINOMA PENIS

91. True about verrucous carcinoma is all except: *(Punjab 2009)*
    a. Locally aggressive form of condyloma acuminate
    b. Also known as Buschke-Lowenstein Tumor
    c. They frequently metastasize
    d. Wide excision is the treatment of choice

92. Buschke-lowenstein tumor is: *(MHCET 2016)*
    a. Malignant transformation in plantar wart
    b. Malignant transformation in anogenital wart
    c. Malignant transformation in common wart
    d. Malignant transformation in seborrheic wart

93. What is the name of this penile tumor?

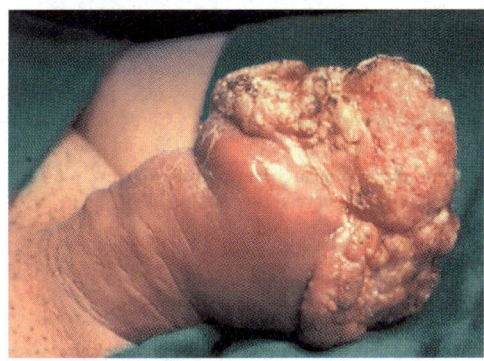

    a. Bowen's disease
    b. Erythroplasia of Queyrat
    c. Buschke-Lowenstein tumor
    d. None of the above

94. In CA penis, soft tissue planes are best delineated by:
    a. MRI
    b. CT scan *(GB Pant 2011)*
    c. X-ray
    d. USG

95. The most common cause of death in carcinoma penis: *(MHPGMCET 2008, AIIMS Nov 94)*
    a. Uremia
    b. Urinary sepsis
    c. Lung metastases
    d. Erosion of femoral vessels

96. Cabana procedure is done in: *(GB Pant 2010)*
    a. CA testis
    b. RPLND
    c. Sentinel LN biopsy in penile carcinoma
    d. None

97. Sentinel lymph node of carcinoma penis: *(MHSSMCET 2006)*
    a. Cabana
    b. Virchow
    c. Delphian
    d. Darwins

98. Erythroplasia of Queyrat occurs in: *(MCI Sept 2008)*
    a. Scrotum
    b. Testes
    c. Penis
    d. Bladder

99. Not true about carcinoma penis is: *(AIIMS Nov 2001)*
    a. Erythroplasia of Queyrat is a precancerous condition
    b. 40% of patients are under 40 years of age
    c. Circumcision if done any time before puberty provides 100% protection against carcinoma penis
    d. More than 50% patients have inguinal LN enlargement when they present

100. What is true about carcinoma penis? *(AIIMS June 94)*
    a. Metastasis is rare
    b. Occurs more commonly in circumcised male
    c. Arises from corona of glans
    d. Pain is frequent

101. Circumcision is included in management of CA penis at:
    a. Glans *(PGI Dec 98)*
    b. Prepuce
    c. Glandulo prepucial
    d. Shaft of penis

102. Features of carcinoma penis are all except: *(Recent Question 2017)*
    a. Circumcision soon after birth provides total immunity
    b. Metastatic to inguinal nodes
    c. Surgery is treatment of choice
    d. Transitional cell carcinoma

103. Treatment of choice of small preputial penile carcinoma is: *(Recent Question 2016)*
    a. Total penectomy
    b. Partial penectomy
    c. Emasculation
    d. Wide excision

104. Sentinel lymph node biopsy was first done in: *(Recent Question 2017, DNB 2012)*
    a. Carcinoma breast
    b. Carcinoma colon
    c. Carcinoma penis
    d. Melanoma

105. All are true about carcinoma penis except: *(Recent Question 2013)*
    a. Most common type is verrucous
    b. Spreads by blood borne metastasis
    c. Leads to erosion of artery
    d. Slowly progressive

URETHRAL CARCINOMA

106. Most common site of urethral carcinoma in men is: *(Recent Question 2016, All India 2010)*
    a. Bulbomembranous urethra
    b. Penile urethra
    c. Prostatic urethra
    d. Fossa navicularis

MISCELLANEOUS

107. True about congenital short urethra: *(PGI Dec 2003)*
    a. Urethra is short
    b. Opening is always ventral
    c. Prepuce deficient ventrally
    d. Splitting of the two secrotum in the midline
    e. Spatulated penis

108. The posterior urethra is best visualized by: *(AIIMS Nov 2005)*
    a. Static cystogram
    b. Retrograde urethrogram
    c. Voiding cystogram
    d. CT cystogram

109. Length of the male urethra: *(Recent Question 2016)*
    a. 10 cm
    b. 15 cm
    c. 20 cm
    d. 25 cm

110. Length of female urethra: *(Recent Question 2017)*
    a. 2 cm
    b. 4 cm
    c. 6 cm
    d. 8 cm

111. Which part of the male urethra is the widest and most distensible? *(Recent Question 2016, 2015)*
    a. Prostatic
    b. Membranous
    c. Bulbous
    d. Penile

112. The least dilatable part of the urethra:
    a. Prostatic
    b. Membranous
    c. Spongy
    d. All are equally dilatable

113. Bleeding penile ulcer is seen in all except: *(Kerala 94)*
    a. Syphilis
    b. LGV
    c. Chancroid
    d. Granuloma inguinale

114. During urethral catheterization in male patients, resistance is encountered at the following sites except: *(ICS 2005)*
    a. Base of navicular fossa
    b. Mid-penile urethra
    c. Urogenital diaphragm
    d. Bulbomembranous junction

115. Smegma is secreted by: *(DPG 2008)*
    a. Tyson gland
    b. Brenner gland
    c. Cowper's gland
    d. Bartholin's gland

116. There is a high-risk of renal dysplasia in: *(AIIMS June 2003)*
    a. Posterior urethral valve
    b. Bladder exstrophy
    c. Anorectal malformation
    d. Neonatal sepsis

117. Which of the following catheter materials is most suited for long-term is used? *(All India 2005)*
    a. Latex
    b. Silicone
    c. Rubber
    d. Polyurethane

118. All are indications for penile angiography except:
    a. Painful priapism *(AIIMS May 2009)*
    b. Peyronie's disease
    c. Erectile dysfunction
    d. Arterio-venous malformation

119. Narrowest part of urethra: *(PGI SS June 2001)*
    a. External urethral meatus
    b. Membranous urethra
    c. Prostatic urethra
    d. Bladder neck

120. Narrowest part of the urethra is: *(MCI March 2009)*
    a. Prostatic urethra
    b. Bulbar urethra
    c. Penile urethra
    d. Membranous urethra

121. Which of the following is the shortest urethra? *(Recent Question 2017)*
    a. Bulbar
    b. Prostatic
    c. Penile
    d. Membranous

122. Chordee is not seen in: *(MHSSMCET 2005)*
    a. Hypospadias
    b. Chronic urethritis
    c. Priapism
    d. Peyronie's disease

123. In "three glass test" shreds are presents in first glass only. The most probable diagnosis is: *(DNB 2012)*
    a. Urethritis
    b. Cystitis
    c. Prostatitis
    d. Renal pathology

Explanations

HYPOSPADIAS

1. Ans. a. Associated with chordee *(Ref: Smith's 18/e p637; Campbell 11/e p3399-3401; Bailey 27/e p1478)*
2. Ans. a. Defect seen in ventral penis; c. Associated with hooded prepuce; d. Circumcision should be avoided
3. Ans. c. Hypospadias
4. Ans. c. Incidence is 1 in 3000 male births
5. Ans. a. Hypospadias
6. Ans. b. Glandular
7. Ans. b. Avoid surgery till puberty; d. If associated chordee is present, 2 stage operation is done
8. Ans. b. 6–10 months of age
9. Ans. d. Cryptorchidism
10. Ans. b. Dorsal chordee
11. Ans. a. Chordee is reversed after 5 years
12. Ans. a. Glandular
13. Ans. c. Karyotyping
14. Ans. a. Ectopia vesicae
15. Ans. a. Hypospadias
16. Ans. a. It is attributed to failure of complete urethral tubularisation in the fetus
17. Ans. d. Statement A is Correct but Statement R is wrong
18. Ans. b. Hypospadias
19. Ans. a. Before 1 year *(Ref: Campbell 11/e p3401; Smith 18/e p639; Bailey 27/e p1478)*
20. Ans. a. Dennis-Brown *(Ref: Campbell 11/e p3410)*
21. Ans. c. Straightening – Urethroplasty – Balanoplasty

EPISPADIAS

22. Ans. b. Chordee *(Ref: Smith 18/e p639; Campbell 11/e p3221; Bailey 27/e p1478)*
23. Ans. b. Less common

POSTERIOR URETHRAL VALVE

24. Ans. d. Diagnosed by early urethroscopy *(Ref: Smith 18/e p636; Campbell 11/e p2880; Bailey 27/e p1477)*
25. Ans. d. Posterior urethral valve
26. Ans. b. Posterior urethral valves
27. Ans. b. MCU
28. Ans. a. Boys
29. Ans. c. Posterior urethral valve
30. Ans. b. Distal to verumontanum
31. Ans. b. Below verumontanum

PHIMOSIS

32. Ans. a. Wait and watch policy *(Ref: Smith 18/e p640; Campbell 11/e p3370; Bailey 27/e p1486)*
33. Ans. d. Conservative management
34. Ans. a. Both 1 & 2 can be congenital *(Ref: Schwartz 10/e p1664; Bailey 27/e p1486, 1489)*

> Phimosis (1) can be congenital and acquired but paraphimosis (2) is only acquired.

PARAPHIMOSIS

35. Ans. b. Seen in diabetes mellitus *(Ref: Smith 18/e p641; Campbell 11/e p3364-3370; Bailey 27/e p1489)*
36. Ans. c. Only P and R are true
37. Ans. d. All of the above

CIRCUMCISION

38. Ans. d. All of the above *(Ref: Smith 18/e p641; Bailey 27/e p1487)*

Circumcision is indicated in patients with infection, phimosis or paraphimosis.

39. **Ans. c. Carcinoma penis** *(Ref: Smith 18/e p641)*

Indications of Circumcision	
• Phimosis[Q]	• Religion (Jews and Muslims)[Q]
• Paraphimosis[Q]	• Balanitis or balanoposthitis[Q]
• Recurrent UTI[Q]	• BXO (balanitis xerotica obliterans)

40. **Ans. b. Increases sexual drive** *(Ref: Smith18/e p641; Bailey 27/e p1487)*

PRIAPISM

41. **Ans. b. Corpora cavernosa and saphenous vein** *(Ref: Smith 18/e p640; Campbell 11/e p684; Bailey 27/e p1491; Glenn's Urologic Surgery 7/e p489, 490, 491)*

    The **Grayhack shunt** is a surgical **shunt between corpora cavernosa** and **saphenous vein** for the treatment of **ischemic priapism**.

42. **Ans. c. Spinal cord disease** *(Ref: Bailey 27/e p1491; Campbell 11/e p671)*

    Priapism is **rarely seen** as a consequence of **spinal cord disease**.

    ### Persistent Priapism
    - The **penis** remains **erect** and becomes **painful**.
    - This is a **pathological erection** and the **glans penis** and **corpus spongiosum** are **not involved**[Q].
    - The condition is **usually seen as a complication of** a blood disorder such as **sickle cell disease** or **leukaemia**[Q].
    - However, it can sometimes follow **therapeutic injection of papaverine** or even an **abnormally prolonged bout** of otherwise **normal sexual activity**[Q].
    - A **tiny proportion** is caused by **malignant disease** in the **corpora cavernosa** or the **pelvis**.
    - **Priapism** is **rarely seen** as a consequence of **spinal cord disease**[Q].

43. **Ans. a. $PO_2 < 30\%$, $PCO_2 > 60\%$** *(Ref: Campbell 11/e p678)*

Blood Gas Values in Priapism			
Source	PO_2 (mm Hg)	PCO_2 (mm Hg)	pH
• Normal arterial blood • (room air)	> 90	< 40	7.40
• Normal mixed venous • blood (room air)	40	50	7.35
• **Ischemic Priapism** • (first corporal aspirate)	**< 30**[Q]	**> 60**[Q]	**< 7.25**[Q]

44. **Ans. b. Leukemia**

45. **Ans. b. Spinal cord injury**

PEYRONIE'S DISEASE

46. **Ans. d. Peyronie's disease** *(Ref: Smith' 18/e p640; Campbell 11/e p722-725; Bailey 27/e p1490)*

47. **Ans. c. Both of the above** *(Ref: Sabiston 20/e p2019; Schwartz 10/e p1461; Bailey 27/e p1490)*

    The given condition is called Peyronie's disease. Galezia's triad components are Peyronie's disease + Retroperitoneal fibrosis + Dupuytren's contracture.

48. **Ans. b. Condition affects adolescent males**

49. **Ans. b. Medical treatment is effective**

50. **Ans. c. Curved deformity of penis due to fibrous plaque**

51. **Ans. c. Peyronie's disease**

52. **Ans. a. Peyronie's disease**

URINARY TRACT INFECTION

53. **Ans. a. Abdominal ultrasound** *(Ref: Smith 18/e p198; Campbell 11/e p253)*

This patient must be having anatomic genitourinary abnormalitis (VUR), and the next best investigation is USG.

Epidemiology of UTI by Age Group and Sex

Age (years)	Incidence (%) Female	Incidence (%) Male	Risk Factors
< 1	0.7	2.7	Foreskin, **anatomic GU abnormalities**
1–5	4.5	0.5	**Anatomic** genitourinary (**GU**) **abnormalities**
6–15	4.5	0.5	Functional GU abnormalities
16–35	20	0.5	Sexual intercourse, diaphragm use
36–65	35	20	Surgery, prostate obstruction, catheterization
> 65	40	35	Incontinence, catheterization, prostate obstruction

ULTRASOUND

- **Ultrasound study** is an important renal imaging technique because it is **noninvasive, easy to perform,** and rapid and offers **no radiation** or **contrast agent risk** to the patient^Q.

54. **Ans. b. Vesicoureteric reflux**

55. **Ans. c. Cranberry** *(Ref: Smith 18/e p204)*

- **Alternatives to antibiotic therapy** in the **treatment of recurrent cystitis/UTI** include **intravaginal estriol, lactobacillus vaginal suppositories,** and **cranberry juice taken orally**^{Q}.
- **Cranberry juice** is traditionally **used for prophylaxis** and **treatment of UTI**^{Q}.

56. **Ans. a. E. coli** *(Ref: Smith 18/e p199)*

URINARY TRACT INFECTION

- **Most UTIs** are caused **by a single bacterial species**^{Q}.
- At least 80% of the **uncomplicated cystitis** and **pyelonephritis** are due to **E. coli**^{Q}, with most of pathogenic strains belonging to the **O serogroups**.
- Other less common uropathogens include Klebsiella, Proteus, and Enterobacter spp. and enterococci.
- In **hospital acquired UTIs**, a wider variety of causative organisms is found, including **Pseudomonas** and **Staphylococcus** spp^Q.

  - **UTIs** caused by **S. aureus** often result from **hematogenous dissemination**^{Q}.
  - **Group B beta-hemolytic streptococci** can cause **UTIs in pregnant women**^{Q}.
  - In **children**, Klebsiella and Enterobacter spp. are **common causes of UTI**^{Q}.

- **Anaerobic bacteria, lactobacilli, corynebacteria, streptococci** (not including enterococci) and **S. epidermidis** are found in **normal periurethral flora**. They do not commonly cause UTIs in healthy individuals and are considered common **urinary contaminants**^{Q}.

57. **Ans. d. 10^5 or over** *(Ref: Smith 18/e p200)*

Traditionally, > 100,000 CFU/mL (> 10^5) is **used to exclude contamination**.

URINE CULTURE IN UTI

- The **gold standard for identification of UTI** is the **quantitative culture** of **urine** for **specific bacteria**^{Q}.
- The urine should be collected in a **sterile container** and **cultured immediately after collection**. When this is not possible, the urine **can be stored** in the **refrigerator for up to 24 hours**.
- The sample is then diluted and spread on culture plates. Each bacterium will form a single colony on the plates.
- The **number of colonies** is counted and adjusted per milliliter of urine (CFU/mL).
- Traditionally, > 100,000 CFU/mL (> 10^5) ^{Q} is **used to exclude contamination**.

58. **Ans. d. Suprapubic aspiration** *(Ref: Smith 18/e p200)*

Suprapubic aspiration avoids potential contamination.

URINARY TRACT INFECTION

- Most often, the **urine** is often obtained from a **voided specimen**.
- **In children** who are not toilet trained, a **urine collection device**, such as a bag, is placed over the genitalia, and the urine is cultured from the bagged specimen.

  - **Suprapubic aspiration avoids potential contamination**^{Q}; however, due to its invasiveness, it is **rarely used except in children** and **selected patients**.

- **Urine** obtained **from a urinary catheter** is **less invasive** than a suprapubic aspiration and is **less likely to be contaminated than** that from a **voided specimen**^{Q}.

URINARY RETENTION

59. **Ans. d. Meatal ulcer with scabbing** *(Ref: Bailey 27/e p1426)*

    Acute urinary retention in a male child may be due to local inflammatory causes like meatal ulcer with scabbing.

Etiology of Urinary Retention in Children	
• **Neurological** processes (**17%**)	• Locally invading neoplasms (6%)
• **Severe voiding dysfunction** (15%)	• Benign obstructing lesions (6%)
• UTI (13%)	• Idiopathic (6%)
• Constipation (13%)	• Combined UTI and constipation (2%)
• Adverse drug effect (13%)	• Incarcerated inguinal hernia (2%)
• **Local inflammatory causes** (7%)	

60. **Ans. b. Obstructive urinary disease** *(Ref: Bailey 27/e p1426)*

Most Frequent Causes of Acute Urinary Retention		
Male	**Both (Males and Females)**	
• **Bladder outlet obstruction** (MC) • Urethral stricture • Acute urethritis or prostatitis • Phimosis	• **Blood clot** • **Urethral calculus** • **Rupture** of the **urethra** • **Neurogenic** (injury or disease of the spinal cord) • **Smooth muscle cell dysfunction** associated with ageing	• **Fecal impaction** • **Anal pain** (haemorrhoidectomy) • Intensive post-operative analgesic treatment • Some drugs • **Spinal anaesthesia**
Female		
• Retroverted gravid uterus • Bladder neck obstruction (rare)		

    URINARY RETENTION
    - In **acute urinary retention** with significant **bladder distention, rapid drainage** might precipitate **decompression induced hematurea (Ex-vacuo hematurea)**^{Q}
    - Catheter should be **intermittently clamped** and released to permit **gradual** bladder **decompression** over 30–60 minutes^Q.

61. **Ans. c. Herniorrhaphy**
62. **Ans. a. Meatal scab with ulceration**

URETHRAL INJURY

63. **Ans. a. Anterior urethra is the most likely site of injury** *(Ref: Smith 18/e p294; Campbell 11/e p2388; Bailey 27/e p1479)*
64. **Ans. a. Catheterize the patient immediately**
65. **Ans. a. Pass indwelling urethral catheter**
66. **Ans. b. Deep perineal pouch**
67. **Ans. b. Floating prostate on per rectal examination** *(Ref: Smith 18/e p294; Campbell 11/e p2391; Bailey 27/e p1481)*
68. **Ans. d. Catheterize, drain bladder and retain in catheter thereafter**
69. **Ans. c. Treatment of shock and hemorrhage**
70. **Ans. c. Stricture**
71. **Ans. b. Fixity of urethra**
72. **Ans. a. Suprapubic cystostomy**
73. **Ans. a. Ischiorectal fossa** *(Ref: Smith 18/e p292; Campbell 11/e p2391; Bailey 27/e p1479-1481)*

	Bulbar Urethral Injury	Membranous Urethral Injury
Incidence	• **More common**^{Q}	• Less common
Mechanism of injury	• **Direct blow** to the perineum (**Straddle injury**)^Q	• **Blunt pelvic trauma** with **fracture pelvis**^{Q}
Signs and symptoms	• Retention of urine^Q • Blood at urethral meatus^Q • **Perineal** hematoma^Q • Normal prostate^Q	• Retention of urine^Q • Blood at urethral meatus^Q • **Pelvic** hematoma^Q • **High lying prostate**^{Q}
Urine extravasation	• **Superficial extravasation**^{Q}	• **Deep extravasation**^{Q}

74. **Ans. a. Rupture of membranous urethra**
75. **Ans. d. None**
76. **Ans. a. Urethral injury**
77. **Ans. c. True pelvis only**
78. **Ans. b. Suprapubic cystostomy**
79. **Ans. c. Suprapubic cystostomy**

URETHRAL STRICTURE

80. **Ans. a. Magnetic resonance imaging** *(Ref: Smith 18/e p642; Campbell 11/e p918-919)*

STRICTURE URETHRA

- Use of MRI for routine strictures or pelvic fracture urethral distraction defect is not routinely beneficial.

81. **Ans. b. Road-traffic accident with fracture pelvis and rupture urethra**
82. **Ans. b. Bulbar urethra** *(Ref: Sabiston 20/e p2093; Schwartz 10/e p1665; Bailey 27/e p1483)*

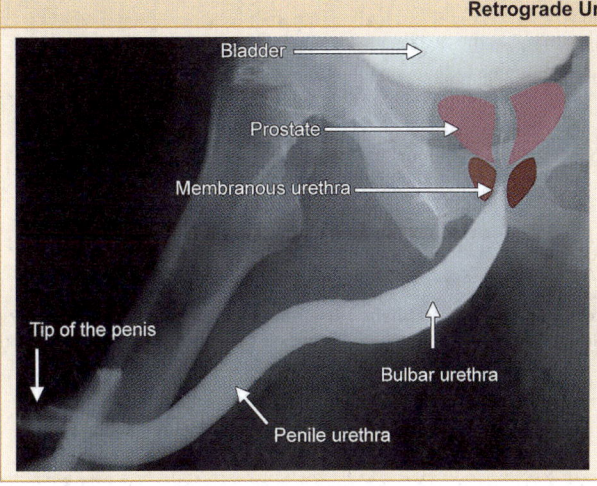
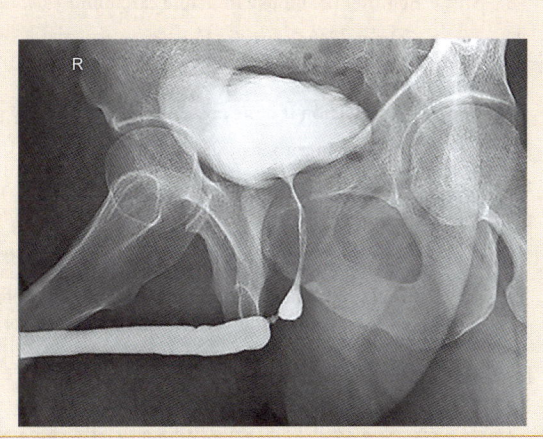

Retrograde Urethrogram

83. **Ans. d. Papilloma of bladder**
84. **Ans. a. Trauma**
85. **Ans. b. Optical internal urethrotomy** *(Ref: Campbell 11/e p921, 10/e p971-972)*

Campbell says "The data show that **strictures at the bulbous urethra** that are **< 1.5 cm in length** and **not associated with dense, deep spongiofibrosis** (i.e. straddle injuries) can be **managed with internal urethrotomy, with a 74% moderately long-term success rate**."

INTERNAL URETHROTOMY

- **Internal urethrotomy** refers to any procedure that **opens the stricture** by **incising it transurethrally**[Q].
- **Internal urethrotomy** is done for **short, soft, passable, bulbar stricture**.
- The urethrotomy procedure **involves incision through the scar to healthy tissue** to allow the **scar to expand (release of scar contracture)**[Q] and the lumen to heal enlarged.
- **MC complication** of **internal urethrotomy** is recurrence of stricture.
- The data show that **strictures at the bulbous urethra** that are **< 1.5 cm in length** and **not associated with dense, deep spongiofibrosis**[Q] (i.e. straddle injuries) can be **managed with internal urethrotomy, with a 74% moderately long-term success rate**[Q].

86. **Ans. a. Congenital stricture of urethra** *(Ref: www.ncbi.nlm.nih.gov › Postgrad Med J › v.82(970); Aug 2006)*

- **Short bulbar strictures** as a result of trauma or otherwise **congenital** are **best treated by anastomotic urethroplasty**[Q].

87. **Ans. d. Urethral stricture**
88. **Ans. a. Bulbar Urethra**
89. **Ans. a. Trauma**
90. **Ans. b. Excision with end-to-end urethroplasty** *(Ref: Campbell 11/e p921)*

"Excision with primary anastomosis has proved to be the gold standard form of repair for anterior urethral strictures. In years past, excision with primary anastomosis was thought to be a relatively limited procedure and applicable only for strictures less than 1.5 to 2.0 cm. However, with better understanding of the anatomy, longer and longer strictures have been successfully addressed with excision and primary anastomosis." –Campbell 11/e p921

CARCINOMA PENIS

91. Ans. c. They frequently metastasize *(Ref: Smith 18/e p389; Campbell 11/e p849; Bailey 27/e p1492)*
92. Ans. b. Malignant transformation in anogenital wart *(Ref: Campbell 11/e p848)*
93. Ans. c. Buschke-Lowenstein tumor *(Ref: Schwartz 10/e p1218; Bailey 27/e p1493)*

> "Buschke–Löwenstein tumour is uncommon. It has the histological pattern of a verrucous carcinoma. It is locally destructive and invasive but appears not to spread to lymph nodes or to metastasise. Treatment is by surgical excision." –Bailey 27/e p1493

94. Ans. a. MRI *(Ref: Campbell 11/e p851)*
95. Ans. d. Erosion of femoral vessels *(Ref: Campbell 11/e p849)*
96. Ans. c. Sentinel LN biopsy in penile carcinoma *(Ref: Campbell 11/e p850)*
97. Ans. a. Cabana *(Ref: Campbell 11/e p850)*
98. Ans. c. Penis *(Ref: Campbell 11/e p848)*
99. Ans. c. Circumcision if done any time before puberty provides 100% protection against carcinoma penis *(Ref: Campbell 11/e p847)*
100. Ans. c. Arises from corona of glans
101. Ans. b. Prepuce
102. Ans. d. Transitional cell carcinoma
103. Ans. d. Wide excision
104. Ans. c. Carcinoma penis *(Ref: Mastery of Surgery 5/e p1531)*

- "The historic contribution by **Cabana** in 1977 (Cancer 1977; 39:456) **established the importance, lymphatic histology with sentinel lymph node mapping** of patients with **penile carcinoma.** This approach identified the **sentinel lymph node** as the **first site of residual nodal metastasis** and is **predictive of the nodal status of the remaining node basin."**

105. Ans. a. Most common type is verrucous

URETHRAL CARCINOMA

106. Ans. a. Bulbomembranous urethra *(Ref: Smith 18/e p322; Campbell 11/e p882)*

MISCELLANEOUS

107. Ans. a. Urethra is short
108. Ans. c. Voiding cystogram *(Ref: Sutton Radiology 7/e p898-899)*

- **Voiding cystourethrography** is the **best method** to visualize the **posterior urethra**[Q].
- **Anterograde techniques** are **best for** visualization of **posterior urethra**[Q].
- **Reterograde techniques** (contrast is injected through tip of urethra) is **best for** visualization of **anterior (penile) urethra**[Q].

109. Ans. c. 20 cm
110. Ans. b. 4 cm
111. Ans. a. Prostatic
112. Ans. b. Membranous
113. Ans. a. Syphilis
114. Ans. b. Mid-penile urethra
115. Ans. a. Tyson gland

- **Tyson's Glands** ultimately produce an **oily substance,** which, when **mixed with shed skin cells,** constitute **smegma**[Q].

116. Ans. a. Posterior urethral valve *(Ref: Cambell 11/e p2880)*

- **Renal parenchymal dysplasia** is the **most important factor** in overall **prognosis**[Q] in posterior urethral valve.

117. Ans. b. Silicone *(Ref: www.nursing-standard..co.uk)*

- **All silicone catheters** are **suitable for use in** patients with **latex allergy** and **can remain in situ for 12 weeks**[Q] or according to manufacturer's instruction.

```
                        ┌─────────────┐
                        │  Catheter   │
                        └──────┬──────┘
              ┌────────────────┴────────────────┐
              ▼                                 ▼
   ┌─────────────────────┐          ┌─────────────────────────┐
   │ Short-Term (14-28 days) │      │   Long-Term (12 weeks)     │
   │ • PVC^Q: 14 days     │          │ • All-silicone^Q: 12 weeks │
   │ • Latex^Q: 14 days   │          │ • Silicone elastomer coated: 12 weeks │
   │ • Teflon^Q: 28 days  │          │ • Hydrogel coated: 12 weeks │
   └─────────────────────┘          └─────────────────────────┘
```

118. **Ans. a. Painful priapism** *(Ref: Campbell 11/e p 678)*

- **Penile angiography** is **indicated in high flow, non-ischemic priapism**, which is painless^Q.
- It is **not indicated in painful (low-flow) priapism**^{Q}.

119. **Ans. a. External urethral meatus**
120. **Ans. d. Membranous urethra**
121. **Ans. d. Membranous** *(Ref: Campbell 11/e p1635; Smith 18/e p14; Bailey 27/e p1477)*
122. **Ans. c. Priapism**
123. **Ans. c. Prostatitis** *(Ref: Bailey 27/e p1475, 26/e p1357)*

THREE GLASS URINE TEST

- The **three glass urine test** is valuable in **diagnosis of chronic prostatitis**
- If the **first glass** with the initial voided sample shows urine containing **prostatic threads, prostatitis** is present.

CHAPTER 25

Testis and Scrotum

UNDESCENDED TESTIS

UNDESCENDED TESTIS

- UDT affects **3%** of **full-term**^{Q} newborns.
- **Incidence** by **1 year** of age is **1%**.
- Approximately **70% to 77%** of UDT will **spontaneously descend**, usually by **3 months**^{Q} of age.

  - **Birth weight**^{Q} may be the **principal determinant** of UDT **at birth** and at **1 year** of life, **independent** of the **length of gestation**.

- In UDT, 80% are **palpable** and 20% are **nonpalpable**^{Q}.
- **MC location** for an ectopic UDT is within the **superficial pouch**^{Q}.

Pathology
- **Germ cell histology** of **both the testes** is abnormal.

The histopathologic hallmarks of UDT are evident between 1-2 years^Q of age:
• **Decreased** numbers of **Leydig cells (Earliest abnormality)**^{Q}
• **Degeneration** of **Sertoli cells**^{Q}
• **Delayed disappearance** of **gonocytes**^{Q}
• **Delayed appearance** of **adult dark spermatogonia**^{Q}
• Failure of primary spermatocytes to develop^Q
• **Reduced total germ cell counts**^{Q}

- **Hypoplasia of the Leydig cells**, observed from the **1st month**^{Q} of life, is the **earliest postnatal histologic abnormality**^{Q} in UDT.
- Adverse effects on **contralateral testes**: Autoantibodies against UDT causes **degenerative changes** in contralateral testis, **germ cell histology** is **abnormal** and **risk of carcinoma**^{Q} is also increased.

Associated Anomalies
- **Epididymal anomalies** and **patent processus vaginalis** up to **90%**^{Q} cases of UDT.
- **Renal Anomalies** in **10% cases** (Renal hypoplasia, agenesis, horse shoe kidney, PUJ obstruction)
- **Hypospadias**

  Hazards: (**SATHI**- Sterility, Atrophy, Trauma, Tumor, Torsion, Hernia, Inflammation)

Neoplasia
• Relative risk of testicular tumor is increased **17 times**.
• MC tumor that develops is **seminoma**^{Q}.
• **Higher the testis, greater the risk**^{Q} (Abdominal testis has higher risk than inguinal)
• **Orchiopexy does not decrease the risk**, it helps in **early detection only**^{Q}.

Infertility
• **Histopathological changes** start at **1 year**^{Q}.
• At **6-8 years**, **spermatogenesis** is **absent**^{Q}.
• **Endocrine functions** are retained as the **Leydig cells** are **less sensitive** to **temperature**^{Q}.
• Surgical repositioning before the onset of histopathological changes decreases the risk of subfertility.
• **Paternity** is significantly **compromised** in men with **bilateral**, but not unilateral UDT.

- **Hernia**: Patent processus vaginalis^Q is seen in **90%** cases of UDT.
- **Torsion**: Increased susceptibility

Diagnosis
- **Inguinal exploration** is **IOC** for UDT^Q.

Diagnostic Laparoscopy

- **IOC** for **'non-palpable' UDT**[Q].
- **MC application** of laparoscopy in children is for UDT.
- **Accuracy** of transperitoneal laparoscopy in locating a non-palpable testis is **100%**[Q] and it subsequently defines the management options.
- **Vas** and **testicular artery** is traced in pelvis.
- **Blind ended vas doesn't conclude** the **absence of testis**[Q], whereas **blind ended testicular artery** is a **definitive investigation** for an **absence of testis**[Q].
- Laparoscopy is also useful in lap. assisted orchiopexy.

Management: Orchiopexy, Ideal time: **6-12 months**[Q] of age. (Best time is **6 months**[Q])

Types of Orchiopexy

1. **Fowler-Stephens** orchiopexy[Q]
2. **Microvascular testicular autotransplantation (Best results)**[Q]
3. **Ladd and Gross** orchiopexy[Q]
4. **Ombridann's** orchiopexy[Q]
5. **Placing testis in Dartos pouch**[Q]
6. **Keetley-Torek** orchiopexy[Q]

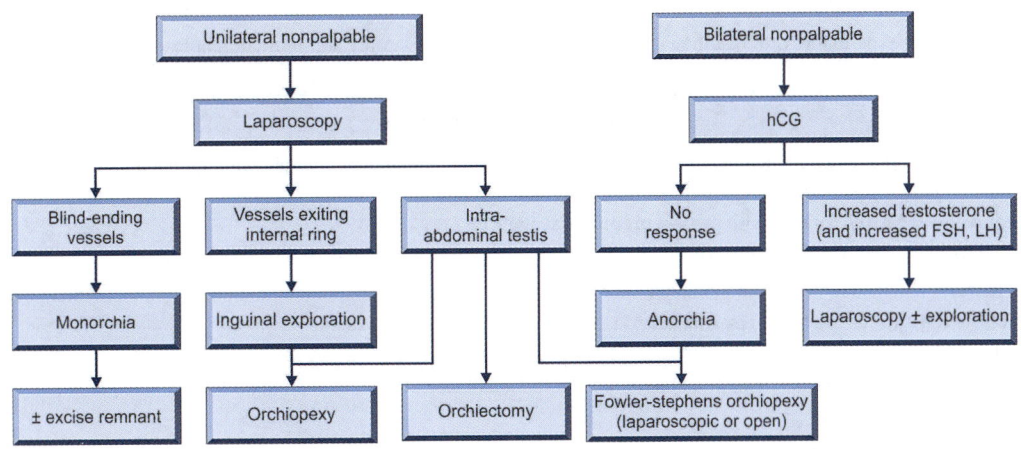

ECTOPIC TESTIS

Ectopic Testis

- An ectopic testicle **descends normally through the inguinal canal** but then **moves into an abnormal position** in the groin area[Q].
- An **ectopic testis** is usually[Q]. **Fully developed**[Q]. The main hazard is **liability to injury**[Q].

Locations of Ectopic Testis

- **Superficial inguinal pouch (MC location)**[Q]
- **Femoral canal**[Q] (the inner portion of the thigh near the groin)
- **Perineum**[Q] (below the scrotum)
- **Suprapubic region**[Q] (above the penis)
- **Contralateral scrotum (Least common)**[Q]

Embryology

- Ectopic testis are likely related to **abnormalities of** the **gubernaculum**[Q], which is a fibrous, cord-like membrane that runs through the inguinal canal from the abdomen to the scrotum.
- The **gubernaculum helps to guide the descent** of the **testicles**[Q] and has branches that attach to these other locations.
- Ectopic testicles usually will not descend into the normal position in the scrotum on their own.
- Most ectopic testicles can be felt (**are palpable**)[Q].

Treatment

- **Surgical treatment** to place an ectopic testicle in its normal position any time **after about age 6 months** but **no later than 2 years of age**[Q].

RETRACTILE TESTIS

Retractile Testis

- **Retractile testis**: Testis has **completed the process of descent** but **found in groin** because of an **overactive cremasteric reflex** or **increased cremasteric muscle tone**Q.

Clinical Features
- **MC age** of presentation: **2-6 years**Q
- Testis can be **manipulated down in scrotum**Q & remain in this location temporarily
- Development of **scrotum is normal**Q (underdeveloped scrotum in UDT)

Treatment
- Retractile testes require **no treatment**Q.

TESTICULAR TORSION

Testicular Torsion

- Twisting of testis on the spermatic cord, resulting in strangulation of the blood supply and infarction of testis.
- Types of testicular torsion: Intravaginal and Extravaginal.

Intravaginal Testicular Torsion

- **Torsion** occurs **within the space of tunica vaginalis**, which is **highly invested**Q, resulting in lack of normal fixation of testis & epididymis to the fascial & muscular coverings (scrotal parietal wall)
- **MC age group** affected is **10-25 years**, with peak in **prepubertal age**Q
- **Cremaster fibers** have a **spiral attachment over the cord**, it favors rotation **when cremaster reflex is strong**Q.

Predisposing Factors
- **Inversion of the testis** (testis lies transversely or upside down) is **MC predisposing factor**Q
- **High investment of tunica vaginalis** causes the **testis to hang within the tunica** like a **clapper in a bell**Q
- **Separation of the epididymis from the body of testis**Q permit torsion of testis without involving cord

Clinical Features
- **Sudden agonizing scrotal pain** with **nausea or vomiting**Q
- **Dysuria** or other **bladder symptoms** are usually **absent**Q
- Affected **testis high-riding in scrotum**, may have **abnormal transverse orientation**Q
- **Cord** is usually **thickened**Q

> - **Absent cremasteric reflux**Q is **highly suggestive** of torsion testis (**present in epididymitis**)

- After several hours massive scrotal edema may obliterate all the findings
- **Prehn's sign** is **negative**Q (On elevation of testis, pain relieved in epididymoorchitis but not in torsion testis)

> - **Deming sign**: Affected testis at **higher level** because of twisting of cordQ
> - **Angel sign**: Opposite testis lies horizontally because of present of mesorchiumQ

Imaging
- **Color Doppler** detects the **decreased blood flow** to the testis in torsion and is **investigation of choice**Q to exclude torsion from epididymoorchitis.
- **Tc99 pertechnate scan** demonstrate **poor radionuclide tracer uptake**Q

Treatment
- Testicular torsion is **urological emergency** as ischemic injury occurs as soon as **4 hours**Q after occlusion of the cord.

> - **Immediate surgical exploration**Q is indicated if testicular torsion is suspected because if treated within first 4 hours, the chances of testicular salvage are high.

- Even if manual detorsion is done, it may not totally correct the rotation and prompt exploration is still indicated.
- Viable as well as testis of marginal viability are preserved, and **orchiopexy** is done either by **placing into dartos pouch without suture fixation** or **suture fixation of tunica albuginea with the parietal wall**Q.

- Exploration of contralateral hemiscrotum must be carried. In almost all cases, a **bell clapper deformity is found.**
- **Contralateral testis** must be fixed to **prevent subsequent torsion**[Q].

- **Risk of autoimmunization** against own sperms is **low in children <10 years**, because there is no blood testis barrier and spermatogenesis is dormant.
- Current recommendation is **preserve a compromised testis in children <10 years**, proceed with orchidectomy in older children.

EXTRAVAGINAL TESTICULAR TORSION

- There is **no anatomical defect**[Q]
- Occurs in **perinatal period**, as there is **no testicular fixation**[Q] (adherence of tunica vaginalis to the dartos layer) by that time, and as a result the spermatic cord and tunica vaginalis **rotate as one unit**[Q]

Prenatal torsion	Postnatal torsion
• A **hard non-tender testis** at birth, **fixed to the overlying skin**[Q]	• **Swelling and tenderness of scrotum**, usually **no fixation**[Q] of the skin
• **Salvage rate** is **nil**[Q]	• **Prompt surgical exploration** is indicated
• **Contralateral scrotal exploration** is **not recommended**[Q] as it is not associated with a testicular fixation defect	• **Exploration of contralateral testis** should be done as **20% cases are associated with bell clapper deformity**[Q]

- **Blue dot sign**: seen in **torsion** of **appendage of testis**[Q].

VARICOCELE

VARICOCELE

- Dilated & tortuous veins of pampiniform plexus (veins draining testis & epididymis)[Q] lying **posterior & above the testis**
- Most common **surgically correctable cause** of male **subfertility**[Q]
- Surgical **correction** can **reverse atrophy** in **adolescents**[Q]

Etiology
- **Absent or incompetent valves** in the internal spermatic or **left testicular vein (MC)**[Q] and it joins left renal vein at right angles.
- Increased venous pressure in left renal vein (**Nutcracker phenomenon**[Q]- caused by compression of left renal vein between aorta and superior mesenteric artery)
- Collateral venous anastomosis
- Compression by sigmoid colon

Clinical Features
- MC seen in **young adults**[Q], **tall thin men**[Q] are frequently affected
- **Painless**, compressible mass lying **posterior and above the testis**
- **Bag of worms** like feel on palpation in standing position[Q]
- Marked **left side predominance**[Q] (90%)
- Varicocele **do not regress spontaneously**[Q], associated with testicular atrophy
- **Suspicious varicoceles:** May be **secondary to RCC**, as growth from renal cell carcinoma **blocks the renal vein by venous permeation**. In RCC, varicocele **does not decompress in supine position**[Q].
  - **Right sided** varicoceles[Q]
  - Varicoceles in **elderly**[Q]
  - **Rapidly evolving** varicoceles[Q]
  - Varicocele that **does not decompress** in supine position[Q]

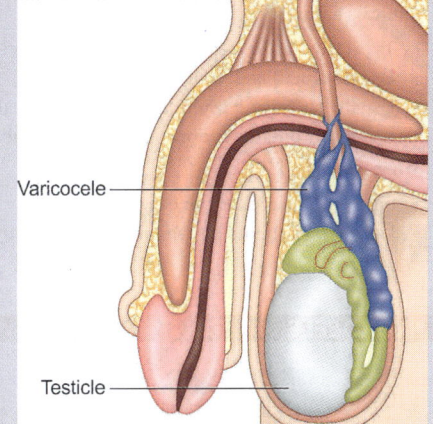

Varicocele Classification	
Subclinical	Not palpable or visible at rest or during Valsalva maneuver, but **demonstrable by special tests**[Q] (**reflux** found on doppler examination)
Grade 1	Palpable during **Valsalva**[Q] maneuver, but not otherwise
Grade 2	Palpable at **rest**[Q], but not visible
Grade 3	**Visible**[Q] and palpable at rest

Effect on Spermatogenesis
- Varicocele **increases the temperature of scrotum**[Q] and this decreases spermatogenesis
- Infertility is observed in higher percentage of individuals.
- Abnormal semen analysis (**decreased sperm motility & number**), normalizes after surgery.
- Improvement in semen quality is seen in up to 65% after varicocele ligation.

Diagnosis
- Diagnosis is made by **clinical examination** and **confirmed by color Doppler analysis** (**reflux/reverse flow** is characteristic of varicoceles)^Q.
- **Venography**: **Most accurate** method of varicocele diagnosis, done for varicocele in the **postsurgical patients**^{Q}.

Indications for surgery	
1. Infertility^Q	4. Significant discomfort
2. Poor testicular growth in adolescents^Q	5. Recruitment to police or armed forces
3. Defective sperm count or motility^Q	

Treatment
- **Ligation** of **testicular vein above** the **inguinal ligament**^{Q} where the pampiniform plexus has coalesced into one or two vessels. (**Venous drainage** after ligation is by **cremasteric veins**^{Q})

> - Best surgical option is microscopic subinguinal ligation^Q.

- Other procedures are open inguinal/subinguinal, laparoscopic or retroperitoneal (**Palomo's operation**) ligation or embolization.
- Complications of surgery:
  - Postoperative hydrocele formation (**least with microscopic ligation** and **embolization**)
  - Testicular atrophy^Q (seen in <1% due to damage of testicular artery).

SPERMATOCELE

Spermatocele

- **Unilocular retention cyst derived from** some portion of the **sperm-conducting mechanism** of the **epididymis**^{Q}.

Clinical Features
- **Typically lies in** the **epididymal head, above** and **behind** the **upper pole** of the **testis**.
- Usually small and unobtrusive^Q.
- Usually **softer** and **laxer than other cystic lesions** in the scrotum but, like them, it **transilluminates**^{Q}
- The **fluid contains spermatozoa**^{Q} and resembles **barley water appearance**^{Q}.

Treatment
- Small spermatoceles can be ignored.
- **Larger ones** should be **aspirated** or **excised** through a scrotal incision.

HYDROCELE

Hydrocele

An accumulation of fluid in layers of tunica vaginalis
Types:
- **Vaginal hydrocele (MC)**^{Q}
  - Abnormal accumulation of serous fluid within the tunica vaginalis.
- **Infantile hydrocele:**
  - Does not necessarily appear in infants.
  - Tunica & processus vaginalis are distended to the inguinal ring **without any connection** with **peritoneal cavity**^{Q}.
- **Congenital hydrocele (Communicating hydrocele):**
  - **Patent processus vaginalis**^{Q} allows peritoneal fluid to freely communicate.
  - Size of hydrocele fluctuates, usually related to activity
  - Congenital hernia has the same defect. UDT are commonly associated.
  - **Wait for 2 years** for **spontaneous closure**^{Q}. Otherwise the treatment is **herniotomy**^{Q}.
- **Funicular hydrocele:**
  - Processus vaginalis remains **patent up to** the **top** of the **testis**^{Q}, where it is shut off from the tunica vaginalis.
- **Hydrocele En bisac or Bilocular hydrocele:**
  - Hydrocele has **2 intercommunicating sacs**, one **above** and one **below** the **neck**^{Q} of the scrotum.
  - The upper sac has **no connection with** the **processus vaginalis**^{Q} and it is in fact the herniated tunica vaginalis.

- **Hydrocele of the cord:**
  - **Central portion** of **processus vaginalis** is **patent**^{Q}, but its upper & lower parts are obliterated.
  - Presents as **painless groin mass** contiguous with cord structures, moves downward and becomes less mobile if testis is pulled gently downwards.
- **Hydrocele of the canal of Nuck:**
  - Female counterpart of Hydrocele of the cord. It is seen in relation to the round ligament.
- **Hydrocele of hernial sac:** Neck of hernial sac becomes **closed by adhesions** or **plugged by omentum** with **retention of fluid secreted by peritoneum of hernial sac**^{Q}

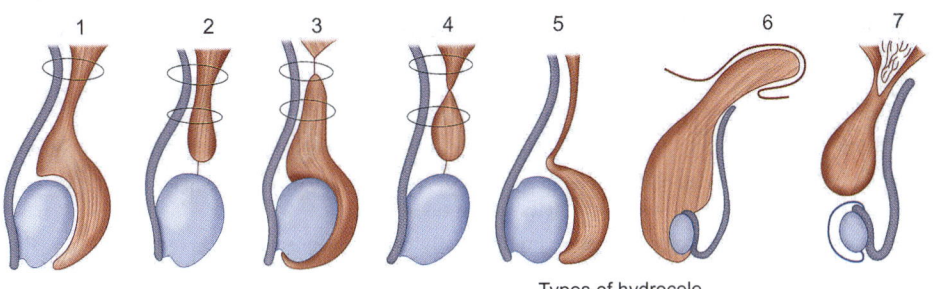

1. Congenital hydrocele
2. Funicular hydrocele
3. Infantile hydrocele
4. Encyted hydrocele of the cord
5. Vaginal hydrocele
6. Bilocular hydrocele
7. Hydrocele of hernial Sae

Types of hydrocele

Secondary Hydrocele
- **Causes** are acute or chronic **epididymo-orchitis (MC)**^{Q}, testicular tumors, torsion of testis
- Usually **lax** and of **small size** with **palpable underlying testis**^{Q}
- Subsides with resolution of epididymoorchitis

Treatment of Vaginal Hydrocele
1. **Small** hydrocele: **Lord's** procedure (**Plication** of sac)^Q
2. **Medium** hydrocele: **Jaboulay's** procedure (**Eversion** of sac)^Q
3. **Large** hydrocele: **Excision** of sac^Q

ACUTE EPIDIDYMOORCHITIS

ACUTE EPIDIDYMOORCHITIS

- **Inflammation** of **epididymis** & **testis**, from an **ascending infection**^{Q} from the lower urinary tract.
- Initially epididymis is involved, after that there is involvement of testis.
- Most cases of epididymitis in **men younger than 35 years** are due to **sexually transmitted organisms** [C. trachomatis (MC)^Q and N. gonorrhoe]
- In **children** and **older men** are due to **urinary pathogens** such as **E. coli**^{Q}.
- In **homosexual men**, **E. coli**^{Q} and other coliform bacteria are common causative organisms.

Clinical Features
- Patient presents with **fever, swollen, red & tender scrotum**^{Q}.
- The epididymis and testis are swollen (**Thickened cord** with **reactive hydrocoele**)^Q
- Symptoms of **urethritis, cystitis or prostatitis**^{Q}
- Urine analysis typically demonstrates **WBCs and bacteria** in the **urine or urethral discharge**^{Q}

Diagnosis
- Scrotal USG showing enlarged epididymis with increased blood flow with reactive hydrocoele.
- **Prepubertal children** diagnosed with epididymitis **require radiologic investigation** for **urinary tract anomalies** such as reflux or ureteral Ectopia^Q.

Treatment
- Antibiotics, rest, scrotal elevation and NSAIDs^Q.

- MC organism causing epididymoorchitis in <35 and sexually active males: **Chlamydia**^{Q}
- MC organism causing epididymoorchitis in **children, elderly, homosexuals: E. coli**^{Q}

FOURNIER'S GANGRENE (IDIOPATHIC SCROTAL GANGRENE)

Fournier's Gangrene (Idiopathic Scrotal Gangrene)

- A form of **necrotizing fasciitis**, with **abrupt onset** of a **rapidly fulminating genital gangrene** of idiopathic origin and **gangrene up to deep fascia**^{Q}.

Predisposing Factors	
• **Diabetes mellitus (MC)** • Local trauma • Paraphimosis	• Anal infections • **Immunosuppression**^{Q}

- **Multiple organisms (aerobes + anaerobes)**^{Q} results in fulminating inflammation of the subcutaneous tissues which results in **obliterative arteritis** of arterioles of the scrotal skin. (**Polymicrobial**)^Q

Clinical Features
- History of **recent perineal trauma, instrumentation,** urethral **stricture** or a **rectal source** of infection is frequently present^Q.
- Infection commonly starts as cellulitis. Involved area swollen, erythematosus and tender as the infection begins to involve the deep fascia.

> • Areas of **purplish** and **blackish** discoloration, **dishwater** like **discharge**, **fetid odour** and **skin necrosis**.
> • **Pain** is predominant with **fever** and **marked systemic toxicity**^{Q}. **Crepitus** is present^Q.

- Skin, superficial fascia, deep fascia is **destroyed**, while **corpora cavernosa, urethra, testis, cord structures** are **preserved**^{Q}.

Management
- Prompt diagnosis and **aggressive treatment**^{Q} is the initial treatment to limit the spread.

> • **IV hydration, antibiotics, surgical debridement** of the necrotic fat and fascia^Q
> • **Mortality** without treatment: **7-75%**^{Q} (Average-20%)

- Surgical debridement is cornerstone, **serial debridement**^{Q} is usually required.
- **Orchidectomy is almost never required**^{Q}, because the testis have their blood supply independent of the compromised fascial and cutaneous circulation of the scrotum.

CLASSIFICATION OF TESTICULAR TUMORS

Classification of Testicular Tumors

- **Germ cell tumors:**
  - Seminomas
  - Non-seminomas:
    - Embryonal cell carcinoma – Yolk sac tumour – Teratoma – Choriocarcinoma
- **Sex cord/gonadal stromal tumors:**
  - Leydig cell tumour – Sertoli cell tumor – Granulosa cell tumor – Thecoma/fibroma
- **Tumors containing both germ cell and sex cord/gonadal stromal elements:**
  - Gonadoblastoma
- **Lymphoid and Hematopoetic tumour:**
  - Lymphoma, Leukemia, Plasmacytoma
- **Miscellaneous:**
  - Carcinoid, Adenoma, Carcinoma

PREDISPOSING FACTORS FOR TESTICULAR GCTS

Predisposing Factors for Testicular GCTs

- **Cryptorchidism**
  - Of the predisposing factors, **cryptorchidism** has the **strongest association** with the **testicular carcinoma**^{Q}.
  - **Higher the testis, greater the risk**^{Q}. Abdominal cryptorchid testis is at higher risk than inguinal cryptorchid testis.

> • **Increased risk** is seen in **both the testis (cryptorchid** and **normally descended testis)**^{Q}
> • **MC tumour seen: Seminoma** > Embryonal cell carcinoma

  - **Orchidopexy does not decrease the risk of malignancy**^{Q}, however it facilitates examination and tumour detection.
- **Testicular feminization syndrome**
- **GCT of one testis** for other testis
- **Testicular carcinoma in sibling**
- **Klinefelter's syndrome** (increases risk of both **testicular** and **mediastinal GCT**) and **male CA breast**^{Q}.
- Administration of DES (**estrogen**) in utero

TESTICULAR TUMORS: MOST COMMON TYPE

TESTICULAR TUMORS

- MC **histological type** of testicular tumour: **Mixed**[Q] (if option is there, otherwise seminoma)

  - MC **tumour** of testis: **Seminoma**[Q]
  - MC **bilateral primary testicular tumour: Seminoma**[Q]
  - **Most radiosensitive** testicular tumor: **Seminoma**[Q]

- MC testicular tumor in **infant & children up to 3 years**: Yolk sac tumour[Q]
- MC testicular tumor in **prepubertal children**: Teratoma[Q]

  - MC **testicular tumor** in patients >60 years: **Lymphoma**[Q]
  - MC **bilateral testicular tumour**: **Lymphoma**[Q]
  - MC **secondary testicular tumour**: **Lymphoma**[Q]

- MC **histologic type** of testicular lymphoma: **Diffuse large B-cell lymphoma (DLBL)**
- Testicular tumour with **best prognosis**: Yolk sac tumour[Q]
- Testicular tumour with **worst prognosis**: Hurricane tumour (Type of **choriocarcinoma**)[Q]

TESTICULAR TUMORS

TESTICULAR TUMORS

- MC **tumour** of testis: Seminoma[Q]
- MC **histological type** of testicular tumour: **Mixed**[Q] (if option is there, otherwise seminoma)
- **Genomic change** found in all **germ cell tumors** is an **isochromosome** of **short arm** of chromosome **12**[Q].

Clinical Features

- MC presentation is a **nodule or painless swelling of one gonad**[Q].
- 10% patients present with acute pain or manifestation due to secondaries like neck or abdominal masses, GI disturbances, respiratory or CNS symptoms, bone pain or lumbar backache due to nerve roots involvement by bulky retroperitoneal disease.
- **Secondary hydrocele** is also seen in **5-10%**[Q] cases.

  - **5% GCT** may present with **gynecomastia**[Q] as a systemic endocrine manifestation.
  - **Gynecomastia** is **more commonly** seen with **sex cord** or **gonadal stromal tumors** (Leydig cell tumor, Sertoli cell tumor, Granulosa/Theca cell tumor)[Q].

- Majority (2/3rd) of seminoma are **confined to testis**[Q] at the time of presentation, whereas majority of **non-seminomatous GCT** have widespread metastasis at presentation.
- Many patients would present with a history of trauma, but trauma merely draws the attention of the patients and has no etiological association with tumour.

  Bilateral Testicular Tumors
  - **Bilateral testicular tumors** are seen in **1-2%** cases.
  - Primary bilateral testicular tumors have tendency of **same histology** on **both sides**[Q].
  - **Seminoma**[Q] is the **MC histological finding** in bilateral **primary** testicular tumor, whereas **malignant lymphoma** is the **MC bilateral testicular tumor**[Q].

- Any patient with a **solid firm intratesticular mass** must be considered to have **testicular tumour** unless proved otherwise.

Investigations

- **USG**: Any hypoechoic area within tunica albuginea is markedly suspicious.

  - **FNAC** is **C**ontraindicated (**Scrotal seedlings** may result in **inguinal LN metastasis**)[Q]

- **Histopathological Diagnosis**: Radical orchiectomy by inguinal canal approach, the **cord is ligated** at **deep inguinal ring (high inguinal orchiectomy)**[Q].
- **Trans-scrotal Orchidectomy** is **contraindicated** as it permits the development of alternate **lymphatic channel pathway** to **inguinal** and **pelvic lymph nodes**.

  Chevassu maneuver[Q]
  - First a **soft clamp** is applied **to** the **cord**, suspicious area is **biopsied** and sent for **frozen section**. If malignant, formally ligate the cord and send the orchiectomy sample for final histopathology.

- **CECT abdomen** for evaluation of **retroperitoneum** and **lymph nodes**[Q].

Spread of Disease

- **Germ cell tumors** of the testis typically **spread** in a **stepwise lymphatic fashion (MC mode)**^{Q}.

  - The **primary landing site for the right testis** is the **interaortocaval area**^{Q} at the level of the right renal hilum, and **for the left testis** is the **para-aortic area**^{Q} at the level of the left renal hilum.
  - In the absence of disease on the left side, no crossover metastases to the right side have ever been identified. However, **right-to-left crossover metastases**^{Q} are common.

- **Retroperitoneum** is the **most commonly involved site**^{Q} in metastatic disease.
- Most **blood borne metastasis** occurs following LN involvement, **Lung is MC organ**^{Q} involved.
- **Choriocarcinoma** is the exception and characterized by **early hematogenous spread**, especially to the **lung**^{Q}.

Chemotherapy

- Chemotherapy for **extragonadal GCT**: Combination of **Bleomycin + Etoposide**^{Q} **+ Cisplatin (BEP)**^{Q}

8th AJCC (2017) TNM Staging for Testicular Tumors	
T: Primary tumor	**N: Regional lymph nodes**
pTis: Intratubular germ cell neoplasia (carcinoma in situ)	**N1**: LN mass ≤2 cm or multiple LN masses, none >2 cm
pT1: Limited to the **testis & epididymis** and no vascular/lymphatic invasion; Tumor may **invade tunica albuginea** but not tunica vaginalis^Q	**N2**: LN mass, **>2 cm** but **<5 cm** or multiple LN masses, any one mass >2 cm but not <5 cm^Q
pT2: Limited to the testis & epididymis **with vascular/lymphatic invasion** or extending through **tunica albuginea** with **involvement** of **tunica vaginalis**^{Q}	**N3**: LN mass >5 cm^Q
pT3: Invades the **spermatic cord** with or without vascular/lymphatic invasion^Q	**M: Distant metastases**
pT4: Invades the **scrotum** with or without vascular/lymphatic invasion^Q	**M1: Non-regional nodal** or **pulmonary metastases**^{Q} **M2: Non-pulmonary visceral masses**^{Q}

Serum Tumor Markers (S)			
	LDH	**hCG (mIU/mL)**	**AFP (ng/mL)**
S0	≤N	≤N	≤N
S1	<1.5 × N	<5,000	<1,000
S2	1.5–10 × N	5,000–50,000	1,000–10,000
S3	>10 × N	>50,000	>10,000

8th AJCC (2017) Staging for Testicular Cancer				
Stage Grouping	**T**	**N**	**M**	**S**
Stage **0**	pTis	N0	M0	S0
Stage **Ia**	**T1**	N0	M0	S0
Stage **Ib**	**T2-T4**	N0	M0	S0
Stage **Is**	Any T	N0	M0	**S1-S3**
Stage **IIa**	Any T	**N1**	M0	S0-**S1**
Stage **IIb**	Any T	**N2**	M0	S0-**S1**
Stage **IIc**	Any T	**N3**	M0	S0-**S1**
Stage **IIIa**	Any T	Any N	**M1**	S0-S1
Stage **IIIb**	Any T	Any N	M0-**M1**	**S2**
Stage **IIIc**	Any T	Any N	M0-**M1a**	**S3**
	Any T	Any N	**M1b**	Any S

Staging and Treatment			
Stage	**Extent of disease**	**Seminoma**	**Nonseminoma**
IA	**Testis only**, without vascular or lymphatic invasion (T$_1$)	Radiation therapy^Q	**RPLND or observation**^{Q}
IB	Testis with **vascular or lymphatic invasion** (T$_2$), or extension through **tunica albuginea** (T$_2$), or involvement of **spermatic cord** (T$_3$), or **scrotum** (T$_4$)	Radiation therapy^Q	**RPLND**^{Q}
IIA	Nodes ≤ 2 cm (N$_1$), S0/S1	Radiation therapy	**RPLND or chemotherapy followed by RPLND**^{Q}

IIB	Nodes >2-5 cm (N$_2$), S0/S1	Radiation therapy^Q	RPLND ± adjuvant chemotherapy or chemotherapy followed by RPLND^Q
IIC	Nodes > 5 cm (N$_3$), S0/S1	Chemotherapy^Q	Chemotherapy followed by RPLND^Q
III	Distant metastasis	Chemotherapy^Q	Chemotherapy followed by surgery (biopsy or resection)^Q
Is	Only serum tumor markers are raised (S$_1$ to S$_3$)^Q	Chemotherapy^Q	Chemotherapy^Q

INTRATUBULAR GERM CELL NEOPLASIA (ITGCN) OR TESTICULAR CARCINOMA IN SITU (CIS)

Intratubular Germ Cell Neoplasia (ITGCN) or Testicular Carcinoma in Situ (CIS)

- **Preinvasive precursor** of all testicular GCTs except:
  - Spermatocytic seminoma^Q
  - Yolk sac tumor^Q
  - Teratoma in children^Q
- Presently, there is **no established tumor marker** for CIS, and **testicular ultrasound** has been shown to be **unreliable** with respect to diagnosing CIS.
- Therefore, **testicular biopsy** remains the **"gold standard"** for **diagnosing CIS**^{Q}.

Risk Factors for ITGCN	
• History of **testicular carcinoma**^{Q} • **Extragonadal GCT**^{Q} • **Cryptorchidism**^{Q} • **Contralateral testis** with unilateral testicular cancer^Q	• **Atrophic contralateral testis**^{Q} with unilateral testicular cancer • **Somatosexual ambiguity**^{Q} • **Infertility**^{Q}

Pathology

- **ITGCN cells** are located on the **basement membrane** of the **seminiferous tubule** and possess morphologic features of malignancy: **Large irregular nucleus, coarse chromatin, and abundant cytoplasm**^{Q}.
- Typically only **one layer** of ITGCN cells is **seen**, but occasionally the **whole tubule** is **filled with ITGCN** cells, which may represent an **early stage** in **progression to GCT**^{Q}.

Clinical Features

- Testis may be **atrophic** but is usually **normal to palpation**
- **Testis biopsy** reliably **diagnoses ITGCN** because the **ITGCN** is almost always **found throughout the testis**^{Q}
- Progression of **ITGCN to invasive disease** may take **15 years**^{Q}.

Treatment

- Treatment options include **observation, radiation therapy,** and **orchiectomy**^{Q}
- **Chemotherapy** so far appears to be **ineffective against ITGCN**.

Tumour Markers	
Oncofetal substances	**Cellular Enzymes**
1. **α-FP:** (Increases in **YET**)^Q - Produced by **trophoblastic cells** - **Increases** in **Yolk sac tumour, embryonal carcinoma and teratocarcinoma. (YET)** - **Does not increase** in pure **choriocarcinoma** and **pure seminoma**^{Q} - Metabolic **half life: 5-7 days**^{Q}	1. **LDH:** - Not a specific tumour marker - Most useful as a marker for **"bulk"** disease - Raised serum LDH has poor prognosis
2. **β-hCG:** (Increases in **CES**MINOMA) - Produced by **syncytiotrophoblastic cells**^{Q} - **Increases in all choriocarcinomas, 50% embryonal carcinoma and 5-10% of pure seminoma** (as they contain syncytiotrophoblast like giant cells). - Serum **half life: 24-36 hours**^{Q}	2. **PLAP** (Placental alkaline phosphatase): - Elevated levels present in as many as 40% patients with advanced disease - Most useful as a marker for **"bulk"** disease - Elevated in **seminoma**^{Q} 3. **GGT** (Gamma glutamyl transpeptidase): - Marker of **seminoma testis**^{Q} - Marker for **"bulk"** disease

YOLK SAC TUMOR

YOLK SAC TUMOR

- MC testicular tumor of **infants** and **children**[Q].
- The terms **endodermal sinus tumor, adenocarcinoma of the infantile testis, juvenile embryonal carcinoma**, and **orchioblastoma** are all used synonymously[Q].

Pathology

- In its pure form, the lesion has a **homogeneous, yellowish, mucinous** appearance[Q].
- **Embryoid bodies**, a common finding in yolk sac tumors, resemble 1- to 2-week-old embryos.

> **Three most common microscopic patterns**
> 1. **Microcystic-** honeycomb appearance, with **hyaline globules**[Q]
> 2. **Endodermal sinus-** perivascular formations known as **Schiller-Duval bodies**[Q]
> 3. **Solid-** small polygonal cells, clear cytoplasm, frequent mitoses

- The pattern of metastatic disease of yolk sac tumors in childhood differs from the pattern in adult germ cell tumors, owing to a higher incidence of hematogenous spread.

Clinical Features

- MC testis tumor in **prepubertal boys**, presents as **slow-growing scrotal mass** in a **young boy**[Q]
- **Hydrocele** is present in **25%** of cases[Q].

Tumor Marker

- **AFP** is elevated in **>90%**[Q].

SEMINOMA

SEMINOMA

- Three subtypes: Classic, anaplastic and spermatocytic.
- **Typical or classic seminoma:**
  - Accounts for **80-85%**[Q] of all seminomas and occurs most commonly in **30 years** of age
  - Histologically, it is composed of **islands or sheets of relatively large cells** with **clear cytoplasm** and **densely staining nuclei**[Q].

  > - **Syncytiotrophoblastic** elements occur in **10-15%**[Q] and **lymphocytic infiltration** occurs in **20%**[Q]. The incidence of **syncytiotrophoblastic** elements corresponds to the frequency of **β-hCG production**[Q].

  - The **slower growth rate of seminomas**[Q] may be inferred from the observation that **treatment failures** may become **evident 2-10 years after** apparently adequate **irradiation** of metastatic sites.
- **Anaplastic seminoma:**
  - Accounts for 5% to 10% of all seminomas
  - Despite its rarity, up to **30% of patients dying with seminoma** have an **anaplastic morphology**[Q].

  > - **More aggressive** and **potentially more lethal**[Q] variant leading to **less favorable results**[Q].
  > - These characteristics include greater mitotic activity, higher rate of local invasion, increased rate of metastatic spread and higher rate of tumor marker (β-hCG) production.

  - **No difference** from classic seminoma when patients are **treated appropriately** and compared **stage for stage**[Q].
  - **Inguinal orchiectomy** plus **radiation therapy** is **equally effective** in controlling both **anaplastic** and **classic seminoma**[Q].
- **Spermatocytic seminoma:**
  - Accounts for 2-12% of all seminomas
  - It is **distinctive tumor both clinically** and **radiologically** as compared to seminoma[Q]

  > - Variants of germ cell tumor that **do not arise from** an **intratubular germ cell neoplasia**[Q] (the other being teratomas of children[Q]).

  - Composed of **cells** that **vary in size** and have **deeply pigmented cytoplasm** and **rounded nuclei** containing **characteristic filamentous chromatin**[Q].
  - Uncommon tumor representing **1-2% of all testicular neoplasms**[Q]
  - Affected individuals are **>65 years**[Q]
  - **Slow growing tumor** that **rarely** if ever **produces metastases**
  - **Only orchidectomy** is required for treatment.
  - **Prognosis** is **excellent**[Q].

TERATOMA

TERATOMA

- Most common testicular tumor in **prepubertal adults**: **Teratoma**[Q]
- Tumor is composed of **two or more** embryonic **germ cell layers**[Q] that may be both mature and immature.
- Tumor is very **heterogeneous** with both **solid** and **cystic**[Q] components.

Teratoma is divided into three subsets
1. **Mature:** Well-differentiated ectodermal, mesodermal, or endodermal tissues
2. **Immature:** Incompletely differentiated tissues
3. **Teratoma with areas of malignant transformation:** sarcoma, squamous carcinoma, adenocarcinoma

- Teratomas are **potentially malignant**[Q]

Clinical Features
- Age range: first, second, and third decades.
- **Mature and immature forms** have **metastatic potential** in **adults** but in **children** are **uniformly benign**[Q].
- The primary tumor generally presents as an **enlarged testis with both solid and cystic components**[Q].
- The **teratoma component** of metastatic GCT is **resistant to chemotherapy** and **radiotherapy**[Q].

Tumor Markers
- **AFP** is **raised in 20-25%**[Q]

TESTICULAR LYMPHOMA

TESTICULAR LYMPHOMA

- **MC testicular tumor** in a patient **>50 years**[Q]
- **MC secondary neoplasm** of the **testis**, accounting for 5% of all testicular tumors.
- It may be seen as **late manifestation** of **widespread lymphoma**; **initial presentation** of clinically **occult disease**; and **primary extranodal disease**[Q].

Pathology
- Grossly, bulging, gray or pink lesion with ill-defined margins. **Hemorrhage** and **necrosis**[Q] are common.
- Diffuse large B cell lymphoma > Burkitt lymphoma

Clinical Findings
- **Painless enlargement**[Q] of the testis is common.
- Generalized **constitutional symptoms** occur in one-fourth of patients.
- **Bilateral testis involvement** occurs in **50%** of patients, usually **asynchronously**.

Treatment
- **FNAC** should be considered in a **known** or **suspected** diagnosis of **lymphoma**[Q]
- **Radical orchiectomy** is reserved for suspected **primary lymphoma**[Q] of the testicle.

LEYDIG CELL TUMORS

LEYDIG CELL TUMORS

- **MC non-germ cell tumors** of **testis** and account for **1-3%** of all testicular tumors.
- **Bimodal age distribution**: **5-9 years** and **25-35** years
- **25%** tumors occur **in childhood**, **bilateral** in **5-10%**.
- **Cause**: **unknown**; unlike germ cell tumors (**no association with cryptorchidism**)[Q]

Pathology
- Small, yellow, well-circumscribed lesion devoid of hemorrhage or necrosis.
- Microscopically, **hexagonally shaped cells** with granular, eosinophilic cytoplasm containing lipid vacuoles are seen.
- **Reinke crystals**[Q] are **fusiform-shaped cytoplasmic inclusions** are **pathognomonic** for **Leydig cells**.

Clinical Features
- **Prepubertal children** present with **virilization**, and tumors are **benign**^{Q}.
- **Adults** are usually **asymptomatic**, although **gynecomastia** may be present in **20–25%**^{Q}.
- **10% of tumors in adults** are **malignant.**
- Laboratory findings include **elevated serum** and **urinary 17-ketosteroids** and **estrogens**^{Q}.

Treatment
- **Initial treatment: Radical orchiectomy**^{Q}
- **RPLND** for **malignant lesions**^{Q}.

Prognosis
- Prognosis is **excellent for benign lesions**, while it remains **poor for disseminated disease.**

CARCINOMA SCROTUM (CHIMNEY SWEEP'S CANCER)

CARCINOMA SCROTUM (CHIMNEY SWEEP'S CANCER)

- **Squamous cell carcinoma of scrotum**^{Q}, most commonly resulted from exposure to environmental carcinogens including **chimney soot, tars, paraffin** and **petroleum products**^{Q}.
- **Superficial inguinal lymph nodes** are the **first lymph nodes involved.**^{Q}

Risk Factors
- Most cases results from **poor hygiene** and **chronic inflammation**^{Q}.

Diagnosis
- **Diagnosis** is established by **biopsy of scrotal skin**^{Q}.

Treatment
- **Wide excision** with **2 cm margins**^{Q} should be performed for malignant tumors.
- **Prognosis** correlates with **presence or absence of nodal involvement**^{Q}.

- MC common **benign lesion** of scrotum: **Sebaceous cyst**^{Q}
- MC common **malignanat tumor** of scrotum: **Squamous cell carcinoma**^{Q}

IMPORTANT TOPICS

IMPORTANT TOPICS

- **Length** of one **seminiferous tubule: 1 meter**^{Q}
- **Length** of **epididymis: 4 meters**^{Q}
- **Total length** of seminiferous tubules: **250 meters**^{Q}

Most Common Lymph Nodes Involved	
CA Penis	Inguinal LN^Q
CA Testis	On **right: Inter-aortocaval**^{Q} **LN** On **left: Paraaortic**^{Q} **LN**
CA Bladder	**Obturator**^{Q} LN
CA Prostate	**Obturator**^{Q} LN

Multiple Choice Questions

UNDESCENDED TESTIS

1. **Best time for surgery of undescended testis is:**
   (Recent Question 2014, 2015; All India 2010)
   a. Just after birth
   b. 6 months of age
   c. 12 months of age
   d. 24 months of age

2. **Surgery for undescended testis is recommended at what age?** *(COMEDK 2014, All India 2011)*
   a. 6 months
   b. 12 months
   c. 24 months
   d. 36 months

3. **Incidence of undescended testis in normal new born:**
   a. 3%
   b. 6% *(DNB 2007)*
   c. 9%
   d. 12%

4. **Most common tumors in undescended testis:**
   (DNB 2005, Punjab 2009)
   a. Seminoma
   b. Teratoma
   c. Embryonal carcinoma
   d. None

5. **Stephen Fowler surgery is done for:** *(GB Pant 2010)*
   a. Ectopic testis
   b. Undescended testis
   c. Hypospadias
   d. Epispadias

6. **All can be prevented by orchiopexy in cryptorchidism except:** *(AIIMS Nov 99)*
   a. Testicular tumor
   b. Epididymoorchitis
   c. Torsion of testis
   d. Sexual ambiguity

7. **Which of the following investigation is used to confirm anorchia?** *(AIIMS Nov 2013)*
   a. PET
   b. MRI
   c. Laparoscopy
   d. USG

8. **Best investigation for undescended testis in 1-year-old child is:** *(Recent Question 2017)*
   a. USG abdomen
   b. CT
   c. MRI
   d. Laparoscopy

9. **Orchidopexy is done in cases of undescended tests at the age of:** *(AIIMS June 2006)*
   a. Infancy
   b. 1-2 years
   c. 5 years
   d. Puberty

10. **What is not seen in undescended testis?** *(AIIMS June 95)*
    a. Hydrocele
    b. Hernia
    c. Teratoma
    d. Seminoma

11. **Incompletely descended testis is commonest on:**
    a. Right side
    b. Left side
    c. Both side
    d. Right sided only

12. **A 5-year-old male child has been brought with a complaint that there is only one testis in the scrotum. On examination, it is found that the testis on the opposite side is felt in the inguinal canal. The patients should be advised:** *(UPSC 96)*
    a. Orchiopexy
    b. To wait till puberty
    c. Orchidectomy
    d. Administration of androgens

13. **Which one of the following statement is true of undescended testis?** *(UPSC 97)*
    a. Usually descends spontaneously at puberty
    b. Orchidopexy to be done if no descent by puberty
    c. Has higher incidence of malignancy
    d. Maintains normal sperm production

14. **True about incompletely descended testis are all of the following except:** *(MCI March 2008)*
    a. Early repositioning can preserve function
    b. It may lead to sterility, if bilateral
    c. Poorly developed secondary sexual characters
    d. May be associated with indirect inguinal. hernia

15. **Testis does not descend beyond:** *(JIPMER 2012)*
    a. 2 months
    b. 4 months
    c. 6 months
    d. 8 months

16. **In cryptorchidism, hallmark histological changes appear in testis at:** *(Recent Question 2016)*
    a. 4 months
    b. 6 months
    c. 8 months
    d. 1 year

17. **Fowler-Stephen surgery is done in:** *(Recent Question 2017)*
    a. Epispadias
    b. Hypospadias
    c. Exstrophy of bladder
    d. Cryptorchidism

ECTOPIC TESTIS

18. **Most common site of ectopic testis:** *(GB Pant 2010)*
    a. Superficial inguinal pouch
    b. Root of penis
    c. Femoral triangle
    d. Perineum

19. **Ectopic testis is found in all location except:**
    (Recent Questions 2016)
    a. Lumbar
    b. Perineal
    c. Intra abdominal
    d. Inguinal

20. **Complication of ectopic testis is:** *(Kerala 94)*
    a. Seminoma
    b. Atrophy
    c. Torsion
    d. All

TESTICULAR TORSION

21. **True about torsion of testis is all except:** *(AIIMS Nov 2001)*
    a. Presents with sudden pain in testis
    b. Commonly associated with pyuria
    c. Doppler U/S shows decreased blood flow to the testis
    d. Simultaneous orchiopexy of the other side should also be done

22. **A 30-year-old male patient presents with sudden onset swelling and pain over the right hemiscrotum. On examination the scrotum is reddened and tender. Which of the following statement about the affecting condition is not true?**
    a. Probable diagnosis is torsion *(All India 2008)*
    b. The right testis is likely to ride high in the scrotal compartment
    c. If torsion confirmed, treat with antibiotics and analgesics and perform corrective surgery immediately
    d. If torsion confirmed, treat with antibiotics and analgesics and perform corrective surgery after 14 days

23. **All of the following abnormalities are predisposing causes for torsion of the testis except:** *(COMEDK 2006)*
    a. Inversion of testis
    b. Low investment of tunica vaginalis
    c. Between 10 to 25 years of age
    d. Separation of the epididymis

24. All are true regarding torsion of the testis, except: *(Orissa 2011)*
    a. Common in adolescents and young adults
    b. Inversion of testis is the most common predisposing cause
    c. Elevation of testis reduces the pain
    d. If diagnosis is doubtful, prompt exploration is the rule
25. A 40-years old man in suffering from fever and pain in scrotum which is not relieved by elevation of testis, 3 days before had sexual contact with a young female: *(All India 97)*
    a. Testicular tumor   b. Acute epididymitis
    c. Torsion of testis   d. Acute orchitis
26. Torsion of testis has to be treated within: *(DNB 2007)*
    a. Immediately   b. 6 hours
    c. 12 hours   d. 15 hours
27. In testicular torsion, surgery within how much time can save viability of testis? *(Recent Question 2013)*
    a. 6 hours   b. 12 hours
    c. 24 hours   d. 1 weeks
28. All the following statements are true regarding torsion of testis except: *(APPG 2015)*
    a. Most common between 10 and 25 years of age
    b. Prompt exploration and twisting & fixation is the only way to save the torted testis
    c. Anatomical abnormality is unilateral and contalateral testis should not be fixed
    d. Inversion of testis is the most common predisposing cause

VARICOCELE

29. Not true about varicocele is: *(AIIMS Nov 2001)*
    a. Common on the right side
    b. Can present as a later sign of renal cell carcinoma
    c. Has bag of worm like feeling
    d. Can lead to infertility
30. Varicocele is common on left testis because: *(All India 98)*
    a. Left testicular vein drains into IVC which has high pressure
    b. Left testicular vein drains into left renal vein which has high pressure
    c. Left testis is lower situated
    d. Compression of testicular vein by rectum
31. What is the grade of given varicocele?

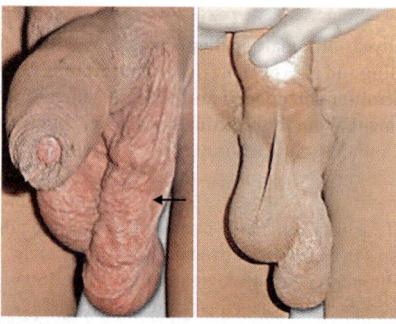

    a. Subclinical   b. Grade I
    c. Grade II   d. Grade III
32. In the treatment of varicocele, testicular vein ligation is done at the level of: *(DPG 96)*
    a. Above inguinal ligament   b. Below inguinal ligament
    c. Neck of the sac   d. Scrotum

33. Which is not true regarding varicocele? *(All India 88)*
    a. Testicular veins involved
    b. More common on the right side
    c. May be the first feature of a renal tumour
    d. Feels like a bag of worms
34. A 58-years old male presenting with acute onset of varicocele on left side most probable cause: *(CMC 98)*
    a. CA testes   b. Epididymitis
    c. Inguinal lymph nodes   d. CA kidney
35. Varicocele of pampiniform plexus of veins has all the following characteristics except: *(MPPG 97)*
    a. Negative transillumination test
    b. Reducible
    c. Cough impulse is present
    d. Frequently on right side
36. Most common cause of surgically treatable male infertility is: *(MAHE 98)*
    a. Varicocele   b. Cryptorchidism
    c. Stricture urethra d. Epididymitis
37. Which of the following is true about varicocele except?
    a. Incompetent valves of testicular vein are responsible for varicocele *(MAHE 2006)*
    b. 90% are on the left side
    c. Asymptomatic cases require surgery
    d. Femoral catheterization with spermatic vein ablation is done in recurrence
38. With reference to varicocele, which one of the following is not true of it? *(UPSC 2007)*
    a. Varicosity of cremastric veins
    b. Left side is affected usually
    c. Feel like a bag of worms
    d. May lead to infertility
39. After varicocele surgery, venous drainage occurs by: *(MHSSMCET 2006)*
    a. Cremasteric veins
    b. Penile veins
    c. Ectopic in the iliac fossa
    d. Present at the usual location
40. True about varicocele is: *(DNB 2007)*
    a. More common on right side
    b. Can cause oligospermia
    c. No effect on valsalva
    d. Lies anterior to testis
41. A young adolescent male came with painless swelling in scrotum since 2-3 months. On palpation, it feels like a bag of worms. What is the possible diagnosis? *(MHSSMCET 2010)*
    a. Varicocele   b. Testicular abscess
    c. Epididymo-orchitis d. Hydrocele
42. True about varicocele due to renal cell carcinoma is:
    a. More common on right side *(MHPGMCET 2003)*
    b. Temperature induced damage to testes occurs
    c. Cough impulse is positive
    d. Does not decompress in supine position
43. Operative managements of varicocele are indicated in which of the following conditions(s)? *(PGI Dec 2008)*
    a. Ipsilateral testis small size
    b. Oligospermia on semen analysis
    c. Grade-3 varicocele (large size)
    d. Signs or symptoms present
    e. Subclinical presentation

44. **Bag of worm like sensation is felt in:** *(Recent Question 2015)*
    a. Varicocele
    b. Hydrocele
    c. Torsion of testis
    d. Congenital hernia

SPERMATOCELE

45. **Regarding spermatocele which is correct?** *(PGI 88)*
    a. Occurs in head of epididymus
    b. Barely water fluid in appearance
    c. Tender
    d. Contain spermatozoa

46. **Chinese lantern on transillumination seen in:**
    (Recent Question 2014)
    a. Spermatocele
    b. Epididymal cyst
    c. Hydrocele of cord
    d. Secondary Hydrocele

47. **Regarding spermatocele all are correct except:**
    a. Occurs in the head of epididymis
    b. Barley water fluid
    c. Tender
    d. Contain spermatozoa

48. **Spermatoceles are most commonly found at:**
    (Recent Question 2017)
    a. Head of epididymis
    b. Testes
    c. Prostate
    d. Seminal vesicle

HYDROCELE

49. **Hydrocele is labeled 'vaginal' when it is:** *(AIIMS 96)*
    a. Limited to scrotum
    b. Upto inguinal canal
    c. Communicating into coelomic cavity
    d. Upto deep inguinal ring

50. **Treatment of a large hydrocele in an infant:** *(Kerala 97)*
    a. Repeated aspirations
    b. Ligation of sac at the opening of inguinal canal
    c. Herniotomy
    d. Eversion of sac

51. **Cause of hydrocele in infants:** *(CMC 98)*
    a. Patent processus vaginalis
    b. Patent gubernaculums
    c. Impaired drainage
    d. Epididymal cyst
    e. Infection

52. **Congenital hydrocele is best treated by:**
    (DNB 2009, 2008, 2005, 2001, Punjab 2011, AIIMS June 2001)
    a. Eversion of sac
    b. Excision of sac
    c. Lords procedure
    d. Herniotomy

53. **Which is false about hydrocele?** *(APPG 2008)*
    a. Almost always fluid is transudate
    b. Get above the swelling
    c. Testis is separate from swelling
    d. Obscures inguinal hernia

54. **Lord's and Jaboulay's operation is done for:** *(AMU 2005)*
    a. Rectal prolapsed
    b. Fistula in ano
    c. Inguinal hernia
    d. Hydrocele

55. **What do these images depict?** *(APPG 2016)*
    a. Jaboulay's operation
    b. Hernia repair
    c. Surgery for Fournier's gangrene
    d. Lord's plication for hydrocele

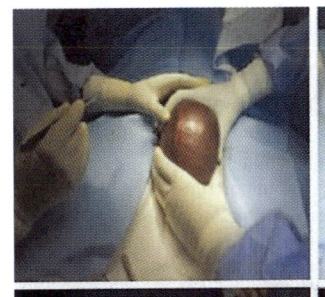 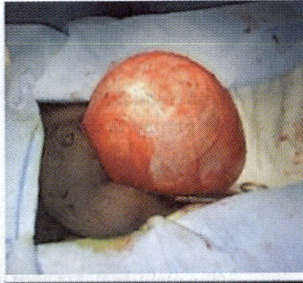
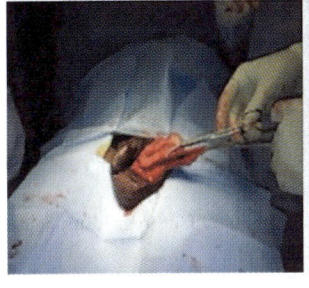 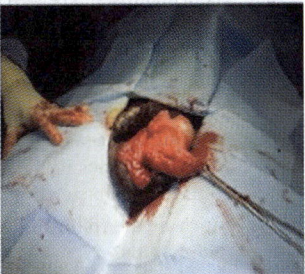

56. **Lords plication is done for:** *(All India 2010)*
    a. Inguinal hernia
    b. Testicular cancer
    c. Hydrocele
    d. Testicular varices

57. **Classical treatment of hydrocele:** *(DPG 2008)*
    a. Aspiration
    b. Aspiration and sclerosant agent
    c. Surgery
    d. Tapping

EPIDIDYMO-ORCHITIS

58. **Most common cause of acute epididymitis in males:**
    (COMEDK 2010, GB Pant 2011)
    a. E. coli
    b. Proteus
    c. Chlamydia trachomatis
    d. N. gonorrhoea

59. **Positive Prehn's sign is:** *(DNB 2010)*
    a. Elevation of testis increases pain of epididymitis
    b. Elevation of testis reduces pain of epididymitis
    c. Depression of testis increases pain of epididymitis
    d. Depression of testis reduces pain of epididymitis

60. **T.B. testis first affects:** *(DPG 95)*
    a. Vas
    b. Epididymis
    c. Body of testis
    d. Tunica vaginalis

61. **True about acute epididymitis is:** *(AIIMS Feb 97, All India 96)*
    a. Associated with urinary infection
    b. Painless
    c. Scrotum size is reduced
    d. Does not mimic with torsion of testes

62. **A 16-year-old boy presents with acute onset pain in the left testis. The following statements about his management are true except:** *(AIIMS Nov 2005)*
    a. The patient should be prescribed antibiotics and asked to come after a week
    b. Colour flow Doppler will be very useful in diagnosis
    c. Scrotal exploration should be done without delay if Doppler is not available
    d. If left testis is not viable on exploration, patient should undergo left Orchidectomy and right orchiopexy

63. Orchitis without epididymitis is seen in: *(All India 92)*
    a. Gonorrhoea
    b. Tuberculosis
    c. Syphilis
    d. Chlamydia infection

64. In differential diagnosis of epididymo-orchitis and torsion it is important that: *(AIIMS 95)*
    a. Elevation of testis in torsion relieves pain
    b. Elevation of testis in epididymoorchitis relieves pain
    c. Tenderness is characteristic of torsion of testis
    d. Fever is characteristic of epididymoorchitis

65. Acute orchitis all are seen except: *(Recent Question 2013)*
    a. Increased local temperature
    b. Decreased blood flow
    c. Etythematous scrotum
    d. Raised TLC

66. Prehn sign is seen in: *(Recent Question 2015; 2013)*
    a. Acute orchitis
    b. Chronic orchitis
    c. Testicular torsion
    d. None

67. Which of the following statements is true regarding acute epididymitis? *(APPG 2016)*
    a. All the statements are true
    b. Mostly bilateral
    c. Absence of blood flow on doppler Examination
    d. Occurs in young sexually active men and is commonly due to C. trachomatis

FOURNIER'S GANGRENE

68. Fournier's gangrene occurs in the: *(JIPMER 90)*
    a. Toes
    b. Scrotum
    c. Fingers
    d. Muscles

69. All are features of Fournier's gangrene except: *(MAHE 2007)*
    a. Testicles are involved
    b. Obliterative arteritis seen
    c. Hemolytic streptococci, isolated
    d. Necrotizing fasciitis

70. All are features of Fournier's gangrene except: *(MAHE 2008)*
    a. Testicles are involved
    b. Obliterative arteritis seen
    c. Hemolytic streptococci
    d. Necrotising fasciitis
    e. E. coli, staphylococci, Cl. welchii can be isolated

71. Fournier's gangrene is seen in: *(MCI Sept 2008)*
    a. Scrotum
    b. Shaft of penis
    c. Base of penis
    d. Glans penis

TESTICULAR CARCINOMA PREDISPOSING FACTORS

72. Predisposing factor of Testicular germ cell tumor:
    a. Cryptorchidism *(PGI Dec 2003)*
    b. Testicular feminization syndrome
    c. Klinefelter's syndrome
    d. Radiation
    e. Trauma

73. Testicular cancer is common in: *(All India 91)*
    a. Ectopic testis
    b. Undescended abdominal testis
    c. Atrophic testis
    d. Anteverted testis

TESTICULAR CARCINOMA

74. Most radiosensitive testicular tumour is: *(MCI March 2008)*
    a. Seminoma
    b. Teratoma
    c. Interstitial tumours
    d. Lymphoma

75. Most common testicular tumour in 4th decade: *(MCI Sept 2008)*
    a. Teratoma
    b. Dermoid
    c. Seminoma
    d. All of the above

76. Which of the following is false about testicular tumor?
    a. Pure seminoma is more aggressive than non-seminoma
    b. Seminoma is radiosensitive *(AIIMS May 2009)*
    c. Seminoma can be treated by orchidectomy with radiotherapy
    d. Seminoma spreads commonly through lymphatics

77. A patient presented with a hard swelling in this right testis. All are true statements except: *(AIIMS Nov 2001)*
    a. Trans scrotal biopsy is needed
    b. Inguinal exploration is done
    c. High inguinal exploration should be done
    d. Scrotal USG is done

78. A 20 years old male presents with hard painless testicular swelling. On investigation, AFP is 3080 ng/ml. No para-aortic or iliac nodes as well as no mediastinal lymph nodes found. Ultrasound shows uniform echotexture and small areas of necrosis. Surrounding structures are normal. What is the next best step?
    a. FNAC *(AIIMS May 2018)*
    b. Trucut biopsy
    c. High inguinal orchidectomy
    d. PET-CT

79. Germ cell tumors of testis are: *(PGI June 2001)*
    a. Seminoma
    b. Teratoma
    c. Leydig cell tumour
    d. Gynandroblastoma
    e. Rhabdomyoma

80. Most common testicular tumor in prepubertal adults is: *(AIIMS May 2008)*
    a. Yolk sac tumor
    b. Embryonal cell Ca
    c. Seminoma
    d. Teratoma

81. Intratubular germ cell tumor found adjacent to: *(PGI May, Dec 2006)*
    a. Spermatocytic seminoma
    b. Dysgerminoma
    c. Yolk sac tumor
    d. Embryonal carcinoma
    e. Choriocarcinoma

82. Which of the following is not seen in testicular carcinoma?
    a. Abdominal lump *(APPG 2006)*
    b. Epididymoorchitis
    c. Inguinal lymphadenopathy
    d. Hydrocele

83. All of the following clinicopathologic features are seen more often in seminomas as compared to non-seminomatous germ cell tumors of the testis except: *(AIIMS May 2005, Nov 2004)*
    a. Tumors remain localized to testis for a long time
    b. They are radiosensitive
    c. They metastasize predominantly by lymphatics
    d. They are often associated with raised levels of serum AFP and HCG

84. Following statements are true about germ cell tumors of testis except: *(AIIMS Nov 2002)*
    a. They constitute 90-95% of pall primary testicular tumors
    b. Seminoma is the most common tumor developing in the patients with cryptorchid testis
    c. AFP is markedly raised in all germ cell tumors
    d. High inguinal orchidectomy is the initial surgical procedure

85. Testicular tumor with best prognosis is: *(PGI Dec 96)*
    a. Teratoma
    b. Seminoma
    c. Choriocarcinoma
    d. All of the above
86. Marker for testicular tumor is: *(AIIMS June 97, PGI June 95)*
    a. Beta-hCG
    b. Acid phosphatase
    c. Alkaline phosphatase
    d. Alpha-fetoprotein
87. A testicular tumor in a man aged 60-years is; most likely to be: *(All India 2001)*
    a. Germ cell tumor
    b. Sertoli cell tumor
    c. Teratocarcinoma
    d. Lymphoma
88. Shyam, a 50-years old male presents with a hard scrotal swelling. All of the following can be done except: *(AIIMS June 2001)*
    a. Testicular biopsy
    b. Chest X-ray
    c. Inguinal exploration
    d. CT abdomen
89. Regarding testicular tumour, the following are false except: *(AIIMS June 2003)*
    a. They are commonest malignancy in older man
    b. Seminomas are radiosensitive
    c. Only 25% of stage I teratomas are cured by surgery alone
    d. Chemotherapy rarely produces a cure in those with metastatic disease
90. Placental alkaline phosphatase is marker of: *(PGI Dec 99)*
    a. Theca cell tumour
    b. Teratoma
    c. Choriocarcinoma
    d. Seminoma
91. Tumor marker for seminoma: *(AIIMS Nov 2013)*
    a. PLAP
    b. LDH
    c. AFP
    d. hCG
92. What % of testicular carcinoma is associated with cryptorchidism? *(PGI Dec 98)*
    a. 10%
    b. 30%
    c. 70%
    d. 90%
93. Which of the following statements is true regarding testicular tumors? *(All India 2006)*
    a. Are embryonal cell carcinomas in 95% of cases
    b. Bilateral in upto 10% cases
    c. Teratomas are more common than seminomas
    d. Usually present after 50-years of age
94. Which of the following is true about seminoma? *(PGI Dec 2005)*
    a. It is radiosensitive
    b. It arises only from cryptorchid testis
    c. AFP is increased
    d. It is chemosensitive
95. Testicular teratoma in adults is: *(DNB 2011)*
    a. Benign
    b. Malignant
    c. Locally aggressive
    d. Border line
96. It is true about seminoma testis that:
    a. It commonly occurs in the 6th decade
    b. An undescended tests is more liable to develop this tumour
    c. Histologically it resembles dysgerminoma of the ovary
    d. It is radioresistant
97. Seminoma testis is seen: *(Assam 96)*
    a. Always in undescended testis
    b. Always bilateral
    c. Occurs in younger
    d. Occurs in elderly
98. Testis tumor is associated with secondary hydrocele in: *(Karnataka 95)*
    a. 1% of cases
    b. 10% of cases
    c. 20% of cases
    d. 30% of cases
99. Most common testicular tumor in prepubertal adults is: *(AIIMS May 2008)*
    a. Yolk sac tumor
    b. Embryonal cell Ca
    c. Seminoma
    d. Teratoma
100. Carcinoma testis, the lymphatic metastasis goes to the first site seen in: *(UPPG 2010)*
    a. Para-aortic lymph nodes
    b. Superficial inguinal nodes
    c. Deep inguinal nodes
    d. Internal iliac nodes
101. A 25-year-old man presents with hydrocele on the left side. Associated condition could be a:
    a. Nephroma
    b. Hepatic malignancy
    c. Testicular tumour
    d. Penile malignancy
102. All are true regarding seminoma except: *(UPPG 2009)*
    a. Common in age between 35 and 45 years
    b. Metastasis to lymphatics
    c. Radioresistant
    d. Not seen before puberty
103. Seminoma of testis has all the following tumour markers except: *(COMEDK 2006)*
    a. AFP
    b. hCG
    c. LDH
    d. Alkaline phosphate
104. Most malignant testicular tumour is: *(DNB 2004)*
    a. Seminoma
    b. Teratoma
    c. Choriocarcinoma
    d. Embryonal carcinoma
105. A 20-year-old male presents with scrotal mass. The first investigation to be done is: *(Recent Question 2014; JIPMER 2011)*
    a. Clinical evaluation (Palpation and transillumination)
    b. USG
    c. Biopsy
    d. AFP
106. Most radiosensitive testicular tumor is: *(UPSC 2005, MHPGMCET 2002)*
    a. Seminoma
    b. Teratoma
    c. Lymphoma
    d. Sertoli cell tumor
107. Testicular tumor, that is rare in childhood: *(MHPGMCET 2006)*
    a. Seminoma
    b. Teratoma
    c. Interstitial cell tumor
    d. None
108. Testicular tumor can simulate: *(PGI SS June 2004)*
    a. Hydrocele
    b. Hematocele
    c. Acute epididymoorchitis
    d. Chronic orchitis
109. Most common testicular tumor in children: *(Recent Question 2017)*
    a. Yolk sac tumor
    b. Leydig cell tumor
    c. Seminoma
    d. Choriocarcinoma
110. A 12-year-old boy presents with serotal mass. The next best things to do in this patent is: *(JIPMER 2011)*
    a. Clinical evaluation
    b. USG
    c. Biopsy
    d. Immenate surgery

TESTICULAR CARCINOMA STAGING

111. High inguinal orchidectomy specimen showed tumor testis with involvement of epididymis without vascular invasion; stage is: *(MAHE 2007)*
    a. T1
    b. T2
    c. T3
    d. T4

112. High inguinal orchidectomy specimen showed teratoma testis with involvement of epididymis; stage is: *(DNB 2011, MAHE 2008)*
    a. T1
    b. T2
    c. T3
    d. T4b

TESTICULAR CARCINOMA TREATMENT

113. Stage I seminoma testis, treatment of choice is:
    a. High inguinal orchidectomy *(AIIMS Nov 2001)*
    b. High inguinal orchidectomy and radiotherapy
    c. Radiotherapy and chemotherapy
    d. Trans-scrotal orchidectomy

114. The treatment of metastatic testicular carcinoma is:
    a. Bleomycin, Etoposide, Cisplatin *(PGI June 99)*
    b. Vinablastine, Etoposide, Cisplatin
    c. Doxorubicin, 5-FU, mercaptopurine
    d. Methotrexate, 5-FU, Vincristine

115. A 27-year-old man presents with a left testicular tumor with a 10 cm retroperitoneal lymph node mass. The treatment of choice is: *(All India 2003)*
    a. Radiotherapy
    b. Immunotherapy with interferon and interleukins
    c. Left high inguinal orchiectomy plus chemotherapy
    d. Chemotherapy alone

116. Treatment of extragonadal germ cell tumour is: *(All India 99)*
    a. Chemotherapy
    b. Radiotherapy
    c. Surgery
    d. Immunotherapy

117. Which one of the following is the treatment of choice for a 4 cm retroperitoneal lymph node mass in a patient with non seminomatous germ cell tumor of the testis? *(AIIMS Nov 2004)*
    a. Radical radiotherapy alone
    b. High orchidectomy + RPLND
    c. RPLND alone
    d. High orchidectomy alone

118. A patient comes with stage III non seminomatous testicular tumor, treatment of choice is: *(AIIMS June 97)*
    a. Radiotherapy
    b. Chemotherapy
    c. Hormonal therapy
    d. Surgery

119. Disseminated seminoma is treated by:
    a. Chemotherapy or radiotherapy and ochidectomy
    b. Only radiotherapy
    c. Only chemotherapy
    d. RPLND

120. Stage-II testicular teratoma is treated by:
    a. Orchidectomy + RPLND *(DNB 2008, 2005, AMU 05)*
    b. Orchidectomy + Chemotherapy
    c. Orchidectomy
    d. Radiotherapy

121. Treatment of stage I teratoma is: *(MCI Sept 2008)*
    a. Chemotherapy
    b. Radiotherapy
    c. Chemotherapy plus Radiotherapy
    d. Observation /RPLND

122. Which of the following is a known complication of modified RPLND (Retroperitoneal lymph node dissection) done for non-seminomatous germ cell tumor of testis? *(MHSSMCET 2005)*
    a. Impotence
    b. Bladder atony
    c. Dry ejaculation
    d. Retrograde ejaculation

123. Which of the following testicular tumor does not require RPLND? *(MHSSMCET 2005)*
    a. Germ cell tumor
    b. Embryonal cell tumor
    c. Seminoma
    d. Teratoma

124. Treatment of Non-seminomatous germ cell tumor of testis with more than 4 cm RPLN includes: *(PGI May 2011)*
    a. RPLND
    b. Inguinal orchidectomy
    c. Chemotherapy
    d. Radiotherapy
    e. Orchidectomy through mid testicular incision

SEX CORD/GONADAL STROMAL TUMORS

125. Not true of sertoli cell tumour: *(Punjab 2009)*
    a. Poor response to radiotherapy
    b. Prominent lymphocytes in section
    c. Common in adults
    d. Can be malignant in 10–20% of cases

CARCINOMA SCROTUM

126. The lymph nodes first involved in cancer of the skin of the scrotum are: *(Karnataka 96)*
    a. Superficial inguinal
    b. External iliac
    c. Para aortic
    d. Gland of Cloquet

ORCHIDECTOMY

127. Subcapsular orchiectomy is done for cancer of: *(DNB 2008, APPG 96)*
    a. Tests
    b. Prostate
    c. Penis
    d. Urethra

128. Ligation of cord in orchidectomy for treatment of testicular tumor is done at: *(PGI 96)*
    a. External ring
    b. Internal ring
    c. Base of scrotum
    d. Just above epididimis

129. Subcapsular orchidectomy is done for cancer of: *(DPG 2005)*
    a. Testis
    b. Prostate
    c. Penis
    d. Male breast cancer

130. Orchidectomy is not done in: *(AIIMS June 2001)*
    a. Prostate cancer
    b. Seminoma testes
    c. Filarial epididemo-orchitis
    d. Male breast cancer

131. Orchiectomy is not indicated in: *(AIIMS Nov 99)*
    a. Seminoma testis
    b. Prostatic carcinoma
    c. Tubercular epididymitis
    d. Male breast cancer

MISCELLANEOUS

132. Dermoid arises from: *(PGI June 97)*
    a. Pluripotent cell
    b. Totipotent cell
    c. Ectoderm
    d. Mesoderm

133. Differential diagnosis of acute funiculitis with a small inguinal swelling is: *(TN 91)*
    a. Undescended testes
    b. Acute orchitis
    c. Lymphadenitis
    d. Small strangulated inguinal hernia

134. Which of the following closely mimics testicular malignancy?
    a. Hydrocele
    b. Hematocele
    c. Spermatocele
    d. Cyst of epididymis

135. The life of preserved semen for artificial insemination is:
    a. One year
    b. Two years
    c. Five years
    d. Ten years
    e. Fifty years

136. Best indication for testicular biopsy in a male is: *(Bihar PG 2014; All India 97)*
    a. Polyspermia
    b. Oligospermia
    c. Necrospermia
    d. Azoospermia

137. Which of the following structure in the spermatic cord is not damaged during vasectomy? *(AIIMS Nov 2012)*
    a. Testicular artery
    b. Ilioinguinal nerve
    c. Autonomic nerves
    d. Pampiniform plexus

138. Young male with history of trauma having left sided testis swollen and erythematous. Other side normal. Diagnosis: *(Recent Question 2013)*
    a. Torsion
    b. Carcinoma
    c. Hematoma
    d. Hernia

Explanations

UNDESCENDED TESTIS

1. **Ans. b. 6 months of age** *(Ref: Smith 18/e p380; Campbell 11/e p3443; Bailey 27/e p1498)*

   If spontaneous testicular descent does not occur, surgical treatment after 6 months of (corrected gestational) age is indicated.

2. **Ans. a. 6 months** *(Ref: Sabiston 20/e p1886; Abdominal wall Hernias- Principle and Management: Springer 2001/176)*

   > **TIMING OF ORCHIOPEXY IN UDT**
   >
   > **Sabiston 20/e p1886, 18/e p2071**
   > - In most pediatric centers, orchiopexy for unilateral UDT is done when patient have reached about **6 months** of age[Q]. This **early intervention** may permit **post-natal germ cell development** to **proceed normally**[Q].
   >
   > **Abdominal wall Hernias- Principle and Management: Springer 2001/176**
   > - In infants with congenital UDT, still undescended after 12 weeks of age, orchiopexy is recommended at **6 months** of age before germ cell development becomes deranged[Q].
   > - Achieve **scrotal placement** ideally by **6 months** of age and by **1 year** of age **at the latest**[Q].

3. **Ans. a. 3%** *(Campbell 11/e p3434)*
4. **Ans. a. Seminoma** *(Campbell 11/e p3451)*
5. **Ans. b. Undescended testis**
6. **Ans. a. Testicular tumor**
7. **Ans. c. Laparoscopy** *(Ref: Smith 18/e p140; Campbell 11/e p3440; Bailey 27/e p1499)*

   Diagnostic laparoscopy is a definitive investigation for an absence of testis (anorchia).

   > - "Impalable undescended testes are either **absent** or **located** in the **abdomen or inguinal canal**. There is **no benefit from imaging** and these are **best managed with a laparoscopy** and usually a staged approach." –Bailey 26/e p111

8. **Ans. d. Laparoscopy** *(Ref: Campbell 11/e p3441; Bailey 27/e p125)*

   > - "Laparoscopy is the procedure of choice to confirm or exclude the presence of a viable or remnant abdominal testis, unless a prominent scrotal nubbin is palpable with other clinical signs of monorchism." –Campbell 11/e p3441

9. **Ans. a. Infancy**
10. **Ans. a. Hydrocele**
11. **Ans. a. Right side** *(Campbell 11/e p3434)*
12. **Ans. a. Orchiopexy**
13. **Ans. c. Has higher incidence of malignancy**
14. **Ans. c. Poorly developed secondary sexual characters**
15. **Ans. b. 4 months**
16. **Ans. d. 1 year**
17. **Ans. d. Cryptorchidism** *(Ref: Campbell 11/e p3447)*

ECTOPIC TESTIS

18. **Ans. a. Superficial inguinal pouch** *(Ref: Smith 18/e p25; Bailey 27/e p1498)*
19. **Ans. a. Lumbar, c. Intra abdominal**
20. **Ans. d. All**

TESTICULAR TORSION

21. **Ans. b. Commonly associated with pyuria** *(Ref: Smith 18/e p707; Campbell 11/e p3391; Bailey 27/e p1500)*
22. **Ans. d. If torsion confirmed, treat with antibiotics and analgesics and perform corrective surgery after 14 days**
23. **Ans. b. Low investment of tunica vaginalis**
24. **Ans. c. Elevation of testis reduces the pain**
25. **Ans. c. Torsion of testis**
26. **Ans. a. Immediately** *(Ref: Campbell 11/e p3391)*
27. **Ans. a. 6 hours** *(Ref: Campbell 11/e p3391)*
28. **Ans. c. Anatomical abnormality is unilateral and contralateral testis should not be fixed** *(Ref: Campbell 11/e p3391)*

VARICOCELE

29. **Ans. a. Common on the right side** *(Ref: Smith 18/e p707; Campbell 11/e p3393; Bailey 27/e p1501)*

30. **Ans. b.** Left testicular vein drains into left renal vein which has high pressure *(Ref: Campbell 11/e p3393)*
31. **Ans. d.** Grade III *(Ref: Sabiston 20/e p2081; Schwartz 10/e p1653; Bailey 27/e p1501)*

The given varicocele is of grade III (visible and palpable at rest).

Varicocele Classification	
Subclinical	Not palpable or visible at rest or during Valsalva maneuver, but **demonstrable by special tests**[Q] (**reflux** found on Doppler examination)
Grade 1	Palpable during Valsalva[Q] maneuver, but not otherwise
Grade 2	Palpable at rest[Q], but not visible
Grade 3	Visible[Q] & palpable at rest

32. **Ans. a.** Above inguinal ligament
33. **Ans. b.** More common on the right side
34. **Ans. d.** CA kidney
35. **Ans. d.** Frequently on right side
36. **Ans. a.** Varicocele
37. **Ans. c.** Asymptomatic cases require surgery *(Ref: Campbell 11/e p3393)*
38. **Ans. a.** Varicosity of cremasteric veins
39. **Ans. a.** Cremasteric veins
40. **Ans. b.** Can cause oligospermia
41. **Ans. a.** Varicocele *(Ref: Campbell 11/e p3393)*
42. **Ans. d.** Does not decompress on lying down position *(Ref: Campbell 11/e p3393)*
43. **Ans. a.** Ipsilateral testis small size, **b.** Oligospermia on semen analysis, **d.** Signs or symptoms present *(Ref: Campbell 11/e p3393)*
44. **Ans. a.** Varicocele *(Ref: Campbell 11/e p3393)*

SPERMATOCELE

45. **Ans. a.** Occurs in head of epididymis, **b.** Barely water fluid in appearance, **d.** Contain spermatozoa *(Ref: Bailey 27/e p1504)*
46. **Ans. b.** Epididymal cyst
47. **Ans. c.** Tender

- Chinese-Lantern pattern on transillumination is more commonly seen in epididymal cyst.

48. **Ans. a.** Head of epididymis

HYDROCELE

49. **Ans. a.** Limited to scrotum *(Ref: Campbell 11/e p3384; Bailey 27/e p1503)*
50. **Ans. c.** Herniotomy
51. **Ans. a.** Patent processus vaginalis *(Ref: Campbell 11/e p3384)*
52. **Ans. d.** Herniotomy
53. **Ans. c.** Testis is separate from swelling
54. **Ans. d.** Hydrocele *(Ref: Campbell 11/e p3384; Bailey 27/e p1503)*
55. **Ans. a.** Jaboulay's operation *(Ref: Campbell 11/e p3384; Bailey 26/e p1382)*

Treatment of Vaginal hydrocele
• **Small** hydrocele: **Lord's** procedure **(Plication** of sac)[Q]
• **Medium** hydrocele: **Jaboulay's** procedure **(Eversion** of sac)[Q]
• **Large** hydrocele: **Excision** of sac[Q]

56. **Ans. c.** Hydrocele
57. **Ans. c.** Surgery *(Ref: Campbell 11/e p3386)*

EPIDIDYMO-ORCHITIS

58. **Ans. c.** Chlamydia trachomatis *(Ref: Smith 18/ep241; Campbell 10/e p3117-3118; Bailey 27/e p1505)*
59. **Ans. b.** Elevation of testes reduces pain of epididymitis
60. **Ans. b.** Epididymis
61. **Ans. a.** Associated with urinary infection
62. **Ans. a.** The patient should be prescribed antibiotics and asked to come after a week
63. **Ans. c.** Syphilis
64. **Ans. b.** Elevation of testis in epididymoorchitis relieves pain *(Ref: Smith 18/e p241; Campbell 11/ep 2913; Bailey 27/e p1505)*

Testicular Torsion	Epididymoorchitis
• Seen in **prepubertal age group (10-25)**^Q • Urine culture is sterile • No fever, **sudden agonizing pain**^Q with affected **testis high-riding**^Q in scrotum • Cremasteric reflex is **absent**^Q • Prehn's sign is **negative**^Q • **Color Doppler: Decreased blood flow**^Q • Treatment: **Immediate surgical exploration**^Q	• **Adults**, age group **20-30**^Q • Evidence of **UTI** • **Fever**, swollen, **red** and **tender scrotum, thickened cord** with reactive **hydrocele**^Q • **Cremasteric reflex is present**^Q • **Prehn's sign is positive**^Q • **Scrotal USG: Enlarged epididymis** with increased blood flow with **reactive hydrocele**^Q. • Treatment: **Antibiotics, rest**, scrotal elevation and **NSAIDs**^Q.

65. Ans. b. Decreased blood flow
66. Ans. a. Acute orchitis
67. Ans. d. Occurs in young sexually active men and is commonly due to C. trachomatis

FOURNIER'S GANGRENE

68. Ans. b. Scrotum *(Ref: Campbell 11/e p403; Bailey 27/e p1509)*
69. Ans. a. Testicles are involved
70. Ans. a. Testicles are involved
71. Ans. a. Scrotum

TESTICULAR CARCINOMA PREDISPOSING FACTORS

72. Ans. a. Cryptorchidism, b. Testicular feminization syndrome, c. Klinefelter's syndrome *(Ref: Smith 18/e p380; Campbell 11/e p784; Bailey 27/e p1506)*
73. Ans. b. Undescended abdominal testis

TESTICULAR CARCINOMA

74. Ans. a. Seminoma *(Ref: Smith 18/e p381; Campbell 11/e p784; Bailey 27/e p1506; CSDT 11/e p1071)*
75. Ans. c. Seminoma
76. Ans. a. Pure seminoma is more aggressive than non-seminoma *(Ref: Smith 18/e p381; Campbell 11/e p788; Bailey 27/e p1506)*
77. Ans. a. Trans scrotal biopsy is needed
78. Ans. c. High inguinal orchidectomy
79. Ans. a. Seminoma, b. Teratoma *(Ref: Smith 18/e p381; Campbell 11/ep786; CSDT 11/e p1071)*
80. Ans. d. Teratoma *(Ref: Smith 18/e p381; Campbell 11/e p788)*

- MC testicular tumour in prepubertal adults: **Teratoma**^Q
- MC testicular tumor of infants and children: **Yolk sac tumor**^Q

81. Ans. b. Dysgerminoma, d. Embryonal carcinoma, e. Choriocarcinoma *(Ref: Smith 18/ep382; Campbell 11/e p797)*
82. Ans. c. Inguinal lymphadenopathy
83. Ans. d. They are often associated with raised levels of serum AFP and hCG *(Ref: Smith 18/e p383; Campbell 11/e p790)*
84. Ans. c. AFP is markedly raised in all germ cell tumors
85. Ans. b. Seminoma *(Ref: Smith 18/e p381; Campbell 11/e p787; Bailey 27/e p1506)*
86. Ans. a. Beta-hCG, d. Alpha fetoprotein
87. Ans. d. Lymphoma *(Ref: Smith 18/e p388; Campbell 11/e p812)*
88. Ans. a. Testicular biopsy
89. Ans. b. Seminomas are radiosensitive
90. Ans. d. Seminoma
91. Ans. a. PLAP *(Ref: Smith 18/e p383; Campbell 11/ep 788)*

- *Tumor marker for seminoma is PLAP (Placental alkaline phosphatase). Though **beta-hCG** is also **raised** in **5-10% of pure seminoma**, as they contain syncytiotrophoblast like giant cells.*

92. Ans. a. 10% *(Ref: Smith 18/e p380)*

The **strongest association** has been with the **cryptorchid testis**. Approximately **7-10%** of **testicular tumors develop in patients** who have a **history of cryptorchidism**; **seminoma is the most common form** of tumor these patients have.

Testis and Scrotum

TESTICULAR TUMORS: EPIDEMIOLOGY AND RISK FACTORS

- Of all primary testicular tumors, **90-95% are germ cell tumors**[Q] (seminoma and nonseminoma)
- **More common** in **whites** and individuals of **higher socioeconomic class**[Q]
- **Slightly more common** on the **right side** than on the left, which parallels the **increased incidence of cryptorchidism** on the **right side**[Q].

  - Of **primary testicular tumors, 1-2% are bilateral**[Q], and about 50% of these tumors occur in men with a history of unilateral or bilateral cryptorchidism.
  - **Seminoma** is the **most common germ cell tumor** in **bilateral primary testicular tumors**[Q], while **malignant lymphoma** is the **most common bilateral tumor of the testis**[Q].

- The **strongest association** has been with the **cryptorchid testis**[Q]. Approximately **7-10%**[Q] of **testicular tumors develop in patients** who have a **history of cryptorchidism; seminoma is the most common form** of tumor these patients have.

  - However, **5-10%** of **testicular tumors** occur in the **contralateral, normally descended testis**[Q].
  - The **relative risk of malignancy is highest for the intraabdominal testis**[Q] (1 in 20) and is significantly lower for the inguinal testis (1 in 80).

- **Orchiopexy does not alter the malignant potential** of the **cryptorchid testis**; however, it does **facilitate examination** and **tumor detection**[Q].

93. Ans. None
94. Ans. a. It is radiosensitive
95. Ans. b. Malignant
96. Ans. b. An undescended testis is more liable to develop this tumour, c. Histologically it resembles dysgerminoma of the ovary
97. Ans. c. Occurs in younger
98. Ans. b. 10% of cases *(Ref: Smith 18/e p791)*

- Approximately **5-10%** of **testicular tumors** may be **associated with hydroceles**[Q].

99. Ans. d. Teratoma
100. Ans. a. Para-aortic lymph nodes
101. Ans. c. Testicular tumour
102. Ans. c. Radioresistant
103. Ans. a. AFP
104. Ans. c. Choriocarcinoma
105. Ans. b. USG
106. Ans. a. Seminoma
107. Ans. a. Seminoma
108. Ans. b. Hematocele
109. Ans. a. Yolk sac tumor *(Ref: Campbell 11/e p3594)*
110. Ans. a. Clinical evaluation

TESTICULAR CARCINOMA STAGING

111. Ans. a. T1 *(Ref: Campbell 11/e p791)*
112. Ans. a. T1

TESTICULAR CARCINOMA TREATMENT

113. Ans. b. High inguinal orchidectomy and radiotherapy
114. Ans. a. Bleomycin, Etoposide, Cisplatin
115. Ans. c. Left high inguinal orchiectomy plus chemotherapy *(Ref: Smith 18/e p384; Campbell 11/e p796; Bailey 27/e p1508)*
116. Ans. a. Chemotherapy
117. Ans. b. High Orchidectomy + RPLND
118. Ans. b. Chemotherapy
119. Ans. c. Only chemotherapy
120. Ans. a. Orchidectomy + RPLND *(Ref: Smith 18/e p385; Campbell 11/e p796; Bailey 27/e p1508)*
121. Ans. d. Observation /RPLND
122. Ans. d. Retrograde ejaculation *(Ref: Smith 18/e p385, 17/e p380)*

RETROPERITONEAL LYMPH NODE DISSECTION (RPLND)

- **RPLND** has been the **preferred treatment** of **low-stage NSGCTs**[Q]
- A **thoracoabdominal** or **midline Transabdominal approach** may be used
- All **nodal tissue between the ureters from the renal vessels** to the **bifurcation of the common iliac vessels is removed**[Q].

  - **RPLND is associated with significant morbidity, especially with respect to fertility in young men**[Q].
  - With a standard RPLND, **sympathetic nerve fibers are disrupted**, resulting in **loss of seminal emission**[Q].

123. Ans. c. Seminoma
124. Ans. a. RPLND, b. Inguinal orchidectomy, c. chemotherapy

SEX CORD/GONADAL STROMAL TUMORS

125. **Ans. b. Prominent lymphocytes in section** *(Ref: Smith 18/e p387; Campbell 11/e p811)*

CARCINOMA SCROTUM

126. **Ans. a. Superficial inguinal** *(Ref: Smith 18/e p391)*

ORCHIDECTOMY

127. **Ans. b. Prostate** *(Ref: Bailey 25/e p1378; Smith 18/e p372)*

Bilateral orchidectomy, whether **total** or **subcapsular**, will **eliminate** the **major source of testosterone** production in patients of **carcinoma prostate**.

CARCINOMA PROSTATE

- **Orchidectomy** is performed **to carry out androgen ablation** in the treatment of **locally advanced** (T3 or T4) disease or of **metastatic disease**[Q].
- In 1941, prostate cancer was shown to be responsive to such treatment by **Charles Huggins**, the only urologist to win a Nobel Prize.
- **Bilateral orchidectomy**, whether **total** or **subcapsular**[Q], will **eliminate the major source of testosterone production**.

128. **Ans. b. Internal ring** *(Ref: Bailey 27/e p1508)*

HIGH INGUINAL ORCHIDECTOMY

- The **cord** must be **ligated as close as possible** to the **internal ring** to facilitate complete removal of cord tissue[Q] in case a later retroperitoneal lymph node dissection is required.

129. **Ans. b. Prostate**
130. **Ans. c. Filarial epididemo-orchitis**
131. **Ans. c. Tubercular epididymitis** *(Ref: Bailey 27/e p1474, 1508)*

INDICATIONS OF ORCHIDECTOMY

- Clotted hydrocele[Q]
- Testicular tumors[Q]
- Prostate cancer[Q]
- Male breast cancer[Q]

MISCELLANEOUS

132. **Ans. b. Totipotent cell**
133. **Ans. d. Small strangulated inguinal hernia**
134. **Ans. b. Hematocele**
135. **Ans. d. Ten years**
136. **Ans. d. Azoospermia** *(Ref: Smith 18/e p699)*

TESTICULAR BIOPSY IN MALE INFERTILITY

- The **testis biopsy** provides **direct information** regarding the **state of spermatogenesis**[Q].
- **Abnormalities of seminiferous tubule architecture** and **cellular composition** are then categorized into several patterns[Q].

  - This procedure is **most useful in** the **azoospermic patient**[Q], in which it is often difficult to distinguish between a failure of sperm production and obstruction within the reproductive tract ducts.
  - A **testis biopsy allows definitive delineation** between these 2 conditions and can **guide further treatment** options **in azoospermic men**[Q].

- **Testis biopsies** may also be **indicated to identify** patients at high risk for **intratubular germ cell neoplasia**. This premalignant condition **exists in 5% of men with a contralateral germ cell tumor of the testis** and is **more prevalent in infertile** than fertile men[Q].

137. **Ans. b. Ilioinguinal nerve** *(Ref: Grays 40/e p1262)*

Ilioinguinal nerve is not a constituent of spermatic cord, hence, it is not damaged during vasectomy.

138. **Ans. c. Hematoma** *(Ref: Schwartz 9/e p1467)*

SECTION 5

Cardiothoracic Vascular Surgery

CHAPTERS

- Arterial Disorders
- Venous Disorders
- Lymphatic System
- Thorax and Lung

SECTION 5

Cardiothoracic Vascular Surgery

CHAPTER 26

Arterial Disorders

ARTERIAL OCCLUSION

Causes of Peripheral Arterial Occlusive Disease

Common
- **Atherosclerosis (MC)**[Q]
- **Buerger's disease**[Q]
- Takayasu arteritis
- SLE
- Post-traumatic
- Radiation injury

Rare
- External compression
- Popliteal entrapment
- Thoracic outlet syndrome
- Retroperitoneal fibrosis
- Coarctation of aorta
- Cystic medial necrosis
- Fibromuscular dysplasia

Causes of Arterial Occlusive Disease

Atherosclerosis
- Seen in patients **>40 years**[Q]
- **MC in 6th or 7th decade**[Q]
- Causes **occlusion of large**[Q] & **medium**[Q] sized vessels (Abdominal **aorta, iliac, femoral, Popliteal, tibial & peroneal arteries**)
- **Symptoms** of peripheral arterial insufficiency is predominantly seen **in lower limbs**[Q]

Buerger's Disease
- Seen in **young males <40 years**[Q]
- Involve **small & medium sized vessels (Tibial, plantar & radial arteries**[Q])
- **Symptoms** of peripheral arterial insufficiency is seen **in both lower & upper limbs**[Q]

Site of Block	Clinical Presentation
Aorto-iliac disease	• **Buttock, thigh & calf** claudication[Q] • Leriche syndrome[Q]
Common femoral disease	• **Thigh & calf** claudication[Q]
Superficial femoral disease	• Calf claudication[Q]
Popliteal artery disease	• Calf claudication[Q]
Crural artery disease	• Calf claudication[Q]

EMBOLIC OCCLUSION

EMBOLIC OCCLUSION

- An embolus is **detached thrombus from heart** or a more **proximal vessel**.
- **MC Source: Left atrium in atrial fibrillation**[Q] >**Mural thrombus following MI**[Q]
- Less common sources: Aneurysms & thrombi formed on atheromatous plaques

Emboli cause Ischemic Symptoms	
Leg	• Pain, pallor, paresis, pulselessness & paraesthesia[Q]
Brain	• TIA or stroke[Q]
Retina	• Amaurosis fugax
Mesenteric vessels	• Possible **gangrene** of corresponding loop of intestine[Q]
Spleen	• Local pain
Kidneys	• Loin pain and hematuria

Clinical Features
- **Embolic arterial occlusion** is an **emergency** that requires **immediate treatment**[Q].
- The leg is often affected, with pain, pallor, paresis, loss of pulsation & paraesthesia (or anesthesia).

> **Diagnosis can be made clinically**[Q] in a patient who has no history of claudication and has a source of emboli, who suddenly develops severe pain or numbness of the limb, which becomes cold & mottled[Q].

- Movement becomes progressively more difficult and sensation is lost[Q].
- Pulses are absent distally[Q] but the femoral pulse may be palpable.

Treatment
- Because of the ensuing stasis, a **thrombus can extend distally** and **proximally**[Q] to the embolus.

> - **Immediate administration of 5000 U of heparin IV** can reduce this extension and maintain patency of the surrounding (particularly the distal) vessels until the embolus can be treated[Q].

- The relief of pain is essential because it is severe & constant.

> - **Embolectomy & thrombolysis**[Q] are the treatments available for limb emboli.

- **Dextran-40 or 70** to reduce plasma viscosity can be given in the management of the ischemic limb for temporary improvement[Q].
- Low molecular weight dextrans are used during acute attack of thromboangitis. They cause hemodilution, decrease viscosity of blood & improve microcirculation. Intra-arterial injection is said to be more effective than intravenous[Q].

BUERGER'S DISEASE (THROMBOANGIITIS OBLITERANS)

BUERGER'S DISEASE (THROMBOANGIITIS OBLITERANS)

- **Segmental inflammatory disease**[Q], affecting **small & medium sized**[Q] arteries in **upper & lower**[Q] extremities
- **Inflammatory process** involves **neighboring veins & nerves**[Q]
- **Definite relationship with smoking**[Q]

Histopathology
- **Sharply segmental acute & chronic vasculitis of small & medium vessels** with **thrombosis of lumen** which may undergo organization & recanalization[Q]
- Thrombus contains microabscesses

> - **Inflammatory process** extends to involve **neighboring veins & nerves**[Q]
> - With time, **all three structures (artery, vein & nerve)** become **incased in fibrous tissue**[Q]

Clinical Features (RIM)
- Characterized **by triad of intermittent claudication, Raynaud's phenomenon & migratory superficial vein thrombophlebitis**[Q]

> - Typically seen in **young (<40 years), male smokers**[Q]

- **Not seen** in **females & non-smokers**[Q]
- Patient initially presents with **foot, leg, arm or hand claudication** progressing to **rest pain and ulcerations** on the toes, feet or fingers

> - **TAO** principally **affects distal (small + medium) vessels**[Q], so **claudication** is usually **confined to calves & feet or forearm & hands**

Diagnosis
- **Angiography of all four limbs**[Q] (multiple limbs may be involved)
- Even if symptoms are not yet present in a limb, angiographic findings may be demonstrated.

> - **Characteristic angiographic findings: Disease confinement to the distal circulation,** usually **infrapopliteal** and **distal to the brachial artery**[Q].
> - **Occlusions** are **segmental** and show "skip" lesions with extensive collateralization, the so-called **"corkscrew collaterals**[Q]**."**

Treatment
- **Abstinence from smoking**[Q] arrests, but does not reverse, the disease.
- **Vasodilators (Xanthinol nicotinate**[Q]**/complamina & Pentoxifylline**[Q]**/trental)**
- **Sympathectomy** for **rest pain** and **ulcerations**[Q]
- **Omental transposition**[Q]
- **Amputations**[Q] in gangrene

> Surgical bypass or revascularization is rarely feasible in Buerger's disease, because of:
> 1. **Occlusion of small & medium sized vessels**[Q]
> 2. Presence of **segmental & skip lesions**[Q]
> 3. **Absence** of **distal target vessel** for **bypass**[Q]

Arterial Disorders

Boyd Classification of Intermittent Claudication	
Grade 1	Pain starts but if the patient continues to walk, the metabolites increase the muscle flow and sweep away substance P produced by exercise and pain disappears[Q].
Grade 2	Pain continues but the patient can still walk with effort[Q]
Grade 3	Pain compels the patient to take rest[Q]
Grade 4	Rest pain[Q]

LUMBAR SYMPATHECTOMY

LUMBAR SYMPATHECTOMY

- **Open sympathectomy** is done preferably **through extraperitoneal approach**[Q].
- **Sympathetic chain** lies on the **sides of body of vertebra**, sometimes inside **psoas muscle sheath.**
    - In **unilateral surgeries**, sympathetic ganglia **L1, L2, L3** and sometimes **L4** are removed[Q].
    - In **bilateral surgeries, L1** of one side is **preserved to avoid retrograde ejaculation**[Q].
- **Lumbar chain** can be **mistaken** with **lymphatic chain, genitofemoral nerve, psoas sheath, psoas minor** leading to technical failure[Q].

Indications of Sympathectomy (BARA CHEF)	
• Buerger's disease[Q]	• Erythrocyanosis[Q]
• Atherosclerosis producing ischemia of limbs[Q]	• Frost bite[Q]
• Raynaud's disease[Q]	• Hyperhydrosis[Q]
• Acrocyanosis[Q]	• Peripheral vascular insufficiency
	• Causalgia[Q]

ANKLE BRACHIAL INDEX (ABI)

ANKLE BRACHIAL INDEX (ABI)

- **ABI** = Systolic **BP** at the **ankle** / Systolic **BP** in the **arms**
- Compared to the arm, **lower blood pressure in** the **leg** is an **indication of blocked arteries (peripheral vascular disease).**
- ABI is calculated by dividing the systolic blood pressure at the ankle by the systolic blood pressures in the arm.

ABI	Interpretation
>1.2	Noncompressible, severely calcified vessel (in DM & ESRD)[Q]
1.0-1.2	**Normal vessels**[Q]
0.5-0.9	**Intermittent claudication**[Q] (mild to moderate ischemia)
0.1-0.4	**Critical limb ischemia**[Q] (Ischemic ulceration, gangrene)

Fontaine Classification of Limb Ischemia	
Stage I	Asymptomatic[Q]
Stage IIa	**Mild** claudication[Q]
Stage IIb	**Moderate to severe** claudication[Q]
Stage III	Ischemic **rest pain**[Q]
Stage IV	**Ulceration** or **gangrene**[Q]

ARTERIAL ULCER

ARTERIAL ULCER

- **Arterial insufficiency ulcers ischemic ulcers** are mostly located on the **lateral surface of** the **ankle** or the **distal digits**[Q].
- **Most common** on **distal ends** of limbs[Q].

Etiology
- Caused by **lack of blood flow** to the capillary beds of lower extremities.
- Most often **endothelial dysfunction** is causative factor in **diabetic microangiopathy & macroangiopathy**[Q]

Characteristic Features
- **Punched-out appearance**[Q]
- **Pulses** are **not palpable**[Q]
- Associated **skin changes (thin shiny skin, absence of hair, brittle nails**[Q])
- **Intensely painful**[Q]

Diagnosis
- The lesion can be easily identified clinically.
- **Arterial doppler & pulse volume recordings** for baseline assessment of blood flow.
- **Radiographs** may be necessary **to rule out osteomyelitis**.

Treatment
- **Vascular surgery** to revascularize the area.
- In **infection: Antibiotics + Debridement**[Q]

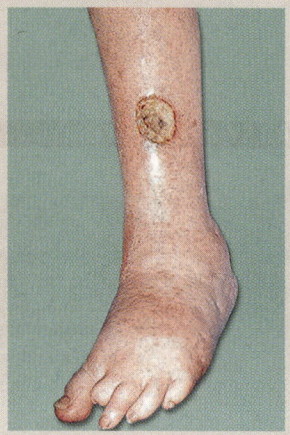

- **Ischemic time for digits is upto 8 hours**[Q].
- **Ischemic time for extremities is 4-6 hours**[Q].
- **Organ containing bag** should be **placed in** a solution of **saline with ice**[Q].

ARTERIOVENOUS FISTULA (AVF)

ARTERIOVENOUS FISTULA (AVF)

- AVF (communication between an **artery & vein**) may be **congenital or acquired** (penetrating trauma or surgically created **for hemodialysis**)

  - **MC type of AVF: Congenital**[Q]
  - **MC cause of acquired AVF: Penetrating trauma**[Q]

- Structural effects on veins: Veins are **arterialized** (become **dilated, tortuous & thick walled**[Q])

Physiological Effects of AVF
- **Increased pulse pressure**[Q] (Increased systolic & decreased diastolic)
- **Increased venous return** leading to **increased HR & increased CO**[Q]
- **Left ventricular enlargement**[Q] and later **cardiac failure**[Q] may occur

  - A congenital fistula in the young patient may cause **overgrowth of** the **limb**[Q]
  - In the leg **indolent ulcers** may result from **relative ischemia below** the **short circuit**[Q]

Clinical Signs
- A pulsatile swelling[Q]
- Thrill on palpation[Q]
- Continuous bruit on auscultation[Q]

  - **Nicoladoni's or Branham's sign: Pressure on artery proximal to fistula** causes the **swelling to diminish in size**, a **thrill** or **bruit to cease**, the **pulse rate** to **fall** & the **pulse pressure** returns to **normal**[Q].

Diagnosis
- **Duplex scan** and/or **angiography** confirm the diagnosis[Q].

Treatment
- Treatment is by **embolization**[Q].
- **Excisional surgery** (rarely) **for severe deformity** or **recurrent hemorrhage**[Q].

Types of Surgically Created Fistula	
Brescia-Cimino Fistula	**Radial** artery & cephalic vein[Q]
Snuffbox Fistula	Posterior branch of **Radial artery & cephalic vein**
Feinberg Fistula	**Radial artery & basilic vein**[Q]

THORACIC OUTLET COMPRESSION SYNDROME (TOS)

THORACIC OUTLET COMPRESSION SYNDROME (TOS)

- **TOS** refers to **compression of subclavian vessels** & nerves of **brachial plexus** in the region of **thoracic inlet**[Q].
- **Divided into**: **Vascular forms** (Arterial and/or Venous) & **Neurogenic forms**
- **Compression** resulting from TOS **is dynamic** & **best evaluated clinically by mechanical provocative maneuvers**[Q]

> - Symptoms most commonly develop secondary to neural compromise[Q]
> - Middle-aged women[Q] are most commonly affected

Neurovascular structures of the upper extremity may be compressed by	
• Cervical rib[Q]	• Trauma (neck hematoma, **bone dislocation**[Q])
• Long transverse process of C7[Q]	• **Fibrous bands**[Q] (congenital and acquired)
• Abnormal first rib[Q]	• Neoplasms[Q]
• Osteoarthritis	• Scalenes muscle[Q]

Clinical Features
- Symptoms vary depending on the anatomic structure that is compressed[Q].
- In > 90% of cases, neurogenic manifestations are reported[Q].

> - **Ulnar nerve (C8-T1) involvement is most common**[Q].
> - It is **associated with**:
>   – **Motor weakness** & **atrophy** of the **hypothenar** & **interosseous muscles**[Q]
>   – **Pain** & **paresthesia** along the **medial aspect** of the **arm, hand, 5th finger** & **medial aspect of 4th finger**[Q].

- Symptoms of **subclavian artery compression**: Fatigue, weakness, coldness, ischemic pain, & paresthesia. **Thrombosis with distal embolization** rarely can occur, producing vasomotor symptoms **(Raynaud's phenomenon)** in the hand or **ischemic changes**[Q].
- **Venous compression**: Edema, venous distention, collateral formation, & cyanosis of the affected limb[Q].

Diagnosis
- **Compression** resulting from TOS **is dynamic** and **best evaluated clinically by mechanical provocative maneuvers**[Q]
- **Specific investigations** (CT scan, MRI, Angiography, X-ray) **are used to exclude other conditions** and to **establish the associated diagnosis**[Q].

Treatment
- Approx. **50-90%** of patients can be **successfully treated** by **improvements** in **postural sitting, standing & sleeping positions, behavior modification** at work and **muscle stretching & strengthening exercises**[Q].

Indications for Surgical Intervention
• Failure of conservative management[Q]
• Progression of sensory or motor symptoms[Q]
• Presence of excessively prolonged ulnar or median nerve conduction velocities[Q]
• Narrowing or occlusion of the subclavian artery[Q]
• Thrombosis of the axillary or subclavian vein[Q]

- **Operation for TOS**: Complete removal of the first rib, with **division of scalenus** anticus & medius[Q].
- **Large aneurysms** or **thrombosis** of the **subclavian artery**: Graft reconstruction[Q]
- **Subclavian vein thrombosis**: Thrombolytic & anticoagulant therapy and simultaneous **surgical decompression**[Q].

Provocative Clinical Tests to establishing the diagnosis of Thoracic Outlet Syndrome (TOS)		
Provocative Test	**Instruction**	**Inference**
Adson's Test[Q] (Scalene Test)	Patient is instructed to: • Take a **deep breath and hold it** • **Extend** the **neck fully** • **Turn face towards** the side	• Maneuver **tightens** the **anterior & middle scalene muscles**, thus decreasing the interscalene space & magnifying any preexisting compression. • **Obliteration** or diminution **of radial pulse** suggests the diagnosis

Surgery Essence

Costoclavicular Test[Q] (Military Position or Halsted Test)	Patient is instructed to: • Draw shoulders downwards and backwards	• Maneuver narrows the costoclavicular space by approximating the clavicle to the first rib thus tending to compress the neurovascular bundle • Obliteration of radial pulse or reproduction of symptoms indicates compression
Hyperabduction Test[Q] (Wright Test)	Patient is instructed to: • **Hyperabduct** (Raise) the **arm to 180°**	• Maneuver causes the neurovascular structures to be pulled around the pectoralis minor tendon, coracoid process and head of humerus • Obliteration or diminution of radial pulse suggests the diagnosis
Roos Test[Q] (Arm Claudication Test)	Patient is instructed to: • Draw shoulders backwards • Rise **arms to horizontal position** with **elbows flexed to 90°** • Exercise the hands	• **Numbness** or **pain in** the **hands with exercise** suggests the diagnosis

RAYNAUD'S PHENOMENON

Raynaud's Phenomenon

- Raynaud's phenomenon is characterized by **episodic digital ischemia** on **exposure to cold** or **emotional stress**[Q]
- Manifested by the **sequential development of digital blanching, cyanosis & rubor** (redness) of **fingers** or **toes**[Q]
- **BCR: B**lanching, **C**yanosis & **R**ubor (redness)

Triphasic Color Response Include Three Stages	
Blanching[Q] (stage of **local syncope**)	• With exposure to cold, digital arterioles goes into spasm • Decreased flow is evidenced by pallor or blanching • Digits may appear white
Cyanosis[Q] (stage of **local asphyxia**)	• Capillaries and venules dilate • Cyanosis results from deoxygenated blood present in these vessels
Red Engorgement[Q] (stage of **recovery**)	• With rewarming or passing of attack, the digital vasospasm resolves • Blood flow into dilated arteries and capillaries increases dramatically • Reactive hyperemia imparts bright red color to the digits • In addition to rubor and warmth, patient often experiences a throbbing, painful sensation during the hyperemic phase

- **Raynaud's phenomenon** is divided into:
  - **Primary** or **idiopathic (Raynaud's disease**[Q]**)**
  - **Secondary** (associated with other diseases)

Associations
- **Raynaud's phenomenon** occurs frequently in patients who also have **migraine** or **variants angina**[Q]. These associations suggest a **common predisposing cause for vasospasm**[Q].
- Occupational groups that **use vibrating tools** are more predisposed
- **Sclerodactyly**[Q] (thickening and tightening of digital subcutaneous tissue) may develop **in few patients**.

RAYNAUD'S DISEASE

Raynaud's Disease

- Diagnosis of **Raynaud's disease** is made when the **secondary causes** of Raynaud's phenomenon are **ruled out**[Q].
- **Majority (70-90%)** of patients are **young women**[Q] <40 years of age.
- Geographic regions located in **cooler, damp climates** have a **higher reported prevalence**[Q].

Characteristic Features
- **Fingers**[Q] are involved **more commonly** than toes.
- On examination, patient is entirely normal.
- Radial, ulnar and **pedal pulses** are **normal**[Q].

Treatment

- There is **no cure**, all **treatments mainly palliate symptoms** and **decrease the severity** and, perhaps, **frequency of attacks**[Q].
- **Majority** (90%) of patients will **respond to avoidance of cold** and **other stimuli**[Q].
- **Remaining** 10% of patients can be **treated with** a variety of **vasodilatory drugs**
- CCBs such as **diltiazem** and **nifedipine** are the **drugs of choice**[Q].

DIABETIC FOOT

Diabetic Foot

- Diabetic foot is related to:
  - **Trophic changes** from **peripheral neuropathy**[Q]
  - **Ischemia** as a result of **microangiopathy** & **macroangiopathy (atherosclerosis)**[Q]
  - **Low resistance to infection**[Q] because of excess sugar in the tissues
- **Neuropathy** (**stocking**-and-**glove** distribution[Q]) **impairs sensation** and favours the **neglect of minor injuries** & **infections**.
- Motor involvement is frequently accompanied by **loss of reflexes & deformities (neuropathic joints)**.
- **Thick callosities** on the sole & **amateur chiropody** may allow the **entry of infection.**
- Any **infection** can **spread proximally with speed in subfascial planes** in diabetic patients.

Clinical Features

- Diabetic ulcers are usually found on the plantar surface of the foot over the metatarsal heads or heel[Q].
- Edema is usually mild with no change in surrounding pigmentation.

Treatment

- Treatment consists of bringing the **diabetes under control** by **diet** & **drugs**[Q].

> - **Necrotic tissue** must **be judiciously débrided**, and **topical antimicrobials** are needed **to control local infection**[Q].

- **In some cases, resection of the underlying bony prominence may improve wound healing.**

AORTIC DISSECTION

Aortic Dissection

- **Aortic dissection is** caused by a **circumferential** or, less frequently, **transverse tear of the intima.**
- **MC site: Right lateral wall** of the **ascending aorta**[Q]
- **Another common site: Descending thoracic aorta** (just below the ligamentum arteriosum).
- **Peak incidence: 6th & 7th decades.**[Q]
- **Men**[Q] are more **commonly affected**

Predisposing Factors	
• **Systemic hypertension**[Q]	• Takayasu's arteritis
• **Cystic medial necrosis**[Q]	• Giant cell arteritis
• Marfan syndrome	• Coarctation of the aorta
• Ehlers-Danlos syndrome	• History of aortic trauma
• Bicuspid aortic valve	• **Third trimester of pregnancy**[Q]

Classification

DeBakey Classification	
Type I	• **Intimal tear in ascending aorta**, involving **descending aorta**[Q]
Type II	• Dissection **limited to ascending aorta**[Q]
Type III	• Intimal tear in **descending aorta** with **distal propagation of the dissection**[Q]

Stanford Classification	
Type A	• Dissection **involves ascending aorta (proximal dissection)**[Q]
Type B	• Limited to the **descending aorta (distal dissection)**[Q]

Clinical Features

- Acute aortic dissection: **Sudden onset of pain**, very severe and tearing, associated with diaphoresis.

> • **Pain** may be localized to the **front** or **back of the chest**, often the **interscapular region**, and typically **migrates with propagation** of the **dissection**[Q].

- **Other symptoms:** Syncope, dyspnea, and weakness[Q].
- **Physical findings:** Hypertension or hypotension, **loss of pulses, aortic regurgitation, pulmonary edema,** and **neurologic findings** due to carotid artery obstruction (hemiplegia, hemianesthesia) or **spinal cord ischemia** (paraplegia)[Q].
- **Signs of aortic regurgitation: Bounding pulses,** a **wide pulse pressure,** a **diastolic murmur** often radiating along the right sternal border, and evidence of CHF[Q].

> - **Ascending aorta dissection:** widened superior mediastinum on Chest X-ray[Q]
> - **Pleural effusion (usually left-sided),** typically **serosanguineous** is seen[Q].

Diagnosis
- IOC for diagnosis in **stable patients: CT angiography**[Q]
- IOC for diagnosis in **unstable patients: Transesophageal echocardiography**[Q]

ANEURYSM

Aneurysm

- **Aneurysm:** Permanent & irreversible localized dilatation of blood vessel with at least **50% increase** in diameter
- **Ectasia:** dilatation <50% of normal diameter
- **AAA** (abdominal aortic aneurysm) is diagnosed if diameter >3 cm in males or >2.6 cm in **females**

> - **MC vessel involved in aneurysm: Circle of Willis**[Q]
> - **MC location of extra-cranial aneurysm: Aorta >Iliac >Popliteal >Femoral (AIPF)**[Q]
> - **MC site of extra-cranial arterial aneurysm is infrarenal aorta**[Q]
> - **MC site of peripheral aneurysm: Popliteal aneurysm**[Q]
> - **Degenerative aneurysms (caused by atherosclerosis) are MC AAA (90%)**[Q]

- **Width of aneurysm** is **most important** predicting **factor** of **rupture**[Q].
- **Juan Parodi**[Q] introduced endovascular aortic aneurysm repair **(EVAR).**

Classification
- **True** (all three layers of vessel are involved), **false** (do not have all three layers of vessel)
- **Infected (mycotic) aneurysm** are false aneurysm
- **Dissecting aneurysm** (dissection with aneurysmal dilatation of false lumen)
- **Fusiform (symmetrical enlargement** involving whole circumference of artery)
- **Saccular** (affect **only part** of the arterial circumference) have **higher risk of rupture**[Q]

ABDOMINAL AORTIC ANEURYSM

Abdominal Aortic Aneurysm

- **MC site** of **aortic aneurysm** is **infrarenal aorta**[Q]
- **Risk Factors:** Age, male gender, white race, smoking and family history[Q]

Clinical Presentation
- **Natural history** of AAAs is **continuous expansion**[Q]

> - **Rupture is MC & most lethal complication**[Q]
> - **Most rupture** occurs **in retroperitoneal space,** others in abdominal cavity, IVC, iliac vein or duodenum **(4th part-MC)**
> - **AAA rupture most commonly in left retroperitoneum**[Q]

- **Growth rate** of AAAs **vary with** aneurysm **size,** more rapid growth seen in aneurysms 5 cm or larger
- **MC symptom: Chronic vague abdominal** or **back pain**[Q]

> - **Triad of aortic rupture: Sudden onset midabdominal or flank pain + shock + pulsatile abdominal mass;** present in **one third** cases only[Q]
> - **Acutely expanding AAA** produce **severe deep back pain** or **abdominal pain radiating to back,** associated with **tenderness** to palpation of aneurysm (this presentation signifies **impending rupture** and **urgent evaluation & treatment** is required)[Q]

- In **aortocaval** or **aortoiliac fistula:** Unilateral or bilateral lower extremity edema, high output CHF & continuous abdominal bruit or palpable thrill is present

Arterial Disorders

- CCBs such as **diltiazem** and **nifedipine** are the **drugs of choice**[Q].
- **Gross hematuria** from **intravesicular venous hypertension** is one of **characteristic sign** of **aortocaval fistula**
- AAA may **rupture into GIT**, MC site is **4th part of duodenum**[Q], producing primary aortoenteric fistula, shock and massive GI bleeding.

  - Occasionally, **microembolization** can occur, resulting in **small patchy areas of ischemia**, usually on the **plantar aspect of** the **foot**, referred to as **trash foot**[Q].

MANAGEMENT OF ABDOMINAL AORTIC ANEURYSM

Diagnosis
- **Plain X-ray** detects AAA in up to **70%** cases by characteristic **"eggshell" pattern of calcification**
- **Negative** abdominal **radiograph doesn't exclude** the diagnosis.

  - **CT is IOC for diagnosis & planning repair in AAA**[Q]
  - **MRI is IOC for diagnosis** and with **MR angiography** planning **repair in AAA** with **renal insufficiency**[Q]

- Advantage of **Percutaneous arteriography** over CT or MRI is its **ability to measure pressure gradient** across occlusive lesions if present, and **potentially to direct treatment**

Screening for Abdominal Aortic Aneurysm
- AAAs remain **asymptomatic for several years, death** from **rupture** occurs in **one third of untreated cases**
- **Ultrasound is preferred method of screening**[Q]

Pre-operative Evaluation
- Patients with major clinical predictors of **cardiac risk** are considered **for pre-operative angiography**

  - Patients with **high grade (70-99%) internal carotid stenosis** are considered for **carotid endarterectomy** before AAA repair[Q]

- **Prompt operative intervention** is indicated in cases of **rupture**[Q]

Medical Management
- **NSAIDs & tetracycline** may have potential to reduce aneurysmal growth by inhibiting MMP.

Indications of repair of AAA	
• Diameter **5.5 cm** or more in men[Q]	• Rate of expansion **>1 cm/year**[Q]
• **Symptomatic** aneurysm[Q]	• **Atypical aneurysms**[Q] (dissecting, pseudoaneurysm, mycotic, saccular and penetrating ulcer) **regardless of size**
• For women and patients with **greater than average rupture risk**, AAA diameter **4.5 to 5.0 cm**	

Treatment
- Open repair: Transperitoneal & Retroperitoneal approach

Indications for Retroperitoneal Approach	
• History of **multiple prior operations**[Q]	• **Horse-shoe kidney**[Q]
• **Hostile abdomen**[Q]	• **Peritoneal dialysis**
• **Radiation treatment**[Q]	• **Inflammatory aneurysm or ascites**[Q]
• **Suprarenal aneurysm extension**[Q]	

- **Advantage:** Reduced GI and pulmonary complications, reduced length of ICU & hospital stay[Q]
- **Disadvantage:** Poor accessibility to distal right arteries and right renal artery

Results of Open Repair
- Mortality rate of **elective open infrarenal AAA repair** is <5% in good risk patients

  - **MC cause of death is myocardial dysfunction**, usually **ischemic in origin**[Q]
  - Complications occur in **10-30%** cases
  - **MC complication is non-fatal MI** followed by **renal failure**[Q]
  - **Renal failure** after repair of **ruptured AAA** carries a **high mortality rate**

- Most serious gastrointestinal complication is **ischemia of the left colon & rectum**[Q]
- **Post-operative hypotension & hemodynamic instability** are contributory factors

- First indication of bowel ischemia may be **substantial IV fluid requirement**^{Q} in the first 8-12 hours after the operation.
- **Diarrhea**, usually **blood** typically follows **within 48 hours**^{Q}
- If necrosis is limited to mucosa: Conservative treatment with bowel rest, antibiotics & fluid resuscitation
- In **full thickness necrosis or peritoneal irritation**: Urgent reoperation with resection of ischemic bowel and **creation of stoma**
- **Mortality rate: 50%**^{Q} (higher when full thickness bowel necrosis & peritonitis occur)

MYCOTIC ANEURYSM

MYCOTIC ANEURYSM

- Mycotic aneurysms are **focal dilatation of arteries** occurring at **points in the arterial wall weakened by infection**

Mycotic aneurysms may originate
1. As a result of **embolization from bacterial endocarditis**^{Q}
2. As an **extension of** an adjacent suppurative process^Q (extravascular source), ex. Osteomyelitis, sinus infection, meningitis etc.
3. By **circulating organisms** directly **infecting arterial wall**^{Q}

- MC location: Femoral artery > Aorta^Q
- MC organisms: Staphylococcus > Salmonella^Q

ILIAC ARTERY ANEURYSM

ILIAC ARTERY ANEURYSM

- Occur in conjunction with aortic aneurysm in 40% cases
- Most isolated iliac aneurysm involve common iliac artery (70%) & internal iliac artery (20%)
- Multiple iliac aneurysms occur in most patients and are bilateral in 33% cases

Etiology
- Occur in association with **atherosclerosis**
- Can also occur in **pregnancy** in absence of atherosclerosis as well as in **Marfan and Ehlers-Danlos syndromes, Kawasaki disease, Takayasu's arteritis, cystic medial necrosis & arterial dissection**

Clinical Features
- More common in **males, right & left sides** are **equally** involved^Q
- Symptoms are caused by **compression** of **adjacent pelvic structures**^{Q} (bladder, colon, ureter, rectum, lumbosacral nerves and pelvic vein)
- Most **common iliac aneurysms** can be palpated on **abdominal exam** whereas **internal iliac artery aneurysm** are more readily palpated on **rectal examination**^{Q}

Treatment
- **Operative mortality rate in** patients with **ruptured iliac aneurysm is 40%.**
- Iliac aneurysms >3.5^Q cm are repaired if possible.

Minimum Size for Surgery (AIPF: All India Police Force)
Abdominal **A**ortic Aneurysm (**5.5 cm**) = **I**liac aneurysm (**3.5 cm**) + **P**opliteal/**F**emoral aneurysm (**2.0 cm**)

Indications of Surgery in Aneurysms on the basis of Size (diameter)	
Descending thoracic aorta	≥6.5 cm^Q
Ascending thoracic aorta	≥5.5 cm^Q
Abdominal aorta	≥5.5 cm^Q
Iliac artery	≥3.5 cm^Q
Femoral & Popliteal artery	≥2.0 cm^Q

Arterial Disorders

POPLITEAL ARTERY ANEURYSM

POPLITEAL ARTERY ANEURYSM

- **MC peripheral aneurysm** and account for **70% cases**[Q]
- **Most patients** are **male** with **bilateral disease in 53% cases**
- **Amputation rate** in **acute thromboembolism** is up to **30%**

Indications for treatment	
• **Symptomatic** patients[Q]	• **Thrombus** in aneurysm[Q]
• Aneurysm **>2 cm**[Q]	• Angiographic evidence of **distal embolization**[Q]

Diagnosis
- Diagnosed by **physical examination and duplex scan**[Q]

FEMORAL ARTERY ANEURYSM

FEMORAL ARTERY ANEURYSM

- **Bilateral in >50% cases** and **92% have a concomitant aortoiliac aneurysm**[Q]
- **True FAA** are almost always degenerative atherosclerotic aneurysms[Q]

Etiology
- **True FAA** are **almost always degenerative** atherosclerotic aneurysms
- **False FAA** may develop as a result of disruption of **graft-artery anastomosis** following surgical revascularization with aortofemoral or femoropopliteal bypass
- **MC organisms** causing mycotic aneurysms are **Staphylococcus aureus, E. coli, Salmonella**[Q].

Diagnosis
- Diagnosis of atherosclerotic FAA is usually made by **physical examination** & confirmed by **USG**[Q].

Treatment
- In patients who present with femoral pseudoaneurysms after catheterization, **USG-guided compression with or without thrombin injection**[Q], can also be used to treat the disease

> - All true FAA >2 cm should be **repaired** because of risk of **thrombo-embolic complications** or **increased risk of rupture**[Q]
> - **High risk of rupture** in cases of **large, false** or aneurysm involving **profunda femoris**[Q]

- Treatment involves **resection & replacement with prosthetic interposition graft** with attempt of revascularization of profunda femoris.

Results of Open Repair
- Asymptomatic patients do well but amputation rate of 10% in symptomatic patients.

> - **Highest amputation rates** in **drug addicts** requiring treatment of infected FAA[Q].
> - **Autologus repair** with a **vein graft** and immediate **coverage with sartorius muscle flap decreases** rate of **reinfection and recurrent bleeding**[Q].

SUBCLAVIAN ARTERY STENOSIS

SUBCLAVIAN ARTERY STENOSIS

- **MC cause of subclavian artery stenosis: Atherosclerotic disease**
- **Left**[Q] subclavian artery stenosis is significantly more common than right

> - **MC site** of stenosis: **First part**[Q] of subclavian artery
> - Stenosis typically occurs just distal to origin of subclavian artery & lies proximal to origin of vertebral artery[Q].

- **Stenosis of first part** of subclavian artery may give rise to **subclavian steal syndrome**[Q]
- **Subclavian steal syndrome** is characterized by **reversed flow in vertebral artery** to compensate for a proximal stenosis in the ipsilateral subclavian artery there by **stealing blood from the 'brain' to feed the 'arm'**[Q].

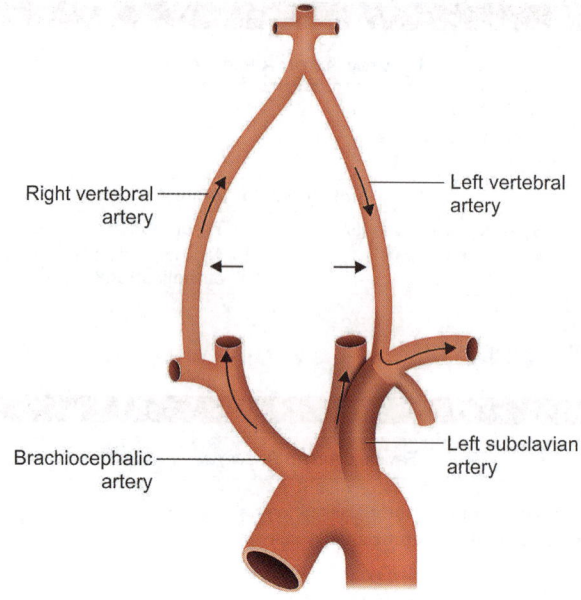

SUBCLAVIAN STEAL SYNDROME

Subclavian Steal Syndrome

- **Occlusion of** either the **innominate (brachiocephalic)** or the **subclavian artery before the origin of vertebral artery reverses the direction of blood flow** in the **ipsilateral vertebral artery**[Q].

  - This **reversal of flow** often is **asymptomatic** but **may cause ischemia** in the **posterior circulation**[Q].
  - **Neurological features** are **weakness, vertigo, visual complaints, & syncope**[Q].
  - Classically **symptoms occur** when **arm exercise increase** the **steal of blood flow from** the **brainstem**[Q].

- The **exercise reduces peripheral resistance** in the affected arm, **lowering blood pressure distal to occlusion**. This in turn results in **increased retrograde flow from** the **vertebral artery**[Q].
- If the contralateral vertebral artery cannot keep up with the demand, the **arm** may **steal blood from the basilar artery,** lowering the pressure in the **posterior cerebral circulation**[Q].
- The result may be transient vertebrobasilar ischemia[Q].

VASCULAR GRAFT

Vascular Graft	
Bioprosthetic	**Synthetic**

- Autograft[Q]
- Homograft (allograft)
- Heterograft (Xenograft)
- Tissue engineered
	- Textile:
	  – Dacron[Q]
	- Non-textile:
	  – ePTFE[Q]
	  – Polyurethane[Q]

Best natural vascular graft: **Reversed saphenous vein**[Q]
Best **synthetic** vascular graft: **Dacron**[Q]
Best vascular graft for **suprainguinal bypass: Dacron**[Q]
Best vascular graft for **infrainguinal bypass: Saphenous vein**[Q]
Best vascular graft for **aorta: Dacron**[Q]
Most preferred graft for **CABG: LIMA (left internal mammary artery) > Saphenous vein**[Q]
MC used graft for **CABG: Saphenous vein**[Q]

TRAUMATIC AORTIC RUPTURE

Traumatic Aortic Rupture

- Traumatic aortic rupture is a **cause of sudden death** after an **automobile collision** or **fall from a great height**^{Q}.
- Vessel is **relatively fixed distal to** the ligamentum arteriosum, just distal to the origin of **left subclavian artery**^{Q}.
- Causes: Trauma to the chest, Rapid deceleration injury^Q
- MC site: Adjacent to ligamentum arteriosum^Q

Clinical Presentation
- Traumatic aortic rupture is lethal in **75-90%** of patients^Q and only **15-20% arrive** at the hospital alive^Q.
- Approx. **90%** of those who arrive alive at the hospital have an **injury** in the region of the **aortic isthmus** >Injuries to the **ascending aorta**^{Q}.
- Usually associated with other injuries like solid organ.

Diagnosis
- X-ray chest: Widened mediastinum^Q
- Aortography: **Gold standard** for diagnosis^Q
- Contrast enhanced CT, Trans-esophageal Echocardiography **(TEE)** are useful in making diagnosis.

Treatment
- Control of systolic BP to less than 100 mm Hg
- Endovascular intra-aortic stenting^Q
- **Direct repair** or **excision & grafting** using **a Dacron graft**^{Q}.

TAKAYASU'S ARTERITIS (AORTOARTERITIS OR PULSELESS DISEASE)

Takayasu's Arteritis (Aortoarteritis or Pulseless Disease)

- Rare but well-recognized **chronic inflammatory arteritis affecting large vessels**, predominantly the **aorta** & its **main branches**^{Q}.
- **Chronic vessel inflammation** leads to **wall thickening, fibrosis, stenosis, & thrombus formation**^{Q}.
- **Symptoms** are related to **end-organ ischemia**.

> - **Pathologic changes** produce **stenosis, dilation, aneurysm formation & occlusion**^{Q}

Clinical Features
- Occurs predominantly in **adolescent girls** and **young women**^{Q}, age of **10-40 years**^{Q}
- More common in **Asia**^{Q}

> - Subclavian artery is MC involved vessel leading to loss or weakening of pulses (Pulseless Disease)^Q.

- Characteristic clinical features: **Hypertension** reflecting renal artery stenosis, **retinopathy, cerebrovascular symptoms**, angina and congestive heart failure, abdominal pain or GI bleeding or **extremity claudication**.

Diagnosis
- Laboratory data: Raised ESR, CRP & WBC count^Q
- IOC for diagnosis: CT angiography^Q
- Gold standard for diagnosis: Angiography^Q

Treatment
- **Steroid therapy** initially, with **cytotoxic agents** in patients **who do not achieve remission**^{Q}.
- **Surgical treatment** is performed **only in advanced stages**, and bypass needs to be delayed during active phases of inflammation.

GIANT CELL ARTERITIS (TEMPORAL ARTERITIS)

Giant cell Arteritis (Temporal Arteritis)

- Predominantly afflicts patients **older than 50 years of age**^{Q}, with a slight (2 : 1) **female preponderance**.
- Incidence **increases for each decade over age 50 years**.
- **Superficial temporal**^{Q}, vertebral, & **major aortic arch branches** may be involved.

Clinical Features
- Ischemic symptoms are common, including **claudication of facial** or **extremity muscles** & **retinal ischemia**^{Q}.
- **Headache** is a common symptom.
- **Blindness, usually irreversible**, is a **dreaded complication**^{Q}.

Treatment
- When the clinical diagnosis is suspected, **treatment** must be **prompt** and **consists of high-dose corticosteroid therapy**^{Q}.
- **Surgery** is **rarely indicated** except in cases of major aortic branch involvement with ischemic symptoms.

CELIAC PLEXUS BLOCK

Celiac Plexus Block

- **Celiac plexus** also known as the **solar plexus** is located behind stomach & omental bursa, and in front of the crura of the diaphragm
- **Location is at** the level of the **first lumbar vertebra.**
- Formed (in part) by the **greater & lesser splanchnic nerves** of both sides, and also parts of the **right vagus nerve.**
- Supplies upper GI organs, lower esophagus, liver & pancreas
- **Done usually bilaterally** using **alchol or phenol**

Indications:

- **Intractable pain** from cancers **(pancreatic cancer)**
- **Intractable pain** related to **chronic pancreatitis**

Side-Effects:

- Most common side effects include **hypotension** & **diarrhea**.
  - **Hypotension:** Because of the sympathetic blockade of splanchnic vasculature
  - **Diarrhea:** Unopposed parasympathetic activity following **celiac plexus block**

Multiple Choice Questions

ARTERIAL OCCLUSION

1. **Acute vascular ischemia manifests as:** *(PGI Dec 2008)*
   a. Pulselessness
   b. Paralysis
   c. Flushing
   d. Anesthesia
   e. Coolness

2. **Clinical feature of acute arterial embolism is:** *(PGI Nov 2017)*
   a. Pulselessness
   b. Pain
   c. Erythema of distal part
   d. Numbness
   e. Sensory loss

3. **The most common cause of peripheral limb ischemia in India is:** *(AIIMS Nov 2005)*
   a. Trauma
   b. Atherosclerosis
   c. Buerger's disease
   d. Takayasu disease

4. **Which among the following is not a feature of peripheral arterial occlusion?** *(Recent Question 2016)*
   a. Shock
   b. Pallor
   c. Pain
   d. Pulselessness

5. **Not a feature of acute arterial occlusion:** *(DNB 2010, AIIMS Nov 98)*
   a. Cyanosis
   b. Pallor
   c. Paralysis
   d. Paraesthesia

6. **What will be the diagnosis of Ramu, who is 45-years old male with history of chronic smoking and pain in lower limb due to blockage of femoral artery?** *(AIIMS Feb 97)*
   a. Thromboangitis obliterans
   b. Atherosclerosis
   c. Embolism
   d. Arteritis

7. **Fogarty's catheter is used for:** *(Recent Question 2015; UPSC 2007)*
   a. Drainage of urinary bladder
   b. Parenteral hyperalimentation
   c. Removal of embolus form blood vessels
   d. Ureteric catheterization

8. **Fogarty's catheter is used for?** *(AIIMS Nov 2010)*
   a. Urethral catheterization
   b. Removal of blood clots from the arteries
   c. Bladder drainage
   d. TPN

9. **Which one of the following is not a symptom of atherosclerotic occlusive disease at the bifurcation of aorta (Leriche syndrome)?** *(UPSC 2008)*
   a. Claudication of buttock and thigh
   b. Claudication of the calf
   c. Sexual impotence
   d. Gangrene localized to the feet

10. **Intermittent claudication is defined as:** *(All India 2009)*
    a. Pain in muscle at rest only
    b. Pain in muscle on first step
    c. Pain in muscle on exercise only
    d. Pain in muscle on last step

11. **Pseudoclaudication is caused by:** *(All India 2009)*
    a. Femoral artery stenosis
    b. Popliteal artery stenosis
    c. Lumbar canal stenosis
    d. Radial artery stenosis

12. **In a subclavian artery block at outer border of 1st rib, all of the following arteries help in maintaining the circulation to upper limb except:** *(AIIMS May 2011)*
    a. Subscapular artery
    b. Superior thoracic artery
    c. Thyrocervical trunk
    d. Suprascapular artery

13. **Both arterial and venous thrombosis occur in:** *(PGI Nov 2011)*
    a. Antiphospholipid antibodies
    b. Antithrombin III deficiency
    c. Hyperhomocysteinemia
    d. Protein C deficiency
    e. Mutation in factor V gene

14. **Maximum tourniquet time for the upper limb is:**
    a. 1/2 hour
    b. 1 hour
    c. 1.5 hours
    d. 2 hours
    e. 2.5 hours

15. **Intermittent claudication at the level of the hip indicates:** *(Recent Question 2016)*
    a. Popliteal artery occlusion
    b. Bilateral iliac artery occlusion
    c. Common femoral occlusion
    d. Superficial femoral artery occlusion

16. **Management of a case of iliac artery embolism requires:**
    a. Embolectomy
    b. Injection
    c. Hypotensive therapy
    d. Sympathectomy

17. **Intermittent claudication is caused by:**
    a. Venous occlusion
    b. Arterial insufficiency
    c. Neural compression
    d. Muscular dystrophy

18. **Treatment of acute femoral embolus is:** *(AIIMS 91)*
    a. Warfarin
    b. Heparin
    c. Immediate embolectomy
    d. Embolectomy after 5 days bed rest

19. **A useful though temporary improvement in a patient's ischemic foot can be attained by giving intravenously:**
    a. 10% Mannitol
    b. 10% Dextrose
    c. Dextran-40
    d. Dextran-100

20. **All are true about embolic arterial occlusion except:** *(JIPMER 95)*
    a. No previous history
    b. Muscles are unaffected
    c. Pulse is absent
    d. Anesthesia is present

21. **Tourniquet time of upper limb:** *(MHSSMCET 2010)*
    a. 1 hour
    b. 2 hours
    c. 3 hours
    d. 4 hours

22. **Which of the following is the most common symptom of aortoiliac occlusive disease?** *(AIIMS November 2016)*
    a. Calf claudication
    b. Gluteal claudication
    c. Impotence
    d. Symptomless

23. **Which of the following is true about Leriche syndrome?** *(Recent Question 2017)*
    a. Caused by aortoiliac occlusion
    b. Erection or impotence problems
    c. Gluteal claudication is seen
    d. All of the above

24. **Fontaine and Rutherford classification of peripheral arterial disease is based on:** *(Recent Question 2017)*
    a. Clinical
    b. Arterial stenosis on imaging
    c. Both clinical and arterial stenosis on imaging
    d. All of the above

BUERGER'S DISEASE

25. Not included in treatment of Buerger's disease:
    (PGI May 2011)
    a. Lumbar sympathectomy   b. Endovascular stent
    c. Rheostatic agent   d. Extra-anatomical bypass

26. All are true about intermittent claudication except:
    a. Most common in calf muscle   *(PGI May 2010)*
    b. Pain in positional
    c. Atherosclerosis is important predisposing factor
    d. Relieved by rest

27. A 45-years old male having a long history of cigarette smoking presented with gangrene of left foot. An amputation of the left foot was done. Representative sections from the specimen revealed presence of arterial thrombus with neutrophilic infiltrate in the arterial wall. The inflammation also extended into the neighboring veins and nerves. The most probable diagnosis is: *(AIIMS May 2006)*
    a. Takayasu arteritis   b. Giant cell arteritis
    c. Hypersensitivity angitis   d. Thromboangitis obliterans

28. True statement of Buerger's disease is/are: *(PGI June 2004)*
    a. Small and medium sized vessels involved
    b. Commonly involves upper limb than lower limbs
    c. Common in male
    d. Common in female

29. Drug used for Buerger's disease: *(MAHE 2005)*
    a. Xanthinol nicotinate   b. Propranolol
    c. GTN   d. All of the above

30. In a patient of vascular disease, angiography was performed and the image is given below. What is the most probable diagnosis?
    a. Popliteal artery aneurysm   b. Leriche syndrome
    c. Buerger disease   d. Aortic stenosis

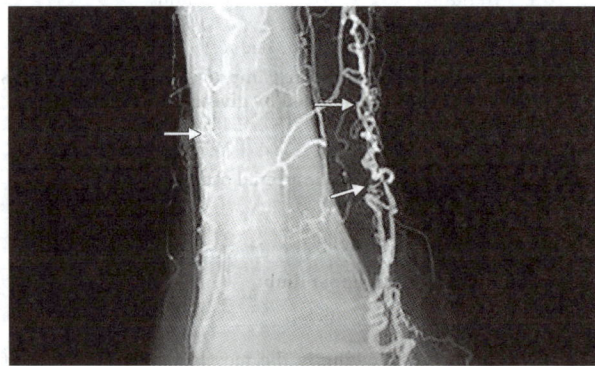

31. Buerger's disease usually affects all of the following except:
    (Recent Question 2014; MCI Sept 2009, 2010)
    a. Small sized arteries   b. Medium sized arteries
    c. Large arteries   d. Deep veins

32. Superficial thrombophlebitis is seen in: *(MCI March 2005)*
    a. AV fistula   b. Raynaud's disease
    c. Buerger's disease   d. Aneurysm

33. Which of the following is true about Buerger's disease?
    a. Atherosclerotic   *(AIIMS Nov 2012)*
    b. Neural involvement present
    c. Ulnar artery and peroneal arteries involved
    d. Only arteriole is involved

34. True about ischemic rest pain: *(PGI May 2010)*
    a. More in night
    b. MC in calf muscle
    c. Increase upon elevation of limbs
    d. Relieved by dependent position
    e. Often associated with trophic changes

35. What is the diagnosis based on the given image?
    (Recent Question 2016)
    a. Dry gangrene   b. Raynaud's disease
    c. Wet gangrene   d. Gas gangrene

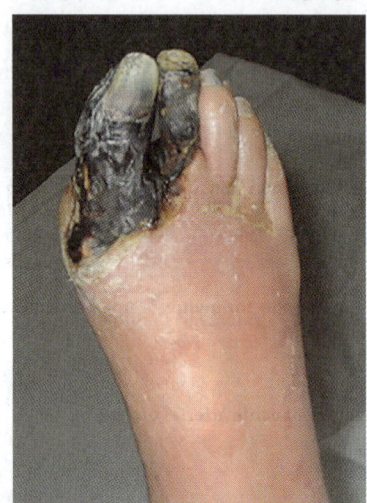

36. Most common cause of gangrene of foot of 30-year-old farmer who is a chronic smoker: *(AIIMS Nov 99)*
    a. Raynaud's disease   b. Myocardial infarction
    c. Atherosclerosis   d. Thromboangitis obliterans

37. Ramu, a 40-year-old male, a chronic smoker presents with claudication and a medial leg ulcer. For the past following procedures would not relieve his rest pain: *(AIIMS June 2001)*
    a. Lumbar sympathectomy   b. Omentoplasty
    c. Conservative amputation   d. Femoropopliteal bypass

38. Which one is not true regarding Buerger's disease?
    a. Men are usually involved   *(AIIMS June 97)*
    b. Occurs below 50 years of age
    c. Smoking is predisposing factor
    d. Veins and nerves are never involved

39. All of the following are the clinical feature of thromboangitis obliterans except: *(All India 2002)*
    a. Raynaud's phenomenon
    b. Claudication of extremities
    c. Absence of popliteal pulse
    d. Migratory superficial thrombophlebitis

40. Buerger's disease affects all except:
    (Recent Question 2015; DNB 2009)
    a. Lymphatics   b. Small vessels
    c. Nerves   d. Veins

41. Most common cause of death in patients with Buerger's disease is: *(AIIMS 87)*
    a. Gangrene
    b. Pulmonary embolism
    c. Myocardial infarction
    d. Carcinoma lung

Arterial Disorders

42. Commonest site of thromboangitis obliterans is:
    (All India 90)
    a. Femoral artery
    b. Popliteal artery
    c. Iliac artery
    d. Pelvic vessels

43. Following are used in treatment of Buerger's disease except:
    a. Trental
    b. Anticoagulation
    c. Sympathectomy
    d. Antiplatelets *(All India 93)*

44. A 40-year-old male, who is a chronic smoker presented with long history of intermittent claudication and blackish discoloration of toes. What is the preferred treatment?
    a. Abstinence from smoking only *(Recent Question 2017)*
    b. Vasodilators
    c. Lumbar sympathectomy
    d. Amputation

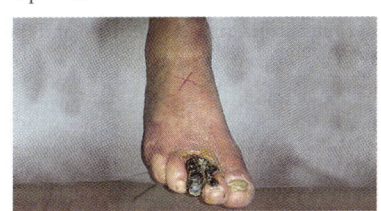

LUMBAR SYMPATHECTOMY

45. Indications for sympathectomy are all except:
    (MHPGMCET 2003)
    a. Intermittent claudication
    b. Ischemic pains
    c. Rest pains
    d. Buerger's disease

46. Lumbar sympathectomy is of value in the management of:
    a. Intermittent claudication *(All India 2009, 2005)*
    b. Distal ischemia affecting the skin of the toes
    c. Arteriovenous fistula
    d. Back pain

47. Sympathectomy is indicated in all following conditions except: *(All India 2009, 2003, Punjab 2007)*
    a. Ischemic ulcers
    b. Intermittent claudication
    c. Anhidrosis
    d. Acrocyanosis

48. Which of the following is spared in lumbar sympathectomy?
    a. L1
    b. L2 *(Recent Question 2015)*
    c. L3
    d. L4 *(JIPMER Nov 2017)*

49. In all of the following, sympathectomy is effective except one: *(AIIMS Sept 96)*
    a. Intermittent claudication
    b. Hyperhydrosis
    c. Raynaud's disease
    d. Causalgia

50. Lumbar sympathectomy is not indicated in: *(AIIMS June 97)*
    a. Healing of ulcer over great toe
    b. Claudication
    c. Rest pain
    d. Buerger's disease

51. Which of the following best responds to sympathectomy?
    (Recent Question 2016)
    a. Buerger's disease
    b. Hyperhydrosis
    c. Raynaud's disease
    d. Acrocyanosis

52. In extraperitoneal approach, to left sympathectomy the following may be injured: *(Recent Question 2016)*
    a. Ureter
    b. Gonadal vessels
    c. A+B
    d. IVC

53. In a lumbar sympathectomy the sympathetic chain in its usual position is likely to be confused with the:
    a. Psoas minor
    b. Genitofemoral nerve
    c. Ilioinguinal nerve
    d. Lymphatics

54. Removal of L1 ganglion in sympathectomy results in:
    (DNB 2006, JIPMER 91)
    a. Impotence
    b. Retention of urine
    c. Sterility
    d. Causalgia

CRITICAL LIMB ISCHEMIA

55. Which of the following statement is not true?
    a. Ankle brachial index <0.5 indicates critical limb ischemia
    b. Ankle brachial index changes during exercise and rest
    c. Ankle brachial index >1 is normal *(AIIMS Nov 2011)*
    d. Smoking is more specific for peripheral vascular disease than coronary artery disease

56. A patient with critical lower limb ischemia presents with:
    a. Intermittent claudication
    b. Intermittent claudication and gangrene
    c. Rest pain and ischemic ulcers *(All India 2009)*
    d. Intermittent claudication and ischemic ulcers

57. An adult patient with leg pain and gangrene of toe. His ankle to brachial arterial pressure ratio would be less than:
    a. 1
    b. 0.3 *(DNB 2011)*
    c. 0.5
    d. 0.8

58. Definition of critical limb ischemia includes:
    a. Rest/Nisht pain *(COMEDK 2014)*
    b. Ankle blood pressure > 50 mm Hg
    c. Intermittent clandication
    d. Well preserved tissues

59. Normal value of ankle brachial index is:
    (Recent Question 2014, 2013)
    a. 0.8
    b. 1
    c. 1.2
    d. 1.4

60. ABPI in imminent necrosis: *(Recent Question 2015)*
    a. < 0.3
    b. < 0.6
    c. < 0.9
    d. > 1.2

61. False elevation of ABPI is seen in: *(Recent Question 2018)*
    a. DVT
    b. Acute limb ischemia
    c. Chronic venous insufficiency
    d. Calcified vessel walls

62. ABPI increases artificially in: *(Recent Question 2018)*
    a. Arteriosclerosis calcified arteries
    b. Ischemic ulcers
    c. Intermittent claudication
    d. DVT

ARTERIAL ULCER

63. One of the following is not indicated for arterial leg ulcer:
    a. Debridement
    b. Elevation of limb *(PGI 96)*
    c. Head end of bed is raised
    d. Low dose aspirin

64. Foot ulcers secondary to arterial insufficiency are successfully treated by all of the following techniques except:
    a. Debridement of devitalized tissue *(COMEDK 2004)*
    b. Elevation of the affected extremity
    c. Antibiotic administration
    d. Bed rest

65. **True regarding leg ulcers & their location is/are:**
    (PGI May 2018)
    a. Arterial insufficiency – tip of the toes
    b. Arterial insufficiency – medial side of leg
    c. Venous insufficiency – above medial malleolus
    d. Diabetic neuropathic ulcer – planter aspect of metatarsal head
    e. Pressure ulcer – heel

AMPUTATION

66. **Re-implantation time for lower limb is:** *(Kerala 97)*
    a. 6 hours   b. 4 hours
    c. 8 hours   d. 10 hours
67. **Stump pain is relieved by:** *(Kerala 97)*
    a. Continuous tapping over the stump
    b. Warming up the stump
    c. Using steroids   d. Using analgesics
68. **For reimplantation surgery, the detached digit or limb is best preserved in cold:** *(Recent Question 2014; UPSC 2000)*
    a. Glycerol   b. Distilled water
    c. Hypertonic saline d. Isotonic saline
69. **Phantom limb is based upon:** *(DNB 2009)*
    a. Law of projection b. Webers law
    c. Munro-Kellie doctrine d. Renshaw cell inhibition
70. **Amputated finger is transported in:** *(Recent Question 2017)*
    a. Plastic bag with wet ice
    b. Plastic bag with dry ice
    c. Plastic bag with cold saline
    d. Plastic bag with cold water

ARTERIOVENOUS FISTULA

71. **Nicoladoni sign is also known as:** *(AIIMS Nov 2008)*
    a. Murray sign   b. Frei sign
    c. Darrier sign   d. Branham sign
72. **All are true about arteriovenous fistula except:**
    (PGI November 2017)
    a. Trauma is most common cause of acquired fistula
    b. Congenital fistula is easier to repair by surgery than acquired fistula
    c. Artificial fistula is surgically created fistulas for hemodialysis access
    d. High blood pressure from artery results in arterialization of vein
    e. Large A-V fistula may cause thrombocytopenia
73. **All of the following are correct regarding AV fistula except:**
    a. Arterialisation of the veins
    b. Proximal compression causes increases in heart rate
    c. Localized gigantism *(MHSSMCET 2005, All India 2001)*
    d. Causes LV enlargement and cardiac failure
74. **A patient presented with local gigantism of the leg and increased pulsations of the lower limb veins. Most probable diagnosis is:** *(AIIMS Nov 2001)*
    a. Tumor
    b. AV fistula
    c. Varicose veins
    d. Incompetence of the saphenofemoral junction
75. **Nicoladoni Branham sign is:** *(PGI Dec 98)*
    a. Compression cause bradycardia
    b. Compression cause tachycardia
    c. Hypotension
    d. Systolic filling

76. **The most common cause of acquired arteriovenous fistula is:** *(All India 2006)*
    a. Bacterial infection   b. Fungal infection
    c. Blunt trauma   d. Penetrating trauma
77. **Commonest cause of A-V fistulae is:**
    (Recent Question 2013, DNB 2000)
    a. Congenital   b. Traumatic
    c. Surgical creation   d. Tumor erosion
78. **Complications arising out of A-V fistula done for renal failure include the following except:** *(JIPMER 2003)*
    a. Infection
    b. Thrombosis
    c. High output cardiac failure
    d. Necrosis of the distal part
79. **Arteriovenous fistula can safely be ligated if the following is positive:** *(COMEDK 2004)*
    a. Allen's test   b. Henle-Coenen sign
    c. Trendelenberg test   d. Schwartz test

THORACIC OUTLET SYNDROME

80. **Thoracic outlet syndrome is primarily diagnosed by:**
    a. Clinical evaluation b. CT scan *(All India 2009)*
    c. MRI   d. Angiography
81. **Which of the following is not a complication of surgery for thoracic outlet syndrome?** *(AIIMS May 2007)*
    a. Pneumothorax
    b. Brachial plexus injury
    c. Lymphocutaneous fistula
    d. Long thoracic nerve injury
82. **Adson's test is positive in:** *(MHSSMCET 2005)*
    a. Cervical spondylosis b. Fracture ribs
    c. Cervical rib   d. All of the above
83. **This is the X-ray of a patient of thoracic outlet syndrome. What is the best management for this patient?**

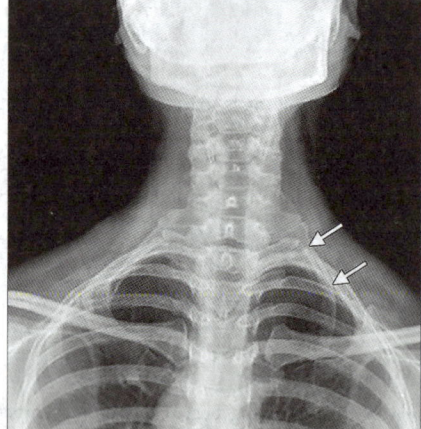

    a. Physiotherapy
    b. Conservative management
    c. Surgical intervention d. None of the above
84. **Which is not true about thoracic outlet syndrome?**
    (Recent Question 2016, AIIMS Nov 98)
    a. Radial nerve is commonly affected
    b. Neurological features are most common
    c. Resection of 1st rib relieves symptom
    d. Positive Adson's test

85. Which is not true regarding thoracic inlet syndrome?
    a. Most commonly radial nerve *(AIIMS Sept 96)*
    b. Resection of 1st rib is effective treatment
    c. Physiotherapy and position exercises relieves symptom
    d. Neurological signs and symptoms are common

86. Commonest symptom associated with thoracic outlet syndrome is: *(Recent Question 2016)*
    a. Intermittent claudication   b. Pain on radial distribution
    c. Pain in ulnar distribution   d. Gangrene

87. All are seen in thoracic outlet syndrome except: *(PGI 97)*
    a. Mass in the neck
    b. Wasting of forearm muscles
    c. Adson's test positive   d. Pallor

88. Adson's test is used for determining vascular insufficiency. It is useful in: *(Recent Question 2013)*
    a. Peripheral vascular disease
    b. Varicose veins
    c. Cervical rib   d. AV fistula

89. Most common age group affected in thoracic outlet obstruction syndrome is: *(DNB 2014)*
    a. 10–25 years   b. 25–45 years
    c. 45–65 years   d. > 65 years

90. All of the following are predisposing factors for thoracic outlet syndrome except: *(Recent Question 2017)*
    a. Scalene muscle
    b. Long transverse process of C7
    c. Spondylosis   d. Cervical rib

RAYNAUD'S DISEASE

91. All of the following are true regarding Raynaud's phenomenon except: *(AIIMS Nov 2012)*
    a. It involves acral parts of fingers
    b. Migratory thrombophlebitis is seen only in Raynaud's phenomenon
    c. Drugs acting by inhibiting the beta receptors in blood vessels also play a role
    d. Emotional stress may also precipitate Raynaud's phenomenon

92. True statement about Raynaud's phenomena: *(PGI Dec 2006)*
    a. Lower limb more commonly involved than upper limb
    b. More common in female
    c. Superficial thrombophlebitis
    d. Associated with migraine

93. Raynaud's syndrome occurs in all of the following except:
    a. SLE   *(DNB 2009, MCI Sept 2007)*
    b. Rheumatoid arthritis
    c. Osteoarthritis   d. Cryoglobulinemia

94. Sequence of colour changes observed in Raynaud's disease: *(MCI Sept 2009)*
    a. Red, blue, white   b. White, blue, red
    c. Blue, red, white   d. White, red, blue

95. If a patient with Raynaud's disease immersed his hand in cold water, the hand will: *(All India 2003)*
    a. Become red   b. Remain unchanged
    c. Turn white   d. Become blue

96. All are true about Raynaud's phenomena except: *(Kerala 95)*
    a. Exposure to cold aggravates
    b. Spasm of vessels
    c. More common in females
    d. Atherosclerosis of vessels

DIABETIC FOOT

97. True regarding management of diabetic foot: *(PGI May 2010)*
    a. Strict diabetic control
    b. Venous system is commonly involved
    c. Topical antibiotics are used
    d. Early amputation should done
    e. Diabetic ulcers are trophic ulcers

98. Site of diabetic foot ulcer: *(PGI June 2005)*
    a. Medial malleolus   b. Lateral malleolus
    c. Heel   d. Head of metatarsal
    e. Head of toes

99. Diabetic gangrene is due to: *(Kerala 94)*
    a. Ischemia
    b. Increased blood glucose
    c. Altered defense by host and neuropathy
    d. All of the above

100. Diabetic gangrene is due to all except: *(TN 86)*
    a. Vasospasm   b. Atherosclerosis
    c. Peripheral neuritis   d. Increased sugar in blood

101. Etiopathogenesis of diabetic foot include the following except: *(UPSC 2007)*
    a. Myelopathy   b. Osteoarthropathy
    c. Microangiopathy   d. Infection

AORTIC DISSECTION

102. The most common site of acute aortic dissection is:
    a. Right lateral wall of ascending aorta
    b. Arch of aorta   *(DNB 2013, COMEDK 2010)*
    c. Suprarenal abdominal aorta
    d. Infrarenal abdominal aorta

103. A 50-year-old male patient, an alcoholic and smoker presents with a 3 hours of severe retrosternal chest pain and increasing shortness of breath. He started having this pain while eating, which was constant and radiated to the back and intersapular region. He was a known hypertensive. On examination, he was cold and clammy with a heart rate of 130/min, and a BP of 80/40 mmHg. JVP was normal. All peripheral pulses were present and equal. Breath sounds were decreased at the left lung base and chest X-ray showed left pleural effusion. What is the most likely diagnosis?
    a. Acute aortic dissection
    b. Acute myocardial infarction
    c. Rupture of the esophagus
    d. Acute pulmonary embolism

104. Dissection of which artery is seen in pregnancy?
    a. Carotid artery   b. Aorta   *(PGI June 2000)*
    c. Coronary artery   d. Femoral artery

AORTIC ANEURYSM

105. Most common cause of abdominal aortic aneurysm is:
    a. Atherosclerosis   b. Trauma   *(All India 2010)*
    c. Syphilis   d. Vasculitis

106. False statement about abdominal artery aneurysm (AAA):
    a. Surgery indicated when size AAA >6 cm   *(PGI Nov 2011)*
    b. 90% of AAA is present below renal artery
    c. Blue toe syndrome may be associated
    d. Mortality rate after surgery is >25%
    e. Commonly causes colon ischemia

107. **The most common site of rupture of abdominal aortic aneurysm is:** *(All India 2009)*
    a. Laterally into the left retroperitoneum
    b. Laterally into the right retroperitoneum
    c. Posteriorly into the posterior retroperitoneum
    d. Anteriorly into the peritoneum (Intraperitoneal)

108. **Most common complication of descending aortic aneurysm surgery:** *(MHSSMCET 2006)*
    a. Renal failure
    b. Distal emboli
    c. Pulmonary infections
    d. Myocardial infarction

109. **The size at which elective surgery is indicated in abdominal aortic aneurysm:** *(MHSSMCET 2008)*
    a. 5 cm
    b. 5.5 cm
    c. 6 cm
    d. 6.5 cm

110. **Abdominal aortic aneurysm is operated when the size is more than:** *(Recent Question 2018)*
    a. 35 mm
    b. 45 mm
    c. 55 mm
    d. 65 mm

111. **Abdominal aneurysm is characterized by all except:** *(PGI June 2000)*
    a. Elective surgery complication should be <5%
    b. Emergency surgery complication <10%
    c. Rarely asymptomatic before rupture
    d. Bigger the size it is more prone to rupture

112. **Mycotic aneurysm is aneurysm infected because of:** *(All India 2006)*
    a. Fungal infection
    b. Blood borne infection (Intravascular)
    c. Infection introduced from outside (Extravascular)
    d. Both intravascular and extra-vascular infection

113. **The procedure of choice for the evaluation of aortic aneurysm is:** *(Recent Question 2013, All India 2006)*
    a. Ultrasonography
    b. Computed tomography
    c. Magnetic resonance imaging
    d. Arteriography

114. **Which of the following is true about coeliac plexus block?**
    a. Located retroperitoneally at the level of L3
    b. Usually done unilaterally *(AIIMS May 2013)*
    c. Useful for the painful conditions of lower abdomen
    d. Most common side effect is diarrhea and hypotension

115. **Most common cause of aneurysm of abdominal aorta is:**
    a. Trauma
    b. Atherosclerosis *(All India 96)*
    c. Syphilis
    d. Cystic medial necrosis

116. **In the abdomen, aneurysms of the commonly occur …… next only to the aorta:** *(Recent Question 2016)*
    a. Internal iliac artery
    b. External iliac artery
    c. Splenic artery
    d. Inferior mesenteric artery

117. **True about visceral aneurysms:** *(JIPMER May 2018)*
    a. Splenic artery is most commonly involved
    b. Hepatic aneurysm is operated irrespective of symptoms
    c. Splenic artery aneurysm is most commonly followed by trauma
    d. True aneurysms are more common nowadays with increasing abdominal trauma

118. **After doing a graft repair of a thoraco-abdominal aneurysm, the patients developed weakness. Most probable cause for this:** *(AIIMS May 2012)*
    a. Decreased blood supply to the lower limbs
    b. Thoraco splanchnic injury
    c. Discontinuation of arteria radicularis magna
    d. Lumbosacral nerve injury

119. **All of the following are true about aortic aneurysm except:** *(JIPMER 2013)*
    a. Saccular aneurysm involves whole circumference
    b. True aneurysm involves all 3 layers
    c. Atherosclerosis is the commonest cause
    d. False aneurysm is not covered by all 3 layers

120. **Dissecting aneurysm is best diagnosed by:** *(WBPG 2015)*
    a. CT
    b. MRI
    c. Angiography
    d. VSG

121. **Oliver's sign is seen in:** *(JIPMER November 2017)*
    a. Ascending aortic aneurysm
    b. Aortic arch aneurysm
    c. Descending aortic aneurysm
    d. Aortic dissection

FEMORAL ARTERY ANEURYSM

122. **Treatment of femoral artery aneurysm:** *(PGI June 2007)*
    a. Ultrasound guided compression of the neck of aneurysm
    b. Thrombin injection
    c. Bypass graft repair
    d. Ligation of involved vessel

123. **Pseudoarterial aneurysm in drug abuser's seen in:**
    a. Radial *(PGI June 2005, June 2007)*
    b. Brachial
    c. Femoral
    d. Carotid
    e. Pedal

POPLITEAL ARTERY ANEURYSM

124. **Most common site of peripheral aneurysm:** *(MCI June 2018, Nov 2017; Recent Question 2015; AIIMS Nov 2008)*
    a. Femoral artery
    b. Radial artery
    c. Popliteal artery
    d. Brachial artery

125. **Popliteal aneurysm-all are true except:** *(SCTIMS 98)*
    a. Presents as a swelling behind the knee
    b. Presents with symptoms due to complication
    c. Surgery is indicated in case of complication
    d. Uncommon among peripheral aneurysm

PSEUDOANEURYSM

126. **Pseudoaneurysms are most commonly due to:** *(Recent Question 2015; JIPMER 93)*
    a. Atherosclerosis
    b. Trauma
    c. Congenital deficiency
    d. Infections

127. **A drug abuser developed pseudoaneurysm. Which of the following is/are should include in the treatment modalities?** *(PGI Dec 2008)*
    a. Ligation of involved vessel and wide surgical debridement
    b. Exposure and ligation with subsequent revascularization
    c. Direct interposition graft with synthetic material in groin for revascularization
    d. Direct interposition graft with autogenous graft
    e. Selective revascularization using remote iliofemoral bypass

SUBCLAVIAN STEAL SYNDROME

128. **Commonest part of subclavian artery to be affected by stenosis is:** *(All India 2009)*
    a. First part
    b. Second part
    c. Third part
    d. Equally affected

129. Which of the following statement is true regarding subclavian steal syndrome? *(AIIMS Nov 2005)*
    a. Reversal of blood flow in the ipsilateral vertebral artery
    b. Reversal of blood flow in the contralateral carotid artery
    c. Reversal of blood flow in the contralateral vertebral artery
    d. Bilateral reversal of the flow in the vertebral arteries

VASCULAR GRAFT

130. Best graft for femoropopliteal bypass:
    (JIPMER May 2018; MHSSMCET 2007)
    a. Autologous vein   b. Dacron
    c. Teflon   d. PTF
131. Best material for below inguinal arterial graft is:
    a. Saphenous vein graft (upside-down)
    b. PTFE   *(WBPG 2015; All India 2009)*
    c. Dacron
    d. Teflon
132. Which of the following is most preferred graft in CABG?

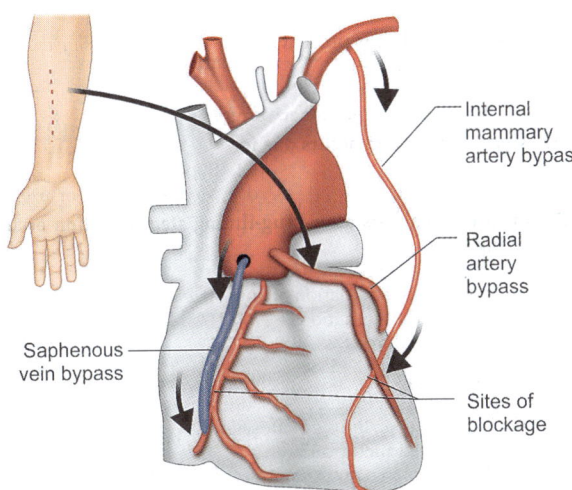

    a. Saphenous vein   b. Radial artery
    c. Internal mammary artery d. Internal jugular vein
133. Neointimal hyperplasia causes vascular graft failure as a result of hypertrophy of: *(All India 2006)*
    a. Endothelial cells   b. Collagen fibers
    c. Smooth muscle cells d. Elastic fibers
134. Dacron vascular graft is: *(Recent Question 2013, All India 2006)*
    a. Nontextile synthetic b. Textile synthetic
    c. Nontextile biologic   d. Textile biologic
135. Preferred material for femoro-popliteal bypass:
    (Recent Question 2018, 2017, 2014)
    a. Dacron   b. PTFE
    c. Saphenous vein   d. Gortex
136. For aortic graft the best material available is:
    a. Dacron   b. Artery   *(DPG 92)*
    c. Vein   d. None
137. Best graft for aortic dissection: *(JIPMER May 2018)*
    a. Dacron   b. Autologous vein
    c. Autologous artery   d. PTFE
138. A knitted dacron artery graft: *(PGI 99)*
    a. Is not porous
    b. Is eventually dissolved by tissue reaction
    c. Never gets infected
    d. Can be easily incised and the opening resutured

139. Not used as graft material in peripheral vascular disease:
    a. Dacron graft   b. Vein   *(PGI 97)*
    c. PTFE   d. PVC
140. Most preferred vascular graft for CABG:
    (Recent Question 2017)
    a. LIMA   b. RIMA
    c. Long saphenous vein d. PTFE

VASCULAR TRAUMA

141. Bullet wounds near major blood vessels should be explored only if:
    a. The extremity is cold
    b. The fingers or toes are paralyzed
    c. The pulse is weakened
    d. There is no pulse
    e. In all cases regardless of physical findings
142. True about aortic transaction: *(PGI June 2008)*
    a. Most commonly associated with deceleration injury
    b. High morality
    c. Surgery definitive treatment
    d. Aortography gold standard
143. Radiological findings of torn thoracic aorta is/are:
    a. Mediastinal widening *(PGI Nov 2011)*
    b. Abnormal aortic contour
    c. Right apical pleural cap
    d. Right paratracheal stripe thickening
    e. Left apical pleural cap
144. Best approach for surgical repair of the injury to abdominal aorta above the level of renal artery involving superior artery, celiac trunk, and the suprarenal branch:
    a. Right medial visceral rotation *(MHSSMCET 2009)*
    b. Left medial visceral rotation
    c. Right Lateral visceral rotation
    d. Left Lateral visceral rotation
145. Management of subclavian artery injury due to inadvertent central catheter insertion include all of the following except:
    (Recent Question 2018)
    a. Closure device   b. Mechanical compression
    c. Covering stent   d. Track embolization
146. What is the name of this maneuver?
    a. Mattox maneuver   b. Kocher's maneuver
    c. Extended Kocher's maneuver
    d. Cattell-Braasch maneuver

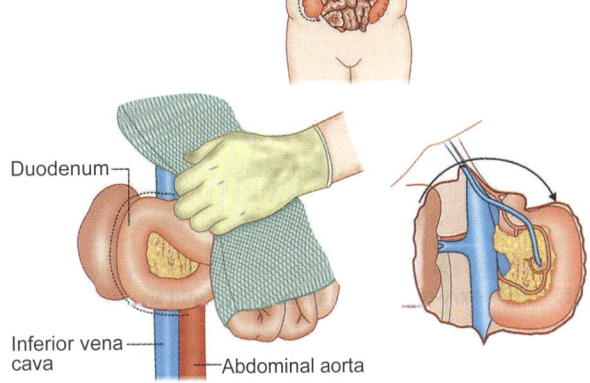

147. What is the name of this maneuver?
    a. Mattox maneuver
    b. Kocher's maneuver
    c. Extended Kocher's maneuver
    d. Cattell-Braasch maneuver

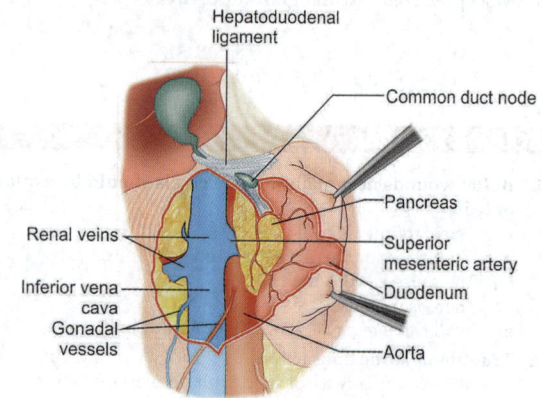

ANGIOGRAPHY AND COMPLICATIONS

148. Seldinger needle is used for: *(MCI March 2010)*
    a. Suturing muscles
    b. Arteriography
    c. Pulmonary biopsy
    d. Lymphangiography

149. All of the following complications may commonly follow lower extremity angiography except:
    a. Renal failure
    b. Dehydration
    c. Arterial occlusion
    d. Intracerebral hemorrhage

150. Most common artery used for cannulation: *(PGI June 97)*
    a. Radial artery
    b. Ulnar artery
    c. Brachial artery
    d. Cubital artery

151. Which is not true about femoral artery cannulation?
    a. Common femoral artery is cannulated *(AIIMS May 2011)*
    b. Single wall puncture is indicated in those with normal coagulation profile
    c. Femoral artery is catheterized at medial third of femoral head
    d. Seldinger technique is used both for femoral artery and vein

TAKAYASU ARTERITIS

152. Bilateral pulseless disease in upper limbs is caused by: *(PGI June 97)*
    a. Aortoarteritis
    b. Coarctation of aorta
    c. Fibromuscular dysplasia
    d. Buerger's disease

153. In Takayasu arteritis most common artery involved is: *(Recent Question 2017, JIPMER 2014)*
    a. Common carotid artery
    b. Subclavian artery
    c. Renal artery
    d. Inferior mesenteric artery

MISCELLANEOUS

154. Allen's test is useful in evaluating: *(APPG 2015, DNB 2011, All India 2006)*
    a. Thoracic outlet compression
    b. Presence of cervical rib
    c. Integrity of palmar arch
    d. Digital blood flow

155. The artery commonly involved in cirsoid aneurysm is: *(Recent Question 2016)*
    a. Occipital
    b. Superficial temporal
    c. Internal carotid
    d. External carotid

156. True about erythrocyanosis except: *(APPG 96)*
    a. Affects young girls
    b. Cold peripheries
    c. Palpable pulses
    d. Ulceration and gangrene of fingers

157. The Hunterian ligature operation is performed for: *(Recent Question 2014; DNB 2003, AIIMS Nov 2008, All India 2003)*
    a. Aneurysm
    b. Varicose veins
    c. AV fistulas
    d. Acute arterial ischemia

158. Popliteal artery pulsations are difficult to feel because:
    a. It is not superficial *(All India 2009)*
    b. It does not cross prominent bone
    c. It is not superficial and does not cross prominent bone
    d. Its pulsations are weak

159. The commonest cause of death following arterial reconstruction of the lower extremity is: *(COMEDK 2004)*
    a. Graft infection
    b. Cerebrovascular accident
    c. Myocardial infarction
    d. Systemic sepsis secondary to skin necrosis

160. Saddle thrombus is present at: *(Punjab 2008)*
    a. Pulmonary artery
    b. Aorta
    c. Pulmonary vein
    d. Bifurcation of pulmonary artery

161. Mycotic aneurysm occurs due to: *(MHSSMCET 2007)*
    a. Fungus
    b. Syphilis
    c. Salmonella
    d. Medial necrosis of arteries

162. In-situ thrombosis after drug-iluting stent insertion occurs owing to: *(MHSSMCET 2008)*
    a. Delayed re-epithelization
    b. Premature termination of anti-platelet therapy
    c. Disturbed coagulation
    d. All of the above

163. Butcher's thigh is: *(DNB 2010)*
    a. Vastus lateral rupture
    b. Subcutaneous lipodermatosclerosis
    c. Bursa in adductor canal
    d. Accidental injury to major vessels in thigh or groin

164. What is the best way to control external hemorrhage? *(DNB 2012)*
    a. Direct pressure
    b. Elevation
    c. Proximal torniquet
    d. Artery forceps

165. Which of the following is a feature of temporal arteritis?
    a. Giant cell arteritis *(AIIMS Nov 2012)*
    b. Granulomatous vasculitis
    c. Necrotizing vasculitis
    d. Leucocytoclastic vasculitis

166. Which of the following is true about coeliac plexus block? *(AIIMS May 2013)*
    a. Located retroperitoneally at the level of L3
    b. Usually done unilaterally
    c. Useful for the painful conditions of lower abdomen
    d. Most common side effect is diarrhea and hypotension

167. Which of the following is the best management for radiation induced occlusive disease of carotid artery? *(MCI Nov 2017)*
    a. Low dose aspirin
    b. Carotid angioplasty and stenting
    c. Carotid endarterectomy
    d. Carotid bypass procedure

168. Not a temporary embolization agent is: *(JIPMER May 2018)*
    a. Collagen
    b. Gel foam
    c. Thrombin
    d. Onyx

Explanations

ARTERIAL OCCLUSION

1. **Ans. a. Pulselessness, b. Paralysis, d. Anesthesia, e. Coolness** *(Ref: Sabiston 20/e p1756, 1777; Schwartz 10/e p872-881; Bailey 27/e p953)*

   ### PERIPHERAL ARTERIAL OCCLUSION
   - Clinical features of peripheral arterial occlusion are classically remembered by 5 Ps: **Pain, Pallor, Pulselessness, Paralysis** and **Paraesthesia** (or anesthesia)^Q
   - Some add 6th P: **Poikilothermia** or **perishing cold**^{Q}
   - **MC presenting symptom** of acute arterial occlusion: **Pain**^{Q}

2. **Ans. a. Pulselessness, b. Pain, d. Numbness, e. Sensory loss**

3. **Ans. b. Atherosclerosis** *(Ref: ASI Surgery/1333)*
   - ASI says **"Most common cause** of **peripheral limb ischemia in adults in India** is **atherosclerosis**^{Q}.

4. **Ans. a. Shock**   5. **Ans. a. Cyanosis**

6. **Ans. b. Atherosclerosis** *(Ref: Sabiston 20/e p1778, 1780; Schwartz 10/e p872-881; Bailey 27/e p887)*

7. **Ans. c. Removal of embolus form blood vessels** *(Ref: Sabiston 20/e p1778; Schwartz 10/e p877, 9/e p755-756; Bailey 27/e p955)*

   ### FOGARTY BALLOON CATHETER
   - **Fogarty balloon catheter** is used for **removal of embolus** form blood vessels^Q
   - **Embolectomy:**
     - Artery (usually the **femoral**), **bulging with clot**, is exposed and held in slings.
     - Through a longitudinal or transverse incision the **clot** begins to extrude and is **removed, together with** the **embolus, with** the help of a **Fogarty balloon catheter**^{Q}.
     - Catheter, with its balloon tip, is introduced both proximally and distally until it is deemed to have passed the limit of the clot.
     - **Balloon is inflated and catheter withdrawn slowly,** together with any obstructing material.
     - **Procedure** is repeated until bleeding occurs.

8. **Ans. b. Removal of blood clots from the arteries**   9. **Ans. d. Gangrene localized to the feet**

10. **Ans. c. Pain in muscle on exercise only** *(Ref: Sabiston 20/e p1765; Schwartz 10/e p828,882; Bailey 27/e p943,947)*
    - **Intermittent Claudication: Crampy pain in muscles induced by exercise** (walking) and **relieved by rest.**

    ### INTERMITTENT CLAUDICATION
    - **Crampy pain in muscles that is:**
      - Brought on by walking^Q (exercise)
      - Relieved by standing still/rest^Q (unlike pseudoclaudication)
      - Not present on taking the first step^Q (unlike osteoarthritis)

11. **Ans. c. Lumbar canal stenosis** *(Ref: Sabiston 20/e p1765; Schwartz 10/e p828,882; Bailey 27/e p943)*
    - When **symptoms mimicking** the symptoms of **intermittent vascular claudication** arise from **lumbar canal stenosis**, the condition is termed as **neurogenic pseudoclaudication.**
    - Pseudoclaudication refers to a variety of conditions that may mimic vascular intermittent claudication. The condition that is **most commonly confused with vascular intermittent claudication** is **neurological pseudoclaudication** due to **lumbar canal stenosis.**

Characteristics	Vascular Claudication	Neurogenic Pseudoclaudication
Age	Old	Old
Gender	**Male**^{Q} >female	Male = female
Current or previous low back pain	Less common	**Very common**^{Q}
Lower Limb Symptoms: • Pain • Numbness, tingling (Paraesthesias) • One or both sides	**Buttock, thigh,** and/or **leg**^{Q} No/Rare Yes (May be **unilateral**)	**Buttock, thigh,** and/or **leg**^{Q} Frequent Yes (Usually **bilateral**^{Q})

Provoking Factors:		
• Walking / Exercise	Yes[Q]	Yes[Q]
• Standing still	No	Yes[Q]
• Up an incline	± More likely[Q]	± Less likely
• Down an incline	± Less likely	± More likely[Q]
Relieving Factors:		
• Stand still	Helps[Q]	No help
• Lean forwards (flexed posture)	No difference	Helps[Q]
Preventive Factor:		
• Time to relief	Slightly **quicker**[Q] (2-5 minutes to disappear)	Slightly **slower**[Q] (15-20 minutes to disappear)
• Pulses	Reduced[Q]	Normal
• Neurological examination	Normal	Minor findings[Q]
• Straight - leg raising test	Negative	Usually negative
Walking distance	Fairly **constant**[Q]	More **variable**

12. **Ans. b. Superior thoracic artery** *(Ref: BDC 4/e pvol I/56, 82)*

A rich anastomosis exists around the scapula between branches of subclavian artery (first part) and the axillary artery (third part). This anastomosis provides a collateral circulation through which blood can flow to the limb when the distal part of subclavian artery or the proximal part of axillary artery is blocked.

Anastomosis around Scapula

• Formed by branches of:
    – **First part** of **subclavian artery**[Q] (**Suprascapular**[Q] and deep branches of **transverse cervical** artery[Q])
    – **Third part** of **axillary artery**[Q] (**Subscapular** and its **circumflex scapular** branch[Q])

13. **Ans. a. Antiphospholipid antibodies, c. Hyperhomocysteinemia** *(Ref: Harrison 20/e p841, 19/e p745; Sabiston 20/e p656, 1809; Schwartz 10/e p886, 9/e p754, 781)*

Abnormality	Arterial Thrombosis	Venous Thrombosis
Factor V Leiden[Q]	-	+
Prothrombin	-	+
Antithrombin III	-	+
Protein C	-	+
Protein S	-	+
Homocystinemia[Q]	+	+
Antiphospholipid syndrome[Q]	+	+

14. **Ans. d. 2 hours** *(Ref: Bailey 25/e p206-207)*

- Excessive tourniquet time causes both local pressure and distal ischemic effects, with nerve damage and even compartment syndrome.
- **Tourniquets** should usually be **let down after 1 hour**[Q] unless close to the end of a procedure.
- They can then be **reinflated after 5-10 min for a further hour**[Q].

• Tourniquet time for upper limb: 1 hour[Q]	• Maximum tourniquet time for upper limb: 2 hours[Q]

15. **Ans. b. Bilateral iliac artery occlusion** *(Ref: Sabiston 20/e p1756-1758; Schwartz 10/e p874, 9/e p753; Bailey 27/e p943-944)*
16. **Ans. a. Embolectomy** *(Ref: Sabiston 20/e p1778; Schwartz 10/e p877, 9/e p752-756; Bailey 27/e p955)*
17. **Ans. b. Arterial insufficiency** 18. **Ans. c. Immediate embolectomy**
19. **Ans. c. Dextran-40.** *(Ref: pmj.bmj.com/content/70/819/5.full.pdf)*

- Dextran-40 or 70 to reduce plasma viscosity can be given in the management of the ischemic limb for temporary improvement[Q].
- Low molecular weight dextrans are used during acute attack of thromboangitis. They cause hemodilution, decrease viscosity of blood and improve microcirculation. Intra-arterial injection is said to be more effective than intravenous[Q].

20. **Ans. b. Muscles are unaffected** 21. **Ans. a. 1 hour**
22. **Ans. b. Gluteal claudication**
23. **Ans. d. All of the above** *(Ref: Sabiston 20/e p1738; Schwartz 10/e p874; Bailey 27/e p943)*
24. **Ans. a. Clinical** *(Ref: Sabiston 20/e p1757; Schwartz 10/e p883)*

Arterial Disorders

BUERGER'S DISEASE

25. Ans. b. Endovascular stent, d. Extra-anatomical bypass *(Ref: Sabiston 20/e p1780; Schwartz 10/e p906, 1822-1823; Bailey 27/e p967)*
26. Ans. b. Pain in positional
    - **Relief of symptoms** is **not dependent upon sitting** or **other positional changes** in **intermittent claudication.**
27. Ans. d. Thromboangitis obliterans
28. Ans. a. Small and medium sized vessels involved, c. Common in male
29. Ans. a. Xanthinol nicotinate *(Ref: en.wikipedia.org/wiki/Xanthinol_nicotinate)*

> **Xanthinol Nicotinate**
> - **Xanthinol nicotinate** (or **xanthinol niacinate** or **complamina**) is **a vasodilator**[Q].
> - It is a combination of **xanthinol** and **niacin (nicotinic acid)**[Q].
> - This vasodilator is **used** in the treatment of Raynaud's phenomenon and **Buerger's** disease.

- Other than the experimental use of **iloprost (prostacyclin or PGI$_2$)** and **thrombolytics**, the use of **antibiotics** to treat infected ulcers, and **palliative treatment of ischemic pain** with **nonsteroidal and narcotic analgesics**, all other forms of pharmacologic treatment have been generally **ineffective** in the treatment of Buerger's disease, including **steroids, calcium channel blockers**, reserpine **pentoxifylline (Trental), vasodilators, antiplatelet drugs.**

30. Ans. c. Buerger disease *(Ref: Sabiston 20/e p1780; Schwartz 10/e p1083, 1822; Harrison 20/e p1925, 19/e p1645)*
31. Ans. c. Large arteries
32. Ans. c. Buerger's disease
33. Ans. b. Neural involvement present *(Ref: Robbins 9/e p512; Sabiston 20/e p1780; Schwartz 10/e p906,1822; Bailey 27/e p567; Harrison 20/e p1925, 19/e p1645)*
34. Ans. a. More in night, b. MC in calf muscle, c. Increase upon elevation of limbs, d. Relieved by dependent position, e. Often associated with trophic changes *(Ref: Sabiston 20/e p1780; Schwartz 10/e p906, 9/e p753; Bailey 27/e p943)*

> **ISCHEMIC REST PAIN**
> - **Ischemic rest pain** is a **grave symptom** caused by **ischemic neuritis**[Q].
> - Indicates advanced **arterial insufficiency** that usually terminates **in gangrene and amputation of the extremity** if arterial reconstruction cannot be performed.
> - **Burning pain** usually **confined to the forefoot, distal to the metatarsals**[Q].
> - It may be localized to the vicinity of an ischemic ulcer or pregangrenous toe.
>   - It is **aggravated by elevation** of the extremity or **by bringing the leg** to the **horizontal position**[Q].
>   - Thus it **appears at bed rest** (hence the name) and **prevent sleep**[Q].
>   - Because **gravity aids** the **delivery of arterial blood**, classically, the patient with rest pain can obtain **relief by** simply **hanging** the **leg over** the **side of the bed**[Q].
>   - This simple maneuver **will not relieve pain caused by peripheral neuropathy**, the **most common cause of foot pain at rest**[Q].
> - If the foot is constantly kept dependent to relieve pain, the leg and foot may be swollen, causing some confusion in diagnosis.
> - **Ischemic neuritis pain** is **severe** and **resistant to opioids** for relief[Q].
> - **Rest pain** occurs when **blood flow is inadequate to meet metabolic requirements**[Q].
> - In the lower extremity, ischemic rest pain is **localized to the forefoot** and generally is easily distinguished from benign nocturnal muscle cramps in the calf, which are also common in older patients.
> - Patients often have **trophic changes**, such as **muscle wasting, thinning of skin, thickening of nails**, and **hair loss** in the **distal affected limb**[Q].

35. Ans. a. Dry gangrene *(Ref: Sabiston 20/e p1780)*
36. Ans. d. Thromboangitis obliterans
37. Ans. d. Femoropopliteal bypass
38. Ans. d. Veins and nerves are never involved
39. Ans. c. Absence of popliteal pulse
40. Ans. a. Lymphatics
41. Ans. c. Myocardial infarction
42. None
43. Ans. b. Anticoagulation
44. Ans. d. Amputation

LUMBAR SYMPATHECTOMY

45. Ans. a. Intermittent claudication *(Ref: Sabiston 20/e p1780; Schwartz 10/e p906, 9/e p771; Bailey 27/e p968)*
    - Lumbar sympathectomy is not of value in the management of intermittent claudication, as blood flow in the skin but not in the muscle is controlled by sympathetic nervous system.

- **Blood flow** in the **skin** but **not in the muscle** is **controlled** by **sympathetic nervous system**^{Q}.
- If the overlying arterial supply is inadequate, ischemic changes in the skin may be relieved by sympathetic blockage but the impaired blood flow to muscles is unlikely to improve^Q.

46. **Ans. b. Distal ischemia affecting the skin of the toes** *(Ref: Sabiston 20/e p1780; Schwartz 10/e p906, 9/e p771; Bailey 27/e p968)*
    - **Lumbar sympathectomy** is **indicated in** the **management of distal ischemia affecting skin of** the **toes.**
    - Arteriovenous fistula, back pain and intermittent claudication are not included amongst the indications for lumbar sympathectomy.
    - **MC indication of sympathectomy** is ischemic disorders mainly of the **limbs**^{Q}.
    - **MC ischemic condition** for which sympathectomy is carried out is **peripheral vascular occlusive disease of** the **young male smokers**^{Q}.
    - **Lumbar sympathectomy** is **not of value in the management of intermittent claudication**^{Q}

47. **Ans. b. Intermittent claudication c. Anhidrosis** *(Ref: Sabiston 20/e p1780; Schwartz 10/e p906, 9/e p771; Bailey 27/e p968)*
    - **Sympathectomy** is **used for** the treatment of **hyperhydrosis.** It would **worsen anhydrosis** rather than treating it.

48. **Ans. a. L1** *(Ref: Sabiston 20/e p1780; Bailey 25/e p924)*
49. **Ans. a. Intermittent claudication**
50. **Ans. b. Claudication**
51. **Ans. b. Hyperhydrosis**
52. **Ans. c. A+B**
53. **Ans. a. Psoas minor, b. Genitofemoral nerve, d. Lymphatics**
54. **Ans. c. Sterility**

CRITICAL LIMB ISCHEMIA

55. **Ans. d. Smoking is more specific for peripheral vascular disease than coronary artery disease** *(Ref: Harrison 20/e p1923, 19/e p1643; Sabiston 20/e p1784,1758; Schwartz 10/e p881-900; Bailey 27/e p945, 946, 947)*
    - **Smoking** is **equally related with coronary artery disease** and **peripheral vascular disease**^{Q}.
    - **Ankle brachial index <0.5** indicates **critical limb ischemia**^{Q}.
    - Exercise normally increases systolic pressure and decreases peripheral vascular resistance. In case of PAD, it augments the pressure gradient across a stenotic lesion. Thus exercise helps in detecting low grade stenotic lesion giving normal ABI at rest (**ABI changes during exercise and rest**^{Q})
    - **ABI >1 is normal**^{Q}.

56. **Ans. c. Rest pain and ischemic ulcers** *(Ref: Harrison 20/e p1923, 19/e p1645; Sabiston 20/e p1784; Schwartz 10/e p881-900; Bailey 27/e p943)*
    - Critical lower limb ischemia is characterized by rest pain. Ulcers and gangrene may occur in patients with critical limb ischemia.

Peripheral Arterial Disease (PAD)

Intermittent Claudication	Critical Limb Ischemia
• **Intermittent claudication** is the **hallmark symptom** of PAD^Q • Results from **mild to moderate arterial occlusive disease**^{Q} • Ischemic symptoms occur typically **during exercise and relieved by rest**^{Q}. • Loss of skin integrity /gangrene is not seen • **Ankle Brachial Index (ABI) >0.5**	• CLI results from **severe arterial occlusive disease**^{Q} in whom resting blood flow cannot provide for basal nutritional needs of tissues • **Ischemic symptoms are present even during rest (rest pain)**^{Q} • **Pain** is **worse** when **legs are horizontal** and may **improve** when legs are **kept in a dependent position**^{Q}. • **Ischemic ulcers, lesions on** the **foot** and **gangrene**^{Q} may be seen • **ABI <0.5**^{Q}

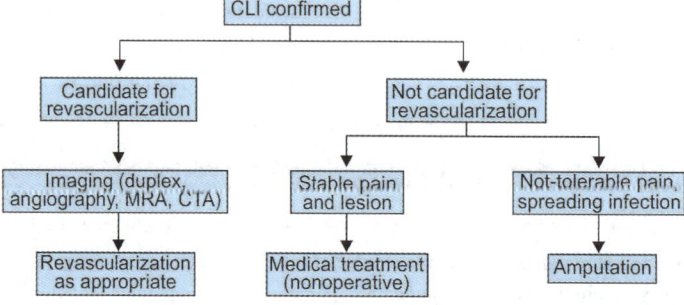

Arterial Disorders

57. Ans. b. 0.3
58. Ans. a. Rest/Night pain
59. Ans. b. 1
60. Ans. a. < 0.3
61. Ans. d. Calcified vessel walls *(Ref: Sabiston 20/e p1758; Schwartz 10/e p830; Bailey 27/e p945)*
62. Ans. a. Arteriosclerosis calcified arteries *(Ref: Schwartz 10/e p829-830; Sabiston 20/e p1784; Bailey 27/e p945-946)*

ARTERIAL ULCER

63. Ans. b. Elevation of limb *(Ref: Schwartz 10/e p259; Bailey 27/e p943)*

    Because **gravity aids** the **delivery of arterial blood**, classically, the patient with rest pain can obtain **relief by** simply **hanging** the **leg over** the **side of** the **bed**.

64. Ans. b. Elevation of the affected extremity
65. Ans. a. Arterial insufficiency....., c. Venous insufficiency......, d. Diabetic neuropathic ulcer..., e. Pressure ulcer – heel

AMPUTATION

66. Ans. a. 6 hours *(Ref: Essential Emergency Trauma by Kaushal Shah, Daniel Egan, Joshua Quaas– 2010/679)*

    - **Ischemic time** for **digits** is **upto 8 hours**[Q].
    - **Ischemic time** for **extremities** is **4-6 hours**[Q].
    - **Organ containing bag** should be **placed in** a solution of **saline with ice**[Q].

67. Ans. None > d *(Ref: Analgesics www.stoppain.org/pain_medicine/content/chronicpain/phantom.asp)*

    ### STUMP PAIN

    - Stump pain is **located at the end** of an amputated limb's stump.
    - It typically is described as a **"sharp," "burning," "electric-like,"** or **"skin-sensitive"** pain.
    - Due to a **damaged nerve** in the **stump region**.

    Treatment
    - **No one treatment** has been **shown to be effective for stump pain**[Q].
    - Because it is a pain due to an injured peripheral nerve, **drugs used for nerve pain may be helpful**.
        - Other approaches also are tried in selected cases, including:
        - Nerve blocks[Q]
        - Transcutaneous electrical nerve stimulation[Q]
        - **Surgical revision** of the stump or **removal of** the **neuroma**[Q]
        - Cognitive therapies

68. Ans. d. Isotonic saline
69. Ans. a. Law of projection *(Ref: Ganong 25/e p171)*

    - A phantom limb is the sensation that an **amputated or missing limb** (even an organ appendix) is **still attached to the body** and is moving appropriately with other body parts based upon **"Law of Projection"**.
    - It states that no matter where a sensory pathway is stimulated along its coure, the sensation produced is referred back to site of receptor.

70. Ans. a. Plastic bag with wet ice *(Ref: Sabiston 20/e p1996; Schwartz 10/e p1800)*

    "If it is anticipated that the amputated part will be considered for replantation, it is critical to transport the patient and the part in an appropriate manner. The amputated part is placed in a clean, dry, plastic bag, which is sealed and placed on top of ice in a Styrofoam container. This keeps the part sufficiently cool at 4° C to 10° C without freezing. The amputated part is wrapped in a lightly moistened saline gauze to prevent tissue drying."- Sabiston 20/e p1996

    "In preparation for replantation, the amputated part and proximal stump should be appropriately treated. The amputated part should be wrapped in moistened gauze and placed in a sealed plastic bag. This bag should then be placed in an ice water bath. Do not use dry ice, and do not allow the part to contact ice directly; frostbite can occur in the amputated part, which will decrease its chance of survival after replantation. Bleeding should be controlled in the proximal stump by as minimal a means necessary, and the stump should be dressed with a non-adherent gauze and bulky dressing."-Schwartz 10/e p1800

ARTERIOVENOUS FISTULA

71. Ans. d. Branham sign *(Ref: Sabiston 19/e p1785-1786; Bailey 26/e p899)*
72. b. Congenital fistula is easier to repair by surgery than acquired fistula

73. Ans. b. Proximal compression causes increases in heart rate
74. Ans. b. AV fistula
75. Ans. a. Compression cause bradycardia
76. Ans. d. Penetrating trauma
77. Ans. a. Congenital
78. Ans. d. Necrosis of the distal part
79. Ans. a. Allen's test *(Ref: Sabiston 20/e p1979; Bailey 27/e p443, 444, 890)*

Allen's Test

- Tests the **adequacy of the blood supply to the hand** from the **radial** and **ulnar arteries** and the **arcade between them**[Q]
- **Allen's test** is used to know the **integrity of palmar arch (patency of radial and ulnar arteries)**[Q]. If these are **patent, AVF** can be safely ligated.

Method of Allen's Test

- Elevate the hand and apply digital pressure on the radial and ulnar arteries to occlude them.
- Ask the patient to make a fist several times.
- The tips of the finger should go pale. Release each artery in turn and observe the return of colour

THORACIC OUTLET SYNDROME

80. Ans. a. Clinical evaluation *(Ref: Sabiston 20/e p1603-1604; Schwartz 10/e p829, 928; Bailey 27/e p991)*
    - **Thoracic outlet syndrome** is **diagnosed primarily by clinical evaluation** and the **diagnosis is based on reproducibility of symptoms** (resulting from compression of neurovascular bundle at the thoracic outlet) **during mechanical provocative maneuvers** (Adson's test or costoclavicular test or Hyperabduction test or Roos Arm Claudication test)
    - **Specific investigations** (CT scan, MRI, Angiography, X-ray) **are used to exclude other conditions** and to **establish** the **associated diagnosis.**

81. Ans. c. Lymphocutaneous fistula *(Ref: Sabiston 20/e p1604; Bailey 26/e p872)*

    Brachial plexus injuries, vascular injuries, pleural effusion, winged scapula, and infection are complications that may arise **secondary to first rib removal.**

Complications of Surgical Treatment of TOS	
• **Brachial plexus injuries**[Q]	• **Pleural effusion**[Q]
• **Winged scapula** due to **long thoracic nerve injury**[Q]	• **Pnemothorax**[Q]
• **Horner's syndrome**[Q]	• **Air embolism**
• **Vascular injuries (subclavian** vessels[Q])	• **Infection**

82. Ans. c. Cervical rib
83. Ans. c. Surgical intervention *(Ref: Sabiston 20/e p1603-1604; Schwartz 10/e p829; Bailey 27/e p991-992)*

    Cervical rib is responsible for the thoracic outlet syndrome and the preferred treatment for cervical rib responsible for thoracic outlet syndrome is surgical resection.

84. Ans. a. Radial nerve is commonly affected
85. Ans. a. Most commonly radial nerve
86. Ans. c. Pain in ulnar distribution
87. Ans. b. Wasting of forearm muscles *(Ref: Sabiston 20/e p1603, 19/e p1594-1595; Schwartz 9/e p704, 790; Bailey 25/e p895)*
88. Ans. c. Cervical rib
89. Ans. b. 25–45 years
90. Ans. c. Spondylosis *(Ref: Sabiston 20/e p1603; Schwartz 10/e p829; Bailey 27/e p991)*

RAYNAUD'S DISEASE

91. Ans. b. Migratory thrombophlebitis is seen only in Raynaud's phenomenon *(Ref: Harrison 20/e p1928, 19/e p1647; Sabiston 20/e p1603-1604; Schwartz 10/e p1823; Bailey 27/e p967)*
92. Ans. b. More common in female, d. Associated with migraine *(Ref: Harrison 20/e p1928, 19/e p1648; Sabiston 20/e p1779-1780; Schwartz 10/e p904; Bailey 27/e p967)*
93. Ans. c. Osteoarthritis
94. Ans. b. White, blue, red
95. Ans. c. Turn white
96. Ans. d. Atherosclerosis of vessels

DIABETIC FOOT

97. Ans. a. Strict diabetic control, c. Topical antibiotics are used, e. Diabetic ulcers are trophic ulcers *(Ref: Harrison 20/e p2882, 19/e p1769; Sabiston 20/e p1767; Schwartz 10/e p1877, 1879; Bailey 27/e p532, 533, 559, 953)*

98. Ans. c. Heel, d. Head of metatarsal
99. Ans. d. All of the above
100. Ans. a. Vasospasm
101. Ans. a. Myelopathy

AORTIC DISSECTION

102. Ans. a. Right lateral wall of ascending aorta *(Ref: Harrison 20/e p1919, 19/e p1640; Sabiston 20/e p1746; Schwartz 10/e p806-816; Bailey 27/e p909-911)*
103. Ans. a. Acute aortic dissection
104. Ans. b. Aorta

AORTIC ANEURYSM

105. Ans. a. Atherosclerosis *(Ref: Harrison 20/e p1919, 19/e p1637; Sabiston 20/e p1722; Schwartz 10/e p850-859; Bailey 27/e p961)*
     - "90% all abdominal aortic aneurysms are related to atherosclerotic disease and most of these aneurysms are below the level of renal arteries."
106. Ans. a. Surgery indicated when size AAA > 6 cm *(Ref: Harrison 20/e p1919, 19/e p1640; Sabiston 20/e p1725; Schwartz 10/e p850-859; Bailey 27/e p961)*

    - **Surgery indicated** when **size of AAA >5.5 cm**^{Q} (Not the 6 cm).
    - After rupture, **mortality rate of emergent operation is 45-50%**^{Q}.
    - **Most serious gastrointestinal complication** is **ischemia of the left colon** and **rectum. Post-operative hypotension** and **hemodynamic instability are contributory factors**^{Q}.
    - Occasionally, **microembolization** can occur, resulting **in small patchy areas of ischemia**, usually on the **plantar aspect of the foot**, referred to as **trash foot**^{Q}.

107. Ans. a. Laterally into the left retroperitoneum
108. Ans. d. Myocardial infarction *(Ref: Harrison 20/e p1919, 19/e p1640; Sabiston 20/e p1741; Schwartz 10/e p850-859; Bailey 27/e p965)*
     - MC complication of descending aortic aneurysm surgery is non-fatal MI >Renal failure.
109. Ans. b. 5.5 cm
110. Ans. c. 55 mm *(Ref: Sabiston 20/e p1725; Schwartz 10/e p852; Bailey 27/e p961)*

    "Surgical treatment is generally recommended for aneurysms more than 5.5 cm in maximal diameter, those demonstrating more than 5 mm of growth in 6 months or more than 1 cm in a year, and aneurysms with a saccular rather than the typical fusiform anatomy."-Sabiston 20/e p1725

111. Ans. b. Emergency surgery complication <10%, c. Rarely asymptomatic before rupture
112. Ans. d. Both intravascular and extra-vascular infection *(Ref: Harrison 20/e p1922, 19/e p1638; Sabiston 20/e p1908)*
     - A mycotic aneurysm is an infected aneurysm resulting from either an extravascular or an intravascular source of infection.
113. Ans. b. Computed tomography
114. Ans. d. Most common side effect is diarrhea and hypotension
115. Ans. b. Atherosclerosis
116. Ans. c. Splenic artery *(Ref: Sabiston 20/e p1788; Schwartz 10/e p1425; Bailey 27/e p961)*

    - MC site of intra-abdominal aneurysm: Aorta >Splenic artery^Q
    - MC site of splanchnic artery aneurysm: Splenic artery^Q

117. Ans. a. Splenic artery is most commonly involved
118. Ans. c. Discontinuation of arteria radicularis magna *(Ref: Sabiston 20/e p1781)*

    ### ARTERIA RADICULARIS MAGNA
    - Arteria radicularis magna **(artery of Adamkiewicz)** is the **main source of blood supply** to the **anterior spinal artery** in the **thoracolumbar segment** of the **spinal cord**^{Q}.
    - It arises from either one of the lower posterior intercostal arteries **(T9-T11)** or of the subcostal artery **(T12)**, or less frequently of the upper lumbar arteries **(L1 and L2)**^{Q}.
    - **Occlusion** or **interruption** is one of the major reasons for **spinal cord ischemia** (leading to **paraparesis/paraplegia**) during **surgery for thoracoabdominal aneurysms**^{Q}.

119. Ans. a. Saccular aneurism involves whole circumference
120. Ans. b. MRI
121. Ans. b. Aortic arch aneurysm *(Ref: Cardiac Surgery by John Norman/p388)*

- *"Oliver's sign: Downward displacement of cricoid cartilage in time with ventricular contraction, in the presence of an aortic arch aneurysm."*– *Cardiac Surgery by John Norman/p388*

FEMORAL ARTERY ANEURYSM

122. **Ans. a. Ultrasound guided compression of the neck of aneurysm, b. Thrombin injection, c. Bypass graft repair** *(Ref: Sabiston 20/e p1782; Bailey 27/e p966)*

123. **Ans. a. Radial, b. Brachial, c. Femoral** *(Ref: Rutherford Vascular Surgery 6/e pvol I/456)*

- "**IV drug abusers** can lead to number of specific vascular complications including **septic thrombophlebitis, Aortic dissection, AV fistula** and **necrotizing fasciitis** with **gangrene of extremity**. The **most frequent vascular complication** in **drug addicts** is **infected pseudoaneurysm** of the **femoral**[Q], **brachial**[Q] or **radial artery**[Q]."

POPLITEAL ARTERY ANEURYSM

124. **Ans. c. Popliteal artery** *(Ref: Sabiston 20/e p1782; Bailey 27/e p966)*
125. **Ans. d. Uncommon among peripheral aneurysm**

Minimum Size for Surgery (**AIPF**: All India Police Force)
Abdominal **A**ortic Aneurysm (**5.5 cm**) = **I**liac aneurysm (**3.5 cm**) + **P**opliteal/**F**emoral aneurysm (**2.0 cm**)

PSEUDOANEURYSM

126. **Ans. b. Trauma**

- **MC cause** of **pseudoaneurysm**: **Trauma** (**Penetrating** trauma or iatrogenic by **catheterization**)[Q]

127. **Ans. a. Ligation of involved vessel and wide surgical debridement** *(Ref: Rutherford Vascular Surgery 6/e pvol II/248-249, 813, 1055-1056)*

Treatment of Pseudoaneurysm

- **USG guided compression** is the **first therapeutic maneuver**[Q] in non-invasive vascular technology. Although it is **safe** but **efficacy is modest** and the procedure is uncomfortable for patient and provider.
- **Injection of thrombin into** the **pseudoaneurysm under duplex ultrasound guidance** has **not replaced compression** as treatment for pseudoaneurysm. This technique is **safe** and **effective**[Q]. It reduces physical effort and time requirements for the technologist and is significantly less uncomfortable for the patient.
- As **spontaneous resolution** of pseudoaneurysm has a **low incidence**, **surgical repair** is the **main therapy** and **gold standard therapy**[Q].

Indications of Surgery	
Absolute	**Relative**
• **Failure** of **other treatment modalities**[Q] • Suspected **secondary infection**[Q] • Evidence of **vascular compromise**[Q] • Ongoing or imminent **hemorrhage**[Q] • **Skin erosion** and **necrosis** due to **false aneurysm expansion**[Q]	• **Femoral neuropathy** • Continuous **anticoagulation** • Concomitant **AV fistula**

Surgical Intervention
• Operative repair can involve **simple stitch** or **replacement** of the entire vessel **with graft**[Q]. • **Mainstays of surgical treatment: Proximal control** (above inguinal ligament of needed, for extensive groin pseudoaneurysm), use of **monofilament suture** for vascular repair and **debridement** of devitalized tissue[Q]. • In the **presence of** any **infection** or when **large residual tissue defect** persists, **muscle coverage** with either **sartorius** or **rectus abdominis flap** over the repaired vessel must be used[Q].

Arterial Disorders

Treatment of Pseudoaneurysm in IV Drug Abusers
- **Ligation** is optional treatment **for infected pseudoaneurysm** because it is **easy, safe** and **cost effective** (in **IV drug abuser** there is **high chance of infection**)[Q]
- **Reconstruction** is **not recommended** because of **extension of infection** at location of pseudoaneurysm and **at artificial graft site**[Q].

SUBCLAVIAN STEAL SYNDROME

128. **Ans. a. First part** *(Ref: Grainger Diagnostic Radiology 4/e p 773; Bailey 27/e p952)*

   MC site of subclavian artery stenosis is the **first part** of the subclavian artery.

129. **a. Reversal of blood flow in the ipsilateral vertebral artery** *(Ref: Bailey 27/e p952)*

VASCULAR GRAFT

130. **Ans. a. Autologous vein**

131. **Ans. a. Saphenous vein graft (upside-down)** *(Ref: Bailey 27/e p890, 949; Washington Manual of surgery 5/e p322)*

   ### INFRA-INGUINAL OCCLUSIVE DISEASE (FEMORAL, POPLITEAL, TIBIAL OCCLUSIVE DISEASE)
   - **Autologous vein** is the **conduit of choice** for **infra-inguinal bypass surgery**[Q]
   - **Great saphenous vein** is the **vein of choice (Lesser saphenous vein** or **arm veins** may be used)[Q]
   - These grafts may be used either **'in situ' after valve destruction** or **reversed conduit**

   #### When Autologous vein grafts are not available PTFE grafts may be used.
   For **above knee grafts, patency rates of PTFE grafts approach** those achieved by autologous venous grafts[Q]
   - For **below knee/distal grafts, patency rates of PTFE grafts** are **substantially lower**[Q].

132. **Ans. c. Internal mammary artery** *(Ref: Sabiston 20/e p1672-1673; Schwartz 10/e p743; Bailey 27/e p890)*

   Most preferred graft for CABG is left internal mammary artery and most commonly used is long saphenous vein.

   "The conduit with the highest patency rate (98% at 5 years and 85%–90% at 10 years) is the internal thoracic artery which is most commonly left attached proximally to the subclavian artery (although occasionally used as a free graft) and anastomosed distally to the target coronary artery."- Schwartz 10/e p743

133. **Ans. c. Smooth muscle cells** *(Ref: Vascular.surgery.duke.edu/files/.../Vascular_Grafts_2-27-09.pdf; Schwartz 9/e p762-764)*

   ### VASCULAR GRAFT FAILURE
   - Smooth muscle cells in the middle layer (media) of the vessel wall become activated, divide, proliferate and migrate into the inner layer (intima)[Q].
   - The resulting abnormal neointimal cells express pro-inflammatory molecules, including cytokines, chemokines, and adhesion molecules that further trigger a cascade of events that lead to occlusive neointimal hyperplasia and eventually graft failure[Q].

134. **Ans. b. Textile synthetic** *(Ref: Sabiston 20/e p234; Schwartz 10/e p4; Bailey 27/e p949, 950, 951)*

135. **Ans. c. Saphenous vein**

136. **Ans. a. Dacron** *(Ref: Schwartz 10/e p4)*
   - **Dacron** is the **favoured material for aortoiliac work**, it **gives excellent results**.

137. **Ans. a. Dacron**

138. **Ans. d. Can be easily incised and the opening resutured**

139. **Ans. d. PVC**   140. **Ans. a. LIMA**

VASCULAR TRAUMA

141. **Ans. c. The pulse is weakened, d. There is no pulse**

142. **Ans. a. Most commonly associated with deceleration injury, b. High morality, c. Surgery definitive treatment, d. Aortography gold standard** *(Ref: Sabiston 20/e p1810, 1818; Schwartz 10/e p214-215; Bailey 27/e p369)*

143. **Ans. a. Mediastinal widening, b. Abnormal aortic contour, d. Right paratracheal stripe thickening, e. Left apical pleural cap** *(Ref: Chapman 4/e p163-164; CSDT 11/e p257-259)*

Traumatic Aortic Rupture

Clinical Features
- History of **high-speed deceleration**[Q] injury
- **Flail chest**[Q]
- **Fractured sternum**[Q]
- **SVC syndrome**
- **Multiple** or 1st or 2nd **rib fractures**
- **Upper extremity hypertension or pulse deficits**[Q]
- **Hematoma** in the carotid sheaths
- **Interscapular bruits**[Q]
- **Hoarseness** with normal larynx

Radiographic Features
- **Widening** of **mediastinum**[Q] (70%)
- **Esophageal deviation** to the **right**[Q]
- **Tracheal deviation** to **right**[Q]
- **Left**[Q] **apical cap** (65%)
- **Downward displacement** of **left main stem bronchus**[Q]
- **Right paratracheal stripe thickening**[Q]
- **Deviation** of NG tube to **right**
- **Left hemothorax**
- **Displaced left paraspinal stripe**[Q]
- **Displaced right** paraspinal stripe

144. **Ans. b. Left medial visceral rotation** *(Ref: Sabiston 20/e p1546, 1815)*
- Left medial visceral rotation exposes entire length of abdominal aorta, celiac axis, proximal part of mesenteric arteries and proximal left renal artery[Q].

145. **Ans. b. Mechanical compression**

Adequate manual compression of the subclavian artery to obtain hemostasis is often **not possible** because of **the interposing subcutaneous tissue** and **bony structure**, as well as **lack of structural support** around subclavian artery.

146. **Ans. d. Cattell-Braasch maneuver** *(Ref: Sabiston 20/e p1546)*

Maneuvers for Retroperitoneal Exposure			
Kocher's Maneuver	**Extended Kocher's Maneuver**	**Mattox Maneuver**	**Cattell-Braasch Maneuver**
• Surgical maneuver to **expose structures** in the **retroperitoneum**[Q] **behind duodenum & pancreas**[Q] • Used for **mobilization of duodenum**[Q]	• **Right sided medial visceral rotation**[Q] • **Right colon** and **duodenum** is **reflected medially**[Q] • **Exposes IVC, Infrarenal aorta, right renal artery** and **iliac vessels**[Q] • Recommended for **drainage** of **infra-mesocolic hematoma**[Q]	• **Left sided medial visceral rotation**[Q] • Left sided viscera (**Left kidney, left colon, spleen** and **pancreas**) are **brought to midline**[Q] • **Exposes** entire length of **abdominal aorta, celiac axis, proximal part** of **mesenteric arteries** and **proximal left renal artery**[Q] • Recommended for **drainage** of **central supramesocolic hematoma**[Q]	• For **extensive retroperitoneal exposure**[Q] • **Right colon** is **fully mobilized** and **reflected medially**[Q] • Good option for **exposure of** the **infrapancreatic segment**[Q]

147. **Ans. b. Kocher's maneuver**

ANGIOGRAPHY AND COMPLICATIONS

148. **Ans. b. Arteriography** *(Ref: Sabiston 20/e p1762; Schwartz 10/e p832-833, 918; Bailey 26/e p190)*
- **Seldinger needle** is **used for angiography** (arteriography).

ARTERIOGRAPHY

- Aortic and lower extremity arteriograms are generally performed by needle puncture of the **femoral**[Q] or brachial arteries[Q] followed by guidewire placement and catheter insertion using the Seldinger technique.

149. **Ans. d. Intracerebral hemorrhage** *(Ref: Sabiston 20/e p1762; Schwartz 10/e p832-833; Bailey 26/e p190)*

Complications of contrast Arteriography

Puncture Site or Catheter Related
- **Hemorrhage**, hematoma[Q]
- **Pseudoaneurysm**[Q]
- Arteriovenous fistula
- **Atheroembolization**[Q]
- **Local thrombosis**[Q]

Contrast Agent Related
- Anaphylactoid or sensitivity reaction
- **Vasodilation**, hypotension[u]
- **Nephrotoxicity**[Q]
- **Hypervolemia**[Q] (osmotic load)

Arterial Disorders

150. **Ans. a. Radial artery** *(Ref: Lee Anesthesia 12/e p25)*
    - Arterial puncture and cannulation is performed to measure PaO_2, $PaCO_2$, SpO_2 and pH to clarify the acid-base and electrolyte status.
    - Any artery that can be compressed after puncture may be used (but **not end arteries**), usually the **radial**[Q] **(preferred)**, brachial or femoral.

151. **Ans. b. Single wall puncture is indicated in those with normal coagulation profile** *(Ref: Mastery of Surgery 5/e p218)*
    - Single wall puncture is indicated in those with coagulopathy as there is more risk of bleeding in double wall puncture technique.

   ### ANGIOGRAPHY
   - **Arterial access** is obtained for **hemodynamic monitoring** and **angiography** and **interventions.**
   - **Femoral artery** is **most frequently cannulated artery** in the body[Q].
     - **Femoral artery** is a **large caliber vessel appropriate for angioplasty** and **stenting** of peripheral vessels[Q].
     - **Radial artery** is **most frequently used site** of arterial cannulation **for hemodynamic monitoring**[Q].
   - Femoral artery is identified in the inguinal region by its pulsation.
   - If fluoroscopy is being used, the **femoral artery** is **typically located over** the **medial third** of the femoral head[Q].
   - Femoral artery cannulation can be done using Seldinger technique.
     - The **Seldinger technique** is a **medical procedure to obtain safe access to blood vessels (both arteries and veins)** and other hollow organs[Q].
   - **Single wall puncture** is indicated **in those with coagulopathy** or **if thrombolysis is planned** because of **increased risk of bleeding in double wall technique**[Q].

TAKAYASU ARTERITIS

152. **Ans. a. Aortoarteritis** *(Ref: Harrison 19/e p2189; Sabiston 20/e p1780; Schwartz 10/e p788, 901; Bailey 27/e p967, 1416)*

153. **Ans. b. Subclavian artery**

MISCELLANEOUS

154. **Ans. c. Integrity of palmar arch**

155. **Ans. b. Superficial temporal**

   ### CIRSOID ANEURYSM
   - A cirsoid aneurysm is the **dilation of a group of blood vessels** due to **congenital malformations** with AV **(arteriovenous) shunting**[Q].
   - **Cirsoid means** resembling a **varix.**
   - **Most commonly occurs over** the **head** usually the **superficial temporal artery.**
   - **Superficial temporal artery** is the **most commonly involved artery**[Q].

156. **Ans. c. Palpable pulses** *(Ref: www.ncbi.nlm.nih.gov Br Med J v.1(3927); Apr 11, 1936)*

   ### ERYTHROCYANOSIS
   - A condition caused by **exposure to cold**[Q]
   - Characterized by **swelling of the limbs** and the appearance of **irregular red-blue patches** on the skin[Q]
   - Occurring especially in **girls** and **women**[Q]

157. **Ans. a. Aneurysm Endovascular Hunterian Ligation**

   ### HUNTERIAN LIGATION
   - **Hunterian ligation** refers to one of the **oldest successful interventions** for **arterial aneurysms: Ligation of** the **femoral artery to treat a popliteal aneurysm**[Q] by **John Hunter** in 1785.

158. **Ans. c. It is not superficial and does not cross prominent bone**
    - The **popliteal pulse** is **difficult to feel** because it is **not superficial** and **does not cross a prominent bone**[Q].

159. **Ans. c. Myocardial infarction** *(Ref: CSDT 11/e p822; Miller's Anesthesia 6/e p2053)*

- Miller says **"Myocardial performance** is the **single most important determinant** of **outcome following a major vascular operation**[Q].**"**
- **Non-fatal** and **fatal MIs** are the **most important** and **specific outcomes** that **determine perioperative cardiac morbidity** in patients for vascular surgery[Q].
- CSDT says **"MI and stroke** are **most common causes of death in vascular surgeries**[Q].**"**

160. **Ans. d. Bifurcation of pulmonary artery** *(Ref: Harrison 20/e p1922, 18/e p2171)*

SADDLE THROMBUS

- A **large thrombus lodged at** an **arterial bifurcation,** where blood flows from a large-bore vessel to a smaller one.
- The **'classic' saddle embolus,** which **occurs at the bifurcation of** the **pulmonary arteries** in **fatal pulmonary embolism** secondary to a centrally migrating venous embolus, is distinctly uncommon[Q].

161. **Ans. c. Salmonella**

162. **Ans. d. All of the above** *(Ref: Harrison 20/e p845, 19/e p296e-1; Schwartz 10/e p431-432, 836)*

STENT THROMBOSIS

- **Clotting suppressant agents** and **anti-clotting agents** should be **continued after drug eluting stents to prevent stent thrombosis**[Q].

  - **Endothelialization** is a hallmark of vascular healing and is **important for the prevention of thrombus formation**[Q].
  - **For drug-eluting stents** (which, by design, delay formation of a new endothelium cover over the stent), **the incidence of clot formation** within the stent **may persist for a longer period of time**[Q].

- **Drug eluting stents** have been associated with **delayed arterial healing** and the **prevalence of latent thrombus** after five years, suggesting that patients may continue to be risk for stent thrombosis for an extended period of time.
- Treatment with the **antiplatelet drugs** appears to be the **most important factor reducing this risk of thrombosis**, and **early cessation of these drugs** after drug-eluting stenting markedly **increases the risk of stent thrombosis** and **myocardial infarction**[Q].

163. **Ans. d. Accidental injury to major vessels in thigh or groin** *(Ref: Bailey 18/e p69, 147)*

BUTCHER'S THIGH

- Butchers thigh is **penetrating wound of femoral triangle** due to **knife slipping while boning meat**.
- Penetrating wound involving main veins in the thigh or groin are **potentially fatal**, as exsanguination may follow the first aid dressing which has apparently controlled the bleeding.

164. **Ans. a. Direct pressure** *(Ref: Advanced Assessment and Treatment of Trauma by Americans (2010)/71)*

EXTERNAL BLEEDING

- Control of external hemorrhage during the early phase (circulation) of resuscitation is imperative.
- **External bleeding is best controlled by direct digital pressure.**
- **Direct pressure assists in** the process of **coagulation** by slowing the flow of blood out of the vessels and **giving clot time to form.**
- In most cases of external bleeding, if pressure is applied quickly to the area of hemorrhage **(direct pressure)** or to the blood vessel supplying the bleed **(indirect pressure)**, the volume of blood escaping will be greatly reduced.
- To be effective, direct pressure must be at least equal to the pressure of the blood attempting to escape.
- Arterial bleeding is often difficult to control and may require upto 5 minutes of firm direct pressure to be successful.

165. **Ans. a. Giant cell arteritis** *(Ref: Harrison 20/e p2583, 19/e p2188)*

Temporal arteritis is also known as Giant cell arteritis.

166. **Ans. d. Most common side effect is diarrhea and hypotension** *(Ref: Anesthesiology Keyword Review by Raj K. Modak 2013/page 130; http://www.ncbi.nlm.nih.gov/pubmed/7818115)*

167. **Ans. b. Carotid angioplasty and stenting**

168. **Ans. d. Onyx** *(Ref: Sabiston 20/e p1733; Embolization by Pascal Chabrot (20130/p3)*

"Temporary embolic agents include absorbable gelatin sponge, Gelfoam sponge powder, starch microspheres, oxidized cellulose, and collagen fiber preparations."

"The **FDA** approved **Onyx (Ethylene-Vinyl Alcohol Copolymer)** in 2005 **for the treatment of arteriovenous malformations.** It is classified as a **liquid, nonadhesive, nonabsorbable, permanent embolic agent** that can be **used off-label for small and large vessels.**"

CHAPTER 27

Venous Disorders

RISK FACTORS FOR HYPERCOAGULABLE STATES/THROMBOSIS

Risk Factors for Hypercoagulable States/Thrombosis	
Inherited	**Acquired**

• **Defective inhibition of coagulation factors:**
  – **Factor V Leiden**^{Q} (resistant to inhibition by activated protein C)
  – **Antithrombin III deficiency**^{Q}
  – **Protein C or S deficiency**^{Q}
  – **Prothrombin gene mutation**^{Q} (G20210A)
• **Impaired clot lysis:**
  – Dysfibrinogenemia
  – **Plasminogen deficiency**^{Q}
  – **t-PA deficiency**^{Q}
  – **PAI-I excess**^{Q}
• **Uncertain mechanism:**
  – **Homocystinuria**^{Q}
  – High **homocysteine** levels due to **MTHFR mutation**^{Q}
	• **Diseases or syndromes:**
	  – Lupus anticoagulant/anticardiolipin syndrome^Q
	  – **Malignancy**^{Q}, **recent MI**^{Q}, **infection**^{Q}
	  – Myeloproliferative disorder
	  – **Thrombotic thrombocytopenic purpura**^{Q}
	  – **Estrogen**^{Q} treatment
	  – Hyperlipidemia, **Diabetes mellitus**^{Q}
	  – Hyperviscocity, **polycythemia**^{Q}
	  – **Nephrotic syndrome**^{Q}
	  – Paroxysmal nocturnal hemoglobinuria^Q
	  – **Inflammatory bowel disease**^{Q}
	  – **Behcet's syndrome**^{Q}
	• **Physiological states:**
	  – **Pregnancy** (especially **post-partum**^{Q})
	  – **Obesity**^{Q}, **Immobilization**^{Q}, **Old age**^{Q}
	  – **Post-operative state**^{Q}

- **MC genetic cause for thrombophilia: Factor V Leiden**
- **MC congenital cause of venous thrombosis: Factor V Leiden**
- **MC genetic hereditary blood coagulation disorder: Factor V Leiden**

Risk of DVT in Relation to Age and Duration of Surgery

High Risk	Moderate Risk	Low Risk
• General **urological surgery** in patient **>40 years**^{Q} • **Extensive pelvic** or **abdominal surgery**^{Q} • **Major orthopaedic surgery**^{Q} of lower limbs	• **General surgery** in patients **≥40 years**^{Q} • Surgery lasting for **≥30 minutes**^{Q} • **General surgery** in patients **<40 years** on **OCPs**^{Q}	• **Uncomplicated surgery** in patients **<40** years **without additional risk** • **Minor surgery (<30 minutes)** in patients **<40 years** without additional risk

Prophylaxis for DVT

Mechanical Prophylaxis	Pharmacological Prophylaxis

• **Early ambulation:**
  – **Simplest method** of prophylaxis^Q
  – Acts by **activating calf-pump** mechanism^Q
• **Pneumatic compression devices:**
  – **MC method** of prophylaxis^Q
  – Pneumatic compression **prevents stasis**^{Q}
	• **Unfractionated heparin:**
	  – Replaced by LMWH
	• **Fractionated low molecular weight heparin (LMWH):**
	  – **Better efficacy**^{Q} than unfractionated heparin
	  – **No laboratory monitoring**^{Q} is necessary

- **Unfractionated heparin & warfarin** are **rarely used in** the **prophylaxis of DVT**^{Q}.

DEEP VENOUS THROMBOSIS

Deep Venous Thrombosis

- DVT of the **leg** is complicated by the **immediate risk of pulmonary embolus** & **sudden death**^{Q}.
- Patients are at **risk of** developing a **post-thrombotic limb** & **venous ulceration**^{Q}.

> **Virchow's Triad**
> - Three factors described by Virchow are important in the development of venous thrombosis. These are:
>   - **Endothelial injury**^{Q} (**vascular injury**)
>   - **Hypercoagulability** of blood^Q (**thrombophilia**)
>   - **Stasis** or turbulence of blood flow^Q

- Most important predisposing factor: **Hospital admission**^{Q} for the treatment of a medical or surgical condition.

Pathology
- MC site of DVT: **Calf or soleal vein**^{Q}
- MC site of DVT leading to pulmonary embolism: **Femoropopliteal vein**^{Q}
- A **thrombus develops in** the **soleal veins** of the calf, this is likely to **extend up** to the next large venous branch and is **more likely to break off** and **embolize**^{Q} to the lung as a pulmonary embolism.
- **Acute right heart obstruction** may lead to **sudden collapse** & **death**^{Q}.

> - **Lung infarction** is **rare**^{Q} as the **lung** has a **dual blood supply** (**bronchial** & **pulmonary arteries**).

Clinical Features
- MC presentation of DVT: **Pain** & **swelling**, especially in the **calf** of one lower limb^Q.
- **Bilateral DVT** is common, occurring in up to **30%**^{Q}.
- Many patients have **no symptoms of thrombosis** and **may first present with** signs of a **pulmonary embolism**, e.g. pleuritic chest pain, hemoptysis & shortness of breath^Q.
- **Physical signs:** Mild pitting edema of the ankle, **dilated surface veins**, a **stiff calf** and **tenderness** over the course of the deep veins.
- **Earliest sign of DVT: Calf tenderness**^{Q}

> - **Low-grade fever** may be present, especially in a patient who is having **repeated pulmonary emboli**^{Q}.

- **Homan's sign:** Resistance (not pain) of the calf muscles to forcible dorsiflexion is not discriminatory and should be abandoned.

Homan's sign	Resistance (not pain) of the **calf muscles to forcible dorsiflexion**^{Q}
Phlegmasia alba dolens	Painful white leg^Q Obstruction of major **deep venous channel**^{Q}
Phlegmasia cerulea dolens	Painful blue leg^Q Obstruction of **both collaterals** & **deep venous channel**^{Q}
Moses sign (Bancroft's sign)	Calf tenderness on **direct pressure on** the **calf**^{Q}
Pratt's sign	Calf tenderness on **squeezing** the **calf** from the sides^Q

Diagnosis
- **D-dimer measurement:** If normal, no indication for further investigation^Q but, if raised, a duplex ultrasound examination of the deep veins should be performed.
- **Duplex ultrasound:** Investigation of choice for diagnosis of DVT (**Filling defects** in flow and **lack of compressibility** indicate the presence of a thrombosis^Q).
- **Ascending venography:** Shows **thrombus as a filling defect**, is now **rarely required**^{Q}.

Treatments
- **Confirmed DVT on duplex imaging:** Start **subcutaneous LMWH** and **rapid anticoagulation with warfarin** unless there is a specific contraindication^Q.

> - **Duration of heparin** should be **at least 5 days**^{Q}.
> - **Warfarin** is usually started at a dose of **10 mg** on **day one**, **10 mg** on **day two** and **5 mg** on **day three**^{Q}.
> - **PT on day 3** guides the **maintenance dose** of warfarin.

- **Thrombolysis:** In iliac vein thrombosis, especially if seen early and limb is **extremely swollen**^{Q}.
- A **minimum treatment time of anticoagulation** advocated **in DVT is 3 months**^{Q}.
- **Palma operation:** Surgical treatment of DVT^Q

VARICOSE VEINS

Varicose Veins

- Varicose veins are **dilated, tortuous elongated superficial veins**^Q ≥3 mm in diameter measured in upright position with demonstrable reflux.
- Most develop in the tributaries of the **greater and lesser saphenous veins**, which are **usually dilated** but rarely varicose themselves.
  - Usual distribution of varicose veins is **below the knee in branches of greater saphenous system**^Q.
- Varicosities in the thigh: **Long saphenous** incompetence^Q
- Varicosities on the back of the leg: **Short saphenous** incompetence^Q

Primary Varicose Veins	Secondary Varicose Veins

• **More common**^Q
• Due to **congenital predisposition** with **occupational reinforcement**^Q
• **Decreased number or defective valves**^Q
	• Less common
	• Arises from **destruction** or **dysfunction of valves** caused by:
	  – **Trauma**^Q – **DVT**^Q – **AV fistula**^Q
	  – Non-traumatic proximal venous obstruction (pregnancy, pelvic tumor)

Risk Factors for Varicose Veins	
• **Female sex**^Q • **Pregnancy** (especially **multiparity**^Q) • **Pelvic tumors**^Q • **Family history**^Q	• **AV fistula**^Q • **DVT**^Q • **Prolonged standing**^Q • **Obesity**^Q

Pathophysiology
- **Defective connective tissue & smooth muscle** in the **vein wall** leading to a **secondary incompetence** of the valves^Q

Clinical Features
- MC symptom: **Dull aching pain in the veins at the end of the day, after prolonged standing**^Q
- Other symptoms: **Ankle swelling**, itching, bleeding, **superficial thrombophlebitis, eczema, lipodermatosclerosis** and **ulceration**^Q.

Diagnosis
- **Duplex ultrasound**: Investigation of choice for diagnosis of **varicose veins**^Q
- **Varicography**: Useful investigation in **recurrent varicose veins** or **complex anatomy**^Q
- **Venography**: Not used as a standard investigation in varicose veins, **useful if the duplex scan indicates, but cannot confirm, the presence of post-thrombotic change**^Q.

Treatment
- **Gold standard** treatment for varicose vein: **Endothermal ablation**^Q
- Patients **without symptoms** or signs of lipodermatosclerosis or ulceration: **Reassurance**^Q
- **Elastic compression stockings**: For **varicose veins with post-thrombotic damage**^Q

  - **Bisgard's Regime**: Limb elevation + Compression stockings + Massage for varicose ulcers^Q

Indications for Varicose Vein Intervention	
• **Cosmesis**^Q • Symptoms **refractory to conservative therapy**^Q • **Bleeding** from a varix	• Superficial **thrombophlebitis**^Q • **Lipodermatosclerosis**^Q • Venous stasis **ulcer**^Q

- A previous **DVT** usually **contraindicates varicose vein surgery**^Q

  - **DVT is a contraindication for** the **treatment of varicose veins**^Q.
  - **Varicose vein surgery** should **never be attempted** in a case **where DVT exists along** with varicose veins, because in these cases, **superficial veins** are the **only valved venous pathway** and excising them will only aggravate the condition^Q.

Endothermal Ablation of Varicose Veins
• **Endothermal ablation (replaced surgical ligation & stripping) is now considered as the gold standard treatment for varicose vein**^Q. • Cost effective & can be performed under local anesthesia. • Methods used: Endovenous laser ablation & RFA^Q

Treatment of Varicose Veins	
Injection sclerotherapy	• **Sodium tetradecyl sulphate** is **most commonly used**[Q] • **Destroys lipid membranes** of endothelial cells causing them to shed, leading to **thrombosis, fibrosis** and **sclerosis**[Q]. • **Not effective** at eradicating varicosities in the presence of **major saphenous incompetence**[Q] • Useful for dealing with **minor varicosities** (**<3 mm**[Q]) and recurrences in the **calf** and **lower leg** • **Tesari method:** Most widely used method for foam sclerotherapy[Q]
Surgical Treatment	• **Ligate** the **saphenofemoral** and/or **saphenopopliteal junctions** and **remove major part of** the **incompetent trunk**[Q]
Radiofrequency ablation	• **Destroy** the **endothelial lining**[Q]
Endovenous laser ablation	• Causes endothelial damage[Q]

Complications of varicose vein surgery
- **Recurrence (MC):** Incidence of recurrence after surgery is upto **10%**[Q].
- **Hematoma** or **Ecchymosis:** MC cause of discomfort[Q] after varicose vein surgery
- Sensory nerve injury

  - **Greater saphenous vein** should only be **stripped** to **just below the knee to avoid damage** to the accompanying **saphenous nerve**[Q]
  - **Sural nerve** must be **carefully dissected off** the lesser saphenous vein at the ankle[Q].

'CEAP' Classification of Chronic Lower Extremity Venous Disease	
C	**Clinical signs** (grade$_{0-6}$), supplemented by **"A"** for **asymptomatic** and **"S"** for **symptomatic** presentation
E	**Etiologic classification** (**c**ongenital, **p**rimary, **s**econdary)
A	**Anatomic distribution** (**s**uperficial, **d**eep, or **p**erforator, alone or in combination)
P	**Pathophysiologic dysfunction** (reflux or obstruction, alone or in combination)

Tests for Varicose Veins	
Morrissey's test	• Cough impulse test[Q]
Perthe's test	• Affected lower extremity is wrapped with elastic bandage and patient is instructed to move around and exercise. • **Increase in size** of the varices indicates **incompetence of deep venous system**[Q] • **Severe crampy pain** is suggestive of **deep venous obstruction**[Q]
Modified Perthes test	• Tourniquet is applied around the upper part of the thigh and patient is asked to walk quickly with tourniquet in the place • **Severe crampy pain** is suggestive of **deep venous obstruction**[Q]
Schwartz test	• In long standing varicose veins if the **lower part of varicosity is tapped**, an **impulse is felt at the saphenous opening**[Q]
Fegans test	• Palpation to find the **fascial defects** to **locate incompetent perforators**[Q]

BRODIE-TRENDELENBURG TEST

BRODIE-TRENDELENBURG TEST

- **Brodie-Trendelenburg test** is **positive** in:
  – Incompetent saphenofemoral junction (SFJ)[Q]   – Incompetent perforators or communicating veins[Q]

Procedure
- Test is performed in two ways.
- In both the methods the patient is first placed in the recumbent position and his legs are raised to empty the veins.
- The SFJ is now compressed with the thumb of the clinician and the patient is asked to stand up quickly.

Components of Brodie-Trendelenburg Test

Component I	Component II
• **Pressure on SFJ** is **released** ↓ • **Varices fill quickly** by a column of blood **from above**[Q] ↓ • Indicates **incompetent SFJ**[Q]	• **Pressure on SFJ** is **not released** ↓ • **Varices fill gradually**[Q] ↓ • Indicates **incompetent perforators**[Q]

TRENDELENBURG OPERATION

> **TRENDELENBURG OPERATION**
>
> - Consists of **saphenofemoral junction flush ligation** & **greater saphenous vein (GSV) stripping**[Q]
>   - All four tributaries (superficial inferior epigastric, superficial circumflex iliac, deep & superficial external pudendal veins) is divided[Q]
> - **Ligate** the **GSV** deep to all tributaries **flush** with the **common femoral vein**[Q]
> - **Greater saphenous vein** should only be **stripped** to **just below the knee to avoid damage** to the accompanying **saphenous nerve**[Q]

VENOUS ULCERS

> **VENOUS ULCERS**

- **Venous disease** is responsible for **60-70% of all ulcers** in the **lower leg**.

Causes of Leg Ulcers	
• **Venous disease**: Superficial incompetence; deep venous damage (post-thrombotic) • **Arterial ischemic ulcers** • Rheumatoid ulcers	• Traumatic ulcers • **Neuropathic ulcers** (diabetes) • Neoplastic ulcers (**SCC** and **BCC**)

Etiology
- **Fibrin cuff theory**: High venous pressure → Pericapillary infiltrate → Fibrin → Fibrosis → Cuffs → Diffusion block → Tissue damage[Q]
- **White cell trapping**: White cell 'trapping' → Reactive oxygen species → Free radicals → Tissue damage[Q].

> - At present, **ambulatory venous hypertension** is the **only accepted cause of ulceration**[Q].

Clinical Features
- **Venous ulcer**: Sloping edge, base contains **granulation tissue**[Q] covered by slough and exudate.
- Any elevation of the **ulcer edge** should indicate the **need for a biopsy** to exclude a carcinoma (SCC or BCC).

> - Venous ulcer of the leg **characteristically develops in** the skin of the **gaiter region**[Q], the **area between** muscles of the **calf & ankle**
> - **Majority of ulcers** develop on the **medial side** of the **calf**[Q]
> - Ulcers associated with lesser saphenous incompetence often develop on the **lateral side** of the leg[Q].

- Almost **all venous ulcers have** surrounding **lipodermatosclerosis** (thickening, pigmentation, inflammation & induration of calf skin[Q])
- **Pigmentation** comes **from hemosiderin & melanin**

> - Presence of an **ankle flare** suggests venous hypertension[Q].
> - **Inverted Champagne bottle leg** is seen in **varicose veins**[Q].

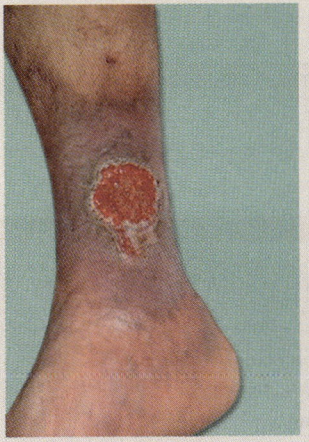 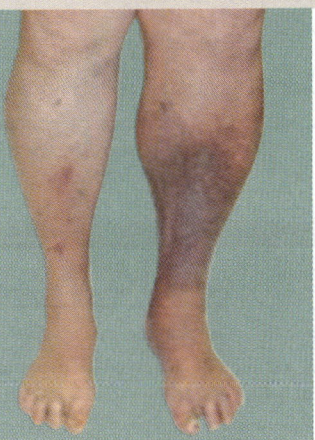 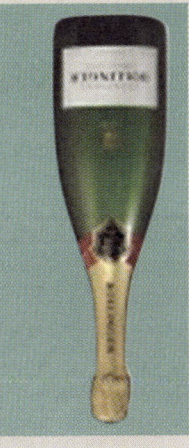

Diagnosis
- **Duplex ultrasound:** Assess the state of deep & superficial veins (**IOC**)[Q]
- **Bipedal ascending phlebography:** Detect obstruction & post-thrombotic changes missed by the duplex scan[Q]

Management
- **Probable venous ulcer:** Patients are initially treated by a **compression bandaging regimen**[Q]
- A **multilayered elastic compression bandaging system** has been shown to be effective (**Charing Cross four-layer bandage**), as has a **rigid multilayered system** (Steripaste three layer bandage)[Q].

Prevention of Recurrence
- **Elastic stockings** should be prescribed for all patients with evidence of **post-thrombotic deep vein damage** and these remain an **alternative treatment** for patients with **superficial venous disease who decline intervention**[Q].

Prognosis
- There is a **20-30% incidence of re-ulceration** by 5 years[Q].
- Greatest risk of re-ulceration is in the **post-thrombotic leg**[Q].

ARTERIO-VENOUS MALFORMATION

Klippel-Trenaunay Syndrome

Characterized by	
• Congenital **AV fistula**[Q]	• **Hypertrophy** of involved **extremity**[Q]
• Cutaneous **hemangioma**[Q]	• **Absence of deep venous system**[Q]
• **Varicose veins**[Q]	

Management
- **Most patients** with Klippel-Trenaunay syndrome should **be treated conservatively with elastic compression** hosiery[Q]
- **Pathological superficial veins should not be removed**[Q] without evidence of an intact deep system.

- **Parkes Weber syndrome:** Multiple AV fistulae causing **venous hypertension, ulceration & high-output cardiac failure**[Q].

Kasabach-Merritt Syndrome

- Characterized by:
  - **Thrombocytopenia**[Q]
  - **Consumptive coagulopathy**[Q]
  - Microangiopathic hemolytic anemia[Q]
  - Enlarging vascular lesion (Hemangioma or AV malformation[Q])

Pathology
- Vascular lesion (**Hemangioma or AV malformation**) triggers an **intravascular coagulation** with **platelet trapping** and consequent **thrombocytopenia**, and an **activation and consumption of coagulation factors**[Q].

Management
- Treatment options: **Embolization, external compression bandages**[Q]
- Drugs: Corticosteroids, vincristine

Malignancies Associated with Migratory Thrombophlebitis	
• **CA pancreas (MC)**[Q]	• **Prostate cancer**[Q]
• **CA lung**[Q]	• **Ovarian** cancer[Q]
• **GI malignancies**[Q]	• **Lymphoma**[Q]

SUPERFICIAL THROMBOPHLEBITIS

Superficial Thrombophlebitis

- This is a **superficial venous thrombosis**, most commonly caused by infusions of IV fluids

Causes of Superficial Thrombophlebitis	
• **Venipuncture** and **IV infusion (MC)**[Q]	• **Buerger's disease**[Q]
• **Trauma**[Q] (especially to varicose veins)	• **Malignancy (Pancreas**[Q])

Clinical Features
- Surface vein feels **solid** and **tender** on palpation.
- **Overlying skin** may be **attached to** the **vein** and in the early stages may be **erythematous** before gradually turning brown.
- A linear segment of vein can be **palpated** once the inflammation has subsided[Q].
  - The **acute inflammation strongly adhere** the **thrombus to the venous wall**, so **no thromboembolic episodes** are seen[Q].

Treatment
- Most patients are treated with **NSAIDs** and **condition resolves spontaneously**[Q].

AXILLARY-SUBCLAVIAN VEIN THROMBOSIS (ASVT)

Axillary-Subclavian Vein Thrombosis (ASVT)

- **Upper extremity DVT** is **much less common** than its lower extremity counterpart
- It is a **serious problem**; pulmonary embolism occurs in up to one third of all patients with an **upper extremity DVT**[Q].
- Upper extremity DVT refers to **thrombosis of** the axillary or subclavian veins[Q].
- ASVT are classified into two forms.

Primary ASVT	Secondary ASVT
• Less common	• More common[Q]
• **No clear cause for** the **thrombosis** is **readily identifiable** at initial evaluation[Q].	• Associated with an **easily identified cause** such as an **indwelling catheter** or a **hypercoagulable state**[Q].
• **History of performing prolonged, repetitive motion activities**[Q], which results in **damage to** the **subclavian vein**, usually where it passes between the **head of** the **clavicle** and **1st rib**[Q].	• Over **30% of patients** with **tunneled subclavian vein access devices** develop **ASVT**[Q].
• Also known as **venous thoracic outlet syndrome, effort thrombosis,** and **Paget-Schroetter syndrome**[Q].	

Clinical Features
- A patient with ASVT **may be asymptomatic** or may present with **varying degrees of upper extremity edema** and **tenderness**[Q].
- Classic findings: Unilateral swelling, pain, extremity discomfort, erythema, and a palpable cord[Q].

Diagnosis
- Duplex ultrasonography confirms the diagnosis[Q].

Treatment
- **Anticoagulation therapy** should **be initiated** once **ASVT is diagnosed to prevent PE** and **decrease symptoms**[Q].
  - Patients presenting with **acute symptomatic primary ASVT** may be candidates for **catheter-directed thrombolytic therapy**[Q].

Adjuvant procedures after thrombolytic therapy may include cervical or first rib resection for thoracic outlet abnormalities, surgical venous reconstruction, and balloon angioplasty for residual venous stenosis[Q].

Multiple Choice Questions

HYPERCOAGULABLE STATES AND DVT RISK FACTORS

1. **All the following disorders are inherited except:**
   a. Protein S deficiency *(Recent Question 2017, JIPMER 2010)*
   b. Antiphospholipid antibody syndrome
   c. Protein C deficiency
   d. Factor V Leiden mutation

2. **Congenital cause of hypercoagulable states are all except:** *(AIIMS Nov 2010)*
   a. Protein C deficiency
   b. Protein S deficiency
   c. MTHFR mutation
   d. Lupus anticoagulant

3. **All of the following are acquired causes of hypercoagulability, except:** *(All India 2009)*
   a. Infection
   b. Inflammatory bowel disease
   c. Myeloproliferative disorders
   d. Prolonged surgery

4. **A patient is admitted with 3rd episode of deep venous thrombosis. There is no history of any associated medial illness. All of the following investigations are required for establishing the diagnosis except:** *(AIIMS Nov 2004)*
   a. Protein C deficiency
   b. Antithrombin II deficiency
   c. Antibodies to factor VIII
   d. Antibodies to cardiolipin

5. **The deficiency of all the following factors increases the incidence of thrombus formation except:** *(DPG 2010)*
   a. Lipoprotein A
   b. Protein-C
   c. Anti-thrombin III
   d. Protein-S

DEEP VENOUS THROMBOSIS

6. **Which of the following is associated with Virchow's triad?**
   a. Hypercoagulability *(MCI Sept 2005)*
   b. Disseminated malignancy
   c. DVT
   d. All of the above

7. **DVT prophylaxis is indicated in all except:** *(PGI May 2011)*
   a. Abdominal surgery for malignant disease and high risk patient
   b. All patients with age more than 40 years
   c. Patient undergoing major orthopedics surgery
   d. Systemic heparin is only method for DVT prophylaxis
   e. 10% of patients of calf vein thrombosis progress to pulmonary embolism

8. **Deep vein thrombosis occurs most commonly after:** *(AIIMS Feb 97)*
   a. Total hip replacement
   b. Gastrectomy
   c. Prostatic operation
   d. Brain surgery

9. **Commonest cause of pulmonary embolism is:** *(All India 99)*
   a. Thrombosis of leg veins
   b. Thrombosis of prostatic veins
   c. IVC thrombosis
   d. Thrombosis of internal pudendal artery

10. **DVT, investigation of choice is:** *(DNB 2005, 2001, PGI Dec 97, June 97)*
    a. Doppler
    b. Plethysmography
    c. Venography
    d. X-ray

11. **The patient falls in hish risk group for DVT and pulmonary embolism after:** *(MHCET 2016)*
    a. Major burns
    b. Major surgery age < 40 years
    c. Major medial illness/cancer
    d. Major orthopedic surgery/fracture pelvis

12. **For prophylaxis of deep vein thrombosis used is:**
    a. Warfarin
    b. Heparin *(PGI June 97)*
    c. Pneumatic shocks garment
    d. Graded stocking

13. **Earliest sign of deep vein thrombosis is:** *(DNB 2005, 2001, 2000, AIIMS 87)*
    a. Calf tenderness
    b. Rise in temperature
    c. Swelling of calf muscle
    d. Homan's sign

14. **White leg is due to:** *(TN 90)*
    a. Femoral vein thrombosis and lymphatic obstruction
    b. Deep femoral vein thrombosis
    c. Lymphatic obstruction only
    d. None of the above

15. **All of the following are seen in deep vein thrombosis except:**
    a. Pain
    b. Discolouration *(All India 90)*
    c. Swelling
    d. Claudication

16. **A 60 years old male has been operated for carcinoma of caecum and right hemicolectomy has been done. On the fourth post-oprative day, the patient develops fever and pain in the legs. The most important clinical entity one should look for is:** *(UPSC 96)*
    a. Urinary tract infection
    b. Intravenous line infection
    c. Chest infection
    d. Deep vein thrombosis

17. **The duration of heparin therapy in deep vein thrombosis is:**
    a. 7-10 days
    b. 15-20 days *(UPPG 96)*
    c. 3-4 days
    d. 1 month

18. **Most common site for venous thrombosis:** *(JIPMER 98)*
    a. Popliteal vein
    b. Soleal vein
    c. Femoral vein
    d. Internal iliac vein

19. **A patient undergoes surgery in pelvic region. Which vein is most likely to result in thrombosis?** *(JIPMER November 2017)*
    a. Iliac vein
    b. Femoral vein
    c. Calf vein
    d. IVC

20. **In DVT all are seen except:** *(CMC 2001)*
    a. High fever
    b. Increased temperature at site
    c. Pain
    d. Tenderenss

21. **Patient had retrograde pelvic thrombophlebitis and it progressed to bilateral ileofemoral occlusion and now the presentation is:** *(Recent Question 2018)*
    a. Blue leg
    b. White leg
    c. Red leg
    d. Purple leg

Venous Disorders

22. In a patient on anticoagulant therapy, the INR is maintained at: *(UPSC 2002)*
    a. 1.5-2.5 times the normal
    b. 2.5-3.5 times the normal
    c. 3.5-4.5 times the normal
    d. 4.5-5.5 times the normal

23. The initial therapy of documented deep venous thrombosis in a post-operative case is:
    a. Subcutaneous heparin therapy
    b. Intravenous heparin therapy
    c. Thrombolytic therapy with urokinase
    d. Aspirin therapy *(Recent Question 2013, Karnataka 2003)*

24. All are done for a case of deep vein thrombosis except:
    a. Thrombolytic therapy
    b. Bandage *(MAHE 07)*
    c. Heparin
    d. Bed rest

25. Which one of the following is the investigation of choice for suspected deep vein thrombosis of the lower extremity?
    a. Radioactive labeled fibrinogen uptake *(UPSC 2007)*
    b. Ascending contrast phlebography
    c. D-dimer estimation
    d. Duplex ultrasonography

26. The device, whose image is given below, used for: *(AIIMS November 2018)*

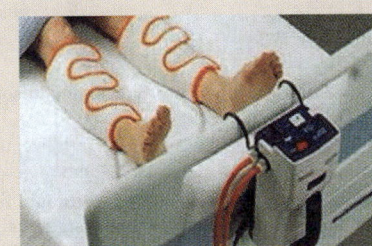

    a. Pneumatic compression stocking to prevention of DVT
    b. Varicose vein
    c. Hypothermia
    d. Cellulites

27. True about compression stocking are: *(PGI May 2018)*
    a. Worn even after ulcer heals to prevent recurrence
    b. Worn in morning & taken off at night before bedtime
    c. Compression occurs maximum at calf
    d. Worn only at edema sites
    e. Provide calf pump

28. All of the following statements are correct about deep venous thrombosis except: *(Recent Question 2019)*
    a. Clinical assessment is highly reliable
    b. Mostly bilateral
    c. Most common clinically presents as pain and tenderness in calf
    d. Some cases may directly present as pulmonary thromboembolism

VARICOSE VEINS

29. 'SEPS' is a procedure used for: *(All India 2009)*
    a. Veins
    b. Arteries
    c. Lymphatics
    d. AV fistula

30. The most common complication of varicose vein stripping is:
    a. Infection
    b. Hemorrhage *(DPG 2011)*
    c. Ecchymosis
    d. Thromboembolism

31. Drug used for sclerotherapy of varicose veins are the following except: *(MCI Sept 2007)*
    a. Ethanolamine oleate
    b. Polidocanol
    c. Ethanol
    d. Sodium tetradecyl sulfate

32. True about venous ulcer: *(PGI Nov 2010)*
    a. Always stripping done
    b. Always examine deep venous system
    c. Biopsy should be taken from chronic ulcer
    d. Associated with Klippel-Trenunay syndrome

33. Treatment of a long-standing non-healing venous leg ulcer with venous leg ulcer with varicose veins in a patient unwilling for surgery or who is inoperable: *(MHPGMCET 2006)*
    a. Antibiotic therapy
    b. Bandaging
    c. Surgical intervention
    d. Haemorhilogogue therapy

34. TRIVEX is a percutaneous technique of: *(MHPGMCET 2009)*
    a. Intravenous intraluminal destruction of vein by ablation catheter
    b. Intravenous intraluminal injection of sclerosant like sodium tetradecyl sulphate
    c. Removal of vein by suction following injection of fluid
    d. Stripping of veins

35. In varicose veins the flow in incompetent perforators is:
    a. From superficial to deep to *(MHSSMCET 2006)*
    b. Form deep to superficial
    c. No flow
    d. Can be to and for

36. Varicose veins of size less than _____ can be best treated by sclerotherapy: *(MHSSMCET 2007)*
    a. 2 mm
    b. 3 mm
    c. 4 mm
    d. 6 mm

37. Amount of sclerosant used in treatment of varicose veins?
    a. 0.5 ml
    b. 2 ml *(MHSSMCET 2008)*
    c. 4 ml
    d. 8 ml

38. Brodie-Tredenlenburg test is positive in:
    (PGI June 2002, MHPGMCET 2001)
    a. Sapheno-Femoral incompetence
    b. Perforator competence above knee
    c. Deep vein incompetence
    d. Perforator competence below knee

39. Most commonly varicose veins are seen with:
    a. Long saphenous vein *(AIIMS June 99)*
    b. Short saphenous vein
    c. Both
    d. Popliteal and femoral vein

40. Regarding varicose veins, which one of the following statements is true: *(AIIMS Nov 2003)*
    a. Over 20% are recurrent varicosities
    b. The sural nerve is in danger during stripping of the long saphenous vein
    c. The saphenous nerve is closely associated with the short saphenous vein
    d. 5% oily phenol is an appropriate sclerosant for venous sclerotherapy

41. Which system is involved in the given image of varicose veins? *(Recent Question 2016)*
    a. Long saphenous vein
    b. Short saphenous vein
    c. Both of the above
    d. None of the above

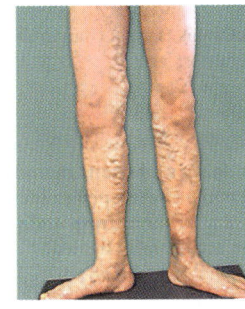

42. Surgery in varicose veins is not attempted in presence of:
    a. Deep vein thrombosis (AIIMS Nov 93, June 2000)
    b. Multiple incompetent perforators
    c. Varicose veins with leg ulcer
    d. All of the above

43. Which is true regarding Trendelenberg operation?
    a. Stripping of the superficial varicose vein (PGI Dec 2001)
    b. Flush ligation of the superficial varicose vein
    c. Ligation of the perforators
    d. Ligation of small tributaries at the distal end of superficial varicose vein
    e. Ligation of short saphenous vein

44. First treatment of rupture of varicose veins at the ankle should be: (All India 2004)
    a. Rest in prone position of patient
    b. Application of a tourniquet proximally
    c. Application of a tourniquet distally
    d. Direct pressure and elevation

45. Perforators are not present at: (AIIMS Nov 2007)
    a. Ankle
    b. Medial calf
    c. Distal to calf
    d. Below inguinal ligament

46. Injection sclerotherapy for varicose veins is by using:
    a. Phenol
    b. Absolute alcohol
    c. 70% alcohol
    d. Ethanolamine oleate

47. The following is the commonest site for venous ulcer: (Recent Question 2014)
    a. Instep of foot
    b. Lower 1/3rd leg and ankle
    c. Lower 2/3rd of leg
    d. Middle 1/3rd of leg

48. The most important perforator of the lower limb is between:
    a. Long saphenous and posterior tibial vein (All India 92)
    b. Short saphenous and posterior tibial vein
    c. Short saphenous and popliteal vein
    d. Long saphenous and femoral vein

49. An operated case of varicose veins has a recurrence rate of:
    a. About 10%
    b. About 25%
    c. About 50%
    d. Over 60%

50. Cocket and Dodd's operation is for: (UPSC 2008, APPG 96)
    a. Saphenofemoral flush ligation
    b. Subfascial ligation
    c. Deep vein thrombosis
    d. Diabetic foot

51. Which of the following test is used to detect perforator incompetence in varicose? (JIPMER 2000)
    a. Trendelenburg test
    b. Fegan's test
    c. Morissey's test
    d. Homan's test

52. Lipodermatosclerosis is most commonly seen at:
    a. Anterior aspect of leg (DNB 2012)
    b. Medial aspect of leg
    c. Anterior aspect of thigh
    d. Posterior aspect of thigh

53. An intern was doing saphenous cannulation for a burn patient. Then the patient developed sudden onset of pain along the medial border of the corresponding foot. Which nerve must have been accidentally ligated? (AIIMS 2000)
    a. Sural nerve
    b. Deep peroneal nerve
    c. Saphenous nerve
    d. Genicular nerve

54. Gold standard diagnostic test in varicose veins is:
    a. Photoplethysmography (JIPMER 2003)
    b. Duplex imaging
    c. Ultrasonography
    d. Radio-labeled fibrinogen study

55. Bisgard treatment is for: (APPG 96)
    a. Arterial ulcer
    b. Venous ulcer
    c. TAO
    d. Raynaud's phenomenon

56. Treatment of choice for a patient presenting with venous ulcer and incompetent perforators: (DNB 2005)
    a. Stripping of saphenous vein
    b. Subfascial ligation of perforators
    c. Saphenofemoral ligation
    d. Conservative

57. Patient presents with varicose vein with sapheno-femoral incompetence and normal perforator. Management options include all of the following except: (AIIMS Nov 2012)
    a. Endovascular stripping
    b. Sclerotherapy
    c. Sapheno-femoral flush ligation
    d. Saphenofemoral flush ligation with striping

58. Contraindication for surgery in varicose veins:
    a. DVT (Recent Question 2015)
    b. Multiple incompetent perforators
    c. Ulcer at ankle
    d. None

59. Inceap classification for chronic venous disorders, CO stands, CO (zero) for: (MHCET 2016)
    a. No signs of venous disease
    b. Reticular veins
    c. Varicose veins
    d. Oedema

60. Elderly male has 0.5 mm dilated tortuous vein in the posterior part of right calf. What is stage as per CEAP classification? (Recent Question 2019)
    a. C0
    b. C1
    c. C2
    d. C3

AV MALFORMATIONS

61. A patient presented with pulsating varicose veins of the lower limb. Most probable diagnosis is: (AIIMS Nov 2001)
    a. Klippel-Trenaunay syndrome
    b. Tricuspid regurgitation
    c. DVT
    d. Right ventricular failure

62. Klippel-Trenaunay syndrome associated with all except: (JIPMER November 2017)
    a. Portwine stain
    b. Varicose veins
    c. Limb lengthening
    d. Fused vertebra

63. True about Kasabach syndrome: (PGI Nov 2009)
    a. May be due to complication of portwine stain
    b. Coagulopathy occurs
    c. Due to complication of hemangioma
    d. Thrombocytopenia present

64. Pulsating varicose vein in young adult is due to: (AIIMS 92)
    a. Arteriovenous fistula
    b. Sapheno femoral incompetence
    c. Deep vein thrombosis
    d. Abdominal tumour

THROMBOPHLEBITIS

65. Migratory thrombophlebitis is seen most commonly with: (PGI June 2002)
    a. Pancreatic carcinoma
    b. Testicular carcinoma
    c. Gastric carcinoma
    d. Breast carcinoma
    e. Liver carcinoma

66. **The most common cause of superficial thrombophlebitis is:**
    a. Intravenous catheters/infusion *(All India 2009)*
    b. DVT
    c. Varicose veins
    d. Trauma

MISCELLANEOUS

67. **All of the following are correct about axillary vein thrombosis except:** *(All India 2001)*
    a. May be caused by a cervical rib
    b. Treated with IV anticoagulant
    c. Embolectomy is done in all cases
    d. May occur following excessive exercise

68. **In obstruction of inferior vena cava there is:** *(All India 97)*
    a. Prominent thoraco epigastric vein
    b. Caput medusa
    c. Hemorrhoids
    d. Esophageal varices

69. **Calf compartment pressure rise to_____ on walking:** *(MHSSMCET 2006)*
    a. 20-30 mm Hg
    b. 60-80 mm Hg
    c. 80-100 mm Hg
    d. 200-300 mm Hg

70. **Harvey's sign is:** *(DNB 2000)*
    a. Transmitted pressure wave on coughing in a varicose vein
    b. Related to the use of venous filling after emptying a length of vein
    c. Loss of hairs from eyebrows
    d. None of the above

71. **May thurner or cockett syndrome involves:**
    a. Common iliac artery obstruction
    b. Internal iliac artery obstruction
    c. Internal iliac vein obstruction
    d. Left iliac vein compression *(Recent Question 2013)*

72. **Venous air embolism is most common in which position in surgery:** *(Recent Question 2013)*
    a. Sitting
    b. Prone
    c. Lateral
    d. Lithotomy

Explanations

HYPERCOAGULABLE STATES AND DVT RISK FACTORS

1. Ans. b. Antiphospholipid antibody syndrome *(Ref: Harrison 20/e p1910, 19/e p743; Sabiston 20/e p1842; Schwartz 10/e p761; Bailey 27/e p987)*
2. Ans. d. Lupus anticoagulant
3. Ans. None
4. Ans. c. Antibodies to factor VIII
5. Ans. a. Lipoprotein A

DEEP VENOUS THROMBOSIS

6. Ans. a. Hypercoagulability *(Ref: Harrison 20/e p1910, 19/e p404-405; Sabiston 20/e p1841; Schwartz 10/e p918-927; Bailey 27/e p986-987)*
7. Ans. d. Systemic heparin is only method for DVT prophylaxis *(Ref: Harrison 20/e p1913, 19/e p1634; Sabiston 20/e p1843; Schwartz 10/e p918-927; Bailey 27/e p989-990)*

> - The patients who has undergone either **major abdominal surgery** or **major orthopedic surgery**, has sustained **major trauma** or has **prolonged immobility** (>3 days) represents an **elevated risk for** the development of **venous thromboembolism**^{Q}.
> - Patients who have undergone **total hip replacement**, **total knee replacement**, or **cancer surgery** will benefit from **extended pharmacologic prophylaxis** for a total of **4-6 weeks**^{Q}.
> - If **untreated**, upto **25% of calf vein thrombosis** may progress to **proximal deep veins** of the leg, where the **incidence of chronic venous insufficiency** is 25% and that of **pulmonary embolism** is 10%^{Q}.

> - **Unfractionated heparin** and **warfarin** are **rarely used** in the **prophylaxis of DVT**^{Q}.

8. Ans. a. Total hip replacement
9. Ans. a. Thrombosis of leg veins
10. Ans. a. Doppler
11. Ans. c. Major medial illness/cancer
12. Ans. b. Heparin; c. Pneumatic shock garments, d. Graded stocking
13. Ans. a. Calf tenderness
14. Ans. b. Deep femoral vein thrombosis
15. Ans. d. Claudication
16. Ans. d. Deep vein thrombosis
17. Ans. c. 3-4 days
18. Ans. b. Soleal vein
19. Ans. c. Calf vein
20. Ans. a. High fever
21. Ans. a. Blue leg
22. Ans. b. 2.5-3.5 times the normal *(Ref: Sabiston 20/e p1844; Schwartz 10/e p921-923)*

Anticoagulant	Parameter	Goal (times control values)
Unfractionated heparin	aPTT^Q	1.5-2.5^Q
Warfarin	PT or INR^Q	2.0-3.0^Q

23. Ans. b. Intravenous heparin therapy *(Ref: Harrison 20/e p1913, 19/e p1634; Sabiston 20/e p1844; Schwartz 10/e p199, 921-923; Bailey 27/e p990)*

ANTITHROMBOTIC THERAPY IN DVT

- **Any venous thrombosis** involving the **femoropopliteal system** is treated with **full anticoagulation**^{Q}.
- Traditionally, the **treatment of DVT centers around heparin treatment** to maintain the PTT at 60 to 80 seconds, followed by **warfarin therapy** to obtain an INR of 2.5 to 3.0^Q.
- This **initial therapy** usually is **continued for at least 5 days**^{Q}, while oral vitamin K antagonists are being simultaneously administered.

Unfractionated Heparin

- **UFH therapy** is **most commonly administered** with an **initial IV bolus of 80 units/kg or 5000 units**^{Q}.
- **Initial bolus** is **followed by a continuous IV drip**, initially at **18 units/kg per hour**^{Q} or **1300 units per hour**^{Q}.
- The **half-life of IV UFH** ranges from **45-90 minutes** and is **dose dependent**^{Q}.
- **Level of antithrombotic therapy** should be **monitored every 6 hours using aPTT**, with the **goal range of 1.5 to 2.5 times control values**^{Q}.

Venous Disorders

24. Ans. d. Bed rest
25. Ans. d. Duplex ultrasonography
26. Ans. a. Pneumatic compression stocking to prevention of DVT *(Ref: Schwartz 10/e p925; Sabiston 20/e p1843; Bailey 27/e p989)*
27. Ans. a. Worn even after ulcer heals to prevent recurrence, b. Worn in morning & taken off at night before bedtime, e. Provide calf pump *(Ref: Schwartz 10/e p925; Sabiston 20/e p1843; Bailey 27/e p989)*
28. Ans. b. Mostly bilateral *(Ref: Schwartz 10/e p919; Sabiston 20/e p1842; Bailey 27/e p986-988)*

VARICOSE VEINS

29. Ans. a. Veins *(Ref: Sabiston 20/e p1841, 19/e p1809; Schwartz 10/e p929-930; Bailey 27/e p982)*

SUBFASCIAL ENDOSCOPIC PERFORATOR VEIN SURGERY (SEPS)

- **SEPS** is a **new endoscopic technique for** the management of **chronic venous insufficiency** due to **incompetent perforator veins**^{Q}.
- SEPS involves **insertion of** a **rigid endoscope** through the skin and superficial fascia to a **plane above** the **muscle**, such that perforator veins are visible as they exit the muscles.
- These **perforator veins** are **dissected** free from surrounding tissue and **closed** with the help of metal clips.

30. Ans. c. Ecchymosis *(Ref: Sabiston 20/e p1836; Schwartz 10/e p929-930; Bailey 27/e p974-982)*
31. Ans. c. Ethanol *(Ref: Sabiston 20/e p1835; Schwartz 10/e p929; Bailey 27/e p979)*

SCLEROSING AGENTS

- These are **irritants** causing **inflammation, coagulation** and ultimately **fibrosis**, when injected into **hemorrhoids** or **varicose veins**^{Q}.
- Used only for **local injection**

Sclerosing Agents	
• **Phenol**^{Q} **(5%)** in **almond** oil or **peanut oil**^{Q} • **Ethanolamine oleate**^{Q} **(5%)** in 25% glycerin and 2% benzyl alcohol • **Polidocanol**^{Q} **(3%)**	• **Sodium tetradecyl sulphate**^{Q} **(3%)** with benzyl alcohol (2%) • **Hypertonic saline**^{Q}

32. Ans. b. Always examine deep venous system; c. Biopsy should be taken from chronic ulcer; d. Associated with Klippel-Trenaunay syndrome *(Ref: Sabiston 20/e p1832; Schwartz 10/e p930-934; Bailey 27/e p982-985)*

- **SCC (Marjolin's ulcer)** may occur **in long standing chronic ulcer**. So, **biopsy** should be taken **to rule out malignancy**^{Q}.
- **DVT** is one of the **main predisposing factors** for **development of venous ulcer**^{Q}.
- **Venous ulcer** is **not always associated with varicose veins**^{Q}.
- Most venous ulcers improve with Bisgard's Regime^Q (Limb elevation + Compression stockings + Massage)
- **Klippel-Trenaunay syndrome** is associated with **varicose veins, limb hypertrophy** and a **cutaneous birthmark (port-wine stain or venous malformation). Deep venous system is anomalous or absent, saphenous vein stripping** can be **hazardous**^{Q}.

33. Ans. b. Bandaging *(Ref: Sabiston 20/e p1832; Schwartz 10/e p931; Bailey 27/e p984)*
34. Ans. c. Removal of vein by suction following injection of fluid *(Ref: Sabiston 20/e p1840)*

TRANSILLUMINATED POWERED PHLEBECTOMY (TIPP) USING TRIVEX

- **TIPP** involves an **irrigated transilluminator**, passed deep to the varicosities, and a powered suction resector, each introduced through a skin incision.
- On activation, the **vein is sucked into** the **resector under direct vision**, morcellated and removed by suction.
- Trivex system uses two components.
- First instrument **illuminates** the **varicose veins** through the skin using advanced fiber optic technology and the **vein resector** is then **guided next to** the **vein** underneath the skin^Q.
- Suction draws the **vein into tip of** the **vein resector** while a rotating blade effectively removes the leg vein^Q.
- With this new varicose vein treatment, **large clusters of varicose veins** can be **accurately removed** through a **minimal number of small incisions** and is far more effective than other forms of varicose vein surgery.

35. Ans. b. Form deep to superficial *(Ref: Bailey 27/e p969)*

- In **varicose veins**, the **flow in** the **incompetent perforators** is **reversed** and goes **from deep to superficial veins**^{Q}.

36. **Ans. b. 3 mm** *(Ref: Sabiston 20/e p1835; Schwartz 10/e p929; Bailey 27/e p979)*
    - **Sclerotherapy** is useful for dealing with **minor varicosities** (<3 mm^Q) and **recurrences** in the **calf** and **lower leg**^{Q}.
    - **Amount of sclerosant used** in treatment of varicose veins is **0.5 ml**^{Q}.

37. **Ans. a. 0.5 ml**

38. **Ans. a. Sapheno-Femoral incompetence** *(Ref: Sabiston 20/e p1831; Bailey 25/e p927-928)*

39. **Ans. a. Long saphenous vein** *(Ref: Sabiston 20/e p1831; Schwartz 10/e p929; Bailey 27/e p975)*
    - The **usual distribution** of **varicose veins** is **below** the **knee in branches of greater saphenous system**^{Q}.

40. **Ans. d. 5% oily phenol is an appropriate sclerosant for venous sclerotherapy**

41. **Ans. a. Long saphenous vein** *(Ref: Sabiston 20/e p1829)*
    - Varicose vein involving long saphenous system is located along anteromedial aspect of lower limb.
    - Varicose vein involving short saphenous system is located along posterolateral aspect of lower limb.

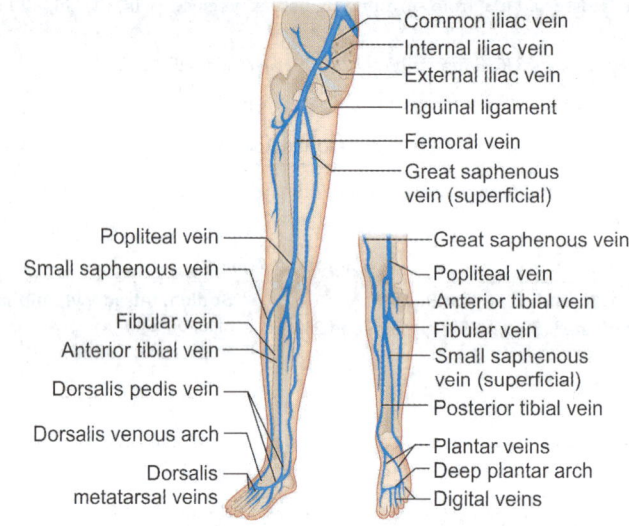

Venous Anatomy of Lower Limb

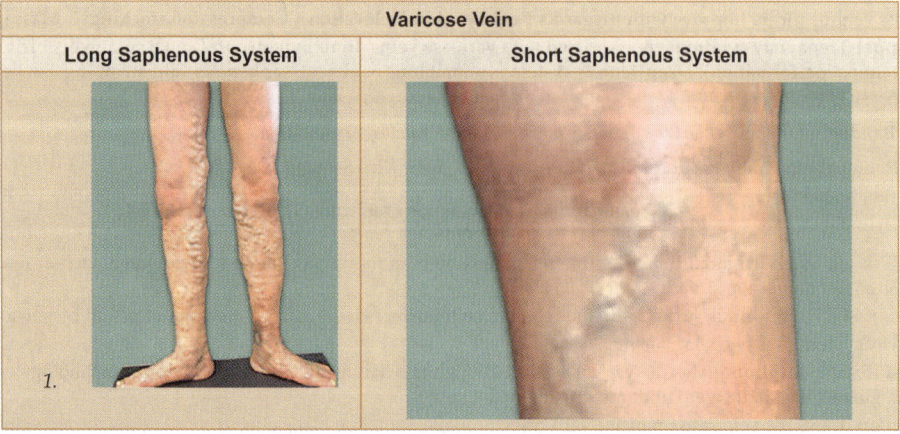

42. **Ans. a. Deep vein thrombosis** *(Ref: Sabiston 20/e p1836; Schwartz 10/e p929; Bailey 27/e p976)*
    - **DVT** is a **contraindication** for the **treatment of varicose veins**^{Q}.
    - **Varicose vein surgery** should **never be attempted** in a case **where DVT exists along** with **varicose veins**, because in these cases, **superficial veins** are the **only valved venous pathway** and excising them will only aggravate the condition^Q.

43. **Ans. b. Flush ligation of the superficial varicose vein** *(Ref: Sabiston 20/e p1836; Schwartz 10/e p917-918; Bailey 27/e p981)*

44. **Ans. d. Direct pressure and elevation** *(Ref: Oxford Textbook of Surgery 2/e p1000)*
45. **Ans. d. Below inguinal ligament** *(Ref: Sabiston 20/e p1828; Schwartz 10/e p915; Bailey 26/e p902)*

> **PERFORATORS LOCATION (IN CBD HUNTERS)**
> - **Below** the **medial malleolus** (**Inframalleolar** perforators/ **May or Kuster**)
> - In the **medial calf** (**Cockett's** perforators[Q])
> - Just **below** the **knee** (**Boyd's** perforators[Q])
> - Just **above** the **knee** (**Dodd's** perforators[Q])
> - At the level of **adductor canal** (**Hunterian** perforators[Q])

46. **Ans. a. Phenol; d. Ethanolamine oleate**
47. **Ans. b. Lower 1/3rd leg and ankle**
48. **Ans. d. Long saphenous and femoral vein**   49. **Ans. a. About 10%**
50. **Ans. b. Subfascial ligation** *(Ref: www.ncbi.nlm.nih.gov/pubmed/4855162)*

> - **Cockett and Dodd Operation: Sub-fascial ligation** of perforators

51. **Ans. a. Trendelenburg test**
52. **Ans. b. Medial aspect of leg** *(Ref: Sabiston 20/e p1832; Bailey 27/e p973, 984, 986)*

> **LIPODERMATOSCLEROSIS**
> - Lipodermatosclerosis is the name given to the **skin changes seen in chronic venous insufficiency.**
> - Components of lipodermatosclerosis:
>   – **Pigmented skin**
>   – **Inflamed subcutaneous tissue**
>   – **Elevated venous pressure** facilitates the extravasation of the RBCs and fluid leading to inflammation
> - The pigmentation is due to **fixation of hemosiderin** in the tissue
> - It is most commonly seen **on gaiter area** (**above medial malleolus**)

53. **Ans. c. Saphenous nerve**   54. **Ans. b. Duplex imaging**
55. **Ans. b. Venous ulcer**
56. **Ans. b. Subfascial ligation of perforators**
57. **Ans. b. Sclerotherapy** *(Ref: Sabiston 20/e p1835; Schwartz 10/e p929-930; Bailey 27/e p979-780)*

> **Injection sclerotherapy** is useful for dealing with **minor varicosities** (**<3 mm**[Q]) and recurrences in the **calf** and **lower leg.** Though it's a treatment option for varicose vein, but for a **patient of varicose vein with sapheno-femoral incompetence and normal perforator**, this will be least preferred amongst the given options.
> **Treatment of Varicose Veins**
> - **Saphenofemoral flush ligation** with **ligation of tributaries** and **stripping of major part of** the **incompetent trunk**[Q]

58. **Ans. a. DVT**   59. **Ans. a. No signs of venous disease**
60. **Ans. b. C1** *(Ref: Sabiston 20/e p1834)*

> **CLINICAL (C OF CEAP) CLASSIFICATION (C0-6)**
> - Any limb with possible chronic venous disease is first placed into one of seven clinical classes (C0-6), according to the objective signs of disease.
>
> | Class | Features |
> |---|---|
> | 0 | • No visible or palpable signs of venous disease |
> | 1 | • Telangiectasia, reticular veins, malleolar flare |
> | 2 | • Varicose veins |
> | 3 | • Edema without skin changes |
> | 4 | • Skin changes ascribed to venous disease (e.g., pigmentation, venous eczema, lipodermatosclerosis) |
> | 5 | • Skin changes as defined above with healed ulceration |
> | 6 | • Skin changes as defined above with active ulceration |

AV MALFORMATIONS

61. Ans. a. Klippel-Trenaunay syndrome *(Ref: Schwartz 10/e p1850; Bailey 27/e p972, 991, 1000)*
62. Ans. d. Fused vertebra
63. Ans. b. Coagulopathy occurs; c. Due to complication of hemangioma; d. Thrombocytopenia present *(Ref: Sabiston 20/e p1903; Schwartz 10/e p1850; Bailey 26/e p598)*
64. Ans. a. Arteriovenous fistula

THROMBOPHLEBITIS

65. Ans. a. Pancreatic carcinoma; c. Gastric carcinoma *(Ref: Sabiston 20/e p1845; Schwartz 10/e p927; Bailey 27/e p990)*
66. Ans. a. Intravenous catheters/infusion

MISCELLANEOUS

67. Ans. c. Embolectomy is done in all cases *(Ref: Sabiston 20/e p1603-1604; Schwartz 10/e p928-929; Bailey 27/e p992)*
68. Ans. a. Prominent thoraco epigastric vein *(Ref: BDC 4/e vol II/197)*

   - **Thoracoepigastric veins** are **important connection between** the **veins of upper and lower limbs** and these get **prominent in IVC obstruction**^{Q}.

69. Ans. d. 200-300 mm Hg *(Ref: Bailey 27/e p971)*

   - **On standing**, the **arterial blood pressure** at the **ankle** rises by **80-100 mm Hg**^{Q}.
   - The **pressure within** the **calf compartment rises** to **200-300 mm Hg**^{Q} **during walking**, which is more than enough to propel the blood in the direction of heart.

70. Ans. b. Related to the use of venous filling after emptying a length of vein

   ### Harvey's Sign
   - Related to the use of venous filling after emptying a length of vein
   - **Delayed venous refilling** is called **Harvey's Sign**

71. Ans. d. Left iliac vein compression

   ### May-Thurner Syndrome/Cockett Syndrome/Iliocaval/Iliac Vein Compression Syndrome
   - Occurs due to compression of left iliac vein by overriding right iliac artery.
   - It result in left iliofemoral deep vein thrombosis.

72. Ans. a. Sitting *(Ref: ncbi.nlm.nih.gov/pmc/articles/PMC 2580000)*

   - *Venous air embolism* is a *potential hazard* whenever the operative site is above the level of patients heart.
   - The *'sitting' position* and its modification *"beach chair"* positions are associated with a *greater incidence of venous air embolism*.

CHAPTER 28

Lymphatic System

LYMPHEDEMA

Lymphedema

Primary Lymphedema
- Occur in **1 of every 1000** individuals
- At birth, **1 in 6000** persons will develop lymphoedema with an **overall prevalence of 0.13–2%**[Q].
- Arise from **congenital malformations** such as **lymphatics**[Q]

Secondary Lymphedema
- **More common**[Q]
- **Filariasis is MC cause worldwide**[Q]
- In Western countries: **Result of neoplasms** and their **surgical treatments** and **radiotherapy**[Q].

Congenital Lymphedema
- Onset **before 1st year** of life[Q]
- Edema is typically present **at birth**[Q]
- Can involve a **single lower extremity, multiple limbs, genitalia** or **face**[Q]
- More likely to be **bilateral** and **involve whole leg**[Q]
- **Familial version** of congenital lymphedema is known as **Milroy disease**[Q].

Lymphedema Precox
- Onset between **1-35 years**[Q]
- **MC type**, seen in **90% cases**[Q]
- More common in **women**[Q]
- Mostly **unilateral**[Q]
- Limited to **foot & calf**[Q]
- **Familial version** of lymphedema precox is known as **Meig's disease**[Q].

Lymphedema Tarda
- Onset **after 35 years**[Q]
- Relatively **rare**

SECONDARY LYMPHEDEMA

SECONDARY LYMPHEDEMA

- Secondary lymphedema is **far more common** than primary lymphedema[Q].
- Secondary lymphedema **develops as a result of lymphatic obstruction** or **disruption**[Q].
- **Axillary node dissection** leading to **lymphedema of the arm** is the **most common cause** of secondary lymphedema **in the United States**[Q].
- Other causes of secondary lymphedema include **radiation therapy, trauma, infection**, and **malignancy**[Q].
- Globally, filariasis (caused by **Wucheriria bancrofti, Brugia malayi**, and **Brugia timori**) is the **most common cause** of secondary lymphedema[Q]

FILARIASIS

FILARIASIS

- **Filariasis: MC cause of lymphedema worldwide**[Q]
- Particularly **prevalent in Africa, India** and **South America**[Q] (affecting 5-10% of the population)
- **Viviparous nematode Wucheria bancrofti**, whose **only host is man**[Q], is responsible for 90% of cases and is spread by the mosquito **(Culex)**[Q].
- Disease is associated with **poor sanitation**[Q].

Pathogenesis
- Parasite **enters lymphatics from** the **blood** and **lodges in lymph nodes**, where it **causes fibrosis** and **obstruction**, due partly to direct physical damage and partly to the immune response of the host[Q].
- **Proximal lymphatics** become **grossly dilated** with adult parasites[Q].
- The degree of edema is often massive **elephantiasis**[Q].

Clinical Features
- Acute: **Fever**, headache, malaise, **inguinal** and **axillary lymphadenitis, lymphangitis,** cellulitis, abscess formation and ulceration, funiculo-epididymo-orchitis[Q]
- Chronic: **Lymphedema of legs** (arm, breast), **hydrocele**[Q], abdominal lymphatic varices, chyluria and lymphuria[Q].

Diagnosis
- **Microfilariae enter the blood at night** and can be identified on a **blood smear,** in a centrifuged specimen of **urine** or in **lymph** itself[Q].
- A **complement fixation test**[Q] is also available and is positive in present or past infection. Eosinophilia is usually present.

Treatment
- **Diethylcarbamazine destroys** the **parasites**[Q] but does not reverse the lymphatic changes.
- Once the infection has been cleared, treatment is as for primary lymphoedema.

BRUNNER'S CLASSIFICATION OF LYMPHEDEMA

\multicolumn{2}{c|}{Brunner's Clinical Classification of Lymphedema}	
Grade	**Clinical Features**
Subclinical (latent)	**Excess interstitial fluid** and **histological abnormalities** in **lymphatics** and **lymph nodes, no clinically apparent lymphedema**[Q]
I	**Pitting edema**, largely or completely **disappears on elevation** and **bed rest**[Q]
II	**Non-pitting edema**, does not significantly reduce upon elevation[Q]
III	Edema associated with **irreversible skin changes**, i.e. **fibrosis, papillae**[Q]

COMPLICATIONS OF LYMPHEDEMA

COMPLICATIONS OF LYMPHEDEMA
- **Limb swelling**: Cause discomfort and aching[Q]
- **Infections**: Recurrent bacterial and **fungal infections, recurrent cellulitis** or **lymphangitis** leading to **skin thickening**[Q]
- **Risk of malignancy**: Lymphangiosarcoma (Stewart-Treves' syndrome[Q])

Malignancies Associated with Lymphedema	
• **Lymphangiosarcoma**[Q] • **(Stewart–Treves' syndrome)** • **Kaposi's sarcoma** (HIV) • Squamous cell carcinoma • Liposarcoma	• Malignant melanoma • Malignant fibrous histiocytoma • Basal cell carcinoma • Lymphoma

Signs in Chronic Lymphedema	
Buffalo hump[Q]	• **Contour of** the **ankle is lost** through infilling of the submalleolar depressions, a 'buffalo hump' forms **on the dorsum of the foot**
Square toes[Q]	• **Toes appear 'square'** because of **confinement of footwear**
Stemmer's sign[Q]	• **Skin on** the **dorsum of the toes cannot be pinched** because of **subcutaneous fibrosis**

LYMPHEDEMA: INVESTIGATIONS

Direct-contrast lymphangiography provides the **finest details** of the lymphatic anatomy. However, it is an invasive study that **involves exposure** and **cannulation of lymphatics** at the **dorsum of the forefoot**, followed by **slow injection of contrast medium** (ethiodized oil). The procedure is tedious, the **cannulation often necessitates aid of magnification optics** (frequently an operating microscope is needed), and the dissection requires some form of anesthetic. **After cannulation of a superficial lymph vessel**, **contrast material is slowly injected** into the **lymphatic system.**

Lymphangiography

Direct Lymphangiography
- Involves the **injection of contrast medium (Isosulfan blue[Q])** into a **peripheral lymphatic vessel** and radiographic visualization of the vessels and nodes[Q].
- **Gold standard** for showing **structural abnormalities** of **larger lymphatics and nodes**[Q]
- **Technically difficult, unpleasant** for the patient
- May cause **lymphatic injury**
- **Reserved for preoperative evaluation of megalymphatics** being considered for **bypass** or **fistula ligation**[Q].

Indirect Lymphangiography
- Indirect lymphangiography involves the **intradermal injection of water-soluble, non-ionic contrast** into **a web space**, from where it is taken up by lymphatics and then **followed radiographically**[Q].
- It will **show distal lymphatics** but **not normally proximal lymphatics and nodes**[Q].

TREATMENT OF LYMPHEDEMA

Treatment of Lymphoedema

- Most (95%) of patients can be **managed non-operatively**[Q]
- **Mainstay of treatment** is nonsurgical measures:
  - Use of **external compressive garments** and **devices**[Q]
  - Limb elevation[Q]
  - Antibiotics for episodes of cellulitis[Q]
  - Specialized complex **physical therapy**[Q]

- **Efficacy** of surgical options is generally poor, and these are **reserved for** cases in which **aggressive nonsurgical measures** have **failed**[Q].

- **Surgical treatment** may be considered in cases of **severe functional impairment**, **recurrent lymphangitis** or **severe pain** despite medical therapy[Q].

Surgical Treatment of Lymphedema

Reconstructive Operations
- Indicated in patients with **proximal** (either primary or secondary) **obstruction** of the extremity, **lymphatic obstruction, dilated lymphatics distal to obstruction**[Q].
- **Bypass procedures:**
  - Omental pedicle
  - **Skin bridge (Gillies**[Q])
  - Anastomosing **lymph nodes** to **veins** (Neibulowitz[Q])
  - **Ileal mucosal patch (Kinmonth**[Q])
  - Direct lymphovenous anastomosis with the aid of operating microscope

Excisional Operations
- Only viable option for patients **without residual lymphatics of adequate size** for reconstructive procedures
- **Sistrunk**[Q]:
  - A **wedge of skin** and **subcutaneous tissue is excised** and wound **closed primarily**[Q]
  - **Most commonly carried out to reduce girth** of the thigh[Q].
- **Kondoleon's or Homan's**[Q]:
  - **Staged subcutaneous excision**[Q] underneath flaps
- **Thompson**[Q]:
  - **Denuded skin flap** is **sutured to deep fascia** and buried beneath the second skin flap ('**buried dermal flap'**[Q])
- **Charles Procedure**[Q]:
  - In **severe lymphedema** with **unhealthy** and **infected skin**[Q]
  - Involves **complete** and **circumferential excision** of **skin, subcutaneous tissue and deep fascia** of the involved leg and dorsum of the foot[Q].

LYMPHANGIOMA

Lymphangioma

- Lymphangiomas are the **lymphatic analogue of** the **hemangiomas** of blood vessels.
- **Divided into two types:**
  - Simple or **capillary lymphangioma**
  - **Cavernous lymphangioma** or **cystic hygroma**

Clinical Features
- Most of these **benign tumors** are **present at birth**, and 90% of them can be **identified by the end of the first year of life**.[Q]
- **Site of cavernous lymphangiomas:** Mainly in **neck** or **axilla**[Q] (rarely in the retroperitoneum)
- **Site of simple capillary lymphangiomas:** Subcutaneously in the **head** and **neck** region and **axilla**.

> - Represent **isolated** and **sequestered segments of** the **lymphatic system**[Q] that retain the ability to produce lymph.
> - As the **volume of lymph inside** the **cystic tumor increases**, they **grow larger** within the surrounding tissues.

Treatment
- **Surgical excision**[Q], taking care to preserve all normal surrounding infiltrated structures.

LYMPHANGIOSARCOMA (ANGIOSARCOMA)

Angiosarcoma (Lymphangiosarcoma)

- Rare tumor that develops as a **complication** of **long-standing** (>10 years) **lymphoedema**[Q].
- Stewart and Treves described **lymphangiosarcoma** of the **upper extremity** in women with **ipsilateral lymphedema** after **radical mastectomy. (Stewart-Treves Syndrome)**[Q]

Clinical Features
- **Acute worsening** of **edema**[Q]
- Appearance of **sub-cutaneous nodules** with propensity towards **hemorrhage and ulceration**[Q]

Treatment
- Pre-operative **chemotherapy** and **radiotherapy** followed by **surgical excision (radical amputation)**[Q]
- Associated with **poor prognosis**.

KIKUCHI DISEASE

Kikuchi Disease

- Rare **subacute necrotizing lymphadenitis**[Q]
- Most commonly seen in **children** and **young adults** of **Asian heritage**[Q]
- **Etiology** is **unknown**

Pathology
- **Necrotizing** and **crescenteric plasmacytoid monocytes**[Q]
- Absence of neutrophils and eosinophils

Clinical Features
- **Most characteristic feature: Painful tender lymphadenopathy**[Q], most commonly **involving cervical LN**
- Less commonly involved LNs include axillary and inguinal LNs
- Deep LNs and extranodal sites are rarely involved
- **Lymphadenopathy** is associated with **fever** and **systemic signs**

Prognosis
- **Self-limiting disease, resolves spontaneously** within **6 months**[Q]

Multiple Choice Questions

LYMPHEDEMA

1. **True about primary lymphedema:** *(PGI Nov 2010)*
   a. Lymphangiosarcoma may occur
   b. Associated with Milroy's disease
   c. Onset between 2-35 years indicates lymphedema tarda
   d. Onset >35 years indicates praecox variety
   e. Prevalence is 2%

2. **Which of the following is not an operation of congenital lymphedema?** *(MHPGMCET 2009)*
   a. Homan's operation
   b. Charles's operation
   c. de Quervain's cross red operation
   d. Sistrunk's operation

3. **In Neibulowitz surgery what is done?**
   a. Skin bridge *(MHSSMCET 2006, 2008)*
   b. Lymph node with vein anastomosis
   c. Ileal mucosal patch
   d. All of the above

4. **Most common type of primary lymphedema is:** *(DNB 2010)*
   a. Lymphedema congenita   b. Lymphedema precox
   c. Lymphedema tarda   d. None

5. **In India, what is the most common cause of unilateral lymphedema of lower limb?** *(UPSC 2007)*
   a. Lymphedema tarda
   b. Carcinoma of penis with metastatic nodes
   c. Filariasis
   d. Tubercular lymphadenopathy

6. **Hydrocele and edema in foot occur in:** *(PGI Nov 2011)*
   a. W. bancrofti   b. B. malayi
   c. B. timori   d. Oncocerca volulus
   e. Guinea worm

7. **Chronic lymphedema of limb is predisposed to all of the following except:** *(All India 2004)*
   a. Thickening of the skin
   b. Recurrent soft tissue infections
   c. Marjolin's ulcer
   d. Sarcoma

8. **Lymphovenous anastomosis is done for:** *(PGI Dec 97)*
   a. Filarial lymphedema   b. Lymphoid cyst
   c. Cystic hygroma   d. Malignant lymphedema

9. **Commonest cause of unilateral pedal edema in India is:** *(All India 90)*
   a. Filariasis   b. Post traumatic
   c. Post irradiation   d. Milroy's disease

10. **All are true about congenital lymphedema except:**
    a. It is bilateral *(Recent Question 2014; All India 91)*
    b. Involve lower limb
    c. Almost always manifests before puberty
    d. Acute lymphangitis may occur

11. **The commonest cause for lymphedema of upper limb is:**
    a. Filariasis *(All India 91, 92)*
    b. Congenital
    c. Neck surgery
    d. Post mastectomy irradiation

12. **Milroy's disease is:** *(JIPMER 92)*
    a. Edema due to filariasis
    b. Post cellulitic lymphedema
    c. Congenital lymphedema
    d. Lymphedema following surgery

13. **Most common bacterial infection in lymphedema is:** *(DNB 2010)*
    a. Staphylococcus   b. Streptococcus
    c. E. coli   d. Pseudomonas

14. **Lymphangiography of the leg is performed by:**
    a. An injection of sodium diatrizoate (Hypaque) subcutaneously between the toes
    b. Injection sodium diatrizoate retrogradely under pressure into a small vein on the dorsum of the foot
    c. Dissecting lymphatics through an incision on the dorsum of the foot
    d. The use of an infusion pump

15. **Finding the cause of unilateral lymphedema of the leg includes:**
    a. Taking a family history
    b. Looking for chronic infection in the foot
    c. Looking for early malignant disease of the testis
    d. Looking for filariasis
    e. Performing a Casoni's test

16. **Treatment of acute lymphangitis requires:**
    a. Antibiotic and rest
    b. Immediate lymphangiography
    c. Immediate multiple incisions
    d. No special treatment

17. **Grade I lymphedema means:** *(JIPMER 2000)*
    a. Pitting edema upto the ankle
    b. Pitting edema upto the knee
    c. Non-pitting edema
    d. Edema disappearing after overnight rest

18. **Chronically lymphedematous limb is predisposed to all of the following except:** *(All India 2004)*
    a. Thickening of the skin
    b. Recurrent soft tissue infections
    c. Marjolin's ulcer
    d. Sarcoma

19. **Stemmer's sign is seen in:** *(Recent Question 2017)*
    a. Lymphedema
    b. Venous disease
    c. Factitious lymphedema
    d. Arterial disease

20. **Diagnosis of lymphedema is usually done by:** *(Recent Question 2017)*
    a. History and clinical examination
    b. Lymphangiogram
    c. MRI
    d. CT scan

21. **Most common cause of lymphedema:**
    a. Filariasis *(Recent Question 2017)*
    b. Lymph node dissection in malignancies
    c. Bacterial infection
    d. Congenital

22. True statement regarding lymphedema is: (PGI May 2018)
a. Can be complicated by cellulitis
b. Familial version of congenital lymphedema is known as Milroy's disease
c. Commonly caused by Wuchereria bancrofti
d. Lymphedema congenital more likely to be unilateral
e. Lymphedema precox is more common in males

LYMPHOMA

23. Popcorn type of Reed-Sternberg cell is seen in the following type of Hodgkin's lymphoma: (COMEDK 2007)
a. Lymphocyte rich
b. Mixed cellularity
c. Lymphocyte predominance
d. Lymphocyte depletion

24. Carcinoma in which surgery is rarely indicated: (PGI Nov 2009)
a. Osteosarcoma
b. Wilms' tumor
c. Neuroblastoma
d. Rhabdomyosarcoma
e. Hodgkin's lymphoma

25. All are poor prognostic factor for Hodgkin's lymphoma except: (PGI Nov 2011, Dec 2001)
a. Young age
b. Involvement of stomach
c. Lymphocyte depletion
d. Extranodal metastasis
e. Large mediastinal mass

26. Commonest presentation of Hodgkin's lymphoma is:
a. Painless enlargement of lymph node (All India 99)
b. Pruritus
c. Fever
d. Leucocytosis

27. The most common site of enlargement of the lymph nodes in Hodgkin's lymphoma is: (All India 95)
a. Mediastinal
b. Axillary
c. Cervical
d. Abdominal

28. Malignant cell in Hodgkin's lymphoma is:
a. Reed Sternberg cell
b. Lymphocytes
c. Histiocyte
d. Reticulum cells

29. Total dose of radiation in Hodgkin's disease is:
a. 500-1000 rad (JIPMER 95)
b. 1000-2000 rad
c. 3000-5000 rad
d. 5000-7000 rad

30. Diagnosis of Hodgkin's disease is confirmed by: (PGI 97)
a. CT scan
b. Bone marrow biopsy
c. Lymph node biopsy
d. Lymphangiography

MISCELLANEOUS

31. A 45 years old man presents with progressive cervical lymph nodes enlargement, since 3 months: most diagnostic investigation is: (All India 2001, 91)
a. X-ray soft tissue
b. FNAC
c. Lymph node biopsy
c. None of the above

32. True about lymphangioma: (PGI June 2003)
a. It is a malignant tumor
b. It is a congenital sequestration of lymphatic channel
c. Cystic hygroma is a lymphangioma
d. Laser excision is done
e. Sclerotherapy is common done

33. True about lymphangioma is:
a. Common in puberty
b. Respond in low doses to radiotherapy
c. Lymphangioma progress slowly and may invade local tissue
d. Predisposes to cancer

34. The most common site of lymphangiosarcoma is: (UPSC 2004)
a. Liver
b. Spleen
c. Post-mastectomy edema of arm
d. Retroperitoneum

35. Lymphangiosarcoma occurs in: (DNB 2010)
a. Lymphangiomas
b. Lymphomas
c. Lymphedema
d. Serous cavity tumour

36. Investigation of choice in detecting small para-aortic lymph node is: (JIPMER 92)
a. Ultra sound scan
b. CT scan
c. Lymphangiography
d. Arteriography

37. In HIV infection, diffuse lymphadenopathy in a person who is clinically well is usually a sign of which of the following?
a. Lymphoma (COMEDK 2004)
b. Kaposi's sarcoma
c. Tuberculosis
d. Persistent generalized lymphadenopathy (PGL)

38. Necrotizing lymphadenitis is characteristically seen in:
a. Kimura disease (All India 2011)
b. Kikuchi disease
c. Hodgkin's disease
d. Castleman disease

39. Lethal midline granuloma is synonym of: (DNB 2007)
a. Wagner's granulomatosis
b. Extra nodal NK cell/T cell lymphoma nasal type
c. Syphilis of nasal septum
d. Tuberculosis of nasal septum

Explanations

LYMPHEDEMA

1. Ans. a Lymphangiosarcoma may occur, b. Associated with Milroy's disease, e. Prevalence is 2% *(Ref: Sabiston 20/e p1849-1850; Schwartz 10/e p934-936, 1879-1880; Bailey 27/e p997-1000)*

   - Primary Lymphedema is uncommon, occurs in 1 of every 1000 individuals. At birth, 1 in 6000 persons will develop lymphoedema with an overall prevalence of 0.13–2%.
   - Lymphangiosarcoma is a rare tumor that develops as a complication of long standing (>10 years) lymphedema.

2. Ans. c. de Quervain's cross red operation *(Ref: Sabiston 20/e p 1852; Schwartz 10/e p934-936, 1879-1880; Bailey 27/e p1007-1012)*

3. Ans. b. Lymph node with vein anastomosis

4. Ans. b. Lymphedema precox

5. Ans. c. Filariasis

6. Ans. a. W. bancrofti; b. B. malayi; c. B. timori *(Ref: Sabiston 20/e p1850, 19/e p1820-1824; Schwartz 10/e p934,1879; Bailey 27/e p1003-1005)*

7. Ans. c. Marjolin's ulcer *(Ref: Sabiston 20/e p1850; Schwartz 10/e p934-936, 1879-1880; Bailey 27/e p998-999)*

8. Ans. a. Filarial lymphedema
9. Ans. a. Filariasis
10. Ans. None
11. Ans. a. Filariasis
12. Ans. c. Congenital lymphedema
13. Ans. b. Streptococcus

   The **most common complication** of both **primary** and **secondary lymphedema is erysipelas** (Acute **Streptococcus bacterial infection** of the deep epidermis with lymphatic spread). Cellulites may occur concurrently in lymphedema because of **pooling of protein rich lymph fluid** makes it easier for the patient to develop an infection.

14. Ans. c. Dissecting lymphatics through an incision on the dorsum of the foot *(Ref: Sabiston 20/e p1850; Schwartz 10/e p935; Bailey 27/e p1006)*

15. Ans. a. Taking a family history; b. Looking for chronic infection in the foot

16. Ans. a. Antibiotic and rest

17. Ans. d. Edema disappearing after overnight rest *(Ref: Sabiston 20/e p1849; Bailey 27/e p998)*

18. Ans. c. Marjolin's ulcer

19. Ans. a. Lymphedema *(Ref: Bailey 27/e p998)*

   "The contour of the ankle is lost through infilling of the submalleolar depressions, a 'buffalo hump' forms on the dorsum of the foot, the toes appear 'square' because of confinement of footwear and the skin on the dorsum of the toes cannot be pinched because of subcutaneous fibrosis (Stemmer's sign)."-Bailey 27/e p998

20. Ans. a. History and clinical examination *(Ref: Bailey 27/e p1006)*

   "It is usually possible to diagnose and manage lymphoedema purely on the basis of history and examination, especially when the swelling is mild and there are no apparent complicating features. In patients with severe, atypical and multifactorial swelling, investigations may help confirm the diagnosis, inform management and provide prognostic information."-Bailey 27/e p1006

21. Ans. a. Filariasis *(Ref: Bailey 27/e p1003)*

22. Ans. a. Can be complicated…, b. Familial version of…., c. Commonly caused by…

LYMPHOMA

23. Ans. c. Lymphocyte predominance *(Ref: Harrison 20/e p780, 19/e p708)*

   ### Hodgkin's Lymphoma

   - Classified into four types according to **Rye's classification**:
     - **Nodular sclerosis (30-60%)**^{Q}
     - **Mixed cellularity (20-40%)**
     - Lymphocyte predominance (<10%)
     - Lymphocyte depleted (<10%)

- **Prognosis:** Lymphocytic predominant[Q] > Nodular sclerosis > Mixed cellularity > Lymphocyte depletion
- **Nodular sclerosis** is MC type all over the world[Q] whereas **mixed cellularity** is MC in India[Q]
- **Nodular sclerosis** is MC in females and **mediastinal involvement**[Q] is particularly common.

Subtypes	Reed Sternberg cells variant
Nodular sclerosis	• Lacunar cells[Q]
Mixed cellularity	• Classic Reed Sternberg cells[Q]
Lymphocyte predominance	• Popcorn cell[Q]
Lymphocyte depleted	• Reticular variant[Q] (more cellular)

24. **Ans. e. Hodgkin's lymphoma** *(Ref: Harrison 20/e p782, 19/e p709)*

- Treatment of **Hodgkin's disease** includes **multiagent combination chemotherapy**, either alone or with **low dose radiation**[Q].
- **Osteosarcoma:** Successful treatment of osteosarcoma requires **multiagent chemotherapy** with **complete surgical resection**.
- **Wilms' Tumor:** Immediate treatment is **nephroureterectomy.** Most of the times all the three modalities of treatment i.e. **surgery, chemotherapy** and **radiotherapy** may be required.
- **Rhabdomyosarcoma:** The optimal therapy of rhabdomyosarcoma involves **multimodality approach**, which includes **chemotherapy, surgery** and **radiotherapy**.
- **Neuroblastoma:** Three main modalities of treatment for neuroblastoma include **chemotherapy, surgery** and **radiation.**

25. **Ans. a. Young age** *(Ref: Harrison 20/e p781, 19/e p708; Anderson Manual of Medical Oncology 2007/p248-258)*

ADVERSE PROGNOSTIC FACTORS FOR HODGKIN'S LYMPHOMA

- Advanced age[Q]
- Mixed cellularity or lymphocyte[Q] depletion histologic type[Q]
- 'B' symptoms[Q]
- Large number of involved nodal regions[Q]
- Anemia[Q]
- Male gender[Q]
- Large mediastinal mass[Q]
- Raised ESR[Q]
- Low serum albumin[Q]

26. **Ans. a. Painless enlargement of lymph node** *(Ref: Harrison 19/e p708-709)*

HODGKIN'S LYMPHOMA

- **Most patients** present with **palpable lymphadenopathy** that is **non-tender**[Q].
- In most patients, these lymph nodes are in the neck, supraclavicular area and axilla.
- **More than half of the patients** will have **mediastinal adenopathy**[Q] at diagnosis and this is sometimes initial manifestation.
- **Diagnosis** is confirmed by LN biopsy[Q].

27. **Ans. a. Mediastinal** *(Ref: Harrison 20/e p781, 19/e p708)*

- In **about 50%** of patients who have both **Hodgkin's** and **Non-Hodgkin's lymphoma**, the **mediastinum** may be the **primary site**[Q].

28. **Ans. a. Reed Sternberg cell**
29. **Ans. c. 3000-5000 rad** *(Ref: Harrison 20/e p781, 19/e p709)*

Moderate **doses** of **30-40 Gray** are usually quite sufficient to take care of localized Hodgkin's disease.

Treatment of Hodgkin's Disease

Stage I (A) and Stage II (A)	Stage III, Stage IV and patients with group 'B' symptoms
• **Treatment of choice** is **brief** course of **chemotherapy** followed by **radiotherapy** to sites of node involvement[Q].	• Cornerstone of treatment is combination chemotherapy. • Chemotherapy with **ABVD** is **first line treatment** and **superior to MOPP**[Q].

ABVD (**A**driamycin, **B**leomycin, **V**inblastine, **D**acarbazine)	• First line treatment[Q] • Most popular regimen in United States[Q] • More effective than MOPP[Q] • Lesser incidence of sterility and secondary malignancies than MOPP[Q]
MOPP (**M**echlorethamine, **V**incristine, **P**rocarbazine, **P**rednisone)	• Less effective and more toxic[Q] • Higher incidence of sterility and secondary malignancies than ABVD[Q]

30. Ans. c. Lymph node biopsy

MISCELLANEOUS

31. Ans. c. **Lymph node biopsy** *(Ref: Harrison 19/e p409)*

    • Harrison says "In cases of **lymphadenopathy**, if the patient history and physical findings are **suggestive of malignancy**, then a **prompt lymph node biopsy** should be done. FNAC is not of much use, as it does not provide enough tissue to reach a diagnosis."

32. Ans. b. **It is a congenital sequestration of lymphatic channel;** c. **Cystic hygroma is a lymphangioma** *(Ref: Sabiston 20/e p1855; Schwartz 10/e p575, 598, 1602-1603; Bailey 27/e p999)*

33. Ans. c. **Lymphangioma progress slowly and may invade local tissue**

34. Ans. c. **Post-mastectomy edema of arm** *(Ref: Sabiston 20/ p766, 842, 19/e p1825; Schwartz 10/e p493, 776, 1468, 1470, 9/e p1285; Bailey 27/e p999-1000, 26/e p931)*

35. Ans. c. **Lymphedema**

36. Ans. b. **CT scan** *(Ref: Sutton 7/e p515)*

    • **Investigation of choice** in detecting **small para-aortic lymph node: CT scan**[Q]

37. Ans. d. **Persistent generalized lymphadenopathy (PGL)** *(Ref: Harrison 19/e p1262, 18/e p466, 1525)*

    ### Persistent Generalized Lymphadenopathy (PGL)

    • **HIV patients** develop **PGL** as an **early clinical manifestation** of HIV infection[Q].
    • PGL is defined as presence of **>1 LN** in **two or three extra-inguinal sites** for **>3 months without an obvious cause**[Q].
    • Enlargement is due to **follicular hyperplasia**[Q].

38. Ans. b. **Kikuchi disease** *(Ref: Nelson 20/e p2414, 18/e p2094)*

39. Ans. b. **Extra nodal NK cell/T cell lymphoma nasal type**

CHAPTER 29

Thorax and Lung

MEDIASTINUM

MEDIASTINUM

Mediastinum is situated **between** the **lungs in** the **center of** the **thorax**.

Mediastinum is divided into 3 compartments		
Anterior or Anterosuperior	**Middle or Visceral compartment**	**Posterior or Paravertebral sulci**
Lies **in front of anterior pericardium** and **trachea**^Q	Lies **within pericardial cavity**^Q including trachea	Lies **posterior to posterior pericardium** and **trachea**^Q.

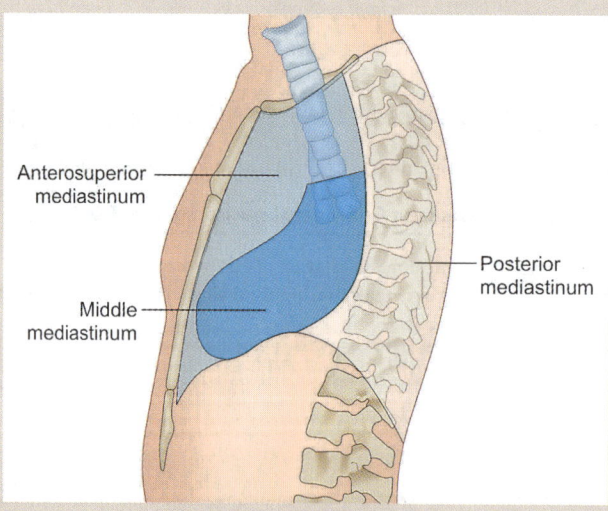

Locations of the Common Mediastinal Masses		
Anterior Mediastinum	**Middle Mediastinum**	**Posterior Mediastinum**

• **Thymoma**^Q (MC in anterior mediastinum)
• **Lymphoma**^Q
• **Germ cell tumors**^Q
• **Thyroid** and **parathyroid masses**^Q
• **Bronchogenic cyst**^Q
• **Aneurysm**^Q
	• **Cysts** (MC in middle mediastinum):
	  – **Pericardial (MC)**^Q
	  – **Bronchogenic**^Q
	  – Enterogenous
	  – **Neuroenteric**^Q
	• Vascular masses (**aneurysm**^Q)
	• LN enlargement and **lymphoma**^Q
	• Mesenchymal tumors
	• Pheochromocytoma
		• **Neurogenic tumors (MC overall**^Q)
		• **Meningoceles**^Q
		• Mesenchymal tumors
		• Pheochromocytoma
		• **Lymphoma**^Q
		• **Bochdalek hernia**^Q
		• **Bronchogenic cyst**^Q
		• **Enterogenous cyst**^Q

Mediastinal Tumors in Adults		
Tumor Type	**Percentage of Total**	**Location**
Neurogenic tumors^Q	21	Posterior
Cysts^Q	20	All
Thymomas^Q	19	Anterior

Tumor Type	Percentage of Total	Location
Lymphomas[Q]	13	Anterior/middle
Germ cell tumors	11	Anterior
Mesenchymal tumors	7	All
Endocrine tumors	6	Anterior/middle

Mediastinal Tumors in Children		
Tumor Type	Percentage of Total	Location
Neurogenic tumors	40[Q]	Posterior[Q]
Lymphomas	18[Q]	Anterior/middle
Cysts	18	All
Germ cell tumors	11	Anterior
Mesenchymal tumors	9	All
Thymomas	Rare	Anterior

MEDIASTINAL MASSES (MM)

- MC anterior MM: Thymoma[Q]
- MC middle MM: Cyst[Q] (Pericardial cyst is MC[Q])
- MC posterior MM: Neurogenic tumors[Q]
- MC MM (overall): Neurogenic tumors[Q]
- MM seen in all three compartments of mediastinum: Lymphoma, bronchogenic cyst & mesenchymal tumors[Q]
- IOC for diagnosis of MM (except neurogenic tumors): CT[Q]
- IOC for diagnosis of neurogenic tumors: MRI[Q]

THYMOMA

THYMOMA

- MC neoplasm of thymus; MC site: Anterior mediastinum[Q]
- Most frequently seen in **40-60 years** of age
- Most thymomas are **completely surrounded by** a **fibrous capsule**[Q]
- On the basis of cell types, divided into:
  - Lymphocytic (25%)
  - Epithelial (25%)
  - Lymphoepithelial (50%)[Q]

Clinical Features

- Mostly asymptomatic[Q], detected incidentally on chest X-ray
- May cause **dysphagia, dyspnea, SVC syndrome** and **paraneoplastic syndromes**[Q]

Paraneoplastic Syndromes		
Autoimmune	Hematological	Neuromuscular
• SLE[Q] • Rheumatoid arthritis • Polymyositis • Sarcoidosis	• Cytopenias[Q] • Red cell aplasia[Q] • Hypogammaglobulinemia[Q] • Erythrocytosis[Q]	• Myasthenia gravis[Q] (MC) • Neuromuscular disorders • Myotonic dystrophy • Myositis

Diagnosis

- **CT: Investigation of choice** for diagnosis of **thymoma**[Q].
- **Definitive diagnosis** is made on **histological study**[Q].

> - **Cytokeratin**[Q] is the **marker** that **best distinguishes thymomas** from lymphomas.
> - **CT scan:** Most lymphomas are associated with **marked lymphadenopathy** and **thymomas** most frequently appear as a **solitary encapsulated mass**[Q].

Staging
- Masaoka staging[Q] system is used.

Treatment
- Treatment of choice: Total thymectomy performed through median sternotomy[Q]
- Large thymoma (>5 cm) with evidence of invasion: Thymectomy + Chemotherapy[Q]
- Myasthenia gravis is treated with thymectomy and anticholinesterase drugs[Q].

BRONCHOGENIC CYST

Bronchogenic Cyst

- **Bronchogenic cysts** originate as **sequestrations** from the **ventral foregut**[Q], the antecedent of the tracheobronchial tree.
- **Cyst wall** is composed **pathognomonic inner layer of ciliated respiratory epithelium**[Q].
- MC location: Middle mediastinum[Q] (65-90%)

Bronchogenic Cyst

Mediastinal	Parenchymal (intrapulmonary)
• Sub-carinal, right paratracheal and hilar locations are most common • **Does not communicate** with the **tracheobronchial tree**[Q]	• Typically **perihilar** with **predilection for lower lobes**[Q] • **Communicate** with the **tracheobronchial tree**[Q]

Clinical Features
- **Two thirds** are **asymptomatic**[Q]
- May produce **symptoms** that **depend** on their **anatomic location**.
- **Paratracheal region**: Airway **compression** and **respiratory distress**
- **Lung parenchyma**: Become infected, present with **fever** and **cough**.

Diagnosis
- **Chest X-ray**: Shows a **dense mass**
- **CT scan** or **MRI**: Delineates the **precise anatomic location**

Treatment
- **Surgical excision** is recommended **in all patients** to **provide definitive histologic diagnosis**[Q], alleviate symptoms, and prevent the development of associated complications.

PULMONARY SEQUESTRATION

Pulmonary Sequestration

- **Malformations** of the lung **without bronchial communication** with an **aberrant systemic blood supply**[Q].
- **MC site**: Posterobasal segment of left lower lobe[Q]
- **Presentation** is with **recurrent chest infection**[Q].

Pulmonary Sequestration

Intralobar	Extralobar
• Reside **within lung parenchyma**[Q] • **Infrequently associated with** other **anomalies**[Q] • Found within the **medial** or **posterior segments** of the **lower lobes** • **Two thirds** occurring **on left side**[Q] • In 85% of cases supplied by an **anomalous systemic vessel** arising from the **infradiaphragmatic aorta**[Q], located within the **inferior pulmonary ligament**. • **Venous drainage** through the **inferior pulmonary vein**. • Because of the **risk for infection** and bleeding, **usually removed**, either by **segmentectomy** or **lobectomy**[Q].	• Surrounded by a **separate pleural covering**[Q] • Occur predominantly in **males**[Q] • More common on the **left side**[Q]. • In 40%, **multiple other anomalies**[Q] are encountered. • **Usually asymptomatic**[Q] • Because there is **usually no bronchial communication**, the **risk for infection is low**. • Many of these malformations may be **observed**[Q].

Diagnosis

- **CT** is **preferred modality** for diagnosis of **pulmonary sequestration**[Q].

  - Historically, angiography was considered an important preoperative study before embarking on resection of a sequestration.
  - More recently, **CT** and **MRI** have **replaced the need for angiography** and **provide excellent mapping of the blood supply**[Q].

PECTUS EXCAVATUM

PECTUS EXCAVATUM

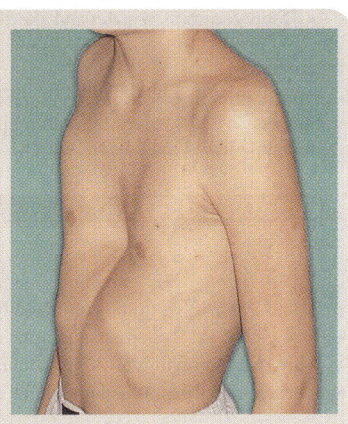

- **Pectus excavatum** (also called **funnel chest**) is the **MC chest wall deformity**[Q]
- Incidence: **1 of 400** children.
- **More common** in **males**
- Arises from **excessive growth** of the **lower costal cartilages**, causing **posterior sternal depression**[Q].

Clinical Features

- **Most patients** are **asymptomatic** at the time of presentation
- **Decrease in respiratory reserve**[Q] or pain along the costal cartilages with exercise.

Diagnosis

- **PFT**: Evaluation of **baseline pulmonary function**[Q]
- **ECHO**: Cardiovascular assessment

  - **In severe cases, decreased stroke volume** and **cardiac output** with a **restrictive pattern** (decreased maximal breathing capacity) on PFT[Q].

- **Chest CT: Haller index**[Q] (Ratio of width of chest wall to depth of sternum to vertebral body

Treatment

- **Early repair** with **best results** between **2-8 years** of age.

Indications for operative intervention	
• Cosmesis[Q] • Psychosocial factors[Q]	• Presence of **respiratory** or **cardiovascular insufficiency**[Q]

- **Ravitch procedure**[Q]: Open surgical procedure for pectus excavatum
- **Nuss procedure**[Q]: Minimal invasive surgery for pectus excavatum

PECTUS CARINATUM

PECTUS CARINATUM

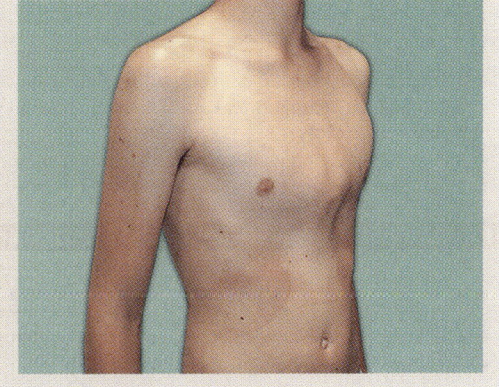

- Also known as **pigeon chest**[Q]
- **Sternum** is **elevated above** the level of **chest**[Q]
- **MC type: Anterior displacement of mid & lower sternum** with adjacent costal cartilages[Q]
- **More common** in **males**
- Associated with **mitral valve disease & coarctation of aorta**[Q]

Clinical Features

- Most patients are **asymptomatic**[Q]
- Treatment is offered for cosmetic reasons

Treatment

- Surgery involves **mobilizing sternum & costal cartilage** close **to its anatomical position**

EVENTRATION OF THE DIAPHRAGM

Eventration of the Diaphragm

- **Abnormally elevated position** of diaphragm from **paralysis** or **atrophy** of the **muscle fibers**.
- May be **congenital anomaly**^{Q} caused by **failure of muscularization**^{Q} of the **dome of** hemidiaphragm, or it may be **acquired** as a result of **dysfunction of** the **phrenic nerve** related to the neuromuscular disease or trauma including operative trauma.
- **Birth trauma**: MC cause of **acquired** diaphragmatic **eventration**, usually related to **breech** presentation.

  - **Most commonly** diagnosed in **pediatric patients**^{Q}
  - **More common in males** and affect **left hemidiaphragm** more frequently.

Treatment
- **Diaphragmatic plication** is **preferred over resection**^{Q}.
- **Surgery to fix** the **diaphragm in inspiration**^{Q} so the paradoxical movement and mediastinal shift are minimized.

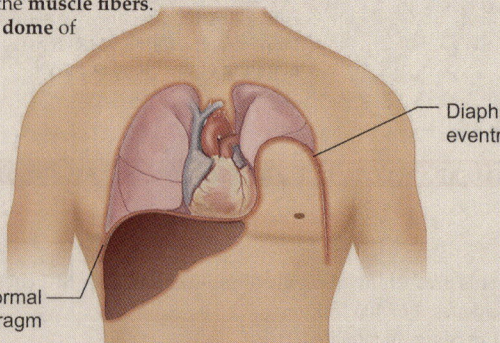

PLEURAL EFFUSION

Pleural Effusion

- About **300 mL**^{Q} of fluid is **required for** the development **of costophrenic angle blunting** seen on an upright chest X-ray.
- At least **500 mL**^{Q} of effusion is necessary **for detection on clinical examination**.
- **Chest tube insertion** is carried out in such a way (angled chest tube, **low insertion site**) that **drainage is as complete as possible**.
- **Chest tube insertion** is done in 5th ICS in midaxillary line.

  - Ideally **chest tube insertion** should be done **through triangle of safety (4th to 6th intercostal space, anterior to mid-axillary line**^{Q}**)**

Boundaries of Triangle of Safety
- **Lateral border** of **pectoralis major**^{Q}
- **Anterior border** of **Lattisimus dorsi**^{Q}
- **Superior border** of 5th or 6th rib^Q

Pleural Effusion

Exudative	Transudative
• **Local factors**^{Q} that influence the formation and absorption of pleural fluid **are altered**. • **Laboratory Features** • Total serum **protein >3 gm/dl**^{Q} • Pleural **fluid protein/serum protein >0.5**^{Q} • Pleural **fluid LDH/serum LDH >0.6**^{Q} • Pleural **fluid LDH >2/3rd** upper limit of serum^Q	• **Systemic factors**^{Q} that influence the formation and absorption of pleural fluid **are altered**. • **Laboratory Features** • Total serum **protein <3 gm/dl**^{Q} • Pleural **fluid protein/serum protein <0.5**^{Q} • Pleural **fluid LDH/serum LDH <0.6**^{Q} • Pleural **fluid LDH <2/3rd** upper limit of serum^Q

PNEUMOTHORAX

Pneumothorax

- Pneumothorax is presence of **air within pleural space**
- **Spontaneous pneumothorax** is also known as **closed pneumothorax**, occurs when **visceral pleura ruptures without an external traumatic or iatrogenic cause**
- **Types**: Primary spontaneous pneumothorax & secondary spontaneous pneumothorax

PRIMARY SPONTANEOUS PNEUMOTHORAX

Primary Spontaneous Pneumothorax (PSP)

- PSP is spontaneous pneumothorax occurring **without underlying lung disease**
- MC cause: **Rupture of apical subpleural bleb**^{Q}

Risk Factors for PSP	
• Male sex^Q	• Family history
• Smoking^Q	• Marfan syndrome^Q (Tall thin body habitus^Q)

Clinical Features
- Sudden in onset, patient presents with **mild dyspnea**^Q

Diagnosis
- Best X-ray film for diagnosis: **Chest X-ray PA view**^Q (expiratory film)
- Best investigation for diagnosis: **NCCT**^Q

Treatment
- Initial treatment: **Simple needle aspiration**^Q
- TOC: **ICD insertion**^Q

Thoracoscopic Management of PSP
• Thoracoscopic management includes **bleb resection** with **pleurodesis by talc** or **pleural abrasion**^Q
• 100% successful in preventing recurrences

Indications of Thoracoscopic Management of PSP	
• Recurrences^Q	• Complete lung collapse in first episode^Q

SECONDARY SPONTANEOUS PNEUMOTHORAX (PSP)

- Occurs in the **setting of underlying lung disease (COPD, asthma, cystic fibrosis**^Q)

Clinical Features
- Symptoms are **more severe**
- Tend to occur in **older patients**
- Patients present with **sharp pleuritic pain & breathlessness**^Q

Treatment
- TOC: **ICD insertion**^Q

OPEN PNEUMOTHORAX ('SUCKING CHEST WOUND')

Open Pneumothorax (Sucking Chest Wound)

- This is due to a **large open defect** in the chest (>3 cm), leading to equilibration between intrathoracic and atmospheric pressure.
- **Air accumulates** in the **hemithorax** (rather than in the lung) with each inspiration, leading to **profound hypoventilation** on the affected side and **hypoxia**^Q.

Clinical Features
- Signs and symptoms are usually **proportionate to the size of the defect**.
- If there is a **valvular effect**, increasing amounts of air will result in a **tension pneumothorax**^Q

Management
- Initial management: **Promptly close the defect**^Q
- A **chest tube** is **inserted as soon as possible** in a site remote from the injury site^Q.
- Definitive treatment: **Formal debridement** and **closure**^Q

TENSION PNEUMOTHORAX

Tension Pneumothorax

- A tension pneumothorax develops when a **'one-way valve'** air leak occurs either **from** the **lung** or **through** the **chest wall**^Q.
- **Air is forced into thoracic cavity** without any means of escape, **completely collapsing the affected lung**^Q.

> • **Mediastinum** is **displaced** to the **opposite side**, **decreasing venous return** and **compressing the opposite lung**^Q.

Common Causes of Tension Pneumothorax	
• Penetrating chest trauma^Q • Blunt chest trauma^Q (with parenchymal injury and air leak that did not spontaneously close)	• Iatrogenic lung punctures (e.g. due to subclavian central venepuncture) • Mechanical positive pressure ventilation^Q

Clinical Features

- Clinical presentation is dramatic.
- The patient is panicky with tachypnoea, dyspnoea and distended neck veins (similar to pericardial tamponade)^Q.
- Clinical examination can reveal tracheal deviation (a late finding – not necessary to clinically confirm diagnosis), hyperresonance and absent breath sounds over the affected hemithorax^Q.

Diagnosis

- Tension pneumothorax is a clinical diagnosis and treatment should not be delayed^Q by waiting for radiologicalconfirmation.

Treatment

- Treatment consists of immediate decompression by rapid insertion of a large-bore needle into the 2nd intercostal space in the mid-clavicular line^Q of the affected hemithorax.
- This is immediately followed by insertion of a chest tube through the 5th intercostal space in the anterior axillary line^Q.

> • If the tension in the pleural space is not relieved, the patient is likely to die from inadequate cardiac output or marked hypoxemia^Q.

HEMOTHORAX

HEMOTHORAX

- Causes: Trauma (MC), tumor, tuberculosis^Q
- Massive hemothorax is usually the result of major pulmonary vascular injuries or major arterial wounds while minor injuries can cause small hemothorax.
- MC cause of massive hemothorax in blunt injury: Torn intercostal vessels because of rib fracture^Q

Diagnosis

- Diagnosis is made by needle aspiration of pleural fluid^Q.
- Chest X-ray: To assess the presence and extent of pleural cavity collection^Q

> • A supine position with horizontal X-ray beam (decubitus position) is better than erect film, as about 400-500 ml of blood may be hidden by diaphragm on upright chest X-ray^Q.

Management

- Most patients with hemothorax should be treated with tube thoracostomy, which allows continuous quantification of bleeding^Q.
- In most of the cases bleeding stops as the lung re-expands^Q.
- Thoracoscopy or thoracotomy: Pleural hemorrhage >200 mL/hour^Q

Indications of Thoracotomy	
• Initial tube thoracostomy drainage of >1000 mL (penetrating injury)^Q or >1500 ml (blunt injury)^Q • Ongoing tube thoracostomy drainage of >200 ml/hr for 3 consecutive hours^Q in non-coagulopathic patients • Caked hemothorax^Q despite of placement of two chest tubes • Tracheo-bronchial injury^Q	• Selected descending torn aorta or great vessel injury^Q • Pericardial tamponade^Q • Cardiac herniation^Q • Massive air leak^Q from chest tube with inadequate ventilation • Open pneumothorax^u • Esophageal perforation^Q

LUNG ABSCESS

Lung Abscess

- **Lung abscess** refers to a **microbial infection** of the **lung** that results in necrosis of the pulmonary parenchyma.
- MC cause of **primary lung abscess**: Anaerobic bacteria[Q]
- Etiology of anaerobic lung abscess: **Aspiration**[Q]

Routes of Infection
- **Aspiration of organisms** that colonize oropharynx (**MC**)[Q]
- **Inhalation** of infection or aerosols
- **Hematogenous** dissemination from extrapulmonary site
- **Direct inoculation** (as in tracheal intubation or stab wounds)
- **Contiguous spread** from an adjacent site of infection

Clinical Features
- **Classic presentation**: An **indolent infection** that **evolves over several days or weeks**, usually in a host who has a **predisposition to aspiration**[Q].
- A **common feature** is **periodontal infection** with **pyorrhea** or **gingivitis**.
- **Symptoms**: Fatigue, cough, sputum production, and **fever**[Q] Chills are uncommon.

Diagnosis
- Lung abscess can be detected by **chest X-ray** and **CT**
- **CT scan**: Investigation of choice for **lung abscess**[Q]

Treatment
- **Treatment** depends on the **presumed** or **established etiology**.
- Infections caused by **anaerobic bacteria**: **Clindamycin**[Q]

- **Persistence of fever beyond 5–7 days** or **progression of the infiltrate** suggests **failure of therapy** and a need to **exclude** factors such as **obstruction, complicating empyema**, and **involvement of antibiotic-resistant bacteria**[Q].

- Lung abscess due to S. aureus: **Vancomycin**[Q]
- **Indications for surgery**: **Failure to respond** to medical management, **suspected neoplasm**, and **hemorrhage**[Q].

Causes of Failures of Medical Management	
• **Failure to drain** pleural collections[Q]	• Giant abscess[Q]
• Inappropriate antimicrobial therapy[Q]	• Resistant pathogen[Q]
• Obstructed bronchus[Q]	• Refractory lesions[Q]

CHYLOTHORAX

Chylothorax

- A chylothorax occurs **when the thoracic duct is disrupted** and **chyle accumulates** in the pleural space.
- MC cause of chylothorax: **Trauma** (most frequently **thoracic surgery**[Q])
- More common on **right side**[Q]

Clinical Features
- Patients with chylothorax present with **dyspnea**, chest pain, fatigue

- **Thoracentesis** reveals **milky fluid**[Q]
- TG level >1.2 mmol/L (110 mg/dL[Q]).

Diagnosis
- **Chest X-ray**: **Large pleural effusion**[Q]
- Patients with chylothorax and no obvious trauma should have a **lymphangiogram** and a **mediastinal CT scan** to assess the **mediastinum for lymph nodes**[Q].

Treatment
- **Treatment of choice**: **Chest tube insertion** + Administration of **octreotide** and **Medium chain triglycerides**[Q].
- If these modalities fail, a **pleuroperitoneal shunt** should be placed unless the patient has chylous ascites.
- An alternative treatment is **ligation of the thoracic duct**[Q].
- Patients with chylothoraxes **should not undergo prolonged tube thoracostomy** with chest tube drainage because this will lead to **malnutrition and immunologic incompetence**[Q].

CHYLURIA

Chyluria

- **Filariasis** is the **MC cause**, with chyluria occurring in 1–2% of cases 10–20 years after initial infestation.

Causes of Chyluria	
• Filariasis[Q]	• Tuberculosis[Q]
• Ascariasis	• Pregnancy[Q]
• Malaria	• Childbirth[Q]
• Tumour	

Clinical Features
- It usually presents as **painless passage** of **milky white urine**, particularly **after a fatty meal**.
- The **chyle may clot**, leading to **renal colic**, and **hypoproteinaemia** may result.

Diagnosis
- **Intravenous urography** and/or **lymphangiography** will often demonstrate the **lymphourinary fistula.**

Treatment
- Treatment includes a **low-fat** and **high protein diet**, **increased oral fluids** to prevent clot colic, and **laparotomy** and **ligation of the dilated lymphatics**.
- Attempts have also been made to **sclerose the lymphatics** either **directly** or **via instrumentation** of the bladder, ureter and renal pelvis.

THORACIC DUCT INJURY

Thoracic Duct Injury

- **Causes:** Iatrogenic trauma[Q] (MC), penetrating and blunt trauma
- **Iatrogenic chylothorax** is a well-known **complication of thoracic operations**[Q]

Clinical presentation
- Most of the patient presents with **chylothorax**
- In **iatrogenic injuries**, **chylous fluid** coming **from drain site**

Complications of Thoracic Duct Injury	
• Dehydration[Q]	• Protein loss[Q]
• Electrolyte losses[Q]	• Impaired immunity[Q] secondary to loss of
• Loss of fat and fat-soluble vitamins[Q]	circulating lymphocytes (lymphopenia[Q])

Management
- **Conservative management:** Low-fat diet with **medium chain triglycerides**[Q], TPN, correction of electrolyte imbalance and **adequate drainage** by **chest tube** or **neck drain**[Q]
- **Octreotide** and recently, **Etilefrine** (an adrenergic agent that acts by causing smooth muscle contraction of the thoracic duct) **are effective**[Q].

> • **Iatrogenic thoracic duct injury** shows **higher rate of spontaneous closure with conservative treatment**[Q] than traumatic injury.

- **Surgery:** Surgery is indicated **after 5 days of conservative treatment, if chyle loss exceeds 1500 ml or if leak persist after 2 weeks**[Q].

> • **VATS guided thoracic duct ligation is surgical treatment of choice**[Q].

Poirier's Triangle
- Thoracic duct is **readily identified within** the confines of **Poirier's triangle**[Q] via left posterolateral thoracotomy.
- **Boundaries:** Arch of aorta, Left subclavian artery and Vertebral column
- The thoracic duct traverses the triangle on **esophagus** that **forms the floor** of the triangle.

POSTOPERATIVE LUNG COLLAPSE (ATELECTASIS)

Postoperative Lung Collapse (Atelectasis)

- **MC postoperative respiratory complication:** Atelectasis[Q]
- As a result of the **anesthetic**, **abdominal incision**, and **postoperative narcotics**, the **alveoli in** the **periphery collapse** and a pulmonary shunt may occur.
- **Aggressive pulmonary toilet** to prevent buildup of secretions and secondary infection High risk in **heavy smokers**, **obese** patients[Q]

Clinical Features
- MC cause of a **postoperative fever** in the **first 48 hours: Atelectasis**[Q]
- **Symptoms:** Low-grade fever, malaise and diminished breath sounds in the lower lung fields.

Management
- **Prevention of atelectasis:** Pain control, deep breaths (spirometry) & cough[Q]
- Rarely, intermittent positive pressure breathing and **chest physiotherapy** may be required.

> - **Encouraging** the patient **to breathe deeply** and **cough** is the **single most valuable management** approach in preventing and resolving atelectasis and pneumonia[Q].

- **Pneumonia:** Managed with **aggressive pulmonary toilet**, induced **sputum for culture** and sensitivity testing, **IV antibiotic therap**y.

ACUTE RESPIRATORY DISTRESS SYNDROME

ACUTE RESPIRATORY DISTRESS SYNDROME

- ARDS is a clinical syndrome of **severe dyspnea** of **rapid onset**, **hypoxemia**, and **diffuse pulmonary infiltrates** leading to **respiratory failure**[Q].
- ARDS is caused by **diffuse lung injury** from many underlying medical and surgical disorders.

> - **Diffuse alveolar damage** is the **most characteristic feature** of ARDS[Q].

Clinical Disorders Associated with ARDS

Direct Lung Injury
- Pneumonia[Q]
- Aspiration of gastric contents[Q]
- Pulmonary contusion[Q]
- Near-drowning[Q]
- Toxic inhalation injury[Q]

Indirect Lung Injury
- Sepsis[Q]
- Severe trauma: Multiple bone fractures, **Flail chest**, Head trauma, Burns[Q]
- Multiple transfusions, Drug overdose
- Pancreatitis[Q]
- Postcardiopulmonary bypass[Q]

Clinical Course and Pathophysiology

Exudative Phase
- **Alveolar capillary endothelial cells** and **type I pneumocytes** are **injured**[Q]
- **Edema** rich in protein accumulates in **interstitial & alveolar spaces**[Q]
- **Neutrophils** traffic into the **pulmonary interstitium & alveoli**[Q]
- **Condensed plasma proteins** aggregate in the **air spaces**[Q] with cellular debris & dysfunctional pulmonary surfactant to **form hyaline membrane whorls**.
- **Alveolar edema** in **dependent portions** of lung
- **Diminished aeration & atelectasis**[Q]
- **Intrapulmonary shunting & hypoxemia**[Q] develop
- **Tachypnea & increased work of breathing** frequently result in **respiratory fatigue** and **respiratory failure**[Q]

Proliferative Phase
- Lasts from **day 7** to **day 21**[Q]
- Most patients recover rapidly and are liberated from mechanical ventilation during this phase[Q].
- Some patients develop **progressive lung injury** and early changes of **pulmonary fibrosis**[Q].
- **First signs of resolution** are evident with initiation of lung repair, organization of alveolar exudates, and **lymphocyte-predominant** pulmonary infiltrate[Q].
- **Proliferation** of **type II pneumocytes** along alveolar basement membranes[Q].
- Presence of **alveolar type III procollagen peptide**, a **marker of pulmonary fibrosis**, is associated with a **protracted clinical course** and **increased mortality from ARDS**[Q]

Fibrotic Phase
- Require **long-term support** on **mechanical ventilators** and/or **supplemental oxygen**.
- **Alveolar edema** and **inflammatory exudates** converted to **extensive alveolar duct** and **interstitial fibrosis**[Q].
- **Acinar architecture** is markedly disrupted, leading to **emphysema-like changes** with large bullae[Q].
- **Progressive vascular occlusion & pulmonary hypertension**.
- Increased risk of **pneumothorax**, reductions in lung compliance, and **increased pulmonary dead space**[Q].

Management of ARDS

- A large-scale, randomized controlled trial sponsored by the National Institutes of Health and conducted by the ARDS Network compared **low VT** (**6 mL/kg**[Q] predicted body weight) ventilation to conventional VT (12 mL/kg predicted body weight) ventilation.
- **Mortality** was **significantly lower** in the **low VT patients** (31%) compared to the conventional VT patients (40%).
- This improvement in survival represents the **most substantial benefit in ARDS mortality**[Q] demonstrated for any therapeutic intervention in ARDS to date.

PULMONARY EMBOLISM

Pulmonary Embolism

- Risk factors for pulmonary embolism are the **risk factors for thrombi formation** within **venous circulation**.
- **Calf venous thrombosis: Low risk** for **embolism**
- **MC form of thromboembolic disease**
- **Thrombosis of larger veins**: High risk for embolism (due to **loosely attached thrombus** to **venous wall**)

> - MC site for DVT: Calf veins[Q]
> - MC source for pulmonary emboli: Proximal vein of lower extremity[Q] (femoro-popliteal and iliac vein)

Risk Factors for Pulmonary Thromboembolism

• Age (Increasing age)[Q]	• Nephrotic syndrome[Q]
• Obesity[Q]	• Inflammatory bowel disease[Q]
• Immobility (bed rest >4 days)[Q]	• Polycythemia[Q]
• Pregnancy[Q] and Puerperium[Q]	• PNH[Q] or Lupus anticoagulant
• High dose estrogen therapy[Q]	• Behcet's syndrome[Q]
• Surgery/trauma (especially of pelvis, hip or lower limb)[Q]	• Homocystinuria[Q]
• Malignancy (especially pelvis, abdominal, metastatic)	• Paralysis of lower limb
• Heart failure/Recent MI[Q]	• Varicose veins, Infection

Clinical Features

- **Most** (60–80%) are **clinically silent** beause they are **small** and there is **dual circulation** in **lungs**.
- **Symptoms: Dyspnea (MC)**[Q], chest pain, hemoptysis and cough
- **Signs: Tachypnea (MC)**[Q], fever, unilateral leg swelling, wheeze, pleural friction rub
- More than **60% obstruction** occurs in **pulmonary circulation** leading to sudden death, COR pulmonale or cardiovascular collapse.
- Multiple emboli over time may cause pulmonary hypertension and right ventricular failure.
- Paradoxical embolus can pass through an inter-atrial or inter ventricular defect. There by entering the systemic circulation.

> - Any patient with **high likelihood** of pulmonary embolism on clinical evaluation **straightaway undergoes imaging tests**, while a patient with **low clinical likelihood** should **first undergo D-dimer test**.

Factors for Clinical Assessment of Pulmonary Embolism

• Clinical signs and symptoms of DVT[Q]	• Immobilization or previous surgery in 4 weeks[Q]
• An alternative diagnosis is less likely than pulmonary embolism	• Previous DVT/PE[Q]
• Heart rate > 100/min[Q]	• Malignancy[Q] (on treatment, treatment in past 6 months)
• Hemoptysis[Q]	

ECG Changes in Pulmonary Embolism
(Sinus tachycardia: MC and non-specific finding on ECG[Q])

Features of Acute Right Heart Strain	Highly predictive of PE

• Acute right axis deviation
• P pulmonale
• Right bundle branch block
• Inverted T waves
• ST segment change
	• $S_1Q_3T_3$[Q]: Seen in <12% patients
	  – S wave in lead I
	  – Q wave in lead III
	  – Inverted T wave in lead III
	  – S wave in lead I, II, and III ($S_1S_2S_3$)

Diagnosis

- **D-dimer: Excellent screening test** for the diagnosis of PE[Q].
- **Best investigation in clinical suspicion of PE: Multidetector CT**[Q]
- Lung scanning is now a 2nd line diagnostic test for PE.
- **Pulmonary angiography: Gold standard for diagnosis of PE**[Q] (but expensive and cumbersome)
- **Modified Well's criteria: Used for predicting PE**[Q]

FAT EMBOLISM SYNDROME

FAT EMBOLISM SYNDROME

Treatment

- Most pulmonary emboli can be treated by **anticoagulation & observation**[Q]
- In cases of **severe right heart strain & shortness of breath, fibrinolytic treatment**[Q] or **radiologically guided catheter embolectomy**[Q] should be performed.

Prophylaxis Against PE

- **IVC filter** in patients with **high risk** of embolism **when anticoagulants are contraindicated**[Q]

Pathophysiology

- Fat embolism is a common phenomenon, more commonly seen in **multiple fracture and in fractures involving lower limbs especially femur**[Q].
- Circulating **fat globules >10 micron**[Q] in diameter occur in most adults after **close fracture of long bones**[Q] and histological traces of fat can be found in the lungs and other internal organs.

Clinical Presentation

- Usually manifests itself **within 24-48 hours**[Q].
- Early **warning signs** (within 72 hours of injury): Slight rise in temperature (**pyrexia**) and pulse rate (**tachycardia**)[Q]

> - In more pronounced cases there is **breathlessness**, mild mental confusion or restlessness, **petechiae on chest, axillae, retina and conjunctival folds**[Q]; progressive to **marked respiratory distress** and coma in severe cases.

Diagnosis

- In addition to the classic clinical features, signs of **retinal artery emboli (Striate hemorrhage** and **exudates**[Q]) may be present.
- **Sputum and urine: Presence of fat globules**[Q].
- Chest X-ray: **Patchy pulmonary infiltration (Snow storm appearance)**[Q]

Laboratory Tests
No characteristic laboratory test, suggestive findings are:
• **Thrombocytopenia**[Q]   • (platelets <1.5 lacks)   • **Tachycardia**[Q]   • **Pyrexia**[Q] • PO_2 <60 mm Hg[Q]   • Fall in hemoglobin value[Q]

Management

- **Supportive pulmonary care, definitive fracture management** and **effective treatment of shock** are the **corner stones** of current fat embolism management.

Respiratory support	Treatment of shock	Fracture stabilization
• Ranges from **oxygen administration** to **full respiratory support** with mechanical ventilation • **Oxygen** is the **only therapeutic tool** of **proven use**[Q]	• Maintain adequate intravascular volume • **Aggressive fluid resuscitation** • **Appropriate CVP monitoring** to avoid fluid overload. • **Albumin** for **fluid resuscitation** along **with a balanced electrolyte solution** because it not only restores blood volume but also binds free fatty acids.	• **Maintain adequate intravascular volume** • Since **movement at** the **fracture site** has been shown to **increase** the **fat emboli** in circulation, **early immobilization of lower extremity fractures**[Q] is advocated

Additional Therapies	
• **Steroids**: Prophylactic corticosteroids benefit high risk patients • **Heparin**: Increase serum **lipase activity** and decrease number of circulating fat globules • **Hypertonic glucose**: Metabolically **decrease production** of **free fatty acids**	• **Dextran**[Q]: To **reduce red cell aggregation, expand plasma volume, decrease blood viscosity** and **reduce platelet adherence** • **Aprotinin**: Decrease platelet aggregation and serotonin release • **Alcohol**: Reduces serum lipase activity

TRACHEOBRONCHIAL FOREIGN BODY

Tracheobronchial Foreign Body

- **Aspiration of foreign bodies most commonly** occurs **in** the **toddler age**^{Q} group.
- **Peanuts** are the object **most frequently aspirated**^{Q}.
- **MC anatomic location** for a foreign body is the **right main stem bronchus** or the **right lower lobe**^{Q}.

Clinical Features
- The child usually will **cough** or **choke while eating** but **may then become asymptomatic**.
- **Total respiratory obstruction** may occur **with a tracheal foreign body**; however, respiratory distress is usually mild if present at all.
- **A unilateral wheeze** is often heard **on auscultation**^{Q}.

Diagnosis
- Chest X-ray: Radiopaque foreign body

> - **Bronchoscopy (rigid) confirms** the **diagnosis** and **allows removal of** the **foreign body**^{Q}.

Complications
- A **solid foreign body** often will cause **air trapping**, with **hyperlucency** of the affected lobe or lung seen especially on expiration.
- **Delay in diagnosis** can lead to **atelectasis** and **infection**^{Q}.

CHRONIC (FIBROSING) MEDIASTINITIS

Chronic (Fibrosing) mediastinitis

- The spectrum of chronic mediastinitis ranges from **granulomatous inflammation** of the **lymph nodes** in the mediastinum **to fibrosing mediastinitis**.
- **Most cases** are due to **TB** or **histoplasmosis**^{Q}, but sarcoidosis, silicosis, and other fungal diseases are at times causative.

Clinical Features
- Patients are **usually asymptomatic**.
- Those with fibrosing mediastinitis usually have **signs of compression of** some **mediastinal structure** such as the **SVC** or **large airways**, **phrenic** or **RLN** paralysis, or obstruction of the pulmonary artery or proximal pulmonary veins.

Treatment
- Other than **ATT for tuberculous mediastinitis**, no medical or surgical therapy has been demonstrated to be **effective for mediastinal fibrosis**^{Q}.

MASSIVE HEMOPTYSIS

Massive Hemoptysis

- Hemoptysis of >200-600 cc in 24 hours^Q
- Massive hemoptysis should be considered a **medical emergency**.

Diagnostic Evaluation
- For most patients, the **next step in evaluation of hemoptysis** should be a **standard chest radiograph**^{Q}.
- If a **source of bleeding** is **not identified** on plain film, a **CT of the chest**^{Q} should be obtained.

> - If all of these studies are unrevealing, **bronchoscopy should be considered.**
> - **Rigid bronchoscopy** with an 8.5 mm or larger bronchoscope is needed.

Treatment
- Large-volume, life-threatening hemoptysis generally requires **immediate intervention regardless of the cause**^{Q}.
- The first step is to establish a **patent airway** usually by endotracheal intubation and subsequent **mechanical ventilation**^{Q}.

> - As most **large-volume hemoptysis arises from an airway lesion**, it is ideal if the site of the bleeding can be identified either by **chest imaging or bronchoscopy (more commonly rigid than flexible)**^{Q}.

> - If the bleeding does not stop with therapies of the underlying cause and passage of time, **severe hemoptysis from bronchial arteries can be treated with angiographic embolization of the culprit bronchial artery**^{Q}.

PULMONARY HAMARTOMA

PULMONARY HAMARTOMA

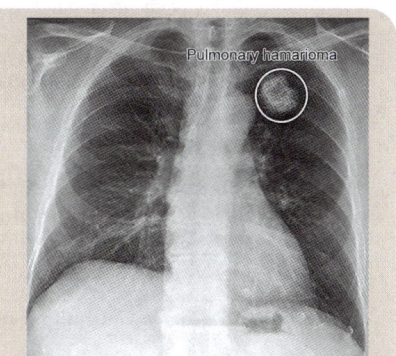

- MC benign tumor of lung: Hamartoma^Q
- Most commonly, **hamartomas** are manifested by **overgrowth of cartilage**^{Q}.

Clinical Features
- Typically seen in **40–60 years** of age, **more common** in males^Q.
- Usually **peripheral**, **grow slowly** in the lung^Q.

Diagnosis
- Chest X-ray: **Popcorn calcification** is diagnostic^Q.
- CT scan: **Coin lesion**^{Q}

Treatment
- Definitive treatment: Excision of lesion^Q

BRONCHIAL ADENOMA

BRONCHIAL ADENOMA

- **Centrally located slow-growing endobronchial lesions** that are **generally carcinoid tumors** (80%), **adenocystic tumors** (so called cylindromas, 10–15%), or **mucoepidermoid tumors** (2–3%).
- Mean age at presentation is **45 years** (range 15–60).

Clinical Features
- MC symptom: **Recurrent Hemoptysis**^{Q}
- History of **chronic cough, intermittent hemoptysis**^{Q}, or **repeated episodes of airway obstruction** with **atelectasis**, or **pneumonias with abscess formation** due to endobronchial lesions obstructing the airway.

Diagnosis
- Usually **visible at bronchoscopy** but are **highly vascular** and may **bleed profusely after a bronchoscopic biopsy**^{Q}.

Treatment
- They are **largely curable by surgical resection (local excision)**, but they **may recur locally** or **become invasive** and **metastasize**^{Q}.
- **Five-year survival after resection** is **95%** for localized disease.

BRONCHIAL CARCINOID

BRONCHIAL CARCINOID

- **Bronchial carcinoids (least malignant)** are the **most indolent** of the spectrum of pulmonary **neuroendocrine tumors**
- Most patients are **<40 years; Not related to smoking**^{Q}

> - Lower respiratory tract (Bronchus, lung, trachea) is the MC site of carcinoid tumor^Q
> - Carcinoid syndrome is uncommon^Q

Pathology
- **Most tumors are confined to main stem bronchus**, commonly **projects into** the **lumen**^{Q}
- Some tumors penetrate the bronchial wall to fan out in the peribronchial tissue producing the **collar-button lesion**^{Q}

Most bronchial carcinoids
• **Do not have secretary activity**^{Q}
• **Do not metastasize** to distant sites^Q
• Are **amenable to resection**^{Q}

MALIGNANT MESOTHELIOMA

MALIGNANT MESOTHELIOMA

- **Malignant mesothelioma is MC tumor of the pleura**^{Q}
- In **20%** of malignant mesotheliomas, the **tumor arises from peritoneum**^{Q}

- **Exposure to asbestos**[Q] is the **major known risk factor**
- More common in **males**[Q], most common **after 40 years** of age.

> - Three types: **Epithelial, sarcomatous**, and **biphasic**[Q]
> - **Epithelial types** are **associated with** a more **favorable prognosis**[Q]

Pathophysiology
- Physical characteristics of **specific fibers** (referred to as **serpentine** or **amphibole**) have been shown to be important.

> - **Serpentine fibers**: Large and curly, **not able to travel beyond larger airways**.
> - **Straight amphibole fibers**: In particular the **crocidolite**[Q] fibers navigate distally into the pulmonary parenchyma, **most clearly associated with mesotheliomas**.

- **Latency period** between asbestos exposure and the development of mesothelioma is **at least 20 years**.

> - **Multicentric tumor** with **multiple pleura-based nodules** coalescing to form sheets of tumor (but **not bilaterally symmetrical**[Q])

- Natural history of the disease in **untreated patients** culminates in **death** due to **local extension**.

Clinical Features
- Most patients present with **dyspnea** and **chest pain**[Q].
- Over 90% have a **pleural effusion**[Q].

Diagnosis
- Results of **thoracentesis** are **diagnostic in <10%** of patients.
- **Chest X-ray**: Pleural effusion, generalized **pleural thickening** and **shrunken hemithorax**[Q].
- **Thoracoscopy** or **open pleural biopsy** with **special staining** of tumor samples is **required to differentiate mesotheliomas from adenocarcinomas**[Q].
- **Butchart**[Q] staging is used for **mesothelioma**

Management
- **No effective therapy**[Q]
- **Treatment options**: Supportive care only, surgical resection, and multimodality approaches (using a combination of surgery, chemotherapy, and radiation therapy).

Differentiation of Mesothelioma from Adenocarcinoma		
	Mesothelioma	Adenocarcinoma
CEA	Negative	Positive[Q]
Cytokeratins (Low molecular weight)	Positive[Q]	Negative
Vimentin	Positive[Q]	Negative
Electron microscopic features	Long, sinuous villi	Short, straight villi with fuzzy glycocalyx

CARCINOMA LUNG (BRONCHOGENIC CARCINOMA)

Carcinoma Lung (Bronchogenic Carcinoma)

- MC type of **lung neoplasm**[Q]
- Arises from **respiratory epithelium** of bronchi, bronchioles and alveoli

> - **MC visceral malignancy** and leading cancer **causing death: CA lung**[Q]

- Mostly arise from lung hilum except bronchoalveolar carcinoma and some adenocarcinoma[Q].
- **Mucinous bronchoalveolar carcinoma** tends to **spread aerogenously** forming **satellite tumors**[Q].

Etiology and Risk factors	
• **Smoking**[Q] (both active and passive) • Air pollution (**Radon**[Q]) • Exposure to **asbestos, uranium** and **nickel**[Q]	• **Old infarct** and **lung scars** (most progress to **adenocarcinoma**[Q]) • Ionizing **radiation exposure**[Q]

Oncogenic abnormality	
Small Cell Carcinoma	Non-small Cell Carcinoma
• Over expression of **bcl-2, myc** and **telomerase**	• Over expression of **bcl-2** and **telomerase** with abnormal **ras gene**[Q] • **K-ras** mutation is **MC mutation** (90%) in **adenocarcinoma**[Q]

Clinical Features

- MC symptoms are cough^Q (MC) > dyspnea > chest pain > hemoptysis.
- Slightly **more common** on **right side**, more frequently occurs in **upper lobes**^{Q}
- **Major source** of **hemoptysis** are **bronchial arteries**^{Q}
- Endobronchial growth of central tumors cause cough, stridor, wheeze and dyspnoea
- **Peripheral tumors** present as **pain** due to pleural or chest wall involvement

Symptoms due to regional spread	
• Tracheal obstruction, esophageal compression, **RLN paralysis**^{Q} • **Pancoast syndrome**^{Q} (involvement of **C8T1 nerves** by pancoast tumor causing pain in **ipsilateral shoulder** and **arm**^{Q})	• Horner's syndrome • SVC syndrome (MC cause is **small cell carcinoma** >SCC)^Q • Malignant pleural effusion^Q

Metastases

- **MC Site of metastasis**: <u>B</u>rain^Q > <u>B</u>one^Q > <u>L</u>iver^Q > <u>A</u>drenal^Q > <u>L</u>ung^Q (**BBLAL**)
- CA lung is MC primary for metastasis to <u>K</u>idney, <u>E</u>sophagus, <u>P</u>ancreas, <u>A</u>drenal, <u>B</u>rain & <u>S</u>kin (**KEPABS**).

Paraneoplastic syndromes	

• **CVS**: Thrombophlebitis, non-bacterial thrombotic endocarditis
• **Metabolic**:
  – Inappropriate **ACTH** and **ADH** secretion (**small cell**)^Q
  – **Hypercalcemia** (**SCC**)^Q
• Acanthosis nigricans (adenocarcinoma), dermatomyositis, icthyosis, erythema gyretum repens
	• **GIT**: Carcinoid syndrome
	• Erythrocytosis
	• **Neuromuscular**:
	  – Dementia, optic neuritis, retinopathy, limbic encephalitis
	  – **Autonomic neuropathy (small cell)**^{Q}
	  – **Lambert-Eaton syndrome**^{Q} (small cell)
	  – Polymyositis, **cerebellar degeneration**^{Q}

Diagnosis and Staging

- **Tissue diagnosis**: Tumor tissue can be obtained by **bronchial** or **transbronchial biopsy**^{Q} through **fiberoptic bronchoscopy**^{Q}; by percutaneous biopsy of enlarge node
- **Integrated PET-CT** scan is the **best imaging modality**^{Q} for diagnosis and staging

8TH AJCC TNM CLASSIFICATION OF LUNG CANCER

8th AJCC (2017) TNM Classification of Lung Cancer
Tis: Carcinoma in situ
T1a: Tumor ≤1 cm in greatest dimension^Q
T1b: Tumor >1 cm but ≤2 cm in greatest dimension^Q
T1c: Tumor >2 cm but ≤3 cm in greatest dimension^Q
T2: Tumor >3 cm but ≤5cm or tumor with any of the following features: Involves **main bronchus**, regardless of **distance to the carina** but **without involvement of carina**^{Q} Invades **visceral pleura**^{Q} Associated with **atelectasis** or **obstructive pneumonitis** that extends to the hilar region either involving part of or the entire lung^Q **T2a**: Tumor >3 cm but ≤4 cm in greatest dimension^Q **T2b**: Tumor >4 cm but ≤5 cm in greatest dimension^Q
T3: Tumor >5 cm but ≤7 cm in greatest dimension or one that **directly invades any of the following**: parietal pleura, chest wall (including superior sulcus tumors), **phrenic nerve, parietal pericardium**; or separate tumor nodule(s) in the same lobe as the primary^Q
T4: Tumor >7 cm or of any size that invades any of the following: **diaphragm, mediastinum, heart, great vessels, trachea, recurrent laryngeal nerve, esophagus, vertebral body, carina**; or Separate tumor nodule(s) in a **different ipsilateral lobe** to that of primary^Q

N1: Metastasis in **ipsilateral peribronchial** and/or **ipsilateral hilar lymph nodes** and **intrapulmonary nodes**, including involvement by direct extension^Q
N2: Metastasis in **ipsilateral mediastinal** and/or **subcarinal lymph node(s)**^{Q}
N3: Metastasis in **contralateral mediastinal, contralateral hilar, ipsilateral or contralateral scalene**, or **supraclavicular lymph node(s)**^{Q}

M1a: Separate tumor nodule(s) in a **contralateral lobe**; tumor with **pleural or pericardial nodules** or malignant pleural (or pericardial) effusion^Q
M1b: Single extra-thoracic metastasis in a single or multiple organs^Q
M1c: Multiple extra-thoracic metastasis in single or multiple organs^Q

8th AJCC (2017) TNM Stage Groupings			
Stage	T	N	M
Occult cancer	TX	N0	M0
0	Tis	N0	M0
IA	T1	N0	M0
IA1	T1mi-T1a	N0	M0
IA2	T1b	N0	M0
IA3	T1c	N0	M0
IB	T2a	N0	M0
IIA	T2b	N0	M0
IIB	T1a-c, T2a-b	N1	M0
	T3	N0	M0
IIIA	T1a-c, T2a-b	N2	M0
	T3	N1	M0
	T4	N0-1	M0
IIIB	T1a-c, T2a-b	N3	M0
	T3, T4	N2	M0
IIIC	T3, T4	N3	M0
IVA	Any T	Any N	M1a/b
IVB	Any T	Any N	M1c

Treatment of Operable NSCCL
- Stage IA, IB, IIA, IIB: Surgical resection^Q
- **Adjuvant chemotherapy** is given in **stage II**^Q
- Stage IIIA with **minimal N2 involvement**: **Neoadjuvant chemotherapy** followed by **surgical resection** with **complete mediastinal LN dissection**^Q
- **Postoperative radiotherapy** for patients found to have **N2 disease**^Q

WHO Classification of Carcinoma Lung

Adenocarcinoma
- **MC** histological **type**^Q
- MC in **non-smokers**, **young** patients, **females**^Q
- Located **peripherally**^Q
- **Slow growth** and propensity to **metastasize** to **opposite lung**^Q
- **Metastasize** more frequently to **CNS**^Q
- Most cells contain **mucin**^Q
- **Noguchi classification**^Q is used for adenocarcinoma

Squamous Cell Carcinoma
- **MC** in **smokers**^Q
- MC type in **India**
- MC variety associated with **hypercalcemia** (produces **PTH-rp**)^Q
- **Central**^Q in distribution
- Prone to undergo **central necrosis** & **cavitation**^Q
- **Pancoast** tumor is histologically **SCC**^Q
- Associated with **best prognosis**^Q

Small Cell Carcinoma
- **Most malignant**, **central**^Q in distribution, strongly related to **smoking**^Q
- Cells are small with little cytoplasm called "**oat cell**"^Q
- Associated with **massive hilar** or **mediastinal lymphadenopathy**, **mediastinal invasion** and **perihilar mass**^Q
- **MC variety** associated with **paraneoplastic syndrome**, **hypokalemia** and **SVC syndrome**^Q
- Most responsive to **chemotherapy** (cisplatin + etoposide)
- Shows response to **radiotherapy**^Q
- Hormones produced by small cell carcinoma: **ACTH**, **AVP** (vasopressin), **calcitonin**, **ANF**, gastrin releasing peptide^Q

Large Cell Carcinoma
- Highly **undifferentiated** with **cavitating** nature
- **Metastasize early** with poor prognosis

BRONCHIOLOALVEOLAR CARCINOMA (BAC)

BRONCHIOLOALVEOLAR CARCINOMA (BAC)

- BAC occurs in the **pulmonary parenchyma** in the **terminal bronchioloalveolar regions**[Q].

Histologically

- Characterized by a **pure bronchioloalveolar growth pattern** with **no evidence of stromal, vascular, or pleural invasion**[Q].
- Key feature: **Growth along preexisting structures**[Q] without destruction of alveolar architecture. This growth pattern has been termed "**lepidic**", and allusion to the neoplastic cells resembling butterflies sitting on a fence.

Two subtypes

- **Nonmucinous**: Columnar, **peg-shaped**, or cuboidal cells
- **Mucinous**: Distinctive, **tall, columnar cells** with cytoplasmic and **intra-alveolar mucin**, growing along the alveolar septa.

Ultrastructurally

- BAC are a heterogeneous group, consisting of **mucin-screting bronchiolar cells**[Q], **Clara cells**[Q], or, rarely, **type II pneumocytes**[Q]

PANCOAST TUMOR (SUPERIOR SULCUS TUMOR)

PANCOAST TUMOR (SUPERIOR SULCUS TUMOR)

- Pancoast's (or superior sulcus tumor) syndrome results **from local extension of** a tumor growing in the **apex of** the lung with **involvement of eighth cervical and 1st and 2nd thoracic nerves**, with **shoulder pain characteristically radiates in** the **ulnar distribution of** the **arm**, often with **radiologic destruction of 1st and 2nd ribs**[Q].
- Often **Horner's syndrome** and Pancoast's syndrome co-exist
- IOC for diagnosis: **MRI**[Q]

Treatment

- **Preoperative RT** followed by **En bloc resection** of lung and **chest wall** with consideration of **postoperative RT** or **intra-operative brachytherapy**[Q].

MYXOMA

MYXOMA

- **MC type** of **primary cardiac tumor** in all age groups: **Myxoma**[Q]
- Occur at all ages, **most commonly in 3rd to 6th decades**, with a **female predilection**.
- Approximately **90%** are **sporadic**
- Remainder are **familial** with **autosomal dominant transmission** (NAME and LAMB syndrome)

Pathology

- Myxomas are **gelatinous structures**, consist of **myxoma cells** embedded in a stroma **rich in glycosaminoglycans**.

  - Most are **solitary,** are located in the atria (**particularly the left atrium**, where they usually arise **from the interatrial septum** in the vicinity of the fossa ovalis), and are **often pedunculated** on a fibrovascular stalk.

- In contrast to sporadic tumors, **familial or syndromic tumors** tend to **occur in younger individuals**, are often **multiple,** may be **ventricular** in location, and are **more likely to recur** after initial resection.

Clinical Features

- **MC clinical presentation** mimics that of **mitral valve disease**: either **stenosis** owing to tumor prolapse into the mitral orifice or **regurgitation** resulting from tumor-induced valvular trauma.
- A characteristic **low-pitched sound**, a "**tumor plop,**" may be appreciated on auscultation during early or mid-diastole
- **Constitutional signs** and **symptoms**: Fever, weight loss, cachexia, malaise

Diagnosis

- IOC for diagnosis: **2D transthoracic or transesophageal echocardiography**[Q]
- **CT and MRI**: Information regarding **size, shape, composition** and **surface characteristics**
- Cardiac catheterization and angiography are **no longer considered mandatory**

Treatment
- **Surgical excision** utilizing cardiopulmonary bypass is **curative**[Q].
- **Recur** in **12–22%** of **familial cases** but in only 1–2% of sporadic cases.
    - **Tumor recurrence** most likely is **due to multifocal lesions** in the **former** and **inadequate resection in the latter**[Q].

CARDIAC TUMORS

Cardiac Tumors

- MC primary cardiac tumor: Myxoma[Q]
- MC malignant tumor of heart in adults: Angiosarcoma[Q]
- MC benign tumor of heart in children: Rhabdomyoma[Q]
- MC malignant tumor of heart in children: Rhabdomyosarcoma[Q]
- MC tumor of cardiac valves: Papillary fibroelastoma[Q]
- MC site of involvement in cardiac metastasis: Pericardium[Q]

CHEST WALL TUMORS

Chest Wall Tumors

- MC chest wall tumor: Metastasis[Q]
- MC benign primary chest wall neoplasm: Osteochondroma[Q]
- MC malignant primary chest wall neoplasm: Chondrosarcoma[Q]

Multiple Choice Questions

MEDIASTINAL TUMORS

1. **Middle mediastinal masses include all the following except:** *(COMEDK 2004)*
   a. Bronchogenic cyst
   b. Ascending aortic aneurysm
   c. Pericardial cyst
   d. Ganglioneuroma

2. **Which of the following is not an anterior mediastinal mass?** *(Recent Question 2018)*
   a. Thymoma
   b. Neurogenic tumor
   c. Thyroid mass
   d. Lymphoma

3. **Common location of thoracic pheochromocytoma:** *(Recent Question 2017)*
   a. Anterior mediastinum
   b. Posterior mediastinum
   c. Middle mediastinum
   d. Superior mediastinum

4. **Middle mediastinal masses include all the following except:** *(COMEDK 2005)*
   a. Bronchogenic cyst
   b. Lymphoma
   c. Pericardial cyst
   d. Ganglioneuroma

5. **Following are the tumors of posterior mediastinum except:** *(COMEDK 2006)*
   a. Neuroblastoma
   b. Ganglioneuroma
   c. Paravertebral abscess
   d. Thymic tumor

6. **The commonest anterior mediastinal tumors is:** *(MCI June 2018, Recent Question 2017, WBPG 2015, Recent Question 2015, COMEDK 2008)*
   a. Aneurysm of descending aorta
   b. Neurogenic tumour
   c. Thymoma
   d. Bronchogenic cyst

7. **During exploration, a patient is found to have a tumor in the thymus that is invading the pericardium and surrounding the left and right phrenic nerves. The pathologist says that appears on frozen section to be a benign thymoma. The surgeon now should:** *(Recent Question 2018)*
   a. Repeat frozen section
   b. Attempt as complete a resection as possible
   c. Close the chest and plan irradiation therapy
   d. Close the chest and await permanent sections

8. **Common tumor of posterior mediastinum are:** *(PGI Nov 2009)*
   a. Lymphoma
   b. Neuroblastoma
   c. Neurogenic tumors
   d. Thymoma
   e. Bronchogenic cyst

9. **D/D of anterior mediastinal mass includes** *(PGI May 2011)*
   a. Teratoma
   b. Thymoma
   c. Lymphoma
   d. Neurogenic tumor
   e. Parathyroid carcinoma

10. **Lymphoma most commonly affects which compartment of the mediastinum?** *(MHPGMCET 2006)*
    a. Anterior
    b. Middle
    c. Posterior
    d. Inferior

11. **The most common mediastinal tumor:** *(MHCET 2016, MHSSMCET 2008)*
    a. Thymoma
    b. Lymphoma
    c. Neurofibroma
    d. Bronchogenic cyst

12. **In thymoma, all are seen except:** *(AIIMS June 2001)*
    a. Hypogammaglobulinemia
    b. Hyperalbuminemia
    c. Red cell aplasia
    d. Myasthenia gravis

13. **Not a posterior mediastinal tumor:** *(AIIMS Nov 98)*
    a. Neurofibroma
    b. Lymphoma
    c. Thymoma
    d. Gastroenteric cyst

14. **Posterior mediastinal tumors:** *(PGI June 2003)*
    a. Neuroblastoma
    b. Bronchogenic cyst
    c. Neuroenteric cyst
    d. Lymphoma
    e. Anterior thoracic meningioma

15. **Majority of lung cysts occur in:** *(AIIMS Nov 94)*
    a. Mediastinum
    b. Near carina
    c. Base of the lung
    d. Peribronchial tissue

16. **Which tumor among the following is not found in anterior mediastinum?** *(AIIMS Nov 95)*
    a. Retrosternal goitre
    b. Thymoma
    c. Teratomatous mass
    d. Neurogenic tumour

17. **Most common tumor in the posterior mediastinum is:** *(Recent Question 2016, DNB 2005, 2000, All India 2008, DPG 2008)*
    a. Neurofibroma
    b. Teratoma
    c. Lymphoma
    d. Bronchogenic cyst

18. **Thymectomy causes:** *(TN 98)*
    a. Failure of rejection of transplanted organs
    b. Myasthenia gravis
    c. Autoimmune disorders
    d. None of the above

19. **The most common primary tumor of mediastinum:**
    a. Lymphoma
    b. Teratoma
    c. Neurogenic tumor
    d. Thymoma

20. **Tumors of anterior mediastinum include the following except:** *(Kerala PG 2015, UPSC 2007)*
    a. Thymoma
    b. Lymphoma
    c. Germ cell tumour
    d. Schwannoma

21. **Which of the following is commonly present in middle mediastinum?** *(PGI November 2017)*
    a. Schwannoma
    b. Thymoma
    c. Bronchogenic cyst
    d. Teratoma
    e. Substernal thyroid

PLEURAL EFFUSION

22. **Most common site for putting chest drain in case of pleural effusion:** *(Bihar PG 2014, AIIMS June 2000, All India 2002)*
    a. 2nd intercostal space mid-clavicular line
    b. 7th intercostal space mid-axillary line
    c. 5th intercostal space mid clavicular line
    d. 5th intercostal space just lateral to vertebral column

23. **Meig's syndrome consist of the following except:** *(Karnataka 94)*
    a. Ascites
    b. Hydrothorax
    c. Benign ovarian tumor
    d. Malignant ovarian tumor

24. **Pseudochylous pleural effusion is most often seen in:**
    a. Tb
    b. Lymphoma
    c. CA lung
    d. Filariasis

25. A rapidly filling hemorrhagic pleural effusion is suggestive of: (COMEDK 2004)
    a. Pneumococcal infection
    b. Tuberculosis
    c. Bronchiectasis
    d. Bronchogenic carcinoma

PNEUMOTHORAX

26. Spontaneous pneumothorax is commonly seen in: (PGI June 2002)
    a. Smokers
    b. Young females
    c. Old age
    d. Short statured men

27. Which of the following is a cause of unilateral hyperluscent lung on chest radiography? (COMEDK 2009)
    a. Poland syndrome
    b. Asthma
    c. Acute bronchiolitis
    d. Pleural effusion

28. Pneumothorax of what size generally needs operative treatment? (MHSSMCET 2010)
    a. >10%
    b. >20%
    c. >30%
    d. >40

29. In a patient with one episode of spontaneous pneumothorax, which is advised? (Jharkhand 2003)
    a. Stop diving
    b. Stop smoking
    c. Stop flying
    d. All

30. For open pneumothorax, which of the following is treatment of choice? (AIIMS June 97)
    a. IPPV
    b. ICD with underwater seal
    c. Thoracostomy and close the rent
    d. Wait and watch

31. A case of spontaneous pneumothorax comes to you. What will be earliest treatment of choice? (AIIMS June 97)
    a. IPPV
    b. Needle aspiration
    c. ICD
    d. Wait and watch

32. Spontaneous pneumothorax exceeding ..... % of chest cavity should have a chest tube inserted:
    a. 10
    b. 25
    c. 45
    d. 60

33. In pneumothorax due to blunt injury, treatment of choice is: (AIIMS 92)
    a. Observation
    b. Pneumonectomy
    c. Thoracotomy
    d. Intercostal drainage

34. A patient presents with sudden onset of breath lessness after subclavian vein cannulation. On examination, breath sounds are absent while the chest is hyper-resonant on percussion on one side. Most likely cause is: (All India 2012)
    a. Iatrogenic pnumothorax
    b. Subclavian vein air embolus
    c. Malposition of cannula
    d. Cardiac arrhythmia

35. While inserting a central venous catheter, a patient develops respiratory distress. The most likely cause is: (Bihar PG 2014, All India 2002)
    a. Hemothorax
    b. Pneumothorax
    c. Pleural effusion
    d. Hypovolemia

36. All of the following are characteristic features of primary spontaneous pneumothorax except: (AIIMS 92)
    a. Male gender
    b. Old age
    c. Tall stature
    d. History smoking

37. Spontaneous pneumothorax is commonly seen in: (PGI June 2002)
    a. Smokers
    b. Young females
    c. Old age
    d. Short statured men

38. Which of the following statements about pneumothorax is true? (AIIMS Dec 94)
    a. Breath sounds are increased
    b. Percussion note is decreased
    c. Always needs chest tube insertion
    d. Often needs chest tube insertion

39. In left sided massive pneumothorax, ECG shows all except: (AIIMS 94)
    a. Left axis deviation
    b. Absent R wave
    c. Peaked P wave
    d. Precordial T wave inversion

40. Intrapleural pressure greater than atmospheric pressure is diagnostic of: (MHPGMCET 2001)
    a. Valvular pneumothorax
    b. Closed pneumothorax
    c. Open pneumothorax
    d. All

41. How will you check the functioning of the ICD tube? (AIIMS November 2017)
    a. By observing for continuous air bubbles coming out of the underwater drain
    b. By observing the movement of air water column in the tube during respiration
    c. By taking X-ray chest repeatedly
    d. By auscultation

TENSION PNEUMOTHORAX

42. A 30-year-old female comes acute breathlessness, neck vein distention, and absent breath sounds and mediastinal shift. Which of the following should be done immediately?
    a. HRCT is the investigation of choice (PGI June 2008)
    b. ABG analysis should be done
    c. CXR
    d. Large bore needle puncture of pleura

43. Tension pneumothorax due to fracture rib is treated by:
    a. Strapping (DPG 2011, PGI 96)
    b. Tube drainage
    c. IPPV
    d. Internal fixation with open reduction

44. Treatment of choice for tension pneumothorax is:
    a. Immediate IC tube drainage (SGPGI 2005)
    b. Continuous aspiration by needle
    c. Intermittent aspiration by needle
    d. Thoracotomy with repair of leakage

45. True regarding management of traumatic pneumothorax is:
    a. Immediate ICD tube insertion (SGPGI 2005)
    b. CT-scan should be done to confirm pulmonary leak
    c. Intermittent needle aspiration
    d. Sealed

46. A patient after road traffic accident presented with tension pneumothorax. What is the first line of management?
    a. Insert wide bore needle in 2nd intercostal space
    b. Immediate chest X-ray (AIIMS Nov 2013)
    c. CT scan
    d. Emergency thoracotomy

47. Condition which builds within hemithorax resulting in collapsed lung, flattened diaphragm, contralateral mediastinal shift and compromised venous return to right side of heart is known as: (MCI Sept 2007)
    a. Open pneumothorax
    b. Flail chest
    c. Massive pulmonary hemorrhage
    d. Tension pneumothorax

48. **Lung injury with bad prognosis is:**
    (DNB 2009)
    a. Open pneumothorax   b. Closed pneumothorax
    c. Tension pneumothorax   d. All have same prognosis

49. **What is the 1st thing to be done to a patient with tension pneumothorax?** *(UPPG 96)*
    a. Insertion of wide bore needle in the inter costal space
    b. Water seal drainage
    c. Leave the patient at rest for air to be absorbed
    d. None

50. **Tensions pneumothorax results in:** *(ICS 98)*
    a. Alkalosis   b. Increased cardiac output
    c. Decreased venous return   d. All of the above

51. **What is the emergent management of tension pneumothorax?** *(AIIMS November 2014)*
    a. Chest X-ray
    b. Emergency room thoracotomy in unstable patients
    c. Insert needle in 2nd intercostal space
    d. Tube thoracostomy in 5th intercostal space

52. **A person met with road traffic accident and came to casualty with contusion on anterior chest wall with Pulse rate-90/minute, BP-120/80 mm Hg, respiratory rate-16/minute. Normal heart sounds are heard but breath sounds were decreased on the left side and trachea was deviated towards right. Which of the following is the first line management?** *(AIIMS May 2017)*
    a. Needle thoracostomy
    b. Pericardiocentesis
    c. Chest tube insertion and drainage
    d. Immediate exploratory thoracotomy

53. **This patient came with acute dyspnea. Which of the following statements is TRUE?** *(APPG 2016)*
    a. It is due to old tuberculosis and fibrosis of left lung
    b. X-ray shows Westermark's sign on right side
    c. A needle should be inserted into the chest wall in the second right intercostal space as an emergency
    d. He needs emergency bronchoscopy to remove possible FB in left side

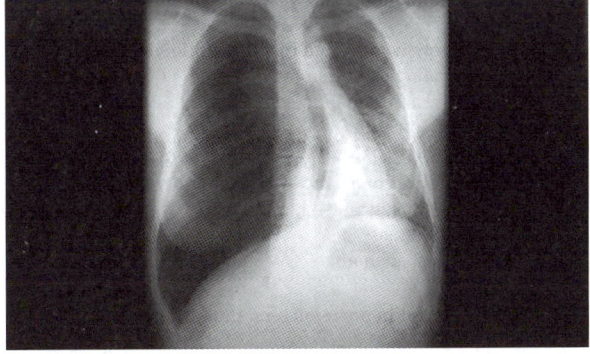

HEMOTHORAX

54. **Decision regarding surgery in a case of hemothorax due to blunt trauma chest should be based on:** *(All India 2008)*
    a. Chest symptoms   b. Hemodynamic status
    c. Nature of chest tube output   d. X-ray finding

55. **The ideal treatment for hemothorax of blood loss greater than 500 ml/hour:** *(PGI June 99)*
    a. Wait and watch
    b. Needle aspiration
    c. Intercostal tube
    d. Open thoracotomy with ligation of vessel

56. **About hemothorax:** *(PGI Dec 2002)*
    a. Seen in choriocarcinoma
    b. Supine posture is better than erect posture
    c. Needle aspiration may be needed for diagnosis
    d. Thoracotomy is always done

57. **Excessive bleeding during hemothorax is caused usually by:** *(AIIMS June 94)*
    a. Vena cava   b. Internal mammary artery
    c. Heart   d. Major artery

58. **Which of the following vessel is injured in hemothorax patient?** *Recent Question 2017)*
    a. Pulmonary artery   b. Pulmonary vein
    c. Bronchial artery   d. Intercostal arteries

LUNG ABSCESS

59. **A 80-year-old male presented with lung abscess in left upper zone. Best treatment modality is:** *(UPPG 2008)*
    a. Antibiotics according to organisms
    b. Surgical drainage
    c. Tube thoracostomy
    d. Wait and Watch

60. **Management of a lung abscess refractory to prolonged antibiotic treatment includes all of the following except:**
    a. Lobectomy   *(COMEDK 2004)*
    b. Open drainage
    c. Tube drainage
    d. Intracavitary antibiotic instillation

61. **Complication of empyema are all except:** *(PGI Dec 99)*
    a. Empyema necessitans
    b. Bronchopleural fistula
    c. Osteomyelitis
    d. Pneumonia

62. **Commonest cause of lung abscess:** *(AIIMS Nov 96)*
    a. Aspiration
    b. Hematogenous spread from distant site
    c. Direct contact
    d. Lymphatic spread

63. **Least common site of lung abscess is:** *(PGI June 99)*
    a. Left upper lobe   b. Left lower lobe
    c. Right upper lobe   d. Right lower lobe

64. **Most common cause of amoebic lung abscess is:** *(AIIMS Nov 94)*
    a. Direct extension from liver   b. Hematogenous spread
    c. Lymphatic spread   d. By inhalation

65. **Failure of adequate drainage in an empyema with a bronchopleural fistula is indicated by:**
    a. Drainage less than 100 cc per day
    b. Hemorrhagic drainage less than 100 cc per day
    c. The development of haemoptysis
    d. Continued productive cough with purulent material
    e. All of the above

66. **Most common cause of cold abscess of chest wall is:** *(TN 95)*
    a. Pott's spine   b. TB abscesses of chest wall
    c. TB of ribs   d. Intercostal lymphadenitis

Surgery Essence

67. **Empyema necessitans is defined as so when:** *(UPSC 2002)*
    a. Plural empyema is under pressure
    b. Pleural empyema has ruptured into bronchus
    c. Pleural empyema has ruptured into the pericardium
    d. Pleural empyema is showing extension to the subcutaneous tissue

68. **Empyema can be caused by the following parasites except:** *(MHSSMCET 2008)*
    a. E. granulosus
    b. Entamoeba coli
    c. Paragonimus westermani
    d. Strongyloides stercoralis

PLEURAL COLLECTIONS

69. **True about chylothorax:** *(DPG 2007)*
    a. Left side more common
    b. Clear fluid
    c. Immediate thoracotomy should be done
    d. TOC is excision and ligation of thoracic duct

70. **Chyluria is caused by all except:** *(MCI Sept 2009)*
    a. Pregnancy
    b. Childbirth
    c. Filariasis
    d. Bile duct stones

SEQUESTRATION OF LUNGS

71. **Intralobar sequestration of lungs takes its blood supply from:** *(Recent Question 2014, AIIMS Nov 94)*
    a. Internal mammary artery
    b. Descending abdominal aorta
    c. Pulmonary artery
    d. None of the above

72. **Lung sequestration occurs most commonly seen in which lobe?** *(AIIMS June 93)*
    a. Apical
    b. Left posterior basal
    c. Left porterosuperior
    d. Right lateral basal

73. **All of the following statements regarding bronchial cysts are true except:** *(MAHE 2005)*
    a. Seen in mediastinum
    b. 50-70% occur in lung
    c. Are commonly infected
    d. Multilocular

74. **True about bronchogenic cyst:** *(Punjab 2007)*
    a. Most of them are located at base of lung
    b. They arise from anomalous development of foregut
    c. They usually communicate with lung
    d. They are lined by pseudostratified epithelium

75. **Intralobar sequestration of lung is commonest in the:**
    a. Apical segment of upper lobe *(Recent Question 2016)*
    b. Medial segment of middle lobe
    c. Lateral basal segment of lower lobe
    d. Posterior basal segment of lower lobe

76. **Extralobar bronchogenic cysts may communicate with the following *except*:**
    a. Esophagus
    b. Stomach
    c. Bronchus
    d. None of the above

77. **Sequestrated lung is supplied most commonly by:** *(Kerala 98)*
    a. Bronchial arteries
    b. Descending aorta
    c. Subclavian artery
    d. Intercostal arteries

78. **Diagnosis of lung sequestration by:** *(JIPMER 2000)*
    a. CT
    b. Angiography
    c. MRI
    d. X-ray

TRACHEOBRONCHIAL FOREIGN BODY

79. **In erect posture, commonest site of foreign body in bronchus:** *(AIIMS June 99)*
    a. Right posterior basal
    b. Right anterior basal
    c. Lateral basal
    d. Medial basal

80. **Foreign body aspiration in supine position causes which of the following parts of the lung commonly to be affected?**
    a. Apical left lobe *(Recent Question 2014, AIIMS June 2002)*
    b. Apical lobe of right lung
    c. Apical part of the lower lobe
    d. Posterobasal segment of left lung

81. **A foreign body completely obstructing the right main bronchus causes:** *(PGI June 99)*
    a. Decreased ventilation perfusion ratio
    b. Increased ventilation in left lung
    c. Perfusion doubles in right lung
    d. Increased VP ratio in right lung

VATS

82. **In Video assisted thoracoscooic surgery for better vision, the space in the operative field is created by:** *(AIIMS June 2002)*
    a. Self retaining retractor
    b. CO_2 insufflations
    c. Collapse of ipsilateral lung
    d. Rib spacing

83. **VATS refers to:** *(Orissa 2011)*
    a. Vacuum assisted thoracic surgery
    b. Video assisted thoracoscopic surgery
    c. Video assisted transplant surgery
    d. None of the above

THORACOTOMY

84. **The following are indications for performing thoracotomy after blunt injury of the chest, *except*:** *(UPSC 2008)*
    a. 1000 ml drainage after placing an intercoastal tube
    b. Continuous bleeding through intercoastal tube of more than 200 ml/hour for three or more hours
    c. Cardiac tamponade
    d. Rib fracture

85. **Thoracotomy is indicated in all the following *except*:**
    a. Penetrating chest injuries *(MHPGMCET 2003)*
    b. Rapidly accumulating hemothorax
    c. Massive air leak
    d. Pulmonary contusion

86. **Surgical indication in the treatment of hemoptysis:**
    a. Profuse uncontrolled bleeding *(PGI Dec 2006)*
    b. Bronchiectasis
    c. Bronchial adenoma
    d. Bronchial fistula

87. **Muscle not cut in posterolateral thoracotomy is:** *(PGI Dec 98)*
    a. Serratus anterior
    b. Latissimus dorsi
    c. Rhomboides major
    d. Pectoralis major

88. **Which is not an indication of thoracotomy?** *(AIIMS Nov 98)*
    a. Massive pneumothorax
    b. Pulmonary contusion
    c. Bleeding more than 200 ml/hour in thoracotomy tube
    d. Esophageal rupture

89. During emergency thoracotomy, the incision is made > 1 cm lateral to sternal margin to preserve: *(All India 2012)*
    a. Intercoastal artery
    b. Superior epigastric artery
    c. Internal mammary artery
    d. Intercostal vein

90. Emergency thoracotomy is indicated following chest trauma in the following conditions *except*: *(APPG 2016)*
    a. Scapular and sternal fractures
    b. Esophageal perforation
    c. Penetrating injury with cardiac tamponade
    d. Massive hemothorax

BENIGN LUNG TUMORS

91. The most common benign tumor of the lung is: *(COMEDK 2008)*
    a. Hamartoma
    b. Alveolar adenoma
    c. Teratoma
    d. Fibroma

92. Image of CT chest is given below. Which of the following statement is incorrect about this condition? *(Recent Question 2016)*
    a. Most common benign tumor of lung
    b. More common in females
    c. Usually peripheral
    d. Grow slowly

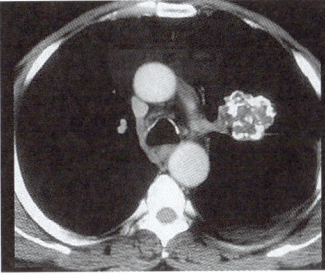
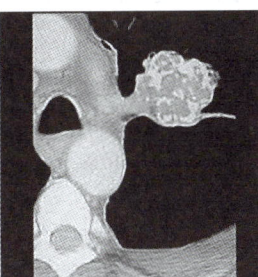

93. Most common symptom of bronchial adenoma is:
    a. Chest pain
    b. Cough *(All India 96)*
    c. Recurrent hemoptysis
    d. Weight loss

94. True about bronchial adenoma: *(All India 98)*
    a. 10-15% of all lung tumour
    b. Mostly malignant
    c. Recurrent hemoptysis
    d. Peripherally located

95. The following is true about bronchial carcinoids:
    a. Highly radiosensitive *(JIPMER 2011)*
    b. Metastasis common
    c. Carcinoid syndrome does not manifest
    d. Commonly arises from terminal bronchioles

96. Blood stained sputum may be the only symptom in: *(Kerala 90)*
    a. Bronchiectasis
    b. Carcinoma bronchus
    c. Adenoma bronchus
    d. Pulmonary T.b.

MESOTHELIOMA

97. All are true regarding mesothelioma except: *(AIIMS May 2011)*
    a. Bilaterally symmetrical
    b. Associated with asbestos exposure
    c. Histopathology shows biphasic pattern
    d. Occurs in late middle age

98. Pleural mesothelioma is associated with: *(PGI Dec 2005)*
    a. Asbestosis
    b. Berylliosis
    c. Silicosis
    d. Baggasosis

99. In a patient of mesothelioma, one often finds:
    a. Hypoglycemia
    b. An association with asbestosis
    c. Hemorrhagic pleural effusion
    d. Clubbing of fingers
    e. All of the above

100. Which of the following is true about Mesothelioma?
    a. Pleural effusion is exudative *(Recent Question 2017, 2016)*
    b. Butchart staging is used
    c. Manganese exposure is a predisposing factor
    d. Cough and dyspnoea are common late features

SQUAMOUS CELL CARCINOMA

101. Cavity formation in bronchogenic carcinoma occurs in: *(Recent Question 2016)*
    a. Oat cell carcinoma
    b. Squamous cell carcinoma
    c. Adenocarcinoma
    d. Bronchoalveolar

ADENOCARCINOMA

102. True statement about adenocarcinoma lung are:
    a. Common in females *(PGI June 2005)*
    b. Not associated with smoking
    c. Central cavitation is a characteristic feature
    d. Peripheral involvement is common
    e. Upper lobe involvement is common

103. A patient presented with 1cm coin lesion over right upper lobe of lung on X-ray not suggestive of metastasis. FNAC revealed adenocarcinoma, no lymphadenopathy. Treatment is:
    a. Surgery *(JIPMER 2010)*
    b. Surgery + chemotherapy
    c. Surgery + Radiotherapy
    d. Surgery + chemoradio therapy

104. What is true regarding adenocarcinoma lung? *(AIIMS Dec 94)*
    a. Causes 50% of lung cancers
    b. Unlikely histological variant in young patients
    c. Associated with subcutaneous angiomyolipoma
    d. Peripheral location

105. Commonest type of lung carcinoma in nonsmokers is: *(Kerala PG 2015, AIIMS Dec 94)*
    a. Squamous cell carcinoma
    b. Adenocarcinoma
    c. Alveolar cell carcinoma
    d. Small cell carcinoma

106. Lung to lung metastasis is seen in:
    a. Adenocarcinoma of lung
    b. Squamous cell carcinoma
    c. Small cell carcinoma
    d. Neuroendocrine tumor of lung

SMALL CELL CARCINOMA

107. Which of the following statements about small cell carcinoma is true? *(All India 2009)*
    a. Bone metastasis is uncommon
    b. Peripheral in location
    c. Chemosensitive tumor
    d. Paraneoplastic syndrome with PTH is common

108. Poorest prognosis in lung cancer is associated with: *(COMEDK 2005)*
    a. Small cell carcinoma
    b. Adenocarcinoma
    c. Squamous cell carcinoma
    d. Adenosquamous cancer

109. Marker of small cell cancer of lung is: (DNB 2011)
    a. Synaptobrevin   b. Chromogranin
    c. Cytokeratin   d. Vimentin
110. All are elaborated by small cell carcinoma lung, except:
    a. ADH   b. ACTH   (PGI June 2000)
    c. 5-HT   d. Noradrenaline
111. The lung tumour responding best to radiotherapy: (UPPG 96)
    a. Small cell anaplastic   b. Squamous cell carcinoma
    c. Adenocarcinoma   d. All respond equally well
112. In small cell carcinoma of the lung, one of the following is not seen: (Kerala 97)
    a. Hypercalcemia   b. Hyponatremia
    c. Watery diarrhea   d. Hypokalemia
113. All of the following statements about small cell carcinomas are true, except: (PGI June 2006)
    a. Commonest malignancy of lung
    b. Associated with paraneoplastic syndrome
    c. Cause SVC obstruction
    d. Chemosensitive
    e. Commonly metastasizes to brain
114. Which of the following statements about small cell carcinoma is true? (All India 2009)
    a. Bone metastasis is uncommon
    b. Peripheral in location
    c. Chemosensitive tumor
    d. Paraneoplastic syndrome with increase PTH is common
115. In a chronic smoker, a highly malignant aggressive and metastatic lung carcinoma is: (AIIMS May 2001)
    a. Squamous cell carcinoma
    b. Small cell carcinoma
    c. Adenocarcinoma   d. Large cell carcinoma
116. Following hormonal levels are increased in small cell carcinoma of lung except: (All India 97)
    a. ACTH   b. Growth hormone
    c. ANF   d. AVP
117. Carcinoma lung responding best to chemotherapy:
    a. Squamous cell carcinoma
    b. Oat cell type
    c. Adenocarcinoma
    d. All respond equally
118. Clubbing is least common in: (AIIMS Dec 97)
    a. Squamous cell carcinoma
    b. Adenocarcinoma
    c. Small cell carcinoma of lung
    d. Mesothelioma
119. Most cases of paraneoplastic syndrome are associated with which type of lung carcinoma: (JIPMER 2013)
    a. Small cell carcinoma
    b. Bronchogenic carcinoma
    c. Bronchoalveolar carcinoma
    d. Adenocarcinoma

CARCINOMA LUNG

120. Which of the following statements about lung carcinoma is true? (All India 2010)
    a. Squamous cell variant accounts for 70% of all lung cancers
    b. Oat cell variant typically present with cavitation
    c. Oat cell variant is typically associated with hilar adenopathy
    d. Adenocarcinoma variant is typically central in location
121. All of the following statements about non-small cell carcinoma of lung (NSCCL) are true except: (All India 2012)
    a. Contralateral mediastinal nodes are contraindication to surgical resection
    b. Single agent chemotherapy is preferred for patients >70 years with advanced disease
    c. Squamous cell carcinoma is the most common NSCCL among Asian population
    d. Geftinib is most effective for female smokers with adenocarcinoma histology
122. Ramesh, 40-year-male patient presenting with polyuria, pain abdomen, nausea, vomiting, altered sensorium was found to have bronchogenic carcinoma. The electrolyte abnormality seen in him would be: (AIIMS May 2002)
    a. Hypokalemia   b. Hyperkalemia
    c. Hypocalcaemia   d. Hypercalcemia
123. A 60-year-old male presented to the emergency with breathlessness, facial swelling and dilated veins on the chest wall. The most common cause is: (All India 2003)
    a. Thymoma
    b. Lung cancer
    c. Hodgkin's lymphoma
    d. Superior vena caval obstruction
124. Which of the following tumor is most commonly associated with superior vena cava syndrome? (All India 2011)
    a. Lymphoma   b. Small cell carcinoma
    c. Non small cell carcinoma   d. Metastasis
125. In a 56-year-old chronic smoker there was a mass in bronchus which is successfully resected. This mass is most likely to be positive for: (AIIMS Nov 2009)
    a. Cytokeratin
    b. Vimentin
    c. Epithelial membrane cadherin
    d. Leukocyte
126. A 60-year-old male presents to the clinic with complaints of abdominal pain, constipation and coin pain radiating to the groin of over a week duration. He has 25-pack year smoking history and is currently being evaluated for a hicar mass picked UP on chest radiography. As part of this laboratory work-up, the serving calcium was found to be elevated. The elevated serum calcium level is most likely linked to:
    a. Paratharoid adenoma   (COMEDK 2014)
    b. Parathoroid hyperplasia
    c. Vitamin D intoxication
    d. Secretion of PTH-related peptic
127. Which of the following has no infectious etiology?
    a. Nasopharyngeal carcinoma   (AIIMS Nov 2009)
    b. Hepatocellular carcinoma
    c. Non-small cell lung carcinoma
    d. Gastric carcinoma
128. Most common site of metastasis in lung carcinoma:
    a. Liver   b. Adrenal   (AIIMS May 2007)
    c. Bone   d. Brain
129. True about lung carcinoma: (PGI June 2009)
    a. Adenocarcinoma most common
    b. Squamous cell carcinoma is most common
    c. Originates for type-II pneumocytes
    d. Oat cell (Neuroendocrine cells)
    e. Squamous cell carcinoma peripherally located

130. Histological variants of bronchoalveolar carcinoma includes: *(PGI Nov 2011)*
    a. Clara cells
    b. Adenosquamous
    c. Mucin secreting cells
    d. Type II pneumocytes
    e. Neuroendocrine cell

131. Superior sulcus tumor of the lungs characteristically present with: *(JIPMER 2011)*
    a. Horner syndrome
    b. Breathlessness
    c. Hemoptysis
    d. Pancoast syndrome

132. Superior vena cava syndrome is caused most commonly by: *(MCI Sept 2009, AIIMS Nov 95)*
    a. Adenocarcinoma
    b. Squamous cell carcinoma
    c. Small cell carcinoma
    d. Large cell carcinoma

133. A 60-year-old male was diagnosed as carcinoma right lung. On CECT chest there was tumour of 5 × 5 cm in upper lobe and another 2 × 2 cm size tumour nodule in middle lobe. The primary modality of treatment is: *(DPG 2010, All India 2004)*
    a. Radiotherapy
    b. Chemotherapy
    c. Surgery
    d. Supportive treatment

134. A 65-year-old miner has lost 7 kg weight within two months, has presented with cough, and blood streaked sputum. He was treated for pulmonary tuberculosis 10 years ago. He also has drooping of his left eyelid for one month. On physical examination, there is ptosis of the left eye and papillary miosis. Chest X-ray revealed round opacification in the left upper apical lobe. What is the most probable diagnosis? *(AIIMS May 2006)*
    a. Secondary tuberculosis
    b. Adenocarcinoma
    c. Squamous cell carcinoma
    d. Asbestosis

135. Hoarseness secondary to bronchogenic carcinoma is usually due to extension of the tumor into: *(UPSC 2002)*
    a. Vocal cord
    b. Superior laryngeal nerve
    c. Left recurrent laryngeal nerve
    d. Right vagus nerve

136. All seen in pancoast syndrome except: *(HPU 2005)*
    a. Brachial plexus involvement
    b. Dyspnoea
    c. Clubbing
    d. Myasthenia gravis

137. Most common site of metastasis of carcinoma bronchi:
    a. Liver + Bones
    b. Prostate *(HPU 2005)*
    c. Kidney
    d. Breast

138. Clinical manifestations of bronchogenic carcinoma include of the following except: *(ICS 2005)*
    a. Hoarseness of voice due to involvement of left recurrent laryngeal nerve
    b. Horner's syndrome
    c. Diaphragmatic palsy due to infiltration of phrenic nerve
    d. Gastroparesis due to vagal involvement

139. The site of temporal bone metastasis is most commonly seen with: *(UPPG 2010)*
    a. Carcinoma breast
    b. Carcinoma bronchus
    c. Carcinoma kidney
    d. Carcinoma prostate

140. Carcinoma responding maximally to radiotherapy is: *(MCI Sept 2006)*
    a. Squamous cell carcinoma
    b. Adenocarcinoma
    c. Small cell carcinoma
    d. Large cell carcinoma

141. Most common type of carcinoma lung is: *(AIIMS May 93)*
    a. Small cell carcinoma
    b. Adenocarcinoma
    c. Squamous cell carcinoma
    d. Large cell carcinoma

142. All of the following are true regarding oat cell carcinoma of lung, except: *(AIIMS June 99)*
    a. Variant of large cell anaplastic carcinoma
    b. Chemotherapy is effective
    c. Paraneoplastic syndrome may be present
    d. Causes SIADH

143. In pancoast tumor, following is seen except: *(PGI June 98)*
    a. Horner's syndrome
    b. Rib erosion
    c. Hemoptysis
    d. Pain in shoulder and arm

144. Pancoast's syndrome is due to: *(Recent Question 2017)*
    a. C4-5 invasion
    b. C8-T1 invasion
    c. Lower trunk involvement
    d. C5-6 invasion

145. In case of CA lung, which among the following will be contraindication for surgical resection? *(AIIMS Nov 2000)*
    a. Malignant pleural effusion
    b. Hilar lymphadenopathy
    c. Consolidation of one lobe
    d. Involvement of visceral pleura

146. A 50-year-old-smoker male presents with pain along the left arm and ptosis. His chest radiograph shows a soft tissue opacity at the left lung apex with destruction of adjacent ribs. The picture is suggestive: *(AIIMS Nov 2003)*
    a. Adenocarcinoma lung
    b. Bronchial carcinoid
    c. Pancoast tumour
    d. Bronchoalveolar carcinoma

147. The first step when doing a penumononectomy for cancer of the bronchus is to: *(UPPG 97)*
    a. Ligate the pulmonary vein
    b. Ligate pulmonary artery
    c. Divide the bronchus
    d. Perform lymph node clearance

148. A 60 years old man presents with non productive cough and haemoptysis for 4 weeks; He has grade III clubbing, and a lesion in the apical lobe on X-ray most likely diagnosis here is: *(All India 2001, AIIMS June 2000)*
    a. Small cell carcinoma
    b. Non-small cell carcinoma
    c. Fungal infection
    d. Tuberculosis

149. A patient presents with secondaries to the adrenals. The most common site of primary is: *(WBPG 2012, All India 2000)*
    a. Lung
    b. Kidney
    c. Breast
    d. Stomach

150. Most common symptom of lung carcinoma: *(AIIMS 90)*
    a. Cough
    b. Dyspnea
    c. Weight loss
    d. Chest pain

151. The commonest intrabronchial cause of hemoptysis is: *(AIIMS May 95)*
    a. Carcinoma lung
    b. Adenoma lung
    c. Emphysema
    d. Bronchiectasis

152. A 60-year-old chronic smoker presents with complaints of hemoptysis. Her chest X-ray appears to be normal. What is the next best investigation? *(All India 2001)*
    a. Bronchoscopy
    b. High resolution CT
    c. Sputum cytology
    d. Pulmonary function test

153. A 60-year-old man is suspected of having bronchogenic carcinoma. TB has been ruled out in this patient. What should be the next investigation? *(All India 2001)*
    a. CT guided FNAC
    b. Bronchoscopy and biopsy
    c. Sputum cytology
    d. X-ray chest

154. A patient presents with a cavitatory lesion in right upper lobe of lung. The best investigation is: *(All India 2000)*
    a. Bronchoscopy, lavage and brushing
    b. CT scan
    c. X-ray
    d. FNAC

PULMONARY EMBOLISM

155. All of the following conditions may predispose to pulmonary embolism except: *(All India 2003)*
    a. Protein S deficiency
    b. Malignancy
    c. Obesity
    d. Progesterone therapy

156. A 23-year-old boy, a badminton player, sustained injury of left ankle. He was immobilized for 3 months, the cast was removed and patient was able to walk normally. Later he complained of pain and swelling in the left calf, left ankle and foot. His mother massaged him for 30 minutes. After a while he developed acute onset of breathlessness and was brought to emergency and died. Most likely cause of death is: *(AIIMS May 2017)*
    a. Pulmonary thromboembolism
    b. Congestive cardiac failure
    c. Massive stroke
    d. Hypovolemic shock

157. A patient had a femur fracture for which internal fixation was done. Two days later, the patient developed sudden onset shortness of breath with low-grade fever. What is the likely cause? *(AIIMS May 2017)*
    a. Pneumothorax
    b. Fat embolism
    c. Pleural effusion
    d. Congestive heart failure

158. A patient with history of trauma, presented with bilateral femoral fracture, respiratory distress & red urine. For evaluation of patient all the following are included in major criteria of Gurd's criteria except: *(PGI May 2018)*
    a. Unexplained decrease in platelets
    b. Tachycardia
    c. Petechiae
    d. CNS depression
    e. Pulmonary edema

159. In acute pulmonary embolism, the most frequent ECG finding is: *(AIIMS May 2006)*
    a. S1Q3T3 pattern
    b. 'P' pulmonale
    c. Sinus tachycardia
    d. Right axis deviation

160. Most common symptom in pulmonary embolism: *(MCI Sept 2007)*
    a. Dyspnea
    b. Pleuritic chest pain
    c. Cyanosis
    d. Hemoptysis

161. Ventilation perfusion imaging is most useful for the diagnosis of: *(COMEDK 2004)*
    a. Pulmonary thromboembolism
    b. Asthma
    c. Interstitial lung disease
    d. Hypersensitivity pneumonitis

162. Gold standard to diagnose pulmonary embolism is:
    a. Chest X-ray *(MHCET 2016)*
    b. Pulmonary angiography
    c. Ventilation purfusion scintiscan
    d. CT chest

163. Early and reliable indication of air embolisms during anesthesia can be obtained by continuous monitoring of: *(COMEDK 2008)*
    a. ECG
    b. Blood pressure
    c. End-tidal CO_2
    d. Oxygen saturation

164. A mill-wheel type of murmur during laparoscopy suggests:
    a. Tension pneumothorax *(COMEDK 2009)*
    b. Intra-abdominal bleeding
    c. Gas embolism
    d. Pre-existing valvular disease

165. Radiographic features of pulmonary embolism include all except: *(COMEDK 2011)*
    a. Westermarck's sign
    b. The Fleischner sign
    c. Hampton's hump
    d. Virchow sign

166. CT angiographic finding of acute pulmonary thromboembolism includes: *(PGI Nov 2011)*
    a. Filling defect of main pulmonary artery
    b. Pleural fibrosis
    c. Lobar and segmental oligemia
    d. Pleural effusion
    e. Peripheral, wedge-shaped consolidations

167. Patient admitted with fracture shaft of femur in a few days developed respiratory distress, ↓SPO_2 and petechial rashes. Diagnosis: *(JIPMER 2011)*
    a. Fat embolism
    b. Pulmonary embolism
    c. Hemolytic anemia
    d. Crush syndrome

168. Investigation of choice in pulmonary embolism:
    a. Ventilation perfusion scan *(JIPMER 2010)*
    b. MRI
    c. CECT
    d. X-ray

169. A patient with fracture pelvis is admitted in ICU after surgery. Postoperatively he develops sudden dyspnea and chest. The likely cause is: *(AIIMS Nov 99)*
    a. Pulmonary thromboembolism
    b. Shock
    c. Respiratory infection
    d. ARDS

170. All are true about pulmonary embolism, except: *(AIIMS May 94)*
    a. Chest pain is the most common symptom
    b. Most commonly presents within 2 weeks
    c. More is the survival time, more is the chance of recovery
    d. Arises from leg veins

171. The most common source of pulmonary embolism is:
    a. Amniotic fluid embolism *(AIIMS May 95)*
    b. Calf vein thrombi
    c. Large veins of leg
    d. Cardiothoracic surgery

172. A 55-year-old man who has been on bed rest for the past 10 days complains of breathlessness and chest investigation should be: *(All India 2004, 2003)*
    a. Lung ventilation-perfusion scan
    b. Pulmonary arteriography
    c. Pulmonary venous angiography
    d. Echocardiography

173. The most definitive method of diagnosing pulmonary embolism is: *(AIIMS Nov 2005)*
    a. Pulmonary arteriography
    b. Radioistope perfusion pulmonary scintigraphy
    c. EKG
    d. Venography

174. A young patient presents to the emergency with acute pulmonary embolism. Patients blood pressure is normal but echocardiography reveals right ventricular hypokinesia and compromised cardiac output. The treatment of choice in this patient is: *(AIIMS Nov 2001)*
    a. Thrombolytic therapy
    b. Anticoagulation with low molecular weight heparin
    c. Anticoagulation with warfarin
    d. Inferior vena cava filters

175. In pulmonary embolism, fibrinolytic therapy is responsible for: *(PGI Dec 97)*
    a. Risk of hemorrhage
    b. Prognosis good
    c. Massive emboli
    d. All of the above

176. IVC filter is used in following except: *(PGI Dec 97)*
    a. Massive emboli
    b. Negligible size of emboli
    c. Repeated emboli
    d. None

177. D-Dimer is the most sensitive diagnostic test for:
    a. Pulmonary embolism *(DPG 2011)*
    b. Acute pulmonary edema
    c. Cardiac tamponade
    d. Acute myocardial infarction

178. The sequence of symptoms in pulmonary embolism is:
    a. Fever, pain, dyspnea *(DNB 90)*
    b. Fever, dyspnea
    c. Dyspnea, pain, hemoptysis
    d. Dyspnea, cough, purulent sputum

179. The commonest site of lodgment of pulmonary embolus is in the territory of: *(UPSC 95)*
    a. Right lower lobe
    b. Right upper lobe
    c. Left Lower lobe
    d. Left upper lobe

180. A young male presented with dyspnea, bleeding and petchial hemorrhage in the chest after 2 days following fracture shaft of the femur right side. Most likely cause is: *(UPPG 2008)*
    a. Air embolism
    b. Fat embolism
    c. Pulmonary thromboembolism
    d. Amniotic fluid embolism

THORACIC INJURY

181. True regarding presentation(s) of thoracic duct injury: *(PGI June 2009)*
    a. Electrolyte imbalance
    b. Lymphopenia
    c. Dehydration
    d. Lymphedema
    e. Chylothorax may be present

182. True about chest trauma: *(PGI June 2008)*
    a. ECG done in all cases associated with sternal fracture
    b. Under water seal drainage if associated with pneumothorax
    c. X-ray chest investigation of choice
    d. Urgent surgery needed in all cases

183. Interstitial emphysema may be found in the following conditions: *(Kerala 98)*
    a. Chest injury
    b. Tracheostomy
    c. Surgical wound
    d. All

ADULT RESPIRATORY DISTRESS SYNDROME

184. Most common abnormality associated with ARDS:
    a. Hypoxemia *(JIPMER 2011)*
    b. Hypercapnea
    c. Diffuse alveolar damage
    d. Bilateral alveolar infiltrates

185. The ideal tidal volume in a patient ventilated for ARDS is: *(COMEDK 2010)*
    a. 6 mL/kg
    b. 10 mL/kg
    c. 14 mL/kg
    d. 20 mL/kg

186. Adult respiratory distress syndrome is defined by all except:
    a. PCWP >18 mm Hg *(COMEDK 2005)*
    b. PaO_2/FiO_2 <200
    c. Diffuse bilateral air space edema on chest X-ray
    d. All the above

187. Which of the following is most characteristic feature of ARDS?
    a. Diffuse alveolar damage *(All India 2012)*
    b. Hypoxia and hypoxemia
    c. Surfactant deficiency
    d. Hypocapnia

188. Acute lung injury is characterized by all, *except*:
    a. Alveolar infiltrates *(PGI Dec 2004)*
    b. Hypoxemia
    c. Pulmonary shunting
    d. PaO_2/FiO_2 <200 mm of Hg
    e. None of the above

189. All are seen in ARDS, *except*: *(AIIMS May 95)*
    a. Pulmonary edema
    b. Decreased tidal volume
    c. Hypercapnia
    d. Decreased compliance

190. Which of the following is not seen in ARDS? *(All India 96)*
    a. Pulmonary edema
    b. Hypoxemia
    c. Stiff lung
    d. Hypercapnia

PULMONARY TUBERCULOSIS

191. A young man with pulmonary tuberculosis presents with massive recurrent hemoptysis. For angiographic treatment, which vascular structure should be evaluated first? *(All India 2004)*
    a. Pulmonary artery
    b. Bronchial artery
    c. Pulmonary vein
    d. Superior vena cava

192. Indications of surgery in pulmonary TB: *(PGI Dec 2006)*
    a. Suspicion of malignancy
    b. Cavitary lesion with aspergilloma
    c. Massive hemoptysis
    d. All of the above

CARDIAC TUMORS

193. The most common primary cardiac tumor is: *(Recent Question 2016, COMEDK 2004)*
    a. Rhabdomyoma
    b. Myxoma
    c. Leiomyoma
    d. Lipoma

HEART TRANSPLANTATION

194. Absolute contraindications of heart transplantation:
    a. HIV infection *(PGI Dec 2000)*
    b. Age >60 years
    c. Irreversible pulmonary hypertension
    d. Significant pulmonary vascular disease
    e. Malignancy

PECTUS EXCAVATUM AND CARINATUM

195. Regarding pectus excavatum all are true *except*:
    a. Gross CVS dysfunction *(PGI Dec 97)*
    b. Decrease in lung capacity
    c. Cosmetic deformity
    d. Depression in chest

MISCELLANEOUS

196. CABG is done for all of the following indications *except*:
    a. To reduces symptoms *(All India 99)*
    b. To prevent further catastrophics
    c. To prolong life
    d. To prevent progress of native blood vessel disease

197. Valvoplasty is done in following *except*: *(PGI Dec 97)*
    a. Coarctation of aorta   b. PS
    c. MS   d. AS

198. Treatment of choice in postoperative lung collapse is all *except*: *(AIIMS June 95)*
    a. Needle drainage
    b. Corticosteroids
    c. Pulmonary resection
    d. Endoscopic suction

199. Following is true of eventration of diaphragm:
    a. It is a development defect *(Recent Question 2016)*
    b. Early surgery is treatment
    c. Defect is usually muscular
    d. Diagnosed mostly clinically

200. Broncholithiasis means: *(Kerala 96)*
    a. Calcified lymph nodes eroding into bronchus
    b. Foreign body calcified in bronchus
    c. Lithium deposition in bronchial wall
    d. A hamartoma

201. Complication to PEEP include all *except*:
    a. Pulmonary edema   b. Emphysema
    c. Cardiogenic shock   d. Pneumonia

202. The greatest incidence of bronchopleural fistula is following:
    a. Segmental resection   b. Lobectomies
    c. Pneumonectomies   d. Thorocotomy

203. The most important consideration in a patient with borderline pulmonary function requiring lung resection is: *(Karnataka 2003)*
    a. The amount of nonfunctioning lung tissue to be removed
    b. The amount of functioning lung tissue to be removed
    c. Experience of the surgical team
    d. Elevated pulmonary artery pressure

204. Which needle is used for pleural biopsy? *(COMEDK 2007)*
    a. Vin silvermann's   b. Abram's
    c. Abraham's   d. Osgood's

205. Heimlich valve is used for drainage of: *(COMEDK 2008)*
    a. Pneumothorax
    b. Hemothorax
    c. Emphysema
    d. Malignant pleural effusion

206. The organism most frequently related to mediastinal fibrosis is: *(DPG 2010)*
    a. Actinomycosis   b. Histoplasma
    c. Hansen's bacillus   d. Staphylococcus

207. Which is true regarding hydatid cyst of lung?
    a. Never ruptures *(AIIMS June 2002)*
    b. Calcification is common
    c. Always associated with cyst in the liver
    d. More common in lower lobes

208. The commonest site for extragonadal germ cell tumour is: *(COMEDK 2009)*
    a. Retroperitoneum
    b. Sacrococcygeal region
    c. Pineal gland
    d. Mediastinum

209. The most popular incision for open general thoracic surgical procedures is: *(COMEDK 2010)*
    a. Anterior thoracotomy
    b. Median sternotomy
    c. Lateral thoracotomy
    d. Transverse thoracosternotomy

210. Pleura ends at which level in the posterior axillary line: *(Punjab 2007)*
    a. Medial border of 11th rib
    b. Lateral border of 11th rib
    c. Medial border of 12th rib
    d. Lateral border of 12th rib

211. All are indications for surgery in bronchiectasis *except*:
    a. Hemoptysis *(JIPMER 2010)*
    b. Copious symptoms
    c. Bleeding
    d. Recurrent infections

212. Bastio surgery for refractory LV hypertrophy is: *(MHSSMCET 2006)*
    a. Patch repair   b. MR repair
    c. Ventriculectomy   d. Ventriculoplasty

213. Resting intrapleural pressure: *(MHSSMCET 2007)*
    a. -2 to -6 mm Hg
    b. +2 to +6 mm Hg
    c. -5 to -10 mm Hg
    d. -10 to +10 mm Hg

214. True about chest wall tumor: *(PGI November 2017)*
    a. Fibrous dysplasia is the most common malignant soft tissue tumor
    b. Lipomas are the most common benign tumors
    c. Desmoid is low-grade sarcomas of soft tissue of chest wall
    d. Lung metastasis with direct chest wall extension should be treated with radical en-bloc resection of the chest wall and underlying lung
    e. Rhabdomyosarcoma is the second most common chest wall tumor in children

215. Topical application of mitomyin C is recommended for:
    a. Endoscopic treatment of angiofibroma *(All India 2012)*
    b. Sturge-Weber syndrome
    c. Skull bone osteomyelitis
    d. Laryngotracheal stenosis

216. CXR of industrial worker exposed to asbestos over 20 years shows an ill-defined round opacity in the lower lobe with a comet tail appearance on PA-view. Which of the following is the most likely diagnosis? *(All India 2012)*
    a. Mesothelioma
    b. Bronchogenic carcinoma
    c. Round atelectasis
    d. Pulmonary infarct

217. Coronary graft is most commonly taken from: *(DNB 2012)*
    a. Femoral vein
    b. Saphenous vein
    c. Axillary vein
    d. Cubital vein

218. Patient can safely undergo major lung resection without increased risk of post operative complication if: *(DNB 2006)*
    a. FEV1 > 1L, Normal DLCO
    b. FEV1 > 1L, Decreased DLCO
    c. FEV1 > 2L, Normal DLCO
    d. FEV1 > 2L, Decreased DLCO

219. Which of the following is false about hemoptysis? *(AIIMS Nov 2013)*
    a. Massive hemoptysis is bleeding >600 mL in 24 hours
    b. In 90% cases, bleeding from bronchial arteries
    c. CT chest is the first investigation done
    d. In an unstable patient, rigid bronchoscopy is done to identify the lesion

220. Hamman's sign is seen in: *(APPG 2016)*
    a. Pneumomediastinum
    b. Diaphragmatic paralysis
    c. Empyema thoracis
    d. Subphrenic abscess

221. A 44 years old male underwent a VATS thymectomy for myasthenia graves. During surgery, the pleura was accidentally injured. The surgeon decided to put a drain in the pleural cavity. Which of these statements is correct about the timing of removal of intercostal chest tube? *(AIIMS November 2016)*
    a. After partial expansion of lungs and <50 mL output from drain for 2 consecutive days
    b. After complete expansion of lungs and <30 mL output from drain for 2 consecutive days
    c. After complete expansion of lungs and <200 mL output from drain for 2 consecutive days
    d. On 4th day, irrespective of the output from the drain and lung expansion

222. A 56-year-old patient came to casualty with history of massive hemoptysis. His routine investigations and chest X-ray was normal. Which of the following is not done to prevent hemoptysis? *(AIIMS May 2017)*
    a. Bronchial artery embolization
    b. Pulmonary artery embolization
    c. Bronchoscopic laser cauterization
    d. Lobectomy of the affected segment

Explanations

MEDIASTINAL TUMORS

1. Ans. d. Ganglioneuroma *(Ref: Sabiston 20/e p1608; Schwartz 10/e p670-680; Bailey 27/e p935)*
2. Ans. b. Neurogenic tumor *(Ref: Sabiston 20/e p1608; Schwartz 10/e p673; Bailey 27/e p936)*
3. Ans. b. Posterior mediastinum *(Ref: Imaging in Oncology by Michael A. Blake (2008)/p165)*

   - "The posterior mediastinum is the usual site of intrathoracic pheochromocytoma. They have also rarely been reported to occur in the middle mediastinum, with involvement of the left atrial wall or interatrial septum and aortic arch." –*Imaging in Oncology by Michael A. Blake (2008)/p165*

4. Ans. d. Ganglioneuroma
5. Ans. d. Thymic tumor
6. Ans. c. Thymoma
7. Ans. b. Attempt as complete a resection as possible
8. Ans. a. Lymphoma, b. Neuroblastoma, c. Neurogenic tumors, e. Bronchogenic cyst
9. Ans. a. Teratoma, b. Thymoma, c. Lymphoma, e. Parathyroid carcinoma
10. Ans. a. Anterior *(Ref: Sabiston 20/e p1608; Schwartz 10/e p1259; Bailey 27/e p935-936)*

    ### LYMPHOMA
    - **Anterior mediastinum is MC site**^{Q}
    - Occasional involvement of middle compartment and rare involvement of posterior mediastinum
    - **Chemotherapy** and/or **radiotherapy** results in a **cure rate of up to 90%** for **early-stage** Hodgkin's disease and up to **60% for** more advanced stages^Q.

      - MC tumor of middle mediastinum: Lymphoma^Q
      - MC mass of middle mediastinum: Pericardial cyst^Q

11. Ans. c. Neurofibroma *(Ref: Schwartz 10/e p677-678)*
12. Ans. b. Hyperalbuminemia *(Ref: Sabiston 20/e p1610; Schwartz 10/e p675-676; Bailey 27/e p935)*
13. Ans. c. Thymoma
14. Ans. a. Neuroblastoma, b. Bronchogenic cyst, c. Neuroenteric cyst, d. Lymphoma
15. Ans. a. Mediastinum *(Ref: Sabiston 20/e p1580; Schwartz 10/e p679, 1018, 1607)*
16. Ans. d. Neurogenic tumor
17. Ans. a. Neurofibroma
18. Ans. a. Failure of rejection of transplanted organs *(Ref: www.ncbi.nlm.nih.gov/pmc/articles/PMC2974301)*

    - In **adult life, thymectomy has no demonstrable effect on antibody response** or upon homograft survival.
    - However, it has been shown that **thymectomy in adult mice, combined with total body irradiation**, can **result in homograft tolerance of a high degree.**
    - This finding suggests that the **thymus gland may resume its perceptor function in adult life** under circumstances in which there is **temporary suppression of the lymphopoietic system.**

19. Ans. c. Neurogenic tumor
20. Ans. d. Schwannoma
21. Ans. c. Bronchogenic cyst

PLEURAL EFFUSION

22. Ans. b. 7th intercostal space mid-axillary line *(Ref: Sabiston 20/e p1605; PJ Mehta 13th/361)*
23. Ans. d. Malignant ovarian tumour *(Ref: Harrison 20/e p2008, 19/e p593)*

    ### MEIG'S SYNDROME
    - Triad of **ascites, pleural effusion** and **benign ovarian tumor (fibroma)**^{Q}
    - It **resolves after the resection of the tumor**^{Q}.
    - Because the **transdiaphragmatic lymphatic channels are larger in diameter on** the **right**, the **pleural effusion is classically on** the **right side**^{Q}.

24. **Ans. a. TB** *(Ref: http://radiology.rsna.org/content/216/2/478.long)*

    Most common cause of **pseudochylous pleural effusion** is **tuberculous pleurisy**.

    ### CHYLIFORM PLEURAL EFFUSION (PSEUDOCHYLOUS OR CHOLESTEROL EFFUSION)

    - Chyliform pleural effusion, often called **pseudochylous** or cholesterol effusion, is a **high-lipid effusion** that is not chylous.
    - The **most common cause** of this pleural reaction is **tuberculous pleurisy**[Q], but it has **also been described in** association with **rheumatoid arthritis**.
    - The presence of a **fat-fluid level within the pleural space** is **unique to pseudochylous effusion**[Q].

25. **Ans. d. Bronchogenic carcinoma** *(Ref: Sabiston 20/e p1605; Schwartz 10/e p680; Bailey 27/e p921)*

    A **rapidly filling hemorrhagic pleural effusion** is suggestive of **malignancy**, most commonly **bronchogenic carcinoma**.

    ### MALIGNANT PLEURAL EFFUSION

    - Malignancy is a common cause of pleural effusion.
    - Most malignant pleural effusions are **exudative**[Q].
    - They are the **second most common exudative effusive process**.
    - **Metastatic breast** and **lung cancers** are the **most common malignancies**[Q] that cause malignant effusions.

PNEUMOTHORAX

26. **Ans. a. Smokers** *(Ref: Harrison 20/e p2009, 19/e p1719; Sabiston 20/e p1607; Schwartz 10/e p649-650; Bailey 27/e p919)*
27. **Ans. a. Poland syndrome** *(Ref: Wolfgang Radiology/271)*

    Hyperlucent Lung

Unilateral	Bilateral
Chest wall defects: • Mastectomy • **Poland syndrome**[Q] (absent pectoralis muscle) • Endobronchial obstruction **Pulmonary vascular causes:** • Pulmonary arterial hyperplasia • Pulmonary embolism • Congenital lobar emphysema	**Decreased soft tissue:** • Thin body habitus • **Bilateral mastectomy** **Cardiac causes** of decreased pulmonary blood flow: • Right to left shunt • **Eisenmenger's syndrome** **Pulmonary causes** of decreased pulmonary blood flow: • **Pulmonary embolism** • **Emphysema** • Bulla or bleb • **Interstitial emphysema**

28. **Ans. b. >20%**
29. **Ans. d. All** *(Ref: http://en.wikipedia.org/wiki/Pneumothorax)*

    ### AFTERCARE OF PNEUMOTHORAX

    - **Smoking cessation**[Q]
    - **Air travel is discouraged for** up to **7 days**[Q] after complete resolution of a pneumothorax if recurrence does not occur.
    - **Underwater diving is considered unsafe**[Q] after an episode of pneumothorax unless a preventative procedure has been performed.

30. **Ans. c. Thoracostomy and close the rent** *(Ref: Bailey 27/e p368)*
31. **Ans. b. Needle aspiration**   32. **Ans. b. 25**   33. **Ans. d. Intercostal drainage**
34. **Ans. a. Iatrogenic pneumothorax** *(Ref: Complications in Anesthesiology by Kirby (2007)/169)*

Common causes of Iatrogenic Pneumothorax (in decreasing order)	
• **Transthoracic needle lung biopsy**[Q] • **Subclavian vein cannulation**[Q] • **Thoracentesis**[Q]	• **Pleural biopsy**[Q] • **Positive pressure ventilation**[Q]

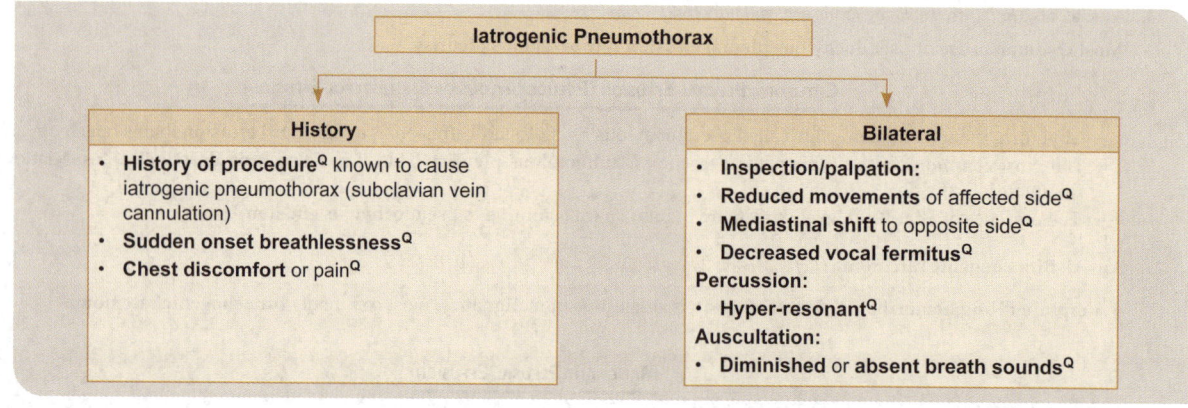

35. Ans. b. Pneumothorax
36. Ans. b. Old age
37. Ans. a. Smokers
38. Ans. d. Often needs chest tube insertion
39. Ans. a. Left axis deviation *(Ref: http://www.ncbi.nlm.nih.gov/pubmed/21320674)*

Common ECG Changes Associated with Left-sided Pneumothorax	
• Right axis deviation^Q	• QRS alterations^Q (amplitude changes)
• Reduced R-wave amplitude^Q in precordial leads	• T-wave inversions^Q

40. Ans. a. Valvular pneumothorax *(Ref: Sabiston 20/e p428; Schwartz 10/e p163-164; Bailey 27/e p367)*

TENSION PNEUMOTHORAX

- **Tension pneumothorax** occurs when the **opening** that allows **air to enter** the pleural space **functions as a one-way valve**, allowing more **air to enter** with every breath but **none to escape**^Q.
- There is **built up of positive pressure within hemithorax**, to the extent that **intrapleural pressure is greater the atmospheric pressure** causing lung to collapse^Q.

41. Ans. b. By observing the movement of air water column in the tube during respiration *(Ref: Pleural Diseases By Richard W. Light 5/e p400)*

"When the patient is not receiving suction, the patency of the chest tube can be assessed by observing the oscillations in the water seal chamber with respiratory movements." –Pleural Diseases By Richard W. Light 5/e p400

TENSION PNEUMOTHORAX

42. Ans. d. Large bore needle puncture of pleura *(Ref: Sabiston 20/e p428; Schwartz 10/e p163-164; Bailey 27/e p367)*
43. Ans. b. Tube drainage
44. Ans. a. Immediate IC tube drainage
45. Ans. b. CT-scan should be done to confirm pulmonary leak *(Ref: Bailey 27/e p366)*

TRAUMATIC PNEUMOTHORAX

- Traumatic pneumothoraxes can result **from penetrating** and **nonpenetrating chest trauma**.
- Traumatic pneumothoraxes should be **treated with tube thoracostomy** unless they are very small.

  - **Iatrogenic pneumothorax** is a **type of traumatic pneumothorax** that is becoming more common.
  - **Leading causes** are **transthoracic needle aspiration, thoracentesis**, and the **insertion of central intravenous catheters**^Q.
  - Most can be **managed with supplemental oxygen** or **aspiration**^Q, but if these measures are unsuccessful, a tube thoracostomy should be performed.

46. Ans. a. Insert wide bore needle in 2nd intercostal space *(Ref: Sabiston 20/e p428; Schwartz 10/e p164, 9/e p138; Bailey 27/e p367)*

- First line of management in tension pneumothorax: Insert wide bore needle in 2nd intercostal space.
- *"Treatment of tension pneumothorax consists of immediate decompression by rapid insertion of a large-bore needle into the 2nd intercostal space in the mid-clavicular line*^Q *of the affected hemithorax."*

47. Ans. d. Tension pneumothorax
48. Ans. c. Tension pneumothorax
49. Ans. a. Insertion of wide bore needle in the inter costal space
50. Ans. c. Decreased venous return
51. Ans. c. Insert needle in 2nd intercostal space
52. Ans. c. Chest tube insertion and drainage *(Ref: Sabiston 20/e p230-231; Schwartz 10/e p164; Harrison 20/e p2009, 19/e p1719)*
53. Ans. c. A needle should be inserted into the chest wall in the second right intercostal space as an emergency

HEMOTHORAX

54. Ans. b. Hemodynamic status, e. Nature of chest tube output *(Ref: Bailey 27/e p366, 368; Trauma Manual: Companion to trauma 4th/165)*

- Nature of chest tube drainage and Hemodynamic status both provide vital clues that may form an indication of surgery (Thoracotomy). However a deteriorating **hemodynamic status despite adequate volume resuscitation** should form the **most important guide, for urgent emergency thoracotomy** and is the **single best answer of choice.**

    - Bailey says "If the patient is **in extremis** with a **falling systolic blood pressure**, despite volume resuscitation, there is no choice but to proceed **immediately with a left anterolateral thoracotomy**".

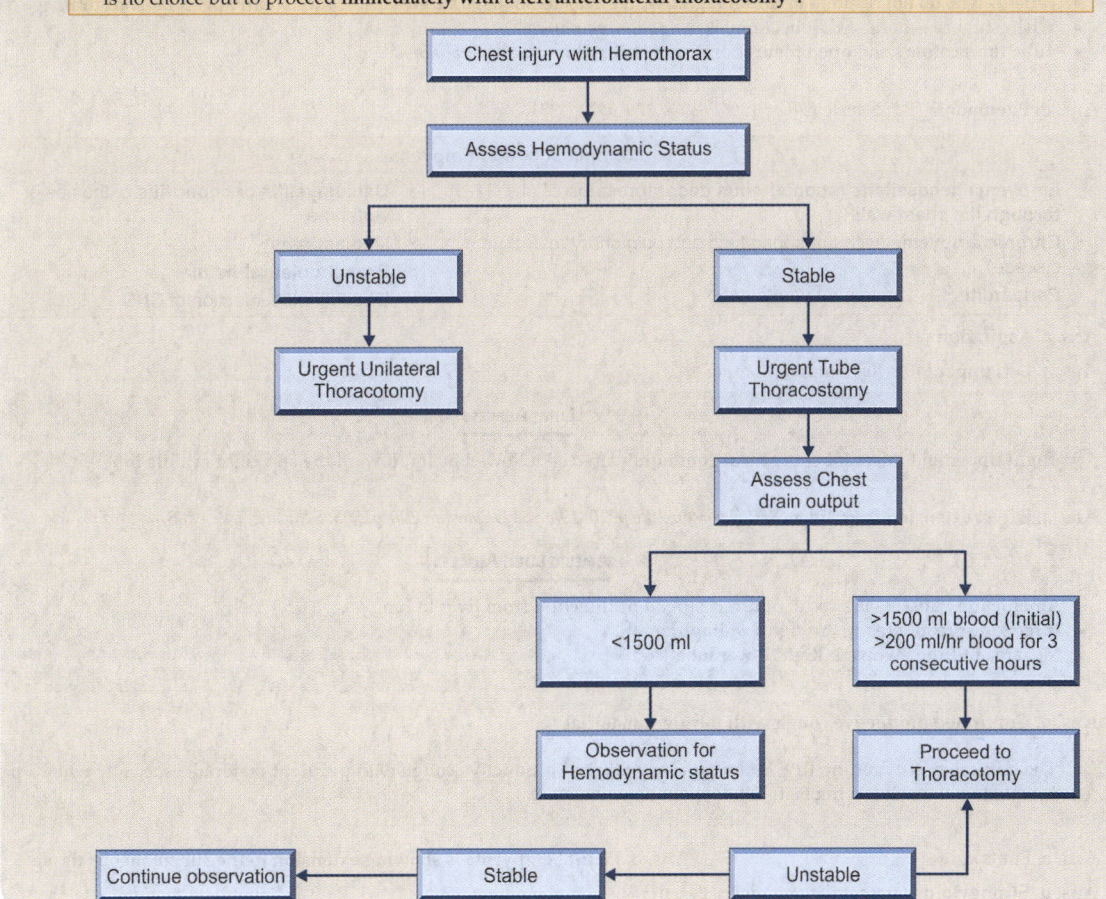

55. Ans. d. Open thoracotomy with ligation of vessel
56. Ans. a. Seen in choriocarcinoma, b. Supine posture is better than erect posture, c. Needle aspiration may be needed for diagnosis *(Ref: Harrison 20/e p2008, 19/e p1718; Schwartz 10/e p200; Bailey 26/e p355)*
57. Ans. d. Major artery
58. Ans. d. Intercostal arteries *(Ref: Schwartz 10/e p166; Bailey 27/e p368)*

"The most common cause of massive haemothorax in blunt injury is continuing bleeding from torn intercostal vessels or occasionally from the internal mammary artery secondary to the fracture of ribs." –*Bailey 27/e p368*

> "After blunt trauma, a major hemothorax usually is due to multiple rib fractures with severed intercostal arteries, but occasionally bleeding is from lacerated lung parenchyma which is usually associated with an air leak. After penetrating trauma, a great vessel or pulmonary hilar vessel injury should be presumed." –Schwartz 10/e p166

> "Hemothorax usually derives from bleeding of intercostal and internal mammary arteries and is caused by vessel wall injury from fractured ribs. Very rarely, hemothorax can be caused by traumatic laceration of diaphragmatic vessels from broken ribs." –Emergency Radiology: Imaging and Intervention edited by Borut Marincek, Robert F. Dondelinger (2007)/p187

LUNG ABSCESS

59. Ans. a. Antibiotics according to organisms *(Ref: Harrison 20/e p921, 19/e p815; Sabiston 20/e p1595; Schwartz 10/e p650-651; Bailey 27/e p937)*
60. Ans. d. Intracavitary antibiotic instillation *(Ref: Harrison 20/e p921, 19/e p815; Sabiston 20/e p1595; Schwartz Schwartz 10/e p650-651; Bailey 27/e p937)*

TREATMENT OF LUNG ABSCESS
- Patients who **do not respond to initial regimen** and who **do not have surgical indications**, **early percutaneous drainage** is done[Q].
- When surgery is indicated, **lobectomy** is the **preferred choice**[Q].
- **Tube thoracotomy** and **open pleural drainage** is also done for lung abscess[Q].

61. Ans. d. Pneumonia *(Ref: Sabiston 20/e p1605; Bailey 27/e p922, 923)*

Complications of Empyema

Empyema necessitans (**spontaneous decompression** of pus **through** the **chest wall**[Q])	**Osteomyelitis** or **chondritis** of the ribs or vertebrae
Chronic empyema (with entrapped lung and pulmonary restrictive disease)	**Mediastinitis**[Q]
Pericarditis[Q]	**Bronchopleural fistula**[Q]
	Disseminated infection of CNS

62. Ans. a. Aspiration
63. Ans. a. Left upper lobe *(Ref: Schwartz 10/e p650)*

LUNG ABSCESS
- **Right upper** and **lower lobes** are **most commonly affected** followed by **left lower lobe** and **right middle lobe**[Q].

64. Ans. a. Direct extension from liver *(Ref: Harrison 20/e p920, 19/e p814; Sabiston 20/e p1595; Schwartz 10/e p285)*

AMEBIC LUNG ABSCESS
- **Amebic lung abscess** is a result of **direct spread of infection from liver to lung**[Q].
- **Infection spread** directly **through** the **diaphragm**[Q].
- **MC area of lung** involved: **Right lower lobe**[Q]

65. Ans. d. Continued productive cough with purulent material
- The **clinical sign** of getting BPF is outlined as **continued productive cough** with **purulent material**, especially **when a patient is rolled** on the **side having Fistula**[Q].

66. Ans. a. Pott's spine
67. Ans. d. Pleural empyema is showing extension to the subcutaneous tissue
68. Ans. d. Strongyloides strecoralis *(Ref: Bailey 24/e p117)*

Parasitic Causes of Empyema

Paragonimus wetermani[Q]	**Entamoeba coli**[Q]
E. granulosus[Q]	

PLEURAL COLLECTIONS

69. Ans. d. TOC is excision and ligation of thoracic duct *(Ref: Sabiston 20/e p1606; Schwartz 10/e p685-687; Bailey 27/e p1013)*
70. Ans. d. Bile duct stones *(Ref: Bailey 27/e p1003, 1004, 1013)*

SEQUESTRATION OF LUNGS

71. Ans. b. Descending abdominal aorta *(Ref: Sabiston 20/e p1581; Schwartz 10/e p1607; Bailey 27/e p937)*
72. Ans. b. Left posterior basal
73. Ans. b. 50-70% occur in lung, c. Are commonly infected, d. Multilocular
74. Ans. b. They arise from anomalous development of foregut)
75. Ans. d. Posterior basal segment of lower lobe
76. Ans. c. Bronchus
77. Ans. b. Descending aorta
78. Ans. a. CT

TRACHEOBRONCHIAL FOREIGN BODY

79. Ans. a. Right posterior basal *(Ref: Schwartz 10/e p1607-1608; Bailey 27/e p924)*
80. Ans. c. Apical part of the lower lobe
81. Ans. a. Decreased ventilation perfusion ratio

VATS

82. Ans. c. Collapse of ipsilateral lung *(Ref: Sabiston 20/e p355; Schwartz Schwartz 10/e p704; Bailey 27/e p370, 922-923, 931, 934)*

> **VIDEO ASSISTED THORACOSCOPIC SURGERY (VATS)**
> - In contrast to most laparoscopic techniques, the **working space for VATS** is created not by adding an insufflating gas but rather by **removing air from the ipsilateral lung parenchyma** causing **collapse of the ipsilateral lung**^{Q}.
> - Used for **pulmonary decortication, pleurodesis,** and **lung** or **pleural biopsies**

83. Ans. b. Video assisted thoracoscopic surgery

THORACOTOMY

84. Ans. d. Rib fracture *(Ref: Sabiston 20/e p427, 429; Schwartz 9/e p159; Bailey 27/e p371, 930, 931)*

Indications of Thoracotomy	
• Initial tube thoracostomy drainage of **>1000 ml (penetrating injury)**^{Q} or **>1500 ml (blunt injury)**^{Q} • Ongoing tube thoracostomy drainage of **>200 ml/hr for 3 consecutive hours**^{Q} in non-coagulopathic patients • **Caked hemothorax**^{Q} despite of placement of two chest tubes • **Tracheo-bronchial injury**^{Q}	• Selected **descending torn aorta** or **great vessel injury**^{Q} • **Pericardial tamponade**^{Q} • **Cardiac herniation**^{Q} • **Massive air leak**^{Q} from chest tube with inadequate ventilation • **Open pneumothorax**^{Q} • **Esophageal perforation**^{Q}

85. Ans. d. Pulmonary contusion
86. Ans. a. Profuse uncontrolled bleeding, c. Bronchial adenoma, d. Bronchial fistula *(Ref: Tuberculosis by William N. Rom/519; Harrison 18/e p1371-1373)*

Indications of Pulmonary Resection in TB (Hemoptysis)

Absolute (Massive BDS)	Relative (Phobia)
• **M**assive hemoptysis^Q (600 ml/24 hours) • **B**ronchopleural fistula^Q • **D**estroyed lung, positive sputum • **S**uspicion of carcinoma^Q	• **P**ersistent positive sputum • **H**emoptysis • **O**pen, negative cavity; TB empyema • **B**ronchial stenosis • **A**typical tubercular infection • **A**spergillosis (fungal balls)

87. Ans. c. Rhomboides major *(Ref: Sabiston 20/e p1579; Farquharson's Operative Surgery 9/e p132)*

> **POSTEROLATERAL THORACOTOMY**
> - **Posterolateral thoracotomy** is the **most frequently used operation** to access the **thorax**^{Q}.
> - **Incision** is made through **5th intercostal space**^{Q}.

Following muscles may be cut in Posterolateral Thoracotomy	
• Lattissimus dorsi^Q • Serratus anterior^Q	• Trapezius^Q • Intercostal muscles^Q

88. Ans. b. Pulmonary contusion
89. Ans. a. Internal mammary artery
90. Ans. a. Scapular and sternal fractures

BENIGN LUNG TUMORS

91. Ans. a. Hamartoma *(Ref: Schwartz 10/e p622, 9/e p526; Bailey 27/e p934)*
92. Ans. b. More common in females *(Ref: Schwartz 10/e p622; Bailey 27/e p934)*
    Popcorn calcification is diagnostic of pulmonary hamartoma, which is more common in males.
93. Ans. c. Recurrent hemoptysis *(Ref: Harrison 18/e p753)*   94. Ans. c. Recurrent hemoptysis
95. Ans. c. Carcinoid syndrome does not manifest *(Ref: Robbins 9/e p719; Harrison 20/e p602, 19/e p563)*
96. Ans. c. Adenoma bronchus

MESOTHELIOMA

97. Ans. a. Bilaterally symmetrical *(Ref: Sabiston 20/e p1607; Schwartz 10/e p688; Bailey 27/e p146, 922)*
98. Ans. a. Asbestosis   99. Ans. e. All of the above   100. Ans. b. Butchart staging is used

SQUAMOUS CELL CARCINOMA

101. Ans. b. Squamous cell carcinoma

ADENOCARCINOMA

102. Ans. a. Common in females, d. Peripheral involvement is common *(Ref: Harrison 20/e p538, 19/e p511; Sabiston 20/e p1583; Schwartz 10/e p679,1018,1607; Bailey 27/e p925)*
103. Ans. a. Surgery *(Ref: Harrison 20/e p547, 19/e p516; Sabiston 20/e p1590)*
104. Ans. d. Peripheral location   105. Ans. b. Adenocarcinoma   106. Ans. a. Adenocarcinoma of lung

SMALL CELL CARCINOMA

107. Ans. c. Chemosensitive tumor *(Ref: Harrison 20/e p538, 19/e p522)*
Small cell carcinomas are **highly chemosensitive** with an overall **90% regression rate with chemotherapy.**

Property	Small cell carcinoma	Non small cell carcinoma
Location	• Central location^Q	• Peripheral location^Q
Metastasis	• **Highly metastatic** lesion with widespread metastasis at time of diagnosis. • **Common site** of metastasis include **brain, bone, liver** and **adrenals**^{Q}	• Less metastatic than small cell carcinoma
Paraneoplastic syndrome	• ACTH^Q • AVP (Vasopression)^Q • Calcitonin^Q • ANF^Q • Gastrin Releasing peptide	• PTH-rp^Q
Response to chemotherapy	• Superior response^Q • Overall regression rate 90%^{Q} • Rate complete regression in 30%	• Inferior response • Objective shrinkage in 30-50% • Complete response: uncommon

108. Ans. a. Small cell carcinoma   109. Ans. b. Chromagranin   110. Ans. d. Noradrenaline
111. Ans. a. Small cell anaplastic   112. Ans. a. Hypercalcemia, c. Watery diarrhea
113. Ans. a. Commonest malignancy of lung   114. Ans. c. Chemosensitive tumor   115. Ans. b. Small cell carcinoma
116. Ans. b. Growth hormone   117. Ans. b. Oat cell type
118. Ans. c. Small cell carcinoma of lung   119. Ans. a. Small cell carcinoma

CARCINOMA LUNG

120. Ans. c. Oat cell variant is typically associated with hilar adenopathy *(Ref: Sabiston 20/e p1583; Schwartz 10/e p623-645; Bailey 27/e p925; Harrison 20/e p538, 19/e p511)*

- Small cell carcinoma or oat cell variant is associated with **massive hilar** or **mediastinal lymphadenopathy, mediastinal invasion** and **perihilar mass**

121. **Ans. d. Geftinib is most effective for female smokers with adenocarcinoma histology** *(Ref: Harrison 19/e p521; Davidson 21/e p703)*

- **Geftinib** is an oral small molecule tyrosine kinase inhibitor **approved for treatment of** patients with **NSCCL**. Data to support the use of Geftinib in NSCCL are however diminishing and **Geftinib is most effective in females** who have **never smoked** with **adenocarcinoma** histology.
- **Single agent chemotherapy** is **preferred** for **elderly patients (>70 years)**.

Contraindication to Surgical Resection in NSCCL (Severe CID FM)	
• **Severe** or **unstable cardiac** or other **medical conditions**[Q]	• **Distant metastasis** (M1)[Q]
• **Contralateral mediastinal nodes (N3)**[Q]	• **FEV1 <0.8 L**[Q]
• **Invasion** of **central mediastinal structures** including **heart, great vessels, trachea** and **esophagus (T4)**[Q]	• **Malignant pleural effusion (M1)**[Q]

122. **Ans. d. Hypercalcemia**
123. **Ans. d. Superior vena caval obstruction** *(Ref: Harrison 20/e p541, 19/e p1787)*
124. **Ans. b. Small cell carcinoma**
125. **Ans. a. Cytokeratin** *(Ref: Fishman Pulmonary Disease 4/e p848)*

- **Cytokeratin positivity** is seen in **almost all NSCCL** (Non small cell carcinoma lung) due to their **epithelial origin**.
- **Chromagranin and synaptophysin positivity** is seen in **small cell carcinoma**.

126. **Ans. d. Secretion of PTH-related peptic**
127. **Ans. c. Non-small cell lung carcinoma**
128. **Ans. b. Adrenal**
129. **Ans. a. Adenocarcinoma most common, d. Oat cell (Neuroendocrine cells)**
130. **Ans. a. Clara cells, c. Mucin secreting cells, d. Type II pneumocytes** *(Ref: Robbins 9/e p716-717, 8/e p725)*
131. **Ans. d. Pancoast syndrome** *(Ref: Harrison 19/e p519; Sabiston 20/e p583; Schwartz 10/e p623, 641-642; Bailey 27/e p926)*
132. **Ans. c. Small cell carcinoma**
133. **Ans. c. Surgery** *(Ref: Sabiston 20/e p1591)*

Best treatment is induction chemoradiotherapy followed by surgery.

134. **Ans. c. Squamous cell carcinoma**

Squamous Cell Carcinoma	
• **MC** in **smokers**, MC type in **India**[Q]	• **Central** in distribution and prone to undergo **central necrosis** and **cavitation**[Q]
• MC variety associated with **hypercalcemia**[Q] (produces PTH-rp)	• Associated with **best prognosis**[Q]
• **Pancoast** tumor is histologically **SCC**[Q]	

135. **Ans. c. Left recurrent laryngeal nerve**
136. **Ans. d. Myasthenia gravis**
137. **Ans. a. Liver + Bones**
138. **Ans. d. Gastroparesis due to vagal involvement**
139. **Ans. b. Carcinoma bronchus** *(Ref: www.ncbi.nlm.nih.gov v.63(Suppl 1); Jul 2011)*

TEMPORAL BONE METASTASIS
• Metastatic tumors to the temporal bone are **uncommon**
• Usually seeded by the **hematogenous route**
• **MC metastatic lesion** in the temporal bone: **CA Breast**[Q]
• **Lung, prostate** and **renal carcinomas** are all **well documented for** their **metastatic potential** to the **temporal bone**[Q].

140. **Ans. c. Small cell carcinoma**
141. **Ans. b. Adenocarcinoma**

Adenocarcinoma	
• **MC** histological **type**, MC in **non-smokers, young patients, females**[Q]	• **Metastasize** more frequently to **CNS**
• Located **peripherally** with slow growth and propensity to **metastasize** to **opposite lung**[Q]	• Most cells contain **mucin**[Q]
	• **Noguchi classification** is used for **adenocarcinoma**[Q]

142. **Ans. a. Variant of large cell anaplastic carcinoma**
143. **Ans. c. Hemoptysis**
144. **Ans. b. C8-T1 invasion** *(Ref: Sabiston 20/e p355; Schwartz 10/e p623)*
145. **Ans. a. Malignant pleural effusion**
146. **Ans. c. Pancoast tumour**
147. **Ans. b. Ligate pulmonary artery** *(Ref: Bailey 27/e p932-933)*

PNEUMONECTOMY

- **Pneumonectomy** is anatomically **more straightforward than lobectomy** (in carcinoma bronchus):
- The **pulmonary artery** is **first dissected**, **divided** and **sutured**[Q].
- The **pulmonary veins** are then isolated, **divided** and sutured.
- The **main bronchus** is **divided** so that no blind stump remains. The technique of **stump closure** is important if a bronchopleural fistula is to be avoided. The tissues are carefully handled and the **stump** is **usually stapled**.

148. Ans. b. Non-small cell carcinoma
149. Ans. a. Lung
150. Ans. a. Cough
151. Ans. a. Carcinoma lung
152. Ans. a. Bronchoscopy
153. Ans. b. Bronchoscopy and biopsy
154. Ans. a. Bronchoscopy, lavage and brushing *(Ref: Bailey 27/e p923)*

Uses of Bronchoscopy	
Diagnostic	Confirmation of disease: • Carcinoma of the bronchus[Q] • Inflammatory and Infective process
Investigative	• Tissue biopsy[Q]
Preoperative assessment	• Before lung resection[Q] • Before esophageal resection • Persistent hemoptysis[Q]
Therapeutic	• Removal of secretions • Removal of foreign bodies[Q] • Stent placement, endobronchial resection

PULMONARY EMBOLISM

155. Ans. d. Progesterone therapy *(Ref: Harrison 20/e p1910, 19/e p1631; Sabiston 20/e p294-296; Schwartz 10/e p924-925; Bailey 27/e p987)*

- **Estrogen**, not the **progesterone** therapy **predisposes to thrombosis** and **pulmonary embolism**.

156. Ans. a. Pulmonary thromboembolism *(Ref: Harrisons 20/e p1910, 19/e p1632)*
157. Ans. b. Fat embolism *(Ref: Harrison 20/e p1910, 19/e p1632; Robbins 9/e p128; Apley's 9/e p681; Rockwood 6/e p553)*
158. Ans. a. Unexplained decrease in platelets, b. Tachycardia *(Ref: Textbook of Orthopedics (2018)/p237)*

Gurd's Criteria for Diagnosing Fat Embolism		
Major Criteria	**Minor Criteria**	**Laboratory Features**
• Petechial rash • Respiratory symptoms (Tachypnea, dyspnea, bilateral inspiratory crepitations, hemoptysis, bilateral diffuse patchy shadowing on chest X-ray) • Neurological sign (confusion, drowsiness, coma)	• Tachycardia (>120/min) • Pyrexia (>34.90C) • Retinal changes (fat or petechiae) • Jaundice • Renal changes (anuria or oliguria)	• Thrombocytopenia (>50% decrease on admission value) • Sudden decrease in hemoglobin level >20% of admission value • Raised ESR • Fat macroglobulinemia

159. Ans. c. Sinus tachycardia
160. Ans. a. Dyspnea
161. Ans. a. Pulmonary thromboembolism
162. Ans. b. Pulmonary angiography
163. Ans. c. End-tidal CO_2

CAPNOGRAPHY

- It is the **continuous measurement** of end tidal CO_2 and its waveforms.
- It works on the **principle** that **infrared light** is **absorbed** by CO_2.
- Useful in **diagnosing pulmonary embolism** by **air, fat** or **thrombus** (sudden fall in End-tidal CO_2 occurs). It **may become zero** if the **embolus** is **large enough to block pulmonary circulation**[Q].

164. Ans. c. Gas embolism
165. Ans. d. Virchow sign
166. Ans. a. Filling defect of main pulmonary artery, c. Lobar and segmental oligemia, d. Pleural effusion, e. Peripheral, wedge-shaped consolidations *(Ref: Harrison 20/e p1913-1914, 19/e p1632-1633; Danhert Radiology 5/e p51; Bhadury radiology 2/e p32)*
167. Ans. a. Fat embolism *(Ref: Apley's 8/e p535-536, Rockwood 6/e p553)*
168. Ans. c. CECT
169. Ans. a. Pulmonary thromboembolism

170. Ans. a. Chest pain is the most common symptom
171. Ans. c. Large veins of leg
172. Ans. a. Lung ventilation-perfusion scan
173. Ans. a. Pulmonary arteriography
174. Ans. a. Thrombolytic therapy *(Ref: Harrison 19/e p1634; Sabiston 20/e p296; Schwartz 10/e p924-925; Bailey 27/e p990)*

TREATMENT OF PULMONARY EMBOLUS

- Most pulmonary emboli can be **treated by anticoagulation** and **observation**
- **Severe right heart strain** and **shortness of breath** indicates the need for **fibrinolytic treatment**^{Q}.
  - **Thrombolysis** (or embolectomy) is **treatment of choice** in **massive PE** or **high risk (hypotension ± Right ventricular dysfunction)**^{Q}

Prophylaxis Against Pulmonary Embolism
- In patients who are considered at **high risk of embolism** or **when anticoagulants are contraindicated**, a **vena cava filter** may be inserted to prevent the onward passage of any emboli.
- **Filters** can also be placed **in patients** who **continue to have pulmonary emboli** despite **adequate anticoagulation**Q.
- **Greenfield filter: Most commonly used**^{Q}

175. Ans. a. Risk of hemorrhage
176. Ans. b. Negligible size of emboli
177. Ans. a. Pulmonary embolism
178. Ans. c. Dyspnea, pain, hemoptysis
179. Ans. d. Left upper lobe
180. Ans. b. Fat embolism

THORACIC INJURY

181. Ans. a. Electrolyte imbalance, b. Lymphopenia, c. Dehydration, e. Chylothorax may be present *(Ref: Sabiston 20/e p428; Schwartz 10/e p177-179, 200-203; Bailey 27/e p756)*
182. Ans. a. ECG done in all cases associated with sternal fracture, b. Under water seal drainage if associated with pneumothorax, c. X-ray chest investigation of choice *(Ref: Bailey 27/e p366, 938)*

CHEST TRAUMA

- **Sternal fracture** also constitute a **marker for serious associated injuries**, including **myocardial contusion, myocardial rupture**, esophageal perforation, airway injuries and thoracic aortic rupture.
- In **blunt cardiac injuries**, **ECG** is the **first diagnostic test**^{Q}.
- **Routine investigation** in the **emergency department** of **injury to** the **chest** is based on **clinical examination**, supplemented by **chest radiography**.
- In the **unstable patient**, **chest radiography** is the **investigation of first choice**^{Q}, provided that it does not interfere with resuscitation.

183. Ans. d. All

ADULT RESPIRATORY DISTRESS SYNDROME

184. Ans. a. Hypoxemia *(Ref: Harrison 20/e p2031, 19/e p1736; Sabiston 20/e p1599)*
185. Ans. a. 6 mL/Kg *(Ref: Harrison 20/e p2033, 19/e p1736)*

MANAGEMENT OF ARDS

- A large-scale, randomized controlled trial sponsored by the National Institutes of Health and conducted by the ARDS Network compared **low VT** (**6 mL/kg**Q predicted body weight) ventilation to conventional VT (12 mL/kg predicted body weight) ventilation.
- **Mortality** was **significantly lower** in the **low VT patients** (31%) compared to the conventional VT patients (40%).
- This improvement in survival represents the **most substantial benefit in ARDS mortality**^{Q} demonstrated for any therapeutic intervention in ARDS to date.

186. Ans. a. PCWP >18 mm Hg *(Ref: Harrison 19/e p1736, 18/e p2205)*

Diagnostic Criteria	Acute Lung Injury (ALI)	ARDS
PaO_2/FiO_2	• ≤300 mm Hg^Q	• ≤200 mm Hg^Q
Onset	• Acute^Q	• Acute^Q
Chest X-ray	• Bilateral alveolar or interstitial infiltrates^Q	• Bilateral alveolar or interstitial infiltrates^Q

Contd...

Contd…

Absence of Left Atrial Hypertension	• PCWP ≤18 mm Hg^Q • No clinical evidence of increased left atrial pressure^Q	• PCWP ≤18 mm Hg^Q • No clinical evidence of increased left atrial pressure^Q

187. Ans. a. Diffuse alveolar damage
188. Ans. d. PaO$_2$/FiO$_2$ <200 mm of Hg
189. Ans. c. Hypercapnia
190. Ans. d. Hypercapnia

PULMONARY TUBERCULOSIS

191. **Ans. b. Bronchial artery** *(Ref: Grainger Radiology 4/e p609)*

    Brochial arteries are the major source of hemoptysis.

192. **Ans. d. All of the above** *(Ref: Tuberculosis by William N. Rom/519; Harrison 18/e p1371-1373)*

CARDIAC TUMORS

193. **Ans. b. Myxoma** *(Ref: Harrison 20/e p1847, 19/e p289e-1)*

HEART TRANSPLANTATION

194. **Ans. a. HIV infection, c. Irreversible pulmonary hypertension, e. Malignancy** *(Ref: Bailey 27/e p1556, 25/e p1428; Harrison 19/e p1518, 18/e p1916)*

PECTUS EXCAVATUM AND CARINATUM

195. **Ans. a. Gross CVS dysfunction** *(Ref: Sabiston 20/e p1601; Bailey 27/e p939, 940)*

MISCELLANEOUS

196. **Ans. d. To prevent progress of native blood vessel disease** *(Ref: Sabiston 20/e p1674)*

    - A successful **CABG reduces symptoms, prevents catastrophies** and **prolongs survival.**
    - It **does not prevent progress of native blood vessel disease**. Infact Restenosis of the grafted vessel is noted with the time.

197. **Ans. a. Coarctation of aorta**

    Valvoplasty is done in valvular disease like MS, MR, AS or AR. It is not done in coarctation of aorta.

198. **Ans. d. Endoscopic suction** *(Ref: Sabiston 20/e p291-292)*

    Endoscopic suction is not used in postoperative level collapse.

199. **Ans. a. It is a development defect, c. Defect is usually muscular** *(Ref: www.ncbi.nlm.nih.gov › ... Lung India › v.26(2); Apr-Jun 2009 by AP Kansal)*

200. **Ans. a. Calcified lymph nodes eroding into bronchus** *(Ref: www.ncbi.nlm.nih.gov/pubmed/12376611)*

    ### BRONCHOLITHIASIS

    - **Calcified** or **ossified material** is **present within** the **bronchial lumen**^{Q}
    - **Radiographic findings: Airway obstruction**^{Q} such as atelectasis, mucoid impaction, bronchiectasis, and expiratory air trapping.
    - Broncholithiasis is **strongly suggested at CT** (when an **endobronchial** or **peribronchial calcified nodule** is associated with bronchial obstruction)

201. Ans. b. Emphysema
202. Ans. b. Lobectomies
203. Ans. d. Elevated pulmonary artery pressure
204. **Ans. b. Abram's** *(Ref: Bailey 27/e p922)*

    ### NEEDLES FOR PLEURAL BIOPSY

    - Abrams' needle
    - Cope's needle

205. **Ans. a. Pneumothorax** *(Ref: thorax.bmj.com ›Volume 58, Issue suppl 2)*

    ### HEIMLICH VALVE

    - **Heimlich chest drain valve** is a specially designed flutter valve used to replace underwater bottles in chest drainage.
    - The valve allows **unidirectional flow**^{Q}.
    - In clinical situations like **spontaneous pneumothorax, open thoracotomy, recurrent pleural effusion**^{Q}, chest drainage can be simplified with Heimlich chest drain valve.

206. **Ans. b. Histoplasma** *(Ref: Sabiston 20/e p1596; Schwartz 10/e p679-680)*

The organism most frequently related to mediastinal fibrosis is Histoplasma.

207. **Ans. d. More common in lower lobes**
208. **Ans. d. Mediastinum**
209. **Ans. c. Lateral thoracotomy** *(Ref: Bailey 27/e p930)*

The **standard route into thoracic cavity** is through a **posterolateral thoracotomy**.

210. **Ans. d. Lateral border of 12th rib** *(Ref: BDC 4th/vol-I/220)*

Level of ↓	Inferior margin of pleural reflection	Lung lower border (Pleural level-2)
Mid-clavicular line	8th rib^Q	6th rib^Q
Mid-axillary line	10th rib^Q	8th rib^Q
Posterior axillary line (Lateral border of sacrospinalis/erector spinae)	12th rib^Q	10th rib^Q

211. **Ans. a. Hemoptysis** *(Ref: Bailey 27/e p936)*

BRONCHIECTASIS

- **Chronic irreversible dilatation** of the **medium-sized bronchi**^{Q}, which may occur following a suppurative pneumonia or bronchial obstruction.
  - **If generalized** it is almost never considered for surgical resection^Q.

Treatment
- **Removal of** the **bronchiectatic part** of the lung for symptoms of **bleeding**^{Q}, **recurrent infection**^{Q} or **copious symptoms**^{Q} can be **very effective** when the **disease is localized**.

212. **Ans. c. Ventriculectomy**

Bentall's operation	For **aortic root aneurysm repair** **Reimplantation of coronary ostia** into composite graft
Bastio surgery	For **Left ventricular hypertrophy** **Ventriculectomy** is done^Q

213. **Ans. a. -2 to -6 mm Hg**
214. **Ans. b. Lipomas are the…, c. Desmoid is low-grade…., d. Lung metastasis…, e. Rhabdomyosarcoma…..**
215. **Ans. d. Laryngotracheal stenosis** *(Ref: Dhillon 3/e p67)*

- **Topical Mitomycin C** is the **drug of choice** used to aid the treatment of **laryngeal stenosis**^{Q}.
- **Topical Mitomycin C** can **inhibit fibroblast activity** and **restenosis**^{Q}.

216. **Ans. c. Round atelectasis** *(Ref: Thoracic Imaging by Golanski (Thieme) 2010/Atelectasis/Chapter 2)*

ROUND ATELECTASIS

- **Rounded subpleural opacity**, most commonly in **lower lobes**^{Q}
- **Comet tail sign positive**^{Q}
- **Typical history of asbestos exposure**^{Q} is often present

217. **Ans. b. Saphenous vein** *(Ref: Bailey 27/e p890)*

- **Saphenous vein** are the **most commonly employed conduits in coronary vascularization**.
- Most preferred graft for CABG: LIMA (left internal mammary artery) > Long saphenous vein^Q

218. **Ans. c. FEV1 >2L, Normal DLCO** *(Ref: Bailey 27/e p916-918)*

> **PULMONARY FUNCTION TEST**
>
> - Pulmonary function studies are routinely performed when any resection greater than a wedge resection will be performed.
> - Of all the measurements available, the **two most valuable are FEV1 and DLCO**.
> - For every 10% decline in patients DLCO, the risk of any pulmonary complications (As estimated by odd ratio) increased by 42%.
> - Patients with **FEV1 >2.0 L can tolerate pneumonectomy**, and those with an **FEV1 of >1.5 L can tolerate lobectomy.**

219. **Ans. c. CT chest is the first investigation done** *(Ref: Harrison 20/e p517, 19/e p246; Sabiston 20/e p1598)*

> - "**Massive hemoptysis** may be defined as **greater than 500 to 600 mL of blood loss from the lungs in 24 hours**."-Sabiston 19/e p1589
> - "Massive hemoptysis is one of the most dreaded of all respiratory emergencies and can have a variety of underlying causes. **In 90% of cases,** the **source of massive hemoptysis** is the **bronchial circulation."**
> - "For most patients, the **next step in evaluation of hemoptysis** should be a **standard chest radiograph**. If a **source of bleeding** is **not identified** on plain film, a **CT of the chest** should be obtained."
> - "If all of these studies are unrevealing, **bronchoscopy should be considered**. Rigid **bronchoscopy** with an 8.5-mm or larger bronchoscope is needed."
> - "As most **large-volume hemoptysis arises from an airway lesion**, it is ideal if the site of the bleeding can be identified either by **chest imaging or bronchoscopy** (more commonly rigid than flexible)."

220. **Ans. a. Pneumomediastinum**

221. **Ans. c. After complete expansion of lungs and <200 mL output from drain for 2 consecutive days** *(Ref: http://www.modernmedicine.com/content/chest-tube-removal)*

    It is recommended to remove the drain after checking the lung for full expansion & drain output is <200 mL for 2 consecutive days.

Ideal Time to Remove Drain	
Surgery	**Post-operative Time to Remove the Drain**
Thyroidectomy	24 hours[Q]
ICD drain	<200 mL in 24 hours[Q]
Mastectomy	5 days[Q]
Colorectal anastomosis	5-7 days[Q]
T-Tube Drain	10 days[Q]

222. **Ans. d. Lobectomy of the affected segment** *(Ref: Harrison's 20/e p517, 19/e p247; Sabiston 20/e p1598; Schwartz 10/e p662, 663)*

SECTION 6

Plastic Surgery

CHAPTERS

- Burns
- Plastic Surgery and Skin Lesions
- Wound Healing, Tissue Repair and Scar

CHAPTER 30

Burns

PATIENTS WITH THE FOLLOWING CRITERIA ARE REFERRED TO A DESIGNATED BURN CENTER

PATIENTS WITH THE FOLLOWING CRITERIA ARE REFERRED TO A DESIGNATED BURN CENTER

- Partial-thickness **burns >10% TBSA**[Q]
- Burns involving the **face, hands, feet, genitalia, perineum,** or **major joints**[Q]
- Any **full-thickness burn**[Q]
- **Electrical burns,** including **lightning injury**[Q]
- **Chemical burns**[Q]
- **Inhalation injury**[Q]
- Burns in patients with **preexisting medical disorders**[Q] that could complicate management, prolong recovery, or affect outcome
- Any patient with burns and **concomitant trauma**[Q] (e.g., **fractures**) in which the burn injury poses the greater immediate risk for morbidity and mortality.
- **Burned children in hospitals without qualified personnel** or equipment to care for children
- Burns in patients who will **require special social, emotional,** or long-term rehabilitative intervention

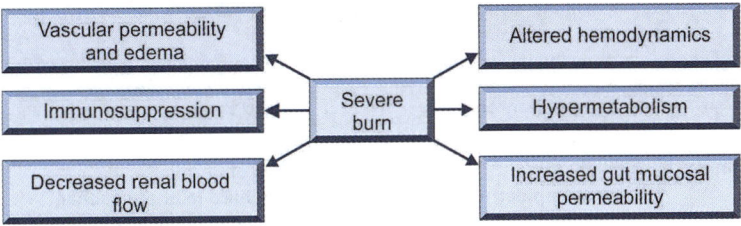

PATHOPHYSIOLOGY OF BURNS

- **Radiant heat loss** is increased from the burn wound **secondary to increased blood flow & integumentary loss**[Q].
- Heat loss also occurs because of **evaporation of water from** the **burn wounds**[Q]. This leads to significant fluid loss also.

> - **Significant burns** are associated with **massive release of inflammatory mediators**, both in wound and in other tissues.
> - These mediators produce vasoconstriction and **vasodilatation, increased capillary permeability** and **edema** locally and in distant organs.

- **Immune System:** Global depression in immune function (depressed cellular function in all parts of the immune system, including activation and activity of neutrophils, macrophages, B and T lymphocytes).
- **Metabolism:** Increased release of catabolic hormones like **catecholamines, corticosteroids** and **glucagon** leads to **hypermetabolic state**[Q].

> - Stress ulcers (**Curling ulcers**[Q]) of burns are due to **decrease in mucosal defenses**[Q] (**acid secretion is not increased**[Q])

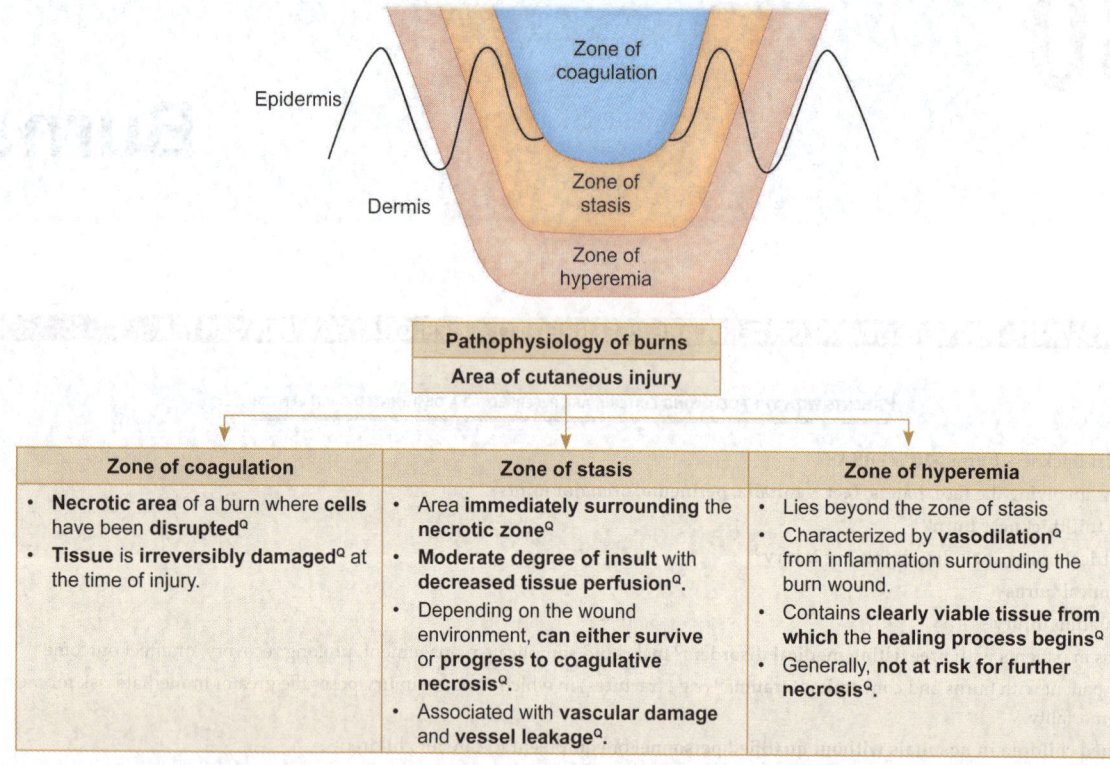

Pathophysiology of burns
Area of cutaneous injury

Zone of coagulation
- **Necrotic area** of a burn where **cells have been disrupted**[Q]
- **Tissue is irreversibly damaged**[Q] at the time of injury.

Zone of stasis
- Area **immediately surrounding** the **necrotic zone**[Q]
- **Moderate degree of insult** with **decreased tissue perfusion**[Q].
- Depending on the wound environment, **can either survive** or **progress to coagulative necrosis**[Q].
- Associated with **vascular damage and vessel leakage**[Q].

Zone of hyperemia
- Lies beyond the zone of stasis
- Characterized by **vasodilation**[Q] from inflammation surrounding the burn wound.
- Contains **clearly viable tissue from which the healing process begins**[Q]
- Generally, **not at risk for further necrosis**[Q].

BURN CLASSIFICATION

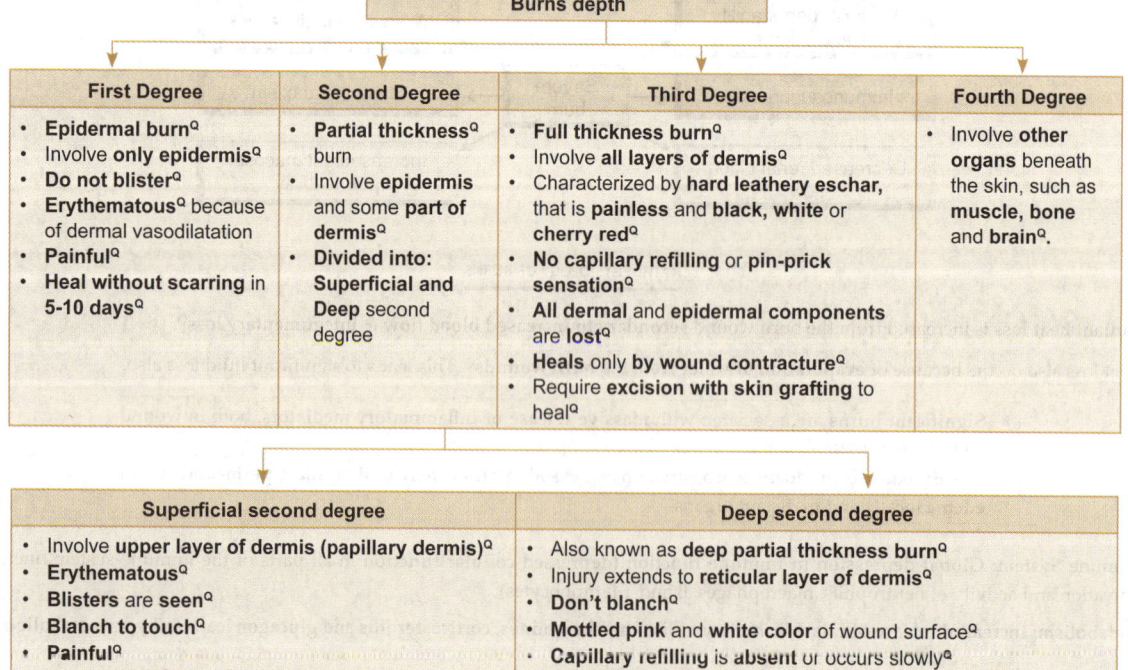

Burns depth

First Degree
- **Epidermal burn**[Q]
- Involve **only epidermis**[Q]
- **Do not blister**[Q]
- **Erythematous**[Q] because of dermal vasodilatation
- **Painful**[Q]
- **Heal without scarring in 5-10 days**[Q]

Second Degree
- **Partial thickness**[Q] burn
- Involve **epidermis** and some **part of dermis**[Q]
- **Divided into: Superficial and Deep** second degree

Third Degree
- **Full thickness burn**[Q]
- Involve **all layers of dermis**[Q]
- Characterized by **hard leathery eschar**, that is **painless** and **black, white** or **cherry red**[Q]
- **No capillary refilling** or **pin-prick sensation**[Q]
- **All dermal** and epidermal components are **lost**[Q]
- **Heals only by wound contracture**[Q]
- Require **excision with skin grafting** to heal[Q]

Fourth Degree
- Involve **other organs** beneath the skin, such as **muscle, bone and brain**[Q].

Superficial second degree
- Involve **upper layer of dermis (papillary dermis)**[Q]
- **Erythematous**[Q]
- **Blisters are seen**[Q]
- **Blanch to touch**[Q]
- **Painful**[Q]
- **Heals without scarring in 7-14 days**[Q]

Deep second degree
- Also known as **deep partial thickness burn**[Q]
- Injury extends to **reticular layer of dermis**[Q]
- **Don't blanch**[Q]
- **Mottled pink** and **white color** of wound surface[Q]
- **Capillary refilling is absent** or occurs slowly[Q]
- **Pain is absent**[Q]
- **Pin-prick sensation is preserved**[Q]
- **Heals in 3-9 weeks** with **scar formation**[Q]

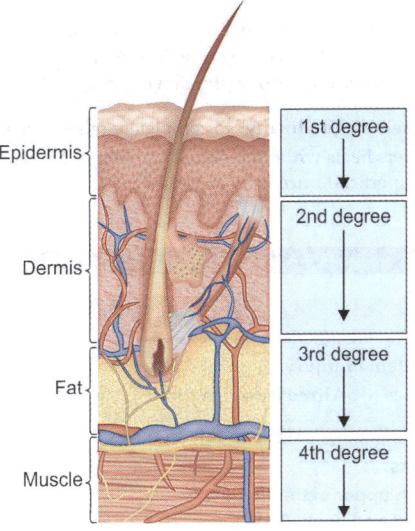

ESCHAROTOMY

Escharotomy

- **Circumferential full thickness burns to the limbs** require emergency surgery to avoid **compartment syndrome**.
- **Incising the whole length of full thickness burns** treats tourniquet effect of this injury.

Levels of Escharatomy	
Upper limb	• **Mid-axial, anterior to elbow medially** to avoid the ulnar nerve
Hand	• **Midline in the digits**
Lower limb	• **Mid-axial, posterior to the ankle medially** to avoid saphenous nerve
Chest	• Down the chest lateral to nipple, across the chest below clavicle & across the chest at the level of xiphisternum

FEVER IN BURN PATIENTS

Fever in Burn Patients

- Many of the **physiological criteria** that has been **claimed to reflect sepsis** are **non-infectious manifestations** of **post injury hypermetabolism**^{Q}.
  - **Hyperthermia** (39°C or greater) is occasionally **a febrile a response to infection,** particularly in **children,** but **episodic elevation in temperature** are **common in uninfected burn patients**^{Q}.
- The **hypermetabolic phase**^{Q} mediated by greatly **increased levels of catecholamines, prostaglandins, glucagon** and **cortisol** occurs after the **acute phase** and also produces pathophysiological changes.
- Burn patients exhibit **increased blood flow** to organs and tissues, **an increased internal core temperature, hypoproteinemia** and **edema formation**^{Q}.

CARE OF BURN PATIENTS

Care of Burn Patients

Cool the burn wound

- This **provides analgesia** and **slows the delayed microvascular damage** that can occur after a burn injury.
- Cooling should occur **for a minimum of 10 min** and is **effective up to 1 hour after** the **burn injury.**
- It is a **particularly important first aid step in partial-thickness burns**, especially **scalds.**
- In temperate climates, cooling should be at **about 15°C,** and hypothermia must be avoided.

- **Room temperature water** can be **poured** on the wound **within 15 minutes of injury** to decrease the depth of wound, but **any subsequent measures to cool** the **wound** are **avoided to prevent hypothermia**^{Q}.

> - Iced water should never be used, even on the smallest of burns^Q.
> - If ice or cold water is used on larger burns, systemic hypothermia often follows, and the associated cutaneous vasoconstriction can extend the thermal damage.

- The **entire constricting eschar** must be **incised longitudinally**^Q to completely relieve the impediment to blood flow.
- **Superficial partial thickness burn** with blisters **heals without residual scarring in 2 weeks** irrespective of the dressing. Treatment is **non-surgical**. The simplest method of **treating superficial burn** is **by exposure**^Q.

BURN SIZE (% BSA)

Burn Size (% BSA)

- Determination of **burn size estimates** the **extent of injury**.
- **Burn size** is assessed by **Wallace rule of nines** (By **Alfred Russel Wallace**^Q)

> **Wallace rule of nines**
> - **In adults:**
>   - Each **upper extremity: 9%**^Q
>   - **Head and neck: 9%**^Q
>   - **Lower extremities: 18%**^Q
>   - **Anterior** and **posterior** aspects of the **trunk: 18%**^Q
>   - **Perineum** and genitalia: **1%**^Q

- **Children** have a relatively **larger proportion** of body surface area **in their head and neck**, which is compensated for by a relatively smaller surface area in the lower extremities.
  - In infants: Head and neck- **21%**^Q ; Each leg- **13%**^Q
- **Berkow formula**^Q is used to **accurately determine burn size in children**.
- **For estimating smaller burns:** Area of open hand^Q (including palm and extended fingers) of the patient is approximately **1%**^Q of TBSA
- This method is helpful in **evaluating splash burns** and burns of **mixed distribution**.

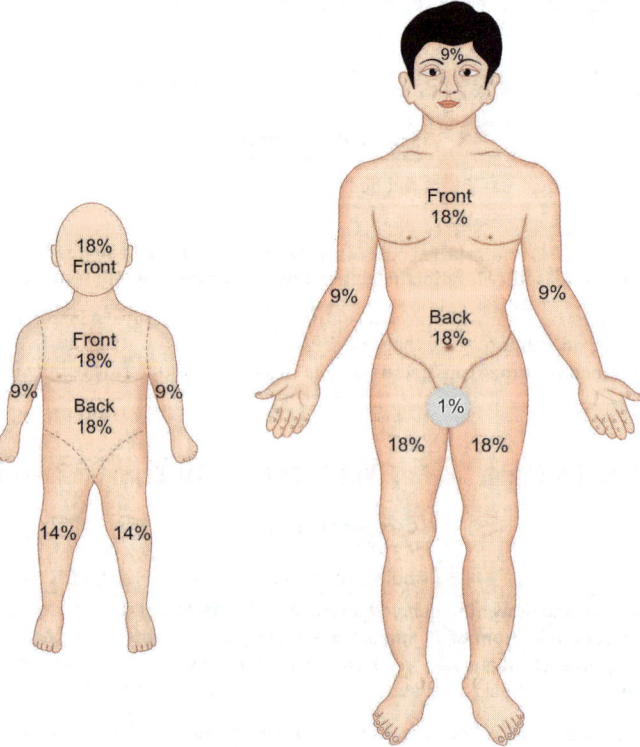

Estimation of burn size using the rule of nine

FLUID RESUSCITATION

FLUID RESUSCITATION

- **IV fluid resuscitation**: In **children** with burn >10%[Q] TBSA & **adult** with burn >15%[Q] TBSA
- **Regimen** of **fluid resuscitation follows** the **fluid loss**, which is at its **maximum in first 8 hours** and slows such that by 2-36 hours the patient can be maintained on her/his normal daily requirement.

Fluids used in resuscitation
• **Ringer Lactate** is **most commonly used**[Q].
• Some centers use **human albumin, FFP** or **hypertonic saline**[Q]

- If **oral resuscitation** is to be commenced, it is important that the **water given is not salt free**. Hyponatremia and **water intoxication can be fatal**[Q].
- In **children, maintenance fluid** must be given, usually **dextrose-saline.**[Q]
- **Simplest** and **most widely used formula: Parkland formula**[Q]

• **Hypertonic saline** has been **effective in treating burn shock**[Q].
• It produces **hyperosmolality** and **hypernatremia.**
• This reduces the shift of intracellular water to the extracellular space.
• Advantage includes **less tissue edema** and a resultant **decrease in escharotomies** and **intubation**[Q].

- **Protein** should be given **after the first 12 hours** of burn.
- The commonest **colloid based formula** is **Muir and Barclay formula**[Q].

Monitoring of Resuscitation

- The key to monitoring is **urine output**[Q].

• **Urine output** should be **0.5-1.0 mL/kg/hour**[Q] (i.e. 30-60 ml per hour[Q]).

- Other measures for monitoring:
  - Acid base balance and Hematocrit
  - In **cardiac dysfunction**: Transesophageal USG and **Central line**[Q]

Venous Access for Infusion

- In adults: Ideal sites are **veins in hand, antecubital fossa** or **neck**.
- **Saphenous vein cut down** is useful **in patient with difficult access** and is used in preference to central venous cannulation.
- **CVP line** is used for **CVP monitoring**, helps in **estimating fluid overload**[Q].

Resuscitation Formulas			
Formula	Crystalloid Volume	Colloid Volume	Free water
Parkland[Q]	4 mL/kg per % TBSA burn	None	None
Brooke[Q]	1.5 mL/kg per % TBSA burn	0.5 mL/kg per % TBSA burn	2.0 L
Galveston[Q] (pediatric)	5000 mL/m² burned area + 1500 mL/m² total area	None	None

Topical Antimicrobials used in Burn

Silver sulphadiazine cream (1%)	Silver nitrate solution (0.5%)	Mafenide acetate cream (5%)	Silver sulphadiazine and cerium nitrate
• This gives **broad-spectrum prophylaxis**[Q] against bacterial colonization • **Particularly effective** against **Pseudomonas** and **MRSA**[Q] • **MC** used	• **Highly effective** as a prophylaxis **against Pseudomonas** colonization[Q] • **Not as active** as silver sulphadiazine cream **against** some of the **Gram -ve aerobes.** • It **needs to be changed** or the wounds **resoaked every 2-4 hours**[Q]. • Produces **black staining** of all the **furniture** surrounding the patient.	• Popular in the **USA** • **Painful to apply**[Q] • Associated with **metabolic acidosis**[Q].	• Useful for **full-thickness burns.** • Induces a **hard effect on** the **burned skin**[Q] • In **elderly patients**, to reduce cell-mediated immuno-suppression[Q] • **Cerium nitrate** forms a **sterile eschar and** boost cell mediated immunity

- MC cause of death at the site of burn: Asphyxia
- MC cause of death in burns: Septicemia^Q
- MC cause of early death in burns: Hypovolemic shock^Q
- MC cause of late death in burns: Septicemia^Q
- MC organism responsible for sepsis in burns: Pseudomonas^Q

POST BURN NECK CONTRACTURE

Post Burn Neck Contracture

- **Cervical contractures** are major problems in **burns involving** the **chest, neck & face**^Q.
- **Severe neck flexion contracture** in the acute phase often **require early reconstruction**^Q to aid in airway management
- **Neck contractures** should usually be **dealt with prior to facial burn reconstruction**^Q as the extrinsic contractile forces from the neck can cause facial deformities and can adversely affect the maturation of scars on the face.

  - When **split-thickness skin grafting** is **unsuccessful** because of recurrent contracture or does not provide a satisfactory aesthetic result, **local flap reconstruction of anterior neck** is an **excellent technique**^Q.

- **Perioral Deformities**: Microstomia, macrostomia, irreversible damage to dentition & loss of jawline definition^Q
- **Anterior neck contractures** in the acute period are **best prevented by aggressive splinting** and **incisional releases** & **grafting**^Q when indicated.

  - **Deep second** & **third degree burns do not heal** in timely fashion **without autografting**^Q
  - **Escharotomies** is done in case of **deep second** & **third degree buns** wounds **to decrease constriction of eschar**^Q

LOW-TENSION INJURIES

Low-tension injuries

- **Low-tension** or **domestic appliance injuries do not have enough energy to cause destruction** to significant amounts **of subcutaneous tissues**^Q when the current passes through the body.
- **Resistance** is **too great.**
- **Entry & exit points,** normally **in the fingers,** suffer **small deep burns**; these may cause underlying **tendon** and **nerve damage,** but there will be little damage between.
- The **alternating current creates a tetany** within the muscles, and thus patients often describe how they were **unable to release the device** until the power was turned off.
- A common finding in patients with electric burns is **myoglobinuria** manifested as **highly concentrated** and **pigmented urine.**

  - **Main danger** with these injuries is from the **alternating current interfering with normal cardiac pacing.** This can cause **cardiac arrest**^Q.
  - The **electricity** itself **does not** usually **cause significant underlying myocardial damage,** so **resuscitation, if successful, should be lasting.**

Multiple Choice Questions

BURNS: % BSA

1. According to "rule of nines", burns involving perineum are:
   a. 1%   b. 9%   *(MCI March 2009)*
   c. 18%   d. 27%

2. A five years old child presents to the emergency department with burns. The burn area corresponding to the size of his palm is equal to: *(All India 2011)*
   a. 1% BSA   b. 5% BSA
   c. 10% BSA   d. 20%

3. In a 6 years old child with burns involving the whole of head and trunk, estimated body surface area of burns is:
   a. 44%   b. 52%   *(COMEDK 2008)*
   c. 55%   d. 58%

4. Rule of nine of estimate surface area of a burnt patient was introduced by: *(Recent Question 2016)*
   a. Mortix Kaposi   b. Wallace
   c. Joseph Lister   d. Thomas Barclay

5. Best method to assess burns in 5 years old child caused by boiling water: *(AIIMS May 2013)*
   a. Palm method   b. Rule of 9
   c. Lund and Browder chart   d. Rule of one

6. A child has circumferential burn of both of thighs and buttocks, face and scalp with singeing of hairs. Calculate the percentage of burns: *(JIPMER 2014, AIIMS May 2013)*
   a. 24   b. 27
   c. 37   d. 45

7. Head and face burn in infant is: *(Recent Question 2014, 2013)*
   a. 15%   b. 18%
   c. 12%   d. 32%

8. Percentage of burn in children is best assessed by:
   a. Rule of 9   b. Rule of palm = 1%
   c. Lund and Browder chart   d. Wallace rule *(DNB 2014)*

9. Percentage of body surface area involved in the burns involving scalp and face in an adult using Berkow formula: *(Recent Question 2017)*
   a. 7%   b. 8%
   c. 9%   d. 10%

BURNS

10. A burn patient is referred when: *(PGI June 2004)*
    a. 10% superficial burn in child
    b. Scald in face
    c. 25% superficial burn in adult
    d. 25% deep burn in adult
    e. Burn in palm

11. In burns heat loss is by/due to:
    a. Dilatation of veins
    b. Shock
    c. Exposed area by evaporation
    d. None of the above

12. Metabolic derangements in severe burns are all except:
    (PGI June 2000)
    a. ↑corticosteroid secretion   b. Hyperglycemia
    c. ↑secretion of HCl   d. Neutrophil dysfunction

13. Pus in burns form in:
    a. 2-3 days   b. 3-5 days
    c. 2-3 weeks   d. 4 weeks

14. Fever in burnt patient is caused by:
    a. Septicemia   *(PGI Nov 2009, June 2009)*
    b. Due to hypermetabolism
    c. Decreased sweating
    d. Release of pyrogens from dead product
    e. Dehydration

15. True about thermal burn injury: *(PGI June 2009)*
    a. Outermost layer is zone of stasis
    b. Middle layer is zone of hyperemia
    c. Inner layer is zone of coagulation
    d. Hyperemia is due to vasodilatation
    e. Zone of stasis is associated with vascular damage

16. Undue restlessness in a patient during the immediate post burn period is often a manifestation of: *(Karnataka 95)*
    a. Hypoxia   b. Hypovolemia
    c. Hyperkalemia   d. Anxiety

17. All require hospitalization except: *(DNB 2002, All India 91)*
    a. 5% burns in children   b. 10% scalds in children
    c. Electrocution   d. 15% deep burns in adults

18. True about burns: *(PGI 2000)*
    a. Hyperglycemia is seen in early burns
    b. Child with burns should have damp dressing
    c. Chemical powder burns should be kept dry
    d. 3rd degree burns are painfull

BURNS DEPTH

19. True regarding burns: *(PGI Dec 2007)*
    a. Only 2nd and 3rd degree is considered in the classification
    b. 2nd degree-Epidermis + papillary dermis
    c. Blisters-2nd degree
    d. Curling ulcer can occur
    e. Classified according to depth of invasion

20. In a patient with the burn wound extending into the superficial epidermis without involving the dermis would present all of the following except: *(SGPGI 2005)*
    a. Healing of the wound spontaneously without scar formation
    b. Anesthesia at the site of burn
    c. Blister formation   d. Painful

21. A third degree circumferential burn in the arm and forearm region, which of the following is most important for monitoring?   *(UPPG 2004)*
    a. Blood gases
    b. Carboxy-oxygen level
    c. Macroglobinuria cryoglobinuria
    d. Peripheral pulse and circulation

22. True statement regarding 2nd degree deep burn:
    (PGI Dec 2008)
    a. Blanch on pressure   b. Erythema
    c. Dry white colour   d. Painless
    e. Predispose to hypothermia

23. Degree of burns in a patient with prominent vessels with decreased needle prick sensation and dryness:
    a. Superficial partial thickness burns
    b. Deep partial thickness burns (MHSSMCET 2006)
    c. Electric burns   d. Full thickness burns

24. Burn involving epidermis and full thickness of dermis:
    a. First degree burns   (MHSSMCET 2008)
    b. Partial-thickness second degree burns
    c. Full-thickness second degree burns
    d. Third degree burns

25. True about burn is: (UPPG 2010)
    a. Full thickness burn feels, leathery, painless
    b. Electric burn are superficial
    c. IV fluid formula used Curreri and Brooke
    d. Skin grafting done after 48 hours
    e. 1 year of age in head and neck region covers 18%

26. Which of the following is not seen in 3rd degree burns?
    (MCI March 2009)
    a. Loss of skin appendages   b. No vesicles
    c. Red color   d. Extremely painful

27. In second degree burns, re-epithelialisation occurs around:
    a. 1 week   b. 2 weeks   (MCI Sept 2009)
    c. 3 weeks   d. 4 weeks

28. Which of the following is false regarding deep 2nd degree burns?   (MCI Sept 2009)
    a. Heal by scar deposition   b. Painless
    c. Damage to deeper dermis   d. Less blanching

29. Superficial burns; true is/are: (PGI June 2001)
    a. Always requires skin grafting
    b. Dry and inelastic   c. Blister formation
    d. Painless   e. Can be healed within 7-10 days

30. Burns with vesiculation, destruction of the epidermis and upper dermis is: (PGI June 99)
    a. 1st degree   b. 2nd degree
    c. 3rd degree   d. 4th degree

31. Blisters are seen in which type of burns? (DNB 2009)
    a. Superficial first degree   b. Superficial second degree
    c. Third degree   d. Deep first degree

32. 2nd degree burns indicate involvement of: (JIPMER 2013)
    a. Epidermis   b. Dermis
    c. Subcutaneous tissue   d. Deep fascia

33. False regarding deep second-degree burns: (MCI June 2018)
    a. Heal by scar deposition   b. Painless
    c. Damage to deeper dermis   d. Less blanching

34. Which layer is involved in blister formation in a superficial partial thickness burn?   (AIIMS November 2017)
    a. Epidermis   b. Dermis
    c. Papillary dermis   d. Reticular dermis

TREATMENT OF BURNS

35. Parkland formula is: (JIPMER 2010)
    a. Percentage of burns × weight (kg) × 4 = volume in ml
    b. Percentage of burns × weight (kg)/2 = 1 volume in ml
    c. Percentage of burns × weight (kg) × 9 = volume in ml
    d. 500 ml/m2 BSA + 1500 ml/m^2 = volume in ml

36. In a 50 kg adult, how much of fluid should be given in first 8 hours in burns of 40%? (Recent Question 2018, MCI Nov 2017)
    a. 2 litres   b. 4 litres
    c. 8 litres   d. 6 litres

37. A woman was brought to the casualty 8 hours after sustaining burns on the abdomen, both the limbs and back. What will be the best formula to calculate amount of fluid to be replenished?   (AIIMS May 2017)
    a. 2 mL/kg × %TBSA   b. 4 mL/kg × %TBSA
    c. 8 mL/kg × %TBSA
    d. 4 mL/kg × % TBSA in first 8 hours followed by 2 mL/kg/hour × % TBSA

38. A 1.5-years-old child was brought to emergency with history of burn by hot water on both hands and palms. The lesion was pink, oozing and painful to air and touch. Which of the following is the best management for this patient?
    a. Paraffin gauze and dressing   (AIIMS May 2017)
    b. Collagen dressing   c. Excision and grafting
    d. Apply 1% silver sulfasalazine ointment and keep the wound open

39. During fluid resuscitation in a burns patient using Parkland's formula, volume of fluid given in first 8 hours:
    a. 25%   b. 50% (Recent Question 2017)
    c. 75%   d. 100%

40. IV formula for burn is: (Recent Question 2015, UPPG 2009)
    a. Total % body surface area x weight x 4 = volume in ml
    b. Total % body surface area x weight x 5 = volume in ml
    c. Total % body surface area x weight x 6 = volume in ml
    d. Total % body surface area x weight x 7 = volume in ml

41. Which of the following formula for fluid administration in a patient with burns is not correct? (MHSSMCET 2008)
    a. Parkland: 4 ml kg/% TBSA burn of RL
    b. Brooks: 1.5 ml kg/% TBSA burn of RL + 0.5 ml kg% burn + 2000 ml D5W
    c. Shrine: 5000 ml m^2 TBSA burn + 2000 ml m^2 TBSA
    d. Evans: 8 ml kg/% TBSA burn of RL

42. Treatment of burns includes: (PGI June 2008)
    a. No bandage to head and neck
    b. Immediate application of ice cold water
    c. Superficial burns without blister-no need of dressing
    d. Escharotomy done for peripheral circumscribed lesions

43. What should be the ideal temperature of the cool water to be applied over burns?   (MHPGMCET 2006)
    a. Ice cold   b. 3-4°C
    c. 8-10°C   d. 14-15°C

44. Safest strategy of treatment for a patient of inhalational burn injury who has presented within 4-5 hours:
    (MCI Nov 2017, MHPGMCET 2007)
    a. Binasal catheter O2 inhalation
    b. O2 therapy with well-fitting face mask
    c. Elective cricothyroidotomy
    d. Elective endotracheal intubation

45. In burns management, which of the following is the fluid of choice?   (Recent Question 2014, DNB 2012, 2005)
    a. Dextrose 5%   b. Normal saline
    c. Ringer lactate   d. Isolyte-M

46. A 50 kg female has second degree deep burn involving 45% total body surface area (TBSA). Regarding her management which of the following statement (s) is/are true: (PGI Dec 2008)
    a. Give rapid normal saline infusion
    b. Half of the calculated fluid should be given in initial 8 hours
    c. 9 liters of Ringer's lactate should be given in first 24 hours
    d. Urine output should be maintained at 25–30 ml/hour
    e. CVP line should be inserted

47. All of the following are true regarding fluid resuscitation in burn patients except: *(MCI March 2008)*
    a. Consider intravenous resuscitation in children with burns greater than 15% TBSA
    b. Oral fluids must contain salts
    c. Most preferred fluid is Ringer's lactate
    d. Half of the calculated volume of fluid should be given in first 8 hours
48. What is the most important aspect of management of burn injury in the first 24 hours? *(UPSC 2007)*
    a. Fluid resuscitation   b. Dressing
    c. Escharotomy   d. Antibiotics
49. In excessive burns, least useful is: *(AIIMS June 94)*
    a. Blood   b. Dextran
    c. Ringer lactate   d. Nasogastric intubation
50. True statement about burn resuscitation: *(PGI Dec 2003)*
    a. Colloid preferred in initial 24 hours
    b. Colloid preferred if burnt area is >15% of total BSA
    c. Half of the calculated fluid given in initial 8 hours
    d. Urine output should be maintained at 50-60 mL/hour
    e. Diuretics should be given to all patients of electric burn
51. Which of the following is true about burns? *(PGI Dec 2005)*
    a. 3rd generation cephalosporin is drug of choice
    b. S. aureus is most common infection of burn
    c. Toxic shock syndrome is most common in burns patients
    d. Pseudomonas is most common infection in dry wound
    e. Moist dressing is done
52. Which of the following is true about burn management?
    a. Intravenous access fluid is done and antibiotics is not given in children *(PGI Dec 2005)*
    b. Escharotomy should be done for peripheral circumscribed lesion
    c. Moist dressing is done
    d. Parkland formula is used with 8 ml/kg body weight
    e. Prognosis depend on the time of resuscitation of the patient
53. Exposure treatment is done for burns of the:
    a. Upper limb   b. Lower limbs
    c. Thorax   d. Abdomen
    e. Head and neck
54. Deep skin burn is treated with: *(AIIMS 91)*
    a. Split thickness graft   b. Full thickness graft
    c. Amniotic membrane   d. Synthetic skin derivatives
55. The cold water treatment of burns has the disadvantage that it increase the chances of:
    a. Pain   b. Exudation
    c. Infection   d. None of the above
56. The best guide to adequate tissue perfusion in the fluid management of a patient with burns, is to ensure a minimum hourly urine output of: *(Karnataka 2004)*
    a. 10-30 ml   b. 30-50 ml
    c. 50-70 ml   d. 70-100 ml
57. Burns in which part of body are nursed without occlusive dressing? *(DPG 2005)*
    a. Hands   b. Legs
    c. Head and Neck   d. Chest
58. Which of the following is effected against Pseudomonas and is used in burns patients? *(DNB 2009)*
    a. Silver sulphadiazine   b. Silver sulphazine
    c. Sulphamethoxazole   d. Sulphadoxine
59. True regarding opsite dressing is: *(PGI May 2018)*
    a. Wound can be seen   b. Vapor permeable
    c. Impermeable to bacteria d. Water permeable
    e. Increased chances of maceration
60. In children with burns, maintenance IV fluid normally given is: *(MHCET 2006)*
    a. Ringer lactate   b. 5% dextrose
    c. Normal saline   d. Dextrose saline

COMPLICATIONS OF BURNS

61. Late deaths in burns is due to: *(PGI Dec 99)*
    a. Sepsis   b. Hypovolemia
    c. Contractures   d. Neurogenic
62. Most common cause of death due to burns in early period is:
    a. Sepsis   b. Hypovolemic shock
    c. Both   d. None *(APPG 2008)*
63. Most common carcinoma after burns is: *(DPG 2008)*
    a. Squamous cell carcinoma b. Adenocarcinoma
    c. Melanoma   d. Mucoid carcinoma
64. Most common cause of death in burns is: *(Punjab 2008)*
    a. Primary shock   b. Secondary shock
    c. Hemorrhagic shock   d. Septicemic shock
65. Burns shock is: *(Punjab 2011)*
    a. Hypovolemic   b. Neurogenic
    c. Endotoxic   d. Cardiogenic
66. Which of the following statement(s) is/are true about post-burn neck contracture? *(PGI June 2009)*
    a. Occur because of conservative management of deep burn
    b. Treated by flaps
    c. Obliteration of cervicomental angle
    d. Dental abnormalities may be present
    e. Never develop in deep dermal burn
67. Death from burns in first 10 days is due to all except:
    a. Shock   b. Infection *(DNB 2005)*
    c. Renal failure   d. Respiratory distress

MISCELLANEOUS

68. Domestic low-voltage electric supply can cause all the following except: *(MHPGMCET 2007)*
    a. Contact wound
    b. Cardiac arrest
    c. Cardiac fibrillation
    d. Deep subcutaneous tissue damage
69. Main danger with low tension (Domestic) electric AC current: *(MHPGMCET 2009)*
    a. Renal injury (ARF)   b. Cardiac arrest
    c. Muscle necrosis   d. Paralysis
70. Operation theatre fire is most commonly due to: *(DNB 2010)*
    a. Argon beam coagulators
    b. Lasers
    c. Fibre optic illumination
    d. Electrosurgical equipment
71. Myoglobinuria is seen in which type of burn? *(DNB 2012)*
    a. Flame burn   b. Scald burn
    c. Electric burn   d. Contact burn

Explanations

BURNS: % BSA

1. **Ans. a. 1%** *(Ref: Sabiston 20/e p507; Schwartz 10/e p227-236, 1820-1822; Bailey 27/e p621)*
2. **Ans. a. 1% BSA**
3. **Ans. a. 44%** *(Ref: Sabiston 20/e p508)*

Berkow Formula to Estimate Burn Size (%)			
Body Part	0-1 year	1-4 years	5-9 years
Head	19^Q	17^Q	13^Q
Neck	2	2	2
Anterior trunk	13	13	13
Posterior trunk	13	13	13

4. **Ans. b. Wallace**
5. **Ans. c. Lund and Browder chart** *(Ref: Schwartz 19/e p199-200)*

> "In children younger than 3 years old, the head accounts for a larger relative surface area and should be taken into account when estimating burn size. Diagrams such as the **Lund and Browder chart** give a **more accurate accounting of the true burn size in children**."- *Schwartz 10/e p199*
>
> "For children and infants, the Lund-Browder chart is used to assess the burned body surface area. Different percentages are used because the ratio of the combined surface area of the head and neck to the surface area of the limbs is typically larger in children than that of an adult." *http://en.wikipedia.org/wiki/Total_body_surface_area*

6. **Ans. c. 37** *(Ref: Sabiston 20/e p507)*
7. **Ans. b. 18%** *(Ref: Sabiston 20/e p508)*

    A Child Has
    - Circumferential burn of both of thighs = 6.5 + 6.5 = 13
    - Buttocks = 2.5 + 2.5 = 5
    - Face and scalp with singeing of hairs = 17

    Total burn = 13 + 5 + 17 = 35%

Berkow Diagram to Estimate Burn Size (%) Based on Area of Burn in an Isolated Body Part						
Body Part	0-1 yr	1-4 yr	5-9 yr	10-14 yr	15-18 yr	ADULT
Head	19	17	13	11	9	7
Neck	2	2	2	2	2	2
Anterior trunk	13	13	13	13	13	13
Posterior trunk	13	13	13	13	13	13
Right buttock	2.5	2.5	2.5	2.5	2.5	2.5
Left buttock	2.5	2.5	2.5	2.5	2.5	2.5
Genitalia	1	1	1	1	1	1
Right upper arm	4	4	4	4	4	4
Left upper arm	4	4	4	4	4	4
Right lower arm	3	3	3	3	3	3
Left lower arm	3	3	3	3	3	3
Right hand	2.5	2.5	2.5	2.5	2.5	2.5
Left hand	2.5	2.5	2.5	2.5	2.5	2.5
Right thigh	5.5	6.5	8	8.5	9	9.5
Left thigh	5.5	6.5	8	8.5	9	9.5
Right leg	5	5	5.5	6	6.5	7
Left leg	5	5	5.5	6	6.5	7
Right foot	3.5	3.5	3.5	3.5	3.5	3.5
Left foot	3.5	3.5	3.5	3.5	3.5	3.5

8. **Ans. c. Lund and Browder chart**
9. **Ans. a. 7%** *(Ref: Sabiston 20/e p508)*

BURNS

10. Ans. a. 10% superficial burn in child; b. Scald in face; c. 25% superficial burn in adult; d. 25% deep burn in adult; e. Burn in palm
    (Ref: Sabiston 19/e p521-522; Schwartz 10/e p227-236; Bailey 27/e p620)
11. Ans. c. Exposed area by evaporation *(Ref: Sabiston 20/e p508; Bailey 26/e p386-387)*
12. Ans. c. ↑secretion of HCl
13. Ans. b. 3-5 days
14. Ans. a. Septicemia; b. Due to hypermetabolism *(Ref: Total Burn Care by David N. Herndon 3/e p158; Sabiston 20/e p509; Bailey 27/e p627)*
15. Ans. c. Inner layer is zone of coagulation; d. Hyperemia is due to vasodilatation; e. Zone of stasis is associated with vascular damage: *(Ref: Sabiston 20/e p506; Schwartz 10/e p197-199; Bailey 26/e p386-387)*
16. Ans. d. Anxiety
17. Ans. a. 5% burns in children
18. Ans. a. Hyperglycemia is seen in early burns

BURNS DEPTH

19. Ans. b. 2nd degree-Epidermis + papillary dermis; c. Blisters-2nd degree; d. Curling ulcer can occur; e. Classified according to depth of invasion *(Ref: Sabiston 20/e p506-57; Schwartz 10/e p229; Bailey 26/e p389-390)*
20. Ans. b. Anesthesia at the site of burn; c. Blister formation
21. Ans. d. Peripheral pulse and circulation *(Ref: Sabiston 20e p515; Schwartz 10/e p234, 1820; Bailey 27/e p624)*

> **ESCHAROTOMIES**
>
> - When deep **second-** and **third-degree burn wounds** encompass the **circumference** of an **extremity**, **peripheral circulation** to the limb can be **compromised**[Q].
>   - Development of **generalized edema** beneath a non-yielding eschar **impedes venous outflow** and **affects arterial inflow** to the distal beds.
>   - This can be **recognized by numbness** and **tingling** in the limb and **increased pain in digits**[Q].
> - **Arterial flow** can be **assessed by determination** of **Doppler signals** in the digital arteries and the palmar and plantar arches in affected extremities.
> - **Capillary refill** can also be **assessed**.
>   - **Extremities at risk** are identified either **on clinical examination** or by measurement of **tissue pressures >40 mm Hg**[Q].
>   - These extremities **require escharotomies (release of** the **burn eschar** by **incising** the **lateral** and **medial aspects** of the extremity)[Q]

22. Ans. c. Dry white colour; d. Painless; e. Predispose to hypothermia
23. Ans. b. Deep partial thickness burns
24. Ans. d. Third degree burns
25. Ans. a. Full thickness burn feels, leathery, painless; e. 1 year of age in head and neck region covers 18% *(Ref: Bailey 27/e p622, 631; CSDT 11/e p/273)*

- **Electric burns** are both **superficial** and **deep**, depending upon the thickness involved.
- **Curreri, Sutherland and Davies formulas** are **feeding formulas of burn patients**[Q].

26. Ans. d. Extremely painful
27. Ans. b. 2 weeks
28. Ans. d. Less blanching
29. Ans. c. Blister formation; e. Can be healed within 7-10 days
30. Ans. b. 2nd degree
31. Ans. b. Superficial second degree
32. Ans. b. Dermis
33. Ans. b. Painless
34. Ans. c. Papillary dermis *(Ref: Sabiston 20/e p506; Schwartz 10/e p229; Bailey 27/e p622)*

TREATMENT OF BURNS

35. Ans. a. Percentage of burns × weight (kg) × 4 = volume in ml *(Ref: Sabiston 20/e p514; Schwartz 10/e p232; Bailey 27/e p624)*
    - **Half of fluid** is given in **first 8 hours** and **other half** in **next 16 hours**[Q]
36. Ans. b. 4 litres *(Ref: Sabiston 20/e p514; Schwartz 10/e p230; Bailey 27/e p624)*
37. Ans. b. 4 mL/kg × %TBSA *(Ref: Sabiston 20/e p514; Schwartz 10/e p230; Bailey 27/e p624)*
38. Ans. a. Paraffin gauze and dressing *(Ref: Kirk General Surgical Operations 6/e p548)*
39. Ans. b. 50% *(Ref: Sabiston 20/e p514; Schwartz 10/e p230; Bailey 27/e p624)*

40. **Ans. a. Total % body surface area x weight x 4 = volume in ml**
41. **Ans. c. Shrine: 5000 ml m² TBSA burn + 2000 ml m² TBSA; d. Evans: 8ml Kg/% TBSA burn of RL**
42. **Ans. a. No bandage to head and neck; c. Superficial burns without blister-no need of dressing; d. Escharotomy done for peripheral circumscribed lesions** *(Ref: Sabiston 20/e p513; Schwartz 10/e p200-204; Bailey 27/e p624)*

Management of Burn Wound

Exposure Method
- **No dressings** are applied **over wound**^{Q} after application of the agent to the wound 2-3 times a day
- Used for **face** and **head**^{Q}
- Disadvantages:
  - Increased **pain, heat loss**^{Q}
  - Risk of **cross-contamination**^{Q}

Closed Method
- **Occlusive dressing** is applied over the agent and changed twice daily^Q
- Generally **closed method** is **preferred**^{Q}
- Advantages:
  - Less pain, less heat loss^Q
  - Less risk of cross contamination^Q
- Disadvantages:
  - Potential **increase in bacterial growth**^{Q} if dressing is not changed twice daily.

43. **Ans. d. 14-15°C**
44. **Ans. d. Elective endotracheal intubation** *(Ref: Bailey 27/e p620)*

INITIAL MANAGEMENT OF THE BURNED AIRWAY
- **Early elective intubation** is **safest**^{Q}
- **Delay** can make **intubation very difficult** because of **swelling**^{Q}
- Be ready to **perform an emergency cricothyroidotomy** if **intubation is delayed**^{Q}

45. **Ans. c. Ringer lactate**
46. **Ans. b. Half of the calculated fluid should be given in initial 8 hours; c. 9 liters of Ringer's lactate should be given in first 24 hours; e. CVP line should be inserted**
47. **Ans. a. Consider intravenous resuscitation in children with burns greater than 15% TBSA**
    - **IV fluid resuscitation:** In **children** with burn **>10%** TBSA and **adult** with burn **>15%** TBSA
48. **Ans. a. Fluid resuscitation**
49. **Ans. a. Blood** *(Ref: Sabiston 20/e p514; Schwartz 10/e p230; Bailey 27/e p624)*

- **RL is preferred agent for resuscitation** for the initial 24 hours^Q.
- **Nasogastric intubation** is done to **decrease the risk of emesis** and **possible aspiration** (as paralytic ileus develops in the patients of burn).
- **Dextran** is a **colloid** and **can be used after 24 hours** however, **albumin** is the **preferred** and **most widely used colloid**^{Q}.

50. **Ans. c. Half of the calculated fluid given in initial 8 hours; d. Urine output should be maintained at 50-60 mL/hour**
51. **Ans. d. Pseudomonas is most common infection in dry wound** *(Ref: Sabiston 20/e p516; Schwartz 10/e p202; Bailey 27/e p625)*

- In **burn management, topical antimicrobials** are used.
- **Pseudomonas** is the **most common infection**^{Q} in burn patients. It has replaced streptococci and staphylococci because of availability of good antibiotics.
- **Toxic shock syndrome** is most commonly associated with **tampon use** in **menstruating females**. It is caused by **Staphylococcus** infection producing **TSST-1.**
- **Damp dressing** should **not be used.**

52. **Ans. b. Escharotomy should be done for peripheral circumscribed lesion; e. Prognosis depend on the time of resuscitation of the patient**
53. **Ans. e. Head and neck**
54. **Ans. a. Split thickness graft**
55. **Ans. c. Infection** *(Ref: CSDT 11/e p1272)*
56. **Ans. b. 30-50 ml**
57. **Ans. c. Head and Neck**
58. **Ans. a. Silver sulphadiazine**
59. **Ans. a. Wound can be seen, b. Vapor permeable, c. Impermeable to bacteria** *(Ref: Sabiston 20/e p517)*

"*OpSite Dressing: Provides a moisture barrier; inexpensive; decreased wound pain; use complicated by transudate and exudate requiring removal; no antimicrobial properties*"- Sabiston 20/e p517

60. Ans. d. Dextrose saline

COMPLICATIONS OF BURNS

61. **Ans. a. Sepsis** *(Ref: Sabiston 20/e p516; Schwartz 10/e p233; Bailey 26/e p394-395)*
    - Following successful resuscitation, most acute morbidity and virtually all mortality in severely burned patients are related to infection[Q].
    - This is because thermal injury causes profound immunosuppression that is proportional to the TBSA of the burn[Q].
    - Inspite of burn patients at significant risk to infection, prophylactic systemic antibiotics are not part of modern care, as they do not reduce septic complications and only lead to increased bacterial resistance[Q].

    - MC cause of **death at the site of burn: Asphyxia**[Q]
    - MC cause of **death in burns: Septicemia**[Q]
    - MC cause of **early death in burns: Hypovolemic shock**[Q]
    - MC cause of **late death in burns: Septicemia**[Q]

62. Ans. b. Hypovolemic shock
63. Ans. a. Squamous cell carcinoma
64. Ans. d. Septicemic shock

CARCINOMA IN BURNS
- **Squamous cell carcinoma** is MC carcinoma in burns[Q].
- SCC commonly occurs in **long standing (Marjolin's ulcer), old scar** or **keloid**[Q].
- Both **Marjolin's ulcer** and **keloid** are **complications** that arise **after burns**[Q].

65. **Ans. a. Hypovolemic** *(Ref: Sabiston 20e p514; Schwartz 10/e p204; Bailey 27/e p618-619)*
    - **Proper fluid management** is **critical to survival**[Q] in burn patient.
    - The **hypovolemic shock**[Q] in burn patient is special in the sense that total body water remains unchanged in a burn patient.
    - The **thermal injury** leads to a **massive shift from** the **intravascular compartment** to the **extravascular compartment** leading to **edema formation**[Q].

66. **Ans. a. Occur because of conservative management of deep burn; b. Treated by flaps; c. Obliteration of cervicomental angle; d. Dental abnormalities may be present** *(Ref: Total Burn Care by David N. Herndon 3/e p714-715; Sabiston 19/e p534-535; Schwartz 10/e p182; Bailey 27/e p628)*

67. Ans. c. Renal failure

MISCELLANEOUS

68. **Ans. d. Deep subcutaneous tissue damage** *(Ref: Bailey 27/e p631)*
69. Ans. b. Cardiac arrest
70. **Ans. d. Electrosurgical equipment** *(Ref: British Journal of Anesthesia, vol 50, Issue 7, Page 659-664)*

OPERATION THEATRE FIRE
- The **two most common source of operation theatre fire** is **electrosurgical unit (ESU)** and **lasers**.
- ECRI's analysis of case reports show that the **most common ignition sources** are **electrosurgical instruments (68%)** and **lasers (13%)**.
- **Most common fire location is airway (35%),** head or face (28%), and elsewhere on or inside the patient (38%).
- An oxygen-enriched atmosphere was a contribution factor in 74% of all cases.

71. Ans. c. Electric burn

CHAPTER 31
Plastic Surgery and Skin Lesions

GRAFT TAKE

Graft Take

- Skin graft take occurs in three phases, imbibition, inosculation, & revascularization.

Plasma Imbibition	Inosculation	Revascularization
• Graft survives up to **first 48 hours**[Q] because of plasma imbibition • Involves **free absorption of nutrients** into the graft	• **Donor** and **recipient capillaries are aligned** during inosculation[Q] • Inosculation **completes by 4–5 days**[Q]	• **After 5 days**[Q], revascularization occurs • Graft demonstrates **both arterial and venous outflow**[Q]

- During these initial few days the graft is most susceptible to deleterious factors such as **infection, mechanical shear forces and hematoma or seroma**[Q].

SKIN GRAFT

Partial Thickness (Thiersch) or Split Skin Graft

- Consist of **epidermis & variable portion of dermis**[Q]
- **Large size of graft can be taken**[Q]
- **Site: Thigh (MC)**[Q] upper arm, flexor aspect of forearm and abdominal wall
- Grafts are **hairless** and **do not sweat**[Q] (these structures are not transferred)

  - Skin graft must be **applied to a well-vascularized recipient wound bed**. It will **not adhere to exposed bone, cartilage, or tendon** devoid of periosteum, perichondrium, or peritenon, respectively, or devoid of its vascularized perimembranous envelope.

- MC causes of **skin graft failure: Hematoma** (or seroma), **infection**, & **movement** (shear).
- **Pie crusting: Stab incisions** in the graft preemptively **to create small outlets for fluid to drain** from beneath the graft

  - **Beta hemolytic Streptococci** can **destroy split skin grafts completely, presence** of this organism is a **contraindication** to grafting[Q].

- **Graft immobilization is critical to the graft take** and can be accomplished with bolster dressing, light compression wraps or a vacuum assisted closure device.

Skin Grafts

Partial Thickness (Thiersch) Graft	Full Thickness (Wolfes) Graft
• It includes **all epidermis & part of dermis**[Q]. • Partial thickness **grafts are thin, uptake of graft is easy (easy survival)**[Q]. • **Large grafts could be taken** as the donor site is left with a **part of dermis** which will cause **easy regeneration of epidermis**[Q]. • **Contract upto 40%**, not useful for **cosmetic surgeries**[Q]. • **Donor site** will **heal well**[Q] without any contraction, and is reusable.	• It includes **all epidermis & dermis**[Q]. • **Uptake is difficult** because of thickness • Less chances of survival • **Small grafts** could be **taken**[Q] as the donor site does not have epidermal or dermal remnants to allow epithelialization • **Very minimal contraction** making it **suitable** for **cosmetic surgeries** on **face**[Q]. • **Donor site** will have to be **closed primarily** or **left open to granulate** and **contract**[Q].

Contraction of Graft
- **Primary:** Occurs when the graft is harvested, **depends upon** amount of **dermis** present, **more in full thickness graft**
- **Secondary:** Occurs after the surgery, **more in partial thickness graft**

MESHED SKIN GRAFTS

Meshed Skin Grafts

- **Split grafts** may be **meshed to expand** the **surface area** that can be covered^Q.
- This technique is **particularly useful** when a **large area must be resurfaced**, as **in major burns**.

> - **Meshed grafts** usually also have **enhanced reliability of engraftment**, because the **fenestrations allow for egress of wound fluid** and **excellent contour matching** of the wound bed by the graft^Q.

- **Fenestrations** in meshed grafts **re-epithelialize by secondary intention** from the surrounding graft skin.

> - **Major drawbacks** of meshed grafts are **poor cosmetic appearance** and **high secondary contraction**^Q.

- **Meshing ratios** used usually range from **1:1.5 to 1:6**, with higher ratios associated with magnified drawbacks.

PEDICEL GRAFT OR FLAP

Pedicel Graft or Flap

- **Flap: Partially** or **completely isolated segment** of tissue with its **own blood supply**^Q

Absolute Indications for Flaps	
• **Exposed bone**^Q	• **Open joint** or **non-biological**^Q **implant materials**^Q
• **Radiated vessel**^Q	• **Pressure sores** at bony prominences
• **Brain**^Q	

For **critical** and **small areas** such as an **eyelid**, a **full thickness graft** is selected, so that contraction of the grafted material is minimum.

Type of Flaps on the basis of source of Vascular Supply

Random	Axial	Free
• Random flaps **rely on** the **low perfusion pressures** found in **subdermal plexus**^Q to sustain the flap • Used to **reconstruct relatively small, full-thickness defects** that are not amenable to skin grafting.	• Axial flap is **based on** a **named blood vessel**^Q • Provide a **reproducible** and **stable skin** or **skin-muscle (myocutaneous) flap**^Q. • Can be used to provide much needed length and bulk • **Axial flap** that **remains attached to its proximal blood supply** and **transposed to a defect** is known as a **pedicled flap**^Q.	• **Autogenous transplantation**^Q of vascularized tissues. • **Complete detachment** of the **flap**, with **devascularization**, from the **donor site**^Q • **Revascularization** of the flap with **anastomoses to blood vessels** in the **recipient site**^Q

MARJOLIN'S ULCER

Marjolin's Ulcer

- **Low grade SCC**^Q, which develops on a **chronic benign ulcer** or a **long standing scar** tissue.
- **Arises from** the **edge**^Q of the ulcer

Marjolin's ulcer may develop in	
• **Post burn scar**^Q	• Chronically **discharging osteomyelitis sinus**^Q
• Long standing **venous ulcer**^Q	
• **Chronic ulcer**^Q due to trauma	• **Post-radiation ulcer**

Characteristic Features

- **Slow growing**^Q as scar tissue is **relatively avascular**
- **Painless** as there **no nerves in** the **scar tissue**^Q
- **No secondary deposits**^Q in regional lymph node, as there are **no lymphatic vessels** in scar tissue
- If the ulcer invades the normal tissue, then only lymph node may be involved by lymphatic spread
- **Radioresistant**^Q due to **avascularity**

Diagnosis

- IOC for diagnosis: **Biopsy**^Q

Treatment

- Wide local excision followed by flap cover^Q
- **Radiotherapy is avoided**^Q

BOWEN'S DISEASE

Bowen's Disease

- This is an **SCC in situ**^{Q}, of which 3–11% progress to SCC.
- **Etiological agents:** Chronic solar damage, inorganic arsenic and **HPV16**^{Q}
- This is rare, **slow-growing intraepidermal SCC** that often **mimics a chronic dermatosis**^{Q}.
- It should now be considered as a **form of AIN III** (Anal intraepithelial neoplasia).

Clinical Features
- It usually **presents with pruritus**^{Q} and on examination looks like **psoriasis** or **senile keratosis**.
- Presents as a **slowly enlarging, erythematous, scaly patch** or **plaque**^{Q}.

Treatment
- **Topical therapy** with **5-fluorouracil** or **imiquimod** is an effective treatment^Q.
- Alternatives: **Surgical excision** with a 4-mm margin or **Mohs' micrographic surgery**^{Q} for larger or recurrent lesions.

BASAL CELL CARCINOMA (RODENT ULCER)

Basal Cell Carcinoma (Rodent Ulcer)

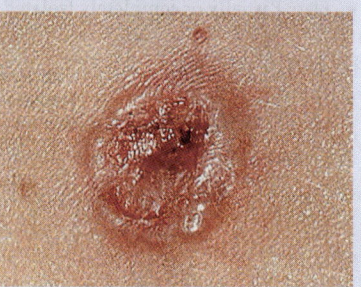

- **Locally invasive** carcinoma, **arises from** the **basal layer**^{Q} of the epidermis
- **MC type of skin cancer**^{Q}
- **90%** of **BCC** are seen **in the face**^{Q}, above a **line from** the **corner of mouth to lobule of ear**.
- **MC site: Nose >Inner canthus**^{Q} of the eye, also known as **Tear cancer**^{Q}.

Types of BCC
- **Nodular: MC type of BCC**^{Q}, characterized by small slow growing **pearly nodules**, often with **telangiectatic vessels** on its surface. **Central depression** with **umbilication**^{Q} is a classic sign.
- **Pigmented:** Mimic malignant melanoma
- **Cystic**
- **Superficial**

Characteristic Features of BCC	
• Low grade malignancy^Q • More common in fair and dry skinned people • Nuclear palisading^Q on histology	• Exposure to sunlight^Q is an important etiological factor • Has been seen following prolonged administration of Arsenic^Q

Spread
- BCC usually spreads by **local invasion**^{Q}, rarely metastasizes
- **Rodent ulcer:** It gradually **destroys the tissues**, it comes **in contact with**.
- **Lymphatic spread** is **not seen**^{Q} (Regional lymph nodes are not enlarged)
- Blood spread is extremely rare.

Diagnosis
- Diagnostic procedure for BCC is **wedge biopsy**^{Q}.

Treatment
- **Non-aggressive tumor** on **trunk** or **extremities**: Excision or electrodissection and curettage^Q
- **Large, aggressive,** located at **vital areas** or recurrent: Moh's micrographic surgery^Q

SQUAMOUS CELL CARCINOMA (EPITHELIOMA OR EPIDERMOID CARCINOMA)

Squamous Cell Carcinoma (Epithelioma or Epidermoid Carcinoma)

- It is a carcinoma of the cells of epidermis that usually migrate outwards to the surface.
- Originate from **prickle cell layer**^{Q}; Seen in > 40 years of age

• MC skin cancer in darkly pigmented races^Q
• 2nd MC skin cancer in light skinned races^Q
• MC causative factor: Sunlight^Q
• MC site: Ears, cheeks, lower lip and back of hands^Q

Predisposing Factors for SCC	
• Senile or **actinic keratosis**[Q]	• Contact with **tars** and **hydrocarbons**[Q]
• Chronic skin lesions (**lupus vulgaris**[Q], cutaneous TB)	• **Erythroplasia of Queyrat**[Q]
• **Sunlight** or **irradiation**[Q]	• **Immunosuppression**[Q]
• Chronic irritation; **HIV, HPV-16**[Q]	• **Psoralens, Arsenic exposure**[Q]

Pathology
- Microscopically mass of keratin is surrounded by normal looking squamous cells, presenting with characteristic **prickle cell appearance**[Q], which are arranged in concentric manner as seen in '**onion skin**'. This whole appearance is called "**cell nest** or **epithelial pearl**[Q]".
- MC type of SCC: Ulcerative type[Q]

Clinical Features
- MC symptom: **Nodule** or **ulcer**[Q]
- **Edge** of ulcer: **Raised** and **everted** with **indurated base (pathognomonic)**[Q]

Diagnosis
- Diagnosis is made by **wedge biopsy**[Q] (taken from **edge of ulcer**)

Treatment
- **Small (< 1 cm)** or **non-invasive** SCC: Excision with **1 cm margin**[Q]
- **Large, aggressive**, located at **vital areas** or **recurrent**: Moh's micrographic surgery[Q]

MOH'S MICROGRAPHIC SURGERY FOR SCC AND BCC

Moh's Micrographic Surgery for SCC and BCC

- **Mohs' technique** uses **serial excision** in small increments coupled with **immediate microscopic analysis to ensure tumor removal**, yet limit resection of aesthetically valuable tissue[Q].
- **Advantage**: All specimen margins are evaluated[Q].

> - **Major benefit**: Ability to remove a tumor with **minimal sacrifice** of **uninvolved tissue**[Q].
> - **Particular value** in managing tumors of the **eyelid, nose**, or **cheek**[Q]
> - Indicated in **large, aggressive tumors** located at **vital areas** or **recurrent tumors**[Q]

- **Major drawback**: **Procedure length** (Total lesion excision may require multiple attempts at resection, and many procedures may be carried out over several days)
- **Recurrence & metastases** rates are **comparable to** those of **wide local excision**[Q].

MALIGNANT MELANOMA

Malignant Melanoma

- Melanoma is neoplastic disorder produced by **malignant transformation of normal melanocytes**[Q].

> - **Site most commonly associated** with melanocytic transformation in the skin, where **melanocytes reside at the dermo-epidermal junction (Junctional melanocytes)**[Q].
> - **MC site of MM in men**: Back & trunk[Q]
> - **MC site of MM in women**: Lower extremity[Q]

- **Most susceptible individuals**: Fair complexions, red or **blonde hair, blue eyes** and **freckles** and who **tan poorly** and **sunburn easily**.
- MM is positive for **S-100, HMB-45, vimentin** but **negative for cytokeratin-20**[Q].

Risk factors for Malignant Melanoma	
• **Xeroderma pigmentosum**[Q]	• **Giant** congenital melanocytic nevus
• **Actinic damage (UVR)**[Q]	
• **Family history** of melanoma[Q]	• **Increased number** of ordinary melanocytic naevi
• Presence of **dysplastic naevus**[Q]	• **History** of sunburn[Q]

Types of Malignant Melanoma: (In order of decreasing frequency)	
Superficial spreading	• MC type of MM^Q • MC site: Torso
Nodular	• Most malignant^Q • MC site: Head, neck and **trunk** • Vertical growth phase only
Lentigo maligna	• Least malignant^Q • MC site: Face
Acral lentiginous	• Least common, worst prognosis^Q, • MC site: Sole, under great toe nail

Characteristic Features

- Classic appearance of melanoma: **ABCD** (**A**symmetry, **B**order irregularity, **C**olor variation, **D**iameter >6 mm)^Q
- MC route of metastasis: Through **Lymphatics**^{Q}
- MC site of systemic metastasis: **Liver**^{Q}
- Other common visceral sites of metastasis: Lung, brain, GIT (small intestine), bone, adrenal.

> • **Microsatellites:** Discrete tumor nests > 0.05 mm in diameter, **separated from main body of tumor by normal dermal collagen** or **subcutaneous fat**^{Q}.
> • **Microsatellites** are associated with **increased risk** of **regional LN metastasis**^{Q}.

Diagnosis

- Confirmed by **'full thickness excisional biopsy'**^{Q}
- Incisional biopsy for large lesions and lesions in proximity to important structures (eye, nose, ear)

Treatment

- Treatment: **Surgical excision**^{Q} with **sentinel LN biopsy** (Margin: **1 cm** for < 1 mm thickness, **2 cm** for **1–4 mm** thickness, **2–3 cm** for **> 4 mm** thickness)
- **LN dissection** if LN is palpable or positive on sentinel LN biopsy
- MM is **radioresistant tumor; Chemotherapy: IFN-alpha 2b**

Clark's levels^Q (on the basis of depth of invasion): EPIRS	
I	• Melanoma restricting to **Epidermis** and appendages^Q
II	• Invading **Papillary dermis** without filling it^Q
III	• Reach **Interface** of papillary and reticular dermis^Q
IV	• Invading **reticular dermis**^{Q}
V	• Invading **subcutaneous tissue**^{Q}

- MM is **sub-classified into 5 Clark levels**, to indicate their **depth of invasion** and **prognosis**^{Q}.
- **Breslow's depth of invasion:** Actual measurement of the deepest invasion from the granular layer^Q.

Breslow's Thickness	
Stage I	• < 0.75 mm^Q
Stage II	• 0.75–1.5 mm^Q
Stage III	• 1.6–4.0 mm^Q
Stage IV	• > 4.0 mm^Q

Prognostic Factors (**Depends** most importantly **on staging**^{Q})	
• **Depth of invasion** (most important prognostic factor)^Q • **Ulceration**^{Q} (presence of ulceration carries worst prognosis)	• **Lymph node status**^{Q} • **Satellite lesion**^{Q} • **Distant metastasis**^{Q}

VASCULAR ANOMALIES

Vascular Anomalies

Port-wine Stain
- A vascular malformation
- **Present at birth**[Q]
- **Grows along with** the **child**[Q]
- **Do not regress**[Q]
- **Face involvement** in areas supplied by **5th cranial nerve**[Q]

Strawberry Angiomas
- Type of **capillary hemangioma**
- **Baby** is **normal at birth**[Q]
- **Appears at** the age of **1–3 weeks**[Q]
- **Grows with** the **child upto 1 year** of age and then cease to grow[Q]
- By the age of **9 years, 90%** demonstrate **complete involution**[Q]
- **Emptying sign**[Q] is demonstrable

Salmon Patch
- Also known as **Macular stain** or **stork bite**[Q]
- **Present at birth**[Q]
- Seen over **forehead in** the **midline** and **over** the **occiput**[Q]
- **Disappears by** the age **1 year**[Q]

HEMANGIOMA

- Benign, abnormally dense collections of dilated small blood vessels
- Occurs in the skin or internal organs
- Hemangioma is a compressible swelling

- **Calcification** is seen **in congenital hemangioma** and **GLUT-1** is **negative**[Q]

Clinical Types of Hemangioma

According to Depth of Invasion
- **Capillary hemangioma:**
  - **Best cosmetic results** obtained **by laser ablation**[Q]
- **Cavernous hemangioma**

According to Rate of Involution
- Rapidly Involuting Congenital Hemangioma (**RICH**):
  - **Grow** at a **rapid rate for 4–6 months,** then growth ceases[Q]
  - **Spontaneous involution** begin and **completed by 5–7 years** of age[Q]
- Non-Involuting Congenital Hemangioma (**NICH**):
  - Mostly **present at birth**[Q]
  - Undergo **rapid growth** during **first 4–6 months**[Q]
  - **Grow in proportion to** the **growth of the child**[Q]

Treatment
- Treatment of hemangiomas: Observation with reassurance[Q] of parents that regression and involution will occur.
- Local wound care, topical application of lidocaine for pain and laser cauterization may be beneficial treatment modalities.

- **Laser therapy** has been **effective in lightening affected skin**[Q]

EPIDERMOID CYST (SEBACEOUS OR EPIDERMAL CYST)

EPIDERMOID CYST (SEBACEOUS OR EPIDERMAL CYST)

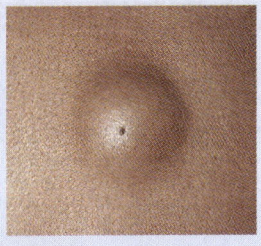

- Epidermoid cyst results from **proliferation of epidermal cells** within a circumscribed space of dermis (which had got **implanted within the dermis**[Q])
- **Sebaceous cyst** is a **misnomer** as the cysts are **not of sebaceous origin** and the **white creamy material** filled within is not sebum, but is **keratin (desquamated epithelial cells**[Q])
- **Type of retention cyst** (secretions are pent up in a gland owing to blockage of the duct)

Pathology
- **Cyst wall** consist of a **layer of epidermis** oriented with the basal layer superficial and more matured layers are deep.
- **Desquamated cells (keratin)** collect in the centre and form creamy substance of the cyst.

Clinical Features
- **Usually asymptomatic**[Q], unless get infected or inflamed and become painful
- **Firm, round, flesh colored** to yellow or white subcutaneous nodules of variable size.

- **Central punctum**^{Q} may teether the cyst to the overlying epidermis, from which the white creamy material can be expressed.
- **Rarely malignancies**^{Q} **(BCC, SCC)** can develop in epidermoid cyst.

> - **No punctum** in **scrotal** and **scalp sebaceous cyst**^{Q}.

Treatment

- **Excision with** the **wall** is treatment of choice^Q.
- **Infected cyst: Incision and drainage** (After resolution of the abscess, **cyst wall** must be **excised to prevent recurrence**)^Q

LIPOMA

Lipoma

- MC subcutaneous neoplasm: **Lipomas**^{Q}
- MC site: **Trunk**^{Q} (may appear anywhere)
- Also known as **universal tumor**^{Q}
- Can be **encapsulated** or **diffuse**
- Other sites: Subcutaneous, Subfascial, subsynovial, intra-articular, intramuscular, subserous, submucous, CNS, intraglandular and reteroperitoneal

Pathology

- **Lobulated tumor** composed of **normal fat cells**

Clinical Features

- Typically **soft** and **fleshy** on palpation
- May grow to a **large size** and become substantially deforming.

> - **Bracket calcification** is seen in lipoma of corpus callosum^Q

Treatment

- **Surgical excision**^{Q} is required for tumor removal

ADIPOSIS DOLOROSA (DERCUM'S DISEASE)

Adiposis Dolorosa (Dercum's Disease)

- A **rare condition** characterized by **multiple, painful lipomas**^{Q}.
- These lipomas **mainly occur on** the **trunk, upper arms** and upper legs.
- Mostly occur between **35–50 years,** more common in **women**

Clinical Features

- **Multiple lipomas** and **neuropathic pain** are the **cardinal symptoms**^{Q}

Treatment

- Treatment is usually targeted towards **pain relief**^{Q} rather than lipoma removal.

RETROPERITONEAL LIPOMA

Retroperitoneal Lipoma

- These swellings sometimes reach an **immense size**^{Q}.
- Retroperitoneal lipoma is often malignant (liposarcoma) and **may increase rapidly in size**^{Q}.

> - A **retroperitoneal lipoma** sometimes undergoes **myxomatous degeneration**^{Q}
> - A complication that **does not occur in** a lipoma in any other part of the **body**^{Q}

Clinical Features

- Swelling or **indefinite abdominal pain**
- More common in **women**

Diagnosis

- Diagnosis is usually by ultrasound and **CT scanning**.

HIDRADENITIS SUPPURATIVA

HIDRADENITIS SUPPURATIVA

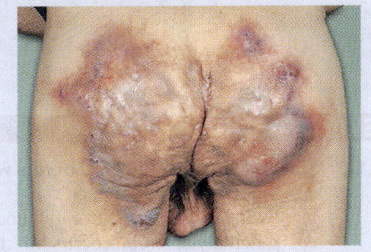

- Hidradenitis suppurativa is a **defect** of the **terminal follicular epithelium**[Q]
- Follicular defect **results in apocrine gland blockage, obstructed infection** leads to **abscess formation** throughout affected **axillary**[Q], **inguinal**[Q] and **perianal regions**[Q].
- Following spontaneous rupture of these localized collections, **foul-smelling sinuses** form and **repeated infections** create a **wide area of inflamed, painful tissue**[Q].

Treatment
- **Acute infections:** Application of **warm compresses, antibiotics** and **open drainage**[Q]
- **Chronic Hidradenitis:** Wide excision and **skin grafting**[Q]

KERATOACANTHOMA

KERATOACANTHOMA

- Keratoacanthoma is **self healing nodular lesion** with **central ulceration**[Q]
- More common in **men**, usually found **on the face** of 50–70 years old.
- Lesions can **grow to 1–3 cm over 6 weeks** and typically **resolve spontaneously** over the **subsequent 6 months**[Q].

Etiopathogenesis
- Classically a **cup-shaped growth** that exhibits symmetry about its middle.
- **Central crater** is **filled with a plug of keratin**[Q].
- **Unclear etiology** (may be caused by **HPV infecting a hair follicle**)
- Associated with smoking and **chemical carcinogen exposure**.

Treatment
- **Removal of central keratin plug** may **speed resolution**[Q].
- **Excision** is recommended **for persistent lesions**[Q]
- **Excision scar** is often **better** than that which remains after resolution.

Cocks Peculiar Tumour	• Infected or ulcerated sebaceous cyst of the scalp[Q] • Resembles fungating epithelioma[Q]
Potts Puffy Tumour	• Osteomyelitis of the Frontal bone of skull[Q] • Associated with subperiosteal swelling & edema[Q]
Pilomatrixoma	• Also known as Calcifying epithelioma of Malherbe[Q] • Benign hair follicle derived tumor[Q]
Cylindroma	• A malignant epithelial tumour also known as Turban tumor[Q] • Known as cylindroma because of histological appearance

Multiple Choice Questions

SKIN GRAFTING

1. 'Take in' of split skin graft occurs when? *(PGI Dec 2008)*
   a. Tight dressing is applied
   b. Excessive discharge from wound
   c. β-hemolytic streptococcus infection is present
   d. Wound bed not vascularised

2. Thiersch graft is which type of graft?
   (JIPMER 2012, MHPGMCET 2008, 2001, DPG 2005)
   a. Partial thickness b. Full thickness
   c. Pedicle d. Patch

3. Which of the following statements about mesh skin grafts is not correct? *(UPSC 2006)*
   a. They permit coverage of large areas
   b. They allow egress of fluid collections under the graft
   c. They contract to the same degree as a grafted sheet of skin
   d. They "take" satisfactorily on a granulating bed

4. Split skin grafts in young children should be harvested from: *(UPSC 2007)*
   a. Buttocks b. Thigh
   c. Trunk d. Upper limb

5. Which of the following is not a wound closure technique? *(UPSC 2008)*
   a. Partial thickness skin graft
   b. Composite graft
   c. Vascular graft
   d. Musculocutaneous graft

6. Who said: "Skin is the best dressing"? *(Karnataka 2004)*
   a. Joseph Lister b. John Hunter
   c. James Paget d. Mc Neill Love

7. Within 48 hours of transplantation, skin graft survives due to: *(AIIMS Nov 2000, AIIMS Nov 99)*
   a. Amount of saline in graft
   b. Plasma imbibition
   c. New vessels growing from the donor tissue
   d. Connection between donor and recipient capillaries

8. Ideal graft for leg injury with 10 × 10 cm exposed bone: *(AIIMS Nov 99)*
   a. Amniotic membrane graft
   b. Pedicle graft
   c. Full thickness graft
   d. Split thickness skin graft

9. Wolfe Graft is: *(APPG 2015)*
   a. Thin split thickness graft
   b. Thick split thickness skin graft
   c. Medium thickness split thickness skin graft
   d. Full thickness skin graft

10. Skin grafting is absolutely contraindicated in which skin infection? *(AIIMS June 97)*
    a. Staphylococcus b. Pseudomonas
    c. Streptococcus d. Proteus

11. What does "Take in" means in case of skin grafting?
    a. Revascularization of the graft *(AIIMS June 97)*
    b. Return of the sensation
    c. When the graft becomes adherent to recipient site
    d. Non adherent graft is shed off

12. All can take split thickness graft except:
    (MCI March 2005, AIIMS Sept 96)
    a. Fat b. Muscle
    c. Skull bone d. Deep fascia

13. All are true about skin grafting, except: *(All India 2000)*
    a. Partial thickness graft involves epidermis and part of dermis
    b. Full thickness graft includes epidermis, dermis, without subcutaneous tissue
    c. For large areas, full thickness graft is used
    d. Full thickness graft has cosmetic value

14. The given instrument is used for harvesting the graft from healthy area in split skin thickness graft:

    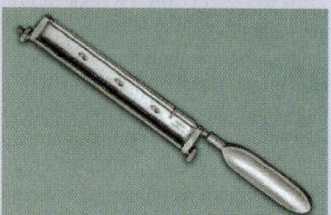

    a. Dermatome b. Silver's knife
    c. Catlin amputating knife d. Humby knife

15. Split skin graft can be applied over: *(PGI June 99)*
    a. Muscle b. Bone
    c. Cartilage d. Eyelid

16. Skin graft for facial wounds is taken from: *(AIIMS 92)*
    a. Medial aspect of thigh b. Cubital fossa
    c. Groin d. Postauricular region

17. Full thickness skin graft can be taken from the following sites except: *(AIIMS 87)*
    a. Elbow b. Back to neck
    c. Supraclavicular area d. Upper eyelids

18. Skin graft stored at 4°C can survive up to: *(DNB 2009)*
    a. 1 week b. 2 weeks
    c. 3 weeks d. 4 weeks

19. The best skin graft for open wounds is: *(All India 93)*
    a. Isograft b. Homograft
    c. Allograft d. Autograft

20. All are advantages of split thickness skin grafting except:
    a. Good uptake *(Recent Question 2013)*
    b. Reusable donor site
    c. Less contraction
    d. Large grafts can be harvested

21. Identify the correct statement regarding skin grafts & flaps: *(APPG 2016)*
    a. Grafts are tissues that are transferred without their blood supply and they revascularise at the new site
    b. In pedicle flaps, various tissues, often with bone or muscle, are transferred
    c. Full thickness grafts are useful for rebuilding missing elements of nose etc.
    d. Split thickness grafts have limited durability and are called Wolfe grafts

FLAPS

22. **True statement for axial flap is:** *(All India 97)*
    a. Carries its own vessels within it
    b. Kept in limb
    c. Transverse flap
    d. Carries its own nerve in it

23. **Best procedure to be done after an injury to leg associated with exposure of underlying bone and skin loss:** *(AIIMS Nov 98)*
    a. Pedicle flap
    b. Split skin grafting
    c. Full thickness grafting
    d. Skin flap

24. **Skin flap is used in all except:**
    a. Bone
    b. Tendon
    c. Burn wound
    d. Cartilage

25. **The subdermal plexus forms the vascular basis for:** *(JIPMER 2002)*
    a. Randomised flaps
    b. Axial flaps
    c. Mucocutaneous flaps
    d. Fasciocutaneous flaps

26. **Myocutaneous flap includes which tissues?** *(DPG 2007)*
    a. Muscle only
    b. Muscle and vascular pedicle
    c. Muscle and skin
    d. Skin, muscle and vascular pedicle

27. **Best heal flap is:** *(Recent Question 2017)*
    a. Medial plantar artery flap
    b. Lateral plantar artery flap
    c. Reversed sural artery flap
    d. Anterolateral thigh flap

28. **A 3-6 cm scalp defect is closed by:** *(Recent Question 2017)*
    a. Primary simple closure
    b. Split skin grafting
    c. Secondary closure
    d. Local flaps

29. **In the patient as shown below, chest wall closure has been achieved by using which flap?** *(AIIMS May 2017)*

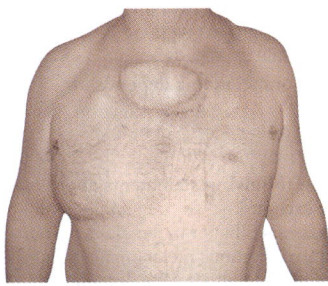

    a. Transversely oriented rectus abdominis muscle flap
    b. Vertically oriented rectus abdominis muscle flap
    c. Pectoralis major myocutaneous flap
    d. Serratus anterior muscle flap

30. **Split thickness skin graft is not taken up by:** *(MCI June 2018)*
    a. Fat
    b. Muscle
    c. Deep fascia
    d. Skull bone

MARJOLIN'S ULCER

31. **The most common malignancy found in Marjolin's ulcer is:** *(MCI June 2018, DPG 2009 Feb)*
    a. Basal cell carcinoma
    b. Squamous cell carcinoma
    c. Malignant fibrous histiocytoma
    d. Neutrophic malignant melanoma

32. **True about Marjolin's ulcer:** *(PGI June 2007)*
    a. The associated cancer is squamous cell carcinoma
    b. May occur due to chronic venous insufficiency
    c. Progress to basal cell carcinoma
    d. Arise from base of the ulcer

33. **A tumour arising in a burns scar is likely to be:** *(Recent Question 2014, COMEDK 2009, PGI June 2006, June 97)*
    a. Basal cell carcinoma
    b. Squamous cell carcinoma
    c. Malignant melanoma
    d. Fibrosarcoma

34. **Which of the following is true about Marjolin's ulcer?** *(Orissa 2011, PGI Dec 97)*
    a. Ulcer over scar
    b. Rapid growth
    c. Rodent ulcer
    d. Painful

PREMALIGNANT LESIONS OF SKIN

35. **Bowen's disease is:** *(DPG 2005)*
    a. Mimics chronic dermatosis
    b. Premalignant condition
    c. Presents with pruritus
    d. All of the above

36. **All the following are premalignant conditions except:** *(MHSSMCET 2008)*
    a. Actinic Keratosis
    b. Steatoma multiplex
    c. Erythroplakia of Queyrat
    d. Keratosis of lip

SQUAMOUS CELL CARCINOMA

37. **Squamous cell carcinoma can arise from:**
    a. Long standing venous ulcers
    b. Chronic lupus vulgaris
    c. Rodent ulcer
    d. All of the above

38. **Margins of squamous cell carcinoma is:** *(Recent Question 2016)*
    a. Inverted
    b. Everted
    c. Rolled
    d. Undermined

39. **Buschke-Lowenstein tumor is:** *(TN 2003)*
    a. Molluscum contagiosum
    b. Condyloma lata
    c. Giant condyloma accuminata
    d. Metastasis

40. **Moh's micrographic surgery is done for:**
    a. Cutaneous melanoma *(Recent Question 2016)*
    b. Dermatofibrosarcoma protuberans
    c. Squamous cell carcinoma
    d. None of the above

BASAL CELL CARCINOMA

41. **The commonest clinical pattern of basal cell carcinoma is:** *(COMEDK 2008, MCI March 2005)*
    a. Nodular
    b. Morpheaform
    c. Superficial
    d. Keratotic

42. **Most common site of basal cell carcinoma is:** *(All India 94, MHPGMCET 2001)*
    a. Face
    b. Trunk
    c. Neck
    d. Extremities

43. What is the most probable diagnosis based on the given image? *(AIIMS November 2017)*

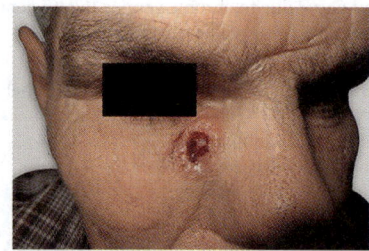

   a. Basal cell carcinoma b. Malignant melanoma
   c. Squamous cell carcinoma d. Marjolin's ulcer

44. A 48 years old sports photographer has noticed a small nodule over the upper lip from four months. The nodule is pearly white with central necrosis, telangiectasia. The most likely diagnosis would be:
   a. Basal cell carcinoma b. Squamous cell carcinoma
   c. Atypical melanoma d. Kaposi sarcoma

45. Which of the following cutaneous malignancies do not metastasize through the lymphatics? *(All India 94)*
   a. Squamous cell carcinoma
   b. Basal cell carcinoma
   c. Melanoma d. Kaposi's sarcoma

46. Diagnostic procedure for basal cell carcinoma:
   a. Wedge biopsy b. Shave
   c. Incisional biopsy d. Punch biopsy

47. All of the following are true about basal cell carcinoma except: *(DNB 2009)*
   a. Most common site is upper eyelid
   b. Locally invasive
   c. Rarely metastasizes
   d. Associated with exposure to sun

48. In pigmented basal cell carcinoma, treatment of choice is:
   a. Chemotherapy b. Radiotherapy *(PGI 98)*
   c. Cryosurgery d. Excision

49. Moh's micrographic excision for basal cell carcinoma is used for all of the following except: *(Karnataka 2006)*
   a. Recurrent Tumor
   b. Tumor less than 2 cm in diameter
   c. Tumors with aggressive histology
   d. Tumors with perineural invasion

50. Basal cell carcinoma spreads by: *(MAHE 2007)*
   a. Lymphatics b. Hematogenous
   c. Direct spread d. None of the above

51. About basal cell carcinoma, false is: *(DPG 2006)*
   a. Spreads to local lymph nodes
   b. Seen on face
   c. Seen on exposure of sunlight to skin
   d. Responds well to radiation

52. Characteristic feature of basal cell carcinoma is: *(AIIMS May 2012)*
   a. Keratin pearls b. Foam cells
   c. Nuclear palisading d. Psammoma bodies

53. Reconstruction of tip of nose after excision of basal cell carcinoma is done by: *(DNB 2014)*
   a. Bipedicled flap b. Bilobed flap
   c. Full thickness skin graft d. Split skin graft

MALIGNANT MELANOMA

54. In the Clarke's level of tumor invasion for malignant melanoma level 3 refers to: *(COMEDK 2006)*
   a. All tumor cells above basement membrane
   b. Invasion into reticular dermis
   c. Invasion into loose connective tissue of papillary dermis
   d. Tumors cell at junction of papillary and reticular dermis

55. True about malignant melanoma: *(PGI June 2008)*
   a. Lymphatic spread
   b. Lymph node biopsy is always done
   c. Biopsy to be done when sentinel node is involved
   d. Microsatellitism

56. Common features of melanoma, which of the following is not the part of mnemonic ABCDE? *(MHSSMCET 2009)*
   a. Elevation b. Asymmetric outline
   c. Variation in color d. Diameter < 6 mm

57. In malignant melanoma, change seen is all except:
   a. Ulceration b. Bleeding *(DPG 2006)*
   c. Satellite lesions d. Hair in mole

58. Treatment of choice for melanoma is: *(DPG 2006)*
   a. Chemotherapy b. Surgical excision
   c. Radiotherapy d. Surgery and chemotherapy

59. Most common origin of melanoma is from:
   (Bihar PG 2014, AIIMS Nov 2001)
   a. Junctional melanocytes b. Epidermal cells
   c. Basal cells d. Follicular cells

60. Most common type of malignant melanoma is:
   a. Superficial spreading *(AIIMS Nov 2001, UPPG 2009)*
   b. Lentigo maligna melanoma *(JIPMER 2014, 2012)*
   c. Nodular d. Acral lentiginous

61. Most common site of lentigo maligna melanoma is:
   (DNB 2013, AIIMS Nov 2001)
   a. Face b. Legs
   c. Trunks d. Soles

62. The most malignant form of malignant melanoma is:
   a. Nodular *(PGI June 99)*
   b. Hutchinson's melanotic freckle
   c. Acral lentiginous type
   d. Superficial spreading

63. Prognosis of melanoma depends on: *(PGI June 98)*
   a. Stage
   b. Depth of melanoma of biopsy
   c. Duration of growth d. Site

64. All of the following statements about malignant melanoma are true except: *(All India 97)*
   a. Prognosis is better in female than in male
   b. Acral lentiginous melanoma carries a good prognosis
   c. Stage IIa shows statelite deposits
   d. Most common type is superficial spreading melanoma

65. Biopsy from a mole on the foot shows cytologic atypia of melancytes and diffuse epidermal infiltration by anaplastic cells, which are also present in the papillary and reticular dermis. The most likely diagnosis is: *(All India 2004)*
   a. Melanoma, Clark level IV
   b. Congential melanocytic nevus
   c. Dysplastic nevus
   d. Melanoma, Clark level III

66. Which of the following is true about melanoma?
   a. Amelanotic melanoma is associated with worst prognosis
   b. Complete excisional biopsy is the management
   c. Thinner melanoma has good prognosis
   d. Back in MC site is females *(PGI Dec 2005)*
   e. Congenital giant nevus is associated with minimal risk of malignancy

67. Melanoma should be excised with a margin of: *(UPSC 88)*
    a. 2 cm   b. 5 cm
    c. 7 cm   d. 10 cm
68. Most severe form of malignant melanoma is: *(Kerala 94)*
    a. Superficially spreading
    b. Nodular infiltrating type
    c. Those arising in lower type
    d. Those in choroid
69. Melanoma staging is based on which classification?
    a. Breslow   b. Clark's   *(DNB 2009)*
    c. Both   d. Bethesda
70. Worst prognosis in melanoma is seen in the subtype:
    a. Superficial spreading   *(Kerala 2001)*
    b. Nodular melanoma
    c. Lentigo maligna melanoma
    d. Amelanotic melanoma
71. Least common site for spread of melanomas: *(DNB 2012)*
    a. GIT   b. Lungs
    c. Liver   d. Renal
72. Which one of the following is not included in the treatment of malignant melanoma? *(UPSC 2005)*
    a. Radiation   b. Surgical excision
    c. Chemotherapy   d. Immunotherapy
73. A 40 years old man presented with al flat 1 cm × 1 cm scaly, itchy black mole on the front of thigh. Examination did not reveal any inguinal lymphadenopathy. The best course of management would be: *(UPSC 2007)*
    a. FNAC of the lesion
    b. Incision biopsy
    c. Excisional biopsy
    d. Wide excision with inguinal lymphadenectomy
74. Inguinal lymph node enlargement is seen in: *(MPPG 97)*
    a. Seminoma testis   b. Malignant melanoma foot
    c. CA cervix   d. None
75. Risk factor for malignant melanoma all the following are risk factors foe malignant melanoma except: *(DNB 2014)*
    a. Giant congenital nevi
    b. Family history melanoma
    c. Exposure to UV light
    d. HPV infection
76. All of the following are marker of melanoma except: *(Recent Question 2016)*
    a. S-100   b. Cytokeratin-20
    c. HMB-45   d. Vimentin
77. Immunotherapy is effective in: *(Recent Question 2016)*
    a. SCC   b. BCC
    c. Malignant melanoma   d. None
78. Pigmented lesion suspicious of melanoma of size 1 cm with ulceration and features of ABCD. What is the next step? *(Recent Question 2017)*
    a. Wide local excision with 1 cm margin
    b. Excision biopsy with 1-2 mm margin
    c. Punch biopsy at the edge of the lesion
    d. Incisional biopsy

SKIN PATCH/STAIN/HEMANGIOMA

79. Which of the following is a regressing tumor? *(DPG 2011)*
    a. Portwine stain   b. Strawberry angioma
    c. Venous angioma   d. Plexiform angioma
80. True about congenital hemangioma:
    a. Congenital variety stops growing after birth
    b. Fully mature at birth   *(PGI June 2007, Dec 2007)*
    c. NICH variety persists
    d. RICH variety involutes   e. Calcification can occur
81. Following is regressive tumor: *(MHPGMCET 2007)*
    a. Venous angioma   b. Strawberry angioma
    c. Port-wine stain   d. Juvenile angioma
82. Which of the following statement is correct?

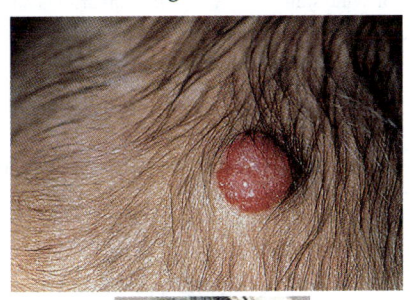

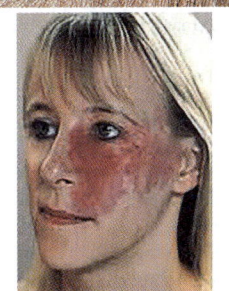

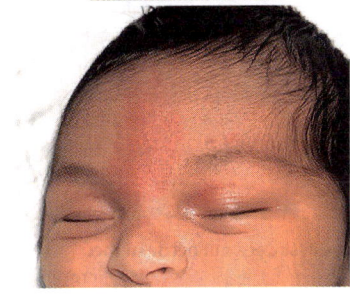

   a. 1-Strawberry angioma, 2-Portwine stain, 3-Salmon's patch
   b. 1-Strawberry angioma, 2- Salmon's patch, 3- Portwine stain
   c. 1- Salmon's patch, 2- Strawberry angioma, 3-Salmon's patch
   d. 1- Portwine stain, 2- Strawberry angioma, 3-Salmon's patch
83. Treatment for strawberry angioma: *(MHSSMCET 2006, JIPMER 95)*
    a. Steroids   b. Local excision
    c. Masterly inactivity   d. Antibiotic coverage
84. The best results in treatment of capillary nevus have been achieved by: *(AIIMS 84)*
    a. Full thickness skin graft   b. Dermabrasion
    c. Tatooing   d. Argon laser treatment
85. Spontaneous regression is seen in all except: *(All India 93)*
    a. Salmon patch
    b. Small cavernous hemangioma
    c. Portwine stain   d. Strawberry angioma

86. Salmon patch usually disappears by age:
    (Recent Question 2016)
    a. One month b. One year
    c. Puberty d. None of the above

87. Eleven months old child presents with erythematous lesion with central clearing which has been decreasing in size:
    (All India 97)
    a. Strawberry angioma b. Nevus
    c. Portwine stain d. Cavernous hemangioma

88. Regarding hemangiomas following are true:
    a. Salmon patch disappears after the age of one
    b. Port wine stain present throughout life
    c. Salmon patch-on forehead midline and over occiput
    d. All are correct

89. The best cosmetic results for large capillary (port wine) hemangiomas are achieved by: *(UPSC 2005)*
    a. Excision and split-thickness skin
    b. Laser ablation
    c. Chemotherapy d. Immunotherapy

90. Best method to treat a large port-wine hemangiomas:
    a. Radiotherapy *(DNB 2010)*
    b. Tattooing
    c. Excision with skin grafting
    d. Pulsed eye laser

91. Which is not true about Sturge Weber syndrome?
    (AIIMS Sept 96)
    a. Portwine stain b. Calcification in brain
    c. Cortical atrophy d. Intracranial hamartoma

92. Which of these does not change or remains same throughout life?
    (AIIMS Nov 2001)
    a. Salmon patch b. Strawberry angiomas
    c. Portwine stain d. Capillary hemangiomas

93. Spontaneous regression is seen in: *(Recent Question 2016)*
    a. Portwine hemangioma b. Strawberry hemangioma
    c. Cavernous hemangioma d. Arterial angioma

SEBACEOUS CYST

94. Sebaceous cyst does not occur in the:
    a. Scalp b. Scrotum
    c. Back d. Sole

95. True about epidermoid cyst: *(PGI Dec 2005)*
    a. Punctum is present b. Keratin is present
    c. Sebaceous material present d. Autosomal inheritance
    e. May turn malignant

96. What is the most probable diagnosis based on the given image:
    (Recent Question 2017)

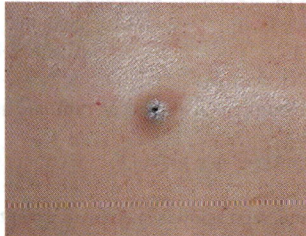

    a. Dermoid cyst b. Sebaceous cyst
    c. Lipoma d. Hemangioma

97. Cystic lesion over scalp as shown in the image:
    (Recent Question 2019)

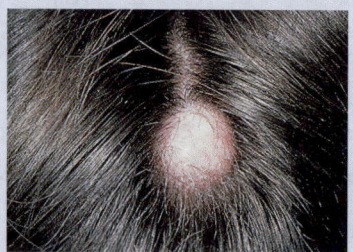

    a. Sebaceous cyst b. Dermoid cyst
    c. Neural tumor d. Meningioma

98. Sebaceous cyst is: *(DNB 2004)*
    a. Distention cyst b. Retention cyst
    c. Implantation dermoid d. Mucus cyst

99. Cock's peculiar tumor is: *(DNB 2009, MCI Sept 2007)*
    a. Infected sebaceous cyst b. Osteomyelitis of skull
    c. Cyst in the skull d. Tumor of the skull

100. Cock's peculiar tumor is:
    (MCI June 2018, Recent Question 2014, AIIMS Nov 2010)
    a. Basal cell carcinoma b. Squamous cell carcinoma
    c. Ulcerated sebaceous cyst d. Cylindroma

LIPOMA

101. The term universal tumor refers to:
    a. Adenoma b. Papilloma
    c. Fibroma d. Lipoma

102. Dercum's disease is commonest in the: *(Recent Question 2016)*
    a. Face b. Arm
    c. Back d. Thigh

103. Lipoma becomes malignant commonly at which site:
    a. Subcutaneous b. Retro-pertioneal
    c. Sub-aponeurotic d. Intermuscular

104. Dercum's disease is characterized by: *(DNB 2008)*
    a. Lipodermatosclerosis
    b. Tender subcutaneous lipoma
    c. Morbid obesity d. None

105. Myxomatous degeneration is lipoma is seen in those occurring in: *(MHSSMCET 2006)*
    a. Breast b. Pancreas
    c. Intramuscular d. Retroperitoneum

HIDRADENITIS SUPPURATIVA

106. Hidradenitis suppurativa is found to occur in:
    (Recent Question 2016)
    a. Axilla b. Circumanal
    c. Scalp d. Groin

KERATOCANTHOMA

107. Keratocanthoma is:
    a. A type of basal cell carcinoma
    b. Infected sebaceous cyst
    c. Self healing nodular lesion with central ulceration
    d. Pre-malignant disease

108. **True about keratocanthoma:** *(PGI 2000)*
    a. Benign tumor
    b. Malignant skin tumor like squamous cell carcinoma
    c. Treatment same as for squamous cell carcinoma
    d. Easy to differentiate from squamous cell carcinoma histologically
    e. Treatment is masterly inactivity

MISCELLANEOUS

109. **Cause of persistence of a sinus or fistulae includes:**
    a. Foreign body
    b. Non dependent drainage
    c. Unrelieved obstruction
    d. Presence of malignancy
    e. All of the above

110. **The best dressing is:**
    a. Opsitie
    b. Amnion
    c. Tulle grass
    d. Skin

111. **Hydrocele is a type of ……cyst:**
    a. Retention
    b. Distension
    c. Exudation
    d. Traumatic

112. **Calcifying epithelioma is seen in:** *(JIPMER 95)*
    a. Dermatofibroma
    b. Adenoma sebaceum
    c. Pyogenic granuloma
    d. Pilomatrixoma

113. **Which of the following statement is correct?**

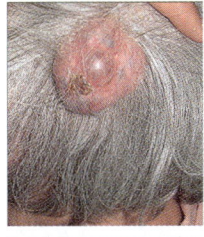
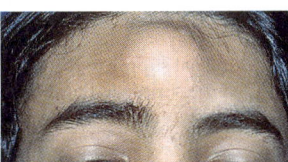
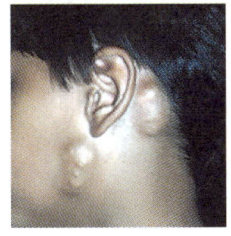
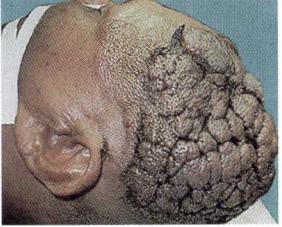

    a. 1-Cock's peculiar tumor, 2-Pott's puffy tumor, 3-Pilomatrixoma, 4-Cylindroma
    b. 1-Cock's peculiar tumor, 2-Pott's puffy tumor, 3-Cylindroma, 4- Pilomatrixoma
    c. 1- Pilomatrixoma, 2-Pott's puffy tumor, 3- Cock's peculiar tumor, 4-Cylindroma
    d. 1- Cylindroma, 2-Pott's puffy tumor, 3-Pilomatrixoma, 4- Cock's peculiar tumor

114. **Boil can occur at all sites except:** *(TN 95)*
    a. Pinna
    b. Skin
    c. Scalp
    d. Palm

115. **Frost bite is treated by:** *(AMC 2000)*
    a. Rapid rewarming
    b. Slow rewarming
    c. IV pentoxyphyllin
    d. Amputation

116. **Which is true regarding frostbite injury?** *(PGI November 2017)*
    a. In first and second degree frostbite, affected part shows redness & edema
    b. Spontaneous recovery without any treatment is rule
    c. Extensive involvement in frostbite is called chilblain
    d. Initial treatment is rewarming
    e. Autoamputation may occur in severe cases

117. **Treatment for pyoderma gangrenosum is:** *(Jharkhand 2003)*
    a. Steroids
    b. I.V. antibiotics
    c. Surgery + antibiotics
    d. Surgery alone

118. **Which of the following materials for implants will evoke least inflammatory tissue response?**
    a. Polypropylene
    b. Bovine collagen
    c. Polyaglactin
    d. Cotton

119. **Cylindroma is:** *(DPG 2007)*
    a. Appendage tumor
    b. Acinic cell carcinoma
    c. Pleomorphic adenoma
    d. Warthin's tumour

120. **Pyogenic granuloma, true statements is/are:** *(PGI June 2007)*
    a. Vascular pathology
    b. Bleeds rarely
    c. Increased in pregnancy
    d. Local excision
    e. Recurrent and malignant

121. **Lines of Blaschko represent:** *(All India 2011)*
    a. Lines along lymphatics
    b. Lines along blood vessels
    c. Lines along nerves
    d. Lines of development

122. **Bedsore is an example of:** *(All India 99)*
    a. Tropical ulcer
    b. Trophic ulcer
    c. Venous ulcer
    d. Post thrombotic ulcer

123. **Ainhum is seen in:** *(Recent Question 2014, All India 99)*
    a. Base of great toe
    b. Base of fingers tips
    c. Base of toe
    d. Ankle

124. **The given condition is most commonly seen in:**

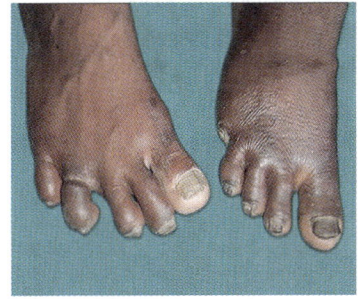

    a. Great toe
    b. Little toe
    c. Third toe
    d. Fourth toe

125. **Trophic ulcers are caused by:** *(PGI June 2002)*
    a. Leprosy
    b. Buerger's disease
    c. Syringomyelia
    d. DVT
    e. Varicose veins

126. **Which of the following is true?** *(PGI Dec 2005)*
    a. Viral warts spontaneously resolve
    b. Plantar warts should not be excised
    c. Callosity are formed occupationally
    d. Corns are viral in etiology

127. **Ulcer with undermined edges is seen in:** *(MHPGMET 2005)*
    a. Malignant ulcer
    b. Tubercular ulcer
    c. Venous ulcer
    d. Trophic ulcer

128. **Which of the following is not a true cyst?**
 (MHPGMCET 2006)
 a. Sebaceous cyst
 b. Dermoid cyst
 c. Bone cyst
 d. Apoplectic cyst

129. **What is the most probable diagnosis based on the given image?**
 (Recent Question 2017)

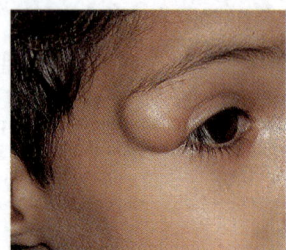

 a. Dermoid cyst
 b. Sebaceous cyst
 c. Lipoma
 d. Hemangioma

130. **Pilomatrixoma is:** (MHPGMCET 2006)
 a. A fleshy skin mass
 b. A type of skin tag
 c. A benign epithelial tumor
 d. A malignant skin neoplasm

131. **Sinus is lined by:** (MHPGMCET 2007)
 a. Simple squamous epithelium
 b. Columnar epithelium
 c. Granulation tissue
 d. Fibrous tissue

132. **A swelling which is variable in consistency with diffuse margins is likely to be:** (MHSSMCET 2005)
 a. Inflammatory
 b. Benign
 c. Malignant
 d. Non-specific

133. **Zadek's procedure is:** (MHSSMCET 2005)
 a. Resection of part of nail with nail bed
 b. Resection of complete nail with part of nail bed
 c. Injection phenol at base of toe nail
 d. Wide excision of nail

134. **Which of the following is a compressible swelling:**
 (DNB 2013, 2010)
 a. Lipoma
 b. Hernia
 c. Hemangioma
 d. Sebaceous cyst

135. **Which of the following flap is used for eye lid surgery?**
 (MHSSMCET 2010)
 a. Bilope flap
 b. Rhomboid flap
 c. Bipedicle flap
 d. Transposition flap

136. **Bilobed graft is used in:** (Recent Question 2017)
 a. Nose
 b. Eyelid
 c. Cheek
 d. Fingertips

137. **Radiotherapy is the treatment of choice of which one of the following tumors?** (UPSC 2008)
 a. Verrucous carcinoma
 b. Malignant melanoma
 c. Marjolin's ulcer
 d. Rodent ulcer

138. **Pott's Puffy tumor refers to:** (COMEDK 2014)
 a. Osteomyelitis of the frontal bone
 b. Tuberculosis of the spine
 c. Actionomycosis of maxilla
 d. Osteonecrotic tumor of Jaw

139. **Potts puffy tumor is:** (Recent Question 2019, 2018)
 a. Subperiosteal abscess of ethmoid bone
 b. Subperiosteal abscess of frontal bone
 c. Mucocele of ethmoid bone
 d. Mucocele of frontal bone

140. **Manchot, Salmon, Taylor names are related to:**
 (Recent Question 2017)
 a. Free-flap
 b. Arterial supply to the skin
 c. Nerve supply to the skin
 d. Arterial supply to muscle

Explanations

SKIN GRAFTING

1. **Ans. None** *(Ref: Sabiston 20/e p1939; Schwartz 10/e p264-265, 266; Bailey 27/e p639-640)*
   Light compression wraps favor 'take in' of split skin graft, not the tight dressing.
2. **Ans. a. Partial thickness** *(Ref: Sabiston 20/e p1939; Schwartz 10/e p264-265, 266; Bailey 27/e p639)*
3. **Ans. c. They contract to the same degree as a grafted sheet of skin** *(Ref: Sabiston 20/e p1939; Schwartz 10/e p264-265; Bailey 27/e p635,636,639,640)*
4. **Ans. b. Thigh**
5. **Ans. c. Vascular graft**
6. **Ans. a. Joseph Lister**

   - **Joseph Lister said "Skin is the best dressing".**

7. **Ans. b. Plasma imbibition**
8. **Ans. b. Pedicle graft** *(Ref: Sabiston 20/e p1939; Schwartz 9/e p1651; Bailey 27/e p635, 637)*

   - Skin graft must be **applied to a well-vascularized recipient wound bed**. It will **not adhere to exposed bone^Q, cartilage^Q, or tendon^Q** devoid of periosteum, perichondrium, or peritenon, respectively, or devoid of its vascularized perimembranous envelope.
   - Radiation damaged tissues are poor recipient sites.
   - So an exposed bone surface is covered by a graft which has its own blood supply. Such grafts are known as flaps or pedicle grafts.

9. **Ans. d. Full thickness skin graft**
10. **Ans. c. Streptococcus**
11. **Ans. a. Revascularization of the graft**
12. **Ans. c. Skull bone**
13. **Ans. c. For large areas, full thickness graft is used**
14. **Ans. d. Humby knife**
15. **Ans. a. Muscle** *(Ref: CSDT 12/e p1211)*

   For **critical** and **small areas** such as an **eyelid**, a **full thickness graft** is selected, so that contraction of the grafted material is minimum.

16. **Ans. d. Postauricular region** *(Ref: CSDT 12/e p1211)*

Donor Sites for Full Thickness Grafts	
• Eyelids^Q	• Inguinal area^Q
• Postauricular skin^Q	• Genital area^Q
• Supraclavicular skin^Q	• Submammary skin^Q
• Antecubital skin^Q	• Subgluteal skin^Q

17. **Ans. b. Back to neck**
18. **Ans. b. 2 weeks** *(Ref: Facial Plastic and Reconstructive Surgery by Ira D. Papel/44)*

   Excess split-skin autografts harvested and meshed during a surgical session are often stored at short-term for later burn surgery or graft failure.

   The current procedure in **skin storage involves wrapping the meshed autograft** on a piece of **ringer lactate** or **normal saline moistened gauze**, transferring it into a sterile container and **storing it in a 40 C for 2 weeks.** The graft should never be totally immersed in saline because it will become macerated. After 14 days of storage the respiratory activity of skin graft reduced by 50%.

19. **Ans. d. Autograft**
20. **Ans. c. Less contraction**
21. **Ans. a. Grafts are tissues that are transferred without their blood supply and they revascularise at the new site**

FLAPS

22. **Ans. a. Carries its own vessels within it** *(Ref: Sabiston 19/e p1917-1919; Schwartz 9/e p1651-1654; Bailey 27/e p637)*
23. **Ans. a. Pedicle flap**
24. **Ans. c. Burn wound**

25. **Ans. a. Randomised flaps**
26. **Ans. d. Skin, muscle and vascular pedicle**
27. **Ans. c. Reversed sural artery flap** *(Ref: Sabiston 20/e p1969; Schwartz 10/e p1877)*
28. **Ans. d. Local flaps** *(Ref: Sabiston 20/e p1950; Schwartz 10/e p1860)*

"*Scalp flaps are elevated at the subgaleal level, and many possible designs exist. In theory, defects as large as 30% of the scalp can be closed with scalp flaps elevated on major vessels.*"-*Sabiston 20/e p1950*

29. **Ans. c. Pectoralis major myocutaneous flap** *(Ref: Sabiston 20/e p1953; Schwartz 10/e p1873; Grabb and Smith Plastic Surgery 7/e p921)*

In the patient as shown in the question, chest wall closure has been achieved by using pectoralis major myocutaneous flap. Pectoralis major myocutaneous flap is one of the most commonly used flaps in chest wall reconstruction. Flaps frequently used for chest wall reconstruction include one or both the pectoralis major muscles, latissimus dorsi muscles, and rectus abdominis muscles, as well as the greater omentum.

"*Reconstruction of the Chest Wall: The choice of muscle depends on the location of the defect; options include the latissimus dorsi, serratus anterior, and pectoralis major muscle flaps. Other muscle flaps with limited but specific uses are the trapezius and superiorly based rectus abdominis. The greater omentum can be transposed on the right gastroepiploic artery as a pedicle flap to provide well-vascularized tissue with the bulk and pliability to obliterate dead space, but it is a secondary choice because of the risks of intra-abdominal complications.*" -*Sabiston 20/e p1953*

"*The pectoralis major muscle is the workhorse pedicled flap for coverage of the sternum, upper chest, and neck.*" -*Schwartz 10/e p1873*

Type of Flap	Uses
Pectoralis Major Myocutaneous (**PMMC**) flap	Head & neck reconstruction[Q] Sternal & chest wall reconstruction, especially **anterior & superior central chest**[Q]
Transverse Rectus Abdominis Muscle (**TRAM**) flap	**Breast reconstruction**[Q]
Vertical Rectus Abdominis Muscle (**VRAM**) flap	Used to cover **defects of sternum, chest wall, pelvis & perineal areas**[Q]
Latissimus dorsi flap	**Breast reconstruction**[Q] Chest wall reconstruction especially **lateral or anterolateral defects of upper 1/3rd of chest wall**[Q]
Serratus anterior flap	Head & neck reconstruction[Q] **Non-sternal & lower chest wall defects**[Q]

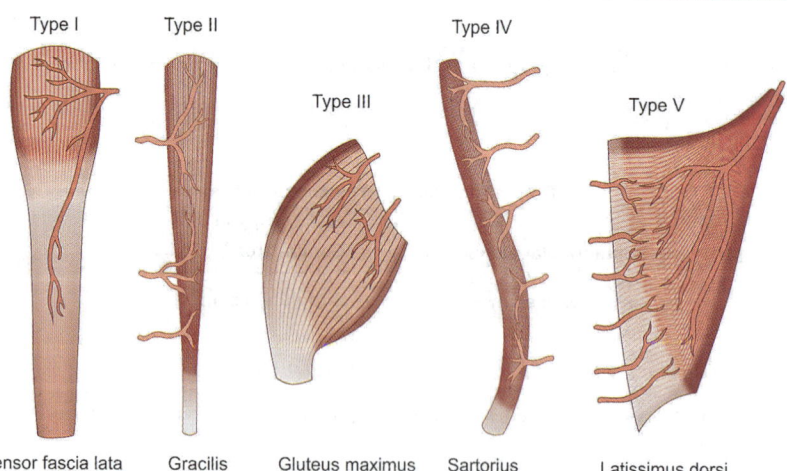

Mathes & Nahai Classification of muscles flap

Mathes & Nahai Classification of Muscles Flap (According to vascular supply)		
Type	Description	Example
I	**Single dominant pedicle**[Q]	• Tensor fascia lata
II	**Single dominant** pedicle with **minor pedicles**[Q]	• Gracilis • Trapezius
III	**Two dominant** pedicles[Q]	• Gluteus maximum • Rectus abdominis • Serratus anterior

| IV | Multiple segmental pedicles without a single dominant pedicle[Q] | • Sartorius
• External Oblique |
| V | Single dominant pedicle with secondary segmental pedicles[Q] | • Pectoralis major
• Latissimus dorsi
• Internal oblique |

30. Ans. d. Skull bone

MARJOLIN'S ULCER

31. Ans. b. Squamous cell carcinoma *(Ref: Schwartz 10/e p259, 1817; Bailey 27/e p605)*
32. Ans. a. The associated cancer is squamous cell carcinoma, b. May occur due to chronic venous insufficiency
33. Ans. b. Squamous cell carcinoma
34. Ans. a. Ulcer over scar

PREMALIGNANT LESIONS OF SKIN

35. Ans. d. All of the above *(Ref: Sabiston 20/e p748; Schwartz 10/e p847, 1217-1218; Bailey 27/e p606, 607)*
36. Ans. b. Steatoma multiplex *(Ref: Sabiston 20/e p747; Schwartz 10/e p847, 1217, 1218; Bailey 27/e p606-607)*

Premalignant Skin Lesions	
• Senile or actinic keratosis[Q] • Bowen's disease[Q] • Erythroplasia of Queyrat[Q]	• Chronic scars[Q] • Radiodermatitis[Q] • Prokeratosis[Q]

SQUAMOUS CELL CARCINOMA

37. Ans. a. Long standing venous ulcers, b. Chronic lupus vulgaris *(Ref: Sabiston 20/e p747; Schwartz 10/e p1218; Bailey 27/e p605)*
38. Ans. b. Everted
39. Ans. c. Giant condyloma accuminata *(Ref: Bailey 27/e p1368, 1493)*

GIANT CONDYLOMA ACUMINATUM

- **Giant condyloma acuminatum** (also known as a **Buschke-Löwenstein tumor**)[Q]
- Rare cutaneous condition characterized by an **aggressive, wart-like growth** that is a **verrucous carcinoma**[Q].
- It is attributed to **HPV**[Q].

40. Ans. c. Squamous cell carcinoma

BASAL CELL CARCINOMA

41. Ans. a. Nodular *(Ref: Sabiston 20/e p748; Schwartz 10/e p486-487; Bailey 27/e p604-605)*
42. Ans. a. Face
43. Ans. a. Basal cell carcinoma *(Ref: Harrison 19/e p500; Robbins 9/e p1157)*

Lesion near inner canthus with raised, pearly borders and central crust and with telangiectasia on surface of the lesion is highly suggestive of basal cell carcinoma.

44. Ans. a. Basal cell carcinoma
45. Ans. b. Basal cell carcinoma
46. Ans. a. Wedge biopsy
47. Ans. a. Most common site is upper eyelid
48. Ans. d. Excision
49. Ans. b. Tumor less than 2 cm in diameter *(Ref: Sabiston 20/e p735; Schwartz 10/e p486-487; Bailey 27/e p605)*
50. Ans. c. Direct spread
51. Ans. a. Spreads to local lymph nodes
52. Ans. c. Nuclear Palisading
53. Ans. b. Bilobed flap *(Ref: Bailey 27/e p641)*

Bilobed flap is used to cover a convex defect as on tip of nose. The bilobed flap is widely used for small nasal defects because it allows one to distribute tensions further from he primary defect, thus controlling the degree of tension along the alar margin

MALIGNANT MELANOMA

54. Ans. d. Tumors cell at junction of papillary and reticular dermis *(Ref: Sabiston 20/e p728; Schwartz 10/e p488-492; Bailey 27/e p608)*
55. Ans. a. Lymphatic spread, b. Lymph node biopsy is always done, c. Biopsy to be done when sentinel node is involved, d. Microsatellitism
56. Ans. d. Diameter < 6 mm
57. Ans. d. Hair in mole
58. Ans. b. Surgical excision
59. Ans. a. Junctional melanocytes
60. Ans. a. Superficial spreading
61. Ans. a. Face
62. Ans. a. Nodular
63. Ans. a. Stage, b. Depth of melanoma of biopsy, d. Site
64. Ans. b. Acral lentiginous melanoma carries a good prognosis, c. Stage IIa shows statelite deposits

   According to latest staging, presence of satellites is included in stage III.
65. Ans. a. Melanoma, Clark level IV
66. Ans. a. Amelanotic melanoma is associated with worst prognosis, b. Complete excisional biopsy is the management, c. Thinner melanoma has good prognosis *(Ref: Bailey 27/e p610)*

AMELANOTIC MELANOMA

- **Amelanotic melanoma** is a type of skin cancer in which the **cells do not make melanin.**
- They can be **pink, red, purple** or of **normal skin color,** hence **difficult to recognize**[Q].
  - It has an **asymmetrical shape** and an **irregular faintly pigmented border**[Q].
  - **Atypical appearance** leads to **delay in diagnosis,** the **prognosis is bad**[Q].
  - **Recurrence rate** is **high**[Q].

DESMOPLASTIC MELANOMA

- **Desmoplastic melanoma** is mostly found on the **head** and **neck region**[Q].
- It has a **propensity for perineural infiltration**[Q] and often **recurs locally**[Q] if not widely excised.
- It may be **amelanotic clinically**[Q].

67. Ans. a. 2 cm
68. Ans. b. Nodular infiltrating type
69. Ans. c. Both
70. Ans. d. Amelanotic melanoma
71. Ans. d. Renal
72. Ans. a. Radiation
73. Ans. c. Excisional biopsy
74. Ans. b. Malignant melanoma foot
75. Ans. d. HPV infection
76. Ans. b. Cytokeratin-20
77. Ans. c. Malignant melanoma
78. Ans. b. Excision biopsy with 1-2 mm margin *(Ref: Devita 10/e p1354; Sabiston 20/e p734; Schwartz 10/e p490)*

SKIN PATCH/STAIN/HEMANGIOMA

79. Ans. b. Strawberry angioma *(Ref: Schwartz 10/e p485; Bailey 27/e p613)*
80. Ans. a. Congenital variety stops growing after birth, b. Fully mature at birth, c. NICH variety persists, d. RICH variety involutes, e. Calcification can occur *(Ref: Schwartz 10/e p485; Bailey 26/e p598-599)*
81. Ans. b. Strawberry angioma
82. Ans. a. 1-Strawberry angioma, 2-Portwine stain, 3-Salmon's patch *(Ref: Schwartz 10/e p1849; Bailey 27/e p613)*

Strawberry Angiomas	Port-wine Stain	Salmon Patch
- Type of **capillary hemangioma** - **Baby** is **normal at birth**[Q] - **Appears at** the age of **1–3 weeks**[Q] - **Grows with** the **child upto 1 year** of age and then cease to grow[Q] - By the age of **9 years, 90%** demonstrate **complete involution**[Q] - **Emptying sign**[Q] is demonstrable	- A vascular malformation - **Present at birth**[Q] - **Grows along with** the **child**[Q] - **Do not regress**[Q] - **Face Involvement** In areas supplied by **5th cranial nerve**[Q]	- Also known as **Macular stain** or **stork bite**[Q] - **Present at birth**[Q] - Seen over **forehead in** the **midline & over** the **occiput**[Q] - **Disappears by** the age **1 year**[Q]

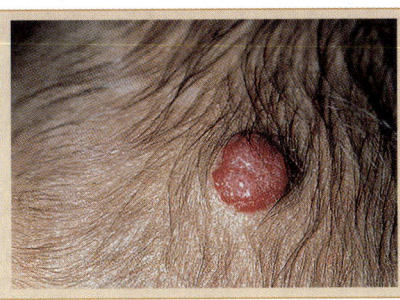 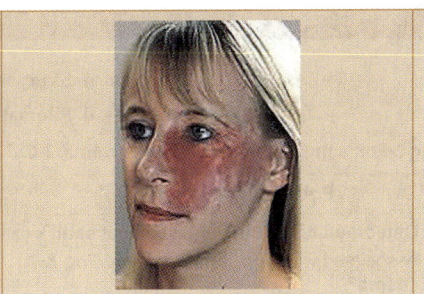 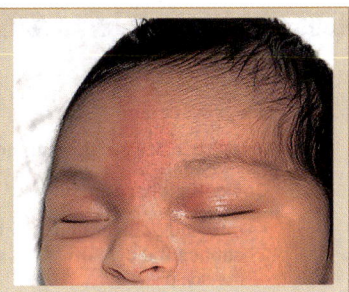

83. Ans. c. Masterly inactivity
84. Ans. d. Argon laser treatment
85. Ans. c. Portwine stain
86. Ans. b. One year
87. Ans. a. Strawberry angioma
88. Ans. d. All are correct
89. Ans. b. Laser ablation
90. Ans. d. Pulsed eye laser *(Ref: Roxburgh 17/e p194, 205)*

> Selective photothermolysis or pulsed eye laser is the treatment of choice for portwine hemangioma.
> Excellent results have been obtained with careful and time-consuming treatment with a 585-nm flash lamp-pumped pulsed eye laser. Treatment sessions can begin in babies and anesthesia is not always necessary.

91. Ans. d. Intracranial hamartoma *(Ref: Bailey 26/e p599)*

STURGE-WEBER SYNDROME / ENCEPHALOTRIGEMINAL SYNDROME

- Usually sporadic, characterized by:
  - Large **unilateral cutaneous angioma**^{Q} (port-wine stain)
  - **Angiomas** in **brain** involving **ipsilateral cerebral hemisphere** and **meninges**
  - **Focal seizures**^{Q} typically occurs **opposite to** the **side of lesion**^{Q}
  - Adrenal **pheochromocytoma**
  - Cerebral angiomas lead to **cortical atrophy**^{Q}

  - Angiomas are visible radiologically as **Tram-track** or **rail track calcification** mainly in **occipital region**^{Q}

92. Ans. c. Portwine stain
93. Ans. b. Strawberry hemangioma

SEBACEOUS CYST

94. Ans. d. Sole *(Ref: Schwartz 10/e p1218, 9/e p411; Bailey 27/e p598-599)*
95. Ans. a. Punctum is present, b. Keratin is present, e. May turn malignant
96. Ans. b. Sebaceous cyst *(Ref: Sabiston 20/e p1860; Schwartz 10/e p486; Bailey 27/e p598)*
97. Ans. a. Sebaceous cyst
98. Ans. b. Retention cyst
99. Ans. a. Infected sebaceous cyst
100. Ans. c. Ulcerated sebaceous cyst

LIPOMA

101. Ans. d. Lipoma *(Ref: Sabiston 20/e p2011; Schwartz 10/e p486; Bailey 27/e p544, 936)*
102. Ans. c. Back
103. Ans. b. Retro-pertioneal *(Ref: Sabiston 20/e p2011-2012; Schwartz 9/e p413; Bailey 27/e p1065)*
104. Ans. b. Tender subcutaneous lipomas
105. Ans. d. Retroperitoneum

HIDRADENITIS SUPPURATIVA

106. a. Axilla, b. Circumanal, d. Groin *(Ref: Sabiston 20/e p1410; Schwartz 10/e p476,506,1233; Bailey 27/e p595-596,1367-1368)*

KERATOACANTHOMA

107. Ans. c. Self healing nodular lesion with central ulceration *(Ref: Bailey 27/e p606)*
108. Ans. a. Benign tumor, e. Treatment is masterly inactivity

MISCELLANEOUS

109. Ans. e. All of the above
110. Ans. d. Skin
111. Ans. c. Exudation
112. Ans. d. Pilomatrixoma
113. Ans. a. 1-Cock's peculiar tumor, 2-Pott's puffy tumor, 3-Pilomatrixoma, 4-Cylindroma *(Ref: Bailey 27/e p657, 602, 603)*

Cocks Peculiar Tumour	Potts Puffy Tumour	Pilomatrixoma	Cylindroma
• **Infected** or **ulcerated sebaceous cyst of the scalp**^{Q} • Resembles **fungating epithelioma**^{Q}	• **Osteomyelitis** of the frontal bone of **skull**^{Q} • Associated with **subperiosteal swelling & edema**^{Q}	• Also known as **Calcifying epithelioma of Malherbe**^{Q} • **Benign hair follicle derived tumor**^{Q}	• A **malignant epithelial tumour** also known as **Turban tumor**^{Q} • Known as cylindroma because of its appearance

114. Ans. d. Palm
115. Ans. b. Slow rewarming *(Ref: Bailey 27/e p953, 422)*

FROSTBITE

- **Frostbite** injuries affect the **peripheries in cold climates.**
- The initial treatment is with **slow rewarming**^{Q} in a bath at 42 °C.
- The cold injury produces **delayed microvascular damage.**
- Level of damage is difficult to assess.
- **Surgery** usually **does not play a role** in its management, until there is absolute demarcation of the level of injury.

116. Ans. a. In first and second….., d. Initial treatment…., e. Autoamputation may occur….
117. Ans. a. Steroids *(Ref: Bailey 27/e p596)*

PYODERMA GANGRENOSUM

- Relatively uncommon **destructive cutaneous lesion.**
- Clinically, a **rapidly enlarging, necrotic lesion** with **undermined border** and **surrounding erythema** characterize this disease.
- Commonly associated with **IBD, rheumatoid arthritis, hematologic malignancy** and **monoclonal immunoglobulin A gammapathy.**

Treatment
- **First-line therapy:** Systemic treatment by **corticosteroids and cyclosporine**^{Q}.
- **If ineffective, alternative therapeutic procedures** include systemic treatment with **corticosteroids** and **mycophenolate mofetil;** mycophenolate mofetil and cyclosporine.

118. Ans. a. Polypropylene
119. Ans. a. Appendage tumor
120. Ans. a. Vascular pathology, c. Increased in pregnancy, d. Local excision *(Ref: Bailey 27/e p614; Roxburgh 17/e p197)*

PYOGENIC GRANULOMA

- Relatively common **vascular lesion of skin** and **mucosa**
- The name is **misnomer** (it is neither a granuloma, nor pyogenic in origin)
- Most are **small** (0.5–1.5 cm), **raised, pedunculated, soft, red nodular lesions** showing **superficial ulceration** and a tendency to **bleed after trivial trauma**^{Q}.
- Often arise in **pregnancy** particularly **on gingiva**^{Q} or elsewhere in oral mucosa

Treatment
- Local excision with a minimal margin.

121. **Ans. d. Lines of development** *(Ref: Neurocutaneous Disorders by Ruggieri (2008)/364)*
    Lines of Blaschko represents random line of development of skin.
122. **Ans. b. Trophic ulcer**
123. **Ans. c. Base of toe** *(Ref: Bailey 25/e p914)*

Ainhum

- Ainhum is a disease of **unknown etiology**
- Usually **affects black men**^{Q} (and occasionally women) who have **run barefoot in childhood**^{Q}.
- It is recorded in **central Africa, central America** and the **Orient**.
- A **fissure appears** at the level of the **interphalangeal joint of a toe**, usually of the **little toe**^{Q}.
- **Fissure is followed by** a **fibrous band** that **encircles** the **digit** and **causes necrosis**^{Q}.

Treatment
- Early stage: **Z-plasty**^{Q}; Later stage: **Amputation**^{Q}

124. **Ans. b. Little toe**
125. **Ans. a. Leprosy, c. Syringomyelia** *(Ref: Sabiston 19/e p1943-1945; Bailey 27/e p69-70)*
126. **Ans. a. Viral warts spontaneously resolve, c. Callosity are formed occupationally** *(Ref: Sabiston 19/e p1402; Schwartz 10/e p485, 1233; Bailey 27/e p599,1368,1486,1496)*
    Corn and callosities are hyperkeratosis due to chronic excessive pressure or friction on the skin.

Warts

- Warts are epidermal growths associated with **HPV infection**^{Q}
- Histologically characterized by: **Hyperkeratosis, acanthosis, papillomatosis** and **koilocytes**
- **Recurrences** are common
- Some **warts** are **risk factors for SCC**^{Q}.

Treatment
- Removed by number of chemical including **formalin, podophyllin** etc^Q.
- **Surgical excision** or **curettage with electrodissection**^{Q} can also be done.
- Treatment of extensive areas of skin requires surgical excision under GA.

127. **Ans. b. Tubercular ulcer**
128. **Ans. d. Apoplectic cyst** *(Ref: Bailey 24/e p209)*

Cyst

- Cyst is a sac that is filled with a fluid or semi-fluid material.
- Two of the most common types of cyst that occur under the skin surface are **sebaceous cyst** and **dermoid cyst**. These are **true cyst, line by epithelium**.
- **Pseudocyst of pancreas** and **apoplectic cyst** are **not lined by epithelium**, and are **not true cyst**^{Q}.

129. **Ans. a. Dermoid cyst** *(Ref: Sabiston 20/e p1860; Schwartz 10/e p1737; Bailey 27/e p667)*
130. **Ans. c. A benign epithelial tumor**
131. **Ans. c. Granulation tissue** *(Ref: Bailey 27/e p616)*

- A **sinus** is **a blind-ending tract** that **connects a cavity lined with granulation tissue** (often an abscess cavity) with an epithelial surface.

132. **Ans. c. Malignant**
133. **Ans. b. Resection of complete nail with part of nail bed** *(Ref: Orthopedics and Fractures by T. Duckworth, C. M. Blundell (2010)/215)*
    Zadek's procedure is resection of complete nail with part of nail bed in ingrowing toe-nail.

Zadek's Procedure

- **For recurrent problems** in ingrowing toe-nail, the **toenail** and its **growing point removed** so that the **nail does not ever re-grow** (Zadek's procedure)^Q.

134. **Ans. c. Hemangioma**
135. **Ans. c. Bipedicle flap** *(Ref: Bailey 27/e p641)*
136. **Ans. a. Nose** *(Ref: Sabiston 20/e p836)*

LOCAL FLAPS

- A local flap is raised next to a tissue defect in order to reconstruct it.

Basic Patterns of Local Flaps	
Transposition flap	• **Most basic design,** leaving a graftable donor site
Z-plasty	• For **lengthening scars** or **tissues**
Rhomboid flap	• For **cheek, temple, back** and **flat surface defects**
Rotation flap	• For **convex surfaces**
Advancement flap	• For **flexor surfaces;** may need triangles excised at the base to make it work (commonly called **Burrow's triangles**)
V-to-Y advancement	• Commonly used for **fingertips** and **extremities**
Bilobed flap	• For convex surfaces, especially the **nose**[Q]
Bipedicle flap	• For **eyelids,** rarely elsewhere[Q].

137. **Ans. d. Rodent ulcer** *(Ref: http://emedicine.medscape.com/article/276624-treatment#aw2aab6b6b4)*

  - Among the given options, only rodent ulcer (BCC) is radiosensitive, rest all are not responsive to radiotherapy.

138. **Ans. a. Osteomyelitis of the frontal bone**
139. **Ans. b. Subperiosteal abscess of frontal bone**
140. **Ans. b. Arterial supply to the skin** *(Ref: Grabb & Smith /p29)*

CHAPTER 32

Wound Healing, Tissue Repair and Scar

WOUND

Wound

- **Wound**: Breach in continuity of skin or surface epithelium
- **Simple wound**: Only **skin & subcutaneous tissue** is involved[Q]
- **Complex wound**: Involves underlying **nerves, vessels, tendons** with **devitalized tissue**[Q]

WOUND HEALING

Wound Healing

- Mechanism by which body attempts to restore the integrity of injured part

Phases of Wound Healing

Inflammatory Phase	Proliferative Phase	Remodeling Phase
• Begins **immediately after wounding**[Q] • Last for **2-3 days**[Q] • **Bleeding → Vasoconstriction & thrombus formation** to limit blood loss → **Platelets stick** to damaged **endothelial linings**[Q]	• Last from **3rd day to 3rd week**[Q] • Consist of **fibroblast activity** with **production of collagen, glycosaminoglycans & proteoglycans** • **Angioneogenesis**[Q]: Growth of new vessels as capillary loops • **Re-epithelialization**[Q] of wound surface • **Increase in tensile strength** of wound due to **increased type III collagen**, deposited in random fashion[Q] • **Wound contraction**[Q]: Reduces the surface area of wound	• Characterized by **maturation of collagen**[Q] • **Type I collagen replacing type III** until a **ratio of 4:1 is achieved**[Q] • **Realignment of collagen fibers** along the line of tension[Q] • **Decreased wound vascularity**[Q] • **Wound contraction**[Q] • **Maturation of collagen**: Increased tensile strength of wound[Q] • **Wound strength is maximum at 12th week post injury**[Q] (represents approximately **80% of uninjured skin strength**[Q])

FACTORS ADVERSELY AFFECTING WOUND HEALING

Factors that Inhibit Wound Healing

Local Factors	Systemic Factors
• **Infection**[Q] • **Ischemia**[Q] • **Foreign body**[Q] • **Hematoma**[Q] • Movement • Mechanical stress • Necrotic tissue	• **Diabetes mellitus**[Q] • **Ionizing radiation**[Q], **temperature**[Q] • **Advanced age**[Q], **Malnutrition**[Q] • Vitamin **C** and **A deficiency**[Q] • Mineral (**Zinc** and **Iron**[Q]) deficiencies • Drugs (**Steroids**[Q], **Doxorubicin**) • **Jaundice**[Q], **Uremia**[Q], **Malignancy**[Q]

CLASSIFICATION OF SURGICAL WOUNDS

Wounds Class	Definition
I: Clean	• Uninfected operative wound without inflammation^Q • Respiratory, alimentary, genital or infected urinary tract is not entered^Q • Wounds are closed primarily^Q, if necessary drained with closed drainage^Q **Examples of Clean Wound** • Inguinal hernia^Q • Mastectomy^Q • Joint replacement^Q • Abdominal aortic aneurysm (AAA) repair^Q • Thyroidectomy^Q
II: Clean contaminated	• Operative wound in which respiratory tract, GIT or genitourinary tract is entered under controlled condition without unusual contamination^Q **Examples of Clean Contaminated Wound** • Cholecystectomy^Q • Elective GI surgeries (elective colonic resection^Q, gastrectomy^Q) • CBD exploration^Q
III: Contaminated	• Open, fresh accidental wounds^Q • Operations with major break in sterile techniques^Q • Gross spillage from GIT^Q • Incision in which acute non-purulent inflammation is encountered^Q **Examples of Contaminated Wound** • Spill during elective GI surgery^Q • Enterotomy during bowel obstruction^Q • Perforated gastric ulcer^Q • Human bite^Q • Appendicular perforation^Q • Open fracture^Q • Penetrating abdominal trauma^Q
IV: Dirty	• Old traumatic wound with retained devitalized tissue^Q • Wound with clinical infection or perforated viscera with high degree of contamination^Q • Organism causing post-op infection is already present^Q in the wound before operation • Associated with severe inflammation^Q **Examples of Dirty Wound** • Perforated diverticulitis^Q • Fecal peritonitis^Q • Frank pus^Q • Necrotizing soft tissue infection^Q

Wounds Class	Risk of Infection	Need for Prophylaxis
Clean	5%^Q	• Usually not required^Q
Contaminated	10%^Q	• Usually required^Q
Clean-contaminated	20–30%^Q	• Required^Q
Dirty	30–40%^Q	• Treatment required^Q (not the prophylaxis)

CLASSIFICATION OF WOUND CLOSURE & HEALING

Healing by Primary Intention	Healing by Secondary Intention	Healing by Tertiary Intention
• Also known as healing by first intention^Q • Occurs when there is: 　– Apposition of wound edges^Q 　– Minimal surrounding tissue trauma & least inflammation^Q 　– Associated with best scar^Q	• Occurs in the wounds that are: 　– Left open^Q 　– Allowed to heal by granulation, contraction & epithelialization^Q	• Also known as "delayed primary intention healing"^Q • Occurs when wound edges are not opposed immediately, in contaminated or untidy wounds^Q • Delayed closure of wound^Q is done when inflammatory & proliferative phase of healing is well established • Results in less satisfactory scar^Q as compared to healing by primary intention

CHRONIC WOUND

CHRONIC WOUND

- Wounds that **do not heal within 3 months**^{Q}
- **Delay in healing** can occur at any phase but **most often occur in inflammatory phase**^{Q}

Treatment
- **Surgical treatment** is only indicated if **non-operative treatment has failed** or patient suffers from **intractable pain**^{Q}

DEGLOVING INJURY

DEGLOVING

- Skin & subcutaneous fat are stripped by avulsion from the underlying fascia^Q
- Leaving neurovascular structures, tendon or bone exposed^Q

COMPARTMENT SYNDROME

COMPARTMENT SYNDROME

- Typically occur in **closed lower limb injuries**^{Q}

Clinical Features
- Characterized by **severe pain**^{Q}; **Pain on passive movement** of affected compartment muscle^Q
- **Distal sensory disturbance**^{Q}
- Finally by **absence of pulses distally**^{Q} (a late sign^Q)

Diagnosis
- **Compartment pressure** is measured by using a **pressure monitor & catheter placed in muscle compartment**^{Q}

Treatment
- **Fasciotomy** if **pressure is constantly > 30 mm Hg** or presence of **clinical signs of compartment syndrome**^{Q}
- In fasciotomy: Longitudinal incision is given over **skin, subcutaneous fat & fascia**; muscle should **bulge through fasciotomy opening**^{Q}

PRESSURE SORE

PRESSURE SORE

- Also known as **Bed sores/Pressure ulcer/Decubitus ulcer/Pressure sore/Trophic ulcer/Penetrating ulcer**^{Q}
- Definition: Tissue necrosis with ulceration due to prolonged pressure^Q
- Preventable
- Incidence: **5% of hospitalized patients**; **Higher incidence** in: **Paraplegic**^{Q} patients, **elderly & severely ill**^{Q} patients
- MC site: **I**schium^Q > **G**reater trochanter^Q > **S**acrum^Q > **H**eel^Q > **M**alleolus^Q > **O**cciput^Q (Indira Gandhi Stadium inauguration by HM Office)
- Mechanism: External pressure exceeds the capillary occlusive pressure (>30 mm Hg) → Blood flow to the skin stops → Tissue hypoxia, necrosis & ulceration^Q
- Other mechanisms: Due to impaired nutrition, defective blood supply, neurological deficit^Q

Neurological Causes (SPL DPT)	
Syringomyelia, **S**pina bifida, **S**pinal injury^Q	**D**iabetic neuropathy^Q
Peripheral neuritis, **P**eripheral nerve injury^Q	**P**araplegia^Q
Leprosy^Q	**T**abes dorsalis^Q

Clinical Features
- Painless punched out ulcer^Q; Base formed by bone^Q

	Staging of Pressure Sore
Stage	**Description**
1	**Non-blanchable erythema without a breach** in epidermis (**early superficial ulcer**^{Q})
2	**Partial thickness skin loss** involving **epidermis & dermis** (Late superficial ulcer^Q)
3	**Full thickness skin loss extending into subcutaneous tissue** but not through underlying fascia (**Early deep ulcer**^{Q})
4	**Full thickness skin loss through fascia with extensive tissue destruction**, maybe **involving muscle, bone, tendon or joint (Late deep ulcer**^{Q})

Management

- **Prevention is the best treatment**^{Q} with: Good skin care; special **pressure dispersion cushions or foams**; Use of **low air-loss & air-fluidized beds**^{Q}; Urinary or fecal diversion in selected case
- **Bed bound patients: Turned** at least **every 2 hours**^{Q}
- **Wheel chair bound patients: Lift** themselves **off** their seat for **10 second every 10 minutes**^{Q}
- **Surgical treatment**: Reserved for the patient with **no improvement after conservative management**; includes **adequate debridement, vacuum assisted closure** or **Flap closure**

> - Large skin flaps with muscle & intact sensory innervations is preferred^Q (Example: Extensor fascia lata with lateral cutaneous nerve of thigh^Q)

VACUUM ASSISTED CLOSURE/ NEGATIVE PRESSURE WOUND THERAPY

Vacuum Assisted Closure/Negative Pressure Wound Therapy (NPWT)

- NPWT promotes wound healing by **applying a vacuum through a special sealed dressing.**
- Continued **vacuum draws out the fluid** from wound & **increases blood flow** to the area.
- **Vacuum** may be **applied continuously or intermittently**, depending upon the types of wound being treated & clinical objectives.
- **Negative pressure** of **–125 mm Hg**^{Q} is used.
- **Dressing** should be **changed 2-3 times/week**^{Q}

Primary Effects of NPWT on Wound Healing	
Macrodeformation^Q	Drawing the wound edges together leading to contraction
Stabilization of wound environment^Q	Wound protected from outside micro-organisms in a warm & moist environment
Reduced edema^Q	With removal of soft tissue exudates
Microdeformation^Q	Leading to cellular proliferation on the wound surface

Contraindications for NPWT Use	
• Malignancy in the wound^Q	• Non-enteric & unexplored fistula^Q
• Untreated osteomyelitis^Q	• Necrotic tissue with eschar^Q

SCAR

Scar

- **Maturation phase** of wound healing **leads to formation of scar**^{Q}
- **Immature scar (Pink, raised, hard & itchy**^{Q}**)** → As the **collagen matures & becomes denser, scar** becomes almost **acellular**, as fibroblast & blood vessels reduce → Scar becomes **paler, flattens, softer & itching diminishes**^{Q} → Tensile strength of scar increases; maximum at **12th week**^{Q} (after 3 months) post-injury; represent approx. **80% of uninjured skin strength**^{Q}
- Types of scar: Atrophic scar, hypertrophic scar & keloid

ATROPHIC SCAR

Atrophic Scar

- **Pale, flat & stretched** in appearance; Appear on the **back & in areas of tension**^{Q}
- **Easily traumatized** as epidermis & dermis are thinned; **Excision & resuturing rarely improves such scar**^{Q}

HYPERTROPHIC SCAR

Hypertrophic Scar

- **Excessive scar tissue** that **does not extend beyond the boundaries of original incision or wound**^{Q}
- Results from **prolonged inflammatory phase**^{Q} of wound healing and/or **unfavorable scar citing**^{Q} (across the lines of skin tension)

Histology
- Excess collagen & hypervascularity[Q] (more marked in keloid with more type III collagen)
- Contains well organized type III collagen; Improves spontaneously with time[Q]

Treatment
- **Linear hypertrophic scar**: Treated with **pressure therapy** or **silicone gel sheet application**[Q]
- **Ongoing hypertrophy**: Treated with **intralesional steroids (Triamcinolone**[Q]**)**
- **Scars persist after 1 year**: Surgical **excision + primary closure** of wound[Q]

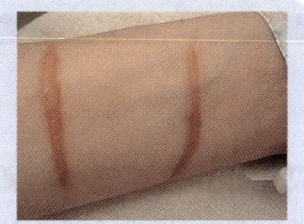

KELOID

KELOID

- Excessive scar tissue that **extends beyond the boundaries of original incision or wound**[Q]
- **Etiology**: Unknown; Genetic predisposition, more common in blacks[Q]
- **Associated with**: Elevated levels of growth factors; deeply pigmented skin[Q]
- **Common in certain areas of body**: Above clavicle[Q], upper extremities[Q], on the trunk[Q], face[Q] (Especially seen in **triangle** whose boundaries are **xiphisternum & each shoulder tip**[Q])

Histology
- Excess collagen & hypervascularity; Contain **disorganized type I & III collagen**[Q]
- **Thicker collagen bundles**[Q] form acellular node like structures

Treatment
- **Keloids rarely regress with time**, often **refractory to medical & surgical intervention**[Q]
- **First line treatment**: Silicones in combination with **pressure therapy & intralesional corticosteroid** injection[Q]
- **Refractory cases** (after 12 months of therapy): **Excision + Post-op radiotherapy**[Q] (external beam or brachytherapy)
- **New treatment modalities**: Internal cryotherapy[Q] & 5% Imiquimod[Q]

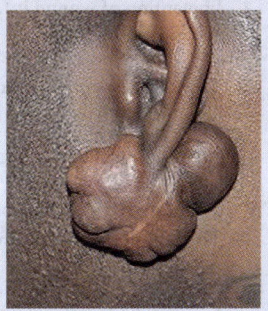

Feature	Hypertrophic Scar	Keloid
Genetic	Not familial[Q]	May be **familial**[Q]
Race	Not race related[Q]	**Black**[Q] >white
Sex	Female = male	**Female**[Q] >male
Age	Children[Q]	10-30 years[Q]
Border	Remains **within wound**[Q]	**Outgrows** wound area
Natural history	**Subsides** with time	Rarely subsides
Site	Flexor surfaces[Q]	**Sternum (MC**[Q]**)**, shoulder, face
Etiology	Related to **tension**[Q]	Unknown
Develop	Within 4 weeks	3 months to year after trauma
Symptoms	**Raised**, some pruritus **Respect wound confines**	**Pain, pruritus, hyperesthesia** **Growth beyond wound margins**
Histology	**Parallel orientation** of collagen fibers	**Thick wavy** collagen fibers in **random orientation**

CONTRACTURE

CONTRACTURE

- A **tight web restricting the range of movement** at the joint[Q]
- When the **scar crosses joints or flexion creases** is known as contracture[Q]

Clinical Features
- It can cause **hyperextension or hyperflexion deformity**[Q]
- In **neck**, may **interfere with head extension**[Q]

Treatment
- **Multiple Z-plasties**[Q]; Inset of **grafts or flaps**[Q]
- **Splintage & intensive physiotherapy** in post-op period[Q]

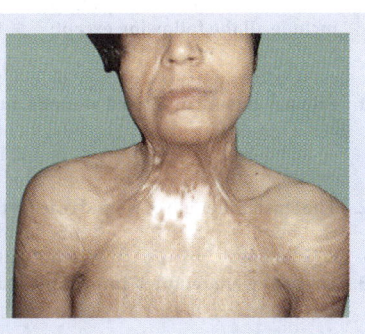

Multiple Choice Questions

WOUND HEALING

1. **Wound healing is affected by:** *(PGI Dec 2007)*
    a. Age
    b. Nutrition
    c. Dryness or wetness of wound
    d. Drugs
    e. Temperature

2. **Prevention of wound infection is done by:** *(PGI June 2005)*
    a. Pre-op shaving
    b. Pre-op antibiotic therapy
    c. Monofilament suture
    d. Wound apposition

3. **True about wound healing:** *(PGI June 2009)*
    a. Infected wound heal by primary intention
    b. Deep dermal wound heal by scar formation
    c. Wound contraction is found in healing by secondary intention
    d. More intense inflammatory response in primary intention

4. **True about chronic wound:** *(PGI Nov 2009)*
    a. Found in DM
    b. Always require surgical treatment
    c. May be associated with vascular compromise
    d. Monofilament sutures prevent infection
    e. Any wound that does not heal within 3 month

5. **Cell not involved in healing of clean wound:** *(PGI Nov 2011)*
    a. Macrophages
    b. Platelet
    c. Fibroblasts
    d. Polymorphonuclear leukocytes
    e. Myofibroblasts

6. **Management of an open wound seen 12 hours after the injury:** *(DPG 2011)*
    a. Suturing
    b. Debridement and suture
    c. Secondary suturing
    d. Heal by granulation

7. **The vitamin which has inhibitory effect on wound healing is:** *(MAHE 2005)*
    a. Vitamin A
    b. Vitamin E
    c. Vitamin C
    d. Vitamin B-complex

8. **The tensile strength of the wound starts and increases after:**
    a. Immediate suture of the wound *(WBPG 2012, MAHE 2005)*
    b. 3–4 days
    c. 7–10 days
    d. 6 months

9. **In a sutured surgical wound, the process of epithelialization is completed within:** *(UPSC 2007)*
    a. 24 hours
    b. 48 hours
    c. 72 hours
    d. 96 hours

10. **Factors that may adversely affect the healing of wounds include all the following except:**
    a. Exposure to UV light
    b. Exposure to radiation
    c. Obstructive jaundice
    d. Advanced neoplasia

11. **Primary closure of incised wounds must be done within:**
    a. 2 hours
    b. 4 hours
    c. 6 hours
    d. 12 hours
    e. 16 hours

12. **The tensile strength of wound reaches that of normal tissue by:**
    a. 6 weeks
    b. 2 months
    c. 4 months
    d. 6 months

13. **Following are required for wound healing except:**
    a. Zinc
    b. Copper *(All India 93)*
    c. Vitamin C
    d. Calcium

14. **Patient has lacerated untidy wound of the leg and attended the casualty after 2 hours. His wound should be:**
    a. Sutured immediately *(Recent Question 2016)*
    b. Debrided and sutured immediately
    c. Debrided and sutured secondarily
    d. Cleaned and dressed

15. **When is the maximum collagen content of wound tissue?**
    a. Between 3rd to 5th day
    b. Between 6th to 17th day
    c. Between 17th to 21st day
    d. None of the above

16. **A patient with grossly contaminated wound presents 12 hours after an accident, his wound should be managed by:**
    a. Thorough cleaning and primary repair *(UPSC 96)*
    b. Thorough cleaning with debridement of all dead and devitalized tissue without primary closure
    c. Primary closure over a drain
    d. Covering the defect with split skin graft after cleaning

17. **Delayed wound healing is seen in all except:** *(APPG 96)*
    a. Malignancy
    b. Hypertension
    c. Diabetes
    d. Infection

18. **In the healing of clean wound the maximum immediate strength of the wound is reached by:**
    a. 2–3 days
    b. 4–7 days
    c. 10–12 days
    d. 13–18 days

19. **A clean incised wound heals by:** *(DPG 92)*
    a. Primary intention
    b. Secondary intention
    c. Excessive scaring
    d. None of the above

20. **Which one of the following surgical procedures is considered to a have a clean-contaminated wound?**
    a. Elective open cholecystectomy for cholelithiasis
    b. Herniorrhaphy with mesh repair
    c. Lumpectomy with axillary node dissection
    d. Appendectomy with walled off abscess

21. **Fibroblasts in healing wound are derived from:** *(UPSC 2008, PGI 98)*
    a. Local mesenchyme
    b. Epithelium
    c. Endothelium
    d. Vascular fibrosis

22. **Tensile strength of wound becomes normal after:** *(Recent Question 2013)*
    a. 6 weeks
    b. Never
    c. 4 months
    d. 6 months

23. **In classification of contaminated wound, which of the following are included?** *(PGI May 2018)*
    a. Resection of unprepared bowel
    b. Perforated appendix resection
    c. Resection of intestinal fistula
    d. Inguinal hernia repair
    e. Hysterectomy

KELOID AND HYPERTROPHIC SCAR

24. **True statement(s) regarding hypertrophic scar:**
    a. Grow beyond wound margin *(PGI Dec 2008)*
    b. More common in female
    c. Not familial
    d. Rarely subsides
    e. Not race related

25. **True statement regarding hypertrophic scar:**
    a. Usually occurs across the flexural areas
    b. Does not improve with time
    c. Overgrows its boundaries
    d. Develops months after surgery *(JIPMER May 2018)*

Wound Healing, Tissue Repair and Scar

26. **Which of the following is true about keloid?**
    (Recent Question 2018, 2017)
    a. Wide local excision is treatment of choice
    b. Collagen is same but arranged haphazardly
    c. Will not spread beyond wound site
    d. More amount of growth factors

27. **All are true about keloid except:** *(PGI Dec 2007)*
    a. Grows beyond would margin
    b. Excess collagen deposition
    c. Precancerous leading to cancer
    d. More common in female e. Whites are at high risk

28. **Which one of the following statements is true regarding the picture depicted here?** *(APPG 2016)*
    a. Commonly seen on eyelids, genitalia, palms and soles
    b. Tend to occur 3 months to one year after initial insult
    c. All these statements are true
    d. Commonly extend into underlying subcutaneous tissue

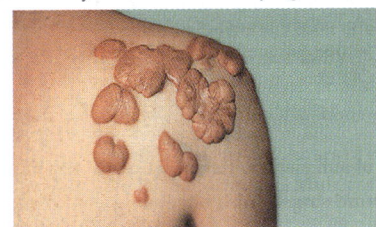

29. **The following statement about keloid is true:**
    (Recent Question 2018)
    a. Elevated levels of growth factor is not seen
    b. Extended excision is the treatment of choice
    c. It do not extend beyond the wound
    d. It will have more collagen and vascularity

30. **Most common site of hypertrophic keloid is:**
    a. Face   b. Leg   *(AIIMS Nov 93)*
    c. Presternal area   d. Arm

31. **First line treatment for keloid is:**
    a. Intralesional injection of keloid
    b. Local steroid   c. Radiotherapy
    d. Wide excision   *(Recent Question 2015, AIIMS Dec 94)*

32. **Drug used for intralesional injection keloid is:**
    (AIIMS June 95)
    a. Prednisolone   b. Triamcinolone
    c. Androgen   d. Hydrocortisone

33. **Keloid scar is made up:** *(Recent Question 2016)*
    a. Dense collagen   b. Loose fibrous tissue
    c. Granulomatous tissue   d. Loose areolar tissue

34. **What is true about keloids?** *(JIPMER 95)*
    a. It appears immediately after surgery
    b. It appears a few days after surgery
    c. It is limited in its distribution
    d. It is common in old people

35. **Keloid is best treated:** *(UPSC 95, 2001)*
    a. Intralesional injection of trimacinolone
    b. Wide excision and grafting
    c. Wide excision and suturing
    d. Deep X-ray therapy

36. **The following statement about keloid is true:**
    (Recent Question 2016)
    a. They do not extend into normal skin
    b. Local recurrence is common after excision
    c. They often undergo malignant change
    d. They are more common in whites than in blacks

37. **The worst position for scars is:**
    a. Back   b. Shoulder
    c. Sternum   d. Abdomen

38. **Keloid formation is not seen over:** *(Recent Question 2016)*
    a. Ear   b. Face
    c. Eyelids   d. Neck

VACUUM ASSISTED CLOSURE

39. **Vacuum assisted closure is contraindicated in:**
    a. Chronic osteomyelitis   *(Recent Question 2017)*
    b. Large amount of necrotic tissue with eschar
    c. Abdominal wound
    d. Surgical wound dehiscence

40. **All of the following are principles of negative pressure wound therapy except:** *(Recent Question 2017)*
    a. Stabilization of wound environment
    b. Clearance of infection
    c. Macrodeformation of the wound
    d. Decreased edema

41. **Negative pressure wound therapy (NPWT) is used in:**
    (Recent Question 2018)
    a. Bedsore in sacrum after debridement
    b. After amputation negative suction
    c. Osteomyelitis
    d. Unexplored fistulas

MISCELLANEOUS

42. **The best scars are seen in:**
    a. Infants   b. Children
    c. Adults   d. Very old people

43. **If suture marks are to be avoided, skin sutures should be removed by:** *(JIPMER 81, AMC 89)*
    a. 72 hours   b. 1 week
    c. 2 weeks   d. 3 weeks

44. **Degloving injury is:** *(Kerala 2000)*
    a. Surgeon made wound   b. Lacerated wound
    c. Blunt injury   d. Avulsion injury
    e. Abrasive wound

45. **In treatment of hand injuries, the greatest priority is:**
    (All India 96)
    a. Repair of tendons   b. Restoration of skin cover
    c. Repair of nerves   d. Repair of blood vessels

46. **'Limb salvage' primarily depends on:** *(AIIMS 97)*
    a. Vascular injury   b. Skin cover
    c. Bone injury   d. Nerve injury

47. **In an open injury during toileting and debridement, muscle viability is detected by:** *(PGI June 2003)*
    a. Colour of the muscle   b. Muscle size
    c. Muscle function   d. Muscle contractility
    e. Punctate bleeding spots on cut edge

48. **Criteria for viability of muscle are all except:**
    (Recent Question 2014)
    a. Colour   b. Intact fascia
    c. Contractibility   d. Bleeding on cutting

49. **Degloving injury:** *(Recent Question 2019, 2018)*
    a. Separation of skin only
    b. Separation of skin + subcutaneous tissue
    c. Separation of skin + subcutaneous tissue + fascia exposing tendons
    d. Separation of tendon exposing the bone

Explanations

WOUND HEALING

1. **Ans. a. Age; b. Nutrition; d. Drugs; e. Temperature** *(Ref: Sabiston 20/e p130-134, 19/e p151-164; Schwartz 10/e p241-268; Bailey 27/e p24)*
2. **Ans. b. Pre-op antibiotic therapy; c. Monofilament suture; d. Wound apposition** *(Ref: Bailey 27/e p52)*

   - Bailey says **"Preoperative shaving should be avoided except for aesthetic reasons** or to **prevent adherence of dressings**^{Q}. If it is to be undertaken, it **should be undertaken immediately before surgery** as the **SSI rate** after clean wound surgery may be **doubled if it is performed the night before**, because **minor skin injury enhances superficial bacterial colonization**^{Q}. Cream depilation is messy and **hair clipping is best**, with the **lowest rate of infection**^{Q}."

   > **Avoiding Surgical Site Infections**
   > - **Staff** should always **wash** their **hands between patients**^{Q}
   > - Length of **patient stay** should be **kept** to a **minimum**^{Q}
   > - **Preoperative shaving** should be **avoided if possible**^{Q}
   > - **Antiseptic skin preparation**^{Q} should be standardized
   > - **Bowel preparation for intra-abdominal surgeries**^{Q}
   > - **Pre-operative antibiotics** given **IV** at the time of **induction**^{Q}
   > - Attention to theatre technique and discipline
   > - **Avoid hypothermia** perioperatively and **ensure supplemental oxygenation** in recovery^Q
   > - **Monofilament sutures** are used over polyfilament sutures to **prevent infection**^{Q}
   > - **Proper apposition** of the wound and **prevention of** any **dead space** and **hematoma**^{Q}

3. **Ans. b. Deep dermal wound heal by scar formation; c. Wound contraction is found in healing by secondary intention** *(Ref: Sabiston 20/e p130-134; Schwartz 10/e p234, 1820; Bailey 27/e p24-25; Robbins 9/e p106)*
4. **Ans. a. Found in DM; c. May be associated with vascular compromise; d. Monofilament sutures prevent infection; e. Any wound that does not heal within 3 month** *(Ref: Bailey 27/e p29)*
5. **Ans. b. Platelet; e. Myofibroblasts** *(Ref: Sabiston 20/e p130-134; Schwartz 10/e p234,1820; Bailey 27/e p24-25)*

   > **CUTANEOUS WOUND HEALING**
   > - **Wound contraction:** Most clearly **differentiates primary from secondary healing**^{Q}
   > - **Permanent wound contraction** requires the **action of myofibroblasts, altered fibroblasts** that have the ultrastructural characteristics of smooth muscle cells^Q.
   > - **Contraction of these cells** at the wound site **decreases the gap** between the dermal edges of the wound.

6. **Ans. b. Debridement and suture** *(Ref: Sabiston 19/e p245; Schwartz 10/e p234,1820; Bailey 27/e p24-26, 89; Robbins 9/e p109)*

   - If the **blood supply to** the **wound is adequate** and **bacterial invasion is absent, wound** can be **safely closed anytime following proper debridement** and **irrigation**^{Q}.
     - If there is **established infection** and **tissue is of doubtful viability** has been left in-situ, then the **wound is left open** and **re-explored after 48 hours**^{Q}.
     - If there is **infection**, and the **doubtful viable tissue** is **now healthy**, the **deep tissues can be repaired** and the **wound is closed**^{Q}.
     - If however there is **further necrosis** and **infection**, the wound is **again debrided** and **left open**^{Q}.

7. **Ans. b. Vitamin E**
8. **Ans. b. 3–4 days**
9. **Ans. b. 48 hours**
10. **Ans. a. Exposure to UV light**
11. **Ans. c. 6 hours** *(Ref: Sabiston 19/e p245; Schwartz 9/e p219; Bailey 27/e p24-25,89; Robbins 9/e p109)*

WOUNDS CAN BE CLOSED BY

- **Primary suture:**
  - Clean wounds[Q]
  - Selected contaminated wounds after thorough **wound toileting** and **debridement**[Q]
- **Delayed primary suture:**
  - Heavily contaminated wounds[Q]
  - Wounds in which **wound toileting** has been **delayed for 6–8 hours**[Q]
- Left open to heal by secondary closure

12. **Ans. None** *(Ref: Sabiston 20/e p141; Schwartz 10/e p245; Robbins 9/e p109)*

The tensile strength of wound never equals that of unwounded skin.

WOUND STRENGTH

- **At the end of** the **1st week, wound strength** is approximately **10%** of that unwounded skin[Q].
- **Strength increases rapidly over** the **next 4 weeks**[Q].
  - This rate of increase then slows at approximately the **third month** after the original incision, and reaches a plateau at about **70–80%** of the **tensile strength**[Q] of unwounded skin, a condition that may persist for life.
- The **recovery of tensile strength** results from the **excess of collagen synthesis** over collagen degradation during the first two months of healing and later from **structural modification of collagen fibres**[Q] (cross linking, increased fiber size) after collagen synthesis ceases.

13. **Ans. None**
14. **Ans. b.** Debrided and sutured immediately
15. **Ans. c.** Between 17th to 21st day

- Over the **first three weeks, strength** and **collagen content both increases** but **after 21 days collagen content** remain **static and only wound strength increases**[Q].

16. **Ans. b.** Thorough cleaning with debridement of all dead and devitalized tissue without primary closure
17. **Ans. b.** Hypertension
18. **Ans. d.** 13–18 days
19. **Ans. a.** Primary intention
20. **Ans. a.** Elective open cholecystectomy for cholelithiasis
21. **Ans. a.** Local mesenchyme
22. **Ans. b.** Never
23. **Ans. a.** Resection of unprepared bowel, **b.** Perforated appendix resection

KELOID AND HYPERTROPHIC SCAR

24. **Ans. c.** Not familial; **e.** Not race related *(Ref: Sabiston 20/e p142-143; Schwartz 10/e p261-263; Bailey 27/e p31; Robbins 9/e p109)*
25. **Ans. a.** Usually occurs across the flexural areas
26. **Ans. d.** More amount of growth factors *(Ref: Bailey 27/e p31)*

"A keloid scar is defined as excessive scar tissue that extends beyond the boundaries of the original incision or wound. Its aetiology is unknown, but it is associated with elevated levels of growth factor, deeply pigmented skin, an inherited tendency and certain areas of the body (e.g. a triangle whose points are the xiphisternum and each shoulder tip). The histology of both hypertrophic and keloid scars shows excess collagen with hypervascularity, but this is more marked in keloids where there is more type III collagen."- Bailey 27/e p31

27. **Ans. c.** Precancerous leading to cancer; **e.** Whites are at high risk *(Ref: Sabiston 20/e p143; Schwartz 10/e p261-263; Bailey 27/e p31; Robbins 9/e p109)*
28. **Ans. b.** Tend to occur 3 months to one year after initial insult *(Ref: Sabiston 20/e p143; Schwartz 10/e p261; Bailey 27/e p31)*
29. **Ans. d.** It will have more collagen and vascularity
30. **Ans. c.** Presternal area

31. Ans. a. Intralesional injection of keloid *(Ref: Bailey 27/e p31)*
32. Ans. b. Triamcinolone
33. Ans. a. Dense collagen
34. Ans. b. It appears a few days after surgery
35. Ans. a. Intralesional injection of triamcinolone
36. Ans. b. Local recurrence is common after excision
37. Ans. c. Sternum
38. Ans. c. Eyelids

VACUUM ASSISTED CLOSURE

39. Ans. b. Large amount of necrotic tissue with eschar *(Ref: Long, Mary Arnold; Blevins, Anne (2009). "Options in negative pressure wound therapy". Journal of wound, ostomy and continence nursing 36 (2): 202-11)*
40. Ans. b. Clearance of infection
41. Ans. a. Bedsore in sacrum after debridement

MISCELLANEOUS

42. Ans. d. Very old people
43. Ans. b. 1 week *(Ref: Bailey 27/e p31-32)*

- **Suture marks** may be **minimised by** using **monofilament sutures** that are **removed** early **(3–5 days)**[Q].
- Sutures **inserted under tension** will **leave marks**[Q].
- The wound can be strengthened post suture removal by the use of sticky strips.
- **Fine sutures** (6/0 or smaller) placed **close to** the **wound margins** tend to **leave less scarring**[Q].
- **Subcuticular suturing avoids suture marks** either side of the wound or incision[Q].

44. Ans. d. Avulsion injury *(Ref: Bailey 27/e p27)*
45. Ans. d. Repair of blood vessels
46. Ans. a. Vascular injury
47. Ans. a. Colour of the muscle; d. Muscle contractility; e. Punctate bleeding spots on cut edge *(Ref: Bailey 25/e p354-356)*

Muscle Viability is Detected by '4C'

- **Colour**[Q]: Dead muscle has **dark unhealthy colour**, has **lost its sheen**
- **Contractility**[Q]: **Dead muscles do not twitch** when held by forceps.
- **Consistency**[Q]: Dead muscle has **lost** its **turgor** and is **mushy** in consistency
- **Capillary bleeding**[Q]: Dead muscle **does not bleed** at cut ends.

48. Ans. c. Intact fascia
49. Ans. b. Separation of skin + subcutaneous tissue *(Ref: Bailey 27/e p27)*

SECTION 7

Neurosurgery

CHAPTERS

- Cerebrovascular Diseases
- CNS Tumors

CHAPTER 33: Cerebrovascular Diseases

ARNOLD-CHIARI MALFORMATION

Arnold-Chiari malformation

Type I Chiari malformation
- Displacement of **cerebellar tonsil into cervical canal**[Q]
- Associated with **syringomyelia** of cervical canal
- Typically produces symptoms **during adolescence or adult life**[Q]
- **Not associated with hydrocephalus.**[Q]
- Patients complain of **recurrent headache, neck pain, urinary frequency, and progressive lower extremity spasticity**[Q].

Type II Chiari malformation
- Lesion represents an **anomaly** of the **hindbrain**
- Characterized by **elongation of** the **4th ventricle** and **kinking** of the **brainstem**, with **displacement** of the **inferior vermis, pons,** and **medulla** into the cervical canal[Q].
- Type II Chiari malformation is characterized by **progressive hydrocephalus** with a **myelomeningocele**[Q].
- Plain skull radiographs show a **small posterior fossa** and a **widened cervical canal**[Q].
- CT scanning with contrast and MRI display the **cerebellar tonsils protruding downward** into the **cervical canal** and the **hindbrain abnormalities**.
- The anomaly is treated by **surgical decompression**[Q].

VERTEBRAL BODY ANOMALIES

Vertebral Body Anomalies

- **Spina Bifida Occulta**
- **Spina Bifida Aperta**
  - Meningocele
  - Myelomeningocele
  - Myeloschisis

MENINGOCELE

MENINGOCELE

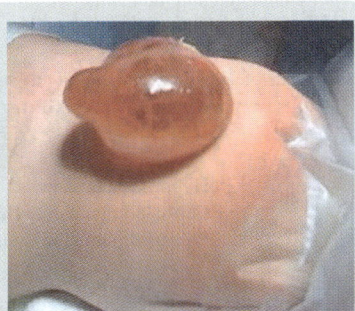

- **Herniation** of **meninges** through a **defect** in the **posterior vertebral arches**[Q].
- **Spinal cord** is **usually normal** and assumes a **normal position** in the spinal canal
- There may be tethering, syringomyelia, or diastematomyelia.

Clinical Features
- A **fluctuant midline mass,** that may transilluminate occurs along the vertebral column, in the **lower back**[Q].
- Most meningoceles are **well-covered with skin** and pose no threat to the patient.

Diagnosis
- **Plain roentgenograms** demonstrate a defect[Q].

Treatment
- **Asymptomatic children** with **normal neurologic findings** and **full-thickness skin** covering the meningocele may have **surgery delayed**[Q].
- Patients with **leaking CSF** or a **thin skin** covering should undergo **immediate surgical treatment** to prevent meningitis[Q].

MYELOMENINGOCELE

MYELOMENINGOCELE

- **Most severe form of dysraphism** involving the vertebral column
- **Incidence: 1/4,000 live births**[Q]
- MC site of myelomeningocele: **Lumbosacral region (75%)**[Q]

Etiology

- **Genetic predisposition** exists; the risk of recurrence after **one affected child** increases to **3-4%** and increases to **10%** with **two** previous abnormal pregnancies.

  - **Nutritional** and **environmental factors: Folate**[Q] is intricately involved in the prevention and etiology of NTDs.
  - **Maternal peri-conceptional use** of folic acid supplementation **reduces** the **incidence** of **neural tube defects** in pregnancies at risk by at least **50%**[Q].
  - To be effective, folic acid supplementation should be **initiated before conception** and **continued until** at least the **12th week of gestation** when neurulation is complete[Q].

Prevention

- All women of childbearing age and who are capable of becoming pregnant take 0.4 mg of folic acid daily.

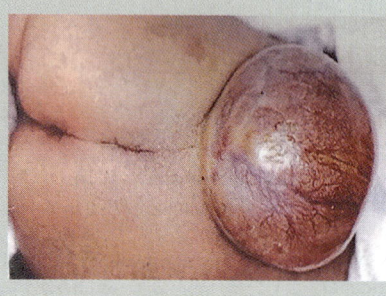

Drugs increasing the risk of myelomeningocele	
• Trimethoprim[Q]	• Phenobarbital[Q]
• Carbamazepine[Q]	• Primidone[Q]
• Phenytoin[Q]	• Valproic acid[Q]

Clinical Features

- Produces **dysfunction of skeleton, skin, gastrointestinal** and **genitourinary tracts**, in addition to the **peripheral nervous system** and **CNS**[Q].
- **Extent** and **degree** of the **neurologic deficit** depend on the **location** of the myelomeningocele, as well as the **associated lesions**.

Location	Manifestation
Low sacral region	**Bowel** and **bladder incontinence** associated with **anesthesia** in the **perineal area** but with no impairment of motor function.
Midlumbar region	Flaccid paralysis of lower extremity, absence of deep tendon reflexes, lack of response to touch and pain
Thoracic region	**Increasing neurologic deficit** as the myelomeningocele **extends higher** into the thoracic region.
Upper thoracic and **cervical region**	Very minimal neurological deficit and no hydrocephalus

DANDY-WALKER MALFORMATION

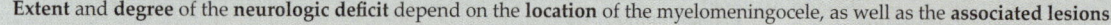

Dandy-Walker Malformation

- **MC posterior fossa malformation**[Q]
- **Prevalence:** 1 per 30,000 live births
- Consists of a **cystic expansion** of **4th ventricle** in the posterior fossa & **midline cerebellar hypoplasia**[Q]
- Results from a **developmental failure** of the **roof** of the **4th ventricle**[Q] during embryogenesis.

Dandy-Walker Malformation is characterized by the triad of
• Hypoplasia of vermis[Q]
• Cephalad rotation of the vermian remnant & cystic dilatation of 4th ventricle extending posteriorly[Q]
• Enlarged posterior fossa with torcular-lambdoid inversion[Q]

Clinical Features

- **MC manifestation: Macrocephaly**[Q] (80% cases); Associated with **hydrocephalus**[Q] (90% cases)
- Infants present with a **rapid increase** in **head size** & **prominent occiput**[Q].
- Transillumination of the skull may be positive.
- Most children have evidence of **long-tract signs**, **cerebellar ataxia**, and **delayed motor** & **cognitive milestones**, probably due to the **associated structural anomalies**[Q].

Associations

- **CNS abnormalities** are present in **70% cases** (i.e, **Agenesis** of the **posterior cerebellar vermis** & **corpus callosum**[Q], cortical dysplasia, polymicrogyria)

Diagnosis

- **IOC for diagnosis: MRI**[Q]

Treatment
- Managed by **shunting** the **cystic cavity**^Q (and on occasion the ventricles as well) in the presence of hydrocephalus.

Prognosis
- **High (~70%) mortality rate** due to associated abnormalities
- **Poorer prognosis** if diagnosed **prior to 21 weeks** of gestation

CAUSES OF CEREBROVASCULAR ACCIDENTS

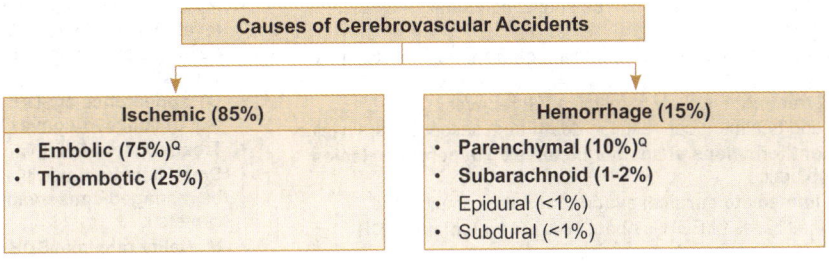

Intracerebral (Parenchymal) Hemorrhage	Subarachnoid Hemorrhage
• MC type of **intracranial hemorrhage**^Q • MC cause is **hypertension**^Q, causing rupture of small perforating arteries or arterioles^Q • MC site: Basal ganglia (**Putamen**^Q)	• **2nd MC cause** of intracranial hemorrhage^Q • MC cause: **Trauma** > Spontaneous rupture of **Berry aneurysm**^Q • MC site of Berry aneurysm is **anterior circulation** of "circle of willis"^Q

BERRY ANEURYSM (SACCULAR OR CONGENITAL ANEURYSM)

BERRY ANEURYSM (SACCULAR OR CONGENITAL ANEURYSM)

- **Berry aneurysms:** MC intracranial aneurysm^Q, **saccular** in appearance, arising at the **bifurcation of intracranial arteries**.
- About **85%** aneurysms occur in the **anterior circulation**, on the **circle of willis**^Q.

Occurrence of Berry aneurysm in order of frequency
• **Anterior communicating artery-Anterior Cerebral junction (29%)**^Q • Posterior communicating artery-Internal carotid junction (28%) • Middle cerebral bifurcation (18%) • Intracranial carotid bifurcation (8%) • Vertebrobasilar or basilar bifurcation (3%)

- **MC type** of intracranial aneurysm^Q; Multiple in 20-30% cases
- **Predisposing factors:** Smoking and **hypertension**^Q
- **Wall of Berry aneurysm** is made up of **thickened hyalinized intima**^Q. The adventitia covering the sac is continuous with that of parent artery.

Increased Risk of Berry Aneurysm in (FM)	
• ADPKD^Q • Ehlers-Danlos syndrome • NF-1^Q	• Marfan's syndrome • Fibromuscular dysplasia • Coarctation of aorta

- **Rupture of aneurysm** usually occurs **at the apex**^Q (dome) resulting in **subarachnoid hemorrhage**^Q or **intraparenchymal hemorrhage** or both^Q.
- **Unruptured aneurysms** are **usually completely asymptomatic**^Q.

Treatment
- Treatment consists of **coiling, coiling through a stent, or surgical clipping**
- **Endovascular coil occlusion is preferred over surgical clipping**^Q
- **Open craniotomy & clipping** is reserved for lesions not to be amenable to endovascular coiling^Q.

EXTRADURAL HEMATOMA AND SUBDURAL HEMATOMA

Extradural Hematoma	Subdural Hematoma (Acute)
• EDH is a **neurosurgical emergency**[Q]. • Nearly always **associated with** a **skull fracture**[Q]. • More common in **young male patients**[Q]. • Associated with **tearing of a meningeal artery**[Q]. • Hematoma accumulates in the space between **bone & dura**. • MC site: **Temporal**[Q] (pterion is **thinnest part** of skull & **overlies middle meningeal artery**) • **Not always arterial**: disruption of a major dural venous sinus can result in an EDH. • **Force required to sustain a skull fracture can be surprisingly small**[Q] – a fall from standing or a single blow to the head. • **Classical presentation**: Initial injury followed by a **lucid interval**[Q] (occurring in <1/3rd of cases) • **Early recognition & treatment** is likely to result in **full recovery** • Delays in diagnosis and treatment can result in **death** from secondary brain injury. • **EDH on CT scan**: **Lentiform** (**lens shaped** or **biconvex**[Q]) hyperdense lesion between the skull and brain. • **Treatment of EDH**: **Immediate surgical evacuation**[Q] via a craniotomy. • **Overall mortality** for all cases of EDH is about **18%** but for **isolated EDH** it is about **2%**.	• **SDH** accumulates in the space **between dura** and **arachnoid**[Q]. • **Disruption** of a **cortical vessel** or **brain laceration**[Q] • Nearly **always associated with** a **significant primary brain injury**[Q]. • Patients present with an **impaired conscious level** from the time of injury, but further deterioration can occur as the hematoma expands. • **CT appearance** of SDH: **Hyperdense** (acute blood) **concavo-convex appearance**[Q]. • **Treatment** of SDH: **Evacuation** via craniotomy. • **Small hematomas** with little mass effect may be **managed conservatively** in neurosurgical centers. • **Mortality rate** from **SDH** is **much higher** than for EDH and is as high as **40%** in some series[Q].

CLASSIFICATION OF SDH

Classification of SDH

- **Acute SDH: < 3 days**[Q]
- **Subacute SDH: 4-21 days**[Q]
- **Chronic SDH: >21 days**[Q]

CHRONIC SUBDURAL HEMATOMA

Chronic Subdural Hematoma

- Chronic SDH: Collection of blood breakdown products that is **at least 2-3 weeks old**[Q].
- Chronic SDHs often occur in patients without a clear history of head trauma, as they may arise from minor trauma[Q].

Clinical Features

- **Alcoholics**, the **elderly**, and **patients on anticoagulation** are at **higher risk** for developing **chronic SDH**[Q].
- Patients may present with **headache, seizure, confusion**, **contralateral hemiparesis**, or **coma**[Q].

Treatment

- A chronic SDH >1 cm or any symptomatic SDH should be surgically drained.
- **Chronic SDH** typically consists of a **viscous fluid**, with a texture and **dark brown color** reminiscent of **motor oil**.
- A simple **burr hole** can effectively **drain most chronic SDHs**.

  - The procedure is **converted to open craniotomy** if the SDH is **too congealed for irrigation drainage**, the complex of membranes **prevents effective drainage**, or **persistent hemorrhage** occurs that cannot be reached with bipolar cautery through the burr hole[Q].

- **Follow-up head CT scans**: Approximately **1 month later** to document resolution.
- Harrison says "Epidural hematomas occur in **upto 10% of severe head injury** cases and are **less often associated with** underlying **cortical damage than subdural hematomas.**"[Q]

SUBARACHNOID HEMORRHAGE

Subarachnoid Hemorrhage

- MC cause: Trauma >Spontaneous rupture of **Berry aneurysm**[Q]

Clinical Features

- **Sudden transient loss of consciousness**[Q] (occurs in nearly half of the patients)
- **Excruciating severe headache**[Q]: presenting complaint in 45% of cases (worst headache of patients life) more common upon regaining consciousness when loss of consciousness is associated

- Neck stiffness and vomiting^Q: are common associations
- Focal neurological deficit: uncommon.
- Sudden headache in the absence of focal neurological deficit is the hallmark of aneurysmal rupture.^{Q}

- Associated prodromal symptoms (suggest **location** of progressively enlarging unruptured aneurysm):
  - **Third cranial nerve palsy**^{Q}: Aneurysm at junction of **PCA** and **ICA**
  - **Sixth nerve palsy**^{Q}: Aneurysm in **cavernous sinus**
  - Occipital and posterior cervical pain: **Inferior cerebellar artery aneurysm**
  - **Pain in or behind the eye**^{Q}: **MCA aneurysm**

Diagnosis
- **Noncontrast CT scan: Investigation of choice** (Lumbar puncture is not indicated prior to an imaging procedure)
- **CSF picture: Hallmark** of aneurysmal rupture is **blood in CSF (Xanthochromic spinal fluid**^{Q})

  - **Lumbar puncture** should be performed, **if the CT scan fails to establish the diagnosis of SAH** and **no mass lesion** or **obstructive hydrocephalus** is found to establish the presence of subarachnoid blood.^{Q}

Treatment
- **Traumatic subarachnoid hemorrhage** is **managed conservatively**^{Q}.

DIFFUSE AXONAL INJURIES (DAI)

Diffuse Axonal Injuries (DAI)

- **DAI** represents the **presence of widespread axonal damage (white matter)** in **both hemispheres secondary to severe head injury**^{Q}.
- Results from application of **severe acceleration/deceleration** or **angular strain** to the brain (**injuries to axons by shearing force**^{Q})
- **MC location: Lobar white matter** at the **junction of grey and white matter**^{Q} > Corpus callosum > Brain stem

Pathology
- **Hemorrhagic** or **non-hemorrhagic white matter tears** in both hemispheres.

Clinical Features
- Clinical presentation vary from concussion to coma
- **Loss of consciousness** is a common finding^Q
- **DAI: MC cause of post-traumatic vegetative state**^{Q}
- **Raised ICT may or may not be associated**^{Q}

Diagnosis
- **MRI is IOC for DAI**^{Q} (better than CT scan).

Prognosis
- **DAI** carries an **extremely poor prognosis**^{Q}.

Brain Injury	
Primary Brain Injury	**Secondary Brain Injury**

• Primary brain injury occurs **at the time of impact**
• Includes injuries such as:
  – **Brainstem and hemispheric contusions**^{Q}
  – **Diffuse axonal injury**^{Q}
  – **Cortical lacerations**^{Q}
	• Secondary brain injury occurs at **some time after** the **moment of impact**^{Q}
	• **Preventable**^{Q}
	• **Principle causes**: Hypoxia, hypotension, raised ICP, reduced cerebral perfusion pressure and pyrexia^Q

CEREBRAL CONTUSIONS

Cerebral Contusions

- **Cerebral contusions** result from the **brain being damaged by:**
  - Impacting against the skull either at the **point of impact** (the **'coup'**) or on the **other side of** the head (**'contre-coup'**)^Q
    - As the **brain slides forwards and backwards over** the **ridged cranial fossa floor** (most often affecting the **inferior frontal lobes** and **temporal poles**)^Q

Diagnosis

- **CT scan: Heterogeneous** with **mixed areas of high** and **low density**[Q].
  - There may be an associated mass effect. Contusion appears uniformly hyperdense.

Treatment

- Cerebral contusions **rarely require immediate surgical treatment**.

> - Patient with **cerebral contusions** must be **admitted for observation** as these lesions will **tend to mature** and **expand for 48–72 hours** following injury[Q].

- **Small proportion** of cerebral contusions will require **delayed surgical evacuation to reduce** the **mass effect**[Q].

SKULL BASE FRACTURES

Skull Base		
Anterior Cranial Fossa	**Middle Cranial Fossa**	**Posterior Cranial Fossa**
• Formed by frontal bone[Q]	• Formed by temporal & sphenoid bone[Q]	• Formed by occipital bone[Q]
Cribriform plate: Sieve like structure between anterior cranial fossa & nasal cavity		

Anterior Cranial Fossa Fracture	Middle Cranial Fossa Fracture	Posterior Cranial Fossa Fracture

• **MC type** of skull base fracture[Q]
• Caused by **fracture of cribriform plate**[Q]
• Clinical features:
  – Subconjunctival hematoma[Q]
  – CSF rhinorrhea[Q]
  – Epistaxis[Q]
  – Anosmia[Q]
  – Periorbital hematoma or **"Raccoon eyes"**[Q]
  – Carotico cavernous fistula[Q]
  – Frontal lobe contusion[Q]
	• Caused by **fracture of petrous part of temporal bone**[Q]
	• Clinical features:
	  – CSF otorrhea[Q]
	  – Paradoxical rhinorrhea[Q]
	  – Hemotympanum[Q]
	  – **Battle sign**[Q]: Bruising or ecchymosis behind ear
	  – Ossicular disruption[Q]
	  – VII & VIII cranial nerve palsies[Q]
	  – Temporal lobe contusion[Q]
		• Caused by **fracture of occipital bone**[Q]
		• Clinical features:
		  – Visual disturbances[Q]
		  – VI cranial nerve injury[Q]
		  – Jugular foramen syndrome (**Vernet syndrome**[Q]): Paresis of IX, X, XI cranial nerves[Q]
		  – Basilar artery injury[Q]
		  – Occipital contusion[Q]

STEPWISE APPROACH TO TREATMENT OF ELEVATED INTRACRANIAL PRESSURE

Stepwise Approach to Treatment of Elevated Intracranial Pressure

- Insert ICP monitor—**ventriculostomy**[Q] versus parenchymal device
- **General goals**: maintain ICP <20 mm Hg and CPP 60 mm Hg[Q]
- For ICP >20–25 mm Hg for >5 min:
  - Drain CSF via **ventriculostomy**[Q] (if in place)
  - **Elevate head of the bed**[Q]; midline head position
  - Osmotherapy—**mannitol**[Q] 25–100 g q4h as needed (maintain serum osmolality <320[Q] mosmol) or hypertonic saline[Q] (30 mL, 23.4% NaCl bolus)
  - **Glucocorticoids**—dexamethasone 4 mg q6h for vasogenic edema from tumor, abscess[Q] (**avoid glucocorticoids** in head **trauma, ischemic** and **hemorrhagic stroke**[Q])
  - **Sedation**[Q] (e.g., morphine, propofol, or midazolam); add neuromuscular paralysis, if necessary (patient will require endotracheal intubation and mechanical ventilation at this point, if not before)
  - **Hyperventilation**[Q]—to $PaCO_2$ 30–35 mm Hg
  - **Pressor therapy**[Q]—phenylephrine, dopamine, or norepinephrine to maintain adequate MAP to ensure CPP 60 mm Hg (maintain euvolemia to minimize deleterious systemic effects of pressors
  - Consider **second-tier therapies** for **refractory elevated ICP**:
    a. High-dose barbiturate therapy (**"pentobarb coma"**)[Q]
    b. **Aggressive hyperventilation** to $PaCO_2$ <30 mm Hg[Q]
    c. **Hypothermia**[Q]
    d. **Hemicraniectomy**[Q]

BRAIN ABSCESS

BRAIN ABSCESS

- Intracerebral abscess may occur as a result of **direct spread from air sinus infection**, following **surgery** or from **hematogenous spread** especially associated with **respiratory infection, endocarditis** or **dental infection**^{Q}.
- **Increased risk** of abscess in: **Cyanotic heart disease, immunocompromised** (diabetes, solid organ transplant, hematological malignancy or long-term steroids)^Q

Etiology	Location
Otitis media, mastoiditis	Temporal lobe^Q >Cerebellum
Paranasal sinusitis, dental infections	Frontal lobes^Q
Hematogenous	Parietal lobe^Q

Clinical Features
- Presentation is with **focal signs, seizures** and **raised ICP**, as with other mass lesions, but the **time course is often short**^{Q}
- Patients may be febrile or have a raised peripheral white cell count or inflammatory markers.

Diagnosis
- IOC for diagnosis: **MRI**^{Q}
- CT scan: Ring-enhancing mass lesion (may be **multiple** in case of **hematogenous spread**)^Q

Treatment
- **Surgical drainage + IV antibiotics** for at least 6 weeks^Q.
- **Multiple small abscesses** may be **treated medically** with antibiotics targeted against organisms
- Steroids are **reserved for** cases with **significant edema** or **mass effect**^{Q}
- Owing to the **high risk of seizures**, patients should also be **treated with anticonvulsants**.

NORMAL-PRESSURE HYDROCEPHALUS (NPH)

NORMAL-PRESSURE HYDROCEPHALUS (NPH)

- Characterized by the **clinical triad** of:
  - **Abnormal gait** (ataxic or apractic)^Q
  - **Dementia**^{Q} (usually **mild to moderate**, with an emphasis on executive impairment)
  - **Urinary urgency** or **incontinence**^{Q}
- This syndrome is a **communicating hydrocephalus**^{Q} with a patent aqueduct of Sylvius

- NPH may be caused by **obstruction to normal CSF flow over the cerebral convexities** and **delayed resorption** into the venous system.
- The indolent nature of the process results in **enlarged lateral ventricles** with relatively **little increase in CSF pressure**^{Q}.

Diagnosis
- MRI: Enlarged lateral ventricles (hydrocephalus) with little or **no cortical atrophy**^{Q}
- **Lumbar puncture opening pressure** falls in the **high normal range**^{Q}
- **CSF protein, glucose** and **cell counts** are **normal**.

Multiple Choice Questions

BERRY ANEURYSM

1. **The most common site of Berry aneurysm is:** *(All India 94)*
   a. Junction of anterior communication artery with anterior cerebral artery
   b. Junction of posterior communicating artery with internal carotid artery
   c. Bifurcation of middle cerebral artery
   d. Vertebral artery

2. **All are common sites of berry aneurysm, except:** *(AIIMS June 93)*
   a. Posterior cerebral artery   b. Vertebral artery
   c. Anterior cerebral artery   d. Middle cerebral artery

3. **True about berry-aneurysm is following except:**
   a. Associated with familial syndrome   *(PGI June 2000)*
   b. Most common site of rupture is apex which causes SAH
   c. Wall contains smooth muscle fibroblasts
   d. 90% occurs at anterior part of circulation at branching point

4. **Most common presentation of intracranial aneurysm is:** *(PGI June 98)*
   a. Coarctation of aorta   b. Systemic hypertension
   c. Hypotension   d. Intracranial hemorrhage

5. **Which is least common site of Berry aneurysm?** *(AIIMS Dec 95)*
   a. Basilar artery   b. Vertebral artery
   c. Anterior cerebral artery   d. Posterior cerebral artery

CEREBROVASCULAR ACCIDENTS

6. **All are predisposing causes of cerebral venous thrombosis except:** *(COMEDK 2005)*
   a. Hypotension   b. Oral contraceptives
   c. Pregnancy   d. Aplastic anemia

7. **The most common site of hypertensive intracranial hemorrhage is:** *(COMEDK 2010)*
   a. Putamen   b. Midbrain
   c. Medulla   d. Cerebrum

8. **Most common cause of cerebrovascular accident is:** *(AIIMS 96, All India 98)*
   a. Embolism   b. Arterial thrombosis
   c. Venous thrombosis   d. Hemorrhage

9. **Most common cause of stroke young women in India among OCP users:** *(PGI Dec 98)*
   a. Cortical vein thrombosis   b. Moyamoya disease
   c. Atherosclerosis   d. HT

10. **Most common cause of intracranial hemorrhage is:** *(AIIMS Nov 98)*
    a. Subarachnoid hemorrhage
    b. Intracerebral hemorrhage
    c. Subdural hemorrhage
    d. Extradural hemorrhage

11. **The commonest cause of intracerebral bleed is:**
    a. Thrombocytopenia   b. Diabetes   *(All India 95)*
    c. Hypertension   d. Berry aneurysm

12. **Which of the following is the most common location of hypertensive hemorrhage?** *(KERALA PG 2015; All Indian 2003, 94, AIIMS Nov 2002)*
    a. Pons   b. Thalamus
    c. Putamen/external capsule   d. Subcotrical white matter

13. **Commonest cause of subarachnoid hemorrhage is:**
    a. Rupture of circle of Willis aneurysm   *(All India 98)*
    b. Rupture of vertebral artery aneurysm
    c. Rupture of venecomitants of corpus striatum
    d. Rupture of dural sinuses

14. **Which of the following is the most common cause of late neurological deterioration in case of cerebrovascular accident?** *(AIIMS Nov 2000)*
    a. Rebleeding   b. Vasospasm
    c. Embolism   d. Hydrocephalus

15. **A patient known to have mitral stenosis and arterial fibrillation presents with acute onset of weakness in the left upper limb which recovered completely in two weeks. The most likely diagnosis is:** *(All India 2010)*
    a. Transient ischemic attack   b. Ischemic stroke
    c. Hemorrhagic stroke   d. Vasculitis

16. **'Duret hemorrhages' are seen in:** *(AIIMS May 2008)*
    a. Brain   b. Kidney
    c. Heart   d. Lung

17. **Denver criteria is used for:** *(Recent Question 2017)*
    a. Blunt cerebrovascular trauma
    b. Blunt trauma chest
    c. Blunt trauma abdomen
    d. Penetrating trauma abdomen

EDH AND SDH

18. **Subdural hematoma is caused by injury of:** *(Recent Question 2017)*
    a. Cortical vessels   b. Venous sinus
    c. Middle cerebral artery   d. Middle meningeal artery

19. **Lucid interval is classically seen in:** *(MCI June 2018, DNB 2010, COMEDK 2007, PGI Dec 97)*
    a. Intracerebral hematoma
    b. Acute subdural hematoma
    c. Chronic subdural hematoma
    d. Extradural hematoma

20. **Middle meningeal vessel damage results in:** *(COMEDK 2011)*
    a. Subdural hemorrhage   b. Subarachnoid hemorrhage
    c. Intracerebral hemorrhage   d. Epidural hemorrhage

21. **Common site for extradural hemorrhage:** *(DNB 2012)*
    a. Frontal   b. Temporoparietal
    c. Occipital   d. Brainstem

22. **A 15 days duration SDH is:** *(MHSSMCET 2009)*
    a. Hyperacute   b. Acute
    c. Subacute   d. Chronic

23. **For chronic SDH the duration should be more than:** *(MHSSMCET 2010)*
    a. 3 days   b. 7 days
    c. 15 days   d. 1 months

24. Best treatment of subdural hematoma in a deteriorating patient: *(HPU 2005)*
    a. By I/V Mannitol
    b. Oxygenation
    c. Use of steroids
    d. Surgical evacuation
25. This is the plain CT scan of a male who sustained an injury with a baseball bat. Which of the following statements are TRUE regarding this condition? *(APPG 2016)*
    P. Middle meningeal artery is the vessel commonly injured
    Q. Usually occurs several weeks after a trivial injury, often forgotten
    R. Lucid interval is classical but seen only in 1/5 t0 1/3 patients
    S. May be associated with a Hutchinson pupil:

    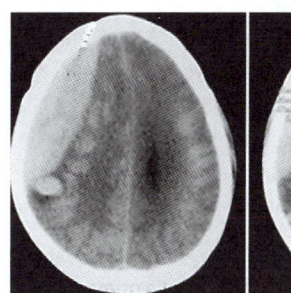 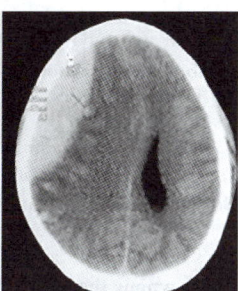

    a. Only P, R are correct
    b. Only P, R, S are correct
    c. Only Q,R,S are correct
    d. P,Q,R,S all are correct
26. Chronic subdural hematoma refers to collection present for a period of: *(Karnataka 2006)*
    a. 7 days
    b. 6 months
    c. 1 year
    d. 21 days
27. Extradural hematoma is associated with what % of severe trauma? *(PGI Dec 98)*
    a. 36%
    b. 10%
    c. 77%
    d. 96%
28. A person has been brought in casualty with history of road accident. He had lost consciousness transiently and gained consciousness but again became unconscious. Most likely, he is having brain hemorrhage of: *(AIIMS Nov 2005)*
    a. Intracerebal
    b. Subarachnoid
    c. Subdural
    d. Extradural
29. Management of extradural hemorrhage is: *(AIIMS 93)*
    a. Antibiotics
    b. Immediate evacuation
    c. Evacuation after 24 hours
    d. Observation
30. Features of extradural hemorrhage include in all *except*:
    a. Severe hypotension
    b. Deteriorating consciousness
    c. Fixed dilated pupil on the same side
    d. Fracture line crossing the temporal bone
31. An elderly man who has had a trivial history of head injury three months ago, develops headache and turns unconscious. On examination, he is found to have fixed left dilated pupil and right hemiplegia. What is the most likely diagnosis?
    a. Contusio-cerberi *(UPSC 96)*
    b. Extradural hematoma
    c. Chronic subdural hematoma
    d. Brain abscess
32. Most common cause of sub-dural hematoma: *(SCTIMS 98)*
    a. Middle meningeal artery tear
    b. Rupture of superior cerebral vein
    c. Internal carotid artery tear
    d. None of the above
33. A patient presents with sudden headache and vomiting and unconsciousness. The diagnosis is: *(DPG 2009 Feb)*
    a. Subarachnoid hemorrhage
    b. Intracerebral hemorrhage
    c. Subdural hemorrhage
    d. Extradural hemorrhage
34. Subdural hematoma most commonly results from:
    a. Rupture of intracranial aneurysm *(AIIMS May 2004)*
    b. Rupture of cerebral AVM
    c. Injury to cortical bridging veins
    d. Hemophilia
35. Which of the following will manifest as "pachymeningitis heamorrhagica interna"? *(MAHE 2006)*
    a. Epidural hematoma
    b. Subdural hematoma
    c. Subarachnoid hemorrhage
    d. Brain infraction
36. Immediate surgery is indicated in: *(Kerala 95)*
    a. Extradural hemorrhage
    b. Subdural hemorrhage
    c. Intracerebral hemorrhage
    d. Brain laceration
37. A 62-years-old diabetic female patient presented with history of progressive right-sided weakness of one month duration. The patient was also having speech difficulty. Fundus examination showed papilledema. Two months ago, she also had a fall in her bathroom and struck her head against a wall. The most likely clinical diagnosis is: *(AIIMS Nov 2004)*
    a. Alzheimer's disease
    b. Left parietal glioma
    c. Left MCA territory stroke
    d. Left chronic subdural hematoma
38. An elderly female presented with history of progressive right-sided weakness and speech difficulty. She gives a history of a fall in her bathroom two months back. The most likely clinical diagnosis is: *(All India 91)*
    a. Progressive supranuclear palsy
    b. Left cerebral tumor
    c. Left sided stroke
    d. Left chronic subdural hematoma
39. You are a surgeon posted at CHC. A patient of head injury comes to you with rapidly deteriorating sensorium and progressive dilatation and fixation of pupil. Neurosurgeon and CT scan is not available. You decide to make a burr hole to emergently relieve the intracranial pressure. Which of the following sites will you choose? *(AIIMS November 2014)*
    a. In the temporal region contralateral to the side of pupillary dilatation
    b. In the midline if both pupils are equal or it is not known which side dilated first
    c. In the left temporal region if no localizing sign is found
    d. Refer to higher centre if both pupils are equal or it is not known which side dilated first

SUBARACHNOID AND INTRACRANIAL HEMORRHAGE

40. The common cause of subarachnoid hemorrhage is:
    a. Arteriovenous malformation *(All India 2006)*
    b. Cavernous angioma
    c. Aneurysm
    d. Hippocampus
41. A patient comes to ER with headache describing it as worst headache in his life. What is the next step?
    a. CT brain
    b. Lumbar puncture
    c. MRI brain *(AIIMS November 2017)*
    d. Observation and analgesics
42. Most common cause of subarachnoid hemorrhage is: *(Recent Question 2016, 2014, AIIMS Nov 98, All India 1999)*
    a. Hypertension
    b. AV malformation
    c. Berry aneurysm
    d. Tumors

Surgery Essence

43. A female presented with severe headache of sudden onset. On CT scan a diagnosis of subarachnoid hemorrhage is made. The most common site of subarachnoid hemorrhage is: *(AIIMS June 2001)*
    a. Middle meningeal artery
    b. Berry aneurysm rupture
    c. Basilar artery
    d. Subdural venous sinuses

44. Which of the following grading methods is used to evaluate the prognosis/outcome after subarachnoid hemorrhage?
    a. Glasgow coma scale *(All India 2010)*
    b. Hess and Hunt scale
    c. Glasgow - Blatchford bleeding score
    d. Intracerebral hemorrhage score

45. Identify the condition shown in the CT scan below: *(Recent Question 2018)*
    a. Extradural hemorrhage
    b. Subdural hemorrhage
    c. Subarachnoid hemorrhage
    d. Intraventricular hemorrhage

46. A 45-year-old hypertensive male presented with sudden onset most severe headache, vomiting and neck stiffness. On examination he didn't have any focal neurological deficit. His CT scan shoed blood in the Sylvain fissure. The probable diagnosis is: *(AIIMS May 2003)*
    a. Meningitis
    b. Ruptured aneurysm
    c. Hypertensive bleed
    d. Stroke

47. A 45-year-old male patient presented in the casualty with two hours history of sudden onset of severe headache associated with nausea and vomiting, on clinical examination the patient had necks stiffness and right sided ptosis. Rest of the neurological examination was normal. What is the clinical diagnosis? *(AIIMS Nov 2003)*
    a. Hypertensive brain hemorrhage
    b. Migraine
    c. Aneurysmal subarachnoid hemorrhage
    d. Arteriovenous malformation

48. An adult hypertensive male presented with sudden onset severe headache and vomiting. On examination, their is marked neck rigidity and no neurological deficit was found. The symptoms are most likely due to:
    a. Intracranial parenchymal hemorrhage
    b. Ischemic stroke *(AIIMS May 2013, AIIMS May 2012)*
    c. Meningitis
    d. Subarachnoid hemorrhage

49. A young female presents with severe headache and neck stiffness of abrupt onset. She says, she has never had such severe headache before. She also complains of associated nausea and photophobia. Likely diagnosis is: *(AIIMS May 2009)*
    a. Subarachnoid hemorrhage (SAH)
    b. Migraine
    c. Viral encephalitis
    d. Hydrocephalus

50. A patient presented with thunder clap headache followed by unconsciousness and progressive III cranial nerve pasty. Which of the following is the most likely diagnosis:
    a. Extradural hemorrhage *(AIIMS Nov 2010)*
    b. Aneurysmal subarachnoid hemorrhage
    c. Basilar migraine
    d. Cluster headache

51. Triple H therapy for subarachnoid hemorrhage consists of all except: *(DNB 2014)*
    a. Hypertension
    b. Hypervolaemia
    c. Hemodilution
    d. Hypothermia

HEAD INJURY

52. In a head injury patient, mannitol should not be used for control of increase intracranial pressure when:
    a. Serum osmolality >320 mOsmol/kg *(COMEDK 2010)*
    b. Arterial $PaCO_2$ <35 mm Hg
    c. Arterial PaO_2 >100 mm Hg
    d. Arterial pH 7.4

53. Which of the following is not correct about head injury? *(Recent Question 2018)*
    a. MRI needed to assess hemorrhage
    b. GCS assessment helps in prognosis
    c. Hematoma must be operated
    d. All of the above

54. Cerebral edema is not caused by: *(Punjab 2011)*
    a. Lead toxicity
    b. Craniosynostosis
    c. Corticosteroids administration
    d. Vitamin A intoxication

55. Not a primary brain injury: *(Punjab 2011)*
    a. Diffuse axonal injury
    b. Contusion
    c. Concussion
    d. Intracerebral hematoma

56. Which among the following is a not a primary brain injury? *(JIPMER 2010)*
    a. Cortical lacerations
    b. Brainstem herniation
    c. Diffuse axonal injury
    d. Brainstem contusion

57. About cranial trauma false is: *(AIIMS Nov 2010)*
    a. Raccoon eyes seen in subgaleal hemorrhage
    b. Depressed skull fracture is associated with brain injury at the immediate area of impact
    c. Caroticocavernous fistula occur in base skull fracture
    d. Post traumatic epilepsy seen in 15%

58. Which is an ominous sign in case of severe head injury?
    a. Development of diabetes insipidus *(PGI Nov 2010)*
    b. Anisocoria
    c. New focal deficit
    d. Depressed skull fracture
    e. Decorticate posturing

59. A 25 years old male of head injury was brought to emergency in unconscious state. What is the name of sign seen in this image?

    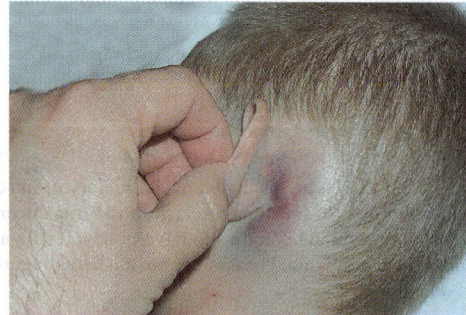

    a. Duret hemorrhage
    b. Battle sign
    c. Kernohan's phenomenon
    d. Raccoon sign

60. Battle's sign is present in: *(MHSSMCET 2006, 2005)*
    a. Anterior cranial fossa fracture
    b. Middle cranial fossa fracture
    c. Posterior cranial fossa fracture
    d. Fracture lesser wing of sphenoid

61. In a vehicular accident, extensive contusions of brain due to acceleration and deceleration injury indicate what kind of injury? *(MHSSMCET 2006)*
    a. Penetrating injury
    b. Coup-Countercoup injury
    c. Second impact syndrome
    d. Crush injury
62. The most common neurologic abnormality that occurs with head injury is: *(Karnataka 2005)*
    a. Hemiplegia
    b. Ocular nerve palsy
    c. Altered consciousness
    d. Convulsion
63. Cushing reflex is: *(UPPG 2007)*
    a. ↑Mean arterial pressure with increased intracranial pressure
    b. ↑Mean arterial pressure with decreased intracranial pressure
    c. ↓Mean arterial pressure with increased intracranial pressure
    d. ↓Mean arterial pressure with decreased intracranial pressure
64. Raised intracranial pressure will cause: *(MCI March 2007)*
    a. Tachycardia
    b. Hypotension
    c. Papilloedema
    d. Normal looking anterior fontenalle in infants
65. True statement regarding fracture base of the skull are all of the following except:
    a. Prophylactic antibiotics are usually not required
    b. Associated with 8th cranial nerve palsy
    c. Early surgery is indicated for optimal outcome
    d. May present with CSF otorrhoea
66. The cause of systemic secondary insult to injured brain include all of the following except: *(AIIMS May 2006)*
    a. Hypercapnia
    b. Hypoxemia
    c. Hypotension
    d. Hypothermia
67. In a patient with head injury damage in the brain is aggravated by: *(All India 2010)*
    a. Hyperglycemia
    b. Hypothermia
    c. Hypocapnia
    d. Serum osmolality
68. Best prognostic factor for head injury is: *(All India 2007)*
    a. Glasgow coma scale
    b. Age
    c. Mode of injury
    d. CT
69. A 25 years old male was brought to casualty with history of RTA. NCCT was done. What is the diagnosis?
    (Recent Question 2017)
    a. EDH
    b. SDH
    c. Subarachnoid hemorrhage
    d. None of the above

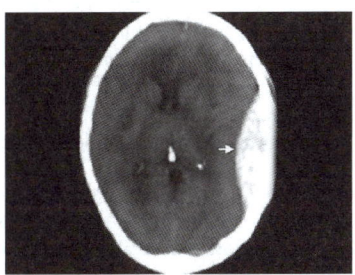

70. True regarding epidural hematoma is/are: *(PGI May 2018)*
    a. Arterial bleed
    b. On CT scan it gives biconvex lenticular hyperdense appearance
    c. Located on lateral side of hemisphere
    d. Common after injury at pterion

71. The earliest manifestations of increased intracranial pressure following head injury is: *(All India 2005)*
    a. Ipsilateral papillary dilatation
    b. Contralateral papillary dilatation
    c. Altered mental status
    d. Hemiparesis
72. A 65 years old male was brought to casualty with history of RTA. NCCT was done. What is the diagnosis?
    (Recent Question 2017)
    a. EDH
    b. SDH
    c. Subarachnoid hemorrhage
    d. None of the above

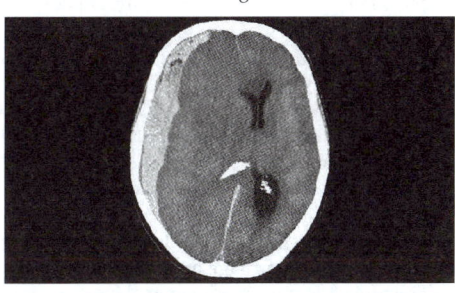

73. False statement regarding subdural hematoma:
    (JIPMER May 2018)
    a. Occurs on both sides
    b. Not visible on X-ray
    c. Surgery can be done
    d. Unilateral surgery
74. Transtentorial uncal herniation causes all except:
    (AIIMS May 2001)
    a. Ipsilateral dilated pupils
    b. Ipsilateral hemiplegia
    c. Cheyne stokes respiration
    d. Decorticate rigidity
75. A patient present with unilateral painful ophthalmoplegia. Imaging revealed an enlargement of cavernous sinus on the affected side. The likely diagnosis is: *(AIIMS May 2008)*
    a. Gradenigo syndrome
    b. Cavernous sinus thrombosis
    c. Tolosa-Hunt Syndrome
    d. Orbital Pseudotumor
76. Non-noxious stimuli perceived as pain is termed as:
    (AIIMS May 2008)
    a. Allodynia
    b. Hyperalgesia
    c. Hyperesthesia
    d. Hyperpathia
77. Spontaneous CSF leaks may be associated with all except:
    a. Increased Intracranial Tension *(AIIMS Nov 2008)*
    b. Pseudotumor cerebri
    c. Empty Sella Syndrome
    d. Encephalocele
78. All of the following statements about Diffuse Axonal Injury (DAI) are true except: *(All India 2008)*
    a. Caused by shearing force
    b. Predominant white matter hemorrhages, in basal ganglion and corpus callosum
    c. Increased intracranial tension is seen in all cases
    d. Most common at junction of grey and white matter
79. Retraction ball is seen in: *(Recent Question 2015)*
    a. Burns
    b. Acute pancreatitis
    c. Diffuse axonal injury
    d. Tracheobronchial injury
80. Neurosurgery is indicated for all except: *(Recent Question 2013)*
    a. SDH
    b. EDH
    c. Depressed fracture
    d. Diffuse axonal injury

Surgery Essence

81. A 24-year-old man falls on the ground when he is struck in the right temple by a baseball. While being driven to the hospital, he lapses into coma. He is unresponsive with the dilated right pupil when be reaches the emergency department. The most important step in initial management is: *(BIHAR PG 2014; All India 2002)*
    a. Craniotomy
    b. CT scan of the head
    c. X-ray of the skull and cervical spine
    d. Doppler ultrasound examination of the neck

82. All of the following lower intracranial pressure except:
    a. Mannitol
    b. Furosemide *(All India 98)*
    c. Corticosteroids
    d. Hyperventilation

83. In skull fracture, the condition in which an operation is not done immediately is: *(All India 96)*
    a. Depressed fracture
    b. Compound fracture
    c. CSF leak
    d. Increased size of head

84. Surgery is not useful in:
    a. Cerebral edema
    b. Depressed fracture
    c. Extradural hemorrhage
    d. Subdural hemorrhage

85. In a patient with head injury black eye associated with subconjunctival hemorrhage occurs when there is:
    a. Fracture of floor of anterior cranial fossa
    b. Bleeding between the skin and galea aponeurotica
    c. Hemorrhage between galea aponeurotica and pericranium
    d. Fracture of greater wing of sphenoid bone

86. Patient with a history of fall presents weeks later with headache and progressive neurological deterioration. The diagnosis is: *(Recent Question 2016)*
    a. Acute subdural hemorrhage
    b. Extradural hemorrhage
    c. Chronic subdural hemorrhage
    d. Fracture skull

87. The treatment of post traumatic epilepsy is:
    a. Mannitol infusion
    b. Immediate corticosteroids
    c. Long term anticonvulsants
    d. Long term corticosteroids

88. Following are the features of raised intracranial tension *except*:
    a. Altered sensorium
    b. Papilloedma
    c. Convulsions
    d. Tachycardia

89. Facial nerve palsy is seen in the following fracture:
    a. Anterior cranial fossa
    b. Middle cranial fossa
    c. Cranial vault
    d. Posterior cranial fossa

90. The most important clinical finding in a case of head injury is: *(JIPMER 91)*
    a. Pupillary dilatation
    b. Level of consciousness
    c. Focal neurological deficit
    d. Fracture skull

91. Signs of cerebral compression are all *except*: *(Recent Question 2016)*
    a. Bradycardia
    b. Hypotension
    c. Papilloedma
    d. Vomiting

92. In patient of head injury with rapidly increasing intracranial tension without hematoma, the drug of choice for initial management would be: *(UPSC 2000)*
    a. Lasix
    b. Steroids
    c. 20% Mannitol
    d. Glycine

93. All of the following are indications of CT scan in head injured patient except: *(DNB 2014)*
    a. GCS < 13
    b. Vomiting 1 episode
    c. Focal neurological deficit
    d. Mild head injury in patient Age > 65 years

94. All of the following are the components of Cushing triad except: *(Recent Question 2017)*
    a. Bradycardia
    b. Hypertension
    c. Pupillary dilatation
    d. Respiratory irregularity

95. Management of raised ICP are all except: *(Recent Question 2017)*
    a. Hypothermia
    b. Hypercapnia
    c. Decompressive craniectomy
    d. Barbiturate

GLASGOW COMA SCALE

96. True about Glasgow coma scale: *(JIPMER 2011)*
    a. Includes verbal response
    b. Includes papillary reflex
    c. High score means poor prognosis
    d. Includes measurement of intracranial pressure

97. A patient who had traumatic head injury has spontaneous eye opening, tries to remove examiners hands on painful stimuli and irrelevant talks/stances. What is the GCS score? *(AIIMS November 2017)*
    a. 11
    b. 13
    c. 3
    d. 1

98. A patient of motor vehicle accident was admitted to the casualty. He does not speak but moans every now and then, eyes are closed but opens to pain, the right limb is not moving but the left limb shows movement to pain. Both the legs are in extended posture. What will be the GCS score? *(AIIMS May 2017)*
    a. 5
    b. 7
    c. 9
    d. 11

99. Glasgow outcome score of vegetative state: *(Recent Question 2017)*
    a. 2
    b. 3
    c. 5
    d. 8

100. Best predictor in the GCS: *(Recent Question 2017)*
    a. Eye opening
    b. Motor response
    c. Verbal response
    d. All

101. A patient with head injury opens eyes to painful stimulus, uses inappropriate words, and localizes pain, what is his GCS score? *(MHCET 2016, All India 2011)*
    a. 8
    b. 10
    c. 12
    d. 14

102. Minimal Glasgow coma scale is: *(Recent Question 2015, DNB 2012, UPPG 2010, MCI March 2007)*
    a. 0
    b. 1
    c. 2
    d. 3
    e. 4

103. Mild head injury is having Glasgow coma scale of:
    a. 3-5
    b. 5-8 *(SGPGI 2005)*
    c. 8-10
    d. 13-15

104. Which of the following is not a component of Glasgow coma scale? *(DNB 2009, All India 2006)*
    a. Eye opening
    b. Motor response
    c. Pupil size
    d. Verbal response

105. Total score in Glasgow coma scale of a conscious person is:
    a. 8
    b. 3 *(All India 2006)*
    c. 15
    d. 10

106. Regarding Glasgow coma scale, which is not true?
    a. Ranges from 6-12 *(AIIMS Nov 94)*
    b. Low score indicates deteriorating brain function
    c. Based on eye opening, verbal response and motor response
    d. Score below 5 shows poor prognosis

107. All are true about Glasgow coma scale, *except:*
    a. Score between 3 and 15   (AIIMS June 94)
    b. Obeying motor command is given maximum score
    c. Consists of eye opening, motor and verbal response
    d. Increased score indicates poor prognosis

108. A person with inappropriate words evaluated by GCS will have a verbal score of: (All India 2012)
    a. 4   b. 3
    c. 2   d. 1

109. Prognostic factor in head injury: (Recent Question 2013)
    a. Age of patient   b. Glasgow coma scale
    c. Mode of injury   d. Presence of facial trauma

110. What are the minimum and maximum possible values of Glasgow Coma Score?   (AIIMS November 2015)
    a. Minimum = 3, Maximum = 15
    b. Minimum = 0, Maximum = 13
    c. Minimum = 0, Maximum = 15
    d. Minimum = 3, Maximum = 18

111. Glasgow coma scale of a patient with head injury, who is confused, able to localize on right side and does flexion on left side and opens eye for painful stimuli on sternum: (Recent Question 2018)
    a. 6   b. 11
    c. 12   d. 7

BRAIN ABSCESS

112. Management of epidural abscess is: (DNB 2011)
    a. Immediate surgical evaluation
    b. Conservative management
    c. Antibiotics
    d. Aggressive debridement

113. Brain abscess in cyanotic heart disease is commonly located in: (All India 2006)
    a. Cerebellar hemisphere   b. Thalamus
    c. Temporal lobe   d. Parietal lobe

114. Brain abscess may be due to the following:
    a. Chronic suppurative otitis media
    b. Chronic lung abscess
    c. Trauma
    d. Any of the above

115. Subdural collection of pus in a head injury patients after 3 days, the responsible organism is: (UPPG 2009)
    a. Staph aureus   b. B hemolytic streptococcus
    c. H. influenza   d. Pneumococcus

116. A young female patient with long history of sinusitis presented with frequent fever along with personality changes and headache of recent origin. The fundus examination revealed papilledema. The most likely diagnosis is: (AIIMS Nov 2004)
    a. Frontal lobe abscess
    b. Meningitis
    c. Encephalitis
    d. Frontal bone ostemomyelitis

CNS CONGENITAL ANOMALIES

117. Meningomyelocele patient after being operated developed hydrocephalus due to: (PGI Dec 98)
    a. Arnold Chiari malformation
    b. Injury to absorptive surface
    c. Central canal injury
    d. Arachnoidal block

118. Commonest site of meningocele is:
       (BIHAR PG 2014, DNB 2005, 2001, All India 89)
    a. Lumbosacral   b. Occipital
    c. Frontal   d. Thoracic

119. Which of the following statement is correct?

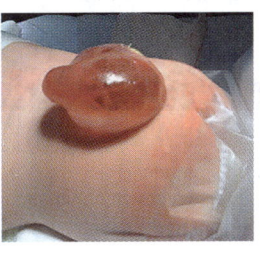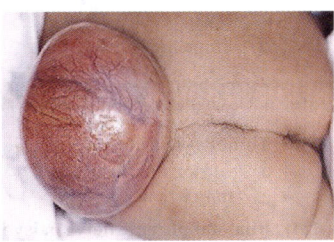

    a. 1-Meningocele, 2-Meningomyelocele
    b. 1-Meningocele, 2-Encephalocele
    c. 1- Encephalocele, 2-Meningomyelocele
    d. 1- Encephalocele, 2- Meningocele

120. Not true regarding Dandy-Walker cyst: (AIIMS June 98)
    a. Cerebellar vermis hypoplasia
    b. Hydrocephalus
    c. Arachnoid cyst   d. Posterior fossa cyst

121. What will be the diagnosis of the child with pulsatile swelling on medial side of the nose?   (AIIMS June 98)
    a. Teratoma   b. Meningocele
    c. Dermoid cyst   d. Carcinoma of ethmoid bone

122. A new born presents with swelling in base of the spine in which meninges herniates through bony defect cause is?
    a. Defect in pedicle   (UPPG 2009)
    b. Defect in body
    c. Defect in fusion of vertebral arches
    d. Defect is transverse process

123. A new born with meningomyelocele has been posted for surgery. The defect should be immediately covered with:
       (AIIMS May 2013, All India 2012)
    a. Normal saline guaze   b. Povidone iodine guaze
    c. Tincture benzoin guaze   d. Methylene blue guaze

HYDROCEPHALUS

124. In normal pressure hydrocephalus, all are seen *except:*
       (PGI Dec 97)
    a. Convulsion   b. Ataxia
    c. Dementia   d. Incontinence

125. Most commonly performed shunt for hydrocephalus is:
       (AIIMS May 2015)
    a. Ventriculoperitoneal   b. Ventriculopericardial
    c. Ventriculopleural   d. Lumboperitoneal

NERVE COMPRESSION SYNDROME

126. Carpal tunnel syndrome is due to the compression of:
    a. Median nerve   (JIPMER 2011, COMEDK 2006)
    b. Anterior interosseous nerve
    c. Radial nerve   d. Ulnar nerve

127. Carpel tunnel syndrome is caused by all except:
       (Recent Question 2016, AIIMS May 2011)
    a. Amyloidosis   b. Hypothyroidism
    c. Addison's disease   d. Diabetes mellitus

128. In causalgia, the nerve most commonly affected are:
    a. Radial and ulnar   b. Median and sciatic
    c. Radial and peroneal   d. Ilioinguinal and sural
129. Commonest cause of carpal tunnel syndrome is:
    a. Malunited Colle's fracture   (All India 95)
    b. Rheumatoid arthritis involving flexor retinaculum
    c. Myxedema
    d. Pregnancy

NERVE INJURIES

130. Tinnel's sign indicates: (Kerala 91)
    a. Atrophy of nerves   b. Neuroma
    c. Injury to nerve   d. Regeneration of nerves
131. Bilateral phrenic nerve palsy is caused by:
    a. Carcinoma bronchus
    b. Polio
    c. Medullary carcinoma thyroid
    d. Paget's disease
132. After an open injury, the optimum time for nerve suture is:
    a. Immediately   b. Within one moth
    c. 1-2 month   d. 2-4 month
    e. When wound is free from infection
133. In Erb-Duchene paralysis, the injury is limited to the:
    a. 2nd and 3rd cervical nerves   (COMEDK 2008)
    b. 3rd and 4th cervical nerves
    c. 4th and 5th cervical nerves
    d. 5th and 6th cervical nerves
134. Peripheral nerves can withstand ischemia up to: (JIPMER 93)
    a. 30 minutes   b. 1 hour
    c. 2 hours   d. 4 hours

MISCELLANEOUS

135. Which of the following is the most common location of intracranial neurocysticercosis?   (AIIMS Nov 2005)
    a. Brain parenchyma   b. Subarachnoid space
    c. Spinal cord   d. Orbit
136. The nerve of Kuntz is an important landmark in:
    a. Lumbar sympathectomy
    b. Cervicodorsal sympathectomy
    c. Obturator neurectomy d. Splanchnicectomy
    e. Herniorraphy
137. A dome shaped skull with a high forehead in the infant with slight hydrocephalus (Olympian brow) is seen in:
                                              (Recent Question 2016)
    a. Marasmus   b. Congenital syphilis
    c. Rickets   d. Arnold Chiari syndrome
138. The parasitic infection capable of producing spinal cord compression is/are:
    a. Leishmaniasis   b. Wuchereriasis
    c. Echinococcosis   d. Amoebiasis
139. The following are CNS findings of CO_2 narcosis: (PGI 90)
    a. Excitement   b. Increased pH of CSF
    c. Decreased pH of CSF   d. Papilledema
140. All of the following conditions are known to cause diabetes insipidus except: (AIIMS 2004)
    a. Multiple sclerosis   b. Head injury
    c. Histiocytosis   d. Viral encephalitis
141. Cells from the neural crest are involved in all except:
    a. Hirschprung's disease   (AIIMS June 2003)
    b. Neuroblastoma
    c. Primitive neuroectodermal tumor
    d. Wilms' tumor
142. All can commonly occur in a patient who suffered decelerating injury in which pituitary stalk was damaged. except one:
    a. Diabetes mellitus   (AIIMS Nov 2000)
    b. Thyroid insufficiency
    c. Adrenocortical insufficiency
    d. Diabetes insipidus
143. The defective migration of neural crest cells results in:
    a. Congenital megacolon
    b. Albinism   (PGI June 2006)
    c. Adrenogenital hypoplasia
    d. Dentinogenesis imperfect
144. Premature filling of veins is a manifestation in cerebral angiography of:
    a. Trauma
    b. Brain tumor
    c. Arteriovenous malformation
    d. Arterial occlusion
145. Neurosurgical treatment of epilepsy usually involves, removal of epileptic focus from which lobe: (Karnataka 2003)
    a. Frontal lobe   b. Temporal lobe
    c. Occipital lobe   d. Parietal lobe
146. Blow out fracture refers to: (JIPMER 2011)
    a. Fracture of orbit   b. Fracture of nasal septum
    c. Fracture base of skull d. Fracture of mandible
147. The 'Phenomenon of Kernohan's notch' is associated with:
                                              (MHSSMCET 2006)
    a. Third nerve palsy with contralateral hemiplegia
    b. Subfalacine herniation
    c. Transtentorial herniation
    d. Foramen magnum fracture
148. Signs of base of skull fracture are following except:
    a. Raccoon eyes   (MHSSMCET 2011)
    b. Battle's sign
    c. Constricted pupil
    d. Hemotympanum
149. A newborn present with congestive heart failure. On examination has bulging anterior fontenalle with a bruit on auscultation. Trans-fontenallar USG shows a hypoechoic midline mass with dilated lateral ventricles. Most likely diagnosis: (AIIMS Nov 2011, May 2010, Nov 2006)
    a. Medullloblastoma
    b. Encephalocele
    c. Vein of Galen malformation
    d. Arachnoid cyst

Explanations

BERRY ANEURYSM

1. Ans. a. Junction of anterior communication artery with anterior cerebral artery *(Ref: Harrison 20/e p1904; Sabiston 20/e p1904; Schwartz 9/e p1534; Bailey 26/e p311)*
2. Ans. b. Vertebral artery
3. Ans. c. Wall contains smooth muscle fibroblasts *(Ref: Harrison 19/e p01784)*
4. Ans. d. Intracranial hemorrhage
5. Ans. b. Vertebral artery

CEREBROVASCULAR ACCIDENTS

6. Ans d. Aplastic anemia
7. Ans. a. Putamen *(Ref: Harrison 20/e p3092, 19/e p2582)*
8. Ans. a. Embolism *(Ref: Harrison 20/e p3069, 19/e p2560)*
9. Ans. a. Cortical vein thrombosis *(Ref: Harrison 19/e; p2566)*

- Young women on OCPs are predisposed to stroke due to venous thrombosis of lateral saggital sinus or small cortical veins (cortical vein thrombosis)[Q].

10. Ans. b. Intracerebral hemorrhage
11. Ans. c. Hypertension
12. Ans. c. Putamen/external capsule
13. Ans. a. Rupture of circle of Willis aneurysm
14. Ans. b. Vasospasm *(Ref: Harrison 20/e p2086, 19/e p1785)*

VASOSPASM

- Narrowing of the arteries at the base of the brain following SAH occurs regularly.
- This vasospasm causes symptomatic ischemia and infarction in approximately 30% patients and is the major cause of delayed morbidity or death[Q].
- Sign of ischemia appear 4-14 days after the hemorrhage, most frequently at about 7 days[Q].

Major Causes of Delayed Neurological Deficit after CVA	
Re-rupture[Q]	Vasospasm[Q]
Hydrocephalus[Q]	Hyponatremia[Q]

15. Ans. b. Ischemic stroke
16. Ans. a. Brain *(Ref: Robbins 9/e p1255)*

DURET HEMORRHAGE

- In case of increased ICP down ward herniation of brainstem occur, which cause stretching of perforators of basilar artery and may results in bleed (Duret hemorrhage)[Q].
- Duret hemorrhage is small area of bleeding in ventral and paramedian part of upper brainstem (midbrain and pons)[Q].
- It usually indicates a fatal outcome, however survival has been reported.
- Diagnosis is made on CT or MRI.

17. Ans. a. Blunt cerebrovascular trauma *(Ref: Sabiston 20/e p424; Schwartz 10/e p198)*

"Digital subtraction angiography subsequently confirmed blunt cerebrovascular injuries (BCVI) in 30% of this high-risk cohort. Commonly referred to as the Denver criteria, these risk factors are used to screen patients and to prompt further evaluation."-*Sabiston 20/e p424*

EDH AND SDH

18. Ans. a. Cortical vessels *(Ref: Sabiston 20/e p1916; Schwartz 10/e p1719; Bailey 27/e p334)*
19. Ans. d. Extradural hematoma
20. Ans. d. Epidural hemorrhage
21. Ans. b. Temporoparietal
22. Ans. c. Subacute *(Ref: Bailey 27/e p334,335; Schwartz 10/e p1719-1720)*

CLASSIFICATION OF SDH

- Acute SDH: <3 days[Q]
- Subacute SDH: 4-21 days[Q]
- Chronic SDH: >21 days[Q]

23. Ans. c. 15 days
24. Ans. d. Surgical evacuation
25. Ans. b. Only P, R, S are correct
26. Ans. d. 21 days *(Ref: Harrison 19/e p457e-3; Sabiston 19/e p439-441; Schwartz 10/e p1719-1720; Bailey 27/e p335)*
27. Ans. b. 10% *(Ref: Harrison 19/e p441e-3)*

- Harrison says "**Epidural hematomas** occur in **upto 10% of severe head injury** cases and are **less often associated with** underlying **cortical damage than subdural hematomas.**"[Q]

28. Ans. d. Extradural
29. Ans. b. Immediate evacuation
30. Ans. a. Severe hypotension
31. Ans. c. Chronic subdural hematoma
32. Ans. b. Rupture of superior cerebral vein
33. Ans. a. Subarachnoid hemorrhage *(Ref: Harrison 20/e p2084, 19/e p1784-1785; Sabiston 20/e p1916; Schwartz 10/e p1730-1731; Bailey 27/e p335,658,661)*
34. Ans. c. Injury to cortical bridging veins
35. Ans. b. Subdural hematoma *(Ref: www.ncbi.nlm.nih.gov/pubmed/11915757 by M Guénot - 2001)*

Chronic Subdural Hematoma

- Virchow, in 1857, denied a traumatic origin, and gave the name of **"pachymeningitis hemorrhagica interna"**[Q] to this pathology which he explained by inflammatory processes.
- The traumatic etiology of chronic subdural hematoma was recognized in the 20th century, especially by Trotter in 1914.

36. Ans. a. Extradural hemorrhage
37. Ans. d. Left chronic subdural hematoma
38. Ans. d. Left chronic subdural hematoma
39. Ans. c. In the left temporal region if no localizing sign is found *(Ref: Ramamurthi and PN Tandon's Textbook of Neurosurgery 3/e Vol-1/ p442)*

Burr hole to emergently relieve the intracranial pressure should be done in the left temporal region if no localizing sign is found, to evaluate and decompress the dominant hemisphere.

Choice of Side for Initial Burr Hole

Start with a temporal burr hole on the side:
- **Ipsilateral to a blown pupil:** This will be on the **correct side in >85% of epidural hemorrhages** and **other extra- axial mass lesions.**
- **If both pupils are dilated**, use the side of the first dilating pupil (If known).
- If pupils are equal, or it is **not known which side dilated first**, place on **side of obvious external trauma.**
- **If no localization clues**, place hole on left side (to evaluate and decompress the dominant hemisphere).

SUBARACHNOID AND INTRACRANIAL HEMORRHAGE

40. Ans. c. Aneurysm
41. Ans. a. CT brain *(Ref: Harrison 20/e p2084, 19/e p1785, 1786)*
42. Ans. c. Berry aneurysm
43. Ans. b. Berry aneurysm rupture
44. Ans. b. Hess and Hunt scale *(Ref: Harrison 20/e p2085, 19/e p1785; Sabiston 20/e p1906)*

- **Hess and Hunt Scale:** Most widely used scale to grade the severity of subarachnoid hemorrhage, predict the prognosis / outcome of hemorrhage and thereby **plan further intervention**[Q].

Grading Scale for Subarachnoid Hemorrhage	
Grade	Hunt – Hess Scale
1	**Mild headache**, normal mental status, no cranial nerve or motor findings
2	**Severe headache**, normal mental status, may have cranial nerve deficit
3	**Somnolent, confused**, may have cranial nerve or **mild motor deficit**
4	**Stupor, moderate to severe motor deficit**, may have intermittent reflex posturing
5	Coma, reflex posturing or flaccid
Good grade: Grade 1, 2 and 3; **Poor grade:** Grade 4 and 5	

45. Ans. c. Subarachnoid hemorrhage
46. Ans. b. Ruptured aneurysm
47. Ans. c. Aneurysmal subarachnoid hemorrhage
48. Ans. d. Subarachnoid hemorrhage
49. Ans. a. Subarachnoid hemorrhage (SAH)
50. Ans. b. Aneurysmal subarachnoid hemorrhage

Cerebrovascular Diseases

51. **Ans. d. Hypothermia** *(Ref: Comprehensive Board Review in Neurology by Mark K. Borsody (Thieme) p63)*

TRIPLE H THERAPY

- Triple H therapy of subarachnoid hemorrhage used to ameliorate cerebral perfusion, consists of:
  1. **Hypervolemia**
  2. **Hypertension**
  3. **Haemodilution**

HEAD INJURY

52. **Ans. a. Serum osmolality >320 mOsmol/kg** *(Ref: Harrison 20/e p2077, 19/e p1779-1780; Schwartz 10/e p195-197, 575-578, 1715-1721; Bailey 26/e p318)*

MANNITOL

- Mannitol is widely used to **reduce ICP**^{Q}
- Commonly used preparation: 20% solution, 0.25-1 gm/kg is given IV as bolus^Q
- **Serum osmolality** should **not** be **allowed to go >320 mOsm/L,** to **avoid systemic acidosis** and **renal failure**^{Q}.

Uses of Mannitol
- To reduce increased ICT or intraocular tension^Q
- To maintain GFR and urine flow in impending renal failure^Q
- Forced diuresis in hypnotic or other poisoning^Q
- To counteract low osmolality of plasma/ECF^Q due to rapid hemodialysis or peritoneal dialysis

Contraindication of Mannitol	
Acute tubular necrosis^Q	Acute left ventricular failure^Q
Anuria^Q	CHF^Q
pulmonary edema^Q	Cerebral hemorrhage^Q

53. **Ans. c. Hematoma must be operated**
54. **Ans. c. Corticosteroids administration**

    Steroids are used in treatment of cerebral edema

55. **Ans. d. Intracerebral hematoma** *(Ref: Bailey 27/e p331-332)*
56. **Ans. b. Brainstem herniation**
57. **Ans. a. Raccoon eyes seen in subgaleal hemorrhage** *(Ref: Schwartz 10/e p174)*

   - Otorrhea, rhinorrhea, raccoon eyes and Battle's sign suggest a **basilar skull fracture**^{Q}.

58. **Ans. b. Anisocoria, e. Decorticate posturing** *(Ref: Harrison 19/e p1774)*

HEAD INJURY

- A sudden enlargement (dilation) of one pupil (anisocoria) is an **ominous sign**^{Q}.
- Abnormal posturing (decorticate posturing) a characteristic positioning of the limbs **caused by severe diffuse injury** or **high ICP**, is an **ominous sign**^{Q}.

59. **Ans. b. Battle sign** *(Ref: Schwartz 10/e p174; Bailey 27/e p332)*

   "Battle's sign: A skull base fracture may be associated with bruising over the mastoid process."-Bailey 27/e p332

60. **Ans. c. Posterior cranial fossa fracture**
61. **Ans. b. Coup-Countercoup injury** *(Ref: Bailey 27/e p336, 26/e p317)*
62. **Ans. c. Altered consciousness**
63. **Ans. a. ↑Mean arterial pressure with increased intracranial pressure** *(Ref: Schwartz 10/e p1580-1583; Bailey 27/e p328-329)*

CUSHING REFLEX

- The **Cushing reflex** classically presents as an **increase in systolic blood pressure, reduction of the heart rate (bradycardia)**, and **irregular respiration**^{Q}.
- It is **caused by increased intracranial pressure**^{Q}.
- These symptoms can be **indicative of insufficient blood flow** to the **brain (ischemia)** as well as **compression of arterioles**^{Q}.

64. **Ans. c. Papilloedema**

65. **Ans. c. Early surgery is indicated for optimal outcome** *(Ref: Bailey 27/e p333)*

BASE OF SKULL FRACTURES

- **Base of skull fractures** may be associated with **7th** or **8th nerve palsies**^{Q}.
- **CSF otorrhoea** or **rhinorrhoea** often resolves spontaneously^Q.
- **Antibiotics are not required prophylactically** unless for concomitant facial fractures^Q.
- A **delayed craniotomy**^{Q} and **anterior fossa dural repair** is **occasionally required**^{Q} for persistent CSF leak to prevent meningitis.

66. **Ans. d. Hypothermia** *(Ref: Bailey 25/e p299-300; Harrison 19/e p457e-1)*

Causes of Secondary Brain Injury	
Hypoxia^Q: PO_2 <8 kPa	**Hypercapnia**^{Q}
Hypotension^Q: SBP< 90 mm Hg	**Pyrexia (hyperthermia)**^{Q}
Raised ICP^Q: ICP >20 mm Hg	**Seizures**^{Q}
Low cerebral perfusion pressure^Q: CPP <65 mm Hg	**Metabolic disturbance (Hypergycemia**^{Q}**)**

67. **Ans. a. Hyperglycemia** *(Ref: Harrison 19/e p457e-1)*

- **Hyperglycemia** is **associated with a poor outcome after traumatic brain injury** and has been shown to be **associated with increased mortality**^{Q}.
- **Hyperglycemia injures** the **microvasculature** and **worsens ischemia**^{Q}.

68. **Ans. a. Glasgow coma scale**
69. **Ans. a. EDH**
70. **Ans. a. Arterial bleed, b. On CT scan…, c. Located on lateral side…., d. Common after injury**
71. **Ans. c. Altered mental status**
72. **Ans. b. SDH**
73. **Ans. a. Occurs on both sides**
74. **Ans. d. Decorticate rigidity** *(Ref: Harrison 20/e p2069, 19/e p1772; Sabiston 20/e p417-418; Schwartz 10/e p1713; Bailey 27/e p329, 26/e p312)*

Decorticate rigidity is seen in central herniation, not in uncal herniation.

Brain Herniation

Uncal Herniation	Central Herniation
• **Uncus** and **temporal lobes** are **forced through** the **cerebellar tentorium**^{Q} • Sequential **compression of ipsilateral 3rd nerve**, contralateral **brainstem** (later) and whole brainstem (eventually) occurs^Q. • **Physical Signs:** – **Early**: **ipsilateral dilated pupils**, signs of supratentorial mass lesion^Q – **Late**: **Ipsilateral hemiplegia**, progressive **ptosis** and **3rd nerve palsy**, **Cheyne-stokes respiration**^{Q} – **Very late**: Quadriparesis, bilateral fixed and **dilated pupils**, erratic respiration and death	• **Diencephalon** (**thalamus** and related structures that lie between upper brainstem and cerebral hemispheres) are **forced through** the **tentorium**^{Q} • Sequential **compression of upper midbrain (first), pons (later) and medulla (finally)**^{Q} • **Physical Signs:** – **Early**: Erratic respiration, **small reactive pupils**, increased limb tone and **bilateral extensor plantar**^{Q} – **Late**: Cheyne-stokes respiration, **decorticate rigidity**^{Q} – **Very late**: fixed and **dilated pupils**, **decerebrate posturing**^{Q}

75. **Ans. c. Tolosa-Hunt Syndrome** *(Ref: Harrison 20/e p191, 3172, 19/e p207, 1352)*

TOLOSA-HUNT SYNDROME/ORBITAL APEX SYNDROME

- One of the **lesion of orbital apex**^{Q}
- Characterized by **painful, acute ophthalmoplegia**, with or without **involvement of** the **optic nerve** and **ophthalmic division (V_1)** **of trigeminal nerve**^{Q}
- Responds promptly to **steroid treatment**^{Q}

  - Tolosa described a case in which a **mass of granulation material** was found **around the carotid artery in** the **cavernous sinus** and **asymmetrical enlargement of cavernous sinus**, now referred as **Tolosa-Hunt syndrome**^{Q}.

76. **Ans. a. Allodynia** *(Ref: Harrison 20/e p139, 19/e p87, 158)*

Terminology	Sensory Disturbance
Allodynia	• Situation in which a **non-painful stimulus**, once perceived, is **experienced as painful, even excruciating**[Q]. • An example is elicitation of a painful sensation by application of a vibrating tuning fork.
Hyperalgesia	• **Severe pain** in response to a **mildly noxious stimulus**
Hyperpathia	• **Threshold for a sensory stimulus is increased** and **perception is delayed**, but once felt, it is **unduly painful**. • Broad term **encompasses all** the phenomena described by **hyperesthesia, allodynia, and hyperalgesia**.

77. **Ans. None.** *(Ref: Diagnostic Nuclear Medicine 4/e p838)*

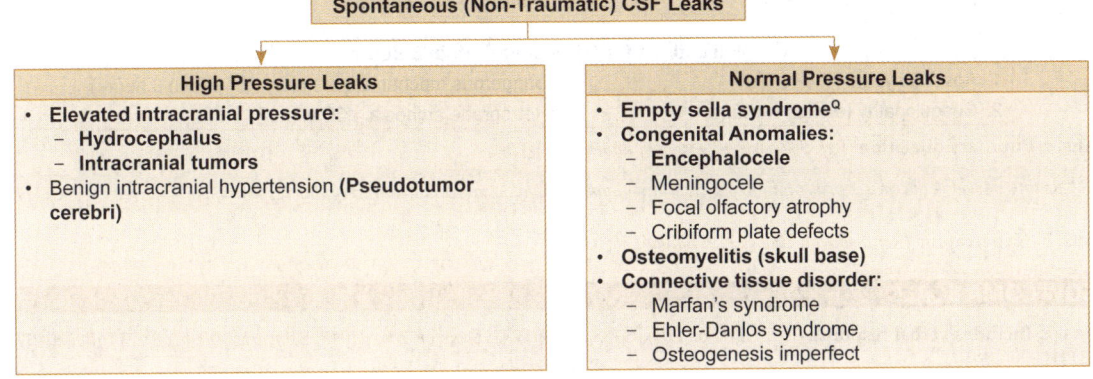

78. **Ans. c. Increased intracranial tension is seen in all cases** *(Ref: Harrison 20/e p2077, 19/e p457e-2; Sabiston 20/e p1916-1916)*

79. **Ans. c. Diffuse axonal injury**   80. **Ans. d. Diffuse axonal injury**   81. **Ans. a Craniotomy**

82. **Ans. b. Furosemide** *(Ref: Harrison 20/e p2077, 19/e p1780; Sabiston 20/e p1919)*

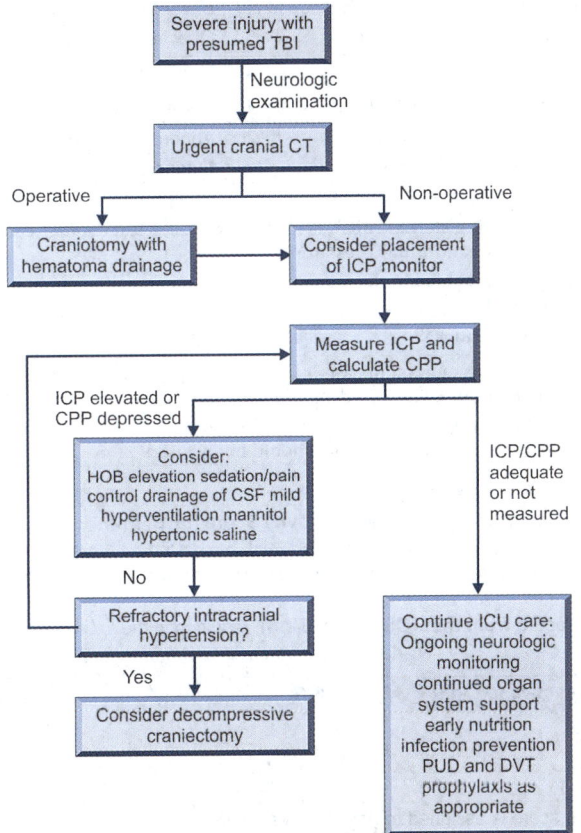

Traumatic brain injury (TBI)

83. Ans. c. CSF leak
84. Ans. a. Cerebral edema
85. Ans. a. Fracture of floor of anterior cranial fossa
86. Ans. c. Chronic subdural hemorrhage
87. Ans. c. Long-term anticonvulsants
88. Ans. d. Tachycardia
89. Ans. b. Middle cranial fossa
90. Ans. b. Level of consciousness
91. Ans. b. Hypotension
92. Ans. c. 20% Mannitol
93. Ans. b. Vomiting 1 episode *(Ref: Bailey 27/e p330)*

NICE Guidelines for CT Imaging within 1 Hour	
1. GCS < 13 at any point	4. Suspected open, depressed or basal skull fracture
2. GCS 13 or 14 at 2 hours	5. Seizures
3. Focal neurological deficit	6. Vomiting > one episode

Indications for CT Imaging within 8 Hours	
1. Age > 65 years	3. Dangerous mechanism of injury (CT within 8 hours)
2. Coagulopathy (e.g. on warfarin)	4. Retrograde amnesia > 30 min

94. Ans. c. Pupillary dilatation *(Ref: Schwartz 10/e p1713; Bailey 27/e p328)*

"Cushing's triad is the classic presentation of intracranial hypertension, bradycardia, and irregular respirations."- *Schwartz 10/e p1713*

95. Ans. b. Hypercapnia *(Ref: Sabiston 20/e p1919; Bailey 27/e p336)*

GLASGOW COMA SCALE

96. Ans. a. Includes verbal response *(Ref: Harrison 20/e p3183, 19/e p1777; Sabiston 20/e p1918; Schwartz 10/e p168,1711; Bailey 27/e p331, 26/e p312)*

REVISED GLASGOW COMA SCALE 2014

Revised GCS (2014)					
Eye Opening (E)		Verbal Response (V)		Best Motor Response (M)	
Spontaneous	4	Oriented	5	Obeying commands	6
To **Speech**^{Q}	3	Confused	4	Localizing	5
To **Pressure**^{Q}	2	**Words**^{Q}	3	Normal flexion (withdrawal)	4
None	1	**Sounds**^{Q}	2	Abnormal flexion	3
		None	1	Extension	2
				None	1

- GCS specifically **recommends avoiding sternal rubs**^{Q} as it causes bruising & responses can be difficult to interpret. They also **do not recommend routine use of retromandibular pressure**^{Q}.
- **Revised GCS (2014)** changes are highlighted in the above table.
- Maximum score-15^Q, minimum score-3^Q.
- Best predictor of outcome: Motor response^Q

  - Reporting of Non-testable Score Aspects: In cases of a non-testable aspect, the new GCS should only be noted in its components. Any element that cannot be tested should be marked as NT, for "not testable".
  - For intubated patients or patients with tracheostomy, VNT is used. It is no longer recommend to assign 1 point to non-testable elements, therefore a combined score should not be used.

GCS-P	GCS-PA CT
• **GCS-P** is calculated by **subtracting the Pupil Reactivity Score (PRS) from the Glasgow Coma Scale (GCS) total score: GCS-P = GCS – PRS**^{Q} • **Pupil reactivity score** represents the **number of nonreactive pupils (0, 1, or 2)**^{Q}. • This **number is subtracted from the GCS score (3–15)**, resulting in the **GCS-P (1–15)**^{Q}.	• **GCS-PA CT: GCS, Pupils, Age & CT findings**^{Q} • **Probability of mortality 6 months after head injury based on** the patient's admission **GCS-P** and **age with no CT abnormality (A), exactly 1 CT abnormality (B),** and **2 or more CT abnormalities (C).** • **Potential CT abnormalities** include **intracranial hematoma, absent cisterns & SAH**^{Q}.

Pupils Unreactive to Light	PRS
Both pupils	2
One pupil	1
Neither pupil	0
Note: Higher score is assigned to non-reactive pupils.	

Cerebrovascular Diseases

97. Ans. b. 13 *(Ref: Sabiston 20/e p1918; Schwartz 10/e p1712; Bailey 27/e p331)*
98. Ans. c. 9 *(Ref: Sabiston 20/e p1918; Schwartz 10/e p1712; Bailey 27/e p331)*
99. Ans. b. 3 *(Ref: Sabiston 20/e p1918; Schwartz 10/e p1712; Bailey 27/e p331)*
100. Ans. b. Motor response *(Ref: Sabiston 20/e p1918; Schwartz 10/e p1712; Bailey 27/e p331)*
101. Ans. b. 10
102. Ans. d. 3
103. Ans. d. 13-15
104. Ans. c. Pupil size
105. Ans. c. 15
106. Ans. a. Ranges from 6-12
107. Ans. d. Increased score indicates poor prognosis
108. Ans. b. 3
109. Ans. b. Glasgow coma scale
110. Ans. a. Minimum = 3, Maximum = 15
111. Ans. b. 11

BRAIN ABSCESS

112. Ans. a. Immediate surgical evacuation *(Ref: Bailey 27/e p656-657)*
113. Ans. d. Parietal lobe *(Ref: Harrison 20/e p1014, 19/e p900; Sabiston 20/e p1934-1935; Schwartz 10/e p1745; Bailey 26/e p609-610)*

> Brain abscess in congenital heart diseases occur due to hematogenous seeding of blood borne bacteria. These blood borne bacteria bypass the capillary bed due to right to left shunt. They commonly infect parietal and frontal lobes (territory of middle cerebral artery).

114. Ans. d. Any of the above
115. Ans. a. Staph aureus
116. Ans. a. Frontal lobe abscess

CNS CONGENITAL ANOMALIES

117. Ans. a. Arnold Chiari malformation *(Ref: Sabiston 20/e p1932; Schwartz 10/e p1745; Bailey 27/e p484, 668)*

Type II Chiari malformation is characterized by progressive hydrocephalus with a myelomeningocele.

118. Ans. a. Lumbosacral *(Ref: Sabiston 20/e p1932; Schwartz 10/e p1750; Bailey 27/e p484, 667)*
119. Ans. a. 1-Meningocele, 2-Meningomyelocele *(Ref: Sabiston 20/e p1931-1932; Schwartz 10/e p1750; Bailey 27/e p667)*
120. Ans. c. Arachnoid cyst *(Ref: Sabiston 20/e p1932; Schwartz 9/e p1553)*
121. Ans. b. Meningocele
122. Ans. c. Defect in fusion of vertebral arches
123. Ans. a. Normal saline guaze *(Ref: Sabiston 20/e p1931-1932; Schwartz 10/e p1645; Bailey 27/e p484, 667)*

Meningomyelocele should be covered with a non-sticking sterile saline soaked guaze and plastic shield wrap to maintain moisture.

HYDROCEPHALUS

124. Ans. a. Convulsion *(Ref: Harrison 20/e p3112, 19/e p2606; Sabiston 20/e p1930)*
125. Ans. a. Ventriculoperitoneal *(Ref: Bailey 27/e p653-656; Nelson 19/e p2008-2011)*

Most common shunt used for hydrocephalus is ventriculoperitoneal shunt.

> *"Therapy for hydrocephalus depends on the cause. Medical management, including the use of acetazolamide and furosemide, can provide temporary relief by reducing the rate of CSF production, but long-term results have been disappointing. Most cases of hydrocephalus require extracranial shunts, particularly a ventriculoperitoneal shunt. Endoscopic third ventriculostomy (ETV) has evolved as a viable approach and criteria have been developed for its use, but the procedure might need to be repeated to be effective." - Nelson 19/e p2011*

NERVE COMPRESSION SYNDROME

126. Ans a. Median nerve *(Ref: Harrison 20/e p3444, 19/e p2221; Sabiston 20/e p2006; Schwartz 10/e p1791; Bailey 27/e p 508)*

CARPAL TUNNEL SYNDROME

- Carpal tunnel syndrome is an **entrapment median neuropathy**[Q]
- Causing **paresthesia, pain, numbness** in the distribution of the median nerve due to its **compression** at the wrist **in the carpal tunnel.**[Q]

Risk Factors for Carpal Tunnel Syndrome	
Pregnancy[Q]	Rheumatoid arthritis[Q]
Diabetes[Q]	Colle's fractures[Q]
Obesity[Q]	Amyloidosis[Q]
Hypothyroidism[Q]	Acromegaly[Q]
Heavy manual work or work with vibrating tools[Q]	Use of **steroids** and **estrogens**[Q]

Clinical Features

- **Main symptom**: **Intermittent numbness** of the **thumb, index, long** and **radial half** of the **ring finger**. **Numbness** often occurs **at night**[Q].
- **Long-standing CTS** leads to **permanent nerve damage** with **constant numbness, atrophy** of some of the muscles of the **thenar eminence and weakness of palmar abduction.** [Q]
- **Pain** is **primarily numbness** that is **so intense** that it **wakes one from sleep**[Q].

Diagnosis

- **Specific clinical tests include:**
    - Tinel's[Q] percussion over the carpal tunnel
    - Phalen's test[Q] (reproduction of paraesthesia with full wrist flexion)
    - Carpal tunnel compression with full wrist flexion

> - **Rarely** does **electrophysiological testing add to** the **clinical tests**, but it is a good tool for tracking changes.

Treatment

- **Conservative treatments:** Use of **night splints** and **corticosteroid injection**[Q].
- Disease modifying treatment: **Surgery to cut** the **transverse carpal ligament**[Q] (creating space for the nerve)

127. Ans. c. Addison's disease
128. Ans. b. Median and sciatic
129. Ans. d. Pregnancy

NERVE INJURIES

130. **Ans. d. Regeneration of nerves** *(Ref: Schwartz 10/e p1798-1799,1805; Bailey 27/e p385)*

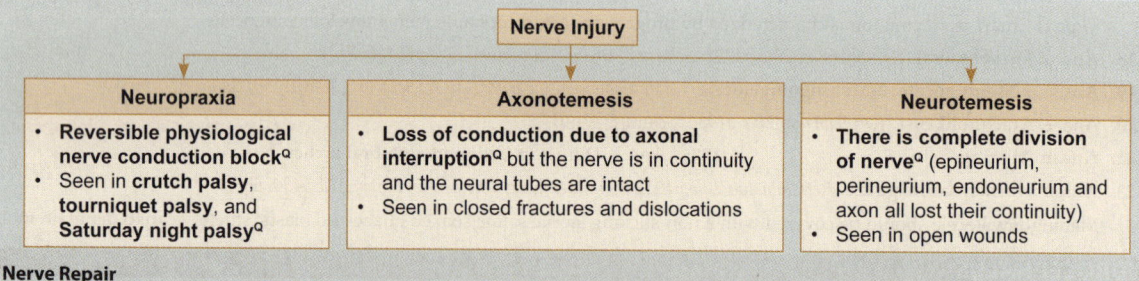

Nerve Repair

- A **clean cut nerve** is **best repaired as soon as** this **can be done safely**[Q].
- The **higher (proximal)** the **lesion**, the **worse the prognosis**[Q].
- Pure motor or pure sensory nerves recover better than mixed, because there is less chances of axonal confusion.

> - **Tinel's sign** indicate **regeneration of nerve**[Q].
> - Rate of regeneration of nerve is **1 mm/day**[Q].

Prognosis after Nerve Suturing

- **Radial nerve (best)**[Q] >Median nerve >Ulnar nerve >Peroneal nerve >Sciatic and femoral nerve (worst prognosis)[Q]

131. Ans. b. Polio
132. Ans. e. When wound is free from infection
133. Ans. d. 5th and 6th cervical nerves
134. Ans. d. 4 hours

MISCELLANEOUS

135. Ans. a. Brain parenchyma

136. **Ans. b. Cervicodorsal sympathectomy** *(Ref: http://www.ncbi.nlm.nih.gov/pmc/articles/PMC1468385/)*

NERVE OF KUNTZ

- **Nerve of Kuntz: Thoracic origin** of a **sympathetic supply to** the **upper limb**[Q]
- An **inconstant intrathoracic ramus** which joined the 2nd intercostal nerve to the ventral ramus of the 1st thoracic nerve, proximal to the point where the latter gave a large branch to the brachial plexus, has become known as the 'nerve of Kuntz'
- These **variant sympathetic pathways** may be **responsible for** the **recurrence of symptoms after sympathectomy surgery**[Q].

Cerebrovascular Diseases

137. Ans. b. Congenital syphilis
138. Ans. c. Echinococcosis
139. Ans. c. Decreased pH of CSF
140. Ans. a. Multiple sclerosis
141. Ans. d. Wilms' tumor
142. Ans. a. Diabetes mellitus
143. Ans. a. Congenital megacolon, b. Albinism

> Defective migration of neural crest results in Hirschprung's disease (congenital megacolon), albinism, melanoma and oropharyngeal teratoma.

144. Ans. c. Arteriovenous malformation

- Diagnosis of AVM is made **by conventional catheter cerebral angiography**^{Q}
- **Diagnosis** is based on **demonstration of arteries** and **veins** on the same conventional angiographic image, proving the **high-flow shunting of blood (leading to early filling of veins**^{Q}**)** through the **nidus network** or **fistulous vessels**.
- In the **typical AVM**, there is a **cloudlike nidus**, or **network of smaller vessels**, well seen **on angiography**.

145. Ans. b. Temporal lobe *(Ref: Harrison 20/e p3065, 19/e p2556; Sabiston 20/e p1925; Schwartz 10/e p1746-1747)*

NEUROSURGICAL TREATMENT OF EPILEPSY

- The **most common surgical procedures** performed **for epilepsy** are **anterior temporal lobectomy**^{Q}, **focal cortical resection, multiple subpial transection, hemispherectomy**, and **corpus callosotomy**.

146. Ans. a. Fracture of orbit
147. Ans. c. Transtentorial herniation *(Ref: Harrison 19/e p1772; Bailey 25/e p624)*

KERNOHAN'S NOTCH PHENOMENON

- **Kernohan's notch** is a **cerebral peduncle indentation** associated with some forms of **transtentorial herniation (uncal herniation)**^{Q}.
- **Compression of** the **contralateral cerebral peduncle** against the **free edge of** the **tentorium (Kernohan's notch)** causes an **ipsilateral hemiparesis** with **ipsilateral 3rd nerve palsy**^{Q}.

KERNOHAN-WOLTMAN SIGN

- **Lateral displacement of** the **midbrain** may **compress** the **opposite cerebral peduncle**, producing a **Babinski's sign** and **hemiparesis contralateral to** the **original hemiparesis (the Kernohan-Woltman sign**^{Q}**)**.

148. Ans. c. Constricted pupil
149. Ans. c. Vein of Galen malformation *(Ref: Sabiston 19/e p1876)*

Diagnosis of **Vein of Galen malformation** should be suspected in any **newborn** presenting **with unexplained congestive heart failure** and **hydrocephalus**.

- **Vein of Galen** is **formed by** the confluence of the **two internal cerebral veins** and receives the **entire deep venous drainage** of the **cerebrum**.
- Vein of Galen then **joins the inferior saggital sinus** and **empties** the **venous drainage into** the **straight sinus**.

VEIN OF GALEN MALFORMATION

- Vein of Galen malformation is characterized by **aneurysmal dilatation** and **arteriovenous malformation** of Galen^Q.
- Most commonly presents in the **neonatal period**^{Q}

Clinical Features
- **High output failure, bounding carotid pulse, hydrocephalus**^{Q}
- **Increased intra-cranial pressure, intraventricular hemorrhage from rupture**.
- **Cerebral ischemia** from **intracranial 'steal' phenomenon** and **CHF**^{Q}.
- **Marked continuous cranial bruit**^{Q}

Diagnosis
- **Cranial ultrasonography: Initial investigation of choice**^{Q}
- **MRI and Angiography:** Used to define the lesion better

CHAPTER 34

CNS Tumors

WHO CLASSIFICATION OF BRAIN TUMORS

WHO Classification of Brain Tumors

1. **Neuroepithelial tumours**:
   – **Glioma**: Astrocytomas, Oligodendrogliomas, Ependymoma, Choroid plexus tumour
   – **Pineal tumours**
   – **Neuronal tumours**: Ganglioglioma, Gangliocytoma, Neuroblastoma
   – **Medulloblastoma**

2. **Nerve sheath tumours**: Vestibular schwannoma
3. **Meningeal tumours**: Meningioma
4. **Pituitary tumours**
5. **Germ cell tumours**: Germinoma, Teratoma
6. **Lymphomas**
7. **Tumour-like malformations**: Craniopharyngioma, Epidermoid tumours, Dermoid tumour, Colloid cyst
8. **Metastatic tumours**
9. **Contiguous extension from regional tumours**: Glomus tumour

BRAIN TUMOR

MC primary brain tumor	Meningioma^Q (35%) > glial tumors^Q (30%)
MC brain tumor	Metastasis^Q
MC malignant BT of childhood Most radiosensitive BT	Medulloblastoma^Q
BT associated with calcification (COM)	Craniopharyngioma^Q (most) > ODG^Q (90%) > Meningioma^Q (20–25%)

BRAIN TUMOR

- Most brain tumors occur **sporadically**^{Q}
- **Radiation exposure** & **genetic abnormalities** are the risk factors^Q

Genetic abnormalities associated with brain tumors (RL not in MTV GT)	
• **R**etinoblastoma^Q • **L**i-Fraumeni^Q • **N**F-1 & 2^Q • **M**EN 1^Q	• **T**urcot's syndrome^Q • **V**HL syndrome^Q • **G**orlin syndrome^Q • **T**uberous sclerosis^Q

Clinical Features
- Three cardinal symptoms: Seizures, Raised ICT & focal neurological deficit^Q (FND)
- **Raised ICT** leads to **headache (worse in morning & straining**^{Q}, associated with nausea & vomiting)
- FND: Progressive over time, characteristic of location^Q
- Pituitary adenoma may also present with **endocrine abnormalities**^{U}

Diagnosis
- IOC for diagnosis: MRI^Q

Treatment:
- **Dexamethasone:** Reduces peritumoral edema^Q
- **Anti-epileptics:** For tumors close to sensorimotor strip^Q
- **Mannitol:** Administered before dural opening & operative resection^Q
- **Surgery:** Primary goals of surgery includes **histologic diagnosis & reduction of mass effect** by removal of as much as tumor with preservation of neurological function^Q
- **Radiotherapy:** In cases of **positive margins & tumor infiltrating surrounding brain**^Q
- **Craniospinal irradiation:** For tumors associated with **CSF spread**

ASTROCYTOMA

Astrocytoma

- Astrocytomas arise from **astrocytes**^Q
- Mostly **supratentorial in adults** & **infratentorial in children**^Q
- Astrocytoma is **MC posterior fossa tumor in children**^Q
- **Majority** of astrocytoma are **low grade in children & high grade in adults**^Q
- **MC astrocytoma in children: Pilocytic astrocytoma**^Q
- **MC astrocytoma in adults: Glioblastoma multiforme**^Q **(GBM)**

Pathology
- Majority of **astrocytomas infiltrate** adjacent **brain**. Juvenile pilocytic astrocytomas & pleomorphic xanthoastrocytomas are exceptions^Q
- Histologic features associated with higher grade tumors: **Hypercellularity, nuclear atypia & endovascular hyperplasia**^Q.
- **Necrosis**^Q is present **only** with **GBMs**; it is required for the diagnosis.

WHO Classification of Astrocytoma			
Grade I or Pilocytic Astrocytoma	**Low-grade, or grade II Astrocytomas**	**Grade III or Anaplastic**	**Grade IV or Glioblastoma Multiforme**
• **Discrete** appearing, **contrast enhancing** and often **cystic** with a **mural nodule**^Q. • **Mean age: First two decades** of life. • Curable by **radical resection**^Q (no infiltration of surrounding brain) • **Radiation therapy and chemotherapy have no role** • **Median survival time: 8-10 years.**	• Occur in **children** and **young adults**^Q. • Most patients present with **seizures**^Q. • Typically demonstrate **nuclear atypia**; have a **low degree of cellularity** • **Treatment: Observation and follow-up, radiation** with or without **chemotherapy**, and **surgery.** • **Surgery** is **not curative** because most of these tumors are **infiltrative** with **no clear margins**^Q. • The **median survival** time is **7–8 years.**	• **Irregular enhancement** on **MRI** • **Treatment: Cytoreductive surgery** followed by **EBRT**^Q. • **Median survival** time for anaplastic astrocytoma: **2–3 years**	• **Endothelial proliferation** or **necrosis**^Q on histology makes the tumor **grade IV**. • Know as **butterfly tumor** as it crosses midline^Q • Seen in **older patients (>50 years)**. • GBMs: **Ring enhancement** with **central necrosis** on **MRI**^Q. • Treatment: Cytoreductive surgery followed by **EBRT**^Q. • The **extent of tumor resection** has a **significant effect** on time to tumor **progression** and median **survival**^Q. • **Carmustine** and **cisplatin** have been the primary agents used against **malignant gliomas**^Q. • **Temozolomide**^Q has shown some promise in the management of **newly diagnosed** and **recurrent GBM**, with an overall survival time of 13.6 months. • Median survival time for GBM is **<1 year**.

OLIGODENDROGLIOMA (ODG)

Oligodendroglioma (ODG)

- ODG accounts for approximately **10% of gliomas**
- Predilection for the **cortex** and **white matter** of cerebral hemispheres **(frontal lobe in 50–65%)**
- **MC genetic alterations** include **loss of heterozygosity** on chromosome **19q >1p**^Q. These alterations are usually associated with a **better prognosis**.

> • **Characterized by** classic histologic feature of **"fried egg" cytoplasm, "chicken wire" vasculature,** and **microscopic calcifications**^Q.

Clinical Feature
- This tumor frequently presents with **seizures**

Diagnosis
- **Calcifications** and **hemorrhage** on CT or MRI **suggest** the **diagnosis**^{Q}.
- **Calcifications** is seen in **28-60%** in ODGs on **plain radiographs**, and on **90%** of **CT**^{Q}.

Treatment
- Primary modality of treatment: **Surgical resection + Chemotherapy**^{Q}
- Respond to procarbazine, lomustine (CCNU), vincristine (**PCV**) **chemotherapy**.
- Chromosomal deletion, **1p** and **19q**, has been associated with **robust response** to **temozolomide**^{Q}.

Prognosis
- **Median survival time** ranges from **3 to 5 years**

EPENDYMOMA

Ependymoma

- Arise from **ependymal lining** of **cerebral hemispheres** & remnants of **central canal** of **spinal cord**.
- Manifest predominantly in **children** (within the **fourth ventricle**) and **young adults**.
- MC histologic type in **adults**: Myxopapillary ependymoma^Q, which typically **arises from filum terminale**^{Q} of spinal cord and appears in **lumbosacral region**^{Q}.

Diagnosis
- On CT or MRI, ependymomas typically appear as **diffusely enhancing masses**^{Q} relatively well demarcated from adjacent neural tissue.
- **MRI findings** include a **well-circumscribed** lesion with varying degrees of enhancement. **Ventricular** or **brainstem displacement** and **hydrocephalus** are frequent features.

Treatment
- Optimal treatment includes **maximal possible resection** without causing neurological deficits followed by **EBRT**.
- Ependymomas have the potential to **spread through** the **neuraxis** by **seeding** of **CSF**; **craniospinal radiation**^{Q} is recommended in this case.

MEDULLOBLASTOMA

Medulloblastoma

- MC malignant brain tumor of childhood: Medulloblastoma
- Turcot syndrome (A variant of FAP) is associated with increased incidence of medulloblastoma
- **Highly malignant tumor** found in **cerebellum**^{Q} and **infratentorial** location
- Occur predominantly in **children**^{Q} (peak incidence at **3-4 years**^{Q})
- Medulloblastoma is **most radiosensitive brain tumor**^{Q}

| • MC site: Vermis (75%) | • MC site in adults: Lateral cerebellar hemisphere |

Clinical Characteristics
- **Child** usually presents with features of **increased intracranial tension**^{Q}.
- **Adults** present with **ataxia** and **unilateral dysmetria** as lateral origin is more common^Q.

Metastasis
- **Dissemination through CSF** is common leading to **drop metastasis**^{Q}.
- Metastasis outside CNS^Q affects **bone, lymph node** and **liver**.
- Tumor dissemination is **most important prognostic factor**^{Q}.

Treatment
- Despite of extreme radiosensitivity, it should be **surgically excised**^{Q}.
- Surgical excision should be **followed by radiotherapy** and **chemotherapy**^{Q}.

> • **Carmustine (BCNU)** and **vincristine** are primarily used for recurrences, in **poor-risk patients**, and in **children <3 years to avoid radiation therapy**^{Q}

Prognosis
- Patients **without a residual tumor** and **negative CSF seeding** have **5-year survival rate >75%**.

MENINGIOMA

MENINGIOMA

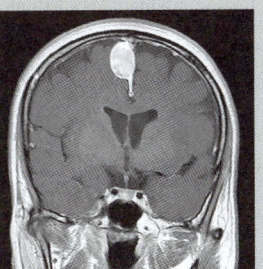

- MC primary brain tumor: Meningioma (35%) >Glial tumors (30%)
- Meningiomas are the **MC intracranial, extra-axial dural-based neoplasm**[Q].
- Predominantly benign tumors of **adults**[Q], more common in **women**[Q].

  - Derived from **meningomesothelial cells** of **arachnoid**[Q]
  - Mostly occur **along** the **superior sagittal sinus**[Q]
  - **Most** are **slow growing** & **encapsulated**[Q]

Pathology:
- **Round encapsulated mass** showing characteristic **enplaque pattern of growth**[Q]
- Tumor may range from firm to fibrous to finely gritty and may show extreme **calcification** & **psammoma bodies**[Q]

Clinical Presentation:
- Motor deficit in 90% (spasticity & lower limb weakness), **sensory deficit** in 60% or **sphincter dysfunction** of bladder[Q].

Radiological findings in Meningioma	
• Nearly all meningiomas **enhance intensely**[Q] following contrast administration. • **Abnormal vascular markings**[Q] • **Enlarged foramen spinosum**[Q] on the side of lesion • **Dural tail** • **Calcification (20-25%)** in the tumor[Q]	• Invasion of bone cause localized **bony hyperostosis**/mixed osteoblastic & osteolytic response less commonly. It may show **'sun ray spicules'** & local bone expansion with pneumatization so called **'blistering'** • Signs of increased intracranial tension[Q]

Treatment:
- **Surgery** is the **treatment of choice** for **symptomatic meningiomas**.
- **Extent of resection** is the **most important factor** in the prevention of **recurrence**.
- **Simpson grading system** is used for **meningioma resection**[Q]
- **Recurrence** after gross total resection occurs in **11-15%** of cases.

CNS Tumors	
Intra-axial (LANe)	**Extra-axial (PSM)**
• Neuronal • Astrocytoma (Glioma)[Q] • Lymphoma	• Pituitary[Q] • Schwannoma[Q] • Meningioma[Q]

PITUITARY ADENOMA

PITUITARY ADENOMA

- Pituitary adenomas arise primarily from **anterior pituitary gland**[Q]
- **MC cause** of hyperpituitarism: **Pituitary adenoma**[Q]
- Classified as either **functional** (secreting) or **nonfunctional** (nonsecreting) tumors
- Former presenting **earlier with symptoms** caused by **physiologic effects** and the latter presenting when of **sufficient size** to cause **neurologic deficits** by mass effect on the chiasm with consequent **bitemporal hemianopsia**[Q].
- Incidence is increased in **MEN-1**[Q]

  - **Pituitary adenoma** can be **differentiated from hyperplasia by reticulin stain**[Q]
  - **Absence of reticulin stain** in pituitary adenoma[Q]

Clinical Features
- Occur commonly in **third** & **fourth decades** and affect **both sexes equally**[Q].
- **MC functional tumor** is **prolactinoma**[Q], which causes **amenorrhea** & **galactorrhea** in women[Q].

Diagnosis
- MRI is IOC for pituitary tumors[Q]
- Typically, the **pituitary gland enhances rapidly** owing to lack of blood-brain barrier.

- Microadenoma may appear as a **nonenhancing area within the gland**.
- Diagnostic workup includes a **full endocrinologic profile** and a **formal visual fields test**[Q].

Treatment

- **Dopamine agonist, bromocriptine**[Q], can **shrink prolactinomas** in **75%** of patients with **macroadenomas** in **6-8 weeks**, but only as long as therapy is maintained.
- Bromocriptine may also work on **GH-secreting tumors** with tumor **shrinkage** in **<20%**.
- **Octreotide**[Q] can **reduce GH levels** in 71% of patients, with a **significant reduction** in tumor **volume** in **30%** of cases.

Indications of Surgery as an Initial Treatment	
• GH-secreting tumors[Q] • Primary Cushing's disease[Q] • Any adenoma causing acute visual deterioration[Q]	• Nonprolactin-secreting macroadenomas causing symptoms by mass effect[Q]

- **Surgical approach** of choice: **Sublabial** or **intranasal trans-sphenoidal**[Q] approach
- **Recurrence rate: 12%** (most recurrences occur 4-8 years after surgery)
- **Radiosurgery** can also be used either as **primary therapy**, as an **adjuvant therapy** after subtotal resection, or **for recurrent disease**.
- **Main dose-limiting structure** is proximity to the **optic chiasm** & **optic nerves** (within 3-5 mm). In this case, **fractionated EBRT** may be indicated as an adjuvant therapy

> - **MC suprasellar mass in children: Craniopharyngioma**[Q]
> - **MC suprasellar mass in adults: Pituitary adenoma**[Q]

CRANIOPHARYNGIOMA

CRANIOPHARYNGIOMA

- Craniopharyngiomas are **benign cystic lesions** that occur **most frequently** in **children**[Q].
- There is a **second peak** of incidence around **50 years** of age.
- Derived from **Rathke's pouch**[Q] and arise near the pituitary stalk, commonly extending into the suprasellar cistern.

> - Craniopharyngiomas are often **large, cystic**, and **locally invasive**[Q].

Clinical Features

- **More than half** of all patients present **before 20 years**[Q]
- Presents with signs of **increased intracranial pressure**[Q], including headache, vomiting, papilledema, and hydrocephalus.
- Associated symptoms include **visual field abnormalities**[Q], personality changes and cognitive deterioration, cranial nerve damage, sleep difficulties, and weight gain.

> - Associated with **hypopituitarism (90%), diabetes insipidus (10%) & growth retardation (50%)**[Q]

Diagnosis

- **Calcification** occurs in **all pediatric** and roughly **half** of **adult** craniopharyngiomas[Q].
- **MRI** is superior to CT for **evaluating cystic structure** and **tissue components** of craniopharyngiomas[Q].
- **CT** is useful to define **calcifications** and evaluate **invasion** into surrounding **bony structures** & **sinuses**.

Treatment

- Treatment involves transcranial or **transsphenoidal**[Q] surgical resection followed by **postoperative radiation** of residual tumor.

> - **Surgery alone** is **curative** in **less than half** of patients because of **recurrences** due to **adherence to vital structures** or because of **small tumor deposits in hypothalamus** or **brain parenchyma**[Q].
> - In the **absence** of **radiotherapy**, about **75%** of **craniopharyngiomas recur**, and 10-year survival is **<50%**[Q].

- In patients with **incomplete resection, radiotherapy improves** 10-year **survival** to 70–90% but is associated with **increased risk** of **secondary malignancies**[Q].
- Most patients require **lifelong pituitary hormone replacement**[Q].

> - **Cortisol (hydrocortisone)** is the **first hormone to be replaced**[Q] in patients with **panhypopituitarism after craniopharyngioma surgery.**

PRIMARY CNS LYMPHOMA

Primary CNS Lymphoma

- PCNSL is a rare **non-Hodgkin's lymphoma**[Q] accounting for **<3%** of primary brain tumors.
- The **incidence** is **rising** due to the **high frequency** of CNS lymphoma in **AIDS** patients and **transplant recipients**[Q].

> - PCNSL in **immunocompetent patients** usually consists of **diffuse large B-cell lymphomas**[Q].
> - PCNSL in **immunocompromised patients** is typically **large cell** with **immunoblastic** and more **aggressive features**[Q].
> - Also known as **ghost-cell tumor** because of its tendency for **partial** to **complete resolution on CT** after the administration of **steroids**[Q].

- **Epstein-Barr virus** frequently plays an **important role** in the pathogenesis of **HIV-related PCNSL**[Q].
- A **stereotactic needle biopsy** is indicated when the index of suspicion for CNS lymphoma is high because these lesions are **highly sensitive** to **radiation**[Q].

Clinical Features
- PCNSL usually presents as a **mass lesion**, with **neuropsychiatric symptoms**, symptoms of **increased intracranial pressure**, lateralizing signs, or **seizures**[Q].
- Median age at diagnosis: **52 years** (younger in the immunocompromised).

Diagnosis
- On contrast-enhanced MRI: **Densely enhancing tumor**[Q]
- **Immunocompetent** patients have **solitary lesions** more often than immunosuppressed patients.
- Frequent **involvement** of the **basal ganglia, corpus callosum,** or **periventricular region**[Q].
- **Stereotactic biopsy** is necessary for **histologic diagnosis**[Q].

> - **Glucocorticoids** should be **withheld** before **biopsy** due to **cytolytic effect** on **lymphoma cells** leading to nondiagnostic tissue (**Ghost cell tumor**)[Q]

Treatment
- PCNSL is relatively sensitive to glucocorticoids, chemotherapy and radiotherapy.
- **High-dose methotrexate**[Q] produces **response rates** of **35-80%** and median survival up to 50 months.
- Combination of **methotrexate** with other chemotherapeutic agents such as **cytarabine**, as well as **whole-brain radiotherapy**, increases the **response rate** to **70–100%**[Q].

> - In **non-AIDS cases**, chemotherapy + EBRT prolongs survival compared with EBRT alone.
> - **AIDS patients** are treated with **whole-brain radiotherapy, high-dose methotrexate,** and initiation of **highly active antiretroviral therapy**[Q].

Prognosis
- **Without therapy**, median survival time is **1.8–3.3 months**.
- In **AIDS-related cases**, the median survival time is only **3–5 months**.
- **With radiation**, median survival time is **10 months**.

SPINAL TUMORS

Spinal Tumors

- MC spinal tumor: **Metastasis**[Q]
- MC primary spinal tumor: **Nerve sheath tumor**[Q]
- MC intramedullary tumor: **Astrocytoma**[Q]
- MC site of primary spinal tumor: **Intradural extramedullary**[Q]

ACOUSTIC NEUROMA

Acoustic Neuroma

- Acoustic neuroma is a **benign, encapsulated**, extremely **slow growing** tumor of **8th nerve**.
- MC site of origin: Inferior vestibular > superior vestibular nerve
- Age group of **40-60 years**. (M:F = 1:1)

Clinical Features
- Presenting symptom: **Progressive unilateral sensorineural hearing loss**[Q] accompanied by **tinnitus**
- **Cochleo-vestibular symptoms** are the **earliest symptoms**[Q].

Cranial Nerve Involvement		
V	VII	IX and X
Reduced corneal sensitivity and numbness of face[Q]	Hypoesthesia of posterior meatal wall[Q] Loss of taste[Q] Decreased lacrimation[Q]	Dysphagia/hoarseness[Q]

- Brainstem involvement, Cerebellar involvement, Raised intracranial tension

Diagnosis
- **MRI with gadolinium contrast** is the **gold standard** for diagnosis of acoustic neuroma^Q.

> - Acoustic neuroma **can arise from any nerve except Optic** and **Olfactory** because they are **myelinated by oligodendroglia** rather than Schwann cells^Q.

Tumors that spread through CSF (CPM germ CAP)	
• **C**NS Lymphomas^Q	• **C**horoid plexus carcinoma
• **P**inealoblastomas^Q	• **A**naplastic ependymomas
• **M**edulloblastoma^Q	• **P**rimitive neuroectodermal tumors
• **G**erm cell tumors^Q	

STEREOTACTIC RADIOSURGERY

STEREOTACTIC RADIOSURGERY

- SRS is a **non-surgical radiation therapy used to treat functional abnormalities** & **small tumors** of brain^Q.
- Deliver precisely-targeted concentrated dose of radiation in fewer high-dose treatments to a defined volume in the brain^Q.
- When **SRS** is **used to treat body tumors**, it's called **stereotactic body radiotherapy**^{Q} (SBRT).

> **Two methods** of **frame-based stereotactic radiosurgery** are currently **widely used.**
> - **Gamma knife uses cobalt-201**^{Q} radiation sources focused on one point.
> - **Modified linear accelerators**^{Q} deliver **high-energy x-rays (photons)** in multiple arcs, thereby minimizing the effect on surrounding brain tissue.

- **Primary risks** of stereotactic radiosurgery are **radiation necrosis** & **radiation injury** to surrounding structures.

Common uses of Stereotactic Radiosurgery (BAT)	
Brain tumor^Q (Benign, malignant, primary & metastatic tumors, single & multiple)	**A**rteriovenous malformations^Q
Benign lesions of cranial nerves^Q	**T**rigeminal neuralgia^Q

> - **SBRT** is currently used and/or being investigated for use in **treating malignant or benign small-to-medium size tumors** of lung, liver, abdomen, spine, prostate, head & neck^Q.

METASTATIC BRAIN TUMORS

METASTATIC BRAIN TUMORS

- **Metastatic brain tumors** are the **MC tumors** of the **brain**^{Q}.
- They outnumber primary brain tumors by **10 to 1.**

> - **Location:** Cerebral hemispheres (80%) mainly the **frontal lobes**^{Q}, cerebellum (**15%**) and brainstem (**5%**).
> - **MC primary sites: CA lung**^{Q} (50%) > **breast cancer**^{Q} (15-20%)

- Metastases to the brain are **multiple** in >70% of cases.

Diagnosis
- **IOC: MRI** with **gadolinium enhancement**^{Q}
- Lesions are at the **gray-matter** and **white-matter junction, well circumscribed**, surrounded by **edema**^{Q}.

Treatment
- **Surgery** is recommended for accessible lesions (**up to 3**) causing mass effect followed by **whole-brain radiation therapy (WBRT) to eradicate micrometastases**^{Q}.
- **Stereotactic radiosurgery** followed by **WBRT** has also been shown to be as effective as surgery in the management of metastatic brain tumors (< 3 cm).
- **Chemotherapy** is not useful in most brain metastases except **small cell lung cancer** and **seminomas**.

Prognosis
- **Median survival time** with optimal treatment: **7–12 months**

Multiple Choice Questions

CNS TUMORS PREDISPOSING FACTORS

1. **All of the following hereditary conditions predispose to CNS tumors, except:** *(DPG 2010, AIIMS 2005)*
   a. Neurofibromatosis 1 and 2
   b. Tuberous sclerosis
   c. Von-Hippel-Lindau syndrome
   d. Xeroderma pigmentosum

2. **All of the following statements about Neurofibromatosis are true, except:** *(All India 2009)*
   a. Autosomal recessive inheritance
   b. Cutaneous neurofibromas
   c. Cataract
   d. Scoliosis

3. **Which of the following is the most common tumor associated with type-1 neurofibromatosis?** *(AIIMS Nov 2007, May 2003)*
   a. Optic nerve glioma
   b. Meningioma
   c. Acoustic schwannoma
   d. Low grade astrocytoma

4. **Neurofibromatosis type-2 is associated with:** *(PGI Dec 2000)*
   a. Bilateral acoustic schwannoma
   b. Multiple care-au-lait spots
   c. Chromosome-22
   d. Lisch nodule
   e. Posterior subcapsular lenticular cataract

5. **Widened neural foramina is frequently seen in:** *(All India 2012)*
   a. Neurofibromatosis
   b. Tuberous sclerosis
   c. Sturge-Weber syndrome
   d. Klippel-Fiel syndrome

6. **All of the following may be associated with Von-Hippel Lindau syndrome, except:** *(All India 2009)*
   a. Retinal and cerebella hemangioblastomas
   b. Gastric carcinoma
   c. Pheochromocytoma
   d. Renal cell carcinoma

7. **In Von-Hippel Lindau syndrome, the retinal vascular tumours are often associated with intracranial hemangioblastoma. Which one of the following regions is associated with such vascular abnormalities in this syndrome?** *(All India 2005)*
   a. Optic radiation
   b. Optic tract
   c. Cerebellum
   d. Pulvinar

8. **Which of the following statement about VHL syndrome is true?** *(All India 2012)*
   a. Multiple tumors are rarely seen
   b. Craniospinal hemangioblastoma are common
   c. Supratentorial tumors are common
   d. Tumors of Schwann cells are common

9. **Neurofibromatosis-2 is/are associated with:** *(PGI Nov 2011)*
   a. Meningioma
   b. Schwannoma
   c. Glioma
   d. Lisch nodule
   e. Hearing loss

10. **A child presents to the clinic with history of seizures and mental retardation. Clinical examination reveals multiple hypopigmented macules. What is the likely diagnosis?** *(All India 2010)*
    a. Tuberous Sclerosis
    b. Neurofibromatosis
    c. Sturge Weber Syndrome
    d. Linear epidermal nevus syndrome

11. **The diagnosis of a patient presenting with seizures, mental retardation and sebaceous adenoma is:** *(All India 95)*
    a. Hypothyroidism
    b. Tuberous sclerosis
    c. Toxoplasmosis
    d. Down syndrome

12. **Triad of tuberous sclerosis includes all, except:** *(All India 2009)*
    a. Epilepsy
    b. Adenoma sebacium
    c. Low intelligence
    d. Hydrocephalus

13. **Adenoma sebacium is a feature of:** *(AIIMS 2005)*
    a. Neurofibromatosis
    b. Tuberous sclerosis
    c. Xanthomatosis
    d. Incontinentia pigmenti

14. **CNS tumor seen in Von Hippel Lindau syndrome is:** *(PGI Dec 99)*
    a. Meningioma
    b. Cerebellar hemangioblastoma
    c. CNS lymphoma
    d. Glioma

15. **Neurofibromatosis is associated with:** *(PGI Dec 98)*
    a. Papillary carcinoma
    b. Islet cell tumor
    c. Pheochromocytoma
    d. Glucagonoma

16. **Plexiform neurofibromatosis commonly affects:**
    a. Facial nerve
    b. Trigeminal nerve
    c. Peripheral nerve
    d. Glossopharyngeal nerve

17. **Musculoskeletal abnormality in neurofibromatosis is:**
    a. Hypertrophy of limb
    b. Scoliosis
    c. Café au lait spots
    d. Pseudo arthrosis
    e. All

18. **Neurofibromatosis presents as all of the following except:** *(UPSC 2001)*
    a. Elephantiasis neuromatosa
    b. Plexiform neuroma
    c. Von Recklinghausen's disease
    d. Lymphadenovarix

19. **Brain tumor is associated with all except:** *(PGI Dec 99)*
    a. Tuberous sclerosis
    b. Von Hippel landau syndrome
    c. Neurofibromatosis
    d. Sturge-Weber syndrome

20. **What is not a feature of Sturge-Weber syndrome?**
    a. Rail track appearance
    b. Hemiatrophy of the brain
    c. Convulsion
    d. Empty sella

CNS TUMORS: CLINICAL FEATURES AND TREATMENT

21. **A 55-years old female presents with grade I Ependymoma extending from C7-T1 with no neural defect. Surgery is done, next management is:** *(DPG 2008)*
    a. Post-op chemotherapy
    b. Post-op chemoradiation
    c. Imaging, regular follow-up, chemotherapy if required
    d. Imaging, regular follow-up, radiotherapy if required

22. **All of the following are features of brain tumor except:** *(Recent Question 2017)*
    a. Pin point pupil
    b. Seizures
    c. Headache
    d. Focal neurological deficit

23. Most common brain tumour: *(Recent Question 2017)*
    a. Meningioma b. Glioma
    c. Metastasis d. Astrocytoma

24. Psychiatrics symptoms, true except: *(PGI 2000)*
    a. More common with supra than infra tentorial tumors
    b. More common with slow growing
    c. More with temporal than frontal lobe tumours
    d. More with brain stem lesions

25. Which of the following tumor is not known to increase in pregnancy? *(All India 2006)*
    a. Glioma b. Pituitary adenoma
    c. Meningioma d. Neurofibroma

26. Which one of the following tumors shows calcification on CT scan? *(All India 2005)*
    a. Ependymoma b. Medulloblastoma
    c. Meningioma d. CNS lymphoma

27. A 35 years old patient presented to hospital with headache, ataxia and imbalance. On laboratory evaluation, RBC count was very high. MRI brain was performed and the image is given below. What is the most probable diagnosis?
    a. Medulloblastoma b. Pilocytic astrocytoma
    c. Hemangioblastoma d. Craniopharyngioma

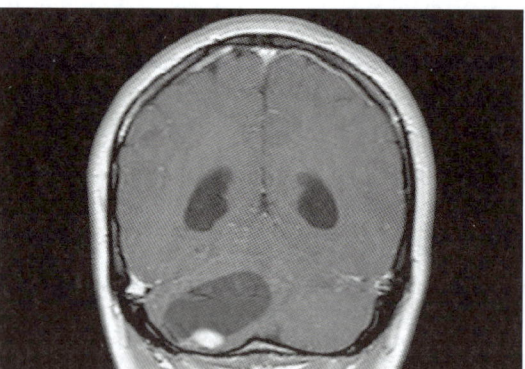

28. Stereotactic radiosurgery is done for: *(JIPMER 2002)*
    a. Glioblastoma multiforme
    b. Medulloblastoma spinal cord
    c. Ependymoma
    d. AV malformation of brain

29. Which of the following brain tumors doesn't spread via CSF? *(DPG 2011, All India 2004)*
    a. Germ cell tumor b. Medulloblastoma
    c. CNS Lymphoma d. Craniopharyngioma

30. The characteristic feature of a frontal lobe tumor is:
    a. Abnormal gait b. Aphasia *(All India 94)*
    c. Distractibility d. Antisocial behavior

31. Prophylactic craniospinal irradiation is recommended in:
    a. Gemistocytic astrocytoma *(PGI 2007)*
    b. Posterior fossa ependymoma
    c. Meningioma
    d. Medulloblastoma

32. All of the following tumors may be malignant except:
    a. Glioma b. Astrocytoma *(All India 97)*
    c. Hemangioblastoma d. Ependymoma

33. The CNS tumor present with calcification: *(PGI June 99)*
    a. Oligodendroglioma b. Astrocytoma
    c. Medulloblastoma d. pheochromocytoma

34. Lowest incidence of cerebral tumours is seen in:
    a. Occipital b. Frontal
    c. Temporal d. parietal

35. Cerebellar hemangioblastoma and retinal tumours are seen in: *(JIMPER 2012)*
    a. VHL syndrome b. NF-1
    c. Tuberous selerosis d. NF-2

BRAIN METASTASIS

36. Which of the following carcinoma most frequently metastasizes to brain? *(MCI June 2018; AIIMS 2005)*
    a. Small cell carcinoma lung b. Prostate cancer
    c. Rectal carcinoma d. Endometrial cancer

37. Most common site of brain metastasis: *(DNB 2011)*
    a. Brainstem b. Cerebellum
    c. Cerebral cortex d. Thalamous

ASTROCYTOMA

38. Which of the following is the most common type of glial tumors? *(All India 2006)*
    a. Astrocytomas b. Medulloblastomas
    c. Neurofibromas d. Ependymomas

39. In children most common posterior fossa tumour is: *(AIIMS Dec 95)*
    a. Meningiomas b. Astrocytoma
    c. Medulloblastoma d. Glioblastoma multiforme

40. A 25-year-old male presented with morning headache, projectile vomiting and seizures. MRI was done. What is the diagnosis on the basis of radiological findings?
    a. Meningioma b. Glioblastoma
    c. Medulloblastoma d. Oligodendroglioma

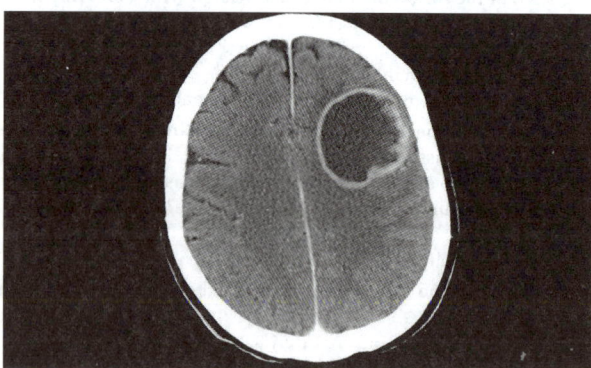

41. Glioblastoma multiforme may occur in the following except: *(DPG 93)*
    a. Cerebrum of adult b. Brain stem of child
    c. Spinal cord of adult d. Adrenal medulla of child

42. Which of the following brain tumors is highly vascular in nature? *(AIIMS May 2006)*
    a. Glioblastoma b. Meningiomas
    c. CP angle epidermoid d. Pituitary adenomas

43. Most common intracranial neoplasm in adults is: *(AIIMS May 93, May 94)*
    a. Meningioma b. Astrocytoma
    c. Posterior fossa tumor d. Ganglioneuroma

CNS Tumors

44. What is the most probable diagnosis based on the given MRI image? *(Recent Question 2016)*
    a. Pilocytic astrocytoma
    b. Glioblastoma multiforme
    c. Oligodendroglioma
    d. Meningioma

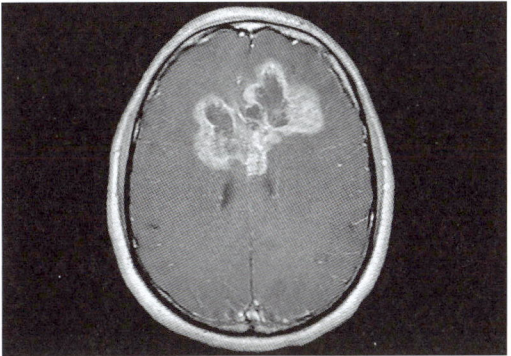

45. Which of the following statements about cerebellar astrocytomas in pediatric age group is false? *(All India 2008)*
    a. These are usually low grade tumors
    b. These are more commonly seen in the 1st and 2nd decades
    c. These tumors have a good prognosis
    d. These tumors are more common in females

46. Most common site of sub ependymal astrocytoma (Giant cell): *(AIIMS Nov 2007)*
    a. Trigone of lateral ventricle
    b. Foramen of Monro
    c. Temporal horn of lateral ventricle
    d. 4th ventricle

47. Glioblastoma multiforme is a variant of: *(COMEDK 2005)*
    a. Medulloblastoma
    b. Meningioma
    c. Astrocytoma
    d. Neuroblastoma

48. A 10 years old child was brought to the hospital by mother with history of headache, nausea, vomiting, irritability, difficulty to coordinate movements and visual complaints. MRI was performed and the image is given below. What is the most probable diagnosis? *(Recent Question 2016)*
    a. Medulloblastoma
    b. Pilocytic astrocytoma
    c. Hemangioblastoma
    d. Craniopharyngioma

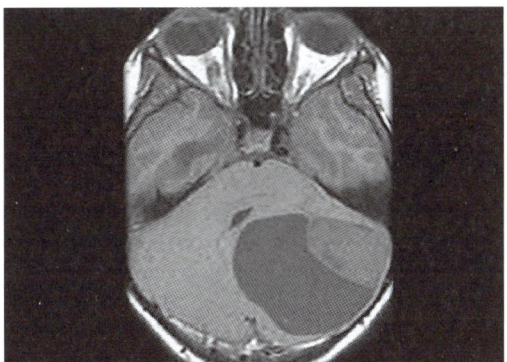

49. All are true regarding pilocytic astrocytoma, except:
    a. Seen in elderly above 80 years *(AIIMS May 2009)*
    b. Seen in posterior fossa
    c. Good prognosis
    d. Most common primary brain tumor in children

50. A child present with raised ICT. On CT scan, a lesion is seen around foramen of Monroe and multiple periventricular calcific foci. What is the most probable diagnosis?
    a. Central neurocytoma *(AIIMS Nov 2011)*
    b. Ependymoma
    c. Subependymal giant cell astrocytoma
    d. Gangioganglioma

MEDULLOBLASTOMA

51. Which of the following is true about medulloblastoma?
    a. Radiosensitive tumor *(PGI Dec 2005)*
    b. Spreads through CSF
    c. Surgical treatment is not done
    d. Occurs in young age group
    e. It is a supratentorial tumor

52. Chang staging is used for? *(AIIMS May 2010)*
    a. Retinoblastoma
    b. Medulloblastoma
    c. Ewing's sarcoma
    d. Rhabdomyosarcoma

53. Long term effect of craniospinal irradiation for medulloblastoma is: *(JIPMER 2011)*
    a. Secondary malignancy
    b. Neuro endocrine abnormalities
    c. Neurocognitive effects
    d. Hearing loss

54. Medulloblastoma exclusively occurs in the:
    a. Medulla
    b. Cerebellum
    c. Cerebral hemisphere
    d. Spinal cord

55. True about medulloblastoma is: *(AIIMS Nov 95)*
    a. Highly radiosensitive
    b. Surgery is the only treatment
    c. Occurs in adult age group
    d. Chemotherapy is useful

MENINGIOMA

56. A 45-years old female complains of progressive lower limb weakness, spasticity, urinary hesitancy. MRI shows intradural enhancing mass lesion. Most likely diagnosis is: *(AIIMS Nov 2011, Nov 2006, All India 2007)*
    a. Dermoid cyst
    b. Intradural lipoma
    c. Neuroepithelial cyst
    d. Meningioma

57. Radiological features of meningioma: *(PGI 2009)*
    a. Calcification
    b. Erosion
    c. Sutural diastasis
    d. Osteosclerosis
    e. Vascular erosion

58. A 40-year-old female presented with weakness of lower limbs with bladder dysfunction. On the basis of MRI findings, what is the diagnosis?
    a. Astrocytoma
    b. Meningioma
    c. Pituitary adenoma
    d. Oligodendroglioma

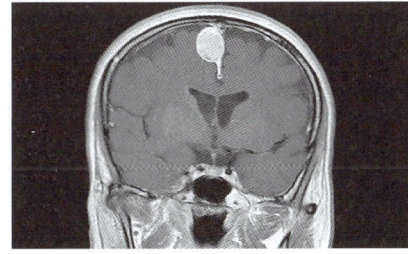

59. A 48-years old woman comes with bilateral progressive weakness of both lower limbs, spasticity and mild impairment of respiratory movements. MRI shows an intradural mid-dorsal midline enhancing lesion. What is the diagnosis?
    (AIIMS May 2010)
    a. Intradural lipoma
    b. Meningioma
    c. Neuroenteric cyst
    d. Dermoid cyst

60. Best prognosis among following is seen in: *(DNB 2007)*
    a. Astrocytoma
    b. Oligodendroglioma
    c. Meningioma
    d. Medulloblastoma

61. Extra-axial intracranial lesion showing contrast enhancement on MRI: *(All India 2012)*
    a. Meningioma
    b. Ependymoma
    c. Arachnoid cyst
    d. Astrocytoma

62. A lady had meningioma with inflammatory edematous lesion. She was planned for surgery. Junior resident mistake in writing pre-op notes is: *(AIIMS May 2012)*
    a. Stop steroids
    b. Wash head with shampoo
    c. Antibiotic sensitivity
    d. Continue antiepileptics

63. All of the following tumors usually show psammoma bodies except: *(MHCET 2016)*
    a. Papillary carcinoma of thyroid
    b. Meningioma
    c. Serous cystadenoma of ovary
    d. Hepatocellular carcinoma

CRANIOPHARYNGIOMA

64. Suprasellar calcification with polyuria seen in:
    (PGI Dec 2002)
    a. Langerhan cell histocytosis
    b. Medulloblastoma
    c. Pinealoma
    d. Craniopharyngioma
    e. Astrocytoma

65. A 6-years old boy has been complaining of headache, ignoring to see the objects on the sides for four months. On examination, he is not mentally retarded, his grades at school are good, and visual acuity is diminished in both the eyes. Visual charting showed significant field defect. CT scan of the head showed suprasellar mass with calcification. Which of the following is the most probable diagnosis?
    (AIIMS Nov 2004, 2005)
    a. Astrocytoma
    b. Craniopharyngioma
    c. Pituitary adenoma
    d. Meningioma

66. A 15 years old boy was brought to the hospital with the chief complaints of headache, vomiting and visual complaints. On examination, there were signs of growth retardation. MRI image is given below. What is the most probable diagnosis?
    a. Medulloblastoma
    b. Pilocytic astrocytoma
    c. Hemangioblastoma
    d. Craniopharyngioma

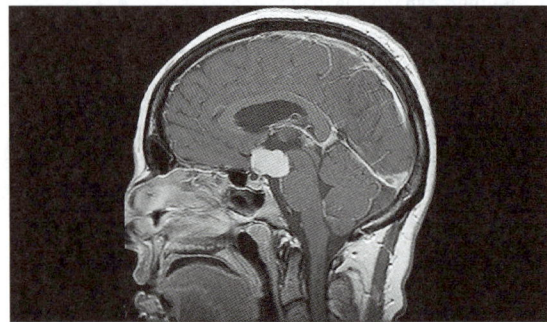

67. A six year old child managed by complete surgical removal of craniopharyngioma developed multiple endocrinopathies. Which of following hormones should be replaced first?
    (All India 2011)
    a. Hydrocortisone
    b. Growth Hormone
    c. Thyroxine
    d. Prolactin

68. Which of the following is the most common cause of a mixed cystic and solid suprasellar mass seen on cranial MR scan of a 10 years old child? *(AIIMS 2005)*
    a. Pituitary adenoma
    b. Craniopharyngioma
    c. Optic chiasmal glioma
    d. Germinoma

69. All the following are true of craniopharyngioma except:
    a. Derived from Rathke's pouch *(All India 94)*
    b. Contains epithelial cells
    c. Present in sella or infra-sellar location
    d. Causes visual disturbances

PITUITARY ADENOMA

70. Which of the following is true about pituitary adenoma?
    a. Accounts for 10% of brain tumors *(PGI Dec 2005)*
    b. Erodes the sellar and extends into surrounding area
    c. Prolactinoma is least common
    d. It is differentiated by reticulin stain

71. The most preferred approach for pituitary surgery at the present time is: *(JIPMER November 2017; All India 2006)*
    a. Transcranial
    b. Transethmoidal
    c. Transphenoidal
    d. Transcallosal

72. A 35 years old female with amenorrhea, galactorrhea has bitemporal hemianopia. The most probable diagnosis is:
    a. GnRH adenoma *(JIPMER 2010)*
    b. Sellar chordoma
    c. Craniopharyngioma
    d. Prolactin secreting pituitary microadenoma

73. A 30 years old male complains of loss of erection; he has low testosterone and high prolactin level in blood; what is the likely diagnosis? *(All India 2001)*
    a. Pituitary adenoma
    b. Testicular failure
    c. Craniopharyngioma
    d. Cushing's syndrome

74. Most common cause of hypersecreting pituitary tumour is:
    a. Pituitary adenoma *(DNB 2009)*
    b. Pituitary carcinoma
    c. Autoimmue disease of pituitary
    d. Transection of stalk

SPINAL TUMORS

75. The commonest extradural spinal tumor is:
    a. Neurofibroma
    b. Glioma
    c. Meningioma
    d. Metastasis

76. Commonest spinal tumour is: *(SCTIMS 98)*
    a. Meningioma
    b. Ependymoma
    c. Neurofibroma
    d. Neuroblastomas

77. Most common location of spinal tumors: *(AIIMS Nov 2007)*
    a. Intramedullary
    b. Intradural extramedullary
    c. Extradural
    d. Equally distributed

CNS LYMPHOMA

78. True about primary CNS lymphoma: *(PGI 2009)*
    a. Reticulin staining done
    b. Essentially B-cell type
    c. Associated with EBV
    d. Indolent disease with good prognosis
    e. Chemotherapy highly effective

79. All are true regarding Primary CNS lymphoma except:
    a. Radiotherapy and chemotherapy is of no value
    b. Occurs in AIDS patient   (AIIMS Feb 97)
    c. Commonly occurs in immune-compromised persons
    d. EBV may be a cause

SCHWANNOMA AND NEUROFIBROMA

80. Dumbbell tumor is seen in: (GB Pant 2011)
    a. Meningioma   b. Neurofibroma
    c. Ependymoma   d. Thymoma

81. Vestibular schwannoma arises most frequently from:
                                      (All India 2011)
    a. Superior vestibular nerve
    b. Inferior vestibular nerve
    c. Cochlear nerve
    d. Facial nerve

MISCELLANEOUS

82. Commonest orbital tumour causing exophthalmos is:
                                      (Recent Question 2016)
    a. Glioma   b. Meningioma
    c. Hemangioma   d. Neuroblastoma

83. Which of the following is primary neurogenic tumour?
                                      (JIPMER 90)
    a. Meningioma   b. Glioblastoma
    c. Acoustic neuroma d. Neuroblastoma

84. Witzelsucht syndrome (i.e. "Pathological Joking") is seen in:
                                      (All Inida 90)
    a. Frontal lobe tumours   b. Parietal lobe tumours
    c. Temporal lobe tumours   d. Intra Ventricular tumours

85. MRI is the investigation of choice in all of the following except: (COMEDK 2007, 2004)
    a. Syringomyelia   b. Brain stem tumors
    c. Skull bone tumors d. Multiple sclerosis

86. All of the following are neuronal tumors, except:
                                      (All India 2011)
    a. Gangliocytoma   b. Ganglioglioma
    c. Neurocytoma   d. Ependymoma

87. A 20-year female patient with 6th cranial nerve palsy on T2 weighted MRI shows a hyperintense lesion in cavernous sinus which shows homogenous contrast enhancement. Most probable diagnosis is: (AIIMS Nov 2010)
    a. Schwannoma
    b. Meningioma
    c. Cavernous sinus hemangioma
    d. Astrocytoma

88. Imaging modality of choice for detecting radiation induced cerebral necrosis: (AIIMS Nov 2009, 2005)
    a. PET scan   b. Biopsy
    c. MRI   d. CT

89. Not a neuroglial tumor: (Kerala 95)
    a. Shwannoma
    b. Astrocytoma
    c. Medulloblastoma
    d. Ependymoma

90. Investigation of choice for leptomeningeal carcinomatosis:
                                      (AIIMS Nov 2011)
    a. PET Scan   b. SPECT
    c. Gd enhanced MRI d. CT scan

91. A patient was diagnosed with intracranial cavernous angioma on MRI. MRI finding chracteristic of this lesion is:
                                      (AIIMS Nov 2011)
    a. Well defined nidus
    b. Definite arterial feeders
    c. Phlebectasis
    d. Popcorn like lesion

92. All of the following are true about long terms sequel of cranio spinal radiothreapy for children with CNS tumors except:
    a. Neurocognitive dysfunction   (All India 2012)
    b. Endocrinologic dysfunction
    c. Musculoskeletan hypoplasia
    d. Neuropsychological sequel are independent of radiation dose

93. Enlargement of pituitary tumour after adrenalectomy is called as: (DNB 2009)
    a. Nelson syndrome
    b. Steel-Richardson syndrome
    c. Hamman-Rich syndrome
    d. Job's syndrome

94. Stereotactic surgery is used for treatment of:
                                      (AIIMS Nov 2012)
    a. Brain tumor   b. Lungs carcinoma
    c. Cervix cancer   d. Renal carcinoma

95. Highly vascular tumor of brain and spinal cord in adults:
                                      (AIIMS May 2013)
    a. Metastasis
    b. Pilocytic astrocytoma
    c. Hemangioblastoma
    d. Cavernous malformation

Explanations

CNS TUMORS PREDISPOSING FACTORS

1. **Ans. d. Xeroderma pigmentosum** *(Ref: Harrison 20/e p645, 19/e po599; Bailey 27/e p145)*
2. **Ans. a. Autosomal recessive inheritance** *(Ref: Harrison 20/e p649, 19/e p604; Sabiston 20/e p754; Schwartz 10/e p677; Bailey 27/e p145)*

Neurofibromatosis	
Neurofibromatosis-1	**Neurofibromatosis-2**

• Also known as **peripheral** neurofibromatosis or **von-Recklinghausen's syndrome**^{Q}
• **Most prevalent** type (**90%**^{Q})
• **NF-1 gene**: Chromosome **17**^{Q}
• **Autosomal dominant**^{Q}
• **Diagnostic Criteria for NF-1** (Diagnosed when **any two** of the following are present):
  1. **≥6 *café-au-lait* macules**^{Q} >5 mm in greatest diameter in prepubertal individuals and >15mm in greatest diameter in post-pubertal individuals.
  2. **Axillary** or **inguinal freckling**^{Q}
  3. **≥2 iris Lisch nodules**^{Q}
  4. **≥2 neurofibromas** or **one plexiform neurofibroma**^{Q}
  5. Sphenoid dysplasia or cortical thinning of long bone, with or without pseudoarthrosis
  6. **Optic gliomas**^{Q}
  7. A **first degree relative** with NF-1 whose diagnosis was based on the aforementioned criteria.
	• Also known as **central** neurofibromatosis or **bilateral acoustic neurofibromatosis**^{Q}
	• Less prevalent (10%)
	• **NF-2 gene**: Chromosome **22**^{Q}
	• **Autosomal dominant**^{Q}
	• **Diagnostic Criteria for NF-2**^{Q} (Diagnosed when **any one** of the following is present):
	  1. **Bilateral 8th nerve masses** consistent with **acoustic neuromas**^{Q}
	  2. A parent, sibling, or child with NF-2 and either
	  3. **Unilateral 8th nerve mass** or **any two** of the following:
	    – Neurofibroma^Q
	    – Meningioma^Q
	    – Glioma^Q
	    – Schwannoma^Q
	• Bilateral acoustic neuromas are the most distinctive tumors in patients with NF-2^Q.

3. **Ans. a. Optic nerve glioma**
4. **Ans. a. Bilateral acoustic schwannoma, c. Chromosome -22, e. Posterior subcapsular lenticular cataract**
5. **Ans. a. Neurofibromatosis** *(Ref: Differential Diagnosis in Conventional Radiology (Thieme) 2007/260)*
6. **Ans. b. Gastric carcinoma** *(Ref: Harrison 20/e p649, 19/e p599; Sabiston 20/e p693; Bailey 27/e p145)*

Von Hippel Lindau Syndrome (AD)	
Characteristic Tumors/Cysts	**Other Tumors/Cysts**

• **Hemangioblastomas:**
  – **Cerebellar** hemangioblastoma^Q
  – **Retinal** hemangioblastoma^Q
  – **Spinal** hemangioblastoma^Q
	• RCC^Q
	• Pheochromocytoma^Q
	• Pancreatic endocrine tumors
	• Adrenal carcinomas
	• **Benign cysts** in kidney, epididymis, liver or pancreas^Q

• **Polycythemia** is a **characteristic feature in VHL** due to **erythropoietin production** by **hemangioblastoma** and/or **RCC**^{Q}.

7. **Ans. c. Cerebellum**
8. **Ans. b. Craniospinal hemangioblastoma are common**
9. **Ans. a. Meningioma, b. Schwannoma, c. Glioma, e. Hearing loss**
10. **Ans. a. Tuberous Sclerosis** *(Ref: Roxburgh's 17/e p201; Harrison 20/e p649, 19/e p604)*

Tuberous Sclerosis/Epiloia/Bourneville's Disease		
Skin Lesion	**Neurological**	**Benign Neoplasm**
• **Adenoma sebacium**^{Q} (facial angiofibroma) • **Ash leaf** shaped hypopigmentd **macules**^{Q} • **Shagreen Patch**^{Q}- yellow thickening of lumbosacral skin • Depigmented nevi	• Seizure^Q • Mental retardation^Q • Subependymal nodules^Q which may calcify • Hydrocephalus^Q	• Rhabdomyoma^Q • Angiomyoma^Q of liver, kidney, pancreas etc. • Ependymoma^Q • Astrocytoma^Q

11. Ans. b. Tuberous sclerosis
12. Ans. d. Hydrocephalus
13. Ans. b. Tuberous sclerosis
14. Ans. b. Cerebellar hemangioblastoma
15. Ans. c. Pheochromocytoma
16. Ans. b. Trigeminal nerve
17. Ans. e. All
18. Ans. d. Lymphadenovarix

- Elephantiasis neuromatosa is the most impressive manifestation of NF-1.

19. Ans. d. Sturge-Weber syndrome
20. Ans. d. Empty sella *(Ref: Bailey 26/e p599)*

STURGE-WEBER SYNDROME / ENCEPHALOTRIGEMINAL SYNDROME

- Usually sporadic, characterized by:
  - Large unilateral cutaneous angioma^Q **(port-wine stain)**
  - **Angiomas** in brain involving **ipsilateral cerebral hemisphere** and **meninges**
  - **Focal seizures**^{Q} typically occurs **opposite to the side of lesion**^{Q}
  - **Adrenal pheochromocytoma**
  - Cerebral angiomas lead to **cortical atrophy**^{Q}

  - Angiomas are visible radiologically as **Tram-track** or **rail track calcification** mainly in **occipital region**^{Q}

CNS TUMORS: CLINICAL FEATURES AND TREATMENT

21. Ans. d. Imaging, regular follow-up, radiotherapy if required *(Ref: Harrison 20/e p643, 19/e p601; Sabiston 20/e p1912; Schwartz 10/e p1734, 1738; Bailey 27/e p664)*

    - Harrison says "Following the gross total excision of an Ependymoma, the prognosis is excellent. The five year disease free survival is >80%. However, **many ependymoma cannot be totally excised**, and **postoperative focal external beam radiation** or **stereotactic radiosurgery is used.**"

22. Ans. a. Pin point pupil *(Ref: Sabiston 20/e p1909; Schwartz 10/e p1732; Bailey 27/e p662-663)*
23. Ans. c. Metastasis *(Ref: Sabiston 20/e p1915; Schwartz 10/e p1732; Bailey 27/e p663)*
24. Ans. b. More common with slow growing, c. More with temporal than frontal lobe tumours *(Ref: Kaplan and Sadock's Concise Textbook of Clinical Psychiatry (2008)/74)*

PSYCHIATRIC SYMPTOMS IN BRAIN TUMORS

- **Mental changes** are likely to occur in patients with **supratentorial tumors**, and more commonly among patients with tumors of the **frontal** and **temporal lobes**.

  - **Psychiatric symptoms** are **more common in frontal lobe tumors**^{Q}.
  - **Depression**: More common in frontal lobe tumors^Q
  - **Psychosis**: More common in **temporal lobe tumors**^{Q}

- **Left sided frontal tumors** are more commonly associated with **akinesia** and **depression**, while **right sided lesions** are more often associated with **euphoria**.
- **Delirium** is most often a component of **rapidly growing**^{Q}, **large**, or **metastatic tumors**.

25. Ans. a. Glioma *(Ref: CGDT 9/e p429)*

    - Although brain tumors are not specifically related to gestation, **meningiomas**, **angiomas**, and **neurofibromas** are thought to **grow more rapidly with pregnancy**^{Q}.

26. Ans. c. Meningioma *(Ref: Sutton Radiology 7/e p1739)*

    - **Meningioma** range from **firm** and **fibrous to finely gritty** or they may be **extremely calcified** with **Psammoma bodies**^{Q}.
    - **Calcification** is also **seen in ependymoma**, but **more common in meningioma**^{Q}.

27. **Ans. c. Hemangioblastoma** *(Ref: Harrison 20/e p2754, 19/e p578; Sabiston 20/e p1913)*

Hemangioblastoma

- MC primary intra-axial tumor in the **adult posterior fossa**[Q]
- Occur almost **exclusively** in the **posterior fossa (cerebellum**[Q])
- **Solid** or **cystic** with a **mural nodule**[Q]
- May occur sporadically, and **20% of cases may be associated with von Hippel-Lindau disease** (hemangioblastomas, retinal angiomas, RCC, pheochromocytoma, renal and pancreatic cysts)[Q].

Pathology
- Histologically **benign**[Q], and may be associated with **erythrocytosis**[Q].
- Appear as **cystic tumors** with an enhancing tumor on the cyst wall known as the **mural nodule**
- Pathology reveals **abundant thin-walled vascular channels**[Q]

Clinical Features
- Most patients present with **headache, hydrocephalus**, symptoms of **raised ICT and cerebellar dysfunction**[Q]
- Polycythemia due to **increased erythropoietin production** occurs in ~20% cases[Q]

Diagnosis
- **Sharply demarcated homogeneous masses** composed of **cyst with non-enhancing walls**, except for a **mural nodule which vividly enhances**[Q]

Treatment
- **Surgical resection** is **curative** for sporadic (non-VHL associated) tumors[Q].
- **En-bloc resection** of the **mural nodule alone**, leaving the cyst wall, is **sufficient**[Q].

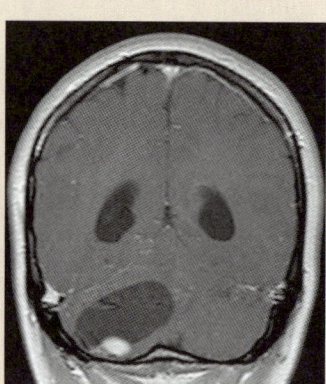

28. **Ans. d. AV malformation of brain** *(Ref: Sabiston 20/e p1923; Schwartz 10/e p1749)*
29. **Ans. d. Craniopharyngioma** *(Ref: Harrison 20/e p648, 19/e p0599-601)*
30. **Ans. d. Antisocial behavior**

Frontal Lobe Tumors

- **Personality changes** are **common symptom** of frontal lobe tumor.
- **Frontal lobe controls behavior** and judgment[Q].
- Patients may be **socially disinhibited, display antisocial behavior**, shows **severe impairment of judgment, insight** and **foresight**[Q].

  - **Witzelsucht syndrome:** Self amusement from poor jokes and puns, also known as **pathological joking**, is seen in **frontal lobe tumors**[Q]

31. **Ans. d. Medulloblastoma** *(Ref: Harrison 20/e p647, 19/e p601, 603)*

Prophylactic Craniospinal Irradiation

- Prophylactic craniospinal irradiation is useful in **CNS malignancy** which **disseminate via CSF** or any **malignancy** with **high risk of CNS spread**[Q].

Common Manifestations	Less Common Manifestation
• Medulloblastoma[Q]	• ALL[Q]
• Glioblastoma[Q]	• Non hodgkin's lymphoma[Q]
• Germinoma[Q]	• Leptomeningeal Rhabdomyosarcoma[Q]
• Small cell Ca of lung[Q]	

32. **Ans. c. Hemangioblastoma** *(Ref: Harrison 20/e p2754, 19/e p578; Sabiston 20/e p1913; Schwartz 10/e p1735-1736)*
33. **Ans. a. Oligodendroglioma** *(Ref: Harrison 20/e p646, 19/e p600; Sabiston 20/e p1911; Schwartz 10/e p1733; Bailey 27/e p664)*

Tumors with Calicification: (COM) Craniopharyngioma (Most) > Oligodenoroglioma (90%) > Meningioma (20–25%)

34. **Ans. a. Occipital**
35. **Ans. a. VHL syndrome**

BRAIN METASTASIS

36. **Ans. a. Small cell carcinoma lung** *(Ref: Harrison 20/e p649, 19/e p604)*
37. **Ans. c. Cerebral cortex**

ASTROCYTOMA

38. **Ans. a. Astrocytomas** *(Ref: Harrison 20/e p644, 19/ep599; Sabiston 20/e p1911; Schwartz 10/e p1733, 1738-1739; Bailey 27/e p664)*
39. **Ans. b. Astrocytoma**
40. **Ans. b. Glioblastoma**
    - Glioblastoma multiforme: Ring enhancement with central necrosis on MRI^Q.
41. **Ans. d. Adrenal medulla of child**
42. **Ans. a. Glioblastoma** *(Ref: Harrison 20/e p645, 18/e p3384-3386; Osborn Neuroradiology (1994)/541, 591)*
    - Osborn says "**Glioblastoma** is **highly vascular,** sometimes so vascular that it **resembles an AV malformation on angiography**."
43. **Ans. a. Meningioma** *(Ref: Harrison 20/e p643, 19/e p602)*

    Harrison says "meningiomas are diagnosed with increasing frequently as more people undergo neuroimaging for various indications. They are now the most common primary brain tumor, accounting for approximately 35% of total.

    - **MC primary brain tumor: Meningioma (35%) > glialtumors (30%)**
    - MC malignant brain tumor of childhood: Medulloblastoma
    - MC brain tumor: Metastasis

44. **Ans. b. Glioblastoma multiforme** *(Ref: Sabiston 20/e p1911; Harrison 20/e p645, 19/e p91e-4; Robbins 9/e p1307)*
45. **Ans. d. These tumors are more common in females** *(Ref: Nelsons 20/e p2455)*

    Cerebellar astrocytomas do not show any clear gender predilection and are **equally common** in both **males** and **females**.

46. **Ans. b. Foramen of Monro** *(Ref: Neurology in Clinical Practice 4/e p428; Sutton Radiology 7/e p1735)*

    ### SUBEPENDYMAL GIANT CELL ASTROCYTOMA

    - **Most common site** of **subependymal giant cell astrocytoma** is the **ependymal wall of lateral ventricle near** the **foramen of Monro**^{Q}.
    - Causes **obstruction at** the **foramen of Monro** leading to **ventricular enlargement** and **raised ICT**.

        - Presence of **multiple periventricular calcific foci (calcified subependymal nodules)** suggest the diagnosis of **Tuberous sclerosis** with **subependymal giant cell astrocytoma**^{Q}

47. **Ans. c. Astrocytoma**
48. **Ans. b. Pilocytic astrocytoma** *(Ref: Sabiston 20/e p1911; Harrison 20/e p644, 19/e p441e-39f; Robbins 9/e p1340)*
49. **Ans. a. Seen in elderly above 80 years**   50. **Ans. c. Subependymal giant cell astrocytoma**

MEDULLOBLASTOMA

51. **Ans. a. Radiosensitive tumor, b. Spreads through CSF, d. Occurs in young age group** *(Ref: Harrison 20/e p647, 19/e p602; Sabiston 20/ep,; Schwartz 10/e p1734)*
52. **Ans. b. Medulloblastoma**
53. **Ans. c. Neurocognitive effect** *(Ref: www.ncbi.nlm.nih.gov/pubmed/9121399)*

    ### CRANIOSPINAL IRRADIATION (CSI)

    - **Hypothyroidism**: One of the **earliest late side effects of CSI** and **2nd MC (after GH disturbance**^{Q})
    - **Prevalence of hypothyroidism is 40–80% after CSI**^{Q}
    - Significantly increased risk of development of **benign thyroid nodules** and **papillary carcinoma of the thyroid** many years later^Q.

54. **Ans. b. Cerebellum**   55. **Ans. a. Highly radiosensitive**

MENINGIOMA

56. **Ans. d. Meningioma** *(Ref: Harrison 20/e p648, 19/e p602; Chapman 4/e p 431; Sabiston 20/e p1913; Schwartz 10/e p1735,1738; Bailey 27/e p665)*
57. **Ans. a. Calcification, d. Osteosclerosis, e. Vascular erosion**
58. **Ans. b. Meningioma** *(Ref: Chapman 4/e p431)*
59. **Ans. b. Meningioma**
60. **Ans. c. Meningioma**
    - Meningioma is slow growing and encapsulated tumor having best prognosis among the given options.

61. Ans. a. Meningioma
62. Ans. a. Stop steroids

- **Sudden withdrawal of steroids** may lead to **adrenal insufficiency,** particularly during period of stress such as surgery.

63. Ans. d. Hepatocellular carcinoma

CRANIOPHARYNGIOMA

64. Ans. d. Craniopharyngioma *(Ref: Harrison 20/e p648, 19/ep 603, 18/e p3389; Schwartz 10/e p1736-1737)*
65. Ans. b. Craniopharyngioma
66. Ans. d. Craniopharyngioma *(Ref: Harrison 20/e p648, 19/e p2262)*
67. Ans. a. Hydrocortisone
68. Ans. b. Craniopharyngioma
69. Ans. c. Present in sella or infra-sellar location

PITUITARY ADENOMA

70. Ans. a. Accounts for 10% of brain tumors, b. Erodes the sellar and extends into surrounding area, d. It is differentiated by reticulin stain *(Ref: Harrison 20/e p2673, 19/e p603; Sabiston 20/e p1914; Schwartz 10/e p1735; Bailey 27/e p665-666,841,842)*

CUSHING DISEASE

- **Pituitary dependent cause** of **Cushing syndrome** (pituitary adenoma secreting **excessive ACTH)**

71. Ans. c. Transphenoidal
72. Ans. d. Prolactin secreting pituitary microadenoma
73. Ans. a. Pituitary adenoma
74. Ans. a. Pituitary adenoma

SPINAL TUMORS

75. Ans. d. Metastasis *(Ref: Scott Atlas, MRI of the Brain and Spine 3rd/1742; Sabiston 20/e p1913; Schwartz 10/e p1737-1739)*
76. Ans. c. Neurofibroma
77. Ans. c. Extradural

CNS LYMPHOMA

78. Ans. a. Reticulin staining done, b. Essentially B-cell type, c. Associated with EBV *(Ref: Harrison 20/e p647, 19/e p601; Sabiston 20/e p1914; Schwartz 10/e p1736; Bailey 25/e p630)*
79. Ans. a. Radiotherapy and chemotherapy is of no value

SCHWANNOMA AND NEUROFIBROMA

80. Ans. b. Neurofibroma
    - The term **"dumbbell"** lesion is used to describe **neurofibroma.**
81. Ans. b. Inferior vestibular nerve *(Ref: Harrison 20/e p648, 19/e p220; Sabiston 19/e p1889; Schwartz 9/e p1541; Bailey 26/e p616)*

MISCELLANEOUS

82. Ans. a. Glioma
83. Ans. d. Neuroblastoma
84. Ans. a. Frontal lobe tumours
85. Ans. c. Skull bone tumors *(Ref: Bailey 27/e p197-198,199)*

MAGNETIC RESONANCE IMAGING

- MRI was discovered by **Lauterbeur**[Q] in 1973.
- MRI is **best for soft tissues**[Q].

86. Ans. d. Ependymoma *(Ref: Robbins 9/e p601)*

- **Ependymomas** are **glial tumors,** derived from the **ependymal cells** that line the ventricular surface. These tumors **do not originate from neurons**[Q].

87. Ans. a. Schwannoma *(Ref: Osborn Radiology/501)*
    - **Schwannoma** is **hypointense** on **T1** and **hyperintense** on **T2.**

CNS Tumors

88. **Ans. a. PET scan**
89. **Ans. c. Medulloblastoma**
90. **Ans. c. Gd enhanced MRI**
91. **Ans. d. Popcorn like lesion** *(Ref: Osborn Neuroradiology/313)*

   MRI appearance of cavernous angioma is highly characteristic, showing **"popcorn like lesion"** [Q].

92. **Ans. d. Neuropsychological sequelae are independent of radiation dose** *(Ref: Tumors of Pediatric CNS (Thieme) 2001/141)*

   - **Total radiation dose** is the **strongest factor** determining the **magnitude of white matter changes** as well as **neuropsychological effects**[Q].

93. **Ans. a. Nelson syndrome** *(Ref: Harrison 20/e p2682, 19/e p2273)*

   ### Nelson Syndrome
   - Nelson syndrome refers to a spectrum of symptoms and signs arising from an **adrenocorticotropin (ACTH)–secreting pituitary macroadenoma after a therapeutic bilateral adrenalectomy.**
   - The spectrum of clinical features observed relates to the **local effects of the tumor on surrounding structures**, the **secondary loss of other pituitary hormones**, and the **effects of the high serum concentrations of ACTH on the skin.**

94. **Ans. a. Brain tumor** *(Ref: Sabiston 20/e p1923; Schwartz 10/e p1749)*

   Stereotactic surgery is used for treatment of brain tumors

95. **Ans. c. Hemangioblastoma** *(Ref: Harrison 20/e p2754, 19/e p578; Sabiston 20/e p1913; Schwartz 10/e p1735-1736)*

   - *Highly vascular tumor of brain and spinal cord in adults Hemangioblastoma.*

SECTION 8

Head and Neck

CHAPTERS

- ☐ Oral Cavity
- ☐ Salivary Glands
- ☐ Neck
- ☐ Facial Injuries and Abnormalities

CHAPTER 35

Oral Cavity

RISK FACTORS FOR CANCER OF ORAL CAVITY

Risk Factors for Cancer of Oral Cavity

- Tobacco[Q]
- Alcohol[Q]
- Areca nut/pan masala[Q]
- Sharp or jagged tooth[Q]
- Ill-fitting dentures[Q]
- Syphilitic glossitis[Q]
- Human papilloma virus[Q]
- Epstein-Barr virus[Q]
- Plummer-Vinson syndrome[Q]
- Poor nutrition

Conditions Associated with Malignant Transformation

High-risk Lesions
- Erythroplakia[Q]
- Speckled Erythroplakia[Q]
- Chronic hyperplastic candidiasis[Q]

Medium-risk Lesions
- Oral submucous fibrosis[Q]
- Syphilitic glossitis[Q]
- Sideropenic dysphagia[Q] (Paterson-Kelly syndrome)

Low-risk or Equivocal-risk Lesions
- Oral lichen planus
- Discoid lupus erythematosus
- Discoid keratosis congenita

ORAL SUBMUCOUS FIBROSIS

ORAL SUBMUCOUS FIBROSIS

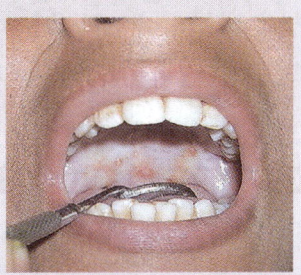

- Oral submucous fibrosis is a **progressive disease** in which **fibrous bands form beneath the oral mucosa**[Q].
- Almost **entirely confined to the Asian population**[Q]
- Risk factor for **oral cavity malignancies** (squamous cell carcinoma[Q])

Risk Factors
- Research strongly indicates that oral submucous fibrosis is **significantly associated** with the use of **pan masala areca nut, with or without concurrent alcohol use**[Q].
- Tobacco smoking alone is **not associated** with oral submucous fibrosis.

Pathology
- Characterised by **epithelial fibrosis** with **associated atrophy & hyperplasia** of overlying **epithelium**[Q].
- **Epithelium** shows changes of **epithelial dysplasia**[Q].

Clinical Features
- Scarring produces contracture, resulting in **limited mouth opening & restricted tongue movement**[Q].

Treatment
- Restricted mouth opening can be treated with either **intralesional steroids** or **surgical excision & skin grafts**[Q].

IMPORTANT POINTS ABOUT CARCINOMA ORAL CAVITY

- MC gene mutated in CA oral cavity: **p53**[Q]
- MC site of CA oral cavity: **Tongue >Lip**[Q]
- MC histological type of CA oral cavity: **Squamous cell carcinoma**[Q]
- MC type of cancer in India: **CA oral cavity**[Q]
- MC site of CA oral cavity in India: **Buccal mucosa**[Q] (38%) > Anterior tongue (16%) > Lower alveolus (15.7%)
- MC pattern of spread: **Local extension & regional lymphatic spread**[Q]
- LN metastasis is most common in: **CA tongue**[Q] > Floor of mouth > Lower alveolus > Buccal mucosa > Upper alveolus > **Hard palate > Lip**[Q].

- **Bilateral lymphatic spread** is common in: **Lower lip**^{Q}, **supraglottis**^{Q} & **soft palate**^{Q}.
- **MC site of metastasis: Lung**^{Q}
- **Edge biopsy** is recommended for **diagnosis of oral cavity malignancies**^{Q}.
- **MRI: IOC** for **staging of head & neck malignancies**^{Q}.
- **MC flap used** for reconstruction of **head & neck malignancies: PMMC (pectoralis major myocutaneous)** flap based on pectoral branch of **Thoracoacromial vessels**^{Q}

8th AJCC (2017) TNM Classification of Carcinoma Lip & Oral Cavity			
Primary Tumor (T)		**Regional Lymph Nodes (N)**	
Tis	Carcinoma in situ.	N1	Metastasis in a **single ipsilateral LN, ≤3 cm** in greatest dimension without extranodal extension^Q
T1	Tumor **≤2 cm** in greatest dimension & **≤5 mm** depth of invasion^Q	N2a	Metastasis in **single ipsilateral LN, >3 cm** but **≤6 cm** in greatest dimension without extranodal extension^Q
T2	Tumor **≤2 cm** in greatest dimension & **>5 mm** but **≤10 mm** depth of invasion or tumor **>2 cm** but **≤4 cm** in greatest dimension & **depth of invasion ≤10 mm**^{Q}	N2b	Metastases in **multiple ipsilateral LN,** none >6 cm in greatest dimension without extranodal extension^Q
T3	Tumor **>4 cm** in greatest dimension **>10 mm** depth of invasion^Q	N2c	Metastases in **bilateral** or **contralateral LN,** none >6 cm in greatest dimension without extranodal extension^Q
T4a	**Lip:** Tumor invades through **cortical bone, inferior alveolar nerve, floor** of mouth, or **skin (of chin or nose)**^{Q}	N3a	Metastasis in a **LN >6 cm** in greatest dimension without extranodal extension^Q
		N3b	Metastasis in **a single or multiple LNs with clinical extranodal extension**^{Q}
	Oral cavity: Tumor invades through **cortical bone** mandible or maxillary sinus or invades the **skin of face**^{Q}.	**Distant Metastasis**	
T4b	Tumor invades **masticator space, pterygoid plates,** or **skull base** and/or encases **internal carotid artery**^{Q}.	M0	No distant metastasis.
		M1	Distant metastasis.

Stage Grouping							
0	**I**	**II**	**III**	**IVA**	**IVB**	**IVC**	
Tis N0M0	T1 N0M0	T2 N0M0	T3 N0M0 T1-3 N1 M0	T4a N0-1 M0 T1-4a N2 M0	Any T N3 M0 T4b Any N M0	Any N Any T M1	

CARCINOMA LIP

Carcinoma Lip

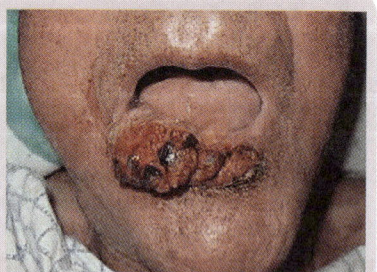

- **MC site of CA lip: Vermillion of lower lip**^{Q}
- Typically seen in **males of 40-70 years**^{Q}
- Definite correlation between **CA lip** and **exposure to sunlight** (UV radiations^Q)
- **MC presentation: Non-healing ulcer** or growth^Q
- **LN metastasis is rare** and **develops late,** mainly to **submental** and **submandibular** LNs^Q.
- **Bilateral lymphatic spread** is seen in **CA lower lip**^{Q}.

Treatment of Carcinoma Lip	
• T1 and T2	• **Surgery is TOC**^{Q} • If **1/3rd or less of lip is involved:** 'V' or 'W' shaped **full thickness excision** with lateral margin of 5 mm + **Primary closure**^{Q} • If **more than 1/3rd of lip is involved:** Flap reconstruction (**Abbe-Estlander flap**)^Q
• T3 and T4	• **Combined radiation** and **surgery**^{Q} (vermilonectomy or lip shave)

Prognosis
- CA lip has the **best prognosis**^{Q} in CA oral cavity.

Lip Reconstruction	
Cross-lip Flaps	Circumoral Advancement Flaps
• Lip-Switch (Abbe-Estlander) flap[Q] used to repair defects of either upper or lower lip, based on superior labial artery[Q]	• Karapandzic flap[Q]: Uses a sensate, neuromuscular flap based on labial artery[Q]. • Webster-Bernard repair[Q]: Use lateral nasolabial flap with buccal advancement

CARCINOMA BUCCAL MUCOSA (CHEEK)

Carcinoma Buccal Mucosa (Cheek)

- **MC site** of CA oral cavity in India: Buccal mucosa[Q]
- Related to chewing a combination of **tobacco mixed with betel leaves, areca nut** and **lime shell**[Q]
- Most malignant tumors are **low grade SCC**[Q]
- Frequently appearing on background of leukoplakia
- **Lymphatic spread** is first to **level I and II LNs**[Q].

Clinical Feature
- **Pain is minimal**, obstruction of Stenson's duct can lead to parotid enlargement.

Treatment
- **T1: Excision** with primary closure[Q]
- **T2: Surgery ± Radiotherapy**[Q]
- **T3 and T4: Surgery + Radiotherapy** or **chemoradiation**[Q]

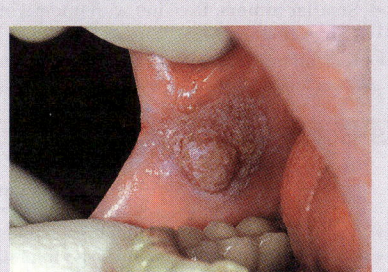

CARCINOMA TONGUE

Carcinoma Tongue

- **MC site** is **middle of lateral border**[Q] or ventral aspect of the tongue.
- **MC histological type** is **squamous cell carcinoma**[Q].
- **MC associated risk factors** are **tobacco** and **alcohol**[Q].
- **MC variety** is **ulcerative**[Q].
- **30% patients** presents with **cervical node metastasis**[Q].

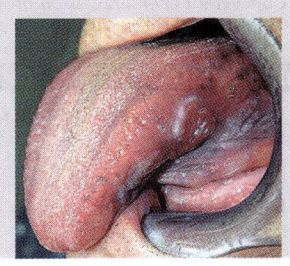

CARCINOMA ORAL TONGUE

Carcinoma Oral Tongue

- The intrinsic tongue musculature provide little restriction to tumour growth, thus it may enlarge considerably before producing symptoms.
- Presents as **painless mass** or **ulcer** that **fails to heal** after minor trauma[Q].
- **MC complaint**: Mid-irritation of tongue[Q].
- **MC site**: Lateral border of the **junction of middle & posterior third**[Q].
- **Primary basin** for **cervical metastasis** is superior deep jugular nodes (Level II)[Q].
- For diagnosis, **wedge biopsy** is taken **from** the **edge of ulcer** but in proliferative growth, **punch biopsy** is taken[Q].

	Treatment of Carcinoma Oral Tongue
T1	• **Partial glossectomy** with primary closure[Q]
T2	• **Hemiglossectomy** for **small well-circumscribed** and **well differentiated** lesion[Q] • **Radiotherapy** for **large, poorly differentiated** lesion[Q]
T3	• **Total glossectomy** followed by **radiation**[Q]
T4	• **Surgery** (Total glossectomy, **mandibulectomy**, MRND, laryngectomy) + **Postoperative radiation**[Q]

Management of Recurrence
- **Most recurrences** occur within **2 years.**
- **Radiation failure** is managed by **glossectomy**[Q].
- **Surgical failure** is managed by **radiation**[Q].
- If **recurrence** is **limited to mucosa**, it is best managed by **surgery**
- If **recurrence** is in the **soft tissue of** the **neck, palliation** is indicated.

CANCER OF HARD PALATE

Cancer of Hard Palate

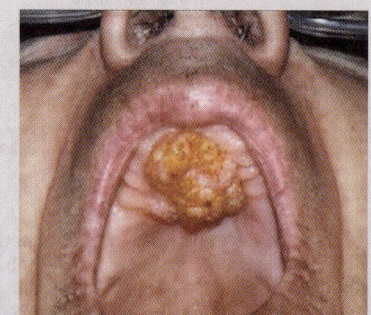

- SCC of hard palate is **rare, Associated with reverse smoking**
- Minor salivary gland tumors occur in the hard palate.
- Most cancers are **well differentiated** and of **ulcerative variety**[Q].

Clinical Features
- Presents as painless mass[Q] in the roof of the mouth
- Lymphatic metastasis is **uncommon**, mainly to level I and II.

Treatment
- **Smaller tumors:** Excision with underlying bone.
- **Larger tumors:** Maxillectomy
- **Radiotherapy** is used in advanced lesions.

CHEMOTHERAPY IN CANCERS OF ORAL CAVITY, HEAD AND NECK

Chemotherapy in Cancers of Oral Cavity, Head and Neck

- Adjuvant **chemotherapy** has been reported to **improve the rate of organ preservation** with **no change in overall survival**[Q].
- Chemotherapy is often **employed in palliative setting** in patients with **recurrent, unresectable** or **distant metastases**[Q].
- **Drugs used:** Cisplatin[Q], Methotrexate, 5-FU, Docetaxel and Paclitaxel

> - **Cisplatin** is the **cornerstone drug** in the modern management of head & neck cancer[Q].
> - **Most beneficial** is concurrent chemotherapy[Q].

- The addition of **concurrent chemotherapy** (cisplatin) to conventional radiation **significantly improved survival over radiation alone**[Q].
- **Concurrent chemoradiation** protocols have **improved locoregional control** and **reduce** the **development of distant disease**[Q].

CARCINOMA OF POSTERIOR THIRD OR BASE OF TONGUE

Carcinoma of Posterior Third or Base of Tongue

- Remains **asymptomatic for long time** and patient **present with metastasis in cervical nodes**[Q].
- **First node involved** is superior deep jugular nodes (Level II), spread is then along the jugular chain to the mid-jugular (Level III) and lower jugular (Level IV)[Q].

Clinical Features
- **Early symptoms:** Sore throat, feeling of lump in throat, and slight discomfort on swallowing
- Because many **lesions** are **silent, level II neck mass** is often the **first sign**[Q].

RADIOTHERAPY IN CANCERS OF ORAL CAVITY

Radiotherapy in Cancers of Oral Cavity

- SCC is **vascularized** and **well-oxygenated** tends to be **most radiosensitive**[Q].
- Deep invasion of muscle or bone tends to decrease the response to radiotherapy
- **Large cervical metastatic nodes** are **best managed by** a combination of surgery and **radiation therapy** rather than by radiation alone[Q].
- Mostly given as **EBRT** (External Beam Radiotherapy), **60 Gray** over **6 weeks**[Q].

Complications of Radiotherapy
1. **Xerostomia (MC)**[Q]
2. **Mucositis**[Q]
3. Temporary or permanent dysgeusia
4. **Osteoradionecrosis (ORN)**[Q]:
   - Related to **carries tooth** in the radiation field[Q]
   - Results from **decreased production of saliva** and **damage to microvasculature** of mandible and maxilla[Q]
   - Best managed with **prophylactic dental care**[Q]
   - ORN may require daily **hyperbaric oxygen treatments** for 4-6 weeks, either alone or in conjunction with surgical intervention[Q]

MALIGNANT NEOPLASMS OF PARANASAL SINUSES

MALIGNANT NEOPLASMS OF PARANASAL SINUSES

- Most frequently involved: **Maxillary sinuses**^{Q} > Ethmoids > Frontal > Sphenoid.
- **Ethmoidal tumors** mainly spread to **jugulodiagastric** and **subdiagastric nodes**^{Q}.
- **Maxillary tumors** mainly spread to **mandibular nodes**^{Q}.

> - People working in **hardwood furniture industry, nickel refining, leather work and manufacture of mustard gas** have shown higher incidence of sinonasal cancer^Q.
> - Cancer of the maxillary sinus is common in **Bantus of South Africa** where locally made **snuff** is used, which is found **rich in nickel and chromium**^{Q}.

- Workers of **furniture industry** develop **adenocarcinoma of the ethmoids** and upper nasal cavity^Q
- Those engaged in **nickel refining** develop **SCC and anaplastic carcinoma**^{Q}.
- More than 80% of the malignant tumors are of **SCC** variety^Q.

CARCINOMA OF MAXILLARY SINUS

CARCINOMA OF MAXILLARY SINUS

- Common in **40-60** years of age, more common in **males**^{Q}
- Systemic metastasis are **rare**, may be seen in **lungs (MC)**^{Q} and occasionally in bone.

Clinical Features
- Early features of maxillary sinus malignancy are **nasal stuffiness, blood stained discharge, facial paraesthesia, or pain and epiphora**^{Q}.
- Nodal metastasis is **uncommon** and occurs only in the late stage of disease.
- **Maxillary tumors** mainly spread to **mandibular nodes**^{Q}.

Diagnosis
- **CT scan:** Best non-invasive method to find the extent of disease.

Treatment
- For SCC, combination of **radiotherapy** and **surgery**^{Q} gives better results than either alone.
- Radiotherapy can be given before or after surgery.

MANDIBULECTOMY

Mandibulectomy

Marginal Mandibulectomy	Segmental Mandibulectomy

• **Conservative mandibulectomy**^{Q}
• Refers to **partial excision** of the **superior portion** of mandible in vertical phase^Q
• **Inner cortical surface** and a portion of **underlying medullary cavity is excised**^{Q}
• **Preserve mandibular continuity**^{Q}
• Indicated **when tumor lies within 1 cm** of the mandible or **abuts the periosteum** without evidence of direct bony invasion^Q
	• **Entire through and through segment of mandible is resected.**
	• Results in **mandibular discontinuity**^{Q}
	• Requires **major reconstructive procedure** for cosmetic and functional purposes^Q
	• **Indications:**
	  1. **Invasion of medullary space** of mandible^Q
	  2. **Tumor fixation to occlusal surface** of mandible in **edentulous patient**^{Q}
	  3. **Invasion** of tumor into the mandible **via mandibular** or **mental foramen**^{Q}
	  4. **Tumor fixed** to the mandible^Q

TRISMUS

TRISMUS

- **Restriction to mouth opening**, including **restrictions caused by trauma, surgery** or **radiation**^{Q}.
- **Implications: Reduced nutrition** due to impaired mastication, **difficulty in speaking**, and **compromised oral hygiene**^{Q}.
- Often observed in **persons** who have **received radiation** to the **head and neck**, in conjunction with difficulty in swallowing^Q.
- **Limited jaw mobility** can result from **trauma, surgery, radiation treatment,** or **even TMJ problems**^{Q}.

> - **Radiation**^{Q} that affects the **temporomandibular joint**, the **pterygoid muscles**, or the **masseter muscle**, is **most likely to result in trismus**.
> - Some patients who have not received radiation treatment may develop **trismus secondary to scarring** and **edema after surgery**^{Q}.

CANCRUM ORIS (NOMA DISEASE OR GANGRENOUS STOMATITIS)

CANCRUM ORIS (NOMA DISEASE OR GANGRENOUS STOMATITIS)

- Cancrum oris or gangrenous stomatitis, is a **gangrenous disease** leading to **tissue destruction** of the **face**, especially the **mouth and cheek**^{Q}
- Rapidly progressive, polymicrobial, opportunistic infection that occurs during periods of **compromised immune function**^{Q}.
- Main organisms implicated: Fusobacterium, Prevotella and Borrelia vincentii^Q

Predisposing Factors	
• **Malnutrition** or **dehydration**^{Q}	• **Recent illness**^{Q}
• **Poor oral hygiene**^{Q}	• **Malignancy**^{Q}
• **Poor sanitation**^{Q}	• Immunodeficiency disorder (**AIDS**)^Q
• Unsafe drinking water	

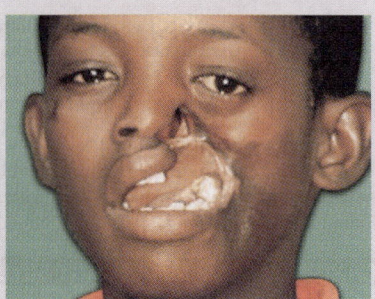

Clinical Features
- Mainly affects **children <12 years** in the **poorest countries** of Africa^Q.
- **Most children** are between **2 and 6 years**
- Mucous membranes of the **mouth develop ulcers**
- **Rapid, painless tissue degeneration**, can **degrade tissues** of the **bones** in the **face**.
- Associated with **high morbidity** and **mortality**^{Q}

Treatment
- Improvement in **hygiene** and **nutrition**^{Q}
- Progression can be halted by **antibiotics** and improved nutrition^Q
- **Reconstructive plastic surgery**^{Q} to repair its permanent physical effects

APHTHOUS ULCER

APHTHOUS ULCER

- Also known as a **canker sore**^{Q}
- A type of mouth ulcer that presents as a **painful open sore** inside the **mouth** or **upper throat** characterized by a break in the **mucous membrane**^{Q}.
- Its **cause is unknown**, but they are **not contagious**.
- Also known as **aphthous stomatitis** and alternatively as **Sutton's Disease**, especially in the case of **major, multiple,** or **recurring ulcers**^{Q}.

Types of Aphthous Ulcer		
Minor Ulceration	**Major Ulcerations**	**Herpetiform Ulcerations**
• Size **3-10 mm**	• Size **>10 mm**^{Q}	• Characterized by **small, numerous, 1-3 mm lesions** that **form clusters**.
• **MC aphthous ulcers**^{Q}	• Appearance similar to minor ulcerations	• Most severe form^Q
• Appear as **erythematous halo**^{Q} with yellowish or grayish color.	• More painful	• Occurs more frequently in **females**
• **Pain**^{Q} is the characteristic symptom	• Take **>1 month to heal** and **leave a scar**^{Q}.	• Onset is often **in adulthood**.
• May last about **2 weeks**	• Typically develop **after puberty** with **frequent recurrences**^{Q}.	• Typically **heal in <1 month without scarring**^{Q}.

Etiology
- **Exact cause** is **unknown**^{Q}
- Citrus fruits, physical trauma, lack of sleep, sudden weight loss, food allergies, immune system reactions, and deficiencies in vitamin B_{12}, iron, and folic acid may contribute to their development.
- **MC trigger: Trauma** to the **mouth**^{Q}

Multiple Choice Questions

CARCINOMA ORAL CAVITY PREDISPOSING FACTORS

1. **Regarding premalignant oral lesions:** *(COMEDK 2005)*
   a. Leukoplakia should be proved by biopsy
   b. Leukoplakia does not disappear after cessation of smoking
   c. Erythroplakia has a higher risk for malignancy
   d. Oral submucous fibrosis is seen in all parts of the world

2. **All of the following are precancerous lesions for carcinoma oral cavity except:** *(Recent Question 2017)*
   a. Erythroplakia
   b. Speckled erythroplakia
   c. Discoid lupus erythematosus
   d. Chronic hyperplastic candidiasis

3. **The most strongly implicated premalignant condition of the oral cavity is:** *(COMEDK 2010)*
   a. Fordyce spots
   b. Erythroplakia
   c. Median rhomboid glossitis
   d. Erythema multiforme

4. **Treatment of leukoplakia:** *(JIPMER 2011)*
   a. Local excision
   b. Excision and radiotherapy
   c. Topical chemotherapy
   d. Repositioning of ill fitting dentures

5. **Treatment of erythroplakia:** *(MHSSMCET 2007)*
   a. Excision
   b. Stoppage of alcohol and tobacco
   c. Vitamin supplementation
   d. Laser ablation

6. **All of the following predisposes to oral cancer, except:** *(Orissa 2011, PGI Dec 99)*
   a. Erythroplakia
   b. Leukoplakia
   c. Submucosal fibrosis
   d. Lichen planus

7. **Saroj, a 32-years-old female, from rural background presented with a history of chronic tobacco chewing since 14 years of age. Now she has difficulty in opening her mouth. On oral examination, no ulcers are seen. Most probable diagnosis is:** *(AIIMS June 2001)*
   a. Submucous oral fibrosis
   b. Carcinoma of buccal mucosa
   c. TM joint arthritis
   d. Trigeminal nerve paralysis

8. **Virus causing head and neck cancer:** *(PGI Nov 2011)*
   a. EBV
   b. HSV
   c. HPV
   d. HBV
   e. HCV

9. **All of the following predispose to squamous cell carcinoma, except:** *(AIIMS June 93)*
   a. Lichen planus of mouth
   b. Bowen's disease
   c. Inverted papilloma of nose
   d. Chronic irritation of oral mucosa by jagged teeth

10. **The pre-malignant condition with the highest probability of progression to malignancy is:** *(Bihar PG 2014, All India 2002)*
    a. Dysplasia
    b. Hyperplasia
    c. Leukoplakia
    d. Erythroleukoplakia

11. **The commonest pre-malignant condition of oral cancer is:** *(All India 95)*
    a. Leukoplakia
    b. Aphthous ulcer
    c. Lichen planus
    d. Erthro-leukoplakia

12. **A 70-year-old male presented with asymptomatic white patch on oral cavity following application of the denture. Treatment of choice is:** *(UPPG 2008)*
    a. Low does radiotherapy
    b. Biopsy of the all the tissues
    c. Ascertaining that denture is fitted properly
    d. Antibiotics

13. **Which of the following is the cause of submucosal fibrosis?** *(MCI November 2017)*
    a. Alcohol
    b. Candidiasis
    c. Betel nut chewing
    d. Pan leaf chewing

CARCINOMA ORAL CAVITY

14. **Second primary tumor of head and neck is most commonly seen in malignancy of:** *(AIIMS May 2012)*
    a. Oral cavity
    b. Larynx
    c. Hypopharynx
    d. Paranasal sinuses

15. **The commonest site of oral cancer among Indian population is:** *(Kerala PG 2015, All India 2004)*
    a. Tongue
    b. Floor of mouth
    c. Alveobuccal complex
    d. Lip

16. **Most common site of oral cavity carcinoma is:** *(All India 96)*
    a. Lip
    b. Cheek
    c. Tongue
    d. Palate

17. **Areas of carcinoma of oral mucosa can be identified by staining with:** *(Recent Question 2016)*
    a. 1% zinc chloride
    b. 2% silver nitrate
    c. Gentian violet
    d. 2% toluidine blue

18. **SCC in the oral cavity and lips tend to metastasize to lymph nodes at which levels:** *(MHCET 2016)*
    a. I, II, III
    b. I, II, VI
    c. III, IV, V
    d. I, II, retropharyngeal nodes

19. **Most common site of oral cancer:** *(Recent Question 2017)*
    a. Lips
    b. Tongue
    c. Buccal mucosa
    d. Alveolus of teeth

20. **All of the following are indications for adjuvant radiotherapy in head and neck cancers except:** *(Recent Question 2017)*
    a. Multiple lymph node disease
    b. Extranodal involvement
    c. Lymphovascular invasion
    d. Lymph node >3 cm

CARCINOMA LIP

21. **Abbe-Estlander flap is used for:** *(All India 2008)*
    a. Lip
    b. Tongue
    c. Eyelid
    d. Ears

22. **Abbey Estlander flap is based on:** *(AIIMS May 2008)*
    a. Lingual artery
    b. Facial artery
    c. Labial artery
    d. Internal maxillary artery

23. **Carcinoma of lip is characterized by the following except that:** *(UPSC 2007)*
    a. 90% of the lip cancers occurs on the lower lip
    b. The most common site of origin is the vermillion border
    c. 2 cm x 2 cm cell carcinomas can be treated by V-shaped excision and primary closure
    d. Since lymph node metastases are common after a radical dissection of neck is mandatory

24. Stain used to diagnose premalignant lesions of lip is: *(DNB 2011, 2006)*
    a. Crystal violet b. H and E
    c. Toluidine blue d. Giemsa

25. Treatment of choice for carcinoma of lip of less than 1 cm is:
    a. Radiation *(All India 90)*
    b. Chemotherapy c. Excision
    d. Radiation and chemotherapy

26. Neuromuscular preserving flap in lip: *(Recent Question 2017)*
    a. Abbe flap b. Webster flap
    c. Karpandzic flap d. Johansen flap

CARCINOMA BUCCAL MUCOSA AND CHEEK

27. True statement(s) about oral cancer is/are: *(PGI June 2004)*
    a. Most common in buccal mucosa
    b. Metastasis uncommon
    c. Respond to radiotherapy
    d. Surgery done
    e. Syphilis and dental irritation predisposes

28. Metastasis of CA buccal mucosa goes to: *(AIIMS Nov 96, All India 97)*
    a. Regional lymph node b. Liver
    c. Heart d. Brain

29. In carcinoma cheek, what is the best drug for single drug chemotherapy? *(AIIMS June 93)*
    a. Vincristine b. Cyclophosphamide
    c. Cisplatin d. Daunorubicin

30. An old man who is edentulous developed squamous cell carcinoma in buccal mucosa that has infiltrated to the alveolus. Following is not indicted in treatment:
    a. Radiotherapy *(All India 2002)*
    b. Segmental mandibulectomy
    c. Marginal mandibulectomy involving removal of the outer table only
    d. Marginal mandibulectomy involving removal of upper half of mandible

31. A patient with cheek cancer has a tumour of 2.5 cm located close to and involving the lower alveolus. A single mobile ipsilateral lymph node measuring 6 cm is palpable. The TNM stage is: *(Recent Question 2013, COMEDK 2008)*
    a. T1N1M0 b. T2N2M0
    c. T2N1M0 d. T4N2M0

32. In the reconstruction following excision of previously irradiated cheek cancer, the flap will be:
    a. Local tongue b. Cervical
    c. Forehead
    d. Pectoralis major myocutaneous

CARCINOMA PALATE

33. All are true about carcinoma palate, except: *(AIIMS June 94, Nov 93)*
    a. Slow growing b. Bilateral lymphatic spread
    c. Adenocarcinoma d. Presents with pain

CARCINOMA TONGUE

34. A patient has carcinoma of tongue in the right lateral aspect with lymph node of 4 cm size in level 3 on the left side of neck, what is the stage? *(AIIMS Nov 2006)*
    a. N0 b. N1
    c. N2 d. N3

35. A patient presented with a 1 X 1.5 cms growth on the lateral border of the tongue. The treatment indicated would be:
    a. Laser ablation *(Recent Question 2014, AIIMS June 2002)*
    b. Interstitial brachytherapy
    c. External beam radiotherapy
    d. Chemotherapy

36. A patient with CA tongue is found to have lymph nodes in the lower neck. The treatment of choice for the lymph nodes is:
    a. Lower cervical neck dissection *(All India 2005)*
    b. Suprahyoid neck dissection
    c. Tele radiotherapy
    d. Radical neck dissection

37. Carcinoma of tongue most commonly occur at:
    a. Dorsum *(Recent Question 2013 MCI March 2009)*
    b. Lateral border of anterior 2/3rd
    c. Lateral border of posterior 1/3rd
    d. Tip

38. Tongue ulcer with everted edges is: *(MHPGMCET 2005, 2001)*
    a. Aphthous ulcer b. Tubercular
    c. Malignant d. Dental

39. A 60-year-old man presents with an ulcer on lateral margin of tongue also complains of ear pain, most probable diagnosis is: *(PGI 96)*
    a. Dental ulcer b. Carcinomatous ulcer
    c. Tuberculosis ulcer d. Syphilitic ulcer

40. Carcinoma of the tongue:
    a. Occurs most commonly on the lateral border of the middle third of tongue
    b. Metastasize readily to cervical lymph nodes
    c. Is usually radiosensitive
    d. Treated surgically should include homolateral neck dissection except for very small lesion
    e. All of the above

41. The commando operation is: *(Recent Question 2016)*
    a. Abdomino-perineal resection of the rectum for carcinoma
    b. Disarticulation of the hip for gas gangrene of the leg
    c. Extended radical mastectomy
    d. Excision of carcinoma of the jaw and lymph nodes enbloc

CARCINOMA MAXILLA

42. Treatment for stage T3N1 of carcinoma maxilla is: *(DNB 2012, AIIMS June 96)*
    a. Radiation therapy only b. Chemotherapy only
    c. Surgery and radiation
    d. Chemotherapy and radiation

43. The lymph not to be involved first in maxillary carcinoma:
    a. Superior deep cervical nodes *(DNB 2007)*
    b. Jugulodigastric nodes
    c. Submandibular d. Subdigastric nodes

MANDIBLE AND MANDIBULECTOMY

44. A 80-year-old patient presents with a midline tumor of the lower jaw, involving the alveolar margin. He is edentulous. Treatment of choice is: *(All India 2001)*
    a. Hemimandibulectomy
    b. Commando operation
    c. Segmental mandibulectomy
    d. Marginal mandibulectomy

TRISMUS

45. Trismus in oral cancer patients is severe in those treated with: *(Karnataka 99)*
    a. Surgery and Radiotherapy
    b. Chemotherapy alone
    c. Surgery alone
    d. Not related to treatment

CANCRUM ORIS

46. All are true about cancrum oris *except*: *(PGI Dec 97)*
    a. Associated with malnutrition and vitamin deficiency
    b. Follows chronic infection
    c. Involves jaw
    d. Treatment is excision and skin grafting with tubed pedicle graft

LUDWIG'S ANGINA

47. Which of the following statements best represent Ludwig's angina? *(AIIMS May 2005)*
    a. A type of coronary artery spasm
    b. An infection of the cellular tissues around submandibular salivary gland
    c. Esophageal spasm
    d. Retropharyngeal infection

DENTAL CYST AND ABNORMALITIES

48. The most frequent tooth to be impacted is: *(UPSC 2007, Karnataka 98)*
    a. Lower third molar
    b. Lower canine
    c. Upper third molar
    d. Upper premolar

49. Impacted wisdom teeth may produce referred pain via: *(Orissa 99)*
    a. Lingual nerve
    b. Facial nerve
    c. Branch of the auriculotemporal nerve
    d. None of the above

50. Radiographic finding of floating teeth can be seen in: *(Karnataka 2002)*
    a. Ectodermal dysplasis
    b. Cleidocranial dysplasia
    c. Osteopetrosis
    d. Histiocytosis-X

51. The most common cyst of the oral region is: *(DPG 2008)*
    a. Dentigerous cyst
    b. Keratosis cyst
    c. Dermoid cyst
    d. Periapical cyst

52. Dentigerous cyst arises from: *(DPG 2009 Feb, MHPGMCET 2003)*
    a. The root of a caries tooth
    b. The periosteum of the fractured mandible
    c. An unerupted permanent tooth
    d. The sequestrum of osteomyelitis of mandible

53. Which jaw cyst is premalignant? *(AIIMS May 2012)*
    a. Nasopalatine cyst
    b. Radicular cyst
    c. Odontogenic keratocyst
    d. Dentigerous cyst

54. What are Rushton bodies? *(DNB 2012)*
    a. Hyaline bodies of odontogenic cyst
    b. Refractile bodies of radicular cyst
    c. Bodies seen in ameloblastoma
    d. Hyaline bodies seen in dentigerous cyst

55. Which of the following is correct about ameloblastoma? *(Recent Question 2016)*
    a. Highly malignant
    b. Occurs in children <5 years
    c. Most common odontogenic tumour
    d. Mandible is not the most common site

EPULIS

56. Epulis arises from: *(Recent Question 2013, PGI Dec 99)*
    a. Enamel
    b. Root of teeth
    c. Gingiva
    d. Pulp

57. Epulis is: *(DNB 2014)*
    a. Benign
    b. Malignant
    c. Reactive process
    d. Precancerous

58. Which of the following statement is incorrect about the given condition?

    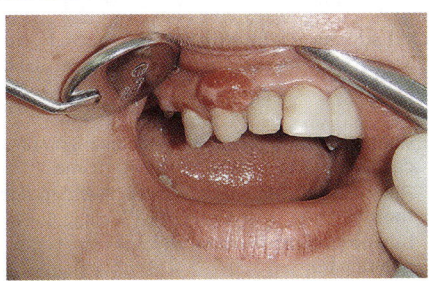

    a. Arise from gingiva
    b. Benign
    c. Types are fibromatous, ossifying and acanthomatous
    d. None of the above

MISCELLANEOUS

59. Asymptomatic hemangioma on ventral surface of the tongue in a 10 years old boy is treated by:
    a. Watchful expectancy
    b. Surgical Excision
    c. Radiotherapy
    d. Laser

60. Pharyngocutaneous fistula is seen in all *except*: *(AIIMS June 99)*
    a. Chemotherapy
    b. Surgery
    c. No wound care
    d. Radiotherapy

61. Gum tumour with 2 contralateral mobile lymph nodes in neck come under: *(PGI Dec 99)*
    a. $T_3 N_2 M0$
    b. $T_2 N_2 M0$
    c. $T_4 N_2 M0$
    d. $T_3 N_3 M0$

62. A patient has small, oval multiple ulcers in oral cavity with red erythematous margins. The diagnosis is: *(AIIMS Nov 93)*
    a. Carcinoma
    b. Aphthous ulcer
    c. Tubercular ulcer
    d. Syphilitic ulcer

63. Multiple painful ulcers on tongue are seen in all except: *(All India 96)*
    a. Aphthous ulcer
    b. Tuberculous ulcers
    c. Herpes ulcers
    d. Carcinomatous ulcers

64. Painless ulcer of the tongue is due to:
    a. Dyspepsia
    b. Syphilis
    c. Tuberculosis
    d. None of the above

65. Reparative granuloma of jaw is treated by: *(DPG 2009 Feb)*
    a. Antibiotics
    b. Wedge resection
    c. Resection and bone grafting
    d. Curettage

66. Treatment of T4N0M0 stage of head and neck carcinoma is: *(DNB 2009)*
    a. Surgery alone
    b. Radiotherapy alone
    c. Chemoradiation
    d. Surgery and radiotherapy

67. N-3 TNM staging of head and neck tumors shows: *(Recent Question 2018)*
    a. Metastasis in lymph nodes >2 cm
    b. Metastasis in lymph nodes >5 cm
    c. Metastasis in a lymph node >6 cm
    d. None

Explanations

CARCINOMA ORAL CAVITY PREDISPOSING FACTORS

1. **Ans. c. Erythroplakia has a higher risk for malignancy** *(Ref: Bailey 27/e p761-762; Devita 9/e p564; Cancer of the Head and Neck by Suen and Myer 4/e p284-285)*
   - **Oral submucous fibrosis** is almost **entirely confined to** the **Asian population** and is characterized pathologically by **epithelial fibrosis** with associated **atrophy** and **hyperplasia** of the overlying **epithelium**.

Leukoplakia	Erythroplakia
• **White keratotic plaque** or patch that **cannot be rubbed off**[Q] and cannot be given another diagnostic name	• **Red mucosal plaque,** most commonly found on the **soft palate** and **tonsillar pillars**[Q]
• **Risk factors: Smoking, alcohol, ill-fitting dentures, jagged tooth**[Q]	• Does not arise from an obvious mechanical or inflammatory cause
• **Key pathologic features: Hyperkeratosis, parakeratosis, acanthosis**[Q]	• Cannot be ascribed to another clinical or pathological condition
• In **most cases,** lesions **regress spontaneously** after stopping alcohol or tobacco consumption or correction of underlying cause[Q].	• **Key pathologic features: severe cellular dysplasia**[Q]
• **Baseline biopsy** should be done[Q]	• Because of **increased malignant potential, all erythroplakic lesions** must be **biopsied**[Q].
• Lesions with **moderate to severe dysplasia** should be **excised**[Q].	• **Higher risk (17 times)** of **malignant transformation than leukoplakia**[Q].
• Oral leukoplakia has **low potential for malignancy**[Q].	

2. **Ans. c. Discoid lupus erythematosus** *(Ref: Sabiston 20/e p789; Schwartz 10/e p580; Bailey 27/e p761)*
3. **Ans. b. Erythroplakia**
4. **Ans. d. Repositioning of ill fitting dentures**

LEUKOPLAKIA

- In **most cases,** lesions **regress spontaneously** after stopping alcohol or tobacco consumption or **correction of underlying cause**[Q].

5. **Ans. a. Excision**
6. **Ans. d. Lichen planus**
7. **Ans. a. Submucous oral fibrosis** *(Ref: Bailey 27/e p763; Devita 9/e p729)*
8. **Ans. a. EBV, c. HPV**
9. **Ans. a. Lichen planus of mouth**
10. **Ans. d. Erythroleukoplakia**
11. **Ans. a. Leukoplakia**
12. **Ans. c. Ascertaining that denture is fitted properly**
13. **Ans. c. Betel nut chewing**

CARCINOMA ORAL CAVITY

14. **Ans. a. Oral cavity** *(Ref: Second primary malignancies in patients with head and neck cancers by Sandeep Samant, Head and Neck 2005; 27; 1042)*
    - "The site of index cancer influences the most likely site of a second primary malignancy, as an example, in a series of 1257 patients with SCC of the head and neck, patients with an index malignancy arising in the **larynx** were more like to develop a **second primary cancer in the lung**, while those arising in the **oral cavity** were more likely to develop a **second primary in** the **head and neck** or **esophagus**. This relationship has been observed in other studies as well."

    - Patients with **head and neck SCC** are at **increased risk for** the **development of second primary malignancies** compared with general population[Q].
    - These second primary malignancies **typically develop in the aerodigestive tract** (lung, head and neck, esophagus)[Q].
    - MC second primary malignancy: Lung cancer[Q]
    - **Highest** relative **increase in risk** is for a **second head and neck cancer**[Q].

15. **Ans. c. Alveobuccal complex** *(Ref: Bailey 26/e p709-710; Devita 9/e p729; Cancer of the Head and Neck by Suen and Myer 4/e p297-304)*
16. **Ans. c. Tongue**
17. **Ans. d. 2% toluidine blue** *(Ref: www.headandneckoncology.org/content/1/1/5)*

TOLUIDINE BLUE

- Toluidine blue is a **basic metachromatic dye** with **high affinity for acidic tissue** components, thereby **staining tissues rich in DNA** and **RNA**[Q].
- **Wide applications** both as **vital staining in living tissues** and as a **special stain** used in vivo to **identify dysplasia** and **carcinoma of** the **oral cavity**[Q].

18. **Ans. a. I, II, III.**   19. **Ans. b. Tongue** *(Ref: Sabiston 20/e p796; Schwartz 10/e p582; Bailey 27/e p765)*
20. **Ans. d. Lymph node >3 cm** *(Ref: Devita 10/e p430)*

CARCINOMA LIP

21. **Ans. a Lip:** *(Ref: Bailey 27/e p769; Devita 9/e p744-745; Cancer of the Head and Neck by Suen and Myer 4/e p301-302)*
22. **Ans. c. Labial artery** *(Ref: Bailey 27/e p769; Devita 9/e p744; Cancer of the Head and Neck by Suen and Myer 4/e p301-302)*

Lip Reconstruction	
Cross-lip Flaps	**Circumoral Advancement Flaps**
• **Lip-Switch (Abbe-Estlander) flap**[Q] used to repair defects of either upper or lower lip, based on superior **labial artery**[Q]	• **Karapandzic flap**[Q]: Uses a sensate, **neuromuscular flap** based on **labial artery**[Q]. • **Webster-Bernard repair**[Q]: Use lateral nasolabial flap with buccal advancement

23. **Ans. d.** Since lymph node metastases are common after a radical dissection of neck is mandatory
24. **Ans. c. Toluidine blue** *(Ref: Indian Journal od Dental Research 2007; vol-18; Issue 3; p103-105)*

   • **Toluidine blue detects efficiently and rapidly mitotic figures** in sections of paraffin embedded human tissues **especially in oral cavity.**

25. **Ans. c. Excision**   26. **Ans. c. Karpandzic flap** *(Ref: Grabb & Smith/p378)*

CARCINOMA BUCCAL MUCOSA AND CHEEK

27. **Ans. b. Metastasis uncommon, c. Respond to radiotherapy, d. Surgery done, e. Syphilis and dental irritation predisposes** *(Ref: Bailey 27/e p772; Devita 9/e p749; Cancer of the Head and Neck by Suen and Myer 4/e p302-305)*
28. **Ans. a. Regional lymph node**
29. **Ans. c. Cisplatin** *(Ref: Bailey 27/e p155; Devita 9/e p749; Cancer of the Head and Neck by Suen and Myer 4/e p291-292)*
30. **Ans. c. Marginal mandibulectomy involving removal of the outer table only**

   • Whenever **SCC of oral cavity involve** the **mandible** (or **within 1 cm** of mandible), **mandibulectomy** becomes necessary[Q].
   • In **marginal mandibulectomy, inner cortical surface** and a portion of **underlying medullary cavity** is **excised** (not only the outer table)[Q].

31. **Ans. d. T4N2M0**
32. **Ans. d. Pectoralis major myocutaneous** *(Ref: Bailey 26/e p716; Devita 9/e p749; Cancer of the Head and Neck by Suen and Myer 4/e p302-305)*

RECONSTRUCTION OF CHEEK

   • For cheek reconstruction, **mucosal flaps** are used.
   • **PMMC (pectoralis major myocutaneous) flap**: **Most widely used flap** for **head and neck reconstruction**[Q].

Males	Females
• **Forehead flap** based on **anterior branch** of **superficial temporal artery** can be used[Q].	• **Deltopectoral flap** based on **perforating branch** of **internal mammary artery** is used[Q].

CARCINOMA PALATE

33. **Ans. d. Presents with pain** *(Ref: Bailey 27/e p774; Devita 9/e p750; Cancer of the Head and Neck by Suen and Myer 4/e p311-313)*

CARCINOMA TONGUE

34. **Ans. c. N2**
35. **Ans. b. Interstitial brachytherapy:** *(Ref: Bailey 27/e p769; Devita 9/e p747-749, 752-754; Cancer of the Head and Neck by Suen and Myer 4/e p297-301)*

   • Suen and Myer says "**Radiation therapy** may be **curative in early cancer** (T1 and some T2) and may **preserve maximal normal anatomy** and **function. Brachytherapy** allows delivery of a **large radiation boost** to the **primary tumor bed.**"

36. **Ans. d. Radical neck dissection** *(Ref: Bailey 27/e p769; Devita 9/e p748; Cancer of the Head and Neck by Suen and Myer 4/e p299)*

Lymph Node Metastasis in CA Tongue

- **Elective or therapeutic treatment** of the **cervical lymphatics** is recommended for virtually all patients with cancer of the oral tongue.
- It is recommended that patients with **bulky metastatic deposits** undergo **standard radical dissection** or **MRND**^{Q}.

37. **Ans. b. Lateral border of anterior 2/3rd**

38. **Ans. c. Malignant** *(Ref: Bailey 27/e p616)*

Type of Ulcer	Edge
• Septic ulcer	• **Sloping** edges^Q
• Tuberculous ulcer	• **Undermined** edges^Q
• Carcinomatous ulcer	• **Everted hard** edges^Q
• Rodent ulcer	• Barely visible **pearly edges**^{Q}
• Syphilitic ulcer	• **Punched-out** appearance with **raised indurated edges**^{Q}

39. **Ans. b. Carcinomatous ulcer**
40. **Ans. e. All of the above**
41. **Ans. d. Excision of carcinoma of the jaw and lymph nodes en-bloc** *(Ref: Cancer of the Head and Neck by Suen and Myer 4/e p291)*

Commando's Operation (Combined Mandibulectomy and Neck Dissection Operation)

- **Commando's operation:** Total glossectomy hemimandibulectomy + Removal of floor of mouth + Radical lymph node dissection^Q
- Indicated when **carcinoma** is **fixed to mandible** with **infiltration of floor of mouth**^{Q}.

CARCINOMA MAXILLA

42. **Ans. c. Surgery and radiation:** *(Bailey 27/e p774; Devita 9/e p768-771; Cancer of the Head and Neck by Suen and Myer 4/e p179)*
43. **Ans. c. Submandibular nodes** *(Ref: Grays 39/e p577)*

MANDIBLE AND MANDIBULECTOMY

44. **Ans. c. Segmental mandibulectomy** *(Ref: Devita 9/e p746; Cancer of the Head and Neck by Suen and Myer 4/e p293-294)*

TRISMUS

45. **Ans. a. Surgery and Radiotherapy:** *(Ref: Bailey 25/e p750)*

CANCRUM ORIS

46. **Ans. b. Follows chronic infection** *(Ref: www.ncbi.nlm.nih.gov)*

LUDWIG'S ANGINA

47. **Ans. b. An infection of the cellular tissues around submandibular salivary gland:** *(Ref: Bailey 27/e p756)*

Ludwig's Angina

- Ludwig's angina is **infection of submandibular space**^{Q}.
- **Bacteriology: Mixed infections**^{Q} involving **both aerobes and anaerobes**^{Q} are common.

Etiology:
- **Dental infections** are responsible for **80% of cases**^{Q}.

Clinical Features:
- Marked difficulty in swallowing (**odynophagia**)^Q, with varying degree of **trismus**.

Treatment:
- **Systemic antibiotics**^{Q} with **incision** and **drainage of abscess**^{Q}.

DENTAL CYST AND ABNORMALITIES

48. **Ans. a. Lower third molar** *(Ref: Scott-Brown's Otorhinolaryngology 7/e p1924-1925)*

Impacted Tooth

- Tooth that has failed to erupt completely or partially to its correct position in the dental arch and its eruption potential has been lost.
- **MC affected tooth**: Lower 3rd molar[Q] >Upper 3rd molar >Upper canine

49. **Ans. c. Branch of the auriculotemporal nerve:** *(Ref: Scott-Brown's Otorhinolaryngology 7/e p1924-1925)*

- **Unerupted wisdom teeth**, **erupting teeth**, and **malocclusion** can cause **ear pain** secondary to direct impingement of the **auriculotemporal nerve**[Q].

50. **Ans. d. Histiocytosis-X** *(Ref: Sutton 7/e p1542)*

Floating Tooth Sign

- On radiographic examination of mandible, **erosion of the bony alveoli around** the **teeth**, so that they seem to be floating in space[Q]
- Seen in **histiocytosis X**[Q]

51. **Ans. d. Periapical cyst** *(Ref: Scott-Brown's Otorhinolaryngology 7/e p1924-1925)*

Periapical Cyst (Radicular Cyst)

- MC type of jaw cyst[Q]
- Periapical cyst is **inflammatory in origin**[Q].
- Extremely common lesions found at the **apex of teeth**[Q].
- Develop as a result of **long-standing pulpitis**, caused by advanced carious lesions or by trauma to the tooth.
- **Periapical inflammatory lesions** persist as a result of the **continued presence** of **bacteria** or other offensive agents in the area.
- **Treatment**: Complete removal of offending material and appropriate restoration of the tooth or extraction.

52. **Ans. c. An unerupted permanent tooth** *(Ref: Scott-Brown's Otorhinolaryngology 7/e p1924-1925)*

- Dentigerous cyst arises from an unerupted permanent tooth.

Dental Abnormalities

Dental Cyst	Dentigerous Cyst	Ameloblastoma
• Develops at the **apices of caries tooth**[Q] with necrotic pulp • More common in **upper jaw**[Q] **X-rays shows:** • **Circular radioluscent area**[Q] in relation to root of normally erupted tooth • **Margins** may be **sclerotic**[Q]	• Arises from **unerupted teeth**[Q] • MC in **lower 3rd molars** • **Cyst** also **contain unerupted teeth**[Q] **X-ray shows:** • **Unilocular cyst** or **soap bubble appearance**[Q]	• Benign neoplasm **arising** from **ameloblast (odontogenic epithelium)**[Q] • **MC odontogenic tumour**[Q] • Most ameloblastoma occur in mandible **near angle** and **ramus** of **mandible**[Q]

53. **Ans. c. Odontogenic keratocyst** *(Ref: Scott-Brown's Otorhinolaryngology 7/e p1924, 1925)*

Odontogenic Keratocyst

- Odontogenic keratocyst is **locally aggressive** and has a **high rate of recurrence**[Q].
- Most often diagnosed in patients between **10-40 years**.
- Occur most commonly **in males** within the **posterior mandible**, particularly in the region of **3rd molar tooth**[Q].
- Radiographically present as **well-defined unilocular** or **multilocular radiolucencies**.

> - Odontogenic keratocysts are characterized by an epithelial lining that is parakeratinized & stratified.
> - It is characterized by basal layer of neatly arranged, palisaded, columnar and cuboidal cells above which are several layers of squamous epithelium. This **lining** has a **high mitotic rate** and **rarely** may become **dysplastic** and **develop into squamous cell carcinoma**[Q].

Treatment:

- **Aggressive** and **complete removal** of the lesion
- **Recurrence rates** for **inadequately removed lesions** can reach **60%**[Q].

54. **Ans. a. Hyaline bodies of odontogenic cyst** *(Ref: Shafers 6/e p268)*

RUSHTON BODIES

- **Rushton bodies** or **hyaline bodies of odontogenic cysts** feature as **eosinophilic, straight or curved, irregular or rounded structure within the epithelial lining of odontogenic cyst.**
- Rushton bodies occur almost **exclusively within odontogenic cyst.**

55. **Ans. c. Most common odontogenic tumour**

EPULIS

56. **Ans. c. Gingiva**

EPULIS

- **Epulis** is any **benign lesion** situated on the **gingiva.**
- Three types: fibromatous, ossifying and acanthomatous.

57. **Ans. a. Benign**
58. **Ans. d. None of the above)**

Epulis arises from gingiva, is benign and types are fibromatous, ossifying and acanthomatous.

MISCELLANEOUS

59. **Ans. a. Watchful expectancy** *(Ref: Bailey 25/e p716, 717)*

    Asymptomatic hemangioma on ventral surface of the tongue in 10 years old boy is treated by watchful expectancy.

HEMANGIOMA

- Mucosal hemangiomas can occur in **oral cavity** or **oropharynx**^{Q}.
- **Mostly** seen in **children**^{Q}
- When hemangiomas are **present at birth** or **in young children**, they should be **only observed** for some period as **spontaneous regression can occur**^{Q}.

60. **Ans. a. Chemotherapy** *(Ref: http://www.ncbi.nlm.nih.gov/pmc/articles/PMC2640019/)*

PHARYNGOCUTANEOUS FISTULA

- **Pharyngocutaneous fistula (PCF)** is the MC complication after total laryngectomy^Q.
- Reported incidence: **3-65%**
- Appears in the **early post-operative period** after total laryngectomy^Q (3rd- 8th post-operative day).
- Risk Factors:
  – **Wound closure under tension**^{Q} – Concurrent neck dissection^Q – Prior radiation therapy^Q

61. **Asn. a. $T_3 N_2 M_0$, b. $T_2 N_2 M_0$, c. $T_4 N_2 M_0$, d. $T_3 N_3 M_0$**   62. **Ans. b. Aphthous ulcer** *(Ref: Robbins 9/e p728)*
63. **Ans. d. Carcinomatous ulcers**

    Aphthous ulcers, tubercular and herpetic ulcers are painful.

CARCINOMATOUS ULCER

- Carcinomatous ulcers are **painless** but may become painful in advanced stages, with extension into surrounding tissues.

64. **Ans. b. Syphilis** *(Ref: Robbins 9/e p379)*
    - **Syphilis** chancres can occur in the mouth and they are **painless.**
65. **Ans. d. Curettage** *(Ref: medind.nic.in/ibn/t06/i4/ibnt06i4p677)*
    - Reparative granuloma of Jaw is treated by curettage.

Giant Cell Reparative Granuloma

- Giant cell reparative granuloma is an apparently **reactive intraosseous lesion** of the **mandible** and **maxilla** following **trauma induced intraosseous hemorrhage**^{Q} and containing prominent giant cells.
- Also known as **Central giant cell granuloma**^{Q}
- MC site: Anterior part of **mandible**^{Q} (2/3rd of cases) between the 2nd **premolar** and 2nd **molar**^{Q} with extension across the midline.
- 2nd MC site: Small bones of **hands** and **feet**^{Q}

Clinical Features

- It is a **disease of the young** presenting as a **painless swelling** in the anterior jaw and
- Radiographically appearing as a **lytic expansile lesion** with a characteristic **tendency of resorbing the root tips** of adjacent unerupted teeth.

Treatment

- **Curettage** or **local excision**^{Q}
- **Recurrence rate: 22-50%**
- Lesion eradication typically **does not require >2 excisions**.
- **Chemical cautery, electrocautery, cryotherapy,** calcitonin, Interferon alpha and intralesional steroids are used **for more aggressive** and **recurrent lesions**.

66. Ans. d. Surgery and radiotherapy *(Ref: Mastery of Surgery 5/e p308; Bailey 27/e p767)*
67. Ans. c. Metastasis in a lymph node >6 cm

CHAPTER 36

Salivary Glands

ETIOLOGY OF SALIVARY GLAND TUMORS

ETIOLOGY OF SALIVARY GLAND TUMORS

- **Radiotherapy** to head and neck (for mucoepidermoid carcinoma)^Q
- **EBV** infection (for lymphoepithelial carcinoma)^Q
- Exposure to **silica dust, nitrosamines**^{Q}
- Increased risk in females with **early menarche** and **nulliparity**^{Q}
- **Trisomy 5** in primary mucoepidermoid carcinoma of **minor** salivary glands
- Polysomy of **3 and 17** especially in **adenoid cystic carcinoma**

  - **Translocation** involving chromosome 11 in mucoepidermoid carcinoma
  - MC neoplasm of **salivary gland**: Pleomorphic adenoma^Q
  - MC malignant tumor of salivary gland: Mucoepidermoid carcinoma^Q
  - MC neoplasm of salivary gland **in children**: Hemangioma^Q
  - MC malignant tumor of salivary gland **in children**: Mucoepidermoid carcinoma^Q
  - MC malignant tumor of minor salivary glands: Adenoid cystic carcinoma^Q
  - Best diagnostic modality for parotid swelling: FNAC^Q
  - Open incisional biopsy is **contraindicated**^{Q} due to **tumor cell implantation** and formation of **parotid fistula**^{Q}.
  - Best imaging investigation for **salivary gland neoplasms: MRI**^{Q}

IN SALIVARY GLAND TUMORS

IN SALIVARY GLAND TUMORS

- MC site of minor salivary gland tumors are oral cavity (**hard palate**)^Q
- There are no minor salivary glands in the anterior half of the palate, so tumors arise on **posterolateral hard palate** and all of the **soft palate**^{Q}
- **Malignancy varies inversely with** the size of gland^Q (most of minor salivary gland tumors are malignant)

  - **Parotid** gland: 25%^{Q} malignant, **Submandibular and Sublingual gland: 50%**^{Q} malignant, **Minor salivary glands: 75%**^{Q} malignant

- **Open** surgical **biopsy** is **contraindicated**^{Q}, as it can cause **tumor seeding** of the track

  - Most salivary gland tumors are **radioresistant**^{Q}
  - **Neutron therapy** has been used in the management of **unresectable** salivary gland **tumors**^{Q}
  - Name of incision for parotidectomy: **Sistrunk incision**^{Q}

Indications of Radiotherapy in Salivary Gland Tumors	
• High grade tumors^Q	• Bone invasion^Q
• Large primary lesions^Q	• Cervical LN metastasis^Q
• Perineural invasion^Q	• Positive surgical margins^Q

PLEOMORPHIC ADENOMA

PLEOMORPHIC ADENOMA

- It is **MC benign** salivary gland tumor and **MC** tumor of **major salivary glands**^{Q}.
- MC site is **parotid tail (superficial lobe)**^{Q}
- Less common in the submandibular glands and sublingual glands, relatively rare in minor salivary glands.

- Known as **mixed tumor**^{Q} as it is composed of both **epithelial** & **mesenchymal** components
- Encapsulated but sends **pseudopodia (finger-like projections)**^{Q} into surrounding glands, **enucleation is not done** to avoid recurrence.

- Pleomorphic adenoma is **unicentric** but **recurrences are multicentric**^{Q}
- Usually **not involve** the **facial nerve**.

Clinical Features
- Presents as **painless swelling** without any appreciable change in size, with typical site at **below, in front** and **behind** the **ear lobule**^{Q}.
- Slow growing lobular tumor affecting **women** around **40 years**.
- Pleomorphic adenoma involving deep lobe may push the tonsil and pillars of fauces towards midline and known as **dumbbell tumor**^{Q} with component both in neck and oral cavity.

Diagnosis
- **FNAC** is diagnostic^Q

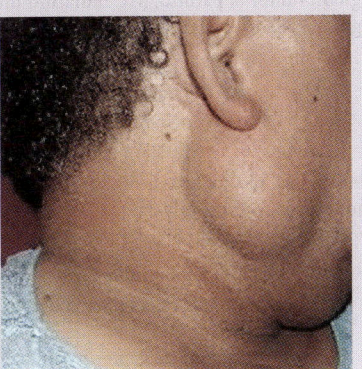

Treatment
- Superficial parotidectomy (**Patey's operation**)^Q
- Excision of whole gland in cases of pleomorphic adenoma of submandibular gland
- Name of incision for parotidectomy: **Lazy 'S', modified Blairs or Sistrunk incision**

Complications
- **Malignant change (3-5%)**
  - Known as **carcinoma ex pleomorphic adenoma** or **malignant mixed tumor**
  - **Rapid growth, pain,** paraesthesia, **enlarged cervical LN** and restriction of jaw movements, **facial weakness** or skin invasion and **fixation of mastoid tip** is suggestive of malignant transformation
  - Histological findings suggestive of malignant change are microscopic foci of **necrosis, hemorrhage, calcification** and **excessive hyalinization**^{Q}
  - Prognosis for invasive carcinoma depends on degree of local infiltration
- **Recurrence**^{Q}, particularly after enucleation

WARTHIN'S TUMOR (PAPILLARY CYSTADENOMA LYMPHOMATOSUM)

WARTHIN'S TUMOR (PAPILLARY CYSTADENOMA LYMPHOMATOSUM)

- **Second MC benign tumor** of the **parotid gland**^{Q}
- Derived from **salivary tissues inclusion** in **lymph nodes**^{Q} (so can arise from cervical nodes)
- Occurs **exclusively in parotid gland**^{Q} and almost always occur in the **lower portion of parotid**^{Q} overlying the angle of mandible.

  - Consists of **both epithelial & lymphoid elements**^{Q} thus known as **adenolymphoma** (probably arises from remnants of parotid tissue trapped in lymph nodes within the parotid gland)
  - More common in **males**^{Q}, in **5th to 7th decade**^{Q}.
  - Associated with **smoking**^{Q}, **bilateral in 10%**^{Q} cases, never involves facial nerve.
  - It is **well encapsulated, cystic**, extremely slow growing tumor, **never turns malignant**^{Q}.

- Peculiar feature of Warthin's tumor: **'hot' spot in 99mTc-pertechnate scan**^{Q}. (Other tumors of the parotid show 'cold' spot)

Histopathology
- **Papillary cystic pattern** lined with columnar oncocytes and cuboidal cells with **marked lymphoid component**^{Q}
- **Lined by a double layer of neoplastic epithelial cells**^{Q} resting on a dense lymphoid stroma sometimes bearing germinal centers.

  - The **double layer of lining cells distinctive**^{Q}, with a surface palisade of columnar cells resting on a layer of cuboidal to polygonal cells

Diagnosis
- **FNAC** is best diagnostic modality

Treatment
- **Superficial parotidectomy**^{Q}

MUCOEPIDERMOID CARCINOMA

Mucoepidermoid Carcinoma

- MC malignant tumor of **parotid**, MC radiation induced neoplasm^Q of parotid
- MC malignant salivary gland tumor in children^Q

> - Consist of admixture of **squamous cells, mucous secreting cells, intermediate cells** and **clear** or **hydropic cells**^{Q}
> - Include two major elements- **mucin producing cells** and **epithelial cells**^{Q} of epidermoid variety

- Greater the epidermoid content, more malignant is the behavior
- Usually **not causes facial paralysis**^{Q}
- Of two types: Low grade and high grade

Low-grade Type	High-grade Type
• Well circumscribed mass having **cystic mucinous**^{Q} material	• Grossly **infiltrative** and has less tendency to cyst formation (**hard tumor**)
• **Mucin producing**^{Q} cells predominate	• **Squamous cells** predominate
• Well differentiated	• **Poorly differentiated**^{Q}
• More common in **children**	• Less common
• TOC: **Superficial** or **total** parotidectomy^Q	• TOC: **Total parotidectomy +/- radical neck dissection**

ACINIC CELL CARCINOMMA

Acinic Cell Carcinoma

- Rare tumors composed of cells resembling the normal **serous acinar cells**^{Q} of salivary glands
- Occur almost **exclusively** in **parotid glands**^{Q}

> - **Low grade** malignancy, mostly affecting **women**
> - Present as round or ovoid solitary **encapsulated** tumor

- Histologically tumor is characterized by **highly cellular structure** with relative **absence** of **stroma**
- Tumor tends to involve the regional **lymph nodes**
- Treatment: **Radical excision**^{Q}

ADENOID CYSTIC CARCINOMA

Adenoid Cystic Carcinoma

- **Second MC malignant tumor** after mucoepidermoid carcinoma^Q
- **MC malignant tumor** in submandibular, sublingual and minor salivary glands^Q

> - **MC site of origin** is in **minor salivary glands** located in **oral cavity (hard palate)** followed by **sinonasal tract**^{Q}
> - MC type is **Cribiform pattern**^{Q}, and is characterized by "Swiss-Cheese" appearance^Q
> - It has **neurotropic properties**, MC involved nerves are **facial nerve**^{Q}, mandibular (V3) and maxillary branches of trigeminal nerve.

- **Skip lesions**^{Q} along nerves are common, leading to treatment failure, because of difficulty in treating full extent of invasion.
- May grow along **haversian system** of bone without showing bone destruction
- It is **tracherous tumor** as it appears benign even when it is malignant

Clinical Features

- Characterized by its **tendency to invade perineural tissues** and **lymphatics**, thus causes **pain** (which may be prominent and early symptom) and **facial nerve paralysis**^{Q}
- High incidence of **distant metastasis** but **indolent growth**^{Q}

> - Incidence of **distant metastasis** is correlated with **stage of disease** (size of primary tumor and status of LNs)
> - MC site of metastasis is **lung**, lung metastasis are **usually multiple** and **prolonged survival** without treatment is **not unusual**^{Q}

Diagnosis
- Best diagnostic modality is **FNAC**[Q]
- MRI is **radiological IOC** as it detects **early perineural spread** and **intracranial extension**[Q]

Treatments
- **Radical excision** (irrespective of benign appearance) with **largest cuff of normal tissues** around the boundaries of tumor (poorly incapsulated with infiltrating nature)[Q].
- **Post-op radiotherapy** should be given if **margins are positive**[Q].

SIALOLITHIASIS

SIALOLITHIASIS

- 80% of all salivary gland stones occur in **submandibular gland**[Q], 10% occur in parotid, 7% in sublingual and the remainder in minor salivary glands.

> **MC site** is **Wharton's duct**[Q] > submandibular gland substance

- **Composition of stone: Calcium and magnesium phosphate** or **carbonate**[Q]
- Due to deposition of **calcium salts**, 80% stones are **radio opaque**[Q]

> **Submandibular Salivary Gland Calculi** are **More Common** than Parotid Because
> - **Wharton's duct** has **long, curved and upward course** and is **hooked** by **lingual nerve** leading to **inadequate drainage**[Q]
> - Secretion is **more viscid**[Q] than parotid gland secretion

Clinical Features
- **Pain** and **swelling**[Q] of submandibular region, aggregated by food, classically by sucking a lemon
- **Stone impacted** in the **duct** may produce the referred **pain** in the **tongue** due to irritation of **lingual nerve**, as it hooks around the submandibular duct[Q]

Diagnosis
- IOC for diagnosis of sialolithiasis: **NCCT**[Q]

Treatments
- Stone in the duct is removed by giving **incision directly over** the **stone**[Q] in long axis
- **Excision** of **submandibular gland**[Q] when stone is in the gland substance.

COMPLICATIONS OF PAROTIDECTOMY

COMPLICATIONS OF PAROTIDECTOMY

- Facial nerve paresis or paralysis[Q]
- Frey's syndrome[Q]
- **Sensory abnormalities** associated with sacrifice of **greater auricular nerve**[Q]
- Salivary fistula[Q]

FREY'S SYNDROME OR AURICULOTEMPORAL SYNDROME (GUSTATORY SWEATING)

FREY'S SYNDROME OR AURICULOTEMPORAL SYNDROME (GUSTATORY SWEATING)

- It results from **damage** of **auriculotemporal**[Q] nerve during dissection in parotidectomy
- **Aberrant cross innervations** between **secretomotor parasympathetic fibers** of parotid gland and **sympathetic fibers** supplying the **sweat gland**[Q]

Clinical Feature
- **Sweating** and **erythema** over the region of parotid glands as a consequence of autonomic stimulation of salivation by smell or taste of food.

Diagnosis
- Minor's starch iodine test[Q]

Treatment
- **Antiperspirant (aluminium chloride)** application
- **Botulinum toxin** treatment is used for symptomatic **Frey's syndrome**
- **Surgical interruption** of secretary fibers by **tympanic neurectomy**, in non-responding cases

PAROTID FISTULA

Parotid Fistula

- Internal fistula opens inside the mouth and doesn't give rise to symptoms
- **External fistula:** gland fistula or duct fistula

Causes
- Rupture of parotid abscess[Q]
- Penetrating injury
- Inadvertent incision during drainage of parotid abscess[Q]
- After superficial parotidectomy[Q]

Clinical Presentation
- When the external fistula is **connected** to the **gland, external opening** is **pinpoint**, though discharge is present for several months, usually **closes spontaneously.**
- When external fistula is **connected** with **major duct**, there is **outpouring** of **parotid secretions** onto cheek during meals with **excoriation** of surrounding skin

Diagnosis
- **Sialograply** or **sialogram**

Treatment
- **Newman** and **Seabrock's operation**[Q] (in cases of fistula connected with main duct, this operation reconstructs the duct)

RANULA

Ranula

- A **cystic swelling in** the **floor of mouth** that resembles a **frog belly**[Q].
- Term ranula should only be applied to a **mucous extravasation cyst** that arises from the **sublingual gland**[Q]

Etiology
- **Commonly** the lesion is induced by **local trauma** and **duct rupture,** followed by mucin spillage into the surrounding soft tissues (**mucous extravasation phenomenon**)[Q]
- Uncommonly, it is due to **obstruction**, probably caused by mucous plug or a sialolith

Histopathology
- Mucin accumulation surrounded by granulation and fibrous tissue (**mucous extravasation phenomenon**)[Q]
- A cyst cavity, filled with mucin and lining by the ductal epithelium (mucous retention cyst)[Q]
- Chronic inflammation of the cyst wall is present. Infiltration by numerous neutrophils, histiocytes, and plasma cells are common[Q].

Clinical Features
- **Exclusively** present on the **floor of mouth**[Q]
- **Usually unilateral,** lateral to midline[Q]
- **Smooth, dome shape, fluctuating** and **painless** swelling[Q]
- The color is usually **bluish**, but deep lesions may have a normal color.
- The size varies from a few to several centimeters in diameter. Very large lesions which may occupy the floor of mouth can also occur.

Diagnosis
- Diagnosis is usually made **clinically**[Q].

Treatment
- **Surgical removal** or **marsupialization**[Q].
- MC structure injured during ranula surgery: Submandibular duct[Q]

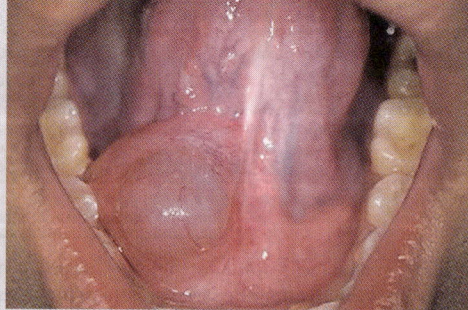

PLUNGING RANULA

Plunging ranula

- **Intraoral ranula** with **cervical prolongation**[Q].
- Plunging ranula **extends from** the **floor** of the mouth below the mylohyoid **into** the **neck**.
- This is nearly always an **extravasation pseudocyst.**
- Presents as **soft painless, ballot table mass** with **cross fluctation**[Q].

SJÖGREN SYNDROME

SJÖGREN SYNDROME

- Chronic disease characterized by **dry eyes (keratoconjunctivitis sicca)** and **dry mouth (xerostomia)** resulting from **immunologically mediated destruction** of the **lacrimal** and **salivary glands**[Q].
- It occurs as an **isolated disorder (primary form)**, also known as the **sicca syndrome** or more often **in association with another autoimmune disease (secondary form)**[Q].
- **Rheumatoid arthritis** is the **MC** associated disorder[Q]

Pathology
- Characterized by **lymphocytic infiltration** and **fibrosis** of the **lacrimal** and **salivary glands**[Q].
- **Earliest histologic finding** in both the major and minor salivary glands is **periductal** and **perivascular lymphocytic infiltration**[Q].

> - **Most important antibodies:** Directed against **SS-A (Ro)** and **SS-B (La)**[Q], which can be detected in 90% of patients (**serologic markers**[Q] of the disease)
> - Patients with **high titers of antibodies to SS-A** are more likely to have early disease onset, longer disease duration, and **extraglandular manifestations**[Q].

Clinical Features
- Occurs **most commonly in women**[Q] between the ages of **50 and 60**.
- **Characteristic symptoms:** Keratoconjunctivitis and xerostomia[Q]
- **Parotid gland enlargement** is present in **half of the patients**[Q]
- **Extraglandular disease** are seen **in one third** of patients

Diagnosis
- **Biopsy** of the **lip (to examine minor salivary glands)** is **essential for** the **diagnosis of Sjögren syndrome**[Q].

Multiple Choice Questions

SALIVARY GLAND TUMORS

1. Which among the following is most common neoplasm of salivary gland? *(Recent Question 2014, WBPG 2012, AIIMS June 98, All India 2002)*
   a. Pleomorphic adenoma
   b. Adenoid cystic carcinoma
   c. Mucoepidermoid carcinoma
   d. Mixed tumor

2. Most common tumor of parotid gland is: *(DNB 2008, 2000, AIIMS June 93)*
   a. Squamous cell carcinoma b. Pleomorphic adenoma
   c. Adenolymphoma d. None of the above

3. Best diagnostic modality for parotid swelling is: *(AIIMS Nov 94)*
   a. Enucleation
   b. FNAC
   c. Superficial parotidectomy
   d. Excisional biopsy

4. Swelling of deep lobe of parotid gland presents as swelling in: *(DNB 2001)*
   a. Parapharyngeal space
   b. Cheek
   c. Temporal region
   d. Below the ear

5. What is the name of this incision given for parotidectomy?
   a. Battle incision b. Modified Blairs incision
   c. Maylard incision d. Cherney incision

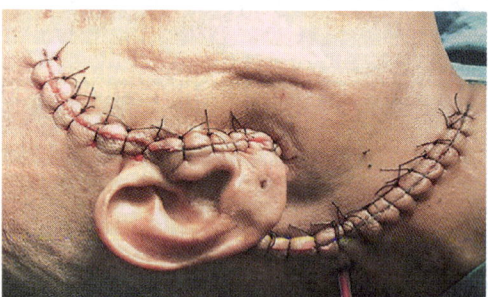

6. True about parotid tumor: *(PGI Nov 2010)*
   a. Facial nerve involvement indicates malignancy
   b. Pleomorphic adenoma is MC variety
   c. Malignant disease is MC variety
   d. Superficial parotidectomy is the treatment of choice

7. About 50% the tumors are benign and even malignant tumors of this salivary gland are slow growing:
   a. Parotid gland b. Sublingual gland
   c. Submandibular gland d. All of the above

8. Most common site of minor salivary gland tumor:
   a. Cheek b. Palate *(MHSSMCET 2005)*
   c. Sub-lingual gland d. Tongue

9. Open biopsy is done for salivary gland tumor unless they are arising from: *(Recent Question 2015)*
   a. Palate b. Buccal
   c. Sublingual d. Parotid

10. Surgical treatment of parotid tumor involving the deep lobe is: *(Recent Question 2016)*
    a. Total parotidectomy with facial nerve preservation
    b. Total parotidectomy with facial nerve sacrifice
    c. Subtotal parotidectomy
    d. Subtotal parotidectomy with facial nerve sacrifice

11. Treatment of pleomorphic adenoma without facial nerve infiltration and limited to superficial lobe:
    a. Superficial parotidectomy *(Recent Question 2016)*
    b. Total parotidectomy
    c. Parotidectomy followed by radiotherapy
    d. Observation

PLEOMORPHIC ADENOMA

12. Regarding pleomorphic adenoma of salivary gland true statement(s) is/are: *(PGI Dec 2008)*
    a. Parotid gland is most commonly involved
    b. Malignant transformation does not occur
    c. Also called mixed tumor
    d. More commonly found in men than women
    e. Superficial parotidectomy is treatment of choice

13. A patient presented with gradually progressive painless mass since 10 years. It is firm to nodular & variable in consistency at each site. Most probable diagnosis is: *(Recent Question 2019)*

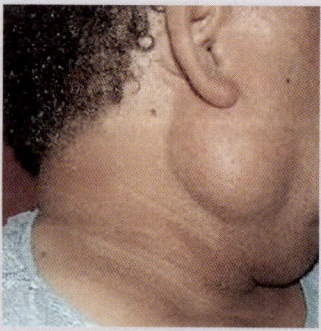

   a. Dermoid cyst b. Sebaceous cyst
   c. Pleomorphic adenoma d. Malignancy

14. True regarding benign mixed parotid tumour is: *(DNB 2005)*
    a. Slow growing and lobular b. Firm and capsulated
    c. 50% of parotid tumour d. All of the above

15. Most common tumor of parotid gland: *(MCI June 2018, MHPGMCET 2007)*
    a. Warthin's tumor b. Pleomorphic adenoma
    c. Adenocarcinoma d. Hemangioma

Salivary Glands

16. **Treatment of choice for pleomorphic adenoma:**
    (Recent Question 2015, 2014, DNB 2008, DPG 2008, MCI Sept 2010, 2007, AIIMS Nov 2001, Nov 95, All India 97)
    a. Superficial parotidectomy   b. Radical parotidectomy
    c. Enucleation   d. Radiotherapy

17. **Ramavati, a 40-year-old female presented with a progressively increasing lump in the parotid region. On oral examination, the tonsil was pushed medially, Biopsy showed it to be pleomorphic adenoma. The appropriate treatment is:**
    (AIIMS June 2001)
    a. Superficial parotidectomy
    b. Lumpectomy
    c. Conservative total parotidectomy
    d. Enucleation

18. **All are true for pleomorphic adenoma except:** *(PGI Dec 99)*
    a. Arises from parotid
    b. May turn into malignant
    c. Minor salivary glands involved
    d. None

19. **Mixed tumors of the salivary glands are:** *(All India 2006)*
    a. Most common in submandibular gland
    b. Usually malignant
    c. Most common in parotid gland
    d. Associated with calculi

20. **Which of the following is an indication of radiotherapy in pleomorphic adenoma of parotid?** *(All India 2004)*
    a. Involvement of deep lobe
    b. 2nd histologically benign recurrence
    c. Microscopically positive margins
    d. Malignant transformation

21. **Mixed parotid tumour arises from:**
    a. Epithelium   b. Epithelium + Mesenchymal
    c. Mesenchymal   d. None of the above

22. **All are true about pleomorphic adenoma except:** *(DNB 2014)*
    a. Malignant transformation risk is high
    b. Mixed tumor
    c. Benign tumour
    d. Encapsulated

WARTHIN'S TUMOR

23. **True statement regarding Warthin's tumor:**
    a. Common in females *(Recent Question 2016, JIPMER 2010)*
    b. Most malignant
    c. Hot spots on Tc-99 scan
    d. Most common tumor of minor salivary gland

24. **Exclusively found in parotid gland:** *(PGI May 2011)*
    a. Warthin's tumor   b. Acinic cell
    c. Pleomorphic   d. Adenocarcinoma
    e. Mucoepidermoid

25. **Warthin's tumour is:** *(DNB 2012, AIIMS May 2005, June 2003)*
    a. An adenolymphoma of parotid gland
    b. A pleomorphic adenoma of parotid
    c. A carcinoma of the parotid
    d. A carcinoma of submandibular salivary gland

26. **Treatment of choice for Warthin's tumour:**
    (AIIMS Nov 2001, All India 98, 96)
    a. Superficial parotidectomy   b. Enucleation
    c. Radiotherapy   d. Injection of a sclerosant agent

27. **Hot spot on Tc-99 is seen in which parotid tumour?**
    (Recent Question 2016, JIPMER 2014, 2010; AIIMS May 2013)
    a. Adenolymphoma   b. Adenoid cystic carcinoma
    c. Acinic cell tumour   d. Adenocarcinoma

28. **Cystic spaces lined by double layer of neoplastic epithelial cells resting on dense lymphoid tissue is a feature of:**
    (Recent Question 2016, APPG 2015)
    a. Dermoid cyst   b. Warthin tumor
    c. Aneurysmal bone cyst   d. Hashimoto's thyroiditis

MUCOEPIDERMOID CARCINOMA

29. **Most common malignant tumour of parotid is:**
    (Recent Question 2016, DNB 2011, 2010, DPG 2008)
    a. Epidermoid carcinoma
    b. Mucoepidermoid carcinoma
    c. Squamous cell carcinoma
    d. Adenocarcinoma

30. **Mucoepidermoid carcinoma of parotid arises from:**
    (PGI June 99)
    a. Secretory cells   b. Excretory cells
    c. Myoepithelial cells   d. Myofibril

31. **Mucoepidermoid carcinoma is seen in:** *(MHSSMCET 2005)*
    a. Sebaceous gland   b. Pancreas
    c. Parotid gland   d. All

ADENOID CYSTIC CARCINOMA

32. **The most common tumour of the minor salivary gland is:**
    (DNB 2013, WBPG 2012, COMEDK 2008)
    a. Mucoepidermoid carcinoma
    b. Acinic cell carcinoma
    c. Adenoid cystic carcinoma
    d. Pleomorphic adenocarcinoma

33. **Tumor with perineural invasion:**
    (Recent Question 2015, DNB 2009, AIIMS Nov 2010, MHSSMCET 2007)
    a. Adenocarcinoma   b. Adenoid cystic carcinoma
    c. Basal cell carcinoma   d. Squamous cell carcinoma

34. **All the following tumors can spread perineurally except:**
    (MHSSMCET 2007)
    a. Adenoid cystic carcinoma of salivary gland
    b. Carcinoma gallbladder
    c. Hilar cholangiocarcinoma
    d. None of the above

35. **Which among the following parotid tumor spreads through neural sheath?**
    (Karnataka 2013, NEET Pattern, DNB 2013, AIIMS June 97, 96)
    a. Mixed parotid tumor   b. Adenoid cystic carcinoma
    c. Squamous Cell carcinoma   d. Oxyphilic lymphoma

36. **Swiss cheese pattern is seen in:** *(DPG 2007)*
    a. Warthin's tumor
    b. Adenoid cystic carcinoma
    c. Pleomorphic adenoma
    d. Mucoepidermoid carcinoma

37. **Adenoid cystic carcinoma of parotid gland all are true except:**
    (UPPG 2010)
    a. Most common malignant tumour of minor salivary gland
    b. Most common submandibular gland tumor
    c. Spreads perineurally
    d. Local recurrence is common
    e. Radiotherapy is the treatment of choice

ACINIC CELL CARCINOMA

38. Acinic cell tumor is tumor of: (MHPGMCET 2002)
    a. Parotid gland
    b. Breast
    c. Parathyroid
    d. Thyroid

39. Acinic cell carcinomas of the salivary gland arise most often in the: (All India 2006)
    a. Parotid gland
    b. Minor salivary glands
    c. Submandibular gland
    d. Sublingual gland

CARCINOMA PAROTID

40. Which of the following is false about salivary gland tumors? (DPG 2008, 2007)
    a. Pleomorphic adenoma is MC tumor of parotid
    b. Adenoid cystic carcinoma MC occurs in minor salivary glands
    c. Warthin's tumor is MC malignant tumor of salivary glands
    d. Perineural invasion is seen is adenoid cystic carcinoma

41. True statement(s) about salivary gland tumors: (PGI June 2004)
    a. Pleomorphic adenoma can arise in submandibular gland
    b. Warthin's tumour arises from submandibular gland
    c. Pleomorphic adenoma is most common tumour of submandibular gland
    d. Acinic cell carcinoma is most malignant
    e. Frey's syndrome is due to injury of auriculotemporal nerve

42. All of the following statements about lymphoepithelioma of the parotid gland are true, except: (All India 2009)
    a. Parotid gland is the most common site of lymphoepithelioma in the head and neck region
    b. It is associated with EBV infection
    c. It is highly radiosensitive
    d. It is a type of squamous cell carcinoma

43. Most of the parotid tumor are managed by: (All India 97)
    a. Total parotidectomy
    b. Radical parotidectomy
    c. Superficial parotidectomy
    d. Radical parotidectomy and neck dissection

44. All of the following are true regarding malignant salivary gland tumours except: (DNB 2010)
    a. Painful
    b. Present with skin ulceration
    c. Cervical lymphadenopathy
    d. Simple enucleation is treatment of choice

SALIVARY GLAND STONES

45. Commonest salivary gland to get stones: (APPG 2015, Recent Question 2014, NEET 2013, DNB 2011, 2003, DPG 2006, MCI March 2005, 2007, AIIMS Nov 99, June 99)
    a. Parotid
    b. Submandibular
    c. Minor salivary gland
    d. Sublingual

46. In which one of the following conditions the sialography is contraindicated? (All India 2005)
    a. Ductal calculus
    b. Chronic parotitis
    c. Acute parotitis
    d. Recurrent sialadenitis

47. Treatment of submandibular salivary gland duct calculi is: (TN 90)
    a. Excision of submandibular gland
    b. Opening the duct at the frenulum
    c. Opening the duct and removal of calculus
    d. Excision of gland and duct

48. All of the following statement regarding stones in the submandibular gland are true except: (MCI March 2007)
    a. 80% of stones occur in the submandibular gland
    b. Majority of submandibular stones are radiolucent
    c. Stones are the most common cause of obstruction within the submandibular gland
    d. Patient presents with acute swelling in the region of the submandibular gland

49. Investigation using dye to find out stone in salivary gland: (Recent Question 2013)
    a. Sialography
    b. Mammography
    c. MR angiography
    d. USG

50. What percent of submandibular salivary gland stones are radiopaque? (MHCET 2016)
    a. 10%
    b. 70%
    c. 80%
    d. 90%

51. What are the three cranial nerves that are at risk during the removal of submandibular salivary gland? (APPG 2016)
    a. Marginal mandibular branch of facial nerve, glossopharyngeal nerve and spinal accessory nerve
    b. Lingual nerve, marginal mandibular branch of facial nerve & spinal accessory nerve
    c. Hypoglossal nerve, facial nerve & glossopharyngeal nerve
    d. Marginal mandibular branch of facial nerve, lingual nerve & hypoglossal nerve

PAROTIDECTOMY AND COMPLICATIONS

52. After removal of parotid gland, patient is having sweating on the cheeks while eating. In this complication seen after parotidectomy, the auriculotemporal nerve which contains parasympathetic secretomotor fibers to parotid gland is fused with which nerve? (AIIMS May 2012)
    a. Greater petrosal nerve
    b. Facial nerve
    c. Greater auricular nerve
    d. Buccal nerve

53. Frey's syndrome occurs due to aberrant misdirection of fibers from salivary glands to sweat glands. These fibers come from which of the following? (Recent Question 2019)
    a. Facial nerve
    b. Trigeminal nerve
    c. Auriculotemporal nerve
    d. Glossopharyngeal nerve

54. All of the following statements are true about Frey's syndrome except: (Recent Question 2019)
    a. Gustatory sweating
    b. Aberrant misdirection of sympathetic fibers of auriculotemporal nerve
    c. Botulinum toxin is one of the treatments suggested
    d. Less chances with enuculeation than parotidectomy

55. Management of Frey's syndrome include following except: (MHSSMCET 2010, 2008)
    a. Botulinum toxin
    b. Temporal fascial graft
    c. Aluminum chloride
    d. Antiperspirants

56. The 'Starch iodine test' is useful to diagnose: *(MHSSMCET 2011)*
    a. Wegener's granulomatosis b. Cat scratch disease
    c. Sarcoidosis d. Frey's syndrome
57. Which of the following is not true regarding radical parotidectomy? *(MHSSMCET 2009)*
    a. In radical parotidectomy the facial nerve is preserved
    b. Anesthesia of the ear lobe due to sectioning of the great auricular nerve can occur
    c. Gustatory sweating (Frey's syndrome) can occur
    d. None
58. Which of the following group constitute Frey's syndrome?
    a. Hyperhidrosis, enophthalmos and miosis *(Karnataka 94)*
    b. Anhidrosis, enophthalmos and miosis
    c. Redness and sweating over the auriculotemporal region during meal
    d. Pain over the distribution of the auriculotemporal nerve during meal
59. The nerve sacrificed in parotid surgery: *(DNB 2013, APPG 98)*
    a. Auriculotemporal b. Facial
    c. Buccal d. Cervico facial
60. Incision for superficial parotidectomy: *(WBPG 2015)*
    a. L-shaped b. Y-shaped
    c. S-shaped d. Z-shaped

PAROTID FISTULA

61. Newman and Seabrook's operation is used for:
    a. Repair of parotid fistula *(Recent Question 2016)*
    b. For parotid calculi
    c. For carcinoma of tongue
    d. For treatment of recurrent chronic parotitis
62. Seabrook's operation is done for: *(MHSSMCET 2006)*
    a. Parotid duct fistula b. Thyroglossal fistula
    c. Thyroglossal cyst d. Branchial fistula

RANULA

63. Which of the following best represents 'ranula'? *(AIIMS May 2005)*
    a. A type of epulis
    b. A thyroglossal cyst
    c. Cystic swelling in the floor of mouth
    d. Forked uvula
64. What is the most probable diagnosis based on the given image?

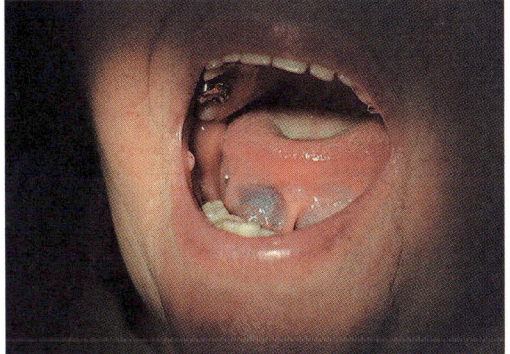

    a. Pleomorphic adenoma b. Ranula
    c. Warthin's tumor d. Adenoid cystic carcinoma

65. What is ranula? *(DNB 2007, 2005)*
    a. Retention cyst of sublingual gland
    b. Retention cyst of submandibular gland
    c. Extravasation cyst of sublingual glands
    d. Extravasation cyst of submandibular glands
66. Which of the following is not true about ranula? *(MHSSMCET 2010)*
    a. Arises from sublingual salivary glands
    b. Pseudocyst
    c. Appearance is like "Frog's belly"
    d. None
67. Excision of ranula is associated with injury to: *(DNB 2010, MHSSMCET 2007, PGI 96)*
    a. Lingual nerve b. Lingual artery
    c. Parotid gland d. Submandibular duct
68. Which of the following statements about 'ranula' is most correct? *(All India 2011)*
    a. It is type of epulis
    b. It is a cystic swelling in the floor of mouth
    c. It is a type of thyroglossal cyst
    d. It is a type of mucus retention cyst
69. Plunging ranula is: *(Recent Question 2015)*
    a. Cystic growth of sublingual gland
    b. Lymph node
    c. A tumor in floor of mouth
    d. None

SALIVARY GLANDS ANATOMY AND PHYSIOLOGY

70. True about salivary gland: *(PGI Dec 2006)*
    a. There are more than 400 minor glands
    b. 90% of all parotid tumors are malignant
    c. 90% of minor salivary tumors are malignant
    d. Superficial parotidectomy done in parotid tumors
    e. Warthin's tumor common in parotid
71. Which of the following is not a landmark for facial nerve during parotid surgery? *(All India 2008)*
    a. Digastric muscle
    b. Inferior belly of omohyoid
    c. Tragal pointer
    d. Retrograde dissection of distal branch
72. The parotid duct is known as:
    a. Wharton's duct b. Stenson's duct
    c. Duct of Santorini d. Duct of Wirsung
73. Nerve which lies in association to Wharton's duct is:
    a. Hypoglossal b. Lingual
    c. Facial d. Spinal accessory
74. Inflammatory enlargement of deep lobe of parotid gland is seen in:
    a. Posterior pharyngeal wall b. Supratonsillar area
    c. Anterior tonsillar pillar d. Tonsillar fossa/bed
75. Which of the following nerves lies closest of the Whartson's duct? *(COMEDK 2007)*
    a. Hypoglossal b. Lingual
    c. Chorda tympani d. Facial
76. Structure exposed after parotid surgery is: *(DPG 2008)*
    a. Internal jugular vein b. Facial nerve
    c. Muscles d. Facial artery

77. **All of the following are anatomical markers for localization of facial nerve during parotid surgery, except:** *(DPG 2008)*
    a. Posterior belly of digastric
    b. Mastoid process
    c. Inferior belly of omohyoid
    d. Bony external auditory meatus

78. **In submandibular gland surgery, the nerve least likely to be injured is:** *(DPG 2011, JIPMER 93)*
    a. Inferior alveolar nerve
    b. Hypoglossal nerve
    c. Lingual nerve
    d. Mandibular branch of facial nerve

79. **Most common location of ectopic submandibular salivary gland tissue is:** *(MCI Sept 2009, UPPG 2002)*
    a. Cheek
    b. Palate
    c. Angle of mandible
    d. Tongue

80. **In surgery of submandibular salivary gland, nerve often involved:** *(PGI June 97)*
    a. Hypoglossal
    b. Glossopharyngeal
    c. Facial
    d. Lingual

SJOGREN'S SYNDROME

81. **True regarding Sjogren's syndrome are all of the following except:** *(MCI Sept 2009)*
    a. Autoimmune condition
    b. Males are commonly affected
    c. Progressive destruction of lacrimal and salivary gland
    d. No single laboratory investigation is pathognomonic

82. **Sjogren's syndrome refers to disease of:**
    a. Parotid glands
    b. Thyroid disease
    c. Parathyroid glands
    d. Multiple endocrine neoplasia

83. **Biopsy of the parotid gland in a patient with Sjogren's disease shows:** *(JIPMER 2011)*
    a. Neutrophils
    b. Lymphocytes
    c. Eosinophils
    d. Basophils

MISCELLANEOUS

84. **Bacterial pyogenic parotitis affecting the parotid gland is most common after:** *(MCI March 2008)*
    a. Uveo-parotid fever
    b. Mumps
    c. Debilitation after major surgery
    d. After administration of iodine

85. **Bilateral parotid enlargement does not occur in:** *(AIIMS Nov 96)*
    a. Sjogren's syndrome
    b. Sarcoidosis
    c. SLE
    d. Chronic pancreatitis

86. **A bacterial pyogenic parotitis is found most commonly in which of the following?** *(Orissa 99)*
    a. Mumps
    b. Debilitation after major surgery
    c. Drug reaction (iodine mumps)
    d. Uveoparotid fever

87. **Sialosis refers to:** *(Karnataka 2006)*
    a. Bilateral parotitis
    b. Sjogren's syndrome
    c. Non-inflammatory parotid enlargement
    d. Bilateral salivary duct ectasia

88. **Ackerman's tumour is:** *(DPG 2008)*
    a. Mucoepidermoid carcinoma
    b. Epidermoid carcinoma
    c. Squamous cell carcinoma
    d. Adenocarcinoma

89. **Bilateral parotid enlargement is seen in:** *(DNB 2008)*
    a. Wegner's granulomatosis
    b. Sjogren's syndrome
    c. Kimura's disease
    d. All of the above

90. **True regarding acute sialadenitis is/are:** *(PGI May 2018)*
    a. Most common in submandibular glands
    b. Most common type is viral
    c. Can present with stasis of saliva
    d. There may be tender pre-auricular nodes
    e. Stone removal may be done by probing through oral route

Explanations

SALIVARY GLAND TUMORS

1. **Ans. a. Pleomorphic adenoma** *(Ref: Bailey 27/e p787; Devita 9/e p774; Cancer of the Head and Neck by Suen and Myer 4/e p480-490)*

   - MC neoplasm of **salivary gland**: **Pleomorphic adenoma**^{Q}
   - MC malignant tumor of salivary gland: **Mucoepidermoid carcinoma**^{Q}
   - MC neoplasm of salivary gland **in children**: **Hemangioma**^{Q}
   - MC malignant tumor of salivary gland **in children**: **Mucoepidermoid carcinoma**^{Q}
   - MC malignant tumor of **minor salivary glands**: **Adenoid cystic carcinoma**^{Q}

   <u>**ALL SALIVARY GLAND TUMORS ARE MOST COMMON IN PAROTID EXCEPT**</u>

   - **Adenoid cystic carcinoma**: MC malignant tumor of **minor salivary glands**^{Q}
   - **Squamous cell carcinoma**: Mostly seen in **submandibular gland**^{Q}

2. Ans. b. Pleomorphic adenoma
3. Ans. b. FNAC
4. Ans. a. Parapharyngeal space
5. Ans. b. Modified Blairs incision
6. **Ans. a. Facial nerve involvement indicates malignancy, b. Pleomorphic adenoma is MC variety, d. Superficial parotidectomy is the treatment of choice**

   In **parotid tumors, rapid growth, pain**, paraesthesia, **enlarged cervical LN** and restriction of jaw movements, **facial weakness** or skin invasion and **fixation of mastoid tip** is suggestive of malignant transformation.

7. **Ans. b. Sublingual gland, c. Submandibular gland** *(Ref: Bailey 27/e p783; Devita 9/e p774-778; Cancer of the Head and Neck by Suen and Myer 4/e p480-490)*

8. **Ans. b. Palate** *(Ref: Bailey 27/e p776; Devita 9/e p777-778; Cancer of the Head and Neck by Suen and Myer 4/e p487-489)*

   - MC malignant tumor of minor salivary glands: **Adenoid cystic carcinoma**^{Q}
   - MC site of origin is in **minor salivary glands** located in **oral cavity (hard palate)** followed by **sinonasal tract**^{Q}

9. Ans. d. Parotid
10. Ans. a. Total parotidectomy with facial nerve preservation
11. Ans. a. Superficial parotidectomy

PLEOMORPHIC ADENOMA

12. **Ans. a. Parotid gland is most commonly involved, c. Also called mixed tumour, e. Superficial parotidectomy is treatment of choice** *(Ref: Bailey 27/e p787; Devita 9/e p774; Cancer of the Head and Neck by Suen and Myer 4/e p414)*

13. **Ans. c. Pleomorphic adenoma** *(Ref: Bailey 27/e p787)*
14. Ans. d. All of the above
15. Ans. b. Pleomorphic adenoma
16. Ans. a. Superficial parotidectomy
17. Ans. c. Conservative total parotidectomy
18. **Ans. d. None** *(Ref: Robbins 9/e p787, 8/e p758)*

    - Pleomorphic adenoma arises most commonly from the parotid gland^Q.
    - Pleomorphic adenoma is **less common** in the **submandibular gland** and **sublingual glands; relatively rare** in the **minor glands**^{Q}.

19. Ans. c. Most common in parotid gland
20. **Ans. c. Microscopically positive margins** *(Ref: Devita 9/e p776; Cancer of the Head and Neck by Suen and Myer 4/e p499-501)*
21. Ans. b. Epithelium + Mesenchymal
22. Ans. a. Malignant transformation risk is high

WARTHIN'S TUMOR

23. **Ans. c. Hot spots on Tc-99 scan** *(Ref: Bailey 27/e p789; Devita 9/e p774; Cancer of the Head and Neck by Suen and Myer 4/e p414)*
24. Ans. a. Warthin's tumor, b. Acinic cell
25. Ans. a. An adenolymphoma of parotid gland

26. Ans. a. Superficial parotidectomy
27. Ans. a. Adenolymphoma
28. Ans. b. Warthin tumor

MUCOEPIDERMOID CARCINOMA

29. Ans. b. Mucoepidermoid carcinoma *(Ref: Bailey 27/e p788; Devita 9/e p774-777; Cancer of the Head and Neck by Suen and Myer 4/e p489)*
30. Ans. a. Secretory cells
31. Ans. c. Parotid gland

ADENOID CYSTIC CARCINOMA

32. Ans. c. Adenoid cystic carcinoma *(Ref: Bailey 27/e p727,778; Devita 9/e p777-778; Cancer of the Head and Neck by Suen and Myer 4/e p487-489)*
33. Ans. b. Adenoid cystic carcinoma
34. Ans. d. None of the above *(Ref: Bailey 25/e p752; Devita 9/e p778, 1021, 1037; Cancer of the Head and Neck by Suen and Myer 4/e p488)*

Perineural Spread is seen in	
• Adenoid cystic carcinoma^Q	• Ductal adenocarcinoma of pancreas^Q
• CA GB^Q	• Cholangiocarcinoma^Q

35. Ans. b. Adenoid cystic carcinoma
36. Ans. b. Adenoid cystic carcinoma
37. Ans. b. Most common submandibular gland tumour

ACINIC CELL CARCINOMA

38. Ans. a. Parotid gland
39. Ans. a. Parotid gland *(Ref: Devita 9/e p774; Cancer of the Head and Neck by Suen and Myer 4/e p489-490)*

CARCINOMA PAROTID

40. Ans. c. Warthin's tumor is MC malignant tumor of salivary glands
41. Ans. a. Pleomorphic adenoma can arise in submandibular gland, c. Pleomorphic adenoma is most common tumour of sub mandibular gland, e. Frey's syndrome is due to injury of auriculotemporal nerve
42. Ans. a. Parotid gland is the most common site of Lymphoepethelioma in the Head and Neck region *(Ref: Devita 9/e p729, 752, 774)*
    - The **most common site** of **lymphoepethelioma** is the **nasopharynx^Q**. Lymphoepethelioma occurs **rarely in** the **parotid** and **submandibular glands.**

LYMPHOEPETHELIOMA

- Lymphoepethelioma: Undifferentiated carcinoma of the nasopharyngeal type
- Lymphoepethelioma is a **variant of squamous cell carcinoma^Q** that arises in lymphoid bearing areas
- Found **most commonly in** the **nasopharynx^Q**
- Rarely occur in **parotid** and **submandibular glands^Q**

Common sites of Lymphoepethelioma in Head and Neck		
• Nasopharynx (MC site)^Q	• Faucial tonsils	• Lingual tonsils (base of tongue)

- Histologically the squamous component is highly undifferentiated while the lymphoid component is essentially benign (non-neoplastic lymphocytes)
- **EBV** is **commonly linked** when this tumor is located in the **nasopharynx^Q**
- **High tendency to metastasize** and is **exquisitely radiosensitive^Q**

Important characteristic features	
• High tendency to metastasize^Q	• Extreme radiosensitivity^Q

43. Ans. c. Superficial parotidectomy *(Ref: Bailey 27/e p789; Devita 9/e p775-777; Cancer of the Head and Neck by Suen and Myer 4/e p494-501)*

TREATMENT OF CHOICE FOR PLEOMORPHIC ADENOMA	
• In parotid gland: superficial parotidectomy^Q	• In other salivary glands: excision of the affected gland^Q

TREATMENT OF SALIVARY GLAND TUMORS

- **Surgery**
  - Principal treatment of cancer of salivary glands is **surgical excision**, used either as a single modality or **in most cases**, in conjunction **with adjuvant radiation therapy.**

Parotid malignancies	• Superficial parotidectomy^Q with preservation of facial nerve • Total parotidectomy^Q with nerve preservation if **deep lobe** is **involved**
• Other salivary glands	• En-bloc excision^Q of tumor (involved gland)

- **Neck dissection for lymph nodes:** In clinically palpable nodes and High grade malignancies
- **Radiotherapy**

Indications of radiotherapy in Salivary Gland Tumors

• **High grade** tumors^Q	• **Bone invasion**^Q
• **Large primary** lesions^Q	• Cervical **LN metastasis**^Q
• **Perineural invasion**^Q	• **Positive surgical margins**^Q

- **No role of chemotherapy** in salivary gland tumors due to **incomplete** and **short lived response without** any **survival advantage.**

44. **Ans. d. Simple enucleation is treatment of choice**

SALIVARY GLAND STONES

45. **Ans. b. Submandibular** *(Ref: Bailey 27/e p780)*
46. **Ans. c. Acute parotitis** *(Ref: Bailey 27/e p786)*

SIALOGRAPLY (PTYALOGRAPHY)

- Contrast X-ray examination of salivary glands and duct

Indications	Contraindications
• Salivary duct **stones** and **strictures**^Q • **Chronic sialedenitis**^Q • **Tumors** of salivary glands	• **Contrast allergy**^Q • **Acute sialedenitis**^Q

47. **Ans. c. Opening the duct and removal of calculus**   48. **Ans. b. Majority of submandibular stones are radiolucent**
49. **Ans. a. Sialography** *(Ref: Sutton's radiology 7/e p535, Bailey & Love 25/e p760)*
50. **Ans. c. 80%**   51. **Ans. d. Marginal mandibular branch of facial nerve, lingual nerve & hypoglossal nerve**

PAROTIDECTOMY AND COMPLICATIONS

52. **Ans. c. Greater auricular nerve** *(Ref: Grays 40/e p436; Bailey 27/e p792)*
    - "**Cross innervation** between **somatic sensory supply (greater auricular)** and **parasympathetic secretomotor fibers** to the parotid is considered to be part of the anatomical basis for the phenomenon of **gustatory sweating (Frey's syndrome)** seen after parotid surgery, when the nerve is at risk of injury."

COMPLICATIONS OF PAROTIDECTOMY

- Facial nerve paresis or paralysis^Q
- Frey's syndrome^Q
- **Sensory abnormalities** associated with sacrifice of **greater auricular nerve**^Q
- Salivary fistula^Q

53. **Ans. c. Auriculotemporal nerve** *(Ref: Bailey 27/e p792)*
54. **Ans. b. Aberrant misdirection of sympathetic fibers of auriculotemporal nerve** *(Ref: Bailey 27/e p792)*
55. **Ans. b. Temporal fascial graft** *(Ref: Bailey 27/e p795; Cancer of the Head and Neck by Suen and Myer 4/e p498)*
56. **Ans. d. Frey's syndrome**
57. **Ans. a. In radical parotidectomy the facial nerve is preserved** *(Ref: Bailey 27/e p792; Cancer of the Head and Neck by Suen and Myer 4/e p495)*
    - **Radical parotidectomy: Facial nerve is sacrificed,** particularly if there is a reasonable prospect of cure.

RADICAL PAROTIDECTOMY

- **Radical parotidectomy** envolves **resection of all parotid gland tissue** and **elective sectioning of facial nerve** usually through the main trunk.

Surgery Essence

58. Ans. c. Redness and sweating over the auriculotemporal during meal
59. Ans. b. Facial
60. Ans. c. S-shaped

PAROTID FISTULA

61. Ans. a. Repair of parotid fistula
62. Ans. a. Parotid duct fistula *(Ref: Cancer of the Head and Neck by Suen and Myer 4/e p498)*

RANULA

63. Ans. c. Cystic swelling in the floor of mouth *(Ref: Bailey 27/e p779)*
64. Ans. b. Ranula *(Ref: Bailey 27/e p779)*
65. Ans. c. Extravasation cyst of sublingual gland
66. Ans. d. None
67. Ans. d. Submandibular duct *(Ref: Clinical Surgery by Rob's and Smith vol-9/56)*

> The **treatment of ranula** constitutes a problem, owing to technical **difficulty of complete excision without damage to adjacent structures such as submandibular duct.**

68. Ans. b. It is a cystic swelling in the floor of mouth
69. Ans. a. Cystic growth of sublingual gland

SALIVARY GLANDS ANATOMY AND PHYSIOLOGY

70. Ans. a. There are more than 400 minor glands, c. 90% of minor salivary glands are malignant, d. Superficial parotidectomy done in parotid tumors, e. Warthin's tumor common in parotid *(Ref: Bailey 27/e p776)*

MINOR SALIVARY GLANDS

- The mucosa of the oral cavity contains approximately **750 minor salivary glands**^{Q}.
- They are distributed in the mucosa of the **lips, cheeks, palate, floor of the mouth** and **retromolar area**^{Q}.
- These minor salivary glands also appear in other areas of the **upper aerodigestive tract**^{Q} including the oropharynx, larynx and trachea as well as the sinuses.
- Overall, they **contribute to 10%** of the **total salivary volume**
- Their **secretion is mainly mucous**^{Q} in nature and has many functions such as coating the oral cavity with saliva.

71. Ans. b. Inferior belly of omohyoid *(Ref: Bailey 27/e p790)*

MAJOR SURGICAL LANDMARKS TO THE FACIAL NERVE

- **Tympanomastoid suture line (most constant** landmark)^Q
- **Tragal pointer**^{Q}
- **Posterior belly of digastric**^{Q}
- **Retromandibular vein**^{Q}
- **Styloid process**^{Q}

72. Ans. b. Stenson's duct *(Ref: Bailey 27/e p778,780,785; Cancer of the Head and Neck by Suen and Myer 4/e p495)*

SALIVARY GLANDS ANATOMICAL FEATURES

- Parotid gland: **Serous acini**^{Q}
- Submandibular gland: **Mucus + Serous acini**^{Q}
- Sublingual + minor salivary glands: **Mucinous acini**^{Q}

  - Parotid gland: **Stenson's duct**^{Q} (opens at upper **2nd molar** tooth^Q)
  - Submandibular gland: **Wharton's duct**^{Q} (opens into the papilla just **lateral** to the **frenulum**^{Q})
  - Sublingual gland: **Ducts of Rivinus**^{Q}, Bartholin duct^Q

- Sublingual gland secretes via tiny openings, **ducts of Rivinus** directly into the floor of mouth or via several ducts which unite to form the common **sublingual duct of Bartholin**, which then **merges with Wharton's duct.**

73. Ans. b. Lingual *(Ref: Bailey 27/e p780)*

Lingual **nerve** lies in a **close association with submandibular duct** and **most prone to damage during submandibular gland surgery.**

SUBMANDIBULAR GLAND

- The **deep part of the gland lies on** the **hyoglossus muscle closely related to the lingual nerve** and **inferior** to **the hypoglossal nerve**^{Q}.
- **Submandibular duct lies between** the **lingual** and **hypoglossal nerves** on hyoglossus, but, at the **anterior border** of the muscle, it is **crossed laterally by the lingual nerve**^{Q}, terminal branches of which ascend on its medial side.

Salivary Glands

MANAGEMENT OF SIALOLITHIASIS

- If the **stone is lying within** the **submandibular duct** in the **floor of the mouth** anterior to the point at which the **duct crosses the lingual nerve** (second molar region), the **stone** can be **removed** by **incising longitudinally over** the **duct**[Q].
- Once the stone has been delivered, the wall of the duct should be left open to promote free drainage of saliva.
- Suturing the duct will lead to stricture formation and the recurrence of obstructive symptoms.
- Where the **stone** is **proximal to the lingual nerve**, i.e. at the hilum of the gland, **stone retrieval via an intraoral approach** should be **avoided** as there is a **high risk of damage** to the **lingual nerve**[Q] during exploration in the posterior lingual gutter. **Treatment** is by **simultaneous submandibular gland excision** and **removal of the stone** and **ligation of the submandibular duct** under direct vision[Q].

74. **Ans. d. Tonsillar fossa/bed** *(Ref: BDC 4/e pvol III/136, 217)*
    - Parotid gland is related to lateral pharyngeal wall. Tonsillar fossa is present in lateral pharyngeal wall.

75. **Ans. b. Lingual**

76. **Ans. b. Facial nerve** *(Ref: Bailey 27/e p789)*

    Structure exposed after parotid surgery is facial nerve.

    - **Superficial parotidectomy:** The dissection is made in the **Patey's facio-venous plane** and commenced at the **postero-inferior border of the parotid gland**, where the **main trunk of the facial nerve is found out**[Q].
        - **Radical parotidectomy: Facial nerve is sacrificed**, particularly if there is a reasonable prospect of cure[Q].

77. **Ans. c. Inferior belly of Omohyoid**

78. **Ans. a. Inferior alveolar nerve** *(Ref: Bailey 27/e p780)*

Important anatomical relationships of the submandibular glands	
• Lingual nerve[Q]	• Facial artery[Q]
• Hypoglossal nerve[Q]	• Marginal mandibular branch of the facial nerve
• Anterior facial vein[Q]	

79. **Ans. c. Angle of mandible** *(Ref: Bailey 27/e p780)*

    ### ECTOPIC/ABERRANT SALIVARY GLAND TISSUE

    - **MC ectopic salivary tissue** is the **Stafne bone cyst**.
    - This presents as an **asymptomatic**, clearly demarcated radiolucency of the **angle of the mandible**, characteristically **below the inferior dental neurovascular bundle**[Q].
    - It is formed by **invagination into the bone** on the lingual aspect of the mandible **of an ectopic lobe** of the **juxtaposed submandibular gland**[Q].
    - **No treatment** is required[Q].

80. **Ans. a. Hypoglossal, c. Facial, d. Lingual**

SJOGREN'S SYNDROME

81. **Ans. b. Males are commonly affected** *(Ref: Robbins 9/e p227; Bailey 27/e p796; Harrison 20/e p2561, 19/e p2166)*

82. **Ans. a. Parotid glands**   83. **Ans. b. Lymphocytes**

MISCELLANEOUS

84. **Ans. c. Debilitation after major surgery** *(Ref: Bailey 27/e p786)*

    ### ACUTE SUPPURATIVE PAROTITIS

    - Characterized by **presence of pus** and seen in **debilitated/dehydrated/or in patients with poor oral hygiene**[Q].
    - **MC organism** (responsible for): **Staph. aureus**[Q]

    Treatment
    - Initial treatment is **proper hydration/antibiotics/improving oral hygiene**[Q].
    - If **abscess** develops then it is **drained**[Q] by giving a J shaped incision.

85. **Ans. c. SLE** *(Ref: Harrison 20/e p2561, 224)*

Causes of Bilateral Parotid Enlargement	

• Viral infections:
  – Mumps[Q]
  – Influenza
  – Epstein-Barr virus[Q]
  – Coxsackie virus A[Q]
  – Cytomegalovirus[Q]
  – HIV[Q]
• Sarcoidosis[Q]
• Amyloidosis[Q]
• Kimura's disease
	• Wagner's Granulomatosis
	• Sjögren's syndrome[Q]
	• Metabolic:
	  – Diabetes mellitus[Q] – Hyperlipoproteinemias
	  – Chronic pancreatitis[Q] – Hepatic cirrhosis[Q]
	• Endocrine:
	  – Acromegaly[Q] – Gonadal hypofunction

86. **Ans. b. Debilitation after major surgery**

87. **Ans. c. Non-inflammatory parotid enlargement** *(Ref: Bailey 27/e p795)*

SIALOSIS

- **Sialosis** is an uncommon **non-neoplastic** and **non-inflammatory disorder** causing **bilateral non-painful enlargement of** the **major salivary glands**[Q].

88. **Ans. c. Squamous cell carcinoma** *(Ref: Oxford textbook of oncology, Vol. I/1995/1046)*

Ackerman's tumour is a distinct variant of well-differentiated squamous cell carcinoma.

ACKERMAN'S TUMOUR

- Ackerman's tumour is a **distinct variant** of **well-differentiated SCC** that may develop **in any mucosal surface in** the **upper respiratory** and **digestive tract**[Q].
- It is also called as **verrucous carcinoma**[Q].

  - Most verrucous carcinoma are reported within the **oral cavity**[Q] but they make up 1-2% of malignant laryngeal tumours within the larynx.
  - Verrucous carcinomas occur **mainly in the elderly patients**[Q].
  - Verrucous carcinomas may be **multifocal** and **warty** in their **appearance**[Q].

- The **pushing infiltrating margins** are characteristic of verrucous carcinomas.
- Lymphatic spread is rare.

Risk Factors for Verrucous Carcinoma

- Frequent use of **tobacco (MC)**[Q+]
- **HPV infection**[Q]

Histology

- Well-differentiated, keratinising epithelium, with few mitotic figures and no cellular atypia.

Treatment

- **Surgery** is the **treatment of choice**.

89. **Ans. d. All of the above**

90. **Ans. b. Most common type is viral, c. Can present with stasis of saliva, e. Stone removal may be done by probing through oral route....** *(Ref: Bailey 27/e p796)*

CHAPTER 37

Neck

CAROTID BODY TUMOR

Carotid Body Tumor (Chemodectoma)

- Arises from **chemoreceptor cells**^Q on the **medial side** of carotid bulb
- Histologically it is a **non-chromaffin paraganglioma**^Q
- Usually **benign, unifocal** and **nonhereditary, Schamblin classification** is used for **carotid body tumour**
- Associated with **pheochromocytoma**^Q

  - **Higher incidence** in areas where **people live at high altitudes** because of **chronic hypoxia** leading to **carotid body hyperplasia**.

Clinical Features
- Present most commonly in the **5th decade**^Q
- Approximately **10%** have **family history**^Q.
- Patient presents with a **long history** of several years of a **slowly enlarging painless lump** at the **carotid bifurcation**.
- Mass is **firm, rubbery, pulsatile** and is **mobile from side to side** but not up and down
- A **bruit**^Q may also be present

Diagnosis
- Doppler study
- **Carotid angiogram: Lyre sign**^Q (**splaying** of **internal & external** carotid arteries)
- **FNAC & biopsy** are **contraindicated**^Q because of their **highly vascular nature**

Treatment
- Because these tumors **rarely metastasize**^Q and their **overall rate of growth** is **slow**, the need for **surgical removal** must be **considered carefully** as complication of surgery are potentially serious.
- **Operation** is **best avoided in elderly patients**^Q.
- **Preoperative embolization** is performed for tumors >3 cm.
- Tumors >5 cm are associated with a need for **concurrent carotid artery replacement**.

Complications
- Most frequent sequela from resection: Cranial nerve injury (MC-superior laryngeal nerve^Q)
- **First-bite syndrome**^Q: Pain with the **initiation of mastication**
- **Excision of bilateral carotid body tumors** may lead to **baroreceptor failure**, with **wide fluctuations in BP**.

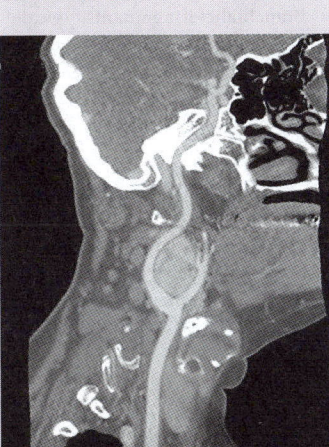

CYSTIC HYGROMA

Cystic Hygroma

- Cystic hygromas are **multiloculated cystic spaces**^Q lined by endothelial cells
- It results due to **sequestration of** a portion of **jugular lymph sac from** the **lymphatic system**^Q.
- Cysts are **filled with clear lymph** and are **lined by endothelium**^Q.
- **Turner's syndrome** is associated with cystic hygroma^Q.
- **Most** cystic hygromas **involve** the **lymphatic jugular sacs**

- MC site: Posterior neck region^Q (Posterior triangle^Q)
- Other common sites: Axilla, mediastinum, inguinal & retroperitoneal regions^Q
- Approximately 50% of them present at birth^Q
- It may show spontaneous regression^Q

Clinical Features

- Usually present as **soft cystic masses** that distort the surrounding anatomy, can result in acute airway obstruction.
- Usually **manifests in** the **neonates** or in **early infancy**^Q (50% present **at birth**).
- Prone to **infection & hemorrhage** within the mass.
- Swelling is **soft & partially compressible** and invariably increases in size when the child coughs or cries.

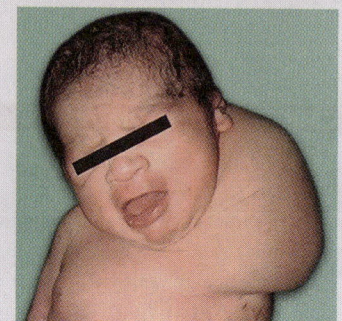

- Characteristic features: Brilliantly translucent^Q

Diagnosis

- IOC for diagnosis: MRI^Q
- MRI play a **crucial role in preoperative planning**^Q

Treatment

- **Complete surgical excision** is the **preferred treatment**^Q.
- **Injection of sclerosing agents**^Q such as **bleomycin** or **OK-432 (Picibanil)**, derived from **Streptococcus pyogenes** may eradicate the cystic hygroma.

BRANCHIAL CLEFT REMNANTS

Branchial Cleft Remnants

- **Branchial cleft remnants** typically present as a **lateral neck mass**^Q on a toddler.
- Structures of the head & neck are derived from **6 pairs of branchial arches**, their intervening **clefts & pouches**.
- **Congenital cysts, sinuses, or fistulas** result from **failure of these structures to regress, persisting in** an **aberrant location**.

- All branchial remnants are **present at the time of birth**; however, they are **often not recognized** until later in life.
- These lesions may present as **sinuses, fistulas, or cartilaginous rests in infants**^Q.
- They occur **more commonly as cysts** in older children and **adolescents**^Q.

- Clinical presentation may range from a continuous mucoid drainage from a fistula or sinus to the development of a **cystic mass**^Q that may become infected.
- **Branchial remnants** may also be palpable as **cartilaginous lumps** or **cords**^Q corresponding with a fistulous tract. Dermal pits or skin tags may also be evident.

Branchial Cleft Remnants

First Branchial Cleft Remnants
- Typically located in the **front** or **back of** the **ear** or in the **upper neck near** the **mandible**^Q.
- **Fistulas** typically **course through** the **parotid gland**, deep or **through branches of the facial nerve, and end in the external auditory canal**^Q.

Second Branchial Cleft Remnants
- **Most common**^Q
- **External ostium** is **located along** the **anterior border** of the **SCM muscle**, in the vicinity of the **upper half to lower third** of the muscle^Q.
- **Stepladder counterincisions** are often necessary to excise the fistula completely^Q.
- Typically, the **fistula penetrates platysma, ascends along** the carotid sheath to the level of hyoid bone, and turns medially to extend between carotid artery bifurcation^Q.
- The fistula then **courses behind** the **posterior belly of digastric** and **stylohyoid muscles** to end in the **tonsillar fossa**^Q.

Third Branchial Cleft Remnants
- Third branchial cleft remnants usually **do not have associated sinuses** or **fistulas**
- Located in the **suprasternal notch** or **clavicular region**^Q.
- Most often contain **cartilage**^Q
- **Present** clinically as a **firm mass** or **subcutaneous abscess**^Q.

BRANCHIAL ABNORMALITIES

Branchial Abnormalities

Branchial Cyst
- Develops from **vestigial remnants of 2nd branchial cleft**[Q]
- Lined by **squamous epithelium**[Q]
- Contains **thick, turbid fluid** full of **cholesterol crystals**[Q].
- Cyst usually **presents in** the **upper neck** in **early or middle adulthood**[Q]
- Found at the **junction of upper third & middle third** of the **SCM muscle** at its **anterior border**[Q].
- **Fluctuant swelling** that may transilluminate and is often **soft** in its early stages[Q].
- **USG** and **FNAC** aid diagnosis
- **Treatment** is by **complete excision**[Q]

Branchial Fistula
- Branchial fistula may be **unilateral** or **bilateral**[Q]
- Thought to represent a **persistent 2nd branchial cleft**[Q].
- Tract is **lined by ciliated columnar epithelium**[Q]
- There may be a small amount of **recurrent mucous** or **mucopurulent discharge** onto the neck[Q].
- **External orifice** is nearly **always** situated in the **lower third** of the **neck** near anterior border of SCM[Q]
- **Internal orifice** is located on the **anterior aspect** of **posterior faucial pillar** just behind the **tonsil**[Q].
- **Internal aspect** of the tract **may end blindly** at or close to the lateral pharyngeal wall, **constituting a sinus rather than a fistula**.
- The **tract follows the same path** as a branchial cyst and **requires complete excision**, often by **more than one transverse incision** in the neck[Q].

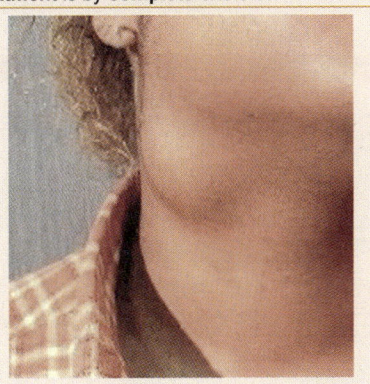 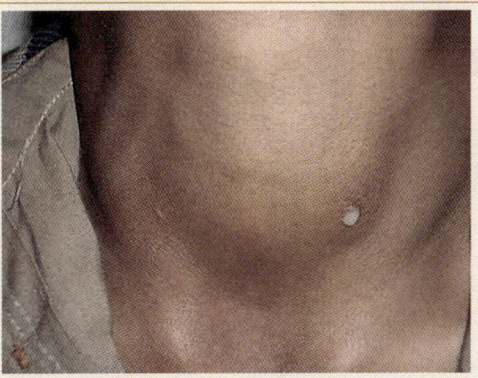

CERVICAL RIB

CERVICAL RIB

- Rib arising from 7th cervical vertebra[Q]
- MC on right side[Q]

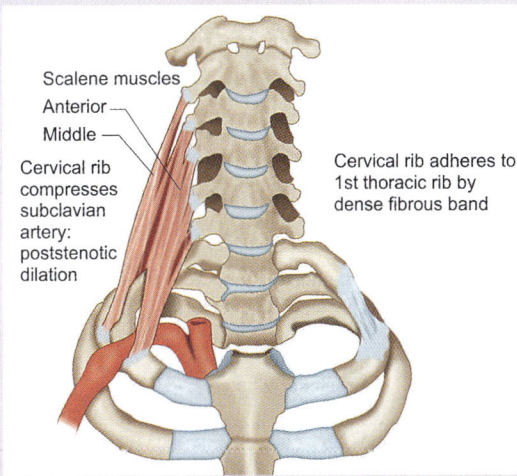 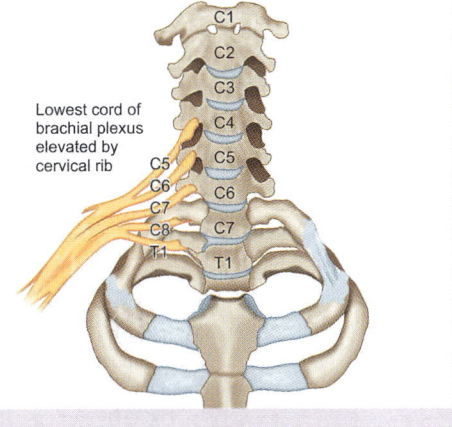

Types:
1. **Complete:** Reaches **up to 1st thoracic rib**[Q]
2. **Bulbous end:** Has a **bulbous end**
3. **Tapering end:** Rib **tapers**
4. **Fibrous band:** Rib is represented by thick fibrous band

Clinical Features
- Cervical rib with **local symptoms: Lump & tenderness** in supraclavicular fossa[Q]
- Cervical rib with **vascular symptoms: Pain, pallor & pulselessness**[Q]
- Cervical rib with **nerve pressure symptoms: Pain & paraesthesia** along medial aspect of forearm & hand[Q]

Diagnosis
- Diagnosed by **X-ray of neck**[Q]

Treatment
- **Mild cases:** Sling exercise
- **In severe cases:** Scalenotomy (resection of scalenus anterior muscles)
- **In troublesome cases:** Removal of cervical rib[Q]

CERVICAL LYMPH NODES

CERVICAL LYMPH NODES

- **Cervical lymphatic nodal basins** contain 50-70 lymph nodes per side
- **Virchow or left supraclavicular nodes** are included in **level IV**[Q].
- Divided into seven levels

Level	Lymph Node
IA	• **Submental**[Q]
IB	• **Submandibular**[Q]
II	• **Upper**[Q] jugular
III	• **Middle**[Q] jugular
IV	• **Lower**[Q] jugular
V	• **Posterior triangular**[Q]
VI	• **Anterior compartmental or central**[Q]
VII	• **Superior mediastinal**[Q]

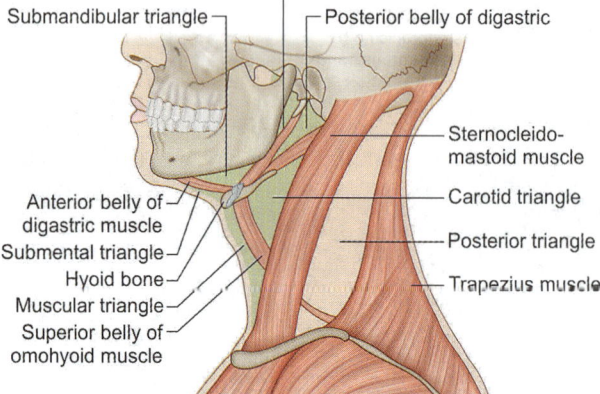

Cervical lymph node levels

NECK DISSECTION

Neck Dissection

Comprehensive Neck Dissection
- **Radical Neck Dissection**: Removal of lymph nodes **I-V** + **spinal accessory nerve** + **internal jugular vein** + **sternocleidomastoid muscle**^{Q}
- **Extended Radical Neck Dissection**: Radical Neck Dissection + removal of **one or more groups** of lymph nodes, **non-lymphatic structures** or both
- **Bilateral Radical Neck Dissection**
- **Modified Radical Neck Dissection**: Removal of level **I-V lymph nodes** with- (Mnemonic: **SISm**)
  - **Type I**: preserves only **spinal accessory nerve**^{Q}
  - **Type II**: preserves both **spinal accessory nerve** and **internal jugular vein**^{Q}
  - **Type III**: preserves **spinal accessory nerve, internal jugular vein** and **sternocleidomastoid muscle**^{Q} (**Functional neck dissection**^{Q})

Selective Neck Dissection
- **Supraomohyoid Neck Dissection**: Removal of level **I-III** LNs^Q
- **Extended supraomohyoid Neck Dissection**: Removal of level **I-IV** LNs^Q
- **Posterolateral Neck Dissection**: Removal of level **II-V** LNs + **suboccipital** LNs + **retroauricular** LNs
- **Lateral Neck Dissection**: Removal of level **II-V** LNs + **internal jugular vein**
- **Central Compartment Neck Dissection**: Removal of level **VI** LNs

CARCINOMA LARYNX

CARCINOMA LARYNX

- More common in **males**^{Q}, seen in **40-70 years**^{Q}
- **Tobacco**^{Q} and **alcohol**^{Q} are well established risk factor
- **Cigarette smoke**: Benzopyrene and hydrocarbons are carcinogenic in man.
- About 90-95% of laryngeal malignancies are **squamous cell carcinoma**^{Q} with various grades of differentiation.
- **Cordal lesions** are often **well-differentiated**^{Q} while **supraglottic ones** are Anaplastic.

Carcinoma Larynx

Supraglottic Cancer
- Supraglottic cancer is **less frequent than glottic cancer**^{Q}.
- **Nodal metastases occur early**^{Q}, upper and middle jugular nodes are often involved.
- **Bilateral metastases** may be seen in cases of epiglottic cancer.
- **Pain on swallowing is the most frequent initial symptom**^{Q}.
- **Mass** in the neck may be the **first sign**.
- **Hoarseness** is a **late symptom**.
- **Pain** may be **referred to ear** by way of **vagus nerve** and **auricular nerve of Arnold**^{Q}.

Glottic Cancer
- **MC site of CA Larynx**^{Q}.
- Mostly originates from **free edge and upper surface of anterior 1/3rd of true vocal cord**^{Q} followed by middle third 1/3rd.
- Spread locally to anterior commissure than to opposite cord (**conus elasticus** initially **acts as barrier for subglottic spread**^{Q}).
- **Fixation** of vocal cord **indicates spread of disease to thyroaretenoid** muscle and is a **bad prognostic sign**^{Q}.
- As vocal cord **is free of lymphatics, nodal metastases** is **never seen in cordal cancer**^{Q}, unless the disease spread beyond membranous cord.
- **Hoarseness is MC and the earliest symptom**^{Q} because of this glottic cancer is **detected early**.

Subglottic Cancer
- **Least common site**^{Q}.
- Subglottic region extends from glottic area to lower border of cricoid cartilage.
- Spreads locally around anterior wall to opposite side or downwards to trachea, upward spread to vocal cord is late and **hoarseness is not an early symptom**^{Q}.
- Lymphatic metastases to prelaryngeal, pretracheal (**Delphian node**^{Q}) and lower jugular nodes.
- **Earliest** and **most prominent symptom is stridor**^{Q}, but it appears only in advanced stage.
- **Hoarseness** is **late feature**.

Treatment of CA Larynx

Stage	Site	Treatment
T_1	All site	• External beam radiotherapy^Q
T_2	Glottic and Subglottic lesion Supraglottic lesion	• Radiotherapy^Q • Supraglottic laryngectomy^Q
T_3 and T_4	All sites	• **Total laryngectomy with neck dissection**^{Q} for clinically positive nodes with postoperative radiotherapy if nodes are not palpable

NASOPHARYNGEAL CARCINOMA

Nasopharyngeal Carcinoma

- Nasopharyngeal cancer is **most common in China** particularly in **southern states** and **Taiwan**^{Q}.
- People in **Southern China, Taiwan and Indonesia** are more prone to this cancer^Q.
- **MC tumor** to produce **cervical LN metastasis**^{Q}
- **MC tumor** responsible for **secondaries in the neck** with **no obvious primary malignancy**^{Q}

> - **Burning of incense** or **wood (Polycyclic hydrocarbon)**, use of **preserved salted fish (Nitosamines)** along with **vitamin C deficient diet** (vitamin C blocks nitrosification of amines and is thus protective) may be other factors operative in China^Q.

Etiology

- Exact etiology is not known. The **factors responsible are**:
  - **Genetic**: Chinese
  - **Viral**: Epstein-Barr virus^Q
  - **Environmental**: Air pollution, smoking of tobacco and opium, nitrosamines from dry salted fish, smoke from burning of incense and wood

Pathology

- **Squamous cell carcinoma**^{Q} in various grades of its differentiation or its variants as transitional cell carcinoma and **lymphoepithelioma**, is the most common.

> - **MC site of origin**: Fossa of Rosenmuller in the lateral wall of **Nasopharynx**^{Q}.
> - **LN involvement** is **common** because of **rich lymphatic network in** the **nasopharynx**^{Q}.

Clinical Features

- **Age**: It is mostly seen in **fifth to seventh decades** but may involve younger age groups.
- **Sex**: **Males** are three times more prone than females.
- **Cervical lymphadenopathy** is MC presenting symptom (60-90%)^Q.

> - **Nasal**: Nasal obstruction, nasal discharge, denasal speech (rhinolalia clausa) and epistaxis.^{Q}
> - **Otologic**: Due to obstruction of Eustachian tube, there is conductive hearing loss, serous or suppurative otitis media.^{Q}

- Presence of **unilateral serous otitis media** in an **adult** should raise suspicion of nasopharyngeal growth.
- Involvement of **IX, X and XI cranial nerves** may occur, constituting **jugular foramen syndrome**.

> - Can cause **conductive deafness** (Eustachian tube blockage), **ipsilateral temporoparietal neuralgia** (involvement of CN V) and **palatal paralysis** (CN X)-collectively called **Trotter's triad**.

- **Cervical nodal metastases** may be the **only manifestation** of **nasopharyngeal cancer**^{Q}.
- **Nodal metastases** are seen **in 75%** of the patients, when first seen, **about half of them** with **bilateral nodes**.
- **Distant metastases** involve **bone, lung, liver** and other sites.

> - **Jaccods's triad**: Ipsilateral **ophthalmoplegia** + **Amaurosis** + Ipsilateral **neuralgia**^{Q}

Diagnosis

- **CT scan**: Demonstrate **erosion of bone** at the base of skull and the **extent of tumor**.
- **Biopsy** is **essential** to show the **exact histology** of the malignancy.

> - In **absence of nasopharyngeal lesion** but with **strong suspicion of malignancy, nasopharynx** is **exposed by transpalatal approach** and a **strip of mucosa** and **submucosa** from the region of **fossa of Rosenmuller** should be **taken** and subjected to **histology**.

Treatment

- **Irradiation**^{Q} is treatment of choice.
- **Chemotherapy** for stage **III** and **IV** cancers

Multiple Choice Questions

CAROTID BODY TUMOR

1. **True about carotid body tumour is:** *(UPPG 2010)*
   a. Origin from non chromaffin tissue
   b. Most commonly is seen with people live at high altitude
   c. Family history positive
   d. FNAC is diagnostic
   e. Painful non mobile lump in the neck

2. **A 40-years old patient is suffering from carotid body tumor. Which of the following is the best choice of treatment for him?** *(AIIMS Nov 2004)*
   a. Excision of tumor
   b. Radiotherapy
   c. Chemotherapy
   d. Carotid artery ligation both proximal and distal to the tumor

3. **A 60-year-old male presented with painless, compressible swelling in right side of neck. What is the diagnosis on the basis of given image findings?**
   a. Branchial cyst
   b. Cystic hygroma
   c. Chemodectoma
   d. Branchial fistula

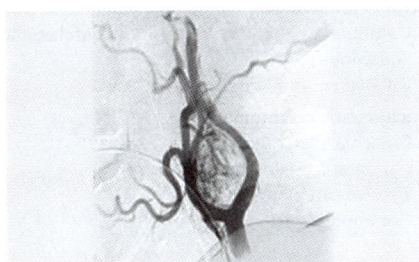

4. **True statement about carotid body tumor is:** *(PGI June 2002)*
   a. Non-chromaffin paraganglioma
   b. Good prognosis
   c. Rarely metastasizes
   d. Similar to mixed parotid tumor

5. **True about carotid body tumour is:** *(DPG 2006)*
   a. Arises from Schwann cell
   b. Causes hypertension
   c. Arises from endothelial cell
   d. None of the above

6. **Main problem associated with carotid body tumor operation is:** *(MHPGMCET 2001)*
   a. The tumor blends with jugular vein
   b. The tumor blends with bifurcation of carotid artery
   c. Recurrence
   d. Vasovagal shock

7. **Which one is not true regarding carotid body tumour?**
   a. Unilateral *(Recent Question 2016, AIIMS June 97)*
   b. Surgical resection is the treatment
   c. Non-chromaffin paraganglioma
   d. Middle age group is affected

8. **Carotid body tumor most commonly presents at:** *(Recent Question 2015)*
   a. 20-30 years
   b. 40-50 years
   c. 60-70 years
   d. Early childhood

CYSTIC HYGROMA

9. **Cystic hygroma may be associated with:** *(MCI March 2005)*
   a. Turner's syndrome
   b. Klinefelter's syndrome
   c. Down's syndrome
   d. All of the above

10. **Brilliantly translucent swelling in the neck region in a 2 years child diagnosis is:** *(UPPG 2009)*
    a. Lipoma
    b. Teratoma
    c. Cystic hygroma
    d. Thyroglossal cyst

11. **This is the image of a newborn baby. The swelling is:**
    a. Transilluminant
    b. Brilliantly transilluminant
    c. Translucent
    d. Brilliantly translucent

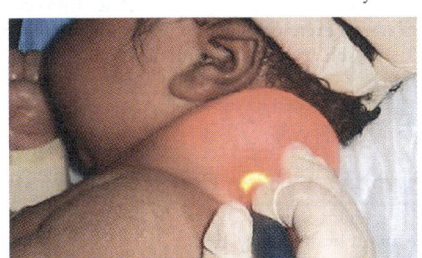

12. **Which is incorrect about cystic hygroma?** *(APPG 2008)*
    a. Brilliantly translucent
    b. Radiotherapy
    c. Sclerotherapy with bleomycin
    d. Sclerotherapy with actinomycin

13. **All are true about cystic hygroma except:** *(AMU 95, DPG 2010)*
    a. Pulsatile
    b. May cause respiratory obstruction
    c. Common in neck
    d. Present in birth

14. **True about cystic hygroma:** *(DPG 2008)*
    a. Present in anterior triangle of neck
    b. Sclerosing agents are not useful
    c. Pre-operative MRI is crucial
    d. Surgery is always indicated

15. **Treatment of cystic hygroma includes:** *(PGI May 2011)*
    a. Complete excision
    b. Marsupialization
    c. Repeated aspiration
    d. Injection of sclerosing agents
    e. Observation or regular follow up

16. **Cystic hygroma is known to occur in all except:** *(Karnataka 2005, MHPGMCET 2002)*
    a. Calf
    b. Neck
    c. Axilla
    d. Mediastinum

17. **Treatment of choice for cystic hygroma:**
    a. Percutaneous aspiration *(DNB 2013, MHPGMCET 2007)*
    b. Intralesional sclerosant injection
    c. En-bloc resection
    d. Surgical excision

18. **Which of the following is false regarding cystic hygroma?**
    a. Brilliantly translucent lesion *(MHPGMCET 2008)*
    b. Surgical excision is treatment of choice
    c. Recurrence is common with percutaneous Picibanil therapy
    d. A cystic lesion containing blood filled spaces

19. **True regarding cystic hygroma is:** *(AIIMS Nov 93)*
    a. Non transilluminant
    b. Lined by columnar epithelium
    c. Lined by stratified squamous epithelium
    d. Develops from jugular lymphatic sequestration

20. **All are true about cystic hygroma except:**
    a. Aspiration is diagnostic *(Punjab 2009, PGI Dec 99)*
    b. 50% present at birth
    c. Presents as posterior cervical swelling
    d. Sequestration of lymphatic tissue

21. **Cystic compressible, translucent swelling in the posterior triangle of neck:** *(DNB 2008, All India 89)*
    a. Cystic hygroma
    b. Branchial cyst
    c. Thyroglossal cyst
    d. Dermoid cyst

22. **The following are examples of Retention cysts due to blockade of excretory duct except one which is an example of Distension cyst due to exudation. Which is the one?** *(APPG 2016)*
    a. Cystic hygroma
    b. Sebaceous cyst
    c. Bartholin's cyst
    d. Ranula

BRANCHIAL CYST AND FISTULA

23. **True about branchial cyst:** *(PGI Nov 2011)*
    a. Arise from lower third of sternocleidomastoid
    b. Peak age of presentation is 3rd decade
    c. Cyst wall consists of lymphoid tissue
    d. Fluid contains cholesterol crystal
    e. Lined by squamous epithelium

24. **Most frequent site of branchial cyst is at:** *(MHSSMCET 2005)*
    a. Upper third of posterior border of Sternocleidoma-stoid
    b. Lower third of anterior border of Sternocleidoma-stoid
    c. Upper third of anteromedial border of Sternocleidomastoid
    d. Supraclavicular fossa

25. **True about branchial anomaly:** *(AIIMS Nov 2006)*
    a. Cysts are more common than sinuses
    b. For sinuses surgery is not always indicated
    c. Cysts present with dysphagia and hoarseness of voice
    d. Most commonly due to 2nd branchial remnant

26. **The given swelling develops from the remnant of:**

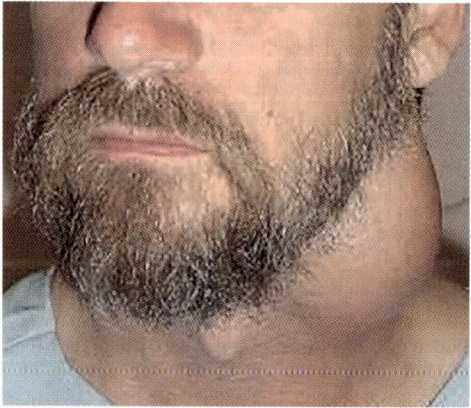

    a. 1st branchial cleft
    b. 2nd branchial cleft
    c. 3rd branchial cleft
    d. 4th branchial cleft

27. **True about branchial cyst:** *(PGI June 2007)*
    a. Seen deep to lower 1/3rd of sternocleidomastoid
    b. Wall consists of lymphoid tissue
    c. Filled with straw colored fluid with cholesterol crystals
    d. Presents at birth

28. **What is true about branchial cyst?** *(DPG 2007)*
    a. Present in anterior triangle of neck
    b. Cauterization is done
    c. Arises from 2nd cleft
    d. Present in lower 3rd of neck

29. **Branchial cyst arises from which branchial cleft?**
    a. First
    b. Second *(MCI Sept 2009)*
    c. Third
    d. Fourth

30. **The commonest site of branchial cysts is:** *(MCI June 2018, All India 94)*
    a. Upper 1/3rd of the SCM
    b. Lower 1/3rd of the SCM
    c. Upper 2/3rd of the SCM
    d. Lower 2/3rd of the SCM

31. **The most common site of the internal opening of a branchial fistula is at the:** *(UPSC 95)*
    a. Lateral nasopharyngeal wall
    b. Fossa of Rosenmuller
    c. Gingivo-labial sulcus
    d. Tonsillar fossa

32. **Commonest treatment of branchial cyst:** *(HPU 2005)*
    a. Cystectomy
    b. Aspiration
    c. Excision
    d. Nothing done

33. **Brachial cyst is lined by:** *(Recent Question 2017)*
    a. Columnar epithelium
    b. Cuboidal epithelium
    c. Squamous epithelium
    d. Ciliated columnar epithelium

34. **Branchiogenic carcinoma:** *(Recent Question 2017)*
    a. Branchial cyst cancer
    b. Carcinoma arising from bronchus
    c. Type of carcinoma lung
    d. Commonly seen in young adults

THYROGLOSSAL CYST AND FISTULA

35. **Excision of the hyoid bone is done in:** *(HPU 2005)*
    a. Branchial cyst
    b. Branchial fistula
    c. Thyroglossal cyst
    d. Sublingual dermoids

36. **Which is never a cause of thyroglossal fistula?**
    a. Infection of thyroglossal cyst
    b. Inadequate removal of thyroglossal cyst
    c. Congenital
    d. None of the above

37. **Thyroglossal fistula develops due to:** *(Kerala 91)*
    a. Developmental anomaly
    b. Injury
    c. Incomplete removal of thyroglossal cyst
    d. Inflammatory disorder

CERVICAL RIB

38. **Regarding cervical rib, which statement is correct?**
    a. It always connects to the scalene tubercle by a fibrous band
    b. It passes through the apex of the supraclavicular triangle
    c. It causes pressure on the ulnar nerve
    d. Pain is often located in the forearm

39. **Adson's test is positive in:** *(Kerala 89)*
    a. Cervical rib
    b. Cervical spondylosis
    c. Cervical fracture
    d. Cervical dislocation

NECK DISSECTION

40. Structures not removed in radical neck dissection: *(PGI June 2007)*
    a. X nerve
    b. XI nerve
    c. Tail of parotid
    d. Parotid and post-auricular nerve

41. Structures preserved in radical neck dissection is: *(Recent Question 2017, All India 2000)*
    a. Vagus nerve
    b. Submandibular gland
    c. Sternocleidomastoid
    d. Internal Jugular Vein

42. Which structure is preserved during modified radical neck dissection? *(DNB 2004)*
    a. Phrenic nerve
    b. Submandibular gland
    c. Sternocleidomastoid
    d. Thoracic duct

43. In post radical neck dissection shoulder syndrome, all are seen except: *(AIIMS Nov 2008)*
    a. Restricted range of movement
    b. Pain
    c. Shoulder drooping
    d. Normal electromyographic finding

44. Modified radical dissection of neck all structures are preserved except: *(UPPG 2010)*
    a. Sternomastoid
    b. External jugular vein
    c. Internal jugular
    d. Spinal accessory

45. Level V cervical nodes includes: *(MCI Sept 2007)*
    a. Upper jugular nodes
    b. Middle jugular nodes
    c. Lower jugular nodes
    d. Posterior triangle nodes

46. In radical neck dissection, which structure is not removed? *(MCI March 2005)*
    a. Cervical group of lymph nodes
    b. Sternocleidomastoid muscle
    c. Internal jugular vein
    d. None of the above

47. Kallu, 60 years old male presented with carcinoma stomach and palpable LN in left supraclavicular region. What is the level of this lymph node?
    a. III
    b. IV
    c. V
    d. VI

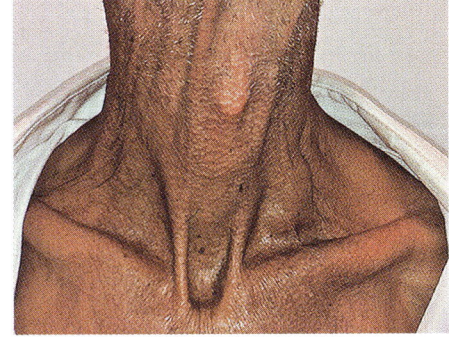

48. Radical neck dissection included all except: *(MHSSMCET 2005)*
    a. Sternocleidomastoid
    b. Accessory nerve
    c. Level III lymph nodes
    d. Jugular vein

49. Posterior triangle LN is what level? *(MHSSMCET 2009)*
    a. Level I
    b. Level II
    c. Level V
    d. Level IV

50. In extended supraomohyoid neck dissection, lymph lode dissection is done up to: *(Recent Question 2016, MHSSMCET 2010)*
    a. 2
    b. 3
    c. 4
    d. 5

51. Structures preserved in modified radical neck dissection: *(PGI May 2011)*
    a. Accessory nerve
    b. Sternocleidomastoid muscle
    c. Submandibular gland
    d. Internal jugular vein
    e. Omohyoid muscle

52. Structures not removed in functional neck dissection is: *(AIIMS Nov 93)*
    a. Carotid artery, vagus nerve
    b. Sternomastoid muscle, internal jugular vein
    c. Spinal accessory nerve, submandibular salivary gland
    d. Neck nodes

53. Structures preserved in functional radical dissection of the neck: *(Recent Question 2017)*
    a. Internal jugular vein
    b. Sternomastoid
    c. Lymph nodes
    d. Accessory nerve

54. Radical dissection of neck includes all except: *(Recent Question 2017)*
    a. Cervical lymph nodes
    b. Sternocleidomastoid
    c. Phrenic nerves
    d. Internal jugular vein

55. A nerve injured in radical neck dissection leads to loss of sensation in medial side of the arm, nerve injured is:
    a. Long thoracic nerve *(DNB 2014)*
    b. Thoracodorsal nerve
    c. Dorsal scapular nerve
    d. Medial cutaneous nerve of arm

56. In MRND type-II, structures preserved are: *(MHCET 2016)*
    a. Spinal accessory nerve + SCM
    b. Spinal accessory nerve + internal jugular vein
    c. SCM + internal Jugular vein
    d. Level I-V LN + SCM

57. Removal of level I, II, III, IV lymph node in neck is called: *(Recent Question 2016)*
    a. Extended supraomohyoid dissection
    b. Supraomohyoid dissection
    c. Anterolateral dissection
    d. Posterolateral dissection

CA LARYNX

58. Precancerous lesion of the larynx include:
    a. Keratosis laryngis
    b. Pachydermia laryngis
    c. Laryngis sicca
    d. Sclerma

CA NASOPHARYNX

59. Trotters triad is seen in: *(Recent Question 2017)*
    a. Angiofibroma
    b. Nasopharyngeal carcinoma
    c. Laryngeal carcinoma
    d. Growth in fossa of Rosenmuller

60. Which of the following is the most common tumour to produce metastasis to cervical lymph nodes? *(UPSC 2008)*
    a. Glottic carcinoma
    b. Nasopharyngeal carcinoma
    c. Carcinoma base of tongue
    d. Carcinoma lip

61. Secondaries in the neck with no obvious primary malignancy is most often due to: *(JIPMER 93)*
    a. CA Stomach
    b. CA Larynx
    c. CA Nasopharynx
    d. CA Thyroid

MISCELLANEOUS

62. True about superior sulcus tumor: *(DPG 2007)*
    a. Anhidrosis in thoracic region
    b. Pain in upper aspect of arm
    c. Flexor atrophy
    d. 2nd and 3rd rib erosion

63. A 30-year-old lady presented with cystic neck swelling as shown in the picture below. What could be the possible diagnosis? *(Recent Question 2019)*

    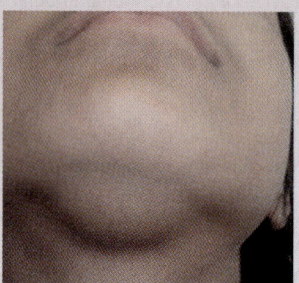

    a. Dermoid cyst
    b. Sebaceous cyst
    c. Branchial cyst
    d. Secondaries neck

64. In which of the following head and neck cancers, is lymph node metastasis least common? *(AIIMS May 2008)*
    a. Tongue
    b. Buccal mucosa
    c. Hard palate
    d. Lower alveolus

65. Blow out carotid is characteristically seen with: *(AIIMS Nov 98)*
    a. Thyroidectomy
    b. Radical neck dissection
    c. Flap necrosis
    d. Sistrunk operation

66. Which of the following does not move on deglutition? *(All India 91)*
    a. Subligual dermoid
    b. Thyroid nodule
    c. Pretracheal lymph node
    d. Thyroglossal cyst

67. An elderly male presents with 4 × 5 cm lump in right neck. FNAC revealed it to be squamous cell carcinoma. No primary was found. A diagnosis of unknown primary was made. According to AJCC system or classification, the TNM staging of tumour would be: *(JIPMER 2014, AIIMS May 2013)*
    a. T1N2M0
    b. T0N2aM1
    c. T1N2cM0
    d. T0N2aMx

Explanations

CAROTID BODY TUMOR

1. b. Most commonly is seen with people live at high altitude; c. Family history positive *(Ref: Sabiston 20/e p810, 19/e p814-815; Schwartz 10/e 678, 849; Bailey 27/e p757; Devita 9/e p772-773)*
2. Ans. a. Excision of tumor
3. Ans. c. Chemodectoma *(Ref: Sabiston 20/e p810; Schwartz 10/e p678; Bailey 27/e p757)*
4. Ans. a. Non-chromaffin paraganglioma; b. Good prognosis; c. Rarely metastasizes
5. Ans. d. None of the above
6. Ans. b. The tumor blends with bifurcation of carotid artery
7. Ans. None
8. Ans. b. 40-50 years

CYSTIC HYGROMA

9. Ans. a. Turner's syndrome *(Ref: Sabiston 20/e p1861, 19/e p1819; Schwartz 10/e 598, 1852; Bailey 27/e p754)*
10. Ans. c. Cystic hygroma
11. Ans. b. Brilliantly transilluminant
12. Ans. b. Radiotherapy
13. Ans. a. Pulsatile
14. Ans. c. Pre-operative MRI is crucial
15. Ans. a. Complete excision, d. Injection of sclerosing agents
16. Ans. a. Calf
17. Ans. d. Surgical excision
18. Ans. d. A cystic lesion containing blood filled spaces
19. Ans. d. Develops from jugular lymphatic sequestration
20. Ans. a. Aspiration is diagnostic
21. Ans. a. Cystic hygroma
22. Ans. a. Cystic hygroma

BRANCHIAL CYST AND FISTULA

23. Ans. b. Peak age of presentation is 3rd decade; c. Cyst wall consists of lymphoid tissue; d. Fluid contains cholesterol crystal; e. Lined by squamous epithelium *(Ref: Sabiston 20/e p1862, 19/e p834; Schwartz 10/e p598,1602; Bailey 27/e p753-754)*
24. Ans. c. Upper third of anteromedial border of Sternocleidomastoid
25. Ans. d. Most commonly due to 2nd branchial remnant *(Ref: Sabiston 20/e p1862, 19/e p834; Schwartz 10/e p598,1602; Bailey 27/e p753-754)*
26. Ans. b. 2nd branchial cleft *(Ref: Sabiston 20/e p1862; Schwartz 10/e p598; Bailey 27/e p753)*

> "**A branchial cyst, thought to develop from the vestigial remnants of the second branchial cleft, is usually lined by squamous epithelium, and contains thick, turbid fluid full of cholesterol crystals. The cyst usually presents in the upper neck in early or middle adulthood and is found at the junction of the upper third and middle third of the sternomastoid muscle at its anterior border.** It is a fluctuant swelling that may transilluminate and is often soft in its early stages so that it may be difficult to palpate."
> -Bailey 27/e p753

27. Ans. b. Wall consists of lymphoid tissue; c. Filled with straw colored fluid with cholesterol crystals
28. Ans. c. Arises from 2nd cleft
29. Ans. b. Second
30. Ans. a. Upper 1/3rd of the SCM
31. Ans. d. Tonsillar fossa
32. Ans. c. Excision
33. Ans. c. Squamous epithelium *(Ref: Sabiston 20/e p1862; Schwartz 10/e p598; Bailey 27/e p753)*
34. Ans. a. Branchial cyst cancer

> "Branchiogenic carcinoma, which is squamous cell carcinoma arising in a branchial cyst, is extremely rare and a highly contentious clinicopathologic entity."

THYROGLOSSAL CYST AND FISTULA

35. Ans. c. Thyroglossal cyst
36. Ans. c. Congenital *(Ref: Sabiston 20/e p1861, 19/e p814; Schwartz 10/e p598,1521-1522,1602; Bailey 27/e p755)*

THYROGLOSSAL FISTULA

- A thyroglossal fistula usually presents as **discharging sinus** in the **midline**[Q] of the neck in the line of thyroid descent.
- It is **never congenital** but **follows infection** or **inadequate removal** of a **thyroglossal cyst**[Q]
- **Acquired condition**[Q]

Clinical Features
- Presentation is with a **fistulous opening near to** the **midline** of the **neck**[Q]
- Fistula may become **infected** & **discharge pus**[Q]

Treatment
- Fistula should be **excised along with** the **thyroglossal tract upto** the **base of** the **tongue.**
- This requires **removing the central (middle one third)** of the **hyoid bone**[Q].

37. Ans. c. Incomplete removal of thyroglossal cyst

CERVICAL RIB

38. Ans. c. It causes pressure on the ulnar nerve; d. Pain is often located in the forearm *(Ref: Sabiston 20/e p1604, 19/e p1595; Bailey 27/e p939, 952, 992)*
39. Ans. a. Cervical rib

NECK DISSECTION

40. Ans. a. X nerve; c. Tail of parotid; d. Parotid and post-auricular nerve *(Ref: Sabiston 20/e p794; Schwartz 10/e p595; Bailey 27/e p758-759; Cancer of the Head and Neck by Suen and Myer 4/e p416-418)*

Radical Neck Dissection	Modified Radical Neck Dissection

• Removal of lymph nodes **I-V + spinal accessory nerve + internal jugular vein + sternocleidomastoid muscle**[Q]	• Removal of level **I-V lymph nodes** with (Mnemonic: **SISm**):
	  – **Type I:** preserves only **spinal accessory nerve**[Q]
	  – **Type II:** preserves both **spinal accessory nerve** and **internal jugular vein**[Q]
	  – **Type III:** preserves **spinal accessory nerve, internal jugular vein and sternocleidomastoid muscle**[Q] (**Functional neck dissection**[Q])

41. Ans. a. Vagus nerve
42. Ans. c. Sternocleidomastoid
43. Ans. d. Normal electromyographic finding *(Ref: Surgical Management of Neck Metastasis by Jack L Gluckman, Jonas T Johnson/53)*

SHOULDER SYNDROME

- In **radical neck dissection**, the **most crippling complication** is the **"Shoulder syndrome"** arising from **denervation** and **atrophy of** the **trapezius** muscle due to **sacrifice of** the **spinal** accessory nerve[Q].

Shoulder syndrome is characterized by
- **Inability to abduct** the shoulder **beyond 90°** cephalad[Q]
- **Long standing pain** in the shoulder[Q]
- **Deformity** of the shoulder girdle (**drooping** of the shoulder with **abduction** and external **rotation**)[Q]

44. Ans. b. External jugular vein
45. Ans. d. Posterior triangle nodes *(Ref: Sabiston 20/e p792; Schwartz 10/e p595-597; Bailey 27/e p728,729,764,800,801)*
46. Ans. d. None of the above
47. Ans. b. IV
48. Ans. None
49. Ans. c. Level V
50. Ans. c. 4 *(Ref: Sabiston 20/e p794; Schwartz 10/e p595; Bailey 27/e p758-759; Cancer of the Head and Neck by Suen and Myer 4/e p416-418)*
51. Ans. a. Accessory nerve; b. Sternocleidomastoid muscle; d. Internal jugular vein
52. Ans. a. Carotid artery, vagus nerve; b. Sternomastoid muscle, internal jugular vein
53. Ans. a. Internal jugular vein; b. Sternomastoid; d. Accessory nerve

54. Ans. c. Phrenic nerves
55. Ans. d. Medial cutaneous nerve of arm *(Ref: Bailey 25/e p733)*
56. Ans. b. Spinal accessory nerve + internal jugular vein
57. Ans. a. Extended supraomohyoid dissection

CA LARYNX

58. Ans. a. Keratosis laryngis; b. Pachydermia laryngis *(Ref: Schwartz 10/e p589-591; Scott-Brown 5/e p106)*

   - **Localized area** of **thickening** of the epithelium which appear as **single** or **multiple chalky white elevations** on the upper surface and edge of one or both the cords usually with **involvement of the membranous portion** are not uncommon.
   - These have been designated as **keratosis**, hyperkeratosis, leukoplakia, **pachydermia laryngis** or by other terms by laryngologist and pathologist.
   - **Laryngeal keratosis** or **pachydermia laryngis** is a **precursor of laryngeal cancer** that **bears great similarity to oral leukoplakia**^{Q}.

CA NASOPHARYNX

59. Ans. b. Nasopharyngeal carcinoma *(Ref: Sabiston 20/e p804-805; Schwartz 10/e p580, 593-594; Bailey 27/e p733-735; Devita 9/e p764-766)*
60. Ans. b. Nasopharyngeal carcinoma
61. Ans. c. CA Nasopharynx

MISCELLANEOUS

62. Ans. d. 2nd and 3rd rib erosion *(Ref: Sabiston 20/e p1591, 1592; Schwartz 10/e p623, 641-642)*
63. Ans. a. Dermoid cyst *(Ref: Sabiston 20/e p1860)*
64. Ans. c. Hard palate *(Ref: Bailey 27/e p764-765; Devita 9/e p750; Cancer of the Head and Neck by Suen and Myer 4/e p288-289)*

   - **LN metastasis** is **most common in: CA tongue**^{Q} >Floor of mouth >Lower alveolus >Buccal mucosa >Upper alveolus >**Hard palate** > Lip^Q.

65. Ans. b. Radical neck dissection *(Ref: www.ajnr.org/content/28/1/181)*

   History of radiation exposure followed by radical neck dissection increases the risk of carotid blowout in head and neck cancers.

   ### CAROTID BLOWOUT

   - Carotid blowout refers to **rupture of** the **carotid** and its **branches**
   - It is **one of the most devastating complications** associated with **therapy for head and neck cancers**^{Q}
     - **Carotid blowout** tends to occur **in head and neck cancer**^{Q}, **radiation induced necrosis**^{Q}, **recurrent tumors**^{Q} or **pharynocutaneous fistulas**^{Q}.
   - The **clinical signs** and **symptoms** related to rupture of carotid artery have been referred as **carotid blowout syndrome**
   - Reported **morbidity** and **mortality rates** are **40%** and **60%** respectively.

66. Ans. a. Sublingual dermoid *(Ref: Schwartz 9/e p1344-1345)*

Structures Moving with Deglutition	
• Thyroid gland^Q	• Pre and paratracheal nodes^Q
• Thyroglossal cyst^Q	• Sub-hyoid bursa^Q

67. Ans. d. T0N2aMx

CHAPTER 38

Facial Injuries and Abnormalities

CLEFT LIP AND CLEFT PALATE

CLEFT LIP AND PALATE

- Clefts of the **lip, alveolus & hard and soft palate** are the **MC congenital abnormalities** of the **orofacial structures**[Q].
- Frequently **occur as isolated deformities** but **can be associated with** other medical conditions, particularly **congenital heart disease**[Q].

  - **Incomplete clefts** affect only a portion of the lip and contain a **bridge of tissue connecting** the **central & lateral lip elements**, referred to as **Simonart's band**[Q].
  - **Cleft lip** is due to **non-fusion of maxillary process** with **medial nasal process**[Q].
  - **Unilateral cleft lip** is associated with **posterior displacement of alar cartilage**[Q].

Incidence
- **Highest incidence** reported for **cleft lip & palate** occurs in the **Indian tribes of Montana**, USA (1:276).
- **Cleft lip/palate** predominates **in males**[Q].
- **Cleft palate alone** appears to be **more common in females**[Q].

  - Incidence of **cleft lip & palate is 1:600 live births**[Q]
  - Incidence of isolated **cleft palate is 1:1000 live births**[Q].

Distribution
- In **unilateral cleft lip** the deformity affects the **left side**[Q] in **60%** of cases.

Typical Distribution of Cleft Types
- Cleft lip alone: 15%
- Cleft lip & palate: 45% (MC)[Q]
- Isolated cleft palate: 40%

Etiology of cleft lip and palate
- **Etiology of cleft lip & palate**: Genetic predisposition & a contributory environmental component[Q].
- **Environmental factors**: Maternal epilepsy[Q] & drugs (steroids, diazepam & phenytoin[Q]).

Associated syndromes
- Although most clefts of the lip and palate occur as an isolated deformity, **Pierre Robin sequence** remains the **most common syndrome**[Q].
- **Other associated syndromes**: **Stickler's** (ophthalmic and musculoskeletal abnormalities), **Shprintzen's** (cardiac anomalies), **Down's, Apert's** and **Treacher-Collins' syndromes**.

Types of Cleft Lip	Types of Cleft Palate
• **Unilateral** cleft lip	• **Incomplete**: Cleft of the **hard palate** remains **attached to** the **nasal septum and vomer**[Q]
• **Bilateral** cleft lip	• **Complete**: Nasal septum and vomer are completely separated from the palatine processes[Q]

Antenatal diagnosis
- All but **isolated cleft palate** can be **diagnosed by ultrasound** after **18 weeks**[Q] gestation

Problems immediately after birth
- Some babies are able to feed normally but **some** will **need assistance**
- **Breathing problems** in **Pierre Robin sequence** may be **life threatening**

Management

- Surgical techniques are aimed at **restoring normal anatomy**.

• Cleft lip	• Repaired between **3 and 6 months** of age[Q]
• Cleft palate	• Repaired between **6 and 18 months** of age[Q]

Principles of Surgery

- **Cleft lip surgery attaches** and **reconnects** the **muscles** around the **oral sphincter**[Q]
- **Cleft palate surgery** aims to **bring together mucosa** and **muscles** with **minimal scarring**[Q]
- **Two-stage procedures** attempt to **minimize dissection**[Q]

Secondary Management

- Following primary surgery, **regular review by** a **multidisciplinary team** is essential[Q].
- Many aspects of cleft care require long-term review: **Hearing, speech, dental development, facial growth**[Q].

LAHSAL SYSTEM OF CLASSIFICATION

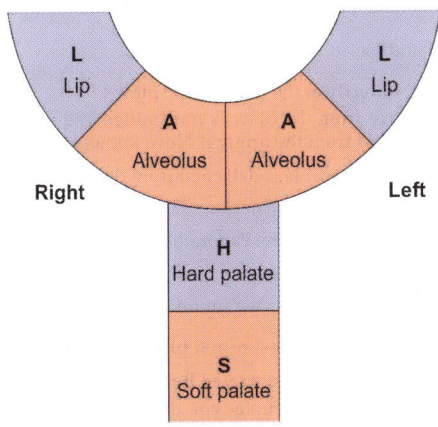

LAHSAL System of Classification

- **LAHSAL system** is a **diagrammatic classification of cleft lip & cleft palate**.
- In this classification system, **mouth is divided into 6 parts**. i.e. LAHSAL
- Right Lip; right Alveolus; Hard palate; Soft palate; left Alveolus; left Lip
- **First character** is for **patients right lip** & **last character** for **patients left lip**
- **Complete cleft** is indicated with a **capital letter** & an **incomplete cleft** with **small letter**.
- **No cleft** is represented with a **dot**.

Examples of LAHSAL System of Classification	
Bilateral complete cleft lip & palate	LAHSAL
Left complete cleft lip	L
Right incomplete cleft lip & alveolus	la....
Incomplete hard palate, complete soft palate defect	..hS..

CLEFT LIP REPAIR TECHNIQUES

Cleft Lip Repair Techniques

- Millard Rotation Advancement Technique: Most widely used[Q]
- Le Muserier[Q]
- Thompson[Q]
- Tennison-Rendall[Q]

TIMING OF PROCEDURES FOR CLEFT LIP AND CLEFT PALATE

Timing of Primary Cleft Lip and Palate Procedures (After Delaire)

Cleft lip alone	Cleft palate alone	Cleft lip and palate

• **Unilateral** (one side): One operation at **5-6 months**
• **Bilateral** (both sides): One operation at **4-5 months**
	• **Soft palate only**: One operation at **6 months**Q
	• **Soft and hard palate**: Two operations
	  – Soft palate at **6 months**Q
	  – Hard palate at **15-18** months
		• **Unilateral**: Two operations
		• Cleft lip and **soft palate** at **5-6 months**
		• **Hard palate** and **gum pad** with or without lip revision at **15-18 months**
		• **Bilateral**: Two operations
		  – **Cleft lip** and **soft palate** at **4-5 months**
		  – **Hard palate** and **gum pad** with or without lip revision at **15-18 months**

MANDIBULAR FRACTURE

Fractures of the Mandible

- **Condylar neck**Q is the **weakest part** of the mandible and MC site of fractureQ

  - Mandible may fracture directly at the **point of** the **blow**Q
  - **Indirectly** where the **force from** the **blow is transmitted** and the **mandible fractures at a point of weakness distant from the original blow**, known as **'guardsman' fracture**Q.

- **'Butterfly' fracture** of the mandible: A **segment of mandible** is **detached from** the **rest of** the **mandible** in the canine regionsQ.

Diagnosis

- Recommended radiographic evaluation of a **mandible fracture**: **Panoramic radiograph (Panorex)** and **Towne's view X-ray**Q.

Treatment

- As in midface fractures, **restoration of dental occlusion** forms the **foundation for fracture management**Q.

  - **Intermaxillary fixation before fracture exposure** and **plating is necessary**Q.

- **Condylar** and **subcondylar mandible fractures** are most often **treated by IMF alone**Q.
- **Medical management** of mandibular fractures involves a **purée-type diet, interdental fixation** for several weeks, **1% chlorhexidine** mouth rinses, and **antibiotics**Q.

MIDFACE FRACTURE

Midface Fractures

- **Midface fractures** involving the **maxilla** can be classified by fracture patterns know as **Le Fort I, II, and III**.

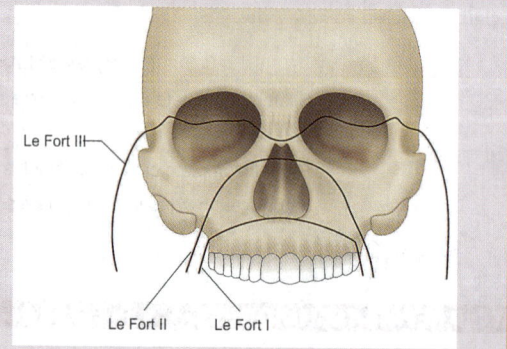

Le Fort I	• **Fracture line runs above and parallel to palate**Q • Effectively **separates alveolus** and **palate** from the **facial skeleton above**Q
Le Fort II	• **Pyramidal** in shapeQ • Passes through the **root of nose, lacrimal bone, floor of orbit, upper part** of **maxillary sinus** and **pterygoid plate**Q • **Orbital floor is always involved**Q
Le Fort III	• **Complete disjunction** of the **facial skeleton** from the **skull base**Q • **Fracture line runs high** through the **nasal bridge, septum** and **ethmoids**, and through the **bones of orbit** to the **frontozygomatic suture**Q.

Management

- **Interdental** or **intermaxillary fixation** is **necessary** to reestablish the **proper dentoskeletal relationships, immobilize the fractured bones**, and **ensure normal postoperative occlusion**Q.

ZYGOMATIC BONE FRACTURE

Zygomatic Bone Fracture

- MC fracture of the **middle third of the face**: **Nose > zygomatic bone**[Q]
- Also known as **Tripod fracture**[Q], because the zygoma is fractured at its 3 processes:
  1. **Zygomatico-frontal** fracture[Q]
  2. **Zygomatico-temporal** fracture[Q]
  3. **Infraorbital** fracture[Q]

Clinical Features of Zygomatic Bone Fracture

- **Flattening** of **malar prominence**[Q]
- **Step-deformity** of infraorbital margin
- **Epistaxis**[Q]
- **Restricted ocular movements** due to entrapment of **inferior rectus muscle**[Q] (may lead to **diplopia**[Q])
- **Anesthesia** in the distribution of **infraorbital nerve**[Q]
- **Oblique palpebral fissure**, due to entrapment of lateral palpebral ligament
- **Periorbital emphysema** due to escape of air from the maxillary sinus

Diagnosis
- **X-ray Water's view**[Q]
- **CT scan**: Best for diagnosis of zygomatic bone fracture[Q]

Treatment
- Only **displaced fractures** require **treatment**[Q]
- **Treatment of choice**: Open reduction and internal fixation[Q]

BLOW OUT FRACTURE OF ORBIT

Blow-out Fractures of the Orbit

- **Direct trauma to** the **globe of the eye** may push it back within the orbit.
- Occur when a **blunt object strikes** the **globe**[Q].
- **Weakest plate of bone**, most commonly the **orbital floor**, fractures, and the **orbital contents herniate down into** the **maxillary antrum**[Q].
- **Tear-drop sign**[Q] is seen

  - **Soft-tissue herniation** lead to **muscular dysfunction**, particularly the **inferior oblique** and **inferior rectus**, leading to **failure of** the eye to rotate upwards.
  - **Enophthalmos** and **diplopia** can follow[Q]
  - **Paraesthesia** in the distribution of the **infraorbital nerve** is an important clue to the blow-out fracture[Q].

Treatment
- Significant **delay in treatment** may be associated with **less success** than early diagnosis and planned treatment.
- **Orbital floor exploration** allows for **release of displaced** or **entrapped soft tissue**, **correcting** any **extra-ocular motility disturbances**[Q].

Multiple Choice Questions

CLEFT LIP AND PALATE

1. True about cleft palate: *(PGI Nov 2010)*
   a. Surgery should be done at 1 year
   b. 50% recover speech after operation
   c. Associated with hearing loss
   d. Associated with cleft lip in 45%

2. Surgical correction in cleft palate primarily aims at all of the following except: *(MCI March 2010)*
   a. Control of regurgitation
   b. To promote normal dentition and facial growth
   c. To get a normal speech
   d. Normal appearance of lips, nose and face

3. Ideal time for cleft lip repair surgery: *(MHPGMCET 2006, JIPMER 97)*
   a. 3-6 weeks
   b. 6-12 weeks
   c. 1-1.5 years
   d. 3-4 years

4. Ideal time for surgery in case of unilateral cleft lip: *(MHPGMCET 2008)*
   a. <3 months
   b. 3 to 6 months
   c. 6 to 9 months
   d. >12 months

5. Unilateral cleft lip is best repaired at: *(Recent Question 2017)*
   a. 4-5 months
   b. 5-6 months
   c. 6-9 months
   d. 9-12 months

6. All are do about submucosal cleft palate except: *(DNB 2012)*
   a. Bifid uvula
   b. Notched hard palate
   c. Lip pits
   d. Zona pellucida

7. Which is the appropriate age for repair of cleft palate? *(All India 98, 94, AIIMS June 98)*
   a. 6 months to 1 year
   b. 12-15 months
   c. At puberty
   d. Just after birth

8. With respect to repair of cleft palate, the soft palate is first repaired, ideal time for which is? *(Recent Question 2016)*
   a. 12 months
   b. 9 months
   c. 6 months
   d. 3 months

9. Commonest type of cleft lip is: *(AIIMS 91)*
   a. Bilateral
   b. Midline
   c. Combined with cleft palate
   d. Unilateral

10. In cleft lip operation all the stitches are removed on: *(Recent Question 2016)*
    a. 2nd day
    b. 4th day
    c. 10th day
    d. 14th day

11. Unilateral clefts are most common on:
    a. Left side
    b. Right side
    c. Median
    d. None of the above

12. The following is the method for operating cleft lip except: *(Recent Question 2016)*
    a. Le Muserier's method
    b. Tennison's method
    c. Millard's method
    d. Wardill's method

13. Cleft lip is due to non fusion of: *(PGI 2001)*
    a. Maxillary process with lateral nasal process
    b. Maxillary process with medial nasal process
    c. Maxillary process with mandibular process
    d. All of the above

14. Unilateral cleft lip is associated with: *(PGI 99)*
    a. Posterior displacement of alar cartilage
    b. Columella elongated
    c. Always cleft palate
    d. Defective sucking

15. Most common congenital anomaly of the face is:
    a. Cleft lip alone *(MCI March 2008)*
    b. Isolated cleft palate
    c. Cleft lip and cleft palate
    d. All have equal incidence

16. Millards 'Rule of Ten' includes all except: *(AMU 95)*
    a. 10 lbs
    b. 10 weeks of age
    c. 10 gm% hemoglobin
    d. 10 months of age

17. In LAHSHAL terminology for cleft lip and cleft palate, LAHSHAL denotes: *(Recent Question 2013)*
    a. Bilateral cleft palate only
    b. Bilateral cleft lip only
    c. Bilateral cleft lip and palate
    d. No cleft

18. Which of the following is the ideal time for the repair of cleft palate? *(Recent Question 2014, AIIMS November 2014)*
    a. 9-12 months
    b. 18-24 months
    c. 2-3 years
    d. 5-6 years

19. Pierre Robbin's sequence includes: *(PGI Dec 2008)*
    a. Glossoptosis
    b. Airway obstruction
    c. Cleft lip
    d. Micrognathia
    e. Heart anomaly

20. Which one of the following is the primary defect in Pierre Robbin's syndrome? *(UPSC 2006)*
    a. Micrognathia
    b. Glossoptosis
    c. High arched palate
    d. Cleft palate

21. Pierre Robbin's syndrome is:
    a. Cleft palate with syndactyly
    b. Cleft palate with mandibular hypoplasia and respiratory obstruction
    c. Cleft lip with mandibular hypoplasia
    d. Cleft lip

22. Hynes pharyngoplasty is used to improve a child's:
    a. Appearance
    b. Teething
    c. Speech
    d. Feeding

23. Rhinoplasty is usually done at the age (years) of until the nose is fully grown:
    a. 6 years
    b. 12 years
    c. 16 years
    d. 25 years

24. Rhtidectomy operation involves: *(JIPMER 92)*
    a. Correction of nasal defects
    b. Removal of wrinkles in forehead
    c. Straightening of curved penis
    d. Correction of protruding lips

Facial Injuries and Abnormalities

MAXILLOFACIAL INJURY

25. Fracture mandible with edentulous jaw is best treated with:
    a. External fixator *(UPPG 2004)*
    b. Minerva-plaster
    c. Interdental wiring
    d. Intermaxillary elastic traction

26. Most common site of mandible fracture: *(Recent Question 2017)*
    a. Condyle   b. Angle
    c. Ramus   d. Body

27. Best view for mandible is: *(UPPG 2007)*
    a. Antero-posterior   b. Lateral
    c. Oblique   d. Orthopentomogram

28. A man sustained injury and presented with fluid coming out through nose. What could be the possible fracture? *(MCI March 2007)*
    a. Fracture base of skull   b. Fracture of mandible
    c. Fracture of maxilla   d. None of the above

29. A 20-year-old man is hit on the eye with a ball. On examination there is restriction of lateral and upward gaze and diplopia. There is no obvious visible sign of enophthalmos, the likely diagnosis is:
    a. Zygoma fracture
    b. Maxillary fracture
    c. Blow out fracture of the orbit
    d. Injury to lateral rectus

30. Best treatment of above condition will be:
    a. Do nothing and assurance
    b. Explore the orbit
    c. Ophthalmic exercise to correct diplopia
    d. Reinsertion of lateral rectus muscle

31. Clinical feature of fracture of zygomatic bone include all of the following except: *(All India 97)*
    a. Diplopia   b. Trismus
    c. Bleeding   d. CSF rhinorrhea

32. What is the type of fracture?
    a. Le Fort I   b. Le Fort II
    c. Le Fort III   d. Le Fort IV

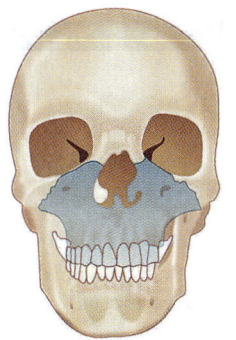

33. Mandible is commonly fractured: *(Recent Question 2016)*
    a. At the neck of the condyle
    b. Through the angle
    c. Through the cannine fossa
    d. At the middle

34. Le Forte II facial fracture implies: *(Recent Question 2016)*
    a. Fracture running through alveolar ridge
    b. Fracture running through midline of the palate and zygomatico maxillary suture
    c. Fracture running through zygomatic process of the maxilla, floor of orbit, root of nose on one side only
    d. Similar to C but on both sides

35. Le-Forte fracture is for: *(Recent Question 2017)*
    a. Facial skeleton   b. Lower limb bone
    c. Spinal injury   d. Pelvis fracture

36. Tripod fracture is seen in: *(DNB 2010)*
    a. Zygomatic bone   b. Temporomandibular joint
    c. Maxilla   d. Frontal bone

37. Costen's syndrome refers to neurological pain associated with: *(DNB 2010)*
    a. Sphenopalatine ganglion
    b. Temporomandibular joint
    c. Glossopharyngeal nerve
    d. Lingual nerve

38. In Kernahan Striped Classification, the main reference point is: *(Recent Question 2018)*
    a. Incisive foramen   b. Soft palate
    c. Hard palate   d. Alveolus

Explanations

CLEFT LIP AND PALATE

1. **Ans. a. Surgery should be done at 1 year, c. Associated with hearing loss, d. Associated with cleft lip in 45%** *(Ref. Sabiston 20/e p1946-1947; Schwartz 10/e p1840-1844; Bailey 27/e p688-700)*
2. **Ans. d. Normal appearance of lips, nose and face** *(Ref. Sabiston 20/e p1947; Schwartz 10/e p1840-1844; Bailey 27/e p692, 25/e p662-668)*

> **OBJECTIVES OF THE CLEFT PALATE REPAIR**
> - To produce **anatomical closure** of the defect^Q.
> - To create an apparatus for **development** and **production** of **normal speech**^{Q}.
> - To **minimize** the **maxillary growth disturbances** and **dento-alveolar deformities**^{Q}.

3. **Ans. b. 6-12 weeks**
4. **Ans. b. 3 to 6 months**
5. **Ans. b. 5-6 months** *(Ref: Sabiston 20/e p1946; Schwartz 10/e p1844; Bailey 27/e p692)*
6. **Ans. c. Lip pits** *(Ref. Cleft Palate and Craniofacial abnormalities by Ann W. Kummer/51)*

> **SUBMUCOSAL CLEFT PALATE**
> - A congenital defect that affects the underlying structure of the palate, while the **oral surface mucosa is intact**
> - Most children with submucosal cleft palate are asymptomatic and this is often not diagnosed until later
> - Identification of submucosal cleft palate requires intraoral examination for:
>   1. Bifid uvula
>   2. **Zona pellucida** (submucosal absence of muscularis uvulae)
>   3. **Notching of posterior border of hard palate**
>   4. **Nasopharyngeal regurgitation during feeding** (only finding of occult submucosal cleft palate)

7. **Ans. a. 6 months to 1 year**
8. **Ans. c. 6 months** *(Ref. Bailey 27/e p692)*
9. **Ans. c. Combined with cleft palate**
10. **Ans. b. 4th day** *(Ref. Sabiston 18/e p2134)*

Guidelines for Day of Suture Removal by Area			
Body Regions	**Removal**	**Body Regions**	**Removal**
Eyelid	3-4	Chest, abdomen	8-10
Eyebrow	3-5	Ear	10-14
Nose	3-5	Back	12-14
Lip	3-4^Q	Extremities	12-14
Face (other)	3-4^Q	Hand	10-14
Scalp	6-8 days	Foot, sole	12-14

11. **Ans. a. Left side**
12. **Ans. d. Wardill's method** *(Ref. Sabiston 20/e p1947; Schwartz 10/e p1840-1844; Bailey 27/e p692)*
13. **Ans. b. Maxillary process with medial nasal process**
14. **Ans. a. Posterior displacement of alar cartilage**
15. **Ans. c. Cleft lip and cleft palate**
16. **Ans. d. 10 months of age**

> **"RULE OF 10s" BY SURGEONS WILHELMMESEN AND MUSGRAVE**
>
> **Surgery is done in cleft lip in a child when**
> - Age ≥10 weeks^Q
> - Weight ≥10 pounds^Q
> - Hemoglobin ≥10 gm^Q

17. **Ans. c. Bilateral cleft lip and palate** *(Ref: Bailey 26/e p637)*

18. **Ans. a. 9-12 months**

19. **Ans. a. Glossoptosis, b. Airway obstruction, d. Micrognathia** *(Ref. Schwartz 10/e p1848; Bailey 27/e p689, 691, 701)*

PIERRE ROBIN SEQUENCE

- **Pierre Robin sequence** remains the **most common syndrome** in clefts of the lip and palate
- **Pierre Robin** sequence is **characterized by three pathognomonic findings**:
  1. Microretrognathia (primary defect)[Q]
  2. Glossoptosis[Q]
  3. Respiratory distress[Q]

> - **Pierre Robin** sequence **may** or **may not be associated with a palatal cleft**[Q].

- **Micrognathia prevents** the **natural caudal migration of** the **tongue** resulting in the deformity[Q].
- Functional consequences include **intermittent respiratory obstruction** and **obstructive sleep apnea** that may **affect feeding, growth**, and **safety of the airway**[Q].

> - **Posteriorly displaced tongue (glossoptosis)**, which is associated with **early respiratory** and **feeding difficulties**[Q].
> - **Treatment: Beverly-Douglas procedure (Tongue is fixed anteriorly**[Q])

20. **Ans. a. Micrognathia**

21. **Ans. b. Cleft palate with mandibular hypoplasia and respiratory obstruction**

22. **Ans. c. Speech** *(Ref. Bailey 25/e p663)*

HYNES PHARYNGOPLASTY

- Used for the treatment of **Velopharyngeal incompetence** leading to **speech problems**[Q]

23. **Ans. c. 16 years** *(Ref. Bailey 27/e p699, 701, 702)*

ORTHOGNATHIC SURGERY

- **Orthognathic surgery** is to correct conditions of the jaw and face related to structure, growth
- Orthognathic surgery is **usually performed** when **facial growth is complete** (16 years in **female patients**, 19 years in **male patients**[Q]).
- It's suggested to get **rhinoplasty** (correcting and reconstructing the form, restoring the functions, and aesthetically enhancing the nose) done after **16 years**[Q] of age, when **natural bone structure** is "settled".

24. **Ans. b. Removal of wrinkles in forehead** *(Ref. Dorland's Dictionary 28/e p1463)*

RHYTIDECTOMY

- A **facelift operation** by **surgical removal of wrinkles**[Q]
- Type of **cosmetic surgery** procedure used to **give a more youthful facial appearance.**

MAXILLOFACIAL INJURY

25. **Ans. a. External fixator** *(Ref. Sabiston 20/e p422; Schwartz 10/e p197; Bailey 27/e p358)*

26. **Ans. a. Condyle** *(Ref. Sabiston 20/e p1949; Schwartz 10/e p1853; Bailey 27/e p358)*

27. **Ans. d. Orthopentomogram**

28. **Ans. a. Fracture base of skull** *(Ref. Sabiston 20/e p420; Schwartz 10/e p576; Bailey 27/e p333)*

BASILAR SKULL FRACTURE

- **Fracture** of **the base of the skull**, typically involving the **temporal** bone, **occipital** bone, **sphenoid bone**, and/or **ethmoid** bone[Q].
- **Such fractures** can cause **tears in the** meninges, with resultant **leakage of** the CSF[Q].

  - **Leaking fluid** may accumulate in the **middle ear space**, and **dribble out through** a **perforated eardrum** (**CSF otorrhea**[Q]) or into the **nasopharynx via** the **eustachian tube**, causing a **salty taste**.
  - **CSF** may also **drip from the nose** (**CSF rhinorrhea**[Q]) in fractures of the **anterior skull base**, yielding a **halo sign**[Q].
  - These signs are **pathognomonic for basilar skull fracture**[Q].

29. Ans. c. Blow out fracture of the orbit *(Ref. Sabiston 20/e p421; Schwartz 10/e p577; Bailey 27/e p677)*
30. Ans. b. Explore the orbit
31. Ans. d. CSF rhinorrhea *(Ref. Sabiston 20/e p421; Schwartz 10/e p577, 1854-1855; Bailey 27/e p359)*
32. Ans. b. Le Fort II *(Ref: Sabiston 20/e p810; Schwartz 10/e p678; Bailey 27/e p757)*
33. Ans. a. At the neck of the condyle
34. Ans. d. Similar to C but on both sides *(Ref. Sabiston 20/e p422; Schwartz 27/e p577; Bailey 27/e p360)*
35. Ans. a. Facial skeleton *(Ref: Schwartz 10/e p577; Bailey 27/e p360)*
36. Ans. a. Zygomatic bone
37. Ans. b. Temporomandibular joint *(Ref. Dhingra 4/e p400)*

COSTEN'S SYNDROME

- **Abnormality of temporomandibular joint due to defective bite**
- Characterized by **otalgia, feeling of blocked ear, tinnitus** and sometimes vertigo
- **Pain also radiates to frontal, parietal and occipital region**

38. Ans. a. Incisive foramen (Ref: Classification in Facial Plastic Surgery By Paul James (2009)/p49

Kernahan Striped Y Classification
• **Incisive foramen** is taken as reference[Q]   • The 'Y' is divided into three sections: **Lip, alveolus & palate**[Q]

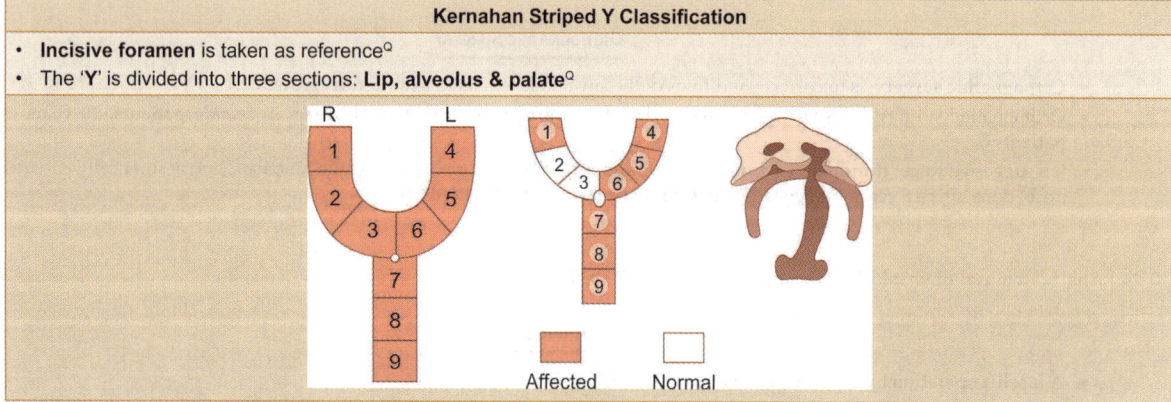

SECTION 9

Oncology

CHAPTERS

- Oncology
- Sarcoma

CHAPTER 39

Oncology

SCREENING IN MALIGNANCY

Well-established Benefit of Screening in			
• Colorectal cancer[Q]	• CA cervix[Q]	• CA oral cavity[Q]	• CA breast[Q]

American Cancer Society Recommendations for Early Detection of Cancer in Average-Risk, Asymptomatic Individuals			
Cancer Site	Population	Test or Procedure	Frequency
• Breast	Women aged ≥ 20 years	• Breast self-examination • Clinical breast examination • Mammography	• **Monthly**, starting at age **20** • **Every 3 years**, ages 20–39; **Annual**, starting at age **40**[Q] • **Annual**, starting at age **40**[Q]
• Colorectal	Men and women aged ≥ 50 years	• Fecal occult blood test (**FOBT**) or fecal immunochemical test (**FIT**) • Flexible sigmoidoscopy[Q] • FOBT and flexible sigmoidoscopy[Q] • Double-contrast barium enema (**DCBE**)[Q] • Colonoscopy[Q]	• **Annual**, starting at age **50**[Q] • **Every 5 years**, starting at age **50** • **Annual FOBT** (or FIT) and **flexible sigmoidoscopy** every **5 years**, starting at age **50**[Q] • DCBE every 5 years, starting at age 50[Q] • Colonoscopy every 10 years[Q], starting at age 50
• Prostate	Men aged ≥50 years	• Digital rectal examination (**DRE**) and prostate-specific antigen (**PSA**) test[Q]	• Offer PSA test and DRE annually, starting at **age 50**, for men who have life expectancy of at least 10 years
• Cervix	Women aged ≥18 years	• Pap test[Q]	• Cervical cancer screening beginning **3 years after first vaginal intercourse**, but no later than age 21 years
• Endometrial	Women at **menopause**	—	• At the time of menopause, women at average risk should be informed about the risks and symptoms of endometrial cancer

SCREENING IMMUNOHISTOCHEMISTRY

Screening Immunohistochemistry

- **Epithelial Markers:** Cytokeratin (positive in **carcinomas**)[Q]
- **Lymphoid Markers:** CD-45 (positive in **lymphoma**)[Q]
- **Melanocytic Markers:** S-100 (positive in **melanoma**)[Q]
- **Mesenchymal Markers:** Vimentin (positive in **sarcoma**)[Q]
- **Neuroendocrine Markers:** Chromagranin and **neuron specific enolase**[Q]

TUMOR MARKERS

Tumor Markers

- Tumor markers are **indicators of cellular, biochemical, molecular, or genetic alterations** by which neoplasia can be recognized[Q].
- These **surrogate measures of** the **biology** of the cancer provide insight into the **clinical behavior** of the tumor[Q].
- This is particularly **useful when** the **cancer is not clinically detectable**[Q].
- The information provided may:
  - Be **diagnostic** and **distinguish benign from malignant disease**[Q]
  - **Correlate with** the amount of tumor present (so-called **tumor burden**[Q])
  - **Allow subtype classification** to more **accurately stage** patients[Q]
  - Be **prognostic**, either by the **presence or absence** of the marker or by its **concentration**[Q]
  - **Guide choice of therapy** and **predict response to therapy**[Q]

Markers	Associated Cancers	Non-neoplastic Conditions
Hormones		
• **Human chorionic gonadotropin** • **Calcitonin** • **Catecholamines**	• **Trophoblastic tumors**[Q], **nonseminomatous** testicular tumors • **Medullary carcinoma**[Q] of thyroid • **Pheochromocytoma**[Q]	• Pregnancy
Oncofetal Antigens		
• Alpha-Fetoprotein • **CEA**	• **Liver**[Q] cell cancer, **nonseminomatous**[Q] germ cell tumor of testis, **lung**[Q] cancer • Adenocarcinoma of the **colon**[Q], **pancreas**[Q], **lung**[Q], **breast**[Q], **ovary**[Q], **prostate**[Q]	• Cirrhosis, hepatitis • Pancreatitis, hepatitis, inflammatory bowel disease, smoking
Isoenzymes		
• Prostatic acid phosphatase • **Neuron-specific enolase** • Lactate dehydrogenase	• Prostate cancer • **Small cell** cancer of lung[Q], **Neuroblastoma**[Q] • Lymphoma, Ewing sarcoma	• Prostatitis, prostatic hypertrophy • Hepatitis, hemolytic anemia, many others
Specific Proteins		
• **Immunoglobulins** • PSA and prostate specific membrane antigen	• **Multiple myeloma**[Q] and other gammopathies • **Prostate cancer**[Q]	• Infection, MGUS • **Prostatitis, prostatic hypertrophy**[Q]
Mucins and Other Glycoproteins		
• CA-125 • CA-19-9 • CD30 • CD25	• **Cancer of ovary**[Q], fallopian tube, **endometrium**[Q], **cervix, breast**[Q], **lung**[Q], **pancreas**[Q] and **colon**[Q] • **Colon**[Q] cancer, **pancreatic**[Q] cancer • **Hodgkin's disease**[Q], anaplastic large cell lymphoma • **Hairy cell leukemia, adult T cell leukemia/lymphoma**[Q]	• **Pregnancy**[Q], **endometriosis**[Q], **PID**[Q], **uterine fibroids**[Q] • **Pancreatitis,** Ulcerative colitis

SENTINEL LYMPH NODE BIOPSY

Sentinel Lymph Node Biopsy

- Sentinel LN: First LN which **receives lymph directly from tumor**[Q]
- **Cabana** demonstrated the **concept of SLN first** in **carcinoma penis**[Q]
- SLN biopsy in carcinoma penis is known as Cabana procedure[Q]
- **SLN biopsy is usually done in: CA breast**[Q]**, CA penis**[Q] **& Malignant melanoma**[Q]
- SLN biopsy is also **applied successfully in cancers of head & neck**[Q] **and vulva**[Q]
- **No special OT is required**[Q]
- Indication of SLN biopsy in breast cancer: Clinically non-palpable axillary LN[Q]
- SLN biopsy is usually **done intra-operatively** by using **isosulphan blue dye**[Q] (1% lymphazurin) or **radioactive (Tc-99 labeled sulphur**[Q]) colloid. Accuracy of detection of SLN biopsy is **best when both** of the methods **are combined**[Q].
- When **radioactive colloid** is used, the **SLN is detected by gamma-camera**[Q]
- **Blue dye colors the afferent lymphatics & SLN, hence aids in the identification**[Q]
- Most of the times >1 SLN in carcinoma breast[Q]

Contraindication of SLN Biopsy in CA Breast		
• Palpable lymphadenopathy[Q]	• Prior axillary surgery, chemotherapy or radiotherapy[Q]	• Multifocal breast cancer[Q]

Complications of SLN Biopsy in CA Breast		
• Skin tattooing[Q] (MC) • Necrosis[Q]	• Urine discoloration • Anaphylaxis	• Intercostobrachial nerve palsy[Q] (MC injured nerve in SLN biopsy)

LYMPH NODE METASTASIS

Important Lymph Nodes	
Rotter's nodes[Q]	• Interpectoral nodes (CA breast)[Q]
Rouvier nodes[Q]	• Retropharyngeal nodes (CA Nasopharynx)[Q]
Delphian nodes[Q]	• Pre-cricoid/Pre-tracheal/Pre-laryngeal lymph nodes[Q]
Irish nodes[Q]	• Nodes in left axilla (CA stomach)[Q]
Sister Mary Joseph nodes[Q]	• Periumbilical metastatic cutaneous nodules
Virchow nodes[Q]	• Left supraclavicular node[Q]
Cloquet node[Q]	• Femoral canal node[Q]
LN of Lund[Q]	• Cystic lymph node[Q]
Krouse lymph node	• Jugular fossa lymph node[Q]

BONE METASTASIS

- MC site of primary for bone metastasis: CA Breast > CA prostate > RCC > CA lung > CA thyroid > CA bladder
- MC cause of osteoblastic secondaries in males: CA Prostate[Q]
- MC cause of osteoblastic secondaries in females: CA Breast[Q]
- MC tumor metastasize to bone in females: CA Breast[Q]
- Lytic expansile metastasis is seen in: RCC follicular carcinoma thyroid
- MC site of bone metastasis: Dorsal spine (Thoracic vertebra[Q])

BONE METASTASIS

- Metastatic tumors of bone are **more common than primary bone tumors**[Q].
- Tumors usually **spread to bone hematogenously**, axial skeleton is seeded **more than appendicular skeleton** partly due to **persistence of red marrow**[Q].

  - In order of decreasing frequency, the **sites most often involved** are **vertebrae (most common)**[Q] >proximal femur >pelvis >ribs > sternum >proximal humerus >skull.
  - **Extremities distal to elbow** and knee are **least commonly involved sites**[Q], but if distal extremity is involved there is **high probability of myeloma**[Q].
  - Metastasis to small bones originate from: Lung, kidney or colon[Q].

- Bone is a **common site of metastasis** for carcinoma of the **prostate, breast, lung, kidney, bladder, thyroid, lymphomas and sarcomas**[Q].
- **Bateson's vertebral plexus** allow cells to enter the vertebral circulation without first passing through the lungs and is responsible for **high rate of prostate cancer metastasis to bone**[Q].

Diagnosis

- **Bone scan is investigation of choice** for bone metastasis[Q].

  - **Purely osteolytic lesions** are **best detected by plain radiography**, but they are not apparent until they are **>1 cm** and have **destroyed 30-50% of bone**[Q].
  - These are associated with **hypercalcemia** and with the **excretion of hydroxyproline** containing peptides[Q].

Treatment

- Treatment options: **Bisphosphonates, corticosteroids, radiotherapy (EBRT) and radionuclides.**
- **EBRT is given in symptomatic bony metastasis**[Q].
- **Samarium-153**, is a **beta emitter**, very effective in **relieving pain of bone metastasis**[Q].

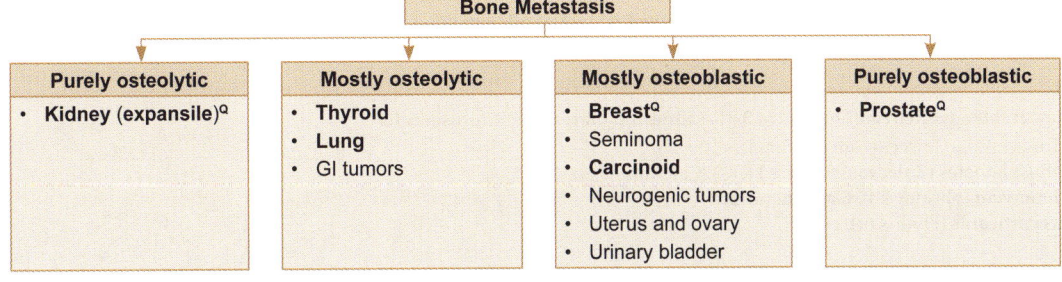

ONCOLOGICAL EMERGENCY

	Oncologic Emergencies	
Structural-obstructive Oncologic Emergencies (Space Occupying Lesion) (PSM HAS Obstruction IN Urine)	**Metabolic or Hormonal Emergencies** (Paraneoplastic Syndromes) (HAS)	**Treatment Related Emergencies** (HT PNH)
• **P**ericardial tamponade^Q • **S**VC syndrome^Q • **M**alignant biliary obstruction • **H**emoptysis • **A**irway obstruction • **S**pinal cord compression^Q • Intestinal **obstruction** • **I**ncreased intracranial pressure • I**n**tracerebral leukocytostasis • **N**eoplastic meningitis • **U**rinary obstruction	• **H**ypercalcemia^Q • **A**drenal insufficiency • **S**IADH	• **H**emolytic-Uremic syndrome • **H**uman antibody infusion reactions • **T**umour lysis syndrome^Q • Ty**p**hlitis^Q • **P**ulmonary infiltrate • **N**eutropenia and infection • **H**emorrhagic cystitis

TUMOR LYSIS SYNDROME

Tumor Lysis Syndrome

- Caused by **destruction of** large number of **rapidly proliferating neoplastic cells**^Q
- Frequently, **acute renal failure** develops as a result of the syndrome^Q.
- **Most frequently associated with** the treatment of **Burkitt's lymphoma, ALL** and other **high grade lymphomas**^Q, **chronic leukemias** and rarely with solid tumors.

Pathophysiology
- **Hyperuricemia:** Due to destruction of malignant cells and rapid turnover of nucleic acid
- **Hyperkalemia:** Due to release of intracellular K leading to arrhythmia.
- **Hyperphosphatemia** and **Hypocalcemia:** Due to **release of intracellular phosphate,** which combines with calcium into bone, **calcium phosphate gets deposited in renal tubules** causing **renal failure**^Q.
- **Lactic acidosis:** Due to **deranged oxidative metabolism**^Q

Characteristic Abnormalities of Tumor Lysis Syndrome	
• Hyperuricemia^Q • Hyperkalemia^Q • Hyperphosphatemia^Q	• Lactic acidosis^Q • Hypocalcemia^Q

Treatment
- **Hydration**, NaHCO$_3$, **Allopurinol, Rasburicase** (recombinant urate oxidase), **Hemodialysis**^Q

HYPERCALCEMIA OF MALIGNANCY

Hypercalcemia of Malignancy

- **Main factor** leading to hypercalcemia is either **increased release of calcium form bone** or **increased calcium reabsorption** from DCT^Q.
- Mostly **underlying cause** is **secretion of PTH-rp**^Q.

Treatment
- **Mainstay of therapy: Rehydration** with a **0.9% saline** and diuresis with **furosemide**^Q
- Other drugs used to lower serum calcium levels:
  - **Bisphosphonates (Zoledronic acid is DOC), Calcitonin**^Q
  - **Mithramycin** (plicamycin), **Gallium nitrate**^Q
  - **Glucocorticoids** (Hydrocortisone)^Q

TYPHLITIS (NEUTROPENIC ENTEROCOLITIS)

Typhlitis (Neutropenic Colitis)

- Also referred to as **necrotizing colitis, ileocecal syndrome** and **cecitis**[Q]
- Classically seen in **neutropenic patients after chemotherapy**[Q] with cytotoxic drugs.
- More common among **children**[Q] than among adults
- More common among patients with **acute myelocytic leukemia** (AML) or **ALL**[Q]

Clinical Features
- Clinical syndrome of **fever** and **right-lower-quadrant tenderness** in an **immunosuppressed host**[Q].
- Associated **diarrhea** (often bloody) is common

Diagnosis
- Diagnosis can be confirmed by the finding of a **thickened cecal wall** on **CT** or **USG**[Q].

Treatment
- Most cases resolve with medical therapy alone[Q].
- Surgical intervention: If there is **no improvement by 24 hours** after start of antibiotic treatment and in **perforation**[Q]

SUPERIOR VENA CAVA SYNDROME

Superior Vena Cava (SVC) Syndrome

- Clinical manifestation of SVC obstruction, with severe reduction in venous return from head, neck and upper extremities.
- MC cause is **Lung cancer (small cell and squamous cell carcinoma)**[Q], alongwith **lymphoma** and **metastatic tumors** responsible for more than 90% of all SVC syndrome.
- In young adults, **malignant lymphoma** is the **leading cause** of SVC syndrome[Q].

Clinical Features
- Patients present with **neck and facial swelling** (especially around the eyes), **dyspnoea**, and **cough**[Q].
- Other symptoms include hoarseness, tongue swelling, headache, nasal congestion, epistaxis, dysphagia, pain, dizziness, syncope.
- Characteristic physical findings are dilated neck veins, increased number of collateral veins covering the anterior chest wall, cyanosis, and edema of the face, arms and chest[Q].

Diagnosis
- Most significant chest radiographic finding is **widening of the superior mediastinum (MC right side)**[Q]
- CT scan: Investigation of choice[Q].

Treatment
- Potentially life threatening complication of **superior mediastinal mass** is **tracheal obstruction**[Q].
- Diuretics with low salt diet, head elevation and oxygen may produce temporary symptomatic relief.

Treatment	Underlying cause
Radiation Therapy[Q]	Non-small cell lung cancer, Metastatic solid tumors
Chemotherapy[Q]	Small cell carcinoma or lymphoma
Surgery[Q]	All other cases

RADIOSENSITIVITY OF TUMORS

Most radiosensitive **ovarian** tumor	• Dysgerminoma[Q]
Most radiosensitive **brain** tumor	• Medulloblastoma[Q]
Most radiosensitive **testicular** tumor	• Seminoma[Q]
Most radiosensitive **lung** tumor	• Small cell CA[Q]
Most radiosensitive **kidney** tumor	• Wilms tumor[Q]
Most radiosensitive **bone** tumor	• Ewing's Sarcoma[Q] and Multiple myeloma[Q]

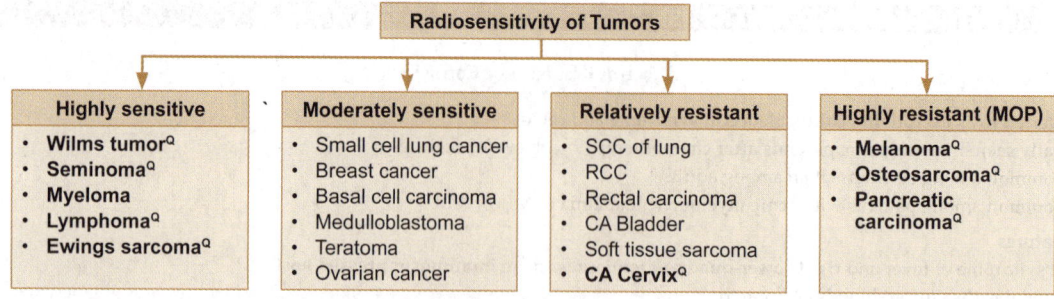

In Radiotherapy

- **Most radiosensitive tissue** of body: **Bone marrow**[Q]
- **Least** radiosensitive tissue of body: **Nervous tissue / Brain**[Q]
- **Most radiosensitive blood cell: Lymphocyte**[Q] (That's why Lymphocytic predominant Hodgkins lymphoma has best prognosis)
- **Least radiosensitive blood cell: Platelet**[Q]
- **Most common organ** to be affected by radiation: **Skin**[Q] (Erythema earliest change, layer most commonly affected stratum basalis)
- Sebaceous gland function does not recover after radiotherapy.
- **Pinna** and **axillae** are common sites of **radionecrosis** i.e. for skin doses.
- Most **radio resistant** organ: **Vagina**
- Most common **mucosa** to be affected by radiation: **Intestinal mucosa**[Q] (Earliest symptom is **diarrhea**)
- **Most sensitive abdominal organ: Kidney**

IONIZING RADIATIONS

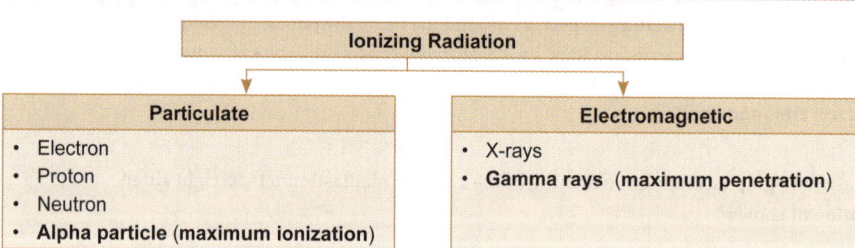

SYSTEMIC RADIONUCLIDES

Systemic Radionuclides

- **Systemic radionuclides** are **non-sealed** radionuclides which are administered orally, intravenously or intracavitary.
- Before administering it, **pregnancy** should be **ruled out**
- **Breastfeeding** should be **discontinued for 1–2 weeks**.

Types	T½ (Days)	Decay Particles	Use
Sodium iodide (I¹³¹)[Q]	8[Q]	Gamma, beta[Q]	**Hyperthyroidism** (diffuse toxic goiter, toxic multinodular goiter, or solitary toxic thyroid nodule), **thyroid carcinoma**[Q]
Sodium phosphate (P³²) Colloidal chromic Phosphate	14.3	Beta[Q]	Myeloproliferative disorders (**Polycythemia** and **thrombocytosis**[Q]) Intra-cavitary therapy of **malignant ascites**, **malignant pleural effusion** and **brain cyst**[Q]
Samarium-153 (Sm) chloride	1.9	Beta[Q]	Painful bone metastases[Q]
Strontium-89 (Sr) chloride	50.5	Beta[Q] Never gamma	Painful bone metastases[Q]
Rhenium (Re)	3.8	Beta and Gamma	Painful bone metastases[Q]

RADIOTHERAPY

RADIOTHERAPY

- **X-rays** and **gamma rays** are the **most common radiations used** to treat cancers.
- X-rays are **generated by linear accelerators**
- Gamma rays are generated **from decay of atomic nuclei** in radio-isotopes like **cobalt**.
- **Cobalt**-60 is a synthetic radioactive isotope of cobalt with a **half-life** of 5.27 years
- **Cobalt-60** is **used only in teletherapy**
- **Radiation energy** is absorbed by tissue causing **ionization** or **excitation**^{Q}, which are responsible for various biological effects.
- Susceptibility of various phases of cell cycle to radiation: $G_2M^Q > G_2 > M > G_1 >$ Early S > Late S Phase^Q.

Phase of Cell Cycle	Comment
$G_2M > G_2$	• **Most sensitive**^{Q} to radiation
End of S phase	• **Most resistant**^{Q} to radiation
G_1	• Radiation exposure leads to **chromosomal aberration**
G_2	• Radiation exposure leads to **chromatid aberration**

Techniques to Reduce the uncertainty due to Respiratory Motion in Radiotherapy

Respiratory gating	Active breathing control	Deep inspiration breath holding technique
• Patient **respiration during radiotherapy** can **cause significant motion of** the **tumor volume,** which can be **mitigated by gating** the **accelerator beam to the patient respiration.**^{Q} • **Respiratory gating** is one of the **latest techniques in radiation therapy** and involves **matching radiation treatment to a patient** own **respiratory pattern.**^{Q} • This approach **decreases possible complications** and **side effects,** while **using higher doses** and **getting better outcomes.**	• Patient nose is clamped • Patient breathes through an ABC apparatus, which simultaneously control radiation dose.	• **Patient** is asked to **hold** the **breath in deep inspiration.** • **Breath hold minimizes tumor motion** • It **expands** the **lung to its maximum volume** putting the **healthy lung tissue out of** the **radiation field**

Radiotherapy

Teletherapy	Brachytherapy	Systemic Therapy
• Beams of **radiation generated at a distance** and **aimed at the tumor** within the patient • **Most commonly used form** of radiation therapy	• **Encapsulated sources** of radiation **implanted directly into** or **adjacent to tumor** tissues	• **Radionuclides targeted** in some fashion **to a site of tumor**

BRACHYTHERAPY

BRACHYTHERAPY

- **Radiation therapy with encapsulated source** of radiation **implanted directly into** or adjacent to **tumor tissue.**
- It is delivered in two ways (1) **Intracavitary implants**^{Q} (2) Interstitial implants
- **Interstitial implantation** is of two types:
  1. **Permanent implants (PGI)**^{Q}: Pd-103^Q, Gold (Au)-198^Q, I-125^Q
  2. **Temporary implants (ICT)**^{Q}: Ir-192^Q, Cs-137^Q (Temporary)
- Normal tissues are spared from radiation injury^Q.

Interstitial implants

Permanent Interstitial Implants (PGI)
- Performed when the **tumor to be treated is inaccessible** making the **removal of radioisotope impossible** or impractical.
- These implants have usually **short half lives**.
- Isotopes used (PGI):
  - Palladium (Pd) 103^Q
  - Gold (Au) 198^Q
  - Iodine 125^Q
- Used in deep seated lesion in **pelvis, abdomen, lung, colorectum**

Temporary Interstitial Implants (ICT)
- Temporary **removable implants** are used in anatomic areas where there is **no body cavity** or **orifice to accept radioactive sources**.
- Isotopes used (ICT):
  - Iridium 192 (MC)^Q
  - Cesium 137^Q (ICT: Iridium cesium temporary)
- Used in **breast** and **chest wall irradiation**, anterior, lateral and posterior wall of **vagina**

INTENSITY MODULATED RADIOTHERAPY

Intensity Modulated Radiation Therapy (IMRT)

- The radiation dose is designed to **conform to the three dimensional (3-D) shape of** the **tumour** by modulation or controlling the intensity of the radiation beams to **focus a higher radiation dose to the tumour** while **minimizing radiation exposure to surrounding normal tissues**^{Q}.

Indications of IMRT
- Prostate cancer^Q
- Pancreatic tumors
- Head and neck cancers
- Primary and metastatic brain tumors
- Liver tumors (HCC and metastasis)

RADIOSENSITIZER AND RADIATION PROTECTOR

Radiotherapy

Radiosensitizer
- Oxygen^Q (most effective Radiosensitizer)
- Metronidazole^Q, misonidazole, tinidazole
- 5-FU^Q (non-hypoxic cell sensitizer)
- Hydroxyurea^Q (non-hypoxic cell sensitizer)
- BUDR and IUDR^Q (non-hypoxic cell sensitizer)
- Cisplatin^Q, paclitaxel, gemcitabine
- Mitomycin^Q, topotecan, vinorelbine
- Dactinomycin (Actinomycin D)^Q

Radiation Protectors
- Amifostine
- IL-1
- GM-CSF

- Hypoxic cells are **resistant** to radiotherapy^Q.
- **Augmentation of oxygen** is the **basis of radiosensitization**^{Q}.

CHEMOTHERAPY

Chemotherapy

Highly Chemosensitive Tumors
- Hodgkin's lymphoma
- Wilms' tumor
- Ewing's sarcoma
- ALL
- Teratoma (testis)
- Embryonal Rhabdomyosarcoma
- Choriocarcinoma

Chemoresistant Tumors
- Melanoma
- SCC of lung
- HCC
- Thyroid carcinoma

Chemotherapy in Cancers of Oral Cavity, Head and Neck

- Adjuvant **chemotherapy** has been reported to **improve the rate of organ preservation** with **no change in overall survival**^{Q}.
- Chemotherapy is often **employed in palliative setting** in patients with **recurrent, unresectable or distant metastases**^{Q}.
- Drugs used: Cisplatin^Q, Methotrexate, 5-FU, Docetaxel and Paclitaxel

  - Cisplatin is the **cornerstone drug** in the modern management of head and neck cancer^Q.
  - Most beneficial is concurrent chemotherapy^Q.

- The addition of **concurrent chemotherapy** (cisplatin) to conventional radiation **significantly improved survival over radiation alone**^{Q}.
- Concurrent chemoradiation protocols have **improved locoregional control** and reduce the **development of distant disease**^{Q}.

Multiple Choice Questions

TUMOR MARKERS

1. The following is a marker of Paget's disease of the mammary gland: *(All India 2007)*
   a. S-100
   b. HMB-45
   c. CEA
   d. Neuron specific enolase

2. In which of the following tumors alpha-feto protein is elevated? *(AIIMS Nov 2005)*
   a. Choriocarcinoma
   b. Neuroblastoma
   c. Hepatocellular carcinoma
   d. Seminoma

3. Which of the following tumor secretes erythropoietin? *(PGI June 2010)*
   a. Pheochromocytoma
   b. Hepatoma
   c. RCC
   d. Adrenal adenoma
   e. Breast cancer

4. Uses of tumor marker are: *(PGI June 2001)*
   a. Screening of a cancer
   b. Follow-up a cancer patient, especially for knowing about recurrence
   c. Confirmation of a diagnosed cancer
   d. For monitoring the treatment of a cancer

5. Erythropoietin secreting tumor: *(PGI June 2001)*
   a. Cerebellar hemangioblastoma
   b. Hepatoma
   c. Renal cell carcinoma
   d. Adrenal adenoma
   e. Fibromyoma of uterus

6. CA-125 is associated with: *(PGI June 2002)*
   a. Colon carcinoma
   b. Breast carcinoma
   c. Ovarian carcinoma
   d. Bronchogenic carcinoma
   e. Pancreatic carcinoma

7. CA-125 is associated with: *(PGI Dec 2007)*
   a. Pregnancy
   b. Breast carcinoma
   c. TB
   d. Endometrial carcinoma
   e. Endometriosis

8. CEA is associated with: *(PGI June 2002)*
   a. Adenocarcinoma of colon
   b. Pancreatic carcinoma
   c. Neuroblastoma
   d. Ovarian carcinoma
   e. Prostatic carcinoma

9. AFP is raised in: *(PGI Dec 2003)*
   a. CA Prostate
   b. HCC
   c. CA Lung
   d. CA Breast
   e. CA Colon

10. Which one of the following is frequent cause of serum alpha-fetoprotein level greater than 10 times the normal upper limit? *(UPSC 2004)*
    a. Seminoma
    b. Metastatic carcinoma of liver
    c. Cirrhosis of liver
    d. Oat cell tumor of lung

11. Which of the following is marker for carcinoma?
    a. Cytokeratin
    b. Vimentin *(All India 2012)*
    c. Calcitonin
    d. CD-45

12. α-fetoprotein increase in all of the following except: *(All India 94)*
    a. Hepatocellular carcinoma
    b. Seminoma of the testes
    c. GI neoplasms
    d. Embryonal cell carcinoma

13. All are recognized tumor markers except: *(PGI Dec 99)*
    a. Beta hCG
    b. Beta-2 microglobulin
    c. Alpha fetoprotein
    d. Acid phosphatase

14. CEA is increased in all *except*: *(AIIMS May 2007)*
    a. Lung cancer
    b. Breast cancer
    c. Colon cancer
    d. Osteogenic sarcoma

15. Regarding CEA-false is: *(AIIMS 97)*
    a. Prognostic indicator
    b. Glycoprotein
    c. Elevated in colorectal carcinoma
    d. Elevated only when there is hepatic metastasis

SCREENING IN MALIGNANCY

16. In which of the following diseases, the overall survival is increased by screening procedure? *(All India 2005)*
    a. Prostate cancer
    b. Lung cancer
    c. Colon cancer
    d. Ovarian cancer

17. Screening increase life span in which of the following carcinoma? *(PGI June 2007)*
    a. Breast
    b. Colon
    c. Prostate
    d. Lung

18. Screening is useful for: *(PGI Nov 2011)*
    a. Carcinoma Lung
    b. Carcinoma Breast
    c. Carcinoma Skin
    d. Carcinoma Cervix
    e. Carcinoma Ovary

19. Least amenable to screening is: *(AIIMS June 94)*
    a. Breast
    b. Cervix
    c. Oral cavity
    d. Lung

LYMPH NODE METASTASIS

20. Which one of the following is the most common tumor to produce metastasis to cervical lymph nodes? *(UPSC 2008, AIIMS June 2002)*
    a. Glottic carcinoma
    b. Nasopharyngeal carcinoma
    c. Carcinoma base of tongue
    d. Carcinoma lip

21. In which of the following head and neck cancers, is lymph node metastasis least common? *(AIIMS May 2008)*
    a. Tongue
    b. Buccal mucosa
    c. Hard palate
    d. Lower alveolus

22. Delphian nodes are: *(COMEDK 2008)*
    a. Pretracheal
    b. Paratracheal
    c. Supraclavicular
    d. Posterior triangle

23. A 55-year-old chronic smoker presents with complaints of hoarseness of voice, and single enlarged painless lymph node in left supraclavicular region. Next step to be done:
    (AIIMS Nov 2000)
    a. CT Scan of chest
    b. Sputum examination for AFB
    c. Laryngoscopy and chest X-ray
    d. Excision biopsy of the node

24. A patient comes with stony hard, painless lymph node in left supraclavicular fossa. A biopsy report states squamous cell carcinoma. What is the diagnosis? *(AIIMS Nov 99)*
    a. Stomach carcinoma   b. Breast carcinoma
    c. Lung carcinoma   d. Pancreatic carcinoma

25. A 65-year-old smoker presents with hoarseness, hemoptysis and a hard painless lump in the left supraclavicular fossa. Which of the following is the most appropriate diagnostic step? *(AIIMS June 2004)*
    a. Undertake an open biopsy of the neck lump
    b. Undertake a radical neck dissection
    c. Do fine needle aspiration cytology
    d. Give a trial of Anti tuberculous therapy

26. Which carcinoma most commonly metastasizes to cervical lymph nodes? *(AIIMS June 93)*
    a. Maxillary sinus   b. Posterior tongue
    c. Cheek   d. Hard palate

27. Lymph node metastasis is a common feature with the following variant of soft tissue sarcoma: *(All India 97)*
    a. Fibrosarcoma   b. Angiosarcoma
    c. Liposarcoma   d. Neurofibrosarcoma

BONE METASTASIS

28. Most common cause of skeletal metastasis is: *(UPPG 2009)*
    a. Kidney   b. Prostate
    c. Breast   d. Thyroid

29. Treatment of bony metastasis is by: *(JIPMER 2011)*
    a. Samarium-153   b. I-131 with tositumumab
    c. P-32   d. Yttrium

30. Best investigation for bone metastasis is:
    (All India 2012, 2011)
    a. MRI   b. CT
    c. Bone scan   d. X-ray

31. Bony metastasis is common with all of the following except:
    (All India 98)
    a. CA breast   b. CA lung
    c. CA testis   d. CA prostate

32. Not true about bone metastasis: *(AIIMS June 98)*
    a. Uncommon distal to elbow and knee
    b. Breast secondary may be osteoblastic
    c. Renal cell carcinoma secondary are expansile
    d. Soft tissue sarcoma causes bony metastasis

33. Secondaries of all following cause osteolytic lesions except:
    (All India 95)
    a. Prostate   b. Kidney
    c. Bronchus   d. Thyroid

34. Expansile lytic osseous metastases are characteristic of primary malignancy of:
    a. Kidney   b. Bronchus
    c. Breast   d. Prostate

35. A malignant tumor of childhood, that metastasizes to bones most often is: *(All India 2006)*
    a. Wilms tumor   b. Neuroblastoma
    c. Adrenal gland tumors
    d. Granulosa cell tumor of ovary

36. All of the following produce osteoblastic secondaries except: *(DNB 2012, All India 94)*
    a. CA Prostate   b. Carcinoid tumors
    c. CA Breast   d. Multiple myeloma

37. Which of the following is rare site for metastasis?
    (SGPGI 2004)
    a. Vertebrae   b. Skull
    c. Pelvis   d. Forearm and leg bones

38. Pulsating tumors include all except: *(PGI 88)*
    a. Bone sarcoma   b. Osteoclastoma
    c. Secondaries from hypernephromas
    d. Secondary from prostate

39. Most common primary of metastatic bone tumor in a male is: *(DNB 2009)*
    a. Lung   b. Liver
    c. Bone   d. Brain

ONCOLOGICAL EMERGENCIES

40. Features of tumor lysis syndrome:
    (PGI May 2011, PGI Dec 2006)
    a. Hyperuricemia   b. Hypercalcemia
    c. Hypophosphatemia   d. Hyperphosphatemia
    e. Hyperkalemia

41. Tumor lysis syndrome is associated with all of the following laboratory feature except: *(DNB 2012, AIIMS Nov 2003)*
    a. Hyperkalemia   b. Hypercalcemia
    c. Hyperuricemia   d. Hyperphosphatemia

42. Tumor lysis syndrome is characterized by all except:
    (AIIMS November 2017)
    a. Hyperuricemia   b. Hypercalcemia
    c. Hyperkalemia   d. Hyperphosphatemia

43. Hypercalcemia associated with malignancy is most often mediated by: *(All India 2005)*
    a. PTH   b. PTH-rp
    c. IL-6   d. Calcitonin

44. Hypercalcemia of malignancy treatment consist of all except:
    (PGI May 2011)
    a. Dexamethasone   b. Saline infusion
    c. Pamidronate   d. Furosemide
    e. Phosphate

45. A patient with leukemia on chemotherapy develops acute lower abdominal pain associated with anemia, thrombocytopenia and leucopenia. Which of the following is clinical diagnosis?
    (All India 2006)
    a. Appendicitis   b. Leukemic colitis
    c. Perforation peritonitis d. Neutropenic colitis

46. Which of the following tumor is most commonly associated with superior vena cava syndrome?
    (Recent Question 2014, WBPG 2012, All India 2011)
    a. Lymphoma
    b. Small cell carcinoma
    c. Non small cell carcinoma
    d. Metastasis

47. A 53 years old patient was admitted complains of dyspnea. On examination he has puffy face with engorged veins over the chest. SVC obstruction is suspected. Chest X-ray shows mediastinal enlargement. What is the next step?
    (AIIMS November 2017)
    a. Total blood count with peripheral smear
    b. CT thorax
    c. Start cyclophosphamide
    d. Urgent referral to RT

48. Which of the following is not an oncological emergency?
    a. Spinal cord compression *(AIIMS June 2003)*
    b. Superior vena cava syndrome
    c. Tumor lysis syndrome
    d. CA cervix stage IIIb with pyometra

LYMPHOMA

49. The commonest site of lymphoma in the gastrointestinal system is: *(COMEDK 2007)*
    a. Small bowel   b. Stomach
    c. Large intestine   d. Esophagus

50. In neuroblastoma the most common presentation is:
    a. Lytic lesion in skull with suture diastasis *(All India 98)*
    b. Lung metastasis
    c. Renal invasion
    d. Secondaries in brain

51. Commonest tumor of lumbar region in children is:
    (AIIMS June 98)
    a. Dermoid cyst   b. Neuroblastoma
    c. Wilms' tumour   d. Appendix

SENTINEL LYMPH NODE BIOPSY

52. Sentinel lymph node biopsy is an important part of the management of which of the following conditions?
    (All India 2002)
    a. Carcinoma prostate   b. Carcinoma breast
    c. Carcinoma lung   d. Carcinoma nasopharynx

53. The given image shows methylene blue being injected in the peritumoral region. Which of the given procedure is being performed? *(AIIMS May 2018)*

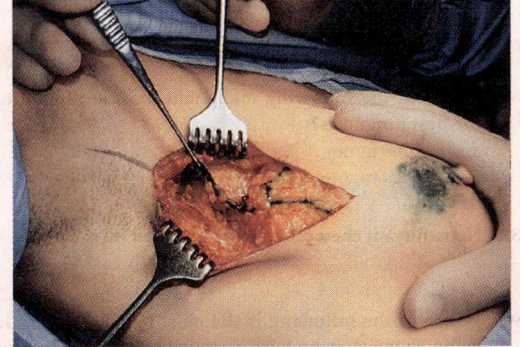

    a. Sentinel lymph node biopsy
    b. Tumor painting
    c. Breast tattooing
    d. Peritumor marking with dye

54. Which of the following technique has been depicted in the image? *(AIIMS November 2018)*

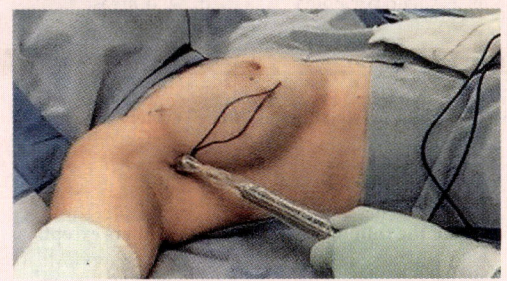

    a. Brachytherapy
    b. USG
    c. Sentinel lymph node biopsy
    d. Lateral pectoral nerve block

55. True about sentinel lymph node biopsy: *(PGI June 2004)*
    a. Special OT is required   b. Blue dyes injected
    c. Contraindicated if axillary LN is involved biopsy
    d. It is done to avoid inadvertent axillary LN biopsy
    e. Radioactive dye is used

56. Sentinel lymph node biopsy is most useful for:
    (AIIMS November 2018)
    a. Carcinoma cervix   b. Carcinoma endometrium
    c. Carcinoma vulva   d. Carcinoma vagina

57. Sentinel lymph node biopsy is done in all except:
    a. CA breast   b. CA penis *(DNB 2012)*
    c. Malignant melanoma   d. CA colon

GI MALIGNANCY

58. Upper GI endoscopy and biopsy from lower esophagus in a 48-year-old lady with chromic heart burn shows presence of columnar epithelium with goblet cells. The feature is most likely consistent with: *(AIIMS June 2003)*
    a. Dysplasia   b. Hyperplasia
    c. Carcinoma in-situ   d. Metaplasia

59. By mucosal resection which carcinoma can be diagnosed early? *(AIIMS June 98)*
    a. Esophageal carcinoma   b. Anal carcinoma
    c. Colon carcinoma   d. Pancreatic carcinoma

60. In which case immunoguided surgery is done?
    (AIIMS June 98)
    a. CA colon   b. CA pancreas
    c. CA jejunum   d. CA anal canal

SPONTANEOUS REGRESSION

61. In which case spontaneous regression is not seen?
    (AIIMS Sept 96, All India 98)
    a. Malignant melanoma   b. Osteosarcoma
    c. Neuroblastoma   d. Choriocarcinoma

62. Spontaneously regressing tumors are: *(PGI June 2006)*
    a. Malignant melanoma   b. Neuroblastoma
    c. Ewing's sarcoma   d. Wilms' tumour

63. Spontaneous regression of malignant tumor is feature of:
    (AIIMS June 93)
    a. Neuroblastoma   b. Renal cell carcinoma
    c. Burkitt's lymphoma   d. Wilms' tumor

64. **Tumor known to regress is:** *(PGI Dec 97)*
   a. Neuroblastoma   b. Retinoblastoma
   c. Adenocarcinoma   d. CA breast

RADIOTHERAPY

65. **Most radio resistant phase in cell cycle:**
   (Recent Question 2014, JIPMER 2011)
   a. G_1 b. Early S
   c. Late S   d. G_2

66. **All of the following are pure beta emitters except:**
   (AIIMS May 2011)
   a. Yttrium-90   b. Phosphorus-32
   c. Strontium-90   d. Samarium-153

67. **All of the following radioisotopes are used as systemic radionuclide, except:** *(All India 2006)*
   a. Phosphorus-32   b. Strontioum-89
   c. Iridium-192   d. Samarium

68. **Phosphorus-32 emits:** *(All India 2006)*
   a. Beta particles   b. Alpha particles
   c. Neutrons   d. X-rays

69. **Which one of the following has the maximum ionization potential?** *(All India 2006)*
   a. Electron   b. Proton
   c. Helium ion   d. Gamma photon

70. **Which of the following malignant tumors is radioresistant?**
   (All India 2006; AIIMS 2007)
   a. Ewing's sarcoma   b. Retinoblastoma
   c. Osteosarcoma   d. Neuroblastoma

71. **The most radiosensitive tumor among the following is:**
   (Recent Question 2014, All India 2006)
   a. Bronchogenic carcinoma   b. Carcinoma parotid
   c. Dysgerminoma   d. Osteogenic sarcoma

72. **Which of the following imaging techniques gives maximum radiation exposure to the patient?** *(All India 2006)*
   a. Chest X-ray   b. MRI
   c. CT scan   e. Bone scan

73. **The technique employed in radiotherapy to counteract the effect of tumor motion due to breathing is known as:**
   a. Arc technique   b. Modulation *(All India 2005)*
   c. Gating   d. Shunting

74. **Which one of the following radioisotope is not used as permanent implant?** *(All India 2005)*
   a. Iodine-125   b. Palladium-103
   c. Gold-198   d. Cesium-137

75. **Which of the following elements is obsolete in radiotherapy?**
   (AIIMS 2009)
   a. Cesium-137   b. Cobalt-60
   c. Radium-226   d. Iridium-192

76. **Craniospinal irradiation is employed in the treatment of:**
   a. Oligodendroglioma   *(KGMC 2011, PGI 2009)*
   b. Pilocytic astrocytoma   c. Mixed oligoastrocytoma
   d. Medulloblastoma   e. Glioblastoma

77. **Which of the following is the most radiosensitive phase of the cell cycle?** *(MHCET 2016, AIIMS Nov 2012, All India 2008, PGI 2009, 2008)*
   a. G_2M b. G_2
   c. S   d. G_1

78. **Amifostine protects all of the following except:**
   (All India 2009)
   a. CNS   b. Salivary glands
   c. Kidneys   d. GIT

79. **Which of the following is the most radiosensitive tumor?**
   a. Ewing's sarcoma *(Recent Question 2014, AIIMS Nov 2005)*
   b. Hodgkin's disease
   c. Carcinoma cervix
   d. Malignant fibrous histiocytoma

80. **Which of the following radioactive isotopes in not used in brachytherapy?** *(AIIMS 2005)*
   a. Iodine-125   b. Iodine-131
   c. Cobalt-60   d. Iridium-192

81. **High energy linear accelerators use:** *(PGI 2006)*
   a. X-rays   b. Gamma-rays
   c. Alpha-rays   d. Infrared-rays
   e. β-rays

82. **Ionizing radiation cause maximum damage in:** *(PGI 2005)*
   a. Hypoxic cells   b. Cells in S phase
   c. Cells in G_2M phase   d. Dividing cells
   e. Neurons

83. **Which radionuclide is commonly used in teletherapy units?**
   (Orissa 2011)
   a. Radium-226   b. Cobalt-60
   c. Caesium-137   d. Iridium-192

84. **The half life of radioactive Cobalt-60 is:** *(Orissa 2011)*
   a. 2.26 years   b. 3.26 years
   c. 5.26 years   d. 7.26 years

85. **Amifostine is:** *(AIIMS May 2012)*
   a. Radiosensitiser   b. Radioprotector
   c. Radiomodifier   d. Radiomimetic

86. **Which of the following is radioprotective agent?**
   a. Cisplatin   *(Recent Question 2016, All India 2012)*
   b. Amifostine
   c. Methotrexate
   d. Colony stimulating factor

87. **For which malignancy, intensity modulated radiotherapy (IMRT) is the most suitable?** *(AIIMS Nov 2005)*
   a. Lung   b. Prostate
   c. Leukemia   d. Stomach

MISCELLANEOUS

88. **Which of the following malignant disease of children has the best prognosis?** *(AIIMS Nov 2003)*
   a. Wilms' tumor   b. Neuroblastoma
   c. Rhabdomyosarcoma
   d. Primitive neuroectodermal tumor

89. **Neoadjuvant chemotherapy is not used in:** *(AIIMS Feb 97)*
   a. CA thyroid   b. CA breast
   c. CA esophagus   d. CA lung

90. **Which of the following is the most beneficial technique of using chemotherapy with a course of radiotherapy in head and neck malignancies?** *(AIIMS Nov 2004)*
   a. Neo adjuvant chemotherapy
   b. Adjuvant chemotherapy
   c. Concurrent chemotherapy
   d. Alternating chemotherapy and radiotherapy

91. What is the name of the given instrument?

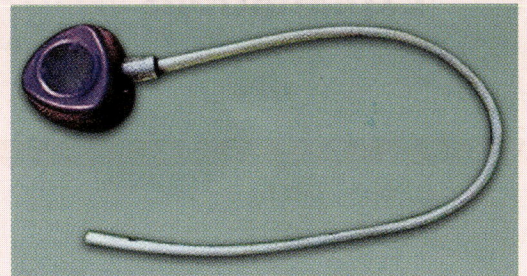

    a. Gamma camera   b. Chemoport
    c. IVC filter   d. Pacemaker

92. Drug of choice for chemotherapy induced vomiting: *(Recent Question 2019)*
    a. Granisetron   b. Prazosin
    c. Clonidine   d. Dimenhydrinate

93. Migratory thrombophlebitis is associated with the following malignancies except: *(AIIMS Nov 2004)*
    a. Lung cancer   b. Prostate cancer
    c. Pancreas cancer   d. Gastro-intestinal cancer

94. Small deposits of neuroendocrine cell hyperplasia in scarred lungs are known as: *(JIPMER 2014)*
    a. Teratoma   b. Tumor let
    c. Carcinoid   d. Hamartoma

95. The most common malignant tumor of adult males in India is: *(All India 2004)*
    a. Oropharyngeal carcinoma
    b. Gastric carcinoma
    c. Colo-rectal carcinoma
    d. Lung cancer

96. Most common cancer in India: *(All India 97)*
    a. CA cervix   b. CA breast
    c. CA lung   d. CA oral cavity

97. Trousseau's sign is seen in all the following except:
    a. CA lung   b. CA Stomach *(All India 94)*
    c. CA Pancreas   d. Liposarcoma

98. Pseudolymphoma is seen in: *(PGI Dec 97)*
    a. Sjogren's syndrome   b. SLE
    c. Mixed connective tissue disease
    d. Behect's syndrome

99. Pancoast tumor is seen with cancer of: *(PGI Dec 99)*
    a. Apical lobe of lung   b. Lingual lobe
    c. Thyroid   d. Pyriform fossa

100. Erythema chronicum migrans is seen in: *(PGI June 99)*
    a. Lyme's disease   b. Glucagonoma
    c. Gastrinoma   d. Pheochromocytoma

101. All of the following are examples of round cell tumor, except: *(AIIMS Nov 2005)*
    a. Neuroblastoma   b. Ewing Sarcoma
    c. Non hodgkin's lymphoma
    d. Osteosarcoma

102. RET proto-oncogene mutation is a hallmark of which of the following tumors?
    a. Medullary carcinoma thyroid
    b. Astrocytoma   c. Paraganglioma
    d. Hurthle cell tumor thyroid

103. All are correctly matched except: *(PGI June 2006)*
    a. BRCA-1: Lung   b. BCL-2: Apoptosis
    c. Chromosome 16: Philadelphia chromosome
    d. APC gene: Colon

104. Adjuvant chemotherapy is of definite value in: *(AIIMS Nov 2006)*
    a. CA colon   b. CA pancreas
    c. CA gallbladder   d. CA esophagus

105. Which of the following tumors are surgically curative?
    a. Pheochromocytoma   b. Insulinoma
    c. Glucagonoma   d. Appendicular carcinoid
    e. All

106. Which is not having underlying malignancy? *(APPG 2008)*
    a. Paget's disease of bone   b. Paget's disease of nipple
    c. Paget's disease of vulva   d. Paget's disease of anal region

107. Glomus tumor is seen in: *(Recent Question 2014, AIIMS Nov 2008)*
    a. Liver   b. Adrenals
    c. Pituitary   d. Finger

108. BRCA-1 gene is located on: *(Recent Question 2014, AIIMS May 2011)*
    a. Chromosome 13   b. Chromosome 11
    c. Chromosome 17   d. Chromosome 22

109. A 24-year-old man presented with retroperitoneal, necrotic, heterogenous enhancing mass on CT near the hilum of the left kidney. What is the most probable diagnosis?
    a. Metastatic germ cell tumor *(AIIMS Nov 2010)*
    b. Metastatic melanoma
    c. Lymphoma
    d. Metastatic transitional cell tumor

110. Octreotide is used in all except: *(AIIMS May 2011)*
    a. Insulinoma   b. Glucagonoma
    c. Glioma   d. Carcinoids

111. Feature(s) of hamartoma is/are: *(PGI Nov 2011)*
    a. Benign   b. Malignant
    c. Malformation   d. Mostly Asymptomatic

112. Most common site of carcinoma in India: *(MHPGMCET 2001)*
    a. Lung   b. Oral cavity
    c. Breast   d. Uterus

113. National Cancer Control Programme (NCCP) launched in India in the year: *(Orissa 2011)*
    a. 1975   b. 1982
    c. 1985   d. 1992

114. Acanthosis nigricans is seen in: *(DNB 2009)*
    a. GI malignancy   b. Lung cancer
    c. Breast cancer   d. All of the above

115. Smoking is a risk factor for all cancer except: *(DNB 2007)*
    a. Esophagus   b. Urinary bladder
    c. Pancreas   d. Gallbladder

116. Most common Non-Hodgkin's lymphoma of orbit:
    a. B cell   b. T cell *(AIIMS May 2013)*
    c. NK cell   d. Plasma cell

117. Most common malignant chest wall tumor: *(Recent Question 2017)*
    a. Chondrosarcoma   b. Osteosarcoma
    c. Synovial sarcoma   d. Rhabdomyosarcoma

118. Reddish firm swelling which bleeds on touch in a 20 years old female is: *(Recent Question 2018)*
    a. Hemangioma'   b. Fibroadenoma
    c. Pyogenic granuloma   d. Lipoma

Explanations

TUMOR MARKERS

1. **Ans. c. CEA** *(Ref: Harrison 20/e p532, 19/e p473; Schwartz 10/e p301-302; Sabiston 20/e p698-702)*
   Paget's disease of nipple is differentiated by superficial spreading melanoma by **CEA positivity**[Q].

2. **Ans. c. Hepatocellular carcinoma**

3. **Ans. b. Hepatoma, c. RCC** *(Ref: Harrison 20/e p666, 19/e p400)*

Erythropoietin Secreting Tumors	
• Renal cell carcinoma[Q]	• Cerebellar hemangioblastoma[Q]
• Hepatocellular carcinoma[Q]	• Massive uterine leiomyoma[Q]

4. **Ans. a. Screening of a cancer, b. Follow up a cancer patient, especially for knowing about recurrence, d. For monitoring the treatment of a cancer** *(Ref: Harrison 20/e p447, 19/e p473; Sabiston 20/e p697-702)*

5. **Ans. a. Cerebellar hemangioblastoma, b. Hepatoma, c. Renal cell carcinoma, e. Fibromyoma of uterus**

6. **Ans. a. Colon carcinoma, b. Breast carcinoma, c. Ovarian carcinoma, d. Bronchogenic carcinoma, e. Pancreatic carcinoma**

7. **Ans. a. Pregnancy, b. Breast carcinoma, d. Endometrial carcinoma, e. Endometriosis**

8. **Ans. a. Adenocarcinoma of colon, b. Pancreatic carcinoma, d. Ovarian carcinoma, e. Prostatic carcinoma**

9. **Ans. b. HCC, c. CA Lung**

10. **Ans. b. Metastatic carcinoma of liver**

11. **Ans. a. Cytokeratin** *(Ref: Robbins 9/e p334)*

12. **Ans. b. Seminoma of the testes**

13. **Ans. None**

14. **Ans. d. Osteogenic sarcoma**

15. **Ans. d. Elevated only when there is hepatic metastasis**

SCREENING IN MALIGNANCY

16. **Ans. c. Colon cancer** *(Ref: Harrison 20/e p449, 19/e p481; Schwartz 10/e p298, 9/e p252; Bailey 27/e p146-147)*

    Schwartz says "Because the **majority of colorectal cancers** are thought to **arise from adenomatous polyps**, preventive measures focus upon identification and removal of these premalignant lesions. In addition, **many cancers** are **asymptomatic** and **screening** may **detect** these **tumors at** an **early** and **curable stage**."

17. **Ans. b Colon**

18. **Ans. b Carcinoma Breast, d. Carcinoma Cervix**

19. **Ans. d. Lung**

LYMPH NODE METASTASIS

20. **Ans. b. Nasopharyngeal carcinoma** *(Ref: Sabiston 20/e p803-805; Schwartz 10/e 580, 593-594; Bailey 27/e p733-735; Devita 9/e p764-766)*

    ### Nasopharyngeal Carcinoma
    - MC tumor to produce **cervical LN metastasis**[Q]
    - MC tumor responsible for **secondaries in the neck** with **no obvious primary malignancy**[Q]

21. **Ans. c. Hard palate** *(Ref: Bailey 27/e p764-765; Devita 9/e p750; Cancer of the Head and Neck by Suen and Myer 4/e p288-289)*

    - **LN metastasis** is **most common in:** CA tongue[Q] >Floor of mouth >Lower alveolus >Buccal mucosa >Upper alveolus >**Hard palate >Lip**[Q].

22. **Ans. a. Pretracheal** *(Ref: Bailey 27/e p800, 801)*

23. **Ans. d. Excision biopsy of the node** *(Ref: Harrison 20/e p412, 19/e p409)*

- Harrison says "In cases of **lymphadenopathy**, if the patient history and physical findings are **suggestive of malignancy**, then a **prompt lymph node biopsy** should be done. FNAC is not of much use, as it does not provide enough tissue to reach a diagnosis."

24. **Ans. c. Lung carcinoma** *(Ref: Harrison 20/e p538, 18/e p738; Sabiston 20/e p1583; Schwartz 10/e 623-645; Devita 9/e p799-812)*

- SCC is a variant of lung cancer, rest three options are most commonly adenocarcinoma.

25. **Ans. a. Undertake an open biopsy of the neck lump**   26. **Ans. b. Posterior tongue**
27. **Ans. b. Angiosarcoma** *(Ref: Harrison 20/e p654, 19/e p119e-2; Sabiston 20/e p766)*

BONE METASTASIS

28. **Ans. c. Breast** *(Ref: Harrison 20/e p471-472, 19/e p119e-4; Devita 9/e p2512-2513; CSDT 12/e p1202; Apley 9/e p216)*
29. **Ans. a. Samarium-153**   30. **Ans. c. Bone scan** *(Ref: Sutton 7/e p1251)*
31. **Ans. c. CA testis**   32. **Ans. d. Soft tissue sarcoma causes bony metastasis**
33. **Ans. a. Prostate**   34. **Ans. a. Kidney**

PULSATING SECONDARIES

- Follicular carcinoma thyroid^Q
- RCC^Q

35. **Ans. b. Neuroblastoma** *(Ref: Schwartz 10/e p678,1639-1640; Sabiston 20/e p1887-1888; Bailey 27/e p847; Harrison 20/e p454, 19/e p618)*

NEUROBLASTOMA

- **Metastasis** is present in **60–70%** of patients **at the time of diagnosis**^{Q}
- **Common sites of metastasis: Long bones (MC)**^{Q}, Liver, Lymph nodes and Skin
- **Lung metastasis** is rare in **neuroblastoma**^{Q}
- Neuroblastoma is the MC extracranial solid tumor in **childhood**^{Q}
- Neuroblastoma is the **2nd MC solid malignancy** of childhood **after brain tumors**^{Q}
- **MC intra abdominal solid tumor** in childhood: **Neuroblastoma**^{Q}

36. **Ans. d. Multiple myeloma**   37. **Ans. d. Forearm and leg bones**
38. **Ans. d. Secondary from prostate**
39. **Ans. a. Lung** *(Ref: Bailey 24/e p1330)*

- "**Prostate, breast** and **lung** primaries account for 80% of all bone metastasis."

ONCOLOGICAL EMERGENCIES

40. **Ans. a. Hyperuricemia, d. Hyperphosphatemia, e. Hyperkalemia**   41. **Ans. b. Hypercalcemia**
42. **Ans. b. Hypercalcemia** *(Ref: Harrison 20/e p519, 19/e p1795; Sabiston 20/e p90; Schwartz 10/e p81)*

"Tumor lysis syndrome (TLS) is characterized by hyperuricemia, hyperkalemia, hyperphosphatemia, and hypocalcemia and is caused by the destruction of a large number of rapidly proliferating neoplastic cells. Acidosis may also develop. Acute renal failure occurs frequently."-Harrison 20/e p519

43. **Ans. b. PTH-rp** *(Ref: Harrison 20/e p663, 19/e p313, 609, 717, 2476, 2477)*   44. **Ans. None**
45. **Ans. d. Neutropenic colitis** *(Ref: Harrison 20/e p521, 19/e p488; Schwartz 10/e 1236, 1241; Bailey 27/e p1307)*
46. **Ans. b. Small cell carcinoma** *(Ref: Harrison 20/e p511, 19/e p1787)*
47. **Ans. b. CT thorax** *(Ref: Harrison 20/e p511, 19/e p1787-1788)*

"Computed tomography (CT) provides the most reliable view of the mediastinal anatomy. The diagnosis of SVCS requires diminished or absent opacification of central venous structures with prominent collateral venous circulation. Magnetic resonance imaging (MRI) has no advantages over CT."- Harrison 20/e p511, 19/e p1788

48. **Ans. d. CA cervix stage IIIb with pyometra** *(Ref: Harrison 20/e p511, 19/e p1787)*

LYMPHOMA

49. Ans. b. Stomach *(Ref: Sabiston 20/e p1278, 19/e p1218-1219; Schwartz 10/e 1259; Bailey 27/e p1140-1141)*

GI LYMPHOMA

- MC site for **lymphoma**[Q] in the **GIT: Stomach >Ileum**
- MC site of **gastric lymphoma: Antrum**[Q]
  - MC type of gastric lymphoma: Diffuse large B-cell lymphoma[Q] (55%) > MALToma (40%)
  - DLBL is MC type of NHL, extranodal lymphoma and GI lymphoma.

50. Ans. a. Lytic lesion in skull with suture diastasis   51. Ans. b. Neuroblastoma

SENTINEL LYMPH NODE BIOPSY

52. Ans. b. Carcinoma breast *(Ref: Harrison 20/e p559, 19/e p497, 103e-3; Schwartz 10/e 305-306, 545-547; Sabiston 20/e p849-851)*
53. Ans. a. Sentinel lymph node biopsy *(Ref: Harrison 20/e p559; Sabiston 20/e p849-851; Schwartz 10/e p305-306)*
54. Ans. c. Sentinel lymph node biopsy *(Ref: Harrison 20/e p559; Sabiston 20/e p849-851; Schwartz 10/e p305-306)*
55. Ans. b. Blue dyes injected
56. Ans. c. Carcinoma vulva *(Ref: Harrison 20/e p559; Sabiston 20/e p849-851; Schwartz 10/e p306-306)*   57. Ans. d. CA colon

GI MALIGNANCY

58. Ans. d. Metaplasia *(Ref: Sabiston 20/e p1050; Schwartz 10/e 1017-1018; Bailey 27/e p1081)*

BARRETT'S ESOPHAGUS

- **Metaplasia** of esophageal **squamous epithelium into columnar** in **distal**[Q] esophagus
- It is consequence of **severe reflux esophagitis**[Q]
- **MC type** of columnar epithelium is **intestinal epithelium (Intestinal metaplasia**[Q])

59. Ans. a. Esophageal carcinoma *(Ref: Schwartz 10/e 1008-1009; Sabiston 20/e p1034-1035)*

ENDOSCOPIC MUCOSAL RESECTION (IN CA ESOPHAGUS)

- EMR provides essential staging information that **guides treatment**[Q].
- It may also be used as a **therapeutic modality for premalignant** and **early malignant conditions**[Q].

60. Ans. a. CA colon *(Ref: www.ncbi.nlm.nih.gov/pubmed/11775180)*

RADIO-IMMUNOGUIDED SURGERY FOR COLORECTAL CANCER

- The **intra-operative detection** of metastatic disease in **colorectal cancer** depends on **tumor-associated antigen** and **antibodies** as well as **detection technology** (A hand-held gamma detecting probe)[Q].

SPONTANEOUS REGRESSION

61. Ans. b. Osteosarcoma *(Ref: Robbins 9/e p477, 1041, 955, 1339, 1149)*

Tumors with Spontaneous Regression (NCR MR)	
• Neuroblastoma[Q]	• Malignant melanoma[Q]
• Choriocarcinoma[Q]	• Retinoblastoma[Q]
• Renal cell carcinoma[Q]	

62. Ans. a. Malignant melanoma, b. Neuroblastoma   63. Ans. a. Neuroblastoma, b. Renal cell carcinoma
64. Ans. a. Neuroblastoma, b. Retinoblastoma

RADIOTHERAPY

65. **Ans. c. Late S** *(Ref: Harrison 19/e p103e-4; Schwartz 10/e 313-314)*
66. **Ans. d. Samarium-153** *(Ref: Harrison 20/e p657, 19/e p103e-4)*

Pure Beta Emitters	
• Strontium (Sr)-90 ^{Q}	• H-3 (Tritium) ^{Q}
• Yttrium (Y)-90 ^{Q}	• Phosphorus (P)-32 ^{Q}

67. **Ans. c. Iridium-192** *(Ref: Principle and Practice of Radiation Oncology (Lippincott) 4/e p637; Harrison 19/e p103e-4)*
68. **Ans. a. Beta particles**
69. **Ans. c. Helium ion** *(Ref: Harrison 19/e p103e-4)*

Alpha particles (**helium ion**) and **low energy neutrons** are **densely ionizing**; X-rays and gamma rays are sparsely ionizing.

70. **Ans. c. Osteosarcoma** *(Ref: Essentials of Radiology by Bhaduri/502)*
71. **Ans. c. Dysgerminoma**   72. **Ans. c. CT scan** *(Ref: Bailey 25/e p130)*

Diagnostic procedure	Typical effective dose (mSv)	Equivalent no. of chest radiographs
Radiographic examinations		
Limbs and joints (except hip)	< 0.01	< 0.5
Chest (single PA film)	**0.02**	**1**
Skull	0.07	3.5
Thoracic spine	0.7	35
Lumbar spine	**1.3**	**65**
Hip	0.3	15
Pelvis	0.7	35
Abdomen	1.0	50
Intravenous urography	**2.5**	**125**
Barium swallow	1.5	75
Barium meal	3	150
Barium follow-through	3	150
Barium enema	**7**	**350**
CT head	**2.3**	**115**
CT chest	**8**	**400**
CT abdomen or pelvis	10	500
Radionuclide studies		
Lung ventilation (133Xe)	0.3	15
Lung perfusion (99mTc)	1	50
Kidney (99mTc)	1	50
Thyroid (99mTc)	**1**	**50**
Bone (99mTc)	**4**	**200**
Dynamic cardiac (99mTc)	6	300
PET head (18F-FDG)	**5**	**250**

73. **Ans. c. Gating** *(Ref: Radiation oncology by Leibe Phillips 2/e p192-192)*

The technique employed in radiotherapy to counteract the effect of tumor motion due to breathing is known as Gating.

74. **Ans. d. Cesium-137** *(Ref: Washington and Lever Principle of Radiotherapy 2/e p326; Harrison 19/e p103e-4, 18/e p691-692)*
    - Cs-137 is not used as permanent implant, it is used as temporary interstitial implant.

75. **Ans. c. Radium-226** *(Ref: Text Book of Radiation Oncology by Leibel Philips 2nd/231)*

RADIUM-226

- **Radium-226 is not used anymore because of:**
    - **Longest half life** among all isotopes
    - Emits **alpha** and **gamma rays,** which is the **most dangerous combination**
    - Produces **radon,** a radioactive inert gas, which is **difficult to remove**

76. Ans. d. Medulloblastoma, e. Glioblastoma *(Ref: Harrison 20/e p648, 19/e p599-602)*

77. Ans. a. G_2M

78. Ans. a. CNS *(Ref: Radiation Oncology 8/e p41; Harrison 19/e p839-840)*

AMIFOSTINE

- Amifostine offers **no protection to CNS**, as it **doesn't cross blood brain barrier**
- Amifostine is a radiation protector
- Amifostine provide **protection against hematologic** and **non-hematologic toxicity of cisplatin** also

Mechanism of action:
- Amifostine **scavenge free radicals** produced by ionizing radiations

Tissue Protected:
- **Gut lining, hematopoietic system** and **salivary glands**

79. Ans. a. Ewing's sarcoma

80. Ans. c. Cobalt-60 *(Ref: Text Book of Radiation Oncology by Leibel Philips 2nd/231)*

81. Ans. a. X-rays *(Ref: Harrison 19/e p103e-4)*

82. Ans. c. Cells in G_2M phase, d. Dividing cells   83. Ans. b. Cobalt-60

84. Ans. c. 5.26 years   85. Ans. b. Radioprotector *(Ref: Radiation Oncology 8/e p41)*

86. Ans. b. Amifostine   87. Ans. b. Prostate *(Ref: Text Book of Radiation Oncology by Leibel Philips 2/e p315, 334)*

MISCELLANEOUS

88. Ans. a. Wilms' tumor *(Ref: CSDT 11/e p1345; CPDT 16/e p807-809)*

- **5-year survival** in **localized Wilms' tumor** of **favorable histology: >97%**

89. Ans. a. CA thyroid *(Ref: Harrison 20/e p2716, 19/e p2303)*
- Thyroid carcinoma is poorly responsive to chemotherapy.

90. Ans. c. Concurrent chemotherapy *(Ref: Bailey 27/e p151, 155; Devita 9/e p749; Cancer of the Head and Neck by Suen and Myer 4/e p291-292)*

91. Ans. b. Chemoport

"Chemoports are totally implantable venous access devices used to facilitate chemotherapy administration. Internal jugular veins and subclavian veins are the commonly used venous access for port placement. These devices are usually retained over a period of 1 to 2 years or more after which the device is explanted. Some of the long-term complications include catheter embolism, catheter or port occlusion, catheter breakage, device rotation, and vascular thrombosis."

92. Ans. a. Granisetron *(Ref: Harrison 20/e p256)*

"5-HT3 antagonists like ondansetron and granisetron prevent postoperative vomiting, radiation therapy–induced symptoms, and cancer chemotherapy– induced emesis, but also are used for other causes of emesis."-Harrison 20/e p256

93. Ans. b. Prostate cancer *(Ref: Sabiston 20/e p1845, 19/e p1816-1817; Schwartz 10/e p927; Bailey 27/e p990)*

Malignancies associated with Migratory Thrombophlebitis	
• CA pancreas (MC)[Q]	• Prostate cancer[Q]
• CA lung[Q]	• Ovarian cancer[Q]
• GI malignancies[Q]	• Lymphoma[Q]

- **Trousseau's syndrome:** Migratory thrombophlebitis[Q]
- **Trousseau's sign:** Carpopedal spasm in hypocalcemia[Q]
- **Troisier's sign:** Palpable left supraclavicular LN (Virchow's node)[Q]

94. Ans. b. Tumor let   95. Ans. a. Oropharyngeal carcinoma *(Ref: Bailey 27/e p740; Devita 9/e p729)*

96. Ans. d. CA oral cavity

97. Ans. d. Liposarcoma

98. **Ans. a. Sjögren's syndrome** *(Ref: Harrison 20/e p340, 352, 19/e p353,365)*

PSEUDOLYMPHOMA

- Group of disorders having a **benign course** but exhibiting **clinical** and **histological features** suggestive **of malignant lymphoma**.
- Characterized by **benign infiltration of lymphoid cells** or **histiocytes** which microscopically resembles a malignant lymphoma.

Pseudolymphoma is seen in	
Autoimmune Disorders	**Drug-induced**
• Sjogren syndrome • Dysgammaglobulinemia	• Phenytoin and phenobarbital • Primidone

99. **Ans. a. Apical lobe of lung**

100. **Ans. a. Lyme's disease** *(Ref: Harrison 20/e p1008, 19/e p1150)*

Condition	Seen in
Necrolytic erythema migrans	• Glucagonoma
Erythema chronicum migrans	• Lyme's disease
Erythema infectiosum (fifth disease)	• Parvovirus B19
Erythema marginatum	• Acute rheumatic fever

101. **Ans. d. Osteosarcoma** *(Ref: Robbins 9/e p476-479)*

Small Round Blue Cell Tumors (WEL PNR)	
• Wilms' tumor^Q • Ewing's sarcoma^Q • Lymphoma^Q • Medulloblastoma^Q • Small cell variant of osteosarcoma^Q	• Primitive neuroectodermal tumor^Q • Neuroblastoma^Q • Rhabdomyosarcoma^Q • Askin tumor^Q • Desmoplastic small cell tumor^Q

102. **Ans. a. Medullary carcinoma thyroid** *(Ref: Sabiston 20/e p691)*

103. **Ans. a. BRCA-1: Lung, c. Chromosome 16: Philadelphia chromosome**

104. **Ans. a. CA colon** *(Ref: Harrison 20/e p585, 19/e p543)*

- Harrison says "**Chemotherapy** can be administered **as an adjuvant** (i.e. in addition to surgery or radiation) after all clinical apparent disease has been removed. This use of chemotherapy may have **curative potential in breast** and **colorectal neoplasms**, as it attempts to **eliminate clinically unapparaent tumor** that may have **already disseminated**."

105. **Ans. a. Pheochromocytoma, b. Insulinoma, d. Appendicular carcinoma** *(Ref: Sabiston 20/e p957; Schwartz 10/e 1574,1585-1588; Bailey 27/e p846,850,1315)*

Glucagonoma are **mostly malignant** and **metastatic** at the time of presentation.

106. **Ans. a. Paget's disease of bone**

107. **Ans. d. Finger** *(Ref: Bailey 27/e p614, 711, 712)*

GLOMUS TUMOUR

- These arise from **subcutaneous arteriovenous shunts (Sucquet–Hoyer canals)** especially in the **corium of** the **nail bed.**
- Typically, they are **small, purple nodules** measuring a few millimetres in size, which are **disproportionately painful in response to insignificant stimuli (including cold exposure)**.
- **Subungual varieties** may be **invisible** causing **paroxysmal digital pain.**

108. **Ans. c. Chromosome 17**

109. **Ans. a. Metastatic germ cell tumor** *(Ref: Harrison 19/e p588; Computed Body Tomography by Lee Sagel 4/e p1207)*

The necrotic retroperitoneal mass represents necrotic lymph nodes. Necrotic lymph nodes usually suggest malignant metastasis, most likely due to testicular (germ cell) tumor.

Testicular Tumors

- **Testicular tumors** tend to **metastasize via** the **lymphatic system**.
- In general, the **testicular lymphatics** which **follow** the course of the **testicular vessels**, drain directly into the **lymph nodes in** or **near** the **renal hilus**.
- After involvement of these sentinel nodes, the **lumbar paraaortic nodes become involved** (unilaterally or bilaterally), followed by **spread to the mediastinal** and **supraclavicular nodes** or hematogenous dissemination to lungs, liver and brain.
- **Seminoma** is c-kit positive tumor[Q]

110. **Ans. c. Glioma** *(Ref: KDT 6/e p577)*

- **Somatostatin** is a 'universal switch off'. Somatostatin analogue **octreotide decreases secretion of** various **hormones**.

Uses of Octreotide	
• **Pancreatic neuroendocrine tumors** (**insulinoma**, glucagonoma, VIPoma)[Q]	• **Acromegaly**[Q]
• **Carcinoid tumors** and **syndrome**[Q]	• **Bleeding varices**[Q]
	• **Enterocutaneous fistula**[Q]

111. **Ans. a. Benign, c. Malformation, d. Mostly Asymptomatic** *(Ref: Robbins 9/e p267)*

Hamartoma

- **Hamartoma** refers to an **excessive, focal overgrowth of cells** and **tissues native to** the **organ** in which it occurs[Q].
- **Cellular elements** are **mature** and **identical to** those **found in** the remainder of the **organ**[Q]
- **Do not reproduce** the **normal architecture** of the surrounding tissue[Q].
- **Benign nature**[Q]
- **Mostly asymptomatic,** rarely presents with life-threatening clinical problems[Q]

Heterotopia (or Choristoma)

- **Choristoma** is applied to **microscopically normal cells** or **tissues** that are **present in abnormal locations**[Q].
- **Examples:** Rest of **pancreatic tissue** found **in** the **wall of** the **stomach** or **small intestine**, or a small mass of adrenal cells found in the kidney, lungs, ovaries, or elsewhere[Q].

112. **Ans. b. Oral cavity**

113. **Ans. a. 1975** *(Ref: www.nihfw.org/.../NationalHealthProgramme)*

National Cancer Control Programme

- To control the problems associated with cancer the Govt. of India has launched a **National Cancer Control Programme in 1975** stressing on **primary prevention** and **early detection of cancer**[Q].

Males	Females
• **MC cancer** in **males** (**PLC**): **Prostate >Lung >Colorectal**[Q]	• **MC cancer** in **females** (**BLC**): **Breast >Lung >Colorectal**[Q]
• **Cancer deaths** in **males** (**LPC**): **Lung >Prostate >Colorectal**[Q]	• **Cancer deaths** in **females** (**LBC**): **Lung >Breast >Colorectal**[Q]

114. **Ans. d. All of the above**

"**Acanthosis nigrican** can be a **reflection of an internal malignancy**, most commonly the **adenocarcinoma of GIT, lung, uterus and breast**."

115. **Ans. d. Gallbladder**

116. **Ans. a. B cell** *(Ref: http://www.mdanderson.org/patient-and-cancer-information/cancer-information/cancer-types/eye-cancer/orbit.html)*

Orbital Lymphoma

- MC type of cancer of the orbit in adults^Q
- Usually a form of **B-cell non-Hodgkin's lymphoma**^{Q}.

Clinical Features

- It may show up as a **nodule in the eyelid** or **around** the **eye**, or it may cause the **eye** to be **pushed out**^{Q}.
- This type of eye cancer **usually does not cause pain**^{Q}.

Diagnosis

- **First step in diagnosis** of orbital lymphoma may be a **CT scan of the orbit** followed by a **surgical biopsy**^{Q}.
- Making the correct diagnosis of the biopsy is very important.

Treatment

- **Radiation therapy, monoclonal antibody** therapy, **chemotherapy** or a combination of these, depending on type of lymphoma the stage of the tumor.

117. **Ans. a. Chondrosarcoma** *(Ref: Sabiston 20/e p1602; Schwartz 10/e p667)*

"Chondrosarcomas are the most common primary chest wall malignancy. As with chondromas, they usually arise anteriorly from the costochondral arches. CT scan shows a radiolucent lesion often with stippled calcifications pathognomonic for chondrosarcomas."-Schwartz 10/e p667

118. **Ans. c. Pyogenic granuloma** *(Ref: Sabiston 20/e p2012; Bailey 27/e p614)*

"Pyogenic granuloma is a misnomer for an exuberant outburst of highly vascular granulation tissue at the site of previous relatively trivial trauma. These lesions are friable, bleed easily, and may grow rapidly. They respond to curettage or simple excision. They usually occur on the fingertips."-Sabiston 20/e p2012

CHAPTER 40

Sarcoma

SOFT TISSUE SARCOMA

SOFT TISSUE SARCOMA

- Rare unusual neoplasm of soft tissues
- MC site: Extremity^Q **(lower >upper)** > Trunk > Retroperitoneum >Head & Neck
- MC type: Liposarcoma >Leiomyosarcoma >Synovial sarcoma >Malignant peripheral nerve sheath tumor >**Malignant fibrous histiocytoma^Q** > GIST
- MC pediatric soft tissue sarcoma: Rhabdomyosarcoma^Q
- Hematogenous spread is typical of sarcomas^Q

Histopathological Type of STS is Site Dependent	
Extremity	Malignant fibrous histiocytoma^Q >Liposarcoma
Retroperitoneum	Liposarcoma^Q
Viscera	GIST^Q

Pathology

- STS tends to **grow along fascial planes^Q**, with the surrounding soft tissue compressed to **form a pseudocapsule^Q**.
- Clinical behavior of STS is determined by: **Anatomic location (depth), grade & size^Q**
- **MC route of spread** in soft tissue sarcoma: **Hematogenous^Q**
- MC site of metastasis: Lung^Q; Lymphatic metastasis is rare^Q

Clinical Features

- MC symptom of STS: **Painless mass^Q**
- Size at presentation is **dependent on the location of tumor^Q**.

> - **Smaller tumors** are located **in distal extremities^Q**
> - **Larger tumors** are detected **in proximal extremity** and **retroperitoneum^Q**.
> - **Retroperitoneal STS** almost always present as **large asymptomatic mass^Q**

Diagnosis of Soft Tissue Sarcoma

- **Core-cut** or **true-cut biopsy (CT or USG guided)** is diagnostic^Q
- **Incisional biopsy** is done **if core-cut biopsy is non-diagnostic^Q**
- **FNAC: To confirm** or **rule out** presence of **metastatic focus** or **local recurrence^Q**
- **MRI:** IOC for assessing extremity STS^Q
- **CECT:** IOC for assessing retroperitoneal sarcoma^Q

Treatment

- **Adequate excision + adjuvant radiotherapy** with or without adjuvant chemotherapy^Q.
- **Two most active chemotherapy agents** against STS: **Doxorubicin & ifosfamide^Q**

Prognosis

- Best prognostic factor of soft tissue sarcoma:

Grade

- Best prognosis is seen in: Extremity STS^Q
- Most important predictor of metastasis in STS: Grade^Q
- MC cause of death in STS: **Metastasis^Q**; 5-year survival rate for STS (all stages): **50–60%**

SARCOMAS WITH LN METASTASIS

- MC site of metastasis in sarcomas of extremity: Lungs^Q
- MC site of metastasis in retroperitoneal sarcomas: Liver^Q > Lungs^Q
- LN metastasis is uncommon in soft tissue sarcoma^Q.

Sarcomas with Lymph Node Metastasis (MARCES)	
• **M**alignant fibrous histiocytoma^Q	• **C**lear cell sarcoma^Q
• **A**ngiosarcoma^Q	• **E**pithelial sarcoma^Q
• **R**habdomyosarcoma^Q	• **S**ynovial sarcoma^Q

RHABDOMYOSARCOMA

RHABDOMYOSARCOMA

- **Rhabdomyosarcoma** arises from **mesenchymal tissues.**
- MC sites of origin: Head & neck^Q (parameningeal^Q) > Extremities > Genitourinary tract > Trunk
- MC pediatric soft tissue sarcoma: Rhabdomyosarcoma^Q
- Associated with: NF, Beckwith-Weidman syndrome, Li-fraumeni and Fetal alcohol syndrome

Pathology
- MC histological type: Embryonal rhabdomyosarcoma^Q; MC type in adults: Pleomorphic variant^Q
- Diagnostic cell: Rhabdomyoblast^Q
- May contain **tadpole cells** or **strap cells**^Q
- **Embryonal type** consist of spindle cell variant and **sarcoma botryoides**^Q (tumor cells resemble **tennis racket**^Q and tumor cells form submucosal zone of hypercellularity known as **cambium layer**^Q)
- Best & most special marker for RMS: Myogenin^Q > MYOD–1^Q > Desmin^Q

Clinical Features
- MC presenting symptom: Mass^Q (may or may not be painful)
- **Bimodal, first peak** between **2–5 years, second peak** between **15–19 years**
- **Extremity RMS** are **more common** in **lower extremity**^Q
- MC site of metastasis: Lung^Q

Diagnosis
- **Diagnosis** is **confirmed by biopsy**^Q
- **MRI:** IOC for diagnosing **extent of disease**^Q
- **CT:** Used to rule out **lung metastasis**^Q

Treatment
- **Wide-local excision**^Q of tumor with surrounding involved tissue
- Tumor **not amenable to primary excision: Neoadjuvant chemotherapy,** after the tumor has decreased in size, **resection of gross residual disease**
- **Radiation therapy:** When **microscopic** or **gross residual disease** exists after initial treatment.

Prognosis
- Prognosis is related to the **site of origin, resectability, presence of metastases, number of metastatic sites,** and **histopathologic features**^Q.
- **Embryonal variant** is a **favorable**^Q and **alveolar type** has an **unfavorable prognosis**^Q.

Favorable Primary Sites	Unfavorable Primary Sites
• Orbit^Q	• Extremity^Q
• Nonparameningeal head & neck^Q	• Parameningeal^Q
• Paratestis^Q	
• Vagina^Q	

LEIOMYOSARCOMA

LEIOMYOSARCOMA

- Leiomyosarcomas are malignant tumors composed of cells showing **smooth muscle features**.
- **MC site: Uterus**^{Q}
- **Desmin** and **actin** are the **MC positive stains**^{Q}.

> - Grading of leiomyosarcomas is difficult, and **mitotic activity**^{Q} appears to be the best indicator of subsequent prognosis when combined with location and size.

- Common major vascular sites: **Pulmonary artery** and **IVC**^{Q}
- **Large tumor size** and **high mitotic rate/high grade** are factors in **poorer outcome**.
- **Complete excision** remains the **primary therapeutic choice**^{Q}.

ANGIOSARCOMA

ANGIOSARCOMA (LYMPHANGIOSARCOMA)

- Rare tumor that develops as a **complication** of **long-standing** (>10 years) **lymphoedema**^{Q}.
- Stewart and Treves described **lymphangiosarcoma** of the **upper extremity** in women with **ipsilateral lymphedema** after **radical mastectomy. (Stewart-Treves Syndrome)**^{Q}

Clinical Features
- **Acute worsening** of **edema**^{Q}
- Appearance of **subcutaneous nodules** with propensity towards **hemorrhage and ulceration**^{Q}

Treatment
- Preoperative **chemotherapy** and **radiotherapy** followed by **surgical excision (radical amputation)**^{Q}
- Associated with **poor prognosis**

SYNOVIAL SARCOMA

SYNOVIAL SARCOMA

- Synovial sarcoma usually occurs in **young adults**^{Q}.
- **Typically found** in the **para-articular areas of tendon sheaths & joints**^{Q}.
- At least **50% of cases** are in the **lower limbs**^{Q} (especially the **knee**^{Q}), and most of the remainder are seen in the upper limbs.
- It generally **does not originate from synovial tissue**^{Q}.
- Composed of two morphologically distinct types of cells that form a **characteristic biphasic pattern**^{Q}.

> - Characteristic chromosomal translocation, **t(X;18)(p11.2;q11.2)**^{Q}
> - **These hallmark translocations** have become the **gold standard in diagnosing synovial sarcoma**^{Q}
> - **100% of biphasic and 96% of monophasic synovial sarcomas** possess the **specific t(X;18)(p11.2;q11.2) translocation**^{Q}.

Treatment
- Adequate excision + adjuvant radiotherapy with or without adjuvant chemotherapy^Q.

KAPOSI SARCOMA

KAPOSI'S SARCOMA

- Kaposi's sarcoma appears as **rubbery bluish nodules** that occur **primarily on the extremities**^{Q} but **may appear anywhere** on the **skin and viscera**^{Q}.
- Classically, KS is seen in people of **Eastern Europe** or **sub-Saharan Africa**^{Q}.

AIDS-RELATED KAPOSI'S SARCOMA

- **AIDS-related KS** occurs **primarily in male homosexuals** and **not in IV drug abusers** or **hemophiliacs**^{Q}
- **Lesions spread rapidly** to the **nodes** and GI and **respiratory tract often are involved**^{Q}.
- Development of AIDS-related KS is **associated with concurrent infection** with a **herpes-like virus (HHV-8)**

Pathology
- Usually multifocal^Q rather than metastatic.
- Histologically, the lesions are composed of **capillaries lined by atypical endothelial cells**^Q.
- **Early lesions** may **resemble hemangiomas**, while **older lesions** contain more spindle cells and **resemble sarcomas**.
- Lesions are **locally aggressive** but **undergo periods of remission**^Q.

Treatment
- Treatment for all types of KS consists of **radiation**^Q to the lesions.
- **Combination chemotherapy** is effective in controlling the disease, although most patients develop an opportunistic infection during or shortly after treatment^Q.
- **Surgical treatment** is **reserved for lesions** that **interfere with vital functions**:, such as
  - Bowel obstruction and Airway compromise^Q
- Most common malignancy in HIV positive individuals: NHL > Kaposi sarcoma^Q

DERMATOFIBROSARCOMA PROTUBERANS

Dermatofibrosarcoma Protuberans (DFSP)

- DFSP is a **low-grade sarcoma** because it **may recur locally** but **rarely metastasizes**^Q.
- Monomorphous, mononuclear, **spindle cell lesion involving** both **dermis & subcutis**^Q.
- MC site: **Trunk**^Q (50%) >Extremities (30%) >Head & neck (20%)

Pathology
- **Large lesions** often are associated with **satellite nodules; Positive** for **CD34**^Q
- Have **unpredictable radial extensions**^Q of tumor **permeating through** the **subcutaneous tissue** large distances from the primary nodule.
- More than 75% of DFSP have a **ring chromosome**^Q, composed of translocated portions of chromosomes **17 & 22**^Q

Clinical Features
- Typically **presents in early** or **mid-adult life**, beginning as a **nodular cutaneous mass**^Q.
- **Pattern of growth: Slow** and **persistent**^Q
- Lesion enlarges over many years, it **becomes protuberant**^Q

Diagnosis
- IOC for diagnosis: Incisional biopsy

Treatment
- **Aggressive resection (2-4 cm margin)** with removal of underlying fascia with **special attention** to **radial margins** (local recurrence rate <5%)
- Up **to 50% recur after simple excision**^Q.
- **Imatinib**: First line of treatment for **advanced disease**^Q.
- **Neoadjuvant imatinib for unresectable tumors**^Q

Multiple Choice Questions

SOFT TISSUE SARCOMA

1. **Most common sarcoma in a child is:** *(JIPMER 98)*
   a. Fibrosarcoma
   b. Rhabdomyosarcoma
   c. Leiomyosarcoma
   d. Liposarcoma

2. **Most common site of lymphangiosarcoma:** *(MHPGMCET 2007, JIPMER 91)*
   a. Spleen
   b. Liver
   c. Retroperitoneum
   d. Post irradiated postmastectomy limb

3. **The most common sarcoma in childhood:**
   a. Malignant histiocytoma *(MHSSMCET 2008)*
   b. Rhabdomyosarcoma
   c. Osteosarcoma
   d. Liposarcoma

4. **With regard to the malignant behavior of leiomyosarcoma, the most important criterion is:** *(All India 2006)*
   a. Blood vessel penetration by tumour cells
   b. Tumour cells is lymphatic channels
   c. Lymphocyte infiltration
   d. The number of mitoses per high power field

5. **Synovial sarcoma all are true except:** *(All India 2010)*
   a. Originates in synovium
   b. Seen in young age group
   c. Occurs at extra-articular sites more often
   d. Seen in sites such as knee and foot

6. **In which case lymph nodes are resected prophylactically?** *(AIIMS Nov 98, Feb 97)*
   a. Embryonal rhabdomyosarcoma
   b. Liposarcoma
   c. Fibrosarcoma
   d. Neurofibroma

7. **All of the following soft tissue sarcoma has propensity for lymphatic spread except:** *(AIIMS Nov 2005)*
   a. Neurofibrosarcoma
   b. Synovial sarcoma
   c. Rhabdomyosarcoma
   d. Epitheloid sarcoma

8. **M.C. retroperitoneal tumour is:** *(DNB 2011, AIIMS June 98)*
   a. Fibrosarcoma
   b. Liposarcoma
   c. Dermoid cyst
   d. Rhabdomyosarcoma

9. **True about soft tissue sarcoma:** *(PGI Dec 2002)*
   a. Lymphatic spread
   b. Enlarged size
   c. Pseudoencapsulated
   d. Spread though musculoaponeurotic plane

10. **True statement about soft tissue sarcoma is/are:** *(PGI June 2004)*
    a. Liposarcoma is MC retroperitoneal sarcoma
    b. Incisional biopsy is needed when size >5 cm
    c. FNAC is diagnostic
    d. TNM staging done
    e. Radiosensitive

11. **Which of the following is best indicator of prognosis of soft tissue sarcoma?** *(AIIMS Nov 2000, Feb 97, Nov 96, All India 98)*
    a. Tumor size
    b. Histological type
    c. Nodal metastasis
    d. Tumor grade

12. **Malignant neoplasm arising from mesenchymal tissue are:** *(COMEDK 2004)*
    a. Carcinoma
    b. Sarcoma
    c. Adenomas
    d. Teratomas

13. **Which of the following sites of soft tissue sarcoma carries the best prognosis?**
    a. Head and neck
    b. Extremity
    c. Visceral
    d. Reteroperitoneal

14. **Most common site of rhabdomyosarcoma is:** *(DNB 2011)*
    a. Orbit
    b. Nasopharynx
    c. Extremities
    d. Hypopharynx

15. **Most common soft tissue tumour of adults is:** *(DNB 2010)*
    a. Embryonal rhabdomyosarcoma
    b. Liposarcoma
    c. Synovial sarcoma
    d. Malignant fibrous histiocytoma

16. **Sarcoma botryoides is also known as:**
    a. Embryonal rhabdomyosarcoma *(WBPG 2012, DNB 2010)*
    b. Alveolar rhabdomyosarcoma
    c. Leiomyosarcoma
    d. Lipoblastomatosis

17. **Blood borne spread is a feature of:** *(DNB 2010)*
    a. Carcinoma
    b. Sarcoma
    c. Dysplasia
    d. Metaplasia

18. **Malignant change in lipoma of retroperitoneum may present with:** *(DNB 2009)*
    a. Asymptomatic
    b. Renal failure
    c. Abdominal pain
    d. All of the above

19. **Which of the following immunohistochemical marker can be used for the diagnosis of rhabdomyosarcoma?** *(JIMPER 2014, AIIMS May 2013)*
    a. Myeloperoxidase
    b. Desmin
    c. Cytokerartin
    d. Synaptophysin

20. **Commonly done surgery in sarcoma is:** *(JIMPER 2012)*
    a. Wide excision
    b. Compartmental exlision/exenteration
    c. Excision
    d. Enucleation

21. **In which of the following malignancies, histological grade is a good prognostic indicator?** *(JIMPER 2011)*
    a. Soft tissue sarcoma
    b. RCC
    c. Malignant melanoma
    d. All

22. **Which one of the following statements is true regarding soft tissue sarcoma?** *(APPG 2016)*
    a. Most common location is retroperitoneal
    b. Fibrosarcoma is the commonest histological variety of soft tissue sarcoma
    c. Death is mostly due to lung metastases
    d. Account for <1% of pediatric malignancies

23. **Most common site of metastasis in extremity sarcoma:** *(Recent Question 2017, 2016)*
    a. Lung
    b. Liver
    c. Kidney
    d. Lymph node

DERMATOFIBROSARCOMA PROTUBERANS

24. Maximum margin of excision is needed for:
    (Recent Question 2016)
    a. Malignant melanoma
    b. BCC
    c. SCC
    d. Dermatofibrosarcoma protuberans

KAPOSI SARCOMA

25. The tissue of origin of Kaposi sarcoma is: *(AIIMS 2005)*
    a. Lymphoid
    b. Neural
    c. Vascular
    d. Muscular

26. Commonest malignancy in HIV patient: *(AIIMS Nov 99)*
    a. Kaposi sarcoma
    b. Adenoma of stomach
    c. Astrocytoma
    d. CNS lymphoma

27. All are true regarding Kaposi sarcoma except:
    a. Predominant in male *(AIIMS Feb 97)*
    b. Multicentric origin
    c. Chemotherapy is treatment of choice
    d. Occurs in AIDS patients only

28. Kaposi's sarcoma: *(SGPGI 2004)*
    a. Does not occur in non HIV positive persons
    b. Has increasing incidence among AIDS patients
    c. No GI bleeding
    d. Uncommon among homosexual HIV positive

29. Kaposi sarcoma is commonly seen in: *(AMU 95)*
    a. Upper limbs
    b. Lower limbs
    c. Head and Neck
    d. Trunk

30. Kaposi sarcoma is caused by: *(Recent Question 2016)*
    a. HHV 17
    b. HHV 8
    c. HPV 16
    d. Human simian virus 40

Explanations

SOFT TISSUE SARCOMA

1. Ans. b. Rhabdomyosarcoma *(Ref: Devita 9/e p1780-1784; Sabiston 20/e p1890, 804, 805; Schwartz 10/e 1465,1470)*
2. Ans. d. Post irradiated postmastectomy limb *(Ref: Sabiston 20/e p842; Schwartz 10/e 493; Bailey 27/e p615,146)*
3. Ans. b. Rhabdomyosarcoma
4. Ans. d The number of mitoses per high power field *(Ref: Devita 9/e p1529-1530)*
   Grading of leiomyosarcomas is difficult, and mitotic activity appears to be the **best indicator of subsequent prognosis** when **combined with location and size.**
5. Ans. a. Originates in synovium *(Ref: Devita 9/e p1545)*
   Synovial Sarcoma: It generally **does not originate from synovial tissue**, and it has been suggested that the name of this sarcoma subtype should be modified.
6. Ans. a. Embryonal rhabdomyosarcoma *(Ref: Harrison 20/e p1849, 18/e p817-820; Schwartz 10/e 1486; Sabiston 20/e p804)*
7. Ans. a. Neurofibrosarcoma
8. Ans. b. Liposarcoma *(Ref: Devita 10/e p1255, 9/e p1534)*

   - MC soft tissue sarcoma in adults: Liposarcoma > Leiomyosarcoma > Malignant fibrous histiocytoma
   - MC retroperitoneal tumor: Liposarcoma^Q

9. Ans. b. Enlarged size, c. Pseudoencapsulated, d. Spread though musculoaponeurotic plane *(Ref: Devita 10/e p1255; Sabiston 20/e p760-764; Schwartz 10/e 666-669)*
10. Ans. a. Liposarcoma is MC retroperitoneal sarcoma, b. Incisional biopsy is needed when size > 5 cm, d. TNM staging done
11. Ans. d. Tumor grade
12. Ans. b. Sarcoma
13. Ans. b. Extremity
14. Ans. a. Orbit
15. Ans. b. Liposarcoma
16. Ans. a. Embryonal rhabdomyosarcoma
17. Ans. b. Sarcoma

    Hematogenous spread is typical of sarcomas and lymphatic spread is typical of carcinoma.
18. Ans. d. All of the above *(Ref: Robbins 8/e p1318)*

   RETROPERITONEAL TUMORS
   - Deep seated mass **in abdomen**
   - When the tumor is **very large** do **symptoms of pain** or functional disturbances occur
   - Retroperitoneal tumors may present themselves with signs of weight loss, emaciation and abdominal pain
   - These tumors may also **compress the kidney** or **ureter** leading to **renal failure**

19. Ans. b. Desmin *(Ref: Devita 9/e p1780-1784; Sabiston 20/e p1890; Schwartz 10/e 666-669,1465-1487)*
    Desmin can be used **for the diagnosis of rhabdomyosarcoma.**
20. Ans. a. Wide excision
21. Ans. a. Soft tissue sarcoma
22. Ans. c. Death is mostly due to lung metastases
23. Ans. a. Lung

DERMATOFIBROSARCOMA PROTRUBERANS

24. Ans. d. Dermatofibrosarcoma protuberans *(Ref: Sabiston 20/e p750, 766)*

KAPOSI SARCOMA

25. Ans. c. Vascular *(Ref: Harrison 20/e p1448, 19/e p1242; Devita 9/e p2101-2104; Sabiston 20/e p750; Schwartz 10/e 485)*
26. Ans. a. Kaposi sarcoma *(Ref: Devita 9/e p2100)*

    - Most common malignancy in HIV positive individuals: NHL>Kaposi sarcoma^Q

27. Ans. d. Occurs in AIDS patients only
28. Ans. b. Has increasing incidence among AIDS patients
29. Ans. b. Lower limbs
30. Ans. b. HHV 8

SECTION 10

Others

CHAPTERS

- Pediatric Surgery
- Trauma
- Transplantation
- Anesthesia and Perioperative Complications
- Robotics, Laparoscopy and Bariatric Surgery
- Sutures and Anastomoses
- Sterilization and Infection
- Fluid, Electrolyte and Nutrition
- Blood Transfusion
- Shock
- Miscellaneous

CHAPTER 41

Pediatric Surgery

Multiple Choice Questions

1. A six years old female presents with constipation and urinary retention. On examination on a presacral mass is noted. Most probable diagnosis is: *(AIIMS May 2008)*
   a. Pelvic neuroblastoma
   b. Rectal duplication cyst
   c. Sacrococcygeal teratoma
   d. Anterior sacral meningocele

2. First meconium is said to be formed during the month of fetal life:
   a. Second   b. Fourth
   c. Seventh   d. Ninth

3. The given tumor is embryological remnant of:

   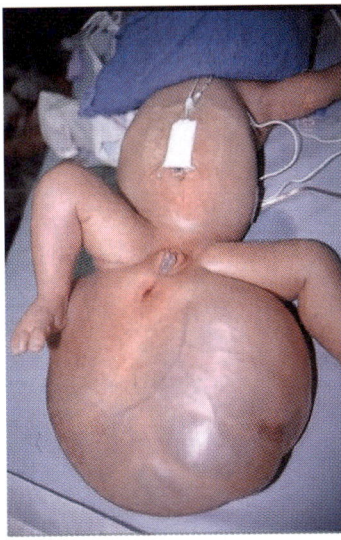

   a. Neural tube
   b. Allantois
   c. Notochord
   d. Primitive streak

4. Sacrococcygeal teratoma is embryological remnant of: *(MHSSMCET 2007)*
   a. Neural tube
   b. Allantois
   c. Notochord
   d. Primitive streak

5. An one month old female child has swelling over the back in the sacral region. There is no cough impulse in the swelling. X-ray examination shows erosion of the coccyx. The most likely clinical diagnosis would be: *(UPSC 95)*
   a. Meningocele   b. Lipoma
   c. Sacrococcygeal teratoma   d. Neurofibroma

6. Most common solid malignant tumor of infancy:
   a. Neuroblastoma   b. Nephroblastoma
   c. Germ cell tumor   d. Rhabdomyosarcoma

7. Most common posterior mediastinal mass in children is:
   a. Hodgkin's disease *(Recent Question 2016)*
   b. Neuroblastoma
   c. Esophageal duplication cyst
   d. Bronchogenic cyst

8. Malignant tumor of childhood that metastasizes to bone most often is: *(Recent Question 2016)*
   a. Neuroblastoma   b. Nephroblastoma
   c. Adrenal gland tumors
   d. Ovarian granulose cell tumor

9. Which of the following is the most common tumor of newborn? *(All India 2012)*
   a. Neuroblastoma   b. Wilms' tumors
   c. Leukemia   d. Sacrococcygeal teratoma

10. Primitive streaks remnants give rise to: *(DNB 2012)*
    a. Neuroblastoma   b. Wilms' tumour
    c. Sacrococcygeal teratoma   d. Hepatoblastoma

11. Currarino triad includes: *(Recent Question 2016)*
    a. Pre-sacral meningocele + Sacral defect + Tethered cord
    b. Ectopia vesicae + Anorectal malformation + Sacrococcygeal osseous defect
    c. Anorectal malformations + Sacrococcygeal osseous defect + Presacral mass
    d. Tethered cord + Anorectal malformations + Ectopia vesicae

12. Most common renal tumor in children: *(Recent Question 2017)*
    a. Renal cyst
    b. Congenital mesoblastic nephroma
    c. Neuroblastoma   d. Nephroblastoma

13. Most common intra-abdominal tumor in infant: *(Recent Question 2017)*
    a. Neuroblastoma   b. Wilms tumor
    c. HCC   d. Hypernephroma

Explanations

1. **Ans. d. Anterior sacral meningocele** *(Ref: Sabiston 20/e p1932; Schwartz 10/e p1750, 9/e p1553)*

   ### ANTERIOR SACRAL MENINGOCELE
   - **Defect of anterior aspect** of **sacrum**[Q] involving one or more segments with herniation of meningeal sac into extra-peritoneal region.
   - More common in **females**[Q]

   Clinical Features
   - **Symptoms** usually occur in **2nd to 3rd decade**[Q]
   - Symptoms are primarily owing to the **mechanical effects**[Q] of a pelvic tumor.
   - **Abdominal pain, constipation, urinary retention**[Q] or incontinence

   Diagnosis
   - **X-ray**: Unilateral sickle shaped distortion of sacral bone (**Scimitar sacrum**[Q]) is **pathognomonic**. This sign is not present in all cases.

2. **Ans. a. Second** *(Ref: Bailey 25/e p85)*

   By **end of 3 months upper small intestine** has become **filled with meconium**. So the answer should be less than 3 months.

   ### MECONIUM
   - Meconium is a sterile mixture of epithelial cells, mucin and bile, formed as the fetus starts to swallow amniotic fluid.
   - By **end of 3 months upper small intestine** has become **filled with meconium**[Q].

3. **Ans. d. Primitive streak** *(Ref: Sabiston 20/e p1893; Schwartz 10/e p1641)*

   Sacrococcygeal teratoma is thought to be a derivative of the primitive streak

4. **Ans. d. Primitive streak** *(Ref: Sabiston 20/e p1893-1894; Schwartz 10/e p1641)*

   ### SACROCOCCYGEAL TERATOMA
   - Teratomas occur most frequently in the **neonatal period**, **sacrococcygeal region** is the **MC site**[Q].
   - More common in **females**[Q]

   - Thought to be a derivative of the **primitive streak**[Q]
   - Most often an obvious **external presacral mass**[Q]

   - **Most** of the **tumor** is **usually external**, with a **minimal intrapelvic presacral component**[Q]
   - These lesions should be **carefully followed** with **serial USG until delivery** because the **blood supply to the tumor** may grow to the point of **stealing a significant proportion of placental blood flow to the fetus**[Q].
   - The development of **hydrops** or **placentomegaly** is associated with a **poor prognosis**[Q].

   - Most neonatal SCTs are **benign**[Q].
   - Incidence of malignancy is **related to age at time of diagnosis** and is most frequently represented as **yolk sac tumors** or **embryonal carcinomas**[Q].

   Treatment
   - **Complete surgical excision**[Q] through a chevron-shaped buttock incision.

   - **Resection of the coccyx is critical**[Q] because **failure to remove** this structure **results in significantly higher local recurrence rates**.

5. **Ans. c. Sacrococcygeal teratoma**

6. **Ans. a. Neuroblastoma** *(Ref: Sabiston 20/e p1887-1888; Schwartz 10/e p678,1639-1640; Bailey 27/e p138)*

7. **Ans. b. Neuroblastoma** *(Ref: Schwartz 10/e p678)*

   Most common posterior mediastinal mass in children is neurogenic tumor (Neuroblastoma among the given options).

8. **Ans. a. Neuroblastoma**

9. **Ans. d. Sacrococcygeal teratoma** *(Ref: Surgery of Childhood Tumors (Springer) 2008/49)*
    - **Sacrococcygeal teratoma** is the **predominant teratoma** as well as the **most common neoplasm** in the **fetus** and **newborn**^{Q} with an estimated incidence of 1:20,000 to 1:40,000 live births and a **female predominance**^{Q} ranging from 2:1 to 4:1.

10. **Ans. c. Sacrococcygeal teratoma**

11. **Ans. c. Anorectal malformations + Sacrococcygeal osseous defect + Presacral mass**
    - **Currarino triad:** Anorectal malformations + Sacrococcygeal osseous defect + Presacral mass

12. **Ans. b. Congenital mesoblastic nephroma** *(Ref: Campbell 11/e p2885)*

    "Although congenital mesoblastic nephroma (CMN) is a rare benign congenital renal tumor it is the most common solid renal tumor in the neonatal period."-Campbell 11/e p2885

13. **Ans. a. Neuroblastoma** *(Ref: Sabiston 20/e p1887; Schwartz 10/e p1639; Bailey 27/e p847)*

CHAPTER 42

Trauma

TRIMODAL MORTALITY MODEL FOR TRAUMA

Trimodal Mortality Model for Trauma		
Immediate Death (Within minutes of injury)	**Early Death** (Death within hours of arrival to hospital)	**Late Death** (Days to weeks after injury)

• Declared **dead at scene** or die shortly after arrival to hospital
• Causes:
   – **Irreversible brain injury**^{Q}
   – **Hemorrhage** from injuries of heart, aorta, liver, lungs & pelvic fracture^Q
	• **Intracranial hemorrhage**^{Q}
	• **Internal hemorrhage** involving **respiratory system & abdominal organs**^{Q}
	• Multiple injuries leading to **severe blood loss**^{Q}
	• **Tension pneumothorax**^{Q}
	• **Cardiac tamponade**^{Q}
		• **Sepsis**^{Q}
		• **Multiple organ failure**^{Q}

TRIAGE

TRIAGE

- **Triage** means **to "sort"**, especially **used for mass-casualties**^{Q}
- **Involves prioritizing** victims into categories based on: **Severity of injury**^{Q}, **likelihood of survival**^{Q} & **urgency of care**^{Q}
- **Triage tags:** Colour codes are used to identify the patients

Categorization of Triage Tags	
Red (immediate)	• **Most critically injured**^{Q} • Includes patients with **major head injury**, injuries to **thorax or abdomen**^{Q} • **Immediate care is required**^{Q}
Yellow (delayed)	• **Less critically injured**^{Q} • Require **in hospital treatment**^{Q}
Green (ambulatory)	• **No life or limb threatening injuries**^{Q}
Black (Expectant)	• **Dead or moribund patients**^{Q}

PRIMARY, SECONDARY AND TERTIARY SURVEY

Primary Survey	Secondary Survey	Tertiary Survey
• Aimed at **detecting & simultaneously treating immediately life threatening injuries**^{Q} • Identified by the mnemonic **'ABCDE'** • **A: Airway maintenance with cervical spine protection**^{Q} • **B: Breathing (ventilation & oxygenation)**^{Q} • **C: Circulation with hemorrhage control**^{Q} • **D: Disability (Brief neurological examination)**^{Q} • **E: Exposure /Environmental control**^{Q}	• Consists of **head to toe systematic assessment** of abdominal, pelvic & thoracic areas^Q • **Complete inspection of body surface** to find all injuries & **neurological examination**^{Q} • Patients & surrogates should be queried to obtain an **AMPLE history** • **A:** Allergies^Q • **M:** Medication^Q • **P:** Past illness or pregnancy^Q • **L:** Last meal^Q • **E:** Events related to injury^Q	• **Comprehensive** patient **evaluation after initial resuscitation period**^{Q} • Usually performed about **24 hours after admission**^{Q} • Include a **thorough physical examination** combined with **targeted radiographic imaging** (X-ray usage or CT) **based on examination finding**^{Q} • **Decreases the delay in diagnosis** of **potentially life-threatening injuries**^{Q}

PRIMARY SURVEY

A: Airway Maintenance with Cervical Spine Protection

- **Cervical spine injury** should be **suspected in all the patients**[Q]
- **All trauma patients** should have **cervical spine immobilization** & **protected through out**[Q]
- **First priority**: Cervical spine followed by airway[Q]
- **Asses the patency of airway**: Elicit the **verbal response**[Q] (simplest way: Ask the patients name; **ability to speak indicates adequate airway protection**[Q])
- **In patients, who cannot speak**, suspect **mental status depression** or airway obstruction. Both are **indication for airway management**[Q]
- Other indications: Noisy breathing[Q], facial trauma[Q] & GCS ≤ 8[Q]

Compromised Airway Require Stepwise Progression
• First **clearing the airway by suctioning** secretions or blood followed by **jaw thrust** or **chin lift**[Q]
• Insertion of **oropharyngeal or nasopharyngeal airway**[Q]
• **Definitive airway of choice** for must injured patients: Oral endotracheal intubation with **cuffed endotracheal tube**[Q]
• **ATLS updates (2018)** recommended **use of video laryngoscope for intubation**[Q]
• **In severe maxillofacial injuries**: Emergency airway (Needle cricothyroidotomy[Q]) & Definitive airway (Tracheostomy[Q])

In Severe Maxillofacial Injuries	
Emergency Airway	**Definitive Airway**
• **Emergency airway: Needle cricothyroidotomy**[Q] • Performed quickly; **High flow O_2** is given **via 4-6 mm tube**[Q] • **Advantage**: Provides time for **definitive airway**[Q] • **Disadvantage**: CO_2 **retention** occurs **within 20-30 minutes**[Q] • **Avoided in children <12 years** of age it can lead to **subglottic stenosis**[Q]	• **Tracheostomy**[Q]

Breathing (Ventilation & Oxygenation)

- **Asses breathing by**: Visualizing chest movements[Q]; Rate & depth of respiration[Q]; Percussion & Auscultation of breath sounds[Q]
- **Limited respiratory effort** or dyspnea requires **support of ventilation & further assessment of chest**[Q]
- **Ventilation problems** are secondary to tension pneumothorax, massive hemothorax or flail chest with pulmonary contusion[Q]

Condition	Management
Tension pneumothorax	• Insertion of **large bore needle in 2nd intercostal space in midclavicular line** followed by ICD insertion in triangle of safety[Q] • **ATLS updates (2018)** says "Recent evidences support insertion of wide bore needle in 5th intercostal space slightly anterior to mid axillary line in adults"[Q]
Massive hemothorax	• **ICD insertion**[Q] • **Optimal size of chest tube** required to drain a hemothorax: **28–32 F**[Q]
Severe pulmonary contusion	• **Aggressive mechanical ventilation**[Q]

Circulation with Hemorrhage Control

- Assess circulation to look for shock; **Primary goal is to rule out shock**[Q]
- **MC cause of shock in trauma**: Hemorrhage[Q]
- **Assess vitals**: Pulse rate & BP[Q]
- **In case of shock** (PR >100/min[Q], BP <100 mm Hg[Q]): Put **two large bore IV cannula**[Q] (**Green cannula**[Q] is preferred); Send **blood for cross match**[Q]

> - **ATLS updates (2018)**: Give **only 1 liter of warm isotonic crystalloids for adults**[Q] (Old edition recommended 1-2 liters of warm crystalloid solution)
> - **ATLS updates (2018)**: In **children <40 kg**, give **20 mL/kg of warm isotonic crystalloids**[Q]

- **Rapid screening** should be done **to identify the cause of life threatening blood loss**[Q]

> - The **source of hemorrhage** is often described as **"on the floor, plus four more"**[Q]
> - **Five major locations** responsible for exsanguination: 1. **External blood loss**[Q]; 2. Thorax; 3. Abdomen; 4. Retroperitoneum (pelvic fracture) 5. Multiple long bone fracture

- **Initial physical examination**: Identifies source of external blood loss & long bone fractures; Managed immediately with direct pressure[Q] or splinting[Q] respectively
- **Chest X-ray**: To evaluate **thoracic blood loss**[Q]; X-ray pelvis: To **identify pelvis fracture**[Q]; FAST: To **evaluate abdomen**

- Two most important X-rays in patients of trauma: Chest X-ray^Q & X-ray pelvis (AP view^Q) as patients is in supine position
- After **initial administration of IV fluid**, patients are **assessed for ongoing signs of shock**^Q
- For **non-responding patients, manage ongoing bleeding + blood transfusion**^Q

> - For trauma resuscitation: Packed cell, plasma & platelets are used in the **ratio 1:1:1**^Q
> - Best indicator of tissue perfusion in trauma: **Urine output**^Q
> - Best indicator to determine amount of fluid required: **CVP**^Q

- **Pediatric mass transfusion protocol (ATLS updates 2018)**: Initial 20 mL/kg bolus^Q of isotonic crystalloid followed by 10-20 mL/kg of packed cells, plasma & platelets in the ration of 1:1:1^Q.

CRASH-2 Trial (ATLS updates 2018)

- **Use of tranexamic acid in hypotensive trauma patients**^Q
- **Tranexamic acid reduces** the risk of **mortality from bleeding** in both **blunt & penetrating trauma**^Q
- **Dose: 1 gm IV over 10 minutes followed by 1 gm over 8 hours**^Q
- **Given to all trauma patients suspected to have significant hemorrhage including SBP <110 mm Hg or PR >110/min**^Q
- Should be **administered within 3 hours of injury**^Q

DISABILITY (BRIEF NEUROLOGICAL EXAMINATION)

- Assess GCS & assess pupils (Size/ equality/ reaction)^Q

Revised Glasgow Coma Scale 2014

Revised GCS (2014)

Eye Opening (E)		Verbal Response (V)		Best Motor Response (M)	
Spontaneous	4	Oriented	5	Obeying commands	6
To **Speech**^Q	3	Confused	4	Localizing	5
To **Pressure**^Q	2	**Words**^Q	3	Normal flexion (withdrawal)	4
None	1	**Sounds**^Q	2	Abnormal flexion	3
		None	1	Extension	2
				None	1

- **GCS** specifically **recommends avoiding sternal rubs**^Q as it causes bruising & responses can be difficult to interpret. They also **do not recommend routine use of retromandibular pressure**^Q.
- **Revised GCS (2014)** changes are highlighted in the above table.
- **Maximum score-15**^Q, **minimum score-3**^Q.
- **Best predictor of outcome: Motor response**^Q

> - **Reporting of Non-testable Score Aspects**: In cases of a non-testable aspect, the new GCS should only be noted in its components. Any **element** that **cannot be tested** should be marked as NT, for **"not testable"**.
> - For **intubated patients** or **patients with tracheostomy**, V_{NT} is used. It is **no longer recommend to assign 1 point to non-testable elements**, therefore a combined score should not be used.

GCS-P	GCS-PA CT
- **GCS-P** is calculated by **subtracting the Pupil Reactivity Score (PRS) from the Glasgow Coma Scale (GCS) total score**: GCS-P = GCS − PRS^Q - **Pupil reactivity score** represents the **number of nonreactive pupils (0, 1, or 2)**^Q. - This **number is subtracted from the GCS score (3-15)**, resulting in the **GCS-P (1-15)**^Q.	- **GCS-PA CT: GCS**, **P**upils, **A**ge & **CT** findings^Q - **Probability of mortality 6 months after head injury based on** the patient's admission **GCS-P** and **age with no CT abnormality (A)**, **exactly 1 CT abnormality (B)**, and **2 or more CT abnormalities (C)**. - **Potential CT abnormalities** include **intracranial hematoma, absent cisterns & SAH**^Q.

Pupils Unreactive to Light	PRS
Both pupils	2
One pupil	1
Neither pupil	0

Note: Higher score is assigned to non-reactive pupils.

EXPOSURE (ENVIRONMENTAL CONTROL)

- **All clothing are removed** for adequate examination
- Core body temperature is obtained & **patient is kept warm**
- **Environmental control** should be maintained with **warm blankets, increased room temperature, heated fluid administration & body warmers.**

ATLS UPDATES (2018) ABOUT LIFE THREATENING INJURIES DURING PRIMARY SURVEY

Life Threatening Injuries During Primary Survey		
Airway	**Breathing**	**Circulation**
• Airway obstruction^Q • Tracheobronchial injuries^Q	• Tension pneumothorax^Q • Open pneumothorax^Q	• Massive hemothorax^Q • Cardiac tamponade^Q • Traumatic circulatory arrest^Q

SECONDARY SURVEY

SECONDARY SURVEY

1. **Head & face:** Rule out skull fracture & laceration
2. **Neck:** Rule out neck injuries
3. **Chest:** Rule out rib fracture
4. **Abdomen:** Rule out abdominal pain, tenderness, bruising; **NG tube insertion** is **contraindicated** in presence of **facial fracture** (**orogastric tube** should be **inserted**), **urinary catheter** should be inserted **if no blood is present at meatus**^{Q}
5. **Back:** Log Roll – **5 people** are required for examination of back, **3 for body, one for head** & **one for examining back**; PR is done at this time^Q
6. **Extremities:** Each limb should be examined for **tenderness, crepitation** or **abnormal movement.**^{Q}
7. **Neurological examination:**
   - Repeat GCS, re-evaluate the pupils
   - Look for any localising/lateralising signs
   - Look for **signs of cord injury**

- For **log roll, ideal number of people** required: **5**^{Q}
- **Minimum number** of people required for log roll: **4**^{Q}

TRAUMA SCORING SYSTEM

	Trauma Scoring System	
Revised Trauma Score	**Trauma and Injury Severity Score (TRISS)**	**Mangled Extremity Severity Score (MESS)**

• RTS combines: (GB Road)
  – **G**lasgow coma scale^Q
  – Systolic **B**lood pressure^Q
  – **R**espiratory rate^Q
	• TRISS combines:
	  – **I**njury Severity Score (ISS)^Q
	  – **R**evised Trauma Score (RTS)^Q
	  – **A**ge^Q
	  – **M**echanism^Q of Injury (Blunt/Penetrating)
		• MESS combines: (ELISA)
		  – **E**nergy that caused the injury^Q
		  – **L**imb **I**schemia^Q
		  – **S**hock^Q
		  – Patient's **A**ge^Q

ABDOMINAL TRAUMA

ABDOMINAL TRAUMA

- MC injured organ in blunt trauma abdomen: **Spleen**^{Q} >**Liver**^{Q}
- MC injured organ in penetrating trauma abdomen (ATLS 2018 update): **Liver**^{Q} (26%) >**Stomach**^{Q} (17%) >**SI**^{Q} (12.9%)
- MC injured organ in gunshot wound: **Small intestine**^{Q} (SI)
- MC injured bowel in blunt trauma abdomen: **Jejunum**^{Q}
- MC injured structure in seat belt injury: **Mesentery**^{Q}
- MC injured site in deceleration injury: **Duodenojejunal junction**^{Q}
- First investigation done in blunt trauma abdomen: **FAST**^{Q}
- Gold standard investigation in stable patients of blunt trauma abdomen: **CECT**^{Q}

FAST

FAST (Focused Assessment with Sonography for Trauma)

- FAST: Emergency USG done very fast, **performed within 2-4 minutes**[Q]
- **Rapid diagnostic examination to assess patients with potential thoracoabdominal injuries**[Q]
- FAST is the **first investigation** done in **blunt trauma abdomen; FAST has replaced DPL**[Q]
- 4 'P's are evaluated **in the sequence: Pericardial sac → Perihepatic region → Perisplenic region → Pelvis**[Q]

Traditional Four Views of FAST	
Subxiphoid transverse view[Q]	• Assess **pericardial sac**[Q]
Right upper quadrant (RUQ) longitudinal view[Q]	• Assess **perihepatic region**[Q]
Left upper quadrant (LUQ) longitudinal view[Q]	• Assess **perisplenic region**[Q]
Suprapubic longitudinal & transverse view[Q]	• Assess **pelvis**[Q]

- **e-FAST (extended FAST)** has **two additional views, right & left thoracic views to rule out pneumothorax or hemothorax**[Q].
- **Stratosphere sign or barcode sign** is seen on **e-FAST** in **pneumothorax**[Q].

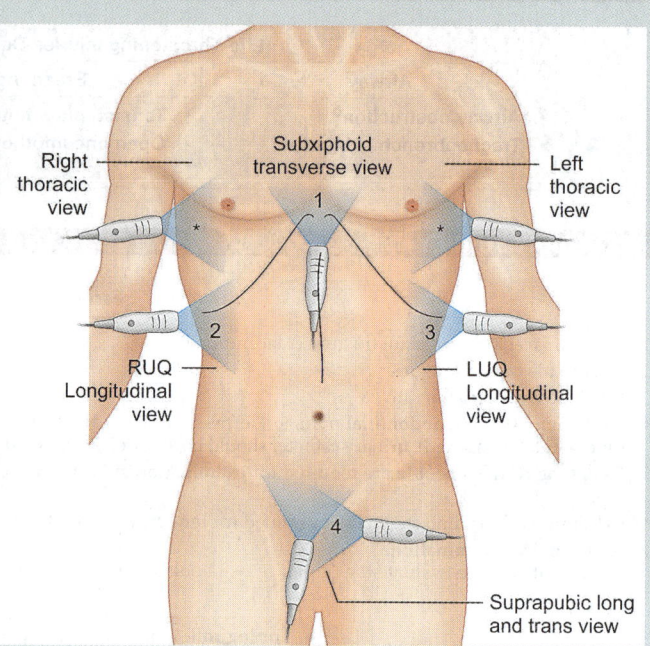

DIAGNOSTIC PERITONEAL LAVAGE

Diagnostic Peritoneal Lavage

- Performed **for blunt trauma abdomen** patients
- DPL is performed through **vertical infra-umbilical midline incision** unless the patient has pelvic fracture or is pregnant[Q]
- Linea alba is sharply incised & **catheter is directed towards pelvis**[Q]
- **Abdominal contents** should initially be **aspirated using a 10-mL syringe**[Q].
- Through the catheter, **one liter of saline or RL is infused into peritoneal cavity**[Q].
- Lavage fluid is sent for assessment

Positive DPL	

• **>10 mL of gross blood is aspirated directly from peritoneal cavity**[Q]	• **Returned effluent contains:**
	  – RBCs >1 lac/mm³[Q] - WBCs >500/mm³[Q]
	  – Demonstrable bacteria or bile[Q] - Amylase >174 IU/dL[Q]

- **Sensitivity of DPL** for detecting significant intra-abdominal injury is **82-96% & specificity 87-99%**.

MANAGEMENT OF BLUNT TRAUMA ABDOMEN

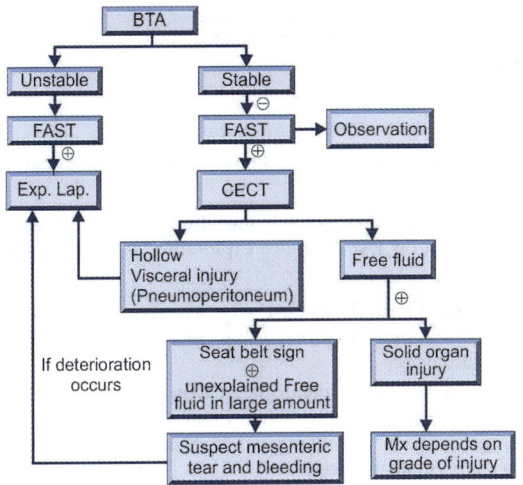

PENETRATING TRAUMA

PENETRATING ABDOMINAL INJURIES

- Gunshot Abdominal Wounds:
  - Chances of **internal injury** is **very high in gunshot wounds**, thus little preoperative evaluation is required and **laparotomy is mandatory**[Q].
- Stab Wounds to Abdomen:
  - **Exploratory laparotomy** is indicated in patients with isolated penetrating abdominal wound if **hypotensive** or **in shock** or **showing peritoneal signs**[Q].

Anterior Stab Wounds	Flank and Back Wounds
• **Local wound exploration** can be performed to determine **if there is any penetration of** the **peritoneal cavity**[Q].	• Risk of injury to **colon, kidney** and **ureter**[Q]
• If the tract terminates without entering the peritoneum, the injury can be managed as a deep laceration[Q] and laparotomy is not needed.	• **Triple contrast CT**[Q] is advised **to detect colon** and **retroperitoneal injuries** and the **need for laparotomy**.
• Otherwise, **penetration of the peritoneum** is assumed and **significant injury** must be **excluded by further diagnostic evaluations**[Q] (FAST, CECT, DPL or laparoscopy)	

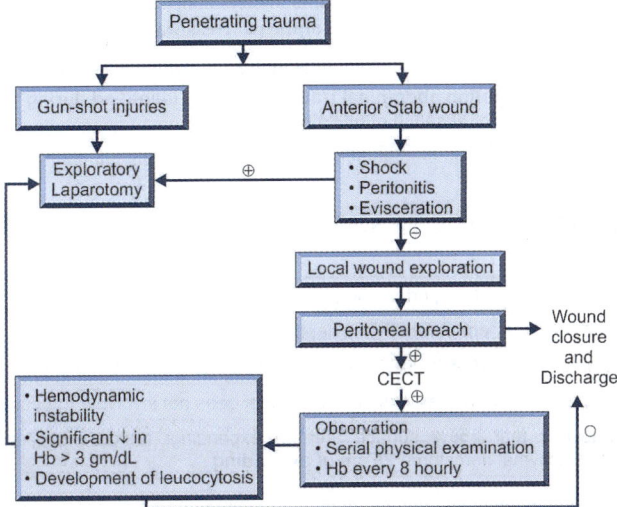

SPLENIC TRAUMA

SPLENIC INJURIES

- MC organ injured in **blunt trauma abdomen**: Spleen[Q]

Pathophysiology
- **Direct compression**[Q] of the organ in the left upper quadrant of the abdomen
- **Deceleration mechanism** that **tears the splenic capsule** or **parenchyma**[Q], mainly at areas fixed or tethered to the retroperitoneum

Diagnosis
- **Identification of splenic injuries** may occur **during laparotomy** in **unstable patients** taken **emergently to the operating room**[Q]
- **Unstable patients** with **intra-abdominal fluid** on **FAST** require **exploration**, with the **spleen** commonly being the **bleeding intra-abdominal organ**[Q]

> - In **stable patients, abdominal CT performed with IV contrast** is the **mainstay for diagnosing & characterizing splenic injuries**[Q]
> - **Images** are typically obtained with the contrast in the **portal venous phase** to enhance the splenic parenchyma maximally while still being able to visualize the vasculature.
> - **Splenic injuries** appear as **disruptions in** the **normal splenic parenchyma**, frequently with **surrounding hematoma & free intra-abdominal blood**[Q]
> - Occasionally, **active extravasation of contrast**, identified as a **high-density blush**, can be identified, **contained within a pseudoaneurysm** or bleeding into the **peritoneal space**[Q]

- **Angiography** has been used **for injuries** that **demonstrate active extravasation by CT**[Q]
- **Angiography** can **identify specific sites of bleeding** from the splenic parenchyma & underlying segmental or trabecular vessels; however, it cannot characterize the splenic parenchymal injury but can be complementary to CT.
- **Advantage of angiography**: Potential to **obstruct sites of bleeding endovascularly** using **angioembolization**[Q]

> - Patients who are candidates for **nonoperative management** of their splenic injury but **demonstrate a blush by CT**, indicating **active extravasation**, may benefit from angiography with embolization to eliminate the splenic pseudoaneurysm[Q]
> - **Angiographic embolization** is considered **only in hemodynamically stable patients**[Q]

Management
- With appropriate patient selection, **many patients with blunt splenic trauma** can be **managed without splenectomy**[Q]
- **No bleeding patient** should go **without splenectomy** or **splenic repair**, especially in an attempt to push the figurative nonoperative envelope[Q]

> - **Hemodynamic stability** is a **prerequisite for nonoperative management** and must **be present without ongoing intravascular volume support**[Q]
> - **Hemodynamic stability** is indicated by a **normal blood pressure** and **lack of tachycardia**, no physical examination findings indicating **shock**, and **absence of metabolic acidosis**[Q]

- Nonoperative management is reserved for **grades I, II** and **isolated** grade III injuries[Q]

Indications of Operative Management of Splenic Trauma
• **Instability** at admission[Q]   • **Exact location of bleeding** is **unknown**[Q]   • Failed nonoperative management[Q]

- Best approach: Midline incision with **packing of all four quadrants** in cases of hemodynamic **instability**[Q]
- Drains should not be placed unless there is concern that the **tail of the pancreas** was also **injured**[Q]

Splenic Injury Secondary to Penetrating Abdominal Trauma
• **Splenic injury** secondary to **penetrating abdominal trauma** is usually **identified during laparotomy** and should be **addressed based on** the presence or absence of **ongoing bleeding**.[Q]
• **Splenectomy** is performed **in cases of ongoing bleeding**[Q]

American Association for the Surgery of Trauma: Spleen Organ Injury Scale		
Grade	Type	Description of Injury
I	Hematoma	Subcapsular tear **<10%** surface area
	Laceration	**Capsular tear <1 cm** parenchymal depth
II	Hematoma	Subcapsular tear, **10–50%** surface area; intraparenchymal, **<5 cm** in **diameter**
	Laceration	Capsular tear, **1–3 cm** parenchymal depth that does not involve a trabecular vessel
III	Hematoma	Subcapsular tear **>50%** surface area or expanding; ruptured subcapsular or parenchymal hematoma; intraparenchymal hematoma **≥5 cm** or **expanding**

Contd...

Contd...

Grade	Type	Description of Injury
	Laceration	>3 cm parenchymal depth or involving trabecular vessels
IV	Laceration	Laceration involving segmental or hilar vessels producing major devascularization (>25% of spleen)
V	Hematoma	Completely shattered spleen
	Laceration	Hilar vascular injury devascularizes spleen

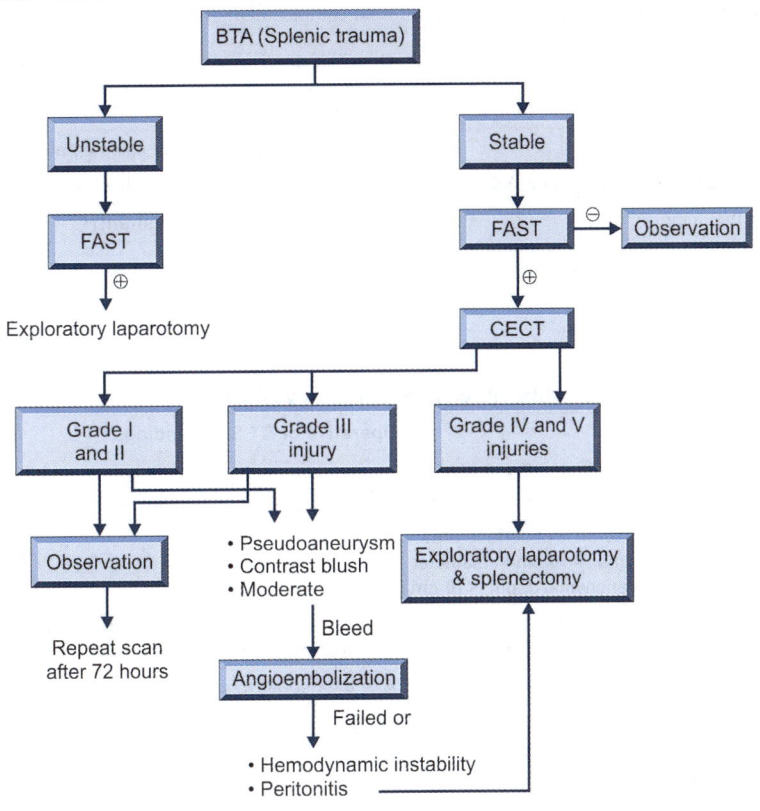

LIVER TRAUMA

HEPATIC INJURY

- MC organ injured in blunt abdominal trauma: Spleen > liver[Q]
- MC injured organ in penetrating trauma: Liver > Stomach > Small Intestine
- **Mechanisms** of blunt hepatic trauma: **Compression** with **direct parenchymal damage** and shearing forces, which tear hepatic tissue and disrupt vascular and ligamentous attachments.
- Most liver injuries (>85%) involve segments **6, 7 and 8** of the liver[Q].
- Most liver injury bleeding is **venous**[Q]; and therefore low pressure, tamponade is readily performed

Diagnosis

- Liver injuries are often **first diagnosed** on **entering the abdomen** in the **unstable patient** explored for the finding of **free fluid on FAST examination**[Q].

  - **Stable patients** with suspected hepatic trauma should undergo **CECT abdomen**[Q].
  - Current **CT modalities** are **excellent** at providing **significant anatomic detail** that allows highly **accurate characterization of injuries**.

- **Contrast extravasation** visualized as a **high-density blush** is identified **indicating** the presence of a **pseudoaneurysm** or **active bleeding** external to the liver capsule[Q].
- **Beer claw laceration:** Multiple Linear laceration of liver on **CECT**
- Liver **injury grading** involves the **extent of parenchymal involvement** and presence of **vascular injury**[Q]

Management

- **Unstable patients: Immediate laparotomy**[Q]
  Conservative criteria for **non-operative management** require
  - Hemodynamically stable patient[Q]
  - Absence of other major injuries[Q]
  - No peritoneal signs on examination[Q]
- **Most treatment failures** occur **within** the **first 24 hours** of **admission**[Q].
- **Failure of nonoperative management** is defined as the development of **hemodynamic instability** or of liver-related **multiple transfusions** despite angiographic embolization, signs of **peritonitis**, or **abdominal compartment syndrome**[Q].

Deep Liver Laceration	Opening the liver wound and directly approaching the bleeding vessel, a procedure known as tractotomy[Q].
Penetrating Liver Tracts	Tractotomy or tamponade using a balloon catheter[Q]
Injuries in the vicinity of retrohepatic IVC	Packing alone, without operative exploration[Q]
Retrohepatic IVC Injury	Atriocaval shunt (Shrock shunt)[Q]

- **Liver parenchymal necrosis** is the **MC complication** of severe liver injury in patients who **undergo operation**[Q].
- **Rebleeding** is the **MC complication** of **nonoperative management**[Q].

Classification of Liver Injury (Moore)

Grade	Types	Operative or CT Scan findings
I	Hematoma Laceration	Subcapsular, **<10%** of surface area Capsular tear, **<1 cm** in parenchymal depth
II	Hematoma Laceration	Subcapsular, **10-50%** of surface area Intraparenchymal, **<10 cm** in diameter **1-3 cm** in parenchymal depth, **<10 cm** in length
III	Hematoma Laceration	Subcapsular, **>50%** of surface area or expanding; ruptured subcapsular or parenchymal hematoma Intraparenchymal, hematoma **>10 cm** or **expanding >3 cm** in parenchymal depth
IV	Laceration	Parenchymal disruption involving **25-75%** of the hepatic lobe or **1-3 Couinauds segments** in a single lobe
V	Laceration Vascular	Parenchymal disruption involving **>75%** of the hepatic lobe or **>3 Couinauds segments** within a single lobe **Juxtahepatic venous injuries**, i.e. retrohepatic **vena cava**/ central **major hepatic veins**
VI	Vascular	**Hepatic avulsion**

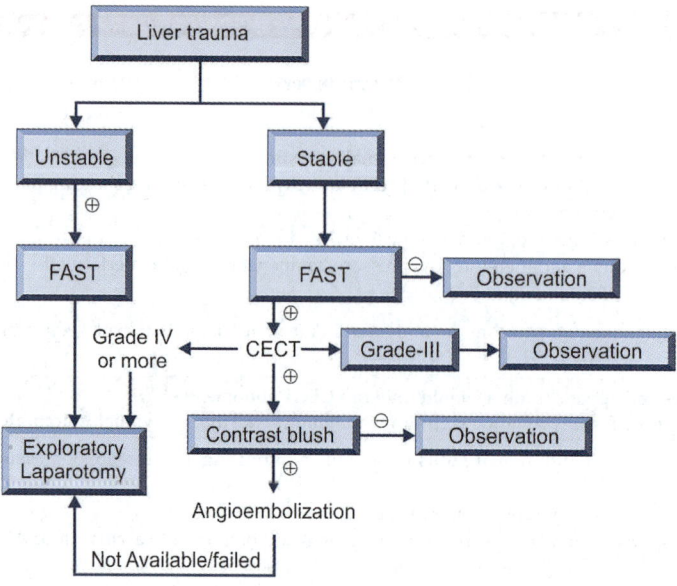

DUODENAL TRAUMA

Duodenal Trauma

- Usually associated with pancreatic injuries^Q

Diagnosis
- IOC for diagnosis: CECT^Q (Only sign is gas or fluid collection in retroperitoneum & leakage of oral contrast^Q)

Management
- Injury to 1st, 3rd & 4th part: Repaired like small bowel with sutures^Q
- Injury to 2nd part: Managed by damage control surgeries & triple tube ostomy is performed (Decompressive gastrostomy, decompressive duodenostomy & feeding jejunostomy^Q)

SEAT BELT INJURY

Seat Belt Injury

- Use of seat belt is associated with injury profile known as seat belt syndrome
- MC injured structure: Mesentery^Q
- Classic seat belt sign: Skin abrasion of neck, chest & abdomen^Q
- Classic seat belt sign is associated with high chances of internal organ injury^Q
- Caused by sudden deceleration → Mesentery tear^Q
- May compress pancreas over vertebral column → Pancreaticoduodenal injury^Q

Longitudinal Tear	Transverse Tear
• Repair the tear as the bowel is perfused by adjacent tissues^Q	• Leads to devascularization of bowel^Q • Resection & anastomosis is done^Q

TRAUMA TRIAD OF DEATH

Trauma Triad of Death

- Trauma triad of death: Hypothermia + Coagulopathy + Metabolic acidosis^Q
- Coagulopathy is most commonly responsible for death^Q

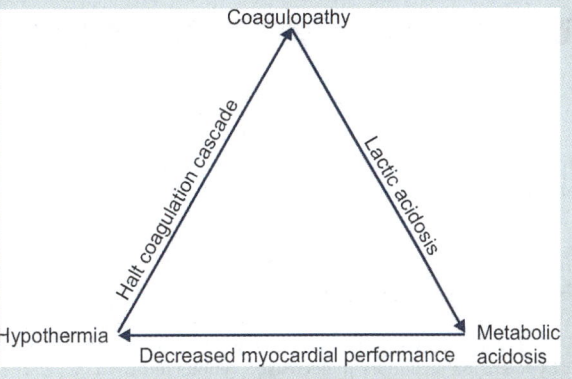

Trauma Triad of Death

DAMAGE CONTROL SURGERY

Damage Control Surgery (DCS)

- DCS centers on coordinating staged operative interventions with periods of aggressive resuscitation to salvage trauma patients sustaining major injuries^Q.
- Damage control includes an abbreviated laparotomy, temporary packing, & closure of the abdomen in an effort to blunt the physiologic response to prolonged shock & massive hemorrhage^Q.

- These patients are often **at limits of their physiological reserve** when they present to operating room and **persistent operative efforts** result in **exacerbation of their underlying hypothermia, coagulopathy & acidosis**, initiating a **vicious cycle** that **culminates in death**^{Q}.
- In these situations, **abrupt termination of** the **procedure** after **control of surgical hemorrhage & contamination**, followed by **ICU resuscitation & staged reconstruction**, can be life saving^Q.

Phases of Damage Control Surgery

Phase I (Initial Exploration)
- This phase consists of an **initial operative exploration** to attain rapid **control of active hemorrhage & contamination**^{Q}
- Abdomen is entered via a **midline incision** and if exsanguinating hemorrhage is encountered **four quadrant packing**^{Q} should be performed
- Any violations of GI tract should be treated with **suture closure** or **segmental stapled resection**^{Q}
- **External drains** are placed to control any major pancreatic or biliary injuries

Phase II (Secondary Resuscitation)
- Following completion of the initial exploration, the **critically ill patient is transferred to the ICU**^{Q}.
- **Invasive monitoring & complete ventilator support**^{Q} are often needed.
- This phase focuses on **secondary resuscitation to correct hypothermia, coagulopathy & acidosis**^{Q}

Phase III (Definitive Operation)
- It consists of **planned re-exploration & definitive repair**^{Q} of injuries
- This phase typically occurs **48 & 72 hours following initial and after successful secondary resuscitation**^{Q}
- Abdomen should be closed primarily if possible
- **Risky GI anastomoses** or **complex reconstruction** should be **avoided**^{Q}

Stages of DCS

Stage	
Stage I	Patient selection^Q
Stage II	Operative control of hemorrhage & contamination^Q
Stage III	ICU resuscitation^Q
Stage IV	Definitive surgery^Q
Stage V	Abdominal closure^Q

ABDOMINAL COMPARTMENT SYNDROME

ABDOMINAL COMPARTMENT SYNDROME

- ACS is defined as increased intra-abdominal pressure (IAP >20 mm Hg) resulting in compression of abdominal structures^Q, producing **fatal complications** due to **pulmonary failure** and **mesenteric vascular compromise**.
- Normal IAP = 5-7 mm Hg; Intra-abdominal hypertension IAP ≥ 12 mm Hg
- ACS occurs **predominantly** in:
  - Patients in profound shock^Q
  - Patients requiring large amounts of resuscitation fluids & blood^Q
  - Those with major visceral or vascular abdominal injuries^Q

- ACS is characterized by a sudden increase in IAP, increased peak inspiratory pressure, decreased urinary output, hypoxia, hypercapnia, & hypotension secondary to **decreased venous return to the heart**^{Q}.

Physiologic Consequences of Increased Intra-abdominal Pressure

Decreased
- Cardiac output^Q
- Central venous return^Q
- Visceral blood flow^Q
- Renal blood flow^Q
- Glomerular filtration

Increased
- Cardiac rate^Q
- Pulmonary capillary wedge pressure^Q
- Peak inspiratory pressure^Q
- Central venous pressure^Q
- Intrapleural pressure
- Systemic vascular resistance^Q

Diagnosis

- Diagnosis is confirmed by **measuring bladder pressure**, which ultimately represents IAP.
- A **urinary bladder catheter** is the **gold standard** indirect method used to measure IAP.

	Abdominal Compartment Syndrome Grading System		
Grade	Bladder Pressure (mm Hg)	Clinical Features	Treatment
I	12–15	None	**Normovolemic** resuscitation
II	16–20	**Oliguria**[Q], splanchnic hypoperfusion	**Hypovolemic** resuscitation
III	21–25	**Anuria**, increased ventilation pressure	**Decompression**
IV	>25	**Anuria**, increased ventilation pressure & decreased PO_2[Q]	**Emergency re-exploration**

Treatment

- Treatment includes **rapid decompression** of elevated IAP **by opening the abdominal wound** & performing a **temporary closure** of abdominal wall with **mesh** or a **plastic bag (Bogota bag)**[Q].

RETROPERITONEAL INJURIES

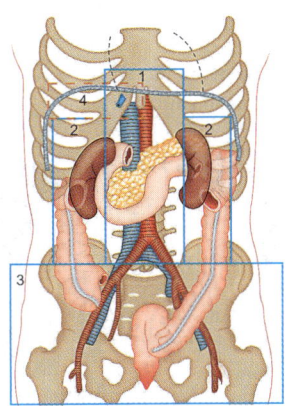

The retroperitoneum is usually divided into three parts based on site of injury. Some authors also describe a 4th zone, i.e. the portal and retrohepatic area. Zone 1 (central) extends from the esophageal hiatus to the sacral promontory. Zone 2 (lateral) extends from the lateral diaphragm to the iliac crest. Zone 3 (pelvic) is confined to the retroperitoneal space of the pelvic bowl.

	Zones of Retroperitoneal Hematoma		
Zone	Extent		Management
Zone 1 (central)	• Extends from **esophageal hiatus to sacral promontory**[Q] • Hematoma or hemorrhage in the **midline** associated with **injuries** to **abdominal aorta, IVC**, their proximal **branches and tributaries**[Q]. • Zone 1 is divided into **supramesocolic and inframesocolic zone** depending on **origin of vascular structure in relation to transverse mesocolon**[Q].		• **Central hematoma** should **always be explored** with **proximal and distal vascular control**[Q]
	Supramesocolic Zone 1	**Inframesocolic Zone 1**	
	• **Suprarenal aorta, IVC, coeliac axis, proximal SMA and vein**, and **proximal renal arteries** and **veins**[Q].	• **Infrarenal aorta & IVC** including their **bifurcations**[Q].	
Zone 2 (lateral)	• Extends from **lateral diaphragm to iliac crest**[Q] • Include distal renal arteries and veins[Q]		• **Lateral hematomas** are **usually renal** in origin and can be **managed nonoperatively**[Q], sometimes with **angioembolization**.
Zone 3 (pelvic)	• Confined to **retroperitoneal space of pelvic bowl**[Q] • Include iliac arteries and veins[Q]		• **Pelvic hematomas** are **exceptionally difficult to control** and should, whenever possible, **not be opened**[Q] • Should be **controlled with packing** (intra- or extrapelvic) and **angioembolization**[Q]
Zone 4	• Include portal and retrohepatic area[Q]		

NECK INJURIES

Neck Injuries

- **Most severe neck injuries** are caused **by penetrating wounds** and may present an immediate threat to life as a result of **airway compromise** or **hemorrhage**^{Q}.

  - **Major vascular & aerodigestive structures** in the neck are located in anterior triangle, & all are deep to the **platysma**^{Q}.
  - **Platysma & SCM** are useful anatomic boundaries^Q.

- Injuries that **do not penetrate** the **platysma** can be considered superficial, and no further investigation is needed. Wounds that **penetrate** the **platysma** must be further evaluated.
- Injuries that are **anterior to SCM** present a high likelihood of significant injury, whereas those that track **posterior to SCM** are unlikely to involve major vascular or aerodigestive structures.
- Penetrating injuries to the **posterior triangle** should raise concern about **trauma to cervical spine & spinal cord**^{Q}.

Neck is divided into Three Horizontal Zones on craniocaudal location	
Zone I	• At thoracic inlet^Q • Extends from **sternal notch to cricoid cartilage**^{Q} • Injuries in this zone carry the **highest mortality** because of the **presence of great vessels**^{Q} & difficult surgical approach.
Zone II	• Midportion of the neck^Q • Extends from **cricoid cartilage to angle of mandible**^{Q}
Zone III	• Extends from **angle of mandible to base of skull**^{Q}

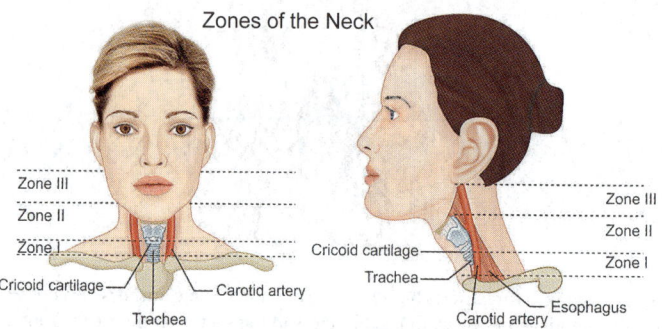

Zones of the Neck

THORACIC INJURIES

Thoracic Injuries

- MC cause of mortality in blunt thoracic trauma: Tracheobronchial injuries^Q
- MC cause of mortality in penetrating thoracic trauma: Hemothorax^Q (secondary to pulmonary laceration)
- MC thoracic injuries: Chest wall injuries^Q

RIB FRACTURE

Rib Fracture

- Occurs secondary to compression of thoracic cage in anteroposterior direction or lateral direction
- **Uncommon** to have **fracture of floating ribs (11th & 12th ribs)** & **first rib fracture**^{Q}
- High velocity impact can cause fracture of 1st rib & **10th-12th** ribs.

  - **MC rib fractured during CPR: 4th-6th rib**^{Q}

- In cases of **1st rib fracture**, suspect injury of subclavian vessels, brachial plexus & apex of lung^Q
- In cases of **10th-12th rib fracture, on right side suspect injury to liver**^{Q} **& on left side suspect injury to spleen**^{Q} (long axis of spleen is related to 10th rib)

Management

- Most rib fractures are **managed conservatively with adequate analgesia. Strapping should not be done**^{Q}

STERNAL FRACTURE

Sternal Fracture

- Uncommon, **typically transverse**[Q]
- Located in **upper & mid portions** of body of sternum[Q]

Clinical Features
- **Tenderness, swelling & deformity** at site of fracture[Q]
- Sternal fracture is associated with severe intrathoracic injuries
- Specific injury to myocardium is common

Diagnosis
- Diagnosed by **chest X-ray**[Q] **(lateral view)**

Treatment
- Management is similar to rib fracture
- **Adequate analgesia & good pulmonary hygiene**[Q]
- **Surgical intervention** is recommended for **displaced fracture**[Q]

PERICARDIAL TAMPONADE

Pericardial Tamponade

- **Rapid accumulation of blood in pericardial space**[Q]
- **Quantity of fluid**: Even **200 mL fluid** which **collets rapidly** can lead to pericardial tamponade[Q]
- Caused by **penetrating trauma**[Q]

Clinical Features
- Characterized by **Beck's triad (MDH)**: **M**uffled heart sounds + **D**istended neck veins + **H**ypotension[Q]

Diagnosis
- IOC for diagnosis: **Echocardiography**[Q]
- Chest X-ray: **Enlarged heart shadow**[Q]

Treatment
- Emergency treatment: **Needle pericardiocentesis**[Q]
- TOC: **Surgical pericardiotomy**[Q]

FLAIL CHEST

Flail Chest

- A flail chest occurs when a **segment of** the **chest wall does not have bony continuity with** the **rest of** the **thoracic cage**[Q].
- This condition usually results from blunt trauma associated with multiple rib fractures, i.e. **two or more consequtive ribs fractured in two or more places**[Q].
- The blunt force required to disrupt the integrity of the thoracic cage typically produces an **underlying pulmonary contusion** as well.

Clinical Features
- On inspiration the **loose segment** of the chest wall is **displaced inwards** and less air therefore moves into the lungs (**Paradoxical respiration**)[Q]
- To confirm the diagnosis the chest wall can be observed for **paradoxical motion of a chest wall segment**[Q] for **several respiratory cycles** and **during coughing**.

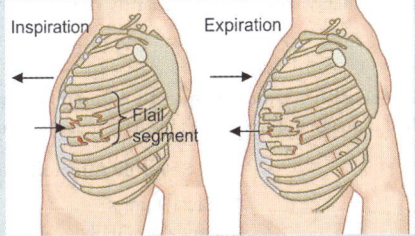

- **Voluntary splinting** as a result of pain, **mechanically impaired chest wall movement** and the **associated lung contusion** are all **causes of** the **hypoxia & respiratory failure**[Q].
- The patient is also at high risk of developing a **pneumothorax or hemothorax**[Q].

Diagnosis
- **Diagnosis** is made **clinically**[Q], not by radiography.

Treatment
- **Chest strapping** or **splinting should be avoided**[Q].
- **Currently, treatment** consists of **oxygen administration**, **adequate analgesia** (including opiates) or **epidural analgesia** & **physiotherapy**[Q].
- **IPPV (Intermittent positive pressure ventilation)** is **reserved for** cases developing **respiratory failure** despite adequate analgesia & oxygen[Q].

DIAPHRAGMATIC INJURIES

DIAPHRAGMATIC INJURY

- **Diaphragmatic injuries** are **often caused by penetrating injuries**[Q].
- Patients **sustaining penetrating injuries below** the **nipples** and **above the costal margins** should be **investigated to rule out diaphragmatic injury**[Q].

Etiology
- **Penetrating trauma** (knife, bullet, repair of hiatus hernia)
- **Blunt trauma** (motor vehicle accident, fall from height, bout of hyperemesis):
  - Caused by **compressive force** applied to the **pelvis** and **abdomen**.
  - Rupture is **usually large**, with herniation of abdominal content into chest

Clinical Features
- **Most diaphragmatic injuries** are **silent** and the presenting features are those of injury to the surrounding organs[Q].
- **Late complication**: Herniation of abdominal contents in to the **chest**[Q].

> - Herniation of organ: Stomach[Q] >Colon >Small intestine >Omentum >Spleen >Kidney and pancreas.

Diagnosis
- There is **no single standard investigation** to diagnose **diaphragmatic injuries**[Q].
- **Chest X-ray** after placement of a nasogastric tune may be helpful (as this may show the **stomach herniated into the chest**)
- Contrast study of upper or lower GIT, CT scan and diagnostic peritoneal lavage all lack positive or negative predictive value.

> - **Most accurate evaluation** is by **video assisted thoracoscopy (VATS)** or **laparoscopy**[Q], offering the **advantage of allowing** the surgeon to proceed to repair and **additional evaluation** of the **abdominal organs**.

Treatment
- **Operative repair**[Q] is recommended **in all cases**.
- All penetrating diaphragmatic injury must be **repaired via the abdomen** and not the chest, to rule out penetrating hollow viscus injury.

> **Bergvist Triad**: Rib fracture + Fracture of **spine/pelvis** + Traumatic rupture of **diaphragm**

BLAST INJURIES

BLAST INJURIES

- **Primary blast injuries** result from the **rapid overpressure** or **shock waves** produced by an explosion
- These injuries result from the **dramatic changes in barometric pressure** projected from the point of detonation
- Primary blast injuries predominantly cause **damage to air filled hollow organs** of the body **from rapid pressure change (barotraumas)**.

> - Damage to air filled organs includes **middle ear, lungs & GIT.**[Q]

- Most sensitive & most frequently injured hollow organ: Tympanic membrane[Q] > Lungs
- Blast damage to the lungs is the MC cause of life threatening injury[Q] following an explosion.

Most Severely Affected Organs	Most Commonly Affected Organs
Air Blast: Lungs[Q]	Air: Tympanic membrane[Q]
Underwater: GIT[Q]	Underwater (Fully submerged): TM[Q]
	Underwater (Head is out): GIT[Q]

CHEST TUBE INSERTION

INTERCOSTAL DRAIN (ICD) INSERTION

- **ICD insertion** is done in **triangle of safety in 5th intercostal space in anterior axially line**[Q].
- Insertion is done over **upper border of lower rib**[Q] & **all eyes of drain** should be **inside pleural space**[Q]

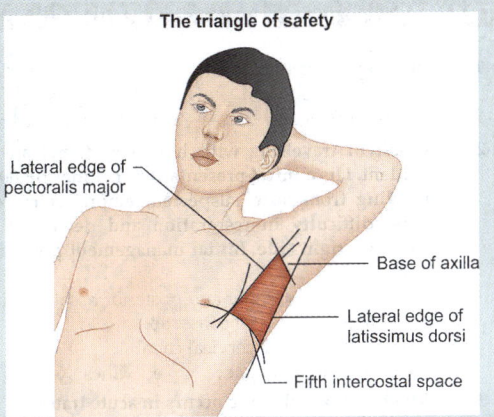

Boundaries of Triangle of Safety	
Anteriorly	• Lateral border of **pectoralis major**[Q]
Laterally	• Lateral border of **latissimus dorsi**[Q]
Inferiorly	• Line of 5th intercostal space[Q]
Superiorly	• Base of axilla[Q]

- Used to provide **evacuation of air or fluid from pleural space**[Q]
- **Under water seal chamber**: Most important element in pleural drainage; **Acts as one-way valve** for evacuation of pleural contents; When **intra-pleural pressure rise**, **free contents** of pleural space are **forced out through chest tube into under water seal**[Q].
- **Re-entry of air** into pleural space is **blocked by underwater seal**[Q]
- Water in the tube is known as water column. The **water column should be moving**[Q].
- **Tip of tube** should be **2-3 cm below the surface of water**[Q].

Follow-up
- Patency of chest tube is assessed by observing oscillations in water seal chamber with respiratory movements[Q].
- Position of chest tube & resolution of intrapleural air or liquid is checked by chest X-ray[Q]

  - **Column movement stops** in blocked tube or **displaced tube**[Q].
  - **Excessive bubbling** in tube suggest bronchopleural fistula[Q]

Removal
- When **lung expands** & air or fluid drainage is **<200 mL in 24 hours**[Q]
- **Chest tube** should be **removed when patient holds the breath at peak of inspiration**[Q].

Multiple Choice Questions

TRAUMA

1. **First step in trauma:** *(Recent Question 2013)*
   a. Blood transfusion
   b. IV fluids
   c. Reconstruction
   d. Maintenance of airways

2. **A patient travelling with high speed met an road traffic accident. His clinical presentation includes BP 80/40 mm Hg, bleeding from nose, suspected femoral fracture, cyanosed body, difficulty in respiration and decreased respiratory sound on right side. Initial management preference will be given to:** *(PGI Nov 2011)*
   a. Hemostatic anterior and posterior nasal packing
   b. Thoracosotomy tube insertion
   c. ETT in line with cervical canal
   d. I.V Fluid immediate
   e. Chest X-ray

3. **Which of the following occurs in acute trauma?** *(JIPMER 2011)*
   a. Increase in insulin
   b. Decrease in glucagon
   c. Decrease in cortisol
   d. Increase in thyroxine

4. **In surgical stress all hormone is increased *except*:**
   a. ADH
   b. ACTH *(PGI June 2009)*
   c. Cortisol
   d. Insulin
   e. Renin

5. **In surgical stress all hormones are increased *except*:**
   a. Adrenaline
   b. ACTH *(PGI Nov 2011)*
   c. Epinephrine
   d. Cortisol
   e. Insulin

6. **Early stage of trauma is characterized by:** *(All India 2003)*
   a. Catabolism
   b. Anabolism
   c. Glycogenesis
   d. Lipogenesis

7. **In case of clearing airway one of the following is not included:** *(AIIMS June 95)*
   a. Neck tilt
   b. Mouth gag
   c. Chin lift
   d. Head lift

8. **First step taken in case of multiple injuries of face and neck:** *(UPSC 2008, AIIMS June 95)*
   a. Blood transfusion
   b. IV fluids
   c. Reconstruction
   d. Maintenance of airways

9. **In severe injury, first to be maintained is:** *(Recent Question 2013, PGI June 97)*
   a. Hypotension
   b. Dehydration
   c. Airway
   d. Cardiac status

10. **Which one of the following veins should be avoided for intravenous infusion in the management of abdominal trauma?** *(UPSC 2001)*
    a. Cubital
    b. Cephalic
    c. Long saphenous
    d. External jugular

11. **Following trauma, which hormone is not released?**
    a. Thyroxine
    b. Glucagon *(All India 92)*
    c. ADH
    d. GH

12. **Protein metabolism after trauma is characterized by all of the following *except*:** *(UPSC 2007)*
    a. Increased liver gluconeogenesis
    b. Inhibition of skeletal muscle breakdown by IL-1 and TNF
    c. Increased urinary nitrogen loss
    d. Hepatic synthesis of acute phase reactants

13. **A female with suspected child abuse was brought to the casualty with severe bleeding from perineum. What should be the first line of management?** *(AIIMS November 2014)*
    a. Airway maintenance
    b. Internal iliac artery ligation
    c. Whole blood transfusion
    d. Inform police before starting the treatment

14. **The first priority in management of a case of head injury with open fracture of shaft of femur is:** *(AIIMS May 2014)*
    a. Neurosurgery consultation
    b. Give IV fluids
    c. Intubation
    d. Splintage of fracture

15. **Back examination of poly-trauma patient is known as:** *(Recent Question 2015)*
    a. Log roll
    b. Barrel role
    c. Chin lift
    d. None

16. **A 45 years old patient presented to you with ongoing massive hematemesis. The patient is alert and hemodynamically stable. What will be the first step in management?** *(AIIMS November 2016)*
    a. Do an urgent upper GI endoscopy
    b. Put the patient in recovery position and secure airway
    c. Insert a cannula and start IV fluids
    d. Send for blood transfusion

17. **An unresponsive patient has been brought to you by the police. What is the first thing you will do?** *(AIIMS November 2016)*
    a. Start chest compressions immediately
    b. Check carotid pulse
    c. Check for response and call help
    d. Start rescue breaths

18. **For the transport of traumatized and conscious patient all the following are done except?** *(AIIMS November 2017)*
    a. On a hard board with head/spine stabilized
    b. In lateral lying position
    c. Talk to patient while he is on board
    d. Rolling without moving the spine

19. **In a school bus accident, which of the following victim you will attend first?** *(AIIMS November 2017)*
    a. A child with airway obstruction
    b. A child with shock
    c. A child with flail chest
    d. A child with severe head injury

20. **Which of the following is the correct sequence?** *(AIIMS November 2017)*
    a. Assess the patient's response, Call for help, check carotid pulse, Start CPR
    b. Check carotid pulse, Start CPR, Call for help, Defibrillate
    c. Defibrillate, Assess response, Check carotid pulse, Maintain airway
    d. Start CPR, Call for help, Defibrillate, Check pulse

21. **Balanced resuscitation in trauma management is:** *(AIIMS November 2017)*
    a. Giving colloids and crystalloids ratio of 1:1
    b. Maintaining pH by ensuring acid base are balanced
    c. Maintaining permissible hypotension to avoid bleeding
    d. Maintaining airway, breathing and circulation simultaneously

22. In trauma transfusion, ratio of RBCs, FFP and platelets is:
    (Recent Question 2017)
    a. 1:1:3
    b. 1:1:1
    c. 1:1:2
    d. 1:1:4

23. All the following are true about imaging in primary survey of a trauma patient except: *(AIIMS May 2017)*
    a. Cervical X-ray is not mandatory
    b. Chest X-ray and pelvic X-ray are taken as a part of primary survey
    c. Hemodynamically unstable patients should not be sent for CT scan
    d. All patients should have chest X-ray-PA view only

24. A patient met with a RTA with paralysis of both upper and lower limb. Patient has not passed urine and tenderness elicited in the cervical region. What will you advise?
    (AIIMS May 2017)
    a. The doctor should order a cervical X-ray and shift the patient from the trolley by himself
    b. The patient should not be shifted and portable X-ray machine should be used after neck stabilization
    c. The doctor will instruct the radiographer to take cervical and chest X-ray
    d. The doctor will instruct the radiographer to take cervical X-ray AP and lateral view without any cervical support

25. Which of the following is an indicator of airway obstruction? *(Recent Question 2017)*
    a. Inability to speak
    b. Poor air exchange
    c. Throat pain
    d. Surgical emphysema

26. Common cause of breathing difficulty in an unconscious patient: *(Recent Question 2017)*
    a. Foreign body
    b. Tongue
    c. Vomitus
    d. Blood

27. Sequence of resuscitation in a trauma patient:
    a. Circulation, airway and breathing *(Recent Question 2017)*
    b. Airway, breathing and circulation
    c. Airway, circulation and breathing
    d. Breathing, airway and circulation

28. Patient with massive hemorrhage presents to the emergency room after road traffic accident. Which of the following should not be done? *(AIIMS November 2018)*
    a. Massive transfusion of fluid challenge
    b. IV crystalloid 2 L, within few minutes
    c. Early tranexamic acid recommended
    d. Check coagulation with thromboelastography, if available

29. Following a RTA, a young man was brought to ER. Due to massive blood loss, 2 units of PRBC and 4 platelets obtained from blood bank. Only one IV line was accessible. What will you do? *(AIIMS November 2018)*
    a. Start PRBC first and store platelet at room temperature
    b. Start platelet and store PRBC at room temperature
    c. Only transfuse PRBC
    d. Transfuse PRBC and store platelet at 2–6 degrees

30. A 42 years old man, intubated after traumatic brain injury (TBI) for decreasing GCS. Currently, he opens his eyes to pressure, is intubated, and withdraws his left arm and leg to pain. What will be his GCS score?
    a. 5
    b. 6
    c. 7
    d. 8

31. Patient had a road traffic accident and put on mechanical ventilation. He is opening his eyes on verbal command, moves all his four limbs spontaneously. What will be his GCS score? *(AIIMS November 2018)*
    a. 12
    b. 11
    c. 9
    d. 10

32. A young patient has been admitted with road traffic accident and had massive haemorrhage. He needs to be transfused with large amounts of fluids. Which IV cannula is preferred?
    (AIIMS November 2018)
    a. Grey
    b. Green
    c. Blue
    d. Pink

TRAUMA SCORING SYSTEM

33. Which one of the following is not a part of the Revised Trauma Score? *(UPSC 2001)*
    a. Glasgow coma scale
    b. Systolic blood pressure
    c. Pulse rate
    d. Respiratory rate

34. Trauma and injury severity score (TRISS) includes:
    (Recent Question 2016, All India 2010)
    a. GCS + BP + RR
    b. RTS + ISS + age
    c. RTS + ISS + GCS
    d. RTS + GCS + BP

35. Mangled Extremity Severity Score (MESS) includes all of the following except? *(Recent Question 2016, AIIMS May 2011)*
    a. Shock
    b. Ischemia
    c. Neurogenic injury
    d. Energy of injury

36. Best assessment score in trauma patients:
    (Recent Question 2017)
    a. Modified trauma score
    b. Revised trauma score
    c. Injury severity score
    d. Mangled extremity severity score

TRIAGE

37. In triage green color indicates: *(COMEDK 2005)*
    a. Ambulatory patients
    b. Dead or moribund
    c. High priority treatment or transfer
    d. Medium priority or transfer

38. Which of the following is colour code and explanantion is matched correctly as per the triage used in disaster management? *(AIIMS November 2017)*
    a. Red-Deceased
    b. Black-Minor injuries
    c. Yellow- Stable patients, observation
    d. Green-Need immediate intervention

39. Triage system is used for:
    (Recent Question 2015)
    a. Burn
    b. Earthquake
    c. Polytrauma
    d. Floods

40. Which colour of triage is given the highest priority?
    a. Red
    b. Green *(AIIMS Nov 2013)*
    c. Yellow
    d. Black

BLUNT TRAUMA ABDOMEN

41. Most common organ involved in blunt injury to the abdomen: *(WB PG 2015, JIPMER 2011, 2014)*
    a. Spleen
    b. Liver
    c. Intestines
    d. Kidney

42. **Investigation of choice for blunt trauma abdomen in unstable patient:** *(PGI Dec 2000)*
    a. X-ray abdomen
    b. USG
    c. Diagnostic Peritoneal lavage (DPL)
    d. MRI
    e. CT scan

43. **Investigation of choice for diagnosing intra abdominal bleeding in an unstable patient:** *(PGI Dec 2001)*
    a. CT scan
    b. MRI scan
    c. USG
    d. Diagnostic peritoneal lavage

44. **Babu is brought to the emergency as a case of road traffic accident. He is hypotensive. Most likely ruptured organ is:**
    a. Spleen
    b. Mesentery *(All India 2001)*
    c. Kidney
    d. Rectum

45. **Commonly injured in blunt abdominal injury is/are:** *(PGI June 2001)*
    a. Mid ileum
    b. Proximal jejunum
    c. Mid jejunum
    d. Distal ileum
    e. Ileocecal junction

46. **A driver wearing seat belt applied brake suddenly to avoid accident. Most common organ injured in seat belt injury:** *(AIIMS May 2013)*
    a. Liver
    b. Spleen
    c. Mesentery
    d. Abdominal aorta

47. **Preferred incision for abdominal exploration in blunt injury abdomen is:** *(All India 2007)*
    a. Always midline incision
    b. Depending upon the organ
    c. Transverse incision
    d. Paramedian

48. **A case of blunt trauma is brought to the emergency, in a state of shock; he is not responding to IV crystalloids; next step in his management would be:** *(All India 2001)*
    a. Immediate laparotomy
    b. Blood transfusion
    c. Albumin transfusion
    d. Abdominal compression

49. **A patient developed hemoperitoneum following RTA, with BP 90/60 and pulse 140/min, which of the following to be done?** *(PGI Dec 2003)*
    a. DPL to be done
    b. Liver is the MC organ to rupture
    c. USG is better than CT scan
    d. X-ray to be taken in supine position
    e. Urgent surgery to be done

50. **A male patient with blunt trauma abdomen is hemodynamically stable. What is the next line of management?** *(All India 2008)*
    a. Observation
    b. Further imaging of abdomen
    c. Exploratory laparotomy
    d. Laparoscopy

51. **Best diagnostic test in stable patient with blunt trauma abdomen is:** *(Recent Question 2016, 2014; DNB 2012)*
    a. CECT scan
    b. MRI
    c. DPL
    d. FAST

52. **A patient with blunt trauma of abdomen at 48 hours, USG shows normal, but patient had tenderness in left lumbar region. Best appropriate diagnosis is by:** *(Recent Question 2018)*
    a. MCU
    b. IVP
    c. CECT abdomen
    d. Repeat USG

53. **Blunt injuries to the abdomen:**
    a. May cause peritonitis
    b. Rarely need urgent laparotomy
    c. May cause intestinal obstruction
    d. May cause gastroduodenal ulceration

54. **Which of the following is not true?** *(DPG 2007)*
    a. Spleen is most commonly injured in the blunt trauma
    b. Small intestine is most commonly injured in penetrating trauma
    c. Thoracic duct injury needs urgent thoracotomy
    d. Conservative treatment is preferred for solid organ injury

55. **FAST stands for:** *(AP PG 2015, AIIMS Nov 2013)*
    a. Focused assessment with sonography for trauma
    b. Focused abdominal sonography for trauma
    c. Fast assessment with sonography for trauma
    d. Fast assignment with sonography and tomography (computed)

56. **Which of the following is not assessed in FAST?** *(Recent Question 2015)*
    a. Right upper quadrant
    b. Left upper quadrant
    c. Hypogastrium
    d. Sub-xiphoid area

57. **A man with blunt injury abdomen after road side accident has a blood pressure of 100/80 mm Hg and a pulse rate of 120/min. Airway has been established and respiration has been stabilized. Next best step in management is:** *(All India 2009)*
    a. Immediate blood transfusion
    b. Blood for cross matching and IV fluids
    c. Ventilate the patient
    d. Rush the patient to the OT

58. **A patient is brought to the emergency as a case of head injury, following a head on collision road traffic accident. His BP is 90/60 mm Hg. Tachycardia is present. Most likely diagnosis is:** *(All India 2001)*
    a. EDH
    b. SDH
    c. Intracranial hemorrhage
    d. Intra-abdominal bleed

59. **A 40-year-old male drive had a car accident in which he got wedged in-between. He complained of severe abdominal pain with radiation to the back. The initial CT on admission was negative except for minimal retroperitoneal hematoma. The diagnosis is:** *(COMEDK 2010)*
    a. Liver injury
    b. Duodenal perforation
    c. Bowel rupture
    d. Pancreatic injury

60. **True about indication of celiotomy in blunt trauma:**
    a. Peritoneal air on imaging *(PGI June 2009)*
    b. Severe hypotension
    c. Grade I spleen damage
    d. Grade II liver damage
    e. Patient with positive diagnostic peritoneal lavage

61. **A patient with abdominal injury presents to the emergency department with signs of signs of peritonitis and shock. Airway and breathing were secured and IV fluids were started with 2 large bore cannulas. The next line of management should be:** *(All India 2011)*
    a. FAST
    b. Exploratory laparotomy under general anesthesia
    c. Insertion of abdominal drain followed by laparotomy
    d. Laparoscopy

62. **The four points of probe placement in Focused Abdominal Sonogram for trauma (FAST) in blunt thoraco-abdominal trauma are:** *(Karnataka 2004)*
    a. Epigastrium, (R) hypochondrium, (L) Lower chest, hypogastrium
    b. Epigastrium, (R) and (L) Hypochondria, (R) Iliac fossa
    c. Epigastrium, (R) and (L) Lumbar regions, hypogastrium
    d. Hypogastrium, (R) and (L) Lumbar regions, (R) lower chest

63. All the following are True regarding fast–except:
    a. It is a focused abdominal sonar for trauma *(APPG 2015)*
    b. It is accurate in detecting < 50 ml of free blood
    c. It cannot reliably exclude injury in penetrating trauma
    d. It detects free fluid in the abdomen or pericardium

64. Isolated splenic/hepatic injury in a child is most commonly managed by: *(Recent Question 2017)*
    a. Conservative management
    b. Laparotomy
    c. Interventional
    d. Splenectomy and liver packing

DAMAGE CONTROL SURGERY

65. Damage control surgery is: *(JIPMER 2014, AIIMS May 2013)*
    a. Minimal intervention done to stabilize the patient and do the definitive surgery later
    b. Maximum possible surgical intervention is done immediately
    c. Done during triage procedure
    d. Done to control damage during surgery

66. Where is the second step of damage control resuscitation carried out? *(AIIMS May 2018)*
    a. In emergency   b. In ICU
    c. In OT   d. Prehospital resuscitation

67. Aim of damage control laparotomy are: *(PGI June 2009)*
    a. Provide fascial closure   b. Arrest hemorrhage
    c. Control contamination   d. Prevent infection
    e. Prevent coagulopathy

68. Aims of abbreviated laparotomy: *(PGI June 2005)*
    a. Decreased change of infection
    b. Early ambulation
    c. Early wound healing   d. Hemostasis

69. Abbreviated laparotomy done for: *(PGI Dec 2007)*
    a. Coagulopathy   b. Hypotension
    c. Early wound healing   d. Early ambulation
    e. Hemostasis

70. A trauma patient was brought to emergency. On evaluation, found to have metabolic acidosis and coagulopathy with liver and duodenal injury. Next step: *(Recent Question 2017)*
    a. Damage control surgery   b. Liver repair
    c. Whipples procedure   d. None of the above

71. A 30 years old young male met with a road traffic accident and came to the trauma center. On examination his BP is 90/56 mm Hg, pulse rate is 150/min, SpO_2 86% and a Glasgow coma score of 8. On examination the patient had multiple injuries and FAST reveals haemorrhage in all quadrants. He was operated upon and the postoperative pictures are shown below. Correctly describe the two pictures. *(AIIMS May 2016)*
    a. Midline laparotomy and meshplasty
    b. Abdominothoracic surgery with abdominal zipping
    c. Damage control surgery and mesh closure of abdomen
    d. Abdominoplasty and primary closure of abdomen

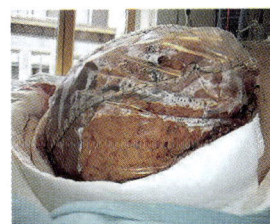 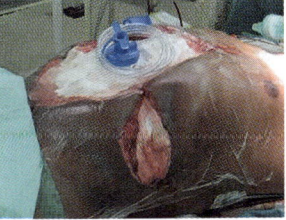

ABDOMINAL COMPARTMENT SYNDROME

72. True about abdominal compartment syndrome:
    a. ↓ Cardiac output   *(PGI June 2009, Dec 2008)*
    b. ↓ Urine output
    c. ↓ Pulmonary capillary wedge pressure
    d. ↓ Venous return
    e. ↓ Systemic vascular resistance

73. True about abdominal compartment syndrome: *(PGI November 2017)*
    a. Normal intra-abdominal pressure is 0-5 mm Hg
    b. Intra-abdominal hypertension is measured by bladder pressure
    c. Earliest sign is renal failure
    d. Management of choice is abdominal opening
    e. Multi-organ failure may occur

74. True about abdominal compartment syndrome include the following except: *(MHSSMCET 2008)*
    a. >15 cm of H_2O
    b. Decreased pulmonary venous pressure
    c. IAP Measured using Foley's catheterization of bladder
    d. With >25-30 mm Hg IAP, life threatening hypoxia and ARDS can occur

75. Abdominal compartment syndrome is characterized by the following except: *(UPSC 2007)*
    a. Hypercarbia and respiratory acidosis
    b. Hypoxia due to increased peak inspiratory pressure
    c. Hypotension due to decrease in venous return
    d. Oliguria due to ureter obstruction

76. Increased intra abdominal pressure is/are associated with:
    a. ↑ Pulmonary capillary wedge pressure *(PGI June 2004)*
    b. ↑ Venous return
    c. ↑ Pulmonary inspiratory pressure
    d. ↑ Renal blood flow
    e. ↑ Cardiac output

77. True about abdominal compartment syndrome:
    a. ↓ Cardiac output   *(PGI Dec 2008)*
    b. ↓ Urine output
    c. ↓ Venous return
    d. ↓ Systemic vascular resistance

78. Which one of the following statements is true regarding Abdominal Compartment Syndrome? *(APPG 2016)*
    a. Reduction in visceral perfusion and increase in intracranial pressure
    b. diagnosis can be reliably made by physical examination
    c. The intraabdominal pressure in grade I ACS is 21-35 cm H320
    d. Definitive surgery is immediately done followed by closure of abdomen

79. Which of the following is best treatment for Grade II abdominal hypertension? *(Recent Question 2016)*
    a. Laparotomy
    b. Immediate decompression
    c. Hypovolemic resuscitation
    d. Normovolemic resuscitation

PENETRATING INJURIES

80. Organ most commonly damaged in penetrating injury of abdomen is: *(WBPG 2014, AIIMS Nov 94, Nov 95)*
    a. Liver   b. Small intestine
    c. Large intestine d. Duodenum

Others

81. Treatment of choice for stab injury caecum: *(All India 89)*
    a. Cecostomy
    b. Ileo-transverse anastomosis
    c. Transverse colostomy
    d. Sigmoid colostomy

82. A man comes to emergency with stab injury to left flank. He has stable vitals. What would be the next step in management: *(AIIMS Nov 2008)*
    a. CECT
    b. Diagnostic peritoneal lavage
    c. Laparotomy
    d. Laparoscopy

83. A patient with stab injury to anterior abdomen presents with a tag of omentum protruding through the abdominal wall near the umbilicus. On evaluation he is hemodynamically stable and shows no signs of peritonitis. Initial management of patient should involve: *(All India 2011)*
    a. FAST
    b. Exploratory Laparotomy
    c. Local Wound Exploration and Suturing
    d. CECT Abdomen

84. Which of the following is not done in case of puncture wound of left colon? *(Recent Question 2015)*
    a. Primary suture
    b. Hemicolectomy
    c. Externalization
    d. Resection and anastomosis

85. In the patient of penetrating injury to the abdomen with shock, next best step is: *(Recent Question 2017)*
    a. USG
    b. FAST
    c. CT
    d. Laparotomy

NECK INJURIES

86. Which of the following is used to define penetrating neck injury? *(AIIMS May 2009, All India 2008)*
    a. 2 cm depth of wound
    b. Injury to vital structures
    c. Breach of platysma
    d. Through and through wound

87. The probable cause of sudden death in a case superficial injury to neck is: *(DNB 2005)*
    a. Injury to phrenic nerve
    b. Air embolism through external jugular vein
    c. Bleeding from subclavian artery
    d. Injury to trachea

88. Zone of neck involving great vessels at thoracic inlet:
    a. I
    b. II *(Recent Question 2016)*
    c. III
    d. IV

BLAST INJURIES

89. In a blast injury, which of the following organ is least vulnerable to the blast wave? *(AIIMS June 2003)*
    a. GI tract
    b. Lungs
    c. Liver
    d. Ear drum

90. Most common organ injured in underwater explosion: *(MHSSMCET 2009)*
    a. TM
    b. GIT
    c. Lungs
    d. Heart

HEPATIC INJURIES

91. A 17-year-old boy is admitted to the hospital after a road traffic accident. Per abdomen examination is normal. After adequate resuscitation, his pulse rate is 80/min and BP is 110/70 mm Hg. Abdominal CT reveals 1 cm deep laceration in the left lobe of the liver extending from the done more than half way through the parenchyma. Appropriate management at this time would be: *(DPG 2011, UPSC 2005)*
    a. Conservative treatment
    b. Abdominal exploration and packing of hepatic wounds
    c. Abdominal exploration and ligation of left hepatic artery
    d. Left hepatectomy

SPLENIC INJURIES

92. A 30-year-old gentleman after sustaining road traffic accident present in emergency with BP 100/60 mmHg, Pulse 120 min and CT scan shows splenic laceration at inferior border after 2 units of blood transfusion, patients conditions are: BP 120/70 mmHg and pulse 84/min; the next line of management is: *(PGI June 2003)*
    a. Laparotomy
    b. Splenorrhaphy
    c. Continue the conservative treatment and take subsequent measures on monitoring the patient
    d. Splenectomy
    e. X-ray abdomen and aspiration

93. A child presents in causality in stable condition after a blunt abdominal trauma associated with splenic trauma. Treatment of choice is: *(Recent Question 2016, AIIMS Nov 2000)*
    a. Observation
    b. Splenectomy
    c. Arterial embolisation
    d. Splenorrhaphy

94. True about blunt abdominal trauma with splenic rupture: *(PGI June 2008)*
    a. Kehr's sign-discoloration around umbilicus
    b. Spleen is most common organ to be involved
    c. Splenectomy is treatment of choice for splenic rupture
    d. Cullen's sign seen

95. A 30-year-old person met with a roadside accident. On admission his pulse rate was 120/minute, BP was 100/60 mmHg. USG examination revealed laceration of the lower pole of spleen and hemoperitoneum. He was resuscitated with blood and fluid. Two hours later, his pulse was 84/minute and BP was 120/70 mm Hg. The most appropriate course of management in this case would be: *(DPG 2011)*
    a. Exploring the patient followed by splenectomy
    b. Exploring the patient followed by excision of the lower pole of spleen
    c. Splenorrhaphy
    d. Continuation of conservative treatment under close monitoring system and subsequent surgery if further indicated

96. About trauma spleen false is: *(DPG 2006)*
    a. Partial splenectomy cannot be done
    b. Post splenectomy infection common
    c. Can cause late onset shock
    d. Mostly managed conservatively

97. Trauma to spleen in a stable patient is best diagnosed by: *(MCI Sept 2005, March 2008)*
    a. X-ray abdomen
    b. USG
    c. CT scan
    d. Diagnostic peritoneal lavage

98. In a RTA patient sustained trauma to left side of chest and abdomen. Fluid in the peritoneum and sign of hypotension was found on physical examination. Most probable diagnosis is: *(DNB 2014)*
    a. Splenic injury
    b. Diaphragmatic injury
    c. Rib fracture
    d. Renal injury

99. A 27 years old patient presented with left sided abdominal pain 6 hours after RTA. He was hemodynamically stable and FAST positive. CT scan showed grade III splenic injury. What will be appropriate treatment? *(Recent Question 2015)*
    a. Splenectomy
    b. Splenorrhaphy
    c. Splenic artery embolization
    d. Conservative management

STOMACH, DUODENUM AND PANCREATIC INJURIES

100. Which of the following statements related to gastric injury is not true? *(All India 2007)*
    a. Mostly related to penetrating trauma
    b. Treatment is simple debridement and suturing
    c. Blood in stomach is always related to gastric injury
    d. Heals well and fast

101. A young patient presents with a massive injury to proximal duodenum, head of pancreas and distal common bile duce. The procedure of choice in this patient should be:
    a. Roux-en-Y anastomosis *(All India 2008)*
    b. Pancreaticoduodenectomy (Whipple's operation)
    c. Lateral tube jejunostomy
    d. Retrograde jejunostomy

CHEST TRAUMA

102. A patient died after a blunt trauma to chest. Most common cause of death in blunt trauma to chest is: *(Recent Question 2016)*
    a. Esophageal rupture
    b. Tracheo-bronchial rupture
    c. Pulmonary laceration
    d. Pneumothorax

103. Commonest cause of death in penetrating injury of chest:
    a. Tracheobronchial injury *(AIIMS Sept 96, June 2000)*
    b. Esophageal rupture
    c. Pulmonary laceration
    d. Chylothorax

104. A 40-year-old man brought to the emergency room with a stab injury to the chest. On examination patient is found to be hemodynamically stable. The neck veins are engorged and the heart sounds are muffled. The following statements are true for this patient except: *(AIIMS Nov 2002)*
    a. Cardiac tamponade is likely to be present
    b. Immediate emergency room thoracotomy should be done
    c. Echocardiogram should be done to confirm pericardial blood
    d. The entry wound should be sealed with an occlusive dressing

105. Following a major trauma a patient presented 54 hours later with raised JVP and CVP of 16 mm of Hg and persistent hypotension. Most probable diagnosis is:
    (PGI Dec 2000, Dec 2003)
    a. Tension pneumothorax
    b. Cardiac tamponade
    c. Head injury
    d. Splenic trauma
    e. Air embolism

106. A male came to the emergency room after car accident. He had dyspnea and chest pain with ecchymosis on anterior chest wall. On examination, pulse rate was 120/min, BP was 80/50 mmHg, the breaths sounds were decreased on left side, JVP was raised and tympanic note was present on percussion. Pelvis and extremities were normal. What is your diagnosis?
    (AIIMS May 2018)
    a. Tension pneumothorax
    b. Massive hemothorax
    c. Cardiac tamponade
    d. Hydropneumothorax

107. Sitaram a 40-year-old man, met with an accident and comes to emergency department with engorged neck veins, pallor, rapid pulse and chest pain. Diagnosis is: *(AIIMS June 99)*
    a. Pulmonary laceration
    b. Cardiac tamponade
    c. Hemothorax
    d. Splenic rupture

108. A patient is brought to casualty with severe hypotension following a road traffic accident. No external injury is evident. The cause of hypotension is: *(AIIMS June 2001)*
    a. Fracture rib
    b. Intrathoracic and abdominal bleed
    c. Iatrogenic shock
    d. Intracranial bleed

109. Which of the following is most common cause of hypotension in fracture ribs (T10-T12)? *(AIIMS Nov 99, June 99)*
    a. Abdominal solid visceral organ injury
    b. Injury to aorta
    c. Inter costal artery damage
    d. Pulmonary contusion

110. Treatment of acutely developing massive left sided hemothorax in a young male after an accident is:
    a. Strapping of chest *(AIIMS Nov 93)*
    b. Tube thoracostomy
    c. Endotracheal intubation + IPPV + pleural fluid aspiration
    d. Conservative, wait and watch

111. Treatment of rib fracture: *(PGI Dec 2002)*
    a. Immediate thoracotomy
    b. IPPV
    c. Strapping
    d. ICWSD

112. Treatment of simple rib fracture include all of the following except: *(Recent Question 2015)*
    a. Analgesic
    b. Physiotherapy
    c. Strapping
    d. Early ambulation

113. In case of blunt injury thorax, most common complication is:
    (AIIMS June 95)
    a. Pneumothorax
    b. Rib fracture
    c. Hemopneumothorax
    d. Aortic rupture

114. Best approach in thoracic trauma is: *(Recent Question 2013)*
    a. Midline sternotomy
    b. Parasternal thoracotomy
    c. Anterolateral thoracotomy
    d. Posterolateral thoracotomy

FLAIL CHEST

115. True about flail chest: *(PGI June 2004)*
    a. Fracture of 3 or 4 ribs
    b. Chest wall moves inwards during inspiration
    c. Mechanical Ventilation always needed
    d. Mediastinal shift
    e. Ultimately leads to respiratory failure

116. What is the treatment of choice in severe fail chest?
    a. IPPV
    b. Strapping *(UPSC 2008)*
    c. Wiring
    d. Nasal Oxygen

117. Steering wheel injury on chest of a young man reveals multiple fractures of ribs and paradoxical movement with severe respiratory distress. X-ray shows pulmonary contusion on right side without pneumothorax. What is the initial treatment of choice? *(UPSC 2007)*
    a. Immediate internal fixation
    b. Endotracheal intubation and mechanical ventilation
    c. Thoracic epidural analgesia and O_2 therapy
    d. Stabilization with towel clips

118. Management of flail chest with respiratory failure is:
    a. Chest tube drainage *(DNB 2008, MCI Sept 2006)*
    b. Oxygen administration
    c. IPPV
    d. Internal operative fixation of the fractures segments

119. Simple rib fracture should be treated with all except:
    (Recent Question 2014, MHPGMCET 2007)
    a. Analgesics   b. Physiotherapy
    c. Early ambulation   d. Strapping of chest

120. A man presented with fractures of 4th to 10th ribs and respiratory distress after RTa. He is diagnosed to have flail chest and a PaO_2 of <60%. Management is: *(AIIMS June 2001)*
    a. Tracheostomy
    b. IPPV with oral intubation
    c. Fixation of ribs
    d. Strapping of chest

121. Treatment of choice of flail chest is: *(Recent Question 2013)*
    a. External fixation of flail segment and mechanical ventilation
    b. Strapping
    c. O_2 administration
    d. Intrapleural local analgesia

DIAPHRAGMATIC INJURY

122. Traumatic diaphragmatic injury except: *(PGI Nov 2009)*
    a. Left side rupture due to weak left hemidiaphragm at point of entry of embryonic origin
    b. Most commonly due to trauma
    c. Smaller tears heal spontaneously and surgery is not required
    d. Abdominal approach is the most favored
    e. Mask ventilation is encouraged in patient with massive visceral herniation

123. True about diaphragmatic injury: *(PGI Dec 2008)*
    a. Advise diagnostic laparoscopy
    b. Chest X-ray is useful
    c. Conservative management is done in most cases
    d. Late complication is herniation of abdominal content
    e. All penetrating diaphragmatic injury must be repaired via chest

124. About diaphragmatic injury, true statement is:
    a. Treatment is conservative *(AIIMS June 98)*
    b. Resolves spontaneously
    c. Left side is more common
    d. Associated with pneumothorax

125. Diagnosis of traumatic rupture of diaphragm: *(PGI June 2007)*
    a. Laparoscopy
    b. Chest X ray
    c. Diagnostic peritoneal lavage
    d. CT

HEAD INJURY

126. Prognosis in head injury is best given by:
    (All India 2007, AIIMS Nov 2006)
    a. Glasgow coma scale   b. Age of patient
    c. Mode of injury   d. CT head

127. Base of the skull fracture presents with involvement of the petrous temporal bone, which of the following important sign is seen? *(UPPG 2007)*
    a. Subconjuctival hematoma
    b. CSF rhinorrhoea
    c. Raccoon eyes   d. Battle sign

128. A 20-years old male come to causality with head injury. Examination reveals normal consciousness and blood in the tympanic membrane. Most likely cause is: *(UPPG 2008)*
    a. Extradural hemorrhage   b. Subdural hemorrhage
    c. Intraventricular hemorrhage
    d. Basilar fracture

129. The earliest manifestation of increased intracranial pressure following head injury is: *(All India 2005)*
    a. Ipsilateral papillary dilatation
    b. Contralateral papillary dilation
    c. Altered mental status
    d. Hemiparesis

130. The term post traumatic epilepsy refers to seizures occurring:
    a. Within moment of head injury *(AIIMS Nov 2002)*
    b. Within 7 days of head injury
    c. Within several weeks to months after head injury
    d. Many years after head injury

131. After 4 weeks of head trauma, patient presents with features of irritability and altered sensorium. Commonest cause will be: *(AIIMS Nov 2000)*
    a. Chronic subdural hematoma
    b. Extradural hematoma
    c. Intraparenchymal bleed
    d. Electolyte imbalance

132. After head injury, biconvex, lenticular shape hematoma in CT scan is characteristic of which of the following:
    a. Extradural hemorrhage *(AIIMS June 99)*
    b. Subdural hemorrhage
    c. Intracerebral hematoma
    d. Diffuse-axonal injury

133. Which of the following is commonest source of extradural hemorrhage? *(AIIMS Nov 98, Feb 97, All India 96)*
    a. Middle meningeal artery b. Subdural venous sinus
    c. Charcot's artery   d. Middle cerebral artery

134. CSF otorrhea is caused by: *(AIIMS Nov 98)*
    a. Fracture of cribriform plate
    b. Fracture of parietal bone
    c. Fracture of petrous temporal bone
    d. Fracture of tympanic membrane

135. Skull base fracture is associated with all of the following except: *(Recent Question 2017)*
    a. Racoon eyes   b. Hemiparesis
    c. CSF Rhino-otorrhea   d. Battle sign

136. Management for CSF rhinorrhoea is: *(AIIMS Feb 97)*
    a. Plain X-ray and packing of nose
    b. Nasal packing only
    c. Antibiotics and observation
    d. Immediate surgery

137. **After rupture of middle meningeal artery bleeding occurs in which region?** *(AIIMS Feb 97)*
   a. Subdural bleed
   b. Extradural bleed
   c. Intracerebral bleed
   d. Subarachnoid bleed

138. **Hemostasis in scalp wound is best achieved by:** *(DGP 2011)*
   a. Direct pressure over the wound
   b. Catching and crushing the bleeders by haemostats
   c. Eversion of galea aponeurotica
   d. Coagulation of bleeders

139. **Abbreviated injury scale score digit for head injury:**
   a. 1
   b. 2 *(Recent Question 2016)*
   c. 3
   d. 4

140. **SDH is caused by injury of:** *(Recent Question 2016)*
   a. Middle meningeal artery
   b. Cortical veins
   c. Superficial temporal artery
   d. None

VASCULAR INJURIES

141. **In traumatic transaction of the femoral artery and vein, which among the following should be done?** *(PGI Dec 2001)*
   a. Femoral artery repair with vein ligation
   b. Repair of artery and vein
   c. Ligation of femoral artery
   d. Below knee amputation
   e. Repair of artery with contralateral sympathectomy

142. **During surgery, both femoral artery and femoral vein injured, next best step:** *(Recent Question 2017)*
   a. Ligate femoral vein & repair femoral artery
   b. Ligate femoral vein & femoral artery
   c. Ligate femoral artery & repair femoral vein
   d. None of the above

143. **A person following a road-traffic accident presented in emergency with laceration of inguinal region. On examination, there was swelling of inguinal region and distal pulsation was felt; internal iliac artery was normal, common iliac and external femoral artery was normal but common femoral vein is transected. Treatment of choice is:** *(PGI June 2003)*
   a. Vein repair with continuity
   b. Sclerotherapy
   c. Ligation of femoral artery and vein
   d. Amputation below knee

144. **In traumatic injury to common femoral vein and external femoral artery, which among the following should be done?** *(PGI Dec 2003)*
   a. Ligation of both artery and vein
   b. Repair of artery and vein
   c. Below knee amputation
   d. Repair of artery and contralateral sympthectomy
   e. Sclerotherapy

145. **True about aortic transaction:** *(PGI June 2008)*
   a. Most commonly due to deceleration injury
   b. High mortality
   c. Surgery definitive treatment
   d. Aortography gold standard

146. **Which of the following causes maximum bleeding?** *(PGI 95)*
   a. Partial arterial severing
   b. Complete arterial severing
   c. Artery caught between fractured end of bones
   d. Intimal tear

SEAT BELT INJURY

147. **Which of the following statement(s) is/are true about trauma injury?** *(PGI June 2009)*
   a. Seat belt can cause pancreato-duodenal injury
   b. Late death is caused by sepsis
   c. Damage Control Surgery (DCS) is used to control major bleeding and to prevent contamination of peritoneal cavity.
   d. In DCS the abdomen is closed in layer to prevent evisceration
   e. In DCS, laparotomy is decided based on patient prognosis

148. **Seat belt causes injury to:** *(MAHE 2004)*
   a. Duodenum
   b. Head injury due to wind screen
   c. Thorax
   d. All

MISCELLANEOUS

149. **A patient presents in emergency with a cervical spine fracture. First thing to do is:** *(AIIMS Nov 99, June 99)*
   a. Locate the fracture by shifting the patient side to side
   b. X-ray of spine
   c. Clear the airway and intubate him
   d. Immobilize the cervical spine

150. **What will be the appropriate management of a patient with a clean wound over forearm with slight loss of tissue? He has received, tetanus toxoid 12 years back:** *(AIIMS June 99)*
   a. Complete course of TT
   b. Only one dose of TT
   c. Full dose of Human tetanus Ig
   d. No treatment needed

151. **Limb salvage can be done in all except:** *(AIIMS Feb 97)*
   a. Nerve injury
   b. Vascular injury
   c. Bone injury
   d. Muscle injury

152. **A patient after sustaining RTA, developed fracture left shaft of femur with guarding and rigidity in the abdomen. Following is to be done:** *(PGI Dec 2003)*
   a. X-ray of left lower limb and USG abdomen
   b. Start IVF, Ryle's tube and catheterization
   c. Stabilize the fracture and monitor the patient and do surgery if necessary later on
   d. Grouping and cross matching of two unit of blood
   e. Stabilize the fracture only

153. **Which one of the following is not a principle followed in the management of missile injuries?** *(UPSC 2004)*
   a. Excision of all dead muscles
   b. Removal of foreign bodies
   c. Removal of fragments of bone
   d. Leaving the wound open

154. **When bullet is shot above pubic symphysis in midline directed backwards, first organ to get injuries is?** *(DPG 2008)*
   a. Bladder
   b. Abdominal aorta
   c. Left renal vein
   d. Spleen

155. **In resection of muscle with history of trauma/crush injury, resection depends on:** *(PGI Dec 2006)*
   a. Contractility of muscle
   b. Color of muscle
   c. Bleeding punctuate spots
   d. Size of muscle
   e. Function of muscle

156. **During reconstruction of an amputated limb which of the following is done first?** *(AIIMS Nov 2010)*
   a. Arterial repair
   b. Venous repair
   c. Fixation of the bone
   d. Nerve anastomoses

157. **Which of the following structures is fixed first during reimplantation of an amputated digit?**
    a. Bone b. Artery
    c. Vein d. Nerve

158. **In treatment of hand injuries, the greatest priority is:**
    (MCI June 2018)
    a. Repair to tendons b. Repair of skin cover
    c. Repair of nerves d. All

159. **Hypotension in acute spinal injury is due to:**
    a. Loss of sympathetic tone *(AIIMS Nov 2006)*
    b. Loss of parasympathetic tone
    c. Orthostatic hypotension
    d. Vasovagal attack

160. **Due to decelerations, aorta can be ruptured at places where it is fixed except:** *(AIIMS May 2012)*
    a. At ligamentum arteriosum
    b. Behind the esophagus
    c. Behind the crura of diaphram
    d. Aortic valve

161. **Criteria for brainstem death includes:** *(All India 2012)*
    a. Positive Doll's eye reflex
    b. Absent pupillary light reflex and dilated pupils
    c. Pinpoint pupils
    d. Positive vestibulo-ocular reflexes

162. **During resuscitation, artefacts of fractured ribs most commonly involve:** *(AIIMS May 2014)*
    a. 2nd–4th ribs
    b. 3rd–5th ribs
    c. 4th–6th ribs
    d. 5th–7th ribs

163. **Definition of degloving injury:** *(Recent Question 2016)*
    a. Separation of skin only
    b. Separation of skin + subcutaneous tissue
    c. Separation of skin + subcutaneous tissue + fascia exposing tendons
    d. Separation up to tendons, exposing bone

Explanations

TRAUMA

1. **Ans. d. Maintenance of airways**
2. **Ans. a. Hemostatic anterior and posterior nasal packing, b. Thoracosotomy tube insertion, c. ETT in line with cervical canal, d. I.V Fluid immediate** *(Ref: Advanced Trauma Life Support (ATLS) Manual 2018; CSDT 11/e p205; Sabiston 20/e p414)*

   The patient in question needs to be managed in accordance with the Advanced Trauma Life Support (ATLS) protocol.

   Always assume all major trauma patients have an injured spine and maintain spinal immobilisation until spine is cleared. Priorties in management are ABCDE.

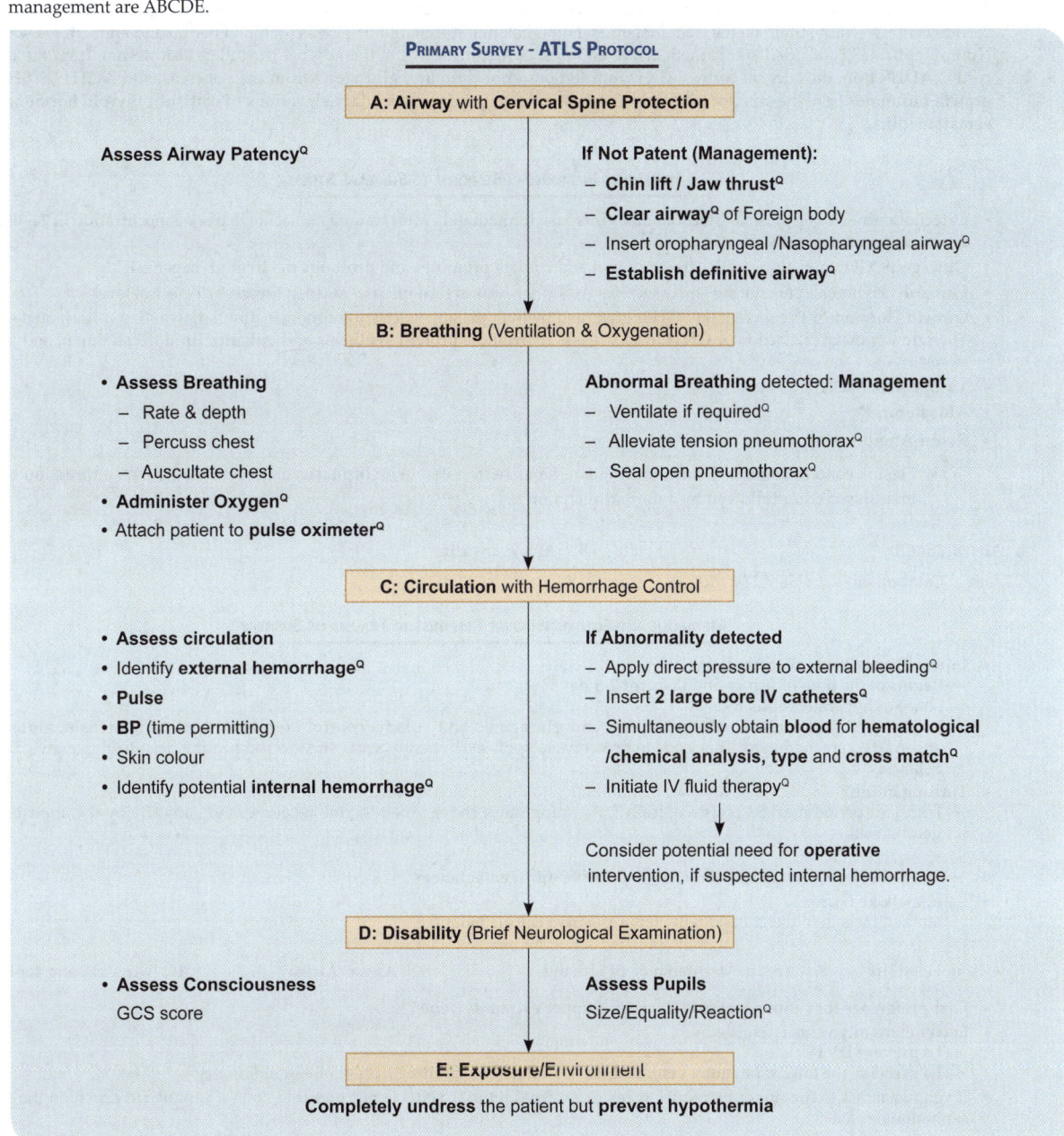

- **Anterior & posterior nasal packing** should be done to **control nose bleeding**^{Q}.
- **Resuscitation** of patient **in hypovolemic shock** begins with making sure that **airway is secure** by ensuring that **ventilation and oxygenation** are **adequate**, and in the case of **hemorrhagic shock**, by **controlling bleeding**^{Q}.
- **External bleeding** is controlled by **application of pressure** over the bleeding areas, **surgical control** or in a rare case, **by tourniquet**^{Q}.
- **Immediately life-threatening pulmonary injuries** that must be **detected** and **treated** (by **chest tube** or **thoracotomy**) include presence of **tension pneumothorax, open pneumothorax, flail chest** and **massive hemothorax**^{Q}.
- **Large bore needle** or **IV cannula** should be in place **while** a **chest tube is inserted** for definitinagement^Q.
- The **chest X-ray** is of utmost importance in thoracic trauma however, the **aforementioned life-threatening injuries preclude the necessity** of chest X-ray for diagnosis and **should be identified clinically**^{Q}.
- **Trauma resuscitation (1:1:1)-** Packed cell, plasma & platelets are used in 1:1:1 ratio^Q.

3. **Ans. d. Increase in thyroxine** *(Ref: Bailey 27/e p7; CSDT 11/e p103-105)*

CSDT says "Following injury, **neural impulses** carried **via spinothalamic pathways** activate the brain stem and thalamic and cortical centers, which stimulate the hypothalamus. Hypothalamic stimulation triggers combined neural and endocrine discharges. **Norepinephrine**^{Q} is released sympathetic nerve endings, **epinephrine**^{Q} from the adrenal medulla^Q, **aldosterone** from the adrenal cortex, **ADH**^{Q} from the adrenal cortex, ADH from the posterior pituitary, **glucagon**^{Q} from the pancreas, and **ACTH**^{Q}, **TSH**^{Q}, and **growth hormone**^{Q} from the anterior pituitary. Theses hormones produce **secondary elevations of cortisol**^{Q}, **thyroid hormone**^{Q}, and **somatomedins**."

HORMONES INCREASED IN RESPONSE TO SURGICAL STRESS

- **Catecholamines**^{Q}: The plasma catecholamines **increase immediately after trauma** and achieve **peak concentration** in **24-48 hours** depending on the severity.
- **Glucagon**^{Q}: Glucagon along with catecholamine and cortisol **promotes** and **prolongs** the **liver glycogenesis.**
- **Cortisol**^{Q}: Hypothalamus during stress secretes ACTH^Q, which in turn initiates sudden increase in cortisol level^Q
- **Growth Hormone**^{Q}: The secretion of GH is governed by hypothalamic factors, autonomic stimulation and non-hormonal signals. The primary metabolic action of **GH** during stress is to **promote protein synthesis** and **enhance lipid break down**, and glucose stores.
- **Vasopressin (ADH)**^{Q}
- **Aldosterone**^{Q}
- **Renin-Angiotensin**^{Q}

> - **Plasma concentration of insulin** during stress has been noted to be **biphasic,** characterized by the **suppression of insulin secretion followed by a normal secretion**^{Q}.

4. **Ans. d. Insulin**
5. **Ans. e. Insulin**
6. **Ans. a. Catabolism** *(Ref: CSDT 11/e p100)*

METABOLIC AND NEUROENDOCRINE RESPONSE TO TRAUMA OR SURGERY

- **Injury Phase (Phase of catabolism):**
  - **Begins at** the **time of injury** and **lasts for 2-5 days**^{Q}
  - Phase of **hypermetabolism**^{Q}
  - Stress hormones (**cortisol, catecholamines and glucagon**^{Q}) and volume control hormones (**renin-angiotensin, aldosterone** and **ADH**^{Q}) are increased. This leads to proteolysis, lipolysis, hyperglycemia and wound healing despite of negative nitrogen balance.
- **Turning Point:**
  - Transient period marked physiologically by turning off of the neuroendocrine response and clinically by the appearance of getting well.
- **Early Anabolic Phase:**
  - Marked by gain in muscular strength or **positive nitrogen balance**^{Q}.
- **Late Anabolic Phase:**
  - Marked by gain in weight and body fat or **positive caloric balance**^{Q}

7. **Ans. d. Head lift**   8. **Ans. d. Maintenance of airways**   9. **Ans. c. Airway**   10. **Ans. c. Long saphenous**

- **First preference for venous access** is always for **upper extremity veins**^{Q}.
- **Lower extremity veins** is **avoided:**
  - To prevent DVT^Q
  - **To preserve** the **long saphenous vein,** as it is used for arterial grafting in case of vascular injury^Q
- If **venous access to the upper extremity veins** or **external jugular veins is not possible,** then a **venous cut down** on the **greater saphenous** is done.

11. **Ans. a.** Thyroxine
12. **Ans. b.** Inhibition of skeletal muscle breakdown by IL-1 and TNF
13. **Ans. a.** Airway maintenance
14. **Ans. c.** Intubation
15. **Ans. a.** Log roll
16. **Ans. b.** Put the patient in recovery position and secure airway *(Ref: BLS/ACLS Guidelines: https://www.resus.org.uk/resuscitation-guidelines/adult-advanced-life-support)*

- As a part of the BLS algorithm, we should start with the airway management in any patient who is collapsed/expected to collapse. Since the patient is hemodynamically stable, the airway is the most important component at risk in this patient and requires immediate attention. The patient should be put in a recovery position i.e. left lateral decubitus position to prevent the risk of aspiration.

17. **Ans. b.** Check carotid pulse
18. **Ans. b.** In lateral lying position *(Ref: Sabiston 20/e p414, 420, 473; Schwartz 10/e p161)*
19. **Ans. a.** A child with airway obstruction *(Ref: Sabiston 20/e p413; Schwartz 10/e p161; Advanced Trauma Life Support (ATLS) Manual 7/e p33-34; CSDT 11/e p205)*

"Following a defined order of assessment, life-threatening conditions are immediately addressed at the time of identification. This initial assessment, also termed the primary survey, follows the mnemonic ABCDE: Airway and cervical spine protection, Breathing, Circulation, Disability or neurologic condition, Exposure and environmental control."- Sabiston 20/e p413

20. **Ans. a.** Assess the patient's response, Call for help, check carotid pulse, Start CPR *(Ref: BLS/ACLS Guidelines: https://www.resus.org.uk/resuscitation guidelines /adult- advanced-life-support; Harrison 19/e p1768; Braunwald's 10/e p844-845)*

According to Adult Basic Life Support (BLS) algorithm, steps followed are: Assess the patient's response, Call for help, check carotid pulse, Start CPR.

\multicolumn{2}{c}{**Adult Basic Life Support (BLS) Algorithm**}	
Safety	• Make sure you, the victim and any bystanders are safe
Response	• Check the victim for a response
Airway	• Open the airway
Breathing	• **Look, listen and feel for normal breathing for no more than 10 seconds**[Q]
Dial 999	• Call an ambulance (999)
Send For AED	• Send someone to get an AED if available
Circulation	• **Start chest compressions** • Place **heel of one hand in lower half of victim's sternum** [Q] • Place **heel of your other hand on top of first hand**[Q] • Interlock the fingers of your hands & ensure that pressure is not applied over the victim's ribs • Keep your arms straight; Position your shoulders vertically above the victim's chest • **Press down on sternum to a depth of 5–6 cm**[Q] • After each compression, release all the pressure on chest without losing contact between your hands & sternum • **Repeat at a rate of 100–120/min**[Q]

Give Rescue Breaths	• **After 30 compressions open the airway again using head tilt & chin lift & give 2 rescue breaths**[Q]
	   • Do not interrupt compressions by more than 10 seconds to deliver two breaths. Then **return your hands without delay to correct position on sternum & give a further 30 chest compressions** [Q]
	   • **Continue with chest compressions & rescue breaths in a ratio of 30:2**[Q]
	• If you are untrained or unable to do rescue breaths, give chest compression only CPR (i.e. continuous compressions at a rate of at least 100–120/min[Q])

If an AED Arrives	• **Switch on the AED** & follow the spoken/visual directions • Ensure that nobody is touching the victim while AED is analyzing the rhythm • **If a shock is indicated, deliver shock** & ensure that nobody is touching the victim • **Immediately restart CPR at a ratio of 30:2**[Q] • **If no shock is indicated, continue CPR**[Q]
Continue CPR	• Do not interrupt resuscitation until: • A health professional tells you to stop ; You become exhausted • The victim is definitely waking up, moving, opening eyes and breathing normally • It is rare for CPR alone to restart the heart. Unless you are certain the person has recovered continue CPR
Recovery Position	• **If you are certain the victim is breathing normally but is still unresponsive, place in the recovery position**[Q]

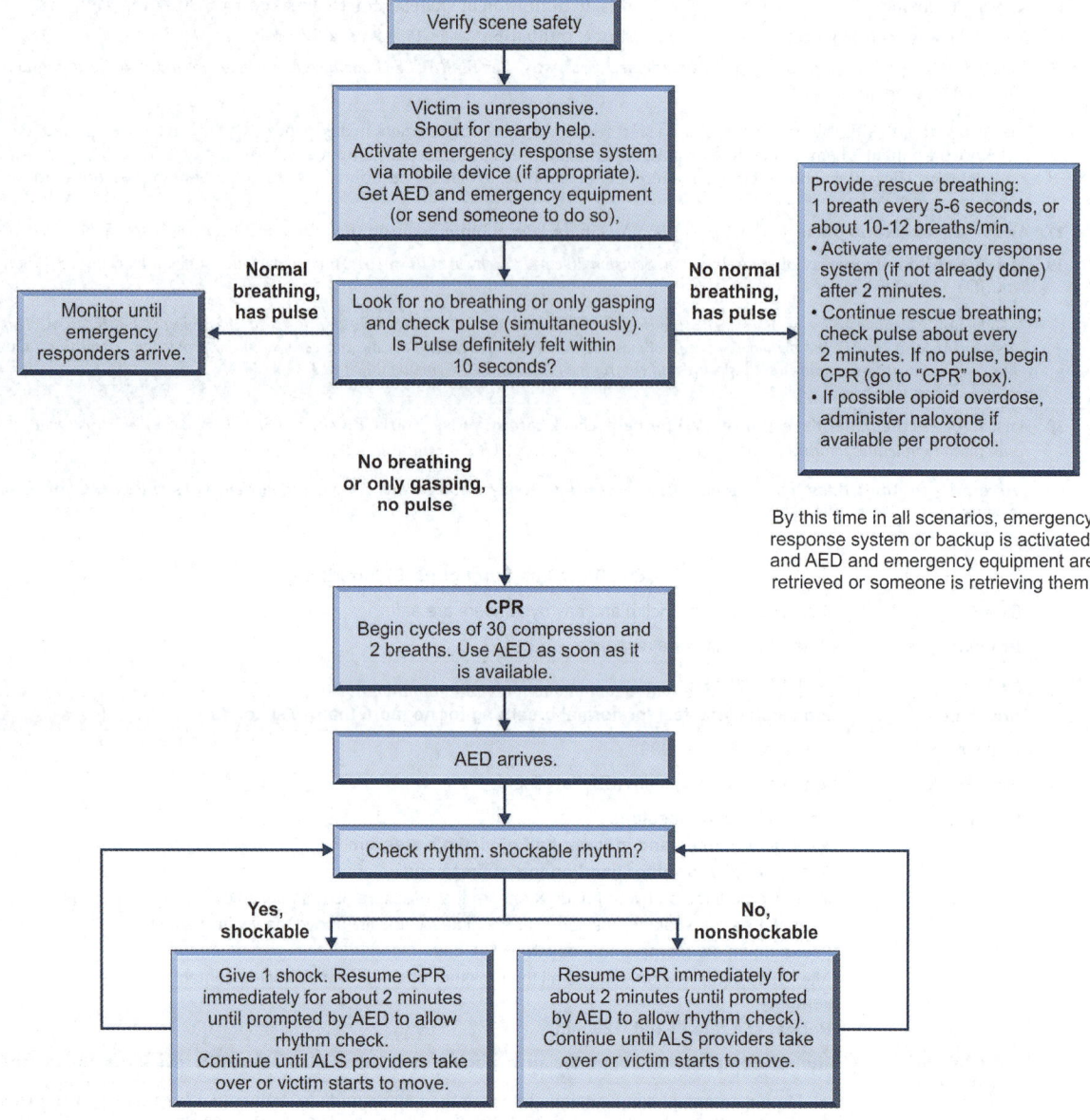

Adult BLS Cardiac Arrest Algorithm 2015 Update

Cardiopulmonary Resuscitation (AHA 2015 Guidelines)

- **"CAB"[Q]** is followed (**not ABC**): Circulation, Airway, Breathing[Q] (**Immediately start chest compressions rather than airway opening[Q]**)
- To allow **full chest wall recoil** after each compression, **rescuer must avoid leaning on the chest** between compressions[Q].

  - Rescuer should not interrupt compressions for >10 seconds[Q].
  - For patients with **ongoing CPR and an advanced airway in place**, a simplified **ventilation rate of 1 breath every 6 seconds[Q] (10 breaths per minute[Q])** is recommended.

- **Routine use of impedance threshold device** (ITD) as an adjunct to conventional CPR is **not recommended[Q]**.
- In **ACLS** (Advanced Cardiac Life Support), **vasopressin does not offer an advantage over the use of epinephrine alone[Q]**. Therefore, **vasopressin has been removed from the Adult Cardiac Arrest Algorithm-2015 Update**. In **2010 update, atropine was removed[Q]** (earlier vasopressin was recommended as an alternative to epinephrine).
- **Low end-tidal carbon dioxide** ($ETCO_2$) in intubated patients **after 20 minutes of CPR** is associated with a **very low likelihood of resuscitation[Q]**.

Trauma

- **Emergency coronary angiography** is recommended for **all patients with ST elevation** and for **hemodynamically or electrically unstable patients without ST elevation** for whom a **cardiovascular lesion is suspected**[Q].

  - During **adult CPR tidal volume of 600 ml (6-7 ml/kg)** should be **adequate to cause the chest to rise**[Q].

- During airway management in an **unconscious trauma patient with possible cervical injury, neck hyperextension** should be avoided.
- The **most widely used waveform** in the automated electrical defibrillators (AEDs) now is the **biphasic truncated exponential (BTE) waveform.**

  - The following **drugs** may be **given through the endotracheal tube during CPR:** **L**ignocaine[Q], **E**pinephrine[Q], **V**asopressin[Q], **A**tropine[Q], **N**aloxone[Q] (LEVAN); (Amiodarone & sodium bicarbonate are not given endotracheally[Q])
  - **Atropine is not recommended for routine use** in the management of **Pulseless Electrical Activity/asystole** and has been removed from the ACLS Cardiac Arrest Algorithm[Q] (Epinephrine, vasopressin & amiodarone are used[Q])

	Adult (>12 years)	Child (1-12 years)	Infant (<1 year)
Compression Depth	At least **2 inches**Q **(5 cm, but not >2.4 inches/6 cm**Q**)**	About **2 inches**Q **(5 cm; 1/3rd of chest depth**Q**)**	About **1.5 inches**Q **(4 cm; 1/3rd of chest depth**Q**)**
Compression: Ventilation ratio	**30:2**Q (one or two rescuer CPR)	**30:2**Q (single rescuer) or **15:2**Q (two rescuer)	
Compression rate	100-120/minQ		

21. **Ans. c. Maintaining permissible hypotension to avoid bleeding** *(Ref: Schwartz 10/e p98; Current Therapy of Trauma and Surgical Critical Care By Juan A. Asensio 2/e p602)*

    Balanced resuscitation in trauma management is maintaining permissible hypotension to avoid bleeding.

    Components of Damage Control Resuscitation
    - **Permissive hypotension**[Q]
    - **Minimizing crystalloid-based resuscitation**[Q]
    - **Immediate release & administration of pre-defined blood products** (red blood cells, plasma & platelets) in ratios similar to those of whole blood[Q].

22. **Ans. b. 1:1:1** *(Ref: Sabiston 20/e p72; Schwartz 10/e p98)*

23. **Ans. d. All patients should have chest X-ray-PA view only** *(Ref: ATLS Guidelines 9/e p6-9, 13; Sabiston 20/e p413-417; Schwartz 10/e p161, 173)*

    In primary survey, cervical X-ray is not mandatory as imaging of the cervical spine can be done later after complete evaluation of spinal cord injuries. Patients with blunt trauma are always sent for plain radiographs of chest and pelvis with anteroposterior (AP) views, as the patient will be in supine position and not the PA views. CT scan is avoided in hemodynamically unstable patients.

    "Transport of a hypotensive patient out of the emergency department for computed tomographic (CT) scanning is hazardous; monitoring is compromised, and the environment is suboptimal for dealing with acute problems. The surgeon must accompany the patient and be prepared to abort the CT scan with diversion to the operating room."- Schwartz 10/e p173

    Advanced Trauma Life Support (ATLS) Guidelines
    - All trauma patients are managed based on **Advanced Trauma Life Support** guidelines.
    - **Steps: Triage → Primary survey → Emergency resuscitation →Adjuncts to primary survey → Secondary survey → Adjuncts to secondary survey**[Q]
    - **Primary Survey includes : Airway & cervical spine stabilization → Breathing & ventilation→ Circulation & blood loss control→ Disability & neurologic evaluation → Exposure/Environment**[Q]
    - **Massive transfusion protocol:** Resuscitation of the patients with **packed red blood cells, fresh-frozen plasma (FFP) & platelets in 1:1:1 ratio** has favorable outcomes[Q].

      - Imaging of cervical spine can be done later after complete evaluation of spinal cord injuries.
      - Patients with blunt trauma are always sent for **plain radiographs of chest & pelvis with anteroposterior (AP) views**, as the patient will be in supine position and **not the PA views.**

    - **CT scan is avoided in hemodynamically unstable patients.** Further contrast induced organ damages also potentiates owing to low circulatory volume.

24. **Ans. b. The patient should not be shifted and portable X-ray machine should be used after neck stabilization** *(Ref: Sabiston 20/e p421; Schwartz 10/e p161; ATLS Manual 9/e p6, 182)*

    In a trauma patient, cervical stabilization is the first step in management along with airway. Hence any imaging should be done after hard neck collar support and long spine board. In fact, a cross table lateral cervical spine X-ray is considered, in the same trolley itself without shifting the patient. A surgeon should accompany the patient if needed, so that patient can be transferred immediately to OT if any hemodynamic instability occurs.

"Simultaneously, all patients with blunt trauma require cervical spine immobilization until injury is excluded. This is typically accomplished by applying a hard collar or placing sandbags on both sides of the head with the patient's forehead taped across the bags to the backboard. Soft collars do not effectively immobilize the cervical spine. For penetrating neck wounds, however, cervical collars are not believed useful because they provide no benefit, but may interfere with assessment and treatment."-Schwartz 10/e p161

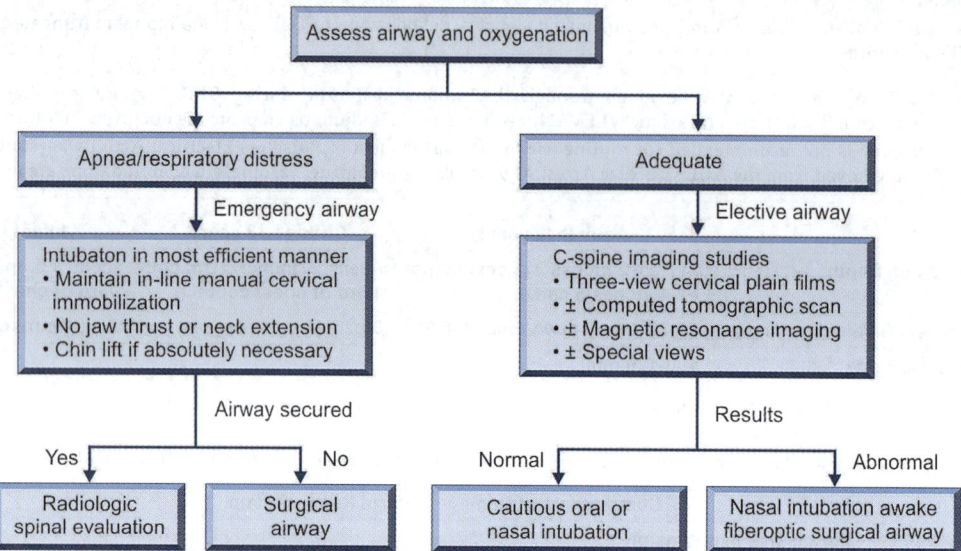

Management of Cervical Spine Injury in a Trauma Patient

Management of Cervical Spine Injury in a Trauma Patient

- The **spine should always be immobilized assuming a spine injury until proven otherwise**
- Blunt & penetrating trauma result in different forms of spinal cord injury.
- **Blunt trauma** causes **cord injury through direct impingement** or **indirect compression due to vertebral fracture or dislocation.**
- **Penetrating trauma** causes **direct cord laceration** or indirectly through **ischemia or fracture**.

  - **Spine immobilization should be done** and after immobilization **X-ray attempted with a portable machine**[Q]
  - **X-rays in the acute trauma are usually taken with the help of portable X-ray machine**, which includes **AP views of cervical, chest & pelvis**, as unnecessary mobilization & shifting of the patient might aggravate injury even with immobilization by cervical collar[Q].

25. Ans. a. Inability to speak
26. Ans. b. Tongue *(Ref: Bailey 27/e p355, 26/e p341)*

"The mouth and nasal passages form part of the upper aero-digestive tract. Lacerations and fractures of the facial skeleton may give rise to immediate or delayed respiratory obstruction. Immediate obstruction may arise from inhalation of tooth fragments, accumulation of blood and secretions, and loss of control of the tongue in the unconscious or semiconscious patient."- Bailey 27/e p341

27. Ans. b. Airway, breathing and circulation *(Ref: Sabiston 20/e p413; Schwartz 10/e p161; Bailey 27/e p323)*
28. Ans. b. IV crystalloid 2 L, within few minutes
29. Ans. a. Start PRBC first and store platelet at room temperature
30. Ans. b. 6

"GCS (2014): E 2, V NT, M 4 = 6. It is no longer recommend to assign 1 point to non-testable elements, therefore a combined score should not be used here as it would imply that the patient is more unwell than they really are."

31. Ans. c. 9

    GCS (2014): E3, V NT, M6 = 9

32. Ans. b. Green

TRAUMA SCORING SYSTEM

33. **Ans. c. Pulse rate** *(Ref: Sabiston 20/e p411; Trauma Manual by Moore and Mattox 4/e p6; The Trauma manual: Trauma and Acute Care Surgery 3/e p5)*
34. **Ans. b. RTS + ISS +age**   35. **Ans. c. Neurogenic injury**
36. **Ans. b. Revised trauma score** *(Ref: Prehospital Trauma Care edited by Eldar Soreide, Christopher M. Grande/p160)*

> "**The RTS is currently the best** and most universal physiological **trauma-scoring** system used for triage purposes." -Prehospital Trauma Care edited by Eldar Soreide, Christopher M. Grande/p160

TRIAGE

37. **Ans. a. Ambulatory patients**
38. **Ans. c. Yellow- Stable patients, observation** *(Ref: Pediatric Emergency Medicine By Jill M. Baren (2008)/p1087)*
39. **Ans. c. Polytrauma**   40. **Ans. a. Red** *(Ref: Sabiston 20/e p409-410)*

BLUNT TRAUMA ABDOMEN

41. **Ans. a. Spleen** *(Ref: Sabiston 20/e p435; Schwartz 10/e p173-174; Bailey 27/e p313)*
42. **Ans. b. USG**
43. **Ans. c. USG** *(Ref: Sabiston 20/e p433; Schwartz 10/e p173-174; Bailey 27/e p372)*

- **Blunt trauma patient** with **hemodynamic instability** should be **evaluated by USG (FAST)** in the resuscitation room, if available^Q.
- **Hemodynamically stable patients** sustaining blunt trauma are adequately **evaluated by CECT**^{Q} (after USG).

44. **Ans. a. Spleen**   45. **Ans. b. Proximal jejunum, e. Ileocecal junction** *(Ref: Sabiston 20/e p441)*

MECHANISM OF INJURY OF SMALL INTESTINE BY BLUNT TRAUMA

- **Crushing of bowel between vertebral bodies** and **blunt object** such as steering wheel or handle bar
- **Deceleration shearing** of the small bowel at points **where it is fixed** such as ligament of Treitz **(duodenojejunal junction)**, the **ileocecal junction** and around the **mesenteric artery**^{Q}.
- Closed loop rupture caused by sudden increase in intra-abdominal pressure.

46. **Ans. c. Mesentery** *(Bailey 27/e p 106)*

   Most common organ injured in seat belt injury is Mesentery.

47. **Ans. a. Always midline incision** *(Ref: Sabiston 20/e p434; 19/e p455; Schwartz 9/e p155; Bailey 27/e p 372, 25/e p275, 287, 1184)*

BLUNT TRAUMA ABDOMEN

- **Preferred incision** for **emergency abdominal exploration** is a **long midline incision**^{Q}.
- Bailey says "The **routine approach for abdominal trauma** is **full midline Laparotomy**"
- Schwartz says "**All emergency abdominal explorations** are performed using a **long midline** incision because of its versatility."^{Q}

48. **Ans. a. Immediate laparotomy** *(Ref: Sabiston 20/e p433; Schwartz 10/e p173-174; Bailey 27/e p 372; CSDT 12/e p228)*
49. **Ans. c. USG is better than CT scan, e. Urgent surgery to be done**
50. **Ans. b. Further imaging of abdomen** *(Ref: CSDT 12/e p228)*

> A **hemodynamically stable patient** after **blunt trauma abdomen** should need **further evaluation by imaging**. Imaging of the abdomen with Ultrasound **(FAST)** is the best **next line of investigation**.

51. **Ans. a. CECT Scan**
52. **Ans. c. CECT abdomen**
53. **Ans. b. Rarely need urgent laparotomy**
54. **Ans. c. Thoracic duct injury needs urgent thoracotomy** *(Ref: Bailey 27/e p 756)*
55. **Ans. a. Focused assessment with sonography for trauma** *(Ref: Sabiston 20/e p415-416)*

   FAST stands for Focused assessment with sonography for trauma.

56. **Ans. c. Hypogastrium**

57. **Ans. b. Blood for cross matching and IV fluids** *(Ref: Advanced Trauma Life Support (ATLS) Manual 7/e p33,34)*

    The patient in question needs to be managed in accordance with the Advanced Trauma Life Support (ATLS) protocol. The **airway** (A) has been **secured** and the respiration / **breathing** (B) have already been **stabilized. Circulation** (C) needs to be established next. This is achieved by **external control of hemorrhage** (no external hemorrhage is present in this patient) and by restoring circulating volume (IV fluids).
    Intravenous access for **fluid resuscitation** should be begun next with **two 16 gauge peripheral catheters**. Blood should be drawn simultaneously and sent for typing and cross matching, at the same time.

58. **Ans. d. Intra-abdominal bleed** *(Ref: CSDT 11/e p252)*

    - CSDT says "Patients with blunt trauma and hypovolemia should be examined first for intra-abdominal bleeding even if there is no overt existence of abdominal trauma."^{Q}

59. **Ans. d. Pancreatic injury** *(Ref: Sabiston 20/e p440-441)*

    This is a typical case of **pancreatic injury** with **minimal retroperitoneal hematoma** and characteristic presentation of **pain radiating to back**.

60. **Ans. a. Peritoneal air on imaging, b. Severe hypotension, e. Patient with positive diagnostic peritoneal lavage** *(Ref: Sabiston 20/e p433; Schwartz 10/e p173-174; Bailey 27/e p373)*

    INDICATIONS OF URGENT LAPAROTOMY IN BLUNT TRAUMA ABDOMEN
    - **Peritonitis**^{Q}
    - **Free** air seen on radiographic examination^Q
    - **Unexplained hypovolemia**^{Q}
    - Positive DPL^Q
    - Presence of other injuries known to be frequently associated with intra-abdominal injuries

61. **Ans. b. Exploratory laparotomy under general anesthesia**
62. **Ans. c. Epigastrium, (R) and (L) Lumbar regions, hypogastrium**
63. **Ans. b. It is accurate in detecting < 50 ml. of free blood**
64. **Ans. a. Conservative management** *(Ref: Sabiston 20/e p433, 1896; Schwartz 10/e p206)*

DAMAGE CONTROL SURGERY

65. **Ans. a. Minimal intervention done to stabilize the patient and do the definitive surgery later** *(Ref: Sabiston 20/e p417; Schwartz 10/e p192-195; Bailey 27/e p318, 319, 326, 327, 378-80)*
66. **Ans. b. In ICU**
67. **Ans. b. Arrest hemorrhage, c. Control contamination, d. Prevent infection, e. Prevent coagulopathy** *(Ref: Sabiston 20/e p417; Schwartz 10/e p192-195)*
68. **Ans. d. Hemostasis**
69. **Ans. a. Coagulopathy, e. Hemostasis**
70. **Ans. a. Damage control surgery** *(Ref: Sabiston 20/e p417; Schwartz 10/e p192; Bailey 27/e p326)*
71. **Ans. c. Damage control surgery and mesh closure of abdomen** *(Ref: Schwartz 10/e p192-195; Bailey 27/e p378)*

    The pictures above are showing minimal abbreviated surgery i.e. damage control surgery in a setting of trauma, and closure of abdomen using meshplasty so as to prevent abdominal compartment syndrome.

ABDOMINAL COMPARTMENT SYNDROME

72. **Ans. a. ↓Cardiac output, b. ↓Urine output, d. ↓Venous return** *(Ref: Sabiston 20/e p555-556; Schwartz 10/e p217-218)*
73. **Ans. a. Normal intra-abdominal..., b. Intra-abdominal hypertension..., d. Management of choice..., e. Multi-organ failure**
74. **Ans. b. Decreased pulmonary venous pressure**
75. **Ans. d. Oliguria due to ureter obstruction**
76. **Ans. a. ↑ Pulmonary capillary wedge pressure, c. ↑ Pulmonary inspiratory pressure**
77. **Ans. a. ↓ Cardiac output, b. ↓ Urine output, c. ↓ Venous return**
78. **Ans. a. Reduction in visceral perfusion and increase in intracranial pressure**
79. **Ans. c. Hypovolemic resuscitation**

PENETRATING INJURIES

80. **Ans. a. Liver**
81. **Ans. b. Ileo-transverse anastomosis** *(Ref: Sabiston 20/e p113)*

    - Sabiston says "**Stab** and **low-velocity wounds** to the colon with **minimal contamination** and **hemodynamic stability** can be **managed by primary repair.**"^{Q}

82. **Ans. a. CECT** *(Ref: Sabiston 20/e p434; Washington Manual of Surgery 5/e p373)*

    According to **EAST Guidelines** "Current recommendations for nonoperative management of penetrating trauma include use of **Triple Contrast CT** (IV, oral and rectal) and **serial examinations**."

    PENETRATING ABDOMINAL INJURIES

    - Gunshot Abdominal Wounds:
      - Chances of **internal injury** is **very high in gunshot wounds,** thus little pre-operative evaluation is required and **laparotomy is mandatory**^{Q}.
    - Stab Wounds to Abdomen:
      - **Exploratory laparotomy** is indicated in patients with isolated penetrating abdominal wound if **hypotensive** or **in shock** or showing peritoneal signs^Q.

Anterior Stab Wounds	Flank and Back Wounds
• **Local wound exploration** can be performed to determine **if there is any penetration of** the **peritoneal cavity**^{Q}. • If the tract terminates without entering the peritoneum, the injury can be managed as a deep laceration^Q and laparotomy is not needed. • Otherwise, **penetration of the peritoneum** is assumed and **significant injury** must be **excluded by further diagnostic evaluations**^{Q} (FAST, CECT, DPL or laparoscopy)	• Risk of injury to **colon, kidney** and **ureter**^{Q} • **Triple contrast CT**^{Q} is advised **to detect colon** and **retroperitoneal injuries** and the **need for laparotomy**.

83. **Ans. d. CECT Abdomen** *(Ref: Practice Management Guidelines for Selective Non-operative Management of Penetrating Abdominal Trauma (Journal of Trauma; Vol 68, No. 3, March 2010)*

    "Omental protrusion in a hemodynamically stable patients without signs of peritoneal irritation is not an absolute indication for exploratory laparotomy"- Injury: volume 18; Issue 2; 87-88

    - **Routine laparotomy** is **not indicated in hemodynamically stable patients** with abdominal stab wounds **without signs of peritonitis** or **diffuse abdominal tenderness** (away from the wound site). ^{Q}
    - Such patients can be **initially managed non-operatively**, but an **abdominopelvic CT scan** should be strongly considered **as a diagnostic tool to facilitate initial management decisions.**^{Q}

84. **Ans. b. Hemicolectomy**
85. **Ans. d. Laparotomy** *(Ref: Sabiston 20/e p434)*

NECK INJURIES

86. **Ans. c. Breach of platysma** *(Ref: Sabiston 20/e p423; Schwartz 10/e p197-200)*
87. **Ans. b. Air embolism through external jugular vein** *(Ref: Bailey 25/e p75, 76, 1381, 1382)*

    When **neck or chest veins are injured**, air may enter the veins and causes **immediate death due to air embolism.**

88. **Ans. a. I** *(Ref: Sabiston 20/e p423; Schwartz 10/e p197-200)*

BLAST INJURIES

89. **Ans. c. Liver** *(Ref: Sabiston 20/e p594-595; Bailey 27/e p430)*
90. **Ans. a. TM**

HEPATIC INJURIES

91. **Ans. a. Conservative treatment** *(Ref: Sabiston 20/e p437-438; Bailey 27/e p 374)*

SPLENIC INJURIES

92. **Ans. c. Continue the conservative treatment and take subsequent measures on monitoring the patient** *(Ref: Trauma Manual by Moore and Mattox 4/e p252)*

    As **the patient is hemodynamically unstable, immediate surgical exploration should be done.**

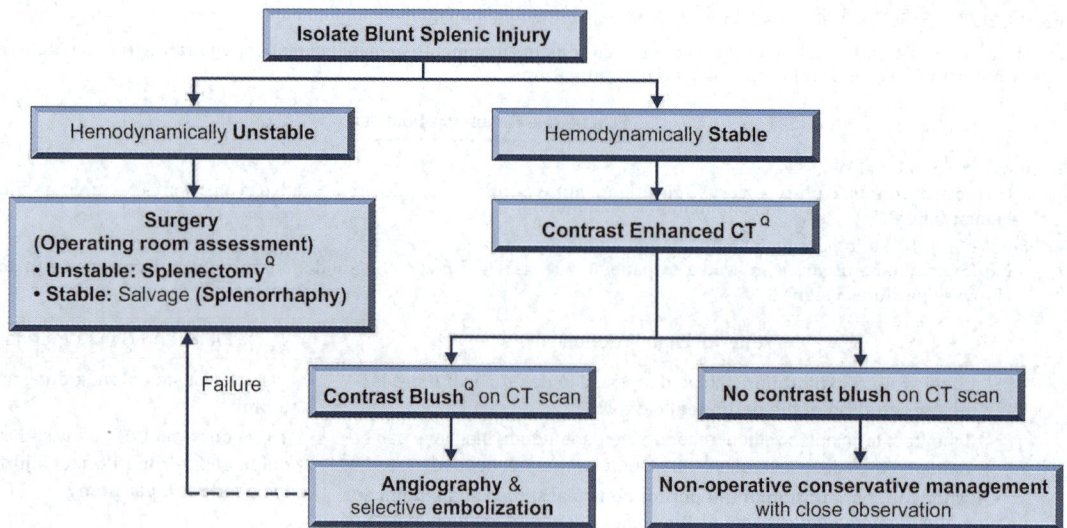

93. Ans. a. Observation
94. Ans. b. Spleen is most common organ to be involved, d. Cullen's sign seen
95. Ans. d. Continuation of conservative treatment under close monitoring system and subsequent surgery if further indicated
96. Ans. a. Partial splenectomy cannot be done

    Splenic trauma is discussed in chapter no. 20 Spleen.
97. Ans. c. CT scan
98. Ans. a. Splenic injury
99. Ans. d. Conservative management

STOMACH, DUODENUM AND PANCREATIC INJURIES

100. Ans. c. Blood in stomach is always related to gastric injury *(Ref: Sabiston 20/e p439; Schwartz 10/e p207, 9/e p178; Bailey 27/e p375)*

     Blood in stomach is suggestive of injury to the stomach but it is not always due to stomach injury.

     Blood in stomach may result from injury to adjacent gastrointestinal tract such as the esophagus or from stress ulcerations.

Gastric Injuries

- **Gastric injuries** are **most commonly** results **from penetrating trauma**[Q].
- **Most common treatment** of penetrating gastric injuries is **simple debridement** and **suturing**[Q].
- **Stomach** has a **rich blood supply**, so healing in gastric injuries is good and poses no special problem.

101. Ans. b. Pancreaticoduodenectomy (Whipple's operation) *(Ref: Sabiston 20/e p1552, 19/e p462-463, 1545; Schwartz 10/e p207, 9/e p179; Bailey 27/e p375, 1236)*

CHEST TRAUMA

102. Ans. b. Tracheo-bronchial rupture
103. Ans. a. Tracheobronchial injury *(Ref: Sabiston 20/e p431)*

     - **Tracheobronchial injuries** are so **fatal** that **most patients die at** the **scene** or **during transport** as a result of poor ventilation.

104. Ans. b. Immediate emergency room thoracotomy should be done *(Ref: Sabiston 20/e p1678; Schwartz 10/e p129,167; Bailey 27/e p367)*

Pericardial Tamponade

- Pericardial tamponade must be differentiated from tension pneumothorax in the shocked patient with distended neck veins.
- It is most commonly the result of **penetrating trauma**[Q].
  - Characterized by **Beck's Triad (MDH): M**uffled heart sounds, **D**istended neck veins & **H**ypotension[Q]

Diagnosis
- Chest X-ray: Enlarged heart shadow[Q]
- Echocardiography: ECHO is **diagnostic**[Q] showing fluid in the pericardial sac
- Central line: Rising central venous pressure[Q]

Treatment
- Needle pericardiocentesis can **buy enough time to move to the operating room**[Q].
- Treatment of choice: Surgical pericardiotomy[Q]

105. Ans. a. Tension pneumothorax, b. Cardiac tamponade *(Ref: Sabiston 20/e p1678; Schwartz 10/e p625; Bailey 27/e p367)*

Cardiac Tamponade	Tension Pneumothorax
• **Hypotension** and **raised JVP & CVP** is seen[Q]	• **Hypotension** and **raised JVP & CVP** is seen[Q]
• More common in penetrating injuries to chest[Q]	• Less common
• **Muffled heart sound** is seen[Q]	• **Respiratory distress** (dyspnea & **T**achypnea), resonant chest, absent breath sounds, mediastinal shift are seen[Q]

106. Ans. a. Tension pneumothorax
107. Ans. b. Cardiac tamponade   108. Ans. b. Intrathoracic and abdominal bleed
109. Ans. a. Abdominal solid visceral organ injury *(Ref: Sabiston 20/e p428; Schwartz 10/e p625)*

- **MC cause of hypotension in trauma** patients: **Hemorrhage**[Q]
- **MC cause of shock** after trauma is **hypovolemia**, and there are **five places** that a patient **can lose large volume of blood**: **Externally**, the **chest**, the **abdomen**, the **retroperitoneum**, and into **muscle compartments** (Blood on the floor and four more).[Q]
- Fracture of lower ribs (T$_9$-T$_{12}$) are usually associated with splenic or hepatic injuries[Q]
- Fracture of upper ribs (T$_1$-T$_3$), clavicle or scapula is usually associated with **major vascular injuries**[Q].

110. Ans. b. Tube thoracostomy
111. Ans. b. IPPV
112. Ans. c. Strapping
113. Ans. b. Rib fracture *(Ref: Schwartz 10/e p625, 9/e p175)*

- Schwartz says "**Most common injury of** the **chest** is **fracture of** one or more **ribs**, including fracture at the costochondral junction."[Q]

114. Ans. c. Anterolateral thoracotomy

FLAIL CHEST

115. Ans. a. Fracture of 3 or 4 ribs, b. Chest wall moves inwards during inspiration, e. Ultimately leads to respiratory failure *(Ref: Sabiston 20/e p1603; Schwartz 10/e p164,203; Bailey 27/e p 368)*
116. Ans. a. IPPV   117. Ans. b. Endotracheal intubation and mechanical ventilation
118. Ans. c. IPPV   119. Ans. d. Strapping of chest
120. Ans. b. IPPV with oral intubation
121. Ans. a. External fixation of flail segment and mechanical ventilation

DIAPHRAGMATIC INJURY

122. Ans. c. Smaller tears heal spontaneously and surgery is not required, e. Mask ventilation is encouraged in patient with massive visceral herniation *(Ref: Sabiston 20/e p432; Schwartz 10/e p202-203; Bailey 27/e p 365, 938)*

With bag and mask ventilation, the air may enter the herniated bowel loops producing more deterioration in respiratory distress.

Bergvist Triad: Rib fracture + Fracture of **spine/pelvis** + **Traumatic rupture** of **diaphragm**

123. Ans. a. Advise diagnostic laparoscopy, b. Chest X-ray is useful, d. Late complication is herniation of abdominal content
124. Ans. c. Left side is more common
125. Ans. a. Laparoscopy, b. Chest X-ray

HEAD INJURY

126. Ans. a. Glasgow coma scale
127. Ans. a. Sub conjunctival hematoma *(Ref: Harrison 20/e p3184, 19/e p 457e-2; Sabiston 20/e p419, 19/e p1894)*
128. Ans. d. Basilar fracture *(Ref: Bailey 27e p333)*
129. Ans. c. Altered mental status *(Ref: Harrison 20/e p2076, 19/e p1779)*

- **Early signs of elevated ICP** includes **drowsiness** and a **diminished level of consciousness**.
- **Coma** and **unilateral papillary changes** are **late signs** and **require immediate intervention**.

130. Ans. d. Many years after head injury *(Ref: Harrison 20/e p3186, 19/e p2547)*

- Harrison says "The **superficial cortical scars** that evolve from contusions are **highly epileptogenic** and may later **manifest as seizures**, even **after many years**."

131. Ans. a. Chronic subdural hematoma *(Ref: Harrison 20/e p3184, 19/e p457e-3-4; Sabiston 20/e p1903, 19/e p439; Schwartz 10/e p1719-1720)*
132. Ans. a. Extradural hemorrhage
133. Ans. a. Middle meningeal artery *(Ref: Sabiston 20/e p417)*
134. Ans. c. Fracture of petrous temporal bone *(Ref: Bailey 27/e p 713-714)*
135. Ans. b. Hemiparesis *(Ref: Schwartz 10/e p1715-1716; Bailey 27/e p333)*
136. Ans. c. Antibiotics and observation
137. Ans. b. Extradural bleed
138. Ans. c. Eversion of galea aponeurotica

Discussed in chapter no. 33 Cerebrovascular disease.

139. Ans. a. 1
140. Ans. b. Cortical veins

VASCULAR INJURIES

141. Ans. a. Femoral artery repair with vein ligation, b. Repair of artery and vein *(Ref: Sabiston 20/e p443-444)*

Vascular Injuries

Arterial Injuries
- Repair of femoral artery is always attempted. Most injuries require end-to-end anastomosis or an interposition graft[Q].
  - Arterial defects of **1-2 cm** can be **bridged**[Q]
  - **Interposition grafts** are employed when **end-to-end anastomosis cannot be accomplished** without tension[Q].

Venous Injuries
- Venous injuries are **more difficult to repair** due their **propensity to thrombose**[Q]
- **Repair** the **venous injuries encountered during exploration** for an associated arterial trauma, but only **in hemodynamically stable** patients if **repair will not jeopardize** or **delay the management** of other significant injuries[Q].
- **Decision to repair** or **ligate** the vein **depends on** the **condition of the patient**[Q]

142. Ans. a. Ligate femoral vein & repair femoral artery *(Ref: Sabiston 20/e p443, 444)*
143. Ans. a. Vein repair with continuity
144. Ans. b. Repair of artery and vein
145. Ans. a. Most commonly due to deceleration injury, b. High mortality, c. Surgery definitive treatment, d. Aortography gold standard *(Ref: Sabiston 20/e p443-444; Schwartz 10/e p214-215; Bailey 25/e p343; CSDT 11/e p257-259)*

Discussed in chapter no. 26 Arterial Disorders.

146. Ans. c. Artery caught between fractured ends of bones

SEAT BELT INJURY

147. Ans. a. Seat belt can cause pancreato-duodenal injury, b. Late death is caused by sepsis, c. Damage Control Surgery (DCS) is used to control major bleeding and to prevent contamination of peritoneal cavity, e. In DCS, laparotomy is decided based on patient prognosis *(Ref: Bailey 27/e p 351, 1061)*

SEAT BELT INJURY

- If a car accident occurs when a seatbelt is worn, **sudden deceleration** can result in a **torn mesentery**[Q].
- Blunt trauma to the abdomen by **seatbelt injury** may **compress the pancreas over the vertebral column** and result in **pancreatico-duodenal injury**[Q]
- If there is any **bruising of the abdominal wall**, or even marks of clothing impressed into the skin, laparotomy may be indicated[Q].

148. **Ans. a. Duodenum**

MISCELLANEOUS

149. **Ans. d. Immobilize the cervical spine**
150. **Ans. b. Only one dose of TT**
151. **Ans. b. Vascular injury** *(Ref: Bailey 27/e p416, 957)*

    Bailey says "**Amputation** should be considered **when part of a limb is dead, deadly** or a **dead loss**. A limb is dead when arterial occlusive disease is severe enough to cause infarction of macroscopic portions of tissue, i.e. gangrene. The occlusion may be in major vessels (atherosclerotic or embolic occlusions) or in small peripheral vessels (diabetes, Buerger's disease, Raynaud's disease, inadvertent intra-arterial injection). If the obstruction cannot be reversed and the symptoms are severe, amputation is required."

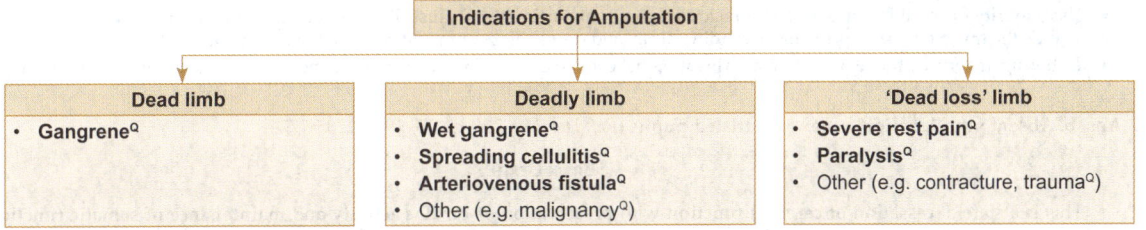

152. **Ans. a. X-ray of left lower limb and USG abdomen, b. Start IVF, Ryle's tube and catheterization, d. Grouping and cross matching of two unit of blood** *(Ref: Sabiston 20/e p414)*
153. **Ans. c. Removal of fragments of bone** *(Ref: http://surgeryonline.wordpress.com/tag/missile-injuries/)*

MANAGEMENT OF MISSILE INJURIES

- In limb wounds, **exploration** is followed by **thorough wound excision**[Q], after which, with very few exceptions, the **wound should be left open**[Q].
- A minimal amount of skin edge (i.e. only that which has been contaminated) should be excised[Q] around the entrance and exit wounds.

  - **Foreign matter** should be **removed** from the wound[Q].
  - **Delayed primary closure** should follow **within 4-7 days** after injury[Q].

- Dead muscle that does not bleed or contract, is mushy in consistency or has an unhealthy colour must be excised. These criteria comprise is the '**4 Cs**' for **muscle excision** (**Colour, Contractility, Consistency, Capillary bleeding**)[Q]

  - **Bone shattered** by high-energy transfer will in many instances **still have attachment to periosteum or muscle**[Q].
  - Such fragments must not be discarded. Loss of bone may result in malunion (e.g. shortening) or nonunion[Q].

154. **Ans. b. Abdominal aorta** *(Ref: Schwartz 10/e p210)*

    When bullet is shot above pubic symphysis in midline directed backwards, first organ to get injuries is abdominal aorta.

    - Penetrating trauma caused by bullet injuries is not limited by elastic properties of the tissue and vascular injuries are far more common[Q].
    - If exsanguinating hemorrhage originates near the midline in the retroperitoneum, direct manual pressure is applied with a laparotomy pad and the aorta is exposed at the diaphragmatic hiatus and clamped.
    - For stable patients with large midline hematomas, clamping the aorta proximal to the hematoma is a wise precaution[Q].

155. **Ans. a. Contractility of muscle, b. Color of muscle, c. Bleeding punctuate spots**
156. **Ans. c. Fixation of the bone** *(Ref: Master Techniques in Orthopedic Surgery Series by Moran and Cooney (2008)/487)*

    Bone is the first structure to be fixed in hand injuries.

SEQUENCE OF REPAIR IN HAND INJURIES (BE FAN OF VEINS)

1. Bone shortening and stabilization/fixation^Q
2. Extensor tendon repair^Q
3. Flexor tendon repair^Q
4. Arterial anastomoses^Q
5. Nerve repair^Q
6. Venous anastomosis^Q
7. Skin/wound closure^Q

157. **Ans. a. Bone**
158. **Ans. a. Repair to tendons**
159. **Ans. a. Loss of sympathetic tone** *(Ref: Sabiston 20/e p420)*

SPINAL CORD INJURIES

- **High spinal cord injuries** can also **result in systemic hypotension** because of **loss of sympathetic tone**^Q.
- The patient will usually have **hypotension** and **relative bradycardia** and will show evidence **of good peripheral perfusion** on physical examination^Q.
- The term **neurogenic shock** is used but is somewhat of a **misnomer** because these patients are **typically hyperdynamic**, with **high cardiac output secondary to loss of sympathetic vascular tone**^Q.

Treatment

- **Hypotension associated with high spinal injury** can be **treated by** alpha-agonist **phenylephrine**^Q.

160. **Ans. b. Behind the esophagus** *(Ref: Sevitt S. The mechanisms of traumatic rupture of the thoracic aorta. Br J Surg 1977; 64; 166)*

- The **majority of blunt injuries to the thoracic aorta** occur **at aortic isthmus just distal to the left subclavian artery**. Other locations include the **transverse arch, proximal ascending aorta**, and **descending aorta just proximal to the diaphragm**^Q.
- **Tethering of aorta by the ligamentum arteriosum** is believed to account for the **high frequency of aortic injury** in the **isthmus region**^Q.

161. **Ans. b. Absent pupillary light reflex and dilated pupils** *(Ref: Harrison 20/e p2073, 19/e p1735-1776)*

BRAIN DEATH

- This is a state of **cessation of cerebral function** with **preservation of cardiac activity** and **maintenance of somatic function by artificial means**^Q.
- It is the only type of brain damage recognized as equivalent to death.

Criteria for Brain Death
• **Widespread cortical destruction** that is reflected by **deep coma** and **unresponsiveness** to all forms of stimulation^Q • **Global brainstem damage** demonstrated by **absent pupillary light reaction** and by the **loss of oculovestibular** and **corneal reflexes**^Q • **Destruction of** the **medulla**, manifested by **complete apnea**^Q.

162. **Ans. c. 4th–6th ribs** *(Ref: https://storify.com/forensicmed/cardiopulmonary-resuscitation-related-rib-fracture)*

During resuscitation, artefacts of fractured ribs most commonly involve 4th – 6th ribs.

- "**The vast majority (90%+) of fractures occur in ribs 2 to 7**; *fractures in the bony parts of rib numbers* **1** *and* **8 to 10** *are possible but probably* **very rare**; *it is* **difficult to see** *how fractures can occur in rib numbers* **11** *and* **12** *following* **standard manual CPR.**"- *https://storify.com/forensicmed/cardiopulmonary-resuscitation-related-rib-fracture.*

163. **Ans. b. Separation of skin + subcutaneous tissue**

CHAPTER 43

Transplantation

HISTORY OF TRANSPLANTATION

History of Organ Transplantation	
First **Renal** transplantation	• Murray[Q] (1954) in identical twins
First **Liver** transplantation	• Starzl[Q] (1963)
First **Pancreas** transplantation	• Kelly & Lillhei[Q] (1966)
First **Heart** transplantation	• Christian Barnard[Q] (1967)
First **Lung** transplantation	• Fritz Derom[Q] (1968)
First **Islet cell** transplantation	• Sutherland[Q] (1974)
First **Heart & Lung** transplantation	• Reitz & Shumway[Q] (1981)
First **successful Intestinal** transplantation	• Deltz[Q] (1988)

TYPES OF GRAFT REJECTION

Types of Graft Rejection		
Hyperacute Rejection	**Acute (cellular) Rejection**	**Chronic Rejection**
• **Immediate** (within minutes to hours) **graft destruction** due to **ABO** or **pre-formed anti-HLA antibodies**[Q]. • Characterised by **intravascular thrombosis**[Q] • **Kidney transplants** are **particularly vulnerable**[Q] to hyperacute graft rejection • **Heart** and **liver transplants** are **relatively resistant**[Q].	• Occurs **during** the **first 6 months**[Q] • Most commonly presents **between 5-30**[Q] **days after transplantation** • **T-cell dependent,** characterized by **mononuclear cell infiltration**[Q] • Usually **reversible**[Q]	• Occurs **after** the **first 6 months**[Q] • **MC cause** of **graft failure**[Q] • **Non-immune factors** may contribute to pathogenesis • Characterized by **myointimal proliferation** in **graft arteries** leading to **ischemia** and **fibrosis**[Q]

Manifestations of Chronic Graft Rejection	
Kidney	• **Glomerular sclerosis & tubular atrophy**[Q]
Pancreas	• **Acinar loss & islet cell destruction**[Q]
Heart	• **Accelerated coronary artery disease** (Cardiac allograft vasculopathy[Q])
Liver	• **Vanishing bile duct syndrome**[Q]
Lungs	• **Obliterative bronchiolitis**[Q]

HLA MATCHING

HLA ANTIGENS

- In organ transplantation, **HLA-A, -B** and **-DR** are the **most important antigens** to take into account when matching donor and recipient in an attempt to reduce the risk of graft rejection
- **HLA matching** has a relatively small but **definite beneficial effect on renal allograft survival** (HLA-DR[Q] >HLA-B >HLA-A).
- Are the **MC cause of graft rejection**[Q]
- Their physiological function is to act as **antigen recognition units**
- Are **highly polymorphic** (amino acid sequence differs widely between individuals)
- **Anti-HLA antibodies** may cause **hyperacute rejection**[Q]

  - In the **case of liver transplants, HLA matching does not confer an advantage**[Q]
  - Although it is **beneficial in cardiac transplantation**, it is **not practicable** because of the **relatively small size of** the **recipient pool** and the **short permissible cold ischemic time**[Q].

TYPES OF GRAFT

Graft			
Autograft	**Isograft**	**Homograft (Allograft)**	**Heterograft (Xenograft)**
• Tissue transplanted **from one site to another** on the **same patient**[Q]	• **Transplant** from a genetically identical donor, such as an **identical twin**[Q]	• **Transplant** from individual of **same species**[Q]	• **Transplant from another species**[Q]

Xenograft	
Concordant Xenograft	**Discordant Xenograft**
• **Transplant between closely related species**[Q] • Example: **For humans, old world monkeys & apes** • Advantage: **Hyperacute rejections is not a threat**[Q] • Disadvantages: Zoonotic transfer of disease (Particularly retroviral transmission)	• Transplant **between distant related or divergent species**[Q] • Example: **For humans, new-world monkeys & other mammals** • For physiologic concern (organ size & availability), **pigs are preferred animal donor**[Q] • Disadvantages: High risk of hyperacute rejection[Q]

COMPLICATIONS OF IMMUNOSUPPRESSION

Complications of Immunosuppression		
Infection	**Malignancy**	**Non-Immune Side Effects**
• **High risk** of opportunistic infection **by viruses**[Q] • **Recipient derived infections**[Q] are more common than donor derived infections • **Risk of bacterial infection** is highest during first month[Q] of transplantation • **Risk of viral infection is highest during first 6 months**[Q] of transplantation; MC problem is **CMV**[Q] Infection • **Viral infection** may result from **reactivation of latent virus** or from **primary infection** • **Chemoprophylaxis** is important in **high risk patients** • **Pre-transplant vaccination** against community acquired infection should be considered	• MC malignancy in transplant recipient: **Skin cancer**[Q] (SCC) • Increased risk of **PTLD & Kaposi sarcoma**	• **Hypertension & chronic allograft nephropathy** caused by **calcineurin inhibitors**[Q] • **New onset diabetes** after transplant is associated with **tacrolimus or steroids**[Q] • **Hyperlipidemia, anemia & accelerated cardiovascular disease**[Q] • **Cardiovascular disease** is the **leading cause of death in transplant survivors**[Q]

Common Infections After Solid Organ Transplantation, by Site of Infection			
	Period after Transplantation		
Infected Site	**Early (<1 Month)**	**Middle (1-4 Months)**	**Late (>6 Months)**
Donor organ	Bacterial and fungal infections of the graft, anastomotic site, and surgical wound	CMV infection[Q]	EBV infection[Q] (may present in allograft organ)
Systemic	Bacteremia and candidemia (often resulting from central venous catheter colonization)	CMV infection[Q] (fever, bone marrow suppression)	CMV infection[Q], especially in patients given **early posttransplantation prophylaxis**; EBV proliferative syndromes (may occur in donor organs)
Lung	Bacterial aspiration pneumonia with prevalent nosocomial organisms associated with intubation and sedation (highest risk in lung transplantation)	*Pneumocystis* infection[Q]; CMV pneumonia[Q] (highest risk in lung transplantation); *Aspergillus* infection[Q] (highest risk in lung transplantation)	*Pneumocystis* infection[Q]; granulomatous lung diseases (nocardiae, reactivated fungal and mycobacterial diseases)
Kidney	Bacterial and fungal (*Candida*) infections (cystitis, pyelonephritis) associated with urinary tract catheters (highest risk in kidney transplantation)	Renal transplantation: BK virus infection (associated with nephropathy[Q]); JC virus infection	Renal transplantation: Bacteria (late urinary tract infections, usually not associated with bacteremia); BK virus (nephropathy[Q], graft failure, generalized vasculopathy)
Liver and biliary tract	Cholangitis	CMV hepatitis[Q]	CMV hepatitis[Q]

Contd…

Contd…

Infected Site	Early (<1 Month)	Middle (1-4 Months)	Late (>6 Months)
Heart	–	*Toxoplasma gondii* infection[Q] (highest risk in heart transplantation)	*Toxoplasma gondii* infection[Q] (highest risk in heart transplantation)
Gastrointestinal tract	Peritonitis, especially after liver transplantation	Colitis secondary to *Clostridium difficile*[Q] infection (risk can persist)	Colitis secondary to **C. difficile** infection (risk can persist)
Central Nervous System	–	*Listeria* (meningitis); *T. gondii* infection	*Listeria* meningitis[Q]; *Cryptococcus* meningitis; *Nocardia* abscess; JC virus-associated PML

CMV INFECTION

CMV INFECTION

- CMV is **most important pathogen** in **clinical transplantation**[Q].
- **CMV infections** usually occur after **30-50 days**[Q] after transplantation.

Clinical Features

- Fever, malaise, arthralgia, leukopenia and thrombocytopenia, hepatitis, **interstitial pneumonitis**[Q], enterocolitis and disseminated disease.

Diagnosis

- **Invasive CMV infection** with **histologic evidence** or a positive **CMV culture** from **deep tissue specimens** is **confirmatory**[Q]
- Chest X-ray: Bilateral diffuse interstitial pneumonia[Q]

Treatment

- **IV ganciclovir**[Q] is the **mainstay** of treatment and is safe and effective for **prophylaxis** and **treatment**.

BK VIRUS INFECTION

BK Virus

- **BK virus** is member of family **Polyoma virus**, associated with nephropathy, typically after 1-4 moths after transplant.
- **High levels of BK virus replication detected by PCR in urine and blood are predictive of pathology**, especially in setting of **renal transplantation**.
- **Urinary excretion of BK virus** and **BK viremia** are associated with the **development of ureteric strictures, Polyoma virus associated nephropathy** (1-10% of renal transplant recipients), and (less commonly) generalized vasculopathy.
- Timely detection and early reduction of immunosuppression are critical and can reduce rates of graft loss related to Polyoma virus associated nephropathy from 90% to 10-30%.

POST-TRANSPLANT LYMPHOPROLIFERATIVE DISORDER

Post-Transplant Lymphoproliferative Disorder (PTLD)

- **PTLD** is associated with **replication of EBV in B cells** induced by **enhanced immunosuppression**, primarily observed in patients who have received **more than one** course of polyclonal antilymphocyte globulin **(ALG)** or **monoclonal OKT3**[Q].

Clinical Features

- Clinical presentation of PTLD includes **fever, malaise** and **lymphadenopathy**[Q]

Diagnosis

- The **diagnosis** is made by **tissue biopsy**[Q].

Treatment

- **Polyclonal PTLD: Discontinuation of immunosuppression** and **antiviral therapy**[Q].
- **Monoclonal PTLD: Radiation, chemotherapy** and occasionally **surgical resection**. Antibody against **CD20**[Q] represents a novel approach in treating monoclonal PTLD with favorable outcome.

CLINICAL TESTING OF BRAINSTEM DEATH

CLINICAL TESTING FOR BRAINSTEM DEATH

- Absence of cranial nerve reflexes: (PCO)
  - **P**upillary reflex[Q]
  - **P**haryngeal (Gag) & Tracheal (Cough) reflex[Q]
  - **C**orneal reflex[Q]
  - **O**culovestibular (Caloric) reflex[Q]
- Absence of motor response:
  - Absence of motor response **to painful stimuli applied to head & face plus**[Q]
  - Absence of motor response **within the cranial nerve distribution to adequate stimulation**[Q]
- Absence of spontaneous respiration[Q]

DONORS

ORGAN DONORS

- Organ donors are of two types: Dead or deceased donors & living donors

Dead or Deceased Donors	Living Donors

• **Brain dead donors** also known as **heart beating donors** or **donation after brain death**[Q] (DBD)
• **Cardiac or circulatory dead** also known as **non-heart beating donors** or **donation after circulatory death**[Q] (DCD)
	• Limited to donation of:
	  – **Kidney**[Q]
	  – **Liver**[Q]
	  – **Lung lobe**[Q]

Donation after Brain Death (DBD) Donors	Donation after Circulatory Death (DCD) Donors
• **Most deceased donors organs** are obtained from **patients with brain-stem death**[Q]. • Brain death occurs when **severe brain injury causes irreversible loss of capacity of consciousness combined with irreversible loss of capacity for breathing**[Q].	• Due to rising demand for organ transplantation, increase in the use of organs from DCD donors • **DCD donors** are grouped according to **Maastricht classification**[Q]

Maastricht Classification for Donation after Circulatory Death (DCD) Donors	
Category	Description (DRACUIa)
1	**D**ead on arrival at hospital[Q]
2	**R**esuscitation attempted without success[Q]
3	**A**waiting cardiac arrest after withdrawal of support[Q] (**Most DCD donors from Category 3**[Q])
4	**C**ardiac arrest while brain dead[Q]
5	**C**ardiac arrest & **U**nsuccessful resuscitation in hospital[Q]

Uncontrolled Donors	Controlled Donors
• Includes category **1, 2 & 5**[Q] • **Warm ischemic time is longer & less predictable**[Q]	• Includes category **3 & 4**[Q] • Death results from **planned withdrawal of life-sustaining cardiorespiratory support**[Q] • **Most DCD donors** are from **controlled donors**[Q]

EXTENDED CRITERIA DONORS (ECD) FOR KIDNEY & LIVER TRANSPLANTATION

Extended Criteria Donors	
Kidney Transplant	Liver Transplant

• Donor **>60 years** of age[Q]
• Donor age **50-59 years** with at least two of the following:
  – **Cerebrovascular accident** as cause of death[Q]
  – **Pre-existing hypertension**[Q]
  – Terminal serum **creatinine >1.5 mg/dL**[Q]
	• **Mild to moderate steatosis**[Q]
	• **Hepatitis C positive**[U]
	• **Hepatitis B—core antibody positive**[Q]

ORGAN PRESERVATION SOLUTION

Organ Preservation Solution

- **Liver, pancreas and kidney** can be successfully preserved for **up to 2 days** by **flushing** the organ **with University of Wisconsin solution** and storing them at hypothermia (0-5°C)[Q].

University of Wisconsin Solution

- **UW solution**: Cationic composition (**high potassium** and **low sodium**) **mimics intracellular levels**[Q] to minimize diffusion down electrochemical gradients.
- UW solution (marketed as **Viaspan**) contains **high level of potassium** and **adenosine**[Q].

Special composition of UW solution	
Lactobionate and raffinose	• Minimizes cell swelling[Q]
Hydroxyethyl starch	• Prevention of the extracellular space expansion[Q]
Glutathione	• Anti-oxidant[Q]
Allopurinol	• Free radical scavenger[Q]
Adenosine	• Precursor for energy metabolism[Q]

MAXIMUM & OPTIMAL COLD STORAGE TIME

Maximum and Optimal Cold Storage Times		
Organ	Optimal storage time (hours)	Safe maximum storage time (hours)
Kidney	<18[Q]	36[Q]
Liver	<12	18
Pancreas	<10	18
Small intestine	<4	6
Heart	<3[Q]	6[Q]
Lung	<3[Q]	8

LIVER TRANSPLANTATION

Liver Transplantation

- **First liver transplantation** was done by **Starzl**[Q] in 1963, in **Denver, University of Colorado**.
- MC cause of death in LT: Sepsis & sepsis-induced multiple organ failure[Q]
- Combined liver & heart transplantation is done in amyloidosis[Q]
- Combined liver & lung transplantation is done in cystic fibrosis[Q]

Indications of Liver Transplantation	
MC indication of LT	• HCV induced cirrhosis[Q]
2nd MC indication of LT	• Alcoholic liver disease[Q]
MC indication of **pediatric LT**	• Biliary atresia[Q]
MC **metabolic disorder** requiring LT	• Alpha-1 antitrypsin deficiency[Q]
MC indication for LT **following acute liver failure**	• Acetaminophen toxicity[Q]

Contraindications of Liver Transplantation	
Absolute	Relative
• Advanced cardiopulmonary disease[Q] • Active untreated sepsis[Q] • Metastatic malignancy to the liver[Q] • Active alcohol abuse[Q] • Severe intractable depression[Q] • Patients with extensive venous thromboses[Q]	• Age >70 years • Obesity (BMI >40 kg/m²) • **Cholangiocarcinoma**[Q] • Chronic or refractory active infections • Ongoing tobacco use or illegal drug use

TYPES OF LIVER TRANSPLANTATION

Types of Liver Transplantation (LT)	
Orthotopic LT	• Graft is **placed at normal anatomical position** after recipient hepatectomy^Q
Heterotopic LT	• Graft is placed **at an alternative site** rather than normal anatomical position^Q
Auxiliary	• Native liver remains in-situ & whole or partial transplant is added^Q
APOLT	• **Left lobe** of recipient liver is **excised** & **donor liver occupies the vacated space**^Q
Auxiliary Heterotopic LT	• Whole liver or lobe placed in subhepatic space^Q
Piggyback LT	• **Orthotopic transplant** that **preserves recipient IVC**^Q
Split LT	• **Cadaveric donor liver** is **divided** & given to **two recipients**^Q
Reduced LT	• **Graft is reduced** to a functional unit of **appropriate size for** the **recipient**^Q

DOMINO LIVER TRANSPLANTATION

- **Explanted liver graft from** liver transplantation **recipient can be reused for transplantation**^Q
- Indications: Familial amyloid polyneuropathy^Q & maple syrup urine disease (MSUD)^Q

SEQUENCE OF ANASTOMOSIS IN ORTHOTOPIC LIVER TRANSPLANTATION (OLT)

SEQUENCE OF ANASTOMOSIS IN ORTHOTOPIC LIVER TRANSPLANTATION (SIPH-B)

- 1. **S**upra hepatic IVC 2. **I**nfra hepatic IVC 3. **P**ortal vein 4. **H**epatic artery 5. **B**ile duct^Q
- Preferred method of biliary drainage:
  - **Direct end-to-end anastomosis** between donor & recipients bile duct^Q
  - **Choledocho-choledochostomy is preferred over choledochojejunostomy**^Q
- Indications of choledochojejunostomy:
  - Diseased recipients extrahepatic bile duct^Q
  - Significant recipient-donor duct size mismatch^Q

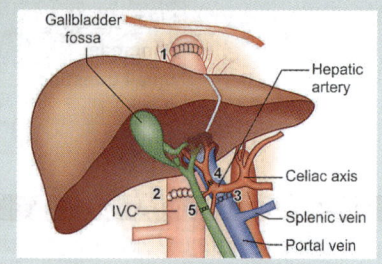

COMPLICATIONS OF LIVER TRANSPLANTATION

COMPLICATIONS OF LIVER TRANSPLANTATION

- **Hepatic artery thrombosis (HAT):**
  - Occur **spontaneously** or part of **acute graft rejection**; Present as **fever, bile leak** or rise in serum transaminase level
  - Requires **immediate re-transplantation**^Q
- **Portal vein thrombosis:** Occur insidiously; **does not require re-transplantation**^Q
- **Chronic liver graft rejection** due to **vanishing bile duct syndrome**^Q

> • **Liver** is **relatively resistant to hyperacute rejection**^Q; **Chronic rejection** is **uncommon in LT**^Q

- Bile leak: MC site of bile leak is choledochal anastomosis^Q
- Biliary stricture^Q

MC Indication for Re-Transplantation (PHARD)

- **P**rimary non-function^Q > **H**AT^Q > **A**cute & chronic rejection > **R**ecurrent **D**isease

RENAL TRANSPLANTATION

RENAL TRANSPLANTATION

- First RT was performed by **Murray in 1954 in identical twins**[Q]

Indication of Renal Transplantation	
End Stage Renal Disease Caused By: (GD for HR POSt at 4 AM)	• Polycystic kidney disease[Q]
• Glomerulonephritis[Q]	• Pyelonephritis[Q]
• Diabetic nephropathy[Q]	• Obstructive uropathy[Q]
• Hypertensive nephrosclerosis[Q]	• SLE[Q]
• Renal vascular disease[Q]	• Analgesic nephropathy[Q]
	• Metabolic disease[Q] (Oxalosis, amyloid)

Contraindication of Renal Transplantation	
Absolute	**Relative**
• Active malignant disease[Q]	• Limited life expectancy
• Active infection[Q]	• History of non-adherence to medication regimen
• Unreconstructable **peripheral vascular disease**[Q]	• History of non-compliance with dialysis
• Severe cardiac or pulmonary disease[Q]	• Financial barrier
• Active IV drug abuse[Q]	• Renal disease with high recurrence rate
• Significant psychosocial barriers	• Morbid obesity

Procedure:
- Renal graft is placed in **iliac fossa in retroperitoneal position**, leaving the **native kidney in-situ**[Q]
- Donor renal vein is anastomosed to external iliac vein[Q]
- Donor renal artery on Carrel's patch (Small portion of surrounding aorta) of donor aorta is **anastomosed to external iliac artery**[Q]
- If **donor renal artery lacks aortic patch** (in cases of **living donor renal transplantation**), graft renal artery is anastomosed to internal iliac artery[Q]
- **Ureter** is kept reasonably short to avoid distal ischemia & **anastomosed to bladder by**:
  - Lich-Gregoir Technique (Preferred[Q]): Direct implantation of ureter into dome of bladder with mucosa to mucosal anastomoses followed by closure over ureter to create a short tunnel
  - Lead-Better Politano technique[Q]

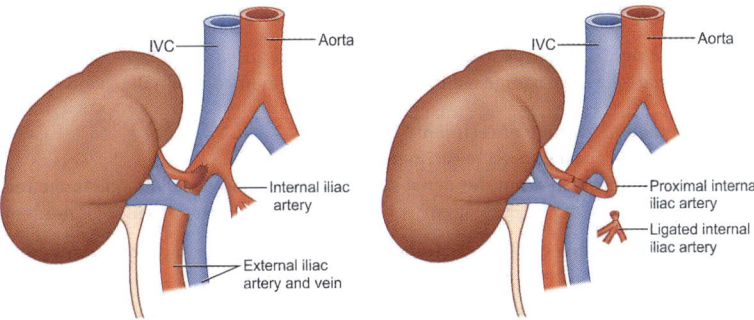

COMPLICATIONS OF RENAL TRANSPLANTATION

Complications of Renal Transplantation	
• MC complication in donor after live kidney donation: **Urinary retention & ileus**[Q]	• **Urinary leak**
• **Renal vein thrombosis**[Q]:	• **Obstruction of transplant ureter**: Best treated by re-implanting the donor ureter into bladder or anastomosis to native ureter
– Diagnosed by **Doppler**	• **Lymphocele**:
– **Urgent surgical exploration** is indicated	– Usually **asymptomatic**
– In most cases, **transplant nephrectomy** is required	– Large lymphocele **can cause ureteric obstruction** or edema of ipsilateral leg[Q]
• **Renal artery stenosis**[Q]:	– Treated by **USG guided percutaneous drainage** or drainage into peritoneal cavity[Q]
– Present late with **increasing hypertension & decreasing renal function**	
– Best treated by **angioplasty** → If not possible → **Open surgery & vascular reconstruction**	

PANCREAS TRANSPLANTATION

Pancreas Transplantation (PT)

- **First PT** was performed by **Kelly & Lillhei**[Q] in 1996.

Types of Pancreas Transplantation
• **SPK** (Simultaneous Pancreas & Kidney) Transplantation: **80% cases**[Q]
• **PAK** (Pancreas after Kidney) Transplantation: **15%** cases
• **PTA** (Pancreas Transplantation alone): **8%** cases (usually done for brittle diabetes)

- **Indications of PT:** Type-1 DM with clear C-peptide deficiency[Q]
- **Indications of SPK:** Insulin therapy with C-peptide level <2 ng/mL[Q] or insulin therapy with C-peptide level >2 ng/mL & BMI <28 kg/m²

Donor Selection

- Organ from **younger, leaner & hemodynamically stable deceased donors are preferred**[Q].
- **Pancreas with significant steatosis** should be **avoided** because of post-op complications (pancreatitis, peripancreatic fat necrosis, infection[Q]).

Contraindications for Procurement	
• Type I DM[Q]	• Chronic pancreatitis[Q]
• Previous pancreatic surgery[Q]	• History of recent malignancy[Q]

- **Procurement Principle, Preparation & Transplant:**
- During the procurement **minimal handling of pancreas is optimal**[Q]
- **Pancreas & liver** are **removed en-bloc** to prevent increased warm ischemic times[Q]

Back-Table Preparation Includes
• Removal of spleen • Suture reinforcement of mesenteric root • Maintaining **at least 1 cm of portal vein**[Q] • Trimming excess distal & proximal duodenum • **Iliac artery** is used as **Y–graft**[Q] in which end-to-end anastomosis of **internal iliac artery to splenic artery** & **external iliac artery to SMA** is done[Q]

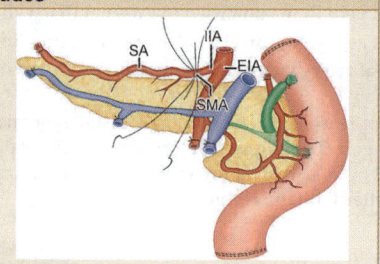

- **Pancreas transplant** is placed on the **right side**[Q] to prevent stretching of venous anastomosis.
- For **systemic venous drainage**, portal vein is **anastomosed to external iliac vein or common iliac vein or distal vena cava** in end-to-side fashion[Q]
- **Iliac artery graft** is sutured to **common iliac artery of recipient**[Q]
- For **portal drainage**, donor portal vein is anastomosed to recipient proximal SMV[Q].
- For **enteric drainage** of exocrine secretions, transplant **duodenal stump** is anastomosed side-to-side **to the recipient mid-jejunum**[Q].
- For **bladder drainage** of exocrine secretions, 4-5 cm cystostomy is made on anterior dome of bladder (**Duodenum is oriented inferiorly**[Q]).

> - In pancreas transplantation, enteric drainage & systemic venous drainage is **most commonly done**[Q].
> - For **bladder drainage**, graft should be oriented with **duodenum inferiorly**[Q]
> - For **enteric drainage**, duodenum can be superior or inferior[Q]
> - **Enteric drainage** is preferred over bladder drainage[Q]
> - **Advantage of bladder drainage:** Allows **monitoring of urinary amylase level** as an **early sign of graft rejection**[Q]

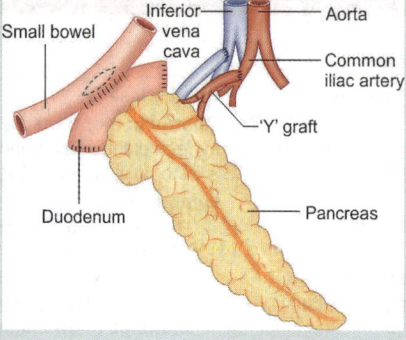
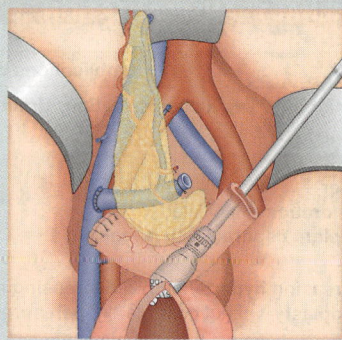

COMPLICATIONS OF PANCREAS TRANSPLANTATION

Complications of Pancreas Transplantation

- **Pancreas graft thrombosis**[Q]:
  - More common as compared to other solid organ due to **relatively low blood flow** through the organ
  - **Venous thrombosis is more common** than arterial thrombosis [Q]
  - Occurs **within first week after transplantation**
  - **Vascular thrombosis is the MC non-immunologic cause of pancreatic graft failure**[Q]
  - **Early pancreatitis**
- **Leak**
  - **Bladder drained transplant** with small leak are managed by **Foley catheter drainage**[Q]
  - **Enteric drained transplant** with leak usually require **operative intervention**[Q]
- **Bleeding**
  - **Immediate post-transplantation bleeding** from **pancreatic parenchyma**[Q]
  - **Delayed GI bleeding** from **enteric anastomosis**[Q]
  - Manifest from **postoperative day 6-10**[Q]; **Self limited**[Q]

ISLET CELL TRANSPLANTATION

ISLET CELL TRANSPLANTATION

- **First human islet cell auto-transplantation** was performed **by Sutherland**[Q] in University of Minnesota, in 1977.

Indications of Islet Cell Transplantation

- **Recurrent, severe hypoglycemia** with **decreased awareness of hypoglycemia**[Q]
- **Severe labile diabetes** with **wide swings of blood glucose** throughout the day[Q]

Principles of Procedure: (Islet cells are infused into portal vein)

- Current transplantation requires **life-long immunosuppression** & limited to most severe forms of diabetes[Q]
- **Edmonton Regimen**: Combination of **induction therapy with daclizumab** (IL-2 receptor antibody) & **maintenance therapy with sirolimus & tacrolimus**[Q] (Avoid steroids)
- **Insulin independence** occurs when **8000-10000 islet cells/Kg** of recipient's body weight is transferred[Q].
- **Four donors pancreas** are needed **for one islet cell transplantation**[Q].

Complications of Islet Cell Transplantation (ICT)

- Most feared complications of ICT: **Bleeding**[Q] (20%) > **Portal vein thrombosis**[Q] (<1%)

SMALL BOWEL TRANSPLANTATION

SMALL BOWEL TRANSPLANTATION

- First successful SBT was performed by **Deltz**[Q] & colleagues in 1988.
- MC indication of SBT in children: **Gastroschisis**[Q] > **Volvulus**[Q] > **Necrotizing enterocolitis**[Q]
- MC indication of SBT in adults: **Mesenteric ischemia**[Q] > **Crohn's disease**[Q] > **Trauma**[Q]

Indications of Small Bowel Transplantation

Short bowel syndrome patients who experience:	
- **IFALD** (Intestinal Failure Associated Liver Disease) - **Parenteral nutrition failure** - **Recurrent catheter related infections** - **Thrombosis of 2 of 6 major** central access veins	- Alteration in growth & development of children - **Severe dehydration & refractory electrolyte changes** - **Impending liver failure** - **Established liver disease** with cirrhosis & portal hypertension

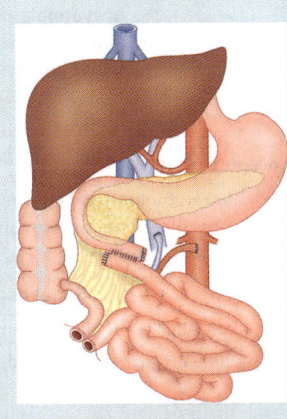

Donor Selection

- **Ideal donor** should have **body weight of 50-75% of the recipient**[Q]
- **Viral serologic testing** of cadaveric donor **for EBV & CMV** is important (Two MC viral infections after SBT[Q])

Types of Intestinal Transplantation

Small bowel with or without a portion of colon	Combined liver & small bowel grafts	Multi-visceral graft

Procedure (Isolated Intestinal Transplant)

- **Graft:** Isolated intestine allograft include **entire jejunum & ileum** with **associated vasculature (SMA & SMV^Q)**
- **Donor jejunum is divided just distal to ligament of Treitz** & ileum is **transected proximal to ileocecal valve^Q**
- **SMA & SMV** are **divided at mesenteric root** at inferior border of pancreas^Q
- In **recipients operation**, donor SMV is **anastomosed to recipient's portal vein** & donor SMA is **anastomosed to infra-renal aorta^Q**.
- Bowel continuity is established proximally & distally by standard techniques of enteric anastomosis
- **Graft jejunum is anastomosed to recipients duodenum** & distal ileum is **brought as an ileostomy^Q**
- **Distal ileostomy** is created for **routine monitoring of graft^Q**

COMPLICATIONS OF SMALL BOWEL TRANSPLANTATION

Complications of Small Bowel Transplantation

- **Technical complications:** Bowel anastomotic leaks, intestine perforations & wound Complications
- MC complication following intestinal transplant: **Bacterial infection (E. coli & Klebsiella^Q) > Viral Infection (CMV Infection^Q)**
- Incidence of PTLD: **SBT recipient^Q (10-20%) > Lung-Heart recipient (5-10%) > Liver recipient (2-5%) > Kidney recipient (1-2%)**
- **GVHD:** Incidence in SBT 0-14% (Because of large amount of lymphoid tissue in small intestine)

> - MC cause of graft loss in SBT: Sepsis >Rejection^Q
> - MC cause of death after SBT: Sepsis^Q

HEART TRANSPLANTATION

Heart Transplantation

- **First HT** was performed by **Christian Barnard^Q** in 1967.

Indications of Heart Transplantation	
• Ischemic dilated cardiomyopathy secondary to CAD^Q (MC)	• Valvular heart disease^Q
• Idiopathic dilated cardiomyopathy^Q	• Myocarditis^Q
	• Congenital heart disease^Q

- Heart transplantation is considered in the patients with **end-stage heart disease** that:
  - **Failed to respond to all other conventional therapy^Q**
  - Predicted **survival without transplantation is only 6-12 months^Q**
  - Patient **<65 years of age without irreversible damage** to other organ systems^Q

Contraindications of Heart Transplantation	
Absolute	**Relative**
• Active infection or HIV +ve^Q	• Age >60 years
• Irreversible pulmonary hypertension^Q	• Significant pulmonary vascular disease
• Malignancy^Q	• Active duodenal ulceration
• Other life-threatening illness^Q	• Creatinine clearance <30 micro mol/Liter
	• Drug or alcohol abuse
	• Psychiatric illness

Procedure of HT

- Median sternotomy is performed; Systemic heparin is given
- Patient is placed on cardiopulmonary bypass & **cooled to 29 °C**.
- After cross-clamping the aorta, **recipient heart is excised at mid-atrial level**

Sequence of anastomosis (LARA → PArA)
• **L**eft **A**trial^Q → **R**ight **A**trial anastomosis^Q → **P**ulmonary **ar**tery^Q → **A**ortic **A**nastomoses^Q

- Patient is rewarmed & weaned from cardiopulmonary bypass.

Domino Procedure
• If **heart-lung transplantation** is undertaken **for isolated respiratory disease, healthy native heart can be used for transplantation^Q**
• **Heart & lung transplantation** is done in: **Primary pulmonary hypertension, idiopathic pulmonary fibrosis, psychiatric illness^Q**

- MC cause of death after heart transplantation: **Infection^Q >Acute rejection^Q > Accelerated CAD^Q**

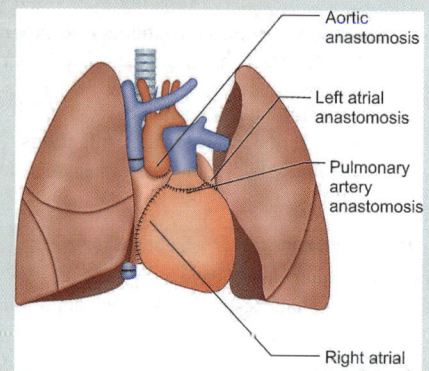

LUNG TRANSPLANTATION

LUNG TRANSPLANTATION

- First lung transplantation was performed by **Fritz Derom**[Q] in 1968

Indications of Lung Transplantation (P-CAB)

- **P**ulmonary fibrosis[Q]
- **P**rimary pulmonary hypertension[Q]
- **C**ystic fibrosis[Q]
- **C**OPD[Q]
- **A**lpha-1 antitrypsin deficiency[Q]
- **B**ronchiectasis[Q]

Types of Lung Transplantation

Single Lung Transplantation (SLT)	Double Lung Transplantation (DLT)

• Benefits two recipients from single donor
• **Advantages:** Shorter extubation time; Less need for cardiopulmonary bypass; Shorter hospitalization
• **Disadvantages:**
  – Quality of life & success rate is lesser as compared to DLT[Q]
  – **Lung hyperinflation** is a common complication following SLT.
  – **Graft compression** by hyperinflated native lung can cause **mediastinal shift & respiratory failure**[Q]
	• **Preferred surgical procedure for** patients with **cystic fibrosis & bronchiectasis**[Q] (Because infection remains in the native lung, if both lungs are not transplanted)
	• Preferred over SLT due to **better quality of life & higher success rate**[Q]

Procedure

- **SLT:** Performed through **posterolateral thoracotomy**[Q] image on left side
- **DLT:** Performed through **bilateral thoracotomy** or **median sternotomy**[Q]
- **Sequence of anastomoses in lung transplantation (PV By BA PA):**
Pulmonary Vein → Bronchial Anastomosis → Pulmonary Artery[Q]
- **Cardiopulmonary bypass** is usually required if **pulmonary hypertension** is present

Complications of Lung Transplantation

- **Dehiscence of airway anastomosis**[Q]
- **Late airway stenosis at bronchial anastomosis** due to ischemia: Treated by dilatation[Q]

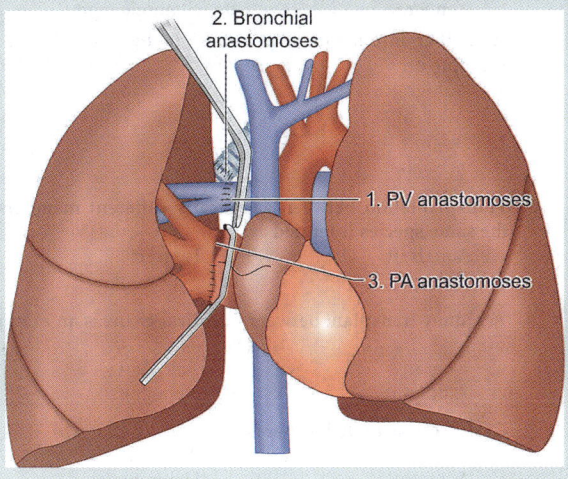

1. PV anastomoses
2. Bronchial anastomoses
3. PA anastomoses

Multiple Choice Questions

FLUIDS USED IN TRANSPLANTATION

1. **Amputated digits are preserved:**
   (AIIMS GIS Dec 2011, All India 92)
   a. Cold saline
   b. Cold Ringer Lactate
   c. Plastic bag in ice
   d. Deep freezer

2. **Allopurinol is used in organ preservation as:**
   a. Antioxidant   *(AIIMS May 2009)*
   b. Preservative
   c. Free radical scavenger
   d. Precursor for energy metabolism

GRAFT

3. **Kidney transplantation is an:** *(DNB 2009, COMEDK 2006)*
   a. Allograft   b. Isograft
   c. Xenograft   d. Synergic graft

4. **If mother is donating the kidney to her son, this is an example of:** *(Recent Question 2019, MCI June 2018)*
   a. Autograft
   b. Allograft
   c. Isograft
   d. Xenograft

5. **Transplantation between genetically different members of the same species is termed as:** *(COMEDK 2009)*
   a. Autograft   b. Isograft
   c. Allograft   d. Xenograft

6. **A kidney transplant between identical twins is an example of:** *(Recent Question 2017, COMEDK 2011)*
   a. Isograft   b. Allograft
   c. Autograft   d. Xenograft

7. **Graft from sister to brother is:** *(JIPMER 90)*
   a. Isograft   b. Allograft
   c. Autograft   d. Heterograft

8. **An isograft indicates transfer of tissues between:** *(All India 93)*
   a. Unrelated donors
   b. Related donors
   c. Mynozygotic twins
   d. From the same individual

9. **Skin grafting done on wound following major skin taken from twin brother:** *(Recent Question 2015, 2013)*
   a. Isograft   b. Allograft
   c. Autograft   d. Xenograft

10. **Concordant xenograft is:** *(Recent Question 2017)*
    a. Between closely related different species
    b. Between same species of different races
    c. Between same species
    d. Between non-identical twins

11. **Least chance of recipient failure in transplant is seen in:** *(Recent Question 2018)*
    a. Allograft
    b. Isograft
    c. Xenograft
    d. Heterotopic graft

MATCHING AND GRAFT REJECTION

12. **Acute cellular rejection following solid organ transplantation occurs:** *(COMEDK 2011)*
    a. Within minutes to hours of transplantation
    b. Within 48 hours of transplantation
    c. Between 5 to 30 days of transplantation
    d. Beyond 30 days after transplantation

13. **Hyperacute rejection is due to:**
    (Recent Question 2016, AIIMS Nov 2012)
    a. Preformed antibodies
    b. Cytotoxic T-lymphocyte medicated injury
    c. Circulating macrophage mediated injury
    d. Endothelitis caused by donor antibodies

14. **Most important HLA for organ transplantation and tissue typing:** *(Recent Question 2016, MAHE 98)*
    a. HLA-A   b. HLA-B
    c. HLA-C   d. HLA-D

15. **HLA matching is not necessary in which of the following organ transplantation?** *(JIPMER 2002)*
    a. Liver   b. Bone marrow
    c. Pancreas   d. Kidney

16. **Immunological rejection is mediated by recipients:**
    a. Eosinophils   b. Lymphocytes
    c. Neutrophils   d. Plasma cells

17. **Transplantation of which one of the following organs is most often associated with hyper-acute rejection?**
    a. Heart   b. Kidney   *(UPSC 2006)*
    c. Lungs   d. Liver

18. **Hyperacute rejection of graft is seen in?**
    (MHSSMCET 2006, 2008, All India 2003)
    a. Lung   b. Liver
    c. Kidney   d. Pancreas

KIDNEY TRANSPLANTATION

19. **Renal transplantation is most commonly done in:**
    a. Chronic glomerulonephritis   *(PGI Dec 97)*
    b. Bilateral staghorn calculus
    c. Horse shoe kidney   d. Oxalosis

20. **Commonest malignancy in renal transplant recipient is:**
    (AIIMS Nov 95)
    a. Skin cancer   b. Renal cell carcinoma
    c. Non-Hodgkin's lymphoma   d. Hodgkin's lymphoma

21. **Most common malignancy in post-transplant individuals:**
    a. PTLD   *(Recent Question 2017)*
    b. Squamous cell carcinoma of skin
    c. Kaposi sarcoma   d. CNS Lymphoma

22. **Highest chance of success in renal transplant is seen when the donor is the?**
    a. Identical twin   b. Father
    c. Mother   d. Sister
    e. Husband

23. **Principal cause of death in renal transplant patients:**
    (Recent Question 2016)
    a. Uremia   b. Malignancy
    c. Rejection   d. Infection

24. Investigation of choice in the early phase of renal transplant: *(Kerala 97)*
    a. IVP
    b. Retrograde cystourethrogram
    c. Ultrasonogram
    d. CT scan

25. Infection in renal transplant patient is usually caused by:
    a. CMV
    b. HIV *(Recent Question 2016)*
    c. Herpes
    d. Salmonella

26. Most common type of renal transplantation in India is:
    a. Allograft
    b. Autograft *(All India 99)*
    c. Isograft
    d. Xenograft

27. A patient had undergone a renal transplantation 2 months back and now presented with difficulty breath. X-ray showed bilateral diffuse interstitial pneumonia. The probable etiologic agent would be: *(AIIMS June 2002)*
    a. CMV
    b. Histoplasma
    c. Candida
    d. Pneumocystis carinii

28. Most common disease caused by CMV in a post renal transplant patients: *(JIPMER 2011)*
    a. Pyelonephritis
    b. Meningitis
    c. Pneumonia
    d. GI ulceration

29. An elderly male presents 2 months after renal transplantation with nephropathy. Which of the following can be a viral etiological agent? *(AIIMS May 2014)*
    a. Polymoa virus BK
    b. Human herpes virus type 6
    c. Hepatitis C
    d. Human papilloma virus, high risk types

30. In renal transplant, graft is placed in? *(Recent Question 2014)*
    a. Upper retroperitoneal space
    b. Iliac fossa
    c. Normal anatomical site
    d. None

31. All of the following are absolute contraindications for renal transplantation except: *(Recent Question 2017)*
    a. Active infection
    b. Active malignancy
    c. Active drug abuse
    d. Reduced life expectancy

32. In renal transplant, transplanted kidney is placed in: *(Recent Question 2018)*
    a. Iliac fossa
    b. Subcostal area
    c. Renal fossa
    d. Loin

33. Immediately after kidney donation, what happens to the creatinine level in the donors? *(Recent Question 2018)*
    a. Remains same
    b. Increases
    c. Decreases
    d. Level is independent of the donation

34. Which of the following is expanded criteria donor (ECD) for kidney transplantation? *(Recent Question 2018)*
    a. Donors with extremes of age
    b. Donors with excess alcohol intake
    c. Donors having cerebrovascular accident
    d. All of the above

35. Long-term complication of live kidney donors: *(Recent Question 2018)*
    a. Hypertension
    b. HPV infection
    c. Renal carcinoma
    d. Pyelonephritis

36. Left kidney is preferred for transplantation because: *(Recent Question 2018)*
    a. Longer renal vein
    b. Higher location
    c. Ease of surgery due to anatomical relations
    d. To prevent damage to liver

LIVER TRANSPLANTATION

37. Expanded criteria for liver donation include all of the following except: *(All India 2012)*
    a. Taken from diseased individual after brain death
    b. Hepatitis B serology positive
    c. Age of donor may be >70 years
    d. Can be taken from individual with mild hepatic steatosis

38. Extended criteria for liver donation include all of the following except: *(All India 2012, AIIMS GIS Dec 2011)*
    a. Donor age > 70 years
    b. HBsAg positive donor
    c. Mild hepatic steatosis
    d. Donor after cardiac death

39. Most common indication of liver transplantation in children: *(Recent Question 2019)*
    a. Biliary atresia
    b. Wilson's disease
    c. Hemochromatosis
    d. Primary biliary cirrhosis

40. Indications of Liver transplantation are all, except: *(PGI June 2005)*
    a. Biliary
    b. Sclerosing cholangitis
    c. Hepatitis A
    d. Cirrhosis
    e. Fulminant hepatic failure

41. Auxiliary orthotopic liver transplant is indicated for:
    a. Metabolic liver disease *(AIIMS May 2008)*
    b. As a standby procedure until finding a suitable donor
    c. Drug induced hepatic failure
    d. Acute fulminant liver failure for any cause

42. Reduced liver transplants: *(GB Pant 2011)*
    a. Given to two recipients after dividing into two parts
    b. Left lateral lobe divided and given to child
    c. Left lateral segment divided from segment 2 and given to child
    d. Part of liver segment transplanted into recipient depending upon requirement

43. All are scoring system used in liver transplant except: *(Recent Question 2016)*
    a. CTP
    b. PELD
    c. MELD
    d. MPI

44. Liver transplantation was first done by: *(Recent Question 2014)*
    a. Starzl
    b. Huggins
    c. Carrel
    d. Christian Bernard

45. All are marginal liver donor except:
    a. Older donor
    b. HBV core antibody positive donors
    c. Moderate steatosis
    d. Severe hepatitis

46. A 65-years old male with cirrhosis would be unsuitable for liver transplantation in the presence of:
    a. CTP 'B'
    b. HCC <5 cm
    c. Ascites
    d. Age >65 years
    e. Active alcohol abuse

47. Which of the following is not an indication for liver transplantation? *(DNB 2002)*
    a. Fatty liver
    b. HIV
    c. Willson's disease
    d. Primary hyperoxaluria

48. Most common indication for liver transplantation is:
    a. HCV induced cirrhosis *(Recent Question 2017)*
    b. HBV induced cirrhosis
    c. Primary sclerosing cholangitis
    d. HCC

49. Most common indication for pediatric liver transplantation is: *(Recent Question 2017)*
    a. Biliary atresia
    b. Metabolic diseases
    c. Alagille's syndrome
    d. HCV

PANCREAS TRANSPLANTATION

50. The advantage of bladder drainage over enteric drainage after pancreatic transplantation is better monitoring of:
    (All India 2009)
    a. HBA₁C levels
    b. Amylase levels
    c. Glucose levels
    d. Electrolyte levels

51. Site of transplantation in islet cell transplant for diabetes mellitus: *(Recent Question 2016)*
    a. Forearm muscles
    b. Pelvis
    c. Thigh
    d. Injected into the portal vein

SMALL INTESTINE TRANSPLANTATION

52. All are true about intestinal transplant except:
    (JIPMER GIS 2011)
    a. Principal barrier to widespread application is vigorous rejection reactions
    b. Severe form of GVHD occurs when T cells of graft respond to foreign HLA cells
    c. Uniquely dangerous complication is loss of protective mucosal barrier, bacterial translocation and severe sepsis
    d. Majority of intestinal grafts are multivisceral grafts

53. Most common cause of death in intestinal transplant:
    (Recent Question 2017)
    a. Sepsis   b. Acute rejection
    c. PTLD   d. GVHD

HEART TRANSPLANTATION

54. Dr. Christian Bernard performed the 1st heart transplant in the year: *(Kerala 97)*
    a. 1962   b. 1965
    c. 1969   d. 1967

55. Human heart transplant was first done by:
    a. Christian Bernard   *(Recent Question 2017)*
    b. Roy Calne
    c. Sutherland
    d. Reitz and Norman Shumway

56. Which of the following is category III for cardiac donation?
    a. Dead on arrival   *(Recent Question 2018)*
    b. Unsuccessful resuscitation
    c. Awaiting cardiac arrest
    d. Cardiac arrest while brain dead

57. Dr. Christian Bernard is associated with: *(DNB 2009)*
    a. Heart transplant   b. Renal transplant
    c. Liver transplant   d. Hair transplant

58. All of the following is true about heart transplantation except: *(Recent Question 2018)*
    a. Immunosuppression is started preoperatively
    b. It is only orthotopic and not heterotopic
    c. A beating heart cadaver/donor is needed
    d. High pulmonary arterial resistance is a contraindication

LUNG TRANSPLANTATION

59. Indications of lung transplantation:
    a. COPD
    b. Alpha-1 antitrypsin deficiency
    c. Cystic fibrosis and brochiectasis
    d. All of the above

60. Order of anastomosis in lung transplant:
    (Recent Question 2017)
    a. Pulmonary artery, pulmonary vein, bronchus
    b. Pulmonary vein, bronchus, pulmonary artery
    c. Pulmonary vein, pulmonary artery, bronchus
    d. Pulmonary artery, bronchus, pulmonary vein

POST-TRANSPLANT INFECTIONS

61. Post-transplant lymphoma is most commonly associated with: *(AIIMS May 2012)*
    a. EBV   b. CMV
    c. Herpes simplex   d. HHV-6

MISCELLANEOUS

62. In which of the following year, the transplantation of human organs act was passed by Government of India?
    a. 1994   b. 1996
    c. 2000   d. 2002

63. Commonest complication of immunosuppression is:
    (Recent Question 2016)
    a. Malignancy   b. Graft rejection
    c. Infection   d. Thrombocytopenia

64. Following drugs are known immunosuppressive agent except:
    a. Prednisolone   b. Cephalosporin
    c. Azathioprine   d. Cyclosporine-A

65. Steroids are used in transplantation: *(TN 2003)*
    a. To prevent graft rejection b. To prevent infection
    c. To speed up recovery   d. To enhance immunity

66. Which of the following organs/tissues are presently not being used for organ/tissue transplantation? *(All India 2011)*
    a. Blood vessels   b. Lung
    c. Liver   d. Urinary bladder

67. Cold ischemic time of the kidney should be ideally below:
    a. 2 hours   b. 6 hours   *(DNB 2010)*
    c. 12 hours   d. 24 hours

68. Length of time for which an organ can be cold stored before transplantation is maximum with: *(MHCET 2016)*
    a. Liver   b. Pancreas
    c. Kidney   d. Small intestine

69. Best temperature to store the procured organ for transplantation is: *(Recent Question 2017)*
    a. –2°C   b. 0°C
    c. 4°C   d. 6°C

70. All of the following nerves are commonly used for grafting except: *(Recent Question 2018)*
    a. Medial antebrachial cutaneous nerve
    b. Dorsal sensory branch of vagal nerve
    c. Musculocutaneous nerve   d. Sural nerve

Explanations

FLUIDS USED IN TRANSPLANTATION

1. **Ans. c. Plastic bag in ice** *(Ref: Sabiston 20/e p1996; Schwartz 10/e p 1800)*

   - The **amputated digits** are **cleansed under saline solution**, **wrapped in saline moistened gauze**, and **placed in a plastic bag**[Q].
   - The **plastic bag containing the part** is then **placed on** (not packed in) a **bed of ice** in a suitable container[Q].
   - The amputated part should never be immersed in nonphysiological solution such as antiseptics or alcohol.

2. **Ans. c. Free radical scavenger** *(Ref: Schwartz 10/e p 332; Bailey 27/e p1546)*

GRAFT

3. **Ans. a. Allograft** *(Ref: Schwartz 10/e p 266; Bailey 27/e p 1533)*
4. **Ans. b. Allograft**
5. **Ans. c. Allograft**
6. **Ans. a. Isograft**
7. **Ans. b. Allograft**
8. **Ans. c. Mynozygotic twins**
9. **Ans. a. Isograft**
10. **Ans. a. Between closely related different species** *(Ref: Sabiston 20/e p631)*

    "Concordant Xenografts: Concordant xenografts refer to transplants between closely related species; for humans, these include Old World monkeys and apes. The critical element defining an animal as concordant is the assembly of carbohydrate antigens on the cell surface. Similar to humans, concordant species lack galactosyl transferase, and as a result, their carbohydrates are the typical blood group antigens and they lack the N-linked disaccharide galactose-α(1-3)-galactose (α-Gal). Thus, the natural antibodies present in the circulation of potential human recipients can be predicted by straightforward blood group typing, thereby avoiding the problem of hyperacute rejection." -Sabiston 20/e p631

11. **Ans. b. Isograft**

MATCHING AND GRAFT REJECTION

12. **Ans. c. Between 5 to 30 days of transplantation** *(Ref: Schwartz 9/e p274-275; Bailey 27/e p 1533-1537)*
13. **Ans. a. Preformed antibodies**
14. **Ans. d. HLA-D** *(Ref: Bailey 27/e p 1534-1538)*
15. **Ans. a. Liver**
16. **Ans. b. Lymphocytes** *(Ref: Bailey 27/e p1534)*

    - The **cellular effectors of graft rejection** include **cytotoxic CD8 T cells**[Q], which **recognize donor HLA class I antigens** expressed by the graft and **cause target cell death** by releasing lytic molecules such as perforin and granzyme.

17. **Ans. b. Kidney**
18. **Ans. c. Kidney**

KIDNEY TRANSPLANTATION

19. **Ans. a. Chronic glomerulonephritis** *(Ref: Campbell 10/e p1226-1227)*

Most Common Cause of End-stage Renal Disease
• Diabetes mellitus >Hypertension >Glomerulonephritis[Q]

20. **Ans. a. Skin cancer** *(Ref: Bailey 27/e p1542)*
21. **Ans. b. Squamous cell carcinoma of skin** *(Ref: Sabiston 20/e p629)*
22. **Ans. a. Identical twin**
23. **Ans. d. Infection** *(Ref: Campbell 10/e p1251-1253)*

Most Common Cause of Death in Renal Transplant Patients
• Heart disease[Q] >Infection[Q] >Stroke

24. **Ans. c. Ultrasonogram:** *(Ref: Bailey 27/e p1550)*

Vascular Complications after Kidney Transplantation
• **Vascular complications** after renal transplantation are low, **presents during the first week** after transplantation with **sudden pain** and **swelling** at the site of the graft.
• **Diagnosis is confirmed by Doppler ultrasonography**[Q].
• **Urgent surgical exploration** is indicated and, in most cases, **transplant nephrectomy**[Q] is required.

25. Ans. a. CMV
26. Ans. a. Allograft
27. Ans. a. CMV *(Ref: Sabiston 20/e p657; Bailey 27/e p1541; Harrison 20/e p1033, 19/e p1192)*
28. Ans. c. Pneumonia
29. Ans. a. Polyoma virus BK *(Ref: Harrison 20/e p508, 19/e p926)*

    Polyoma virus BK can be an etiological agent in an elderly male, who presents 2 months after renal transplantation with nephropathy.

30. Ans. b. Iliac fossa
31. Ans. d. Reduced life expectancy *(Ref: Sabiston 20/e p650)*
32. Ans. a. Iliac fossa
33. Ans. b. Increases

    After kidney donation, both the serum creatinine and creatinine clearance increase.

34. Ans. d. All of the above *(Ref: Sabiston 20/e p651)*
35. Ans. a. Hypertension
36. Ans. a. Longer renal vein

    The left kidney is preferred because of implantation advantage associated with a longer left renal vein making anastomosis easier.

LIVER TRANSPLANTATION

37. Ans. a. Taken from diseased individual after brain death *(Ref: Sabiston 20/e p644)*
38. Ans. b. HBsAg positive donor
39. Ans. a. Biliary atresia
40. Ans. c. Hepatitis A *(Ref: Harrison 19/e p2068)*
41. Ans. a Metabolic liver disease, d. Acute fulminant liver failure for any cause *(Ref: Blumgart 5/e p1689-1693)*
42. Ans. d. Part of liver segment transplanted into recipient depending upon requirement
43. Ans. d. MPI
44. Ans. a. Starzl
45. Ans. d. Severe hepatitis
46. Ans. e. Active alcohol abuse

    Discussed in chapter no. 4 Liver.

47. Ans. b. HIV
48. Ans. a. HCV induced cirrhosis *(Ref: Sabiston 20/e p638)*

    "Chronic hepatitis C virus (HCV) infection is the most common indication for transplantation in the West at present."-Sabiston 20/e p638

49. Ans. a. Biliary atresia *(Ref: Sabiston 20/e p639)*

    "Biliary atresia is the most common indication for liver transplantation in the pediatric patient and is a major concern in the infant with persistent jaundice after birth."-Sabiston 20/e p639

PANCREAS TRANSPLANTATION

50. Ans. b. Amylase levels *(Ref: Sabiston 20/e p660; Schwartz 10/e p340-344; Bailey 27/e p1552)*

    - Bailey: 'Urinary drainage of the pancreas has the advantage that urinary amylase levels can be used to monitor graft rejection'Q

51. Ans. d. Injected into the portal vein *(Ref: Bailey 27/e p1552)*

    - The islets are then purified from the dispersed tissue by density-gradient centrifugation and can be delivered into the recipient liver (the preferred site for transplantation) by injection into the portal veinQ.

SMALL INTESTINE TRANSPLANTATION

52. Ans. d. Majority of intestinal grafts are multivisceral grafts *(Ref: Sabiston 20/e p668-669; Schwartz 10/e p352-354; Bailey 27/e p1555-1556)*
53. Ans. a. Sepsis *(Ref: Sabiston 20/e p672; Bailey 27/e p1556)*

    "The most common reason for mortality after intestine transplantation is infection with sepsis, accounting for 50% of deaths." -Sabiston 20/e p672

HEART TRANSPLANTATION

54. Ans. d. 1967 *(Ref: Bailey 27/e 1556)*

   • **Barnard** performed the **first human heart transplant** in **Cape Town, South Africa**, in **1967**[Q].

55. Ans. a. Christian Bernard *(Ref: Bailey 27/e p1556)*
56. Ans. c. Awaiting cardiac arrest *(Ref: Bailey 27/e p1418)*
57. Ans. a. Heart transplant
58. Ans. b. It is only orthotopic and not heterotopic

LUNG TRANSPLANTATION

59. Ans. d. All of the above *(Ref: Sabiston 20/e p1598)*
60. Ans. b. Pulmonary vein, bronchus, pulmonary artery *(Ref: Bailey 27/e p1557)*

   "Single-lung transplantation is performed through a posterolateral thoracotomy and double-lung transplantation through a bilateral thoracotomy or median sternotomy. During lung transplantation, the donor pulmonary veins on a left atrial cuff are anastomosed to the recipient left atrium. Next, the bronchial anastomosis and the pulmonary arterial anastomosis are completed."
   -Bailey 27/e p1557

POST-TRANSPLANT INFECTIONS

61. Ans. a. EBV *(Ref: Sabiston 20/e p672, 27/e p1542)*

MISCELLANEOUS

62. Ans. a. 1994 *(Ref: www.medindia.net › Health Acts in India)*

   • **Transplantation of Human Organ Act** was passed by Government of India in **1994**[Q].

63. Ans. c. Infection
64. Ans. b. Cephalosporin
65. Ans. a. To prevent graft rejection
66. Ans. d. Urinary bladder *(Ref: Essentials of General Surgery by Lawrence 4/e p475)*

Organs and Tissues that Can be transplanted at Present	
• Kidney[Q]	• Middle ear
• Lung[Q]	• Skin
• Liver[Q]	• Bone/tendons
• Pancreas and islet cells of Langerhans[Q]	• Bone marrow
• Heart and heart valves[Q]	• **Blood vessels**[Q] (most common saphenous vein[Q])
• Cornea[Q]	

67. Ans. None >C (12 hours) *(Ref: Bailey 27/e p1546, 26/e p1421)*
   • Optimal storage time for kidney should be <18 hours.

68. Ans. c. Kidney
69. Ans. c. 4°C *(Ref: Bailey 27/e p1546)*

   "After removal from the donor, the organs may undergo a further flush with chilled preservation solution before they are placed in double or triple sterile bags and stored at 4°C by immersion in ice while they are transported to the recipient centre and await implantation." -Bailey 27/e p1546

70. Ans. c. Musculocutaneous nerve

Most commonly used nerves for grafting:	
• Medial antebrachial cutaneous nerve[Q]	• Greater auricular nerve[Q]
• Dorsal sensory branch of vagus nerve[Q]	• Sural nerve[Q]

CHAPTER 44

Anesthesia and Perioperative Complications

Multiple Choice Questions

1. A young male presented with dyspnea, bleeding and petechial hemorrhage in the chest after 2 days following fracture shaft of the femur right side. Most likely cause is:
   a. Air embolism *(UPPG 2008)*
   b. Fat embolism
   c. Pulmonary thromboembolism
   d. Amniotic fluid embolism

2. Reactionary hemorrhage occurs: *(Recent Question 2016, 2014)*
   a. After 24 hours
   b. After 48 hours
   c. Within 24 hours
   d. After 7 days

3. Secondary hemorrhage is due to: *(DPG 2005)*
   a. Slipped ligature
   b. Occurs 7-16 days after surgery
   c. Due to disconnection of blood transfusion line
   d. None of the above

4. Post-dural puncture headache is typically: *(AIIMS June 2003)*
   a. A result of leakage of blood into the epidural space
   b. Worse when lying down than in sitting position
   c. Bifrontal or occipital
   d. Seen within 4 hours of dural puncture

5. In the immediate post operative period, the common cause of respiratory insufficiency could be because of the following except: *(AIIMS June 2003)*
   a. Residual effect of muscle relaxant
   b. Overdose of narcotic analgesic
   c. Mild hypovolemia
   d. Myocardial infarction

6. A patient undergoing surgery suddenly develops hypotension. The monitor shows that the end tidal CO_2 has decreased abruptly by 155 mm Hg. What is the probable diagnosis? *(AIIMS June 2003)*
   a. Hypothermia
   b. Pulmonary embolism
   c. Massive fluid deficit
   d. Myocardial depression due to anesthetic agent

7. A patient developed respiratory distress and hypoxemia after central venous catheterization through internal jugular vein, reason for this is: *(AIIMS Nov 2000)*
   a. Pneumothorax
   b. Hypovolemia
   c. Septicemia
   d. Cardiac tamponade

8. Commonest artery for cannulation is: *(Recent Question 2013, 2017)*
   a. Radial
   b. Ulnar
   c. Brachial
   d. Cubital

9. An elective surgery is to be done in a patient taking heavy doses of aspirin. Management consists of: *(All India 2000)*
   a. Proceed with surgery
   b. Stopping aspirin for 7 days and then do surgery
   c. Preoperative platelet transfusion
   d. Intraoperative platelet transfusion

10. A two months old infant has undergone a major surgical procedure. Regarding postoperative pain relief which one of the following is recommended? *(All India 2006)*
    a. No medication is needed, as infant does not feel pain after surgery due to immaturity of nervous system
    b. Only paracetamol suppository is adequate
    c. Spinal narcotics via intrathecal route
    d. Intravenous narcotic infusion in lower dosage

11. Air embolism in neural surgery maximum in which position? *(PGI Dec 2007)*
    a. Sitting
    b. Supine
    c. Trendelenberg
    d. Left lateral
    e. Right lateral

12. Most common coagulopathy noted in surgical patients is: *(Recent Question 2016)*
    a. Thrombocytopenia
    b. Afibrinogenemia
    c. Fibrinolysis
    d. Factor VIII deficiency

13. Presence of trifluroacetic acid (TFA) in urine indicates that volatile anesthetic agent used was: *(Recent Question 2016)*
    a. Halothane
    b. Methoxyflurane
    c. Trichloroethylene
    d. None of the above

14. Which of the following is false about Enhanced Recovery Protocol? *(Recent Question 2017)*
    a. IV antibiotics for 72 hours
    b. Pain relief by multimodal analgesia
    c. Early Mobilization
    d. Early nutrition

Explanations

1. **Ans. b. Fat embolism** *(Ref: Apley's 8/e p535-536, Rockwood 6/e p553)*
   - Discussed in chapter no. 29 Thorax and Lung.

2. **Ans. c. Within 24 hours** *(Ref: Bailey 27/e p19)*

Hemorrhage		
Primary Hemorrhage	**Reactionary Hemorrhage**	**Secondary Hemorrhage**
• Hemorrhage occurring **immediately as a result of an injury**^{Q} (or surgery).	• Reactionary hemorrhage is delayed hemorrhage (**within 24 hours**^{Q}). • Usually **caused by dislodgement of clot**^{Q} by resuscitation, normalization of blood pressure and vasodilatation. • May result from **technical failure** such as **slippage of a ligature**^{Q}.	• Secondary hemorrhage is caused by **sloughing of** the **wall of a vessel**. • It usually occurs **7–14 days after injury**^{Q} • **Precipitated by** factors such as **infection, pressure necrosis**^{Q} (such as from a drain) or malignancy.

3. **Ans. b. Occurs 7-16 days after surgery**

4. **Ans. c. Bifrontal or occipital** *(Ref: Harrison 20/e p88 19/e p443e-f)*

   ### POST-LUMBAR PUNCTURE HEADACHE
   - Headache is **positional**^{Q}: it begins when the patient sits or stands upright and **resolves upon reclining.**
   - Location: **Occipitofrontal**^{Q}
   - Nature: usually a **dull ache** but may be **throbbing**^{Q}.
   - **Recumbency** usually **improves** the **headache**^{Q}
   - Post-LP headache usually **begins within 48 hours** but may be **delayed for up to 12 days**^{Q}.
   - Incidence: 10-30%.

   Treatment
   - Beverages with **caffeine** may **provide temporary relief**^{Q}.
   - Initial treatment: **Bed rest**^{Q}
   - Persistent pain: **IV caffeine**^{Q} (500 mg in 500 mL saline administered over 2 hours) can be **very effective**.
   - If a leak can be identified, an autologous blood patch is **usually curative**^{Q}.

5. **Ans. c. Mild hypovolemia** *(Ref: Bailey 27/e p292, 19)*

Causes of Acute Post-Operative Shortness of Breath	
• MI and **heart failure**^{Q} • **Chest infections**^{Q}	• **Pulmonary embolism**^{Q} • **Exacerbation** of **asthma** or **COPD**^{Q}

   - In **mild hypovolemia**, the **systemic blood circulation** is maintained by shifting the blood from splanchnic circulation to the systemic circulation^Q.
   - **Healthy volunteers** could have **10-15% of their blood volume removed** with **no significant change in heart rate, BP, cardiac output** or **blood flow** to the splanchnic bed^Q.

6. **Ans. b. Pulmonary embolism** *(Ref: Harrison 19/e p1631; Sabiston 20/e p230, 294; Bailey 27/e p296, 986-91)*

7. **Ans. a. Pneumothorax** *(Ref: Complications in Anesthesiology by Kirby (2007)/169)*

8. **Ans. a. Radial** *(Ref: Lee Anesthesia 12/e p25)*
   - **Arterial puncture** and **cannulation** is performed to measure PaO_2, $PaCO_2$, SpO_2 and pH to clarify the **acid-base** and **electrolyte status.**
   - Any artery that can be compressed after puncture may be used (but **not end arteries**), usually the **radial**^{Q} (**preferred**), brachial or femoral.

9. **Ans. b. Stopping aspirin for 7 days and then do surgery** *(Ref: www.facs.org › surgerynews › surgerynewsupdat 2012)*

   Aspirin should be **stopped 1 week before surgery**[Q].

10. **Ans. d. Intravenous narcotic infusion in lower dosage** *(Ref: Schwartz 10/e p1601)*

   PAIN MANAGEMENT IN INFANTS

   - For **minor procedures: Pacifiers** dipped in sucrose
   - For **major procedures: IV narcotic agent**[Q] (morphine or fentanyl)
   - **Paracetamol** as **oral suspension** or as **peranal suppositories** can be used for mild to moderate pain.

11. **Ans. a. Sitting** *(Ref: http://emedicine.medscape.com/article/761367-overview)*

   VENOUS AIR EMBOLISM

   - **Venous air embolism** is a well known complication of neurosurgical procedures performed in **sitting position**[Q].
   - **Operative site >5 cm above right atrium** is a risk factor for **VAE**[Q].
   - **More common** in **posterior fossa surgeries**[Q]

   Management

   - Once VAE is suspected, any **central line procedure** in progress should be **terminated immediately**[Q].
   - Administer **100% oxygen**[Q]

     > - Promptly place the patient in **Trendelenberg (Head down) position** and **rotate towards the left lateral decubitus position**[Q]. This maneuver helps trap air in the apex of the ventricle, prevents its ejection into pulmonary arterial system and maintains right ventricular output.

   - Consider transfer to **hyperbaric chamber**[Q].

12. **Ans. a. Thrombocytopenia** *(Ref: Schwartz 10/e, 90-91,1428)*

13. **Ans. a. Halothane** *(Ref: en.wikipedia.org/wiki/Halothane)*

   PHYSICAL PROPERTIES OF HALOTHANE

   - **No analgesia**[Q] and **least pungent (non-irritant)**[Q]
   - **Pleasant to smell**, so **excellent for induction in children**[Q]
   - Halothane has **highest fat/blood coefficient**[Q] 51 (can get deposited in adipose tissues after prolonged exposure)
   - **Trifluoloroacetic acid** is a **metabolite** and **found in urine**[Q].

14. **Ans. a. IV antibiotics for 72 hours** *(Ref: Sabiston 20/e p223; Bailey 27/e p1266)*

   Enhanced Recovery after Surgery (ERAS) Protocols (Fast Track Programs[Q]**)**

   - ERAS refers to **patient-centered, evidence-based, multidisciplinary team developed pathways** for a surgical specialty and facility culture **to reduce the patient's surgical stress response, optimize their physiologic function & facilitate recovery.**
   - These care pathways form an **integrated continuum**, as the patient moves **from home through the pre-hospital / preadmission, preoperative, intraoperative & postoperative phases** of surgery and home again.

Key Elements of an ERAS Program	
• Pre-admission counseling	• Avoidance of opiate analgesia[Q]
• Avoidance of mechanical bowel preparation[Q]	• Maintenance of perioperative temperature
• Preoperative carbohydrate loading[Q]	• Prevention of postoperative nausea and vomiting
• Avoidance of preoperative dehydration[Q]	• Early mobilization[Q]
• No nasogastric tubes[Q]	• Early introduction of oral fluids/diets/ supplements[Q]
• Short, transverse incisions[Q] (or laparoscopic procedure)	• Early removal of urinary catheters[Q]
• Short-acting anaesthetic drugs[Q]	• Continual audit of outcomes
• Avoidance of perioperative fluid/salt overload[Q]	
• Thoracic epidurals[Q]	

CHAPTER 45

Robotics, Laparoscopy and Bariatric Surgery

LAPAROSCOPY

LAPAROSCOPY

- **Needle used** for pneumoperitoneum: **Veress needle**^{Q}
- Most commonly used gas: CO_2^{Q}
- Flow of gas: 1L/min^Q
- Intra-abdominal pressure maintained during laparoscopy: 12-15 mm Hg^Q
- **Trocar** is inserted **at** or **just below** the **umbilicus**^{Q} penetrating **skin, superficial & deep fascia, fascia transversalis & parietal peritoneum.**^{Q}

  - **Post-laparoscopy shoulder pain** is due to CO_2 **retention** causing **irritation of diaphragm** & referred pain to the **shoulder** through **phrenic nerve**^{Q}.

PNEUMOPERITONEUM

PNEUMOPERITONEUM

- Pneumoperitoneum can be created by **closed or open method**.

Closed Method	Open Method
• Uses **veress needle**^{Q}	• Uses **Hasson cannula**^{Q}
• **Low risk of bowel injury**^{Q} due to presence of safety valve at tip	• **Low risk of major vessel injury**^{Q}

GASES USED IN LAPAROSCOPY

GASES USED IN PNEUMOPERITONEUM

- First pneumoperitoneum was created by **filtered room air**^{Q}.
- CO_2 & N_2O are now **preferred** because of **increased risk of gas embolism with room air**^{Q}.
- CO_2: 200 times **more diffusible** than O_2, rapidly cleared from the body & lungs, **does not support combustion**^{Q}
- N_2O: 68% as rapidly absorbed in blood as CO_2, have **mild analgesic effect**, used **for short operative procedures** like sterilization or drilling^Q.
- For prolonged laparoscopic procedures, N_2O **should not be preferred** because it **supports combustion** better than air^Q.

PHYSIOLOGICAL EFFECTS OF LAPAROSCOPY

Physiological Effects of Laparoscopy	
Cardiovascular	• ↑ Intra-abdominal pressure leads to ↑ CVP, ↑ PCWP, ↑SVR and ↑ MAP which further ↓ Preload and ↑ Afterload, ultimately decreasing cardiac output^Q.
Pulmonary	• Cephalad shift of diaphragm decreases FRC, chest wall compliance & tidal volume increasing the work of breathing^Q. • Hypercapnia leading to increase in respiratory rate further adds to this.
Renal	• Increased IAP decreases renal flow, decreasing GFR & reduced urine output. • Raised pCO_2 leads to RAAS stimulation. No long term change in GFR/UO.

Contd…

Contd...

	Physiological Effects of Laparoscopy
Gastrointestinal	• **Decreased perfusion to intestines & stomach** (as a result of increase IAP) **decreases pH**. • Decreased portal and hepatic flow leads to elevation of LFTs
Peripheral vascular	• Incidence of DVT, PE is generally lower post-laparoscopic procedures probably secondary to improved prophylaxis • Risk is increased with longer procedures and reverse Trendelenburg position.

GAS EMBOLISM

Gas Embolism

- **Most commonly** seen **during induction of pneumoperitoneum** at the time of insufflations of gas from **unintended insufflations of gas directly into an open vein**[Q].
- The more soluble a gas in the blood, the lower chances are for gas embolism.
- CO_2 is **preferred for pneumoperitoneum** as it is **highly soluble in blood** and is **rapidly eliminated**[Q].
- CO_2 **Embolism:** An **initial rise in ET-CO_2** due to **pulmonary excretion of absorbed CO_2** is followed by a **sudden decrease due to fall in cardiac output**[Q].

DAY CARE SURGERY

Day Care Surgery or Ambulatory Surgery

- Surgical procedures suitable for ambulatory surgery should be accompanied by **minimal postoperative physiologic disturbances** and an **uncomplicated recovery**[Q].
- The **primary predictors of prolonged stay** or **unanticipated admission after day-care surgery** are related to the **type of surgical procedure** and **associated complications** (e.g. **blood loss, incision pain, postoperative nausea & vomiting**)[Q]
- For **superficial procedures** (e.g. mastectomy,) reductions in both **cost & per-operative complications** have been observed when these procedures are performed on an **outpatient basis**[Q].

Specialty	Types of Surgical Procedures
Dental	• Extraction, restoration, facial fractures
Dermatology	• Excision of skin lesions
General	• Biopsy, **endoscopy**, excision of masses, **hemorrhoidectomy, herniorrhaphy, laparoscopic cholecystectomy, adrenalectomy, splenectomy, varicose vein surgery**[Q]
Gynecology	• Cone biopsy, dilatation & curettage, hysteroscopy, diagnostic laparoscopy, **laparoscopic tubal ligation**[Q], uterine polypectomy, vaginal hysterectomy
Ophthalmology	• Contract extraction, chlazion excision, nasolacrimal duct probing, strabismus repair, tonometry
Orthopedics	• Anterior cruciate repair, knee **arthroscopy**[Q], shoulder reconstructions, bunionectomy, carpal tunnel release, closed reduction, hardware removal, manipulation under anesthesia and minimally invasive hip replacements
Otolaryngology	• Adenoidectomy, laryngoscopy, mastoidectomy, myringotomy polypectomy, **rhinoplasty**, tonsillectomy, tympanoplasty
Pain clinic	• **Chemical sympathectomy, epidural injection, nerve blocks**[Q]
Plastic surgery	• Basal cell cancer excision, cleft lip repair, liposuction, **mammoplasty**[Q] (reductions & agumentations), otoplasty, scar revision, **septorhinoplasty**[Q], skin graft
Urology	• Bladder surgery, circumcision, cystoscopy, lithotripsy, **orchidectomy**[Q], prostate biopsy, vasovasostomy, laparoscopic nephrectomy and prostatectomy

FAST TRACK SURGERY

Fast Track Surgery

- **Coordinated perioperative approach** aimed at **reducing surgical stress & facilitating postoperative recovery**
- Fast track surgery comprises:
  - Preoperative informed consent
  - **Fasting 6 hours for solids & 2 hours for liquids**
  - Atraumatic surgical technique (**avoid drains**)
  - **Reduction of stress**

- Elimination of pain by regional anesthesia (thoracic epidural anesthesia)
- Optimized fluid & temperature management
- Early enteral diet
- Prevention of gastrointestinal atony & postoperative nausea & vomiting
- Rapid postoperative mobilization

MINIMAL ACCESS SURGERY

Minimal Access Surgery (MAS) includes	
• Laparoscopy[Q]	• Perivisceral endoscopy[Q]
• Thoracoscopy[Q]	• Arthroscopy & intra-articular joint surgery[Q]
• Endoluminal endoscopy[Q]	

Advantages of Minimal Access Surgery (MAS)	
• Decrease in wound size[Q]	• Improved mobility[Q]
• Reduction in wound infection, dehiscence, bleeding, herniation & nerve entrapment[Q]	• Decreased wound trauma
	• Decreased heat loss[Q]
• Decrease in wound pain[Q]	• Improved vision[Q]
	• Faster recovery & shorter hospital stay

OBESITY & BMI

Category	BMI
Underweight	<18.5[Q]
Normal	18.5-24.9[Q]
Overweight	25.0-29.9[Q]
Obesity (Class I)	30-34.9[Q]
Severe obesity (Class II)	35-39.9[Q]
Morbid obesity (Class III)	40-49.9[Q]
Superobesity	>50[Q]

PATHOLOGIC CONSEQUENCES OF OBESITY

Pathologic Consequences of Obesity	
System	Pathology
Health	• **Increase in mortality**[Q]
Endocrine	• **Insulin resistance** and type 2 **diabetes mellitus**[Q]
Reproductive	• Male hypogonadism, gynecomastia, menstrual abnormalities, polycystic ovarian syndrome
Cardiovascular	• **Coronary disease,** congestive heart failure
Pulmonary	• Obstructive sleep apnea, "obesity hypoventilation syndrome", **pulmonary hypertension, DVT & pulmonary embolism**[Q]
Heaptobiliary	• Nonalcoholic fatty liver disease, symptomatic **gallstones**
Bone, joint, and cutaneous disease	• Osteoarthritis, acanthosis nigricans, friability of skin, **venous stasis & ulcers**[Q]
Neurologic	• Carpal tunnel syndrome, pseudotumor cerebri, stroke

Increased Cancer Risk in Obese Patients (PEEL CP GO KBC)		
• Prostate[Q]	• Cervix[Q]	• Kidney[Q]
• Endometrial[Q]	• Pancreas[Q]	• Bile duct[Q]
• Esophagus[Q]	• Gallbladder[Q]	• Breast[Q]
• Liver[Q]	• Ovarian[Q]	• Colon & rectum[Q]

BARIATRIC SURGERY

Bariatric Surgery

- Indication for Bariatric Surgery
  - Patients that have a BMI of **35 kg/m²** or more with **comorbidity**[Q]
  - Those with a BMI of **40 kg/m²** or greater regardless of comorbidity[Q]

Bariatric Operation	Mechanism of Action
• Vertical banded gastroplasty • Laparoscopic adjustable **gastric banding (Safest & reversible)**	• **Restrictive**[Q]
• Roux-en-Y gastric bypass (**RYGB**): MC performed procedure now-a-days	• **Largely Restrictive**[Q]/Mildly Malabsorptive
• **Bilopancreatic diversion** • **Duodenal switch**	• **Largely Malabsorptive**[Q]/Mildly Restrictive

VERTICAL BANDED GASTROPLASTY

- **Restrictive operation**: Restricts or decrease food intake[Q]
- **Upper stomach** near esophagus is **stapled vertically** to create a **small pouch along** the **lesser curvature of stomach**[Q]

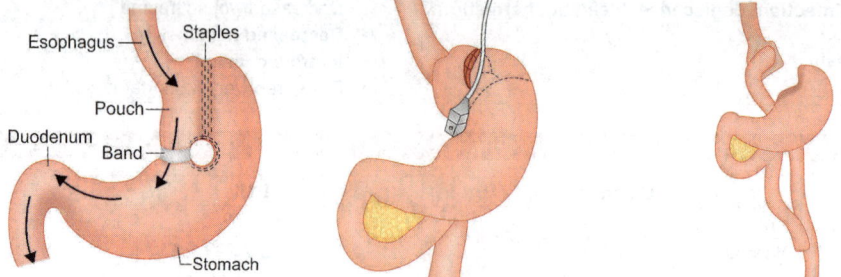

Vertical banded gastroplasty   Laparoscopic adjustable gastric banding   Roux-en-Y gastric bypass

LAPAROSCOPIC ADJUSTABLE GASTRIC BANDING

- Least invasive, safest & reversible[Q]
- Involves placement of **adjustable silicon band around the top part of stomach** & creates a **small stomach pouch**[Q]

ROUX-EN-Y GASTRIC BYPASS

- Most commonly performed bariatric surgery worldwide[Q]
- Upper part of stomach is separated from lower part & connected to Roux-limb of jejunum[Q]
- **Content of gastric pouch: 30-50 mL**[Q]; **Length of Roux-limb of jejunum: 70-100 cm**[Q]

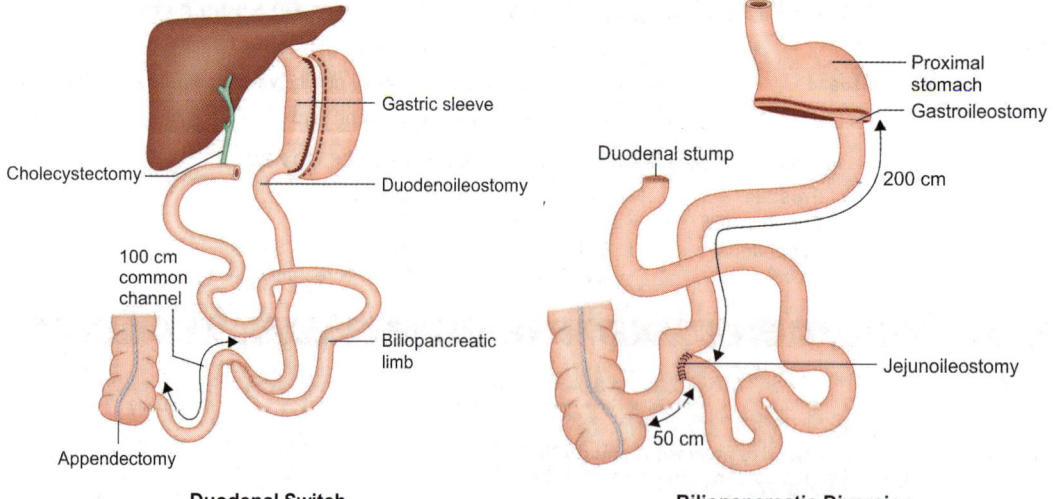

Duodenal Switch   **Biliopancreatic Diversion**

BILIOPANCREATIC DIVERSION

- When the bile is diverted from the intestinal tract so that only the **distal 50 to 100 cm** of **ileum** is **used for bile reabsorption**, the procedure is termed a biliopancreatic diversion.
- **Most effective bariatric surgery**[Q], especially valuable in patients with **severe morbid obesity** or in those who have **failed to maintain weight loss** following gastric bypass surgery or restrictive procedures[Q].
- **Main side effect** with BPD: Patients usually have an increase of **2-4 bowel movements**/day, which in general are **more malodorous**, suggesting fat malabsorption.

DUODENAL SWITCH OPERATION

- It involves a greater curvature **sleeve gastrectomy** with maintenance of the **continuity of** the antrum, pylorus and **first portion** of the duodenum.
- This allows for a **lower marginal ulcer** rate and a lower incidence of **dumping syndrome**.

Components of Duodenal Switch Operation	
• Sleeve gastrectomy[Q]	• Cholecystectomy[Q]
• Duodenoileostomy[Q]	• Appendectomy[Q]
• Jejunoileal bypass[Q]	

PERIOPERATIVE MORTALITY IN BARIATRIC SURGERY

Perioperative Mortality in Bariatric Surgery

- **MC cause of death** within 30 days of bariatric surgery: **Pulmonary embolism**[Q] (36%) > **Cardiac complications** (24%) > **Anastomotic leaks** (20%)
- **MC cause of death** in **immediate postoperative period**: Peritonitis secondary to anastomotic leak[Q] (leak **most commonly** occurs at the gastrojejunostomy)

NEW GUIDELINES OF BARIATRIC SURGERY FOR ASIA

New Guidelines for Asia

- **Overweight** if the BMI is **23 kg/m²** or more[Q] (International Standard is 25).
- **Obese** if the BMI is **25 kg/m²** or more[Q] (I.S. is 30).
- An Indian qualifies for **bariatric surgery** for obesity if the BMI is **32.5 kg/m²** (I.S. 35) **with comorbidity**[Q] or **37.5 kg/m²** without comorbidity (I.S. 40)[Q].

NOTES

Natural Orifice Transluminal Endoscopic Surgery (NOTES)

- **NOTES** is a technique whereby the **peritoneal cavity is entered endoscopically**, via a natural orifice (**mouth, rectum, vagina**) and the surgery is carried out using specialised endoscopic technology and techniques.
- **NOTES cholecystectomy & appendicectomy** have been successfully carried out in humans.
- Additional procedures performed with NOTES: Staging of intra-abdominal malignancy, segmental colectomy, gastrojejunostomy

POEM

Per Oral Endoscopic Myotomy (POEM)

- POEM is the application of esophageal myotomy to the concept of NOTES by **submucosal tunneling** method[Q].
- Used for **treatment of achalasia**[Q]
- Involves creation of **long esophageal myotomy using flexible endoscope**[Q]

ROBOTIC SURGERY

Robotic Surgery

- In 1985 a robot, **The PUMA 560**, was used to place a needle for a brain biopsy using CT guidance.
- In 1987 robotics was used in the first Laparoscopic surgery, a cholecystectomy.
- In 1988, **The PROBOT**, developed at Imperial College London, was used to perform prostatic surgery.
- **The ROBODOC** from Integrated Surgical Systems was introduced in 1992 to mill out precise fittings in the femur for hip replacement.
- Further development of robotic systems was carried out by Computer Motion with the **AESOP** and **ZEUS** Robotic Surgical Systems and Intuitive Surgical with the introduction of **The Da Vinci** Surgical System.

Da Vinci Robot
• It works on **"master-slave" principle**[Q].
• The **surgeon** inserts his hands into a **"master"** that translates motions of his hands into motions of the robotic arms and hand-like instruments. The surgeon acts as the "master" and the robot as the "slave" in this telerobotic "master-slave" system.
• It is commonly used for **prostatectomies, cardiac valve repair** and **gynecological Surgical procedures**[Q]

Multiple Choice Questions

LAPAROSCOPY

1. **The intra-abdominal pressure during laparoscopy should be set between:** *(Recent Question 2017, DNB 2011, AIIMS Nov 2003)*
   a. 5-8 mm of Hg
   b. 10-15 mm of Hg
   c. 20-25 mm of Hg
   d. 30-35 mm of Hg

2. **Gases for pneumoperitoneum:** *(PGI June 2007)*
   a. CO_2
   b. N_2
   c. Room air
   d. N_2O

3. **Which gas is used in laparoscopy?** *(Recent Question 2018, 2015, DNB 2012, AIIMS June 94)*
   a. CO_2
   b. N_2O
   c. O_2
   d. N_2

4. **Layers which are penetrated with trocar and cannula in production of pneumoperitoneum are:** *(PGI June 2005)*
   a. Skin and superficial fascia
   b. Deep fascia
   c. Rectus abdomnis
   d. Transversus abdomnis
   e. Rectus sheath

5. **Shoulder pain post laparoscopy is due to:** *(Recent Question 2014, AIIMS Nov 2007)*
   a. Subphrenic abscess
   b. CO_2 retention
   c. Positioning of the patient
   d. Compression of the lung

6. **A lady presented in the emergency department with a stab injury to the left side of the abdomen. She was hemodynamically stable and a contrast enhanced CT scan revealed a laceration in spleen. Laparoscopy was planned, however, the patients PO_2 suddenly dropped as soon as the pneumoperitoneum was created. What is the most likely cause?** *(All India 2010)*
   a. Gaseous embolism through splenic vessels
   b. Injury to the left lobe of the diaphragm
   c. Inferior vena cava compression
   d. Injury to colon

7. **Day care surgery can be done in:** *(PGI Nov 2010)*
   a. Lateral sphincterotomy
   b. Rhinoplasty
   c. Orchidectomy
   d. Total thyroidectomy
   e. Subcutaneous mastectomy

8. **Advantage of minimal access surgery:** *(Recent Question 2016)*
   a. ↑ Heat loss
   b. Better Hemostasis control
   c. Improved vision
   d. ↓ in wound pain

9. **Advantage of minimally invasive surgery over open surgery are all except:** *(Recent Question 2015)*
   a. Wide/better field of vision
   b. Less operative time
   c. Lest post-operative time
   d. Less post-operative morbidity

10. **Minimal invasive surgery includes all except:** *(MHPGMCET 2002)*
    a. FESS
    b. Lap cholecystectomy
    c. Endoscopic sclerotherapy
    d. PCNL

11. **During laparoscopy, the intra-abdominal pressure is:** *(Recent Question 2014, MHSSMCET 2008)*
    a. 5-10 mm Hg
    b. 12-15 mm Hg
    c. 15-20 mm Hg
    d. 20-25 mm Hg

12. **Instrument used to create artificial pneumoperitoneum in laparoscopy:** *(MHSSMCET 2008)*
    a. Maryland forceps
    b. Veress needle
    c. Trocar
    d. All of the above

13. **Complications of laparoscopy:** *(MHSSMCET 2009)*
    a. Diaphragmatic rupture
    b. Vascular injury
    c. Pneumothorax
    d. All of the above

NOTES

14. **In surgical procedure NOTES, entry point is through:** *(Recent Question 2015)*
    a. Abdomen
    b. Umbilicus
    c. Mouth
    d. Axilla

15. **Which procedure is being performed in the given image?**
    a. Laparoscopic cholecystectomy
    b. NOTES
    c. Percutaneous cholecystectomy
    d. Robotic cholecystectomy

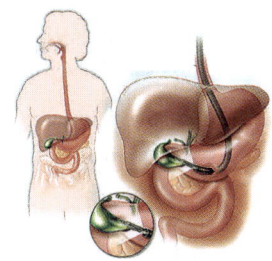

16. **POEM is used for:** *(Recent Question 2018)*
    a. Achalasia cardia
    b. Cancer esophagus
    c. Diffuse esophageal spasm
    d. Nutcracker esophagus

BARIATRIC SURGERY

17. **Cancers associated with excess fat intake are/is:** *(PGI Dec 2000)*
    a. Breast
    b. Colon
    c. Prostate
    d. Lung
    e. Thyroid

18. **Physiological changes seen in laparoscopy include all except:** *(AIIMS May 2015)*
    a. Increased ICP
    b. Decreased FRC
    c. Increased CVP
    d. Increased pH

19. **Bariatric surgical procedures include all except:** *(WBPG 2015, AIIMS Nov 2008)*
    a. Gastric banding
    b. Gastric bypass
    c. Biliopancreatic diversion
    d. Ileal transposition

20. **What is the name of this bariatric procedure?**
    a. LAGB   b. VBG
    c. RYGB   d. Biliopancreatic diversion

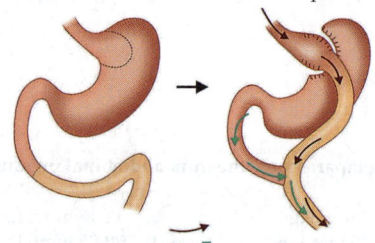

21. **All of the following are primarily restrictive operations for morbid obesity, except:** *(All India 2010)*
    a. Vertical band gastroplasty
    b. Duodenal switch operation
    c. Roux-en-Y operation
    d. Laparoscopic adjustable gastric banding

22. **Complication (s) of obesity is/are:** *(PGI Nov 2010)*
    a. Venous ulcer   b. Pulmonary embolism
    c. ↑Mortality   d. Prostate cancer
    e. Pulmonary hypertension

23. **Morbid obesity is BMI greater than:** *(MHSSMCET 2006)*
    a. 25   b. 30
    c. 40   d. 45

24. **Irrespective of comorbidity, bariatric surgeries should be done when BMI is greater than:** *(MHSSMCET 2008)*
    a. 35   b. 40
    c. 45   d. 50

25. **What is the name of this bariatric procedure?**
    a. Biliopancreatic diversion: Largely malabsorptive, mildly restrictive
    b. Duodenal switch: Largely malabsorptive, mildly restrictive
    c. Biliopancreatic diversion: Mildly malabsorptive, largely restrictive
    d. Duodenal switch: Mildly malabsorptive, largely restrictive

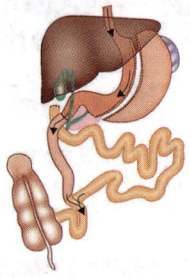

26. **The most effective bariatric surgery with treatment in the form of weight loss for morbid obesity is:** *(MHSSMCET 2008)*
    a. Roux-en-Y surgery   b. Biliopancreatic diversion
    c. Vertical banded gastroplasty
    d. Any of the above

27. **In Duodenal switch operation, which of the following is not done?** *(MHSSMCET 2010)*
    a. Cholecystectomy   b. Appendectomy
    c. Jejunoileal anastomosis   d. Distal gastrectomy

28. **Peterson hernia:** *(MHSSMCET 2010)*
    a. An internal hernia occurring behind Roux-en-Y limb
    b. An internal hernia occurring through window in the transverse mesocolon
    c. Cervical hernia   d. None

29. **What is the name of this surgery?**
    a. Billroth I   b. Billroth II
    c. Subtotal gastrectomy d. Sleeve gastrectomy

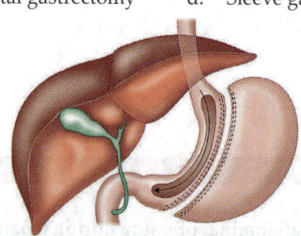

30. **Vertical banded gastroplasty also known as stomach stapling is done for:** *(DNB 2010)*
    a. Gastric carcinoma   b. Achalasia cardia
    c. Perforated gastric ulcer   d. Morbid obesity

31. **What is the name of this bariatric procedure?**
    a. LAGB: Purely restrictive
    b. LAGB: Restrictive + Malabsorptive
    c. VBG: Purely restrictive
    d. VBG: Restrictive + Malabsorptive

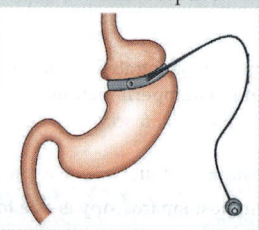

32. **Bariatric surgery which results in maximum weight loss:** *(MHCET 2016)*
    a. Biliopancreatic diversion   b. Gastric sleeve
    c. Gastric banding   d. Gastric bypass

33. **Most commonly performed and acceptable method of bariatric surgery is:** *(AIIMS May 2015)*
    a. Biliopancreatic diversion
    b. Biliopancreatic diversion with ileostomy
    c. Laparoscopic gastric banding
    d. Roux-en-Y gastric bypass

34. **Bariatric surgery with maximum benefits and comorbidity reduction:** *(Recent Question 2017)*
    a. Roux-en-Y gastric bypass
    b. Laparoscopic sleeve gastrectomy
    c. Biliopancreatic diversion
    d. Laparoscopic adjustable gastric banding

ROBOTIC SURGERY

35. **What is the name of most commonly used robot used for the given surgery?**
    a. PUMA 560   b. DaVinci robot
    c. PROBOT   d. ROBODOC

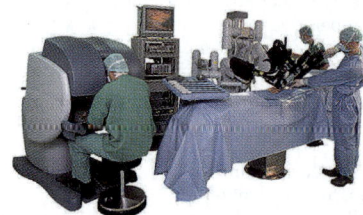

Explanations

LAPAROSCOPY

1. Ans. b. 10–15 mm of Hg *(Ref: Sabiston 20/e p394-396; Schwartz 10/e p417)*
2. Ans. a. CO_2, c. Room air, d. N_2O *(Ref: Sabiston 20/e p396; Schwartz 10/e p417-419)*
3. Ans. a. CO_2
4. Ans. a. Skin and superficial fascia
5. Ans. b. CO_2 retention
6. Ans. a. Gaseous embolism through splenic vessels *(Ref: Laparoscopic Surgery by Garcia & Jacobs/25)*
   - **Sudden drop in pO_2 immediately during induction of pneumoperitoneum** suggest the possibility of **gas embolism** as a result of entry of insufflating gas into circulation through the tear in splenic vessels.
   - **Gas embolism** may also have resulted from **inadvertent insertion of** the **trocar** or **veress needle into a vessel** or **abdominal organ**.
7. Ans. a. Lateral sphincterotomy, b. Rhinoplasty, c. Orchidectomy, e. Subcutaneous mastectomy *(Ref: Bailey 27/e p301)*
8. Ans. c. Improved vision, d. ↓ in wound pain *(Ref: Bailey 27/e p105-108)*
9. Ans. b. Less operative time
10. Ans. d. PCNL *(Ref: Bailey 27/e p105-106)*
11. Ans. b. 12–15 mm Hg
12. Ans. b. Veress needle
13. Ans. d. All of the above

NOTES

14. Ans. c. Mouth *(Ref: Bailey 27/e p117)*
15. Ans. b. NOTES *(Ref: Sabiston 20/e p397; Bailey 27/e p117)*
16. Ans. a. Achalasia cardia

BARIATRIC SURGERY

17. Ans. a. Breast, b. Colon, c. Prostate *(Ref: Sabiston 20/e p1162; Schwartz 10/e p1099-1131)*
18. Ans. d. Increased pH: *(Ref: Bailey 26/e p94; http://www.laparoscopyhospital.com/physiological-changes-laparoscopy.html)*
    Metabolic acidosis (decrease pH) from CO_2 absorption is the primary derangement with laparoscopy.
19. Ans. d. Ileal transposition *(Ref: Sabiston 20/e p1168; Schwartz 10/e p1099-1131)*
20. Ans. c. RYGB
21. Ans. b. Duodenal switch operation
22. Ans. a. Venous ulcer, b. Pulmonary embolism, c. ↑ Mortality, d. Prostate cancer, e. Pulmonary hypertension *(Ref: Sabiston 20/e p1162; Schwartz 9/e p951)*
23. Ans. c. 40 *(Ref: Schwartz 10/e p421-422)*
24. Ans. b. 40
25. Ans. a. Biliopancreatic diversion: Largely malabsorptive, mildly restrictive
26. Ans. b. Biliopancreatic diversion *(Ref: Sabiston 20/e p1171-1172; Schwartz 10/e p1103)*
27. Ans. d. Distal gastrectomy *(Ref: Sabiston 20/e p1172; Schwartz 10/e p1119-1121)*
    - **Sleeve gastrectomy** is done in **duodenal switch operation not the distal gastrectomy**.
28. Ans. a. An internal hernia occurring behind Roux-en-Y limb

Gibbon's hernia	• Hernia with hydrocele[Q]
Borger's hernia	• Hernia into pouch of Douglas[Q]
Beclard's hernia	• Femoral hernia through opening of saphenous vein[Q]
Amyand's hernia	• Inguinal hernia containing appendix[Q]

Ogilive's hernia	• Hernia through the **defect in conjoint tendon** just lateral to where it inserts with the rectus sheath^Q
Stammer's hernia	• **Internal hernia** occurring **through window in** the **transverse mesocolon after** retrocolic gastrojejunostomy^Q
Peterson hernia	• Hernia **under Roux limb** after **Roux-en-Y gastric bypass**^Q

29. Ans. d. Sleeve gastrectomy
30. Ans. d. Morbid obesity
31. Ans. a. LAGB: Purely restrictive
32. Ans. a. Biliopancreatic diversion
33. Ans. d. Roux-en-Y gastric bypass *(Sabiston 20/e p1169; Schwartz 10/e p1102-1103; Harrison 20/e p2849, 19/e p2398)*

    Most commonly performed and acceptable method of bariatric surgery is Roux-en-Y gastric bypass

    "The three restrictive-malabsorptive bypass procedures combine the elements of gastric restriction and selective malabsorption. These procedures are Roux-en-Y gastric bypass, biliopancreatic diversion, and biliopancreatic diversion with duodenal switch. Roux-en-Y is the most commonly undertaken and most accepted bypass procedure. It may be performed with an open incision or by laparoscopy."- Harrison 20/e p2849, 19/e p2398

34. Ans. a. Roux-en-Y gastric bypass *(Ref: Sabiston 20/e p1049, 1178)*

    "In appropriately selected patients, laparoscopic Roux-en-Y gastric bypass is the most durable method of weight loss and control of obesity-related comorbidities, including GERD."-Sabiston 20/e p1049

ROBOTIC SURGERY

35. Ans. b. DaVinci robot *(Ref: Sabiston 20/e p399)*

CHAPTER 46

Sutures and Anastomoses

TYPES OF SUTURES

Suture Materials

Absorbable	Non-absorbable

• These sutures **get absorbed** in the tissues either **by enzymatic digestion** or by **phagocytosis**[Q].
1. **Natural absorbable**:
  – Plain & chromic **catgut**[Q]
2. **Synthetic absorbable: (PVD)**
  – **P**olydioxanone (PDS)[Q], **P**olyglycaprone,
  – Polyglactin (**V**icryl)[Q]
  – Polyglycollic acid (**D**exon)[Q]
	• These sutures **remain in** the **tissues for indefinite period.**
	1. **Natural non-absorbable:**
	  – Linen[Q] – Silk[Q]
	2. **Synthetic non-absorbable: (PEN)**
	  – **P**olypropylene (Prolene)[Q]
	  – **P**olyester[Q] (ethibond)
	  – Monofilament polyamide (**E**thilon)[Q]
	  – **N**ylon[Q]

Depending upon Number of Strands

Monofilament	Polyfilament
• Consist of **single strand**[Q] of fiber • Sutures are **smooth & strong**[Q] • Chances of **bacterial contamination is less**[Q] • **Knot tied** may become **loose**[Q] • Prolene, Ethilon, nylon	• Consist of **multiple strands**[Q] braided together • **Easier to handle** and **knot tied does not slip**[Q] • Bacteria may lodge in the crevices of the suture, so **not suitable in presence of infection**[Q] • **S**ilk, **l**inen, **p**olyglycollic acid (SLIP)

SUTURES: IMPORTANT POINTS

Suture	Types	Raw material	Tensile strength	Absorption rate
Silk	Braided or twisted **multifilament**; Coated (with wax or silicone) or uncoated	Natural protein Raw silk from silkworm	Loses 20% when wet; 80-100% lost by 6 months	Fibrous encapsulation in body at 2-3 weeks; **Absorbed** slowly over **1-2 year**[Q]
Catgut	Plain	Collagen derived from healthy **sheep** or cattle	Lost within 7-10 days	**Phagocytosis** and **enzymatic degradation** within **7-10 days**[Q]
Catgut	Chromic	Tanned with **chromium salts** to **improve handling** and **resist degradation in tissue**[Q]	Lost within 21-28 days	Phagocytosis and enzymatic degradation **within 90 days**
Polyglactin (Vicryl)	Braided multifilament	Copolymer of **lactide & glycolide**[Q] in a ratio of 90:10, coated with polyglactin & calcium stearate	Approx, 60% remains at 2 weeks; 30% remains at 3 weeks	Hydrolysis minimal until 5-6 weeks; Complete absorption **60-90 days**[Q]
Polyglyconate	Monofilament Dyed or undyed	Copolymer of **glycolic acid and trimethylene carbonate**[Q]	Approx, 70% remains at 2 weeks; 55% remains at 3 weeks	Hydrolysis minimal until 8-9 weeks; Complete absorption **180 days**[Q]
Polyglycaprone (Monocryl)	Monofilament	Copolymer of **glycolide & caprolactone**[Q]	21 days maximum	**90-120 days**[Q]
Polyglycolic acid (Dexon)	Braided multifilament Dyed or undyed Coated or Uncoated	Polymer of **polyglycolic acid**[Q]	Approx, 40% remains at 1 week; 20% remains at 3 weeks	**Hydrolysis**[Q] minimal at 2 weeks; significant at 4 weeks; Complete absorption **60-90 days**[Q]
Polydioxanone (PDS)	Monofilament dyed or undyed	**Polyester polymer**[Q]	Approx, 70% remains at 2 weeks; 50% remains at 4 weeks; 14% remains at 8 weeks	Hydrolysis minimal at 90 days; Complete absorption **180 days**[Q]

PRINCIPLES OF SUTURING & ANASTOMOSES

WOUND CLOSURE & ANASTOMOSES

- As a general rule, **each suture** should be **separated by a gap** that is **twice** the **thickness of** the **skin**[Q].
- When **knots are cut short**, the **free ends** or 'ears' should be left **at least 1-2 mm** long[Q]. This is particularly important with **monofilament non-absorbables**[Q].
    - It has been suggested by **Jenkins** that a **suture length to wound length ratio** of 4:1 indicates the **optimum size of tissue bites** and of **suture spacing**[Q].
- **Anastomosis of vessels** was **pioneered by Carrel**[Q].
- **Elliptical incisions** must be **at least 3 times of the width** for the wound **to heal without tension**.
- Length to width ratio: 3:1

TYPES OF SURGICAL KNOTS

Square (Reef) Knot	Surgeons Knot	Granny (Pseudo-square) Knot
• Consist of **two throws** • **Crossing** is done **in each throw** • **Secured knot**	• Consist of **two throws** • **Two wraps** in **first throw** • **Crossing** occurs **in each throw**	• Consist of **two throws** • **Crossing does not occur** in any throw • **Not a secured knot**

NEEDLES: IMPORTANT POINTS

NEEDLES

- **Parts of Needle:** Swaged end (eyeless needle end for suture attachment) or **eye, point & body**
- Best site for holding the needle with needle holder: 1/3rd from swaged end & 2/3rd from pointed end[Q]

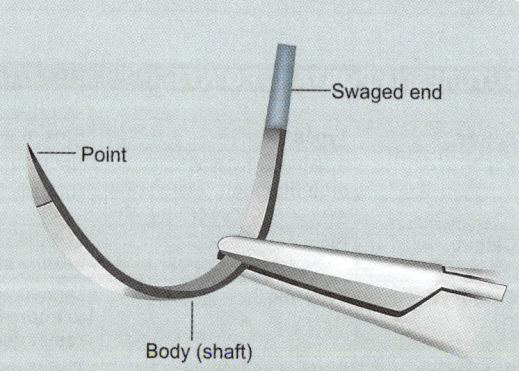

Types of Needle

Round Body	Cutting/Reverse Cutting
• **Taper point & blunt point** • **Round** in cross section Taper point / Blunt point	• **Cutting: Triangular** in cross section **pointing inwards**[Q] • **Reverse Cutting: Triangular** in cross section **pointing outwards**[Q] Conventional cutting / Reverse cutting

SUTURING TECHNIQUES

SUTURING TECHNIQUES

1. **Simple Interrupted Suture:**
- **Needle** is **inserted at right angle, to the incision**
- Pass through the both aspects of suture line, & exit again at right angles
- **Each successive suture** should be **placed at twice the distance from edge of the wound**[Q].

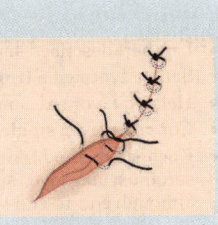

2. **Continuous Suture:**
- First suture is inserted in an identical manner to an interrupted suture
- Rest of the sutures is inserted in a continuous manner, until the far end of wound is reached.
- **At the far end** of the wound suture line should be **secured with Aberdeen knot**[Q] or by tying free end to the loop of cast suture.

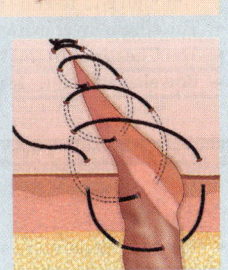

Aberdeen Knot
• Free end of suture is partially pulled through the final loop, several times before being pulled through a final time, completely, prior to cutting.

3. **Mattress Sutures:**
- Used to **produce eversion or inversion** of wound edges[Q]
- Useful in producing **accurate approximation of wound edges**, when the **edges** are **irregular in depth or disposition**[Q]

Horizontal Mattress	Vertical Mattress
• Initial suture is inserted as for an interrupted suture but then **needle moves horizontally & traverses both edges** of the wound once again[Q]	• Initial suture is inserted as for an interrupted suture but then **needle moves vertically & traverses both edges** of wound once again[Q].

4. **Subcuticular Suture:**
- Used in **skin**, where **cosmetic appearance is important**[Q] & skin edges are approximated easily.
- MC used suture is **monocryl**[Q] (**polyglycaprone**[Q])

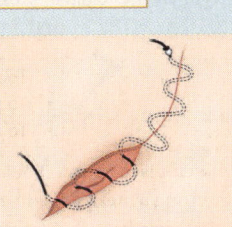

5. **Purse String Suture:**
- **Continuous stitch parallel to a circular wound is applied**[Q]
- Used for **hernia sac & appendectomy**[Q]

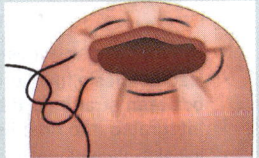

BOWEL ANASTOMOSES

Bowel Anastomoses

- **Lembert** described **seromuscular suture technique** for **bowel anastomosis** in **1826**[Q].
- **Senn** advocated a **two-layer technique for closure**[Q].
- **Halsted** favoured a **one-layer extramucosal closure**[Q].
- **Connell** used a **single layer of interrupted sutures** incorporating all layers of the bowel[Q].
- **Kocher's method**, a two layer anastomosis, first a **continuous all-layer suture using catgut**, then an **inverting continuous** (or interrupted) **seromuscular layer** suture **using silk**, became the standard. There is evidence that **inversion is safest in bowel** (least likely to leak), although end-to-end staplers give an everted anastomosis without complication.
- The **single-layer extramucosal anastomosis**, advocated by **Matheson**[Q], causes the least tissue necrosis or luminal narrowing.
- The **Cheatle split** (making a **cut into** the **anti-mesenteric border**) may help to **enlarge** the **lumen of distal, collapsed bowel**[Q].
- **Bowel anastomotic leaks** are generally occur **on day 7**[Q].

VASCULAR ANASTOMOSES

Vascular Anastomoses

- **Vascular anastomoses** require **more precision** than bowel anastomoses as they must be **immediately watertight**[Q] at the end of the operation when the clamps are removed.
- Suture size depends on vessel calibre:
  - 2/0 for **aorta**[Q]
  - 4/0 for **femoral artery**[Q]
  - 6/0 for **popliteal to distal arteries**[Q]
  - **Microvascular anastomoses** are made using a loupe and an interrupted suture down to **10/0 size**

- **Polypropylene-like sutures** with indefinite integrity give the **best results**[Q]
- **Intimal suture line must be smooth**[Q]
- **Knots** must be **secure**[Q]
- **Needle** must **pass from within outwards**[Q]

TISSUE GLUE

Tissue Glue

- **Tissue glue** is also available based upon a **solution of n-butyl-2-cyanoacrylate monomer**[Q].
- When it is **applied to a wound, it polymerizes to form a firm adhesive bond**[Q]
- **Wound does need to be clean, dry, with near perfect hemostasis and under no tension**[Q].
- **Specific uses**: Closing a laceration on the forehead of a fractious child in Accident and Emergency thus dispensing with local anaesthetic and sutures.
- **Relatively expensive**, it is **quick to use, does not delay wound healing** and is associated with an **allegedly low infection rate**.

MESH

Mesh in Hernia Repair

- Term **'mesh'** refers to **prosthetic material used to strengthen** a hernia repair.

Mesh can be used:
• **To bridge a defect**[Q]: Mesh is **simply fixed over the defect** as a tension-free patch
• **To plug a defect**[Q]: A plug of mesh is **pushed into the defect**
• **To augment a repair**[Q]: Defect is closed with sutures & mesh **added for reinforcement.**

- A well-placed mesh should have **good overlap around all margins of defect, at least 2 cm**[Q] **but up to 5 cm**[Q] if possible.
- Suturing a **mesh edge-to-edge into the defect** (inlay), with no overlap, is **not recommended**[Q].

Types of Mesh

Net meshes	Flat sheets
• **Net meshes** are **woven or knitted**[Q] • **Net meshes allow fibrous tissue in growth between strands** and becoming adherent & integrated into host tissues[Q] within a few months. • Initial fixation of mesh is by glue, sutures or staples.	• **Flat sheets** are **not porous**[Q] but can be perforated with multiple holes. • **'Sheet' meshes do not allow host tissue in growth** but become encapsulated by fibrous tissue[Q]. • Always require **strong, non-absorbable fixation**[Q] to prevent mesh migration.

Types of Mesh			
Synthetic mesh	Synthetic polymers of **polypropylene, polyester** or **polytetrafluoroethylene (PTFE)**. **Non-absorbable** & provoke **little tissue reaction**.		
		Polypropylene	**Strong monofilament mesh**[Q]; **Does not have any antibacterial properties**[Q] **Hydrophobic nature** & **monofilament microstructure impede bacterial in-growth**[Q].
		Polyester	**Braided filament mesh** leading to **increased risk of infection**[Q] **Hydrophilic property** allows **rapid vascular & cellular infiltration within the fibrils** providing **a stronger host–tissue interface**[Q].
		PTFE	**PTFE meshes** are **flat sheets**[Q]; **Do not allow any tissue in-growth**[Q] Used as a **non-adhesive barrier between tissue layers**[Q].
	Synthetic meshes are **very strong**. All meshes **provoke a fibrous reaction**. **More dense or heavyweight meshes** provoke a **greater reaction** leading to **collagen contraction & stiffening**[Q]. **Mesh shrinkage**: Progressive decrease in size of a mesh over time due to **natural contraction of fibrous tissue** embedded in the mesh, reducing the area of mesh itself, leading to **tissue tension & pain**. It can lead to **hernia recurrence** if mesh no longer covers the defect. **Meshes can shrink by up to 50%**[Q]. Meshes with thinner strands & larger spaces between them, **'lightweight, large-pore meshes'**, are preferred as they have **better tissue integration, less shrinkage, more flexibility & improved comfort**[Q].		
	Light weight: weight <40 g/m²[Q]		Heavy weight: Weight >80 g/m²[Q]
Biological mesh	**Sheets of sterilised, decellularised, non-immunogenic connective tissue**[Q]. Derived from **human or animal dermis, bovine pericardium or porcine intestinal submucosa**[Q]. Provide a 'scaffold' to **encourage neovascular in-growth & new collagen deposition**[Q]. **Host enzymes eventually break down** the **biological implant**, which is **replaced & remodelled with 'normal' host fibrous tissue**[Q].		
Absorbable meshes	Made from **polyglycolic acid fibre**[Q]. Used in **temporary abdominal wall closure** & **to buttress sutured repairs**[Q]. **No current role in hernia repair** as they **absorb & induce minimal collagen deposition**.		
Tissue-separating meshes	Designed for **intraperitoneal use**[Q] with **two different surfaces, one being sticky & one being slippery**[Q]. **Good adherence & host–tissue in-growth** is required on **parietal (muscle) side** of mesh but the opposite **(bowel) side** needs to **prevent adhesions to bowel**[Q]. **One side of mesh** is **coated by material which prevents adhesions**, such as polycellulose, collagen, PTFE[Q].		

Limitations to the use of mesh
• Presence of infection limits the use of mesh, particularly **heavyweight types**[Q].
• If a **mesh becomes infected** then it often **needs to be removed**[Q].

Multiple Choice Questions

SUTURES

1. Which of the following is a non-absorbable suture?
   (Recent Question 2016, All India 2008)
   a. Polypropylene   b. Vicryl
   c. Catgut   d. Polydioxanone

2. Absorbable sutures are: *(PGI June 2004)*
   a. Catgut   b. Silk
   c. Polypropylene   d. Polyglycolic acid
   e. Vicryl

3. Surgically used suture material polydioxanone (PDS): *(COMEDK 2014)*
   a. A non-absorbable and remains encapsulated
   b. Undergoes hydrolysis and complete absorption
   c. Undergoes phagocytosis and enzymatic degradation
   d. Is specifically used for heart valves of synthetic grafts

4. Catgut is prepared from submucosal layer of the intestine of: *(Bihar PG 2014, DNB 2005, 2000)*
   a. Cat   b. Sheep
   c. Human being   d. Rabbit

5. Vicryl, the commonly used suture material is a: *(UPSC 2000)*
   a. Homopolymer of polydiozanone
   b. Co-polymer of glycolide and lactide
   c. Homopolymer of glycolide
   d. Homopolymer of lactide

6. PDS is absorbed within: *(WBPG 2012, MAHE 2001)*
   a. 7 days   b. 21 days
   c. 100 days   d. 225 days

7. Surgically used suture material polydioxanone (PDS): *(WBPG 2012, COMEDK 2005)*
   a. Is non-absorbable and remains encapsulated
   b. Undergoes hydrolysis and complete absorption
   c. Undergoes phagocytosis and enzymatic degradation
   e. Is specifically used for heart valves or synthetic grafts

8. The surgeon who introduce catgut in surgery was: *(MAHE 2005)*
   a. Astley Cooper   b. Lord Lister
   c. John Hunter   d. Syme

9. Which of the following is a delayed absorbable synthetic suture material? *(DPG 2009 Feb)*
   a. Chromic catgut   b. Vicryl
   c. Silk   d. Nylon

10. Which of the following is not absorbable suture?
    (DNB 2011, APPG 2008)
    a. Catgut   b. Polyamide
    c. Polyglactin   d. Polyester

11. Which one of the following is used as preservative for packing catgut suture? *(AIIMS Nov 2002)*
    a. Isopropyl alcohol b. Colloidal iodine
    c. Glutaraldehyde   d. Hydrogen peroxide

12. Which of the following is ideal time to removal of scalp suture? *(MHSSMCET 2009)*
    a. 3 days   b. 5 days
    c. 7 days   d. 10 days

13. Suture material used for laparoscopic choledochotomy repair:
    a. Silk   b. Catgut
    c. Polyethylene   d. Vicryl *(MHSSMCET 2010)*

14. Catgut is preserved in: *(Recent Question 2013)*
    a. Glutaraldehyde   b. Isopropyl alcohol
    c. Iodine   d. Cetrimide

15. Raw material used in nylon suture is: *(APPG 2015)*
    a. Polyethylene terephthalate
    b. Polyamide polymer
    c. Polybutylene terephthalate
    d. Polyester polymer

16. Which of the following suture has maximum tensile strength and minimum tissue reaction? *(Recent Question 2015)*
    a. Polyglycaprone   b. Polypropylene
    c. Polyglactine   d. Polydioxanone

17. After a midline laparotomy, you have been asked to suture the incision. What length of suture will you choose?
    (AIIMS November 2016)
    a. 2x incision length b. 4x incision length
    c. 6x incision length d. 8x incision length

18. A woman presents with complete wound dehiscence 4 days after a laparotomy. After prescribing antibiotics for the infection, the surgeon decides to suture the wound. Which of these suture materials should he use? *(AIIMS November 2016)*
    a. Vicryl   b. Mersilk
    c. Catgut   d. Ethilon

19. Which of the following is the preferred suture material for vascular anastomosis? *(Recent Question 2017)*
    a. Non-absorbable, elastic   b. Non-absorbable, non-elastic
    c. Absorbable, elastic   d. Absorbable, non-elastic

20. Maximum tissue reaction is seen with: *(Recent Question 2018)*
    a. Plain catgut   b. Polydioxanone
    c. Silk   d. Chromic catgut

21. Which of the following suture is absorbed in 180 days?
    (Recent Question 2018)
    a. Polydioxanone   b. Catgut
    c. Chromic catgut   d. Nylon

22. Which of the following is not true about Polydioxanone suture?
    a. It is a polymer of ether-ester units
    b. It is biodegradable suture
    c. It is completely absorbed in 9 months
    d. Sterilized by ethylene oxide

23. What type of suture is this? *(APPG 2015)*
    a. Purse string suture   b. Halsted's suture
    c. Pare suture
    d. Mattress interrupted sutures

24. Which of the following statement is correct about the given suture? *(Recent Question 2017)*
    a. Natural absorbable
    b. Synthetic absorbable
    c. Natural non-absorbable
    d. Synthetic non-absorbable

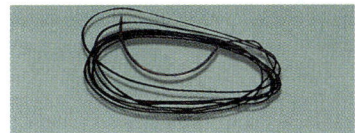

25. Which of the following statement is incorrect about the given suture?
    a. Smooth and strong
    b. Increased risk of bacterial infection
    c. Tied knot may become loose
    d. Consist of single strand

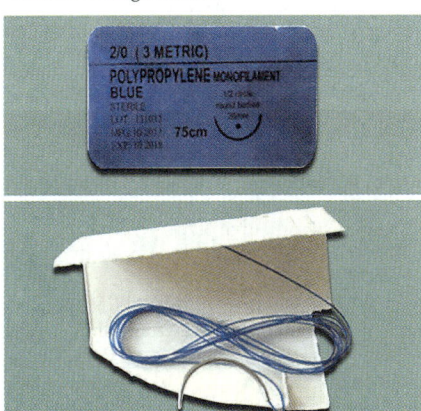

26. What are the copolymers of given suture? *(Recent Question 2016)*
    a. Glycolic acid and trimethylene carbonate
    b. Glycolide and caprolactone
    c. Polyglycolic acid and lactide
    d. Glycolide and lactide

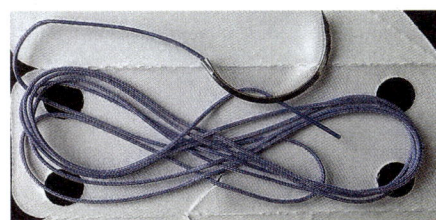

27. What is the preservative used for the given suture?
    a. 2% glutaraldehyde
    b. Peracetic acid
    c. Isopropyl alcohol
    d. Beta-propiolactone

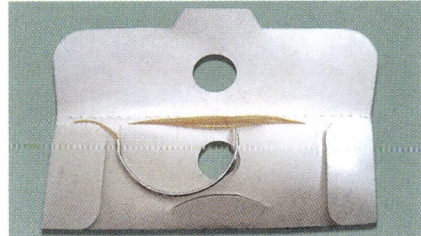

28. A Surgical attending has completed a modified radical mastectomy for a carcinoma breast patient. You have to suture the wound using subcuticular sutures. Which of these sutures will you choose? *(AIIMS May 2016)*

    a.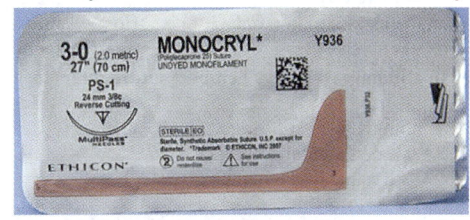

    b.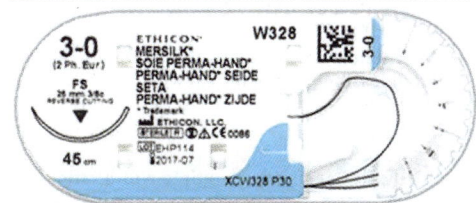

    c.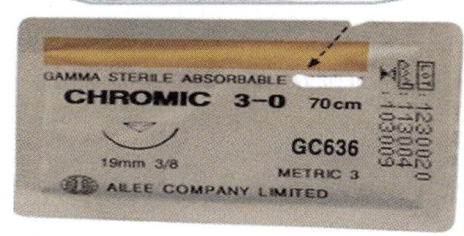

    d.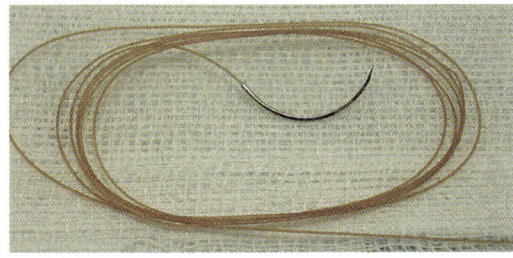

29. Which the following statement is true about the given suture? *(Recent Question 2018)*

    a. It is less reactive
    b. Derived from cat gut mucosa
    c. It is absorbed by phagocytosis and enzymatic dehydration
    d. Made from rabbit gut

30. True regarding 10-0 sutures is? *(PGI May 2018)*
    a. Thicker than 1-0 sutures
    b. Synthetic sutures
    c. Diameter is 0.9 mm
    d. Stronger than 1-0
    e. All of the above

31. Trilene is degraded by: *(Recent Question 2018)*
    a. Enzymatic degradation
    b. Non-enzymatic degradation
    c. Chemical degradation
    d. None

ANASTOMOSIS

32. Disparity of the bowel ends during end to end anastomosis is corrected by: *(Karnataka 2004)*
    a. Cheatle's maneuver
    b. Connell suture
    c. Lambert suture
    d. Czerny technique

33. In abdominal surgery Lembert suture refers to: *(Karnataka 2006)*
    a. Single layer suturing
    b. Sero-muscular sutures
    c. All coat intestinal suturing
    d. Skin suturing

34. Colonic anastomosis is most likely to rupture on which post-operative day? *(MHSSMCET 2005)*
    a. 1-2 days
    b. 3-4 days
    c. After 7 days
    d. After 14 day

35. Regarding vascular surgery distal to popliteal artery, which of the following is true? *(MHSSMCET 2006)*
    a. Suture with polypropylene
    b. 6-0 suture used
    c. Needle pass from within outwards
    d. All the above

36. When knots are cut short, the free ends of 'ears' should be left at least _____ mm long? *(MHSSMCET 2008)*
    a. 1-2 mm
    b. 3-4 mm
    c. 5-6 mm
    d. 7-8 mm

37. In elliptical incisions, length to width ratio: *(Recent Question 2017)*
    a. 4:1
    b. 3:1
    c. 2:1
    d. 1:1

38. Length of suture required closing the incision to the wound length ratio: *(Recent Question 2017)*
    a. 4:1
    b. 3:1
    c. 2:1
    d. 1:1

39. The single layer extramucosal anastomosis was popularized by: *(MHSSMCET 2008)*
    a. Carrel
    b. Antoine Lambert
    c. Norman Matheson
    d. Emil Theodar Kocher

40. On table colonic lavage was used for first time in 1968 by: *(MHSSMCET 2008)*
    a. Muir
    b. Carrel
    c. Connell
    d. Lembert

41. Carrel's triangle is used in: *(MHSSMCET 2008)*
    a. Vascular anastomosis
    b. Bowel anastomosis
    c. Tendon repair
    d. Nerve repair

42. Intestinal anastomosis strength is provided by: *(JIPMER 2015)*
    a. Mucosa
    b. Sub mucosa
    c. Serosa
    d. Muscularis mucosa

43. Stapler used for MIPH: *(Recent Question 2013)*
    a. Linear cutting stapler
    b. Circular cutting stapler
    c. Linear stapler
    d. Circular stapler

44. Tissue suturing glue contains: *(Recent Question 2015)*
    a. Cyanoacrylate
    b. Ethanolamine oleate
    c. Methacrylate
    d. Polychloroprene

45. Six years old child was brought to the hospital with obstructed hernia. On exploration, bowel was found gangrenous. Which of the following is true about anastomosis? *(Recent Question 2018)*
    a. Should be done by continuous layers as it takes less time
    b. Done with catgut
    c. Should be done by using single layer seromuscular lambert sutures
    d. Single layer taking submucosa

46. All of the following are true except: *(PGI November 2017)*
    a. Surgical blade direction should be downward and away from surgeon
    b. During bowel anastomosis, hemostatic forceps are used to grasp intestine
    c. Needle holding forceps damage sutures as it is crushing in nature
    d. Toothed forceps is used to grasp skin, subcutaneous tissue, muscles and sheath
    e. Handle of surgical blade is held with thumb and index finger

MESH

47. Which of the following statement is incorrect about mesh? *(Recent Question 2017)*
    a. Mesh can shrink upto 50%
    b. Weight of light-weight mesh is < 40 gm/m^2
    c. Weight of heavy-weight mesh is > 80 gm/m^2
    d. Flat sheet meshes does not require fixation

48. What is the weight of low-weight mesh? *(Recent Question 2017)*
    a. <40 gm/m^2
    b. <60 gm/m^2
    c. <80 gm/m^2
    d. <90 gm/m^2

KNOTS

49. What is the name of this knot?
    a. Reef knot
    b. Figure of 8 bend
    c. Prusik knot
    d. Overhand knot

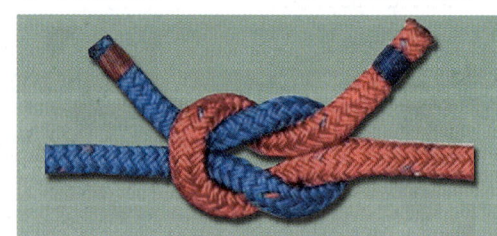

50. What is the name of this knot? *(Recent Question 2019)*

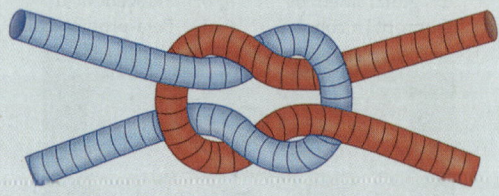

    a. Reef knot
    b. Granny knot
    c. Surgeon's knot
    d. Half-in-half knot

51. What is the name of this knot?
    a. Reef knot
    b. Figure of 8 bend
    c. Prusik knot
    d. Overhand knot

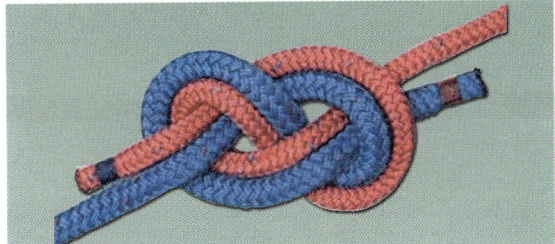

52. What is the name of this knot?
    a. Reef knot
    b. Figure of 8 bend
    c. Prusik knot
    d. Overhand knot

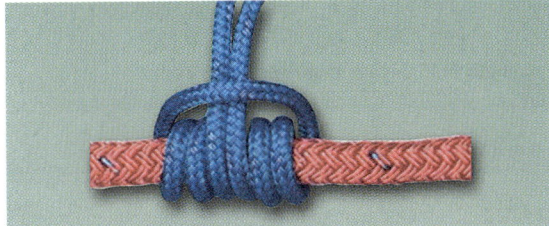

53. What is the name of this knot?
    a. Reef knot
    b. Figure of 8 bend
    c. Prusik knot
    d. Overhand knot

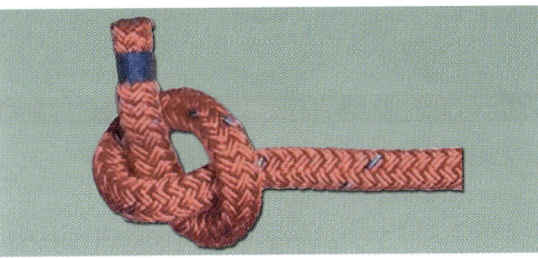

54. What is the name of given knot? *(Recent Question 2016)*
    a. Reef knot
    b. Granny knot
    c. Surgeons knot
    d. Square knot

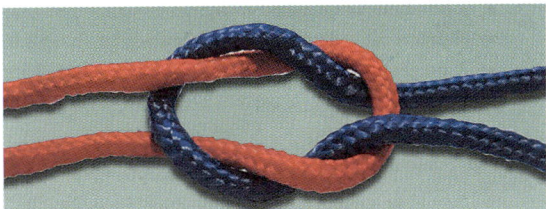

Explanations

SUTURES

1. **Ans. a. Polypropylene** *(Ref. Bailey 27/e p90)*
2. **Ans. a. Catgut, d. Polyglycolic acid, e. Vicryl**
3. **Ans. b. Undergoes hydrolysis and complete absorption**
4. **Ans. b. Sheep** *(Ref. Bailey 27/e p93)*

> **SUTURES**
>
> - **John Hunter** discovered **catgut**^{Q}.
> - **Plain catgut** is derived from **submucosa of sheep's intestine**^{Q}.
> - **Plain catgut** loses **50% tensile strength in 3 days**^{Q} and all tensile strength in 15 days & absorbed in 60 days^Q.
> - **Isopropyl alcohol**^{Q} is used as **preservative for packing catgut sutures**.
>
>> - **Vicryl** (Co-polymer of **glycolide** & **lactide**) maintains **tensile strength for 28-30 days**^{Q} & gets **absorbed in 80-90 days (Delayed absorption)**^{Q}
>> - **Vicryl** is used for **bile duct surgeries**^{Q}.
>
> - **PDS** sutures exhibit the **lowest affinity** to the adherence of E. coli & Staphylococcus aureus; **Dexon sutures** exhibit the **highest affinity** to these species.
> - **Polydioxanone (PDS)** undergoes **hydrolysis** & **complete absorption within 180 days**.
> - Raw material used in nylon suture: Polyamide polymer
> - MC used for subcuticular suturing: **Monocryl (Polyglycaprone)**^{Q}
> - Work-Horse suture for general surgeries: **Vicryl**^{Q}

5. **Ans. b. Co-polymer of glycolide and lactide**
6. **Ans. d. 225 days**
7. **Ans. b. Undergoes hydrolysis and complete absorption** *(Ref. Bailey 27/e p92)*
8. **Ans. c. John Hunter**
9. **Ans. b. Vicryl**
10. **Ans. d. Polyester**
11. **Ans. a. Isopropyl alcohol**
12. **Ans. c. 7 days** *(Ref. Sabiston 18/e p2134)*
13. **Ans. d. Vicryl**
14. **Ans. b. Isopropyl alcohol**
15. **Ans. b. Polyamide polymer**
16. **Ans. b. Polypropylene**
17. **Ans. b. 4x incision length**
18. **Ans. d. Ethilon**
19. **Ans. b. Non-absorbable, non-elastic** *(Ref: Bailey 27/e p99)*

> "Vascular anastomosis: Non-absorbable monofilament suture material should be used, e.g. polypropylene." -Bailey 27/e p99

> "Vascular anastomoses require an extremely accurate closure as they must be immediately watertight at the end of the operation when the vascular clamps are removed. In many cases, some form of prosthetic material or graft may be used which will never be integrated into the body tissues and so the integrity of the suture line needs to be permanent. For this reason, polypropylene is one of the best sutures as it is not biodegradable. It is used in its monofilament form, mounted on an atraumatic, curved, round-bodied needle. Knot security is important, and as polypropylene is monofilament and the anastomosis often depends on one final knot, several throws (between six and eight) of a well-laid reef knot are required. The suture line must be regular and watertight with a smooth intimal surface to minimise the risk of thrombosis and embolus, as well as to avoid any leakage." -Bailey 27/e p99

20. **Ans. c. Silk**
21. **Ans. a. Polydioxanone**
22. **Ans. c. It is completely absorbed in 9 months**

23. **Ans. a. Purse string suture** *(Ref: Jaypee Manual of Surgical Equipments/p 178)*

> **Purse string suture:** A Surgical suture **passed as a running stitch in and out along the edge of a circular wound** in such a way that when the ends of the suture are drawn tight the wound is closed like a purse.

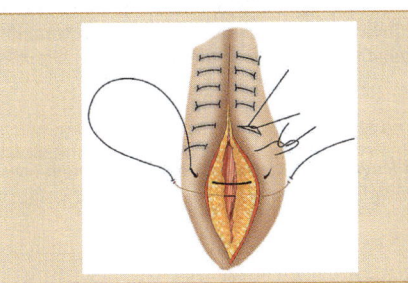

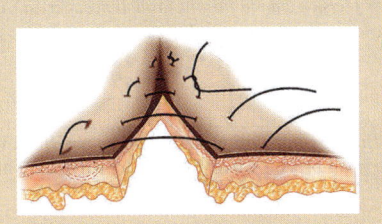

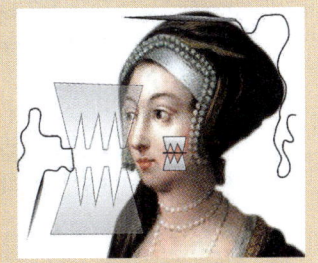

| **Halsted's suture pattern:** An interrupted suture pattern most useful in the suturing of friable tissues. The needle is passed in and out of the skin on one side of the incision, then across the incision and the suture is repeated on the other side. A pass is made at right angles to the suture and then a repeat of the stitch made back across the incision and the two ends tied. | **Mattress interrupted sutures:** A suture made with a **double stitch** that forms a loop about the tissue on both sides of a wound and produces eversion of the edges. | **Pare suture:** The **approximation of the edges of a wound by pasting strips of cloth to the surface and stitching them instead of the skin.** |

24. **Ans. c. Natural non-absorbable** *(Ref: Bailey 27/e p90)*
    Silk suture is natural non-absorbable suture.

25. **Ans. b. Increased risk of bacterial infection** *(Ref: Bailey 27/e p90)*
    Given suture is Polypropylene (Prolene), a monofilament suture, associated with decreased risk of infection.

26. **Ans. d. Glycolide and lactide** *(Ref: Bailey 27/e p93)*

Vicryl
• **Vicryl** (Co-polymer of **glycolide** and **lactide**) maintains **tensile strength for 28-30 days**[Q] and gets **absorbed in 80-90 days (Delayed absorption)**[Q]
• **Vicryl** is used for **bile duct surgeries**[Q].

27. **Ans. c. Isopropyl alcohol** *(Ref: Bailey 27/e p93)*

Catgut
• **John Hunter** discovered **catgut**[Q].
• **Plain catgut** is derived from **submucosa of sheep's intestine**[Q].
• **Plain catgut** loses **50% tensile strength in 3 days**[Q] and **all tensile strength in 15 days** and **absorbed in 60 days**[Q].
• **Isopropyl alcohol**[Q] is used as **preservative for packing catgut sutures.**

28. **Ans. a. Monocryl** *(Ref: Essentials of Breast Surgery by Michael S. Sabel Pg 174)*
    Monocryl sutures 3-0 or 4-0 are used in closure of MRM wounds by subcuticular suturing.

29. **Ans. c. It is absorbed by phagocytosis and enzymatic dehydration** *(Ref: Bailey 27/e p93)*

> • *The given suture is catgut (absorbable suture), which is prepared from sheep gut and absorbed by phagocytosis and enzymatic dehydration.*

30. **Ans. b. Synthetic sutures** *(Ref: Sabiston 20/e p; Schwartz 10/e p; Bailey 27/e p)*

31. **Ans. a. Enzymatic degradation**

ANASTOMOSES

32. **Ans. a. Cheatle's maneuver** *(Ref: Bailey 27/e p98)*
    The **Cheatle split** (making a **cut into** the **anti-mesenteric border**) may help to **enlarge** the **lumen of distal, collapsed bowel**[Q].

33. **Ans. b. Sero-muscular sutures**

34. **Ans. c. After 7 days**

35. **Ans. d. All of the above** *(Ref: Bailey 27/e p99)*

36. Ans. a. 1-2 mm
37. Ans. b. 3:1 *(Ref: Bailey 27/e p85)*

> "Occasionally, it may be necessary to excise a skin lesion with a circular incision in an area when the direction of Langer's lines are not apparent. However, once the circular incision has been made, it can often be observed that the circular incision is converted to an ellipse thus indicating the lines of tension. This circular incision should then be formally converted into an elliptical incision, remembering the **rule of thumb that 'an elliptical incision must be at least three times as long as it is wide'** for the wound to heal without tension." -Bailey 27/e p85

38. Ans. a. 4:1 *(Ref: Bailey 27/e p1041)*

> "It has also been confirmed that the optimal ratio of suture length to wound length is **4:1 (Jenkins' rule).** If less length than this is used, the suture bites are too far apart or too tight and the converse applies if more length than this is used." -Bailey 27/e p1041

39. Ans. c. Norman Matheson
40. Ans. a. Muir *(Ref: www.ncbi.nlm.nih.gov › ... › Ann R Coll Surg Engl › v.75(3); May 1993)*

- **On table colonic lavage** was used for first time in 1968 by **Muir**^Q.

41. Ans. a. Vascular anastomosis
42. Ans. b. Sub mucosa
43. Ans. b. Circular cutting stapler *(Ref: Schwartz 10/e p1224)*

Procedure for prolapse and hemorrhoidectomy —also known as or MIPH — also known as or stapled hemorrhoidectomy

MIPH

- Minimally invasive proctoscopic hemorrhoidectomy (MIPH)
  - In this procudure, a circular cutting stapler (PPH3) is used to excise a short
  - Circumferential segment of rectal mucosa proximal to dentate line, thus ligating venules feeding the hemorrhoides.

44. Ans. a. Cyanoacrylate *(Ref: Bailey 27/e p96)*
45. Ans. d. Single layer taking submucosa *(Ref: Bailey 27/e p98)*

> "Intestinal anastomoses: Interrupted and continuous single-layer suture techniques are adequate and safe." -Bailey 27/e p98

> "However, Halsted favoured a one-layer extramucosal closure, and this was subsequently advocated by Matheson as it was felt to cause the least tissue necrosis or luminal narrowing. This technique has now become widely accepted, although it is essential that this is not confused with a seromuscular suture technique. The extramucosal suture must include the submucosa as this has a high collagen content and is the most stable suture layer in all sections of the gastrointestinal tract." -Bailey 27/e p98

46. Ans. b. During bowel anastomosis, hemostatic forceps are used to grasp intestine
47. Ans. d. Flat sheet meshes does not require fixation *(Ref: Bailey 27/e p1027)*
48. Ans. a. <40 gm/m² *(Ref: Bailey 27/e p1028)*

> "The terms 'light, medium and heavy' are not precisely defined but meshes less than 40 g/m² are generally referred to as light and meshes more than 80 g/m² are heavy." -Bailey 27/e p1028

KNOTS

49. Ans. a. Reef knot
50. Ans. b. Granny knot
51. Ans. b. Figure of 8 bend
52. Ans. c. Prusik knot
53. Ans. d. Overhand knot
54. Ans. b. Granny knot

Granny knot
• **Granny knot** is a binding **knot**, used to secure a rope or line around an object. • It is considered **inferior to the reef knot (square knot)**, which it superficially resembles.

CHAPTER 47

Sterilization and Infection

TECHNIQUES OF STERILIZATION

Techniques of Sterilization	
Steam (121°C for 15 minutes)	• Surgical instruments[Q]
Ethylene oxide	• Heart lung machine[Q], respirators, dental labs
Hot air oven	• Glass syringe[Q], test tubes, flasks[Q], cutting instruments
Irradiation (gamma rays)	• Industrial packaging[Q]
Paracetic acid (STERIS)	• Flexible endoscopes[Q]
Isopropyl alcohol	• Clinical thermometer[Q]
Beta propiolactone >Formaldehyde	• Fumigation of OT, labs, wards[Q]
2% Glutaraldehyde	• Endoscope (cystoscope, bronchoscope)[Q]
Autoclaving	• Culture media, suture materials except catgut[Q]

HOSPITAL ACQUIRED INFECTION

Hospital Acquired Infection (HAI)

- Infection that **follows surgery** or **admission to hospital**
- Common HAI are:

1.	**Respiratory infections**[Q] (including ventilator-associated pneumonia)	10–15%
2.	**UTI**[Q] (mostly related to urinary catheters)	30–40% (MC)[Q]
3.	Bacteremia (mostly related to indwelling vascular catheters)	10–15%
4.	**Surgical site infections**[Q]	15–20% (2nd MC)[Q]
5.	**Antibiotic associated diarrhea**, caused by Clostridium difficile[Q]	5–10%

PREVENTIVE MEASURES FOR HOSPITAL ACQUIRED INFECTION

Preventive Measure for Hospital Acquired Infection

- **Isolation:** Infective patients must be isolated in **room with adequate ventilation** and **negative pressure**[Q]
- **Hospital staff:** Those who are suffering from skin disease, sore throat, common cold, ear infection diarrhea or dysentery and other infections ailments should be **kept away from work until complete cured**[Q].
  - **Handwashing**[Q]: The **most common route of infection is via the hands**[Q]. Hands washing with soap and water may not be sufficient; a **suitable disinfectant must be employed** for handwashing[Q].
- **Dust control:** Hospital dust contains numerous bacteria and virus. Suppression of dust by **wet dusting** and **vacuum (negative pressure) cleaning**[Q] are important control measure.
- **Disinfection:** The article used by the patient as well as patient's urine, feces, sputum should properly disinfect. **Proper sterilization**[Q] of instrument should be enforced.
- **Control of droplet infection:** Use of **face masks**[Q], proper bad spacing, prevention of overcrowding and ensuring adequate lighting and ventilation are important control measure.
- **Nursing technique:** Barrier nursing and task nursing have also been recommended to minimize cross infection.
- **Administrative measures:** There should be a **hospital control infection committee**[Q] to form late policies regarding control of hospital acquired infection.

AREA OF CLEANING & DRAPING IN SURGERIES

Area of Cleaning & Draping in Surgeries	
Cranial surgery	• Depends upon surgeon
Thyroid or neck surgery	• **Chin to nipple** with shoulder & axilla[Q]
Eye surgery	• **Cut eyelashes** of affected eye
Nasal surgery	• No shaving unless with mustache
Ear surgery	• **Two & half inches around ear**[Q]
Chest surgery	• **Base of neck to waist**, axilla & inner arm[Q]
Abdominal & pelvic surgery	• **Nipple to symphysis pubis**, vulva, perineum & thigh[Q]
Kidney-anterior	• **Nipple to perineum**, side to side; supra scapular region to buttocks
Vaginal, scrotal, rectal surgery	• **Waist to perineum** plus **anterior & inner aspect of thigh**[Q] and 6 inches from groin; posterior-entire buttocks & anus
Lower extremities	• **Digits 2 inches above knee**, entire extremity and groin[Q]
Upper extremities	• **Distal arm 2 inches above elbow**, elbow up to axilla[Q]

PROPHYLACTIC ANTIBIOTICS

Prophylactic Antibiotics

- **Antibiotics** should be used **when local wound defenses** are **not established** (the decisive period).
- Ideally, **maximal blood** and **tissue levels** should be **present at the time** at which the **first incision** is made and before contamination occurs.
  - **IV** administration at **induction**[Q] **of anesthesia** is optimal.
  - If induction is not mentioned in the option go for **30 minutes** to **1 hour before surgery**[Q].
- In **long operations**, those involving the **insertion of a prosthesis**, when there is **excessive blood loss** or when **unexpected contamination** occurs, antibiotics may be **repeated 8 and 16 hours later**[Q].
- The use of the newer, **broad-spectrum antibiotics for prophylaxis should be avoided**[Q].
- **Benzylpenicillin**[Q] should be used if **Clostridium** gas gangrene infection is a possibility
- Patients with **heart valve** disease or a **prosthesis** should be **protected** from bacteremia caused by **dental work, urethral instrumentation or visceral surgery**[Q]

Prophylactic systemic antibiotics reduce infection and are clinically beneficial in the following circumstances

- **High-risk gastroduodenal procedures:** Operations for **gastric cancer, ulcer**[Q]**, obstruction**, or **bleeding**
- **High-risk biliary procedures:** Operations in patients **>60 years, CBD stones**, or **jaundice**, previous **biliary tract operations** or endoscopic biliary manipulation
- **Resection** and **anastomosis** of the **colon**[Q] or small intestine
- **Cardiac procedures** through a median sternotomy
- **Vascular surgery** of the **lower extremities** or **abdominal aorta**[Q]
- Operations entering the **oropharyngeal cavity**[Q]
- Implantation of any **permanent prosthetic material**[Q]
- **Amputation** of an extremity with **impaired blood supply**[Q], particularly in the presence of a current or recent ischemic ulcer
- **Craniotomy**
- Any wound with known **gross bacterial contamination**[Q]
- **Accidental wounds** with **heavy contamination** and tissue damage[Q].
- Injuries prone to **clostridial infection** because of **extensive devitalization** of muscle, **heavy contamination,** or **impairment of the blood supply**[Q]

HOW TO AVOID SURGICAL SITE INFECTION?

Avoiding Surgical Site Infections

- **Staff** should **always wash their hands** between patients[Q]
- **Length of patient stay** should be **kept to a minimum**[Q]
- **Preoperative shaving** should be **avoided** if possible[Q]
- **Antiseptic skin preparation** should be standardized[Q]
- Attention to theatre technique and discipline[Q]
- **Avoid hypothermia** perioperatively and ensure **supplemental oxygenation** in recovery[Q]

SURGICAL SITE INFECTION

Surgical Site Infections

- A **major SSI** is defined as a **wound** that either **discharges significant quantities of pus spontaneously** or **needs a secondary procedure to drain it**. The patient may have **systemic signs** such as **tachycardia, pyrexia** and a **raised WBC count** [systemic inflammatory response syndrome (SIRS)]
- Minor wound infections may discharge pus or infected serous fluid but should not be associated with excessive discomfort, systemic signs or delay in return home
- The differentiation between major and minor and the definition of SSI is important in audit or trials of antibiotic prophylaxis.
- There are scoring systems for the severity of wound infection, which are particularly useful in surveillance and research.
- Examples are the **Southampton** and **ASEPSIS systems**[Q].

Southampton Wound Grading System	
Grade/Appearance	Subtype/Appearance
0: Normal healing[Q]	
I: Normal healing with mild bruising or erythema[Q]	• Ia: Some bruising • Ib: Considerable bruising • Ic: Mild erythema
II: Erythema plus other signs of inflammation[Q]	• IIa: At one point • IIb: Around sutures • IIc: Along wound • IId: Around wound
III: Clear or hemoserous discharge[Q]	• IIIa: At one point only (<2 cm) • IIIb: Along wound (>2 cm) • IIIc: Large volume • IIId: Prolonged (>3 days)
IV: Pus[Q]	• IVa: At one point only (<2 cm) • IVb: Along wound (>2 cm)

WOUND DEHISCENCE

Wound Dehiscence (Burst Abdomen)

- **Serous** or **serosanguinous discharge** from the wound is the **first sign**[Q] of dehiscence

  - **Most commonly** observed between 5th and 8th postoperative day[Q] (may occur at any time following wound closure)

- Wound dehiscence is **partial** or **total disruption** of any or all layers of the operative wound.
- **Extrusion** of **abdominal viscera** after rupture of all layers is known as **evisceration**[Q].

Management
- **Wound dehiscence** without evisceration: **Prompt elective closure**[Q] of the wound
- **Wound dehiscence with evisceration:**
  - Wound is **covered with moist towels**
  - Under GA, **any exposed bowel** or **omentum** is rinsed with RL containing **antibiotics** and then **returned to abdomen**
  - Previous sutures are removed, wound is reclosed (**Tension suturing**[Q])

Predisposing Factors for Wound Dehiscence

Local Risk Factors
- **Inadequate closure (Most important)**[Q]
  - Use of **absorbable sutures**
  - **Multilayer closure** (single layer has lower incidence)
- **Midline** and **vertical incisions** are **more prone** than transverse incisions
- **Increased** intra-abdominal **pressure**
- **Deficient wound healing** due to:
  - **Infections**[Q], **Seroma**[Q], **Hematoma**[Q]
  - **Presence of drain**[Q]

Systemic Risk Factors
- **Old age**[Q]
- **Obesity**[Q]
- **Immunosuppression**[Q]
- **Systemic diseases:**
  - Diabetes[Q]
  - Uremia[Q]
  - Jaundice, Sepsis[Q]
  - Cancer[Q]

SEPSIS, SEPTIC SHOCK & MODS

Condition	Definition	Criteria in 2016
Sepsis	• A life threatening **organ dysfunction** caused by a **dysregulated host response to infection**^{Q}	• **Suspected** (or documented) **infection** and an **acute increase in ≥2** sepsis related organ failure assessment **(SOFA) points**^{Q}
Septic Shock	• A subset of sepsis in which **underlying circulatory and cellular/metabolic abnormalities** lead to substantially **increased mortality risk**^{Q}	• **Suspected** (or documented) **infection plus vasopressor therapy** needed to maintain **mean arterial pressure at ≥ 65 mm Hg**^{Q} & **serum lactate > 2.0 mmol/L despite adequate fluid resuscitation**^{Q}

SOFA score is a **24-point measure of organ dysfunction** that uses **six organ systems**^{Q} (renal, cardiovascular, pulmonary, hepatic, neurologic, hematologic^Q), where **0–4 points** are assigned **per organ system.**

MULTIORGAN DYSFUNCTION SYNDROME (MODS)

- **Definition:** Simultaneous **presence of physiologic dysfunction** and/or **failure of two or more organs**^{Q}.
- Occurs in the setting of **severe sepsis**^{Q}, **shock** of any kind^Q, **severe inflammatory conditions** such as **pancreatitis**^{Q} & **trauma**^{Q}.
- Organ failure must persist **beyond 24 hours**^{Q}; mortality risk increases with accrual of failing organs^Q; prognosis worsens with increased duration of organ failure^Q.

CELLULITIS

CELLULITIS

- It is **non-suppurative inflammation, spreading along** the **subcutaneous tissues** and **connective tissue planes** and across intercellular spaces^Q.
- The term is a misnomer, as the **lesion** is one of the **connective** and **interstitial tissue** and not of the cells.

• MC causative organism: Streptococcus pyogenes^Q

Pathology
- The **organism** usually gains **access through a wound** or **scratch or** following **surgical incision**^{Q}.
- There is **wide speared swelling** and **redness** at the area of inflammation, but without definite localization **blebs** and **bullae** form on the skin. **Central necrosis** may occur **at later stage**^{Q}.

Clinical Features
- There is varying degree of **fever** and **toxemia. Affected part** is very much **swollen** and **painful**^{Q}.
- **Diabetic individual** often suffer from cellulitis^Q
- **Examination:** Affected part is warm, swollen and tender, there is **pitting edema** and **brawny induration.** Surrounding lymph vessels may be seen as **red streaks** due to **lymphangitis**^{Q}.

Treatment
- **Rest** and **elevation** of the part to reduce edema; Appropriate **antibiotic** preferably broad spectrum^Q
- **Penicillin** is **still sensitive against streptococci**^{Q}

• **Failure** of inflammatory swelling **to subside after 48 to 72 hours** suggests that an **abscess** has developed. In that case **incision** and **drainage** of the pus should be accomplished^Q.

ERYSIPELAS

ERYSIPELAS

- This is a **sharply demarcated streptococcal infection** of the **superficial lymphatic vessels,** usually associated with **broken skin on the face**^{Q}.

Clinical Features
- Affected area is **erythematous** and **edematous.** Patient may be **febrile** and have a **leucocytosis**^{Q}.

Treatment
- Prompt administration of **broad-spectrum antibiotics after** swabbing the area for **culture and sensitivity** is usually all that is necessary.

CARBUNCLE

CARBUNCLE

- A **carbuncle** is an abscess larger than a boil, usually with one or more openings draining pus onto the skin.
- **Most commonly** caused by **Staphylococcus aureus**^{Q}; MC location: **Nape of the neck**^{Q}.

Etiology
- **Triggers for carbuncle**: **Folliculitis**, **friction** from clothing or shaving, having the **hair pulled out**, generally **poor hygiene, poor nutrition** or **weakening of immunity**^{Q}.
- Persons with **diabetes**^{Q} and **immune system diseases** are **more likely** to develop carbuncles.

Clinical Features
- **Carbuncle**: Made up of several skin boils, infected mass is filled with fluid, pus and dead tissues.
- It may be **red** and **irritated, grow very fast** and have a **white** or **yellow center**^{Q}.

Treatment
- **Proper excision by cruciate incision**^{Q} will usually treat the condition effectively
- **Surgical incision** and **drainage** of **all suppurative collections** with **antibiotics**^{Q}.

NECROTIZING FASCIITIS

NECROTIZING FASCIITIS

- Necrotizing fasciitis is a **rapidly progressive bacterial infection** characterized by involvement and **necrosis of** the **subcutaneous tissue** and **fascia**, with typical **sparing of** the **underlying muscle**^{Q}.
- MC site of infection: **Lower extremities**^{Q}
- May involve trunk, **perineum** (**Fournier's gangrene**) or head and neck and any other site.

Etiological Agents
- MC single etiological agents: **Group A beta hemolytic streptococci**^{Q}

  - More commonly, **necrotizing fasciitis** results from a **polymicrobial synergistic infection**^{Q}

- Microorganism responsible: **Group A beta hemolytic streptococci** + Staphylococcus, E. coli, Pseudomonas, Proteus, Bacteroides/ Clostridium (**Anaerobes**)

Risk Factors for Necrotizing Fasciitis		
• **Diabetes**^{Q} • Pressure sores • **Immunocompromised states**^{Q}	• **Smoking**^{Q} • **Penetrating trauma**^{Q} • **Obesity**^{Q} • **IV drug abuse**^{Q}	• Peripheral vascular disease^Q • **Skin infection / damage**^{Q} (abrasions, bites, boils)

Clinical Presentation
- Pain is the **most important presenting symptom**
- Pain is **disproportionately greater**^{Q} than that expected from degree of cellulites present

  - Without treatment **pain may decrease due to thrombosis of small blood vessels** and **destruction of peripheral nerves** (an **ominous sign**^{Q})

- **Skin Features**: Edema, **erythema**^{Q} (Infected area is red, hot, shiny, swollen and exquisitely tender)
- **Woody hard texture** to subcutaneous tissue
- Inability to distinguish fascial planes and muscle groups on palpation
- **Skin vesicles/cutaneous bullae, soft tissue crepitus** due to **gas production**^{Q} may be seen when necrotizing fasciitis is caused due to mixed flora but not due to group A streptococcus
- **Systemic features**: Fever, **hypotension**, tachycardia, progression to **septic shock, DIC** or **multiple organ failure**^{Q}

Management
- This is a **surgical emergency** and **surgical debridement is mandatory**^{Q}

  - Treatment: Urgent surgical debridement + IV fluids + Broad spectrum IV antibiotics + Supportive treatment^Q

- **Mortality rate** is nearly 100% without surgical debridement^Q
- **Hyperbaric oxygen** helps in **wound healing**^{Q}

GAS GANGRENE

Gas Gangrene

- Caused by **C. perfringens (Gram-positive, anaerobic, spore-bearing** bacilli are widely found in **soil** and **feces)**^{Q}.
- This is relevant to **military, traumatic surgery** and **colorectal operations**^{Q}.

Risk Factors
- **Immunocompromised, diabetics** or patients with **malignant disease**^{Q}
- Wounds containing **necrotic** or **foreign material**, resulting **in anaerobic conditions**^{Q}

Clinical Features
- **Severe local wound pain** and **crepitus (gas in the tissues**, which may also be **noted on plain radiographs)**^{Q}.
- The **wound produces** a **thin, brown, sweet smelling exudate**^{Q}, in which Gram staining will reveal bacteria.

> - **Gas** and **smell** are **characteristic**^{Q} (Myonecrosis)
> - If septicemia occurs, **gas** may be **produced** in the other organ, notably the **liver** known as **'foaming liver'**^{Q}.

- **Edema** and **spreading gangrene** follow the release of **collagenase, hyaluronidase**, other proteases and **alpha toxin**^{Q}.
- **Early systemic complications** with **circulatory collapse** and **multi-organ failure**^{Q} follow if prompt action is not taken

Treatment
- **Antibiotic prophylaxis** in patients at risk, especially when **amputations** are performed **for peripheral vascular disease with open necrotic ulceration**^{Q}.

> - Once a **gas gangrene infection is established, large doses of IV penicillin** and **aggressive debridement** of affected tissues are required^Q.
> - The use of **hyperbaric oxygen** is controversial.

- **Closure of traumatic wounds** or **compound fractures** should be **delayed for 5–6 days**^{Q} until it is certain that these sites are free of infection.

> - **Passive anti-gas gangrene serum** given **IM** or **in emergencies IV**^{Q} used to be common practice in prophylaxis.

TETANUS

Tetanus

- Caused by **Clostridium tetani (anaerobic, terminal spore-bearing, Gram-positive** bacterium)^Q following implantation into tissues or a wound
- **Spores** are widespread in **soil** and **manure**, and so the infection is **more common in traumatic civilian** or **military wounds**.

Clinical Features
- Signs and symptoms of tetanus are mediated by the release of the **exotoxin tetanospasmin**, which **affects myoneural junctions** and the **motor neurons** of the **anterior horn** of the spinal cord.
- **MC initial symptoms: Trismus (lockjaw)**^{Q}, **muscle pain** and **stiffness**, back pain, and difficulty swallowing.

> - A **short prodromal period**, which has a **poor prognosis**, leads to **spasms** in the distribution of the **short motor nerves of** the **face** followed by the **development of severe generalised motor spasms** including **opsithotonus, respiratory arrest** and **death**^{Q}.
> - A **longer prodromal period** of 4–5 weeks is **associated with** a **milder form of** the **disease**^{Q}.

- The **entry wound** may show a **localized small area of cellulitis**; exudate or aspiration may give a sample that can be stained to show the presence of Gram-positive rods.

> - **Risus sardonicus (sardonic grin**^{Q}): Highly characteristic, abnormal, **sustained spasm of** the **facial muscles** that appears to **produce grinning**

Treatment
- **Prophylaxis with tetanus toxoid** is the **best preventative treatment**^{Q}.
- **Established infection: Minor debridement** of the wound with antibiotic **benzylpenicillin**^{Q}
- **Relaxants** may also be required, and the patient may require **ventilation in severe forms**, which may be associated with a high mortality.
- **Anti-toxin using human immunoglobulin** for both **at-risk wounds** and **established infection**^{Q}.

TUBERCULOUS LYMPHADENITIS

TUBERCULOUS LYMPHADENITIS

- Most commonly affects **children** or **young adults**^{Q}, but can occur at any age.
- **Deep upper cervical nodes** are **most commonly affected**^{Q}, but there may be a widespread cervical lymphadenitis with many matting together.
- In most cases, the tubercular bacilli gain entrance through the tonsil of the corresponding side as the lymphadenopathy.
- Both **bovine**^{Q} and **human tuberculosis** may be responsible.

Pathology
- In approximately **80% of patients**, the tuberculous process is limited to the clinically affected group of lymph nodes^Q, but a primary focus in the lungs must always be suspected.
- If **treatment** is **not instituted**, the **caseated node** may **liquefy** and **break down** with the formation of a **cold abscess**^{Q} in the neck.

  - **Collar-stud abscess**^{Q}: Pus is initially confined by the **deep cervical fascia**, but after weeks or months, this may **become eroded at one point, pus flows through the small opening** into the **space beneath the superficial fascia** known as **'collar-stud' abscess**.

Treatment
- Treatment: ATT
- If an **abscess fails to resolve despite ATT**: Excision of the abscess and its surrounding **fibrous capsule** with the **relevant lymph nodes**^{Q}.

SYPHILIS

Congenital Syphilis

Early Congenital Syphilis
- **Snuffles (rhinitis)**^{Q} is **earliest feature**.
- Lesions are **vesicobullous**^{Q}
- **Snail track ulcers** on mucosa

Late Congenital Syphilis
- Characterized by **Hutchinson's triad (interstitial keratitis + 8th nerve deafness + Hutchinson's teeth i.e. pegged central upper incisors)**^{Q}
- **Saddle nose, sabre tibia, mulberry molars**^{Q}
- Bull dog's jaw (protrusion of jaw)
- **Rhagades**^{Q} (linear fissure at mouth, nares)
- Frontal bossing, hot cross bun deformity of skull
- **Clutton's joint**^{Q} (painless swelling of joints, most commonly both knee)
- **Palatal perforation**^{Q}
- **Higaumenakis sign** (periostitis leads to unilateral enlargement of sterna end of clavicle)

Clinical Presentation of Syphilis

Primary Syphilis
- **Painless, indurated, non-bleeding**, usually single **punched out ulcer (hard chancre)**^{Q}
- **Painless, rubbery shotty lymphadenopathy**^{Q}

Secondary Syphilis
- **Bilateral symmetrical asymptomatic** localized or **diffuse mucocutaneous lesion**^{Q} (macule, papule, paulosquamous and rarely pustule)
- **Non-tender generalized lymphadenopathy**^{Q}
- **Highly infectious condylomata lata**^{Q}, in warm moist intertriginous areas
- **Moth eaten alopecia, arthritis, proteinuria**^{Q}

Tertiary Syphilis
- **Gumma, neurosyphilis / tabes dorsalis**^{Q}
- Ostitis, periostitis
- **Aortitis, aortic insufficiency, coronary stenosis and nocturnal angina**^{Q}

ACTINOMYCOSIS

ACTINOMYCOSIS

- Actinomycosis is a **granulomatous suppurative bacterial disease** caused by **Actinomyces**^{Q}.
- Usually **results following tooth extraction, odontogenic infection, or facial trauma**^{Q}.

Clinical Features
- Oral-cervicofacial disease is the MC form^Q, characterized by a painless "lumpy jaw."
- Pelvic actinomycosis is a rare but **proven complication of use of intrauterine devices**^{Q}.

Diagnosis
- Accurate diagnosis depends on **careful histologic analysis.**
- Presence of **sulfur granules within purulent specimen** is **pathognomonic**[Q].

Treatment
- **Penicillin** and **sulfonamides**[Q] are typically effective against these infections.

HAND INFECTIONS

Hand Infection

- **Infections of hand** are most commonly caused by **staphylococcus aureus in 80% of cases**[Q].

Management
- **Elevation, splinting** and **antibiotics** if no pus; **Surgical drainage** if **pus is present**[Q]
- **Tendon sheath pus** needs **irrigation**[Q]
- **Bites** should be **explored**, cleaned and managed with **broad-spectrum antibiotics**[Q]
- All infections need **early mobilization** once inflammation settles[Q]

Infection from	Can spread to
Thumb	• Thenar space[Q]
Index finger	• Thenar space[Q]
Middle finger	• Mid-palmar space[Q]
Ring-finger	• Mid-palmar space[Q]
Little finger	• Ulnar bursa and forearm space of parona[Q]

CHRONIC BURROWING ULCER

Chronic Burrowing Ulcer (Meleney Gangrene)

- Caused by **synergistic infection** of **Microaerophilic non-hemolytic Streptococci** and aerobic hemolytic staphylococci.
- Also known as **burrowing phagedenic ulcer, Meleney's ulcer, progressive synergistic gangrene**
- Associated with the **formation of burrowing cutaneous fissures** and **sinus tracts** that open at distant sites. (**Meleney's burrowing ulcers**)

HILTON'S METHOD OF ABSCESS DRAINAGE

Hilton's Method of Abscess Drainage

- **During drainage** of abscess situated in important areas like **axilla** or **groin**[Q], there is chance **of injury to underlying major vessels and nerves**[Q] if adequate care is not taken.
- In **drainage of abscess** in such locations, the **skin** and **subcutaneous tissue** are **incised with a knife.**
- **Deep fascia is not incised** by sharp knife but **pierced by thrusting a sinus forceps** through the deep fascia and the **sinus forceps** is then **opened up to enlarge the opening in the deep fascia** for **easy drainage of pus**[Q].

> • **Hilton's method protects** underlying important **vessels** and **nerves**[Q].

Multiple Choice Questions

STERILIZATION AND DISINFECTION

1. **Ways to prevent a highly infectious disease transmitted by aerosol; precautions used:** *(PGI Dec 2007)*
   a. Isolation ward
   b. Facemask
   c. Keep isolated in a room with positive pressure
   d. Keep isolated in a room with negative pressure
   e. Cohort nursing

2. **Use of all the following significantly decreases airborne infection in operating room except:** *(UPSC 2000)*
   a. Laminar air flow   b. Air-conditioning
   c. Ultraviolet light   d. Microfilters

3. **A chest physician performs bronchoscopy in the procedure room of the out patient department. To make the instrument safe for use in the next patient waiting outside, the most appropriate method to disinfect the endoscope is by:**
   a. 70% alcohol for 5 min   *(All India 2003)*
   b. 2% glutaraldehyde for 20 min
   c. 2% formaldehyde for 10 min
   d. 1% sodium hypochlorite for 15 min

4. **All the following are sporicidal agents except:** *(JIPMER 2010)*
   a. Ethylene oxide   b. Phenol
   c. Ozone   d. Glutaraldehyde

5. **Flexible endoscopes are best sterilized with:** *(MHSSMCET 2008, MHPGMCET 2007)*
   a. Formaldehyde   b. Ethylene oxide
   c. Gamma irradiation   d. Peracetic acid

6. **Best disinfectant for endoscope is:** *(JIPMER 2014, 2012)*
   a. Hypochlorite   b. Formaldehyde
   c. Glutaraldehyde   d. Chlorohexidine

7. **Blood spills in OT is cleaned with:**
   a. Phenol   *(AIIMS November 2017, Recent Question 2017)*
   b. Alcohol
   c. Quarternary ammonium compound
   d. Chloride compounds

PREVENTION OF INFECTION AND PROPHYLAXIS

8. **What is the best time to give prophylactic antibiotic?**
   a. 1 day before surgery   *(DPG 2007)*
   b. At the time of skin incision
   c. At the time of induction
   d. 2 days before to 3 days after surgery

9. **Regarding antibiotics true statement:** *(PGI June 2006)*
   a. No prophylaxis for clean contaminated surgery
   b. No prophylaxis for gastric ulcer surgery
   c. Prophylaxis for colorectal surgery
   d. Local irrigation with antibiotic

10. **When do we have to start antibiotics to prevent post-operative infection?** *(DPG 2011, JIPMER 2003)*
    a. 2 days before surgery
    b. After surgery
    c. 1 week before surgery
    d. 1 hour before surgery and continue after surgery

11. **Ideally, when should antibiotics be given during a surgery?**
    a. At the time of induction   *(MHSSMCET 2011)*
    b. At the time incision
    c. After the surgery is over
    d. A couple of days prior surgery

12. **Preferred time for prophylactic antibiotic:** *(PGI June 2009)*
    a. 1 day before surgery
    b. At the time of induction of anesthesia
    c. I.V. during surgery
    d. I.M. before 6 hours
    e. Orally given

13. **Optional timing of administration of prophylactic antibiotic for surgical patients is:** *(APPG 2015)*
    a. At the induction of anesthesia
    b. Any time during the surgical procedure
    c. One hour after induction
    d. One hour prior to induction of anesthesia

14. **Preoperative shaving is ideally done at:** *(Recent Question 2016)*
    a. Evening before   b. Morning of operation
    c. Just before operation   d. At operation table

15. **In a postoperative intensive care unit, five patients developed postoperative wound infection on the same wound. The best method to prevent cross infection occurring in other patients in the same ward is to:** *(All India 2003)*
    a. Give antibiotics to all other patients in the ward
    b. Fumigate the ward
    c. Disinfect the ward with sodium hypochlorite
    d. Practice proper hand washing

16. **In a surgical post-operative ward, a patient developed wound infection. Subsequently 3 other patients developed similar infections in the ward. What is the most effective way of preventing the spread of infection?** *(AIIMS Nov 2001)*
    a. Give IV antibiotics to all patients in the ward
    b. Proper hand washing of all ward personnel
    c. Fumigation of the ward
    d. Wash OT instruments with 1% perchlorate

17. **The most effective method of reduction of incidence of institutional pediatric Staphylococcus aureus infection is:** *(COMEDK 2010)*
    a. Mask and gown use with each suspected patient
    b. Meticulous hand washing before and after contact with patients
    c. Treatment of all culture-positive patients with vancomycin
    d. Routine isolation of culture-positive patients

18. **Ampicillin prophylaxis is given in:**
    a. Rectal surgery   b. Splenectomy
    c. Head and neck surgery   d. Biliary surgery

19. **A surgeon decides to operate a patient of carcinoma cecum and perform a right hemicolectomy through a midline laparotomy approach. You have been instructed to prepare the parts of the patient for surgery. What will you do?** *(AIIMS May 2016)*
    a. Clean and drape from the level of nipple to mid thigh
    b. Clean and drape from umbilicus to mid thigh
    c. Clean and drape from chin to knee
    d. Clean and drape from rib cage to inguinal regions

20. Which of the following is preferred for preoperative preparation? *(Recent Question 2017)*
    a. On table clipping of hair
    b. Shaving of hair on the table
    c. Shaving of hair before entry to operation theatre
    d. Shaving of hair one day before surgery

21. Steps taken to prevent postoperative incised wound infection are: *(PGI May 2018)*
    a. Start antibiotics at least 1 day preoperatively
    b. Shaving of hair
    c. One dose of antibiotic just before the incision
    d. Shower preoperatively using an antiseptic
    e. Prevent intraoperative hypothermia

22. Sterile OT zone is: *(PGI May 2018)*
    a. Changing room
    b. Scrub room
    c. Set up room
    d. Cleaner room and stores
    e. Anesthesia inducing room

SIRS AND MODS

23. A 60-year-old lady underwent abdominal surgery and on the 4th post-operative day she was diagnosed to have systemic inflammatory response syndrome (SIRS). What are the features of SIRS? *(UPSC 2004)*
    a. Normal body temperature and normal respiratory rate
    b. WBC >12 × 10⁹/L or <4 × 10⁹/L
    c. Respiratory rate >24 breaths/minute and heart rate >90 beats/minute
    d. Respiratory rate <10 breaths/minute

24. SIRS with established source of infection is known as:
    a. Sepsis   b. Severe sepsis
    c. Septic shock   d. MODS

25. Indicator of hypoperfusion in severe sepsis: *(Recent Question 2016)*
    a. Systolic BP <90 mmHg   b. Lactic acidosis
    c. Oliguria   d. All of the above

26. Q-SOFA score includes: *(PGI May 2018)*
    a. Pulse rate
    b. Respiratory rate
    c. Systolic blood pressure
    d. Altered mental status
    e. Mean arterial pressure

27. Characteristics of SIRS include all of the following except: *(MCI June 2018)*
    a. Leukocytosis
    b. Thrombocytopenia
    c. Infectious or non-infectious cause
    d. Oral temperature more than 38°C

CELLULITIS AND PYOGENIC BACTERIAL INFECTION

28. True about management of necrotizing soft tissue infection: *(PGI Nov 2011)*
    a. Broad spectrum antibiotics should be started
    b. Penicillin is not usually effective due to resistant strains
    c. Immediate debridement + IV antibiotic has main role in treatment
    d. Hyperbaric O₂ is useful
    e. Amputation always indicated

29. False about cellulitis: *(PGI Nov 2010)*
    a. Caused by Strep. pyogenes
    b. Causes SIRS
    c. Localized infection
    d. Abscess if any should be managed conservatively
    e. I and D of abscess should be done

30. What is the most probable diagnosis based on the given image? *(Recent Question 2017)*

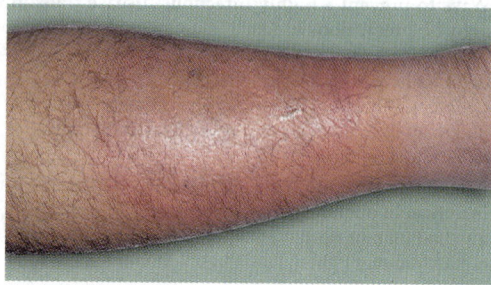

    a. Cellulitis   b. Erysipelas
    c. Ecthyma   d. Erythema nodosum

31. Extensive surgical debridement, decompression or amputation may be indicated in the following clinical setting except: *(UPSC 2007)*
    a. Progressive synergistic gangrene
    b. Acute thrombophlebitis
    c. Acute hemolytic streptococcal cellulitis
    d. Acute rhabdomyolysis

32. Cellulitis is most commonly caused by: *(Recent Question 2014, MCI Sept 2008, 2010)*
    a. Clostridia   b. Staphylococci
    c. Streptococci   d. H. influenza

33. All of the following statements about necrotizing fasciitis are true, except: *(All India 2009)*
    a. Infection of fascia and subcutaneous tissue
    b. Most commonly caused by Group A beta hemolytic streptococci
    c. Most commonly site is perineum followed by trunk and extremities
    d. Surgical debridement is mandatory

34. What is the most probable diagnosis based on the given image? *(Recent Question 2017)*

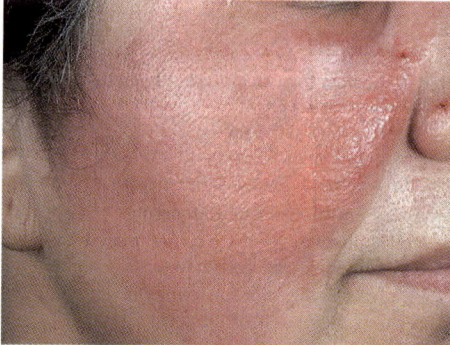

    a. Cellulitis   b. Erysipelas
    c. Ecthyma   d. Erythema nodosum

35. Erysipelas is caused by: *(PGI 88)*
    a. Staph. aureus   b. Staph. albus
    c. Strep. pyogenes   d. Hemophilus

36. Following are true of erysipelas except: (AIIMS 84)
    a. Streptococcal infection
    b. Contagious and infectious
    c. Margins are raised
    d. Common in tropics
37. Chronic thick walled pyogenic abscess may be due to the following except: (AIIMS 84)
    a. Presence of a foreign body
    b. Prolonged antibiotic therapy
    c. Virulent strains of organism
    d. Inadequate drainage
38. Treatment of spreading streptococcal cellulitis is:
    a. Erythromycin
    b. Penicillin
    c. Tetracycline
    d. Chloramphenicol
39. A carbuncle is treated by: (UPSC 95)
    a. Incision and drainage
    b. Cruciate incision and deroofing
    c. Antibiotics alone
    d. Wide excision
40. A boil is due to staphylococcal infection of: (UPPG 97)
    a. Hair follicle
    b. Sweat gland
    c. Subcutaneous tissue
    d. Epidermis
41. True about cellulitis of lower limb: (PGI 2000)
    a. Infection of skin and subcutaneous tissue
    b. Fever and malaise are common
    c. Margins are distinct
    d. Extrnal wound always present
    e. Involved site is red and hot
42. Best management of contaminated wound with necrotic material: (Recent Question 2014, AIIMS Nov 2013)
    a. Debridement
    b. Tetanus toxoid
    c. Gas gangrene serum
    d. Broad spectrum antibiotics
43. Which is not true of carbuncle?
    a. Infective gangrene of subcutaneous tissue
    b. Caused by staphylococcus
    c. Diabetic are more prone
    d. Caused by streptococcus
    e. Penicillin and excision of necrotic tissue is treatment of choice
44. Unlike cellulitis, erysipelas has feature of:
    a. Clearly demarcated margin (PGI November 2017)
    b. Elevated edge
    c. More deeper skin involvement
    d. More generalized spread
    e. More abrupt onset

GAS GANGRENE

45. Gas gangrene is caused by: (JIPMER 2010)
    a. Cl. botulinum
    b. Cl. difficile
    c. Cl. perfringens
    d. Cl. tetani
46. True about treatment of gas gangrene after contaminated road traffic accident: (PGI Nov 2011)
    a. IV administration of anti-gas gangrene serum
    b. Penicillin
    c. Immediate suturing
    d. Surgical debridement
    e. Irrigation of anti-gas gangrene serum
47. Which of the following is not true about gas gangrene?
    a. Caused by Clostridium tetani (MHSSMCET 2011)
    b. Immunocompromised patients are most at risk
    c. Gas and smell are characteristic
    d. Antibiotic prophylaxis is essential when performing amputations to remove dead tissue
48. Hyperbaric oxygen is useful in: (Recent Question 2014, PGI 88)
    a. Tetanus
    b. Gas gangrene
    c. Frostbite
    d. Vincent's angina
49. Which of the following is not true of gas gangrene?
    a. It is caused by clostridium perfringens (AIIMS June 2003)
    b. Clostridium perfringens is a gram-negative spore-bearing bacillus
    c. Gas gangrene is characterized by severe local pain, crepitus and signs of toxemia
    d. High dose penicillin and aggressive debridement of affected tissue is the treatment of established infection
50. Best way to prevent gas gangrene is:
    a. Immunoglobulins (Recent Question 2013, AIIMS Nov 93)
    b. Hyperbaric oxygen
    c. Proper wound debridement
    d. Anti gas gangrene serum
51. Hypotension in a cause of gas gangrene is best treated by: (Recent Question 2016)
    a. Ringer lactate
    b. Normal saline
    c. Plasma
    d. Whole blood
52. Treatment of contaminated wound in gas gangrene is:
    a. Debridement of wound (Recent Question 2016)
    b. Systemic penicillin
    c. Metronidazole administration
    d. Peroxide dressings
53. Foaming liver is seen in: (Recent Question 2016)
    a. Organophosphorus poisoning
    b. Actinomycosis
    c. Gas gangrene
    d. Anthrax
54. Treatment of contaminated wound of leg:
    a. Debridement and antibiotics (Recent Question 2015)
    b. Hyperbaric oxygen
    c. Amputation
    d. None

TETANUS

55. Tetanus is caused by:
    a. Cl. tetani
    b. Cl. welchii
    c. Cl. edematiens
    d. Cl. septicum
56. Following may be premonitory symptoms of tetanus *except*:
    a. Sleeplessness
    b. Anxious expression
    c. Urinary incontinence
    d. Headache
57. Period of onset in tetanus refers to the time between:
    a. First injury to spasm (Karnataka 2006)
    b. First symptom to spasm
    c. First spasm to death
    d. Trismus to laryngeal spasm

TUBERCULOSIS

58. Regarding tuberculous lymphadenitis, which is correct?
    a. Seen in children and young adults
    b. Seen in the aged
    c. History of contact or drinking infected milk
    d. Mostly cervical
    e. All are the correct

59. Commonest cause of acute lymphadenitis in India:
    a. Barefoot walking   (MAHE 2005)
    b. TB
    c. Staphylococcal skin infection
    d. Lymphoma

60. A 10 years old child with pain and mass in right lumbar region with no fever, with right hip flexed and X-ray shows spine changes. Most probable diagnosis is:
    a. Psoas abscess   (AIIMS November 2017)
    b. Pyonephrosis
    c. Retrocecal appendicitis
    d. Torsion of right undescended testis

SYPHILIS

61. Moth eaten alopecia is seen with: (Recent Question 2016)
    a. Leprosy   b. Syphilis
    c. Fungal infection   d. Cylindroma

62. Moon's molars seen with:
    a. Syphilis   b. Leprosy
    c. Amyloidosis   d. Actinomycosis

63. Which of the following about yaws is incorrect?
    a. Caused by Treponema pertenue
    b. Spread by direct contact
    c. Sexually transmitted
    d. Penicillin is used as treatment

64. Painless effusions in joints in congenital syphilis is called:
                                          (All India 95)
    a. Clutton's joints   b. Banton's joints
    c. Charcot's joints   d. Synovitis

65. All are features of gummatous ulcer except: (APPG 96)
    a. Punched out edges b. Syphilitic in nature
    c. Wash leather slough d. Erythematous base

66. Thymus gland abscess seen in congenital syphilis is called:
                                          (Recent Question 2016)
    a. Fouchier's abscess b. Politzeri abscess
    c. Douglas abscess   d. Dubois abscess

67. A mentally retarded child aged 12 years has multiple, painful, discharging shiny white lesions around the anus. Which of the following is the most probable diagnosis: (UPSC 97)
    a. Lupus vlugaris   b. Carcinoma
    c. Syphilitic condyloma d. Hemorrhoids

LEPROSY

68. Globi is seen in leprosy: (Recent Question 2016)
    a. Tuberculoid   b. Lepromatous
    c. Border line   d. Borderline tuberculoid

69. Which of the following parts of the body is not affected by leprosy?   (Recent Question 2016)
    a. Testes   b. Ovary
    c. Nasal mucosa   d. Axilla

70. Leonine facies is seen in leprosy: (Recent Question 2016)
    a. Tuberculoid   b. Borderline
    c. Lepromatous   d. Borderline tuberculoid

71. Most commonly affected peripheral nerve in leprosy is:
    a. Ulnar   b. Radial
    c. Medial   d. Lateral Popliteal

ACTINOMYCOSIS

72. Actinomycosis is sensitive to:
    a. Streptomycin   b. Nystatin
    c. Penicillin   d. Iodox-uridine

73. Most common form of actinomycosis is:
    a. Fascio cervical   b. Thoracic
    c. Right iliac fossa d. Liver

74. A patient with a fistula and chronic pus discharge from lower face and mandible is most commonly suffering from:
                                          (Recent Question 2016)
    a. Dental cyst   b. Vincent's angina
    c. Ludwig's angina   d. Actinomycosis

HIV AND COMPLICATIONS

75. In AIDS, lymphadenopathy is most often due to:
    a. TB   (PGI Dec 97)
    b. Lymphoma
    c. Nonspecific enlargement of lymph node
    d. Kaposi's sarcoma

76. The HIV virus can be transmitted by the following routes, except: (Karnataka 94)
    a. Homosexual contact b. Intact skin
    c. Maternofetal   d. Needle prick

77. The high risk groups for transmission of HIV virus include the following except: (Karnataka 94)
    a. Homosexuals
    b. Hemophiliacs
    c. Children of HIV mothers
    d. Healthcare workers

78. Universal (standard) precautions to be observed by surgeons for the prevention of hospital acquire HIV infection include the following except: (UPSC 2005)
    a. Wearing gloves and other barrier precaution
    b. Washing hands on contamination
    c. Handling sharp instruments with care
    d. Preoperative screening of all patients of HIV

79. Which of the following is not the personal protective equipment?   (Recent Question 2019)
    a. Gloves   b. Lab coat
    c. Face shield   d. Goggles

80. An intern while doing scalp suturing injured his index finger. Which of the following is not correct regarding the management?   (Recent Question 2019)
    a. Should inform authorities
    b. High risk of HIV transmission
    c. Injuries during suturing is more common in non-dominant hand
    d. The part should be washed under running tap water

ANTHRAX

81. Most common form of anthrax is: (Recent Question 2016)
    a. Wool sorters disease b. Alimentary type
    c. Cutaneous type   d. None of the above

82. Malignant pustule occurs in: (KGMC 2011)
    a. Melanoma   b. Gas gangrene
    c. Ovarian tumour   d. Anthrax

HAND INFECTIONS

83. Most common hand infection is due to: *(DPG 2008)*
    a. E. coli
    b. Staph. aureus
    c. Streptococcus
    d. Pseudomonas
84. From the index finger infection goes to: *(AIIMS Nov 96)*
    a. Thenar space
    b. Hypothenar space
    c. Mid-palmar space
    d. Space of parona
85. Felon is: *(Recent Question 2015, DPG 2005)*
    a. Mid palmer space infection
    b. Terminal pulp space infection
    c. Infection of ulnar bursa
    d. Infection of radial bursa
86. Felon most commonly present at: *(Recent Question 2016)*
    a. Index finger
    b. Ring finger
    c. Little finger
    d. Middle finger
87. Pulp space infection is known as: *(MHSSMCET 2009)*
    a. Felon
    b. Paronychia
    c. Perinoychia
    d. Onychonychia
88. Which of the following should not be treated with surgery? *(MHPGMET 2005)*
    a. Felon
    b. Acute paronychia
    c. Herpetic whitlow
    d. Chronic paronychia

INTRA-ABDOMINAL INFECTIONS

89. Sub phrenic abscess, not seen is: *(DPG 2006)*
    a. Air fluid level
    b. Leucopenia
    c. More common on right side
    d. Associated with shoulder pain
90. In which of the following condition burst abdomen is commonly associated? *(PGI Dec 2005)*
    a. Drainage coming out through the wound
    b. Non absorbable sutures
    c. Interrupted sutures
    d. Medial incision is more risk (as compared to transverse incision)
    e. Transverse incision is better than paramedian incision
91. Infection of all the following structures can be cause psoas abscess except: *(DPG 2009 March)*
    a. Vertebrae
    b. Appendix
    c. Hip joint
    d. Ribs
92. All of the following favor postoperative wound dehiscence except: *(Karnataka 2005)*
    a. Malignancy
    b. Vitamin B complex deficiency
    c. Hypoproteinaemia
    d. Jaundice
93. Which of the following is the most pathognomonic sign of impending burst abdomen? *(Recent Question 2015)*
    a. Fever
    b. Shock
    c. Pain
    d. Serosanguinous discharge
94. True regarding wound dehiscence: *(Recent Question 2018)*
    a. If you suspect dehiscence, close with continuous suture of non-absorbable material
    b. Dehiscence happens on 2nd postoperative day
    c. The management of wound dehiscence depends on degree of evisceration and gangrenous bowel
    d. There will sudden gush of fluid just before the dehiscence

NOSOCOMIAL INFECTIONS

95. In a surgical patient, the causes of non-surgical infection:
    a. Lower RTI *(DPG 2010, PGI June 2004)*
    b. Wound infection
    c. Clostridium difficile diarrhea
    d. UTI
96. Most common nosocomial infection: *(Recent Question 2016, Bihar PG 2016)*
    a. Surgical site infection
    b. Respiratory tract infection
    c. Urinary tract infection
    d. Skin & soft tissue infection
97. Most common organism responsible for UTI in hospital: *(Recent Question 2017)*
    a. E. coli
    b. Klebsiella
    c. Proteus
    d. Pseudomonas

HILTON'S METHOD

98. Hilton's method of treatment of an axillary abscess is advised because it: *(Karnataka 94)*
    a. Protects vital structure
    b. Ensures adequate drainage
    c. Hinders the spread of infection
    d. Allows local instillation of antibiotics
99. Hilton's method is best used in: *(Recent Question 2015)*
    a. Breast abscess
    b. Axillary abscess
    c. Paronychia
    d. Pulp abscess
100. Hilton's method is used in: *(MHSSMCET 2005)*
    a. To minimize the scar
    b. To prevent injury to vital structure
    c. To have complete drainage
    d. To drain large abscesses

MISCELLANEOUS

101. Chronic burrowing ulcer is caused by: *(All India 2007, AIIMS May 2008)*
    a. Microaerophilic streptococci
    b. Peptostreptococcus
    c. Streptococcus viridians
    d. Streptococcus pyogenes
102. Mycotic abscesses are due to: *(All India 2006)*
    a. Bacterial infection
    b. Fungal infection
    c. Viral infection
    d. Mixed infection
103. Golden period for treatment of open wound in hours:
    a. 4
    b. 6
    c. 12
    d. 24
104. Sardonic grin is associated with:
    a. Rabies
    b. Tetanus
    c. Bell's palsy
    d. Hemiplegia
105. Scrum pox is seen among players:
    a. Football
    b. Hockey
    c. Rugby
    d. Chess
106. Multiple fistula in ano commonly occurs in: *(TN 91)*
    a. Tuberculosis
    b. Gonococcal protocolitis
    c. LGV
    d. Colloid carcinoma of rectum

107. **Follman's balanitis is caused by:** *(Kerala 2003)*
    a. Trichomonas
    b. Candida
    c. H. Ducreyl
    d. None

108. **All of the following are perils of prolonged antibiotic therapy in intra abdominal sepsis except:**
    a. Masking of general signs
    b. Subacute intestinal obstruction
    c. Malignant change
    d. Frozen pelvis

109. **Pyrexia due to wound infection commonly occurs after:**
    a. Third post operation day *(Recent Question 2017)*
    b. Fifth post operation day
    c. Seventh post operation day
    d. Second post operation day

110. **Antibioma is best treated by:** *(JIPMER 95)*
    a. Partial resection
    b. Complete resection
    c. Aspiration
    d. Administration of antibiotics

111. **True about surgical wounds:** *(PGI Nov 2010)*
    a. No antibiotics required in clean surgery
    b. Incision of abscess is done in contaminated wound
    c. Spillage of stomach content converts a clean/contaminated case to a contaminated case
    d. In clean/contaminated wounds infection rate is 10%
    e. Hernia repair is contaminated wound

112. **Anaerobic infection is precipitated by:** *(MHPGMCET 2001)*
    a. Trauma
    b. Impaired circulation
    c. Tissue necrosis
    d. All of the above

113. **Which of these scoring systems is helpful in assessing severity of wound infection and is used for research and surveillance?** *(AIIMS November 2016)*
    a. Southampton grading scale
    b. ASA classification
    c. Glasgow score
    d. APGAR

114. **Type IIIc Southamton Grading is:** *(Recent Question 2016)*
    a. Erythema along sutures
    b. Large volume of hemoserous discharge
    c. Prolonged hemoserous discharge
    d. Pus at one point

Explanations

STERILIZATION AND DISINFECTION

1. Ans. a. Isolation ward, b. Facemask, d. Keep isolated in a room with negative pressure *(Ref: Prevention of Hospital Acquired Infection by WHO)*
2. Ans. b. Air-conditioning
3. Ans. b. 2% glutaraldehyde for 20 min *(Ref: Bailey 24/e p135)*
4. Ans. b. Phenol *(Ref: Anantnarayan 7/e p31)*

Sporicidal Agents	
• Ethylene oxide^Q	• Halogenes^Q
• Glutaraldehyde^Q	• Ozone^Q

5. Ans. d. Peracetic acid
6. Ans. c. Glutaraldehyde
7. Ans. d. Chloride compounds *(Ref: Infection Control in Clinical Practice By Jennie Wilson (2006)/p173)*

> "High-concentration chlorine-releasing compounds provide the most economical and effective method of treating many spills, especially large spills of blood. Chlorine-releasing granules have the advantage of containing the spill rather than adding to it; they have a longer shelf-life than hypochlorite solutions and are more portable." -Infection Control in Clinical Practice By Jennie Wilson (2006)/p173

PROPHYLAXIS

8. Ans. c. At the time of induction *(Ref: Sabiston 20/e p224, 251; Schwartz 10/e p142; Bailey, 27/e p53)*
9. Ans. c. Prophylaxis for colorectal surgery *(Ref: Sabiston 20/e p251-252)*
10. Ans. d. 1 hour before surgery and continue after surgery
11. Ans. a. At the time of induction
12. Ans. b. At the time of induction of anesthesia
13. Ans. a. At the induction of anesthesia
14. Ans. c. Just before operation
15. Ans. d. Practice proper hand washing *(Ref: Bailey 27/e p52-53)*
16. Ans. b. Proper hand washing of all ward personnel
17. Ans. b. Meticulous hand washing before and after contact with patients
18. Ans. d. Biliary surgery *(Ref: www.ncbi.nlm.nih.gov/pubmed/8526441)*

> **PROPHYLACTIC ANTIBIOTICS IN BILIARY SURGERY**
> - **Prophylactic antibiotics in biliary surgery** are designed to **reduce** the **incidence of postoperative wound infections.**
> - The efficacy of antibiotics in the prevention of wound infections has been demonstrated with first, second and third generation **cephalosporins, ampicillin**^{Q} associated with clavulanate, **ureido-penicillins, aminoglycosides, sulfonamides** and **quinolones.**

19. Ans. a. Clean and drape from the level of nipple to mid thigh
20. Ans. a. On table clipping of hair *(Ref: Sabiston 20/e p232, 286)*

> "Preoperative skin shaving should be undertaken in the operating theatre immediately before surgery as the SSI rate after clean wound surgery may be doubled if it is performed the night before; minor skin injury enhances superficial bacterial colonisation. Cream depilation is messy and hair clipping is best, with the lowest rate of infection." -Bailey 27/e p52

21. Ans. c. One dose of antibiotic just before the incision, d. Shower preoperatively using an antiseptic, e. Prevent intraoperative hypothermia
22. Ans. b. Scrub room, c. Set up room, e. Anesthesia inducing room

SIRS AND MODS

23. Ans. b. WBC $>12 \times 10^9$/L or $<4 \times 10^9$/L, c. Respiratory rate > 24 breaths/minute and heart rate > 90 beats/minute *(Ref: Sabiston 20/e p242, 263; Schwartz 10/e p19,138; Bailey 27/e p51)*

Criteria for Four Categories of the Systemic Inflammatory Response Syndrome

SIRS	Sepsis	Severe Sepsis	Septic Shock
Two or more of the following: • **Temperature** (core) **>38°C or <36°C**[Q] • **Heart rate >90 beats/min**[Q] • **Respiratory rate >20**[Q] breaths/min for patients spontaneously ventilating or a **PaCO$_2$ <32 mm Hg**[Q] • **WBC count >12,000**[Q] cells/mm3 or **<4000**[Q] cells/mm3 or **>10% immature (band) cells** in the peripheral blood smear	• Same criteria as for **SIRS** but **with a** clearly established **focus of infection**[Q]	• **Sepsis** with **organ dysfunction** and **hypoperfusion** **Indicators of hypoperfusion:** • **Systolic BP <90 mm Hg**[Q] • **>40 mm Hg fall** from normal systolic blood pressure[Q] • **Lactic acadosis**[Q] • **Oliguria**[Q] • **Acute mental status changes**[Q]	Patients with **severe sepsis who:** • Are **not responsive to IV fluid infusion** for resuscitation[Q] • **Require inotropic** or **vasopressor agents** to maintain systolic blood pressure[Q]

24. Ans. a. Sepsis
25. Ans. d. All of the above
26. Ans. b. Respiratory rate, c. Systolic blood pressure, d. Altered mental status *(Ref: Sabiston 20/e p; Schwartz 10/e p; Bailey 27/e p)*

Quick Sequential Organ Failure Assessment (SOFA) Score

qSOFA (Quick SOFA) Criteria	Points
Respiratory rate ≥22/min[Q]	1
Change in **mental status**[Q]	1
Systolic BP ≤100 mm Hg[Q]	1

Interpretation

Score	Mortality
0	<1%
1	2-3%
≥2	≥10%

27. Ans. b. Thrombocytopenia

CELLULITIS AND PYOGENIC BACTERIAL INFECTION

28. Ans. a. Broad spectrum antibiotics should be started, c. Immediate debridement + IV antibiotic has main role in treatment, d. Hyperbaric O$_2$ is useful *(Ref: Sabiston 20/e p2035; Bailey 27/e p50, 419)*
29. Ans. c. Localized infection, d. Abscess if any should be managed conservatively *(Ref: Sabiston 20/e p258, 19/e p1740; Schwartz 10/e p151,483; Bailey 27/e p48-49)*
30. Ans. a. Cellulitis *(Ref: Schwartz 10/e p151; Bailey 27/e p596, 597)*
31. Ans. b. Acute thrombophlebitis
32. Ans. c. Streptococci
33. Ans. c. Most commonly site is perineum followed by trunk and extremities

• MC site of necrotizing fasciitis is **extremities**[Q] followed by trunk and perineum (Fournier's gangrene).

34. Ans. b. Erysipelas *(Ref: Schwartz 10/e p151; Bailey 27/e p596, 597)*

Erysipelas can be differentiated from cellulitis by its characteristically raised, advancing edges and sharply demarcated borders, reflecting its more superficial nature. Cellulitis has no lymphatic component and exhibits indiscreet margins.

35. Ans. c. Strep. pyogenes *(Ref: Bailey 27/e p 596-97)*
36. Ans. b. Contagious and infectious, d. Common in tropics
37. Ans. c. Virulent strains of organism
38. Ans. b. Penicillin
39. Ans. a. Incision and drainage, d. Wide excision *(Ref: www.ncbi.nlm.nih.gov)*
40. Ans. a. Hair follicle *(Ref: Schwartz 10/e p474)*

• **Folliculitis, carbuncles** and **furuncles** are all types of localized (superficial) skin infections that fall under the category of **boils**[Q].
• **Hair follicles** serve as **portals for a number of bacteria**, although **S. aureus** is the MC cause of localized **folliculitis**[Q].

41. Ans. a. Infection of skin and subcutaneous tissue, b. Fever and malaise are common, c. Margins are distinct, e. Involved site is red and hot

Sterilization and Infection

42. Ans. a. Debridement
43. Ans. d. Caused by streptococcus
44. Ans. a. Clearly demarcated margin, b. Elevated edge, e. More abrupt onset

GAS GANGRENE

45. Ans. c. Cl. perfringens *(Ref: Harrison 20/e p1109, 19/e p992)*
46. Ans. a. IV administration of anti-gas gangrene serum, b. Penicillin, d. Surgical debridement
47. Ans. a. Caused by Clostridium tetani
48. Ans. b. Gas gangrene, c. Frostbite
49. Ans. b. Clostridium perfringens is a gram-negative spore-bearing bacillus
50. Ans. c. Proper wound debridement
51. Ans. a. Ringer lactate
52. Ans. a. Debridement of wound, b. Systemic penicillin
53. Ans. c. Gas gangrene
54. Ans. a. Debridement and antibiotics

TETANUS

55. Ans. a. Cl. tetani *(Ref: Schwartz 10/e p186,264; Bailey 27/e p50, 417)*
56. Ans. c. Urinary incontinence
57. Ans. b. First symptom to spasm

TUBERCULOSIS

58. Ans. a. Seen in children and young adults, c. History of contact or drinking infected milk, d. Mostly cervical *(Ref: Bailey 27/e p77, 757)*
59. Ans. c. Staphylococcal skin infection *(Ref: Sabiston 20/e p1860, 19/e p1831-1832; Schwartz 10/e p1602; Bailey 27/e p996, 997)*

ACUTE LYMPHADENITIS

- **Enlarged tender lymph nodes** are usually the result of a **bacterial infection** (**staphylococcal**[Q] or **streptococcal**).
- **Treatment of** the **primary cause** (e.g., **otitis media** or **pharyngitis**) **with antibiotics** often is all that is necessary.
- **Fluctuant nodes**: Incision and **drainage**[Q]

60. Ans. a. Psoas abscess *(Ref: Harrison 20/e p958, 19/e p852, 1110; Bailey 27/e p1065)*

"Patients with psoas abscesses frequently present with fever, lower abdominal or back pain, or pain referred to the hip or knee. CT is the most useful diagnostic technique." -Harrison 19/e p852

SYPHILIS

61. Ans. b. Syphilis *(Ref: Rook's 7/e p30.1-30.30, 25.20-39)*
62. Ans. a. Syphilis
63. Ans. c. Sexually transmitted *(Ref: Harrison 20/e p1288, 19/e p207e-2)*

YAWS

- Also known as **pian, framboesia,** or **bouba**; Caused by **Treponema pertenue**[Q]
- **Infection is transmitted by direct contact** with **infectious lesions**[Q].

Clinical Features
- Characterized by the **development of one** or **several primary lesions** ("mother Yaws") followed by **multiple disseminated skin lesions**[Q].
- **All early skin lesions are infectious** and may persist for many months

Treatment
- **Treatment** is normally by a single intramuscular injection of **penicillin**[Q], or by a course of penicillin, **erythromycin** or **tetracycline** tablets

64. Ans. a. Clutton's joints
65. Ans. d. Erythematous base
66. Ans. d. Dubois abscess *(Ref: http://en.wikipedia.org/wiki/Abscess_of_thymus)*

DUBOIS ABSCESSES

- An **abscess of** the **thymus** associated with **congenital syphilis**[Q]
- It can present with **chest pain** behind the sternum.

67. Ans. c. Syphilitic condyloma

LEPROSY

68. Ans. b. Lepromatous *(Ref: Rooks 7/e p29.1-29.19)*

Type of leprosy	Characteristic feature	
Neuritic	• Slit smear negative[Q]	
TT	• Single skin lesion[Q]	• MC type in **India** and **Africa**[Q]
BT	• Satellite lesion[Q]	• MC type in **South East Asia**[Q]
BB>BL	• Inverted saucer lesion[Q]	
LL	• Subepidermal free zone[Q] • Globi[Q] are seen • Lucio phenomenon[Q]	• Lozarine leprosy reaction[Q] • Leonine facies[Q]

LEPROSY

- **MC affected peripheral nerve** in leprosy: **Ulnar nerve**[Q]
- **Organ not involved** in leprosy: **Ovary**[Q]

69. Ans. b. Ovary
70. Ans. c. Lepromatous
71. Ans. a. Ulnar

ACTINOMYCOSIS

72. Ans. c. Penicillin *(Ref: Harrison 20/e p1223, 19/e p1088; Sabiston 20/e p1597-1598)*
73. Ans. a. Fascio cervical
74. Ans. d. Actinomycosis

HIV AND COMPLICATIONS

75. Ans. c. Nonspecific enlargement of lymph node *(Ref: Harrison 20/e p1441, 19/e p1232-1233)*

PERSISTENT GENERALIZED LYMPHADENOPATHY (PGL)

- **HIV patients** develop **PGL** as an **early clinical manifestation** of HIV infection[Q].
- PGL is defined as presence of **>1 LN** in **two or three extra-inguinal sites** for >3 months without an obvious cause[Q].
- Enlargement is due to **follicular hyperplasia**[Q].

76. Ans. b. Intact skin
77. Ans. d. Healthcare workers
78. Ans. d. Preoperative screening of all patients of HIV

UNIVERSAL PRECAUTIONS

- **Universal precautions** refers to the practice, in medicine, of **avoiding contact with patient's bodily fluids**, by means of the wearing of nonporous articles such as **medical gloves, goggles**, and **face shields**[Q].
  - Includes **good hygiene habits**, such as **hand washing** and the **use of gloves** and **other barriers**, **correct handling of hypodermic needles** and **scalpels**, and **aseptic techniques**[Q].
- **Protective clothing include:** Barrier gowns, gloves, eyewear (goggles or glasses) and face shields[Q]
- **Typically practiced against:** Blood, semen, vaginal secretions[Q], synovial fluid, amniotic fluid, CSF, pleural fluid, peritoneal fluid, pericardial fluid

79. Ans. b. Lab coat
80. Ans. b. High risk of HIV transmission

ANTHRAX

81. Ans. c. Cutaneous type *(Ref: Harrison 20/e p936, 19/e p261e-2)*

ANTHRAX

- Caused by **Bacillus anthracis**[Q]
- **Three major clinical forms:** **Cutaneous**[Q] **(MC)**, gastrointestinal and inhalational

Risk Factors for Necrotizing Fasciitis	
Woolsorters' disease	• Occupational hazard for people who sorted wool[Q] • **Most dangerous form** of inhalational anthrax[Q]
Hide porter's disease	• Caused by **contact with contaminated hair, wool, hides** or **products made from them** (Hide porter's disease)[Q]
Malignant pustule	• Commonly seen in **head and neck**[Q] • **Eschar stage** that appears 2-6 days after the hemorrhagic vesicle dries to become a **depressed black scab**[Q] surrounded by redness and extensive edema

82. **Ans. d. Anthrax**

HAND INFECTIONS

83. **Ans. b. Staph. aureus** *(Ref: Sabiston 20/e p2000-2001; 19/e p1977; Bailey 27/e p503-504)*
84. **Ans. a. Thenar space** *(Ref: BDC 4/e vol I/129; Keith and Moore 4/e p765)*
85. **Ans. b. Terminal pulp space infection** *(Ref: Bailey 27/e p503-504)*
86. **Ans. a. Index finger**
87. **Ans. a. Felon**

Hand Infections

Felon	Acute Paronychia	Chronic Paronychia	Herpetic Whitlow
• Felon is **terminal pulp space infection**^{Q} • **Causes severe pain**^{Q} in the finger pulp. • Most commonly involve **index finger**^{Q} • **Pus** is **trapped**^{Q} between fibrous septa which bind the specialized fingertip skin to the underlying bone • **Bone** of the **terminal phalanx** can also become **infected**, resulting in **sequestrum**^{Q}. • An **abscess** should be **drained through** an **oblique incision**^{Q} over the point of greatest tenderness.	• **MC hand infection**^{Q} • Often due to **inappropriate nail trimming** or **skin picking** around the nail fold^Q • After initial inflammation, **pus accumulates beside** the **nail** and **needs to be surgically released**, with or without the **excision** of **outer quarter of** the **nail**^{Q}.	• Appears over several weeks • Usually a **fungal infection**, unrelated to the acute form. • Commonly occurs in **patients** whose **hands** are **frequently immersed**^{Q} • **Microscopy** of scrapings and **fungal cultures** reveals the diagnosis. • Management: Keep the **hand dry** and use of **anti-fungal creams**^{Q} or nail fold surgery.	• Caused by herpes simplex • **Small vesicles** and **crusts** is the **self-resolving** • Seen in **dental workers**^{Q}

88. **Ans. c. Herpetic whitlow**

INTRA-ABDOMINAL INFECTIONS

89. **Ans. b. Leucopenia**

    Leucocytosis is seen in subphrenic abscess, not the leucopenia.

90. **Ans. a. Drainage coming out through the wound, d. Medial incision is more risk (as compared to transverse incision), e. Transverse incision is better than paramedian incision** *(Ref: CSDT 11/e p24)*

91. **Ans. d. Ribs**

Causes of Secondary Psoas Abscess	
• Crohn's disease • **Appendicitis**^{Q} • Ulcerative colitis	• Diverticulitis • Colon cancer • **Vertebral osteomyelitis**^{Q}

• A **prosthetic infection of hip** can give rise to **psoas abscess**^{Q}.

92. **Ans. b. Vitamin B complex deficiency**
93. **Ans. d. Serosanguinous discharge**
94. **Ans. c. The management of wound dehiscence depends on degree of evisceration and gangrenous bowel**

NOSOCOMIAL INFECTIONS

95. **Ans. a. Lower RTI, c. Clostridium difficile diarrhea, d. UTI** *(Ref: Sabiston 20/e p322-323; Harrison 19/e p913-916)*
96. **Ans. c. Urinary tract infection:** *(Ref: Harrison 19/e p913)*

    MC Nosocomial infection: UTI (30–40%) > Surgical Site Infection (15–20%)^Q

97. **Ans. a. E. coli** *(Ref: Bailey 27/e p1441)*

    "UTI: Escherichia coli is the most common organism followed by Proteus mirabilis, Staphylococcus epidermidis and Streptococcus faecalis." Bailey 27/e p1441

HILTON'S METHOD

98. **Ans. a. Protects vital structure** *(Ref: lessons4medicos.blogspot.com/.../hiltons-method-to-drain-abscesses.)*
99. **Ans. b. Axillary abscess**
100. **Ans. b. To prevent injury to vital structure**

MISCELLANEOUS

101. **Ans. a. Microaerophilic streptococci** *(Ref: Dorland's Medical Dictionary 28/e p1770, 1771; Bailey 27/e p5, 419, 597)*
102. **Ans. b. Fungal infection**
103. **Ans. a. 4**
104. **Ans. b. Tetanus**
105. **Ans. c. Rugby**

HERPES GLADIATORUM

- **Herpes Gladiatorum** is one of the most infectious of **herpes-caused diseases** transmitted by **skin-to-skin contact**[Q].
- Strongly associated with **contact sports**, also known as **herpes rugbiorum** or "**scrumpox**" (after **rugby football**), "**wrestler's herpes**" or "**mat pox**" (after wrestling)[Q].

106. **Ans. a. Tuberculosis, c. LGV** *(Ref: Bailey 25/e p1262)*
107. **Ans. d. None**

SYPHILITIC BALANITIS OF FOLLMANN

- **Syphilitic balanitis of Follmann** is a very rare manifestation of **primary syphilis infection**[Q]
- Develop after the appearance of the primary chancre

108. **Ans. c. Malignant change**
109. **Ans. b. Fifth post operation day** *(Ref: Bailey 25/e p265)*

Causes of Post-operative Fever	
Day	**Cause**
2–5 days	**Atelectasis** of the lung[Q]
3–5 days	**Superficial** and **deep wound infection**[Q]
5 days	**Chest infection** including viral respiratory tract infection, **UTI** and **thrombophlebitis**[Q]
>5 days	**Wound infection**, anastomotic leakage, intracavitary collections and abscesses[Q]

110. **Ans. b. Complete resection**

ANTIBIOMA

- **Antibiotic induced swelling**
- When an **abscess occur in** the **breast** and **antibiotic** was **given, without** even **draining** the abscess, the **abscess cavity** next will **become fibrous** and it result in **firm to large lump** in the breast.
- Antibioma can be **confused for malignancy, excision** is done

111. **Ans. a. No antibiotics required in clean surgery, c. Spillage of stomach content converts a clean/contaminated case to a contaminated case, d. In clean/contaminated wounds infection rate is 10%** *(Ref: Sabiston 20/e p224, 251; Schwartz 10/e p 147)*

- **Prophylactic systemic antibiotics** are **not indicated** for patients undergoing **low-risk straightforward clean surgical operations** in which no obvious bacterial contamination or insertion if a foreign body has occurred[Q].
- **SSI risk** has traditionally been **correlated to wound class**. The accepted range of infection rates has been **1-5 % for clean, 3-11% for clean contaminated**[Q], and **>27% for dirty wounds**
- **Contaminated wounds: Open accidental wounds** encountered early after injury, those with **extensive introduction of bacteria** into a normally sterile area of the body due to **major breaks in sterile technique** (e.g. open cardiac massage), **gross spillage of viscus contents** such as from the **intestine**, or incision through **inflamed**, albeit **nonpurulent tissue**[Q].
- **Hernia repair** is **clean wound**[Q].

112. **Ans. d. All of the above**
113. **Ans. a. Southampton grading scale** *(Ref: Bailey's 27/e p48)*

   Southampton grading is used for surgical site infections.

114. **Ans. b. Large volume of hemoserous discharge** *(Ref: Bailey 27/e p48)*

CHAPTER 48

Fluid, Electrolyte and Nutrition

ADJUVANT NUTRITIONAL SUPPORT

ADJUVANT NUTRITIONAL SUPPORT
- Methods of adjuvant nutritional support: Enteral nutrition & total parenteral nutrition

ENTERAL NUTRITION

ENTERAL NUTRITION
- **Enteral feeding** means **delivery of nutrients into the GIT**^{Q}.
- The **alimentary tract** should be **used** whenever **possible**^{Q}.
- This can be achieved with oral supplements (sip feeding) or with a variety of **tube-feeding techniques delivering food into the stomach, duodenum** or **jejunum**^{Q}.

Advantages of Enteral route over Parenteral Route
- **Maintains integrity** of **gastrointestinal tract**^{Q}
- **Reduces translocation of gut bacteria**^{Q} that may lead to infection.
- **Reduces** the **levels of proinflammatory cytokines**^{Q} generated by the gut that contribute to hypermetabolism.

ROUTES OF ENTERAL NUTRITION

ROUTES OF ENTERAL NUTRITION
- Oral supplements by mouth
- Nasogastric tube/Nasojejunal tube: Nasojejunal tube is better due to low risk of aspiration^Q
- Feeding gastrostomy
- Feeding jejunostomy

Gastrostomy	Jejunostomy
• Surgical technique of placing tube into stomach • Common techniques are: **Stamm**^{Q}, **Witzel**^{Q} & **Janeway**^{Q} • Now-a-days **percutaneous insertion under endoscopic control** known as **PEG**^{Q} (**Percutaneous endoscopic gastrostomy**) is preferred • Three methods are used for PEG: **Push** technique, **pull** technique & **introducer** technique^Q	• Usually **preferred over gastrostomy** due to **lower risk of aspiration**^{Q} • Especially useful in **severe pancreatitis**^{Q}, in whom a degree of gastric outlet obstruction may present due to edematous head of pancreas^Q

ENTERAL NUTRITION: INDICATIONS & CONTRAINDICATIONS

Enteral Nutrition

Indications	Contraindications
• **Protein-energy malnutrition** with **inadequate oral intake**^{Q} • **Dysphagia** except for fluids^Q • **Major trauma** (or **surgery**^{Q}) when return to required dietary intake is prolonged • **Inflammatory bowel disease**^{Q} • **Distal, low-output (<200 mL/day) enterocutaneous fistula**^{Q} • To enhance adaptation after massive enterectomy	• Small bowel obstruction or ileus^Q • Severe diarrhea^Q • Proximal small intestinal fistula^Q • Severe pancreatitis^Q

COMPLICATIONS OF ENTERAL NUTRITION

Complications of Enteral Nutrition

Tube-related	Gastrointestinal	Metabolic	Infective
• **Malposition**[Q] • **Displacement**[Q] • **Blockage**[Q] • **Breakage/leakage**[Q] • Local complications (e.g. **erosion of skin/mucosa**)[Q]	• **Diarrhea**[Q] • Bloating, nausea, vomiting • **Abdominal cramps**[Q] • Aspiration[Q] • **Constipation**[Q]	• **Electrolyte disorders**[Q] • **Vitamin, mineral, trace element deficiencies**[Q] • Drug interactions	• **Exogenous** (handling contamination) • **Endogenous** (patient)

TOTAL PARENTERAL NUTRITION (TPN)

TOTAL PARENTERAL NUTRITION (TPN)

- Provision of all nutritional requirements by means of IV route without use of GIT
- Routes of delivery: via **peripheral or central venous access**

Peripheral Parenteral Nutrition/PPN	Feeding via Central Venous Access
• Appropriate for **short-term feeding** of up to **2 weeks**[Q]. • Access can be achieved by: Catheter inserted into a **peripheral vein**[Q] and maneuvered into the central venous system [**peripherally inserted central venous catheter** (PICC) line] or by using a conventional **short cannula**[Q] in the wrist veins. • **PICC lines** have a **mean duration of survival** of **7 days**[Q]. Their disadvantage is that when thrombophlebitis occurs the vein is irrevocably destroyed. • **Advantage:** Avoids the complications associated with **central venous administration**[Q] • **Disadvantage:** Development of **thrombophlebitis**[Q] • **Not indicated** if patients already have an **indwelling central venous line** or in those in whom **long-term feeding** is anticipated.	• Catheter can be inserted via the **subclavian** or **internal** or **external jugular vein**. • **Preferred access site for TPN: Subclavian vein**[Q] > **Internal jugular vein**[Q] > **Femoral vein**[Q] • Most ICU physicians and anesthetists favor **cannulation of internal or external jugular veins** as these vessels are easily accessible. **Disadvantage: Exit site** is situated inconveniently **on the side of the neck**, where repeated movements result in **disruption of the dressing** with the attendant **risk of sepsis**[Q] • **Infraclavicular subclavian**[Q] approach is more suitable for feeding as the catheter then lies flat on the chest wall, which optimizes nursing care. • For **longer term TPN Hickman lines**[Q] are **preferable (minimize line dislodgement** and **reduce** the possibility of line sepsis). • **Post-insertion chest X-ray** is **essential** before feeding is commenced **to confirm** the **absence of pneumothorax** and that the **catheter tip lies in the distal SVC to minimize** the risk of **central venous** or **cardiac thrombosis**[Q].

INDICATIONS OF TPN

Indications for Parenteral Nutrition

Primary Therapy	Supportive Therapy	Areas Under Intensive Study
• **Gastrointestinal cutaneous fistulas**[Q] • **Renal failure**[Q] (acute tubular necrosis) • **Short-bowel syndrome**[Q] • **Acute burns**[Q] • **Hepatic failure** (acute decompensation superimposed on cirrhosis)[Q] • **Crohn's disease**[Q] • **Anorexia nervosa**[Q]	• **Acute radiation enteritis**[Q] • **Acute chemotherapy toxicity**[Q] • **Prolonged ileus**[Q] • **Weight loss**[Q] preliminary to major surgery	• Patients with cancer • Patients with sepsis

TPN FORMULATIONS

TPN Formulations	
Solution with Lipids (3-in-1) **(60/20/20)**[Q]	**Solution without Lipids (2-in-1)** **(75/25)**[Q]
• Calories from **dextrose**: 55-60% • Calories from **amino acids**: 20-25% • Calories from **lipids**: 20%	• Calories from **dextrose**: 75-80% • Calories from **amino acids**: 20-25%

COMPLICATIONS OF TPN

COMPLICATIONS OF TPN

- MC complication of central venous catheterization (CVC): Catheter related sepsis[Q]
- Most dangerous complication following CVC: Pneumothorax[Q]

Complications of Parenteral Nutrition

Related to nutrient deficiency
- Hypoglycemia[Q], hypocalcemia[Q], hypophosphatemia, hypomagnesemia (refeeding syndrome)
- Chronic deficiency syndromes (essential fatty acids[Q], zinc[Q], mineral and trace elements)

Related to overfeeding
- **Excess glucose**: hyperglycemia[Q], hyperosmolar dehydration[Q], hepatic steatosis[Q], hypercapnia, increased sympathetic activity, fluid retention, **electrolyte abnormalities**[Q]
- **Excess fat**: hypercholesterolemia[Q] and formation of lipoprotein X, hypertriglyceridemia[Q], hypersensitivity reactions
- **Excess amino acids**: hyperchloremic metabolic acidosis, hypercalcemia[Q], aminoacidemia, uremia[Q]

Related to sepsis
- Catheter-related sepsis[Q]
- Increased risk of systemic sepsis[Q]

Related to line
- On insertion: pneumothorax[Q], damage to adjacent artery[Q], air embolism,[Q] thoracic duct damage[Q], cardiac perforation or tamponade, **pleural effusion,** hydromediastinum
- Long-term use: occlusion, venous thrombosis[Q]

Electrolyte Abnormalities in TPN
- **Hyponatremia** and **hypernatremia**[Q]
- **Hypokalemia** and **Hyperkalemia**[Q]
- **Hypophosphatemia** and **hyperphosphatemia**[Q]
- **Hypomagnesemia** and **Hypermagnesemia**[Q]
- **Hypocalcemia** and **hypercalcemia**[Q]
- **High zinc** and low **zinc**[Q]
- **High copper** and low **copper**[Q]
- **Hyperchloremic metabolic acidosis**[Q]

REFEEDING SYNDROME

REFEEDING SYNDROME

- Potentially lethal condition
- Occur with **rapid & excessive feeding** of patients with **severe underlying malnutrition** due to: Starvation, alcoholism, delayed nutritional support, anorexia nervosa & massive weight loss in obese patients[Q]

Pathophysiology

- With refeeding, **shift in metabolism** from **fat to carbohydrate substrate** → Increased insulin release → cellular uptake of electrolyte particularly:
  - Phosphate → Hypophosphatemia[Q]
  - Magnesium → Hypomagnesemia[Q]
  - Potassium → Hypokalemia[Q]
  - Calcium → Hypocalcemia[Q]
- Increased risk of arrhythmia, confusion, respiratory failure & death due to dyselectrolytemia[Q]

- Occur with **both enteral & TPN**; More common with **TPN**[Q]
- **Rate of feeding should begin slowly** to prevent metabolic changes[Q]

Treatment
- Treatment involves **matching intake with requirements**[Q]
- **Avoid over feeding**; Calorie delivery should be **increased slowly**[Q]
- Vitamin administration, especially **thiamine before initiation of feeding**[Q]
- **Hypophosphatemia & hypomagnesemia requires treatment**[Q]

NON-ANION GAP ACIDOSIS

Causes of Non-Anion-Gap Acidosis

Tube-related
- External pancreatic or small-bowel drainage[Q]
- Ureterosigmoidostomy, jejunal loop, ileal loop[Q]
- Drugs:
  - Calcium chloride (acidifying agent)
  - Magnesium sulphate (diarrhea)
  - Cholestyramine (bile acid diarrhea)

Gastrointestinal
- Hypokalemia
  - Proximal RTA (type 2)[Q]
  - Distal (classic) RTA (type 1)[Q]
- Hyperkalemia
  - Type 4 RTA[Q]
  - Mineralocorticoid deficiency[Q]
  - Mineralocorticoid resistance[Q]
  - Na delivery to distal Nephron
  - Tubulointerstitial disease
  - Ammonium excretion defect

Metabolic
- Potassium sparing diuretics (amiloride, triamterene, spironolactone)
- Trimethoprim[Q]
- Pentamidine[Q]
- ACE inhibitors and AT-II receptor blockers[Q]
- NSAIDs[Q]
- Cyclosporine[Q]

Infective
- Acid loads (ammonium chloride, hyperalimentation)
- Loss of potential bicarbonate: ketosis with ketone excretion
- Expansion acidosis (rapid saline administration)
- Hippurate
- Cation exchange resins

COMPOSITION OF CRYSTALLOIDS & COLLOIDS

Composition of crystalloid and colloid solutions (mM/L)

Solution	Na$^+$	K$^+$	Ca^{2+}	Cl$^-$	Lactate	Colloid
Hartmann's (RL)	130	4	< 2.7	109	28	
Normal saline (0.9% NaCl)	154			154		
Dextrose saline (4% dextrose in 0.18% saline)	30			30		
Gelofusine	150		< 1	150		Gelatin 4%
Hemacel	145	5.1	< 6.26	145		Polygelin 75 g/L
Hetastarch						Hydroxyethyl starch 6%
Lactated potassium saline injection (Darrow's solution)	121	35		103	53	

HEMODYNAMIC MONITORING

Hemodynamic Monitoring

Central venous Pressure (CVP)
- **Measurement of CVP** and its response to a small fluid challenge may assist in **distinguishing cardiogenic shock and Hypovolemic shock**[Q].
- In **seriously ill patients**, the **CVP is not a reliable indicator of left ventricular function** because of the **wide disparity** that can exist **between left and right ventricular functions**[Q].

Pulmonary Capillary wedge Pressure (PCWP)
- It is a **better indicator** for both **blood volume** and **left ventricular function** than CVP[Q].
- Obtained by **pulmonary artery flotation balloon catheter (Swan-Ganz)**[Q].
- Used to **differentiate left and right ventricular failure, pulmonary embolism, septic shock** and **ruptured mitral valve**[Q]
- **Accurate guide** to therapy with **fluids, inotropic agents** and **vasodilators**[Q].
- May also be used to **measure cardiac output** by thermodilution technique.

Multiple Choice Questions

ENTERAL NUTRITION

1. The length of the feeding tube to be inserted for transpyloric feeding is measured from the tip of: *(AIIMS Nov 2002)*
   a. Nose to the umbilicus
   b. Ear lobe to the umbilicus
   c. Nose to the knee joint
   d. Ear lobe to the knee joint

2. Ramesh met an accident with a car and has been in 'deep coma' for the last 15 days. The most suitable route for the administration of protein and calories is by: *(All India 2002)*
   a. Jejunostomy tube feeding
   b. Gastrostomy tube feeding
   c. Nasogastric tube feeding
   d. Central venous hyperalimentation

3. Contraindications of enteral nutrition: *(PGI Dec 2006)*
   a. Intestinal obstruction
   b. Severe pancreatitis
   c. Severe diarrhea
   d. IBD
   e. Intestinal fistula

4. A patient undergoes a prolonged and complicated pancreatic surgery for chronic pancreatitis. Most preferred route for supplementary nutrition in this patient would be: *(All India 2008)*
   a. Total parenteral nutrition
   b. Feeding gastrostomy
   c. Feeding jejunostomy
   d. Oral feeding

5. Recognized frequent complications of enteral feeding:
   a. Constipation
   b. Diarrhea *(PGI June 2005)*
   c. Aspiration pneumonia
   d. Hypoglycemia
   e. Hypernatremia

6. Not a contraindication of enteral nutrition: *(Punjab 2009)*
   a. Severe diarrhea
   b. Severe pancreatitis
   c. IBD
   d. Intestinal fistula

7. In percutaneous endoscopic gastrostomy (PEG), which of the following is not used? *(MHSSMCET 2008)*
   a. Push technique
   b. Pull technique
   c. Retraction method
   d. Introducer technique

TOTAL PARENTERAL NUTRITION

8. Parenteral nutrition is not used in: *(PGI June 2008)*
   a. Enterocutaneous fistula
   b. Burns
   c. Crohn's disease
   d. Paralytic ileus
   e. Pancreatitis

9. A patient on TPN develops deficiency of: *(PGI Dec 2006)*
   a. Folic acid
   b. Iron
   c. Vitamin B12
   d. Copper
   e. Fatty acids

10. Which of the following nutrients are not included in TPN? *(All India 2011)*
    a. Lipids
    b. Carbohydrates
    c. Proteins
    d. Fibers

11. Side-effect(s) of parenteral nutrition is/are. *(PGI Nov 2011)*
    a. Hypoglycemia
    b. Hyperglycemia
    c. Hypercalcemia
    d. Hypercapnia
    e. Hypophosphatemia

12. Best vein for total parenteral nutrition is: *(MHPGMCET 2002, Recent Question 2017)*
    a. Subclavian vein
    b. Femoral vein
    c. Brachial vein
    d. Saphenous vein

13. One is not indication of total parenteral nutrition: *(AIIMS Nov 95)*
    a. Acute pancreatitis
    b. Enterocolic fistula
    c. Chronic liver disease
    d. Fecal fistula

14. TPN is indicated in all except: *(PGI Dec 2005)*
    a. Short bowel syndrome
    b. Burn
    c. Sepsis
    d. Enterocutaneous fistula

15. True about TPN: *(PGI June 2008)*
    a. Carbohydrate forms about 40% of energy source
    b. In abdominal injury early parenteral nutrition should be started
    c. Proteins forms 60% of energy source
    d. Lipids form 20% of energy source

16. Which of the following is not acomplication of TPN: *(JIPMER 2014, 2013)*
    a. Hyperammonemia
    b. Hypercholesterolemia
    c. Neutrophil dysfunction
    d. Hyperphosphatemia

17. Which of the following is not a complication of Total Parenteral Nutrition? *(AIIMS Nov 2008)*
    a. Metabolic bone disease
    b. Essential fatty acid deficiency
    c. Congestive cardiac failure
    d. Hypophosphatemia

18. Most common complication of parenteral nutrition includes all except: *(MCI Sept 2009)*
    a. Hyperglycemia
    b. Hyperkalemia
    c. Hyperosmolar dehydration
    d. Azotemia

19. Which is best method for supplementing nutrition in patients who have undergone massive resection of the small intestine is? *(MCI Sept 2009)*
    a. Parenteral
    b. Enteral
    c. Gastrostomy
    d. All of the above

20. All of the following are complications in a patient on total parenteral nutrition except: *(MCI Sept 2008)*
    a. Hypercholesterolemia
    b. Hyperglycemia
    c. Hypotriglyceridemia
    d. Hypophosphatemia

21. Which of the following is the most common complication of TPN? *(Recent Question 2016)*
    a. Catheter related complications
    b. Acidosis
    c. Acaculous cholecystitis
    d. Hypokalemia

22. A patient on total parenteral nutrition for 20 days presents with weakness, vertigo and convulsions. Diagnosis is: *(All India 2000)*
    a. Hypomagnesemia
    b. Hyperammonemia
    c. Hypercalcemia
    d. Hyperkalemia

Others

23. **In IV hyperalimentation, we give:** *(PGI June 2002)*
    a. Hypertonic saline b. Fats
    c. Amino acids d. Dextrose
    e. LMW dextran

24. **Complication of TPN include:**
    a. Hyperglycemia b. Hyperkalemia
    c. Hyperosmolar dehydration
    d. Azotemia e. All of the above

25. **Albumin infusion for parenteral use is restricted because:**
    a. It is costly *(Recent Question 2015)*
    b. Carcinogenic
    c. Does not raise oncotic pressure
    d. All of the above

26. **Following TPN, one expects weight gain after:**
    (Recent Question 2016)
    a. 2 days b. 7 days
    c. 4 weeks d. 6 weeks

27. **The minimum amount of proteins needed for positive nitrogen balance is:** *(Recent Question 2016)*
    a. 20-30 gm/day b. 35-40 gm/day
    c. 50 gm/day d. 60 gm/day

28. **Deficiency of following elements is seen with hyperalimentation except:** *(JIPMER 93)*
    a. Calcium b. Phosphates
    c. Zinc d. Magnesium

29. **Following TPN, weight loss is seen:** *(Orissa 99)*
    a. Up to 7 days b. 7-10th day
    c. 10-15th day d. 15th day onwards

30. **TPN may be complicated by:**
    a. Obstructive jaundice b. Hyperosteosis
    c. Hypercalcemia d. Pancreatitis

31. **Complication of total parenteral nutrition is:**
    (Recent Question 2013)
    a. CHF b. Hypochloremia
    c. Metabolic acidosis d. Leukopenia

ELECTROLYTE ABNORMALITIES

32. **Chronic vomiting leads to all except:** *(PGI Nov 2011)*
    a. Hyponatremia b. Hypochloremia
    c. Metabolic alkalosis d. Metabolic acidosis
    e. Hypokalemia

33. **Hypokalemia with alkalosis is found in:** *(Orissa 2011)*
    a. Diarrhea
    b. Vomiting
    c. Ureterosigmoidostomy
    d. Villous adenoma of rectum

34. **Condition which does not cause metabolic acidosis:**
    a. Renal failure *(Recent Question 2016)*
    b. Ureterosigmoidostomy
    c. Pancreatic or biliary fistula
    d. Pyloric stenosis

35. **Following fistulous conditions give rise to maximum fluid and electrolyte imbalance:**
    a. Distal ileal b. Gastric
    c. Duodenal d. Sigmoid

36. **Highest concentration of potassium is seen in:** *(AIIMS 92)*
    a. Jejunum b. Ileum
    c. Duodenum d. Colon

37. **Most common cause of metabolic alkalosis is:** *(Karnataka 94)*
    a. Cancer stomach b. Pyloric stenosis
    c. Small-bowel obstruction d. Diuretics

38. **Hyponatremia in multiple myeloma is:** *(Kerala 95)*
    a. True b. Relative
    c. Absolute d. Pseudo

39. **All of the following are seen in persisting vomiting except:**
    (AIIMS Nov 99)
    a. Hypokalemia b. Decreased K⁺ in urine
    c. Elevated pH of blood d. Metabolic alkalosis

40. **After ureterosigmoidostomy which electrolyte abnormality may occur:** *(AIIMS June 99)*
    a. Hyperchloremic acidosis b. Metabolic alkalosis
    c. Metabolic acidosis d. Hypochloremic acidosis

41. **In post burn patient, true is:** *(AIIMS June 94)*
    a. Hypokalemic alkalosis b. Hyperkalemic alkalosis
    c. Hyperkalemic acidosis d. Hypokalemic acidosis

42. **Which of the following is not an important cause of hyponatremia?** *(All India 2004)*
    a. Gastric fistula
    b. Excessive vomiting
    c. Excessive sweating
    d. Prolonged Ryle's tube aspiration

43. **Metabolic changes associated with excessive vomiting includes the following:** *(All India 99)*
    a. Metabolic acidosis b. Hyperchloremia
    c. Hypokalemia d. Decreases bicarbonates

IV FLUIDS

44. **The highest concentration of potassium is in:**
    a. Plasma b. Isotonic saline
    c. Ringer lactate d. Darrow's solution

45. **Pitting edema indicates an excess of __litres of fluid in tissue spaces:**
    a. 2.5 b. 3.5
    c. 4.5 d. 5.5

46. **In patients depending entirely on parenteral fluids, there is weight loss of daily:**
    a. 50 gm b. 150 gm
    c. 200 gm d. 250 gm

47. **20 mEq (mmol) of potassium chloride in 500 ml of 5% dextrose solution is given intravenously to treat:**
    a. Metabolic alkalosis b. Respiratory alkalosis
    c. Metabolic acidosis d. Respiratory acidosis

48. **Haemacel contains:**
    a. Albumin b. Degraded gelatin
    c. Calcium d. Sodium

49. **In the immediate post operative period, body potassium is:**
    a. Exchanged with calcium
    b. Exchanged with magnesium
    c. Retained in body d. Excreted excessively

50. **Low molecular weight dextran is contra indicated in:**
    a. Fetal distress syndrome *(Recent Question 2016)*
    b. Cerebrovascular accident
    c. Electrical burns d. Thrombocytopenia

51. **C.V.P (Central Venous Pressure) and pulmonary wedge pressure give an accurate assessment of all the following except:** *(UPSC 95)*
    a. Tissue perfusion b. Volume depletion
    c. Volume overload d. Myocardial function

52. **10% dextrose is:** *(DNB 2005)*
    a. Isotonic
    b. Hypotonic
    c. Hypertonic
    d. None

53. **In a patient with multisystem trauma, the presence of hypotension along with elevated central venous pressure is suggestive of:** *(UPSC 97)*
    a. Upper airway obstruction
    b. Major abdominal bleed
    c. Cardiopulmonary problem
    d. Spinal cord injury

54. **Which of the following is the best method to assess the adequacy of replacement?** *(AIIMS 2000)*
    a. Decrease in thirst
    b. Increase in urine output
    c. Blood pressure
    d. Increased PaO_2

55. **In a person who has fasted for 5 days all are seen except:** *(AIIMS 98)*
    a. GH levels decreased
    b. Glucose tolerance decreased
    c. Immunoreactive insulin decreased
    d. Free fatty acids (Plasma) increased

56. **Content of Na+ in ringer lactate is mEq/L:** *(TN 99)*
    a. 154
    b. 12
    c. 130
    d. 144

57. **Fructose is not used in IV infusion as it cause:**
    a. Irritability
    b. Mental retardation
    c. Increased erythrocyte protoporphyrin
    d. Increased urinary coporoporphyrin

58. **Sodium content of one liter of isotonic saline is:** *(DNB 2011)*
    a. 140 mEq
    b. 154 mEq
    c. 40 mEq
    d. 70 mEq

59. **A postoperative patient with pH 7.25, MAP (mean arterial pressure) 60 mm Hg treated with:** *(PGI 2003)*
    a. IV sodium bicarbonate
    b. Only normal saline
    c. Fluid therapy with CVP monitoring
    d. Fluid restriction

60. **Most common cause of water intoxication in surgical patient is due to:** *(COMEDK 2005)*
    a. Colorectal wash with plain water
    b. Syndrome of inappropriate secretion of ADH
    c. Irrigation during transurethral resection of prostate
    d. Excessive infusion of 5% glucose

61. **A young man weighing 65 kg was admitted to the hospital with severe burns in a severe catabolic state. An individual in this state requires 40 kcal per kg body weight per day 1 gm of protein/kg body weight/day. This young man was given a solution containing 20% glucose and 4.25% protein. If 3000 ml of solution in infused per day:** *(AIIMS Nov 2003)*
    a. The patient would not be getting sufficient protein
    b. The calories supplied would be inadequate
    c. Both protein and calories would be adequate
    d. Too much protein is being infused

62. **After 30% loss of blood volume in road traffic accident. What is the next management?**
    a. IV fluids only
    b. IV fluids with cardiac stimulant
    c. Dopamine
    d. Vasopressor drug

63. **Which among the following is best method to assess intake of fluid in polytrauma patient?** *(PGI June 2006, AIIMS Nov 95, AIIMS Nov 94)*
    a. Urine output
    b. CVP
    c. Pulse
    d. BP

64. **Which of the following is hypertonic?** *(DNB 2009)*
    a. 5% dextrose
    b. 0.45% normal saline
    c. 0.9% normal saline
    d. 3% normal saline

65. **All electrolyte abnormalities are seen in immediate postoperative period, except:** *(AIIMS Nov 94)*
    a. Negative Nitrogen balance
    b. Hypokalemia
    c. Glucose intolerance
    d. Hyponatremia

66. **Blood loss during major surgery is best estimated by:** *(PGI June 99)*
    a. Visual assessment
    b. Suction bottles
    c. Transesophageal USG Doppler
    d. Cardiac output by thermodilution

67. **Concentration of sodium in RL is:** *(Recent Question 2013)*
    a. 154
    b. 120
    c. 130
    d. 144

68. **Which of the following is isotonic solution?** *(Recent Question 2017)*
    a. Half normal saline
    b. 1/5th normal saline
    c. Ringer lactate
    d. Dextrose in normal saline

MISCELLANEOUS

69. **The disadvantage of elemental diets in children include:**
    a. Hypertonic dehydration
    b. Lower caloric input
    c. Dumping syndrome
    d. High nitrogen input

70. **During nutritional assessment of a surgical patient, the status of muscle protein is indicated by which one of the following parameters:** *(UPSC 95)*
    a. Serum albumin
    b. Triceps skinfold thickness
    c. Mid-arm circumference
    d. Hb level

71. **Cortisol level returns to normal ____ after hemorrhage:**
    a. 2 weeks
    b. 10 days *(Orissa 98)*
    c. 7 days
    d. 3 days

72. **Body water content in percentage of body weight is lowest in:** *(Orissa 98)*
    a. Well-built man
    b. Fat woman
    c. Well nourished child
    d. Fat man

73. **Water content in infant:**
    a. 60-70%
    b. 75-80%
    c. 80-90%
    d. >90%

74. **Insensible daily water loss is:** *(Recent Question 2016)*
    a. 500-600 ml
    b. 800-1000 ml
    c. 1000-1500 ml
    d. 2000 ml

75. **Critical pH in Mendelson syndrome:** *(Orissa 2004)*
    a. 2.5
    b. 3.0
    c. 3.5
    d. 4.0

76. **The ideal colloidal solution is:** *(MHSSMCET 2005, MHPGMCET 2006)*
    a. Dextran
    b. Plasma
    c. Albumin
    d. Hydroxyethyl starch

77. **Skin fold thickness (for assessment of nutritional status) can be measured at all the following except:** *(MHSSMCET 2006)*
    a. Biceps
    b. Triceps
    c. Suprailiac region
    d. None

78. **In surgical patient malnutrition is best assessed by:**
    a. Serum albumin *(Recent Question 2013)*
    b. Hb level
    c. Mid arm circumference
    d. Triceps skin fold thickness

Explanations

ENTERAL NUTRITION

1. **Ans. b. Ear lobe to the umbilicus**

   - **Feeding tube length** is measured by following the normal route for the tube (**Nasal ala → To ear lobe → To epigastrium**)^Q
   - The distance between the nasal ala and ear lobe is almost equal to the distance between the epigastrium and umbilicus, the length can be measured from **ear lobe to umbilicus**^{Q}.

2. **Ans. a. Jejunostomy tube feeding** *(Ref: Sabiston 20/e p112; Bailey 27/e p284-286)*

   Unless the GI tract is nonfunctional, its use for nutritional support is preferable as compared to TPN. In a patient who is **comatose** either **NG feeding** or **feeding through a gastrostomy tube** may lead to **vomiting** and **aspiration**. This can be **avoided by using a nasoenteric tube** with the **tip placed in jejunum** under fluoroscopic guidance or endoscopic control. Alternatively, a **catheter may be placed directly into the proximal jejunum** through a small upper abdominal incision.

3. **Ans. a. Intestinal obstruction, b. Severe pancreatitis, c. Severe diarrhea, e. Intestinal fistula**

4. **Ans. c. Feeding jejunostomy** *(Ref: Essentials of General Surgery by Lawrence 4/e p80)*

   - A **feeding jejunostomy** is the **preferred procedure to provide supplementary nutrition** in this patient as it **provides protection to the pancreatic anastomosis** and cause **minimal stimulation of pancreatic secretion** thereby **giving rest to the pancreas**^{Q}.
   - After pancreatic surgery, TPN should or only be used when there is intolerance to enteral nutrition or enteral nutrition is contraindicated^Q.
   - Pancreatic surgery does not usually interfere with the function of the gastrointestinal tract and enteral route remains the preferred mode for providing nutrition.

Operations where Early Oral Feeding is not Recommended	

• Major surgery involving upper GI tract:
   – Esophageal resection^Q
   – Gastric resection^Q
	• Major Hepatic Surgery^Q
	• **Major Pancreatic Surgery**^{Q}

5. **Ans. a. Constipation, b. Diarrhea, c. Aspiration pneumonia** *(Ref: Sabiston 20/e p117; Bailey 27/e p286)*

6. **Ans. c. IBD**

7. **Ans. c. Retraction method** *(Ref: Sabiston 20/e p115)*

TOTAL PARENTERAL NUTRITION

8. **Ans. e. Pancreatitis** *(Ref: Sabiston 20/e p118; Bailey 27/e p286)*

9. **Ans. a. Folic acid, b. Iron, c. Vitamin B12, d. Copper, e. Fatty acids** *(Ref: Sabiston 20/e p121; Bailey 27/e p288)*

10. **Ans. d. Fibers** *(Ref: Bailey 27/e p286)*

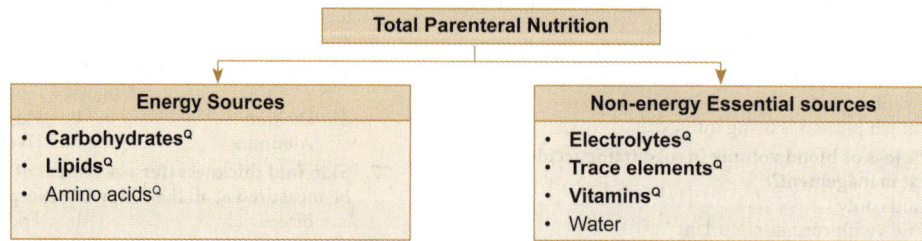

11. **Ans. a. Hypoglycemia, b. Hyperglycemia, c. Hypercalcemia, d. Hypercapnia, e. Hypophosphatemia**

12. **Ans. a. Subclavian vein** *(Ref: Sabiston 20/e p118; Bailey 27/e p287)*

    - **Preferred** site for **central vein infusion: SVC**^{Q}
    - **Preferred access site** for **TPN: Subclavian**^{Q} > **Jugular** > **Femoral vein**

Fluid, Electrolyte and Nutrition

13. Ans. c. Chronic liver disease
14. Ans. c. Sepsis
15. Ans. d. Lipids form 20% of energy source *(Ref: Sabiston 20/e p119)*
16. Ans. d. Hyperphosphatemia
17. Ans. c. Congestive cardiac failure
18. Ans. None *(Ref: CSDT 12/e p161)*
19. Ans. a. Parenteral
20. Ans. c. Hypotriglyceridemia
21. Ans. a. Catheter related complications

- MC complication of central venous catheterization (CVC): Catheter related sepsis[Q]
- Most dangerous complication following CVC: Pneumothorax[Q]

22. Ans. a. Hypomagnesemia *(Ref: Harrison 19/e p88-97)*

Clinical Features

Hypomagnesemia	Hyperkalemia	Hypercalcemia
• **Weakness**, muscle cramps and **tremors**[Q] • **Marked neuromuscular** and **CNS hyperirritability** with jerking and **nystagmus**[Q]	• Interferes with neuromuscular function to produce muscle **weakness** which may progress to **flaccid paralysis**[Q] and **hypoventilation** if respiratory muscles are involved	• **Fatigue, depression, mental confusion**, lethargy[Q] • Anorexia, nausea, **vomiting, constipation and polyuria**[Q]

23. Ans. b. Fats, c. Amino acids, d. Dextrose
24. Ans. e. All of the above
25. Ans. a. It is costly
26. Ans. b. 7 days
27. Ans. d. 60 gm/day
28. Ans. None
29. Ans. a. Up to 7 days
30. Ans. c. Hypercalcemia
31. Ans. c. Metabolic acidosis

ELECTROLYTE ABNORMALITIES

32. Ans. d. Metabolic acidosis *(Ref: Sabiston 20/e p1869, 1205; Schwartz 10/e p73-75, 1599; Bailey 25/e p1065)*

- Chronic vomiting leads to **Hypochloremic, hypokalemic, metabolic alkalosis.**

33. Ans. b. Vomiting *(Ref: Harrison 19/e p320)*

CAUSES OF HIGH ANION–GAP METABOLIC ACIDOSIS

- Lactic acidosis[Q]
- Ketoacidosis[Q] (Diabetic, Alcoholic, Starvation)
- Toxins **(Ethylene glycol, Methanol, Salicylates,** Propylene glycol, Pyroglutamic acid)[Q]
- Renal failure[Q] (acute and chronic)

34. Ans. d. Pyloric stenosis
35. Ans. c. Duodenal *(Ref: Sabiston 20/e p1287)*

ENTEROCUTANEOUS FISTULAS

- **Enterocutaneous fistulas** are classified according to their **location and volume of daily output.**
- These factors **dictate both treatment** and **morbidity** and **mortality rates**[Q].
- In general, the **more proximal** the fistula in the **'intestine'** (but **not** the **stomach**), the **more serious the problem**, with **greater fluid and electrolyte loss**[Q].

- Maximum fluid and electrolyte imbalance occur in duodenal fistulas[Q].

36. Ans. d. Colon *(Ref: Schwartz 10/e p69; Bailey 27/e p281)*

- Maximum K+ concentration: Colon[Q] (30 mEq/L) >Saliva (25 mEq/L)

Composition of GI Secretions					
Type of Secretion	Volume (mL/day)	Na (mEq/L)	K (mEq/L)	Cl (mEq/L)	HCO_3^- (mEq/L)
Stomach	1000–2000[Q]	60–90	10–30	100–130[Q]	0
Small intestine	2000–3000[Q]	120–140	5–10	90–120	30–40

Contd...

Contd…

Type of Secretion	Volume (mL/day)	Na (mEq/L)	K (mEq/L)	Cl (mEq/L)	HCO_3^- (mEq/L)
Colon	—	60	30^Q	40	0
Pancreas	600–800^Q	135–145^Q	5–10	70–90	95–115^Q
Bile	300–800^Q	135–145^Q	5–10	90–110	30–40

37. Ans. b. Pyloric stenosis
38. Ans. d. Pseudo *(Ref: Harrison 19/e p714)*

PSEUDOHYPONATREMIA

- Patients with **multiple myeloma** also have a **decreased anion gap** [i.e., $Na^+ - (Cl^- + HCO_3^-)$] because the **M component** is **cationic**, resulting in **retention of chloride**^{Q}.
- This is **often accompanied by hyponatremia** that is felt to be artificial (**Pseudohyponatremia**) because **each volume of serum has less water** as a **result of the increased protein**^{Q}.

39. Ans. b. Decreased K$^+$ in urine
40. Ans. a. Hyperchloremic acidosis
41. Ans. c. Hyperkalemic acidosis
42. Ans. c. Excessive sweating
43. Ans. c. Hypokalemia

IV FLUIDS

44. Ans. d. Darrow's solution *(Ref: Bailey 27/e p281; www.idruginfo.com/?cat=drug...Darrow's%20Solution)*
45. Ans. c. 4.5
46. Ans. b. 150 g
47. Ans. a. Metabolic alkalosis
48. Ans. b. Degraded gelatin
49. Ans. d. Excreted excessively

- In **immediate post-operative period** due to **increased adrenocortical activity**, there is **Na+ retention and K+ excretion**^{Q}.

50. Ans. d. Thrombocytopenia

- **Dextran interferes with platelet function**^{Q}.

51. Ans. a. Tissue perfusion *(Ref: Sabiston 20/e p555, 52; Bailey 27/e p17)*

- **Urine output** is **best clinical guide of tissue perfusion**^{Q}.

52. Ans. c. Hypertonic
53. Ans. c. Cardiopulmonary problem
54. Ans. b. Increase in urine output
55. Ans. a. GH levels decreased
56. Ans. c. 130
57. None
58. Ans. b. 154 mEq
59. Ans. c. Fluid therapy with CVP monitoring
60. Ans. d. Excessive infusion of 5% glucose
61. Ans. c. Both protein and calories would be adequate *(Ref: Sabiston 20/e p119; Bailey 27/e p282)*

- Calories are calculated by catabolism of glucose (not proteins).

Glucose:
- Amount of glucose in 20% glucose in 3000 ml of solution: 3000 × 20/100 = 600 gms
- 1 gm glucose on catabolism produces: 4.2 kcal
- 600 gms of glucose would produce: 600 × 4.2 = 2520 kcal

Protein:
- Percentage of protein in fluid: 4.25%
- Percentage of protein in 3000 ml of fluid: 3000 × 4.25/100 = 127.5 gms
- Calories required for the patient: 40×65 = 2600 kcal
- Proteins required for the patient: 2 ×65 = 130 gms

	Required Amount	Supplied by Solution
Calories	2600 kcal	2520 kcal
Proteins	130 gms	127.5 gm

Fluid, Electrolyte and Nutrition

62. Ans. a. IV fluids only *(Ref: Sabiston 20/e p553)*
63. Ans. a. Urine output
64. Ans. d. 3% normal saline *(Ref: Fluids and Electrolytes by Lippincott Williams and Wilkins/55)*

Isotonic	Hypertonic	Hypotonic
Dextrose 5% in water	5% dextrose in half normal saline	0.45 normal saline
0.9% normal saline	5% dextrose in normal saline	
Ringer lactate	Dextrose 10% in water	

65. Ans. d. Hyponatremia
66. Ans. b. Suction bottles *(Ref: www.ncbi.nlm.nih.gov/pubmed/16756621)*

Measurement of Blood Loss during Surgery (Gravimetric Method)

- Blood loss during operation is measured by: **Weighing the swabs** after use and subtracting the dry weight and fluid used + **volume of blood collected in suction bottles** (after subtracting irrigating fluid)^Q

67. Ans. c. 130
68. Ans. c. Ringer lactate *(Ref: Schwartz 10/e p76)*

MISCELLANEOUS

69. Ans. a. Hypertonic dehydration, c. Dumping syndrome
70. Ans. c. Mid-arm circumference *(Ref:www.ncbi.nlm.nih.gov/pubmed/1492750)*

Anthropometric Techniques for Nutritional Assessment

- Anthropometric techniques incorporating measurements of **skinfold thicknesses** and **mid-arm circumference** permit estimations of **body fat** and **muscle mass**, and these are **indirect measures of energy** and **protein stores**.

  - **Skinfold thickness** is measured at **ulnar, triceps, subscapular** and **suprailiac region**^{Q}.

71. Ans. d. 3 days *(Ref: adc.bmj.com/content/50/7/555.full.pdf)*

- **The normal** rise in **cortisol** secretion **after** surgery lasts about **3 days.**

72. Ans. b. Fat woman
73. Ans. b. 75-80% *(Ref: Sabiston 20/e p48; Bailey 27/e p280)*
74. Ans. b. 800-1000 mL *(Ref: Bailey 25/e p226)*
75. Ans. a. 2.5 *(Ref: Sabiston 19/e p293)*

Mendelson's Syndrome

- **Critical pH value: 2.5**^{Q}
- **Gastric pH** of 2.5 or less with a **gastric** contents volume greater than **25 ml** are **critical values**^{Q}.
- **Maximum pulmonary damage** is achieved at an aspirate **pH value of 1.5.**

76. Ans. c. Albumin
77. Ans. d. None
78. Ans. c. Mid arm circumference *(Ref: Sabiston 20/e p562)*

CHAPTER 49

Blood Transfusion

TRANSFUSION PROTOCOL

TRANSFUSION PROTOCOLS

- BT should commence within **30 minutes** or removing blood bag from refrigerators because of increased risk of bacterial contamination[Q]
- **Whole blood or packed RBC** transfusion must be completed **within 4 hours**[Q]
- **Platelet and FFP** transfusion should be completed within **20 minutes**[Q]
- **Transfusion set** should have standard filter of **170 μm size**[Q]
- Usual **transfusion needle** size should be of **18-19 gauge**[Q]

CHARACTERISTICS OF SELECTED BLOOD COMPONENETS

Characteristics of Selected Blood Components

Component	Volume (mL)	Content	Clinical Response
Whole Blood	450 ml ± 45	• No elements removed • Contains **RBCs, WBCs, plasma** and **platelets** (**WBCs** and **platelets** may be **non-functional**[Q])	• Not for routine use • Used for **acute massive bleeding, open heart surgery** and neonatal total exchange
Packed RBCs	180–200	• **RBCs** with variable **leukocyte** content and **small** amount of **plasma**	• Increase **Hb 1 gm/dL** and **hematocrit 3%**[Q]
Platelets	50–70	• 5.5×10^{10}/RD unit	• Increase platelet count **5000–10,000/μL**[Q]
FFP	200–250	• **Plasma proteins**: Coagulation factors, proteins C and S, antithrombin[Q]	• Increases **coagulation factors about 2%**
Cryoprecipitate	10–15	• Cold-insoluble plasma proteins, **fibrinogen, factor VIII, vWF**[Q]	• Topical fibrin glue, also **80 IU factor VIII**[Q]

ANTICOAGULANTS

Whole Blood

Anticoagulant used	Maximum storage
ACD/CPD/CP2D	21 days[Q]
CPDA-1 (citrate phosphate dextrose adenine)	35 days[Q]
SAGM (saline adenine glucose mannitol)	42 days[Q]

Actions of Ingredients of anticoagulant solution

Glucose	• ATP generation by glycolysis[Q]
Adenine	• Synthesis of ATP[Q] • Increases shelf life of RBC to 42 days[Q]
Citrate	• Prevents coagulation by chelating calcium[Q]
Sodium diphosphate	• Maintain optimum pH[Q]

MASSIVE BLOOD TRANSFUSION

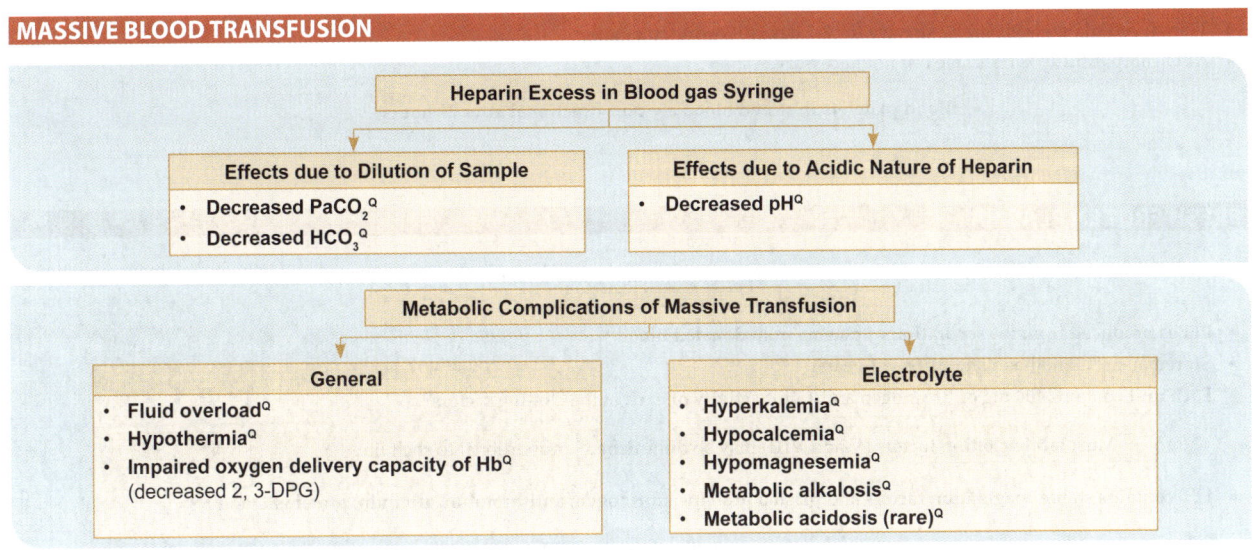

COMPLICATIONS OF BLOOD TRANSFUSION

Complications of Blood Transfusion

Reactions
- Febrile non-hemolytic transfusion reaction (**FNHTR**): **MC**^{Q}
- Allergic
- **Delayed hemolytic**^{Q}
- Transfusion-related acute lung injury (**TRALI**)^Q
- **Acute hemolytic**^{Q}
- Fatal hemolytic
- Anaphylactic

Infections
- Hepatitis **B** and **C**^{Q}
- Hepatitis **G**^{Q}
- **HIV-1 and -2**^{Q}
- **HTLV-I and -II**^{Q}
- Malaria^Q
- **West Nile virus**^{Q}
- **Parvovirus B-19**^{Q}
- **HHV-8**^{Q}
- CMV^Q

Other Complications
- RBC allosensitization^Q
- HLA allosensitization^Q
- Graft-versus-host disease

RED BLOOD CELLS

RED BLOOD CELLS

- RBCs are stored at 1-6°C^Q; Mean life of transfused RBCs is 35 days^Q.

Anticoagulant used	Maximum storage
ACD/CPD/CP2D	21 days^Q
CPDA-1	35 days^Q

PLATELETS

PLATELET CONCENTRATES

- **Volume: 50 ml**^{Q}
- Platelets are the **only blood products** which are **stored at room temperature, 20-24°C**^{Q} (survival is 4-5 days)^Q.
- **1 unit of platelet** increases the count by **5000-10000**^{Q}.

> - The threshold for prophylactic platelet transfusion is 10,000/μL^Q.
> - For invasive procedures, 50,000/μL platelets is the usual target level.
> - Platelet count should be 1,00,000/μL before accepting the patient for surgery.

- **Transfused platelets** generally **survive for 2-7 days** following transfusion.
- **ABO compatibility** is desirable but **not necessary**.

> - **Blood platelets in stored blood** are non-functional after 24 hours^Q.

FRESH FROZEN PLASMA

FRESH-FROZEN PLASMA (FFP)

- **FFP** is produced from the **separation of plasma** from **donated blood**^{Q}.
- Stored at **-18°C** and has a **shelf life** of **1 year**^{Q}.
- **Each unit** contains **400 mg of fibrinogen** and **1 unit activity of each** of the **clotting factors**^{Q}.

> - Most labile clotting factors (**V** and **VIII**) may be **diminished**^{Q} proportional to shelf life.

- **FFP contains stable coagulation factors** and **plasma proteins**: fibrinogen, antithrombin, albumin, proteins C and S^Q.

Indications for FFP	
• **Correction of coagulopathies:** – **Rapid reversal of warfarin**^{Q} – Supplying deficient plasma proteins^Q	• Treatment of **thrombotic thrombocytopenic purpura**^{Q}

- Patients who are **IgA-deficient** and **require plasma support** should receive **FFP from IgA-deficient donors** to prevent anaphylaxis.

> - **FFP should not be** routinely **used to expand blood volume**^{Q}.
> - **FFP:** An **acellular component** and **does not transmit intracellular infections**, e.g., CMV.

CRYOPRECIPITATE

CRYOPRECIPITATE

- **Cryoprecipitate** is a source of **fibrinogen**^{Q}, **factor VIII**^{Q} and **von Willebrand factor (vWF)**^{Q}.
- It is **ideal for supplying fibrinogen** to the volume-sensitive patient.
- Stored at ≤-18°C

> - **1 unit** of cryoprecipitate contains **80-145 units of Factor VIII and 250 mg of fibrinogen**^{Q}.
> - Cryoprecipitate is **pooled from many donors**, so there are **maximum chances of disease transmission** among all blood products^Q.

- Cryoprecipitate may also **supply vWF** to patients with **dysfunctional (type II)** or **absent (type III) von Willebrand disease**.

DEXTRAN

DEXTRAN

- It is a **polysaccharide polymer** of varying molecular weight producing an **osmotic pressure** similar to the plasma
- **Disadvantages:**
  - It induces **rouleaux of RBCs** and this **interferes with blood grouping** and **cross matching**^{Q} procedures, hence need for a blood sample beforehand.
  - It **interferes with platelet function**, hence it is recommended that **total volume** of dextran **should not exceed 1000 mL**.

> - **LMW dextran (short acting)** prevents sludging of RBCs in vessels and **renal shut down in severe hypotension** and it is **less likely to induce rouleaux formation** than HMW dextran (long acting).

Multiple Choice Questions

BLOOD TRANSFUSION

1. MC blood transfusion reaction is: *(All India 2008)*
   a. Febrile non-hemolytic transfusion reaction
   b. Hemolysis
   c. Transmission of infections
   d. Electrolyte imbalance

2. All of the following infections may be transmitted via blood transfusion, except: *(AIIMS May 2009, All India 2002)*
   a. Parvo B-19
   b. Hepatitis G
   c. Dengue virus
   d. Cytomegalovirus

3. Which of the following is the least likely complication after massive blood transfusion? *(AIIMS May 2009)*
   a. Hyperkalemia
   b. Citrate toxicity
   c. Hypothermia
   d. Metabolic acidosis

4. Fresh hold blood transfusion is done with in how much time of collection? *(DNB 2006)*
   a. Immediately
   b. 1 hours
   c. 4 hours
   d. 24 hours

5. Which of the following investigations should be done immediately to best confirm a non matched blood transfusion reaction? *(All India 2010)*
   a. Indirect Coomb's test
   b. Direct Coomb's test
   c. Antibody in patient's serum
   d. Antibody in donor serum

6. Blood components products are: *(PGI Dec 2005)*
   a. Whole blood
   b. Platelets
   c. Fresh frozen plasma
   d. Leukocyte reduced RBC
   e. All of the above

7. A man is rushed to casualty, nearly dying after a massive blood loss in an accident. There is not much time to match blood groups, so the physician decides to order for one of the following blood groups. Which one of the following blood groups should the physician decide: *(AIIMS June 2004)*
   a. O negative
   b. O positive
   c. AB positive
   d. AB negative

8. One unit of fresh blood arises the Hb% concentration by: *(All India 2003, DNB 2012)*
   a. 0.1 gm%
   b. 1 gm%
   c. 2 gm%
   d. 2.2 gm%

9. Which of the following statements about acute hemolytic blood transfusion reaction is true? *(PGI June 2004)*
   a. Complement mediated hemolysis is seen
   b. Type III hypersensitivity is responsible for most cases
   c. Rarely life threatening
   d. Renal blood flow is always maintained
   e. No need for stopping transfusion

10. True about blood transfusions: *(PGI June 98)*
    a. Antigen 'D' determines Rh positivity
    b. Febrile reaction is due to HLA antigens
    c. Anti-d is naturally occurring antibody
    d. Cryoprecipitate contains all coagulation factors

11. Which of the following is better indicator of need for transfusion? *(Recent Question 2016)*
    a. Urine output
    b. Hematocrit
    c. Colour of skin
    d. Clinical examination

12. Massive blood transfusion is defined as: *(PGI 95)*
    a. 350 ml in 5 min
    b. 500 ml in 5 min
    c. 1 litre in 5 min
    d. Whole blood volume

13. How long can blood stored with CPDA? *(JIPMER 2003)*
    a. 12 days
    b. 21 days
    c. 28 days
    d. 48 days

14. Storage period of 35 days for blood is seen with: *(AIIMS November 2017)*
    a. CPD
    b. CPDA-1
    c. ACD
    d. CP2D

15. Massive transfusion in previous healthy adult male can cause hemorrhage due to: *(PGI 98)*
    a. Increased t-PA
    b. Dilutional thrombocytopenia
    c. Vitamin K deficiency
    d. Decreased fibrinogen

16. Arterial blood gas analysis in a bottle containing heparin causes a decrease in value of:
    a. pCO_2
    b. HCO_3
    c. pH
    d. All of the above

17. Massive blood transfusion is defined as: *(Recent Question 2013)*
    a. Whole blood volume in 24 hours
    b. Half blood volume in 24 hours
    c. 40% blood volume in 24 hours
    d. 60% blood volume in 24 hours

BLOOD TRANSFUSION COMPLICATIONS

18. After blood transfusion the febrile non-hemolytic transfusion reaction (FNHTR) occurs due to?
    a. Alloimmunization
    b. Antibodies against donor leukocytes and HLA Ag
    c. Allergic reaction
    d. Anaphylaxis

19. Blood grouping and cross-matching is must prior to infusion of: *(MHPGMCET 2007)*
    a. Gelatin
    b. Dextran
    c. Albumin
    d. FFP

20. Blood grouping and cross matching is must prior to infusion of: *(MHPGMCET 2008)*
    a. Gelatin
    b. Albumin
    c. Dextran
    d. Hemaceal

21. Collection of blood for cross matching and grouping is done before administration of which plasma expander? *(MHSSMCET 2007)*
    a. Hydroxyl ethyl starch
    b. Dextran
    c. Mannitol
    d. Hemacele

22. Mismatched blood transfusion in anesthetic patient presents is: *(PGI June 2000)*
    a. Hyperthermia and hypertension
    b. Hypotension and bleeding from site of wound
    c. Bradycardia and hypertension
    d. Tachycardia and hypertension

23. All of the following are major complications of massive transfusion except: *(All India 2006)*
    a. Hypokalemia
    b. Hypothermia
    c. Hypomagnesaemia
    d. Hypocalcaemia

24. Massive transfusions results in: *(Recent Question 2016)*
    a. DIC
    b. Hypothermia
    c. Hypercalcemia
    d. Thrombocytopenia

RED BLOOD CELLS

25. The maximum life of a transfused RBC is: *(Recent Question 2016)*
    a. One hour
    b. One day
    c. 15 days
    d. 50 days

PLATELETS

26. Platelets can be stored at: *(AIIMS Nov 2005)*
    a. 20-24°C for 5 days
    b. 20-24°C for 8 days
    c. 4-8°C for 5 days
    d. 4-8°C for 8 days

27. Blood platelets in stored blood do not remain functional after: *(Recent Question 2016)*
    a. 24 hours
    b. 48 hours
    c. 72 hours
    d. 96 hours

28. In a patient with thrombocytopenia, what is the target platelet count after transfusion to perform an invasive procedure? *(AIIMS May 2015)*
    a. 30,000
    b. 40,000
    c. 50,000
    d. 60,000

PLASMA

29. Indication of fresh frozen plasma is/are: *(PGI Nov 2011)*
    a. Hypovolemia
    b. Nutritional supplement
    c. Coagulation factor deficiency
    d. Warfarin toxicity
    e. Hypoalbuminemia

30. True about FFP (Fresh frozen plasma) is the following except: *(MHPGMCET 2009)*
    a. Good source of all coagulation factors
    b. Prepared from single unit of blood
    c. Coagulation factor levels are equal to Plasma
    d. None of the above

31. Stored plasma is deficient in: *(Recent Question 2016)*
    a. Factors 7 and 8
    b. Factors 2 and 5
    c. Factors 5 and 8
    d. Factors 7 and 9

32. With reference to fresh frozen plasma (FFP), which one of the following statement is not correct? *(UPSC 2008)*
    a. It is used as volume expander
    b. It is stored at – 40°C to – 50°C
    c. It is a source of coagulation factors
    d. It is given in a dose of 12-15 ml/kg body weight

33. In cholecystectomy, fresh frozen plasma should be given: *(UPPG 2008)*
    a. Just before operation
    b. At the time of operation
    c. 6 hours before operation
    d. 12 hours after operation

34. Half life of factor VIII is: *(Recent Question 2016)*
    a. 4 hours
    b. 8 hours
    c. 34 hours
    d. 48 hours

35. Rosenthal's syndrome is seen in deficiency of factor:
    a. II
    b. V
    c. IX
    d. XI *(DNB 91)*

36. Best blood product to be given in a patient of multiple clotting factor deficiency with active bleeding:
    a. Whole blood *(AIIMS May 2015)*
    b. Packed RBCs
    c. Fresh frozen plasma
    d. Cryoprecipitate

CRYOPRECIPITATE

37. Cryoprecipitate contains: *(MCI March 2009)*
    a. Factor II
    b. Factor V
    c. Factor VIII
    d. Factor IX

38. Cryoprecipitate is a rich source of: *(Recent Question 2016)*
    a. Thromboplastin
    b. Factor VIII
    c. Factor X
    d. Factor VII

39. Which one of the following blood fractions is stored at -40°C? *(UPSC 2006)*
    a. Cryoprecipitate
    b. Human albumin
    c. Platelet concentrate
    d. Packed red cells

40. Cryoprecipitate contains all except: *(MHCET 2016, AIIMS Nov 2007)*
    a. Factor VIII
    b. Factor IX
    c. Fibrinogen
    d. VWF

Explanations

BLOOD TRANSFUSION

1. Ans. a. Febrile non-hemolytic transfusion reaction *(Ref: Harrison 19/e p138e-3, 18/e p954-956)*
2. Ans. c. Dengue virus
3. Ans. d. Metabolic acidosis *(Ref: Harrison 19/e p138e-3, 18/e p954-956)*
4. Ans. d. 24 hours
5. Ans. b. Direct Coomb's test *(Ref: Harrison 19/e p138e-4, 18/e p954)*
6. Ans. e. All of the above *(Ref: Harrison 19/e p138e-2, 18/e p952-954)*
7. Ans. a. O negative *(Ref: Harrison, 19/e p138 e-1, 18/e p951; Bailey 27/e p21-22, 26/e p21-22, 25/e p21-22)*
8. Ans. b. 1 gm%
9. Ans. a. Complement mediated hemolysis is seen *(Ref: Harrison 19/e p138e-3, 18/e p954)*
10. Ans. a. Antigen 'D' determines Rh positivity; b. Febrile reaction is due to HLA antigens *(Ref: Harrison 19/e p138e-1, 138e-4, 18/e p954)*
11. Ans. b. Hematocrit
12. Ans. d. Whole blood volume
13. Ans. c. 28 days *(Ref: Sabiston 19/e p588)*
14. Ans. b. CPDA-1 *(Ref: Wintrobe's 13/e p1278)*
15. Ans. b. Dilutional thrombocytopenia
16. Ans. d. All of the above *(Ref: Clinical Laboratory Medicine 6/e p396)*
17. Ans. a. i.e., Whole blood volume in 24 hours

BLOOD TRANSFUSION COMPLICATIONS

18. Ans. b. Antibodies against donor leukocytes and HLA Ag
19. Ans. b. Dextran
20. Ans. c. Dextran
21. Ans. b. Dextran
22. Ans. b. Hypotension and bleeding from site of wound *(Ref: Schwartz 10/e p119,122,171-172, 9/e p83)*
23. Ans. a. Hypokalemia
24. Ans. a. DIC; b. Hypothermia; d. Thrombocytopenia

RED BLOOD CELLS

25. Ans. d. 50 days *(Ref: Schwartz 10/e p1914-1915, 9/e p78; Bailey 27/e p21, 26/e p21, 25/e p21)*

PLATELETS

26. Ans. a. 20-24°C for 5 days *(Ref: Harrison 18/e p953; Sabiston 19/e p588; Schwartz 10/e p85, 9/e p79; Bailey 27/e p21, 26/e p21)*
27. Ans. a. 24 hours
28. Ans. c. (50,000) *(Bailey 26/e p23; Nelson 20/e p2374)*

PLASMA

29. Ans. c. Coagulation factor deficiency; d. Warfarin toxicity *(Ref: Harrison 19/e p138e-3, 18/e p953; Sabiston 19/e p588)*
30. Ans. a. Good source of all coagulation factors
31. Ans. c. Factors 5 and 8
32. Ans. a. It is used as volume expander
33. Ans. a. Just before operation
34. Ans. b. 8 hours
35. Ans. d. XI *(Ref: http://en.wikipedia.org/wiki/Haemophilia_C)*
36. Ans. c. Fresh frozen plasma *(Harrison 19/e p138 e-3, 18/e p953; Sabiston 20/e p568, 19th/e p588)*

CRYOPRECIPITATE

37. Ans. c. Factor VIII *(Ref: Harrison 18/e p953; Sabiston 19/e p588; Schwartz 10/e p73-75,1599, 9/e p82; Bailey 26/e p21, 25/e p21)*
38. Ans. b. Factor VIII
39. Ans. a. Cryoprecipitate
40. Ans. b. Factor IX

CHAPTER 50

Shock

SHOCK

Shock

- Shock is a **clinical syndrome resulting from inadequate tissue perfusion**
- Shock is MC cause of death among surgical patients[Q]

Classification of Shock	
1. **Hypovolemic**[Q] (MC type)	4. Septic: **Hyperdynamic**[Q] (early) & **Hypodynamic**[Q] (late)
2. Traumatic	5. Neurogenic
3. Cardiogenic	6. Hypoadrenal

Monitoring in Shock
1. The best management of shock is done by putting pulmonary catheter. **PCWP is considered better guide than CVP for fluid titrations**[Q] as it can also determine left ventricular preload.
2. **Invasive arterial pressure** is **mandatory**[Q].
3. **Blood gas analysis**[Q]. There is **metabolic acidosis** in shock.
4. **Mixed venous oxygen saturation** is considered as **best guide for tissue perfusion** (i.e. cardiac output)
5. **Urine output** is **best clinical guide of tissue perfusion**[Q].

HYPOVOLEMIC SHOCK

Hypovolemic Shock

- MC type of shock[Q]
- Causes of **hypovolemic shock**:
  - **Blood loss**[Q] (Trauma, bleeding)
  - **Loss of plasma** due to **extravascular fluid seqestration in burns**[Q]
  - **Loss of body sodium & water** (diarrhea & vomiting[Q])

Pathophysiology of Hypovolemic Shock
• ↓ Intravascular volume → ↓ Venous return → ↓ Ventricular filling → ↓ Stroke volume → ↓ Cardiac output → Inadequate tissue perfusion & compensatory mechanism activation[Q]
• Inadequate tissue perfusion → Cold clammy skin; Oliguria → anuria; Drowsiness & confusion[Q]
• Inadequate tissue perfusion → Lactic acidosis[Q] → Metabolic acidosis[Q] → Tachypnea[Q]
• Compensatory mechanism activation[Q] → Sympathetic stimulation[Q] (↑Adrenaline & ↑Noradrenaline)

Sympathetic stimulation (↑ Adrenaline & ↑ Noradrenaline)	
• **Tachycardia**[Q] (↑Pulse rate)	• **Sweating**[Q]
• **Weak or thready pulse** (↑Total peripheral resistance)	• **Initially maintained BP** followed by **hypotension**

Four Classes of Hemorrhagic Shock (According to the ATLS course)

Parameter	Class I	Class II	Class III	Class IV
Blood loss (%)	0-15^Q	15-30^Q	30-40^Q	>40^Q
CNS	**Slightly** anxious	**Mildly** anxious	**Anxious** or confused	Confused or **lethargic**
Pulse (beats/min)	<100	>100	>120	>140
Blood pressure	Normal	Normal	Decreased^Q	Decreased^Q
Pulse pressure	Normal	Decreased	Decreased^Q	Decreased^Q
Respiratory rate	14-20/min	20-30/min	30-40/min^Q	>35/min^Q
Urine (mL/hr)	>30	20-30	5-15	Negligible^Q
Fluid	Crystalloid^Q	Crystalloid^Q	Crystalloid + blood^Q	Crystalloid + blood^Q
Base deficit	0 to –2 mEq/L	–2 to –6 mEq/L	–6 to –10 mEq/L	–10 mEq/L or less

Clinical Features
- History of trauma, bleeding, burns, diarrhea & vomiting

Class I	Class II	Class III	Class IV
• Compensatory mechanism maintains cardiac output • **Compensated hypovolemic shock**^{Q}	• Hypoxemia^Q • Hypotension^Q • Generalized vasoconstriction • Urine output: 20-30 mL/hour	• **Decompensated shock**^{Q} (↓ CO, ↓ SBP) • Hypotension^Q • Tachycardia^Q (PR >120/min) • Tachypnea^Q • Urine output: 5-15 mL/hour^Q • Patient is **confused**^{Q}	• **Refractory stage**^{Q} • Marked hypotension^Q • Tachycardia & tachypnea^Q • No urine output^Q • Patient is **comatose**^{Q}

CARDIOGENIC SHOCK

Cardiogenic Shock

- Impaired ability of the heart to pump blood

Causes of Cardiogenic Shock

Systolic dysfunction	• Myocardial infarction^Q • Myocardial depressants: Beta-blockers, calcium channel blockers, anti-arrhythmic
Diastolic dysfunction	• Ventricular hypertrophy^Q; Restrictive cardiomyopathy^Q; Cardiac tamponade^Q
Increased after load	• Aortic stenoses^Q; Malignant hypertension^Q
Valvular structural abnormalities	• Papillary muscle rupture^Q • Aortic & mitral regurgitation^Q
Arrhythmias^Q	• Ventricular tachyarrhythmia

Pathophysiology of Cardiogenic Shock

- **Impaired pumping ability of left ventricle** → ↓ Stroke volume & inadequate systolic emptying
- ↓ Stroke volume → ↓ Cardiac output → ↓ BP → ↓ Tissue perfusion^Q
- Inadequate systolic emptying → ↑ Left ventricular filling pressure (↑ preload) → ↑ Left atrial pressure → ↑ Pulmonary artery & capillary pressure → Pulmonary edema^Q

Clinical Features
- Clinical features vary depending on the cause:
  - Signs of myocardial failure: ↑ JVP, reduced pulse volume, hypotension, tachycardia, basal coarse crackles^Q
  - Obstructive (cardiac tamponade): Muffled heart sounds, pulsus paradoxus^Q
  - Pulmonary embolism: Sudden onset dyspnea, tachypnea, tachycardia, hypotension, localized pleural rub^Q, severe central chest pain in massive emboli
  - Other signs: Cold clammy peripheries with pallor, peripheral & central cyanosis^Q

SEPTIC SHOCK

Septic Shock

- **Septic shock** refers to **sepsis accompanied by hypotension** that **cannot be corrected by infusion of fluids**[Q]

Septic Shock	
Definition	A subset of sepsis in which **underlying circulatory and cellular/metabolic abnormalities** lead to substantially **increased mortality risk**[Q]
Criteria in 2016	**Suspected** (or documented) **infection plus vasopressor therapy** needed to maintain mean arterial pressure at ≥65 mm Hg[Q] & serum lactate >2.0 mmol/L despite adequate fluid resuscitation[Q]

- **Refractory septic shock:** Septic shock that lasts for >1 hour & does not respond to fluid or pressure administration

Pathophysiology of Septic Shock
• Initiated by **gram-negative (MC)** or gram-positive **bacteria**, fungi or virus
• **Cell wall** of organisms contain **endotoxins & exotoxins**
• **Endotoxins** → Release of **inflammatory mediators** → Vasodilatation & ↑ capillary permeability → Altered peripheral circulation & massive dilation → Shock[Q]
• Infection → Local inflammatory reaction → Release of inflammatory mediators → Systemic inflammatory response → Diffuse endothelial injury, vasodilatation & ↑ capillary permeability → Progressive vasodilatation & maldistribution of blood flow → Organ hypoperfusion → Multiple organ dysfunction syndrome[Q]

Clinical Features

- **Fever with chills & rigor, warm peripheries** due to vasodilatation[Q]
- **Bounding pulse, rapid capillary refilling & hypotension**[Q]
- Evidence of **infection at local site**[Q]

Treatment

- **First line of treatment: Aggressive volume expansion with crystalloids** & restoration of arterial oxygenation with inspired oxygen & frequently with mechanical ventilation are the **highest priorities**[Q].
- **Second line:** Ionotropic support with dopamine, norepinephrine, or vasopressin in presence of hypotension or dobutamine if arterial pressure is normal[Q].
- **High dose activated protein C**[Q] **(APC)** provides a **survival benefit in** patients with **severe sepsis & septic shock**
- **Plasma expanders** are useful as septic shock is associated with **peripheral vasodilatation causing reactive hypovolemia**[Q]
- **Antibiotics & surgical debridement or drainage** to control infection[Q]

NEUROGENIC SHOCK

Neurogenic Shock

- Result from **loss or suppression of sympathetic tone** → Massive vasodilatation in venous vasculature → ↓Venous return → ↓ Cardiac output → Impaired tissue perfusion & cellular metabolism[Q]

Causes of Neurogenic Shock	
• **High cervical spinal cord injury**[Q]	• **Deep general anesthesia**[Q] (depress vasomotor tone)
• Inadvertent **cephalad migration of spinal** anesthesia[Q]	• **Devastating head injury**[Q]

Clinical Features

- **Paralysis below the level of lesion; Hypotension**[Q]
- **Bradycardia** due to **loss of sympathetic tone**[Q] → Arterial & venous vasodilatation[Q] → Warm & dry skin[Q]
- **Hypothermia**[Q]

Treatment

- Treatment involves a simultaneous approach to **relative hypovolemia** & to **loss of vasomotor tone**.
- **Excessive volumes of fluid**[Q] may be required to restore normal hemodynamics if given alone.
- Once hemorrhage has been ruled out, **norepinephrine** or a **pure alpha-adrenergic agent**[Q] **(phenylephrine)** may be necessary

HYPOADRENAL SHOCK

Hypoadrenal Shock

- In the stress or illness, surgery or trauma, adrenal secretes increased amount of cortisol[Q]
- Unrecognized adrenal insufficiency complicates the host response to stress induced by acute illness or major surgery → Hypoadrenal shock[Q]

Causes of Hypoadrenal Shock
- Chronic administration of high doses of exogenous glucocorticoids[Q]
- Adrenal insufficiency secondary to: Idiopathic atrophy[Q]; Use of etomidate[Q] for intubation; Tuberculosis[Q]; Metastatic disease[Q]; Bilateral adrenal hemorrhage[Q]; Amyloidosis[Q]

CHARACTERISTIC FEATURES OF VARIOUS TYPES OF SHOCK

Physiologic Characteristics of the Various Forms of Shock

Type of Shock	CVP and PCWP	Cardiac Output	SVR	Venous O_2 Saturation
Hypovolemic	↓	↓	↑	↓
Cardiogenic	↑	↓	↑	↓
Septic				
Hyperdynamic	↑↓	↓	↓	↑
Hypodynamic	↑↓	↑	↑	↑↓
Traumatic	↓	↑↓	↑↓	↓
Neurogenic	↓	↓	↓	↓
Hypoadrenal	↑↓	↓	=↓	↓

PARAMETERS FOR SHOCK

Shock Index (SI)	Modified Shock Index (MSI)
• SI is defined as **heart rate divided by systolic BP**[Q]. • **Better marker for assessing severity of shock** than heart rate & BP alone[Q]. • Utility in **trauma patients, sepsis, obstetrics, myocardial infarction, stroke & other acute critical illnesses**[Q]. • **Correlated with need for interventions** such as blood transfusion & invasive procedures including operations. • SI is known as a **hemodynamic stability indicator**[Q]. • SI does **not take into account** the **diastolic BP**	• MSI is defined as **heart rate divided by mean arterial pressure**[Q]. • High MSI indicates a **value of stroke volume & low systemic vascular resistance, a sign of hypodynamic circulation**[Q]. • Low MSI indicates a **hyperdynamic state**[Q]. • MSI has been considered a **better marker than SI for mortality rate prediction**[Q].

Pulse Rate Over Pressure Evaluation (ROPE)

- ROPE = Pulse Rate/Pulse pressure = PR/(SBP–DBP)
- ROPE is useful in the **assessment of compensated hemorrhagic shock.**

DRUG OF CHOICE IN SHOCK

Drug of Choice in Shock	
Anaphylactic shock	• Adrenaline[Q]
Cardiogenic shock	• Noradrenaline or dopamine[Q]
Distributive shock	• Noradrenaline or phenylephrine[Q]
Hypovolemic shock	• Crystalloids[Q]
Shock with oliguria	• Dopamine[Q]
Hypoadrenal shock	• Corticosteroids[Q]
Septic shock	• Broad-spectrum antibiotics[Q]

Multiple Choice Questions

SHOCK

1. Shock is clinically best assessed by: *(Recent Question 2016)*
   a. Urine output
   b. CVP
   c. BP
   d. Hydration

2. Which of the following is the best parameter to assess fluid intake in a poly-trauma patient? *(All India 94)*
   a. Urine output
   b. BP
   c. Pulse
   d. Pulse oximetry

3. Following is the most important factor in the management of shock: *(AIIMS 84)*
   a. Blood pressure
   b. Cardiac output
   c. CVP to 8 cm of water
   d. Deficiency of effective circulation

4. Which of the following is true for shock? *(MCI Sept 2005)*
   a. Hypotension
   b. Hypoperfusion to tissues
   c. Hypoxia
   d. All of the above

5. Best guide for the management of resuscitation is:
   a. CVP *(AIIMS November 2017)*
   b. Urine output
   c. Blood pressure
   d. Saturation of oxygen

6. Modified shock index formula is: *(AIIMS November 2017)*
   a. Heart rate / Systolic BP
   b. Heart rate / Diastolic BP
   c. Heart rate/ Mean arterial pressure
   d. Pulse rate/ Systolic BP

7. First line of therapy in shock in the patients of trauma: *(Recent Question 2017)*
   a. Crystalloids
   b. Colloids
   c. Inotropes
   d. Blood transfusion

8. Optimum urine output in post-operative patient: *(Recent Question 2017)*
   a. 1 mL/min
   b. 2 mL/min
   c. 3 mL/min
   d. 4 mL/min

9. A patient came with profuse diarrhea and dehydration reaches OPD. For examination flow of fluids which cannula can be inserted: *(AIIMS November 2018)*
   a. Green
   b. Blue
   c. Grey
   d. Violet

NEUROGENIC SHOCK

10. Neurogenic shock is characterized by: *(AIIMS May 2014)*
    a. Hypertension and tachycardia
    b. Hypertension and bradycardia
    c. Hypotension and tachycardia
    d. Hypotension and bradycardia

11. A patient with spine, chest and abdominal injury in road traffic accident developed hypotension and bradycardia. Most likely reason is: *(AIIMS Nov 2013)*
    a. Hypovolemic shock
    b. Hypovolemic + neurogenic shock
    c. Hypovolemic + septicemic shock
    d. Neurogenic shock

12. Which of the following are true about neurogenic shock?
    a. Tachycardia *(Recent Question 2016)*
    b. Cold and moist extremity
    c. Due to parasympathetic blockade
    d. Diagnosis of exclusion

HEMORRHAGIC SHOCK

13. Immediate management of a patient with multiple fracture and fluid loss includes the infusion: *(All India 94)*
    a. Blood
    b. Dextran
    c. Normal saline
    d. Ringer lactate

14. Hemorrhage leads to: *(MCI Sept 2005)*
    a. Septic shock
    b. Neurogenic shock
    c. Hypovolemic shock
    d. Cardiogenic shock

15. In traumatic cases, shock is most likely due to: *(Recent Question 2016, DNB 2011, MCI Sept 2007)*
    a. Injury to intra abdominal solid organ
    b. Head injury
    c. Septicemia
    d. Cardiac failure

16. Which of the following is ideal in moderate hemorrhagic shock? *(Karnataka 2012, MCI Sept 2007)*
    a. Dextrose
    b. Ringer lactate
    c. Blood
    d. Dextran

17. Compensatory mechanism in a patient with hypovolemic shock: *(JIPMER 2011)*
    a. Increased renal blood flow
    b. Decrease in cortisol
    c. Decrease in vasopressin
    d. Decreased cutaneous blood flow

18. Features of hypovolemic shock are all *except*: *(NIMHANS 86)*
    a. Oliguria
    b. Bradycardia
    c. Low BP
    d. Acidosis

19. One of the following is earliest indication of concealed acute bleeding: *(All India 95)*
    a. Tachycardia
    b. Postural HT
    c. Oliguria
    d. Cold clammy fingers

20. Blood loss in class II hemorrhagic shock is: *(Recent Questions 2013)*
    a. <15%
    b. 15-30%
    c. 30-40%
    d. >40%

21. Most common type of shock in emergency room is: *(Recent Question 2013)*
    a. Cardiogenic
    b. Hypovolemic shock
    c. Obstructive
    d. Neurogenic

22. Most common type of shock in surgical practice: *(DNB 2014)*
    a. Cardiogenic
    b. Hypovolemic
    c. Neurogenic
    d. Septic shock

23. Most common feature of polytrauma in pediatric age group is: *(Recent Question 2015)*
    a. Hypothermia
    b. Hypovolemic shock
    c. Hypotension
    d. Hypoxemia

24. Which of the following is false about hemorrhagic shock? *(Recent Question 2017)*
    a. Low heart rate
    b. Cold extremity
    c. Due to fluid losses
    d. Vascular resistance high

25. **In traumatic cases, shock is most likely due to:**
    (MCI June 2018)
    a. Injury to intra-abdominal solid organ
    b. Head injury
    c. Septicemia
    d. Cardiac failure

26. **Class III hemorrhagic shock refers to:** *(AIIMS May 2018)*
    a. Blood loss less than 15%
    b. Blood loss between 15%–30%
    c. Blood loss between 30%–40%
    d. Blood loss more than 40%

SEPTIC SHOCK

27. **The most important cause of the death in septic shock is:**
    a. DIC
    b. Respiratory failure
    c. Renal
    d. Cardiac

28. **35-years old Mona developed feature of septicemia. Shock in form of hypotension and low urine output. She was being treated for colonic necrosis. What will be the management?** *(AIIMS June 99)*
    a. IV fluids + dopamine
    b. IV fluids only
    c. Only dopamine
    d. Antibiotic in high dose

29. **Plasma expanders are used in:**
    (Recent Question 2013, DNB 2012)
    a. Septic shock
    b. Vasovagal shock
    c. Neurogenic shock
    d. Cardiogenic shock

30. **All of the following are true about distributive shock *except*:**
    (Recent Question 2017)
    a. Decreased venous return
    b. Decreased cardiac output
    c. Decreased vascular resistance
    d. High mixed venous saturation

MISCELLANEOUS

31. **Blood clot the size of a clenched fist is roughly equal to:**
    (DNB 2010)
    a. 250 mL
    b. 350 mL
    c. 500 mL
    d. 600 mL

32. **What is normal pulmonary capillary wedge pressure?**
    (MHSSMCET 2005)
    a. 4–8 mm of Hg
    b. 8–12 mm of Hg
    c. 12–16 mm of Hg
    d. 15–25 mm of Hg

33. **Patient is on shock. IV cannulation not possible, intraosseous line for IVF should be done within:** *(WBPG 2014)*
    a. 1 minute
    b. 1.5 minutes
    c. 2 minutes
    d. 2.5 minutes

34. **Green coloured IV cannula, the size is:** *(Recent Question 2015)*
    a. 18 Gauge
    b. 20 Gauge
    c. 22 Gauge
    d. 24 Gauge

35. **In a patient with dehydration, which the following color intravenous cannula will you place for rapid fluid resuscitation?** *(AIIMS May 2016)*
    a. Grey
    c. Blue
    b. Pink
    d. Green

36. **22 Gauge IV cannula color is:** *(AIIMS November 2017)*
    a. Green
    b. Grey
    c. Blue
    d. Pink

Explanations

SHOCK

1. **Ans a. Urine output** *(Sabiston 20/e p554; Schwartz 10/e p109-131; Bailey 27/e p17)*

   SHOCK

   - **Shock:** Inadequate delivery of oxygen and **nutrients** due to **poor tissue perfusion**^{Q} to maintain normal tissue and cellular function
   - **Mean arterial pressure <60 mm Hg** in previously normotensive patients
   - **Systemic vascular resistance rises** leading to **decreased cutaneous blood flow**^{Q} and **autoregulation** is **critical in sustaining cerebral** and **coronary blood flow**^{Q}.

Blalock Classification of Shock	
1. **Hypovolemic (MC)**^{Q}	3. Cardiogenic
2. Vasogenic	4. Neurogenic

   - Shock is MC cause of death among surgical patients.

2. **Ans a. Urine output**
3. **Ans d. Deficiency of effective circulation**
4. **Ans d. All of the above**
5. **Ans. b. Urine output** *(Ref: Sabiston 20/e p520; Schwartz 10/e p169; Bailey 27/e p17)*

   "Ultimately, the goal of treatment is to restore cellular and organ perfusion. Ideally, therefore, monitoring of organ perfusion should guide the management of shock. The best measures of organ perfusion and the best monitor of the adequacy of shock therapy remains the urine output." - Bailey 27/e p17

6. **Ans. c. Heart rate/ Mean arterial pressure** *(Ref: Sabiston 20/e p52)*
7. **Ans. a. Crystalloids**
8. **Ans. a. 1 mL/min** *(Ref: Sabiston 20/e p520; Schwartz 10/e p169; Bailey 27/e p17)*

   "Urine output of more than 1 mL/kg is an adequate measure of renal perfusion in the absence of underlying renal disease."- Sabiston 20/e p520

9. **Ans. c. Grey**

NEUROGENIC SHOCK

10. **Ans. d. Hypotension and bradycardia**
11. **Ans d. Neurogenic shock** *(Ref: Harrison 19/e p1750)*

    A patient with **spine, chest and abdominal injury** in road traffic accident developed **hypotension** and **bradycardia**. Most likely reason is **neurogenic shock**.
    *"Neurogenic shock: In addition to **arteriolar dilation, venodilation** causes pooling in the venous system, which **decreases venous return and cardiac output.**"*- Harrison 19/e p1750

12. **Ans d. Diagnosis of exclusion**

HEMORRHAGIC SHOCK

13. **Ans d. Ringer lactate** *(Ref: Schwartz 10/e p109,110,119-123; Bailey 27/e p15)*

    - **Resuscitation following blood loss from multiple fractures** begins with administration of **2-3 liters of isotonic crystalloid** immediately to **restore BP and peripheral circulation**^{Q}.
    - **Lactated ringer (RL) solution** is generally **preferred over 0.9% NaCl** (normal saline) as it is **balanced salt solution** and designed to **mimic extracellular fluid**^{Q}.
    - Resuscitation with **colloids** is **no more effective than crystalloids** but is **more expensive**^{Q}.

14. **Ans c. Hypovolemic shock**
15. **Ans a. Injury to intra-abdominal solid organs**

Shock

16. Ans b. Ringer lactate

- Patients with **blunt trauma** and **hypovolemia** should be **examined first for intra-abdominal bleeding** even if there is no overt existence of abdominal trauma.^{Q}

17. Ans d. Decreased cutaneous blood flow
18. Ans b. Bradycardia
19. Ans a. Tachycardia
20. Ans b. 15-30%
21. Ans b. Hypovolemic shock
22. Ans. b. Hypovolemic
23. Ans. b. Hypovolemic shock
24. Ans. a. Low heart rate
25. Ans. a. Injury to intra-abdominal solid organ
26. Ans. c. Blood loss between 30%–40%

SEPTIC SHOCK

27. Ans d. Cardiac *(Ref: Sabiston 20/e p554; Schwartz 10/e p127,171; Bailey 27/e p13-14)*

- **Hypotension** is the **MC cause of death** in **septic shock**^{Q}.
- **Cardiac output** is **decreased in septic shock,** leading to **hypotension**^{Q}.

28. Ans b. IV fluids only *(Ref: Sabiston 20/e p554; Schwartz 10/e p124-126; Bailey 27/e p15-16)*
29. Ans a. Septic shock
30. Ans. b. Decreased cardiac output *(Ref: Sabiston 20/e p554; Bailey 27/e p13)*

"Distributive shock describes the pattern of cardiovascular responses characterising a variety of conditions, including septic shock, anaphylaxis and spinal cord injury. Inadequate organ perfusion is accompanied by vascular dilatation with hypotension, low systemic vascular resistance, inadequate afterload and a resulting abnormally high cardiac output."- Bailey 27/e p13

MISCELLANEOUS

31. Ans c. 500 mL *(Ref: Bailey 24/e p61)*

- **Blood clot of size of a clenched fist** is roughly equal to **500 ml**^{Q}.

32. Ans b. 8-12 mm of Hg *(Ref: Bailey 26/e p17)*

PULMONARY CAPILLARY WEDGE PRESSURE (PCWP)

- It is a **better indicator** for both **blood volume** and **left ventricular function** than CVP^Q.
- Obtained by **pulmonary artery floatation balloon catheter (Swan-Ganz)** ^{Q}.
- **Normal PCWP: 6-12 mm Hg**^{Q}
- Used to **differentiate left and right ventricular failure, pulmonary embolism, septic shock and ruptured mitral valve**^{Q}
- **Accurate guide** to therapy with **fluids, inotropic agents** and **vasodilators**^{Q}.
- May also be used to **measure cardiac output** by thermodilution technique^Q.

33. Ans b. 1.5 minutes

- Guidelines state that, during CPR in children aged younger than 6 years, intraosseous access should be obtained if there is inability to achieve reliable venous access after **three attempts or 90 seconds,** whichever comes sooner. Intraosseous access has the same benefits in children aged over 6 years but access to the anterior tibial marrow is more difficult and other sites such as the lower femur, iliac crest or sternum should be considered.

34. Ans a. 18 Gauge
35. Ans. a. Grey *(Ref: Bailey 25/e p29)*

    Grey cannula has the **large bore (16 G)** with **flow rate of 180 mL/min** and is the **preferred option for rapid fluid resuscitation** in patients with rehydration.

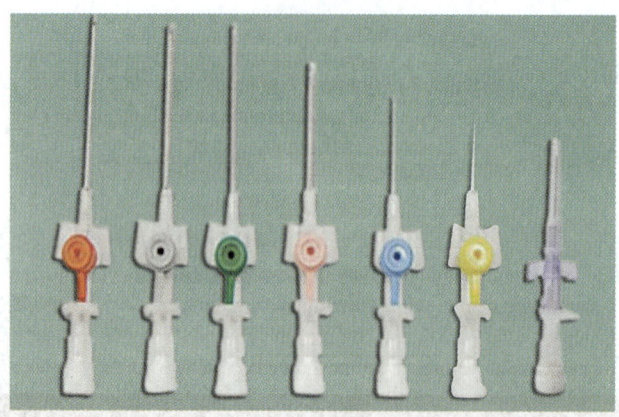

Color code	Gauge	External Diameter (mm)	Length (mm)	Flow Rate (ml/min)	Indications
Orange	14G	2.1	45	240	Trauma, surgical procedures
Grey	16G[Q]	1.8	45	180[Q]	Trauma, surgical procedures
Green	18G[Q]	1.3	32/45	90[Q]	Trauma, quick blood transfusion
Pink	20G[Q]	1.1	32	60[Q]	Normal IV or blood transfusion
Blue	22G[Q]	0.9	25	36[Q]	Children, older adults
Yellow	24G	0.7	19	20	Neonates, children, elderly
Violet	26G	0.6	19	13	Neonates

36. **Ans. c. Blue** *(Ref: Manual of ICU Procedures By Mohan Gurjar (2015)/p240)*

Chapter 51

Miscellaneous

Multiple Choice Questions

1. Most important technical consideration at the time of doing below knee amputation is: *(AIIMS Nov 2000)*
   a. Posterior flap should be longer than the anterior flap
   b. Stump should be long
   c. Stump should be short
   d. Anterior flap should be longer than posterior flap

2. Referred pain from all of the following conditions may be felt along the inner side of right thigh, *except*:
   a. Inflamed pelvic appendix *(All India 2006)*
   b. Inflamed ovaries
   c. Stone in pelvic ureter
   d. Pelvic abscess

3. Following are true about William Halsted: *(PGI June 2008)*
   a. First person to receive nobel prize in surgery
   b. Pioneered introduction of gloves
   c. Promoted radical approach for breast surgery
   d. Pioneered role of antibiotics

4. FNAC needle size: *(AIIMS Nov 2007)*
   a. 18-22   b. 22-26
   c. 27-29   d. 16-18

5. Bee venom can be neutralized by applying:
   a. Soda bicarbonate   b. Vinegar
   c. Lemon juice   d. Dilute HCL

6. The most dangerous injury is: *(Recent Question 2016)*
   a. Snake bite   b. Scorpion bite
   c. Wasp sting   d. Human bite

7. The best site for intramuscular injection is:
   a. Deltoid *(Recent Question 2016)*
   b. Anterolateral part of thigh
   c. Upper outer segment of buttocks
   d. Upper inner segment of buttocks

8. Hereditary spherocytosis is transmitted as:
   (Recent Question 2016)
   a. Autosomal dominant   b. Autosomal recessive
   c. X-linked dominant   d. X-linked recessive

9. Subcutaneous calcification are seen in: *(JIPMER 93)*
   a. Gout   b. Hyperparathyroidism
   c. Onchronosis   d. Malignancies

10. In polycythaemia vera the most common postoperative complication following major surgery is: *(PGI 91)*
    a. Thrombosis   b. Gastric ulcer
    c. Diabetes insipidus d. Haemorrhage

11. Biot's respiration is seen in:
    a. Hypnosedative poisoning
    b. Appendicitis
    c. Cholecystitis
    d. Bulbar poliomyelitis

12. 'Sterile needle test' helps in differentiating: *(Gujrat 2014)*
    a. Healing process   b. Depth of burns
    c. Degenerative process d. Infection

13. Van Buchem's syndrome is characterized by all *except*:
    a. Overgrowth   b. Distortion of mandible
    c. Facial Palsy   *(Gujrat 2014)*
    d. Increased acid phosphatase

14. The stage of myasthenia gravis that best responds to thymectomy is:
    a. Stage 1: active   b. Stage 2: Inactive
    c. Stage 3: burnt out d. Those with thymoma
    e. None of the above

15. Quant's sign (a T-shaped depression in the occipital bone) may be present in: *(Gujrat 2014)*
    a. Down's syndrome   b. Head injury
    c. Rickets   d. Scurvy

16. Nezelof's syndrome is recurrent episodes of: *(Gujrat 2014)*
    a. Appendicitis   b. Cholecystitis
    c. Intestinal obstruction d. Pneumonia

17. Hickey-Hare test is used to diagnose: *(Gujrat 2014)*
    a. Congenital pyloric stenosis
    b. Doudenal atresia
    c. Achlasia cardia   d. Diabetes insipidus

18. Usually employed technique for splanchnic block is:
    (Recent Question 2016)
    a. Braun's method   b. Kappi's method
    c. Wending's method   d. None of the above

19. Secondary amyloidosis occurs in: *(Recent Question 2016)*
    a. Chronic osteomyelitis b. Rheumatoid arthritis
    c. Leprosy   d. Syphilis

20. Arrow headed finger on X-ray is suggestive of:
    a. Acromegaly *(Recent Question 2016)*
    b. Hyperparathyroidism
    c. Down's syndrome
    d. Sarcoidosis

21. A Seldinger needle is used for: *(Recent Question 2016)*
    a. Liver biopsy   b. Suturing skin
    c. Arteriography   d. Lymphography

22. Blongnini's symptom (a feeling of crepitation occurring from gradual increasing pressure on the abdomen) is seen in: *(Gujrat 2014)*
    a. Congenital pyloric stenosis
    b. Gastric polyp
    c. Duodenal atresia
    d. Measles

23. Mauriac's syndrome is characterized by the following *except*:
    a. Diabetes
    b. Obesity *(Gujrat 2014)*
    c. Dwarfism
    d. Cardiomegaly

24. A cricoid hook is used particularly: *(Recent Question 2016; DNB 89)*
    a. In thyroidectomy
    b. In block dissection of the neck
    c. For retracting the superior laryngeal nerve
    d. In tracheostomy

25. Not a premalignant ulcer: *(Kerala 94)*
    a. Bazin's ulcer
    b. Paget's disease of nipple
    c. Marjolin's ulcer
    d. Lupus vulgaris

26. During endotracheal intubation, unilateral breath sounds, no air heard entering the stomach and no gastric distension is suggestive of entry of the endotracheal tube into:
    a. Right main bronchus
    b. Esophagus *(UPSC 96)*
    c. Mid-trachea
    d. Left main bronchus

27. Aminopeptidase is elevated in obstruction of: *(Assam 96)*
    a. Ureter
    b. Urethra
    c. CBD
    d. Bladder

28. Sappey's line denotes a line: *(Karnataka 95)*
    a. Encircling the neck at C6 vertebra level
    b. Encircling the trunk just above the umbilicus
    c. Encircling the salpigian tubes
    d. None of the above

29. Hormonal treatment is given for which of the following malignancy? *(Kerala 96)*
    a. Choriocarcinoma
    b. Carcinoma prostate
    c. Hepatoma
    d. Teratoma
    e. Granulosa cell tumour

30. A female patient complains of periumbilical pain and nausea particularly after taking food. The diagnosis is: *(UPPG 95)*
    a. Meckel's diverticulum
    b. Peptic ulcer syndrome
    c. Lactose intolerance
    d. None

31. Most common tumour among children 1-5 years in South Africa is: *(TN 96)*
    a. Neuroblastoma
    b. Wilms' tumour
    c. Neurofibroma
    d. Burkitt's lymphoma

32. First neurosurgeon of India: *(SCTIMS 98)*
    a. Jacob Chandy
    b. Jacob Abraham
    c. K.V. Mathal
    d. Mathew Chandy

33. Local anesthetics cannot be used at the site of infection because it causes: *(MAHE 2001)*
    a. Spread of infection
    b. Lowered efficiency
    c. Both
    d. None

34. All are true about long flexor tendons *except*: *(Kerala 95)*
    a. Flexor digitorum prefunds inserted to distal phalanx bas
    b. Flexor digitorum superficialis attached to the sides of middle phalanx
    c. Damage to the tendons involves formation of tenoma during repair
    d. Good repair results if tendon sheath is damaged

35. No man's land in palm corresponds: *(Gujrat 2014, MAHE 98)*
    a. Zone I
    b. Zone II
    c. Zone III
    d. Zone IV

36. Failure of migration of neural crest cells is seen in: *(Kerala 2001)*
    a. Albinism
    b. Congenital megacolon
    c. Odonotomes
    d. Adrenal tumour

37. Hypothermia is used in all *except*: *(PGI 98)*
    a. Cardiac surgery
    b. Neonatal ischemia
    c. Heat stroke
    d. Cardiac arrhythmia

38. The commonest symptom post operatively seen is:
    a. Depression
    b. Psychosis *(Kerala 97)*
    c. Euphoria
    d. None of the above

39. The most sensitive qualitative method for detection of air embolism is: *(Gujrat 2014)*
    a. Doppler ultra sound
    b. Elector cardiogram
    c. Arterial pressure
    d. End expiratory carbon dioxide content

40. Fiberoptic endoscopy is contraindicated in: *(Recent Question 2016)*
    a. Children
    b. Aneurysm of arch of aorta
    c. Cervical spondylosis
    d. Hemoptysis

41. Depressed bridge of nose can be due to any of the following *except*: *(Karnataka 2003)*
    a. Leprosy
    b. Syphilis
    c. Thalassemia
    d. Acromegaly

42. In sickle cell anemia sudden onset of pancytopenia with hemolysis and no rise of reticulocyte count occurs in: *(JIPMER 2004)*
    a. Sequestration crisis
    b. Aplastic crisis
    c. Hemolytic crisis
    d. Vaso-occlusive crisis

43. Who said these words: To study the phenomenon of disease without books is to sail an uncharted sea, while to study books without patients is not to go to sea at all? *(Karnataka 2004)*
    a. Hamilton Bailey
    b. Sir Robert Hutchison
    c. Sir William Osler
    d. J.B. Murphy

44. In the acronym "Swelling" used for the history and examination of a lump or swelling, the letter 'N' stands for: *(Karnataka 2004)*
    a. Nodes
    b. Noise (Thrill/bruit)
    c. Numbness
    d. Neurological effects

45. Lamina dura lining the alveolus is: *(Karnataka 2002)*
    a. Cancellous bone
    b. Ligament
    c. Dense cortical bone
    d. Muscle

46. Vidian neurectomy is indicated in: *(MAHE 2005)*
    a. Glossopharyngeal neuralgia
    b. Trigeminal neuralgia
    c. Vasomotor rhinitis
    d. Atrophic rhinitis

47. Orthobaric oxygen in used in: (MAHE 2005)
    a. Carbon monoxide poisoning
    b. Ventilation failure
    c. Anaerobic infection   d. Gangrene
48. 'Tennis elbow' is characterized by: (MAHE 2005)
    a. Tenderness over the medial epicondyle
    b. Tendinitis of common extensor origin
    c. Tendinitis of common flexor origin
    d. Painful flexion and extension
49. Pelvic exenteration is known as: (Gujrat 2014, APPG 2006)
    a. Miles Operation   b. Lyods operation
    c. Finch operation   d. Brunschwigs operation
50. About congenital torticollis all are except: (AIIMS Nov 2006)
    a. Always associated with breech extraction
    b. Spontaneous resolution in most cases
    c. 2/3rd cases have palpable neck mass at birth
    d. Uncorrected cases develop plagicephaly
51. Dye used in chromoendoscopy for detection of cancer: (AIIMS May 2009)
    a. Gentian violet   b. Toluidine blue
    c. Hemotoxiline and eosine   d. Methylene blue
52. Concomitant chemoradiotherapy is indicated in all of the following except: (All India 2009)
    a. Stage IIIB CA cervix   b. T2 N0 M0 anal cancer
    c. T2 N0 M0 glottic cancer
    d. T1 N2 M0 Nasopharyngeal cancer
53. Smoking may be associated with all of the following cancer's except: (All India 2009)
    a. CA Larynx   b. CA Nasopharynx
    c. CA Bladder   d. CA Esophagus
54. Hutchinson and Pepper syndrome is a feature of: (COMEDK 2004)
    a. Von Recklinghausen's   b. Neuroblastoma
    c. Renal cell carcinoma   d. Meningioma
55. What is this sign called? (APPG 2016)

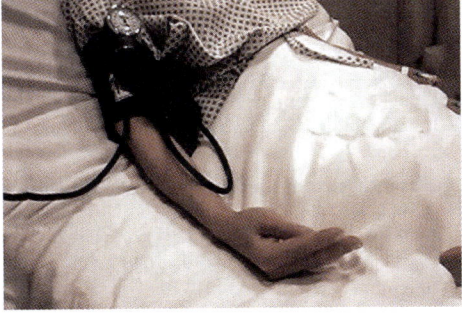

    a. Troisier sign   b. Chvostek's sign
    c. Lhermitte's sign   d. Trousseau's sign
56. Not a submucosal lesion: (Punjab 2009)
    a. Lipoma   b. Ranula
    c. Carcinoid   d. None
57. Frozen section is/are used for: (PGI Nov 2009)
    a. Enzyme
    b. Intraoperative histopathological examination
    c. Fat
    d. Acid fast bacilli
    e. To check surgical margin in tumor surgery
58. Condition associated with panniculitis is/are: (PGI Nov 2009)
    a. Pancreas cancer   b. Chronic pancreatitis
    c. Acute pancreatitis   d. Pancreatic divisum
    e. Post-traumatic pancreatitis
59. True about apocrine gland: (PGI June 2009)
    a. Modified sweat gland
    b. Modified sebaceous gland
    c. Present in axilla and groin
    d. Hidradenitis suppurativa is infection of apocrine gland
60. Not associated with fat necrosis: (PGI June 2009)
    a. Liposuction   b. Radiotherapy
    c. Mammoplasty   d. Carcinoma breast
    e. Following trauma
61. Which of the following is the most commonly used 'fixative' in diagnostic pathology? (Recent Question 2016)
    a. Formaldehyde   b. Ethyl alcohol
    c. Mercuric chloride   d. Picric acid
62. Aflatoxins are produced by: (All India 2011)
    a. Aspergillus flavus   b. Aspergillus niger
    c. Aspergillus fumigates   d. Candida
63. Axillary abscess is safely drained by which approach?
    a. Medial   b. Posterior
    c. Lateral   d. Floor   (AIIMS May 2011)
64. Topical mitomycin C is used in: (AIIMS May 2011)
    a. Basal skull carcinoma   b. Tracheal stenosis
    c. Skull base osteomyelitis   d. Angiofibroma
65. Fixative used in histopathology: (AIIMS May 2012)
    a. 10% buffered neutral formalin
    b. Bouins fixative
    c. Glutaraldehyde   d. Ethyl alcohol
66. Potato nodes are feature of: (DNB 2010)
    a. Sarcoidosis   b. Tuberculosis
    c. Carcinoid   d. Lymphoma
67. Moures sign is seen in: (Recent Questions 2013)
    a. Carcinoma   b. Appendicitis
    c. Varicose vein   d. Pancreatitis
68. Choose the Wrong combination of cancer and its suspected carcinogen: (APPG 2016)
    a. Tobacco - bladder   b. Phenacetin - lung
    c. Arsenic - skin   d. Vinyl chloride - liver
69. French in Foley's catheter refers to: (AIIMS November 2017)
    a. Outer circumference measurement
    b. Inner circumference measurement
    c. Diameter of catheter   d. Lumen size
70. In a pre-operative patient surgical checklist, which of the following is not required? (AIIMS November 2017)
    a. Oral consent   b. Doctor's signature
    c. Site marking
    d. Confirming patient's identity
71. How to measure nasogastric tube length? (AIIMS November 2017)
    a. Tip of nose to ear to xiphisternum
    b. Tip of nose to angle of ear to umbilicus
    c. Mouth to ear to umbilicus
    d. Mouth to ear to midway between xiphisternum and umbilicus
72. Kraissl's lines are: (AIIMS May 2017)
    a. Collagen and elastin lines in stab wounds
    b. Point of maximum tension in a fracture
    c. Point of tension in hanging
    d. Relaxed tension lines in skin

1126 Surgery Essence

73. In fasciotomy the layers that are opened are:
    a. Skin, subcutaneous tissue and superficial fascia
    b. Skin, subcutaneous tissue alone cut
    c. Skin alone cut *(Recent Question 2018)*
    d. Skin, subcutaneous tissue, superficial fascia and deep fascia

74. What are the names of incisions?
    a. 1-Kocher incision; 2-Midline incision; 3-McBurney incision; 4-Lanz incision; 5-Battle incision; 6-Paramedian incision; 7-Transverse incision; 8-Rutherford Morrison incision; 9-Pfannenstiel incision
    b. 1-Kocher incision; 2-Midline incision; 3-McBurney incision; 4-Battle incision; 5-Lanz incision; 6-Rutherford Morrison incision; 7-Transverse incision; 8-Paramedian incision; 9-Pfannenstiel incision
    c. 1-Kocher incision; 2-Midline incision; 3-McBurney incision; 4-Battle incision; 5-Lanz incision; 6-Paramedian incision; 7-Transverse incision; 8-Rutherford Morrison incision; 9-Pfannenstiel incision
    d. 1-Kocher incision; 2-Midline incision; 3-Rutherford Morrison incision; 4-Battle incision; 5-Lanz incision; 6-Paramedian incision; 7-Transverse incision; 8-McBurney incision; 9-Pfannenstiel incision

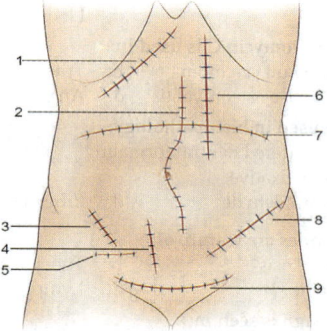

75. Which one of the following statements is TRUE regarding the clinical sign being elicited here? *(APPG 2016)*

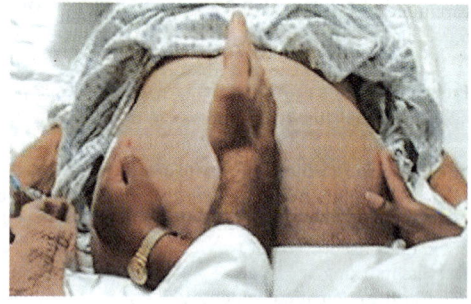

   a. This test is for eliciting shifting dullness
   b. This test helps to detect ascites
   c. The hand on the midline below the umbilicus will feel the vibrations in patients with ascites
   d. All these statements are True

76. What is this position called? *(APPG 2016)*
    a. Trendelenburg position
    b. Lloyd Davis position
    c. Fowler position
    d. Sim's position

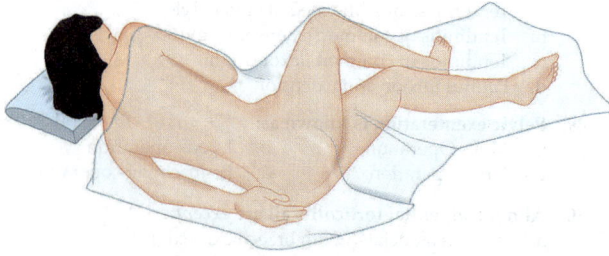

77. Which of the regions marked in the following picture represents the zone 4 of retroperitoneal hemorrhage?
    (AIIMS November 2016)
    a. A   b. C and D
    c. B   d. E

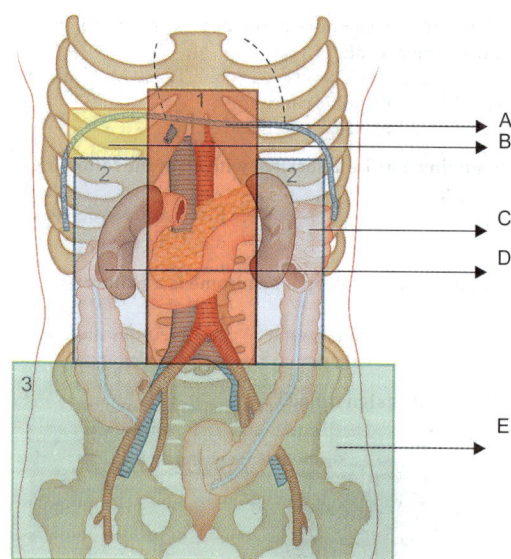

78. One French size of angiographic catheter corresponds to:
    (PGI November 2017)
    a. 0.33 mm   b. 1.67 mm
    c. 0.133 inch   d. 0.013 inch
    e. 0.057 inch

79. Reverse Trendelenburg position is not used for:
    a. Prophylaxis against thromboembolism
    b. High intracranial tension *(PGI November 2017)*
    c. Thyroid surgery
    d. Parathyroid surgery

Explanations

1. **Ans. a. Posterior flap should be longer than the anterior flap** *(Ref: Sabiston 20/e p1769, 19/e p1742; Bailey 27/e p958)*

   ### BELOW KNEE AMPUTATION
   - **Posterior flap** should be **longer than anterior flap** as the **posterior skin** has a **good blood supply** (anterior skin has poor due to lack of muscle an anterior aspect). Good blood supply **helps in easy healing of stump**^{Q}.
   - Equally short anterior and posterior flaps are used only when the long posterior flap technique is not feasible because of previous wounds or extensive tissue ischemia.
     - **Longer stump is better** in general **for amputation at all sites except below knee amputation**^{Q}.
   - **Best level for below knee amputation** (as for prosthetic fitting is concerned): At the **distal musculotendinous junction** of the **gastrocnemius muscle**^{Q}.

2. **Ans. d. Pelvic abscess**
3. **Ans. b. Pioneered introduction of gloves, c. Promoted radical approach for breast surgery**

   ### CONTRIBUTIONS OF WILLIAM STEWARD HALSTED (FATHER OF 'SAFE' SURGERY)
   - **First emergency blood transfusion** was performed on his sister
   - Development of **Halsted radical mastectomy**^{Q}
   - Invention of **surgical gloves**^{Q}

4. **Ans. b. 22-26** *(Ref: www.ncbi.nlm.nih.gov/pubmed/17405171)*
   - **FNAC Needle Size: 21-25 guaze**^{Q}

5. **Ans. a. Soda bicarbonate** *(Ref: Harrison 19/e p2749)*

   Bee venom can be **neutralized** by applying **soda bicarbonate**

6. **Ans. a. Snake bite**   7. **Ans. c. Upper outer segment of buttocks**   8. **Ans. a. Autosomal dominant**
9. **Ans. b. Hyperparathyroidism, d. Malignancies** *(Ref: radiographics.rsna.org/content/19/suppl_1/S11.full)*
   - **Subcutaneous calcifications** are seen in both **hyperparathyroidism** and **malignancies**^{Q}.

10. **Ans. a. Thrombosis** *(Ref: Harrison 20/e p735, 19/e p674 18/e p900)*
    - **Thrombosis: MC postoperative complication** following major surgery in **polycythemia vera**^{Q}.

11. **Ans. None**
    Biot's **respiration** is **seen in raised ICT**.

12. **Ans. b. Depth of burns** *(Ref: Sabiston 20/e p506; Schwartz 10/c p 229, 230)*
    - **'Sterile needle test'** helps in **differentiating depth of burns**.

13. **Ans. b. Distortion of mandible** *(Ref: http://www.ncbi.nlm.nih.gov/pmc/articles/PMC1376897/)*

    ### VAN BUCHEM DISEASE
    - Van Buchem disease (**hyperostosis corticalis generalisata**) is an **autosomal recessive** disorder characterized by **hyperostosis of the skull, mandible, clavicles, ribs,** and **diaphyseal cortices** of the **long bones**^{Q}.
    - **Most striking clinical features** are the **enlargement of the jaw** and **thickness of the skull**, which may lead to **facial nerve palsy, hearing loss,** and **optic atrophy**^{Q}.

14. **Ans. a. Stage 1 active** *(Ref: onlinelibrary.wiley.com/doi/10.1002/bjs.1800650503/pdf)*
    - **Stage I**, the **active stage**, is **characterized by remissions** and **best respond to thymectomy**^{Q}.

15. **Ans. c. Rickets** *(Ref: http://www.kmle.com/search.php?Search=Quant's%20s)*.

Quant's Sign

- A **T-shaped depression in** the **occipital bone** occurring in many cases of **rickets,** especially in **infants lying constantly in bed** with pressure on the **pressure on the occiput**^{Q}.

16. **Ans. d. Pneumonia**

Nezelof Syndrome

- **Nezelof syndrome** (also known as "**Thymic dysplasia with normal immunoglobulins**")
- An **autosomal recessive** congenital immunodeficiency condition due to underdevelopment of the thymus.
- It causes **severe infections** and **malignancies**^{Q}.
- **Treatment:** Antimicrobial therapy, IV immunoglobulin, bone marrow transplantation, thymus transplantation and thymus factors.

17. **Ans. d. Diabetes insipidus** *(Ref: medical-dictionary.thefreedictionary.com/Hickey-Hare+tes)*

Hickey-Hare Test

- **Hickey-Hare test** is **hypertonic saline infusion test** that induces plasma hyperosmolality.
- Used for **distinguishing between different causes** of **polyuria** and **polydipsia**^{Q}.

18. **Ans. a. Braun's method** *(Ref: Lee Anesthesia (2005)/449)*

Splanchnic Block

- **Splanchnic block** can be performed **from the front** (**Braun**^{Q}, Wendling), or **from behind** (**Kappis**).

19. **Ans. a. Chronic osteomyelitis, b. Rheumatoid arthritis, c. Leprosy** *(Ref: Harrison 20/e p805, 19/e p719)*

Amyloidosis

- Amyloidosis is a pathological proteinaceous substance **deposited between cells**^{Q} in various tissues and organs of the body in a variety of clinical settings.

Types of Amyloid Protein

- **AL (Amyloid Light chain):**
  - This is **derived from plasma cells**^{Q} and contains immunoglobulin light chains
  - Associated with **primary amyloidosis** and immunocyte dyscrasias with amyloidosis like **multiple myeloma**^{Q}
- **AA (Amyloid Associate protein):**
  - It is unique non-immunoglobulin protein synthesized by **reticuloendothelial cells of liver**^{Q}.
  - Associated with **secondary amyloidosis** and **reactive systemic amyloidosis**^{Q}.

  > - Chronic inflammatory conditions: Tuberculosis^Q, Bronchiectasis^Q, Osteomyelitis^Q
  > - **Connective tissue disorders: Rheumatoid Arthritis (MC)**^{Q}, Ankylosing spondylitis^Q and Primary biliary cirrhosis^Q
  > - **Non immune derived tumors:** Renal cell carcinoma^Q and Hodgkin's lymphoma^Q

- β_2 microalbumin (Aβ_2m): Hemodialysis associated amyloidosis^Q
- β_2 Amyloid protein: Senile cerebral^Q, Alzheimer's disease^Q
- Transthyretin (ATTR): Familial amyloidotic neuropathies^Q and Systemic senile amyloidosis^Q
- Calcitonin associated amyloid (A cal): Medullary CA thyroid^Q
- Islet amyloid peptide (AIAPP): Type II DM^Q
- Atrial natriuretic factor associated amyloid: Isolated atrial Amyloidosis and Misfolded prion protein (PrPsc) disease

  > - **Common Biopsy sites in Amyloidosis:** Subcutaneous abdominal fat aspirate^Q, Rectum^Q, Skin^Q, Gingiva^Q

20. **Ans. a. Acromegaly** *(Ref: www.acromegalycommunity.com/blog)*
    - **Arrow headed finger** on X-ray is suggestive of **Acromegaly**^{Q}.
21. **Ans. c. Arteriography** *(Ref: Sabiston 20/e p1787; Schwartz 10/e p1051; Bailey 25/e p903)*

    Seldinger **needle** is **used for angiography** (arteriography).

Arteriography

- **Aortic** and **lower extremity arteriograms** are generally performed **by needle puncture** of the **femoral**^{Q} or **brachial arteries**^{Q} followed by **guidewire placement** and **catheter insertion** using the **Seldinger technique.**

22. **Ans. d. Measles**   23. **Ans. d. Cardiomegaly**

MAURIAC SYNDROME

- **Mauriac syndrome** is a rare complication in children and adolescents with **diabetes mellitus type 1,** characterized by **hepatomegaly, growth impairment,** and **cushingoid features**[Q].

24. **Ans. d. In tracheostomy**
    - A **cricoids hook** is **used in tracheostomy**[Q].
25. **Ans. a. Bazin's ulcer**

BAZIN DISEASE

- **Bazin disease** (or "Erythema induratum") is a **panniculitis** on the **back of the calves**[Q].
- It is now considered a panniculitis that is **not associated with a single defined pathogen**[Q].
- It occurs **mainly in women**[Q], but is very rare now.

26. **Ans. a. Right main bronchus**   27. **Ans. c. CBD** *(Ref: American Journal of Gastroenterology; Dec1963, Vol. 41 Issue 6, p620)*

LEUCINE AMINOPEPTIDASE

- **Increased Leucine aminopeptidase (LAP) activity** is seen in:
    - **Carcinoma of the pancreas, choledocholithiasis, acute pancreatitis**[Q]
    - **Viral hepatitis, cirrhosis, carcinoma** with **liver metastases**[Q]
- In **common bile duct obstruction**, whether due to **carcinoma pancreas** or **choledocholithiasis**, the **elevated serum LAP levels returned** to **normal following relief of the obstruction.** This is in agreement with the hypothesis that the increased serum LAP activity in these conditions is the result of bile duct obstruction.

28. **Ans. b. Encircling the trunk just above the umbilicus** *(Ref: Principles and Practice of General Surgery by Kirby I. Bland, Michael G. Sarr, Markus W. Büchler (2008) Volume I/1592)*

SAPPEY'S LINE

- **Sappey's line** defines a **band of skin extending from** the **umbilicus**[Q], along the **iliac crests** over to L1.
- This **line divides sites** which **drain to axilla above, groin below** or **both sites**[Q].

29. **Ans. b. Carcinoma prostate**   30. **Ans. a. Meckel's diverticulum**
31. **Ans. d. Burkitt's lymphoma** *(Ref: www.ncbi.nlm.nih.gov/pubmed/19661660)*
    - Commonest tumour among children 1-5 years in South Africa is Burkitt's lymphoma.
32. **Ans. a. Jacob Chandy** *(Ref: www.cmch-vellore.edu/pdf/jacob.pdf)*
    - **Jacob Chandy: Pioneering Neurosurgeon of India**[Q]
33. **Ans. c. Both**   34. **Ans. d. Good repair results if tendon sheath is damaged**
35. **Ans. b. Zone II** *(Ref: Apley's 8/636-638)*

    Bunnel's no-man's land is Zone II.

ZONE II (NO MAN'S LAND OR DANGEROUS AREA OF HAND[Q])

- Situated **between the opening of** the **flexor sheath** (the **distal palmar crease**) and **insertion of flexor superficialis** (flexor crease of **proximal interphalangeal joint)**[Q]
- Also known as **"No man's land"** or **dangerous area of hand**[Q].
- The **result of flexor tendon repair is worst** in this area because both superficial and deep tendons run together in a tight sheath and passes through three pullies.

36. **Ans. b. Congenital megacolon**   37. **Ans. b. Neonatal ischemia, d. Cardiac arrhythmia** *(Ref: Schwartz 10/e p393, 9/e p674)*
38. **Ans. d. None of the above**

POST-OPERATIVE PSYCHIATRIC SYMPTOMS

- **Delirium**[Q] **(20%)** >Depression (9%) >Dementia (3%) >Functional psychosis (2%).

39. **Ans. d. End expiratory carbon dioxide content** *(Ref: Schwartz 9/e p787-789)*
40. **Ans. b. Aneurysm of arch of aorta**
    - **Fiberoptic endoscopy** is **contraindicated in aneurysm of arch of aorta**.

41. **Ans. d. Acromegaly** *(Ref: Harrison 20/e p1667, 2578, 19/e p1126)*

    Leprosy, **Syphilis** and **Thalassemia** causes **depressed bridge of nose**.

42. **Ans. a. Sequestration crisis** *(Ref: Harrison 20/e p693, 19/e p634)*

43. **Ans. c. Sir William Osler**

    - **Sir William Osler**: "To study the phenomenon of disease without books is to sail an uncharted sea, while to study books without patients is not to go to sea at all"[Q]

44. **Ans. b Noise (Thrill/bruit)**   45. **Ans. c. Dense cortical bone**

46. **Ans. c. Vasomotor rhinitis** *(Ref: www.ncbi.nlm.nih.gov/pubmed/16686388)*

    - **Vidian neurectomy** is indicated in the cases of **vasomotor rhinitis** with **profuse secretion refractory to conservative treatment**[Q].

47. **Ans. a. Carbon monoxide poisoning** *(Ref: www.biomedsearch.com/searchlist.html?p=3101...txt=oxygen...)*

    - Severe **carbon monoxide poisoning** treated by **hyperbaric oxygen therapy**[Q].

48. **Ans. b. Tendinitis of common extensor origin** *(Ref: Bailey 27/e p448)*

    ### TENNIS ELBOW (LATERAL EPICONDYLITIS)

    - This is the **most common cause of elbow pain** excluding traumatic conditions
    - Usually occurs in patients of **30-50 years**; **Etiology** is **unknown**[Q] in most of cases
    - **Strenuous** or **overactivity** may precede symptoms
    - **Anterodistal lateral epicondyle tenderness**[Q]

    Diagnosis
    - **Resisted wrist extension** is a reliable **diagnostic test**[Q]
    - **Local anesthetic injection** is **diagnostically helpful**

    Treatment
    - Vast **majority improve** with **supervised conservative management**[Q]
    - **Open** or **arthroscopic release** yields **good results** in **recalcitrant cases**
    - **Arthroscopic release** also identifies associated pathology

49. **Ans. d. Brunschwig operation.** *(Ref: Medifactsonline blogspot.com/2011/.../1000-eponyms-in-surgery)*

    ### BRUNSCHWIG OPERATION

    - **Pelvic exenteration**[Q]: Surgery to **remove** the **lower colon, rectum** and **bladder**, and **create permanent stoma**.

50. **Ans. a. Always associated with breech extraction** *(Ref: Bailey 27/e p582)*

    ### TORTICOLLIS

    - In torticollis the **head is tilted toward** and **rotated away from the tight sternocleidomastoid muscle**.
    - **Congenital torticollis** is usually **secondary to intrauterine moulding** but may present with fixed **sternocleidomastoid contracture** or with a **palpable mass in the muscle**.
    - Most cases resolve with **stretching** but, occasionally, **surgical release** of the sternocleidomastoid at one or both ends is needed.

51. **Ans. d. Methylene blue**

    ### CHROMOENDOSCOPY

    - **Chromoendoscopy**: Dyes are **instilled** into the **GIT** at the time of **visualization** with **fibre-optic endoscopy**[Q].
    - **Chiefly enhance** the **characterization of tissues**[Q]
    - **Detail achieved** can often **allow for identification of the tissue type** or **pathology**[Q]

    Stains used
    - **Absorptive stains** have an affinity **for particular mucosal elements**, and include **Lugol's iodine, methylene blue** and **gentian violet**[Q].

Lugol's iodine	• Specifically **stains non-keratinized squamous epithelium**[Q] • **Useful for** identifying **squamous tissue, squamous dysplasia & squamous cell carcinomas**[Q].
Methylene blue	• Stains **absorptive epithelium**[Q] • Useful for **identifying** abnormality in **small intestine, colon & Barrett's esophagus**[Q] (intestinal metaplasia)

- **Contrast stains** are **not absorbed** but rather **provide contrast** by **permeating between irregularities in the mucosa to highlight irregularities**. The primary contrast stain is **indigo carmine**[Q].

  - **Chief use** of **Indigo carmine**: **Identification of dysplastic cells** in individuals with **chronic UC**[Q].

- **Reactive stains** undergo an **observable change** due to a **chemical process** related to the function of the gastrointestinal tract. **Congo red** is used as a **test for achlorhydria in the stomach**[Q], as it changes **colour from red to black** at a pH less than 3.

Uses of Chromoendoscopy

- Identification of **squamous cell carcinomas** or **dysplasia** of the esophagus[Q]
- Identification of **Barrett's esophagus** & **dysplasia**[Q]
- identification of **early gastric cancer**[Q]
- Characterization of **colonic polyps** & **colorectal cancer**[Q]
- In **screening for dysplasia** in individuals with **ulcerative colitis**[Q].

52. **Ans. c. T2 N0 M0 glottic cancer** *(Ref: Harrison 20/e p535, 19/e p503, 18/e p735)*

- **Concomitant chemoradiotherapy** is indicated in **advanced cancers of head and neck.**[Q]
- **T2 N0 M0 glottic cancer** represents **stage II cancer** which is defined as **localized disease**, which is not an indication for concomitant chemoradiotherapy.

53. **Ans. None** *(Ref: Harrison 20/e p3293, 19/e p2730)*

Smoking may be associated with all of the above cancers.

Smoking Associated Cancers		
• Lung[Q] • Nasopharynx, oropharynx hypopharynx and Larynx[Q] • Nasal cavity and paranasal sinuses[Q]	• Oral cavity[Q] • Esophagus[Q] • Stomach[Q] • Pancreas[Q] • Liver[Q]	• Kidney[Q] • Ureter and Urinary Bladder[Q] • Uterine Cervix[Q] • Acute Myeloid Leukemia

- **Smoking** is **not** associated with **postmenopausal Breast cancer** and **endometrial cancer.**

54. **Ans. b. Neuroblastoma**

Neuroblastoma

- **Hutchinson and Pepper syndrome** is **skull metastasis** seen in neuroblastoma[Q].

55. **Ans. d. Trousseau's sign**
56. **Ans. b. Ranula** *(Ref: Bailey 27/e p779)*
57. **Ans. a. Enzyme, b. Intraoperative histopathological examination, c. Fat, e. To check surgical margin in tumor surgery** *(Ref: Bailey 25/e p169-170)*

Frozen Section Biopsy

- Biopsy technique in pathology laboratories **for making urgent on-table diagnosis**[Q]
- Frozen section biopsy is a procedure done in a **pathology setup existing adjacent to** the **operation theatre**[Q].
- Surgeons are the main users of this service.

Procedure

- An **unfixed fresh tissue is frozen** (using CO_2 to -25°C) and section are made and stained.

Uses of Frozen Section Biopsy

- It is quick and surgeon can decide the further steps of procedure in the same sitting like **nodal clearance/type of resection** to be done.
- During surgery after resection of the tumor to look for (on table) the **clearance in the margin and depth, also to study the lymph nodes for their positivity**[Q].
- Used for **demonstration of** certain **constituents** which are **lost in processing with alcohol** or **xylene**, e.g., **fat, enzymes**[Q].

58. **Ans. a. Pancreas cancer, c. Acute pancreatitis, d. Pancreatic divisum** *(Ref: Harrison 20/e p352, 19/e p366)*

PANNICULITIS

- **Inflammatory lesions** of the **subcutaneous fat**[Q]
- Divided into the distinct categories:
  - **Septal panniculitis**: Inflammation is confined the **interlobular septa** of the subcutis
  - **Lobular panniculitis**: Inflammation involves the **entire fat lobule** and often the septa as well
  - **Panniculitis secondary to vasculitis**: Involve **large vessels in** the **subcutis,** in which the inflammation is usually restricted to the immediate vicinity of the involved vessel.
- **Pancreatic panniculitis:**
  - Manifests as **painful** or **asymptomatic subcutaneous nodules** or **indurated plaques** on the thighs, buttocks, lower trunk or **distal extremities** usually the lower.
  - Lesions are associated with **acute pancreatitis**[Q] or less commonly, **pancreatic carcinoma**[Q] either of which may be asymptomatic
  - It has also been associated with **low grade pancreatitis** in a patient **with pancreas divisum**[Q].

59. **Ans. a. Modified sweat gland, c. Present in axilla and groin, d. Hidradenitis suppurativa is infection of apocrine gland** *(Ref: Bailey 27/e p593)*

APOCRINE GLANDS

- An **apocrine sweat gland** is a modified **sweat gland**
- In humans, **apocrine sweat glands** are found only in certain locations of the body: **Axilla, areola** and **nipples** of the breast, **perianal region**, and some parts of the **external genitalia**.
- **Hidradenitis suppurative** is **chronic suppurative condition** of apocrine glands bearing skin.

60. **Ans. d. Carcinoma breast** *(Ref: Breast Pathology By Frances P O Malley (2006)/76-78)*

CAUSES OF FAT NECROSIS

- **After surgery/surgical trauma**: Wide local excision, Reduction mammoplasty[Q]
- Following **radiotherapy including iridium implants**[Q]
- Following **trauma**[Q]
- **Autologous fat injection**[Q] using the liposuction technique to fill in irregular contours and small soft tissue defects in the breast may lead to **fat necrosis secondary to poor blood supply** in the injected fat.

61. **Ans. a. Formaldehyde** *(Ref: Surgical Pathology by Rosai and Ackermann 9/e p27)*

FORMALIN

- **Formaldehyde** as a **buffered 10% aqueous solution (formalin**[Q]**)** is the **fixative most commonly used** in **histology**[Q]
- In routine clinical diagnostics it **offers** the **best possible compromise** between a **simple** and a **reliable method** as well as **extremely good structural preservation**[Q].
  - The **strong cross-linking action** of **formaldehyde is essential**, to protect the tissue from the **aggressive effect of concentrated solvents** in the **course of fixation** and **embedding in paraffin**[Q].
- **Fixation of tissue arrests** the **autolysis** and **putrefaction** and **stabilizes the cellular and tissue contents**[Q]

62. **Ans. a. Aspergillus flavus** *(Ref: Ananthnarayan 7/e p625)*

   Primary Aflatoxin Producing Fungi: Aspergillus flavus[Q] and Aspergillus parasiticus[Q]

63. **Ans. d. Floor** *(Ref: BDC 4/e pl/58)*

AXILLARY ABSCESS

- An **axillary abscess** is **incised through** the **floor**[Q] of the axilla, midway between the anterior and posterior axillary folds, and nearer to the medial wall in order **to avoid injury to** the **main vessels running along the anterior, posterior** and **lateral walls.**

64. **Ans. b. Tracheal stenosis** *(Ref: Dhillon 3/e p67)*

- **Topical Mitomycin C** is the **drug of choice** used to aid the treatment of **laryngeal stenosis**[Q].
- Topical Mitomycin C can **inhibit fibroblast activity** and **restenosis**[Q].

65. **Ans. a. 10% buffered neutral formalin**

Miscellaneous

66. **Ans. a. Sarcoidosis** *(Ref: Essentials of Chest Radiology by Janette Collins/165)*

   ### SARCOIDOSIS
   - **Sarcoidosis** is a systemic disease characterized by **non-caseating granulomas in multiple organs**
   - In **90% of cases, symmetrical massive bilateral hilar lymphadenopathy** occur
   - The **cardiac border** (**Potato nodes**) or lung involvement is present and can be revealed by chest X-ray or transbronchial biopsy

67. **Ans. a. Carcinoma**

   - "In normal persons, a click is felt when larynx is moved from side to side over vertebral column, this is called laryngeal click (post cricoid crepitus) It is absent in post cricoid carcinoma" — Moure's sign.

68. **Ans. b. Phenacetin - lung**

69. **Ans. c. Diameter of catheter** *(Ref: The ICU Book By Paul L. Marino 3/e p108)*

   "The size of vascular catheters is expressed in terms of outside diameter of the catheter. Two units of measurements are used to describe catheter size: a metric-based French size and a wire-based gauge size. The French size is a series of whole numbers that increases from zero in increments of 0.33 millimeters (e.g., a size 5 French catheter will have an outside diameter of $5 \times 0.33 = 1.65$ mm). The gauge size was introduced for solid wires and is an expression of how many wires can be placed side-by-side in a given space. The gauge size varies inversely with the diameter of the wire (or catheter)."- The ICU Book By Paul L. Marino 3/e p108

70. **Ans. b. Doctor's signature** *(Ref: Sabiston 20/e p232; Schwartz 10/e p1969)*

Elements of the Surgical Safety Checklist		
Sign In	**Time-Out**	**Sign Out**
• Before induction of anesthesia, members of the team (at least the nurse and an anesthesia professional) state that the following have been done: • **Patient has verified his or her identity, surgical site & procedure and consent.** • The **surgical site is marked** or site marking is not applicable. • **Pulse oximeter** is on the patient & functioning. • All members of the team are aware of whether the patient has a **known allergy**. • **Patient's airway & risk of aspiration** have been evaluated, and appropriate equipment & assistance are available. • If there is a risk of blood loss of at least 500 mL (or 7 mL/kg body weight in children), appropriate access and fluids are available.	• Before skin incision, the entire team (nurses, surgeons, anesthesia professionals, and any others participating in the care of the patient) or specific members state aloud the following: • Team confirms that all team members have been introduced by name & role. • **Team confirms the patient's identity, surgical site & procedure.** • Team reviews the anticipated critical events. • Surgeon reviews critical and unexpected steps, operative duration & anticipated blood loss. • Anesthesia professionals review concerns specific to patient. • Nurses review confirmation of sterility, equipment availability, and other concerns. • **Team confirms that prophylactic antibiotics have been administered ≤60 minutes before incision is made or that antibiotics are not indicated.** • Team confirms that all **essential imaging results for correct patient are displayed in operating room.**	• Before the patient leaves the operating room, the following are done: • Nurse reviews the following aloud with the team: • **Name of procedure**, as recorded • That **needle, sponge, & instrument counts are complete** (or not applicable) • That specimen (if any) is correctly labeled, including patient's name • Whether there are any issues with equipment that need to be addressed • The surgeon, nurse & anesthesia professional review aloud the key concerns for the recovery and care of the patient.

71. **Ans. a. Tip of nose to ear to xiphisternum** *(Ref: Practical Medical Procedures at a Glance By Rachel K. Thomas (2015)/p70)*

   The commonly used method to measure nasogastric tube length is the NEX method. NEX: Nose–Ear–Xiphisternum.

   "To measure the required length of tube, measure from the tip of the patient's nose, to their ear, and then down to the xiphisternum."
   -Practical Medical Procedures at a Glance By Rachel K. Thomas (2015)/p70

72. **Ans. d. Relaxed tension lines in skin** *(Ref: Grabb and Smith's Plastic Surgery 7/e p1-3; Gray's 41/e p157)*

   "Kraissl's lines are essentially exaggerated wrinkle lines obtained by studying the loose skin of elderly faces whilst contracting the muscles of facial expression. These lines for the most part correspond to Relaxed skin tension lines (RSTLs), but slight variation exists on the face, especially on the lateral side of the nose, the lateral aspect of the orbit, and the chin."-Gray's 41/e p157

73. **Ans. d. Skin, subcutaneous tissue, superficial fascia and deep fascia** *(Ref: Bailey 27/e p28)*

   "Fasciotomy involves incising the deep muscle fascia and is best carried out via longitudinal incisions of skin, fat and fascia. The muscle will be then seen bulging out through the fasciotomy opening."-Bailey 27/e p28

74. Ans. c. 1-Kocher incision; 2-Midline incision; 3-McBurney incision; 4-Battle incision; 5-Lanz incision; 6-Paramedian incision; 7-Transverse incision; 8-Rutherford Morrison incision; 9-Pfannenstiel incision

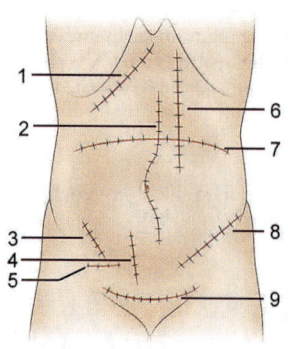

Various abdominal incisions:-
1. Kocher incision
2. Midline incision
3. McBurney incision
4. Battle incision
5. Lanz incision
6. Paramedian incision
7. Transverse incision
8. Rutherford morrison incision
9. Pfannenstiel incision

75. Ans. b. This test helps to detect ascites
76. Ans. d. Sim's position
77. Ans. a. A *(Ref: Bailey 25/e p339-340, Oxford Textbook of Vascular Surgery/ p202)*
78. Ans. a. 0.33 mm, d. 0.013 inch
79. Ans. a. Prophylaxis against thromboembolism